D0599180

FOCUS ON *Pathophysiology*

FOCUS ON
Pathophysiology

BARBARA L. BULLOCK, RN, MSN
Adjunct Professor
Texas Woman's University
Houston Baptist University
Houston, Texas

REET L. HENZE, DSN, RN
Associate Professor, College of Nursing
The University of Alabama in Huntsville
Huntsville, Alabama

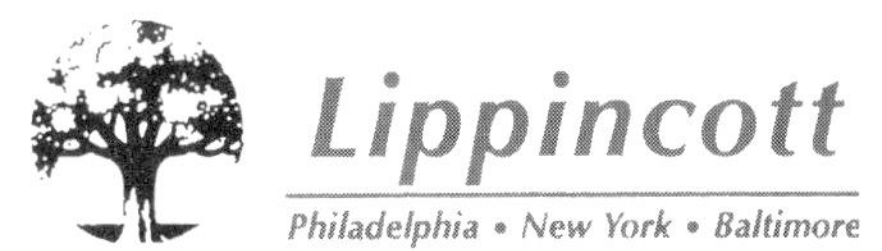

Acquisitions Editor: Lisa Stead
Developmental Editor: Danielle DiPalma
Coordinating Editorial Assistant: Claudia Vaughn
Senior Project Editor: Tom Gibbons
Senior Production Manager: Helen Ewan
Production Coordinator: Nannette Winski
Art Director: Carolyn O'Brien
Indexer: Ellen Murray
Compositor: Circle Graphics
Prepress: Jay's
Printer/Binder: Courier Kendallville

Copyright © 2000 by Lippincott Williams & Wilkins. All rights reserved. This book is protected by copyright. No part of it may be reproduced, stored in a retrieval system, or transmitted, in any form or by any means—electronic, mechanical, photocopy, recording, or otherwise—without the prior written permission of the publisher, except for brief quotations embodied in critical articles and reviews. Printed in the United States of America. For information write Lippincott Williams & Wilkins, 227 East Washington Square, Philadelphia, PA 19106.

Library of Congress Cataloging in Publications Data

Focus on pathophysiology / [edited by] Barbara L. Bullock, Reet L. Henze.
p. cm.
Includes bibliographical references and index.
ISBN 0-7817-1736-1 (paper)
1. Physiology, Pathological. I. Bullock, Barbara L. II. Henze, Reet L.
RB113.F63 1999
616.07'—dc21 99-16400
CIP

Care has been taken to confirm the accuracy of the information presented and to describe generally accepted practices. However, the authors, editors, and publisher are not responsible for errors or omissions or for any consequences from application of the information in this book and make no warranty, express or implied, with respect to the contents of the publication.

The authors, editors and publisher have exerted every effort to ensure that drug selection and dosage set forth in this text are in accordance with current recommendations and practice at the time of publication. However, in view of ongoing research, changes in government regulations, and the constant flow of information relating to drug therapy and drug reactions, the reader is urged to check the package insert for each drug for any change in indications and dosage and for added warnings and precautions. This is particularly important when the recommended agent is a new or infrequently employed drug.

Some drugs and medical devices presented in this publication have Food and Drug Administration (FDA) clearance for limited use in restricted research settings. It is the responsibility of the health care provider to ascertain the FDA status of each drug or device planned for use in their clinical practice.

9 8 7 6 5 4 3 2 1

I would like to dedicate the book to my husband, Pete. I could not have completed this project without his continuing support. He xeroxed and mailed thousands of pages. He also provided encouragement and humor when it was sorely needed.

Barbara L. Bullock

I would like to dedicate the book to the memory of my daughter, Karlin, who died while it was in progress, and to my family who patiently supported me in this endeavor.

Reet L. Henze

Contributors

JANICE STEELE ALWOOD, MS, ARNP, CS
Adult Nurse Practitioner
Burns Center and Skilled Nursing Facility
Tampa General Healthcare
Tampa, Florida
Chapter 28: Normal and Altered Functions of the Skin

ROBERTA H. ANDING, MS, RD/LD, CDE
Faculty
Department of Human Development and Consumer Science
University of Houston
Houston, Texas
Chapter 7: Normal and Altered Nutritional Balance

CAROL ANN BARNETT-LAMMON, RN, MSN
Assistant Professor
Capstone College of Nursing
University of Alabama
Tuscaloosa, Alabama
Chapter 8: Infectious Agents

JUDITH D. BRYAN, RN, MSN, EdD
Associate Professor
School of Nursing
University of Indianapolis
Indianapolis, Indiana
Chapter 9: Inflammation

CHRISTINE CANNON, RN, BSN, MSN, PhD
Associate Professor
College of Health and Nursing Sciences
University of Delaware
Newark, Delaware
Chapter 35: Pain

HELEN A. CARCIO, MS, RN, CS, ANP
Nurse Practitioner
Pioneer Women's Health
Greenfield, Massachusetts
Associate Clinical Professor
University of Massachusetts
Amherst, Massachusetts
Chapter 37: Normal and Altered Female Reproductive Function

KIM CURRY, ARNP, PhD
ARNP Specialist
Hillsborough County Health Department
Tampa, Florida
Chapter 28: Normal and Altered Functions of the Skin

MIGUEL F. da CUNHA, PhD
Professor
The University of Texas–Houston, Health Science Center School of Nursing
Houston, Texas
Chapter 2: Genetic Basis of Human Disease
Chapter 11: Altered Immunity

JOAN PARKER FRIZZELL, RN, PhD
Assistant Professor
School of Nursing
LaSalle University
Philadelphia, Pennsylvania
Chapter 23: Normal Endocrine Function
Chapter 24: Altered Endocrine Function

SUSAN P. GAUTHIER, RN, PhD*
Associate Professor
College of Allied Health Professions
Department of Nursing
Temple University
Philadelphia, Pennsylvania
Chapter 36: Normal and Altered Male Reproductive Function
Chapter 37: Normal and Altered Female Reproductive Function

ROBERT L. ISMEURT, RN, PhD
Associate Professor
Division of Adult Health/Parent–Child Nursing
College of Nursing
Arizona State University
Tempe, Arizona
Chapter 10: Normal Immunology

---

*Deceased

LAURIE A. GASPERI KAUDEWITZ, RN,C, BSN, MSN
Assistant Professor
Family/Community Nursing
East Tennessee State University
Johnson City, Tennessee
Chapter 4: Developmental Stages and Health Alterations

LYNDA MACKIN, RN,C, MS, ANP
Assistant Clinical Professor
Department of Physiological Nursing
University of California, San Francisco
San Francisco, California
Chapter 19: Normal Pulmonary Function
Chapter 20: Altered Pulmonary Function

GRETCHEN McDANIEL, RN, DSN
Associate Professor
Ida V. Moffett School of Nursing
Samford University
Birmingham, Alabama
Chapter 4: Developmental Stages and Health Alterations
Chapter 32: Tumors and Infections of the Central Nervous System

MARTHA A. MULVEY, RN, MS, CNS
Nurse Clinician, Epilepsy Program
University of Medicine and Dentistry of New Jersey
Newark, New Jersey
Chapter 6: Fluid, Electrolyte, and Acid–Base Balance

JENNIFER H. OTTO, MSN, CRNP
Nurse Practitioner
Bone Marrow Transplant
University Medical Center
Tucson, Arizona
Chapter 3: Neoplasia

BARBARA RESNICK, PhD, CRNP
Assistant Professor
Department of Adult Health
University of Maryland
Baltimore, Maryland
Chapter 27: Normal and Altered Functions of the Musculoskeletal System

KAY SACKETT, RN, EdD
Clinical Assistant Professor of Nursing
School of Nursing
State University of New York, University at Buffalo
Buffalo, New York
Chapter 35: Pain

SHARRON P. SCHLOSSER, RN, DSN, CTN
Professor of Nursing
Ida V. Moffett School of Nursing
Samford University
Birmingham, Alabama
Chapter 4: Developmental Stages and Health Alterations

BRENDA K. SHELTON, RN, MS, CCRN, AOCN
Critical Care Clinical Nurse Specialist
The Johns Hopkins Oncology Center
The Johns Hopkins Hospital
Baltimore, Maryland
Chapter 12: Normal and Altered Erythrocyte Function
Chapter 13: Normal and Altered Leukocyte Function

MARIA A. SMITH, RN, DSN, CCRN
Assistant Professor of Nursing
The University of Tennessee at Chattanooga
Chattanooga, Tennessee
Chapter 18: Shock

AMY BETH SOLOMON, RN, BSN
Nurse Clinician II
Department of Oncology
Johns Hopkins Hospital
Baltimore, Maryland
Chapter 12: Normal and Altered Erythrocyte Function

RICHARD A. STRIPP, MS, PhD
Assistant Professor
Pharmacology, Toxicology, and Medical Chemistry
Arnold and Marie Schwartz College of Pharmacy and Health Science
Long Island University
Brooklyn, New York
Chapter 1: Normal and Altered Cellular Function

JULIE N. TACKENBERG, RN, MA, MAOM, CNRN
Manager, Case Management
University Medical Center
Tucson, Arizona
Chapter 33: Chronic and Degenerative Alterations in the Nervous System

ANITA TESCH, BSN, MSN, EdD, RNC
Associate Professor
University of North Carolina at Greensboro
Greensboro, North Carolina
Chapter 21: Normal Renal Function and Urinary Excretion
Chapter 22: Altered Renal Function and Urinary Excretion

DENISE A. TUCKER, RN, BSN, MSN, DSN
Associate Professor in Nursing
School of Nursing
Florida State University
Tallahassee, Florida
Chapter 25: Normal and Altered Function of the Gastrointestinal System
Chapter 26: Normal and Altered Hepatobiliary and Pancreatic Exocrine Function

PATRICIA M. VIDMAR, RN, PhD
Wellness Manager
Provean St. Joseph Medical Center
Joliet, Illinois
Chapter 5: Concepts of Stress, Exercise, and Sleep

THERESA PLUTH YEO, MSN, MPH
Instructor
Johns Hopkins University School of Nursing
Baltimore, Maryland
Chapter 14: Normal and Altered Hemostasis

JOAN E. ZUCKERMAN, PhD
Instructor
Pharmacology and Toxicology
Department of Life Sciences
Long Beach City College
Long Beach, California
Chapter 30: Neurobiology of Psychotic, Anxiety, and Mood Disorders

Reviewers

LINDA C. ANDRIST, PhD, RNC, WHNP
Associate Professor and Coordinator
Adult/Women's Health Nurse Practitioner Track
Graduate Program in Nursing
MGH Institute of Health Professions
Boston, Massachusetts

RUTH BISHOP, RN, BSN, MSN, ACNP
Acute Care Nurse Practitioner
Duke University Medical Center
Durham, North Carolina

KIM R. BOOKOUT, RN, BSN, CETN
Director, Skin and Wound Management Program
Houston, Texas

GAIL A. BREEN, PharmD, BCPS
Assistant Professor of Clinical Pharmacology
Department of Pharmacy Practice
Philadelphia College of Pharmacy and Science
Philadelphia, Pennsylvania

JO ANN BROOKS-BRUNN, DNS, RN, FAAN, FCCP
Assistant Professor
Pulmonary and Critical Care Medicine
Indiana University School of Medicine
Indianapolis, Indiana

MARION E. BROOME
Professor and Research Chair, Nursing of Children
University of Wisconsin, Milwaukee
Milwaukee, Wisconsin

JUDITH BRYAN
Associate Professor
School of Nursing
University of Indianapolis
Indianapolis, Indiana

REITHA CABANISS, RN, MSN
Nurse Faculty
Allied Health and Nursing
Bevill State Community College
Sumiton, Alabama

EDWARD W. CARROLL, BS, MS, PhD
Clinical Assistant Professor
Department of Basic Health Sciences
Marquette University College of Health Sciences
Milwaukee, Wisconsin

ROBERT CONTINO, BSN, MSN, EdD, RN
Associate Professor of Nursing
Wesley College
Dover, Delaware

MARLA J. DeJONG, RN, MS, CCRN, CEN
Assistant Nurse Manager
Coronary Care Unit
Wilford Hall Medical Center
Lackland Air Force Base, Texas

VERONICA DICKERSON, RN, BSN
Director, Vocational Nursing
Panola College
Carthage, Texas

CATHERINE FOSTER, BSN, MSN, CNP
Graduate Faculty
The College of Nursing and Health Sciences
The University of Texas at El Paso
El Paso, Texas

KATHERINE GASPARD, PhD
Senior Lecturer, Department of Health Restoration
School of Nursing
University of Wisconsin, Milwaukee
Milwaukee, Wisconsin

DEBBIE A. GUNTER, RN, BSN, MN, C, FNP
Nurse Practitioner
Duluth, Georgia

GENNELL HILTON, CRNP, CCRN, MS
Nurse Practitioner
Arnold, Maryland

KAREN C. JOHNSON-BRENNAN
Professor and Associate Director of Undergraduate Program
School of Nursing
San Francisco State University
San Francisco, California

MAY PAT KUNERT, BSW, BSN, PhD
Assistant Professor
School of Nursing
Marquette University
Milwaukee, Wisconsin

CAROL ANN LAMMON, RN, MSN
Assistant Professor
Capstone College of Nursing
University of Alabama
Tuscaloosa, Alabama

PATRICIA LANGE-OTSUKA
Academic Coordinator
Assistant Professor of Nursing
Hawaii Pacific University
Kaneoh, Hawaii

PATRICIA GONCE MORTON, RN, PhD
Associate Professor and Coordinator
Acute Care Nurse Practitioner and Clinical Nurse Specialist
Master's Program in Trauma/Critical Care Nursing
University of Maryland School of Nursing
Baltimore, Maryland

OUIDA PATRICIA MURRAY, RN, MA
Assistant Professor of Nursing
York College of the City University of New York
Queens, New York

JOHNNIE NICHOLS, RN, BSN
Nursing Instructor
Panola College
Carthage, Texas

DOROTHY OBESTER, BSNE, MSN, PhD
Professor of Nursing
St. Francis College
Loretto, Pennsylvania

JOAN PLEUSS, MS, RD, CDE
Senior Research Dietician
Clinical Research Center
Medical College of Wisconsin
Froedtert Memorial Lutheran Hospital
Milwaukee, Wisconsin

LEE RICHARD, PhD, RN, CNAA
Instructor
Department of Nursing Education
San Antonio College
San Antonio, Texas

ISABEL S. ROMENA, RN, BSN, MSN, CCRN, MS
Nursing Instructor
San Joaquin Delta College
Stockton, California

JANE C. SHIVNAN, RN, MSN
Nurse Manager
Bone Marrow Transplant
Johns Hopkins Oncology Center
Baltimore, Maryland

LYNN M. SIMKO, MPH, MSN, RN, CCRN
Assistant Professor
School of Nursing
Duquesne University
Pittsburgh, Pennsylvania

STEPHANIE STEWART, RN, PhD
Undergraduate Program Director
College of Nursing
University of Wisconsin, Oshkosh
Oshkosh, Wisconsin

LAURA SUTTON, MS, RN, CS
Associate Professor
Department of Nursing
West Liberty State College
West Liberty, West Virginia

PAM TAYLOR, BSN, M.Ed., PhD
Clinical Assistant Professor
University of Tennessee at Chattanooga
Chattanooga, Tennessee

ANITA TESCH, MSN, EdD, RNC
Assistant Professor of Nursing
University of North Carolina at Greensboro
Greensboro, North Carolina

ELISE VERANSKY, MSN, RNCS
Instructor in Nursing
Penn State, Altoona
Altoona, Pennsylvania

Preface

Pathophysiology is the study of the physiologic and biologic manifestations of disease. It encompasses understanding of the adaptations that the body makes to the alterations produced by disease processes. *Focus on Pathophysiology* truly provides a concentrated study of human disease in a concise, easy-to-use, and logical manner. The intent is to clarify concepts in a user-friendly format. No attempt is made to include treatment regimens or patient care. The reader is referred to appropriate literature for information on treatment and patient care.

Focus on Pathophysiology is based on four previous editions of *Pathophysiology: Adaptations and Alterations in Function.* The basic organization and many of the features of the previous editions have been retained. Since all chapters have been extensively rewritten and refocused, the text has been retitled. The content of this edition reflects current concepts of disease processes, which are continually being updated and clarified by scientific study. Each section is based on the most current research available.

The text is written for undergraduate and graduate students in health-oriented disciplines. It can be used as a supplement to other courses, as a text for a pathophysiology course, or as a reference resource for the practicing clinician.

Built on a solid foundation, this concise, up-to-date pathophysiology text meets the needs of today's diverse readers.

ORGANIZATION OF THE TEXT

The organization of the text is intended to enhance the reader's understanding of the effects of disease on the body and how the body is altered by or adapts to the changes. Normal structure and function provide the basis for understanding the disease effects. Both conceptual and systems approaches have been used.

The text is divided into 12 units:

Unit I provides a basis for understanding cellular alterations in the organs and systems. Normal cellular structure and function is followed by alterations in cellular processes. Genetic disorders and concepts of neoplasia, since they may affect multiple organs and systems, are included. Developmental changes across the life span provide a basis for an understanding of pathophysiologic processes affecting different age levels. The effects of stress, sleep, and exercise on adaptation also are considered. Fluid and electrolyte, acid–base, and nutritional balances and imbalances complete this unit.

Unit II provides essential information for the understanding of bodily defense mechanisms. How infectious agents cause disease and the resulting inflammatory and immune system responses are detailed.

Units III through *XII* examine the physiology and pathophysiology of the major body systems. Beginning with the hematologic system, the text proceeds through circulation, pulmonary, urinary, endocrine, digestion, musculoskeletal and integumentary, nervous, special senses, and reproductive systems.

LEARNING TOOLS

Key Terms: A list of terms, which may be unfamiliar to the student and are considered essential to chapter comprehension, appears at the beginning of each chapter. These terms first appear in **bold** and are defined in the glossary at the end of the text.

Flowcharts: Attractive step-by-step charts throughout the text help the reader map out complex processes. These abundant flowcharts are essential to the study of pathophysiology.

Tables, Boxes and Illustrations: Numerous tables and boxes in every chapter summarize important information and provide ready references for the reader. Many new illustrations have been created to enhance conceptual learning. These important aspects of the text have been reviewed and, where appropriate, revised or replaced.

Focus on Cellular Physiology/Pathophysiology Figure: Special figures throughout the text highlight cellular content. This focus mirrors current research, which analyzes cellular processes as a basis for understanding disease processes.

Chapter Case Studies: To inspire critical thinking, clinical scenarios with related questions are included at the end of relevant chapters. These case studies require the student to incorporate knowledge gained from the chapter and apply it to real-life situations. Discussions of case studies are included at the end of the book.

References: Each chapter includes a listing of the current resources cited in the text, allowing the reader to follow up with more in-depth study.

Changes Across the Life Span: Each unit begins with a developmental summary of the changes occurring during the individual's life span. An individual's vulnerability to particular diseases often is related to his or her age.

Unit Appendices: Each unit concludes with easily accessible appendices. Each appendix includes a detailed unit case study, table(s) of laboratory values and diagnostic tests appropriate to the system, and a unit bibliography.

- The unit case study provides in-depth consideration of a pathophysiologic condition and a method for a clinical focus. These realistic patient scenarios integrate several concepts from the text and challenge readers to apply theory to practice.
- The diagnostic tables summarize current laboratory and diagnostic tests that relate to the unit content. The significance of the test results is included.
- The thorough unit bibliography provides resources that enable the reader to pursue topics in greater depth. Whenever possible, web site addresses have been included.

Glossary: At the end of the book, a descriptive glossary defines key terms presented throughout the text and serves as a quick reference for future readings.

ANCILLARY PACKAGE

Focus on Pathophysiology is accompanied by an Instructor's Manual designed to serve as a complement to the book, with learning materials for students and organizational suggestions for instructors. It has been completely rewritten and contains lecture outline, teaching strategies, and a bank of test questions. Transparency masters of selected illustrations from the text can be used to enhance classroom presentation of material.

Acknowledgments

This project has been greatly enhanced by the addition of many expert contributors from all across the United States. They have rewritten, reorganized, and expanded content with attention to detail. They have also helped us work through multiple revisions and changes. Their diligence is greatly appreciated. The task of including extensive information, yet keeping the text to a reasonable length, is daunting.

We also acknowledge the support and guidance provided by many talented persons at Lippincott Williams & Wilkins, specifically Lisa Stead, Nursing Acquisitions Editor; Danielle DiPalma, Developmental Editor; Renée Gagliardi, Developmental Editor; Maryann Foley, Developmental Editor; Claudia Vaughn, Editorial Assistant; Tom Gibbons, Senior Project Editor; and all of the production staff.

Contributing authors to previous editions were Gaylene Altman, Gloria Anderson, Roberta Anding, Joseph Andrews, Pamela Appleton, Sue Baldwin, Anne Bavier, Cheryl Bean, Carol Bowdoin, Joan Bufalino, Martha Butterfield, Concepcion Castro, Angela Collins, Jules Constant, Miguel da Cunha, Virginia Earles, Ann Edgil, Thomas Fender, Shirley Freeburn, Dorothy Gauthier, Janet Gelein, Darlene Green, Cherry Guinn, Doris Heaman, Reet Henze, Marcia Hill, Pamela Holder, Joan Hurlock, Karen Jones, Bonnie Juneau, June Larrabee, Carla Lee, Marianne Marcus, John Marino, Gretchen McDaniel, M.S. Megahed, Frances Monahan, Jennie Moore, Emilie Musci, Betty Norris, Barbara Norwood, Leah Oakley, Donna Packa, Marilyn Pase, Richard Pflanzer, Helen Ptak, Cammie Quinn, Pearl Rosendahl, Sharron Schlosser, Therese Shipps, Eileen Sjoberg, Carol Stephenson, Camille Stern, Metta Fay Street, Gloria Stuart, Margaret Trimpey, Joan Vitello, Joy Whatley, Linda Williams, and Joan Williamson.

We were saddened by the death of one of our contributors Dr. Susan Gauthier, who died after the completion of the initial draft of the reproductive unit. We were inspired by her enthusiasm and expertise in her contributions to this book.

Our thanks also go to the expert reviewers for their extensive reviews and excellent suggestions for improvement. In many cases, chapters were reorganized and sections rewritten on the basis of their reviews.

Barbara L. Bullock
Reet L. Henze

Contents

Unit 1

Concepts Basic to Pathophysiology 1

Chapter 1

Normal and Altered Cellular Function 3

Richard Stripp

Chapter 2

Genetic Basis of Human Disease 47

Miguel F. da Cunha

Chapter 3

Neoplasia 69

Jennifer H. Otto

Unit 10
Neural Control 875

Chapter 29
Normal Structure and Function of the Nervous Systems 877

Reet L. Henze

Chapter 30
Neurobiology of Psychotic, Anxiety, and Mood Disorders 918

Joan E. Zuckerman

Chapter 31
Traumatic and Vascular Injuries of the Central Nervous System 938

Reet L. Henze

Chapter 32
Tumors and Infections of the Central Nervous System 979

Gretchen McDaniel

Unit
1

Concepts Basic to Pathophysiology

FOCUS ON Musculoskeletal Changes Through the Life Span

INFANT (1–12 MONTHS):

Muscle tissue is almost completely formed at birth, and growth occurs due to the increasing size of the existing fibers under endocrine influence. As muscle size increases, strength increases. Bone growth and hardness increase as increases in calcification of bone occur. All of the bony structures undergo ossification after birth. Bones grow in length and width, and change in the shape is noted.

TODDLER AND PRESCHOOL AGE (1–5 YEARS):

Ossification slows after infancy but continues until early adulthood. Change in the shape of the bones and joints gives rise to clumsiness early in this period and gradual correction later on. Muscles grow faster than bones, and the strength is related to amount of muscle mass. The long bones contain red marrow, which produces blood cells.

SCHOOL AGE (6–12 YEARS):

The long bones increase in length and size. Red marrow is gradually replaced by fatty tissue, and red marrow is found only in the sternum, vertebrae, pelvic bones, and some skull and short-shafted bones. Girls begins to surpass boys in height and weight until the onset of puberty. Growing pains are common due to the bones growing faster than adjacent muscles, which stresses the muscle and ligaments. Posture becomes more like adults as the strength of muscles increases in the thoracic spine area. Muscle mass and strength gradually increase and baby fat decreases. Children double their strength during these years.

ADOLESCENCE (13–19 YEARS):

Maximal growth of muscle mass correlates with the growth of the skeletal system. Growth spurts and muscular strength vary with the person but usually improve in girls through age 15, and boys experience an increase in strength from age 14 to 19. Muscle mass in males exceeds that in females by about twofold. Muscle mass is closely related to amount of androgen secretion. Growth of skeleton occurs with feet and hand elongation and lengthening and broadening of the body frame in both males and females. The epiphyseal plates fuse at a certain point and growth stops. Growth is closely related to maturation of the reproductive system, and males often continue to grow during early adulthood.

YOUNG ADULT AND ADULT (20–45 YEARS):

Female and male muscle mass is influenced by genetic factors, insulin levels, nutrition, growth hormones, testosterone, and exercise. Testosterone increases muscle mass and bone density. Muscle growth is increased in size and not number of muscle fibers. Peak muscular strength occurs around 25 to 30 years and gradually declines about 10% between ages 30 and 60. Bone growth for women usually stops by age 20, whereas in men it may continue through the early 20s. Legs of both males and females usually make up about half of the adult height. Peak bone mass occurs at approximately 35 years of age, and loss after that time is significantly greater in women than men.

MIDDLE-AGED ADULTS (46–64 YEARS):

Bone mass begins to decrease once skeletal growth ceases, and women lose calcium from bone after menopause, with a decrease of 1% to 1.5% each year. There is a significant risk of osteoporotic fractures by age 60 in females. Male bone loss begins later and may not be significant before age 70. Spinal vertebrae are compressed, and cartilage between the vertebrae and hip joints loses water and becomes less elastic, leading to "stiff joints." Muscle mass decreases, with a loss in number and size of the fibers. Muscle strength declines, and fat is often gained over muscle.

LATE ADULTHOOD (65–100+ YEARS):

Bone loss is usual with loss of calcium from bone. The process is accelerated in females, so that by age 70 a woman's skeletal frame may have lost 30% or more of its calcium. A gradual decrease in height is common, with the average being 1.2 cm for each 20 years of life in both men and women. Collapse of the vertebrae and loss of collagen and atrophy in intervertebral disks cause the spinal column to compress and posture to become curved. Bone strength is progressively lost. There is a gradual loss of muscular strength and endurance with atrophy of muscle cells and loss of lean muscle mass.

Chapter 1

Normal and Altered Cellular Function

Richard Stripp

KEY TERMS

allosteric modulation
amphipathic phospholipid molecules
anabolic
anaphase
apoptosis
catabolic
chromatids
chromatin
codon
cotransport (symport)
counter-transport or antiport
covalent modulation
cytosol
desmosomes
diffusion equilibrium
gap (nexus) junctions
hydrophilic
hydrophobic
hypertonic fluid
hypotonic fluid
isotonic fluid
ligands
metaphase
nucleoplasm
osmosis
osmotic pressure
prophase
protons
telophase
tight junctions

The cell is the structural and functional unit of the body that provides the basis for life. Understanding the biology of the human cell is essential to the study of pathophysiology because all pathophysiologic processes reflect changes in normal cell function.

Cells make up the units of tissues, organs, and finally, systems of the human body (Flowchart 1-1). The human body contains more than 75 trillion cells, each of which performs specific functions. These functions are determined by genetic differentiation and are controlled by a highly specific information system that directs the activity of each cellular component.

Although cells have different functions, they are alike in many ways. All cells must perform basic vital functions for their own survival. Cells are the smallest units of life and they are capable of performing the various processes associated with living organisms. These include:

1. Obtaining oxygen and nutrients from their surrounding environment
2. Metabolizing nutrients
3. Eliminating carbon dioxide
4. Synthesizing proteins and other biomolecules
5. Responding to changes in their environment
6. Regulating the movement of materials between external and internal cellular environments
7. Replicating themselves

To perform these functions, cells have certain basic survival needs that are vital to all cells of the body. These needs include oxygen, nutrients, waste elimination, and fluid and electrolyte balance. These survival needs are also points of vulnerability to various stressors. Agents that cause cell injury can be reduced to those that disrupt the cell's basic survival needs. In addition to performing these basic functions, cells of the body also carry out specialized functions that aid other cells in maintaining their internal environments. For example, cells of the kidney have the same basic survival needs as any other cell; in addition, they have specialized characteristics that are important in maintaining fluid and electrolyte balance vital to the basic needs for homeostasis of other cells.

Humans are made up of individual cells, but the arrangement of these cells into tissues and organs provides the whole organism with the ability to cope with the changing environment. This requires specialized coordination of the activities of the individual cells, which in turn depends on the exchange of information between cells and their environment. The control and coordination of the cellular activity involves two basic

FLOWCHART 1-1 **The Human Body**

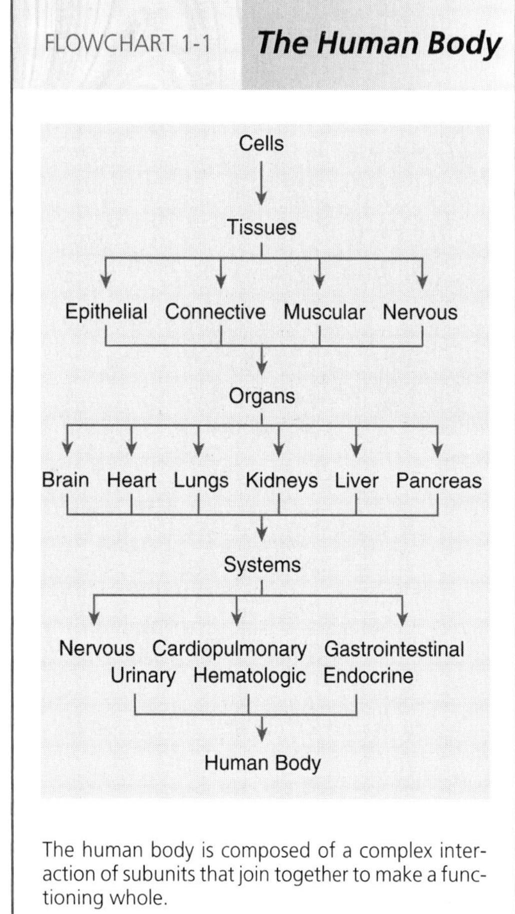

The human body is composed of a complex interaction of subunits that join together to make a functioning whole.

aspects: (1) the regulation of the availability of cellular components needed to carry out various processes (which genes are expressed), and (2) altering the rate at which cellular components carry out physiologic functions (changing the activity of a protein involved in a metabolic reaction or altering the conformation of a protein that is an ion channel).

The cell is composed of many different structures that carry out its complex functions (Fig. 1-1). The outer boundary of the cell is the plasma membrane that functions as a selective barrier that regulates the cellular chemical composition. The interior of the cell is generally divided into two regions: the cytoplasm and the nucleus.

THE CYTOPLASM

The cytoplasm contains two components, the cell organelles and a fluid medium called **cytosol**. This fluid surrounds the organelles and is external to the nucleus of a cell. The intracellular fluid (ICF) refers to all of the fluid inside the cell including the cytosol plus the fluid inside the nucleus (called **nucleoplasm**). The chemical composition of the fluids inside the organelles differs from the cytosol and contributes to the highly complex and organized state of the cell. The nucleus is essentially a storage area for nucleic acid especially deoxyribonucleic acid (DNA), which codes for specific cellular proteins.

Cytosol is composed mostly of water with specific amounts of electrolytes, proteins, lipids, and carbohydrates. The intracellular electrolyte balance is closely regulated and differs from that of extracellular fluid (ECF) (Table 1-1). Proteins maintain structural strength and form, provide for contractility of muscle tissue, and transport vital substances. Proteins also form the enzymes and many of the hormones necessary for regulating many intracellular reactions. Lipids make up a very small portion of the general cell and mainly join with proteins to keep the cell membranes insoluble in water. Carbohydrates constitute a very small amount of the cytoplasm and are used mainly in forming adenosine triphosphate (ATP) for energy.

Organelles

Membrane-bound compartments within the cell make up highly organized physical structures called *organelles* (little organs). Each cell organelle performs specific functions that contribute to the cell's survival and hence the survival of the organism. The function of these complex and diverse organelles is described below and in Table 1-2. Each cell organelle performs specific functions that contribute to the cell's survival and hence the survival of the organism. Organelles include mitochondria, endoplasmic reticulum (ER), free ribosomes, Golgi complex, lysosomes, peroxisomes, the cytoskeleton, centrosomes, and centrioles. The plasma membrane is also considered a cellular organelle and its essential functions are detailed on page 9. The organelles within the cytoplasm have limiting intracellular membranes that keep them separate from each other so they can accomplish their specific purposes. The nucleus, the largest organelle within the cell, is considered a separate entity because it has a specialized function, which is detailed on page 28.

MITOCHONDRIA

Mitochondria (sing., mitochondrion) are membranous, rod-shaped organelles that are the site of ATP synthesis. ATP is a high-energy phosphate compound required by cells when they perform cellular work (such as contraction, secretion, conduction, and transport).

Mitochondria are bounded by a double membrane, the inner one of which is convoluted into a series of shelflike folds called *cristae* that project into the interior of the organelle (Fig. 1-2). The folded inner mem-

FOCUS ON CELLULAR PHYSIOLOGY

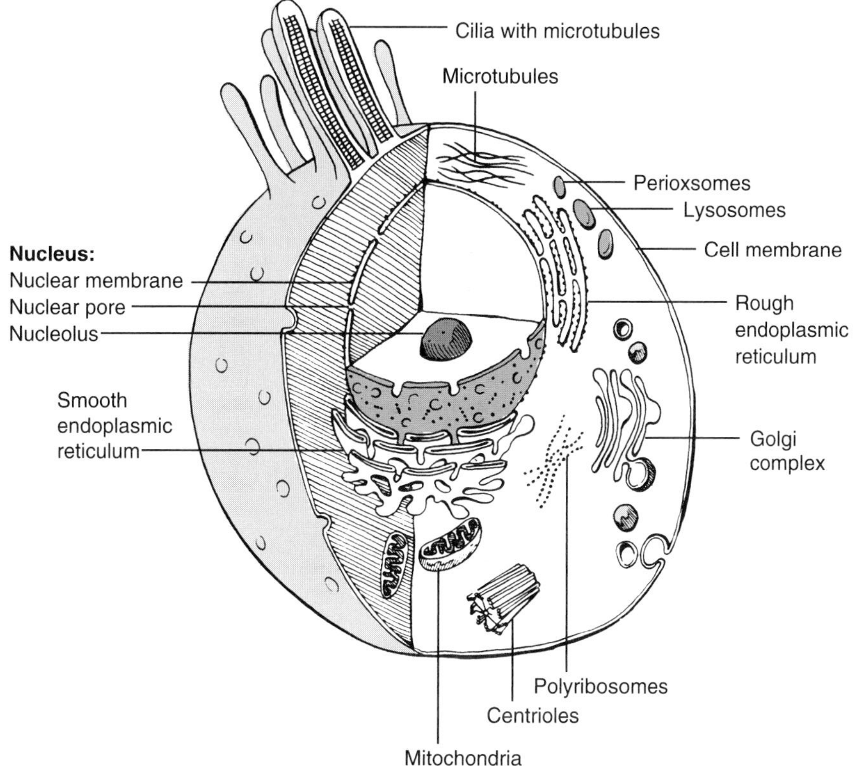

FIGURE 1-1. **The general structure of the cell with its organelles.**

brane presents a large internal surface area on which enzymatic reactions that generate ATP occur. Cells that are very active and have a high energy requirement, such as skeletal muscle cells, have many mitochondria, whereas less active cells, such as bone or cartilage cells, have fewer mitochondria. Usually, within a given cell, mitochondria tend to be most numerous in areas that are highly energy dependent, such as around the contractile elements of the muscle cell or at the terminus of a nerve cell where transmission occurs.

TABLE 1-1

COMPOSITION OF EXTRACELLULAR (ECF) AND INTRACELLULAR (ICF) FLUIDS

CELLULAR CONSTITUENT	ECF	ICF
Sodium (Na^+)	140 ± 5 mEq/L	10 mEq/L
Potassium (K^+)	4 ± 0.5 mEq/L	140 mEq/L
Calcium (Ca^{++})	10 ± 1.0 mg/dL	<1 mg/dL
Magnesium (Mg^{++})	3 mEq/L	58 mEq/L
Chloride (Cl^-)	100 ± 10 mEq/L	4 mEq/L
Bicarbonate (HCO_3^-)	28 ± 3 mEq/L	10 mEq/L
Phosphates	4 ± 1 mEq/L	75 mEq/L
Glucose	90 ± 10 mg/dL	0–20 mg/dL
Amino Acids	30 mg/dL	200 mg/dL
pH	7.4 ± .05	7.0
Proteins	2 g/dL	16 g/dL

* Values are approximate and are meant to show the difference between ECF and ICF.

TABLE 1-2

STRUCTURE AND FUNCTION OF ORGANELLES

ORGANELLE	STRUCTURE	FUNCTION
Plasma cell membrane	• Membrane composed mainly of protein and lipid molecules	• Maintains integrity of cell • Controls the passage of materials into and out of the cell • Provides for signal transduction
Endoplasmic reticulum • Sarcoplasmic reticulum in muscle cells	• Complex of interconnected membrane-bound sacs, canals, and vesicles	• Transports materials within the cell • Provides attachment for ribosomes • Synthesizes lipids and lipoproteins • Contains calcium ions in muscle cells
Ribosomes (polyribosomes)	• Particles composed of protein and RNA molecules	• Synthesize proteins • Polyribosomes are groups or chains that function in complex protein synthesis
Golgi apparatus (complex or body)	• Group of flattened, membranous sacs	• Packages and modifies protein molecules for transport and secretion
Mitochondria	• Membranous sacs with inner partitions	• Release energy from food molecules • Transform energy into usable form
Lysosomes	• Membranous sacs	• Contain enzymes capable of digesting worn out cellular parts or substance that enter cells.
Peroxisomes	• Membranous vesicles	• Contain enzymes called peroxidases to breakdown organic molecules
Centrosome • Centrioles • Cilia • Flagella	• Nonmembranous structure composed of two rodlike centrioles • Motile projections attached to basal bodies beneath the cell membrane	• Help distribute chromosomes to new cells during cell reproduction • Initiate formation of cilia • Propel fluids over cellular surfaces • Enable sperm cells to move
Microfilaments and microtubules	• Thin rods and tubules	• Support cytoplasm and help move substances and organelles within the cytoplasm • Maintain structure (shape) of cell • Microtubules interact with each other to provide movement, such as ciliary and flagellar • Microfilaments constitute myofibrils in muscle cells, necessary for contraction.
Nucleus • Envelope • Nucleolus • Chromatin	• Envelope is double membrane that separates nuclear material from cytoplasm • Nucleolus, dense, non-membranous area of protein and RNA molecules • Chromatin—fibers composed of protein and DNA	• Control center of cell • Envelope controls passage of materials between the nucleus and cytoplasm • Nucleolus is site of ribosome formation • All genetic information for synthesis of proteins needed for carrying on life processes

(Modified from: Shier, D., Butler, J., & Lewis, R. [1996]. *Hole's human anatomy and physiology* [7th ed]. Dubuque, IA: Brown.)

Mitochondria are able to regenerate (replicate) themselves under conditions of increased energy need. They contain a DNA that is part of the mitochondrial structure. The replication process usually occurs at the time of cell division or when there is increased cellular energy need.

ENDOPLASMIC RETICULUM

In some human cells, much of the cytoplasm is filled with an intricate, yet ordered, set of tubular or saclike channels called *cisternae* (Fig. 1-3). All of the channels within the ER are interconnected, giving rise to a netlike structure whose membranes are continuous with the outer membrane of the nuclear envelope.

Much of the surface of the ER may be covered with small particles or granules made up of ribonucleic acid (RNA), which synthesize protein. The particles, called *ribosomes*, give the outer membrane of the ER a rough or granular appearance; therefore, such ER is called *granular or rough ER*. Other surfaces of the ER may be free of ribosomes; hence, they appear relatively smooth. This type of ER is called *agranular* or *smooth ER*.

FOCUS ON CELLULAR PHYSIOLOGY

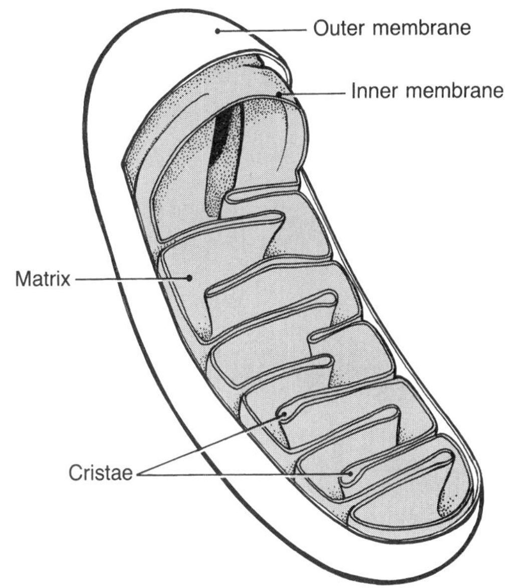

FIGURE 1-2. Appearance and structure of a mitochondrion.

The ER provides a large surface within the cell on which sequences of chemical reactions can occur. Enzymes and other substances are arranged in an assembly-line sequence to provide for efficient production of substances responsible for the metabolic functions of the cell.[13] The granular ER is involved primarily with the production of proteins. Proteins such as hormones, for example, which are destined to be secreted, are put together on the ribosomes of ER. Also, some of the proteins that form structural parts of the cell are produced here. The smooth ER is the site of formation of nonprotein substances, such as the fat-soluble triglycerides, fatty acids, steroids, and phospholipids. Enzymes within the smooth ER are involved in biotransformation of substances such as alcohol, pesticides, and carcinogens.[21] In muscle cells, the smooth ER is called sarcoplasmic reticulum and contains calcium ions (see page 796).

FREE RIBOSOMES

Some of the ribosomes within the cell are not bound to the ER. Instead, a number of ribosomes involved with the production of a specific protein molecule may be linked together, much like pearls on a string, forming a chain structure called a *polyribosome* (see Fig. 1-1). Polyribosomes of several different lengths may be found in the cytoplasm and all are involved with the formation or synthesis of protein molecules. Most of the proteins made on the polyribosomes are for the cell's own use in building cell components (structural proteins) or in regulating cell activities (enzymes).

GOLGI COMPLEX

The Golgi complex, also called the Golgi apparatus or the Golgi body, is a series of concentric, flattened saccules with membranes resembling those of the smooth ER (Fig. 1-4). In some cells, the Golgi membranes appear to be connected to the smooth ER and may be a specialized part of it. Membrane-bound vesicles are frequently observed near the Golgi membranes and represent packaged chemicals arriving at the Golgi complex for further processing or packaged substances leaving the Golgi complex destined for secretion by way of exocytosis (see page 15).

The Golgi complex is predominant in various types of secretory cells, such as the pancreatic acinar cell, and plays several important roles in the process of secretion. Substances destined for secretion (eg, protein

FOCUS ON CELLULAR PHYSIOLOGY

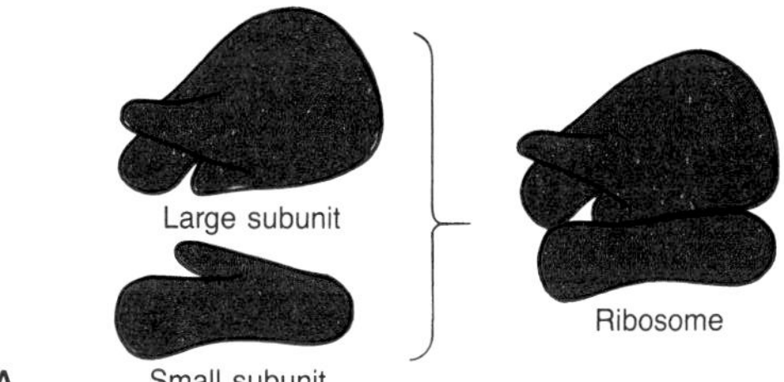

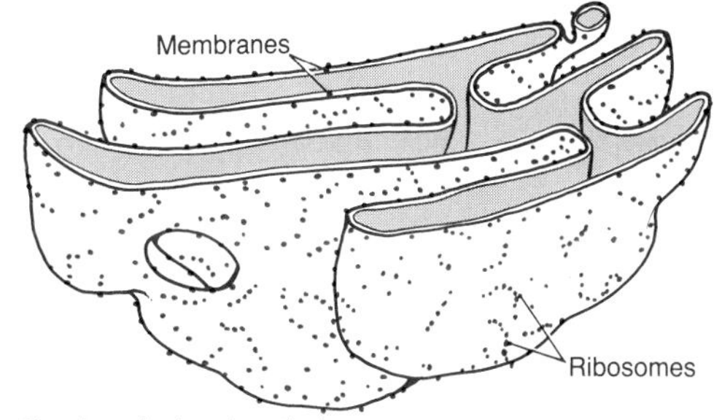

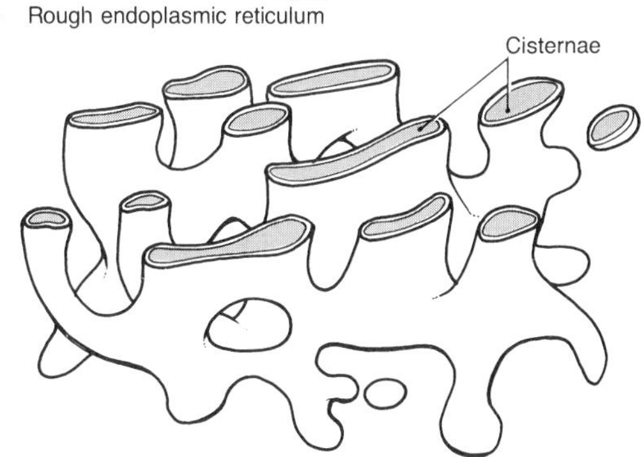

FIGURE 1-3. Appearance of ribosomes and endoplasmic reticulum. **A.** Free ribosomes. **B.** Rough or granular endoplasmic reticulum. **C.** Smooth or agranular endoplasmic reticulum.

FOCUS ON CELLULAR PHYSIOLOGY

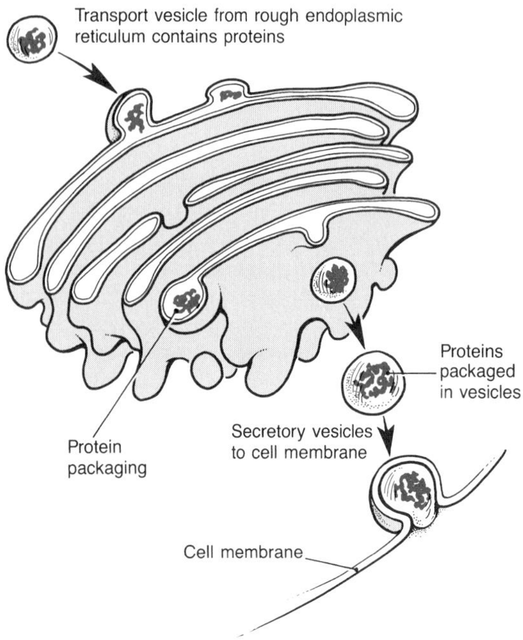

Transport vesicle from rough endoplasmic reticulum contains proteins

Proteins packaged in vesicles

Protein packaging

Secretory vesicles to cell membrane

Cell membrane

FIGURE 1-4. Appearance and function of the Golgi complex.

hormones) may be produced on the granular ER and then transported through the cisternae of the ER to the Golgi apparatus. The Golgi apparatus may then prepare the substance for release by packaging it within a membranous vacuole, which then moves toward the plasma membrane and the substance is released to the exterior of the cell by exocytosis (see page 15).

Other functions of the Golgi complex include producing some substances such as polysaccharides, chemically modifying molecules produced by the ER (eg, activating enzymes), storing synthesized molecules, and producing organelles called lysosomes.

LYSOSOMES

Lysosomes are membrane-bound organelles that are spherical and contain digestive enzymes. They originate from the Golgi complex and ER and participate in intracellular digestive processes.

Lysosomes contain a variety of hydrolytic enzymes that break down protein, nucleic acids, carbohydrates, and lipids. When a cell ingests material by endocytosis, lysosomes fuse their membranes with those of the endocytotic vesicle, forming a common membrane-bound vesicle in which digestion can occur (see page 15). The lysosomal membrane protects the other cellular organelles from the hydrolytic enzymes within the lysosome.

Lysosomes also digest "worn out" or damaged parts of the cell, thereby participating in the recycling of cell constituents, a process called *autophagy*. However, when a cell dies, the lysosomes it contains rupture, releasing enzymes that cause the cell to self-destruct (*autolysis*). Normally the lysosomal enzymes cannot break down the lysosomal membrane.

Numerous lysosomes are present in cells that are very active in ingesting matter by phagocytosis. In some of the leukocytes, for example, lysosomes are so numerous they give the cytoplasm a granular appearance. Lysosomes are a critical part of the body's defensive phagocytic cells that are responsible for destroying foreign proteins (see page 265). Lysosomal enzymes in injured or dead tissue help prepare the affected area for repair.

PERIOXISOMES

These intracellular organelles are smaller than lysosomes and contain oxidative enzymes that form hydrogen peroxide (H_2O_2). The H_2O_2 is involved with detoxification of potentially harmful substances, especially within the liver and kidney.[21]

THE CYTOSKELETON

The complex network of proteins that provide for cellular shape and, in some cases, the ability to carry out coordinated movement is called the cytoskeleton. It is composed of microfilaments, microtubules, and intermediate filaments. Microfilaments are different lengths of rodlike structures composed of actin, the thin filament of muscle tissue. Microfilaments are found both in muscle and nonmuscular tissue.

Microtubules are nonmembranous, cylindrical organelles, the walls of which are composed of 13 filaments of globular proteins called *tubulin*. Microtubules along with microfilaments, function in one or more of the following three ways:

1. To maintain the shape of a cell by providing structural support
2. To act as an internal conduit for the movement of materials from one part of the cell to another
3. To provide for certain forms of cellular movement, such as ciliary motion

Intermediate filaments are strong tough proteins that provide structural reinforcement within cells. They also hold organelles in place and assist the microtubules in giving shape to the cell.[14]

CENTROSOMES AND CENTRIOLES

Near the nucleus of many cells is a dense area of cytoplasm called the *centrosome*. It contains two hollow, cylindrical structures called *centrioles*, which are composed of nine sets of microtubules arranged in a radial fashion, but without the central pair of tubules (9 + 0 pattern). Centrioles are often found near the nuclear envelope with the long axis of one lying at right angles to the other (Fig. 1-5). The function of the centrioles is to form and organize a complex array of microtubules in nondividing cells. In dividing cells, it forms the spindle apparatus, a structure needed to separate a single cell into two daughter cells when the cell divides (see page 31). The microtubules that make up the wall of the centriole are arranged in sets of three, lying in the same plane and embedded in a dense granular substance.

PLASMA AND INTRACELLULAR MEMBRANES

Membranes are major structural components of the cell. The plasma membrane surrounds the entire cell and separates the intracellular and extracellular compartments. Within the cell, membranous organelles are separated from the cytosol by membranes that are similar in structure to the plasma membrane. Membranes perform a variety of functions and have the primary role of regulating the passage of material between compartments. Membranes also have a vital role in cellular communication, are involved in cellular interactions, and are the sites of various biochemical and energy transduction reactions. Hence, membranes are selective barriers that are involved in several important physiologic processes such as metabolism, electrophysiology, and contraction.

The plasma membrane consists of a double layer of lipid molecules (the lipid bilayer) with proteins bound to each layer as well as within the layers (Fig. 1-6). Lipids account for about half the mass of the plasma membrane and consist of phospholipids, glycolipids, and others such as cholesterol. The most abundant of the lipids are **amphipathic phospholipid molecules**, which have a polar end and a nonpolar end. Phospholipids in the bilayer are arranged so their polar region points toward the interior or exterior of the cell and their nonpolar regions are buried in the interior of the membrane.[15] The polar region is **hydrophilic** and tends to associate with water, but the nonpolar fatty acid tails are **hydrophobic** and repel water. This arrangement allows the membrane to behave as a barrier, restricting the loss of intracellular material and governing material entry. The lipid bilayer behaves as a liquid crystal (fluid nature) and gives the membrane the ability to change shape and fuse with other membranes. The plasma membrane exists in a fluid state at body temperature, and the protein and lipid components move within the membrane; that is, the structure of the plasma membrane is dynamic, not static. Because the membrane is fluid and resembles a patch-

FOCUS ON CELLULAR PHYSIOLOGY

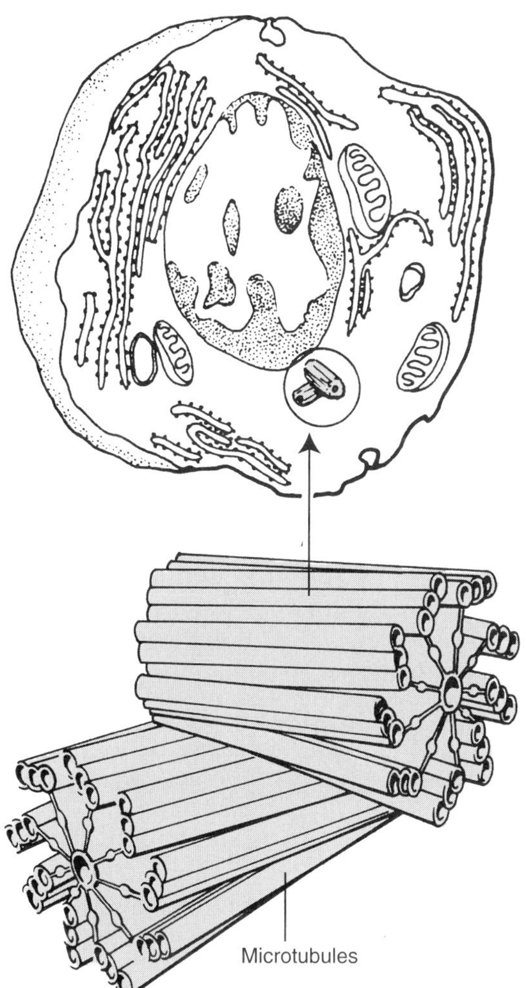

FIGURE 1-5. Centrioles. **A.** Placement in relationship to the nucleus. **B.** Appearance and composition of the centriole.

FOCUS ON CELLULAR PHYSIOLOGY

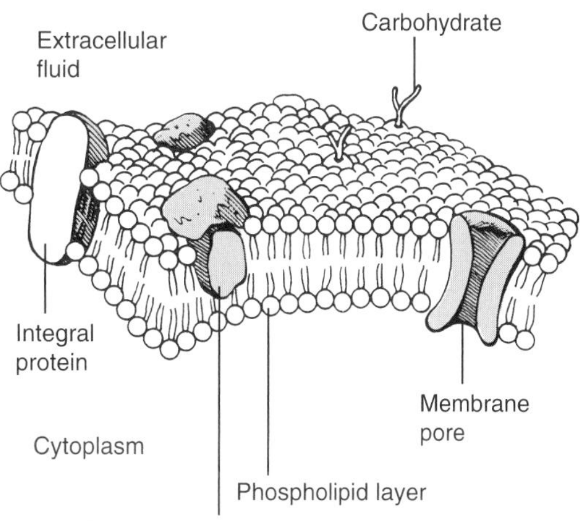

FIGURE 1-6. The structure and components of the lipid bilayer.

work or mosaic of protein and lipid, this concept is often called the *fluid mosaic model* of membrane structure.

Proteins are anchored in or on the lipid bilayer. Those bound to the inner or outer membrane surface are called *peripheral proteins*. Those partially or completely embedded in the lipid bilayer are called *integral proteins*. Membrane proteins may have other types of molecules attached to them. Proteins on the outer membrane surface, for example, may have carbohydrates attached. These are called *glycoproteins*. Carbohydrates may also be attached to the polar region of the phospholipid molecules, forming *glycolipids*. Membrane proteins not only form part of the molecular structure of the plasma membrane, but they also have many functional roles, such as transporting and exchanging materials between the cell and its environment. Other proteins are enzymes that speed up or act as catalysts in chemical reactions.

The intracellular membranes allow for different constituents within the organelles. Lysosomes, for example, are filled with proteolytic enzymes for their specific purposes. In some cells, the ER is called the sarcoplasmic reticulum and contains large amounts of calcium. The membranes of the organelles allow for separation of the compartments within the cells.

Functions of Membrane Components

The various components of the plasma membrane are responsible for carrying out the different functions of the membrane. In general, the lipid bilayer gives the membrane its physical characteristics, and the proteins give it its biologic features.

The lipid bilayer has at least three important functions: (1) it forms the structure of the membrane; (2) the hydrophobic interior serves as a barrier to the passage of water-soluble substances between the intracellular and ECF; and (3) it gives the membrane fluidity.

Proteins within the plasma membrane serve multiple functions. They:

1. Act as channels across the lipid bilayer allowing small water-soluble substances such as ions to pass through the membrane. Most of these channels are highly selective and cells vary in the number, kind, and activity of the channels that they possess. Some channels are regulated and can be "opened" or "closed" to a specific ion. This results from changes in the shape of the channels in response to a stimulus or controlling mechanism. These protein ions channels are referred to as "gated channels."
2. Serve as carrier molecules that transfer materials across membranes that are not capable of traversing the membrane on their own
3. Bind with specific molecules or chemical messengers such as hormones or neurotransmitters
4. Orchestrate the signal transduction mechanisms that are important carrying messages to the interior of the cell (see page 23)
5. Catalyze various biochemical reactions that occur in the membrane
6. Provide energy transduction and ATP synthesis in mitrochondrial membranes
7. Form cellular structure or specialized membrane junctions

MEMBRANE TRANSPORT

For the cell to produce its own cytoplasm, synthesize chemicals for export, or derive energy from chemicals and convert the energy into useful work, the cell must acquire chemicals from the ECF. Cell metabolism also produces waste products that must be eliminated from the cell into the ECF. Because the plasma membrane separates the ICF from the ECF, all substances that either enter or leave the cell must pass through the plasma membrane.

In general, the mechanisms of cellular exchange can be divided into passive and active movement across the cell membrane. *Passive movement* includes the process of diffusion, osmosis, filtration, and carrier-mediated facilitated diffusion. *Active movement* involves energy driven carrier-mediated transport systems as well as endocytosis and exocytosis. Epithelial transport moves substances across epithelial cells and may use active or passive mechanisms.

Diffusion

Diffusion is defined as the net movement of a substance from a region of higher concentration to a region of lower concentration or down a concentration gradient. With the cell membrane as a barrier, lipid-soluble molecules of any size can dissolve through the lipid bilayer and simply diffuse into or out of the cell. If the substance is equally distributed between two regions, no concentration gradient exists and **diffusion equilibrium** is said to be present. The rate of net diffusion of a given substance, or the time that it takes for diffusion equilibrium to occur, is directly proportional to the concentration gradient, the cross-sectional or surface area of the diffusion pathway, and the temperature of the diffusing substance. The rate of net diffusion is determined by the amount of substance available, by kinetic motion, and by cell membrane openings through which the substance can move.[13] Additional factors include the atomic or molecular size and configuration, the ability of the diffusing solute to dissolve in lipids, and the presence or absence of an electrical charge on the diffusing solute particles.

The plasma membrane presents a barrier to the movement of materials into and out of the cell. Substances that diffuse through the membrane must either dissolve in the fluid structure of the plasma membrane and then diffuse from one side to the other, or they must pass through interruptions in the membrane called *membrane channels* or *pores.* Pores are fluid-filled channels formed by proteins within the membrane. Small substances may diffuse in or out through the pores. Some examples include small amounts of sodium (Na^+), potassium (K^+), calcium (Ca^{++}), chloride (Cl^-), and bicarbonate (HCO_3^-) and large amounts of water.[21] In general, molecules whose molecular weights are greater than 200 are unable to, or else have difficulty in, passing through plasma membrane channels.[3] How readily an ion or molecule diffuses in or out of a cell, therefore, depends on both its physical and chemical properties, as well as the physical and chemical properties of the plasma membrane that the molecule or ion is attempting to cross.

The movement of oxygen molecules into cells and carbon dioxide molecules out of cells is an example of the process of diffusion. Metabolic process occurring within the cell are continually consuming oxygen molecules, so that the concentration gradient favors diffusion of this gas into the cell. Carbon dioxide molecules are being continually produced during cellular metabolism, so the concentration gradient favors diffusion of this gas out of the cell. Other substances that diffuse through the membrane include nitrogen, steroids, and fat-soluble vitamins (Fig. 1-7).

FOCUS ON CELLULAR PHYSIOLOGY

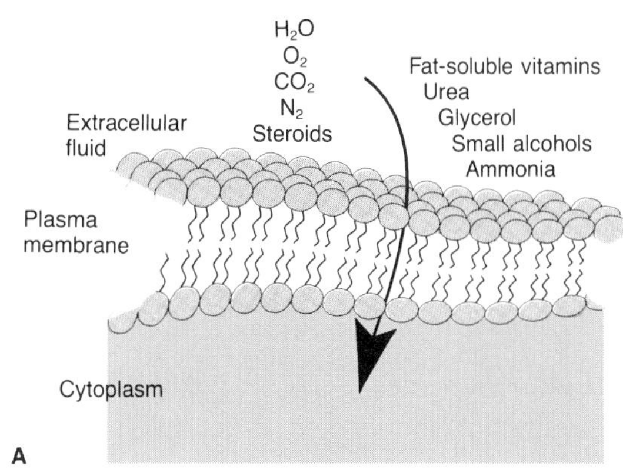

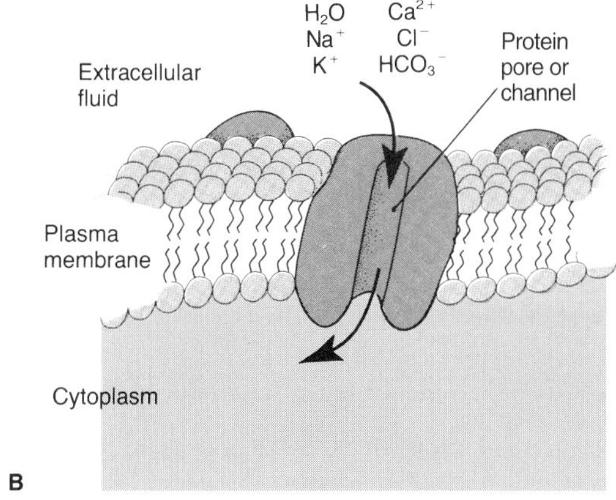

FIGURE 1-7. Passive diffusion across the cell membrane occurs down a concentration gradient. **A.** Substances that can pass directly through the cell membrane. **B.** Substances that diffuse through a protein channel.

Osmosis

Osmosis is the net diffusion of water through a selectively permeable membrane that separates two aqueous solutions with different solute concentrations. The membrane is impermeable to one or more of the solutes. If the concentration of nondiffusible solutes (substances dissolved in water that cannot diffuse through the membrane) is greater on one side of the membrane than the other, net diffusion of water (osmosis) occurs through the membrane toward the area of greater solute concentration until the solute/solvent ratio is equal on both sides of the membrane, or until a force of equal magnitude opposing the force created by the movement of water is applied. Water molecules diffuse from an area of greater water concentration through a selectively permeable membrane to an area of lesser water concentration (Fig. 1-8).

During osmosis, pressure is created on the membrane as water moves from an area of higher concentration, through the membrane, to an area of lesser concentration. This pressure is called **osmotic pressure.** The magnitude of osmotic pressure depends on the number of particles (solute particles) in the solution toward which water is moving. The greater the number of nondiffusible particles in that solution, the greater its osmotic pressure.

Fluids that contain osmotically active particles in the same concentration as found in the plasma of blood are **isotonic.** If a human erythrocyte is placed in an isotonic solution, it neither swells nor shrinks because the net diffusion of water in or out of the cell is zero. An example of an isotonic solution is 0.9% sodium chloride in water (normal saline). Normally, the net volume of the cell remains constant. If a concentration difference for water occurs, the water will move, causing the cell to shrink or to swell.[13] Fluids that contain a higher concentration of osmotically active particles than blood plasma are termed **hypertonic fluids.** Erythrocytes that are placed in a hypertonic solution shrink and shrivel (*crenation*) because net diffusion of water out of the cell occurs. **Hypotonic fluids** contain a lower concentration of osmotically active particles than does plasma; therefore, erythrocytes swell and hemolyze when placed in hypotonic

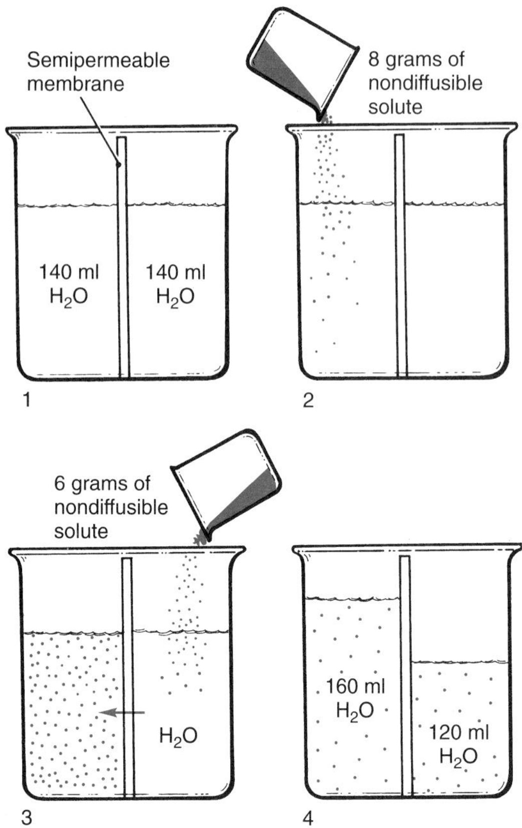

FIGURE 1-8. **Osmosis. A.** A beaker of water with superimpermeable membrane separating the sides. **B.** Add 8 g of a nondiffusible substance to one side. **C.** Add 6 g of a nondiffusible substance to the other side. **D.** The water moves toward the more concentrated side and makes the concentrations equal, with more fluid on one side than the other.

solutions because the net diffusion of water is into the cell (Fig. 1-9). In the body, osmosis is important in maintaining plasma volume, interstitial and ICF volumes, and the volumes of other fluid compartments.

FOCUS ON CELLULAR PHYSIOLOGY

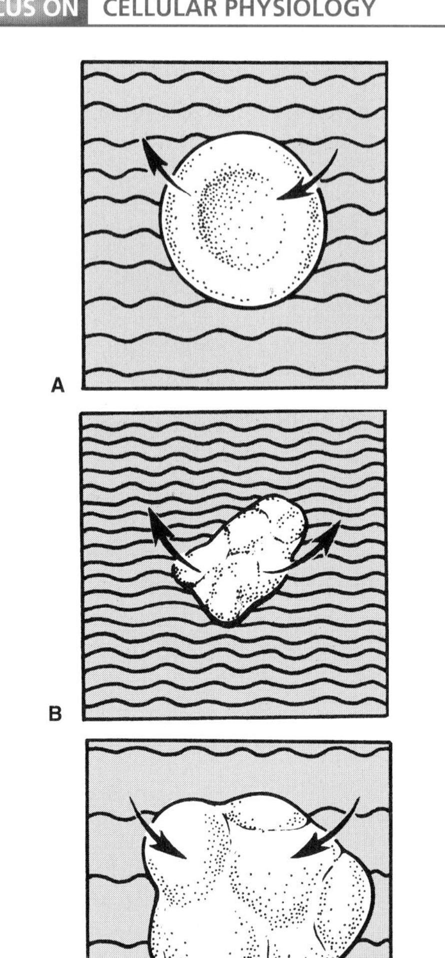

FIGURE 1-9. **A.** Isotonic solution (cell volume unchanged). **B.** Hypertonic solution (cell volume decreased). **C.** Hypotonic solution (cell volume increased).

Filtration

Substances, especially water, will move across a membrane because of pressure differences, always moving from greater to lesser pressure areas. Filtration is an important concept in the kidneys in the formation of glomerular filtrate. Larger particles remain in the capillaries due to their size and the impermeability of the glomerular basement membrane (see page 591).

Carrier-Mediated Transport Systems

The transport systems described above produce a net movement of molecules down their concentration gradients via their ability to pass through the membrane due to their lipid solubility or small size. The cell needs to be able to also transport materials that are not lipid-soluble and are larger in size. Many types of solutes such as glucose, amino acids, and various inorganic ions (eg, Na^+, Cl^-, K^+) are transported across plasma membranes by carrier molecules. Some of these transport systems are active and require metabolic energy, whereas others are passive, requiring no energy. Carrier-mediated transport systems often display one or more of the following protein-binding characteristics:

SPECIFICITY. Carrier systems are generally specific for a particular solute. For example, the system that transports glucose will not transport other organic solutes such as amino acids.

SATURATION. Many systems have a maximum rate (called *transport maximum*, or *Tm*) at which a solute can be transported. If more solute is present than the system can handle, the system is said to be saturated and transporting solute at maximum rate. Below saturation level, the rate of transport varies directly with solute concentration (ie, the higher the solute concentration, the faster the rate of transport).

COMPETITION. If the same carrier system transports two different solutes in the same direction, the rate of transport of each will be diminished by the presence of the other. In other words, the solutes compete for transport by the carrier, and some of each solute will be transported at the carrier's maximum rate.

ENERGY DEPENDENCY. Many carrier systems require energy to function. Substances (metabolic inhibitors) that interfere with energy-producing reactions of the cell often stop transport processes.

SPEED. Substances transported by mediated transport are usually moved more rapidly than are those moving by simple diffusion.[3]

FACILITATED DIFFUSION

Facilitated diffusion uses a carrier protein to assist the movement of a molecule not capable of diffusing across the membrane. Although not an example of diffusion in the strictest sense, the movement is down the concentration gradient and is passive. Because the molecule is being moved from a region of high concentration to one of lower concentration, energy is not required. Facilitated diffusion is subject to the protein-binding characteristics described above. The system is saturable and specific and can be subjected to competition. The binding of the solute particle to the carrier protein results in a conformation change that translocates the solute to the other side of the membrane (Fig. 1-10). The affinity of the solute particle for the carrier protein is the same on the two sides of the membrane; therefore, when the concentration is equal on either side of the membrane (equilibrated), there would be no net flow.

This process of assisted diffusion is especially important in moving glucose across membranes of erythrocytes, muscles, and adipose cells. Normally, there is a very small reserve of glucose for energy metabolism within the cell, so the cell is dependent on the transport of glucose from the ECF. Glucose is not soluble in the lipid of the cell membrane and is too large to pass through the membrane pores. After combining with the carrier molecule, forming the glucose–carrier complex, the conformation of the complex changes and permits glucose to dissociate from the carrier on the cytoplasmic side of the membrane. The carrier is now free to bind another solute particle. Because there are limited numbers of binding sites the system is *saturable* and subject to *competition*.

FOCUS ON CELLULAR PHYSIOLOGY

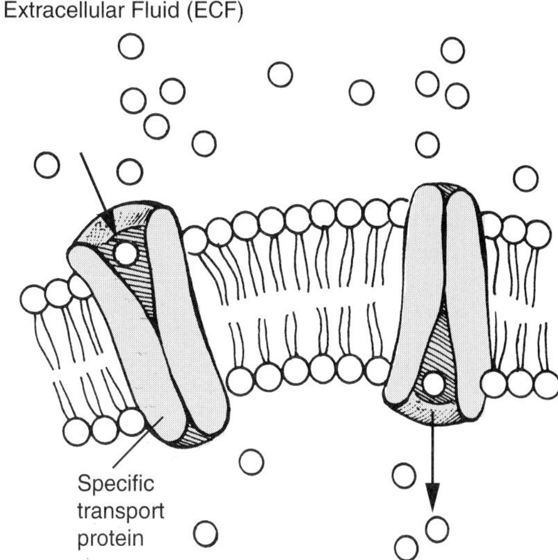

FIGURE 1-10. **In facilitated diffusion, a specific transport protein binds a substance (in this case, glucose) and carries it from a higher concentration in the ECF to a lower concentration in the ICF. A conformational change in the transport protein allows the molecule to enter.**

The mechanism of facilitated passive transport involves combining glucose with specific carrier molecules that are in the cell membrane. The hormone insulin has a major effect on glucose transport and has been shown to increase the rate of glucose transport sevenfold to tenfold in some cells. Insulin increases the number of glucose transport proteins available and also increases the rate of glucose metabolism in cells, thus increasing the magnitude of the concentration gradient.[3] An example of saturation is demonstrated with the appearance of glucose in the urine in uncontrolled diabetes mellitus. As the filtered load of glucose increases (due to excessive blood glucose) at the kidney, the glucose transporters in the kidney are saturated and glucose, which is normally completely reabsorbed back into the blood, appears in the urine. This, then, creates an osmotic gradient that increases the water content of the urine and the characteristic polyuria (excretion of large amounts of urine) seen with diabetes mellitus.

ACTIVE TRANSPORT

Active transport is a carrier-mediated process that is capable of transferring solute particles against their concentrations gradients. Active transport systems reverse the effects of diffusion and are therefore capable of doing work. These systems always require the expenditure of energy and are called "active transport" systems, or simply "pumps." All of the body's cells are capable of active transport in one way or another. The ability of a cell to carry out active transport depends on energy derived from metabolism. The two classes of active transport systems are based on how they derive energy. *Primary active transport* uses energy directly derived from metabolism (directly from ATP). *Secondary active transport* couples the energy from the downhill movement of charged particles and depends on primary active transport to maintain an ion gradient.

Primary Active Transport Systems

The four primary active transport systems include sodium–potassium adenosine triphosphatase (ATPase), calcium ATPase, hydrogen ion ATPase, and hydrogen–potassium ATPase. The ATPase (carrier protein) groups of proteins are capable of hydrolyzing ATP. Therefore, the same protein that binds is also capable of hydrolyzing ATP and using the chemical energy released to move the ions against their concentration gradients. For an ion to be moved from a region of low concentration to a region of higher concentration requires that the binding of the ion to the carrier protein be asymmetrical.[11] The transporter breaks down ATP and in the process phosphorylates itself. The phosphorylation of the transporter maintains the protein in a high-affinity state for the transported solute on the low concentration side of the membrane (see page 24). The transport protein changes conformation in such a way that it exposes the binding site on the opposite side (higher concentration) of the membrane and the solute is released.

The *sodium–potassium pump* (Na^+, K^+–ATPase) is an important example of active transport present in all cells (Fig. 1-11*A*). The pumping of the Na^+, K^+–ATPase protein maintains the characteristic distribution of sodium and potassium ions in the ICF and ECF. The ICF normally contains a much higher concentration of potassium than the ECF. Also, the ECF contains a much higher concentration of sodium ions than the ICF (see Table 1-1). These balances must be rigidly maintained for proper cellular function. Many cellular functions depend on the ion gradients maintained by the Na^+, K^+–ATPase. The Na^+, K^+–ATPase transports three sodium ions out of the cell, thereby preventing their accumulation inside. It also returns two potassium ions to the inside of the cell. This requires direct energy from ATP. The result is a net transfer of a positive charge to ECF and the transport process is not electrically neutral.

The Na^+, K^+–ATPase is important for cell volume regulation.[11] The Na^+–K^+ pump prevents accumulation of sodium ions within the cell; by doing so, it also minimizes water influx and cellular swelling. Accumulation of sodium ions in ICF tends to cause osmosis of water toward the interior of the cell. The pumping of sodium ions out of the cell overcomes the continual tendency for water to enter the cell. If cellular metabolism ceases or decreases (as seen with hypoxia), adequate ATP is not produced and sodium will diffuse into the cell and not be removed, increasing the solute concentration in the ICF. This will create an osmotic gradient, water moves into the cell, and cellular swelling begins immediately.[13]

Calcium (Ca^{++}–ATPase is found in the plasma membrane and the ER membrane and Ca^{++}–ATPase maintains lower calcium concentrations in the cytoplasm (Fig. 1-11*B*).[9] Hydrogen$^+$–ATPase is located in the plasma membrane and in several organelle mem-

FOCUS ON CELLULAR PHYSIOLOGY

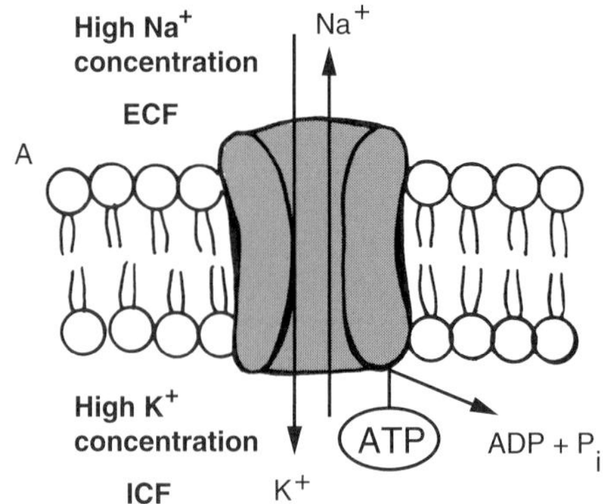

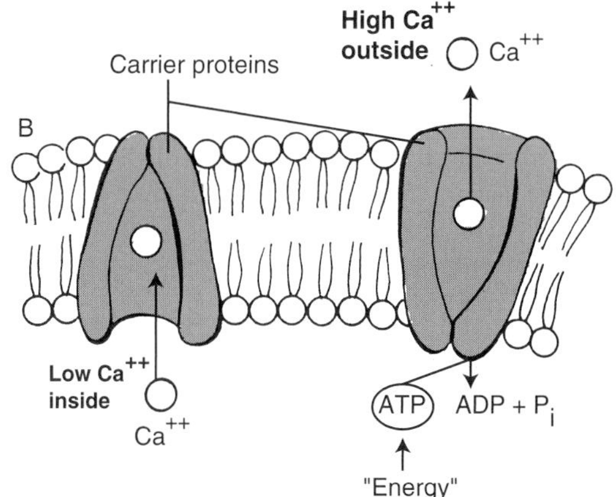

FIGURE 1-11. During active transport a molecule combines with a transport or carrier protein, and the carrier transports the molecule from an area of low concentration to an area of high concentration. Energy is always required. **A.** The sodium–potassium pump is an important example that maintains the characteristic sodium and potassium ionic distribution. **B.** Calcium ions also may be moved by active transport through the cell membrane or into the sarcoplasmic reticulum in muscle cells.

branes. H^+–ATPase has several important roles such as energy transduction in mitochondrial membranes and for acid–base balance by the kidneys. H^+,K^+–ATPase is located in the membrane of acid-secreting cells of the stomach and kidneys.[1]

Secondary Active Transport Systems

Secondary active transport uses the ion gradients created by primary active transport as an energy source (Fig. 1-12). This can be illustrated by visualizing a dam. Water builds up on one side of the dam and if allowed to move to the other side, energy is released and can be harnessed for other purposes. The ion gradient is similar, with ions in a high-energy state due to their separation across the membrane. If the ions are allowed to flow down their gradient to the lower energy state, the energy released can be used to drive the other uphill reactions. For example, the energy stored in an ion gradient can be used to phosphorylate adenosine diphosphate (ADP) to synthesize ATP during oxidative phosphorylation (see page 20) or it can be coupled to the pumping of another solute molecule against its concentration gradient as in secondary active transport.[19] The most common ion used in secondary active transport is sodium. Sodium binds to the transporter, resulting in a change in affinity of the binding site for the transported solute. The changes in the transporters are brought about by **allosteric modulation**, which refers to the binding of a ligand to a protein or changing the conformation of the protein (see page 25). Sodium moves down its concentration gradient while the transported solute moves against the concentration gradient. The transported solute may move in the same direction as sodium in a process known as **cotransport** or **symport** through coupling of two different molecules, or in the opposite direction called **counter-transport** or **antiport** (two different molecules travel in the opposite directions through a common carrier mechanism). A variety of organic molecules are transported by secondary active transport.

FOCUS ON CELLULAR PHYSIOLOGY

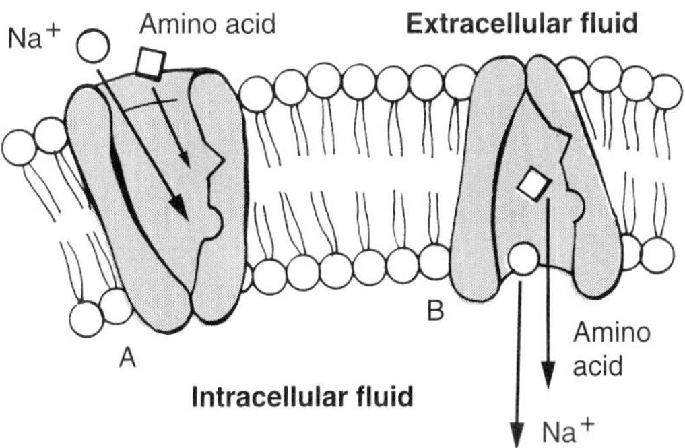

FIGURE 1-12. Secondary active transport. The electrochemical gradient is provided by the sodium pump, and the amino acid (as well as glucose and other molecules in specific circumstances) is moved uphill, against its concentration gradient (see text).

Endocytosis and Exocytosis

Endocytosis and exocytosis are methods for bringing particles into the cell and releasing secretions to the exterior of the cell. These processes are schematically illustrated in Figure 1-13. Both are essential in carrying out the functional capabilities of specific cells.

Endocytosis refers to the bringing in of protein and other substances through invagination of the outer cell membrane. This process occurs in the following ways:

1. *Pinocytosis* involves movement of water or ECF that adheres to the outer cell membrane stimulating invagination of the membrane. The material is encased or enclosed in a vesicle and floats into the cytoplasm. Lysosomes attach to the vesicle surface, releasing hydrolytic enzymes into the vesicle; the

FOCUS ON CELLULAR PHYSIOLOGY

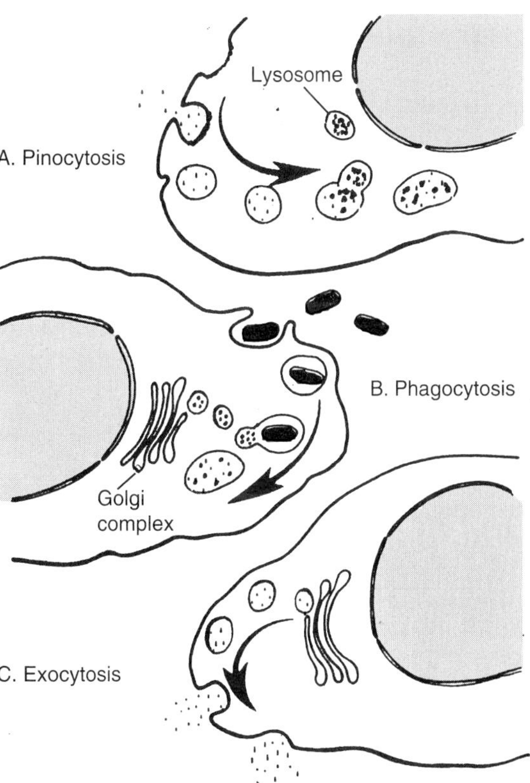

FIGURE 1-13. **A, B.** Endocytosis. Pinocytosis **(A)** allows for intake of certain substances through specific receptors on the cell surface. Phagocytosis **(B)** allows for intake and destruction of bacteria. **C.** Exocytosis is the process by which formed cellular elements are delivered to other areas of the body.

enzymes break down the material. A residual body may be left within the vesicle or excreted through the cell membrane to the ECF.

2. *Phagocytosis* involves the ingestion of particulate material or macromolecular substances. It often refers to the engulfment of a bacterium (see page 264).
3. *Receptor-mediated endocytosis* refers to the movement of substances through cell-surface receptors that stimulate the endocytotic process. Cell membranes have cell-surface receptors that bind specific molecules. Substances, termed **ligands**, bind selectively to these receptors and can be rapidly taken into the cell. In some cases the receptor complexes escape degradation and are recycled to trap more ligand. In other cases the receptor and ligand are both degraded, which leads to a decrease in the number of surface receptors. Important compounds internalized through this process are *low-density lipoproteins*, which provide cholesterol needed for cellular membrane synthesis.[21] After the ligands have been taken into the cell, lysosomes fuse with the vesicles and process the material.

Exocytosis has been termed *reverse pinocytosis* and is an active release of soluble products to the ECF. Secretion granules are formed by the Golgi complex (see page 7). The formed secretion granules move to the inner surface of the cell membrane, adhere, and cause an outpouching of the membrane. The outpouched area ruptures and releases the contents of the secretion granules into the ECF. The secretory products are vital to maintain the steady state of the host and include, for example, secretions necessary for digestion, glandular secretion, and neural transmission.

Both endocytosis and exocytosis require energy and are affected by cellular ability to synthesize ATP. Both processes require enzymatic activity to enhance the rate of the reactions.

Epithelial Transport

Various molecules must cross epithelial cells. This may happen by two mechanisms: (1) they may simply pass through the extracellular spaces between the cells in a process known as the paracellular pathway, or (2) they may pass through the cell via transcellular pathways (the more common route). To cross the epithelial barrier, the molecule must cross both the basal and luminal membranes and this may involve active and passive processes.

ELECTRICAL PROPERTIES OF CELLS

Differences in electrical potential across the plasma membrane are characteristic of all living cells and are called *membrane potentials*. The membrane potential exists because of unequal distribution of ions between the inner and outer surfaces of the cell membrane, the differences in membrane permeability to various ions, and active transport systems that maintain ionic imbalance across the membrane. The electrical charge for the inside of the cell is more negative than the outside and the membrane is said to be polarized.

Some cells are "excitable" cells and can generate impulses at their membranes, which can be used to transmit signals along the membranes.[13] The *resting membrane potential* in electrically excitable cells normally is about −70 to −85 mV from the inside to the outside of the cell when the cell is in the resting state (Fig. 1-14). There is a small excess of negatively charged ions inside the ICF and excess positive ions in the ECF. The opposite charges are attracted to one another and the membrane separates them. The major determinant of the resting membrane potential is that the membrane is more permeable to potassium at rest than sodium. More potassium leaks out of the cell because there are 50 to 75 times more open potassium channels in the plasma membrane than open sodium channels.[13] As potassium diffuses down its concentration gradient, some of the positively charged potassium ions move into the cell because of the electric gradient. When the magnitude of the flow of an ion is equal but in opposite directions, due to the electric and concentration gradients, an equilibrium potential for that ion exists. The value of the equilibrium potential depends on the concentration gradient of the ion across the membrane. The larger the magnitude of the gradient, the greater the equilibrium potential. The potassium equilibrium potential is approximately −90 mV and +60 mV for sodium. The resting membrane potential for a nerve cell is approximately −70 mV because some positively charged sodium ions are leaking into the cell, making it slightly more positive than the potassium equilibrium potential. Neither sodium nor potassium is at its equilibrium potential so the flow of the ions continues; however, the resting membrane potential is much closer to the potassium equilibrium potential. The gradients are maintained by the action of the Na^+, K^+–ATPase, which pumps the Na^+ that leaks in back out of the cell and the potassium that leaks out back into the cell. The Na^+, K^+–ATPase unequally distributes the ions (three sodiums ions out for every two potassium ions in) resulting in a net movement of charge across the membrane, which contributes to the membrane potential and accounts for the name "electrogenic pump." Transient changes in the membrane's permeability to ions alter the voltage across the membrane and represent a major mechanism by which cells can communicate.

Some cells have the ability to respond to various types of stimuli, especially electrochemical stimuli. This response is called *cell excitability* and refers to the changing or altering of the electrical potential across

FOCUS ON CELLULAR PHYSIOLOGY

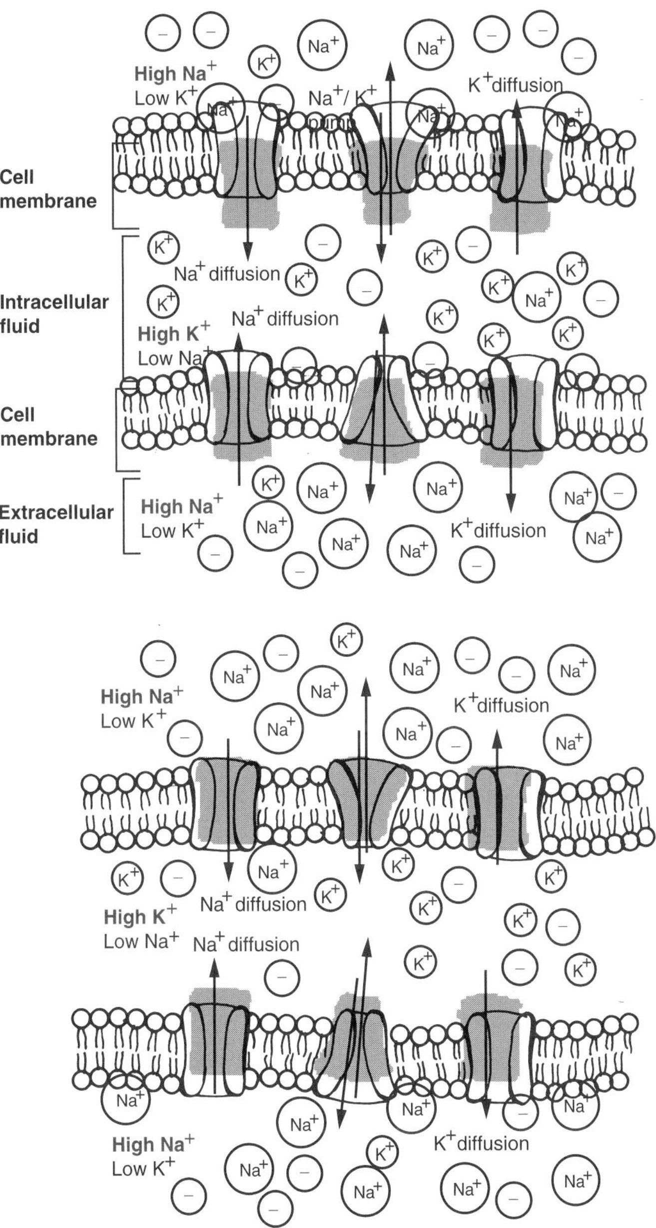

FIGURE 1-14. Development of the resting membrane potential. **A.** Active transport creates a concentration gradient across the cell membrane for sodium ions (NA^+) and potassium ions (K^+). K^+ diffuses out of the cell rather slowly but nonetheless faster than Na^+ can diffuse in. **B.** This unequal diffusion results in a net loss of positive charge and a resultant excess of negative charge inside the membrane. (Adapted from Shier, D., Butler, J., & Lewis, R. [1996]. *Hole's human anatomy and physiology* [7th ed.]. Dubuque, IA: W. C. Brown.)

the cell membrane. Nerve and muscle cells are considered to be excitable cells because they can change membrane potential, effect an action or response, and return to the resting state. The excitable tissue or cell receives a stimulus that rapidly changes its resting membrane potential.

Neurons signal information by changes in membrane potentials called graded potentials and action potentials. *Graded potentials* are local potentials that vary in amplitude and are conducted decrementally. An *action potential* is a rapid reversal of polarity in electrically excitable cells.[19]

Action Potentials

Action potentials bring about various responses in target cells, mainly those of contraction of a muscle and transmission of the impulse to the next neuron. The cell then returns to the normal resting state, characterized by reestablishment of the resting membrane potential. Many changes occur in cell membranes, when an action potential is elicited. Figure 1-15 represents the eliciting of an action potential.

The following discussion of the action potential refers to a neuron but applies with minor variation to other excitable cells, such as skeletal and cardiac muscle cells.

1. When an adequate positive stimulus is applied to the neuron, a rapid and marked change occurs in the *membrane potential* at the point on the membrane at which the stimulus was applied. The positive stimulus increases the sodium permeability of the membrane, allowing sodium to begin entering the cell at a faster rate than it can be pumped out.
2. As more sodium passes through the membrane, the membrane potential becomes less negative. After the membrane potential has been reduced to a critical value called the *threshold*, voltage-sensitive sodium channels are activated. At approximately −45 mV, the voltage gated sodium channels open and sodium rapidly diffuses into the cell down its electric and concentration gradients. At this point, the membrane is much more permeable to sodium than potassium and the membrane potential begins to approach the sodium equilibrium potential as the inside of the membrane becomes more positive.
3. The positively charged sodium reverses the polarity of the membrane potential resulting in a depolarization (the inside of the cell becomes positive to the outside of the cell) of the membrane. The increase in membrane permeability is transient and lasts for less than 1 msec. At this point inactivation gates in the sodium channel begin to close, blocking sodium entry into the cell.
4. At the peak of the action potential, the potassium channels that were activated by the threshold stimulus begin to open, thus increasing the membrane permeability to potassium ions. Almost immediately after sodium influx begins to depolarize the membrane, an increase in potassium diffusion out of the cell begins and it accelerates as the movement of sodium causes the inside of the membrane to become positive. Potassium leaves the cell for the same reasons that sodium entered—favorable electrical and chemical gradients coupled with an increase in membrane permeability.
5. As potassium efflux accelerates, further diffusion of sodium into the cell is inhibited by a decrease in sodium permeability, and the net loss of positive charges (K^+) from the inside causes the membrane potential to return to zero and then become negative once again, reestablishing the resting potential. More potassium leaves the cell than is actually required to restore the resting potential.
6. For a short time, the inside of the membrane is more negative than it normally is at rest. This increased internal negativity is termed *hyperpolarization*. The return of the membrane potential to resting level is completed by the sodium–potassium pump, which exchanges internal sodium for external potassium, thereby restoring the normal internal/external ratios of these ions.
7. The activities that restore the resting membrane potential after depolarization of the membrane collectively characterize the phenomenon of repolarization.[13]

The action potential (membrane depolarization and repolarization) can be graphically represented as

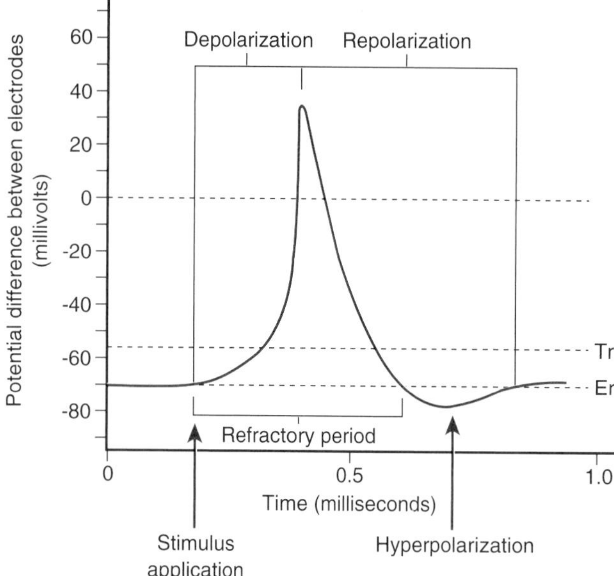

FIGURE 1-15. Representation of an action potential showing voltage versus time during depolarization and restoration of the resting potential. (Tr, threshold; Er, resting potential.)

change in voltage versus time (see Fig. 1-15). The duration of the action potential for a neuron is less than 0.5 msec. The action potential represents the change in membrane potential only in the region of the membrane where an adequate depolarizing stimulus has been applied. The entire plasma membrane does not simultaneously depolarize and then repolarize in response to an adequate stimulus. Once an action potential is generated, however, it spreads from one area of the membrane to another, resulting in the propagation of a nerve impulse.

A nerve impulse is a wave of depolarization followed by a wave of repolarization that travels along a nerve fiber away from the point of stimulation (Fig. 1-16). The sequence of one area of depolarization inducing depolarization in an adjacent area results in a wave of

FOCUS ON CELLULAR PHYSIOLOGY

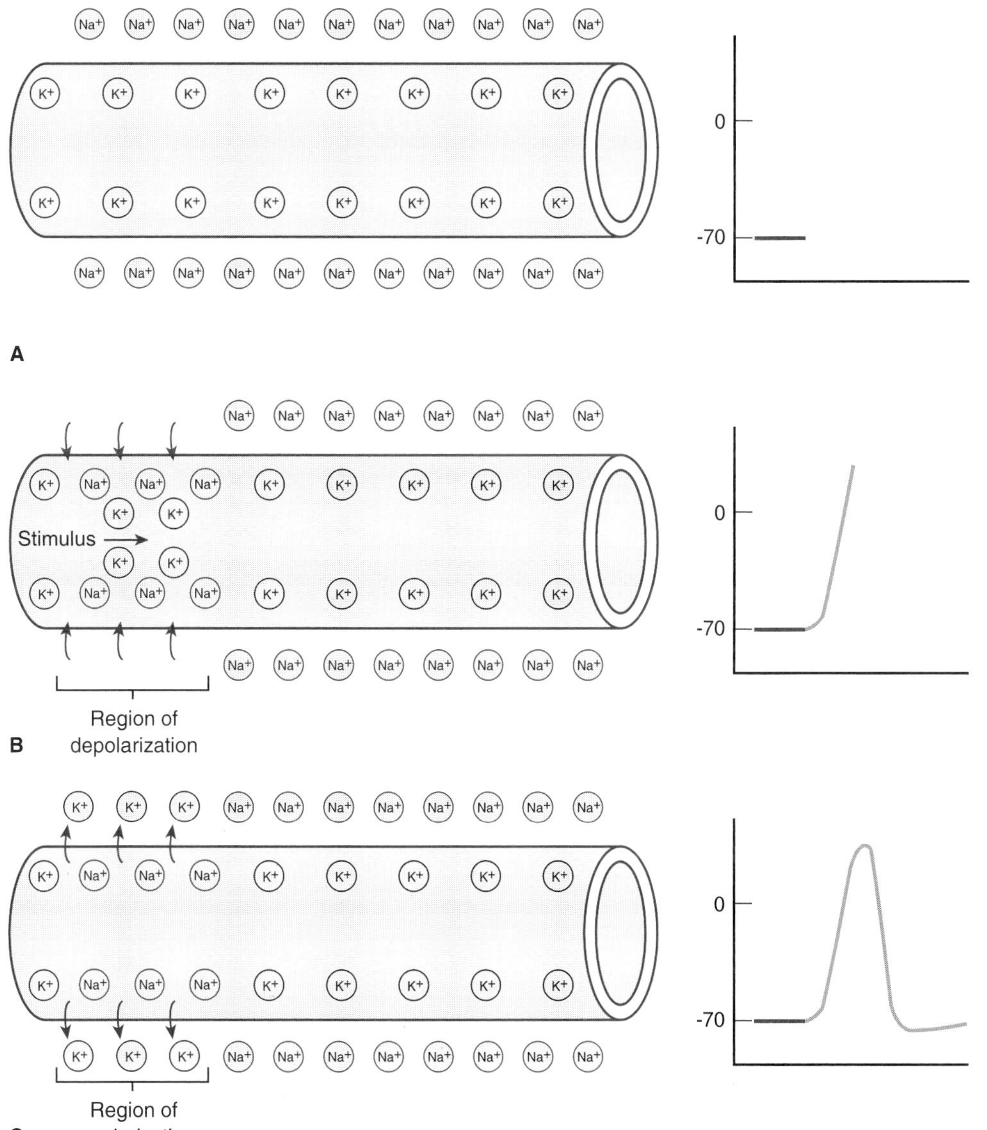

FIGURE 1-16. **A.** At rest the membrane potential is about –70 millivolts. **B.** When the membrane reaches threshold sodium channels open, some Na^+ diffuses inward, and the membrane is depolarized. **C.** Soon afterward potassium channels open, K^+ diffuses out, and the membrane is repolarized. (Shier, D., Butler, J., & Lewis, R. [1996]. *Hole's human anatomy and physiology* [7th ed.]. Dubuque, IA: W. C. Brown.)

depolarization that is propagated along the nerve fiber in a manner similar to the burning of a gunpowder fuse. The action potential is generated at the site of stimulus and propagated away from the site. As soon as the wave of depolarization passes a segment of the fiber, that segment is repolarized and its ability to respond to another stimulus is soon restored.[21]

Once generated, each impulse is conducted in an identical manner without change in magnitude or velocity. Stimuli that fail individually or collectively to reduce the membrane potential to threshold fail to generate an action potential and therefore produce no nerve impulse. The response of a nerve fiber to a stimulus is either maximal or zero. In other words, weak stimuli do not generate weak impulses and strong stimuli, strong impulses. This property is called the *all-or-none law*.

On reaching the axon terminal, the action potential activates voltage-sensitive calcium ion channels in the presynaptic membrane. Calcium ions diffuse into the cell and trigger vesicles containing neurotransmitters to fuse with the cell membranes and release their contents into the synapse. The neurotransmitter diffuses across the synapse and binds to receptors on the postsynaptic cell membrane ultimately triggering a response.[4]

After an action potential has been generated, a minimum amount of time is required before that area of the membrane becomes capable of responding in an identical manner to a second stimulus. This minimum period is called the *refractory period*. The length of the refractory period determines the maximum number of impulses that the fiber can conduct each second. Fibers with short refractory periods can conduct impulses at a higher frequency than fibers with long refractory periods. Nerve fibers conduct impulses at a much higher rate or frequency than do myocardial muscle fibers; therefore, their refractory periods differ considerably.

CELLULAR ENERGY METABOLISM

Cellular metabolism is the sum of all the biochemical reactions (**catabolic** and **anabolic**) in the cell. Many of these reactions would not occur spontaneously and thus require energy. The major cellular energy currency is ATP, which is required for numerous cellular functions such as active transport, biosynthetic reactions, and cellular movement to name just a few. ATP is a nucleic acid derivative that contains high-energy phosphate bonds that, when broken, release energy that can be coupled to other "uphill" reactions such as pumping ion against their concentration gradient. All cells generate ATP from the transfer of energy from the catabolism of fuel molecules, carbohydrates, lipids, and proteins to ADP as a phosphate group. Energy is then transferred to various cell functions via the hydrolysis of ATP to ADP and phosphate. The normal production of ATP occurs in a cycle involving three metabolic pathways: (1) glycolysis, (2) the Krebs cycle, and (3) oxidative phosphorylation.

Glycolysis

Glycolysis is the breakdown of the hexose glucose to two three-carbon pyruvate molecules. The enzymes for glycolysis are located in the cytoplasm and carbohydrates are the only fuel molecules that enter the glycolytic pathway. Glycolysis is catalyzed by 10 enzymes in a linear pathway (Fig. 1-17). In the presence of oxygen, glycolysis is the first step in the complete oxidation (aerobic metabolism) of glucose to carbon dioxide and water. Glycolysis generates four molecules of ATP for each glucose molecule; however, two molecules of ATP are spent in the early stages of glycolysis to phosphorylate glucose and fructose-6-phosphate, resulting in production of two ATPs. Therefore, a small yield of ATP is formed by glycolysis in the absence of oxygen (anaerobic glycolysis). Figure 1-17 shows that glycolysis itself is an anaerobic process. Glycolysis proceeds to produce pyruvic acid (pyruvate). Without available oxygen, pyruvate is reduced to lactic acid. The glycolytic, anaerobic system is inefficient, but it can keep certain cells viable for short periods of time. In the normal, unstressed cell, anaerobic metabolism provides less that 5% of the ATP requirements of the cell; the lactic acid that is formed diffuses out of the cell into the tissues and plasma.

The glycolytic process occurs during periods of intense muscular exertion in which oxygen consumption exceeds oxygen supply. Cellular respiration does not produce enough ATP, and the resulting accumulation of lactic acid in the muscle causes pain. The process produces an *oxygen debt* of the muscle that requires deep breathing after exercise to restore the balance of ATP. The recovery time may be very short or up to several hours. This process has been termed *recovery oxygen consumption*. The lactic acid remaining in the muscle cell can be reconverted to glucose or pyruvic acid in the presence of oxygen. Lactic acid that leaves the cell during exercise is carried to the liver, where it is converted to glycogen and carbon dioxide.[13]

Krebs Cycle

Although carbohydrates are the only fuel molecules that enter the glycolytic pathway, several nutrients (products of carbohydrate, lipid, and protein metabolism) are capable of fueling the next step in aerobic metabolism, the Krebs cycle (Fig. 1-18). The enzymes of the Krebs cycle, also known as the citric acid cycle, are located in the mitochondrial matrix. Acetyl coenzyme A (acetyl CoA) is

FOCUS ON CELLULAR PHYSIOLOGY

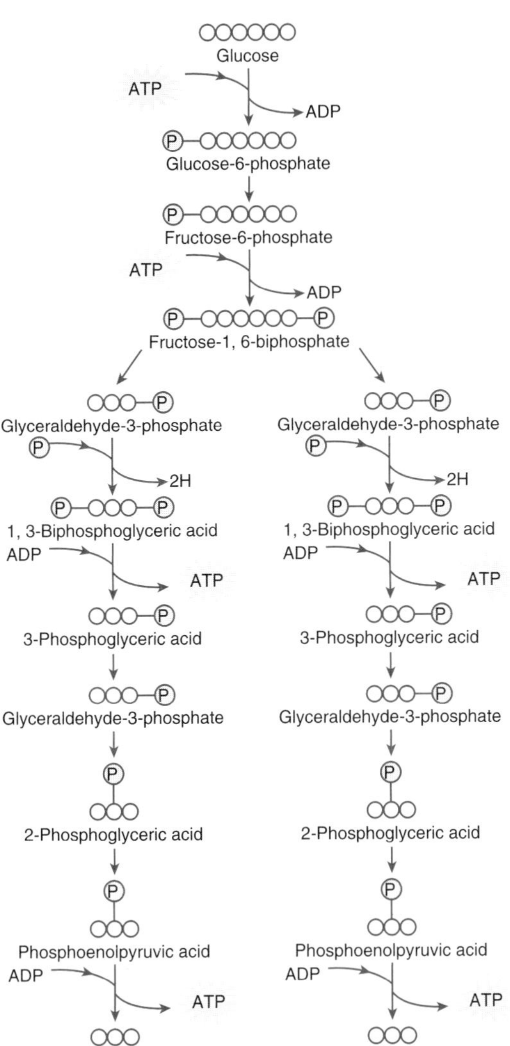

FIGURE 1-17. **Chemical reactions of glycolysis. There is a net production of two ATP molecules from each glucose molecule. The four hydrogen atoms released provide electrons that may be used to generate ATP in the electron transport system. (Shier, D., Butler, J., & Lewis, R. [1996]. *Hole's human anatomy and physiology* [7th ed.]. Dubuque, IA: W. C. Brown.)**

the major substrate, derived from the fuel molecules, that enter the Krebs cycle. The predominant fuel molecule is the pyruvate formed during glycolysis, which then enters the mitochondria and is converted to acetyl CoA. Acetyl CoA, synthesized from lipid and protein metabolism, also enters the Krebs cycle at this point and amino acids are capable of entering the cycle at other points in the cycle. The cycle begins with the combination of the two carbon acetyl group with the four carbon oxaloacetate molecules to form citrate. In eight sequential steps of the cycle, two molecules of carbon dioxide are produced, and four pairs of hydrogen atoms are transferred to coenzymes, flavin adenine nucleotide (FAD) and nicotinamide adenine dinucleotide (NAD) to form one $FADH_2$ and three NADH. Each complete cycle produces one substrate level phosphorylation of guanosine diphosphate (GDP) to guanosine triphosphate (GTP), which can be transferred to ADP to form ATP. The transfer of the hydrogens to the coenzymes represents a transfer of energy, and these molecules are used in the next and final step of aerobic ATP synthesis, oxidative phosphorylation.

Oxidative Phosphorylation

Oxidative phosphorylation is the last step in aerobic metabolism. The synthesis of ATP from ADP and phosphate uses the energy released when molecular oxygen (hence aerobic) combines with hydrogen atoms to form water. The enzymes involved with oxidative phosphorylation are located in the inner mitochondrial membrane. The hydrogen atoms, or more specifically the electrons of the hydrogen atoms, from glycolysis and the Krebs cycle are transferred by the reduced coenzymes to a series of metal-containing enzyme complexes known as the electron transport chain (ETC) (Fig. 1-19). As the electrons flow through this complex, with molecular oxygen being the final acceptor molecule, a series of energy transfers occur. Each protein complex in the ETC that accepts the electrons from the previous protein has a greater affinity for the electrons.[3] The electrons flow from higher to lower energy states; therefore, as the electrons are passed along the chain, energy is released. The reactions of the ETC are used to power the pumping of hydrogen ions across the inner mitochondrial membrane from the matrix to the intermembrane space and sets up an ion gradient. The flow of ions back down their electrochemical gradient provides the energy needed for the oxidative phosphorylation of ATP. The **protons** pass through an enzyme protein channel complex known as ATP synthetase in a process known as the *chemiosmosis model.* The energy released as the protons diffuse across the membrane drives the phosphorylation of ADP to form ATP (Fig. 1-20). Three ATP molecules are formed for each NADH and two for each $FADH_2$ that carry their electrons to the ETC. It follows that 38 ATP molecules can be synthesized aerobically. Clearly aerobic pathways for ATP production are much more efficient than anaerobic pathways.

SPECIALIZED MEMBRANE JUNCTIONS

In many cases, cells are tightly packed and their cell membranes are connected by intercellular junctions

FOCUS ON CELLULAR PHYSIOLOGY

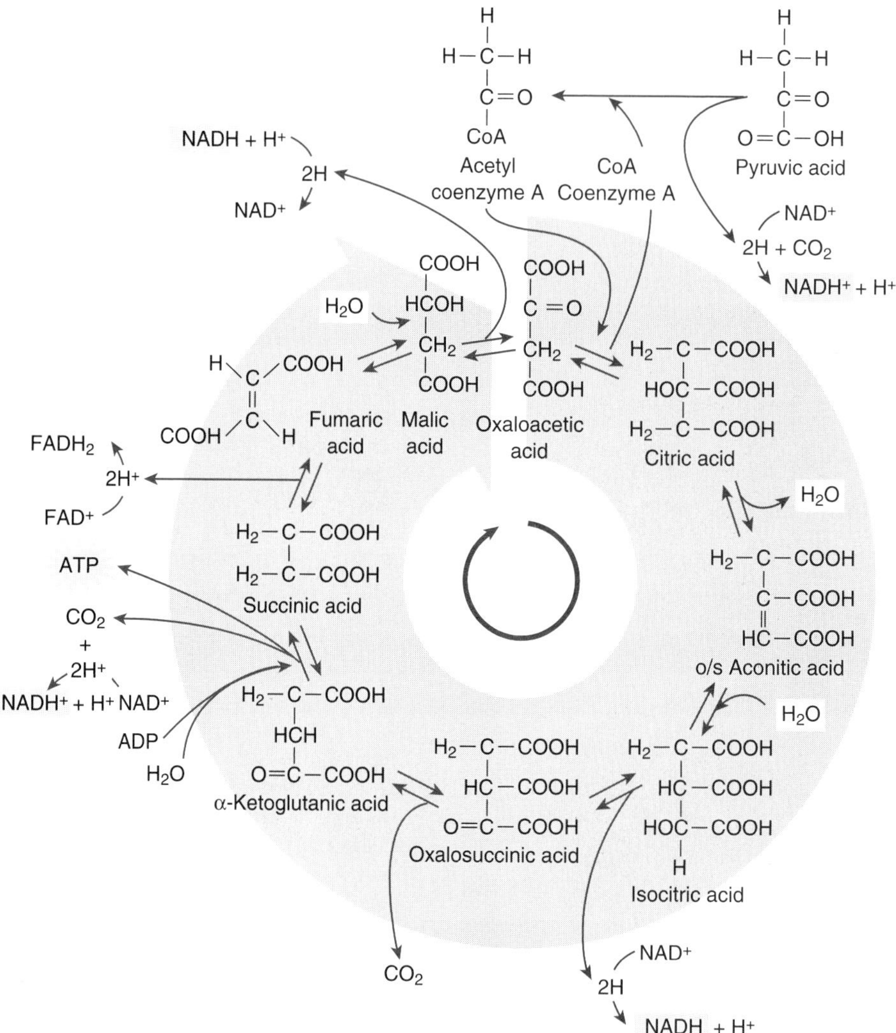

FIGURE 1-18. **Chemical reactions of the citric acid cycle. NADH molecules carrying hydrogen are in *boxes*. (Shier, D., Butler, J., & Lewis, R. [1996]. *Hole's human anatomy and physiology* [7th ed.]. Dubuque, IA: W. C. Brown.)**

or membrane junctions (Fig. 1-21). The three types of membrane junctions are:

1. **Desmosomes**—adhesive junctions found in tissues that are subjected to considerable mechanical stresses (eg, the epithelial cells of the skin). They are often referred to as "spot welds" because they anchor neighboring cells by their extending fibers.
2. **Tight junctions**—literally regions of close association between adjacent membranes, which limit movement of organic molecules through the extracellular spaces. Tight junctions are found in most epithelial tissues that form barriers such as those lining the gastrointestinal tract.
3. **Gap or nexus junctions**—specialized membrane junctions that consist of proteins that form pores connecting adjacent cells. These protein channels, called *connexons*, allow for the rapid exchange of small molecules or ions between the cells.[18,24] These types of membrane junctions are found in cells that have coordinated electrical activity or syncytial functions (eg, cardiac and smooth muscles).

Coordination of Cellular Activity and Signal Transduction

Signal transduction pathways are complex interactions that involve the binding of regulatory substances to plasma membrane receptors that alter the activities of specific cellular proteins and ultimately cause a cellular response.[3] The response of a cell to the primary chemi-

FOCUS ON CELLULAR PHYSIOLOGY

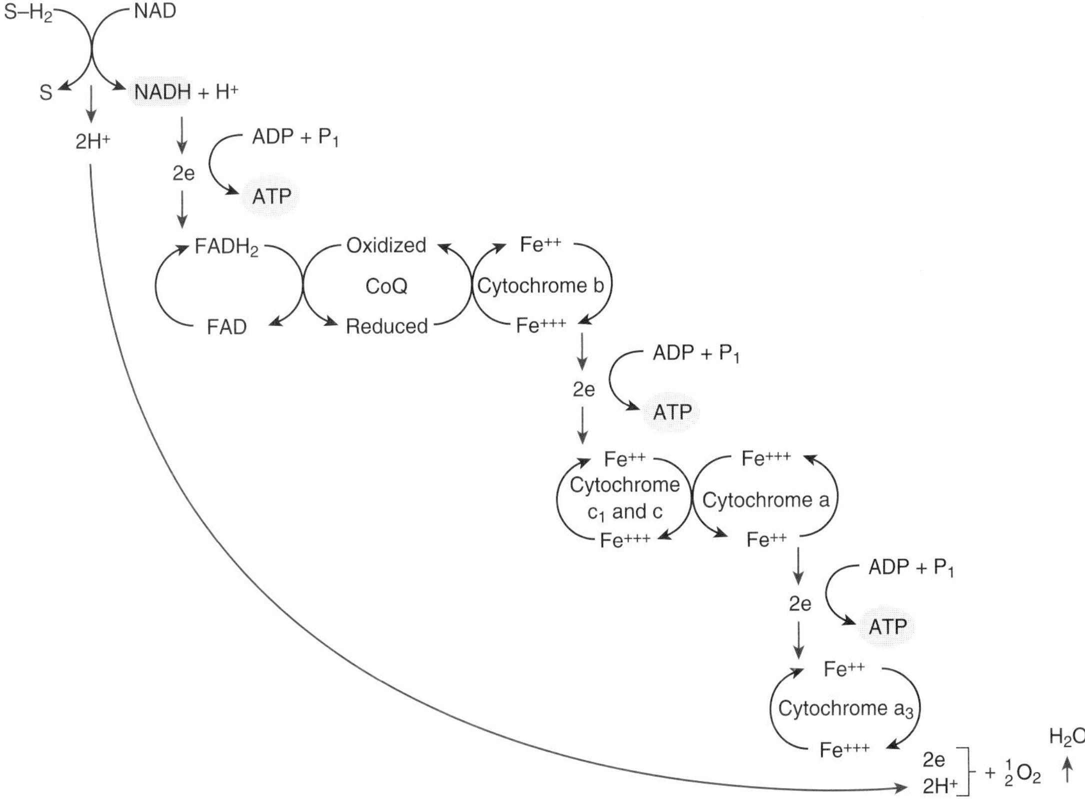

FIGURE 1-19. **Oxidative phosphorylation. Using the electron transport chains, large amounts of energy can be released (see text). (Fox, S.I. [1996].** ***Human physiology*** **[7th ed.]. Dubuque, IA: Times Mirror.)**

cal messenger or first messenger depends on cell type and the receptor activated. For example, activation of a β receptor found on the membrane of specialized cells of the heart, by the neurotransmitter norepinephrine, will result in an increase in heart rate. Similarly, the activation of the same type of receptors on adipose tissue results in lipolysis. The signal transduction pathways triggered by receptor activation may also influence genetic expression. This occurs by activating transcription factors thereby stimulating proliferation or differentiation of the target cells. These pathways are extremely important for homeostasis and often are the target stressors. The most common signal transduction pathways are described in further detail below.

PLASMA MEMBRANE RECEPTORS AND REGULATION OF PROTEIN ACTIVITY

Communication is critical for the survival of cells and the coordination of various physiologic processes. Membranes have a central role in mediating these functions. Homeostatic systems require cell-to-cell communication that is mediated by various chemical messengers such as hormones or neurotransmitters.

Ligand Binding

The initial step in this process is the binding of such messengers (ligand) to a binding site (receptor).[24] Receptors are proteins, or glycoproteins, most commonly located in the plasma membrane or in the cell interior (receptors for lipid-soluble hormones). It is the binding of the chemical messenger to the receptor that initiates the events leading to the cellular response to the message. Such responses include changes in membrane permeability to ions, changes in metabolism, secretion, or contraction. The chemical messenger may come into contact with many different cells; however, it only influences those cells that have receptors for that messenger. Cells that have receptors on their plasma membrane for a chemical messenger are targets for that particular messenger. Because the messenger reaches the target cell via the extracellular fluid they come into contact with many different cells, but they selectively interact with only those cells having appropriate re-

FOCUS ON CELLULAR PHYSIOLOGY

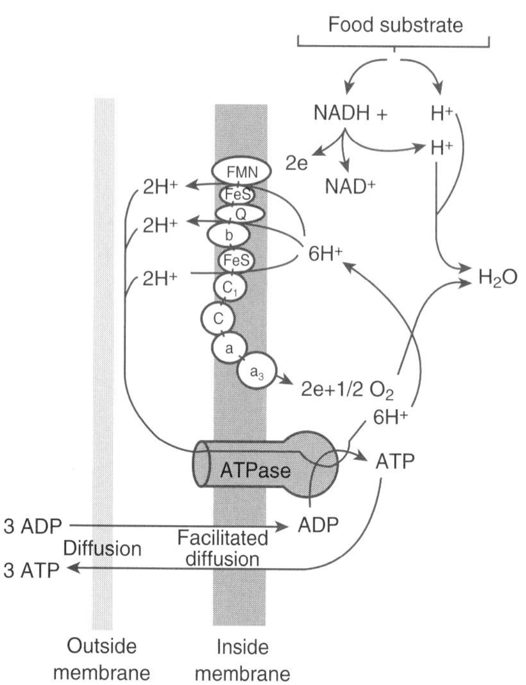

FIGURE 1-20. Chemiosmotic mechanism of oxidative phosphorylation for forming great quantities of ATP. (Guyton, A. & Hall, J. [1996]. *Textbook of medical physiology* [9th ed.]. Philadelphia: W. B. Saunders.)

ceptors to respond.[7] Receptors have binding sites that have characteristics that specifically bind the chemical messenger; that is, they have the property of specificity. Therefore, receptors bind these ligands with high affinity and may be subject to competition as well. The number of receptors a cell has is not fixed and can be regulated. This usually depends on the quantities of messenger available to activate the receptor. Prolonged intense stimulation may decrease the number of receptors for that messenger by a phenomenon known as *downregulation*. This effectively dampens the response to the agonist (stimulus capable of combining with receptors to initiate a reaction). Conversely, exposure to low levels of messenger may cause the number of receptors in the target cell to increase (*upregulation*), increasing the sensitivity of the cell to the agonist.

Regulation of Protein Activity

Proteins mediate many of the functions of the cell and regulation of protein activity is one of the major ways in which the cell controls its functions. The two primary ways in which protein activity is regulated is by control of gene expression and by conformational changes in the protein. Chemical messengers as discussed above often mediate changes in protein activity. Changes in protein conformation are brought about by **covalent modification** via phosphorylation/dephosphorylation and allosteric modulation (Fig. 1-22).

The most common mechanism of altering protein activity is covalent modification. The transfer of a negatively charged phosphate group of ATP to ester linkages results in a change in protein shape and the ability to bind to other substrates. Phosphorylation of proteins is catalyzed by enzymes known as protein kinases. A protein kinase enzyme is one that catalyzes the covalent transfer of a phosphate group from ATP to substrate (protein).[9] The activity of the phosphorylated protein is altered, resulting in the cellular response. The protein that is phosphorylated may be an enzyme that is activated or inactivated, that is, changes its affinity for the substrate thus altering metabolism. It may be an ion channel that is opened or closed via covalent modulation, or it may be a protein involved in secretion or proteins involved in contraction.

Allosteric modulation is another mechanism that may change protein activity. Allosteric modulation involves the binding of a modulator molecule to a regulatory site on a protein thus altering the functional site in some way. The functional site may be a binding site

FOCUS ON CELLULAR PHYSIOLOGY

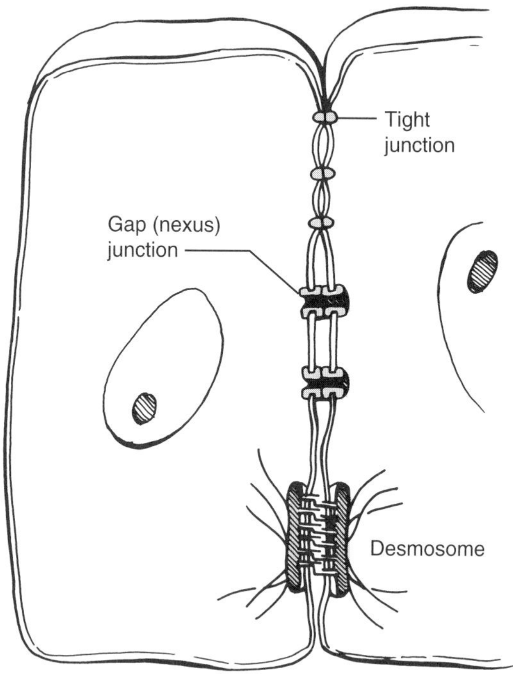

FIGURE 1-21. Specialized membrane junctions. **A.** Desmosomes are adhesive junctions of epithelial cells. **B.** Tight junctions limit movement of molecules and form barriers. **C.** Gap or nexus junctions form pores between adjacent cells to allow for rapid exchange of molecules or ions.

FOCUS ON CELLULAR PHYSIOLOGY

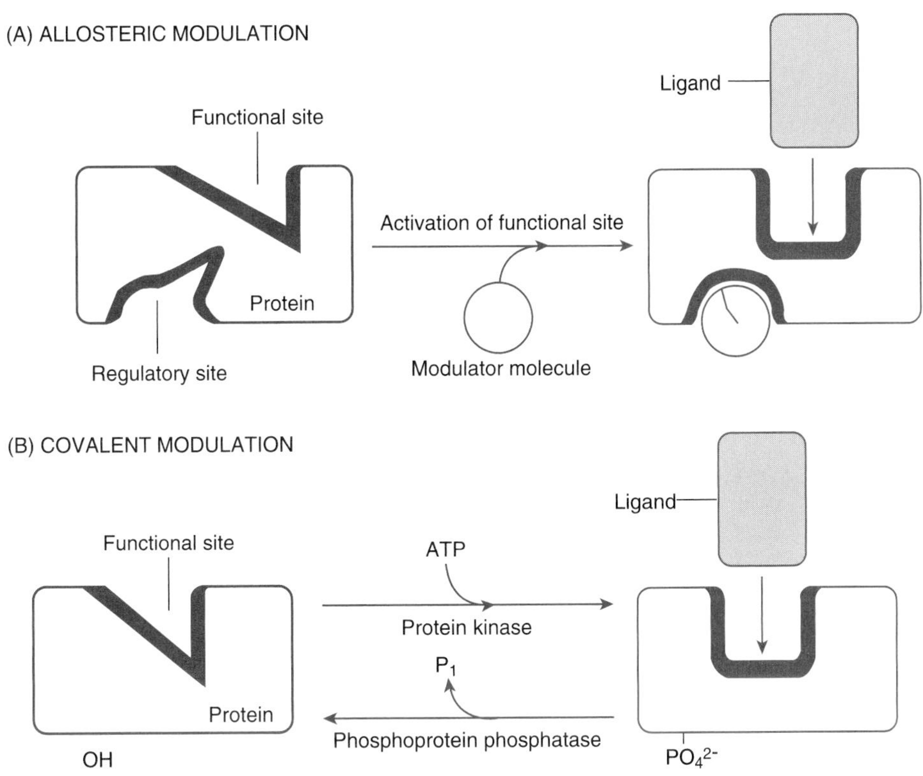

FIGURE 1-22. Allosteric modulation **(A)** and covalent modulation **(B)** of a protein's functional binding site. (Vander, A., Sherman, J., & Luciano, D. [1998]. *Human physiology.* St. Louis: McGraw-Hill.)

of an enzyme, an ion channel, or a protein involved in intracellular signaling.[23] The change is similar to that of covalent modulation with the resulting protein activity altered in some way.

CLASSIFICATION OF SIGNAL TRANSDUCTION MECHANISMS

Considering the amazing number of specialized functions that are regulated in the cell, it is surprising that there are really only three major classes of signal transduction mechanisms that control these responses. The types of cellular responses controlled by primary chemical messengers include: (1) changes in membrane potential (alteration in the membrane's permeability to ions resulting in voltage changes), (2) contraction, if it is a muscle cell, (3) secretion, or (4) changes in metabolism. All of these responses are mediated by changing the activity of proteins involved with these processes. This change in protein activity begins with the binding of a chemical messenger with membrane-associated protein receptors that, in turn, trigger a sequence of events ultimately leading to the response.

Receptors That Are Ion Channels

The simplest way to classify receptors is based on which of the three signal transduction mechanisms they use. The first classification of receptors are those that alter cellular activity by the opening or closing of specific ion channels, thus altering the flux of ions across the membrane. In this example, the receptor is a chemically gated ion channel and the binding of the primary messenger changes the protein conformation thus altering the membrane permeability to an ion. An important example of this type of receptor is the nicotinic receptor that binds the neurotransmitter acetylcholine (Fig. 1-23). Acetylcholine is an important chemical messenger that mediates many cellular functions, such as contraction of skeletal muscle.[19] When acetylcholine binds to the nicotinic receptor there is an allosteric change in the protein conformation that opens the channel, increasing the membrane's permeability to sodium and potassium ions. There is a rapid influx of sodium into the cell that depolarizes the membrane. This is a pivotal event that results in muscle contraction.

FOCUS ON CELLULAR PHYSIOLOGY

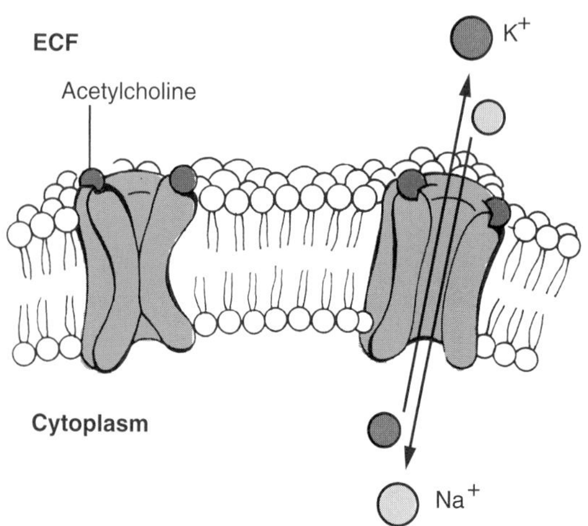

FIGURE 1-23. The nicotinic acetylcholine receptor binds the neurotransmitter acetylcholine. When it binds to the receptor, there is a change in the protein conformation that increases permeability of the membrane to sodium and potassium, causing depolarization of the membrane. (Fox, S. I. [1996]. *Human physiology* [7th ed.]. Dubuque, IA: Times Mirror.)

Receptors That Are Tyrosine Kinase Dependent

Another more complex mechanism is activation of receptors that trigger an enzyme that has protein kinase activity. A large group of chemical messengers, including insulin, various growth factors, and cytokines, signal through receptors that activate tyrosine kinase activity. Agents that excite these types of receptors are usually ligands that promote cell division or differentiation.[23] On activation of this class of receptors, there is a signal through multiple reaction pathways that regulate nuclear or cytosolic events via the phosphorylation of tyrosine residues on proteins.

Receptors Associated with G Proteins

The most common classification of receptors are those that are associated with a class of proteins known as G proteins. They are called G proteins because they avidly bind guanine nucleotides (GTP and GDP). The G proteins are located on the inner face of the plasma membrane and consist of three subunits, alpha (α), beta (β), and gamma (γ). In the unstimulated state, the G proteins are heterotrimer α, β, and γ, and subunits are associated with a GDP bound to the α subunit. The binding of the chemical messenger to the receptor (activation) results in a conformational change in the α subunit that causes it to exchange the GDP for a molecule of GTP. The GTP bound α subunit then dissociates from the β and γ and interacts with various effector proteins ultimately triggering the cellular response. The G protein has GTPase activity and the hydrolysis of the GTP back to GDP permits the reassociation of the α, β, and γ subunits back to the resting state.[3]

SECOND MESSENGERS. Chemical messengers only interact with G protein associated receptors on the cell membrane. Therefore, a mechanism is required that will transmit and amplify the signal to the intracellular targets responsible for carrying out the response. An important mechanism by which this signal transduction system results in the cell response is activation of another set of intracellular messengers (the second messenger). Despite the enormous numbers of messages that use these types of signals, only a few second messengers have been identified that act as intermediates in these processes.[4] The two most common second messengers are cyclic adenosine monophosphate (cyclic AMP or cAMP) and calcium. Once activated, the second messengers initiate a cascade of intracellular changes that result in the cellular response. The receptor, via the G proteins, activate another membrane-associated effector protein, either adenylate cyclase, phospholipase C, or an adjacent G protein gated ion channel changing the membrane potential in the target cell (Fig. 1-24).

The activated adenylate cyclase then catalyzes the conversion of ATP to cAMP (second messenger), which then activates intracellular cAMP-dependent protein kinase A enzymes (Fig. 1-25). Protein kinase A catalyzes the phosphorylation of hydroxyl groups of serine or threonine residues of various proteins that mediate the cellular response. Activated protein kinase A also can migrate to the nucleus where it catalyzes the phosphorylation of transcription factors that enhance or re-

FOCUS ON CELLULAR PHYSIOLOGY

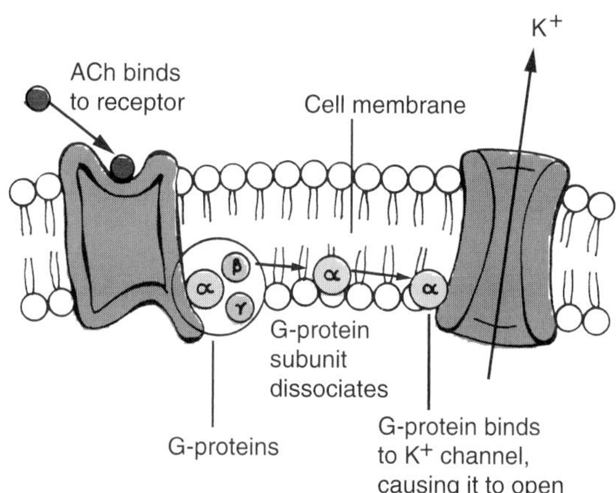

FIGURE 1-24. G-proteins, once activated, activate a membrane-associated effector protein, changing the membrane potential in the target cell. (Adapted from Fox, S. I. [1996]. *Human physiology* [7th ed.]. Dubuque, IA: Times Mirror.)

FOCUS ON CELLULAR PHYSIOLOGY

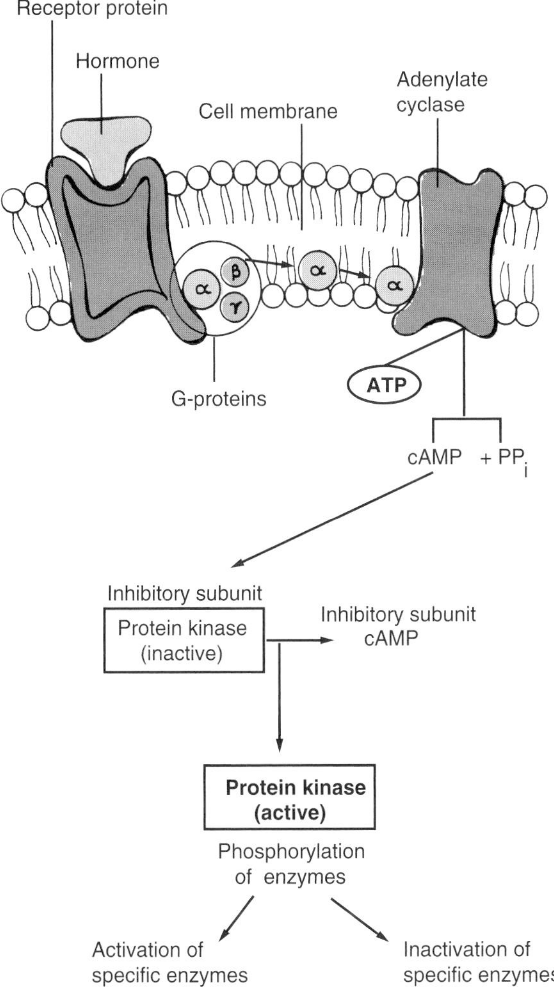

FIGURE 1-25. The response to the protein signal is activation of protein kinase, which allows for the physiologic response (see text). (Adapted from Fox, S. I. [1996]. *Human physiology* [7th ed.]. Dubuque, IA: Times Mirror.)

press gene expression. In addition to activating cAMP-dependent protein kinase, cAMP can also bind to membrane proteins that are ion channels, thereby altering the membrane permeability to those ions. An enzyme, phosphodiesterase that converts cAMP to 5′-AMP restoring the target proteins back to their resting state, removes cAMP.[3] There are many important examples of chemical messengers that use this method of signaling. For example, β receptors that bind the neurotransmitter norepinephrine mediate the cellular responses in the target cell via cAMP second messenger systems.

Another, less understood, second messenger is cyclic 3′,5′ guanosine monophosphate (cyclic GMP or cGMP). Many cells have cGMP-dependent protein kinase proteins; however, few substrates for this enzyme have been identified. This second messenger is the mediator for the effects of the chemical messengers nitric oxide and atrial natriuretic factor.

Some G protein-associated receptors bring about the cell's response by activating a signal transduction cascade through another effector enzyme known as phospholipase C (Fig. 1-26). The activated G protein signals the phospholipase C to catalyze the hydrolysis of a membrane phospholipid, phosphatidylinositol 4,5-bisphosphate (PIP_2) into diacylglycerol (DAG) and inositol 1,4,5-triphosphate (IP_3). DAG and IP_3 are second messengers that mediate various important cellular functions. DAG activates protein kinase C, which then catalyzes the phosphorylation of various cellular proteins changing their activity in a manner similar to that described for protein kinase A. IP_3 increases the permeability of the ER membrane to calcium, increasing cytosolic calcium levels. Extracellular calcium can also enter the cell down its concentration gradient through membrane channels opened by ligand–receptor binding or membrane voltage changes. Calcium is also an extremely important second messenger. The calcium compliments the effects of DAG because protein kinase C is a calcium-dependent enzyme. In addition to facilitating the effects of DAG, some calcium that enters the cytosol also binds with calcium-binding proteins, most often calmodulin, which then mediates the cell response by activating calmodulin-dependent protein kinases.[3] Mechanisms that alter cytosolic calcium concentrations are extremely important in various physiologic processes such as muscle contraction (see page 797).

THE NUCLEUS AND REGULATION OF GENE EXPRESSION

The nucleus is a large membranous organelle frequently located near the center of a cell. It contains large quantities of deoxyribonucleic acid (DNA), which forms the *genes* that control the cell's function. Cellular activities and structure are controlled through the genes by controlling the proteins that are synthesized (see below).

The nucleus is separated from the cytoplasm by a membranous envelope called the *nuclear envelope* (Fig. 1-27). In contrast to the plasma membrane, it consists of two distinct membranes. The membranes are fused together periodically to form circular pores through which material can pass in and out of the nucleus. The pores are about 10 times larger than those of the plasma membrane allowing many protein molecules to pass through with relative ease. Most ions and water-soluble molecules also move easily between the nucleus and cytoplasm. The inner membrane of the nuclear envelope represents the actual nuclear membrane, and

FOCUS ON CELLULAR PHYSIOLOGY

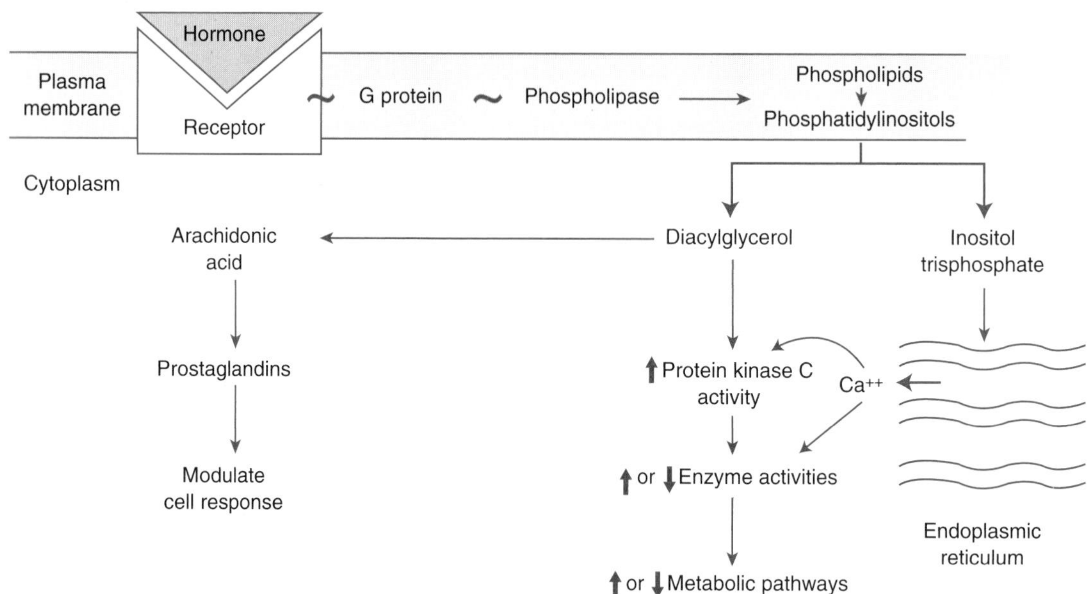

FIGURE 1-26. Mechanism of hormone action via membrane phospholipids. The hormone-receptor complex, via a G protein, activates phospholipase C, which then releases diacylglycerol (DAG) and inositol trisphosphate (IP3) from membrane-bound phosphoinositides. IP3 mobilizes calcium from the endoplasmic reticulum. Calcium with DAG activates protein kinase C, which phosphorylate target enzymes, increasing or decreasing metabolic pathways. DAG also yields arachidonic acid for synthesis of modulating prostaglandins. (Berne, R. M. & Levy, M. N. [1998]. *Physiology* [4th ed.]. St. Louis: Mosby.)

the outer membrane of the envelope gives rise to and is continuous with membranes of the ER.

Distinct nuclear structures may be observed in some cells. Two commonly seen structures are the nucleolus and condensed strands of **chromatin** called *chromosomes.* These are readily identified during cellular mitosis (see page 33).

The *nucleolus* (little nucleus) is a collection of dense fibers and granules forming a small spherical mass that is most visible when the cell is not in the process of mitosis (see Fig. 1-27). The nucleolus is composed primarily of RNA and protein, together with smaller amounts of DNA. These nucleic acids play key roles in the cellular synthesis of proteins. The granules of the nucleolus are precursors of ribosomes, which are the sites of protein synthesis in the cytoplasm.

Chromatin is composed of long molecules of DNA in association with protein. Chromatin fibers are too small to be seen with the light microscope. Before cell division, however, chromatin fibers coil and condense into compact structures that are visible when using the light microscope. These visible, x-shaped structures are called chromosomes. There are 22 pairs of *autosomes* and one pair with either XX or XY for sex determination in the human cell. The pairs of chromosomes differ from one another in size and shape.

FOCUS ON CELLULAR PHYSIOLOGY

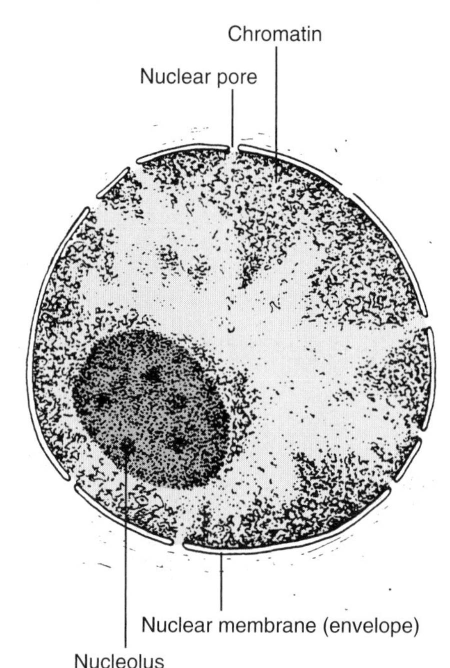

FIGURE 1-27. The nucleus.

Genes

The nucleus directs and controls the activities of the entire cell through the genes. A gene is the linear sequence of nucleotides on DNA that code for the production of a single protein. Genes serve as a master mold for making specific proteins.[21] The sequence is divided into units of three nucleotides, each called a *triplet* or **codon.** The exact sequence of the nucleotide bases (*guanine, thymine, cytosine,* and *adenine*) in each codon determines a unique code and ultimately codes for a single amino acid. The genes determine the specific code that is transcribed as RNA. The gene being transcribed is located on one of the two DNA strands, which serves as the master strand template (pattern) for *messenger RNA (mRNA)* transcription. Other parts of DNA serve as templates for the formation of *transfer RNA (tRNA)* or *ribosomal RNA (rRNA)*. The genetic code, transmitted to the ribosomes, allows for the formation of several thousand types of proteins that are essential to the various functions of human cells (Fig. 1-28). Most proteins contain 100 to 1,000 amino acids.[3]

RNA and Protein Synthesis

Almost all of the chemical reactions associated with normal cellular function are enzyme dependent. All enzymes are proteins, and their synthesis is controlled by nuclear DNA. Therefore, the activity of the cytoplasmic organelles is regulated either directly or indirectly by the nucleus. In addition to enzymes, nuclear DNA contains the blueprints that specify construction of other types of proteins, such as hormones or structural proteins. DNA is envisioned as a twisted ladder, a double helix model, with the sides of the ladder held together by strong bonds. The ends of the ladder terminate in either 3′ or 5′, the labels being derived from the order in which the five carbon atoms composing deoxyribose are numbered. Each DNA subgroup, with one deoxyribose, one phosphate, and one base is called a *nucleotide*.[14] The syn-

FOCUS ON CELLULAR PHYSIOLOGY

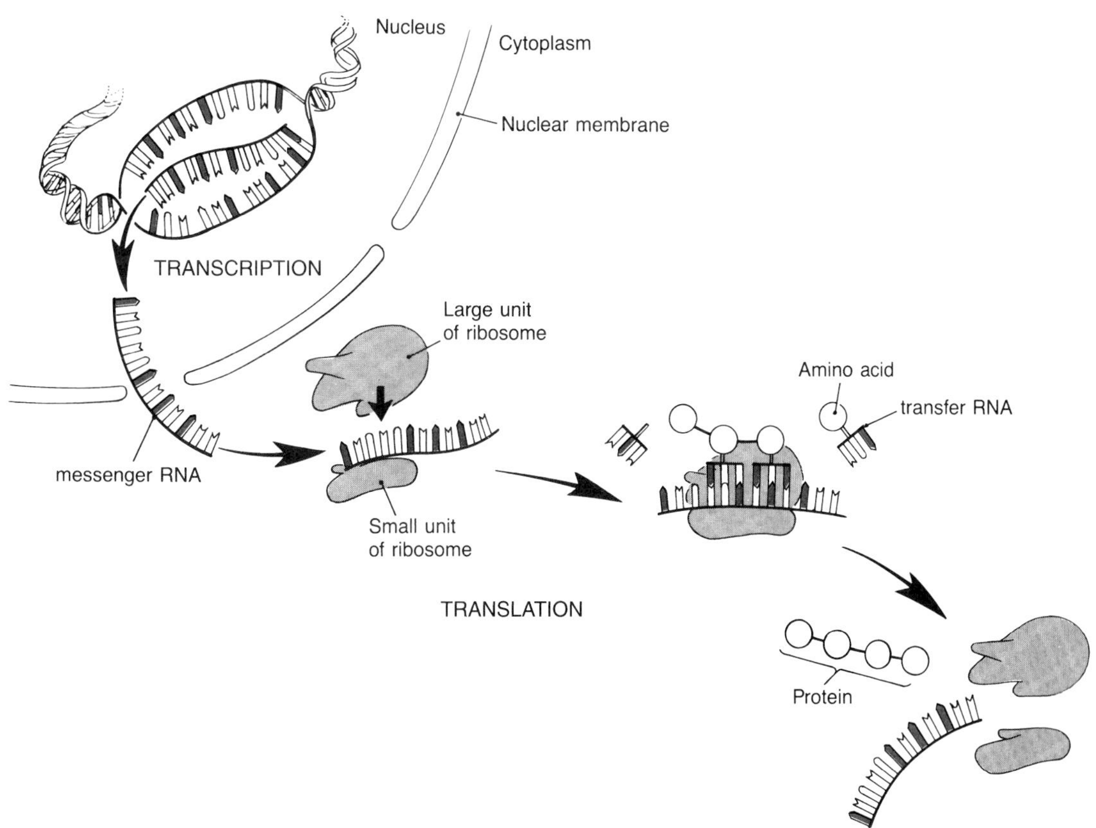

FIGURE 1-28. Mechanism for the production of a protein through the sequencing of specific amino acids. DNA serves as the template for messenger RNA and transfer RNA, which are used in the assembly of the amino acids.

thesis of proteins occurs in two major steps known as *transcription* and *translation* (see Fig. 1-28).

TRANSCRIPTION

Transcription occurs in the nucleus and is the synthesis of RNA from DNA where the code contained in the DNA is "transcribed" to an RNA molecule. During transcription, the DNA molecule partially unwinds into two separate strands. One of the strands acts as a template on which mRNA is synthesized while the other strand is noncoding (Fig. 1-29). The genetic message carried by DNA in the form of a series of *triplets* is transcribed to mRNA by complementary base pairing; thus, the formation of mRNA results in the synthesis of a molecule having a linear sequence of bases that is complementary to that of the DNA from which it was transcribed. Only part of the gene is transcribed. The untranscribed portions of the gene are important for regulation of the transcription.

The promoter is a sequence of nucleotides at the 3′ end of the transcribed portion of the gene that signals the initiation of mRNA synthesis. RNA synthesis on the DNA template is catalyzed by an enzyme called RNA polymerase. Complementary RNA base pairing occurs in a manner similar to DNA except that uracil substitutes for thymine. Transcription factors, which are proteins, help the RNA polymerase recognize the promoter nucleotide sequence and bind to the DNA. Binding of transcription factors aligns the polymerase on the promoter and on phosphorylation of the RNA polymerase begins its movement along the DNA template. Expression of the gene is controlled by the proteins that bind to DNA sequences in the promoter region and also by proteins that bind to regulatory sequences at distant locations of the DNA. Regulatory proteins may act as enhancers or repressors of gene expression.

Transcription continues until the RNA polymerase reaches a terminator sequence on the DNA template. The mRNA molecule separates from the DNA template as fast as it forms and the DNA double helix reforms. The RNA that leaves the nucleus to act as a blueprint for the assembly of the proteins(s) is the messenger RNA. Messenger RNA undergoes various modifications before being dispatched to the cytoplasm. The 5′ end is capped off with a modified form of GTP, which helps protect the mRNA from degradation by hydrolytic enzymes and functions as an attachment signal for ribosomes. The 3′ end is also modified by the addition of 150 to 200 adenine nucleotides called the *poly-A-tail*. The poly-A-tail also helps protect against the hydrolytic degradation of mRNA and may also play a role in facilitating the export of mRNA from the nucleus to the cytoplasm.[1]

Lastly, mRNA processing involves the removal of a large portion of the molecule that is synthesized during transcription by a mechanism known as RNA splicing. Interrupting the coding sequences (known as *exons*) of a gene are regions that do not code for protein called the *introns*. The pre-RNA is edited with the introns being excised and the exons joined by a complex apparatus of RNA and protein called a spliceosome to form an mRNA molecule with a continuous coding sequence. The completed mRNA then carries the code to the ribosomes for protein assembly.

FOCUS ON CELLULAR PHYSIOLOGY

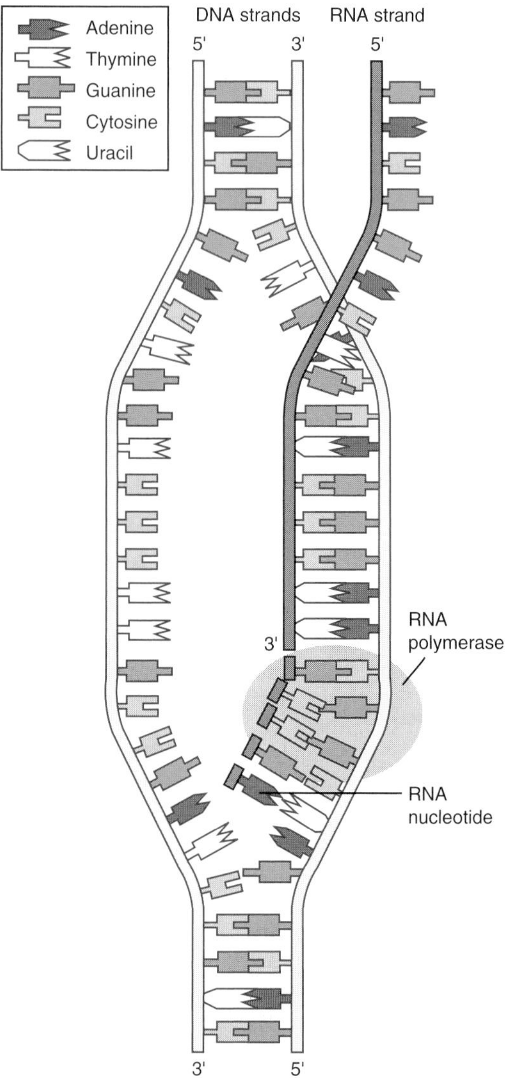

FIGURE 1-29. **Transcription of DNA to mRNA. RNA polymerase II proceeds along the DNA strand in the 3′ to 5′ direction, assembling a strand of mRNA nucleotides that is complementary to the DNA template strand. (Jorde, L. B., Carey, J. C., & White, R. L. [1995]. *Medical genetics.* St. Louis: Mosby.)**

TRANSLATION

Translation (protein assembly) occurs at ribosomes in the cytoplasm. After synthesis, the mRNA leaves the nucleus by way of the pores in the nuclear envelope and enters the cytoplasm, where it becomes associated with ribosomes, the organelles that link amino acids into the polypeptide chains of proteins. Within the ribosomes, the genetic message carried by mRNA in the form of codons is deciphered, and correct amino acids are joined in the proper sequence to form a protein molecule (Fig. 1-30). The process, called translation, involves tRNA. One or more specific tRNA molecules exist for each type of amino acid. Each tRNA molecule binds itself to a specific amino acid and carries it to the site of protein synthesis in the ribosome. The tRNA molecule contains a binding site in the form of an *anticodon*, which recognizes and attaches to the correct codon on mRNA. Thus, as tRNA molecules bearing specific amino acids sequentially bind to mRNA in the ribosome, the amino acids are sequenced into a protein that is then released from the ribosome.

Once the mRNA template becomes associated with the ribosome, the process of peptide synthesis occurs rapidly, taking about 1 second for a new amino acid to be added to the peptide chain. Thus, the synthesis of a protein, such as the hormone insulin (51 amino acids), takes about 1 minute. Several ribosomes may simultaneously translate a single strand of mRNA so protein synthesis may occur more rapidly.

REPRODUCTIVE ABILITY OF CELLS

Most cells have the ability to reproduce themselves through the complex process of *mitosis*. In the adult, new cells take the place of old, worn out or damaged cells in a rigidly defined order that maintains cellular numbers, but allows for the replacement of only the needed cells. The turnover rate is billions of cells per day, but rigid controls inherently limit the number of cells to be reproduced.

Specific controls on the reproductive process produce precisely the correct quantity of cells. For example, if the erythrocyte count decreases, specific stimulating factors cause the bone marrow to increase production of erythrocytes, leading ultimately to increased numbers of circulating red blood cells. When the appropriate level of red blood cells is reached some factor, either diminished stimulation or an inhibitor, suppresses their further production (see page 348).

Regeneration of Cells

The ability of cells to reproduce themselves is called the regenerative capacity of cells. *Labile cells* regenerate frequently and have a life span usually measured in hours or days. Some examples of labile cells are leukocytes (white blood cells) and epithelial cells. Other cells retain the ability to regenerate or reproduce but do so only under special circumstances. These are called *stable cells*, and their life span is measured in years or, sometimes, the entire life span of an organism. Some examples of stable cells are osteocytes of bone, parenchymal cells of the liver, and cells of the glands of the body. In the normal liver cell, for example, mitotic figures are rare, but after injury, mitoses are abundant because the liver has a remarkable ability to repair itself. The third type of cells, the *permanent cells*, live for the entire life of the organism. They include the nerve cell bodies and probably most of the muscle cells. The neuron loses its ability to undergo mitosis at about 6 months of age.[13,21] Myocardial muscle does not regenerate; when it dies, it is repaired by the formation of scar tissue.

Reproduction of Cells

Most of the cells of the body have the ability to reproduce. This property is rigidly controlled with cell regeneration supplying only the needed replacement cells.

THE CELL CYCLE

All human cells have a life cycle, called the cell cycle, that begins when the cell is produced by division of its parent and ends when the cell either divides to give rise to daughter cells or dies. A complete cell cycle consists of four stages labeled growth or gap phase one (G_1), synthesis phase (S), growth (gap) phase two (G_2), and mitosis (M) (Fig. 1-31). All of the stages together between mitotic divisions are called *interphase*.

The G_1 stage is the time interval after the formation of the cell that precedes replication of DNA. The S stage is the time during which DNA replication occurs. The G_2 stage is the time interval after DNA replication and before the beginning of the M stage. The M stage is that period of time in which cell division occurs. Cells not destined for an early repeat of the division cycle are commonly arrested at the G_0 stage. Stable cells can be stimulated from G_0 into G_1 with an appropriate stimulus to provide for regeneration of lost cells.[15]

The process by which a cell divides to form two identical daughter cells is mitosis. Before a cell can undergo mitosis, its chromosomes must duplicate themselves, a process called *replication*.

REPLICATION

Replication of DNA occurs during the S stage of interphase. During this time, the chromosomes appear to be spread out in a tangled mass known as chromatin. In replication, the two strands of the DNA molecule partially uncoil and each serves as a template (pattern) for the formation of another strand (Fig. 1-32). Each template and its complement then form a new DNA

FOCUS ON CELLULAR PHYSIOLOGY

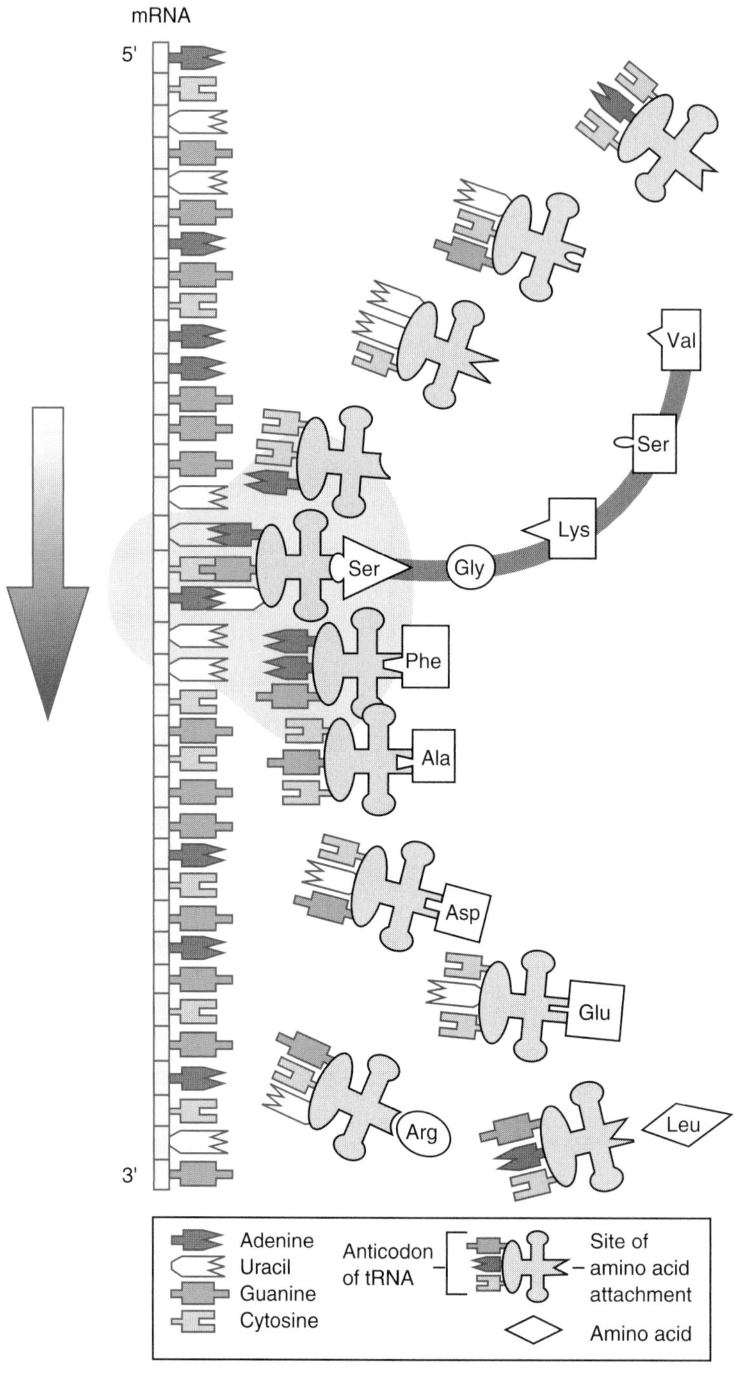

FIGURE 1-30. Translation of mRNA to amino acids. The ribosome moves along the mRNA strand in the 5′ to 3′ direction, assembling a growing polypeptide chain. In this example, the mRNA sequence GUG-AGC-AAG-GGU, UCA has assembled five amino acids—Val, Ser, Lys, Gly, and Ser—into a polypeptide. (Jorde, L. B., Carey, J. C., & White, R. L. [1995]. *Medical genetics.* St. Louis: Mosby.)

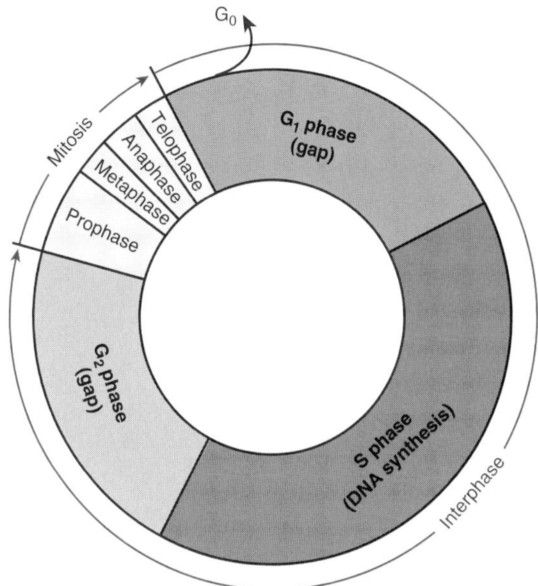

FIGURE 1-31. The cell cycle (see text).

molecule. During mitosis, each daughter cell inherits a DNA molecule that consists of one new strand and one parental strand.

Each chromosome is furnished with a single centromere, an area that holds together the two daughter chromosomes produced when a chromosome replicates (see below). After replication, the two identical, double-stranded molecules of DNA are called **chromatids** as long as they remain attached to each other by the centromere.

MITOSIS

Mitosis is described in terms of phases through which the cell passes as it divides (Fig. 1-33). The phases are defined by the appearance of chromosomes under the light microscope and are designated (in sequence) as *prophase, metaphase, anaphase,* and *telophase.*

PROPHASE. During **prophase**, the chromatin condenses into distinct chromosomes that are visible as pairs of chromatids, joined at the centromere. In prophase, the nuclear membrane and nucleolus disappear and thus appear to be part of the cytoplasm. The centrioles migrate to opposite poles of the cell and a spindle of microtubules forms between the centrioles.

METAPHASE. During **metaphase**, the assembly of the spindle is completed and the chromosomes align in a plane midway between the poles. This plane is called the *equatorial plane.* The chromosomes align at the equatorial plane because they experience an equal pull through the attached microtubules from the two poles of the spindle.

ANAPHASE. **Anaphase** starts with centromere division, which allows the newly divided chromosomes to move to opposite poles of the spindle. They assume a V shape as they are pulled through the cytoplasm by microtubules and filaments of the spindle apparatus.[18]

TELOPHASE. At the beginning of **telophase**, two sets of daughter chromosomes are gathered at opposite poles. A new nuclear envelope is assembled from saccules of ER and surrounds each set of chromosomes. The chromosomes gradually unravel and disperse in the nucleus, disappearing from view. The spindle disintegrates, but the duplicated centrioles remain and nucleoli reappear. As these events of telophase are occurring, a cleft, or cleavage furrow, forms in the plasma membrane. The cytoplasm is divided equally during anaphase or early telophase between the two newly formed daughter cells. This process is called *cytokinesis.* Complete division occurs when the furrow deepens until opposite surfaces make contact and the cell splits.

FOCUS ON CELLULAR PHYSIOLOGY

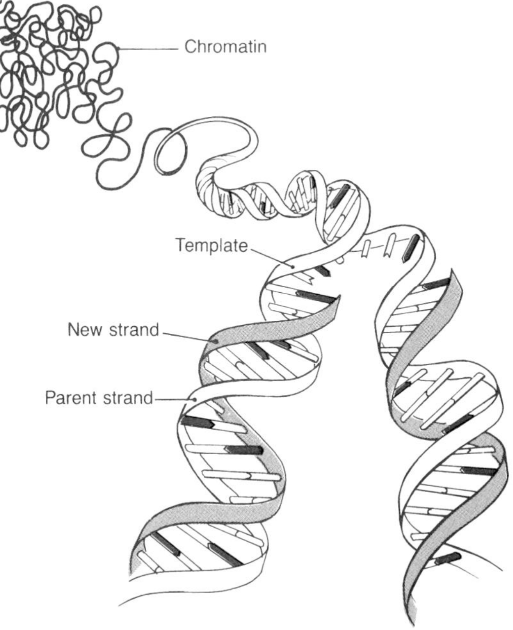

FIGURE 1-32. Replication occurs when the two strands of DNA separate and a new strand is synthesized on each original strand. Each new molecule of DNA is identical to the original molecule.

FOCUS ON CELLULAR PHYSIOLOGY

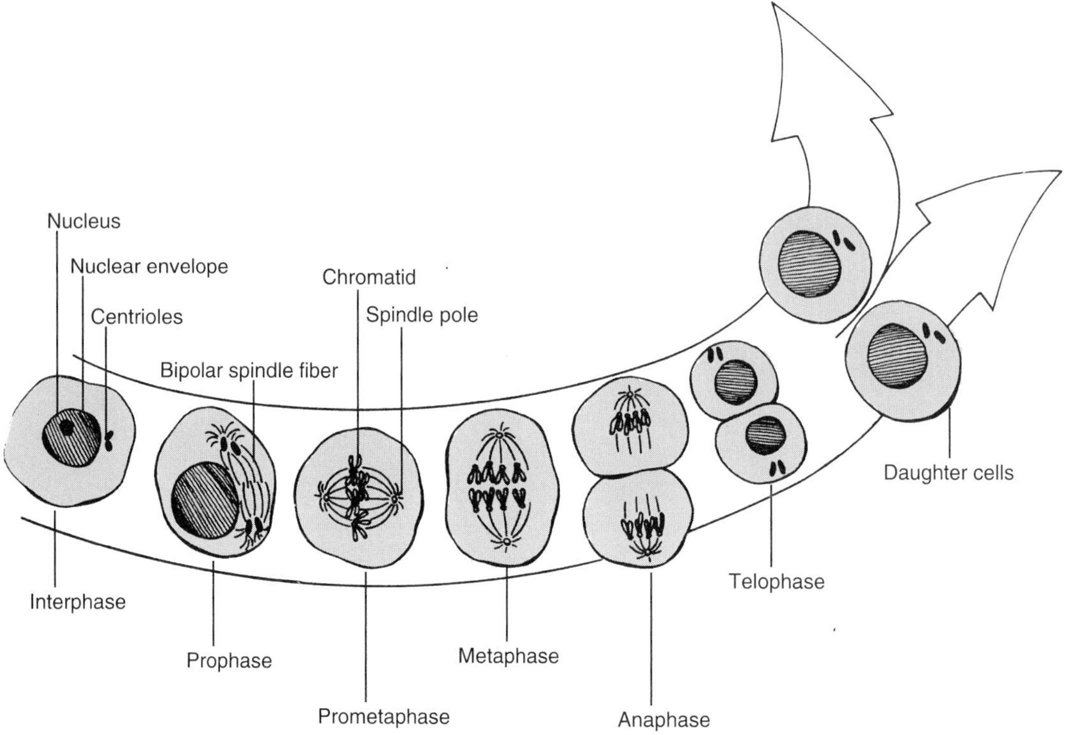

FIGURE 1-33. The stages of mitosis, during which two identical diploid cells are formed from one original diploid cell. (Adapted from Jorde, L. B., Carey, J. C., & White, R. L. [1995]. *Medical genetics.* St. Louis: Mosby.)

MEIOSIS

The process of reproduction of a new organism is through meiosis or reduction division, which is a special nuclear division of the chromosomes that provides 22 autosomes and a single sex chromosome in each sex cell rather than the 23 pairs found in all other somatic cells. The sex cells, called gametes, are the ovum (female egg cell) and sperm (male sex cell). The union of male and female gametes is called fertilization. The resulting *zygote* contains a set of chromosomes from each parent for a total of 23 pairs. Multiple divisions of the zygote eventually produce a new being.

CELLULAR INJURY AND ADAPTATION

The life cycle of a cell exists on a continuum that includes normal activities and adaptation, injury, or lethal changes. Adaptation may be the result of normal life cycle adjustments, such as growth during puberty or the changes of pregnancy. Stress produces physiologic changes that may lead to adaptation or disease. The pathologic changes exhibited may be obvious or difficult to detect. The cell constantly makes adjustments to a changing, hostile environment to keep the organism functioning in a normal steady state. These adaptive adjustments are necessary to ensure the survival of the organism. Adaptive changes may be temporary or permanent. The point at which an adapted cell becomes an injured cell is the point at which the cell cannot functionally keep up with a stressful environment.[17] Injured cells exhibit alterations that may affect body function and be manifested as disease.

Prevention of disease depends on the capacity of the affected cells to undergo self-repair and regeneration. This process of repair prevents cellular injury and death and may prevent the death of the host. Whether a cell adapts to a stressor or is reversibly or irreversibly injured depends on the nature of the stressor and the cell.[8] For example, neurons are highly susceptible to hypoxic injury because they have a greater oxygen requirement than any other cell in the body and little capacity to adapt to oxygen deprivation. They may be irreversibly injured in less than 6 minutes in the absence of oxygen, whereas other cells of the body, such as epithelial cells, may be capable of surviving much longer in the absence of oxygen. The process of adaptation, cell repair, and cell death is a continuum that involves many complex physiologic changes.

Stimuli That Can Cause Cellular Injury or Adaptations

Because the cell is constantly making adjustments to a changing, hostile environment, many agents potentially can cause cellular injury or adaptation. Cellular injury may lead to further injury and death of the cell, or the cell may respond to the noxious stimulation by undergoing a change that enables it to tolerate the invasion (Flowchart 1-2).

Stimuli that can affect the human body are categorized as hypoxia, physical agents, chemical agents, microorganisms, genetic defects, nutritional imbalances, and immunologic reactions (Table 1-3).

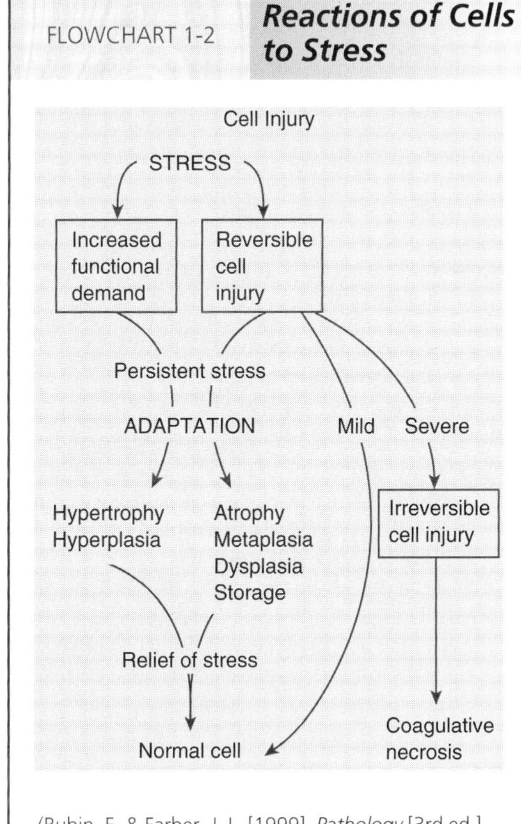

(Rubin, E. & Farber, J. L. [1999]. *Pathology* [3rd ed.]. Philadelphia: Lippincott Williams & Wilkins.)

HYPOXIA

Hypoxia is the most common cause of cellular injury and may be produced by inadequate oxygen in the blood or by decreased perfusion of blood to the tissues, called ischemia. The end results are disturbances of cellular metabolism and local or generalized release of lactic acid. Cellular and organ dysfunction result from lack of oxygen and may lead to cellular, organ, and even somatic death. When cells try to adapt to the lack of oxygen, anaerobic cellular metabolism results in metabolic acidosis (see page 530).

PHYSICAL AGENTS

Physical agents are factors such as mechanical trauma, temperature gradients, electrical stimulation, atmospheric pressure gradients, and irradiation. Physical stimuli directly damage cells, cause rupture or damage of the cell walls, and disrupt cellular reproduction. In addition to the direct damage from the physical agent, hypoxia may increase the extent of the injury.[17] Local swelling may decrease the microcirculation and produce hypoxia to the tissues.

CHEMICAL AGENTS

Chemical agents that can cause injury may include simple compounds, such as glucose, or complex agents, such as poisons. Therapeutic drugs often chemically disrupt the normal cellular balance. Chemicals produce a wide range of physiologic effects. Some chemicals directly damage the cells and cell membranes that they contact. Others may be taken into the cell and disrupt energy production or they may be changed within the cell to toxic metabolites.[17] The end result depends on the degree of disruption.

MICROORGANISMS

Microorganisms cause cellular injury in a variety of ways depending on the type of organism and the innate defense of the human body. Some bacteria secrete exotoxins, which are injurious to the host. Others liberate endotoxins when they are destroyed. Viruses interfere with the metabolism of the host cells and cause cellular injury by releasing viral proteins toxic to the cell (see Chapter 8).

GENETIC DEFECTS

Genetic defects can affect cellular metabolism through inborn errors of metabolism or gross malformations. The mechanisms for cellular disruption vary widely with the genetic defect but may result in intracellular accumulation of abnormal material.

TABLE 1-3

STIMULI THAT CAN CAUSE CELLULAR INJURY

STIMULI	SPECIFIC AGENTS
Physical agents	Trauma, thermal or electrical charges, irradiation
Chemical agents	Drugs, poisons, foods, toxic and irritating substances
Microorganisms	Viruses, bacteria, fungi, protozoa
Hypoxia	Shock, localized areas of inadequate blood supply, hypoxemia
Genetic defects	Inborn errors of metabolism, gross malformations
Nutritional imbalances	Protein-calorie malnutrition; excessive intake of fats, carbohydrates, and proteins
Immunologic reactions	Hypersensitivity reactions to foreign proteins, autoimmune reactions, immune deficiency

NUTRITIONAL IMBALANCES

Nutritional imbalances produce sickness and death in over one-half of the world's population. The imbalances include serious deficiencies of proteins and vitamins especially. Malnutrition may be primary or secondary, depending on whether it is a socioeconomic problem in the underprivileged areas of the world or is self-induced or disease induced. No matter what the cause, nutritional deficiency is a significant cause of cellular dysfunction and death. On the other hand, excessive food intake leads to nutritional imbalances and cell injury through the production of excessive lipids in the body. Excessive fat intake is associated with cancer, cardiovascular diseases, and respiratory and gastrointestinal disorders.[17]

IMMUNOLOGIC REACTIONS

Immunologic agents may cause cellular injury, especially when hypersensitivity reactions occur, causing the release of excess histamine and other substances. The cellular response to immunologic injury is inflammation, production of scar tissue, and even tissue death. Certain structures, such as the renal nephrons, are especially susceptible to immunologic damage (see page 323). Immunodeficiency allows opportunistic organisms to cause disease and dysfunction (see page 292).

Cellular Changes Resulting from Adaptation or Injury

The cell itself will undergo changes that reflect adaptation to a hostile environment or changes that indicate that the cell has been injured. These changes are often manifested as functional changes in the affected cell or organ and may present as clinical signs and symptoms in the affected individual. The manifestations vary according to the cellular change and the degree to which that change has affected the function of a specific organ.

Abnormal intracellular accumulations often result from an environmental change or an inability of the cell to process materials. Normal or abnormal substances that cannot be metabolized may accumulate in the cytoplasm. These substances may be endogenous (produced within the body) or exogenous (produced in the environment) and stored by an originally normal cell. Examples of abnormal exogenous substances include carbon particles, silica, and metals that are deposited and accumulate because the cell cannot degrade them or transport them to other sites.[8]

Common changes in and around cells include swelling, lipid accumulation in organs, liberation of free radicals, glycogen depositions, pigments, calcification, and hyaline infiltration. These changes may be resolved, may become permanent, or may cause death of the host.

CELLULAR SWELLING

Hydropic cellular swelling is the initial response to disruption of cellular metabolism. It occurs most frequently with cellular hypoxia, which impairs the ability of the cell to synthesize ATP. The function of the sodium–potassium pump is decreased allowing sodium to accumulate in the cell and to attract water into the ICF. The resulting shift of ECF to the intracellular compartment causes cloudy intracellular swelling with enlargement of the cell.[17] Ultimately, organs are affected. Cellular swelling is frequently reversible when sufficient oxygen is delivered to the cell and normal ATP synthesis resumes. However, as the cell swells and injury progresses, damage to the cell membrane occurs, causing a true increase in its permeability. When large molecules and enzymes leak out of (or into) the cell, severe injury or death results. Continued accumulation of water in the cells often has the appearance of small or large vacuoles of water, which may represent portions of ER that have been sequestered.[8]

The Ischemia/Hypoxic Model of Acute Cellular Injury

The cellular and biochemical events that occur in acute cellular injury really are a continuous sequence of cellular changes that occur in response to a stimulus. On exposure to lack of oxygen or decreased blood flow the cell will attempt to adapt and assume a new altered steady state to preserve the viability of the cell with some expected changes in function of the cell. If the stimulus exceeds the adaptive capabilities of the cell, the cell may be reversibly injured or it may reach the point of no return and become lethally injured. The result of hypoxic injury is cellular swelling and the effects are described below.

The primary biochemical target of hypoxia is oxidative phosphorylation. With hypoxia, aerobic respiration is compromised and ATP synthesis in the mitochondria stops. Decreases in ATP generated by aerobic metabolism result in the activation of the glycolytic regulatory enzyme, phosphofructokinase (PFK), thus increasing the rate of glycolysis. PFK is an enzyme that catalyzes the phosphorylation of fructose-6-phosphate to fructose-1,6-bisphosphate and is an important allosteric enzyme that regulates glycolysis. With decreases in ATP synthesis and increases in ADP, PFK is activated and glycolysis is stimulated. ATP is generated anaerobically and the pyruvate that is formed is converted to lactic acid reducing intracellular pH. Glycogen phosphorylase is also activated and glycogen synthetase is inactivated; glycogen depletion occurs and further glucose breakdown occurs. Anaerobic ATP synthesis is not efficient and cellular needs are compromised. The loss of ATP has widespread secondary effects on the cell. Active transport fails and cell swelling occurs. The osmotic gain of water results in dilation of the ER and detachment of ribosomes from the ER. This may compromise the synthesis of needed proteins. Membrane integrity is lost with fluid and electrolyte imbalances occurring. The loss of cell volume regulation results in mitochondrial swelling and dysfunction.[8,10]

The events up to this point are considered to be reversible and if oxygen is restored, the cell may return to a normal homeostasis. If the cell has a limited capacity to adapt (as is seen with the neuron or cardiac muscle cell) or the stimulus is prolonged, the cell may reach the point of no return and it becomes lethally injured. Even if oxygen is restored, the cell dies and progresses to the stages described as necrosis (see page 44). This is most often associated with further losses of membrane integrity and calcium influx, mitochondrial damage and loss of ATP, lysosomal swelling, and disruption of lysosomal membranes. Membrane damage is a critical event in lethal cell injury. Calcium accumulation in the cell activates the calcium-dependent phospholipase enzymes that catalyze the breakdown of membrane phospholipid.[12] The degradation products accumulate in the cell and have a detergent effect on membranes, further compromising an already hyperpermeable membrane. Calcium also activates protease enzymes (breakdown proteins) that destroy cytoskeletal proteins. Cytoskeletal abnormalities also may disrupt the membrane. It appears that the intracellular accumulation of calcium is a pivotal event in the destruction of the membrane that is closely associated with lethal cell injury.[12] Furthermore, loss of ATP prevents the new synthesis of phospholipid and proteins so the overall effect is a loss of these biomolecules with no new synthesis occurring (Flowchart 1-3). The lysosomal membranes appear to be affected by the lowering of the intracellular pH and begin to swell. Disruption of lysosomal membranes results in leakage of their contents into the cytoplasm and digestion of the cell from within. The hyperpermeable membrane results in leakage of intracellular proteins into the blood and represents a useful marker of cell death.

LIPID ACCUMULATION

Lipid accumulation refers to a fatty deposition that occurs in the cytoplasm of parenchymal cells of certain organs. Fat droplets accumulate in the intracellular ER and Golgi complex as a result of improper metabolism.[8] The most common location for fatty change is the liver, but the heart and kidneys can also undergo fatty changes when placed under abnormal stimulation.

Cellular Fatty Accumulations

Large, fatty intracellular accumulations have been shown to stimulate progressive necrosis, fibrosis, and scarring of organs. This leads to functional impairment of the involved organ.

Fatty change of the liver is very common. Pathologically, the liver is enlarged, yellow, and greasy looking, with infiltration involving all or only a portion of the organ.[20] Microscopically, the cytoplasm may become filled with lipid, which pushes the nucleus and other cytoplasmic structures to one side. The predominant lipid involved in fatty change of the liver is triglyceride; its presence may be a result of increased synthesis or decreased secretion of this lipid from the cell.[17] This fatty change is the initial change seen in the alcoholic liver because alcohol increases free fatty acid mobilization, decreases triglyceride use, blocks lipoprotein excretion, and directly damages the ER through the liberation of free radicals (see page 38).[8] Protein-calorie malnutrition (PCM) causes a decrease in synthesis of cellular proteins that attach to and transport lipids from the cell, so that fatty change also occurs in PCM.[8] Other hepatotoxins such as carbon tetrachloride (CCl_4) may also cause this change.[17] The fibrous scarring of cirrhosis (see page 761) appears to result from a reaction to the lipid infiltration in the cytoplasm of hepatocytes.

FLOWCHART 1-3 **Acute Cell Injury**

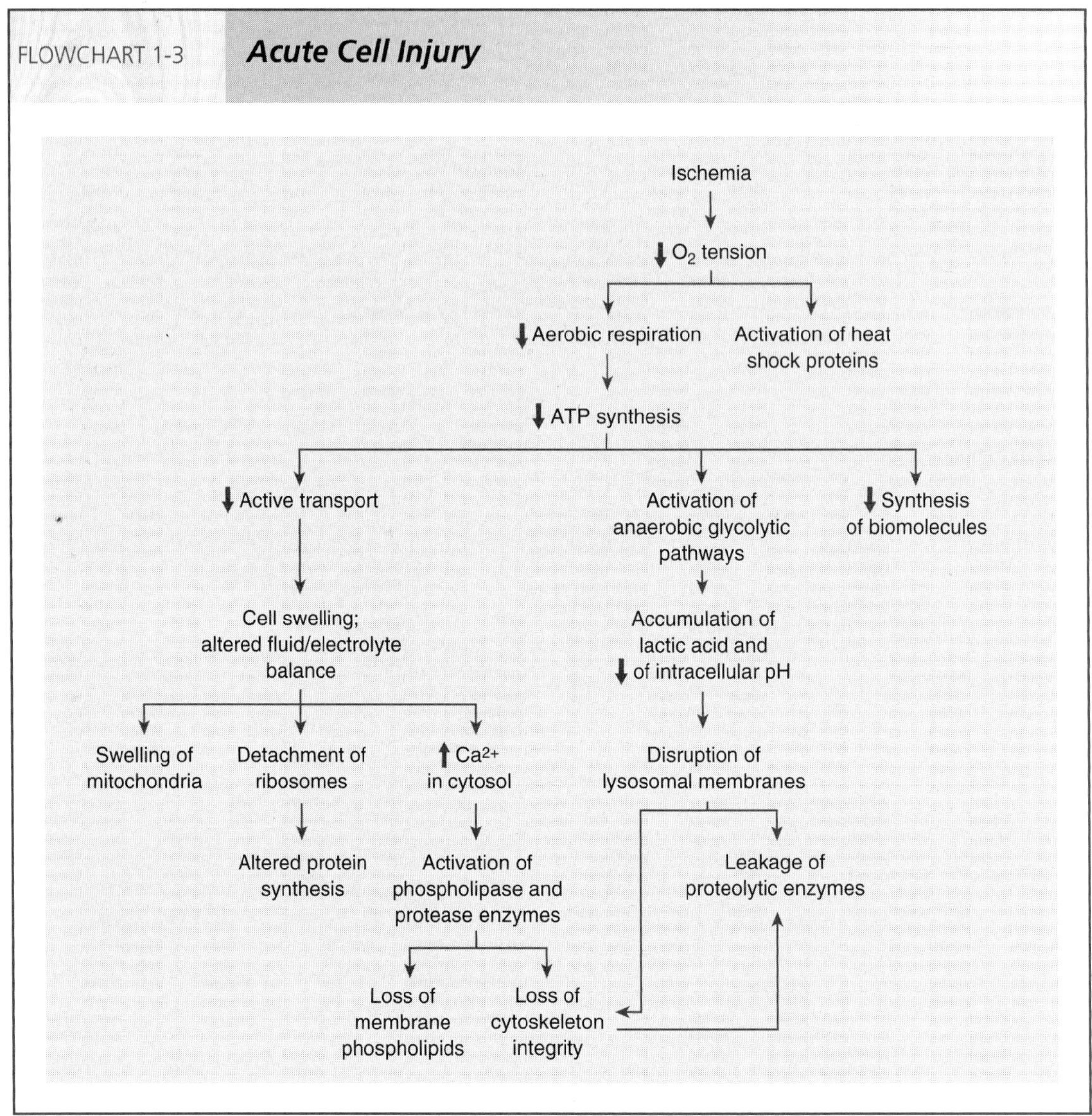

The cells of the heart and kidneys also undergo fatty change under abnormal stimulation. It most commonly occurs in the heart after chronic hypoxia and may be patchy or diffuse. If diffuse, severe infections or toxic states are usually the causative factors. The kidneys show increased fatty change around the proximal convoluted tubules of the nephrons, a change often induced by exposure to certain nephrotoxins or poisons.[5]

Interstitial Fatty Infiltration

Associated with intracellular lipid accumulation is *interstitial fatty infiltration*, a condition that occurs with obesity. Fat cells accumulate between the parenchymal cells of an organ, probably as a result of the transformation of interstitial connective tissue cells to fat cells.[10] This condition rarely seems to affect the function of the organ and localizes most frequently in the heart and pancreas of the extremely obese individual. Other effects of obesity involve fat cells laid down during gestation, during the first year of life, and immediately after puberty. The obese child develops an increased number of fat cells that remain for life but decrease in size after weight loss.[13] Adult-onset obesity, for the most part, occurs when caloric intake exceeds energy requirements and the excess is converted to fat. Areas of subcutaneous fat distribution are related to hereditary characteristics.

FREE RADICALS AND REPERFUSION INJURY

The generation of free radicals has been extensively studied as a mechanism of cell injury. Free radicals arise as a consequence of cellular oxidation–reduction reactions involving enzymatic and nonenzymatic reactions. Damage to cells from these oxygen radicals formed by inflammatory cells has been suggested in diseases of the joints, kidneys, lungs, and heart and also as a reaction to chemicals and ionizing radiation.[17] Flowchart 1-4 shows a variety of free radicals that can be produced by the cell in altered metabolic states. These may be produced by the plasma membrane in the cytoplasm or by the ER. The hydroxyl radical (OH^-) is particularly reactive, especially close to its site of formation. Other free radicals can cause damage at some distance to the initial event. Particularly dangerous is the *lipid peroxidation* process that, in several reactions, results in lipid peroxides, which are unstable and break down to produce aldehydes and organic free radicals. This becomes a self-propagating interaction that can cause widespread membrane damage.[17] The membranes of intracellular organelles are very susceptible to lipid peroxidation. The end result is organelle dysfunction, especially for protein synthesis. Some of the free radicals are oxygen derived (superoxide anion, O_2^-), and these may be released when ischemic tissue is reperfused, causing rapid cell death.[17]

FLOWCHART 1-4 **The Role of Activated Oxygen Species in Human Disease**

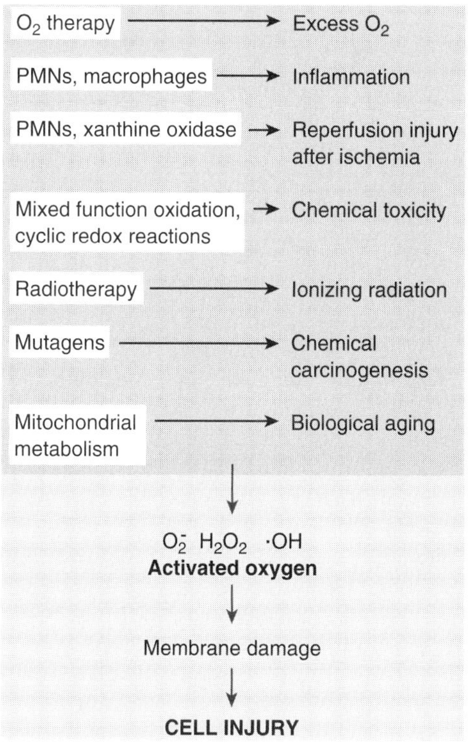

O_2 therapy	→	Excess O_2
PMNs, macrophages	→	Inflammation
PMNs, xanthine oxidase	→	Reperfusion injury after ischemia
Mixed function oxidation, cyclic redox reactions	→	Chemical toxicity
Radiotherapy	→	Ionizing radiation
Mutagens	→	Chemical carcinogenesis
Mitochondrial metabolism	→	Biological aging

↓

O_2^- H_2O_2 ·OH
Activated oxygen

↓

Membrane damage

↓

CELL INJURY

(PMNs = polymorphonuclear leukocytes) (Rubin, E. & Farber, J. L. [1999]. *Pathology* [3rd ed.]. Philadelphia: Lippincott Williams & Wilkins.)

Reperfusion injury has been increasingly noted and studied in ischemic tissue that has been reperfused with activated oxygen. This activated oxygen includes superoxide, hydrogen peroxide (H_2O_2), and hydroxyl radicals. The sources of these activated toxic oxygen species are speculated to be intracellular xanthine oxidase that is released by activated neutrophils (Flowchart 1-5).[22] Macrophages and neutrophils generate large amounts of superoxide anion during phagocytosis. The amount of tissue injury seems to relate to the duration of the ischemia and the tissue affected. With short periods of ischemia, total structural and functional integrity of the cell remains intact. Reperfusion after longer periods of ischemia is associated with deterioration and cellular death. It is the reperfusion with its elaboration of activated oxygen species that causes the cell death rather than the period of ischemia.[17] Lethal injury that occurs during an extended ischemic time is not related to the formation of activated oxygen species but to plasma membrane damage possibly from cellular enzymes or free calcium.[16] Macrophages and neutrophils generate large amounts of superoxide anion during phagocytosis.

Free radicals, once formed, continue a tissue-damaging response until removed by the body or by the body's protection mechanism. Endogenous or exogenous *antioxidants*, such as vitamins C and E, D-penicillamine, and transferrin, block initiation of free radical formation or inactivate free radicals. Vitamin C is a water-soluble vitamin that probably helps to protect other molecules by being oxidized in their place. Vitamin E is a fat-soluble vitamin that prevents the oxidative attack on lipids and other components of the cell and its membranes. Transferrin apparently works by binding free iron.[11] Catalase from peroxisomes decomposes H_2O_2. The tissue-damaging response depends on the balance between formation and factors that terminate formation of free radicals.[8]

GLYCOGEN DEPOSITIONS

Glycogen is a storage form of glucose that is formed and stored in the liver. Normally, it can be quickly degraded to form glucose for energy. Excess deposition of glycogen in organs and tissues occurs with different types of autosomal recessive genetic disorders. One group, called *glycogen storage diseases* or *glycogenoses*, results from specific enzyme deficiencies. Different forms of glycogen accumulate in skeletal and cardiac muscle, as well as in the liver and kidneys. Glycogen disturbances also occur in diabetes mellitus with a greater than normal storage of glycogen in the proximal convoluted tubules of the kidney and in the

FLOWCHART 1-5 **Reperfusion Injury**

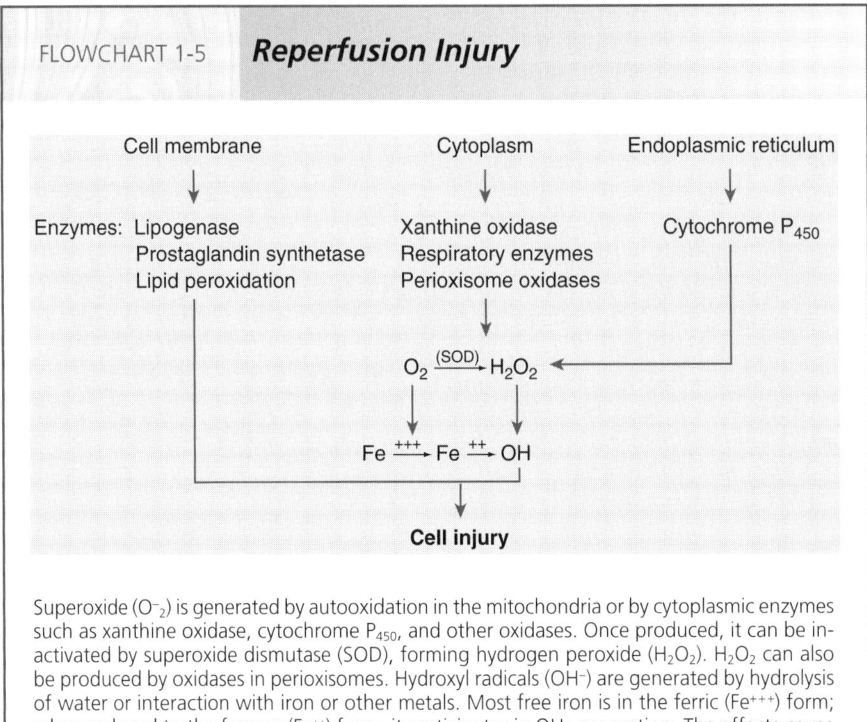

Superoxide (O^-_2) is generated by autooxidation in the mitochondria or by cytoplasmic enzymes such as xanthine oxidase, cytochrome P_{450}, and other oxidases. Once produced, it can be inactivated by superoxide dismutase (SOD), forming hydrogen peroxide (H_2O_2). H_2O_2 can also be produced by oxidases in perioxisomes. Hydroxyl radicals (OH^-) are generated by hydrolysis of water or interaction with iron or other metals. Most free iron is in the ferric (Fe^{+++}) form; when reduced to the ferrous (Fe^{++}) form, it participates in OH^- generation. The effects cause cellular injury through protein, DNA, and plasma membrane breakdown.

liver.[5,20] This disturbance is related to a deficiency in the pancreatic hormone, insulin (see page 664).

PIGMENTATION

Pigments are substances that have color and accumulate within the cells. Many types have been described, some of which are normal components of cells and some of which are abnormal and collect in cells under abnormal stimulation.[1] Pigments are often described as to source or origin: *exogenous* (coming from outside the body) or *endogenous* (produced within the body).

The most common exogenous pigment comes from inhaling organic carbon particulates generated from burning fossil fuels. These particulates accumulate in the macrophages and lymph nodes of the lung tissue. This accumulation produces a blackened appearance of the lungs called *anthracosis*.

Lipofuscin pigmentation of the skin is common in the aging person. The pigment responsible is *lipofuscin* or *lipochrome*, which is visible as golden brown granules. This "wear and tear" pigment is predominant in cells that have atrophied or are chronically injured.[12,22] It also may be present in the brain, liver, heart, and ovaries of an elderly individual. The pigments gradually accumulate with age and apparently do not cause cellular dysfunction.

Melanin is a black-brown pigment that is formed by the melanocytes of the skin. The amount of melanin imparts the degree of color to the skin. It also absorbs light and protects the skin from direct sun rays. Excessive deposition of melanin in the skin is common with Addison's disease (see page 690), many skin conditions, and melanomas that arise from these cells. In the aged person, melanocyte activity is decreased and the skin becomes paler, with areas of hyperpigmentation called "liver spots" or lentigines.[20]

Hemosiderin, a derivative of hemoglobin, is a pigment that is formed from excess accumulation of stored iron. It is often a hemoglobin-derived substance but may be formed due to excess intake of dietary iron or impaired use of iron. One example of localized hemosiderosis is the common *bruise*, which is an accumulation of hemosiderin after the erythrocytes in the injured area are broken down by macrophages. The excess hemoglobin thus released becomes hemosiderin. The colors occur as the hemoglobin is transformed first to biliverdin (green bile), then bilirubin (red bile), and the golden yellow hemosiderin.[17] Deposits of hemosiderin in organs and tissues is called *hemosiderosis*, which may occur with excess of absorbed dietary iron, impaired use of iron, or the hemolytic anemias. For the most part, accumulation of hemosiderin does not interfere with organ function unless it is extreme. Excessive iron storage in some organs is implicated in increased cancer risk.[17] In extreme hemosiderosis of the liver, for example, fibrosis may result.

CALCIFICATION

Normally, calcium is deposited only in the bones and teeth under the influence of various hormones. Pathologic calcification may occur in the skin, the soft tissues, blood vessels, heart, and kidneys. Calcium may precipitate in areas of chronic inflammation or areas of dead or degenerating tissue.

Metastatic calcification can result from excess circulating calcium that comes from bone reabsorption or destruction from conditions such as metastatic tumors or immobilization from fractures or spinal cord injury. Sometimes the cause of this condition is unknown. Calcium precipitates into many areas, including the kidneys, blood vessels, and connective tissue.

Calcium that precipitates into areas of unresolved healing is called *dystrophic calcification.* It may be extracellular, intracellular, or both. It often localizes in the mitochondria and propagates from there. It is often a cause of organ dysfunction such as with atherosclerotic vessels or calcified cardiac valves.[12] Increased uptake of calcium into mitochondria is characteristic of injured cells.[7]

HYALINE INFILTRATION

Hyaline is a word that indicates a characteristic alteration within cells or in the extracellular space that appears as a homogeneous, glassy, pink inclusion on stained histologic section. Because it does not represent a specific pattern of accumulation, different mechanisms are responsible for its formation. Intracellular hyaline changes may include excessive amounts of protein, aggregates of immunoglobulin, viral nucleoproteins, closely packed fibrils, or other substances.[8] Extracellular hyaline refers to the appearance of precipitated plasma proteins and other proteins across a membrane wall. This change is particularly well seen in and around the arterioles and the renal glomeruli. A variety of mechanisms cause the hyaline change, and the implications of this deposition differ depending on the underlying process.[8]

Cellular Changes Caused by Injurious Stimuli

In some cases, the cell undergoes an actual change to adapt to an injurious agent. The changes often manifested are atrophy, dysplasia, hypertrophy, hyperplasia, and metaplasia (Table 1-4). The adaptations are methods by which the cells stay alive and adjust workload to demand.

ATROPHY

Atrophy refers to a decrease in cell size resulting from decreased workload, loss of nerve supply, decreased blood supply, inadequate nutrition, or loss of hormonal stimulation.[20] The word implies previous normal development of the cell and cell loss of structural components and substance.

Physiologic Atrophy

Physiologic atrophy occurs with aging in the parenchyma of organs and allows for survival of cells with decreased function. The cells tend to reproduce less readily. Physiologic atrophy begins in the thymus gland in early adulthood and in the uterus after menopause. Many cells in other glands and muscles also undergo atrophy with aging. These cells may develop an increase in the number of autophagic vacuoles in the cytoplasm that isolate and destroy injured organelles. The triggering mechanism for autophagia is unknown, but it may result in incompletely digested material called *residual* bodies. An example of this is the lipofuscin or brownish pigment seen in the aging cell. Atrophy may progress to cellular injury and death, and the cells may be replaced with connective tissue, adipose tissue, or both.

Disuse Atrophy

Disuse atrophy is common after an extremity has been immobilized in a cast. The decreased workload placed on the affected muscles results in decreased size of the entire muscle. When the workload is again restored, the muscle often enlarges to its preinjury size.

Other Types of Atrophy

Atrophy may also result from starvation, loss of nerve or endocrine stimulation or cellular ischemia. In starvation, cellular atrophy is seen especially in skeletal muscle and in cells not vital to the survival of the organism.[8] Atrophy of target organs of endocrine stimulation often results when the stimulating hormone for the organ hormone secretion is deficient.

Loss of nerve supply, such as when a spinal cord injury interrupts nervous stimulation to the muscles below the level of injury, may cause muscular atrophy. The muscles gradually atrophy, and eventually musculature is replaced by fibrous tissue.

Atrophy of muscles may also be seen with chronic ischemic disease of the lower extremities. The decreased blood supply impairs the metabolism within the cell, and atrophy occurs as a protective mechanism to keep the tissue viable.

DYSPLASIA

Dysplasia refers to the appearance of cells that have undergone some atypical changes in response to chronic irritation. It is not a true adaptive process in that it serves

TABLE 1-4

ADAPTIVE CELLULAR CHANGES

CELLULAR CHANGE	PATHOLOGY	CLINICAL MANIFESTATIONS	CELLULAR EXAMPLE
Atrophy	Decreased cell size Loss of cell size and functions		Atrophy
• Physiologic atrophy	Occurs due to aging and in certain organs such as thymus gland after adolescence	Functional changes in affected organ	
• Disuse atrophy	Decreased workload on muscle will cause shrinkage of entire muscle	Muscle of affected injury becomes shrunken, much smaller than unaffected side	
• Loss of nerve supply	Gradual atrophy of muscles	Muscle becomes wasted and eventually will be replaced with fibrous tissue	
• Chronic ischemia	Impaired muscular metabolism leads to muscle atrophy	Atrophy of muscle seen in tissue	
• Starvation/malnutrition	Skeletal muscle and nonvital tissue atrophies to maintain vital organs	All skeletal muscle atrophied/develops thin, cachectic appearance.	
Dysplasia	Atypical cellular changes in response to chronic irritation may be precancerous	Varies with organ/system affected Frequently seen in respiratory system in person with chronic lung disease	Dysplasia
Hypertrophy	Increase in size of individual cells without an increase in number	Especially seen as response to hypertension or increased cardiac workload in heart Skeletal muscle hypertrophy may be induced with weight lifting or heavy workload	Hypertrophy
Hyperplasia	Increase in numbers of cells due to a normal or abnormal stimulation	*Physiologic* hyperplasia seen during puberty or pregnancy *Pathologic* hyperplasia results with abnormal stimulation of a gland or other organs. May result in hypersecretion such as excessive thyroid hormone and hyperthyroidism	Hyperplasia
Metaplasia	Adaptive substitution of one cell type for another. May be a precancerous lesion	Normally seen in repair of deep wounds, replacing epithelial tissue with connective tissue May be seen with chronic irritation such as calluses on hands or substitution of cells in hostile environment such as with chronic bronchitis	Metaplasia

no specific function. Dysplasia is presumably controlled reproduction of cells, but it is closely related to malignancy in that it may transform into uncontrolled, rapid reproduction.[16,17] The cellular changes often regress on removal of the injurious stimulus. Epithelial cells are the most common types to exhibit dysplasia; changes include alterations in the size and shape of cells, causing loss of normal architectural orientation of one cell with the next. Dysplastic changes are common in the bronchi of chronic smokers and in the cervical epithelium.[8]

HYPERTROPHY

Hypertrophy is an increase in the size of individual cells, resulting in increased tissue mass without an increase in the number of cells. It usually represents the response of a specific organ to an increased demand for work. Hypertrophied cells increase their number of intracellular organelles, especially mitochondria. A good example of *physiologic hypertrophy* is the enlargement of muscles of athletes or weight lifters. The individual muscle cells enlarge but do not proliferate, and this provides increased strength. Physiologic hypertrophy occurs at puberty with enlargement of the sex organs (see page 110). Hypertrophy may also be caused by an increased functional demand such as systemic hypertension in which the myocardium must pump under greater pressure and thus it increases the size of the myocardial muscle cells.

HYPERPLASIA

Hyperplasia is a common condition seen in cells that are under an increased physiologic workload or stimulation. It is defined as increase of tissue mass due to an increase in the number of cells. Cells that undergo hyperplasia are those that are capable of dividing and thus of increasing their number. Whether hyperplasia, rather than hypertrophy, occurs depends on the regenerative capacity of the specific cell.

Physiologic hyperplasia is a normal outcome of puberty and pregnancy. *Compensatory hyperplasia* occurs in organs that are capable of regenerating lost substance. An example is regeneration of the liver when part of its substance is destroyed. *Pathologic hyperplasia* is seen in conditions of abnormal stimulation of organs with cells that are capable of regeneration. Examples are enlargement of the thyroid gland secondary to stimulation by thyroid-stimulating hormone from the pituitary, and parathyroid hyperplasia due to renal failure. Hyperplasia is induced by a known stimulus and almost always stops when the stimulus has been removed. This controlled reproduction is an important differentiating feature of hyperplasia from neoplasia. There is a close relationship between certain types of pathologic hyperplasia and malignancy (see page 78).

METAPLASIA

Metaplasia is a reversible change in which one type of adult cell is replaced by another type. It is probably an adaptive substitution of one cell type more suited to the hostile environment for another.[8] Metaplasia is commonly seen in chronic bronchitis; the normal pseudostratified columnar, ciliated goblet cells are replaced by stratified squamous epithelial cells. The latter cells are better suited for survival in the face of chronic, irritating smoke inhalation or environmental pollution. Metaplasia increases the chances of cellular survival but decreases the protective aspect of mucus secretion. Certain types of metaplasia are closely related to malignancy, which probably indicates that chronic irritation causes the initial change.

Cellular Injury and Death

Cellular injury and death may be caused by microorganisms, lack of oxygen, and physical agents such as extreme temperatures, toxic chemicals, and radiation. The mechanisms by which microorganisms cause cellular injury and death are detailed in Chapter 8. Lack of oxygen (anoxia) is the most common cause of cellular injury and death. The following conditions can produce this problem: ischemia, thrombosis, embolism, infarction, necrosis, and somatic death. **Apoptosis** describes single cell death that occurs due to a "suicide" process in cells that is programmed or initiated by toxins.[17]

In some instances, cellular injury is reversible, or it may progress to a permanent, lethal change. Intracellular changes and their progression are detailed in Flowchart 1-3. Physical agents often induce changes similar to those of anoxia or they may differ depending on the agent and the tissue involved.

ISCHEMIA

Ischemia refers to a critical lack of blood supply to a localized area. It is reversible in that tissues are restored to normal function when oxygen is again supplied to them. Ischemia may precede infarction or death of the tissue, or it may occur sporadically when the oxygen need outstrips the oxygen supply.[2] It is important to differentiate between ischemia, a clinical change, and infarction, a pathologic change.

Ischemia usually occurs in the presence of atherosclerosis in the major arteries. Atherosclerosis is a lipid-depositing process with fibrofatty accumulations, or plaques, on the intimal layer of the artery (see page 433). Atherosclerosis often gives rise to the formation of clots or thrombi on the plaque. These changes compromise blood flow through the artery, which then impairs oxygen supply to the tissues during increased need. In the later stages, the blood supply is impaired even at rest.

The classic conditions resulting from ischemia are *angina pectoris* and *intermittent claudication*. The former refers to pain from ischemia affecting the heart, and the latter refers to pain from ischemia of the extremities usually during activity. Ischemia is often relieved by rest and the tissues return to normal function. It may be progressive, however, and cause *ischemic infarction*, which involves cell death due to lack of blood supply or oxygen. Lack of oxygen supply to the brain, heart, and kidneys can be tolerated for only a short time; damage is irreversible. The fibroblasts of connective tissue, however, have been shown to survive much longer periods of anoxia.

THROMBOSIS

The word *thrombosis* refers to the formation of a clot on the intimal lining of the blood vessels. It may decrease blood flow or totally occlude the vessel. Thrombosis also may occur on the endothelial lining of the heart, called *mural thrombosis*.

The most common factor in thrombosis is disruption of the endothelial lining of the blood vessels, which exposes underlying collagen fibers. Normally the endothelial layer is continuous from the heart throughout the vascular circuit, including the capillaries and veins. When trauma, atherosclerosis, or other factors disrupt this layer, platelets may accumulate, and the intrinsic clotting mechanism is initiated. The body spontaneously initiates its fibrinolytic system to dissolve the clot and reopen the vessel. This may or may not be successful in reestablishing the flow of blood. Stasis of blood and increased blood viscosity also enhance coagulability of blood. Thrombosis most frequently occurs in the deep veins of the legs, and these thrombi may detach, embolize to and lodge in the pulmonary arterial circuit (see page 591). Thrombosis in an artery can disrupt blood flow to the area supplied by the vessel and cause ischemia or infarction of that area.

EMBOLISM

A thrombus may break off and become a traveling mass in the blood. This process is called *thrombotic embolization*. The most common types of emboli are derived from thrombi, but other substances such as fat, vegetations from valves, or foreign particles also may embolize. The obstruction caused by an embolus is called an *embolic occlusion*.

If the embolus arises in the venous circuit, it is carried to and trapped in the vasculature of the pulmonary capillary bed. Depending on the size of the embolus, the clinical result may vary from being asymptomatic to death producing.

If the embolus arises in the left side of the heart, it may travel to any of the arteries branching off the aorta. Arterial embolism may also occur from a larger artery, such as one affected by atherosclerosis, to a smaller artery. When it occludes the arterial tributary, it compromises blood flow to the area supplied.

INFARCTION

Occlusion of the blood supply from an artery causes *infarction*, which is a localized area of tissue death due to lack of blood supply. It is also termed *ischemic necrosis* and may occur in any organ or tissue.

Infarcts may have different pathologic characteristics. They are frequently classified as *pale infarcts, hemorrhagic infarcts*, and *infarcts with bacterial supergrowth*. Pale infarcts are seen in solid tissue deprived of its arterial circulation as a result of ischemia. Red or hemorrhagic infarcts are more frequent with venous occlusion or with congested tissues. The infarcted tissue has a red appearance, due to hemorrhage into the area, that may be poorly defined, causing difficulty in differentiating viable and nonviable tissue.[8] Bacterial supergrowth is common and may be present in the area or may be brought to the area. The classification of *septic infarction* is added when the area shows evidence of bacterial infection. The lesion is converted to an abscess when it is septic and the inflammatory response is initiated. *Gangrene* is an example of infarction in which ischemic cell death is followed by bacterial overgrowth, leading to liquefaction of the tissues. This term is frequently used to describe conditions of the extremities and the bowel.[16]

NECROSIS

The term *necrosis* refers to cell or tissue death characterized by structural evidence of this death.[8] As cells die, the mitochondria swell, functions become disrupted, membranes rupture, and the lysosomal enzymes may be released into the tissues. The nucleus undergoes specific changes that may include shrinking (pyknosis), fragmenting, or gradual fading. Necrosis is commonly described in terms of coagulative, liquefactive, special types, and apoptosis.

Coagulative Necrosis

Coagulative necrosis usually results from lack of blood supply to an area. It is the most common pattern of necrosis and frequently occurs due to infarction in organs such as the heart and kidneys, but it also may result from chemical injury. The cell structure and its architectural outline may be preserved (structured necrosis), but the nucleus is lost.[12] The outline may remain intact with the loss of intracellular organelles (structureless necrosis).

Caseation or *caseous necrosis* has long been described in relation to tuberculosis, but it may be present in a few other conditions. It is an example of structureless necrosis. The central area of necrosis is soft and friable and is surrounded by an area with a cheesy, crumbly appearance. The cellular architecture is destroyed. The area is walled off from the rest of the body and may become rimmed with calcium. Areas of caseous necrosis may localize in areas of tuberculous infestation.[8]

Liquefactive Necrosis

Liquefactive necrosis most frequently occurs in brain tissue and results from fatal injury of the neuron. The breakdown of the neuron causes release of lysosomes and other constituents into the surrounding area. Lysosomes cause liquefaction of the cell and surrounding cells, leaving pockets of liquid, debris, and cystlike structures. Liquefactive necrosis is often described in brain infarction but may be seen with bacterial lesions because of the release of bacterial and leukocytic enzymes. Liquefaction may occur in an area of coagulative necrosis as a secondary change.[8]

Special Types

Fat necrosis is a specific form of cellular death that occurs when lipases escape into fat storage areas. It particularly is seen in acute pancreatic necrosis and causes patchy necrosis of the pancreas and surrounding areas (see page 769). Traumatic fat necrosis most commonly seen in the breast gives rise to a giant cell reaction that can resemble a carcinoma.[8]

Gangrenous necrosis is a combination of coagulative and liquefactive necroses. The term *gangrene* is applied to any black, foul-smelling area that is adjacent to living tissue. The cause of tissue death is ischemia but bacteria and surrounding leukocytes cause liquefaction of the tissues. When the coagulative pattern is dominant, it is called *dry gangrene*. When the liquefactive process is more pronounced, it is called *wet gangrene*.[17]

Gas gangrene (myonecrosis) is a specific type of necrosis that can occur due to *Clostridia* infections. *Clostridia* are gram-positive anaerobes that cause such conditions as tetanus, botulism, and food poisoning.[8,16] Gas gangrene usually occurs in large traumatic wounds in which the organisms cause destruction of the connective tissue framework. Gas bubbles are caused by a fermentative reaction causing a reddish blue appearance of involved tissues. If this material reaches the bloodstream, shock and disseminated intravascular coagulation (DIC) may be produced (see page 393).

Apoptosis

Apoptosis is a distinctive type of cell death in which single or small groups of cells are deleted from their tissue of origin.[6] It can be a normal process or a programmed "suicide" process in cells such as the process seen during embryonic development. Pathologically, the suicide process may be initiated by toxins, irradiation, or large doses of corticosteroids.[6] It is probably initiated by an endogenous endonuclease (enzyme within the cell) that becomes activated and causes destruction of the DNA and nuclear chromatin.

SOMATIC DEATH

Somatic death is death of the body. Irreversible changes occur in cells and organs due to lack of oxygen supply. Individual cells remain alive for different lengths of time. Postmortem changes include rigor mortis, livor mortis, algor mortis, intravascular clotting, autolysis, and putrefaction.

Rigor mortis develops because of depletion of ATP in the muscles. It begins in the involuntary muscles and within 2 to 4 hours it affects the voluntary muscles. The result is stiffening of the muscles, a rigidity that continues for varying periods of time. *Livor mortis* is the reddish blue discoloration of the body that results from gravitational pooling of blood. *Algor mortis* is the term used for the cooling of the body that occurs after death. The rate of cooling depends on the body temperature before death and the postmortem environmental temperature. *Intravascular clotting* results in clots that are not adherent to the lining of the blood vessels and heart. *Autolysis* is the term used to describe digestion of tissues from released substances, such as enzymes from lysosomes. Organs may be swollen and spongy in appearance. *Putrefaction* is caused by saprophytic organisms entering the dead body, usually from the intestines. This results in a greenish discoloration of the tissues and organs, and the organisms may produce gases, leading to foamy or spongy organs.[16]

REFERENCES

1. Alberts, B. et al. (1994). *Molecular biology of the cell* (3rd ed.). New York: Garland.
2. Armstrong, S. C., & Ganote, C. E. (1992). Flow cytometric analysis of isolated rat cardiomyocytes: Vinculin and tubulin fluorescence during metabolic inhibition and ischemia. *Journal of Molecular and Cellular Cardiology, 24,* 149.
3. Berne, R. M., & Levy, M. N. (1998). *Physiology* (4th ed.). St. Louis: Mosby.
4. Bittar, E. E., & Bittar, N. (Eds.). (1995). *Principles of medical biology: Cell chemistry and physiology*. Greenwich, CT: JAI Press.
5. Bonventrue, J. (1993). Mechanisms of ischemic renal failure, *Kidney International, 43,* 1160.
6. Buga, L., et al. (1993). Apoptosis and necrosis: Basic types and mechanisms of cell death. *Archives of Pathology and Laboratory Medicine, 117,* 1208.
7. Byrne, J. H. (1994). *An introduction to membrane transport and bioelectricity: Foundations of general physiology and electrochemistry*. New York: Raven.
8. Chandrasoma, P., & Taylor, C. R. (1998). *Concise pathology* (3rd ed.). Stamford, CT: Appleton & Lange.
9. Creighton, T. E. (1993). *Proteins: Structure and molecular properties* (2nd ed.). New York: Freeman.
10. Das, D. K., et al. (1986). Role of membrane phospholipids in myocardial injury induced by ischemia and reperfusion. *American Journal of Physiology, 251,* H71.

11. Devlin, T. M. (1992). *Textbook of biochemistry with clinical correlations* (3rd ed.). New York: Wiley-Liss.
12. Farber, J. (1982). Membrane injury and calcium homeostasis in the pathogenesis of coagulative necrosis. *Laboratory Investigation, 47,* 114.
13. Guyton, A. C., & Hall, J. E. (1996). *Textbook of medical physiology* (9th ed.). Philadelphia: Saunders.
14. Jorde, L. B., Carey, J. C., & White, R. L. (1995). *Medical genetics.* St. Louis: Mosby.
15. Lodish, H., et al. (1993). *Molecular biology of membranes, structure and function.* New York: Plenum.
16. Mergner, W. J. (1990). *Cell death: Mechanism of acute and lethal cell injury* (Vol. 1). New York: Field and Wood Medical Production.
17. Rubin, E., & Farber, J. L. (1999). *Pathology* (3rd ed.). Philadelphia: Lippincott-Raven.
18. Shier, D., Butler, J., & Lewis, R. (1996). *Hole's human anatomy and physiology* (7th ed.). Dubuque, IA: W. C. Brown.
19. Siegel, G. J., Agranoff, R. W., & Uhler, E. (1998). *Basic neurochemistry: Molecular, cellular, and medical aspects* (6th ed.). Philadelphia: Lippincott-Raven.
20. Szabo, S., & Kovacs, K. (1992). *Functional endocrine pathology.* Oxford, UK: Blackwell Scientific.
21. Tortora, G. J., & Grabowski, S. R. (1997). *Principles of anatomy and physiology* (8th ed.). New York: HarperCollins.
22. Venkatachalam, M. A., et al. (1983). Salvage of ischemic cells by impermeant solute and ATP. *Laboratory Investigation, 49,* 1.
23. Weintraub, B. D. (Ed.). (1995). *Molecular endocrinology: Basic concepts and clinical correlations.* New York: Raven.
24. Yeagle, P. (1993). *The membranes of cells* (2nd ed.). San Diego: Academic Press.

Chapter

2

Genetic Basis of Human Disease

Miguel F. da Cunha

KEY TERMS

acrocentric chromosome
allele
amniocentesis
aneuploidy
autosome
centromere
chromosome
chromosome abnormalities
congenital
cytogenetics
deletion
diploid
DNA
dominant
euploid
gamete
gametogenesis
gene
genetic counseling
genetic engineering
genome
genotype
haploid
hemizygous
heterozygote
homologous
homozygote
karyotype
locus
malformation
meiosis
mendelian inheritance
metacentric chromosome
mitosis
monosomy
mosaicism
multifactorial inheritance
mutation
nondisjunction
oncogene
phenotype
polygenic
polyploidy
recessive
submetacentric chromosomes
syndrome
translocation
trisomy

The knowledge of basic concepts in human genetics is essential to the understanding of genetic disorders. Because genetic diseases are a result of **gene** alterations or **chromosome abnormalities**, the study of genetic diseases requires an understanding of gene function and **chromosome** structure and behavior. Alterations in single genes result in a group of disorders termed **Mendelian**,[1] or single-gene diseases, such as sickle cell disease, galactosemia, and cystic fibrosis. The most thorough and updated collection of mendelian traits is that of McKusick's *Mendelian Inheritance in Man*, which is available in printed[6] and online[11] versions. Changes in multiple but related genes create polygenic and multifactorial disorders, such as cleft lip and palate. Chromosome abnormalities can result from numerical or structural chromosome changes. Numerical (eg, Turner **syndrome**, Down syndrome) or structural (eg, cat's cry disease) chromosomal aberrations will automatically affect large groups of genes. However, alterations in single genes, or even in large groups of genes, will be too small to alter chromosome structure and to be identifiable by **karyotype** analysis.

This chapter summarizes some of the current knowledge in medical genetics and aims to provide the reader with the basic essentials of genetics, in an attempt to awaken an interest in further reading. The general bibliography offers resources on various areas of genetics for a more in-depth pursuit of knowledge in the field. In addition, various glossaries of genetic terms are available online.[15]

GENES

The human **genome** comprises between 50,000 and 100,000 genes, distributed along 46 chromosomes and tightly packed in every nucleated somatic cell. Each human gene has, on the average, 5,000 base pairs, and a single mutation in one base pair ("point mutation") may have devastating effects for the individual. Such is the case of sickle cell disease, in which a single base substitution causes the replacement, in each beta chain of normal human hemoglobin, of one amino acid (glutamic acid) by another (valine). This small alteration will eventually be responsible for the major abnormalities observed in this disease. Details of gene structure and its role in protein synthesis are found in Chapter 1.

Gene Function: A Conceptual Model

Genes are segments of **DNA** that determine a certain biologic function. Some are structural genes that encode for the synthesis of specific polypeptides (proteins); others are regulatory and modulate the function of other genes or groups of genes. Structural genes are described in this chapter and regulatory genes and their effects are found throughout the text. **Mutations** (permanent changes) in structural genes may have significant qualitative and quantitative effects on the synthesis of the corresponding protein, with potential clinical consequences. Proteins can be classified as structural (or constitutive) proteins, and those that affect the metabolism of other molecules or substrates (enzymes). Table 2-1 summarizes the effects of protein disorders on selected genetic diseases.

The genetic regulation of enzymatic activity in a metabolic pathway provides a useful model for gene function. Figure 2-1 illustrates four mechanisms of gene–protein interaction. Panel 1 represents the normal metabolic conversion of a substance **A** into an end-product **K**, via by-products **B**, **C**, **D**, etc. Enzymes **b** and **c**, whose synthesis is controlled by genes **β** and **δ**, catalyze steps **B** → **C**, and **C** → **D**, respectively. A feedback loop ensures physiologic levels of **K**.

On Panel 2, a mutation in gene **β**, prevents normal synthesis of enzyme **b**, creating an interruption of the pathway between **B** and **C**. Assuming a continuous uptake of **A**, two outcomes ensue: accumulation of **B**, and depletion of all products beyond the block, **C, D, . . . K**. An example of this situation is Tay-Sachs disease (or GM_2 gangliosidosis). In this disease, a mutation in the HexA gene (here exemplified by **β**) causes the lack of the enzyme hexosaminidase A (HexA), represented by **b**. Absence of **b** creates an accumulation of ganglioside GM_2 (**B**) in nerve cells, resulting in the clinical manifestations that characterize this progressive neurologic disorder.

Panel 3 depicts a mutation in gene **δ**, which causes depletion of enzyme **c**, and interrupts the metabolic conversion of **C** into **D**. In this instance, an alternative pathway **C** → **E** → **F** is opened. This event may have two outcomes: product **F** may eventually be converted into **K**, with no significant clinical consequences; or **F** may represent the end-point to the alternative pathway. If accumulation of **F** reaches toxic levels, a disease process may occur. Such is the case in phenylketonuria (PKU), an inborn error of metabolism that creates an intolerance to the amino acid phenylalanine. The missing enzyme (**c**, here), which results from mutation in the PKU gene (**δ**), is phenylalanine hydroxylase. The alternative pathway leads to the formation and accumulation of phenylketones (**F**). In combination with phenylalanine deficiency, an excessive amount of phenylketones contributes to the postnatal completion of myelination of nerves resulting in profound mental retardation.

Panel 4 represents a genetic alteration of the enzyme **d**, which is involved in the feedback control of synthesis

TABLE 2-1

PROTEIN CLASSIFICATION AND GENETIC DISEASE

PROTEIN INVOLVED	MECHANISM OF ACTION	RESULTING DISORDER
CONSTITUTIVE PROTEINS		
Globins	Altered oxygen transport	Hemoglobinopathies Sickle cell disease Thalassemias
Dystrophin	Muscle cell defect	Muscular dystrophy
Clotting factors VIIIc and IX	Abnormal clotting activity	Hemophilia A and B
ENZYMES		
Phenylalanine hydroxylase	Interrupted metabolism and accumulation of toxic precursors (phenylalanine and phenylketones)	Phenylketonuria
Hexosaminidase A	Interrupted metabolism and accumulation of precursors (GM_2 ganglioside)	Tay-Sachs disease
Hypoxanthine guanine phosphoribosil transferase	Disruption of metabolic feedback mechanism and accumulation of end-product (uric acid)	Lesch-Nyhan syndrome
3-hydroxy-3methylglutaryl coenzyme A reductase	Disruption of metabolic feedback mechanism and accumulation of end-product (cholesterol)	Familial hypercholesterolemia

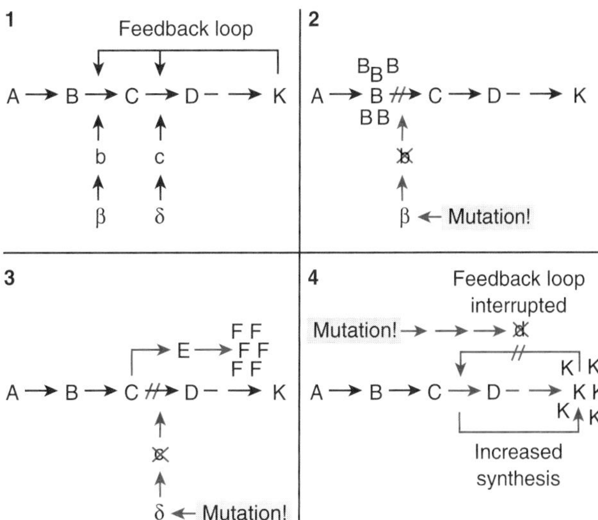

FIGURE 2-1. Gene–protein relationships. **Panel 1.** Normal sequence of events in the metabolic conversion of product A into end product K, mediated by enzymes b and c, which are encoded by genes β and δ, respectively. **Panel 2.** Consequences of a mutation in gene β, resulting in lack of enzyme **b,** interruption of the metabolic pathway, and accumulation of by-product B. **Panel 3.** Consequences of a mutation in gene δ, resulting in lack of enzyme c, interruption of the metabolic pathway, and opening of an alternate pathway. **Panel 4.** Consequences of a mutation in the gene encoding for enzyme d, which is involved in the feedback control loop for end-product K. (Please refer to text for explanation of all panels.)

of **K**. As a result, **K** may accumulate to toxic levels. The prototype genetic disease here is Lesch-Nyhan syndrome, in which **d** is the enzyme hypoxanthine guanine phosphoribosil transferase (HGPRT) and **K** is uric acid. A deficiency in HGPRT and accumulation of uric acid to extremely high levels will result in the development of mental retardation and a tendency for self-mutilation.

Gene Expression

Genetically determined structural and functional features may be under the control of one single gene or may result from the cooperative interaction of several genes (polygenic). In general, traits controlled by a single gene will have a clear threshold for phenotypic expression (eg, "nonaffected" versus "affected"), whereas those controlled by multiple genes will reveal a continuum of phenotypic expression (eg, "mildly affected" to "severely affected"). The vast majority of human characteristics, such as stature, are polygenic.

SINGLE-GENE INHERITANCE

The inheritance of traits controlled by single gene was originally delineated by the works of Gregor Mendel and is based on the principles of segregation and independent assortment of **alleles.**[7] The concept of gene refers to a location (**locus**) on a chromosome that controls a certain biologic function. The genetic constitution of an individual at any given locus is termed **genotype**. For example, the gene involved in Tay-Sachs disease only determines a location in the short arm of chromosome 15 that controls the synthesis of the enzyme HexA. Alternate forms of this gene are represented by its alleles. The normal ("wild-type") allele HexA$^+$, commands the synthesis of HexA, whereas the mutant allele, HexA$^-$, indicates the lack of such command, resulting in the absence of the enzyme. Whether or not a gene is expressed as a certain **phenotype** (measurable or observable features) depends on the arrangements of its alleles and on the concepts of dominance and recessivity.

Dominant Inheritance Pattern

A **dominant** inheritance pattern is evident when the presence of one copy of the mutated allele is sufficient to cause expression of the phenotype. If a gene has only two alleles, one normal (+) and one mutant (–), persons carrying that gene can only have one of three possible allele combinations: (+/+), (+/–), or (–/–) (Fig. 2-2). Persons who display the same alleles (+/+) or (–/–) (individuals **A** and **C**, respectively) are homozygous; those with the (+/–) configuration (such as person **B**) are **heterozygous** for that allele. For a disorder caused by a dominant gene, the homozygote (+/+) would exhibit a normal phenotype, and both the heterozygote (+/–) and the homozygote (–/–) would be affected with the disorder. This means that in the heterozygote, when two outcomes are in question, the ultimate effect of the mutant allele predominates over the effect of the normal allele. Thus, the presence of one copy of the mutant allele is sufficient to cause the phenotype to express, and a double dose of this allele will result in a more accentuated expression.

This dominant pattern applies to genes located on the autosomes. The situation for sex chromosomes in men is different because the X and the Y chromosomes contain very small areas of homology. As such, they do not pair side-by-side during **meiosis**, as do all the autosomes and the X chromosomes in females. Because of this, men are **hemizygous** for all genes on the X chro-

FOCUS ON CELLULAR PHYSIOLOGY

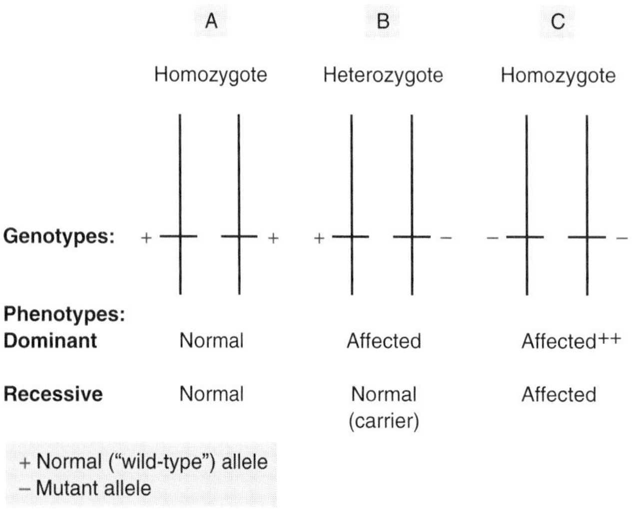

	A	B	C
	Homozygote	Heterozygote	Homozygote
Genotypes:	+ +	+ –	– –
Phenotypes:			
Dominant	Normal	Affected	Affected++
Recessive	Normal	Normal (carrier)	Affected

+ Normal ("wild-type") allele
– Mutant allele

FIGURE 2-2. Single-gene (Mendelian) inheritance. Schematic representation of the three possible allelic arrangements of a gene with two alleles. Represented here are genotypes and possible phenotypes for dominant and recessive inheritance. Note the absence of a carrier state in dominant disease and the occurrence of a heterozygous carrier (**B**) in recessive disease. (See text for details.)

mosome, which do not have a homologous site on the Y, and their alleles are represented as single copies. The character of a single-copy X-linked allele (either + or –) determines its phenotypic expression, respectively as normal or affected. Box 2-1 summarizes characteristics of dominant inheritance.

Recessive Inheritance Pattern

A **recessive** inheritance pattern is evident when two copies of the mutated allele are necessary for the expression of the phenotype. As depicted in Figure 2-2, in the expression of a recessive gene, individuals (**A**) and (**B**) display both a normal (unaffected) phenotype, and only (**C**), who inherited two mutant alleles from both parents, will be affected. This reflects the fact that in the heterozygote, the mutant allele is recessive ("hidden"), and the phenotype expressed will be that of the dominant (normal) allele. In other words, a recessive disease will *only* be phenotypically expressed when a double dose of the mutant allele is present. Because each allele is contributed by one parent, both parents are equally responsible for this outcome. Al-

BOX 2-1

DOMINANT INHERITANCE: CHARACTERISTICS*

Autosomal Dominant Pattern

- Both males and females are equally likely to be affected.
- A single copy of the mutant allele is sufficient to cause the phenotype to express and therefore, a *carrier state does not exist.*
- The homozygote for the mutant allele is usually more severely affected than the heterozygote.
- The phenotype appears in consecutive generations. Affected persons tend to have an affected parent.
- Children of an affected parent have a 50% chance of inheriting the mutant allele and being affected.
- Phenotypically normal persons in a family pedigree are free of the mutant allele and do not transmit the phenotype to their offspring.

X-Linked Dominant Pattern

- Both males and females can be affected, but women are usually less severely affected than men.
- Affected males do not transmit the mutant allele to sons.
- All daughters of an affected male are affected and have a 50% chance to pass the mutant allele to their sons and daughters.

* All partners of affected persons here are considered genotypically normal.

though both individuals **A** and **B** display a normal phenotype, gametes produced by **B** will have a 50% chance of carrying the mutant allele, and therefore **B** is carrier for, and a potential transmitter of, this disease.

Carrier identification is extremely important for **genetic counseling** purposes. Unaffected couples who produce a child with a recessive disease are termed obligate carriers, even if a specific test for this condition is not available. Although testing for heterozygous carriers is available for many diseases, it is not yet practical (or cost effective) to test everyone for all conditions. As such, genetic screening for carriers is usually limited to populations at risk, those who belong to a high-risk group for a certain disorder (eg, Ashkenazi Jews and Tay-Sachs disease), or those who have a positive family history. Box 2-2 summarizes characteristics of recessive inheritance.

POLYGENIC AND MULTIFACTORIAL INHERITANCE

Most known traits are controlled by various genes working in conjunction to express those phenotypes, a type of inheritance termed **polygenic**. When environmental factors also contribute to the expression of the phenotype, the appropriate term is **multifactorial inheritance**. Modern interpretation of genetic control of phenotypes tends to follow a multifactorial model—genetic predispositions exist whose expression is affected by environmental triggers. For example, a person carrying a gene for malignant hyperthermia will only develop this disorder when exposed to environmental stimuli such as certain chemicals and anesthesia gases.

Polygenic and multifactorial traits may be classified into two categories—continuous and discontinuous. Continuous traits are usually normal human characteristics that exhibit a continuous distribution, such as height, number of fingerprint ridges, or skin color. Discontinuous traits are usually pathologic conditions that will manifest above a certain genetic threshold—many birth defects (eg, cleft lip and palate) and various common midlife diseases (eg, peptic ulcer). Box 2-3 lists common discontinuous polygenic and multifactorial traits.

A common characteristic of multifactorial inheritance is a variation in recurrence risks, from pregnancy to pregnancy. Because pregnancies are independent events, in single-gene (or mendelian, after Gregor Mendel[1,7]) inheritance, risk figures remain unchanged and are the same in each and every pregnancy. For example, if a parent is affected with an autosomal dominant gene, the recurrence risk for each pregnancy is 50%. The recurrence risk for a multifactorial trait may increase after the occurrence of an affected pregnancy. Box 2-4 summarizes characteristics of multifactorial inheritance.

In genetic counseling, the geneticist dealing with a single-gene trait will follow a fixed set of mendelian rules, in providing risk figures. In multifactorial inheritance, risk figures are obtained through empirical observation of many cases, after which standardized reference tables are created. These tables usually provide the geneticist with multipliers to be factored into the population risks to obtain the final estimation. For example, if the general risk for a multifactorial disease is 6% (of the general population), the occurrence of a previous case in a family will increase that risk figure by a certain factor or multiplier.

BOX 2-2

RECESSIVE INHERITANCE: CHARACTERISTICS*

Autosomal Recessive Pattern

- Both males and females are equally likely to be affected.
- *A carrier state exists.* Both males and females can be carriers.
- The disease appears to "skip a generation," but members of that generation who have affected children are asymptomatic (heterozygous) carriers.
- Carrier parents have a 25% chance to produce an affected child and a 50% chance of producing a carrier child in each and every pregnancy.
- Parent consanguinity may be a factor when a child is affected with a *rare* recessive disease.

X-Linked Recessive Pattern

- Most affected persons are male. Affected females are extremely rare.
- As in all X-linked inheritance, an affected male never transmits the gene to his sons. (Males give their X chromosomes to their daughters.)
- All daughters of an affected male are (heterozygous) *carriers,* none are *affected* (homozygotes).
- Sons of carrier females have a 50% chance of inheriting the mutant allele and being *affected* (hemizygotes). Daughters have a 50% risk of inheriting the mutant allele and being (heterozygous) *carriers.*

* Unless otherwise specified, all partners of affected or carrier persons here are genotypically normal.

BOX 2-3

MULTIFACTORIAL INHERITANCE: SELECTED EXAMPLES OF DISCONTINUOUS TRAITS

Congenital Abnormalities

- Cleft lip (alone)
- Cleft lip with or without cleft palate
- Club foot
- Congenital cardiac defects
- Diaphragmatic hernia
- Hip dislocation
- Hirschprung disease (aganglionic or toxic megacolon)
- Hypospadias
- Neural tube defects
- Omphalocele
- Pyloric stenosis
- Renal agenesis

Common Midlife Diseases

- Bipolar disease
- Diabetes mellitus (insulin-dependent)
- Epilepsy
- Hyperthyroidism
- Peptic ulcer
- Premature vascular disease
- Rheumatoid arthritis
- Schizophrenia

CHROMOSOMES

In contrast with genes, chromosomes are large structures and can be easily visualized under the microscope with modest magnification. As many as 100,000 human genes are distributed along 46 chromosomes, and the size of human chromosomes varies by approximately 10-fold, from the smallest to the largest; thus, the larger the chromosome involved in a numerical abnormality, the more severe will be the ensuing clinical manifestations.

BOX 2-4

MULTIFACTORIAL INHERITANCE: CHARACTERISTICS

- No clearly defined pattern of inheritance within a single family, even when the disorder is clearly familial in nature.
- The recurrence risk increases when more than one family member has the trait. The closer the relationship, the higher the risk.
- The recurrence risk increases with each occurrence of the event (eg, the recurrence risk is greater after two or more affected pregnancies).
- The recurrence risk increases with increasing severity of the malformation.
- The recurrence risk increases with parents consanguinity.
- For disorders with a sex preference (eg, occurring more often in males), the risk for future occurrence is higher if the previous affected relative belongs to the least susceptible sex (female, in this example).

Normal Chromosome Number and Morphology

Normal human somatic cells contain 46 chromosomes, including 44 autosomes arranged in 22 homologous pairs, and two sex chromosomes, XX in females, XY in males. This is termed the **diploid** (2n) chromosome number; thus in humans, 2n = 46. A **haploid** chromosome number is found in gametes (n = 23). A karyotype is a laboratory-made chart that organizes somatic chromosomes, usually obtained from peripheral small lymphocytes, according to their size and centromere position (Fig. 2-3). Autosomes are classified into seven groups designated groups A through G, in decreasing size:

Group A: pairs 1 through 3
Group B: pairs 4 and 5
Group C: pairs 6 through 12
Group D: pairs 13 through 15
Group E: pairs 16 through 18
Group F: pairs 19 and 20
Group G: pairs 21 and 22

The X chromosome approximates the size and shape of a group C pair, and the Y is similar to a group G chromosome. Short chromosome arms are designated as *p* (for *petit*, or small, in French), long arms as *q*. Each arm is divided into regions, and each region subdivided into bands. As an example, the chromosome constitution found in the *cri-du-chat* (cat's cry) syndrome is represented as: 46,XX,B(5)p^-. This notation translates as: a **deletion** ($^-$) of a portion of the small arm (p) of chromosome pair number 5 of the B group, occurring in a female (XX) with a normal chromosome number (46). In the early 1970s, staining techniques were developed for human chromosomes that caused each homologous chromosome pair to display a different, constant pat-

FOCUS ON CELLULAR PATHOPHYSIOLOGY

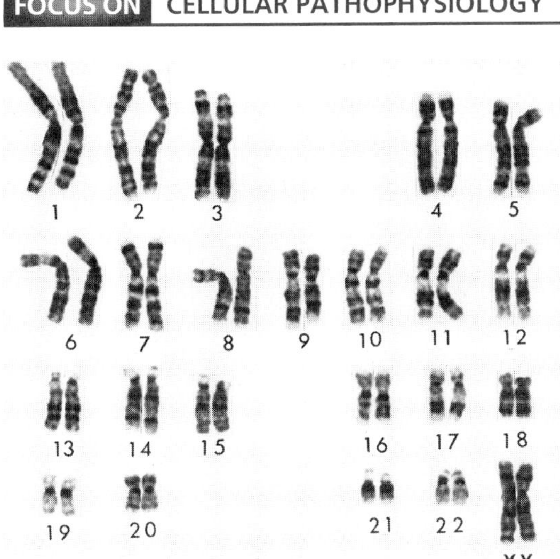

FIGURE 2-3. Karyotype of a human female cell. Chromosomes obtained from a peripheral blood lymphocyte culture. (Courtesy of Dr. David Ledbetter, Department of Human Genetics, University of Chicago.)

tern of banding (eg, Giemsa stain banding depicted in Fig. 2-3). Banding techniques have greatly facilitated the exact placement of chromosomes in groups, as well as the identification of alterations in chromosome structure, such as deletions and translocations.

According to the position of their **centromeres**, chromosomes are classified as **metacentric, submetacentric**, and **acrocentric**. For example, chromosomes A (1 and 3) are metacentric, group B are submetacentric, and groups D and G are the large and small acrocentrics, respectively.

Chromosomal Abnormalities

Chromosome anomalies, studied in the field of **cytogenetics**, are classified as numerical and structural. Virtually all numerical abnormalities and some structural changes may be visually detected by karyotype analysis. Numerical chromosome anomalies can result from the addition of chromosomes to each of the pairs of a diploid cell by exact multiples of the haploid number (23). This will produce cells with chromosome numbers of 69, 92, etc. (**euploidy**). These large alterations in chromosome number (**polyploidy**) result in severe **malformations** seldom compatible with life. In triploid individuals (3n = 69), for example, the genetic imbalance is of such magnitude that their life span will be limited to a few hours or days. However, the addition of one chromosome to one of the pairs (**trisomy**) creates a relatively small **aneuploid** alteration in the total chromosome number (ie, from 46 to 47), which may be compatible with life.

Structural abnormalities result from breakage and atypical rearrangement. Several clastogens (from "clastos," to break, and the suffix "gen" denoting an agent), or chromosome breaking agents, have been identified, and include physical (eg, ionizing radiation), chemical (eg, chlorpromazine), and biologic (eg, viral infections) agents. It must be noted, though, that some breaks are temporary and affect somatic cells, such as those resulting from an infection with the influenza virus. Others are permanent and appear also in germ cells, and therefore have the potential of being transmitted to the offspring. Fig. 2-4 depicts some of the possible consequences of chromosome breakage.

Chromosome breakage may result in loss of the broken fragment–deletion, as observed in the *cri-du-chat* syndrome. In addition, chromosome breakage predisposes to rearrangement of the resulting chromosome fragments. The attachment of a chromosome fragment onto another, nonhomologous chromosome is termed **translocation**, (such as reciprocal translocations and Robertsonian translocations) with potential clinical significance. Reciprocal translocations result from breaks occurring in two different chromosomes, and the fragments are mutually exchanged—derivative chromosomes. Because no loss of genetic material occurred, these translocations are termed balanced, and individuals who are carriers of such exchanges do not exhibit clinical manifestations. Robertsonian translocations occur when the short arms of two acrocentric chromosomes (pairs 13–15 of group D, and pairs 21 and 22 of group G) break off, and the long arms fuse at the centromere, forming what appears to be a single chromosome. Because the short arms of acrocentric chromosomes do not seem to carry a significant number of genes, their loss does not result in clinical manifestations for carriers of this "balanced translocation." However, when carriers of either type of balanced translocation reproduce, the translocated chromosome will be present in a certain percentage of their gametes. On fertilization by a normal gamete, the resulting zygote will have a gene imbalance due to the extra chromosomal (genetic) material. The extra chromosomal material is frequently a source of physical and mental abnormalities in the offspring.

Chromosome Distribution During Cell Division

Somatic cells and early germ cells are diploid (2n = 46) and multiply by **mitosis**, an equational type of cell division that originates two daughter cells with the same chromosome number as the initial cell (see Fig. 1-33). This equitable sharing of chromosomes during anaphase is a result of a phenomenon termed disjunction.

FOCUS ON CELLULAR PATHOPHYSIOLOGY

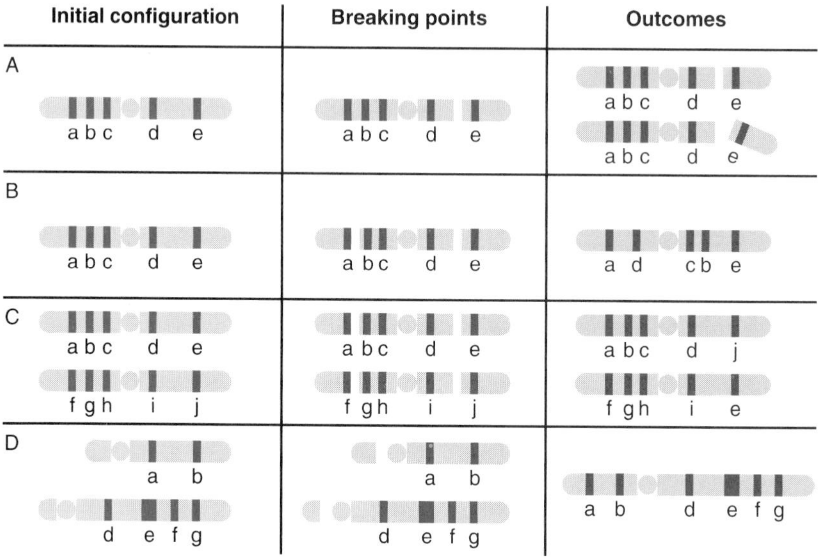

	Initial configuration	Breaking points	Outcomes
A	a b c d e	a b c d e	a b c d e a b c d e
B	a b c d e	a b c d e	a d c b e
C	a b c d e f g h i j	a b c d e f g h i j	a b c d j f g h i e
D	a b d e f g	a b d e f g	a b d e f g

FIGURE 2-4. Examples of structural rearrangements following chromosomal breakage. Shown here are the initial chromosome constitution, breaking points, and outcomes of the breaks and rearrangements. **Panel A.** Break between markers d and e. Three outcomes: deletion on chromosomes, bearing markers a through d; the severed fragment may stay aligned with the rest (*chromosome gap*); or it may be lost (*chromosome break).* **Panel B.** Two breaks (between markers a and b and between d and e). Center portion undergoes a *pericentric inversion;* the newly arranged chromosome bears markers a, d, c, b, and e. **Panel C.** Balanced translocation (no loss of genetic material) between chromosomes a–e and f–j. **Panel D.** balanced Robertsonian translocation (no loss of significant genes) between two acrocentric chromosomes (one from group G, the other from D) following loss of short arms and fusion at the centromere.

Failure of chromatids to separate in anaphase as a result of **nondisjunction**, results in daughter cells that have different chromosome numbers (eg, 45 and 47, instead of 46 and 46). Of the aneuploid cells, those that are **monosomic** will tend to degenerate and die, and the trisomic cells will continue to divide, producing a line of trisomic cells. Mitotic nondisjunction occurring during embryonic development (Fig. 2-5) results in a line of trisomic cells that proliferates concomitantly with the normal cell line, producing a mosaic individual (ie, a person with **mosaicism** for that particular chromosome). For example, a male with mosaicism for Down syndrome will have a chromosomal constitution with dual cell populations—46,XY/47,XY,G(21)$^+$. In this notation, the slash (/) separates the cell line with normal chromosomal number (46,XY), from the line with 47 chromosomes (47,XY,G[21]$^+$), which includes the extra G(21) chromosome.

Nondisjunction can also occur in meiosis I and meiosis II (meiotic nondisjunction) during **gametogenesis** (Fig. 2-6). The result of uneven chromosome distribution is the formation of **gametes** with aneuploid chromosome numbers (eg, 22 and 24, instead of 23 and 23). As it occurs with somatic cells, gametes with an extra chromosome are more likely to survive and to produce an aneuploid zygote. The most common viable aneuploidies are trisomies. In Down syndrome, for example, an aneuploid gamete carrying an extra G(21) chromosome (24,X or Y,G[21]$^+$) fertilizes a normal gamete (23,X or Y) and produces a trisomic zygote [47,XX or XY,G(21)$^+$]. Unlike the mosaic case described above, all somatic cells in this person will contain the extra G(21) chromosome.

CLASSIFICATION OF GENETIC DISORDERS

Genetic diseases are a result of gene alterations or chromosome abnormalities. Alterations in single genes result in a group of disorders termed mendelian, or single-gene diseases, such as sickle cell disease, galactosemia, and cystic fibrosis. Changes in multiple but related genes create polygenic and multifactorial disorders, such as

FOCUS ON CELLULAR PATHOPHYSIOLOGY

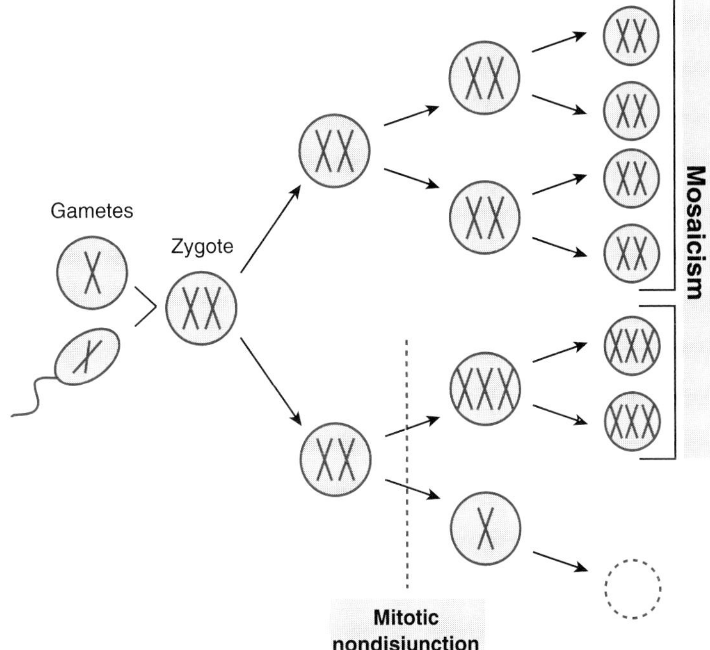

FIGURE 2-5. Mitotic nondisjunction. Nondisjunctional event occurring during embryonic development, after a normal zygote was formed by fertilization of two normal gametes. Only one chromosome pair is represented. Following an initial normal mitosis, the upper cell originates a normal line of cells with the correct chromosome number. The bottom cell undergoes nondisjunction, resulting in a line of cells with one extra chromosome. (The monosomic cell is not viable and there are no further divisions.) The outcome is a *mosaic* individual with two cell lines, one containing the normal chromosome number, the other aneuploid.

FOCUS ON CELLULAR PATHOPHYSIOLOGY

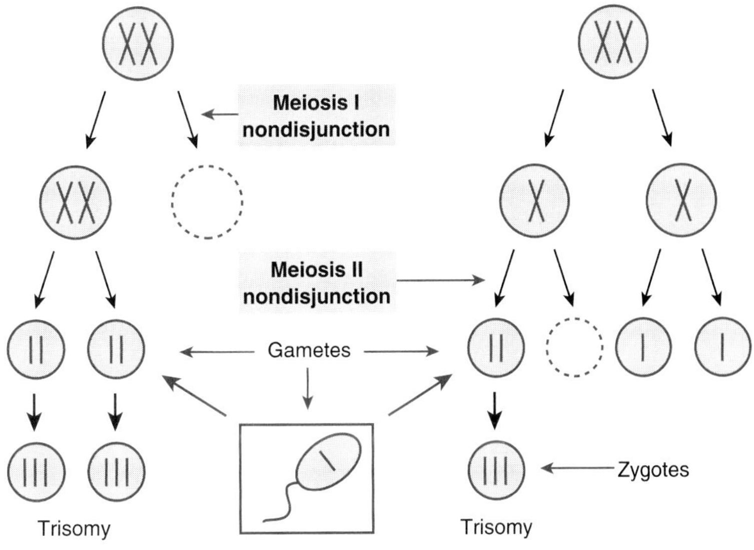

FIGURE 2-6. Meiotic nondisjunction. The cell line at *left* undergoes nondisjunction at meiosis I, the cell on the *right* during meiosis II. Only one chromosome pair is represented. Nondisjunction at meiosis I results in one cell with an extra chromosome and one monosomic cell (which does not survive). Meiosis II will produce two aneuploid gametes, which, upon fertilization by normal, euploid gametes, will produce trisomic zygotes. Likewise, nondisjunction at meiosis II also results in aneuploid gametes and subsequently in trisomic zygotes.

BOX 2-5

INDICATIONS FOR CHROMOSOME ANALYSIS

Multiple independent malformations
Mental retardation
Female with short stature
Family history suggestive of balanced translocation
Advanced maternal age
Multiple miscarriages
Infertility

cleft lip and palate. Gene alterations may be classified using a biochemical approach, according to the type of protein involved (see Table 2-1). To retain the format of the previous section, this chapter classifies genetic disorders by mode of inheritance, as dominant and recessive (autosomal and X-linked).

Chromosome abnormalities are classified here into numerical abnormalities of the autosomes and the sex chromosomes. Chromosome anomalies in a newborn must be suspected when in the presence of (1) growth abnormalities, (2) amniotic fluid volume abnormalities, or (3) **congenital** abnormalities. For genetic counseling purposes, additional indications for chromosome analysis through **amniocentesis** have been identified (Box 2-5). Advanced maternal age has been reported in various studies as a risk factor for many chromosome anomalies, especially free trisomy 21 (Down syndrome), a condition in which the extra chromosome is free and not translocated onto another chromosome. Box 2-6 illustrates the linear increase in such abnormalities as a function of increasing maternal age.

Selected Examples of Single-Gene Disorders

More than 10,000 single-gene (Mendelian) disorders have been catalogued,[6,11] of which 9,772 are autosomal, 584 are X-linked, 37 are Y-linked, and the remaining 60 result from mitochondrial gene action. As genetic research continues, these figures are periodically updated.[10,12] Although not as frequently occurring as multifactorial traits, mendelian disorders have been widely used in genetic research due to the precise understanding of their molecular etiology. Tables 2-2, 2-3, and 2-4 (found at the end of the chapter) summarize characteristics of selected autosomal dominant, autosomal recessive, and X-linked disorders.

Selected Examples of Chromosome Abnormalities

Down syndrome (trisomy 21) is probably one of the most studied and best understood autosomal aneuploidies, perhaps because it is the most common aneuploidy compatible with development to full term and with a reasonable quality of postnatal life. However, shortened life span and reproductive limitations still exist—males with Down syndrome are usually sterile. Some females have reproduced, at times as a result of rape in institutional settings. About one-third of their liveborn also have Down syndrome. Other autosomal aneuploidies are listed in Table 2-5.

Three chromosomal configurations exist in Down syndrome:

FREE TRISOMY [47, XX OR XY,G(21)$^+$]. This represents the majority (95%) of all cases of Down syndrome. The term "free" refers to the fact that the extra chromosome 21 is unattached and segregates freely during meiosis. This is the type of Down syndrome whose frequency increases linearly with increasing maternal age (see Box 2-6).

TRANSLOCATION DOWN SYNDROME [46,XX OR XY,t (Gq/Dq)$^+$ OR t(Gq/Gq)$^+$]. This is the second most frequent type, representing about 4% of all cases. This type results from a Robertsonian translocation occurring between the extra G(21) chromosome and either another small acrocentric [t(Gq/Gq)] or one of the large acrocentrics [t(Gq/Dq)]. About 40% of the cases can be traced to a (normal) parent carrying a balanced trans-

BOX 2-6

MATERNAL AGE AND RISK OF CHROMOSOMAL ABNORMALITIES

Maternal Age	Overall Risk for Abnormalities	Risk for Down Syndrome Births
20	1/526	1/1,667
25	1/476	1/1,250
30	1/417	1/952
35	1/192	1/378
40	1/66	1/106
45	1/21	1/30
49	1/8	1/11

(Modified from Simpson, J. L., & Golbus, M. S. [1998]. *Genetics in obstetrics and gynecology* [3rd ed.]. Philadelphia: Saunders.)

location. The remaining 60% are sporadic occurrences, without a familial connection. In most cases, fathers will be carriers of t(Gq/Gq) and mothers carriers of t(GqDq). It is important to determine the type of translocation carried by a parent because the recurrence risks for future offspring vary in function of the type. When a parent carrying either a t(Gq/Dq) or a t(21q/22q) translocation mates with a normal partner, their chances of producing a child with Down syndrome are 33% (of all liveborn). However, if the translocation carried is t(21q/21q), the risk for Down syndrome among all liveborn is 100%. This latter situation is one of the rare examples in genetics where an abnormality is passed on to *all* living progeny. The incidence of translocation Down syndrome is slightly elevated among mothers who were older than 34 years at conception.

MOSAIC DOWN SYNDROME [46,XX OR XY/47,XX OR XY, G(21)+]. This rarer type of Down syndrome (about 1% of all cases) results from mitotic nondisjunction occurring during early embryonic development of a normal zygote (see Fig. 2-5). Despite the presence of normal cell lines, individuals with Down syndrome mosaicism do not necessarily have a better developmental outcome than those with free trisomy type.

The most common aneuploidies of sex chromosomes are Klinefelter syndrome (47,XXY), Jacob syndrome (47,XYY), Turner syndrome (45,X0), and triple-X female (47,XXX) (Table 2-6). It should be noted here that, in the majority of cases, the presence of the Y chromosome determines a male phenotype. The reason for this is that the Y chromosome contains a region responsible for the organization of testes in a developing embryo, known as TDF, or testis-determining factor.

The notable exception to this rule is the complete androgen insensitivity syndrome (46,XY), which produces the quasi-female phenotype of a tall woman, with well developed breasts; a blind-ending vagina (usually compatible with orgasmic receptive intercourse); absence of uterus, fallopian tubes and ovaries; and presence of well developed bilateral inguinal testes. The defect in this case is an X-linked recessive gene that controls the appearance of receptors for testosterone in embryonic tissues responsible for the organization of male structures. The androgens produced by the developing embryo encounter no responsive tissues, resulting in its development as a female. At birth, external genitalia mimic female organs and the child is raised as a girl. Testicular estrogen production at puberty ensures the development of breasts and confirms the female gender establishment. Intellectual development is normal.

CANCER GENETICS

The possibility that cancer is an inherited disease has been widely investigated and many early observations suggested that at least a genetic component existed in the causation and possible transmission of cancer (Box 2-7). The discovery of **oncogenes**, in the early 1970s, marked the beginning of a new area of understanding of basic cancer mechanisms (Box 2-8). Initially thought to be carried exclusively by retroviruses, oncogenes were later identified as natural mammalian genes that existed in all organisms. Early investigations suggested that oncogenes were found in inactive form (ie, no correlation with cancer could be identified in this state). In reality, even in their so-called inactive form, oncogenes are functional in encoding normal proteins associated with cell division. In their "activated" form, oncogenes trigger malignant transformation of normal cells. Genetic studies have identified "activated" oncogenes in cells of malignant tumors, while their "inactive" counterparts were found in cells of normal surrounding tissue. Oncogenes can be "activated" by a variety of mechanisms. It is thought that the chromosome breakage that results in the translocation t(8/14) in Burkitt lymphoma may be the mechanism that triggers oncogene activation, and therefore, the translocation is not a clinical consequence but a cause of that lymphoma.

The discovery of tumor suppressor genes, in the late 1970s added a new interpretation to cancer causation. One such gene, p53 ("the guardian of the genome"), has acquired scientific notoriety.[4] In its normal, or "wild-type" configuration, p53 is found in normal cells, and its protein product regulates the cell cycle, controls cell proliferation, and helps prevent malignant transformation of those cells. Various mutations of the p53 gene have been identified in more than 50% of cancers.

Other cancer susceptibility genes have been discovered and are under intense research scrutiny. Some

BOX 2-7 CANCER GENETICS: EARLY OBSERVATIONS

- Certain types of cancer occur more frequently within certain families—breast, ovarian, leukemias, colon, etc. Some observations date back to the 19th century.
- Well-defined genetic disorders predispose to various malignancies—Gardner syndrome and colon cancer, Bloom syndrome and lymphomas, etc.
- Certain chromosome abnormalities occur frequently with malignancies—Ph[1] (Philadelphia) chromosome in chronic myelogenous leukemia, translocation t(8/14) in Burkitt lymphoma, etc.
- Certain chromosome aneuploidies predispose to cancer—Down syndrome (trisomy 21) and acute leukemias.

BOX 2-8

CANCER GENETICS: CURRENT KNOWLEDGE

- Genetic predispositions determine risk for malignancies.
- Environmental agents act as triggers, increasing the original risk factor.
- Oncogenes are mammalian genes that activate malignant transformation of normal cells.
- Retroviruses can cause cancer by transmitting an oncogene or by insertional mutagenesis.
- Cancers may be caused by somatic mutations of cancer genes—localized process leading to sporadic (nonhereditary) tumors.
- Germ cell mutations of cancer genes are transmitted to the offspring—hereditary cancers.
- Tumor suppressor genes (eg, *p53*) mutations are found in many cancers.
- Other cancer genes have been identified—BRCA1 (female breast and ovarian cancer), BRCA2 (male and female breast, prostate cancer), APC (colon cancer), etc.

of those are involved in maintaining genome stability, and their mutations permit malignant transformation to occur. Classic examples are BRCA (for breast cancer) types 1 and 2 genes. Discovered in 1994, the BRCA1 gene provided evidence that a genetic predisposition to breast and ovarian cancer existed.[8] Women who carry a germline mutation of the BRCA1, and who have a significant family history of breast or ovarian cancer (or both), will have lifetime risks of approximately 85% for breast cancer and 60% for ovarian cancer. The discovery of BRCA2 in 1995[16] added further evidence of gene-controlled susceptibility to male and female breast cancer and prostate cancer. The effects of BRCA2 are more devastating because resulting male and female breast tumors are more aggressive and have higher metastatic potential than those caused by BRCA1.

Prediction models have been developed to determine cancer risk figures for persons carrying some of the 200 mutations of these genes. However, a precise risk predictability is still uncertain. As an example of the pitfalls of testing for cancer genes, in a recent study, 9 of 10 women with positive family history of breast cancer tested negative for BRCA1.[2] One serious consequence of these results is that women who tested negative may rely on them and become more lax in their early detection methods. In addition, it appears that, with more detailed analysis of discrete groups, some of the previously quoted risks may be overestimated.[14] Because of such difficulty in interpreting their results, many clinicians feel that it is too early to include systematic screening tests for these genes in the general population and would prefer to wait for additional data.[14]

FUTURE TRENDS IN MEDICAL GENETICS

Therapeutic intervention in genetic disorders has always been considered an extremely difficult proposition. Because the systemic consequences of gene disorders are of such high magnitude, only a few metabolic replacement or removal techniques have succeeded. Such current approaches are aimed at correcting the phenotype. Gene therapy (correcting the genotype), although in its early stages of development, presents a more promising approach.[3] The first determinant in genotypic intervention is the identification of the causative gene, determination of its chromosomal location, and its cloning. Knowledge of the order of DNA bases will allow researchers to identify the location of each gene and will be instrumental in understanding their function in disease and in health.

The human genome is represented by approximately 50,000 to 100,000 genes, and each gene has, on the average 5,000 to 10,000 DNA base pairs. The task of obtaining the sequence of all 3 billion human DNA bases was given to the *Human Genome Project*, a heavily-funded (3 billion U.S. dollars), multinational (18 countries), 15-year program initiated in 1990.[9] The project has reached its midpoint, and approximately 10% of the human genome has been mapped. Despite the apparently small percentage, participants in the project are encouraged that the goals appear to be progressing within the planned pace, given the scientific and technological progress in this area of genetics. It has been estimated that structural genes are being mapped at the rate of more than one gene per day, and frequent updates of the numbers of genes mapped in each of the 23 chromosomes are available to researchers around the world.[5,13] The ultimate goals of therapeutic intervention in genetic disorders are to understand the precise gene involvement in the etiology of the disease and to correct dysfunctions at the gene level. By opening the doors for **genetic engineering** and gene therapy, the Human Genome Project is the first step toward the achievement of these goals.

FOCUS ON THE PERSON WITH HEMOPHILIA A

Mr. H is a 30-year-old white man with a long-standing history of severe hemophilia A complicated by hemarthroses of both knees. He presents to the clinic for a routine visit with his pregnant common-law wife and 2-year-old twin daughters.

Mr. H was diagnosed with hemophilia A following profuse bleeding at circumcision. He is an only child. During childhood, Mr. H had repeated bleeding episodes that required multiple hospitalizations and painful treatment. At times he was receiving two to three factor VIII infusions per week. By age 3, swollen and painful knees were evident. Further deterioration of the synovium of both knees continued and he began to have difficulties walking without an obvious limp. A motorcycle accident at age 19 resulted in a compound fracture of his left femur and internal injuries with massive internal bleeding.

Mr. H has a history of massive bleeding after trauma, as well as "spontaneous" hemorrhages in areas of the body subject to trauma, particularly the joints. Recurrent bleeding into the joints has resulted in progressive tissue deterioration and crippling deformities. He is now using crutches, and experiences severe pain at locomotion. Physical exam reveals no petechiae or ecchymoses. His bleeding time is normal, but the clotting time is prolonged. He continues to receive factor VIII concentrate infusions when bleeding occurs.

Questions

1. With respect to the transmission of hemophilia A, what are the possible outcomes of the current and future pregnancies?
2. Is prenatal diagnosis available for this and future pregnancies?
3. What should his daughters be told regarding their hemophilia status?
4. What future manifestations of hemophilia A should be of concern to Mr. H.? How would they affect his quality of life?

TABLE 2-2

SELECTED EXAMPLES OF AUTOSOMAL DOMINANT DISORDERS

DISORDER AND GENERAL CHARACTERISTICS	CLINICAL FEATURES	PRENATAL DIAGNOSIS*	CHROMOSOME LOCATION
ACHONDROPLASIA			
Most common form of dwarfism Adult stature, 48–52 in. Paternal age effect present *Frequency:* 1/26,000	Shortened limbs (rhizomelia) Normal length torso Lordosis Prominent forehead Flattened nasal bridge Short hands, stubby fingers Normal IQ and life span Backaches ↑ risk of spinal cord compression Premature menarche Enlarged breasts Premature menopause	Available (ultrasonography)	4p 16.3
EHLERS-DANLOS SYNDROME			
A group (9 subtypes) of disorders of connective tissue Most common variants are autosomal dominant	Hyperelasticity of skin Hyperflexible joints Vascular fragility Poor wound healing Bruising tendency Predisposition to hemorrhages	Type IV: Possible (lack of type III collagen) Type V: Possible (lysyl oxidase)	Type I: 9q 34.2

(continued)

TABLE 2-2

SELECTED EXAMPLES OF AUTOSOMAL DOMINANT DISORDERS (Continued)

DISORDER AND GENERAL CHARACTERISTICS	CLINICAL FEATURES	PRENATAL DIAGNOSIS*	CHROMOSOME LOCATION
Life span may be limited by vascular events: aneurysms and rupture of large vessels *Frequency:* 1/150,000	Hernias Varicose veins		
FAMILIAL HYPERCHOLESTEROLEMIA			
One of various disorders of lipoproteins One of the most common single-gene disorders Manifestations are sensitive to environmental (dietary) variations (multifactorial?) *Frequency:* 1/200–1/500	Homozygotes tend to develop severe, life-threatening conditions: early onset of atherosclerotic disease of the coronary, cerebral, and peripheral circulation Xanthomas (cholesterol deposits in skin and tendons)	Available (HMG CoA reductase)	19p 13.2
HUNTINGTON DISEASE			
Progressive neurologic deterioration caused by neuron atrophy in discrete areas of the brain Late onset (30–50 years). Few present before age 15 and after age 60. Early onset disease is more severe; late onset disease is more benign, with slow progression. Death occurs approximately 15 y from onset. *Frequency:* 1/18,000–1/25,000 (US and UK) 1/333,000 (Japan)	Psychiatric symptoms Choreoathetoid movements Progressive dementia Secondary findings with early onset disease: —Intellectual decline —Seizures —Rigidity —Dystonia	Available (linked polymorphisms) Presymptomatic testing also available	4p 16.3
MARFAN SYNDROME			
Disorder of connective tissue involving a triad of ocular, skeletal, and cardiovascular abnormalities Average life span: 40–50 y *Frequency:* 1/10,000–1/20,000	Most frequent ocular anomaly: —Subluxation of the lens Common skeletal findings: —Tall stature —Arachnodactyly —Scoliosis Major life-threatening risk: —Aortic fusiform or dissecting aneurysms. —Aortic valve abnormalities	No	15q 21.1
NEUROFIBROMATOSIS TYPE I			
(von Recklinghausen disease) Affected infants born to affected mothers have worse prognosis than those born of affected fathers and those without past family history (fresh mutations). *Frequency:* 1/4,000–1/5,000	Multiple soft tumors of peripheral, nerves, or neurofibromas Abnormal skin pigmentation In early childhood: —Multiple brown (café-au-lait) spots, usually on the torso From adolescence onward: —Neurofibromas Other complications: —Scoliosis —Moderate to severe mental retardation —Learning difficulties —Hypertension —Seizures	Possible (linked polymorphisms)	17q 11.2

(continued)

TABLE 2-2

SELECTED EXAMPLES OF AUTOSOMAL DOMINANT DISORDERS (Continued)

DISORDER AND GENERAL CHARACTERISTICS	CLINICAL FEATURES	PRENATAL DIAGNOSIS*	CHROMOSOME LOCATION
	—Spinal cord/root compression —Optic gliomas —Pheochromocytomas —Malignant changes in the neurofibromas		
OSTEOGENESIS IMPERFECTA TYPE I			
All four types of osteogenesis imperfecta involve osteoporosis and recurrent fractures of long bones with minimal trauma. (Type II results in perinatal lethality with multiple fractures during gestation and birth.) *Life span:* usually normal despite the multiple fractures throughout life *Frequency:* 1/20,000 (all types combined)	Type I disease: —Blue sclera —Conductive deafness (secondary to otosclerosis) —Discolored teeth as a result of dentinogenesis defects	Possible (sulfate incorporation)	17q 21.31
POLYCYSTIC KIDNEY DISEASE, ADULT TYPE			
Renal cysts may remain asymptomatic until third or fourth decades of life. Disease accounts for about 10% of all adult cases of chronic renal failure. *Frequency:* 1/1,000	Development of cysts in: —Kidneys —Liver —Pancreas —Spleen Renal failure Hypertension	Available (linked polymorphism)	4q 21

* Available, diagnosis accomplished; possible, enzyme activity present in normal skin fibroblasts. HMG CoA, 3=hydroxy=3=methylglutaryl coenzyme A

TABLE 2-3

SELECTED EXAMPLES OF AUTOSOMAL RECESSIVE DISORDERS

DISORDER AND GENERAL CHARACTERISTICS	CLINICAL FEATURES	PRENATAL DIAGNOSIS*	CHROMOSOME LOCATION
CYSTIC FIBROSIS			
Most common lethal disease among whites Abnormal exocrine gland function, chronic pulmonary disease, excessive salt in sweat *Carrier detection:* available by DNA analysis *Median life span:* 25 y, but a high percentage of children die before age 10 *Frequency:* 1/2,000–1/2,500 (white) 1/17,000 (African American)	Pancreatic insufficiency: —Lack of trypsin in secretions —Malabsorption Chronic pulmonary disease: —Excessive mucus production —Reduced ciliated epithelium function —Recurrent infections Other manifestations: —Rectal prolapse —Meconium ileus —Liver cirrhosis —Gallbladder tones —Salivary gland obstruction	Available (DNA analysis)	7q 31.2

(continued)

TABLE 2-3

SELECTED EXAMPLES OF AUTOSOMAL RECESSIVE DISORDERS (Continued)

DISORDER AND GENERAL CHARACTERISTICS	CLINICAL FEATURES	PRENATAL DIAGNOSIS*	CHROMOSOME LOCATION
CYSTINURIA			
One of various disorders of amino acid metabolism Condition is diagnosed by decreased intestinal absorption and increased urinary excretion of cystine, lysine, arginine, and ornithine. *Carrier detection:* available *Life span:* normal if treated *Frequency:* 1/10,000	Recurrent renal calculi	Available (labeled cystine incorporation in amniotic fluid cells of chorionic villous samples)	2p 16.3
MUCOPOLYSACCHARIDOSES			
A diverse group (6 syndromes) of mucopolysaccharide accumulation disorders Primary types: —Hurler (type I): (gargoylism) —Hunter (type II): X-linked recessive —Sanfilippo (type III): most common type —Morquio (type IV) *Carrier detection:* available for type II (X-linked recessive) *Life span:* Hurler: death in 2nd decade Hunter: death in 3rd decade Sanfilippo: death in 3rd decade Morquio: death in 3rd decade *Overall frequency:* 1/20,000 (type III most common)	Type I (Hurler): —Coarse facies in infancy —Short stature —Skeletal and joint deformities —Deafness —Corneal clouding —Umbilical hernia —Progressive mental retardation Type II (Hunter) (X-linked): —Similar to type I —Clear corneas Type III (Sanfilippo): —Normal facies, stature, and corneas —Progressive mental retardation in early childhood Type IV: —Normal intelligence, facies, and corneas —Short stature —Scoliosis	Hurler: available (α-L-iduronidase) Hunter: available (L-iduronic acid-2 sulfatase) Sanfilippo: available (Type A: heparin sulfatase) (Type B: *N*-acetyl-α-D-glucosaminidase) Morquio: available (chondroitin sulfate-*N*-acetylhexosaminidase sulfate sulfatase)	Hurler: 4p 16.3 Hunter: Xq 28 Sanfilippo: ? Morquio: 16q 24.3
PHENYLKETONURIA (PKU)			
Disorder of amino acid metabolism resulting from lack of phenylalanine hydroxylase, and accumulation of phenylalanine (phe) and its metabolites. Treatment consists of low phe diet and tyrosine supplementation. Offspring of treated females have increased risk for mental retardation and cardiac malformations if maternal phe levels are not lowered during pregnancy. *Carrier detection:* available by intragenic DNA analysis *Life span:* normal if treated *Frequency:* 1/15,000	Mental retardation if untreated	Available (phenylalanine hydroxylase)	12q 24.1
SICKLE CELL DISEASE			
Serious, chronic hemolytic anemia, due to the production of an abnormal hemoglobin (HbS) with reduced oxygen-carrying capacity	Infarction of: —Lungs —Kidneys —Spleen —Bones	Available (analysis of fetal DNA from chorionic villous sample)	11p 15.5

(continued)

TABLE 2-3

SELECTED EXAMPLES OF AUTOSOMAL RECESSIVE DISORDERS (Continued)

DISORDER AND GENERAL CHARACTERISTICS	CLINICAL FEATURES	PRENATAL DIAGNOSIS*	CHROMOSOME LOCATION
Sickle aspect of red blood cells causes obstruction of small vessels and ischemia distal to blocks. Sickling crises triggered by stress, infection, dehydration. *Carrier detection:* available by Sickledex.test and hemoglobin electrophoresis *Life span:* often fatal in childhood even with treatment, but longer survival is now possible *Frequency:* 1/400–1/600 (African American)	Increased risk for: —Pneumococcal infections —Salmonella osteomyelitis Painful leg ulcers Dactylitis Priapism Renal failure		
TAY-SACHS DISEASE			
Lipid storage disorder caused by lack of hexosaminidase A (HexA) and the resulting accumulation of GM_2 ganglioside in nerve cells. The outcome is a progressive and unrelenting neurologic disease. *Carrier detection:* available by serum β-*N*-acetyl-HexA determination. *Life span:* 100% lethality between ages 3 and 5 y, usually from bronchopneumonia *Frequency:* 1/3,600 (Ashkenazi Jews) 1/360,000 (all other groups)	Normal development to age 3–6 mo, followed by progressive loss of developmental milestones and various mental and motor deficits. Deafness Blindness Seizure activity Generalized spasticity Decerebrate rigidity Cherry-red macular spot	Available (hexosaminidase A)	15q 23–24

* Available, diagnosis accomplished; possible, enzyme activity present in normal skin fibroblasts.

TABLE 2-4

SELECTED EXAMPLES OF X-LINKED DISORDERS

DISORDER AND GENERAL CHARACTERISTICS	CLINICAL FEATURES	PRENATAL DIAGNOSIS*	CHROMOSOME LOCATION
DUCHENNE MUSCULAR DYSTROPHY			
Mode of inheritance: recessive One of two types of X-linked muscular dystrophies (the other is Becker type) resulting from deficiency of dysthrophin Age of onset, < 5 y *Prognosis:* 95% wheelchair-bound by age 12 *Carrier detection:* possible with linked polymorphisms. Carriers (females) exhibit mild manifestations in 2–3% of cases. *Life span:* death in second decade *Frequency:* 1/3,000–1/5,000 male births	Progressive: —Muscular weakening —Atrophy —Contractures Delayed walking Calf pseudohypertrophy Mild mental retardation (1 : 14 cases)	Available (dystrophin deficiency)	Xp 21.2

(continued)

TABLE 2-4

SELECTED EXAMPLES OF X-LINKED DISORDERS (Continued)

DISORDER AND GENERAL CHARACTERISTICS	CLINICAL FEATURES	PRENATAL DIAGNOSIS*	CHROMOSOME LOCATION
GLUCOSE-6-PHOSPHATE DEHYDROGENASE (G6PD) DEFICIENCY			
Mode of inheritance: recessive The most common pathogenic enzyme defect in humans. Triggered by environmental agents (aspirin, sulphonamides, moth balls, fava beans) and infections. High prevalence in the Mediterranean region. *Carrier detection:* carriers (females) are asymptomatic, even when exposed to triggers. *Life span:* normal *Frequency:* 1/10 (African American males) 1/50 (African American females)	Anemia Prolonged neonatal jaundice	Possible (fetal biopsy)	Xq 28
HEMOPHILIA A			
(syn, Classic Hemophilia) *Mode of inheritance:* recessive Common disease of coagulation resulting from factor VIIIc deficiency or defect (10% of patients have normal factor VIIIc levels). Disease expresses as mild, moderate, or severe forms. High frequency of HIV infection among severe hemophiliacs. *Carrier detection:* available (gene has been cloned). *Life span:* limited by disease severity, but usually normal with factor replacement as needed *Overall Frequency:* 1/2,500–1/5,000 male births	"Spontaneous" bleeding in areas of trauma, eg, joints: —Hemarthroses. Petechiae and ecchymoses usually *absent.*	Available (factor VIIIc deficiency)	Xq 28
HEMOPHILIA B			
(syn, Christmas disease) *Mode of inheritance:* recessive Clinically indistinguishable from hemophilia A, but caused by deficiency of a different factor, IX *Carrier detection:* available *Life span:* normal with factor IX replacement as needed *Frequency:* 1/30,000 male births	Similar to hemophilia A	Available (factor IX deficiency)	Xq 27.1
LESCH-NYHAN SYNDROME			
(syn, hypoxanthine guanine phosphoribosil transferase [HGPRT] deficiency) *Mode of inheritance:* recessive Disorder of purine metabolism resulting from HGPRT deficiency and the consequent accumulation of uric acid Onset during infancy *Carrier detection:* available (linked polymorphisms) *Life span:* decreased. *Frequency:* 1/10,000 male births	Spasticity Choreoathetoid movements Self-mutilation Mental retardation Renal calculi Gout Arthritis	Available (HGPRT testing and linked polymorphisms)	Xq 26

(continued)

TABLE 2-4

SELECTED EXAMPLES OF X-LINKED DISORDERS (Continued)

DISORDER AND GENERAL CHARACTERISTICS	CLINICAL FEATURES	PRENATAL DIAGNOSIS*	CHROMOSOME LOCATION
HYPOPHOSPHATEMIC VITAMIN D-RESISTANT RICKETS			
Mode of inheritance: dominant Rare disorder involving a combination of decreased serum phosphate and rickets Treatable with large doses of vitamin D and oral phosphate *Life span:* normal *Frequency:* 1/20,000	Growth retardation Childhood rickets Premature closure of cranial sutures Reduced serum phosphate	Possible (linked polymorphisms) Presymptomatic testing with linked polymorphisms also possible.	Xp 22.2

* Available, diagnosis accomplished; possible, enzyme activity present in normal skin fibroblasts. HIV, human immunodeficiency virus

TABLE 2-5

SELECTED AUTOSOMAL ANEUPLOIDIES

ANOMALY AND CHROMOSOME NOTATION*	FREQUENCY	CLINICAL MANIFESTATIONS	LIFE EXPECTANCY
TRISOMY 21 (DOWN SYNDROME)			
1. Free trisomy: [47, XX, G(21)+] 2. Translocation: [46, XX, t(Dq/Gq)] [46, XX, t(Gq/Gq)] 3. Mosaic: [46, XX/47, XX, G(21)+]	1/650–1/700 births	**MR:** mean IQ 50 **Craniofacial:** —Brachycephaly —Flat occiput —Low-set ears —Oblique palpebral fissures —Epicanthal folds —Brushfield spots (iris) —Broad nasal bones and flattened profile —Open mouth —Protruding tongue **Skeletal:** —Broad, short fingers —Short hand —Clinodactyly (5th finger) **Cardiac:** —Ventricular and atrial septal defects —Patent ductus arteriosus **Other:** —Hypotonia —Respiratory infections —Acute leukemia —Palmar simian crease —Abnormal dermatoglyphics	22% die in 1st decade; 50% by age 60 Primary cause of death: —Hematologic —Malignancies
TRISOMY E (EDWARDS SYNDROME) [47, XX, E(16–18)+]	1/8,000 births	**MR:** severe **Craniofacial:** —Dolichocephaly —Prominent occiput —Low-set, malformed ears —Micrognathia	Overall, 30% die in 1st month, 50% die in 2nd month, < 10% survive 1 y.

(continued)

TABLE 2-5

SELECTED AUTOSOMAL ANEUPLOIDIES (Continued)

ANOMALY AND CHROMOSOME NOTATION*	FREQUENCY	CLINICAL MANIFESTATIONS	LIFE EXPECTANCY
		Skeletal: —Clenched fists —Overlapping fingers —Flexion deformities —Adducted hips —"Rocker-bottom" feet **Cardiac:** —Ventricular and atrial septal defects —Patent ductus arteriosus **Urogenital:** —"Horse-shoe" kidneys —Hydronephrosis —Cryptorchidism —Prominent genitals **Other:** —Hypotonia	
TRISOMY D (PATAU SYNDROME)			
[47, XX, D(13–15)+]	1/20,000 births	**MR:** severe **Craniofacial:** (severe) —Microcephaly —Low set, malformed ears —Micro- or anophthalmia —Coloboma of the iris —Cleft lip and palate **Skeletal:** —Polydactyly —Syndactyly —Overlapping, flexed fingers —Hypoplasia of the pelvis **Cardiac:** —Ventricular and atrial septal defects —Patent ductus arteriosus **Urogenital:** —Malformed kidneys —Hydronephros —Polycystic kidneys —Cryptorchidism —Bicornuate uterus **Other:** —Apneic spells —Seizure activity —Single transverse palmar crease —Single umbilical artery	45% die in 1st month, 70% by the 6th month, <5% survive 3 y

* For convenience, female (XX), and not male (XY) chromosomal constitutions are shown here.
MR, Mental retardation.
(Modified from Simpson, J. L., & Golbus, M. S. [1998] *Genetics in obstetrics and gynecology* [3rd ed.]. Philadelphia: Saunders.)

TABLE 2-6

SELECTED SEX CHROMOSOME ANEUPLOIDIES

ANOMALY AND CHROMOSOME NOTATION	FREQUENCY	CLINICAL MANIFESTATIONS
KLINEFELTER SYNDROME		
47, XXY (or multiple X, Y)	1/1,000 male births	Male phenotype Small testes with decreased androgen production Infertility Well-developed genitalia Sparse facial hair Female pubic hair pattern Slightly taller than normal males (longer legs) Gynecomastia frequent Voice may not change at puberty Infrequent abnormalities: —Scoliosis —Pectus excavatum —5th finger clinodactyly —Dental anomalies —Cardiac anomalies —Pulmonary diseases —Varicose veins Intellectual development: —Normal to borderline (IQ 85) —Language delay
JACOBS SYNDROME		
47, XYY	1/1,000 male births	Male phenotype Tall stature Persistent adult acne Association with aggressive behavior unproven Most offspring are chromosomally normal. Intellectual development is normal.
TURNER SYNDROME		
45, X0	1/10,000 female births	Female phenotype Ovarian dysgenesis (streak gonads) Short stature Decreased estrogens Infertility Delayed sexual development Webbing of the neck Low posterior neckline Neonatal lymphedema Cubitus valgus Short 4th metacarpals "Shield" chest Divergent nipples Sex chromatin negative Coarctation of the aorta Urinary tract abnormalities Fetal cystic hygroma/hydrops Intellectual development: normal
TRIPLE X FEMALE		
47, XXX	1/1,000 female births	No significant anomalies Delayed menarche Premature menopause Most offspring are chromosomally normal. Intellectual development: normal to borderline (5% of cases, approximate IQ 85)

REFERENCES

1. Classic Papers in Genetics—Mendel, Garrod, Hardy, and others: http://www.gdb.org/rjr/history.html
2. Couch, F. J., DeShano, M. L., Blackwood, A., et al. (1997). BRCA1 mutations in women attending clinics that evaluate the risk of breast cancer. *New England Journal of Medicine, 336,* 1409–1415.
3. Cox, T. M., & Sinclair, J. (Eds.). (1997). *Molecular biology in medicine.* Boston: Blackwell Scientific.
4. Culotta, E., & Koshland, D. E. (1993). p53 sweeps through cancer research. *Science, 262,* 1958–1961.
5. Human Genome Project (General Information). http://www.ornl.gov/TechResources/Human_Genome/home.html.
6. McKusick, V. A. (1994). *Mendelian inheritance in man. Catalogs of human genes and genetic disorders* (11th ed.). Baltimore: Johns Hopkins University Press.
7. Mendel Web Introduction. http://www.netspace.org/MendelWeb/MWolby.intro.html
8. Miki, Y., Swensen, J., Shattuck-Eidens, D., et al. (1994). A strong candidate for the breast and ovarian cancer susceptibility gene BRCA1. *Science, 266,* 66–71.
9. National Institutes of Health Gene Sequencing Databases. http://www.ncbi.nlm.nih.gov/genome/seq/index.cgi
10. OMIM, Updated Statistics. http://www.ncbi.nlm.nih.gov/Omim/Stats/mimstats.html
11. *Online mendelian inheritance in man, OMIM*™. Center for Medical Genetics, Johns Hopkins University (Baltimore, MD) and National Center for Biotechnology Information, National Library of Medicine (Bethesda, MD), 1997 World Wide Web URL: http://www.ncbi.nlm.nih.gov/omim/
12. *Online mendelian inheritance in man (OMIM).* Search: http://www3.ncbi.nlm.nih.gov/Omim/searchomim.html
13. Rowen, L., Mahairas, G., & Hood, L. (1997). Sequencing the human genome. *Science, 278,* 605–607.
14. Struewing, J. P., Hartge, P., Wacholder, S., et al. (1997). The risk of breast cancer associated with specific mutations of BRCA1 and BRCA2 among Ashkenazi Jews. *New England Journal of Medicine, 336,* 1401–1408.
15. The University of Edinburgh (Scotland), Biology Teaching Organisation: A Genetics Glossary: http://helios.bto.ed.ac.uk/bto/glossary/
16. Wooster, R., Bignell, G., Lancaster, J., et al. (1995). Identification of the breast cancer susceptibility BRCA2. *Nature, 378,* 789–792.

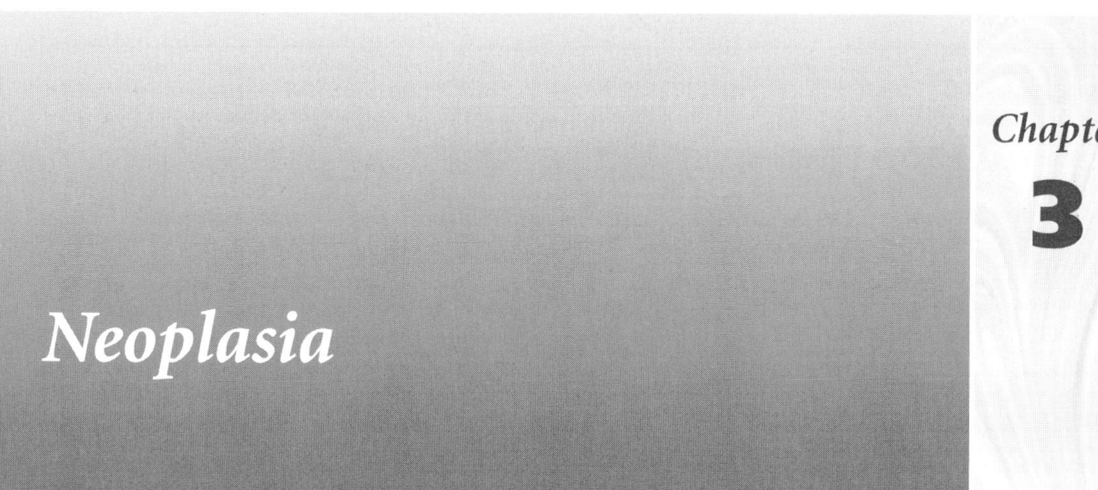

Chapter 3

Neoplasia

Jennifer H. Otto

KEY TERMS

aberrant cellular growth
anaplasia
benign
cancer
carcinogen
carcinogenesis
carcinoma
malignant
metastasis
neoplasia
neoplasm
oncogene
paraneoplastic syndrome
sarcoma
TNM system
tumor (see neoplasm)
tumor suppressor gene

Neoplasia is the development of abnormal cellular growth that is unresponsive to normal growth control mechanisms. A **neoplasm** or **tumor** is a group or clump of neoplastic cells that may be benign or malignant. **Benign** neoplasms do not invade the surrounding tissue. **Malignant** neoplasms grow by invading surrounding tissue and have the ability to travel to and proliferate at a distant site from the primary tumor (**metastasis**). **Cancer** refers to more than 100 distinct malignant entities of uncontrolled cell growth and proliferation. **Aberrant cellular growth** is an alteration in the normal cellular growth, which occurs when the cell escapes the normal controls on growth and differentiation. **Anaplasia** is a term used for the loss of cellular differentiation such that the cell looks less like the parent cell.

The cell is constant confronted by factors that stimulate its inherent capacity for growth and proliferation. Every time a normal cell passes through a cycle of division, the opportunity exists for it to become cancerous. Cancer cells generally contain the full complement of biomolecules necessary for survival, proliferation, differentiation, and expression of many functions specific to the cell type, but they lack the ability to regulate these functions.[11]

EPIDEMIOLOGY

Cancer is the second leading cause of death in the United States. As mortality rates from cardiovascular disease have declined in recent decades, the percentage of deaths due to cancer have concurrently increased.[14] However, some encouraging trends have emerged since the early 1990s, as evidenced by the first sustained decline in cancer mortality since record-keeping began in the 1930s.[8] Despite this positive trend and the advances in the understanding of cell growth and development, many aspects of cancer remain a challenge to clinicians.

Cancer is primarily a disease of the aging; the risk of developing cancer increases significantly with advancing age. However, cancer does strike all age groups, second only to accidents as the leading cause of death in children ages 1 to 14.[19] Figure 3-1 shows the 1998 estimate of new cancer cases and cancer deaths by site and sex. Although prostate cancer and breast cancer are the most common neoplasms in men and women, respectively, for both sexes lung and bronchial cancers are the deadliest.

At least 80% of cancers are related to life-style and environmental **carcinogens**.[5] Combinations of risk factors provide a higher incidence of specific cancers. These factors are briefly discussed in this section, and their mechanisms of **carcinogenesis** are described later in this chapter. The major life-style and environmental risk factors for cancer include tobacco, alcohol, diet, reproductive and sexual behavior, occupation, pollution, industrial products, and medicines. Other risk factors include infectious agents, endogenous hormones, and genetics.[23]

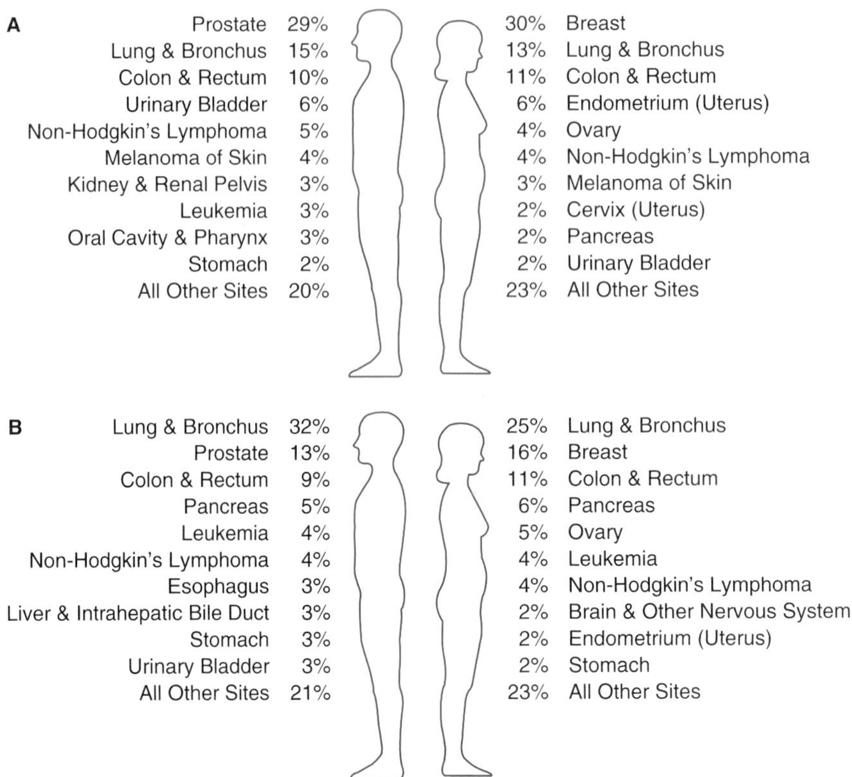

FIGURE 3-1. **A.** Estimated new cancer cases, 1998. **B.** Estimated cancer deaths, 1998. (Landis, S. H., et al. [1998]. Cancer statistics, 1998. *CA: A Cancer Journal for Clinicians, 48*(1), 14.)

Tobacco

Tobacco smoke contains several known carcinogenic agents. Among these agents are polycyclic aromatic hydrocarbons, nitrosamines, aromatic amines, and aldehydes. Studies in many countries have established that the risks of oral cavity, pharyngeal, laryngeal, lung, and esophageal cancers are significantly increased among cigarette smokers.[1] The duration of smoking and the number of cigarettes smoked are positively correlated with cancer risk. Studies also provide evidence of a reduction of cancer risk following cessation of smoking; for example, after 10 years of smoking cessation, the risk of lung cancer is reduced to about 50% the risk experienced by those of similar age and sex who continue to smoke.[1] Chewing tobacco is also associated with oral cancers. Alcohol exhibits a synergistic effect with tobacco, thereby further increasing the risk of oral and esophageal cancers.

Smoking has been linked with cancers of the pancreas, bladder, kidney, and cervix. Compared with nonsmokers, smokers have a two to five times greater risk for developing these cancers, and the risk is also related to duration of use and number of cigarettes smoked. Passive smoking, or inhaling second-hand smoke, probably increases the risk of lung cancer about twofold.[30]

Alcohol

Alcohol plays a role in the induction of cancer in select organs by increasing the effectiveness of carcinogens.[33] A synergistic relationship exists between alcohol and tobacco for cancers of the mouth, pharynx, larynx, and esophagus. Chronic consumption of alcohol commonly induces cirrhosis, a precursor lesion for primary hepatocellular carcinoma.[33] Recent studies have also implicated moderate alcohol ingestion with elevated risk of breast cancer.[13] Alcohol has been linked in some studies with pancreatic cancer.

Diet

Much of the information on dietary linkage to carcinogenesis comes from observational rather than controlled research. Diets high in fat are correlated to a higher risk for cancers of the large bowel, breast, prostate, ovary, endometrium, and pancreas.[33] Numerous studies have linked the incidence of colorectal cancer to high-fat and low-fiber dietary intake.

High-temperature cooking has been associated with the formation of heterocyclic aromatic amines in well-done meats. These amines are potent carcinogens in rats, causing neoplasms in the mammary gland, colon, liver, pancreas, and bladder.[33] Direct ingestion of aflatoxin B, a mold of the genus *Aspergillus flavus* found on corn, barley, peas, rice, soybeans, fruit, some nuts, milk, and cheddar cheese has been linked to liver cancer in humans. Chewing of betel nuts has been directly related to cancers of the oral cavity.

The ingestion of pickled, salt-cured, and smoked foods containing nitrates has been associated with increased risk of gastric cancer. Nitrates are converted in the stomach to nitrites, potent carcinogens in animal studies.[7] Vitamin deficiencies may give rise to altered mucosal integrity, enzyme and metabolic dysfunction, and morphologic abnormalities in certain target organs.[29] Vitamin A and its provitamin, β-carotene, are needed for normal growth in epithelial tissues. Vitamin C is an antioxidant that traps free radicals and reactive singlet oxygen molecules, and blocks the formation of certain carcinogenic compounds.[29] Recent studies have associated vitamin E intake with protection against prostate cancer.

Reproductive and Sexual Behavior

Certain types of malignancies are related to sexual practices. Cervical carcinoma is linked to a history of multiple sexual partners, intercourse at a young age, and multiparity. Cervical cancer is rare in sexually inactive or nulliparous women.[2] Cancer of the penis is rare among men who are circumcised. Human immunodeficiency virus disease is a sexually transmitted disease that permits cancer by decreasing immune resistance.

Occupational, Industrial, and Pollution Links

About 20,000 cancer deaths annually may be due to occupational exposure. Many industries are associated with repeated and prolonged contact with potential carcinogens.[3] Table 3-1 lists a number of suspected

TABLE 3-1

KNOWN OR SUSPECTED CHEMICAL CARCINOGENS IN HUMANS*

TARGET ORGAN	AGENTS	INDUSTRIES	TUMOR TYPE
Lung	Tobacco smoke, arsenic, asbestos, crystalline silica, benzo(a)pyrene, beryllium, bis(chloro)methyl ether, 1,3-butadiene, chromium VI compounds, coal tar and pitch, nickel compounds, soots, mustard gas	Aluminum production, coal gasification, coke production, hematite mining, painters	Squamous, large cell, and small cell cancer and adenocarcinoma
Pleura	Asbestos	—	Mesothelioma
Oral cavity	Tobacco smoke, alcoholic beverages, nickel compounds	Boot and shoe production, furniture manufacturer, isopropyl alcohol production	Squamous cell cancer
Esophagus	Tobacco smoke, alcoholic beverages	—	Squamous cell cancer
Gastric	Smoked, salted and pickled foods	Rubber industry	Adenocarcinoma
Colon	Heterocyclic amines, asbestos	Pattern makers	Adenocarcinoma
Liver	Aflatoxin, vinyl chloride, tobacco smoke, alcoholic beverages	—	Hepatocellular carcinoma, hemangiosarcoma
Kidney	Tobacco smoke	—	Renal cell cancer
Bladder	Tobacco smoke, 4-aminobiphenyl, benzidine, 2-napthylamine	Magenta manufacture, auramine manufacture	Transitional cell cancer
Prostate	Cadmium	—	Adenocarcinoma
Skin	Arsenic, benzo(a)pyrene, coal tar and pitch, mineral oils, soots	Coal gasification, coke production	Squamous cell cancer, basal cell cancer
Bone marrow	Benzene, tobacco smoke, ethylene oxide, antineoplastic agents	Rubber workers	Leukemia

*These carcinogen designations are determined by regulatory or review agencies based on public health needs. They do not imply proof of carcinogenicity in individuals. This table is not all-inclusive.
(From Yuspa, S. H., & Shields, P. G. [1997]. Etiology of cancer: Chemical factors. In V. T. DeVita, Jr., S. Hellman, & S. A. Rosenberg [Eds.], *Cancer: Principles and practice of oncology* (5th ed., p. 191). Philadelphia: Lippincott-Raven.)

chemical carcinogens in humans and their associated target organs, industries, and cancers.

Asbestos, chromium, nickel, and cadmium are notable examples of chemical carcinogens. All are associated with cancer of the lung. Asbestos fibers are thought to function as promoters for other carcinogens such as cigarette smoke and are also linked with cancer of the pleural cavity and gastrointestinal tract. Chromium and nickel also may cause nasal cavity tumors. Cadmium is associated with cancer of the prostate gland.

Environmental pollution through air, soil, and water creates exposure to many chemical carcinogens. In air, polycyclic aromatic hydrocarbons are present in automobile exhaust and other products of combustion, including tobacco smoke. Many potential carcinogens have been identified in water, including inorganic and organic compounds such as metals, nitrates, and vinyl chloride.[3]

Pharmaceutical Agents

Specific pharmaceutical agents used in the past and present have been linked to cancer. Arsenic compounds, used for many years for a variety of conditions, have been associated with squamous cell carcinomas of the skin. Diethylstilbestrol, given to pregnant women in the past for prevention of miscarriage, is linked to a high incidence of adenocarcinoma of the vagina in the female children of exposed women.

Many drugs in common use today have carcinogenic properties. Estrogens have been associated with endometrial and breast cancers; androgens and oral contraceptives have been linked to hepatic tumors. Tamoxifen, an antiestrogenic drug used as a breast cancer preventive agent, has been weakly linked to the development of liver and endometrial cancers. Alkylating agents, widely used antineoplastics, increase the risk for leukemia and lymphoma after solid tumor therapy.[3] Immunosuppressive agents increase the risk of many types of cancer. Other drugs with suspected carcinogenic properties include griseofulvin (cancer in rats), phenacetin (renal cell carcinoma), and coal tar ointments (skin cancer).

Radiation

The mutagenic effects of ionizing radiation became known soon after Roentgen's discovery of the x-ray in 1895. A specific characteristic of ionizing radiation is its ability to penetrate cells and deposit energy within them in a random fashion.[21] Damage to DNA can be direct or indirect. Direct damage results from interaction of the electron within the DNA of the cell. Indirect damage occurs when a secondary electron interacts with a water molecule, giving rise to a free radical, which then damages the DNA. A long latent period often exists between exposure and the development of clinical disease. Firm evidence links exposure to large doses of radiation and development of leukemia. Survivors of the atomic bombings of Hiroshima and Nagasaki in 1945 had a very high incidence of leukemia. Miners of radioactive substances such as uranium have a higher incidence of lung cancer. Low-dose radiation exposure and previous head and neck radiation have been linked to thyroid cancer. The best established etiologic agent in breast cancer is exposure to ionizing radiation, which is thought to induce critical mutations in BRCA1 or perhaps another yet undiscovered gene.[15] Ultraviolet radiation from the sun is a major cause of skin cancers. People with fair complexions are more likely to develop skin cancers than their darker complexioned counterparts because of the lack of protective melanin. Skin cancers are more often seen on sun-exposed areas of the body and in elderly persons.[6]

Infectious Agents

Viral infections account for an estimated one in seven human cancers worldwide.[26] Viruses capable of inducing cancer are called carcinogenic or *oncogenic viruses*, and consist of both DNA viruses and RNA viruses. The DNA viruses are incorporated into the genes of the host and transmitted to subsequent generations. The genes are then expressed without the usual symptoms that accompany infection. The RNA viruses, or *retroviruses*, also contribute genetic information to the host cell. These viruses use an enzyme called reverse transcriptase to develop new DNA sequences that are not attacked and destroyed by the immune system (Fig. 3-2). Table 3-2 lists some carcinogenic viruses and their associated cancers. The DNA virus that causes hepatitis B and the RNA flavivirus that causes hepatitis C are closely linked with the development of hepatocellular carcinoma. The human T-cell leukemia virus type 1 (HTLV-1) is a retrovirus linked to adult T-cell leukemia, a malignancy endemic in parts of Japan, the Caribbean, and parts of Africa.[18] Cervical cancers and anogenital cancers are linked to the human papillomaviruses.

Evidence suggests that some viruses interact synergistically with chemical agents in the carcinogenic process. For example, the high incidence of liver cancer in Africa may be due to interactions between the hepatitis B virus and aflatoxin in the diet; nasopharyngeal cancer in Asia and Burkitt's lymphoma in Africa may be caused by an interaction between the Epstein-Barr virus and nitrosamines in the diet.[32]

Endogenous Hormones

A substantial body of evidence indicates that hormones play a major role in the etiology of several human cancers. Breast tissue exhibits changes with the fluctuations of hormones during the menstrual cycle. Estrogen ap-

FOCUS ON CELLULAR PATHOPHYSIOLOGY

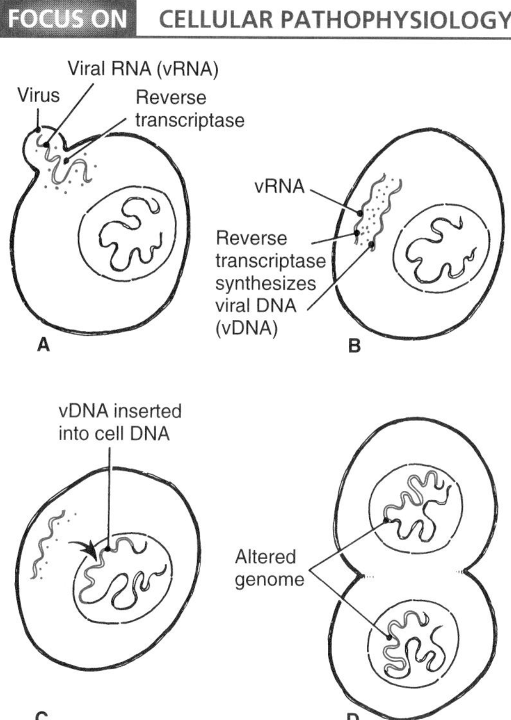

FIGURE 3-2. Schematic showing how RNA viruses change the genome of the cell and cause replication of new cells with altered genome. **A.** Virus infects the cell. **B.** Alteration of cell RNA by virus (vRNA). **C.** Alteration of cell DNA. **D.** Duplication of the cell, with altered DNA going to the progeny.

pears to be the primary stimulant for breast cell proliferation and facilitates mutation or expression of genetic errors leading to breast cancer.[16] High levels of estrogen unopposed by progesterone increase the risk of endometrial cancer by inducing endometrial hyperplasia. Epithelial ovarian cancer is derived from the epithelial cells within the developing follicle or covering the ovarian surface. These cells replicate during or after each ovulation, which is the result of complex hormonal changes. Factors that inhibit ovulation (increased parity, combined oral contraceptives) therefore protect against ovarian cancer.

Prostate cancer depends on androgenic stimulation; the disease does not occur in castrated men. Laboratory evidence indicates that testosterone can cause prostate cancer in rats.[16]

Genetics

A few genetically inherited disorders are directed associated with increased risk for cancer. These include autosomal recessive disorders such as ataxia-telangiectasia, which is closely associated with leukemia, lymphoma, and ovarian cancer. Autosomal dominant disorders such as neurofibromatosis are associated with increased risks of neurofibrosarcoma and acute myelocytic leukemia. Some of the X-linked recessive disorders, especially the immunodeficiency syndromes, are associated with an increased risk of leukemia and lymphoma.

Other examples of inherited cancer syndromes are familial polyposis, a predecessor of colon cancer, and retinoblastoma. Although there appears to be a familial predisposition for specific cancers such as breast, ovarian, and colon, research to isolate genetic markers is ongoing. One example of a genetic link to cancer is the increased risk of breast carcinoma seen in families with the BRCA1 mutation.

THE CELL CYCLE IN NEOPLASIA

The interval from one cell division to the next is called the cell cycle. In a normal cell population, inhibitory controls slow or stop reproduction, whereas stimulating factors cause the process to proceed more rapidly. Therefore, the actual length of a cell life cycle varies. The four phases of the cell cycle are designated G_1, S, G_2, and M (Fig. 3-3). G_0 is a resting phase composed of cells that have left the cell cycle but can be induced to reenter the cycle by specific stimuli. G_1 and G_2 are gap or growth phases. A cell can remain in the G_1 phase for long periods until some key process occurs to signal its entrance into the S phase of DNA synthesis. After the

TABLE 3-2

VIRUSES IMPLICATED IN MALIGNANT NEOPLASIA

VIRUS	ASSOCIATED CANCER
Hepatitis B, hepatitis C	Hepatocellular carcinoma
Herpes simplex type 2	Cervical carcinoma
Epstein-Barr	Burkitt's lymphoma, nasopharyngeal cancer
Human T-cell leukemia virus, type 1	T-cell leukemia
Human papillomaviruses	Cervical carcinoma, anogenital cancers

FOCUS ON CELLULAR PHYSIOLOGY

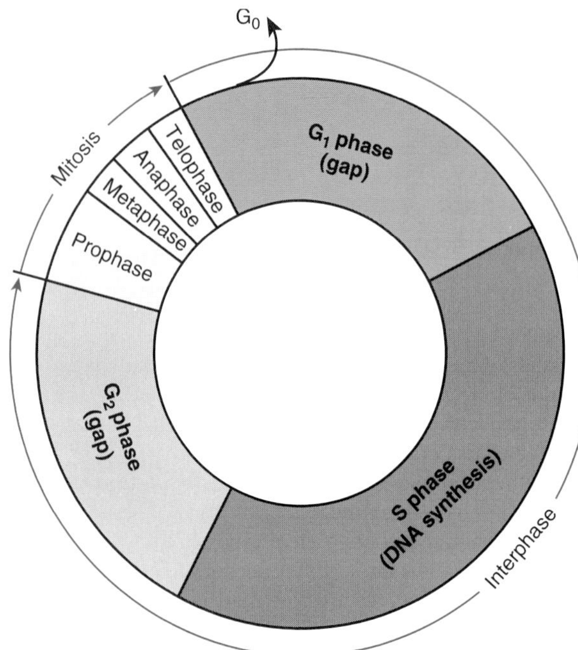

FIGURE 3-3. The cell cycle. Interphase (G_1), DNA synthesis (S), intermediate phase (G_2), and mitosis (M) intervals are shown. The G_0 period may be entered from G_1, and reentry from G_0 to G_1 may occur.

S phase, the cell enters the G_2 phase, during which some residual RNA is synthesized in preparation for mitosis. Mitosis creates two daughter cells that have identical genetic information. The daughter cells may enter into G_1 or G_0, or they may be immediately stimulated to reproduce. Some cells are terminally differentiated and never reenter the cell cycle. These cells (eg, neurons, myocardial cells) do not become neoplastic.

The concept of the cell life cycle has helped in the basic understanding of the process a neoplastic cell goes through in its proliferation. Neoplastic cell populations ignore normal growth limitations and enter the cell cycle repeatedly at different rates. The terms growth fraction, cell cycle time, cell loss, and doubling time are used to describe these neoplastic characteristics. *Growth fraction* refers to the proportion of cells in a given cell population undergoing cell cycle activity at any given time. Rapidly growing neoplasms have a larger number of cells in active reproduction at any given time than do slow-growing neoplasms. The *labeling index* is a measure of cells that are synthesizing DNA, or those in the S phase. This index provides a relatively simple method for estimating proliferative rates of cancerous cells.[11] The labeling index and growth fraction are the parameters that usually differentiate cancer growths from normal tissues. The *cell cycle time* is the time from the onset of one mitosis to the onset of the next mitotic phase. The cell cycle time may actually be slower in cancer growths than in normal tissues. *Cell loss* refers to the number of cells lost in the process of growth. The *doubling time* is the rate at which a neoplasm doubles its cell population. Internal cancers are not often detected before they are about the size of a cubic centimeter, which corresponds to 10^8 to 10^9 cells. The actual rate of doubling varies with the tumor because of host defenses and variable death rates.

CELLULAR CHANGES IN NEOPLASIA

Most of the cell changes in neoplasia relate to those seen with malignant neoplasia. Some concepts also apply to benign neoplasms. The different characteristics are discussed in a later section of this chapter.

Cell Membrane

The outer cell membrane is the point of contact between cells and functions in the control of normal cellular growth. Changes in this membrane have been implicated in the failure of the neoplastic cells to respond to normal growth-control mechanisms. Research in this area has demonstrated aberrant glycosylation in malignancy, which produces abnormal glycolipid and glycoprotein structures in the cell membrane.[4] These structural changes result in alterations of cellular adhesion and intercellular communication. The resulting decrease in cellular adhesion and intercellular communication can lead to loss of contact inhibition and neoplastic change.

CELLULAR ADHESION

Cellular adhesion is a process that involves connections between cells. At least two kinds of connections have described between normal cells in culture: (1) *tight junctions* (membranes of the adjacent endothelial cells are tightly fused) visualized as *desmosomes* by the electron microscopist, and (2) *gap junctions*, which allow passage of small molecules between the two adjoining cells. In tumor cells, tight junctions are usually retained, but gap junctions are frequently reduced or absent[31] (Fig. 3-4).

INTERCELLULAR COMMUNICATION

Intercellular communication is the term used to describe the exchange of information between cells. Contact inhibition, or *density-dependent growth control*, and *anchorage-dependent growth* are observed when normal cells are grown in culture media. Normal cells require a suitable surface for attachment and proliferation. The cells move around freely in the culture media until they touch one another. On contact, they adhere to one another and form parallel lines. They

FOCUS ON CELLULAR PATHOPHYSIOLOGY

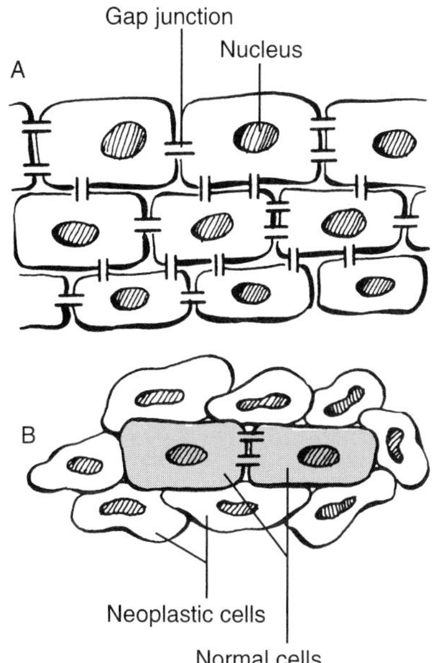

FIGURE 3-4. **A.** Normal cells pass growth control information through the gap junctions. **B.** Neoplastic growth may isolate normal cells from neighboring cells.

then grow on a single layer until they reach the edge of the culture dish, and then growth stops. The cells of a neoplasm, however, respond by continuing to divide and migrate until they are several layers deep. In other words, normal cells respond to a crowded environment, but neoplastic cells do not, because they have lost their ability either to receive or to send the necessary information to stop growth (Fig. 3-5). *Growth factors*, growth-stimulatory and growth-inhibitory substances, play a major role in mediating cell-to-cell communication. Tumor cells display a reduced dependence on growth factors; this autonomy represents a breakdown in the regulatory network maintaining cell growth.[31] The lack of response to growth inhibitor influences accounts for the uncontrolled proliferation characteristic of neoplastic cells.

FOCUS ON CELLULAR PATHOPHYSIOLOGY

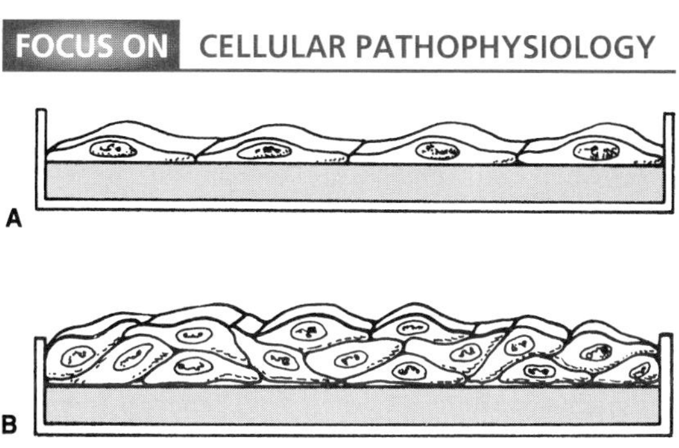

FIGURE 3-5. **A.** Normal cells are inhibited by a crowded environment. **B.** Neoplastic cells continue to grow despite cell contact.

Genetic Changes in Neoplasia

Neoplasia is a multistep process resulting from the accumulation of genetic changes in cells.[28] Two types of genes have been implicated in the neoplastic transformation of cells: **oncogenes** and **tumor suppressor genes**. Their discovery came through the study of retroviruses in tumor induction.

Proto-oncogenes are normal genes that regulate cellular growth processes such as proliferation and differentiation. They are converted into oncogenes by mutation, gene amplification, and chromosomal rearrangement.[28] Oncogenes display a gain in function mechanism; their activation has a positive effect on cell growth. In contrast, tumor suppressor genes normally function to have a negative effect on cell growth. Mutations that inactivate tumor suppressor genes can result in unregulated cell growth. Mutations in the p53 tumor suppressor gene are prevalent in many human cancers.[22] The expression of a malignant phenotype usually requires a combination of oncogene activation and tumor suppressor gene inactivation. Figure 3-6 illustrates mechanisms of growth promotion by an oncogene.

Differentiation and Anaplasia

During fetal development, cells undergo changes in their physical and structural properties as they form the different tissues of the body. This process is called *cellular differentiation*. Differentiated cells become specialized and differ from one another physically and functionally. Nerve cells, for example, are terminally differentiated and do not undergo mitotic division. The more differentiated a cell is, the less likely it is to divide and, therefore, the less susceptible it is to malignant transformation.

The factors that control differentiation are not fully understood but can be divided into extracellular and intracellular regulators. Extracellular regulators of differentiation include the proximity and type of neighboring cells as well as soluble factors like growth factors. Intracellular regulators involve intrinsic programs of gene expression controlled by master regulatory genes.[11] Selective repression of genetic information in cells is probably involved in the control of differentiation.

Cells that look and act like the cell of origin (parent cell) are called *well differentiated cells*. All benign tumors are well differentiated, often being impossible to distinguish from the normal tissue. The cells of a malignant neoplasm are not as well differentiated as the normal tissue. Neoplasms that bear little or no resemblance to the tissue of origin are called *poorly differentiated or undifferentiated tumors*. The lack of differentiation is called

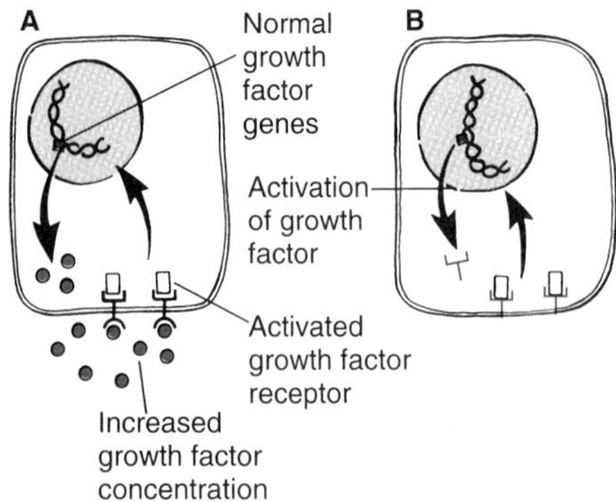

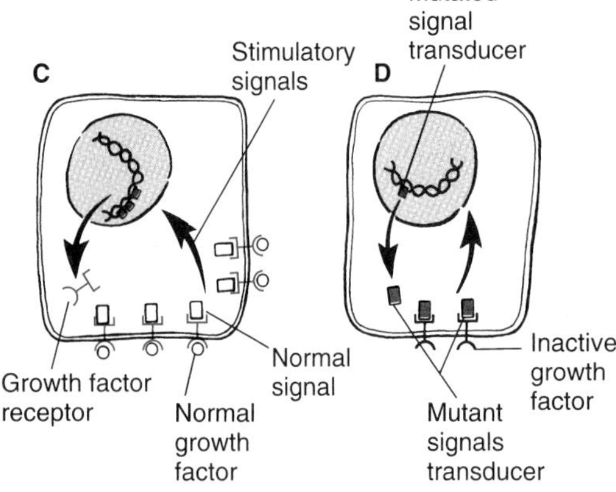

FIGURE 3-6. **Mechanisms of growth promotion by an oncogene. A. The oncogene codes for a growth factor and stimulates tumor cells. B. The growth factor receptor may be defective and constantly activated. C. An increased number of growth receptors may cause amplification of oncogene. D. Defective signal transducers may promote growth without an external trigger.**

anaplasia and is a key feature of malignant tumors. Well differentiated cancer cells may elaborate relatively normal products of the tissue of origin, whereas poorly differentiated cancer cells may lose all specialized functional characteristics. Very anaplastic tumors may elaborate a product that is completely foreign to the tissue of origin. An example is the elaboration of a hormone like the antidiuretic hormone from the oat cell carcinoma of the lung.

CLASSIFICATION OF NEOPLASMS

Neoplasms are customarily classified according to their cell of origin and whether their behavior is benign or malignant. Table 3-3 compares benign and malignant neoplasms. The terminology places the cell or type of tissue of origin as the first part of the name, and the suffix "-oma" (tumor) forms the last portion. Table 3-4 lists classifications of common benign and malignant neoplasms. Epithelial benign tumors of squamous and basal cell origin are called *papillomas*. Glandular epithelial benign tumors are called *adenomas*. Papillomas or adenomas that grow at the end of a stem or pedicle are referred to as polyps, and they may become malignant. Malignant neoplasms of epithelial origin are called **carcinomas**. Those of glandular epithelial origin are called adenocarcinomas. Neoplasms of muscle cell origin are named according to muscle type, such as leiomyoma, which means "smooth muscle tumor." Malignant neoplasms arising from connective tissue such as muscle or bone are called **sarcomas**, an example of which is leiomyosarcoma. Pigmented and embryonic cells are also indicated in the nomenclature of neoplasms. In normal embryologic development, three layers of cells become apparent. The outer layer is the *ectoderm*, which forms the skin and other structures in the adult human. The middle layer, or *mesoderm*, forms the supporting structures of bone, muscle, fat, blood, and connective tissue. Malignant tumors of these mesenchymal structures are called sarcomas. The inner layer is the *endoderm*, which ultimately forms the gastrointestinal tract and other structures. Sometimes *blastoma* is used to denote that the tissue has a primitive or embryonic appearance. A *teratoma* is another embryonic-appearing tumor that comes from all three germ layers but appears as a highly disorganized array of cells. The teratoma is considered to be benign, whereas the *teratocarcinoma* is malignant. Neoplasms of pigmented cells are named for their cell of origin, the melanocyte. Neoplasms of embryonic cell origin also may contain bits of the germinal layers, such as hair or teeth.

TABLE 3-3
COMPARISON OF BENIGN AND MALIGNANT NEOPLASMS

BENIGN	MALIGNANT
Similar to cell of origin	Dissimilar from cell of origin
Edges move outward smoothly (encapsulated)	Edges move outward irregularly
Compresses	Invades
Slow growth rate	Rapid to very rapid growth rate
Slight vascularity	Moderate to marked vascularity
Seldom recur after removal	Frequently recur after removal
Necrosis and ulceration unusual	Necrosis and ulceration common
Systemic effects unusual unless it is a secreting endocrine neoplasm	Systemic effects common

TABLE 3-4

CLASSIFICATION OF COMMON BENIGN AND MALIGNANT NEOPLASMS

CELL	BENIGN	MALIGNANT
EPITHELIAL		
Squamous	Squamous cell papilloma	Squamous cell carcinoma
Basal cell	Basal cell papilloma	Basal cell carcinoma
Glandular	Adenoma	Adenocarcinoma
Pigmented	Benign melanoma	Malignant melanoma
MUSCLE		
Smooth muscle	Leiomyoma	Leiomyosarcoma
Striated muscle	Rhabdomyoma	Rhabdomyosarcoma
NERVE		
Nerve sheath	Neurilemmoma	Neurofibrosarcoma
Glial cells	Glioma	Glioblastoma
Ganglion cells	Ganglioneuroma	Neuroblastoma
Meninges	Meningioma	Malignant meningioma
CONNECTIVE TISSUE		
Fibrous	Fibroma	Fibrosarcoma
Fatty	Lipoma	Liposarcoma
Bone	Osteoma	Osteosarcoma
Cartilage	Chondroma	Chondrosarcoma
Blood vessels	Hemangioma	Angiosarcoma
Lymph vessels	Lymphangioma	Lymphangiosarcoma
Bone marrow		Multiple myeloma Leukemia Ewing's sarcoma
LYMPHOID		
		Malignant lymphoma Lymphosarcoma Reticulum cell sarcoma Lymphatic leukemia Hodgkin's disease
OTHER BLOOD CELLS		
Erythrocytes		Polycythemia vera (?)
Granulocytes		Myelogenous leukemia
Monocytes		Monocytic leukemia
Plasma cells		Multiple myeloma
T or B lymphocytes	Mononucleosis (?)	Lymphocytic leukemia

BENIGN NEOPLASMS

Benign neoplasms consist of cells that are similar in structure to the cells from which they are derived. The cells of benign neoplasms are more cohesive than those of malignant neoplasms. Growth occurs evenly from the center of the benign mass, usually resulting in a well defined border. The edges move outward, smoothly pushing adjacent cells out of the way (Fig. 3-7). As this occurs, many of these tumors become encapsulated. The capsule, composed of connective tissue, separates the tumor from surrounding tissues. A benign neoplasm usually grows slowly and is limited to one area. Its blood supply is less profuse than that of a malignant neoplasm. A benign neoplasm seldom recurs after surgical removal and seldom ulcerates, undergoes necrosis, or causes systemic problems. An exception is a secreting endocrine neoplasm, which causes symptoms resulting from excess hormone secretion.

Benign tumors produce their effects from obstruction, pressure, and secretion. A benign tumor in an enclosed space such as the skull could potentially have serious or lethal effects. Another example is intestinal obstruction resulting from an abdominal benign tumor.

FOCUS ON CELLULAR PATHOPHYSIOLOGY

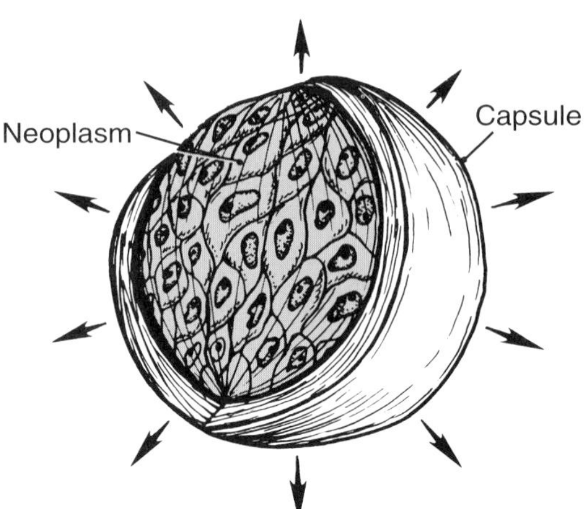

FIGURE 3-7. Encapsulated benign neoplasm. *Arrows* indicate equal expansion from the center.

MALIGNANT NEOPLASMS

Malignant neoplasms have atypical cellular structure, with abnormal nuclear divisions and chromosomes. The malignant cell loses its differentiation or resemblance to the cell of origin. The tumor cells are not cohesive, and, consequently, the pattern of growth is irregular. No capsule is formed, and distinct separation from surrounding tissues is difficult (Fig. 3-8). Malignant cells invade adjacent cells rather than pushing them aside. Tumors have varying growth rates and develop a greater blood supply than normal tissues or benign neoplasms. The hallmarks of malignant neoplasms are the ability to metastasize or spread to distant sites. Box 3-1 summarizes the biologic and cellular characteristics of malignant tumors. They frequently recur after surgical removal and can cause systemic problems.

FOCUS ON CELLULAR PATHOPHYSIOLOGY

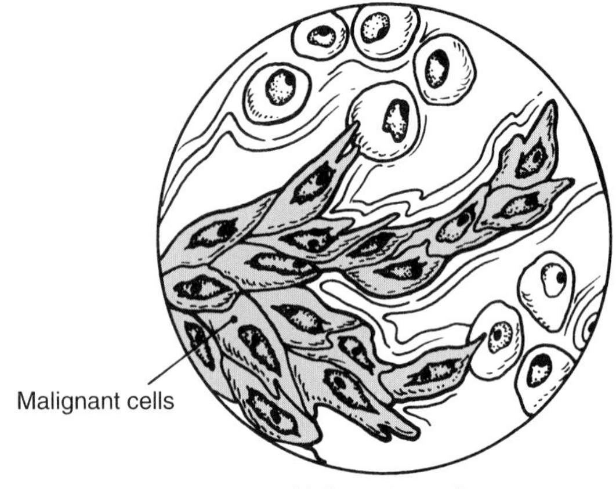

FIGURE 3-8. Malignant neoplasm with irregular borders, indistinct from surrounding tissues.

Mechanisms of Carcinogenesis

Many areas of study have evolved to explain the nature of the different diseases that are cumulatively called cancer. The theory of *somatic cell mutation* was formulated by Bauer in 1928. It supports the concept that genetic abnormalities can be induced by mutational carcinogenic agents and hereditary susceptibility. In the 1940s, Berenblum described a two-step mutational model that involved initiation and promotion. Tumor initiation occurs when a carcinogen causes a mutation by modification of the molecular structure of DNA. Tumor promotion involves the selective expansion of initiated cells, which produces a larger population of cells at higher risk for malignant conversion.[35] The process of initiation and promotion probably goes on for several cycles with subsequent mutations of initiated cells before a tumor is formed.

Carcinogens were described previously as those substances capable of inducing neoplastic growth in sus-

BOX 3-1

BIOLOGIC AND CELLULAR CHARACTERISTICS OF MALIGNANT TUMORS

Pleomorphic—cells and nuclei vary in size and shape
Anaplastic—cells bear little resemblance to the parent cell. *Differentiated cells* appear much like the parent cells and growth pattern is slow; *undifferentiated cells* do not resemble parent cells and are usually rapidly growing tumors.
Abnormal mitoses—products of cell division often result in abnormal cells with a high percentage of cell death
Abnormal or no function—malignant cells rarely function like normal cells and often elaborate products not normally seen in that tissue
Nonencapsulated—tumor invades surrounding tissue rather than compressing it like benign tumors do
Metastatic—tumor has the ability to spread to other sites and establish new growth there

ceptible persons. *Cocarcinogens* increase the activity of carcinogens. *Procarcinogens* are carcinogens that must be activated or modified in the cell to induce cellular changes. It is thought that a number of steps are necessary for the expression of the fully malignant cell. The change in the first cell is a random (carcinogen-induced) mutation. Whether that cell reproduces or dies depends on number of interrelated factors. Carcinogenesis is now being described on the basis of these interrelated mechanisms (Flowchart 3-1). The carcinogenic substances must undergo molecular modification inside the cell to cause the cancer. When they are modified in such a way as to bind to the nuclear DNA, the modification is called activation. In many cases, the DNA disruption is repaired and the process does not progress.

FLOWCHART 3-1 **Simplified Scheme of Cancer Pathogenesis**

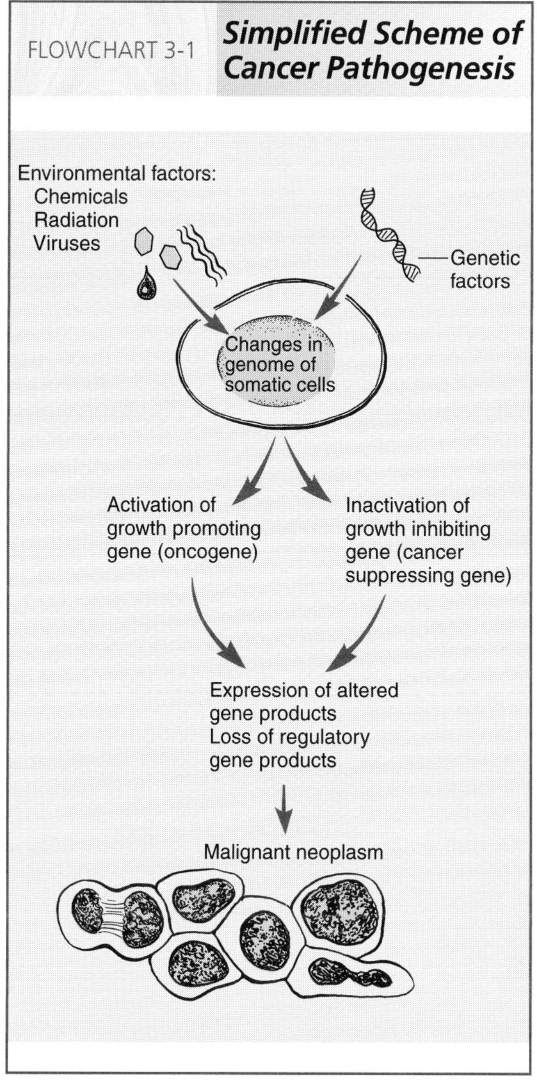

Growth of the Primary Malignant Tumor

The growth rate of malignant tumors tends to correlate with their level of differentiation. Therefore, the more undifferentiated or anaplastic a tumor, the greater is its potential for aggressive growth and dissemination. Each time a cell reproduces, it doubles the tumor mass; it is estimated that a typical tumor has doubled 30 times before it becomes clinically observed. A doubling of 40 times often proves to be fatal to the host. Figure 3-9 depicts tumor growth by the Gompertzian tumor growth curve.[17] The rate of tumor growth is affected by many factors, including blood supply, nutrition, immune responsiveness, and in some tumors, endocrine support. Research has identified endogenous growth factors that promote *angiogenesis*, or blood vessel growth to supply the tumor mass.[12] The increased vascularity of the malignant tumor is critical to providing nutrients and oxygen to sustain its continued growth. In a nutritionally depleted host, the tumor growth may slow because of a decrease in the supply of adequate nutrients. The tumor takes the nutrients from the host, which alters the normal body processes and produces the tumor cachexia syndrome, often called *anorexia-cachexia syndrome.*

Tumor Markers

Tumor markers are substances not normally present in the blood or not present in large quantities that may indicate that a particular type of cancer is present. Table

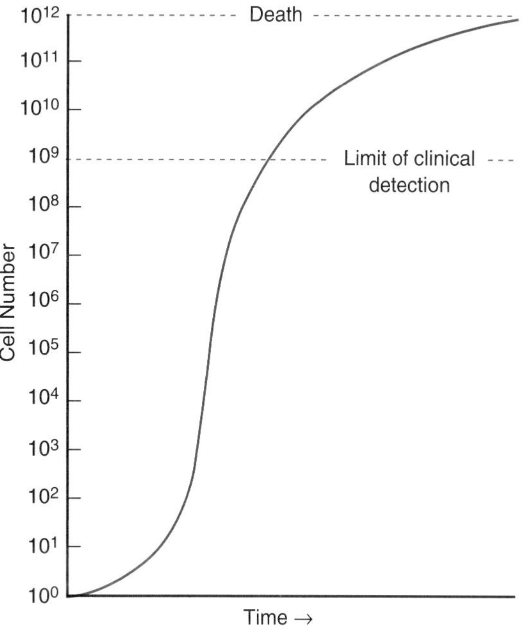

FIGURE 3-9. The Gompertzian growth curve. Early tumor growth is exponential; by the time the tumor is clinically detectable, most of its growth has already occurred.

3-5 lists some examples of tumor markers. In general, tumor markers are not very helpful in establishing a diagnosis or planning therapy because most are not specific for a given tumor; also, they may be present at low levels in the normal physiologic state or in nonmalignant diseases.[25] Markers used in clinical practice include:

- Oncofetal antigens—carcinoembryonic antigen; α-fetoprotein
- Hormones—human chorionic gonadotropin; antidiuretic hormone
- Tumor-specific proteins—immunoglobulins; prostate-specific antigen
- Normal enzymes at elevated levels

The main use for markers is to evaluate response to therapy to detect residual disease or relapse; however, assays of markers may also be used to screen high-risk people for the presence of cancer.

Escape from Immune Surveillance

Histocompatibility antigens are being studied in neoplastic tissue, with the goal being to use a host-versus-tumor reaction to destroy the tumor. If the immune system can recognize the tumor as foreign, immunization prepared from host tumor may cause the host to reject the tumor.

Experimental tumors in animal and cultured cell studies frequently express unique antigens on their cell surfaces. These antigens are capable of being recognized as foreign and subsequently destroyed by T-cell cytotoxic response, by natural killer (NK) cells, by macrophage intervention, or by B cells and complement activation. Immunocompromised individuals do have a much greater risk than the general population of developing malignancies, particularly leukemias and lymphomas. If the immune system is capable of destroying neoplastic tissue, how do tumor cells escape destruction? Most human tumors lack tumor-specific antigens, or the antigen is not expressed at the cell surface to be recognized as foreign. Some tumors can modulate or downregulate the expression of antigens after exposure to the immune system and thereby minimize chances of detection.[31]

Staging

Staging is an effort to describe the extent of a neoplasm in terms that are commonly understood. The purposes of staging are to determine treatment, to evaluate the

TABLE 3-5

SOME SPECIFIC TUMOR MARKERS

MARKER	NORMAL VALUE	SIGNIFICANCE
Alpha-fetoprotein (α FP)	<12.8 IU/mL	Serum globulin normally secreted by liver cells in embryonic life. High levels seen in carcinomas of testicles, pancreas, and liver but may be elevated in acute viral hepatitis.
Carcinoembryonic antigen (CEA)	0.0–3.4 ng/mL	Glycoprotein found in fetal pancreas, liver, and colon. Increased antibody titers found in serum of persons with breast cancer, pancreatic, liver, kidney, and colon cancer. Also may be elevated in pancreatitis, acute renal failure, pneumonia, ulcerative colitis, cigarette smokers, and for no apparent reason.
Prostate-specific antigen (PSA)	Female: <0.5 ng/mL Male: 0.0–4 ng/mL	Protein tumor-specific antigen expressed from prostatic tissues, markedly increased in prostatic cancer, slightly increased in benign prostatic hyperplasia, prostatitis, prostate surgery.
CA 15-3	0–30 u/mL	Glycoprotein elevated in metastatic breast cancer; a smaller percentage is elevated in primary breast cancer, but the marker may be elevated in benign breast disease and gastrointestinal disease.
CA 19-9	0–37 u/mL	Antibody developed against tumor-associated antigens from gastrointestinal and pancreatic cancers. Shows greater specificity for pancreatic cancers than CEA.
CA 125	0–35 u/mL	Antibody developed against tumor-associated antigen; a glycoprotein found on the surface of ovarian cancer cells; also may be elevated during pregnancy, pelvic inflammatory disease; and in endometriosis.
CA 27, 29	0–32 u/mL	Membrane antigen for breast cancer screening; when associated with other marker tests, positive predictive values improve.
Human chorionic gonadotropin (hCG)	<5 mIU/mL	Glycoprotein used in diagnosis and monitoring of gestational trophoblastic diseases such as hydatidiform mole, invasive mole, and choriocarcinoma.

outcome of treatment (patient survival), to estimate prognosis, and to facilitate exchange of information between treatment centers. Although many staging systems have been used over the years, the TNM system is now generally accepted worldwide. The letters in this classification system denote the following: T, the tumor or primary lesion and its extent; N, lymph node involvement; and M, distant metastasis. Tumor in situ, or localized tumor, is abbreviated Tis. TX is used when the extent of the tumor cannot be adequately assessed. Using the letter T and adding ascending numbers indicates increasing tumor size. The degree of cancerous involvement of lymph nodes is indicated by the letter N and either X (cannot adequately assess regional lymph nodes), 0 (no lymph node involvement), or 1 to 3 (ascending numbers indicating increasing numbers of nodal metastases). The absence or presence of distant metastases is designated by an MO or M1, respectively. Box 3-2 shows an example of staging for breast cancer.

Metastasis

The ability of a malignant neoplasm to spread to a distant site is termed metastasis. A clump of malignant cells, no longer attached to the original neoplasm, travels to and becomes established at a new site. The original cancer is the primary neoplasm, tumor, or site. Five phases are involved in metastasis: invasion, cell detachment, dissemination, arrest and establishment, and proliferation (Fig. 3-10). Table 3-6 delineates the process of metastasis from initiation to resistance to therapy.

INVASION

To invade normal adjacent cells, the malignant cells grow out from their original location into the neighboring areas. Three mechanisms explain tumor cell invasion: the rapid growth of malignant cells leading to infiltration induced by mechanical pressure; the decrease in tumor cell cohesiveness accompanied by an increase in cell motility; and the destruction of host tissue by tumor cell-produced degradative enzymes.[10]

The loss of cell-to-cell cohesive forces is associated with the downregulation (or decrease) of the expression of E-cadherin, a cell surface glycoprotein involved in cell-to-cell adhesion. Increased tumor cell motility is associated with the alteration of cytoskeletal elements and the response to various motility-promoting factors.[10]

BOX 3-2 REPRESENTATIVE CLINICAL STAGING SYSTEM FOR BREAST CANCER

T	**Primary Tumors**
TX	Primary tumor cannot be assessed
TO	No evidence of primary tumor
Tis	Carcinoma in situ: intraductal carcinoma, lobular carcinoma, or Paget's disease with no tumor
T1	Tumor 2 cm or less in its greatest dimension a. 0.5 cm or smaller b. Larger than 0.5 cm but not larger than 1 cm in greatest dimension c. Larger than 1 cm but not larger than 2 cm in greatest dimension
T2	Tumor more than 2 cm but not more than 5 cm in greatest dimension
T3	Tumor more than 5 cm in its greatest dimension
T4	Tumor of any size with direct extension to chest wall or to skin (Chest wall includes ribs, intercostal muscles, and serratus anterior muscle but not pectoral muscle) a. Extension to chest wall b. Edema (including peau d'orange), ulceration of the skin of the breast, or satellite skin nodules confined to the same breast c. Both of the above d. Inflammatory carcinoma
N	**Regional Lymph Nodes (Clinical)**
NX	Regional lymph nodes cannot be assessed
NO	No regional lymph node metastases
N1	Metastasis to movable ipsilateral axillary node(s)
N2	Metastases to ipsilateral axillary nodes fixed to one another or to other structures
N3	Metastases to ipsilateral internal mammary lymph node(s)
M	**Distant Metastasis**
MO	No evidence of distant metastasis
M1	Distant metastases (including metastases to ipsilateral supraclavicular lymph nodes)
MX	Presence of distant metastases cannot be assessed.

(Adapted from DeVita V. T., Hellman S., Rosenbeng, S. A. [1997]. *Cancer: Principles and practice of oncology* [5th ed., p. 1569]. Philadelphia: Lippincott.)

To infiltrate a body cavity or blood vessel, the malignant cells must break through the basement cell membrane. A major structural component of the basement cell membrane is type IV collagen; metastatic tumor cells show preferential attachment to this type of collagen and produce enzymes capable of degrading it.

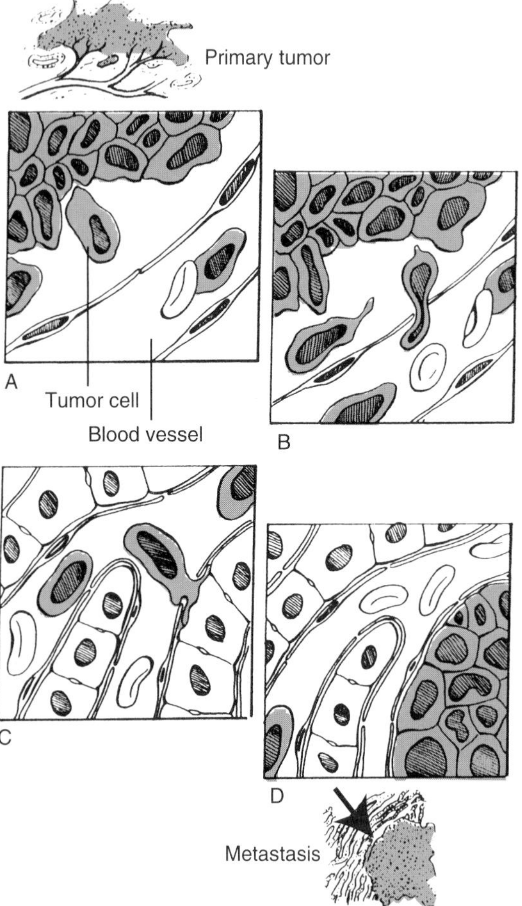

FIGURE 3-10. Metastasis of tumor cells to nonadjacent tissues. **A.** Primary tumor grows and invades the surrounding tissues. Cells are easily shed and can invade the basement membrane of the highly vascular tumor bed. The increased vascularity is caused by the elaboration of tumor angiogenesis factor (TAF) or by procoagulant factors. **B.** The tumor cells move between the endothelial capillary junctions or penetrate the basement membrane of the capillary. **C.** The shed tumor cells become arrested in a capillary bed, often liver, lungs, or brain. At this point they can penetrate the capillary wall and establish in the new environment. **D.** Proliferation at the new site requires a receptive environment, with blood supply and nutrition to encourage tumor growth. Most tumor cells are killed in the process of metastasis.

CELL DETACHMENT

After invading the neighboring tissues, body cavities, and blood vessels, malignant cells separate from the primary neoplasm and penetrate lymphatic or blood vessels. Tumor cells have altered cell-to-cell adhesion properties and are easily shed into the surrounding tissues, blood, and lymph.

DISSEMINATION

Malignant cells travel to distant sites from the primary neoplasm most commonly through the lymphatic and blood vessels. Malignant cells move from lymphatic to blood vessels and vice versa. A malignant neoplasm of just a few grams may shed several million cells into the circulation every day. The vast majority of tumor cells that enter the circulation will not survive. Fibrin deposits, platelet aggregation, and adhesion around tumor emboli are all factors that may protect circulating tumor cells from destruction from mechanical trauma or host immunity.[10]

Lymphatic Dissemination

As the tumor invades surrounding tissue, it penetrates the small lymphatic vessels. Tumor emboli may be trapped in the first lymph node encountered, or may bypass some nodes to form "skip" metastases. The pattern of lymph node involvement depends on the site of the primary tumor and its lymphatic drainage.[10] The lymph node often enlarges, which may be caused by a localized reaction to the tumor cells or by growth of the tumor within the node. Whether lymph nodes can retain tumor cells and prevent their further dissemination remains controversial.[10]

There are numerous venous-lymphatic communications by which tumor cells can pass between the blood and lymph systems. The main communication lies at the thoracic duct, where lymphatic fluid empties directly into the venous circulation.

Hematogenous Dissemination

For a tumor to shed cells into the circulation, the tumor cell must penetrate the capillary basement membrane. This penetration is accomplished by the tumor cell attaching to the basement membrane and then secreting degradative enzymes such as collagenase IV, which induces lysis of the membrane matrix.[20] Tumor then may grow at the site of vascular spread, or it may embolize to other parts of the body. Most tumor cells do not survive the turbulence of circulating blood; chances for survival improve if the tumor cells aggregate with one another or with host cells, such as platelets or leukocytes. The larger the clump of cells, the easier it is to become mechanically wedged into a small vessel. Attachment is also enhanced by localized trauma; tissue damaged physically, chemically, or even by reduction of oxygen tension provides for a better site for tumor cell attachment.[10]

TABLE 3-6

TUMOR–HOST INTERACTION DURING THE METASTATIC CASCADE

METASTATIC CASCADE EVENT	POTENTIAL MECHANISMS
1. Tumor initiation	Carcinogenic insult, oncogene activation or derepression, chromosome rearrangement
2. Promotion and progression	Karyotypic, genetic, and epigenetic instability; gene and amplification; promotion of associated genes hormones
3. Uncontrolled proliferation	Autocrine growth factors or their receptors; receptors for host hormones such as estrogen
4. Angiogenesis	Multiple angiogenesis factors including known growth factors
5. Invasion of local tissues, blood, and lymphatic vessels	Serum chemoattractants, autocrine motility factors, attachment receptors, degradative enzymes
6. Circulating tumor-cell arrest and extravasation	Tumor-cell homotypic or heterotypic aggregation
a. Adherence to endothelium	Tumor-cell interaction with fibrin, platelets, and clotting factors; adhesion to RGD-type receptors
b. Retraction of endothelium	Platelet factors, tumor-cell factors
c. Adhesion to basement membrane	Laminin receptor, thrombospondin receptor
d. Dissolution of basement membrane	Degradative proteases, type IV collagenase, heparanase, cathepsins
e. Locomotion	Autocrine motility factors; chemotaxis factors
7. Colony formation at secondary site	Receptors for local tissue growth factors; angiogenesis factors
8. Evasion of host defenses and resistance to therapy	Resistance to killing by host macrophages, natural killer cells and activated T cells; failure to express or blocking of tumor specific antigens; amplification of drug resistance genes

(From DeVita, V. T., Hellman, S., & Rosenberg S. A. [1997]. *Cancer: Principles and practice of oncology* [5th ed.]. Philadelphia: Lippincott.)

ARREST, ESTABLISHMENT, AND PROLIFERATION

After becoming trapped in the small vessels of the arteries or veins, the aberrant clump of malignant cells must break through the vessel into the interstitial spaces to continue to grow. Cell-free spaces in the endothelial lining of the capillary bed appear to be induced by the malignant cells, a process that involves alterations in cellular adhesion and consequent retraction of the endothelial cells. A new environment conducive to cellular growth must be established after the malignant cells have entered the interstitial spaces.

After the clump of malignant cells has grown to exceed about 2 cm in diameter, it can no longer supply its nutritional needs by diffusion. Its own blood supply becomes essential for further development. The establishment of a blood supply is the factor that changes a self-contained clump of malignant cells into a rapidly growing metastatic tumor. By secreting tumor angiogenesis factor, the tumor causes the blood vessels to send out new capillaries. These new vessels grow toward and eventually penetrate the malignant cell, creating a blood supply to nourish the tumor. Proliferation of metastatic cells depends on the outcome of the tumor's interaction with the host tissues and the net balance of positive or negative regulators, such as stimulatory growth factors or tissue-specific inhibitors.[10] Flowchart 3-2 shows the possible outcomes of metastasis from the primary tumor.

SITES OF METASTASIS

Primary tumors have a tendency to metastasize to and grow in specific organs. For example, cancer of the breast metastasizes to the lungs and brain, whereas cancer of the prostate or adrenals metastasizes to the bone. The site of the metastatic neoplasm is not randomly chosen but may be based on mechanical considerations involving cellular size, pressure, vessel size, and other physical features. Also, the site of metastasis may be similar to the site that fostered the primary growth. Vascularity of the secondary site is essential, and the entrapment of the cells in a capillary network may allow for an environment conducive to secondary growth.

Clinical Manifestations of Neoplasms

In their earliest stages of development, malignant neoplasms are asymptomatic. The mass of cells simply is not large enough to interfere with any bodily functions. As the tumor increases in size, local alterations in function occur. As malignant neoplasms grow and metastasize,

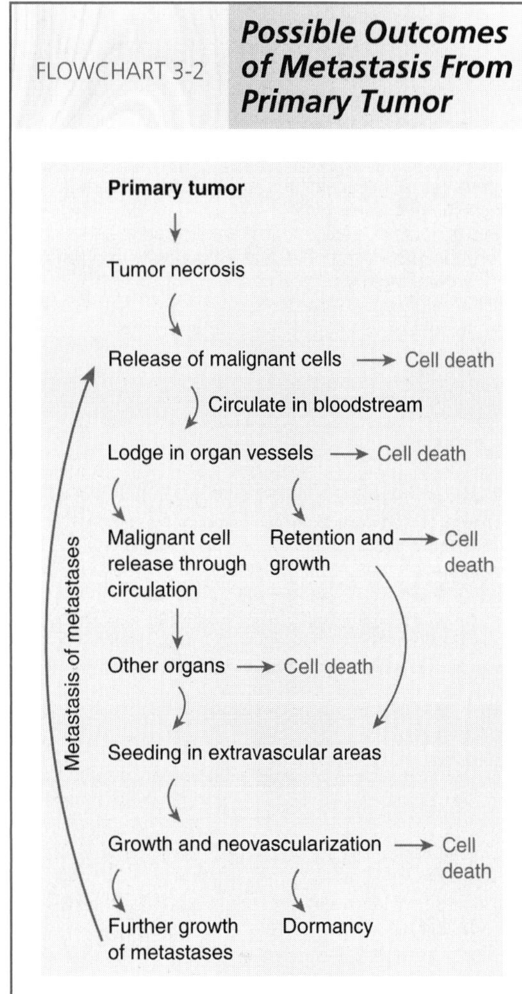

FLOWCHART 3-2 **Possible Outcomes of Metastasis From Primary Tumor**

they interfere with function at distant sites and disrupt the biochemical and nutritional balances of the body.

LOCAL MANIFESTATIONS

The nature and development of local symptomatology depends on the location of the neoplasm and on the size and distensibility of the space it occupies. A neoplasm located in the abdomen, which is large and distensible, may grow to considerable size without producing symptoms. A neoplasm the size of a pea located in the cranial vault, a rigid space controlling vital sensory and motor function, may cause major symptoms.

A tumor can compress surrounding tissues, organs, and their blood supply. The resulting symptomatology is related to interference with blood supply, interference with function, and mobilization of compensatory mechanisms and immune responses. Flowchart 3-3 depicts local manifestations of neoplastic growth.

SYSTEMIC MANIFESTATIONS

Neoplasms have systemic as well as local effects. Systemic symptoms may be the first indication that a person has a malignant neoplasm, and they often accompany advanced metastatic disease. These symptoms include anorexia, nausea, weight loss, and malaise, as well as signs and symptoms of anemia and infection. They reflect system-wide alterations in body processes. The term used to describe these multiple syndromes is **paraneoplastic syndromes**. Significant paraneoplastic syndromes involve the endocrine, nervous, hematologic, renal, and gastrointestinal systems.

ENDOCRINE PARANEOPLASTIC SYNDROME. This results from hormones produced by nonendocrine neoplastic tissues. Symptoms that result vary with the hormone produced.[9] For example, carcinomas of the lung, thymus, and pancreas can produce adrenocorticotropic hormone, causing the person to experience symptoms of Cushing's syndrome.[24] Another example is the hypercalcemia often associated with multiple

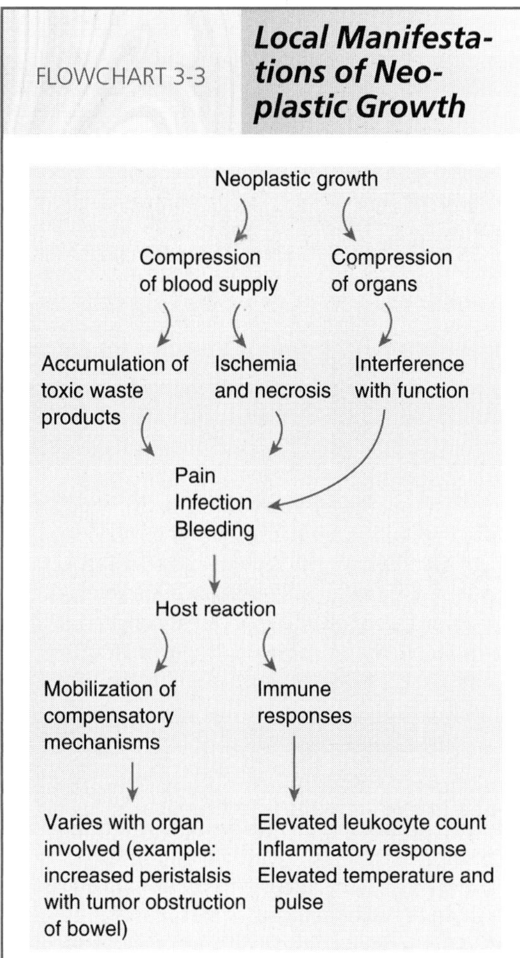

FLOWCHART 3-3 **Local Manifestations of Neoplastic Growth**

myeloma and carcinomas of the lung, kidney, ovary, and other neoplasms. The solid tumors produce hypercalcemia by producing a parathyroid hormone-like agent; in multiple myeloma, the cause is the production of lymphotoxin and tumor necrosis factor, both of which are potent stimulators of bone resorption.[24]

Neurologic Paraneoplastic Syndromes. These are caused by the stimulation of antibody production by the cancer. These antibodies react with neuronal antigens, thereby damaging normal tissue.[24] The symptoms can be grouped according to the area involved: cerebral, spinal cord, or peripheral nerves. Cerebral symptoms include ataxia, dysarthria, hypotonia, abnormal reflexes, dementia, and coma. Spinal cord symptoms include muscle weakness, atrophy, spasticity, hyperreflexia, and paralysis. Peripheral nerve symptoms include sensory loss, weakness, wasting, and depressed reflexes.

Hematologic Paraneoplastic Syndromes. These include polycythemia, which may result from an erythropoietin-secreting tumor; disseminated intravascular coagulation, which is initiated by tumor secretions; and thrombocytopenia, which is possibly related to tumor production of antiplatelet antibodies and may be a manifestation of idiopathic thrombocytopenic purpura or aplastic anemia.

Renal Paraneoplastic Syndromes. These syndromes, such as membranous glomerulonephritis, are most commonly associated with carcinomas of the lung, breast, and gastrointestinal tract.[24] Membranous glomerulonephritis is caused by tumor-associated antigens forming immune complexes that precipitate in the glomeruli; they may cause renal failure.

Gastrointestinal Paraneoplastic Syndromes. These include malabsorption, liver dysfunction, and anorexia-cachexia. More than 90% of persons with advanced disease have a low serum albumin, which may result from the loss of protein into the gut or poor absorption of protein from the intestines. Liver enlargement and decreased function may be associated with the hypoalbuminemia. The anorexia-cachexia syndrome is a common change seen in most persons with advanced malignant disease. This syndrome is manifested by anorexia, loss of body fat, protein loss, depletion of essential nutrients, water and electrolyte imbalance, and major weight loss. A significant loss of taste, competition of the tumor and host for nutrients, and the treatment for cancer contributes to the perpetuation of this syndrome. It is a classic illustration of malnutrition and may manifest as starvation or kwashiorkor.

Generalized Effects. Generalized effects from paraneoplastic phenomena include metabolic alterations such as lactic acidosis, hyperlipidemia, amylase elevation, and muscle and joint alterations. Fever frequently occurs and, in this case, involves an unexplained temperature elevation that subsides with the destruction of the cancer but recurs with its reappearance. Tumor fever occurs with a variety of neoplasms such as Hodgkin's disease and renal adenocarcinoma.[24]

REFERENCES

1. Abeloff, M. D., Armitage, J. O., Lichter, A. S., & Niederhuber, J. E. (1995). *Clinical oncology.* New York: Churchill Livingstone.
2. Averette, H. E., & Nguyen, H. (1995). Gynecologic cancer. In G. P. Murphy, W. Lawrence, Jr., & R. E. Lenhard, Jr. (Eds.), *American Cancer Society textbook of clinical oncology* (2nd ed.). Atlanta, GA: American Cancer Society.
3. Bal, D. G., Nixon, D. W., Foerster, S. B., & Brownson, R. C. (1995). Cancer prevention. In G. P. Murphy, W. Lawrence, Jr., & R. E. Lenhard, Jr. (Eds.), *American Cancer Society textbook of clinical oncology* (2nd ed.). Atlanta, GA: American Cancer Society.
4. Bresnick, E. (1997). Biochemistry of cancer. In J. F. Holland, R. C. Bast, Jr., D. L. Morton, E. Frei, III, D. W. Kufe, & R. R. Weichselbaum (Eds.), *Cancer medicine* (4th ed.). Baltimore: Williams & Wilkins.
5. Casciato, D. A., & Lowitz, B. B. (1995). *Manual of clinical oncology* (3rd ed.). Boston: Little, Brown.
6. Cavalli, F., Hansen, H. H., & Kaye, S. B. (1997). *Textbook of medical oncology.* St. Louis: Mosby.
7. Clinton, S. K., & Giovannucci, E. L. (1997). Nutrition in the etiology and prevention of cancer. In J. F. Holland, R. C. Bast, Jr., D. L. Morton, E. Frei, III, D. W. Kufe, & R. R. Weichselbaum (Eds.), *Cancer medicine* (4th ed.). Baltimore: Williams & Wilkins.
8. Cole, P., & Rodu, B. (1996). Declining cancer mortality in the United States. *Cancer, 78,* 2045–2048.
9. DeVita, V. T., Jr., Hellman, S., & Rosenberg, S. A. (1997). *Cancer: Principles & practice of oncology* (5th ed.). Philadelphia: Lippincott-Raven.
10. Fidler, I. J. (1997). Molecular biology of cancer: Invasion and metastasis. In V. T. DeVita, Jr., S. Hellman, & S. A. Rosenberg (Eds.), *Cancer: Principles & practice of oncology* (5th ed.). Philadelphia: Lippincott-Raven.
11. Fingert, H. J., Campisi, J., & Pardee, A. B. (1997). Cell proliferation and differentiation. In J. F. Holland, R. C. Bast, Jr., D. L. Morton, E. Frei, III, D. W. Kufe, R. R. Weichselbaum (Eds.), *Cancer medicine* (4th ed.). Baltimore: Williams & Wilkins.
12. Folkman, J. (1997). Tumor angiogenesis. In J. F. Holland, R. C. Bast, Jr., D. L. Morton, E. Frei, III, D. W. Kufe, R. R. Weichselbaum (Eds.), *Cancer medicine* (4th ed.). Baltimore: Williams & Wilkins.
13. Frederick, P. L., & Kantor, A. F. (1997). Cancer epidemiology. In J. F. Holland, R. C. Bast, D. L. Morton, E. Frei, III, D. W. Kufe, & R. R. Weichselbaum, (Eds.), *Cancer medicine* (4th ed.). Baltimore: Williams & Wilkins.
14. Garfinkel, L. (1995). Cancer statistics and trends. In G. P. Murphy, W. Lawrence, Jr., & R. E. Lenhard, Jr. (Eds.), *American Cancer Society textbook of clinical oncology* (2nd ed.). Atlanta, GA: American Cancer Society.
15. Haskell, C. M., & Casciato, D. A. (1995). Breast cancer. In D. A. Casciato & B. B. Lowitz (Eds.), *Manual of clinical oncology* (3rd ed.). Boston: Little, Brown.
16. Henderson, B. E., Bernstein, L., & Ross, R. K. (1997). Hormones and the etiology of cancer. In J. F. Holland, R. C. Bast, Jr., D. L. Morton, E. Frei, III, D. W. Kufe, & R. R. Weichselbaum (Eds.), *Cancer medicine* (4th ed.). Baltimore: Williams & Wilkins.
17. Holland, J. F., Bast, R. C., Jr., Morton, D. L., Frei, E., III, Kufe, D. W., & Weichselbaum, R. R. (1997). *Cancer medicine* (4th ed.). Baltimore: Williams & Wilkins, 1997.

18. Howley, P. M. (1995). Viral carcinogenesis. In J. Mendelsohn, P. M. Howley, M. A. Israel, & L. A. Liotta (Eds.), *The molecular basis of cancer.* Philadelphia: Saunders.
19. Landis, S. H., Murray, T., Bolden, S., & Wingo, P. A. (1998). Cancer statistics, 1998. *CA: A Cancer Journal for Clinicians, 48*(1), 6–29.
20. Liotta, L. A., & Kohn, E. C. (1997). Invasion and metastasis. In J. F. Holland, R. C. Bast, Jr., D. L. Morton, E. Frei, III, D. W. Kufe, & R. R. Weichselbaum (Eds.), *Cancer medicine* (4th ed). Baltimore: Williams & Wilkins.
21. Little, J. B. (1997). Ionizing radiation. In J. F. Holland, R. C. Bast, Jr., D. L. Morton, E. Frei III, D, W, Kufe, & R. R. Weichselbaum. (Eds.), *Cancer medicine* (4th ed.). Baltimore: Williams & Wilkins.
22. Mendelsohn, J., Howley, P. M., Israel, M. A., & Liotta, L. A. (1995). *The molecular basis of cancer.* Philadelphia: Saunders.
23. Murphy, G. P., Lawrence W., Jr., & Lenhard R. E., Jr. (1995). *American Cancer Society textbook of clinical oncology* (2nd ed.). Atlanta, GA: American Cancer Society.
24. Odell, W. D. (1997). Paraneoplastic syndromes. In J. F. Holland, R. C. Bast, Jr., D. L. Morton, E. Frei, III, D. W. Kufe, & R. R. Weichselbaum (Eds.), *Cancer medicine* (4th ed.). Baltimore: Williams & Wilkins.
25. Pfeifer, J. D., & Wick, M. R. (1995). The pathologic evaluation of neoplastic diseases. In G. P. Murphy, W. Lawrence, Jr., & R. E. Lenhard, Jr. (Eds.), *American Cancer Society textbook of clinical oncology* (2nd ed.). Atlanta, GA: American Cancer Society.
26. Poeschla, E. M., & Wong-Staal, F. (1997). Etiology of cancer: viruses. In V. T. DeVita Jr., S. Hellman, & S. A. Rosenberg (Eds.), *Cancer: Principles & practice of oncology* (5th ed.). Philadelphia: Lippincott-Raven.
27. Rosenthal, D. S. (1998). Changing trends. *CA: A Cancer Journal for Clinicians, 48*(1), 3–4.
28. Schichman, S. A., & Croce, C. H. (1997). Oncogenes. In J. F. Holland, R. C. Bast, Jr., D. L. Morton, E. Frei, III, D. W. Kufe, & R. R. Weichselbaum (Eds.), *Cancer medicine* (4th ed.). Baltimore: Williams & Wilkins.
29. Schottenfeld, D. (1995). Epidemiology. In M. D. Abeloff, J. O. Armitage, A. S. Lichter, & J. E. Niederhuber (Eds.), *Clinical oncology.* New York: Churchill Livingstone.
30. Tabbarah, H. J., Lowitz, B. B., & Livingston, R. B. (1995). Lung cancer. In D. A. Casciato & B. B. Lowitz (Eds.), *Manual of clinical oncology* (3rd ed.). Boston: Little, Brown.
31. Templeton, D. J., & Weinberg, R. A. (1995). Principles of cancer biology. In G. P. Murphy, W. Lawrence, Jr., & R. E. Lenhard, Jr. (Eds.), *American Cancer Society textbook of clinical oncology* (2nd ed.). Atlanta, GA: American Cancer Society.
32. Weinstein, I. B., Carothers, A. M., Santella, R. M., & Perera, F. P. (1995). Molecular mechanisms of mutagenesis and multistage carcinogenesis. In J. Mendelsohn, P. M. Howley, M. A. Israel, & L. A. Liotta (Eds.), *The molecular basis of cancer.* Philadelphia: Saunders.
33. Weisburger, J. H., & Williams, G. M. (1995). Causes of cancer. In G. P. Murphy, W. Lawrence, Jr., & R. E. Lenhard, Jr. (Eds.), *American Cancer Society textbook of clinical oncology* (2nd ed.). Atlanta, GA: American Cancer Society.
34. Weiss, G. (1993). *Clinical oncology.* Norwalk, CT: Appleton & Lange.
35. Weston, A., & Harris, C. C. (1997). Chemical carcinogenesis. In J. F. Holland, R. C. Bast, Jr., D. L. Morton, E. Frei, III, D. W. Kufe, & R. R. Weichselbaum (Eds.), *Cancer medicine* (4th ed.). Baltimore: Williams & Wilkins.
36. Yuspa, S. H., & Shields, P. G. (1997). Etiology of cancer: Chemical factors. In V. T. DeVita Jr., S. Hellman, & S. A. Rosenberg (Eds.), *Cancer: Principles & practice of oncology* (5th ed.). Philadelphia: Lippincott-Raven.

Chapter 4

Developmental Stages and Health Alterations

Sharron Schlosser / Laurie Kaudewitz / Barbara Bullock / Gretchen McDaniel

KEY TERMS

amphetamine
anorexia nervosa
basal metabolic rate
Bouchard's nodes
bulimia nervosa
chronic fatigue syndrome
cocaine
eclampsia
Heberden's nodes
HELLP syndrome
hyperkeratotic warts
hyperplasia
hypertrophy
kyphosis
morula
opioid
osteoarthritis
osteoporosis
pharmacokinetic factors
preeclampsia
pregnancy-induced hypertension
presbyopia
telangiectasias

This chapter deals with the effect of developmental changes on the susceptibility of the individual to various health problems. These health problems range from those related to growth and development to those dominated by degenerative changes. Throughout the life span, life-styles affect the health of the individual. The chapter is organized into the following major sections: (1) reproduction, (2) infancy through adolescence, (3) adult, and (4) older adult. The focus of the chapter is on health implications of the various stages of life.

BIOPHYSICAL DEVELOPMENT OF REPRODUCTION

Gestation begins with fertilization of the ovum and continues throughout development of the fetus. The duration of gestation is approximately 280 days, or 10 lunar months from the last menstrual period. Typically, the period of gestation is divided into three 3-month periods, termed *trimesters*. During this time, two processes account for the biophysical development of the fetus—**hyperplasia** and **hypertrophy**. Hyperplasia refers to an increased number of cells. whereas hypertrophy indicates increased cell size (see page 43). The early first trimester (first 12 weeks after conception) is characterized by hyperplasia, in which mitotic cellular division accounts for an increase in the number of cells but the size of the cells remains relatively stable. The second trimester (weeks 13–24) is characterized by both hyperplasia and hypertrophy. The process of hypertrophy predominates in the third trimester (week 25 to birth). During this third trimester, the fetus experiences a very rapid period of growth; the number of cells does not change but rather those cells present increase significantly in size.

Fetal Development

The biophysical development of the fetus is traditionally divided into three stages: the germinal period (also referred to as the period of the ovum), the embryonic period, and the fetal period (Table 4-1).

GERMINAL PERIOD

Within hours of fertilization, the process of mitosis begins, usually in the outer third of the fallopian tube. Mitotic cell division continues every 10 to 12 hours throughout the zygote's journey through the fallopian tube. The day-by-day development of the **morula**

(text continues on page 91)

TABLE 4-1

FETAL DEVELOPMENT

PERIOD/TIME	PHYSIOLOGIC DEVELOPMENT	ILLUSTRATION
PERIOD OF THE OVUM Encompasses the first 2 wk following conception		
Within hours of fertilization	Mitosis begins usually in outer third of the fallopian tube.	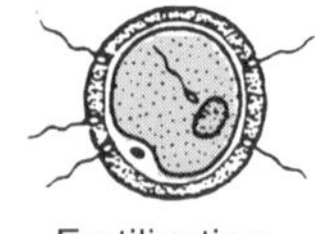 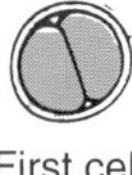
3 days	Fertilized ovum has become 16-cell *morula*.	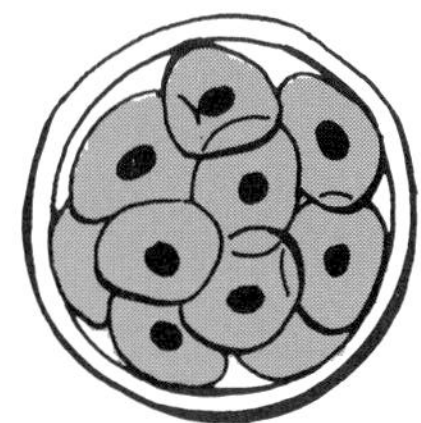
4 days	Cells of morula begin to differentiate into two layers with fluid-filled space. The cell mass is now known as *blastocyst* with the outer layer called the *trophoblast*. Inner cluster of cells is termed inner cell mass or *embryoblast* and eventually becomes the embryo.	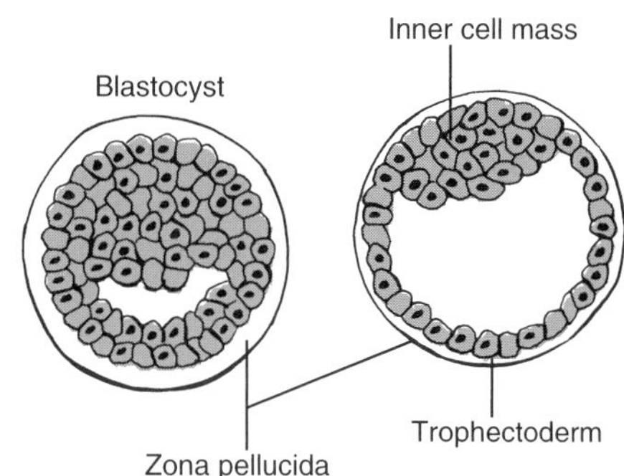
8 days	Implantation process begins. Proteolytic enzymes from trophoblast digest endometrium. Process results in erosion of blood vessels and results in pools of maternal blood, which act as site of exchange between nutrients and waste products.	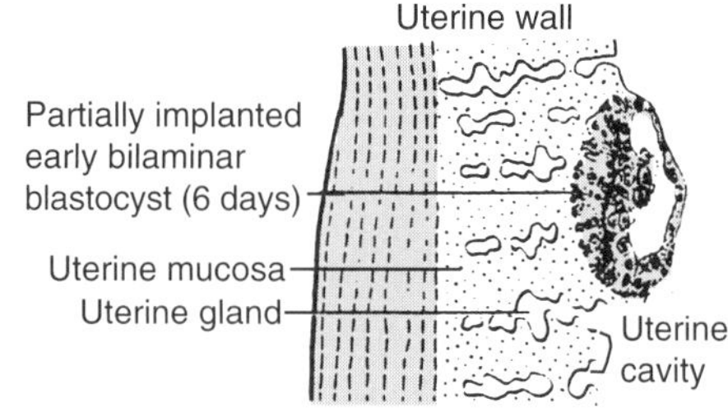
11 days	Implantation process complete. Secretion of human chorionic gonadotropin by implanting trophoblast.	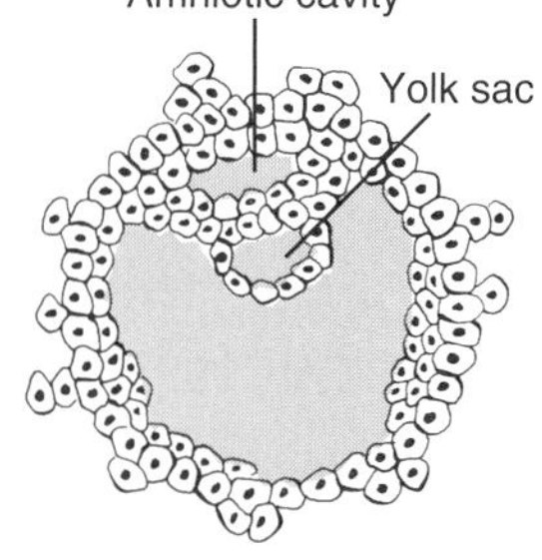

TABLE 4-1

FETAL DEVELOPMENT (Continued)

PERIOD/TIME	PHYSIOLOGIC DEVELOPMENT	ILLUSTRATION
EMBRYONIC PERIOD From complete implantation through 8th wk of development.	Evolution of two germ layers: endoderm, which gives rise to primitive yolk; and the ectoderm, which gives rise to the amniotic sac.	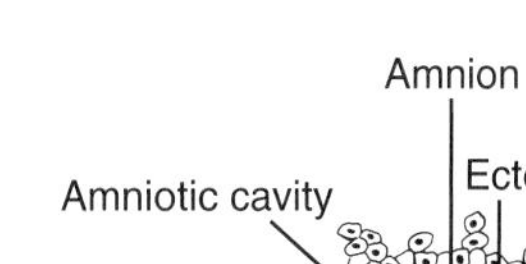
16 days	Differentiation of embryonic disk cells into third primary germ layer—the mesoderm. Chorionic villi begin to form from trophoblasts.	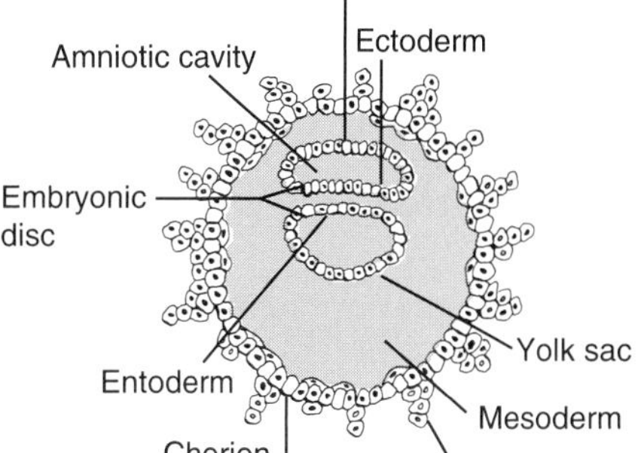
22 days	Ectoderm folds into neural tube, from which brain, head, and spinal cord develop. Two tubes form in mesoderm and fuse to form fetal heart. Eyes, ears, nose, and mouth begin to take shape.	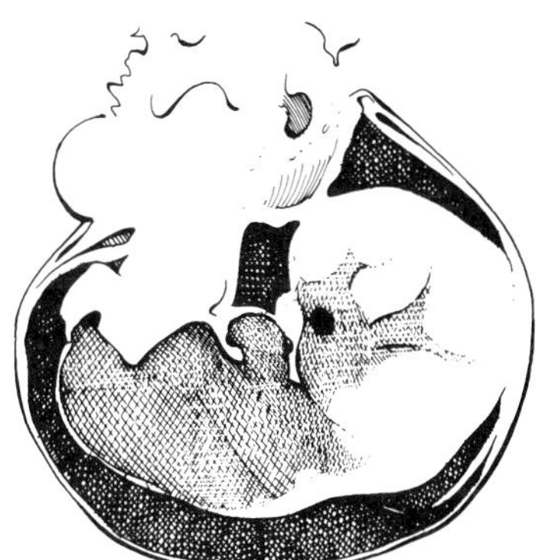
26 days	Arm and leg buds appear, followed by elbows and knees. Fingers and toes lose webbing. External genitalia become evident but are not distinguishable. Embryo measures approximately 3 cm (1.2 in.) from crown to rump and weighs about 2–4 g	
FETAL PERIOD 9th wk to birth of fetus		
9 weeks	Head accounts for 50% of overall body length	
12 weeks	Fetal circulation and placenta complete Distinct fingers and toes Fetus measure 6–9 cm and weighs about 45 g	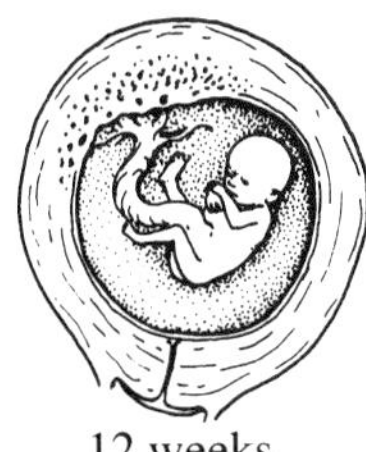 12 weeks
16 weeks	12-cm fetus, weighing about 110 g Distinguishable sex Heartbeat Urine secreted by developing kidneys	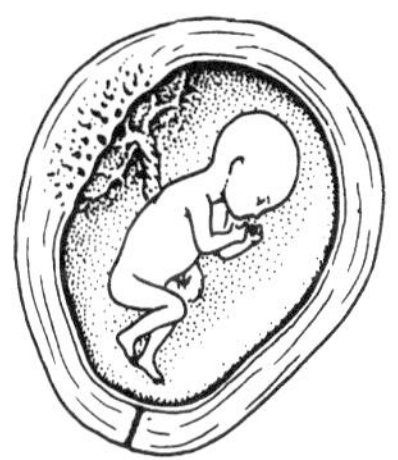 16 weeks

(continued)

TABLE 4-1

FETAL DEVELOPMENT (Continued)

PERIOD/TIME	PHYSIOLOGIC DEVELOPMENT	ILLUSTRATION
20 weeks	Lanugo develops over body Reflexes appear Fetal movement evident to mother 19-cm fetus, weighing 300 g Audible heartbeat with fetoscope	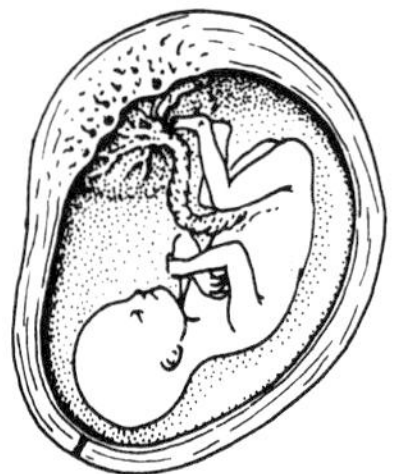 20 weeks
24 weeks	Vernix caseosa appears Skin wrinkled Eyebrows and fingernails present Fetus measures 23 cm and weighs 630 g	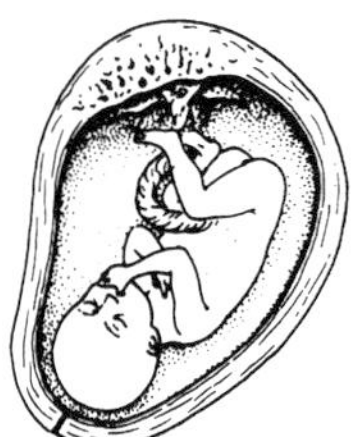 24 weeks
28 weeks	Red skin Eyes free of pupillary membrane 27-cm fetus, weighing 1100 g Increased chance of survival if delivered	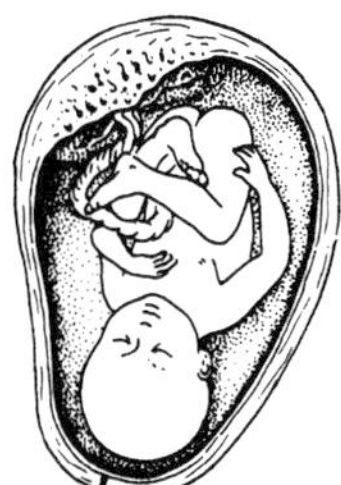 28 weeks
32 weeks	Active fetal movement Open eyelids Viable fetus weighing 1,800 g and measuring 28–30 cm in length	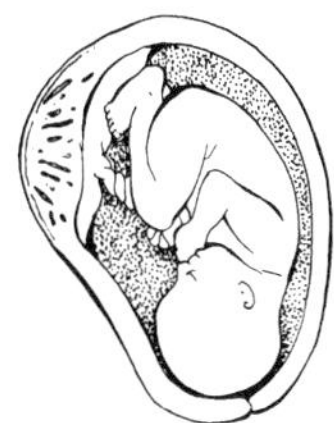 32 weeks
36 weeks	Disappearance of lanugo Decrease in amniotic fluid Lack of subcutaneous fat produces loose wrinkled appearance of face and body Fetus measures about 32 cm and weighs about 2,500 g	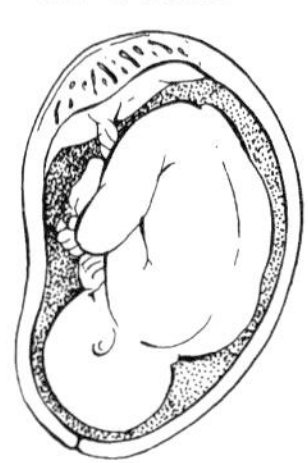 36 weeks

TABLE 4-1

FETAL DEVELOPMENT (Continued)

PERIOD/TIME	PHYSIOLOGIC DEVELOPMENT	ILLUSTRATION
40 weeks	Fully developed fetus measuring approximately 36 cm in length and weighing 3,000–3,600 Smooth skin with slate-colored eyes	40 weeks

into the blastocyst and the implantation process are illustrated in Table 4-1. The secretion of *human chorionic gonadotropin*, which causes a positive pregnancy test, is responsible for the continued functioning of the corpus luteum and resultant production of progesterone.

EMBRYONIC PERIOD

The embryonic period begins with the complete implantation of the blastocyst and extends through the eighth week of prenatal development.[21] Four major accomplishments are associated with this period of development: rapid growth, placenta formation and function, early structural development of organs, and development of a form that is recognizable as a human being. Three primary germ layers—endoderm, ectoderm, and mesoderm—evolve and eventually give rise to all major fetal organs. Table 4-2 lists the structures evolving from each of the three layers.

TABLE 4-2

EVOLUTION OF BODY ORGANS FROM PRIMARY GERM LAYERS

ENDODERM	MESODERM	ECTODERM
Gastrointestinal system	Skin	Epidermis
Liver, pancreas	Bones	Hair, nails
Trachea, lungs	Muscle	Urethra
Pharynx	Heart, blood	Teeth enamel
Thyroid	Spleen	Nervous system
Tonsils	Kidneys, ureters	Mammary glands
	Ovaries, uterus	
	Testes	

FETAL PERIOD

The fetal period begins with the ninth week and terminates with the birth of the fetus, at approximately 40 weeks' gestation. As the embryo enters this stage of biophysical development, the head accounts for about 50% of the overall body length, and human characteristics are evident. Month by month development of the fetus is illustrated in Table 4-1.

Support Structures

The support structures for fetal development include the placenta, the fetal membranes, the yolk sac, and the fetal circulation.

PLACENTA

The blastocyst is covered with a layer of cells known as the trophoblast. Those trophoblasts in direct contact with the endometrium produce finger-like projections called *chorionic villi* that invade and digest the endometrium (see Table 4-1). This invasive process results in erosion of the maternal blood vessels in the endometrium and formation of maternal lakes filled with maternal blood. The placenta is formed from the fusion of the endometrium and enlarging chorionic villi. Tiny blood vessels also form in the chorionic villi. These vessels carry fetal blood that does not mix with the maternal blood.

The processes of diffusion and active transport account for the exchange of nutrients, oxygen, and waste products in the placenta after completion of its development (by the third month). The levels of estrogen and progesterone, originally produced by the corpus luteum (of the ovaries), are now maintained by the placenta. The placenta functions as a barrier to infection, as an endocrine gland in the production of estrogen and progesterone, and as the organ of metabolic and nutrient exchange. The fetal surface of the placenta is covered with the amnion. At term (38–42 weeks) the placenta measures approximately 15 to 20 cm in diameter, 2.5 to 3.0 cm in thickness, and weighs about 400 to 600 g.

The umbilical cord results from the elongation of the body stalk, which connects the embryo to the yolk sac. Tiny blood vessels develop and extend into the chorionic villi. As the body stalk elongates, these tiny vessels merge into the umbilical vein and two umbilical arteries. These blood vessels are protected by a special connective tissue referred to as Wharton's jelly. At term, the umbilical cord measures approximately 2 cm in diameter and is about 50 to 60 cm in length. It coils about 11 times between fetal and placental insertion sites.[55] Straight or noncoiled umbilical vessels have been associated with stillbirth, increased rates of intrapartum fetal heart rate decelerations, meconium staining, fetal anomalies, oligohydramnios, and preterm delivery (see page 101).[55]

FETAL MEMBRANES

The chorion and the amnion are the fetal membranes that constitute the "bag of water." Parts of the trophoblasts not directly involved with the implantation process soon begin to degenerate and form the chorion or outer lining. The amnion is a smooth membrane that evolves from the ectoderm and forms the inner lining of the bag of waters. The amnion secretes amniotic fluid, in volumes of 500 to 1,500 mL. Amniotic fluid functions to regulate temperature, aid in fetal movement, and protect the developing fetus from injury.

YOLK SAC

The yolk sac arises from the endoderm at about the eighth or ninth day after conception. It is responsible for production of red blood cells (RBCs) for about 6 weeks, until the fetal liver is capable of this function. However, it is not responsible for the developing embryo's nutrition. The yolk sac detaches after the end of the sixth week and shrinks.

FETAL CIRCULATION

Three unique structures function during fetal development to provide sufficient blood flow for metabolic and nutritional functions of the placenta: the ductus venosus, the foramen ovale, and the ductus arteriosus. Oxygenated and nourished blood from the placenta enters the fetus through the umbilical vein. Soon after it enters the abdominal wall, the umbilical vain branches. The smaller branch enters the hepatic circulation and later empties into the inferior vena cava through the hepatic vein. The second, larger branch enters the inferior vena cava directly through the ductus venosus. Blood from the inferior vena cava empties directly into the right atrium, where it mixes with blood from the superior vena cava. The majority of this blood passes through the foramen ovale and into the left atrium, where it mixes with deoxygenated blood from the lungs. This blood is then pumped into the left ventricle and out to the fetal body through the aorta. The remaining blood in the right atrium is pumped through the tricuspid valve into the right ventricle and out the pulmonary artery. Only a small portion of this blood continues to the nonfunctioning lungs to nourish them; the remainder passes through the ductus arteriosus and enters the body circulation directly. Deoxygenated blood returns to the placenta through the umbilical arteries, where the process repeats itself. Figure 17-30 illustrates the fetal circulation and direction of blood flow.

Health Alterations: Maternal and Fetal

Alterations of development may occurs during gestation due to maternal illness and infections that affect the intrauterine environment and the development of the fetus. Fetal alterations also may occur due to genetic influences, placental anomalies, and multiple pregnancies. The first 2 months of pregnancy are an especially vulnerable time in embryo development and significant fetal or uterine anomalies often result in spontaneous abortion.

MATERNAL ILLNESSES AND INFECTION

Many conditions can result in disruption of fetal development. The most common ones are: hypertensive disorders, HELLP syndrome, diabetes mellitus, cardiac diseases, acute fatty liver of pregnancy, and sexually transmitted diseases and infections.

Hypertensive Disorders of Pregnancy

Pregnancy-induced hypertension (PIH) occurs in 8% to 11% of all pregnancies.[65] It is the second leading cause of maternal death and a major cause of perinatal mortality in the United States. The term PIH, or **preeclampsia**, is used to describe the combination of hypertension, edema, and proteinuria during pregnancy. The term **eclampsia** is used for this syndrome when the clinical course deteriorates to convulsions or coma.

ETIOLOGY AND PATHOPHYSIOLOGY. The cause of PIH, formerly known as toxemia, is still unknown. Recently two biochemical imbalances have been described, which could account for the clinical manifestations of PIH: (1) increased thromboxane and decreased prostacyclin and (2) increased oxidative stress and lipid peroxidation with antioxidant deficiencies.[61] Thromboxane, a potent vasoconstrictor, stimulates platelet aggregation and uterine contractility, resulting in uteroplacental insufficiency. Prostacyclin, a potent vasodilator, inhibits platelet aggregation and uterine contractility, resulting in increased uteroplacental blood flow. Thus, normal pregnancy is supported by prostacyclin while preeclampsia is supported by thromboxane and decreased uteroplacental blood flow. Flowchart 4-1 illustrates the pathophysiology of the uteroplacental blood flow in PIH. PIH frequently causes the infant to be growth retarded or born prematurely because of decreased placental perfusion. The infant may also suffer from hypoxia and acidosis if the mother experiences eclampsia.

Clinical Manifestations. Hypertension during pregnancy may lead to preeclampsia, eclampsia, cerebral vascular accidents, cardiac failure, aspiration pneumonia, or abruptio placenta. Preeclampsia may occur during pregnancy or early in the postpartal period and is characterized by hypertension, edema, and albuminuria. When convulsions and coma complicate the preeclamptic state, it is termed eclampsia and may be life threatening. Discussions of cerebral vascular accidents, aspiration pneumonia, and congestive heart failure are found in other sections of the text. Abruptio placenta is discussed on pp. 101. The American College of Obstetricians and Gynecologists has developed a classification system based on diagnostic criteria to differentiate and categorize the various types of hypertensive diseases.[2] Criteria for the various types of hypertensive diseases listed in Box 4-1 are based on this classification.

FLOWCHART 4-1 **Pregnancy-Induced Hypertension**

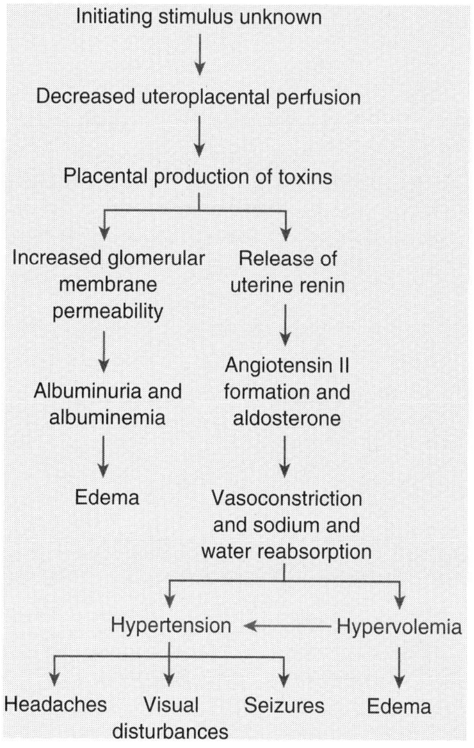

Initiating stimulus unknown
↓
Decreased uteroplacental perfusion
↓
Placental production of toxins
↓ (two branches)

- Increased glomerular membrane permeability → Albuminuria and albuminemia → Edema
- Release of uterine renin → Angiotensin II formation and aldosterone → Vasoconstriction and sodium and water reabsorption

Vasoconstriction and sodium and water reabsorption → Hypertension; Hypervolemia
Hypervolemia → Hypertension
Hypervolemia → Edema
Hypertension → Headaches; Visual disturbances; Seizures

HELLP Syndrome

HELLP syndrome is a variant of PIH that can be fatal for both mother and fetus. It occurs in 2% to 12% of severe preeclampsia and is more frequent in white women and multiparas.[23,51] The characteristics of HELLP are hemolysis (H), elevated liver enzymes (EL), and a low platelet count (LP). HELLP always occurs in association with PIH. Flowchart 4-2 outlines the pathophysiology that occurs in HELLP. Signs and symptoms of HELLP syndrome include nausea and vomiting (50%), malaise over several days (90%), epigastric or right upper quadrant pain (65%), and swelling. Because HELLP syndrome symptoms may be present before the symptoms of PIH, it is often misdiagnosed as disseminated intravascular coagulation, acute hepatitis, gallbladder disease, or other conditions.[51]

Diabetes Mellitus

Diabetes mellitus (DM), either preexisting or gestational, is a challenging condition during pregnancy. Approximately 4% of all pregnancies are complicated by diabetes. Of this number, approximately 90% are gestational (first detected in pregnancy) with the remaining 10% experiencing prepregnant diabetes (either type 1 or type 2; see page 713).[29] Two well known classification systems provide guidelines for understanding the pregnant diabetic. White's classification is summarized in Table 4-3 with associated implications. The National Diabetic Data Group has classified diabetes according to the cause and contributing factors (Box 4-2).

Etiology and Pathophysiology of Gestational Diabetes. Most women who develop gestational diabetes mellitus (GDM) do not have a previous history of carbohydrate intolerance. Risk factors for GDM include obesity, maternal age over 30, hypertension, family history of diabetes mellitus, and previous birth of large (macrosomic) baby.[38] In the first 20 weeks of pregnancy the increases in estrogen and progesterone cause increased insulin production as well as increased glycogen synthesis and tissue glucose use. The actions of insulin are facilitated and significant hypoglycemia can occur. During the last 20 weeks of pregnancy, insulin resistance may be seen and plasma glucose levels elevate.

Clinical Manifestations of Diabetes Mellitus. When the blood glucose levels are controlled, there are fewer problems for both the diabetic mother and fetus. Even with controlled blood glucose levels, however, there is an increase in sudden fetal death and macrosomic neonates.[38] Clinical problems during pregnancy include all of those seen in diabetic women as well as PIH, wide blood glucose swings (from hypoglycemia to hyperglycemia), congenital anomalies, macrosomia, and problems during delivery.[38]

BOX 4-1

CLASSIFICATION OF HYPERTENSIVE DISORDERS OF PREGNANCY WITH DIAGNOSTIC CRITERIA

Pregnancy-Induced Hypertension (PIH)

Gestational hypertension: Blood pressure ≥ 140 mm Hg systolic or ≥ 90 mm Hg diastolic on two occasions at least 6 h apart.

Mild preeclampsia: Development of hypertension; proteinuria ≥ 300 mg in 24-h urine collection or ≥ 1 g/L in at least two random supine specimens collected 6 h or more apart; or edema (> 1+ pitting edema after 12 h of bed rest or weight gain of ≥ 5 lb/in 1 wk); or both proteinuria and edema

Severe: Blood pressure ≥ 160 mm Hg systolic or ≥ 110 mm Hg diastolic on two occasions at least 6 h apart, with the patient on bed rest; proteinuria ≥ 5 g in 24-h urine collection; persistent and severe cerebral or visual disturbances; persistent and severe epigastric pain or right upper-quadrant pain; pulmonary edema or cyanosis; oliguria (< 500 mL of urine in 24-h collection); or HELLP syndrome

Eclampsia: Extension of preeclampsia with tonic-clonic seizures

Chronic Hypertension

Persistent hypertension (blood pressure ≥ 140/90 mm Hg on two occasions more than 25-h apart before 20 wk of gestation or more than 42 d postpartum

Chronic Hypertension With Superimposed PIH

Elevation of systolic pressure > 30 mm Hg and diastolic > 20 mm Hg; proteinuria or generalized edema not previously present

Late or Transient Hypertension

Transient elevations of blood pressure during labor or in the early postpartum period, returning to baseline within 10 days of delivery

(American College of Obstetricians and Gynecologists [1986]. *Management of preeclampsia.* ACOG technical bulletin no. 91. Washington, DC: ACOG.)

FLOWCHART 4-2 **Pathophysiology of HELLP Syndrome**

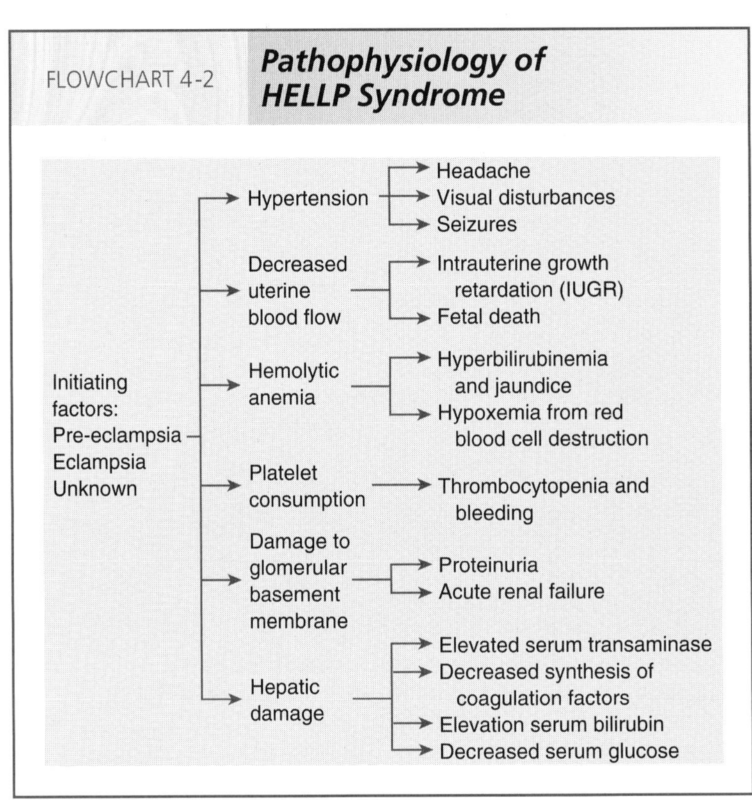

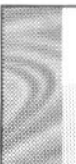

TABLE 4-3

DIABETES IN PREGNANCY WITH IMPLICATIONS

CHARACTERISTICS	IMPLICATIONS
IMPAIRED GLUCOSE HOMEOSTASIS	
Glucose intolerance diagnosed during pregnancy	Treatment with diet is adequate to maintain normal blood glucose levels; normal glucose levels are seen after fetus is born Few complications
Glucose intolerance diagnosed during pregnancy	Treatment requires administration of insulin in addition to diet Risk of fetal macrosomatia Increased risk of developing Type 1 or Type 2 diabetes
Type 2: Onset after age 20	Some endogenous insulin secretion Characterized by insulin resistance Increased risk of PIH, hypertension, fetal anomalies, and macrosomatia
Type 1: Onset between age 10 and 20	Insulin treatment *before* pregnancy Increased risk of PIH, hypertension, fetal anomalies, and macrosomatia
Type 1: Onset before age 10; duration more than 20 y	Fetal growth retardation is possible Retinopathy may accelerate during pregnancy and then regress Increased risk of PIH, hypertension, fetal anomalies, or intrauterine growth retardation possible
Type 1 or 2 with diabetic nephropathy and proteinuria	Anemia, hypertension, PIH, preterm labor common; anomalies and intrauterine growth retardation common
Type 1 or 2 with coronary artery disease	Grave maternal and fetal risk for death

(Adapted from May, K. A., & Mahlmeister, L. R. [1994]. *Maternal & neonatal nursing: Family-centered care* [3rd ed., p. 763]. Philadelphia: Lippincott; and National Diabetes Group Classification.)

COMPLICATIONS OF DIABETES MELLITUS DURING DURING PREGNANCY. Although the maternal mortality rate for the pregnant diabetic patient has decreased in recent years, maternal hyperglycemia and a resultant fetal hyperglycemia place the pregnant diabetic woman at risk for higher mortality and morbidity than the general obstetric population. Fetal anomalies occur in 10% or more of women whose pregnancies are complicated by type 1 DM. Spontaneous abortions also occur more frequently because of compromised placental circulation associated with diabetic vascular complications. Polyhydramnios (increased volume of amniotic fluid) occurs in about 10% to 25% of pregnant diabetics as a result of increased osmotic pressure, increased secretion of amniotic fluid, and diuresis from fetal hyperglycemia. As the pregnancy progresses, fetal hyperglycemia leads to fetal hyperinsulinemia, which results in increased fetal growth, delayed fetal pulmonary maturation, and increased incidence of respiratory distress syndrome (RDS).[17,29] Additionally the presence of vascular involvement, poor glucose control, poor or lack of prenatal care, and PIH further increase the risk to mother and fetus.

After delivery, there is an increase in the rate of infant mortality among infants of diabetic mothers.[38] Complications frequently occurring in infants of diabetic mothers include hypoglycemia, hypocalcemia, hyperbilirubinemia, and RDS. Congenital abnormalities, particularly of the cardiac, renal, and central nervous systems, occur more frequently in these infants. Macrosomia may cause traumatic complications during vaginal delivery. Intrauterine growth retardation (IUGR) in infants occurs as a result of vascular complications.[29]

Cardiac Disease

The increase in blood volume that occurs in pregnancy begins as early as the sixth week of gestation. The blood volume rises slowly in the first trimester, reaching a peak at about 30 to 34 weeks' gestation. A woman who is healthy and without a cardiac disorder can withstand the additional stress from the increased blood volume. However, if she has cardiac pathology, the pregnancy may be complicated. The complications that can occur are related to the degree of dis-

CLASSIFICATION OF DIABETES

Type 1: characterized by beta cell destruction, usually leading to absolute insulin deficiency. It has two forms: immune-mediated diabetes mellitus, which results from a cellular-mediated autoimmune destruction of the beta cells of the pancreas; and idiopathic diabetes mellitus, which refers to forms of the disease that have no known etiologies.

Type 2: diseases of insulin resistance that usually have relative (rather than absolute) insulin deficiency. Can range from predominant insulin resistance with relative insulin deficiency to predominant insulin deficiency with some insulin resistance.

Impaired Glucose Homeostasis: a metabolic stage intermediate between normal glucose homeostasis and diabetes. A risk factor for diabetes and cardiovascular disease.

Gestational Diabetes Mellitus: glucose intolerance in pregnancy.

Other Specific Types: diabetes caused by other identifiable etiologies, including genetic defects of beta cell function; genetic defects in insulin action; diseases of the exocrine pancreas; endocrinopathies; and drug- or chemical-induced, infection, and other uncommon forms

(National Diabetes Group Classification of Diabetes [1997]. *Diabetes Care, 20*(7), 1183–1194.)

ability, as categorized in the New York Heart Association Functional Classification of Heart Disease (see page 475).

Acute Fatty Liver of Pregnancy

Acute fatty liver of pregnancy exhibits a spectrum from mild hepatic dysfunction to hepatic failure, coma, and death.[16,23] The cause is unknown, and although several theories have been proposed, none has been confirmed with clinical studies.[52] The onset of the condition is usually in the latter half of pregnancy and symptoms are those of hepatic failure, including bleeding, nausea and vomiting, jaundice, or coma.[16] Liver function studies, liver biopsy, coagulation studies, and computed tomography scanning may aid in the diagnosis. Table 4-4 provides a comparison of acute fatty liver of pregnancy with other conditions presenting similar clinical manifestations.

Sexually Transmitted Diseases and Other Infections

Sexually transmitted diseases (STDs) are specific diseases or syndromes that are transmitted primarily through sexual contact. The pregnant woman, the unborn fetus, and the neonate suffer severe symptoms and complications as a result of STDs during pregnancy. More than 20 STDs have been identified, and they cause a wide variety of complications during pregnancy, such as spontaneous abortion, premature birth, IUGR, stillbirth, congenital anomalies, and neonatal death.

Other infections also can cause maternal and fetal effects. Table 4-5 lists common infections and their effects on the mother and fetus during pregnancy.

FETAL ALTERATIONS

Multiple factors can cause altered development in the fetus. The more common ones include placenta previa, abruptio placenta, ectopic pregnancy, placental insufficiency, and multiple gestation. Table 4-6 describes placental anomalies and ectopic pregnancy. The impact of genetic abnormalities is discussed in Chapter 2.

Placenta Previa. Placenta previa may cause partial or complete blockage of the birth canal by the placenta. It is often associated with painless vaginal bleeding. The placement of the placenta in the lower segment of the uterus may still allow for vaginal delivery, but placement across the opening of the birth canal requires cesarean section to ensure fetal survival. Ultrasonography is especially helpful in identifying the exact location of the placenta.

Abruptio Placenta. This placental anomaly occurs with premature separation of the placenta from the uterine wall. It is associated with high risk for poor fetal outcome depending on fetal maturity and amount of hemorrhage. Risk factors for abruptio placenta include physical injury, as well as cigarette smoking and the use of cocaine.

Ectopic Pregnancy. Ectopic pregnancy refers to implantation of the fetus outside the uterus. The most common site is the fallopian tube where the fertilized ovum may be caught or become too large to proceed through the tube. The frequency of ectopic pregnancy has increased because of the increased number of women of childbearing age with a history of pelvic inflammatory disease and the use of intrauterine devices for contraception, either of which can cause scarring and alterations within the tube. Ectopic pregnancy is a life-threatening condition for the mother because rupture of the fetal sac can result in hemorrhage. Pregnancy tests and ultrasonography aid in the diagnosis of the presence of a fetal sac outside of the uterus.

TABLE 4-4

DIFFERENTIAL DIAGNOSIS OF ACUTE FATTY LIVER OF PREGNANCY

	ACUTE FATTY LIVER OF PREGNANCY	ACUTE VIRAL HEPATITIS	CHOLESTASIS	SEVERE PREECLAMPSIA
Trimester	Third	Variable	Third	Third
Parity	Nullipara	No association	No association	Nullipara
Clinical manifestations	Malaise, nausea, jaundice, altered sensorium	Malaise, nausea, jaundice, anorexia, altered sensorium	Pruritus, jaundice	Hypertension, edema, proteinuria, oliguria, central nervous system hyperexcitability, coagulopathy
Bilirubin	Increased	Increased	Increased	Normal or increased
Transaminases	Minimal increase	Marked increase	Minimal increase	Normal or minimal to moderate increase
Alkaline phosphatase	Normal for pregnancy	Minimal increase	Moderate increase	Normal for pregnancy
Histology	Fatty infiltration, no inflammation or necrosis	Marked inflammation and necrosis	Biliary stasis, no inflammation	Inflammation, necrosis, fibrin deposition
Perinatal mortality	Marked increase	Minimal increase	Minimal increase	Moderate increase
Maternal mortality	Marked increase	Minimal increase	No increase	Moderate increase
Recurrence in subsequent pregnancy	No	No	Yes	Yes

(From Clark, S. L., Cotton, D. B., Hankins, G. D. V., & Phelan, J. P. [1991]. *Critical care obstetrics* [p. 489]. Cambridge, MA: Blackwell Scientific.)

Placental Insufficiency. Placental insufficiency is a common cause of IUGR. It may result in dysfunction of maternal-placental or fetal-placental circulation that compromises fetal nutrition and oxygenation. Occasionally, the placenta may be too small or inadequately developed to support fetal growth and development. Infarctions, usually found on the maternal side of the placenta, may develop if the blood supply is decreased and necrosis occurs. Fetal risk is greatest if the infarctions occur in the central portion of the placenta and thus interfere with fetal circulation.

Multiple Gestations. The use of fertility drugs in the treatment of infertility has produced an increased incidence in the number of multiple gestations. Multiple gestations constitute a risk factor for fetal growth and development. Because of the limited intrauterine space, prematurity is the most common problem associated with multiple gestations. Monozygotic twins are especially at risk for *transfusion syndrome*, in which one infant is well nourished and developed but the other is pale and anemic and displays evidence of IUGR. In monozygotic twins, the umbilical cords may also become entangled, leading to fetal demise of one twin.

ENVIRONMENTAL FACTORS

Multiple environmental factors can influence the outcome of a pregnancy. These include maternal nutrition and multiple substances that are teratogenic.

Maternal Nutrition

Pregnancy is a unique developmental time. At no other stage in the life cycle does the well-being of one individual, the fetus, depend so directly on the well-being of another individual, the mother. The nutritional status of the mother is a critical determinant of her own well-being and also that of the fetus. Proper nutrition during pregnancy reduces the risks for maternal complications such as PIH and anemia, ensures adequate tissue growth, and promotes optimal infant birth weight.

Inadequate maternal nutrition can cause improper fetal brain development. Inadequate maternal nutrition also has a significant effect on infant birth weight. Infants with low birth weight are at risk for more frequent illnesses, hearing and vision disabilities, behavioral disorders, and learning problems than infants whose weight is within the normal range.

The maternal conditions that indicate those potentially at risk include: (1) adolescence; (2) overweight; (3) underweight; (4) inadequate weight gain; (5) ex-

TABLE 4-5

EFFECTS OF INFECTIONS DURING PREGNANCY

INFECTION	MATERNAL EFFECTS	FETAL EFFECTS
Bacterial vaginosis	Preterm labor; PROM; chorioamnionitis, endometritis, UTI	Prematurity
Chlamydia	Often asymptomatic; infertility; tubal pregnancy	Increased incidence of preterm labor; inclusion conjunctivitis; pneumonitis
Condylomata acuminata	Vulvar warts; may require cesarean birth	None noted
Cytomegalovirus disease	Asymptomatic or mimics mononucleosis	Increase in perinatal mortality; neurologic deficits; sensorineural hearing loss; chorioretinitis; mental retardation, IUGR; microcephaly; hydrocephaly
Gonorrhea	Asymptomatic or vaginal discharge; scarring of fallopian tubes; infertility; endometritis after invasive procedures	Fetal death, mental retardation, ophthalmia neonatorium
Group A streptococcus	Puerperal infection; maternal death	Infection; infant death
Hepatitis A, B, C, D, E	Abortion or preterm labor; fulminant disease; maternal death	Fetal death; fetal deformities; congenital hepatitis; hypothermia; hypoglycemia
Herpes simplex type II	Vulvovaginitis	Increased perinatal mortality; fetal malformations
Influenza	Can produce critical illness if pneumonia develops	Fetal death; congenital anomalies
Monilial vaginitis	Thick, irritating vaginal discharge	Thrush in newborn
Parvovirus	Intrauterine infection	Hydrops fetalis; stillbirth
Rubella	Fever and typical rash, abortion	Increased perinatal mortality; congenital defects of eyes, heart, CNS; sensorineural deafness
Rubeola	Fever and typical rash; abortion	Increased perinatal mortality; congenital or neonatal infection will produce rash
Syphilis	May be asymptomatic or produce primary and secondary lesions	Preterm delivery; congenital syphilis; fetal death
Toxoplasmosis	Asymptomatic	Increased perinatal mortality; congenital anomalies; congenital toxoplasmosis
Trichomoniasis	Often asymptomatic; vaginal bleeding	Possibly an insignificant decrease in birth weight
Urinary tract infections	Asymptomatic; fever, chills, dysuria, urinary frequency, pain; abortion; premature labor	Prematurity, PROM, low birth weight, mental retardation, cerebral palsy; death
Varicella	Typical lesions; may precipitate shingles	Fetal death, growth retardation; fetal malformations

CNS, central nervous system; IUGR, intrauterine growth retardation; PROM, premature rupture of membranes; UTI, urinary tract infection.

cessive weight gain (6) anemia; (7) smoking or use of alcohol or drugs; (8) pica; (9) poor diet; and (10) medical problems such as diabetes.

Teratogens

A teratogen is a substance or agent that produces abnormalities in embryonic or fetal development. The most common teratogens that affect pregnancy and the fetus include: (1) tobacco, (2) alcohol, (3) illicit drugs such as cocaine, (4) possibly caffeine, (5) infections, and (6) radiation.

TOBACCO. Approximately 20% to 46% of pregnant women are smokers.[46,57] Twenty to 25% continue to smoke throughout pregnancy, yet only 60% of these admit to smoking.[9] Maternal smoking during pregnancy results in increased risk for spontaneous abortion, perinatal mortality, low birth weight infants, and

TABLE 4-6

IMPLANTATION ANOMALIES

ANOMALY	INVOLVEMENT	SIGNS/SYMPTOMS	CAUSES/RISK FACTORS
Placenta previa	Lower uterine segment or over cervix	Painless vaginal bleeding in 3rd trimester	Advanced maternal age; increased parity; uterine scarring; multiple gestation; enlarged placenta
Abruptio placenta	Abrupt, premature separation of placenta	Severe abdominal pain; hard, boardlike abdomen	Maternal diabetes; pregnancy-induced hypertension; chronic hypertension; increased parity; overdistention of uterus
Ectopic pregnancy	Implantation outside uterine cavity	Abdominal pain; signs of shock	
Placental Insufficiency	Dysfunctional maternal/placental or fetal/placental circulation		Multiple pregnancy; postmaturity; systemic diseases; hypertension; placental membrane abnormalities

preterm delivery. Furthermore, children of smoking mothers are at increased risk for sudden infant death syndrome (SIDS), asthma, respiratory infection, attention deficit disorder, and delayed development of reading and math skills.[9] *Fetal tobacco syndrome* is a phrase that has been introduced to refer to the specific conditions that result from prenatal exposure to tobacco smoke.

ALCOHOL. Alcohol consumption during pregnancy is a major medical and public health problem due to the accompanying adverse pregnancy outcomes. These adverse outcomes include increased risk of spontaneous abortion and congenital anomalies, low birth weight infants, and infants with neurobehavioral and cognitive deficits. *Fetal alcohol syndrome* includes at least one abnormality in each of the following categories: (1) growth retardation before and after birth; (2) central nervous system (CNS) abnormalities, including microcephaly, abnormal neonatal behavior, and during childhood, attention deficit hyperactivity disorder, as well as mild to moderate mental retardation; and (3) midfacial hypoplasia, including small nose, deep nasal bridge, thin upper lip, and small eyes.[54]

ILLICIT DRUGS. Researchers estimate that 5% to 20% of pregnant women use illicit drugs.[57] These women are at increased risk for abruptio placenta, spontaneous abortion, prematurity, and precipitous labor. Urogenital malformations, cerebrovascular complications, low birth weight, smaller head circumference, respiratory difficulties, drug withdrawal symptoms, and postnatal death are more common in infants of women who use illicit drugs.[57]

Prenatal Diagnostic Studies

Prenatal diagnostic studies of fetal well-being and maturity provide much-needed information regarding pregnancy status. Careful selection of tests can predict placental insufficiency, fetal anomalies, genetic abnormalities, and the ability of the fetus to survive in the existing intrauterine or extrauterine environment. Because maternal morbidity and mortality associated with modern childbearing are low, the focus of prenatal assessment of fetal well-being is to decrease fetal death and disease. Several antenatal diagnostic tests are currently available to assess fetal health and well-being. Unit 1, Appendix A summarizes the use of these diagnostic tests.

Alterations and Adaptations During Labor and Delivery

The accomplishment of a spontaneous delivery requires the interaction of numerous factors. Problems in adaptations can occur as a result of alterations in any of the four Ps—power, passage, passenger, and psyche. *Power* represents the frequency, duration, and intensity of contractions, as well as the pushing effort of the woman. *Passage* refers to the size and type of pelvis and the ability of the cervix and vagina to respond and allow passage of the fetus. *Passenger* is used to refer to the fetus, its head size, position, presentation, attitude, and umbilical. *Psyche*, critical in the birth process, includes the effects of anxiety, tension, and fear, which can lengthen the duration of labor and delivery.

DYSFUNCTIONAL LABOR PATTERNS

The timing, strength, and efficiency of uterine contractions in producing cervical dilatation and effacement are major forces in the timely descent and delivery of the fetus. Alterations in the contraction forces occur when contractions happen continuously, are prolonged, or are insufficient to produce dilatation and effacement. Factors associated with these alterations include fetal malposition, excessive analgesia, fetal postmaturity, cervical rigidity, overdistention of the uterus, and increased maternal age. Any of these alterations may result in dysfunctional labor and may even predispose to additional alterations such as dehydration, exhaustion, infection, and fetal compromise. Four dysfunctional labor patterns are presented in Table 4-7.

PREMATURITY

Premature delivery (before the 37th week of gestation) continues to be the leading cause of perinatal mortality and morbidity.[30] Most neonates who weigh less than 2,500 g at birth are premature but gestational age is a critical determinant in fetal maturity. Preterm labor and delivery may be due to maternal diseases, smoking, acute illnesses during the pregnancy, fetal anomalies, and other conditions. Multiple physiologic problems result from immaturity of the body systems including cardiovascular, pulmonary, gastrointestinal, renal, liver and skin alterations. Early diagnosis is essential if preterm labor is to be interrupted. One promising investigational diagnostic study, fetal fibronectin, may provide the breakthrough needed in dealing with this problem (see Unit 1, Appendix A).

POSTMATURITY

The greatest risks in postterm pregnancy are related to placental aging and a decreased transfer of oxygen and nutrients to the fetus. Amniotic fluid volume may also

TABLE 4-7

COMPARISON OF DYSFUNCTIONAL LABOR PATTERNS

PATTERN	CHARACTERISTICS	MATERNAL IMPLICATIONS	FETAL/NEONATAL IMPLICATIONS
Hypertonic	Occurs in early labor (latent phase)	Exhaustion	Fetal distress
Primary uterine inertia	Occurs most often in nullipara Irregular, ineffective contractions Lack of uterine relaxation between contractions Little to no progress in dilatation of cervix Failure of presenting part to descend	Dehydration Uterine rupture Infection of uterus Vaginal lacerations if delivery is difficult	Sepsis Birth injury
Hypotonic Secondary uterine inertia	Occurs in active labor Established contraction pattern converts to one in which contractions occur less often, decrease in intensity, and decrease in duration	Exhaustion Dehydration Infection of uterus Increased risk of postpartum hemorrhage	Fetal distress Birth injury
Precipitous labor	Labor < 3 h in length	Ruptured uterus Lacerations No one in attendance for delivery	Increased risk for cerebral hemorrhage Fetal hypoxia No immediate care to clear airway, maintain body temperature

be decreased, resulting in umbilical cord compression and fetal death. Postmature neonates usually are pale and have dry, cracked, and peeling skin. The neonate may appear alert but distressed. Both lanugo (fine hair) and vernix (cheesy, fatty material on the skin) tend to be absent. Hair and fingernails are long. If oxygen deprivation occurred during the birth process, the amniotic fluid, umbilical cord, and skin may be stained with meconium (fetal intestinal discharges), with a green to yellow appearance. This neonate is at increased risk for meconium aspiration, asphyxia, hypoglycemia, cold stress, and polycythemia.

PREMATURE RUPTURE OF THE MEMBRANES

Premature rupture of the membranes refers to the spontaneous rupture of the membranes or leakage of amniotic fluid before the onset of labor. Preterm rupture occurs before 37 weeks of gestation. Predisposing factors include multiparity, incompetent cervix, maternal age greater than 35 years, low weight gain during pregnancy, and cervical damage from surgical instrumentation. Diagnosis can usually be confirmed with nitrazine paper, which turns dark blue in the presence of amniotic fluid.

Risk for the development of chorioamnionitis (infection of the chorion and amnion) is increased, especially if delivery does not occur within 24 hours of rupture. Signs of chorioamnionitis include maternal tachycardia and fever, fetal tachycardia, foul-smelling amniotic fluid, and uterine tenderness. If the membranes rupture more than 48 hours before delivery, the fetus is at increased risk for septicemia, pneumonia, and infection of the umbilical cord.

Premature rupture of the membranes early in pregnancy is more threatening because of prematurity of the fetus, possible malposition, risk of prolapsed cord, and infection. Occasionally, corticosteroids are used to increased fetal lung maturity and lessen the chance of RDS in the preterm neonate.

BIOPHYSICAL DEVELOPMENT OF CHILDREN

The biophysical development of a child begins at conception. Further growth and development is a process involving maturation and learning, which is influenced in part by culture, socioeconomic status, and life-style. The following discussion is intended to guide the learner in an understanding of the physiology of development from the transition to extrauterine life through adolescence. The common health alterations from the infancy to adolescence are reviewed.

The Newborn and Extrauterine Adaptation

The fetus must make multiple adjustments to survive in the environment outside the uterus. These include respiratory, circulatory, thermoregulatory, hepatic, renal, immune, and neuromuscular changes. Health alterations in the fetus are commonly related to fetal maturity or congenital defects or both. Most of the common alterations are described in other sections of the text relating to the system affected.

RESPIRATORY AND CIRCULATORY ADJUSTMENTS

Respiratory and circulatory adjustments must be made within minutes after birth to ensure survival. Initiation of respiratory is essential to provide for oxygenation and changes in the pressures in the circulatory system. The circulatory adjustments must move from a placental supply to an independent, intact circulatory system.

Initiation of Respiration

At birth, the loss of the placental connection between the newborn and the mother requires biophysical changes in the infant's respiratory and circulatory systems to support independent, extrauterine functioning. Flowchart 4-3 demonstrates the interaction of chemical, sensory, thermal, and mechanical stimulation in the initiation of respiration at birth. Essentially, changes in blood chemistry, temperature, and the senses stimulate the respiratory center in the medulla. The mechanical force applied to the thoracic cavity with vaginal birth assists with the expulsion of fluid from the newborn lungs through chest compression followed by chest recoil, which allows air to enter the lungs. An infant born by cesarean delivery does not have this mechanical stimulation and may have respiratory difficulties.

Closure of Shunts

Functional closures of fetal shunts are necessary circulatory adaptations that allow appropriate blood flow through the newborn heart. These gradual changes result from pressure changes in the lungs, heart, and major vessels once the oxygen concentration of the blood is increased through respiration. Pulmonary vascular resistance is reduced when inspired oxygen dilates the pulmonary vessels. The resulting increased pulmonary blood flow reduces the pressure in the right side of the heart. Concurrently, there is an increase in the systemic vascular resistance that increases the pressure in the left side of the heart. This process of oxygenation and pressure changes in the circulatory system causes functional closure of the foramen ovale at birth, the ductus arteriosis by the fourth day after birth, and eventually, the ductus venosus at about 1 week (see page 511).[62]

FLOWCHART 4-3 **Interaction of Stimuli in the Initiation of Neonatal Respiration**

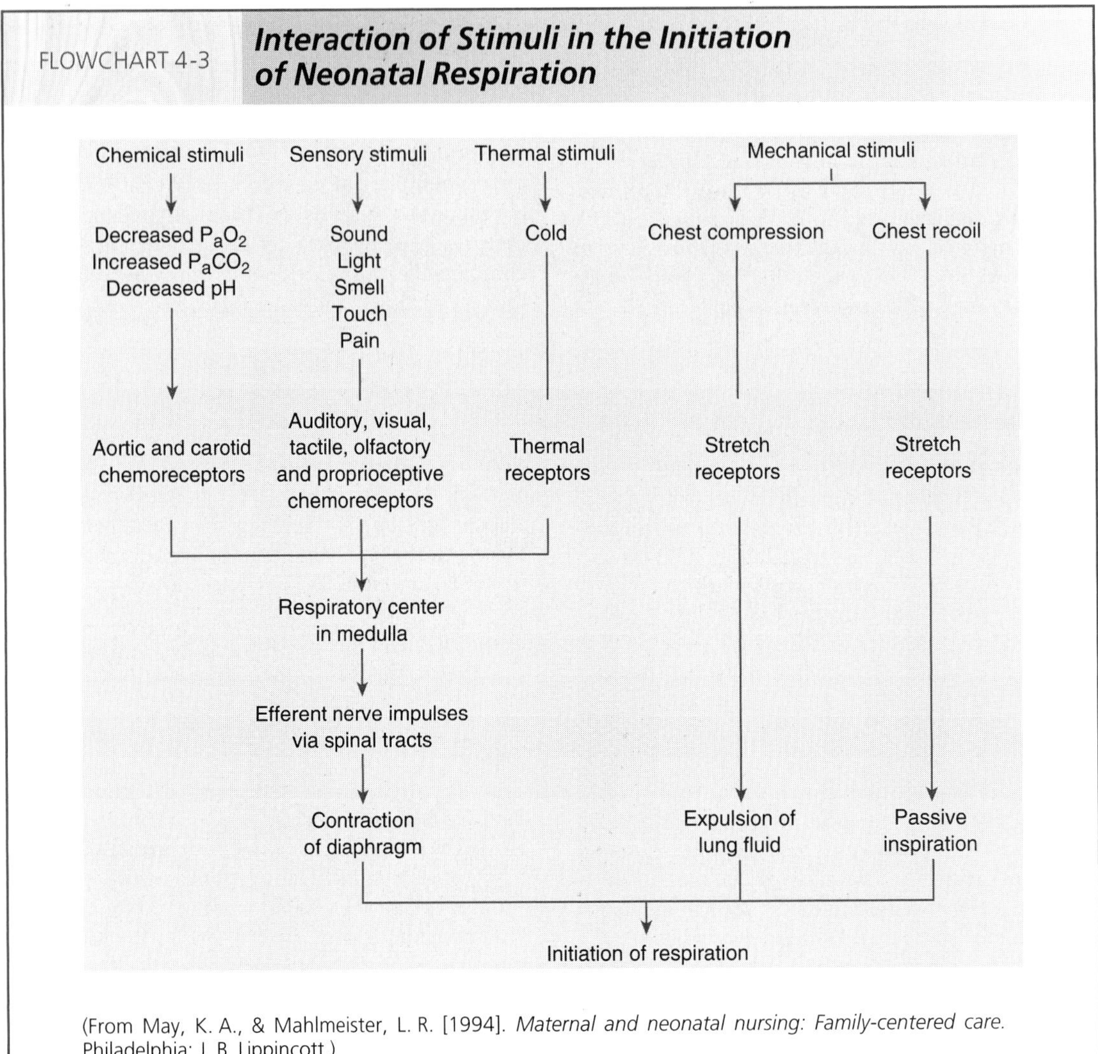

(From May, K. A., & Mahlmeister, L. R. [1994]. *Maternal and neonatal nursing: Family-centered care.* Philadelphia: J. B. Lippincott.)

THERMOREGULATORY ADJUSTMENTS

Thermoregulation is the control of heat production and heat loss through mechanisms activated by the hypothalamus. Newborns are prone to heat loss because of their unique characteristics. Factors that contribute to heat loss are:

- A large body surface area in relation to weight
- Thin skin with little subcutaneous fat
- Immature nervous system causing temperature instability
- Increased metabolic rate
- Heat production through nonshivering thermogenesis

Figure 4-1 illustrates the mechanisms of heat loss in the newborn and the environmental factors that contribute to this loss.

Shivering, a major mechanism of heat production in adults that requires muscular activity, is limited in the newborn. *Nonshivering thermogenesis*, requiring an increase in metabolism and oxygen consumption, is the primary heat production mechanism in the neonate. A full-term newborn has a unique source of adipose tissue called *brown fat*, located behind the sternum, around the neck and between the scapulae. Fat accumulation begins at about 32 weeks' gestation. In response to heat loss, the sympathetic nervous system stimulates the adrenal gland to release norepinephrine at the nerve endings in brown fat. Brown fat is highly vascular and when metabolized, releases heat into the blood, which is then distributed throughout the body, increasing body temperature.

Newborns must also be monitored for hyperthermia because they do not have fully functioning sweat

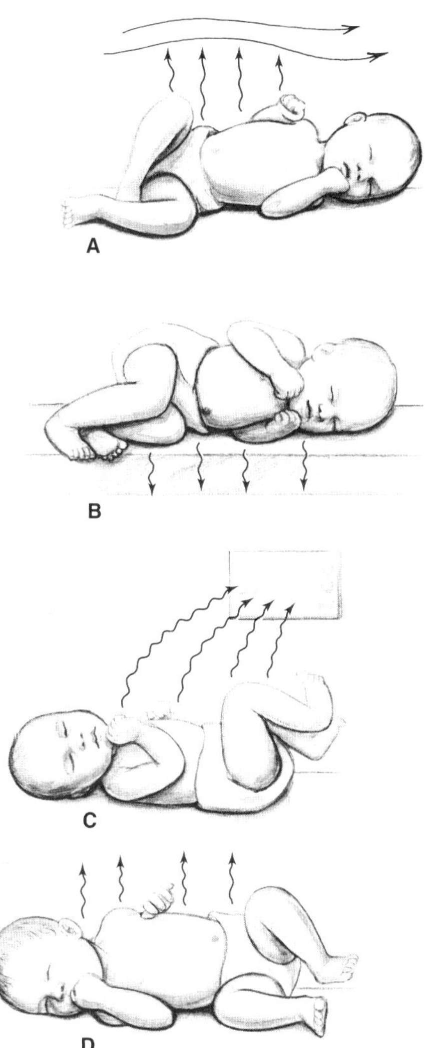

FIGURE 4-1. Heat loss in the newborn. **A.** Convection. **B.** Conduction. **C.** Radiation. **D.** Evaporation.

glands until approximately 1 month of age and cannot effectively release excess body heat. Thermogenesis increases the demand for oxygen and glucose. The normal newborn will meet these demands by an increase in respiratory rate and a release of glucose that has been stored in the liver. The depletion of brown fat and glucose leads to an increase in pulmonary vascular resistance resulting in respiratory distress. An external heat source can significantly reduce the use of brown fat and glucose for thermogenesis in a compromised infant.

HEPATIC ADJUSTMENTS

The liver is the most immature of the gastrointestinal organs at birth. This immaturity results in:

- Decreased plasma protein concentration causing slight edema
- Low prothrombin leading to decreased clotting ability
- Decreased stores of glycogen, which may cause hypoglycemia
- Reduction in glucuronyl transferase, which contributes to physiologic jaundice

Neonatal Jaundice

Neonatal jaundice is a direct result of the inability of the immature neonatal liver to conjugate bilirubin. Approximately 70% of full-term, normal neonates exhibit jaundice.[43] Bilirubin is the end product of the breakdown of RBCs. Before birth, the fetus has more RBCs per ounce than adults.[63] Consequently, at birth, there are more RBCs to break down, resulting in higher levels of bilirubin needing to be excreted by the liver. Flowchart 4-4 illustrates the pathophysiology of neonatal jaundice. Physiologic jaundice appears at

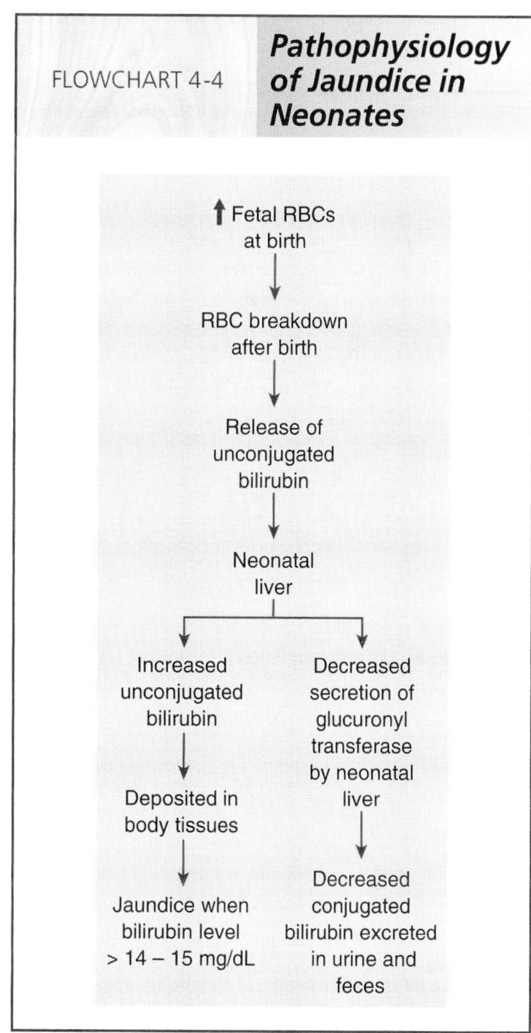

FLOWCHART 4-4 ***Pathophysiology of Jaundice in Neonates***

about 48 hours of age as a result of the breakdown of fetal RBCs.[43] It usually disappears by 1 week of age with bilirubin levels not usually exceeding 12 mg/100 mL.

Jaundice occurring during the first 24 hours of life is often a result of a blood group incompatibility (ABO incompatibility) or an Rh sensitization of the mother. These two pathologic process cause acceleration of the breakdown of RBCs due to an antibody response, increasing the severity of jaundice in the newborn (see page 315).

RENAL ADJUSTMENTS

In utero, urine is formed in the kidneys and excreted into the amniotic fluid. Too much (polyhydramnios) or too little (oligohydramnios) amniotic fluid may be a result of a fetal renal problem. After birth, the newborn will generally void within the first 24 hours and will void approximately 15 to 60 mL/kg per day. The urine of the newborn is usually dilute because the kidney cannot fully concentrate urine until about 3 months of age. Renal thresholds are low, which can lead to acidosis and electrolyte imbalance because bicarbonate concentration and buffering capacity are decreased (see page 178).

IMMUNOLOGIC ADJUSTMENTS

Maternal IgG antibodies are transferred across the placenta to the fetus during the last trimester of pregnancy. In this way, the newborn receives passive immunity to bacterial and viral infections against which the mother has formed specific antibodies. IgA antibodies are passively acquired through breast milk. Passive immunity varies in length from 5 weeks to 3 months.[35] Active immunity begins when the newborn receives immunization injections beginning with the hepatitis B vaccine often administered before the newborn leaves the hospital, followed by the series of newborn immunizations that begin around 8 weeks of age.

NEUROMUSCULAR ADJUSTMENTS

The development of the neuromuscular system progresses in a cephalocaudal direction.[7] This is evident in the fact that newborns and infants first show increased strength with head control followed by control of upper and lower extremities. As they pass into infancy and toddler stages, walking and bowel and bladder controls are begun.

Developmental Stages: Infancy Through Adolescence

Many changes occur from infancy through adolescence. These changes are variable with the individual and the chronological time line varies.

INFANCY

The stages of infant development manifest themselves through very rapid growth in physical and mental areas. Development is not defined along the chronological age line, but more so with the achievement of defined developmental tasks. This foundation is of extreme importance for future growth and maturation.

Biologic Growth. The period of infancy encompasses the first year following birth. During this time there is a rapid, continuous growth pattern that is seen in the month-to-month changes summarized in Table 4-8. Individual variations may be present and may be more evident when dealing with premature infants. In addition to vital signs, infant growth is measured by height, weight, and head and chest circumference.

Dentition. The primary teeth (deciduous or "baby teeth") develop in utero and begin to erupt between 5 and 7 months of age. These teeth stimulate jaw growth and assist with speech development. By 1 year the infant usually has six primary teeth.

Neuromuscular and Sensory Development. Neuromuscular development follows the general principles of cephalocaudal and proximodistal growth. During the first years, the infant refines both gross and fine motor skills. A summary of this development pattern is found in Table 4-9.

Sensory development involves touch, taste, smell, hearing, and sight. Active and passive touch are forms of stimulation that allow the infant to learn about the

(text continues on page 106)

TABLE 4-8

GROWTH PATTERN IN FIRST YEAR OF LIFE

	BIRTH TO 6 MO	6 MO TO 1 Y	AVERAGE
Height	Increase 2.5 cm/mo	Increase 1.5 cm/mo	50% increase in 1st y
Weight	Increase 1.5 lb/mo	Increase 1.5 lb/mo	Doubled by 6 mo Tripled by 1 y
Head circumference	Increase 1.5 cm/mo	Increase 0.5 cm/mo	33% increase in 1st y

TABLE 4-9

GROSS AND FINE MOTOR GROWTH AND DEVELOPMENT OF THE INFANT

DEVELOPMENTAL AREA	1 MO	3 MO	5 MO	7 MO	10 MO	12 MO
Gross motor	Turns and lifts head from prone position (Fig. A)	Pumps arms, shoulders, and head from prone (Fig. B)	Rolls over one or both ways	Sits, may need to lean forward on hands (Fig. D)	Sits with back straight Pulls to standing position	Cruises along furniture or walks alone (Fig. F)
	Reflexive movement of extremities	Moro, stepping and tonic reflexes begin to fade	Sits or possibly stands supported in an exerciser (Fig. C)	Bears weight on legs	Creeps or crawls (Fig. E)	
Fine motor	Uses eyes to track for several feet	Eye–hand balance Grasps object	Turns head when name is called	Reaches and grasps large objects	Uncovers hidden toys	Holds cup and spoon well
	Holds hands fisted	Shakes, waves and throws toy	Explores environment by mouthing objects	Transfers objects from hands	Pincer grasp	Stacks blocks
	May try to reach overhead objects			Palmer grasp		

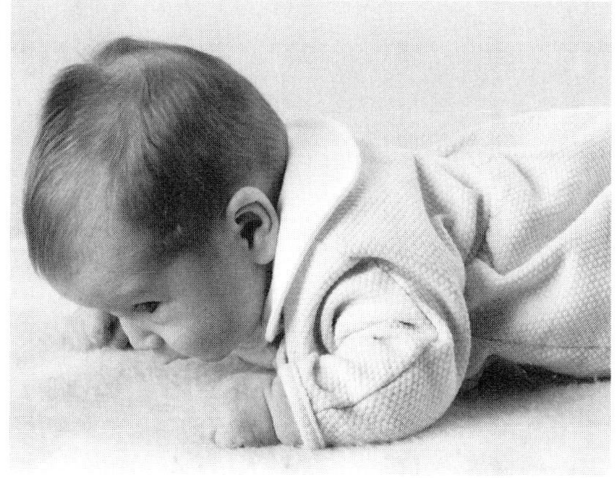

A. This 1-month-old lifts and turns head from prone.

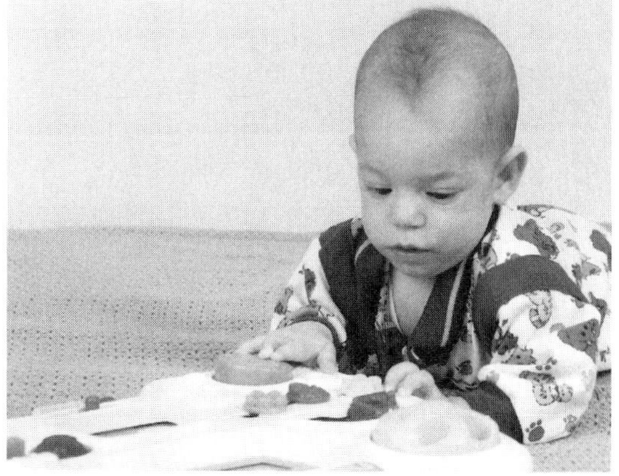

B. This 3-month-old pushes up to look at a toy.

(continued)

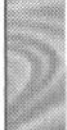

TABLE 4-9

GROSS AND FINE MOTOR GROWTH AND DEVELOPMENT OF THE INFANT (Continued)

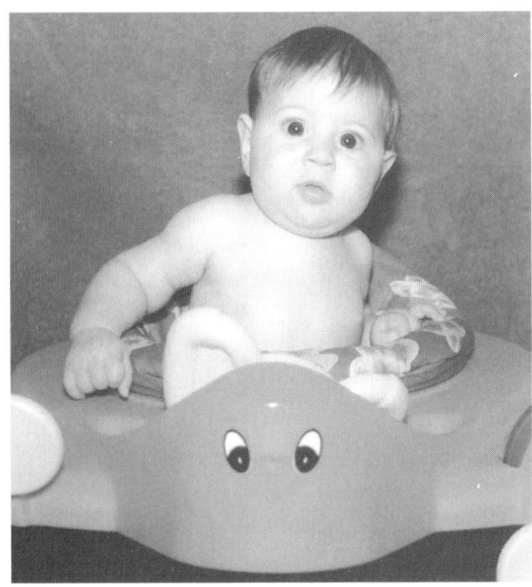

C. This 5-month-old sits supported in an exerciser.

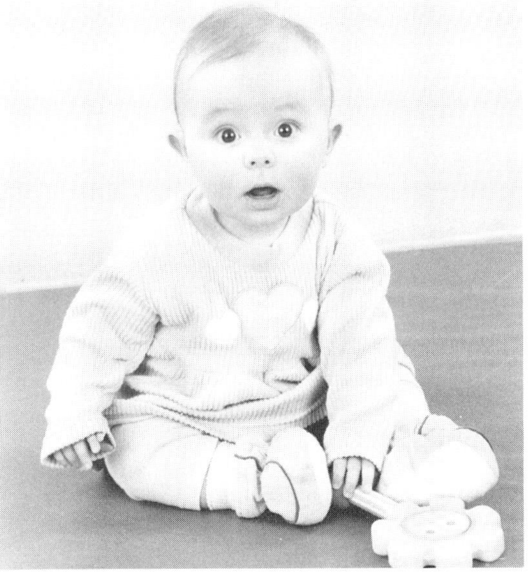

D. This 7-month-old sits well but still tilts slightly forward for balance.

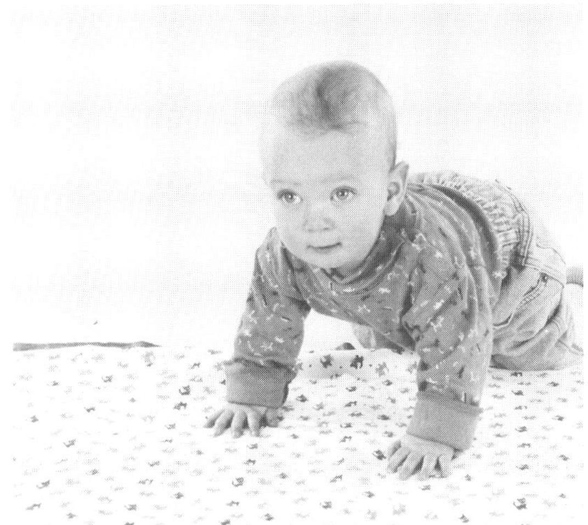

E. This 10-month-old actively crawls around.

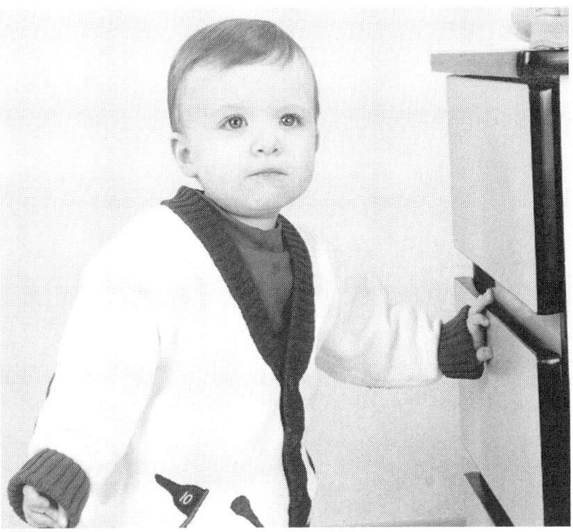

F. This 12-month-old cruises along the furniture.

environment. Infants, like adults, show individual preferences for the taste and small of various things. Taste preferences are quite evident by 7 months of age. Hearing is present at birth but is sometimes limited because of the presence of amniotic fluid or vernix caseosa in the ear canal. Infants respond to loud noises with a startle reflex (Moro reflex) and are quieted by pulsating or rhythmic sounds. The newborn's response to its mother's voice is thought to originate from the prenatal period. Hearing progresses during the first year from listening, to imitating sounds, to responding to its own name, and locating sounds. Sight is one of the infant's first social mechanisms. At birth, the infant can see objects close to its face. By 1 month, the infant can see at a distance of about 18 inches. Depth perception is evident by 6 months. At 8 to 12 months, the infant skillfully uses sight and mobility to explore the surroundings.

COGNITIVE DEVELOPMENT. Piaget (1896–1980), a Swiss psychologist, formulated stages of cognitive development that the infant must achieve level by level. These are similar, yet different, to Freud's (1856–1939) psychoanalytic theory and to Erikson's (1902–1994) psychosocial theory of personality development. A comparison of these three theories is shown in Table 4-10.

SLEEP PATTERNS. Sleep requirements will differ for each infant, but generally the infant will respond to its own needs. For the first 3 to 4 months, the infant's pattern of sleep is one of frequent, short naps, interrupted by crying and fussing. Later the infant will begin to sleep 8 to 10 hours through the night with an average total sleep of 13 to 15 hours each day. Sleep problems are usually physiologic in nature and are rare, with the exception of colic. It is recommended that infants sleep on their backs or sides to decrease the risk of SIDS.

NUTRITION. Adequate caloric intake is essential to support the rapid growth in infancy. As growth decreases in the first year, energy requirements decrease from 120 kcal/kg per day at birth to 100 kcal/kg per day by 1 year.[7] Breast milk or formula provide all the nutrition an infant needs for the first 4 to 6 months. Full-term infants have adequate stores of iron in tissues to meet needs in the first 6 months. Vitamins, iron, and fluoride supplements are not usually necessary until about 6 months of age. Solid foods are introduced one at a time (to detect any food allergies) at about 6 months of age when the gastrointestinal tract is mature enough to digest foods completely and the extrusion reflex disappears.

EARLY CHILDHOOD

Early childhood encompasses both the toddler period (ages 1–3) and the preschool period (ages 3–5). The physical growth spurt seen during infancy slows during early childhood, but motor, cognitive, and psychosocial skills advance and mature. Table 4-11 summarizes biologic growth in early childhood.

BIOLOGIC AND PHYSIOLOGIC GROWTH. The growth pattern of children slows during early childhood with about 12 in. of growth and 5 lb weight gain per year. Physiologic development occurs as the individual systems mature. By the end of the toddler period, all systems are mature with the exception of the endocrine and reproductive systems.

DENTITION. By age 2½ all 20 primary teeth have erupted. Very little change is seen throughout the rest of early childhood.

MOTOR, COGNITIVE AND PSYCHOSOCIAL DEVELOPMENT. Table 4-12 illustrates the maturation of motor, cognitive, and psychosocial skills during early childhood. The child will advance from learning to walk, to riding a bike with training wheels, from saying a few words, to a vocabulary of nearly 2,500 words, and from playing simple games to more cooperative games that require the child to follow rules.

NERVOUS SYSTEM DEVELOPMENT. The total number of brain cells is complete by 1 year of age, with contin-

TABLE 4-10

COMPARISON OF THEORISTS' VIEWS ON COGNITIVE DEVELOPMENT

AGE	PIAGET	FREUD	ERIKSON
Infancy 1–12 mo	Sensorimotor Period —Learns the world through reflexes	Oral stage —Explores world with mouth	Trust vs. mistrust —Learns to love and be loved
Early Childhood 1–3 y	Preconceptual thought —Egocentric	Anal stage —Learns bowel and bladder control	Autonomy vs. Shame and Doubt —Learns independence
3–6 y	Preoperational thought —Includes others	Phallic stage —Learns sexual identity	Initiative vs. Guilt —Learns basic problem solving
Middle Childhood 6–12 y	Concrete operations —Internalized, logical thought	Latent stage —Inactive personality development	Industry vs. Inferiority —Learns how to do things well
Adolescence 12–18 y	Formal Operations —Logical reasoning	Genital stage —Sexual maturity and development of relationships	Identity vs. Role Confusion —Learns who he/she is and adjusts to body image

TABLE 4-11

BIOLOGIC GROWTH FROM EARLY CHILDHOOD THROUGH ADOLESCENCE

AGE (Y)	HEIGHT	WEIGHT
2	34–36 in (86–88 cm) Approximately ½ adult height	26–28 lb (12–13 kg)
3	36–39 in (91–97 cm)	31–33 lb (14–15 kg)
4	38–40 in (97–102 cm)	35–38 lb (16–17 kg)
5	39–41 in (99–104 cm)	40–42 lb (18–19 kg)
6	43–46 in (109–116 cm)	44–46 lb (20–21 kg)
7	45–48 in (114–122 cm)	48–53 lb (22–24 kg)
8	49–51 in (124–130 cm)	55–57 lb (25–26 kg)
9–10	52–54 in (132–137 cm)	59–77 lb (27–35 kg)
11–12	57–59 in (144–150 cm)	77–88 lb (35–40 kg)
13–14	Males 60–68 m (154–172 cm)	84–132 lb (38–60 kg)
	Female 60–66 in (153–167 cm)	88–132 lb (40–60 kg)
15–16	Males 65–71 in (164–180 cm)	110–132 lb (50–60 kg)
	Females 61–66.5 in (155–169 cm)	92–141 lb (42–64 kg)
17–21	Males 64–72 in (163–182 cm)	100–176 lb (50–80 kg)
	Females 61–67 in (156–170 cm)	106–158 lb (48–72 kg)

ued growth in size until about 3 years of age. The maturation of the nervous system, through spinal cord myelinization, accounts for the improved coordination that is evident during early childhood.

Genitourinary Development. Before toilet training can begin, the child must have control of rectal and urethral sphincters and must understand the concept of holding urine and stools until a specific time. Complete myelinization of nerves to sphincters does not occur until 2 years of age, at which time the child can sufficiently concentrate urine, has increased bladder capacity, and has sphincter control.

Nutrition. Caloric requirements range from 100 kcal/kg per day during the toddler period to 85 kcal/kg per day during the preschool period. The diet should contain milk, meat, fruits, vegetables, breads, and cereals. Calcium requirements are about 800 mg/day. Supplemental vitamins are not generally necessary and should not be a substitute for a balanced diet. The meal pattern during early childhood changes. The child is now able to eat three to four small meals per day with between-meal snacks because stomach capacity has increased and there is delayed emptying of the stomach.

MIDDLE CHILDHOOD

Middle childhood (the school-age child) is between 6 and 12 years of age. During this period physical growth slows until the last year (preadolescence). Motor, cognitive, and psychosocial development continues to mature.

Biologic Growth. Growth patterns during middle childhood are more important than individual parameters. Table 4-11 summarizes biologic growth parameters in middle childhood. The child gains an average of 5 to 7 lb and grows an average of 2 to 3 in./year. Boys tend to lag behind girls slightly in height and often do not experience growth spurts in height until adolescence. A growth curve is useful in determining growth patterns and is helpful in early diagnosis of deviations.

During middle childhood, the school-aged child begins to lose the "babyface" image. At the same time the child may appear clumsy because of the growth in height compared to the thinned-down appearance in weight. Fat decreases and there is a lengthening of leg and arm length. This makes the child look tall, thin, and gangly. The center of long bones continues to develop with mature bone marrow activity. Facial structure shows the greatest growth during middle childhood with marked changes in the upper and lower jaws. The sinuses are more pronounced and this allows for more resonance to the voice.

Dentition. Around 6 years of age, the child begins to lose deciduous teeth. By the end of middle childhood, all deciduous teeth are usually gone and have been replaced by permanent teeth. The first molars begin to erupt followed by the second and third into adolescence.

Nervous System and Motor Development. The process of myelinization continues with increase in thickness of the myelin sheath and improved conduction of nerve impulses. The effects of this maturation are seen as the clumsy child of 6 years of age matures into a coordinated sports participant or dancer in later childhood.

TABLE 4-12

PRESCHOOL GROWTH AND DEVELOPMENT

DEVELOPMENTAL AREA	AGE 3	AGE 4	AGE 5
Fine motor skills	Dresses self with simple clothing (Fig. A)	Can lace shoes; can pour from a small pitcher into a glass	Learns to tie shoes
	Copies circles and simple lines with pencil		Draws a 6-part person
Gross motor skills	Runs; climbs steps one at a time	Jumps, skips, walks slowly across a balance beam	Rides a 2-wheel bike with training wheels; hops on one foot (Fig. C)
Intellectual development	Short attention span; eager to learn; pretends to read books	Matches and sorts colors and numbers; enjoys singing and simple riddles	Can learn telephone number and street address
	Vocabulary of 300–1,000 words	Vocabulary of 1,500 words	Vocabulary of 2,000–3,000 words
Psychosocial development	Engages in parallel play	Engages in cooperative and symbolic play (Fig. B)	Has strong attachment to mother; needs frequent approval; is sensitive and responds with hurt feelings to ridicule
	Displays jealous emotions; shows some self-control; attends to toilet needs	Is bossy and talkative; needs positive, firm consistent guidance	

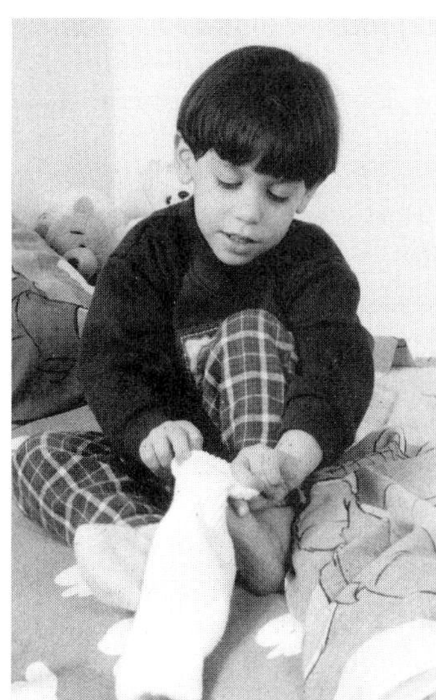

A. This 3-year-old enjoys dressing himself each morning.

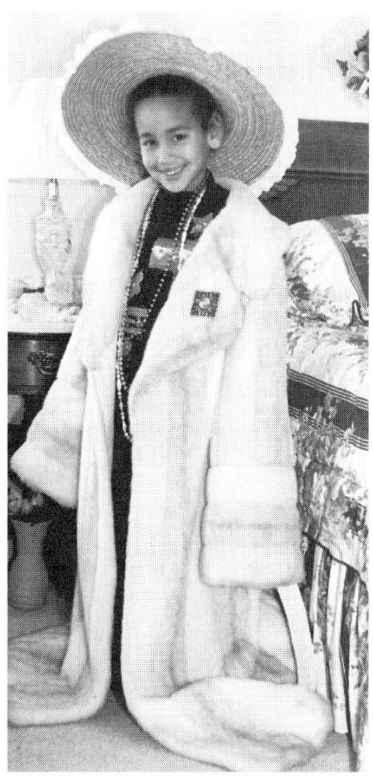

B. This 4-year-old pretends to be a grownup.

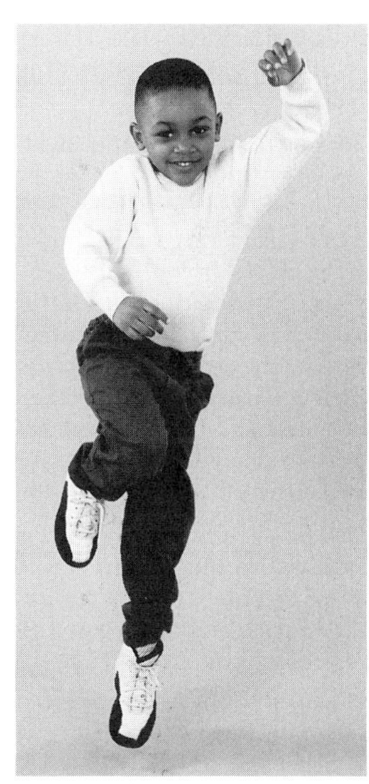

C. This 5-year-old demonstrates his skill of hopping on one foot.

(Adapted from Neff, M. C., & Spray, M. [1996]. *Introduction to maternal and child health nursing*. Philadelphia: Lippincott-Raven.)

Other Systems. Increased kidney size and function allow the child better control of elimination. The development of the immune system helps to account for the period of health associated with middle childhood. Tonsils and adenoids are enlarged and contribute to the production of antibodies when the child is exposed to various diseases. The cardiovascular system matures, cardiac output increases, heart rate decreases, and blood pressure increases. This increases oxygen capacity essential for increased energy needs.

Nutrition. The maturation of the gastrointestinal system allows for increased stomach capacity and intake. The child is also able to go for longer intervals between meals. There is an increased tolerance for food, which, in turn, decreases stomach complaints. The nutritional needs per units of body weight decline from earlier growth spurts until adolescence. Nutrients are important to maintain dental and bone health.

ADOLESCENCE

The period of adolescence begins at about 13 years of age and progresses through rapid physical, intellectual, emotional, and social changes through 19 to 20 years of age. The word adolescence has a Latin derivation meaning, "to grow up." The nervous system development is basically complete. During this time, rapid physical, intellectual, emotional, and social developmental changes occur.

Biologic Growth. As in middle childhood, the pattern of growth rather than individual aspects is most important. Biologic growth changes in adolescence are found in Table 4-11. Overall growth stops with closure of the epiphyseal lines of long bones, which is at about 16 years of age in girls and 19 years in boys. Lean and nonlean body mass doubles during puberty. The increased weight gain in adolescence is attributed to the increase in skeletal mass, muscle mass, and nonlean muscle mass. Androgen is thought to increase the muscle mass that occurs in boys, which might explain the greater strength seen in many boys and young men.[31]

Dentition. The second molars erupt in early adolescence and the third molars or wisdom teeth usually erupt or become problems during late adolescence. Dental caries, braces, and removal of wisdom teeth become problems for the adolescent.

Nutrition. There is an increased need for calories directly associated with the increase in body growth and high **basal metabolic rate** (BMR). Girls need about 2,200 calories per day and boys 2,800 calories per day. These needs will vary depending on the life-style of the adolescent. High-protein and high-calcium diets are necessary during growth of bone and muscle. Girls who have reached menarche should also consume 15 mg of iron daily with either diet or supplement.

Basal Metabolic Rate. During puberty, the thyroid gland increases secretion of thyroxine from the anterior pituitary. This causes an increase in total body metabolism. The BMR increases during periods of growth, reaching a peak at puberty. This increase also causes an increase in body temperature, often causing the adolescent to complain of feeling too warm.

Puberty. Puberty is the period in life when the ability to reproduce begins. The onset of puberty varies from one individual to another. Generally, it occurs between 8 and 14 years of age in girls and lasts about 3 years. In boys, it begins between 9 and 16 years of age and is completed by the end of the adolescent period. The events of puberty are influenced by the anterior pituitary stimulation by the hypothalamus. Gonadotropin-releasing factor stimulates the anterior pituitary to produce follicle-stimulating hormone (FSH), luteinizing hormone, luteotrophic hormone, and prolactin, which stimulate the gonads to begin functioning. FSH stimulates the growth of ova in girls and the Leydig cells in the testes of boys. The adrenal cortex then increases the production of androgen in response to estrogen and testosterone release from the ovaries and the testes respectively. Androgens are antagonistic to pituitary growth hormone, which accounts for the slowed body growth after puberty. Estrogen, testosterone, and androgen are the hormones responsible for the development of the secondary sex characteristics. Figures 4-2 and 4-3 illustrate adolescent sexual maturation and the development of secondary sexual characteristics often referred to as the Tanner staging system. The development of secondary sexual characteristics is orderly, but there are wide variations with each individual.

Health Alterations: Infancy Through Adolescence

Health alterations are those changes that occur in the status of an individual. Certain health alterations occur during specific age periods, but many span more than one period. The following health alterations are listed in approximate order of appearance, but each contains references to when they typically occur.

FEBRILE SEIZURES

Febrile seizures occur in a small percentage of infants when body temperatures rise. The underlying cause is usually an infection that produces the fever. The seizure may result from the rapid rise in temperature or it may be caused by the height that the temperature reaches. Febrile seizures do not develop into epilepsy nor do they usually cause neurologic damage. It is more common with childhood infections and is generally outgrown in early childhood.

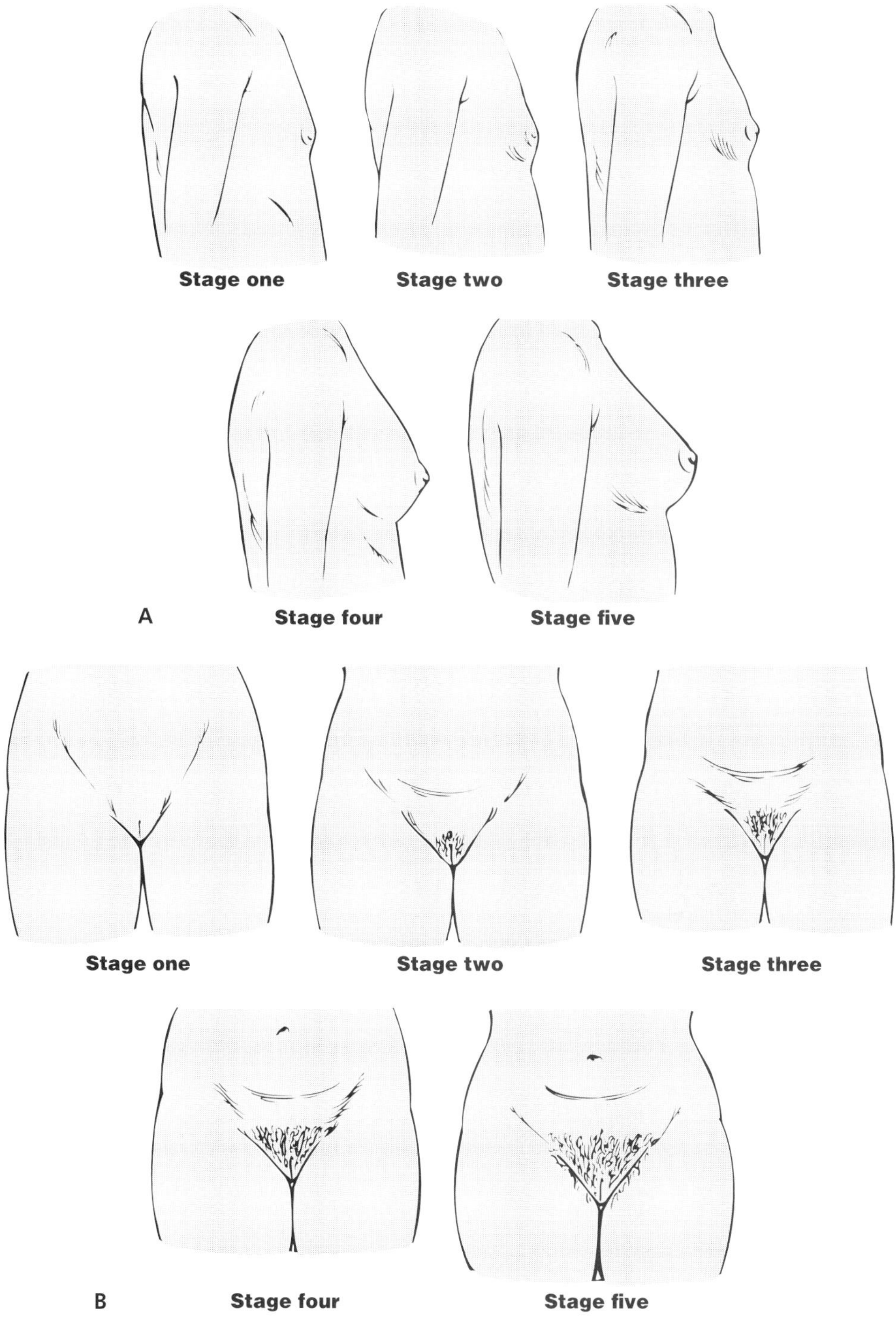

FIGURE 4-2. **A.** Female breast development. Stage 1: prepubertal; elevation of papilla only. Stage 2: breast buds appear; areola is slightly widened and projects as small mound. Stage 3: enlargement of the entire breast with no protrusion of the papilla or the nipple. Stage 4: enlargement of the breast and projection of areola and papilla as secondary mound. Stage 5: adult configuration of the breast with protrusion of the nipple; areola no longer projects separately from remainder of breast. **B.** Female pubic hair development. Stage 1: prepubertal; no pubic hair. Stage 2: straight hair extending along the labia and, between rating 2 and 3, begins on the pubis. Stage 3: pubic hair increased in quantity, darker, and present in the typical female triangle but in smaller quantity. Stage 4: pubic hair more dense, curled, and adult in distribution but less abundant. Stage 5: abundant, adult-type pattern; hair may extend onto the medial part of the thighs.

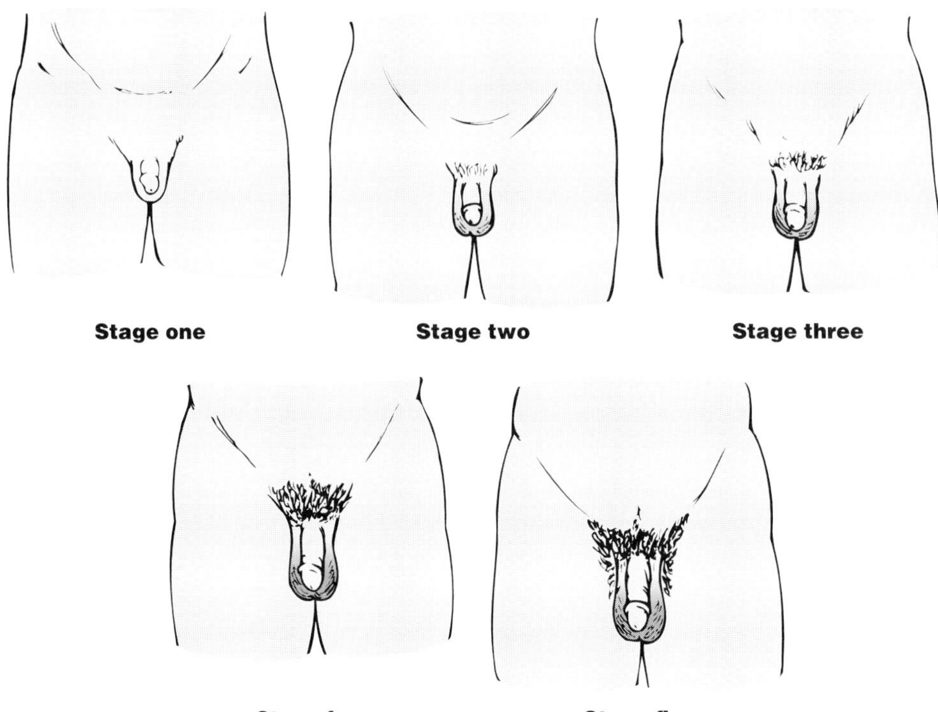

FIGURE 4-3. Male genital and pubic hair development. Ratings for pubic hair and for genital development can differ in a typical boy at any given time, since pubic hair and genitalia do not necessarily develop at the same rate. Stage 1: prepubertal; no pubic hair; genitalia unchanged from early childhood. Stage 2: light, downy hair develops laterally and later becomes dark; penis and testes may be slightly larger; scrotum becoming more textured. Stage 3: pubic hair has extended across the pubis; testes and scrotum are further enlarged; penis is larger, especially in length. Stage 4: more abundant pubic hair with curling; genitalia resemble those of an adult; glans has become larger and broader, scrotum is darker. Stage 5: adult quantity and pattern of pubic hair, with hair present along inner borders of thighs; testes and scrotum are adult in size.

FAILURE TO THRIVE

According to the National Center for Health Statistics, failure to thrive (FTT) is a condition associated with infant growth falling below the fifth percentile for their age. The two primary categories of FTT are:

- Organic failure to thrive (OFTT) resulting from a physical cause such as congenital heart defects, malabsorption syndrome, gastroesophageal reflux, cystic fibrosis, endocrine and renal dysfunction, or acquired immunodeficiency syndrome (AIDS). The manifestations include the growth problems as well as symptoms of the underlying physical problem.
- Nonorganic failure to thrive (NOFTT) results from a condition unrelated to an organic cause or disease. The cause is often related to poor or immature parenting skills, poverty, health beliefs, or family stress. The majority of cases of FTT are NOFTT. Infants exhibiting NOFTT are slow to respond to stimuli, appear listless, and often are unresponsive to nurturing.

COLIC

Colic is a common condition of early infancy. It occurs primarily in the first 3 to 4 months of life and is characterized by paroxysmal intestinal cramping associated with increased gas, abdominal distention, and pain. The cause is unknown, but it is thought to be related to swallowing too much air, overfeeding, or difficulty in digesting a formula too high in carbohydrates. The infant usually exhibits loud crying and pulls its legs up toward its abdomen. Infants with colic will usually continue to thrive, but emotional support of the parents is often needed. Colic usually disappears with decreased gas formation, which occurs when the infant can maintain a more upright posture and the intestinal tract has matured in its ability to digest food.

GASTROESOPHAGEAL REFLUX

Gastroesophageal reflux (GER), a neuromuscular disturbance, occurs when the cardiac sphincter and the lower esophagus relax. This allows gastric contents containing hydrochloric acid to be regurgitated into the esophagus. It is the most common esophageal problem in infants, appearing for no specific reason within the first week after birth, and disappearing by 1 year of age. Delay in growth and development, recurrent respiratory infections from aspiration of stomach contents, and blood in the stools are common complications associated with GER. Children with GER are at higher risk for aspiration pneumonia, SIDS, and FTT.

PYLORIC STENOSIS

A narrowing of the pyloric sphincter at the duodenum due to hypertrophy or hyperplasia of the surrounding muscle is called pyloric stenosis. This obstruction, of unknown etiology, causes delayed emptying of the stomach, an increase in gastric distention, and projectile vomiting. This vomiting predisposes to metabolic alkalosis resulting in weight loss and dehydration.

SUDDEN INFANT DEATH SYNDROME

The unexplained, sudden death, which occurs during sleep of a normal, healthy infant is called SIDS. It is the leading cause of death in infants under 1 year of age.

It is thought that SIDS may be related to a brain stem abnormality of regulation of the cardiopulmonary system. Autopsy often reveals heart, pleural, lung, and thymic petechiae, which are probably terminal events so that an adequate cause of death is not demonstrated on autopsy.[43] Box 4-3 shows the infants who are at risk for SIDS.

OTITIS MEDIA

Acute otitis media is one of the most prevalent childhood diseases after respiratory tract infections. It occurs most frequently in the winter months, in bottle-fed children who maintain a significantly slanted position during feeding, and in children who live with smokers.[14] It is usually seen in children 6 months through 6 years of age, with a slight decline in incidence between 3 and 4 years of age.

Etiology and Pathophysiology. Acute otitis media usually has a rapid onset and lasts approximately 3 weeks. It is especially common in infants and young children because they have short, straight eustachian tubes with undeveloped cartilage within. Otitis media is generally a result of eustachian tube dysfunction. This tube, connecting the middle ear to the nasopharynx, is normally closed. It opens to allow middle ear secretions to drain and to equalize pressure between the middle ear and the outside. Obstruction of the tube will allow secretions to accumulate. This causes a negative pressure within the middle ear. When the tube opens to attempt to equalize the pressure, bacteria may be introduced into the middle ear, causing infection of the mucosal lining.

Clinical Manifestations. Acute otitis media often follows an upper respiratory infection. The child may have a low-grade fever during the respiratory infection, but suddenly spikes a temperature to about 102°F. Young infants will often cry, be very irritable, have a loss of appetite, and may be observed tugging at or rubbing the affected ear. The older child will verbalize the discomfort, will be irritable and lethargic, and have a loss of appetite.

Otitis media is a very serious disease of childhood. If it is untreated, it can cause permanent damage and may result in hearing loss. The condition may become chronic and result in chronic otitis media with a constant buildup of thick, tenacious fluid in the middle ear. This is a long-term condition, often needing treatment until the child is about 10 years old.

BOX 4-3

MAJOR CHARACTERISTICS ASSOCIATED WITH SUDDEN INFANT DEATH SYNDROME

Family background	Highest in low birth weight, premature infants of adolescent mothers; underweight white males; African American infants; and infants of multiple births
Maternal factors	Higher risk with younger than age 20, cigarette smoking during pregnancy and use of illicit drugs; limited education and poor prenatal care
Siblings	Subsequent siblings of SIDS victims
Previous health	Detailed history may show abnormalities, illness within 2 weeks before death. May have had a life-threatening event such as apnea, choking or gagging at some time since birth.
Age	Greatest in 1–6 mo old; peak incidence 2–4 mo
Sex	Males greater risk
Season of year	Fall and winter months
Time of day	Between midnight and 9 AM

RESPIRATORY SYNCYTIAL VIRUS

Respiratory syncytial virus (RSV) is the causative organism in more than half of the cases of bronchiolitis and pneumonia in children under 2 years of age. It is most prevalent during late fall through early spring and usually lasts an average of 1 week. Infants and children who have high risk for RSV are those with bronchopulmonary dysplasia or who were born prematurely, especially before 35 weeks' gestation.[43] Edema of the bronchioles causes increased accumulation of mucus and exudate. Inflammation of the bronchi and bronchioles results in pneumonitis. Dilatation of the air passages on inspiration allows air intake, but obstruction in the small air passages prevents air from being exhaled. This overinflation causes the respiratory distress seen in affected children. Box 4-4 shows the signs and symptoms associated with RSV.

CROUP SYNDROMES

Croup is a general term referring to a group of disease involving inflammation of the larynx, trachea, and major bronchi. It is mainly seen in young children with a higher incidence in boys especially during the fall and early winter respiratory illness season.[64] Croup is usually due to parainfluenza types of viruses, but it can be caused by RSV, adenoviruses, or even bacterial tracheitis due to *Staphylococcus aureus*. Croup syndromes have a characteristic hoarseness, a resonant cough described as "barking," and inspiratory stridor with varying degrees of respiratory distress resulting from obstruction of the larynx. Table 4-13 shows a comparison of two forms of croup syndrome, laryngotracheobronchitis and acute epiglottitis.

BOX 4-4

CLINICAL MANIFESTATIONS OF RESPIRATORY SYNCYTIAL VIRUS

Onset
Fever
Pharyngitis
Coughing/wheezing
Rhinorrhea

Progressive Severity
Progressive tachypnea
Poor air exchange—cyanosis
Apnea
Change in level of consciousness
Pulmonary congestion and pneumonia

ALLERGIC RHINITIS

Allergic rhinitis is an inflammation of the nasal passages characterized by a watery nasal discharge with itchy eyes. It may be seen at any age, but tolerance or milder symptoms may occur over time. The condition is often seasonal and is caused by an allergic reaction to an irritant such as pollen. Antibodies are produced in the tissues in response to the allergen creating an antigen–antibody reaction in the tissues.

ASTHMA

Asthma is the most common medical condition for all children through adolescence but also may be seen in adults. It causes bronchoconstriction, which results in airway obstruction (see page 547). It is often induced by environmental factors and allergens such as air pollution and foods or by physical and psychological factors such as emotional upsets and exercise. The wheezing and resulting respiratory distress are caused by a narrowing of the airways by bronchospasm, mucosal edema, and increased mucus. Status asthmaticus, an attack not responding to conventional treatment, can result in death due to heart failure from exhaustion, atelectasis, or acidosis from bronchial blockage.

CYSTIC FIBROSIS

The lack of the CF protein is called cystic fibrosis. It is an inherited, autosomal recessive disorder affecting the infant or child. It is characterized by (1) chronic pulmonary disease, (2) decreased exocrine pancreatic function, and (3) other complications of inspissated mucus of other organs.[43] It is often diagnosed early in infancy based on clinical findings and a positive sweat chloride test, indicated by high sodium and chloride levels (> 60 mEq/L) in perspiration. The lack of the CF protein causes abnormally thick mucus to become trapped in the lining of the lungs, the pancreatic ducts, and biliary system. Bacteria thrive in this thick mucus and destroy the tissue (see pp. 773). The pathophysiology of the pulmonary features of CF is shown in Flowchart 4-5. Currently the life span of a cystic fibrosis patient is less than 30 years with death usually resulting from pulmonary failure.[43]

DIARRHEA

Diarrhea (frequent passing of loose, watery stools) is not a disease but a symptom of an underlying disorder. Gastrointestinal pathogens, especially bacteria and viruses, cause the production of enterotoxins or unknown pathogenic mechanisms. These pathogens cause especially serious alterations in infants and young children because these youngsters have little fluid volume reserve. These stimulate the secretion of water

TABLE 4-13

COMPARISON OF LARYNGOTRACHEOBRONCHITIS (CROUP) AND EPIGLOTTITIS

ASSESSMENT	LARYNGOTRACHEOBRONCHITIS	EPIGLOTTITIS
Causative organism	Usually viral	Usually *Haemophilus influenzae*
Usual age of child	6 mo–3 y	3–6 y
Seasonal occurrence	Late fall and winter	No seasonal variation
Onset pattern	Preceded by upper respiratory infection; cough becomes worse at night	Preceded by upper respiratory infection; suddenly very ill
Presence of fever	Low grade	Elevated to about 103°F
Appearance	Retractions and stridor; prolonged inspiratory phase of respirations; not very ill appearing	Drooling; very ill appearing; neck is hyperextended to breathe. (Do not attempt to view enlarged epiglottis, or immediate airway obstruction can occur.)
Cough	Sharp, barking	Muffled cough
Radiographic findings	Lateral neck radiograph shows subglottal narrowing	Lateral neck radiograph shows enlarged epiglottis.
Possible complications	Asphyxia due to subglottic obstruction	Asphyxia due to supraglottic obstruction

(From Pillitteri, A. [1999]. *Maternal and child health nursing* [3rd ed.]. Philadelphia: Lippincott Williams & Wilkins.)

and electrolytes and causes dehydration, acid–base imbalances, and circulatory impairment if not treated. Box 4-5 defines the different forms of diarrhea that may be seen.

DEHYDRATION

Fluid volume deficit from excessive loss of water occurs frequently in infants and children as a result of many diseases. There may be loss through vomiting and diarrhea, diabetic ketoacidosis, and extensive burns. Inadequate intake occurs in illnesses associated with fever resulting in greater loss than intake. Often both inadequate intake and excessive loss occur together. Dehydration can be mild, moderate, or life threatening (Table 4-14). There are three types of dehydration;

- Isotonic—most common form; water and electrolyte losses are about equal.
- Hypertonic—there is a greater loss of water than electrolytes, fluid moves from the intracellular to extracellular spaces.
- Hypotonic—electrolyte loss exceeds water loss; fluids move from the extracellular to the intracellular spaces.

SCOLIOSIS

A lateral curvature of the spine is called scoliosis. It is the most common spinal deformity and has its greatest incidence in adolescent girls. A sideways curve of at least 10° is considered scoliosis. Scoliosis requires treatment when the curve exceeds 20°. Scoliosis can be functional, caused by a deformity such as unequal leg length, or it can be structural, causing a loss of spinal flexibility. When the primary curve is accompanied by a secondary curve that puts the head in alignment with the hips, it is called compensated scoliosis. With uncompensated scoliosis, the head and hips are not in alignment. Severe scoliosis can cause respiratory impairment and motor discomfort when activities are performed (see page 823).

ANEMIA

Anemia, the most common hematologic disorder of infants and children, refers to a decreased in the number of RBCs or to a hemoglobin below normal (10–14 g/dL in infants and 12–14 g/dL in older children). Anemia is not considered to be a disease itself but is the result of a pathologic process (see page 353). It may result from: (1) loss of blood, (2) decreased or impaired RBC production, (3) suppressed bone marrow, (4) dietary insufficiencies, or (5) abnormalities of the RBCs such as in sickle cell disease (see page 357). A child with anemia is often pale with complaints of fatigue and lack of energy.

URINARY TRACT INFECTIONS

Urinary tract infections (UTIs) are some of the most common conditions of childhood, occurring most frequently between 2 and 6 years of age and again during adolescence. They occur up to 25 times more frequently in girls than in boys. The causative organism usually is *Escherichia coli*, the bacteria found in stool. The urinary tract structure contributes to the increased incidence in girls. The female urethra is very short, about 2 cm in young girls and 3 cm by young adulthood. This structure allows a ready pathway for organ-

FLOWCHART 4-5 **Basic Pathophysiology of Cystic Fibrosis**

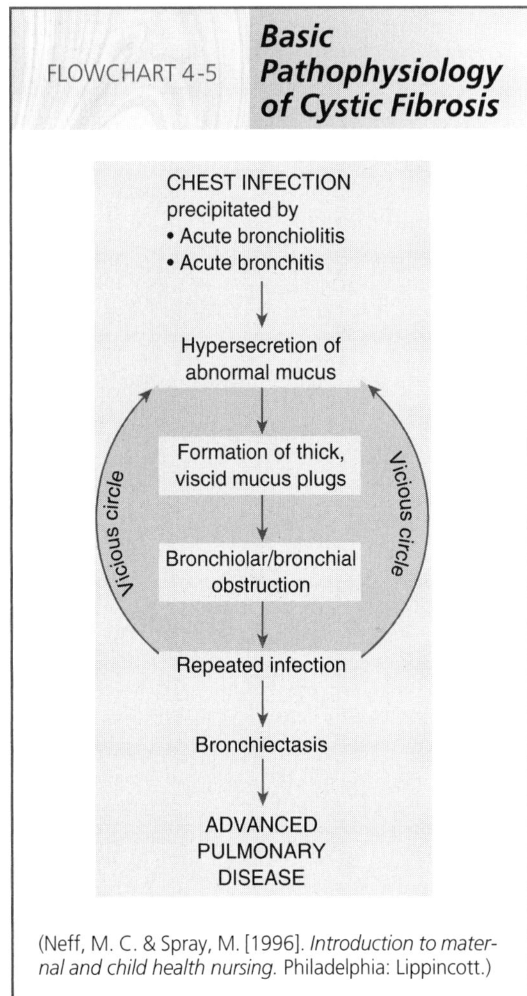

(Neff, M. C. & Spray, M. [1996]. *Introduction to maternal and child health nursing.* Philadelphia: Lippincott.)

ism invasion. The length of the male urethra, 20 cm by adulthood, and the antibacterial properties of the secretions of the prostate gland, inhibit bacterial growth.

The most important factor in the occurrence of UTIs is urinary stasis. Children often avoid emptying the bladder because they are too busy playing to take the time to urinate or because of lack of restroom facilities when they are away from home. Normally, repeated emptying of the bladder rids the bladder of organisms before they can multiply. As the urine remains in the bladder, the body warms it. Bacteria grow rapidly in a warm, moist, dark environment. The clinical manifestations of UTIs include bacteriuria, dysuria, frequency, urgency, and suprapubic pain (see page 606).

DIABETES MELLITUS

Diabetes mellitus (DM), characterized by lack of insulin production (type 1), has it highest incidence in children between 5 and 15 years of age.[43] It is thought to be due to an autoimmune process or perhaps a virus that destroys the insulin-producing cells in the pancreas. Type 1 DM results in a complete lack of insulin production and requires the administration of insulin to sustain life (see page 697). The onset of type 2 DM is much less common in children than in adults and is characterized by an inadequate secretion of insulin for the needs of the body.

ACNE

Acne, an inflammatory skin disorder characterized by papulopustular eruptions, occurs in about 85% of the population. The exact cause is unknown, but the peak incidence is between 16 and 18 years of age, which corresponds to major hormonal changes in the adolescent.[45] It is more common in boys. Inflammation occurs when the oil follicle ruptures and spreads the contents into the skin (see page 346).

MENSTRUAL DISORDERS

Menstrual irregularities are the most frequently reported problem in adolescent girls. *Amenorrhea*, the absence of menses, may be primary or secondary. In primary amenorrhea, menses never begin. This may be caused by structural defects, hormonal imbalances, or physical stress or activity. Secondary amenorrhea oc-

BOX 4-5

TYPES OF DIARRHEA

- *Acute diarrhea*—leading cause of illness under 5 y of age; most often caused by an inflammatory process; most often self-limiting, resolving with little to no treatment; commonly caused by antibiotic therapy
- *Chronic diarrhea*—lasting more than 2 wk; most often associated with malabsorption problems, anatomic defects, or long-term inflammatory processes
- *Bacterial diarrhea*—often caused by *Clostridium difficile;* occurs at any age; seen most often with extended illnesses or after abdominal surgery
- *Viral diarrhea*—most often caused by rotaviruses; high incidence from 6–24 mo of age
- *Parasitic diarrhea*—often caused by *Giardia lamblia* and cryptosporidium; commonly seen in day care centers

TABLE 4-14

ASSESSMENT OF PATIENTS WITH DEHYDRATION

DEGREE OF DEHYDRATION	SYMPTOMS	PERCENT OF WEIGHT LOSS
Mild to moderate	Restless, irritable, sunken eyes, no tears, dry tongue and mouth, thirsty and drinks eagerly	3–9
Severe	Lethargic or unconscious, rapid, thready pulse, cyanosis, cold extremities, rapid breathing, sunken and dry eyes, no tears, dry mouth and tongue, drinks poorly or not able to drink Life threatening unless replacement provided	> 10

(Modified from Neff, M. C., & Spray, M. [1996]. *Introduction to maternal and child health nursing* [p. 581]. Philadelphia: Lippincott-Raven.)

curs after menses has been established and is often associated with stress, physical activity, thyroid problems, marked weight loss or gain, or environmental changes. *Dysmenorrhea*, painful menstruation, is directly related to ovulatory cycles, the amount of prostaglandins secreted, and uterine contractility. *Premenstrual syndrome* has both a physical and an emotional component. It is generally linked to hormonal imbalances and dietary influences. Symptoms include bloating, breast tenderness, fatigue, irritability, food cravings, anxiety, and depression.

EATING DISORDERS AND OBESITY

Although anorexia nervosa and bulimia are thought of as eating disorders, in actuality they are psychological disorders associated with a pathologic fear of gaining weight and a poor self-image (see page 211).

Obesity is a major problem of children and adolescents and is caused by multiple factors, including inactivity, genetic propensity, overeating, and slow metabolism. It may predispose to physical and psychological complications (see page 217).

ADOLESCENT PREGNANCY

The adolescent who becomes pregnant must deal with developmental issues of adolescence at the same time she is dealing with developmental issues of pregnancy. The adolescent is at risk for PIH, iron deficiency anemia, preterm delivery, and cephalopelvic disproportion because her own physical growth may be inadequate to support the growth and delivery of the fetus. In addition, teenage nutrition is typically not balanced and prenatal care may be delayed because of denial.

BIOPHYSICAL DEVELOPMENT OF ADULTS

Adulthood is usually defined as the years from the early twenties to the mid-sixties, which is the largest portion of a person's life span. During this period, human beings are usually their most productive. It is a time of job achievement and recognition, childrearing, and the establishment of values and attitudes that will be transmitted to succeeding generations. Most adults are in relatively good health; however, the prevalence of both chronic disease and fatal illness increases with age. Accidental deaths and suicides/homicides cause a higher percentage of deaths during young adulthood; illness and disability are more frequently seen in later adulthood.[44] Alterations to health may result from self-destructive life-style habits rather than nonpreventable biologic phenomena.[40] Physiologic changes are an ongoing process. Cell death begins even during embryonic development, as does cell renewal. Over the years, cell function and the number of cells gradually decrease. Because of aging, the human passes through stages of immaturity, maturity, and deterioration. Theories regarding the physiologic changes of aging are varied and focus on aging at the cellular level or the wearing out of biologic systems. Cells apparently gradually lose the capacity for self-repair.[16]

This section explores adult developmental changes, destructive life-styles, and some of the related disease processes that are commonly experienced by the adult.

Young Adulthood

Young adulthood usually is described as that period of time following the teenage years until approximately age 30. It is that period of early adult transition and the entrance into the adult world.

For the most part, physical development is complete. Men may experience some physical growth after adolescence as their bodies reach the peak in muscular strength and reproductive ability. Athletic ability may reach a peak due to muscular strength capability during the twenties.[18] Except for accidents and injury, this is normally the healthiest period of life.

Neurologic development is complete by age 20. The young adult continues to refine and develop intellectual and cognitive processes. The potential for improved judgment and problem-solving is influenced by the types of life experiences the individual has. Reaction times to various stimuli usually peak during young adulthood until the late twenties.

Adulthood

The stage of adulthood is variously described as the years between age 30 and age 45.[53] Although there are no major physical changes in adulthood, gradual loss of skin elasticity and a few gray hairs remind the individual that aging is occurring. These changes are a source of stress that are compounded by career pressures and family problems. Good nutrition, proper rest, and physical activity can lessen the effects of aging, but the rate of onset of signs of aging is largely determined by genetic factors.[40]

Physical changes of aging have more variations among adults than children. Aging rarely progresses uniformly throughout the bodily systems. Persons of the same age appear to be of different ages.[40] Gradual physical decline occurs in many systems of the body. The reserve in the systems accounts for continued optimal organ function.

Musculoskeletal System. Muscle growth continues until about the age of 39, and muscle loss begins after that. Active muscles, especially those that are routinely exercised, atrophy more slowly than sedentary muscles.

Sensory System. The gradual changes in the sensory system do not interfere with functioning until late adulthood. Visual acuity often declines early in adulthood, and minute perceptual changes for the colors of blues, greens, and violets occur.[44] Hearing also declines slowly and often becomes a significant problem late in life. Hearing loss may be accelerated by loud, high-pitched sounds such as those of loud rock music.[44]

Cardiopulmonary System. Cardiopulmonary changes are insignificant in adulthood unless these systems are weakened by substance or nicotine abuse. Genetic factors may cause early onset of cardiopulmonary disease. There is normally a gradual functional loss in the lungs, which is accelerated by cigarette smoking. Cocaine abuse produces myocardial weakening and coronary artery spasm.[50]

Endocrine System. The endocrine system is affected by decreased secretion and decreased tissue receptiveness to the hormones. The endocrine system affects all bodily activities including metabolism and sexual functioning.

Reproductive System. The reproductive system is at peak function in the young adult. This is often the period of reproduction and an active sexual life. The woman's reproductive function declines rapidly after age 30; this is evidenced by changing menstrual function with cyclic changes.[50]

Middle Age (Middlescence)

Middle age is a time of usual good health, which is characterized by a group of biophysical changes. Pathologic changes may result if patterns in earlier life were destructive. Illness, disease, and other environmental factors may hasten aging or interrupt a normally healthy period. The physical changes in the forties and fifties are also variable but all persons show signs of aging. These signs are expressed throughout all of the body systems.

Intelligence, memory, and learning do not decrease in the period between ages 45 and 65 years unless there are problems associated with CNS functioning. There is, nevertheless, a gradual slowing of the functional capacity of all organ systems. Of particular concern is the increase of disease processes, such as cardiovascular disease and cancer.

Musculoskeletal and Integumentary Systems. The bony skeleton ceases its growth after full height has been reached. Bone mass rapidly declines after the age of 40, more in women than men. Calcium loss becomes pronounced during the menopausal years in women; however, men also lose calcium but at a later age and a slower rate than do women. Osteoporosis is most common in thin, white women and least common among African Americans.[47] The use of calcium, vitamin D, and estrogen supplements may decrease the rate of demineralization of the bone. Studies are supporting estrogen replacement in early menopause to decrease the rate of bone loss. Loss of height is common during the aging process. It may be due to a change in the normal 130° angle of the hip–femur joint to an angle of 135° or greater.[5]

Muscle strength and mass are directly related to muscle use. Muscle loss is caused by decreased muscle use. Changes in collagen fibers cause a sagging or drooping of muscles, especially those of the face, breast, and abdomen.[5]

The integumentary system shows wrinkling due to collagen fiber changes. Over the life cycle, the water content of the body decreases from about 61% to 53%, and fat content increases from 14% to 30%.[40,44]

Nervous and Sensory Systems. Some individuals experience a gradual decline in CNS function, which may be seen as a decline in mental functioning and mood. Slower reflexes and decreased responsiveness to changes in the environment are common alterations.[5] CNS function is not often impaired (even though brain cell loss is continuous) due to the large reserve of CNS neurons. Middle-aged CNS changes are offset by experience and problem-solving ability.[44]

Visual changes may become marked after age 40. Presbyopia from loss of elasticity in the lens of the eye causes loss of near vision. Hearing and smell loss may become noticeable at around age 50.

Cardiopulmonary System. Cardiopulmonary changes are very dependent on life-style and genetic factors. Middle-aged individuals with high blood pressure and high cholesterol levels and those who smoke are at much higher risk for cardiopulmonary problems than those without these risk factors (see page 466). Maintaining an active life-style prevents loss of myocardial tone. Lung tissue becomes thicker, stiffer, and less elastic with age but this process is markedly accelerated by smoking.[5] Repeated respiratory illnesses such as pneumonia, asthma, and bronchitis alter the lung tissue.

Gastrointestinal System. The gastrointestinal tract exhibits a decline in gastric juice secretion so that total daily acid production decreases.[53] Ptyalin in the saliva decreases sharply after age 40. Stress and life-style changes may affect gastric acid production. Pancreatic enzymes may also gradually decrease from the ages of 20 to 60 years.[53]

Endocrine System. The endocrine system usually exhibits no marked changes, but it is affected by stress and illness, which markedly affect the regulation of blood sugar and electrolyte balance. Middle-aged adults have an increased incidence of type 2 DM, which is related to familial hereditary factors and obesity (see page 714).

Reproductive and Genitourinary Systems. The reproductive system undergoes the most marked changes in middle life, especially in women. During the climacteric period in women the ovaries cease to function and the menstrual cycle ceases either suddenly or erratically. The menopause usually occurs in women at about 51 years of age but may occur earlier or later.[5,53] The resultant estrogen deficiency and pituitary influences cause "hot flashes" and other symptoms (see page 1104). Symptoms are aggravated by stress and family changes that may be occurring at this time. The male climacteric is a much slower process and is related to decline in testosterone production (see page 1074). Male sexual performance declines in middle age, and impotence in men over the age of 50 is a common problem.

Sexual relationships change according to physiologic changes. Women experience menopause and men experience a plateau of sexual responsiveness (stable testosterone levels), which leads to slower response and recovery time. Adaptation to these changes maintains the capacity for satisfying sexual relationships.

Genitourinary problems include stress incontinence or UTIs, which are common problems especially with women. Stress incontinence is caused by a decrease in urethral muscle support and decreased sphincter control.[5] Some problems with incontinence can be improved by changing voiding patterns, treating UTIs, or even surgery.

Destructive Life-Style Patterns and Related Health Alterations

Given proper diet, exercise, rest, and the ability to cope with the stresses of adult living, adulthood should be characterized by peak physical condition and performance. However, a number of destructive life-style patterns place adults at risk for the development of illnesses. Destructive life-styles often have their beginning in adolescence or early adulthood and may continue through older adulthood. The effect of these life-styles, however, are generally manifested during middle or late adulthood. Cigarette smoking, excessive alcohol consumption, illegal drug abuse, risky sexual practices, high-fat or high-cholesterol dietary intake, eating disorders, sedentary life-styles, and fatigue are examples of unhealthful patterns that often originate in response to stress. These behaviors can lead to chronic lung and liver diseases, myocardial infarction, AIDS, neurologic dysfunction, and many other conditions. The use of illegal drugs and alcohol also places individuals at high risk for accidental and homicidal death.

SMOKING

The controversy surrounding the use of tobacco has been evident for a long time. In 1859, Fairholt stated that "tobacco was a comfort to the poor, a luxury for the rich, and . . . united all classes in a common pleasure."[25] The modern period of cigarette manufacture began after the Civil War; however, cigarettes did not begin to be mass manufactured until about 1890. Prior to that time, snuff was the tobacco form of choice in both America and Europe.

The literature is replete with evidence regarding the hazardous effects of smoking. Cigarette smoking has been found to decrease or totally paralyze the mucociliary escalator system (see page 575). It has also been clearly implicated as a major cause of emphysema and chronic bronchitis. The risk of lung cancer increases with the number of cigarettes smoked and the length of time the person smoked. The male smoker is 10 times as likely to develop lung cancer as is the male nonsmoker. The American Cancer Society has estimated that 85% of lung cancer can be attributed to cigarette smoking. The nicotine in cigarettes has been shown to increase the risk of heart disease.[11] Smoking has also been associated with the development of cancer of the bladder.[16] Current focus is on the nonsmoker exposed to environmental tobacco smoke or passive smoke, which may significantly increase the risk to the nonsmoker.

Despite clear evidence that smoking cigarettes is a health hazard, people continue to smoke. It is estimated that 29% of adults in the United States are smokers, but a 0.5% decline per year is being seen.[3] In the past, smoking was seen as an acceptable habit within society. Smoking is a learned behavior that requires practice and becomes a habit. Nicotine in cigarettes is recognized as a substance that is addictive and withdrawal signs are common. These include craving for nicotine, irritability, difficulty in concentrating, and weight gain.[5] True addictive behavior to smoking is indicated when the person must have a cigarette within 30 minutes of awakening and smokes more than 25 cigarettes per day.[3] Otherwise, smoking is a habit and may be seen as purposeful (for such purposes as appetite control) as well as pleasurable. Adolescents view smoking as mature behavior while rationalizing that the health hazards could never happen to them. As a result, the behavior learned at this age is carried with them into adulthood.

SUBSTANCE ABUSE

Many people cope with the stressors of life by the use of substances that alter their mood or perception. The majority use substances that fall into one of the following categories: depressants, narcotics, or stimulants (Table 4-15). A major problem with psychoactive drug use is the potential for abuse and dependence.

Abuse occurs when a person continues using the substance despite the fact that it is creating problems in major areas of his or her life. Individuals are considered dependent on psychoactive substances when (1) they use larger quantities than they originally intended to, (2) they are unable to control or decrease its use, and (3) much of their life revolves around securing or using the substance. When individuals need to increase the amount of the substance to achieve the desired effect,

TABLE 4-15

PROBLEMS WITH PSYCHOACTIVE SUBSTANCE USE

SUBSTANCE	POTENTIAL PROBLEMS
CNS DEPRESSANTS	
Alcohol	Based on alcohol blood levels, CNS depressant effects increase from sedation and anxiety relief to incoordination, slurred speech, ataxia, stupor, unconsciousness, circulatory collapse, and death. Tolerance develops. Chronic use can lead to peripheral nerve injury; polyneuritis; dementia; myocardial lesions; pancreatitis; impaired liver function; nutritional deficiencies, especially B complex; and fetal alcohol syndrome. Withdrawal without treatment can progress from nausea and vomiting, tremors, restlessness, tachycardia, and hypertension to hallucinations, seizures, profound confusion, delirium, and death.
Tranquilizers	Potentiates the effect of alcohol; cross-tolerance with alcohol and sedatives; physical dependence; may accumulate in body with slow excretion by kidneys; may cause fetal deformities. Withdrawal is similar to alcohol.
Barbiturates	Decreases cortical function; ataxia; depresses respiratory centers in medulla; shortens REM sleep; accelerates function of hepatic microsomal enzymes (decreases effectiveness and speeds tolerance); when dependence develops, even temporary abstinence leads to withdrawal symptoms. Withdrawal is similar to that for alcohol.
CNS STIMULANTS	
Amphetamines	Potentiates endogenous catecholamine activity, which elevates mood and increases alertness and concentration. Intoxication produces excitation, hyperactive reflexes, hostility, aggression, convulsions. Prolonged use can lead to dysrhythmias, cerebral vascular spasm, cerebrovascular accident (CVA), paranoidlike state, severe abdominal pain. Physical dependency occurs. Withdrawal leads to fatigue, lethargy, depression.
Cocaine	Immediate and short-lived CNS stimulation similar to amphetamines. Chronic use is associated with multisystem problems including dysrhythmias, CVA, pulmonary edema, perforation of the nasal septum, anorexia, CNS disturbances, and sexual dysfunction. Psychologic dependence can occur.
NARCOTICS	Relieves pain and anxiety and produces a temporary euphoria. CNS depression, pupillary constriction, depressed respirations occur. IV abuse can lead to malnutrition, infection, contaminant toxicity, hepatitis, thromboembolic complications, and AIDS. Tolerance develops with repeated use. Withdrawal includes yawning, tearing, chills and fever, tremors, muscle spasms, and tachycardia. Withdrawal, though uncomfortable, is not life-threatening.

(Adapted from Malseed, R. T., & Harrigan, G. S. [1989]. *Textbook of pharmacology and nursing care.* Philadelphia: Lippincott.)

they have developed tolerance to it.[36] Withdrawal is the term used for the symptoms that result from abstinence from the abused substance. Whether withdrawal will occur depends on the quantity and duration of the use of the substance.[11]

Alcohol

Alcohol is the most frequently abused substance in the United States. Up to 90% of Americans use alcohol, but the frequency of use varies. Of these, it is estimated that 10% of men and 3% to 5% of women meet the criteria for the disease of alcoholism.[11] Alcoholics often do not recognize the impact of alcohol on their lives or the lives of their families. The complications of alcoholism include physiologic impact on the liver and pancreas as well as psychological and social problems (Fig. 4-4). Some of the physical complaints of the alcoholic are sleep disorders, gastrointestinal tract problems, or the results of liver complications (see page 763).

Acute, massive alcohol consumption can have damaging to lethal effects (Fig. 4-5). These may be seen in the individual who consumes massive amounts of alcohol, but they are not frequently seen in the alcoholic individual.

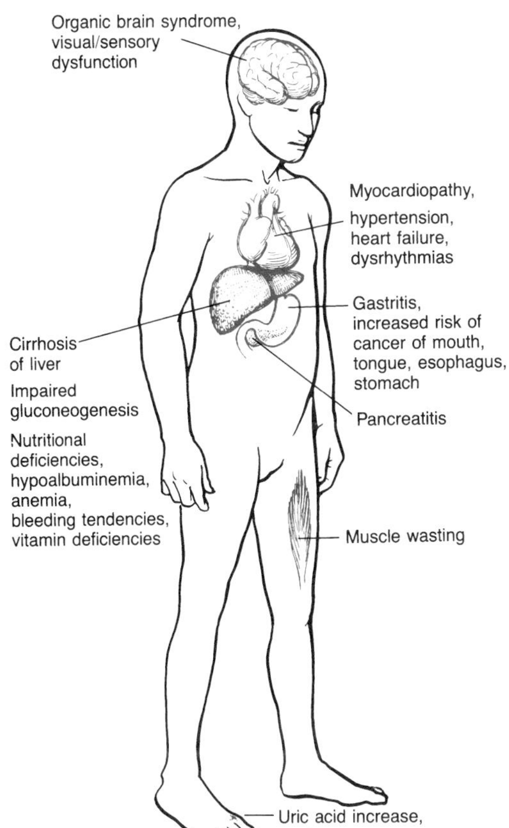

FIGURE 4-4. Alcoholism can have damaging systemic effects.

Withdrawal from alcohol in the alcoholic may be seen within the first 4 to 8 hours after the last drink. Withdrawal is marked by tremor and irritability that progress to agitation, hyperreflexia, and then to visual and auditory hallucinations. Seizures, disorientation, hyperadrenergism, and fever may be seen; these are the hallmark of true delirium tremens and usually resolve within 72 hours. Complications from delirium tremens may claim as many as 10% to 15% fatalities.[11,41] Box 4-6 lists the clinical manifestations of alcohol withdrawal syndrome.

Opioids

Opioids, including morphine, heroin, codeine, oxycodone, and meperidine, are commonly abused drugs. The effects desired by the abuser of these drugs is euphoria, sedation, and analgesia, but overdoses cause respiratory depression, coma, and death. Complications usually result with overdoses or if they are injected in a nonsterile fashion. Systemic reactions to the preparations used causes a high incidence of chronic liver disease especially in heroin abusers. Withdrawal will begin from 2 to 48 hours after the last usage. Especially with heroin, the abrupt stoppage causes rapid onset of restlessness, rhinorrhea, shivering, tachycardia, and hypertension.[42]

Cocaine and Amphetamines

Cocaine is a very commonly abused drug that is usually inhaled nasally but may be smoked, ingested, or injected. Free-basing the drug with diethyl ether produces high serum concentrations and great potential for toxicity. **Amphetamines** are usually taken orally. Both cocaine and the amphetamines produce a sense of euphoria and elation resulting from catecholamine release by the CNS. Over time, with abuse of the drugs, acute and chronic paranoid psychoses have been seen. Physical problems have to do with route of administration and include nasal perforation, rhinitis, renal failure, cerebrovascular accidents, and cor pulmonale.[42] Withdrawal is characterized by lethargy, somnolence, and depression. Craving for the effect of the drug makes it very difficult to stop this addiction. Cocaine can induce many cardiovascular complications such as dysrhythmias, premature myocardial ischemia and infarction, and cardiomyopathy (see page 518).

FOOD-RELATED ABUSE

A significant proportion of adults in the United States have chronic diseases that are caused by nutritional imbalance. Worldwide, nutritional inadequacies are major determinants of resistance to disease and increased mortality. Nutrition is a major environmental factor in the achievement of longevity, in resistance to disease, and in the tolerance and response to stress.

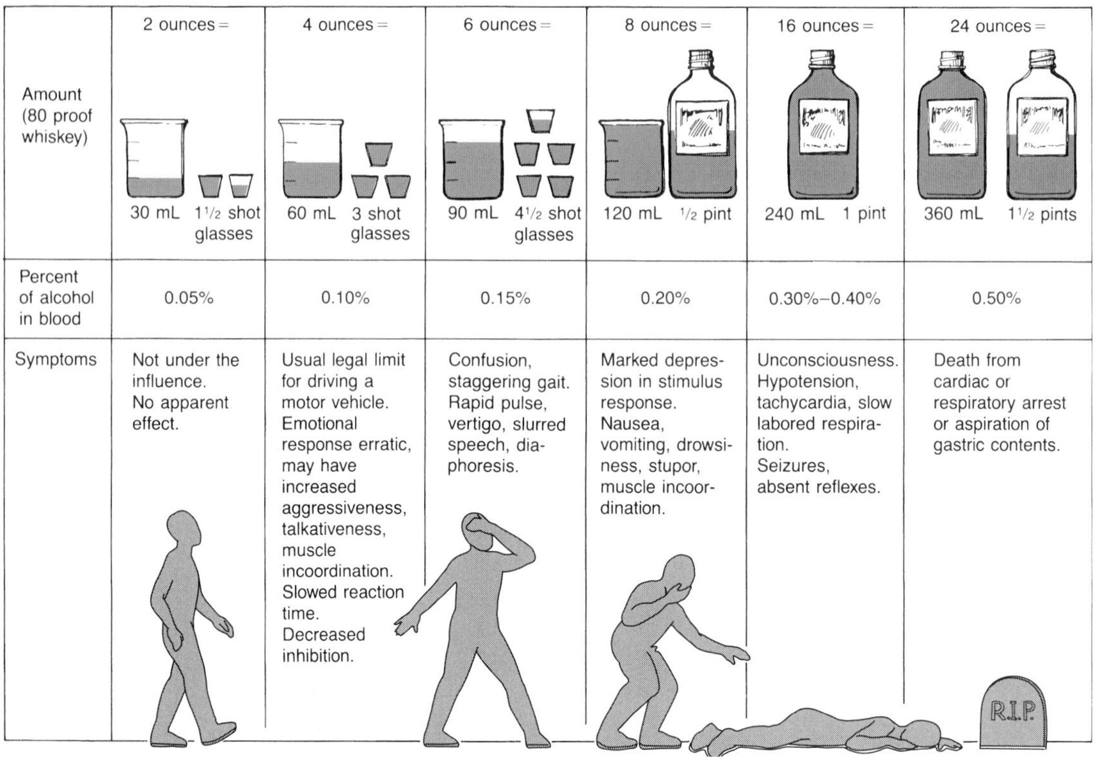

	2 ounces =	4 ounces =	6 ounces =	8 ounces =	16 ounces =	24 ounces =
Amount (80 proof whiskey)	30 mL 1 1/2 shot glasses	60 mL 3 shot glasses	90 mL 4 1/2 shot glasses	120 mL 1/2 pint	240 mL 1 pint	360 mL 1 1/2 pints
Percent of alcohol in blood	0.05%	0.10%	0.15%	0.20%	0.30%–0.40%	0.50%
Symptoms	Not under the influence. No apparent effect.	Usual legal limit for driving a motor vehicle. Emotional response erratic, may have increased aggressiveness, talkativeness, muscle incoordination. Slowed reaction time. Decreased inhibition.	Confusion, staggering gait. Rapid pulse, vertigo, slurred speech, diaphoresis.	Marked depression in stimulus response. Nausea, vomiting, drowsiness, stupor, muscle incoordination.	Unconsciousness. Hypotension, tachycardia, slow labored respiration. Seizures, absent reflexes.	Death from cardiac or respiratory arrest or aspiration of gastric contents.

FIGURE 4-5. Effects of alcohol ingestion on the average 68-kg (150-pound) male. Females usually react earlier to ingestion, even when body sizes are comparable. Symptoms are those generally seen.

ALCOHOL WITHDRAWAL SYNDROME

- Alcohol craving
- Tremor, irritability
- Nausea
- Sleep disturbance
- Tachycardia, hypertension
- Sweating
- Perceptual distortion
- Seizures (12–48 h after last drink)
- Delirium tremens (rare in uncomplicated withdrawal)
  - Severe agitation
  - Confusion
  - Visual hallucinations
  - Fever, tachycardia, profuse sweating, dilated pupils
  - Nausea diarrhea

(From Kelley, W. N. [1997]. *Textbook of internal medicine* (3rd ed.). Philadelphia: Lippincott-Raven.)

Obesity

Obesity is the most common problem in the United States. It is defined as a body mass index of greater than 27.8 kg/m^2 in men and 27.3 kg/m^2 in women. It has been estimated that of adults over the age of 30, 25% to 40% are more than 20% overweight.[56] Obesity is associated with increased incidence of cardiovascular disease, diabetes, pulmonary dysfunction, cancer, and gallstones.[56] Obesity is characterized by a number of metabolic changes related to lipid metabolism. Obese individuals often have elevated serum cholesterol and triglyceride levels and lower high-density lipoprotein concentrations. These changes increase the risk for coronary heart disease.

Anorexia and Bulimia Nervosa

Common eating disorders of early adulthood are **anorexia nervosa** and **bulimia nervosa** (BN) (see page 211). Anorexia nervosa usually begins in adolescence but may continue into adulthood. Bulimia is thought to occur more often in early adulthood. Although treated as two separate disorders, many of the behaviors overlap.

SEDENTARY LIFE-STYLES

The current best estimate is that only about 10% to 20% of adults participate in enough exercise to provide for cardiorespiratory benefit.[10] Recent surveys indicate that fewer than 10% of Americans older than age 18 years meet the criteria for exercise proposed in the 1990 objectives for the nation, and the amount of physical activity at work and in the home has declined steadily with increasing automation and labor-saving aids.[13]

Television viewing is the most pervasive pastime in the United States today. Following sleep and work, it is the nation's third most time-consuming activity. The typical adult watches TV nearly 4 hours daily. When the TV is on, activity ceases and time for exercise is reduced significantly. Due to decreased calorie expenditure, adults who view 3 hours of television or more each day have twice the risk of obesity and an even higher risk of superobesity.[58]

FATIGUE

The term fatigue refers to a loss of power or strength on exertion.[59] It has been described as a feeling of overwhelming tiredness. Fatigue can be emotionally induced when there are extreme stresses or depression in one's life. It also may result when exercise is performed to the extent that liver glycogen stores are depleted and glucose is not available for muscle metabolism. Therefore, fatigue may be a subjective or objective condition. The condition may be temporary or it may occur consistently. It must be differentiated from weakness caused by muscle, neuromuscular, or organic disorders.[59]

Acute fatigue usually occurs due to physical exertion and the extent of the fatigue depends on the physical condition of the person affected. It has a rapid onset and is relieved by varying periods of rest. Individuals also may complain of acute fatigue related to a particularly stressful situation.

Chronic Fatigue Syndrome

Chronic fatigue is often the outcome of chronic illnesses that limit the endurance for activity. It is also one of the main complaints of individuals who seek medical assistance. From the complaints of chronic fatigue a peculiar syndrome, called **chronic fatigue syndrome,** has been identified. It is also *called chronic fatigue and immune dysfunction syndrome (CFIDS)* and is described as disabling fatigue usually associated with low-grade fever that has been present for a period of months.[15] It may be preceded by a flulike illness that leaves the presence of muscle aches and pains, headaches, confusion, depression, sleep disruption, low-grade fever, and sometimes lymph node enlargement or pain.[49]

Chronic fatigue syndrome has been associated with the fungal infection, *Candida albicans*, with chronic mercury poisoning from dental fillings, with anemia, hypoglycemia, hypothyroidism, and sleep disorders. More often it is associated with Epstein-Barr virus (EBV), which is probably a result or complication of CFIDS rather than its cause. Diagnosis of CFIDS is made when there is persistent fatigue over 6 months with associated symptoms and other significant diseases have been ruled out. Not all cases can be linked with EBV and there remains substantial disbelief as to the existence of the condition at all.[15] Research suggests that CFIDS is caused by immune system dysfunction with evidence of immune suppression related to functional deficiencies in natural killer cells (see page 283).

Symptoms of chronic fatigue syndrome are copious, varied, and often elusive but they comprise a syndrome that is extremely debilitating.[28,49] Sleep problems are frequently described despite the complaint of chronic tiredness. These sufferers have symptoms that plateau early in the illness and recur with varying degrees of severity for months to years. Victims describe the good and bad days with the good days contributing to the skepticism of others. The Centers for Disease Control and Prevention (CDC) has recognized chronic fatigue syndrome as a disease that forces individuals to quit work for months or years at a time.[13] The syndrome is felt to represent a major threat to world health and its victims in all countries include teachers, health care workers, clergy, flight attendants, and other individuals who have close contact with the public on a regular basis. Even though the disease apparently does not produce death, 60% to 70% of affected persons remain significantly ill for at least 1 to 3 years. If the illness extends more than 3 years, the chance of total recovery becomes less than 10%.[15]

BIOPHYSICAL DEVELOPMENT OF OLDER ADULTS AND RELATED ALTERATIONS

The phenomenon of aging is variable and complex. It is difficult to define what aging is or to establish the facts about the process. Much of the confusion arises from the difficulty of differentiating between normal aging and changes secondary to disease. Aging leads to a gradual diminution in the functional capacity of the organ systems. Some problems may be attributed to primary structural organ changes and some are secondary, reversible processes (Table 4-16).[60] The aging process is extremely variable among different individuals, making chronological age a poor index of physiologic age or of performance. Advancing years are not

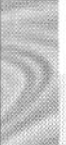

TABLE 4-16

BIOPHYSICAL EFFECTS OF AGING: CHANGES IN BODY SYSTEMS

MUSCULOSKELETAL

Physiologic Alteration	Clinical Consequence
• General skeletal muscle wasting, decreased muscle mass	• Decreased muscle strength, endurance, tone, agility, physical activity
• Reduced capillary circulation results in decreased oxygen supply	• Reduced range of motion, mobility, flexibility, muscle stiffness, slowness
• Loss of minerals	• Brittle bones
• Loss of cortical (compact bone), shortening of the vertebral column, hip and knee flexion	• Reduced height, kyphosis
• Cartilage and joint erosion, overgrowth of bone margins, spurs	• Joint pain, limited motion

SKIN AND DERMAL APPENDAGES

Physiologic Alteration	Clinical Consequence
• Atrophy of all skin layers, water loss, subcutaneous fat loss, less active sebaceous and sweat glands	• Thin, dry skin, reduced turgor, wrinkles; brittle, dry thickened yellowish nails; decreased perspiration
• Reduced capillary circulation	• Injuries slow to heal

NEUROLOGIC

Physiologic Alteration	Clinical Consequence
• Decreased conduction rate of nerve impulses, decreased number of neurons	• Slower reaction time and adaptation to physiologic stressors, slower recover time, memory loss
• Metabolic changes and altered neurotransmitter production	• Insomnia, sleep disturbances, potential depression

SENSORY-VISION

Physiologic Alteration	Clinical Consequence
• Decreased lens elasticity	• Close range reading problems
• Corneal changes	• Cloudy lens
• Loss of soluble proteins with loss of lens transparency	• Cataracts
• Diminished muscle response	• Slow pupil reaction
• Decreased light perception	• Slow light to dark adaptation, poor night vision

SENSORY-HEARING

Physiologic Alteration	Clinical Consequence
• Cerumen (ear wax) contains greater amount of keratin, which is easily impacted	• Temporary hearing loss
• Degenerative changes	• Presbycusis (hearing loss), especially high-pitched sounds

SENSORY-TASTE/SMELL/TOUCH

Physiologic Alteration	Clinical Consequence
• Diminished olfactory function	• Inability to smell, interferes with appetite
• Reduced taste buds	• Decreased appetite, poor nutrition
• Conduction deficits	• Decreased sensitivity to heat, pressure, pain; reduced stereognosis

(continued)

TABLE 4-16

BIOPHYSICAL EFFECTS OF AGING: CHANGES IN BODY SYSTEMS (Continued)

Physiologic Alteration	Clinical Consequence
CARDIOVASCULAR	
• Loss of muscle fiber, increased collagenous material surrounding fibers, loss of myocardial elasticity, diminished baroreceptor response	• Diminished contraction and decreased filling capacity, pulse slow to respond to stress with slow return to normal
• Thickened, rigid valves	• Murmurs (early systolic), fatigue
• Deficient conduction system	• Dysrhythmias, premature beats
• Loss of blood vessel elasticity and increased peripheral resistance	• Increased diastolic and systolic blood pressure, widened pulse pressure, varicose veins, edema
RESPIRATORY	
• Decreased elasticity	• Decreased vital capacity, diminished breath sounds at lung bases, fatigue, breathlessness
• Decreased cilia activity	• Decreased maximal oxygen uptake
• Diminished reflexes	• Difficulty coughing up secretions
• Bone changes in rib cage, respiratory muscle weakness	• Decreased chest expansion and depth of respiration, increased anteroposterior diameter of chest
GENITOURINARY	
• Increased number of abnormal glomeruli, loss of nephrons, reduced renal blood flow	• Decreased creatinine clearance, potential increase in toxic effects of medications, kidneys do not concentrate urine as well
• Decreased bladder capacity	• Frequency, urgency, nocturia, incontinence
• Enlarged prostate in males	• Difficulty initiating urination
• Hormonal changes, diminished vaginal secretions in women	• Delayed erection in men; dryness, painful intercourse in women
GASTROINTESTINAL	
• Loss of teeth, tongue papilla, taste, and smell	• Poor appetite, poor intake, weight loss
• Decreased salivary ptyalin	• Diminished carbohydrate digestion, dry mouth
• Diminished esophageal peristalsis, esophageal waves, poor relaxation of esophageal sphincter	• Delayed emptying, decreased appetite, early satiety
• Diminished gag reflex	• Cough, choking
• Hiatal hernia	• Esophagitis, heartburn, reflux
• Thin gastric mucosa; decreased gastrin, gastric acid, pepsin, and intrinsic factor	• Gastritis, iron deficiency anemia, pernicious anemia, carcinoma
• Diminished colonic muscle tone, decreased intestinal motility	• Constipation, fecal impaction
• Reduced liver weight and blood flow, decreased inducible enzymes of the liver, reduced serum albumin	• Altered drug metabolism, weakness, weight loss

necessarily equated with illness. The appearance of the aging person characteristically is altered. Stature is lost, body proportions are changed, skin is dry and wrinkled, hair is thinning and gray, and changes in body movement are characterized by slowness, stiffness, and diminished coordination and balance.

Variables That Modify Biophysical Effects of Aging

The causes of aging have been investigated for centuries, yet no researcher has been able specifically to identify any single causative factor. Biology, sociology, and psychology have proposed various theories for the changes that occur with the aging process. A discussion of these theories is found in sources in the bibliography. Some current theories include: free radical, waste product, immunologic, cross-linkage, somatic mutation, and genetic aging theories.[19]

Modern health care practices have resulted in an increased life expectancy in the United States. The variability of life span for humans seems to be a function of several factors: heredity, culture, race, nutrition, and environment. Total life span seems to be limited to 90 to 105 years, which supports the belief that aging is an innate process.

In 1958, a group of gerontologists began a comprehensive and ambitious longitudinal study on aging known as the Baltimore Longitudinal Study of Aging. After almost 40 years of investigation, these researchers suggest that the changes of aging are not limited to a single cause. It was found in a number of tests that older people performed as well as younger people, that aging did not always result in gradual loss of intellectual functions, and that in some cases life-style modification improved test performance.[32] These results are part of the emerging body of evidence that suggests that the effects of the changes thought to normally occur with aging can be modified by life-style and environmental variables. An active versus a sedentary life-style is preferred. Physical activity reduces the rate at which aerobic capacity is lost. Moderate weight-bearing activity is beneficial in increasing bone mass.[26] Dietary modifications, such as maintaining a low-cholesterol diet, can influence the occurrence of some age-associated diseases. Discontinuation of cigarette smoking can also decrease the occurrence of disease in the elderly.

Total Body Composition

The total body composition is altered. Lean body mass is reduced, including fat-free body tissues such as nerves, organ parenchyma, and skeletal muscle. Increased amounts of fat are laid down in mesenteric or paranephritic areas rather than in subcutaneous fat. Decreased subcutaneous fat leads to increased skin folding. Amounts of total body potassium, water, and intracellular fluid decrease; however, there is no change in the amount of extracellular fluid. The bone mineral mass is reduced, with increased bone porosity. Figure 4-6 shows the major changes in the body components with aging. The aggregate effect of these losses is reduced total body density.[48]

Weight changes are characteristic. In men, the average maximum weight is 172 lb at ages 35 to 54 years. This falls to 166 lb at ages 55 to 64. In women, the average maximum weight is 152 lb at 55 to 64 years, 146 lb at ages 65 to 74, and 138 lb at ages 75 to 89. The weight of women declines less than that of men.[27]

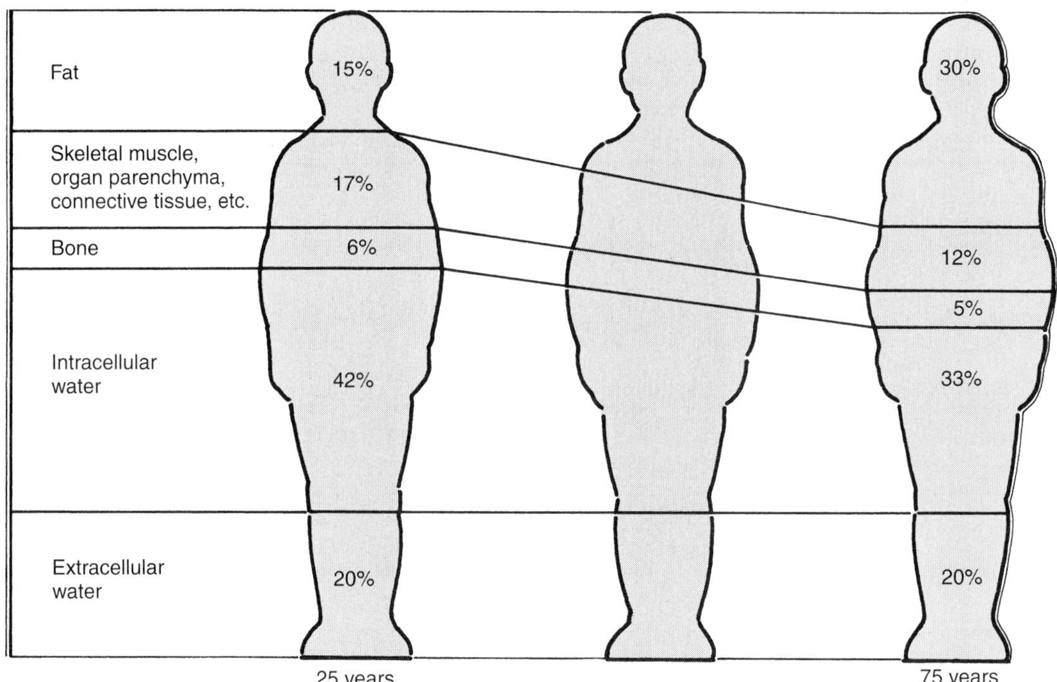

FIGURE 4-6. Changes in major body components with the aging process.

Musculoskeletal System

One of the most visible characteristics of aging is the change in posture and patterns of movement (Fig. 4-7). Successful portrayal of an old person by an actor nearly always includes certain features of body movement, such as stooped posture, muscular rigidity, slow movement, and lack of coordination and stability.

Reduction in height results from hip and knee flexion, **kyphosis** of the dorsal spine, and shortening of the vertebral column. The intervertebral disks become thin, as do the vertebrae themselves, leading to the reduction in height. The thoracic curve of the vertebral column increases, resulting in a kyphosis. This development, along with changes in lung elasticity, results in increased anteroposterior diameter of the chest. The cervical curve increases to compensate for the thoracic curve, causing a tilting of the head. Height loss, therefore, is in the trunk. The length of the long bones is unchanged. The effect is a short trunk and long limbs, which is just the opposite of what is seen in a child (Fig. 4-8).

Joint changes include erosion of the cartilaginous surfaces of the joints, degenerative changes of the soft tissues in the joints, and calcification and ossification of the ligaments resulting in **osteoarthritis**. Osteoarthritic changes in the fingers are easily seen with the development of **Heberden's** and **Bouchard's nodes** (Fig. 4-9). Alterations in neuromuscular function result from the combined effect of changes in the muscles, the peripheral motor neurons, the myoneural synapses, and the CNS. Diet, heredity, and hormonal balances also are influences on the musculoskeletal system.

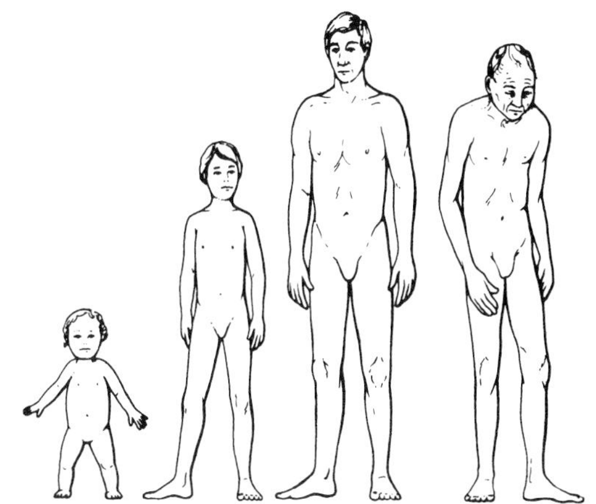

FIGURE 4-8. Changes in body proportions through the life span.

OSTEOPOROSIS

Osteoporosis is basically caused by an increase of bone absorption over bone formation. This primarily affects

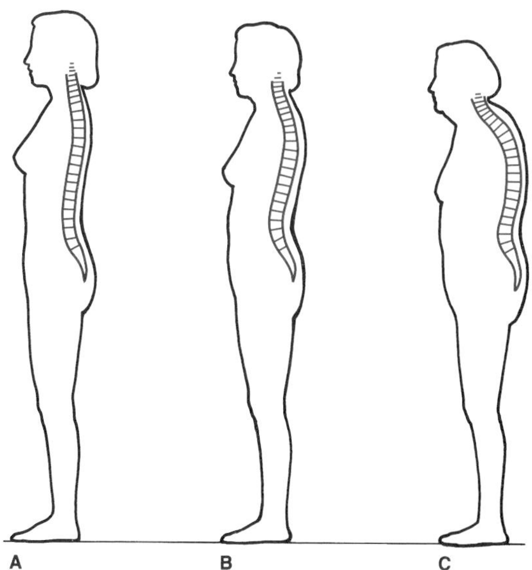

FIGURE 4-7. Posture changes occur gradually as aging occurs. **A.** Early to middle adulthood, spine is straight. **B.** Middle age to early aging with early osteoporosis changes weakening the vertebrae. **C.** Late aging changes may show a height loss of 10 cm or more.

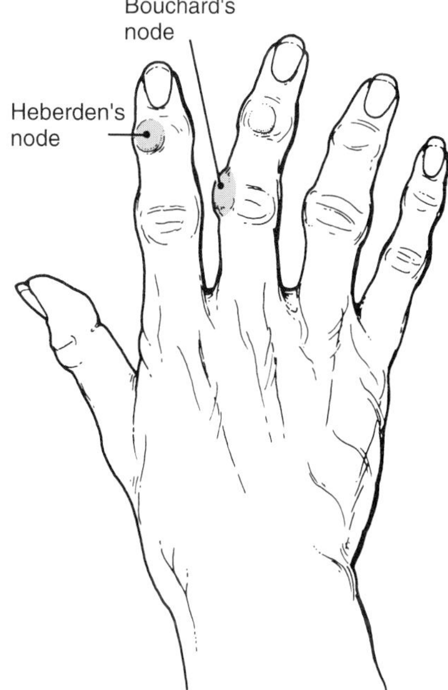

FIGURE 4-9. Heberden's and Bouchard's nodes in an elderly individual. Note the lateral deviation of the third and ring fingers.

trabecular bone and also the cortices of long bones. The outer surfaces of long bones continue to grow slowly throughout life, but with osteoporosis, the inner surfaces are reabsorbed at a slightly faster rate. The end result is a long bone that is slightly longer in external diameter but with thinner walls and with markedly diminished trabecular bone in its ends. Vertebral bodies, which have a larger percentage of trabecular bone, are severely affected by this process.[6]

In osteoporosis, there is evidence of decreased calcium absorption from the gastrointestinal tract. Also, the disease has some relationship with gonad deficiency because its frequency is greatly increased in postmenopausal women. Immobilization and lack of weight-bearing on the skeletal system causes osteoporosis at any age. Elevated levels of cortisone, either exogenous or endogenous, also cause the condition. Regardless of the underlying pathologic process, osteoporosis occurs to a degree in all elderly persons but is much more marked in women.

Of primary concern in osteoporosis is the tendency for bone fracture, most frequently of the vertebrae and the femurs. Studies of elderly persons show that 34% of fractures of the femur are caused by accidents.[8] Twenty-five percent occur because of a "drop attack," which is a sudden fall caused by postural instability that results from changes in the hindbrain and cerebellum. The person suddenly falls to the ground without warning or with a momentary vertigo. Among 384 persons evaluated in one study, the most frequent cause of falls was tripping, followed by loss of balance and drop attack. Forty-three percent of the total sample had neurologic disease.[8]

Kyphosis, or curvature of the spine, in older persons frequently occurs as a result of osteoporosis of the vertebrae. Vertebral atrophy also occurs. Because of the progressive degeneration, the number of cells diminishes, the water content decreases, and the tissues lose turgor and become friable. The combined changes in the vertebrae and disks result in curvature of the spine. Kyphosis causes decreased respiratory capacity of the chest wall and other conditions related to impingement on various spinal nerves as a result of the narrowed disks and vertebral changes. These problems most often occur in the lumbar and cervical spine. Compression fractures of the spine are also common.[4]

FRACTURES RELATED TO CEREBROVASCULAR DISEASE

In the aged individual, the increased risk for falling and bone fractures may be related to cerebrovascular disease, which often causes difficulty in locomotion in elderly persons. Arteriosclerosis of the carotid and vertebral arteries that results in ischemia may cause transient paralysis or light-headedness, poor balance, and falling episodes. If such events occur, the person becomes anxious and tense about moving, and coordination is reduced even further. Older persons who fear falling tend to take fewer and fewer risks; the result is increased immobility. Individuals who have had cerebrovascular accidents tend to have hemiparesis or hemiplegia. Those who recover from such episodes tend to have some motor disability that creates difficulty in walking, postural changes in both sitting and standing, residual spasticity, and footdrop. These factors increase the risk for falling.

Injury from falling is a major problem for the elderly. Fractures of the hip and wrist are frequent, as is head injury. The fractures often result from decreased bone strength related to osteoporosis and the falling result from cerebrovascular insufficiency. Complications also result from immobility during hospitalization and surgical procedures for fractures.

Skin and Dermal Appendages

Next to alterations in the musculoskeletal system, changes in the integument are the most obvious signs of aging. With loss of elasticity, wrinkles, lines, and drooping eyelids occur. Exposed areas, such as the hands, develop age spots or excessive skin pigmentation. The skin becomes dry, thin, fragile, and prone to injury. Nails become dry and brittle. Toenails become susceptible to fungal infection and appear thickened; there is a lifting of the nail plates. The rate of change is very individual and is dependent on such factors as nutrition, genetics, emotions, and environment. Typical changes that occur in the skin are depicted in Figure 4-10.

The skin often reflects other disease conditions such as liver or cardiac disease. Relatively minor skin problems, such as overgrowths of epidermal tissue, cause cosmetic problems but rarely need surgical excision. **Senile telangiectasias,** small scarlet growths scattered over the skin, increase in number after middle age. **Hyperkeratotic warts,** raised brown or black epidermal overgrowths, also develop in increased numbers with age. These two types of lesions, together with others that occur less frequently, have no clinical significance and do not require removal unless irritated by clothing or jewelry. Cancers of the skin are common, especially in fair-skinned individuals or in sun-damaged skin (see page 855).

Nervous System

Visible changes in movement are primarily caused by alterations in the nervous system, with diminished muscle strength and joint mobility contributing only minimally. Movement is an extremely complex activity requiring integration of many portions of the nervous system. Intact sensory information going to the

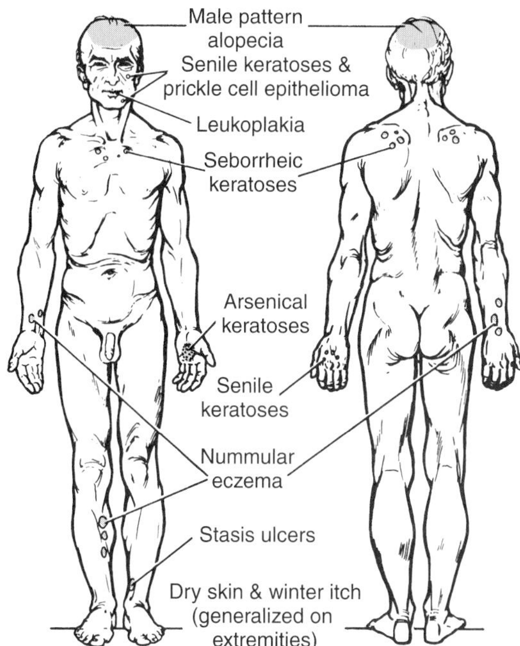

FIGURE 4-10. **Typical skin changes with aging. (Sauer, G. C. [1991].** ***Manual of skin diseases*** **[6th ed.]. Philadelphia: J. B. Lippincott.)**

brain must be coupled with integration of cortical, basal ganglionic, and cerebellar function. The extrapyramidal system is subject to early changes in function owing to diminished presence of neurotransmitters. Vascular supply to all portions of the brain is critical to coordinated function for movement. Locomotion becomes increasingly precarious with aging.

In the aged individual, nerve impulses decrease their rate of conduction by about 10%, which may lead to ischemia, generally lower basal metabolism, and decreased temperature in nerve fibers.[12] The transmission strength of signals from the brain to the body parts decreases as a result of the dwindling number of neurons, the degenerating myelin sheath, and the formation of senile plaque with age. The signals become slightly blurred, and the threshold for arousal of an organ system may be altered. Adaptation to physiologic stressors does not occur as rapidly in the elderly as in younger persons. The increased recovery time within the autonomic system causes an organ to take longer to return to base level activity after stressful situations. The baroreceptors (pressure sensors) in the aorta and carotid arteries become less sensitive to pressure changes, and sudden changes in position may cause dizziness or syncope. Pressure on the carotid sinus may cause serious slowing of the heart rate and may be elicited by twisting and turning of the head.

Because of physiologic and metabolic changes in the brain and reduced oxygen consumption, less intracellular energy is produced; glucose use is diminished, and cerebral blood flow is reduced. The electroencephalogram (EEG) of the older adult remains within the normal limits of other age groups except that it is about one cycle slower (see page 973). Also, physical changes contribute to degeneration of the blood–brain barrier in elderly persons, which has implications for medication administration and may help to explain acute confusional states related to medication administration.

The effects of general changes in the brain are associated with the common characteristics of aging. These include decreasing motor strength; lack of dexterity and agility; difficulties in association, retrieval, and recall; diminished memory and cognitive ability and change in affect; and, often, depression. The behavior resulting from these changes causes concern to both the elderly person and his or her family.

TRANSIENT ISCHEMIC ATTACKS AND STROKES

Transient cerebral ischemic attacks may occur before major cerebrovascular accidents or strokes (see page 952). These attacks are usually caused by arterial occlusion or hypotension. The occlusive phenomena occur most frequently in the carotid artery with signs of hemiparesis, hemianopsia, aphasia, and loss of vision in one eye. The vertebral artery is more often involved with hypotensive states, causing the person to fall forward on the knees (without loss of consciousness), along with vertigo, vomiting, dysarthria, visual blurring, or diplopia.[20]

Sensory System

Few persons escape sensory deficits as they age. They become more vulnerable to injury, more isolated from society, and less able to care for their personal needs as these deficits occur. Deficits are greatest in sight, hearing, taste, smell, and touch, and they interfere with the ability to communicate.

EYES

With age, changes occur in both the structural and functional aspects of the eyes. Eyelids become thinner and wrinkled, and skinfolds result from loss of orbital fat, leading to proptosis. Inversion or eversion of the lids is common, and the conjunctivae are thinner and more fragile.

Arcus senilis, a bluish gray ring, may surround the corneal limbus and be visible against the darker pigments of the eye. Arcus senilis is a harmless change and does not affect visual acuity. Light brown patches may occur in the irides, changing their appearance but not their ability to regulate pupil size. The lenses may develop changes that cause vision problems such as loss of elasticity or **presbyopia**.

EARS

With aging, changes may develop in the functional ability of the ears as well as their external appearance. Population studies indicate that hearing gradually deteriorates beginning in the third decade of life.[33] The external ears undergo very little change other than some slight elongation of the lobes. Cerumen decreases in amount but contains a greater amount of keratin, which easily becomes impacted and difficult to remove. Impacted cerumen can block sound waves and cause temporary hearing loss until it is removed.

The ability to hear high-frequency sounds is reduced first, followed by loss of ability to hear lower frequencies. The term used to describe progressive hearing loss in the aged is *presbycusis*. This bilaterally symmetric perceptive hearing loss starts at about the fourth decade, but the effects are usually not noticeable at their outset.

Exposure to excessive noise, recurrent otitis media in younger years, trauma to the ears, and certain drugs contribute to hearing loss. Persons living or working in highly industrialized areas experience more hearing loss than those in nonindustrial areas.

TASTE, SMELL, AND TOUCH

The aging process does not have as dramatic an effect on taste, smell, and touch as it does on vision and hearing, but these senses are also reduced. There is an obvious decrease in ability to taste sweet and salty flavors, owing to a decrease in the number of taste buds. Diet becomes an important factor because the aging person tends to eat more sweets and to salt food more heavily. The sweets lead to obesity and increased dental problems, and the salt may aggravate existing hypertension. Olfactory function may diminish, resulting in inability to smell, which also interferes with appetite. It also can present a hazard in the case of fire or smoke.

A decrease in tactile sensation may be manifested by difficulty in discriminating between different temperatures. Older persons tend to burn themselves because of this change. Minor injuries occur as a result of occasional unawareness of pain or pressure.

Cardiovascular System

Under normal circumstances, the aging heart adapts and allows the person to maintain an average level of activity. Anatomic and physiologic changes cause reduced stroke volume and cardiac output. The heart begins to have difficulty adapting to the workload, especially when unusual demands are made on it. If the workload is increased by such conditions as hypertension, valvular disease, or myocardial infarction, the result can be altered cardiac adaptation.

Loss of muscle fiber in the heart, with localized hypertrophy of individual fibers, is caused by the increased amount of collagenous material that surrounds every fiber. Anatomic changes in the heart lead to diminished contractility and filling capacity. Thickening of the semilunar and atrioventricular valves causes increased resistance to blood flow. The end result is a heart encased in a more rigid collagen matrix, which leads to diminished contraction and decreased filling capacity of the heart chambers.

The numerous physiologic changes that occur in the heart include alterations in the conduction system, loss of contractile efficiency, and decreased levels of circulating catecholamines. The combination of all these factors results in a heart that no longer has the capacity to meet all the demands that it met in earlier years.

The changes in the conduction systems of the hearts of elderly persons are caused by alterations in the conduction system per se and by ischemia from interrupted blood supply through the coronary arteries. Disturbances of the autonomic nervous system and the local chemical (ionic) environment of the pacemaker cells may initiate dysrhythmias. The conduction impulses may be blocked as a result of increased fibrous tissue and fat in the myocardium, and by loss of fibers in the bifurcating main bundle of His and the junction of the main bundle and its left fascicles.[39]

Blood vessels are markedly affected by degenerative changes in aging, particularly the arteries. Basic to the problems of all arteries is the progressive stiffness caused by the cross-linkage effect on elastin and smooth muscle as the amount of collagen increases. This generalized problem in the arteries leads to increased peripheral resistance.

Changes in the integrity of the veins alters the normal movement of blood toward the heart.[31] Varicose veins occur when the valves of the venous system are destroyed. They are common in older persons, and are usually caused by inactivity, constricting clothing, and crossing the legs at the knees. The venous stasis that occurs with varicose veins further complicates the circulatory problems (see page 454).

ATHEROSCLEROSIS AND HYPERTENSION

Atherosclerosis of the systemic arteries commonly is manifested in the aged. As a person ages, the number of atheromatous plaques increases, resulting in raised areas with a central core of degenerative lipid on the tunica intima. Obstruction to blood flow may impair cardiac, cerebral, or peripheral blood flow. It is associated with hypertension, which apparently accelerates its formation.[16]

Hypertension becomes substantially more common with age, even though it is not an essential aspect of aging. About 40% of whites and more than 50% of African Americans older than 65 years of age have hypertension.[34] The systolic pressure gradually increases with age because of decreased aortic elasticity. The increase in diastolic pressure is less marked and results from increased resistance in the peripheral blood vessels. The diastolic pressure tends to level off in later life. Cardiac output and blood volume are also factors in the regulation of blood pressure. Blood pressure is elevated because of increased resistance to blood flow caused by arteriolar constriction. Blood pressure lowers when arteriolar relaxation reduces resistance to blood flow.

Benign essential hypertension is the most common type in persons older than 70 years of age, with more than 90% of all cases in this category.[31] Elevated pressure usually develops slowly and with little untoward effect, but complications of hypertension occur and account for a significant number of deaths in the United States. Hypertension contributes considerably to diseases of the cardiovascular system. It is associated with increased frequency of coronary artery disease and myocardial infarction and with hemorrhagic problems and infarcts in the brain. It is also associated with major hemorrhage from cerebral arteries and resultant strokes.

Respiratory System

Alterations in the respiratory system in the aged impose many limitations that are not always obvious when the person is at rest but appear with exertion or stress. Under usual circumstances, older persons are capable of maintaining normal daily activities, but various changes make them more susceptible to pulmonary infections. Various consequences of the aging respiratory system are presented in Flowchart 4-6. Among aged individuals, influenza and pneumonia are the fourth leading cause of death, with bronchitis, emphysema, and asthma ranking eighth.[24]

Loss of elasticity affects the older person's pulmonary compliance and results from increased cross-linkage in collagen and elastin fibers around the alveolar sacs. In addition, there is a decrease in the quantity of air that can be taken in during normal breathing. Changes in the costal cartilage result in a diminution of chest wall compliance, which is further complicated by skeletal deformities of the thorax and postural changes such as stooped shoulders. The end result of the loss of elasticity, muscle weakness, and changes in the structure of the chest is difficulty in expiration of air. Although total lung capacity is not changed to a great extent, vital capacity is

FLOWCHART 4-6 **Respiratory System Aging**

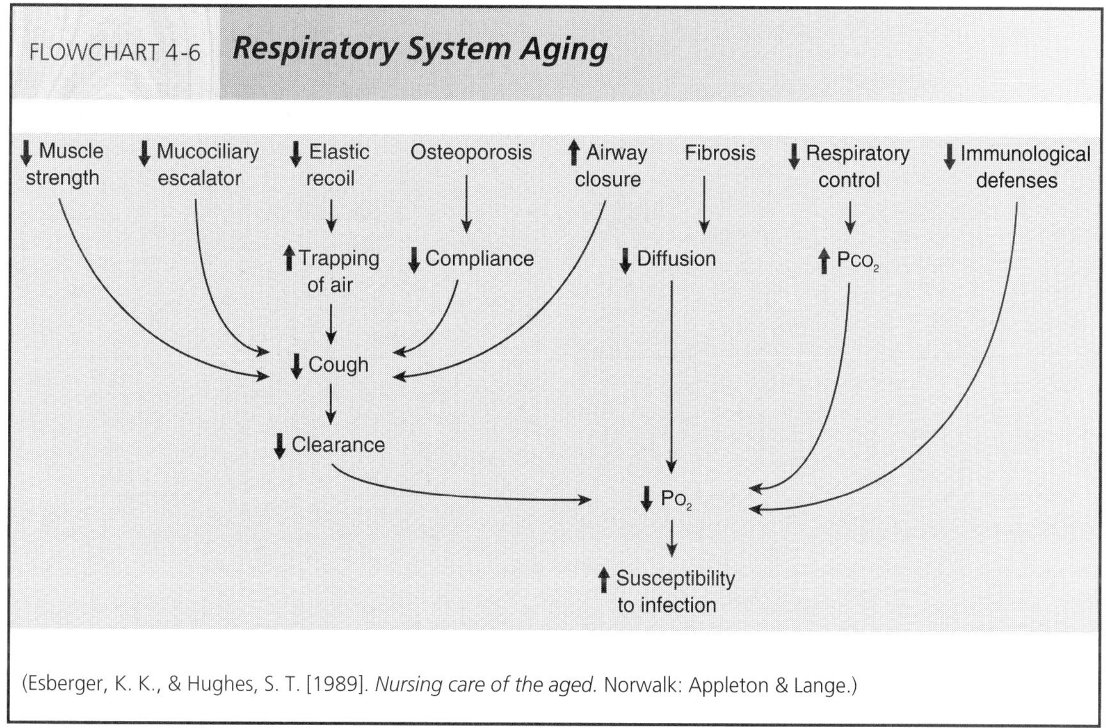

(Esberger, K. K., & Hughes, S. T. [1989]. *Nursing care of the aged.* Norwalk: Appleton & Lange.)

gradually and progressively reduced. The residual volume and functional residual capacity of the lungs are increased.

FUNCTIONAL PROBLEMS AND RESPIRATORY FAILURE

The main functional respiratory problems in the elderly person without pulmonary disease are reduced ventilation of all alveoli, especially at the bases of the lungs, and reduced oxygen partial pressure in the arterial blood. The partial pressure of arterial oxygen (PaO_2) declines with age, averaging 75 mm Hg in the seventh decade. The partial pressure of carbon dioxide ($PaCO_2$), however, remains the same unless disease is superimposed on the diminished ventilation; this constancy is probably a result of the higher rate of diffusion of carbon dioxide. With the structural and mechanical changes that have been described, the bases of the lungs are ventilated less and less. The part of the lungs that is well perfused is the part of the lungs not being ventilated. Blood must be shunted to the ventilated upper portions of the lungs. The redistribution of blood is usually insufficient to compensate, and the PaO_2 falls. The condition becomes worse when the elderly person lies down, and nocturnal hypoxemia may be a major cause of confusion.

An elderly person with little previous difficulty may develop respiratory failure rather rapidly after stress such as surgery, excessive exercise, a sudden rise in environmental pollution (eg, in smog crises), or infection (eg, pneumonia). The assumption must be made that all elderly individuals are at risk for respiratory failure. Respiratory failure is evidenced by a diminishing PaO_2 and a rising $PaCO_2$ associated with a drop in arterial pH.

Potential causes of respiratory failure are surgery, the use of depressant drugs, lung infections, bed rest, pulmonary edema caused by circulatory problems, and pulmonary embolism. Pulmonary embolism occurs frequently in elderly patients who are immobilized because of bone fractures or other conditions requiring bed rest. Any acute condition such as trauma, burns, or myocardial infarction in the elderly may be complicated by respiratory failure. The potential of unrecognized pulmonary changes, particularly those caused by environmental effects, is present in all persons older than age 40.

Genitourinary System

Genitourinary problems in older adults are common conditions that many of these individuals are reluctant to discuss. In addition to causing embarrassment, they are bothersome and are frequently thought of as a sign of growing old. Renal dysfunctions are potentially life-threatening and become more so because of delay in detection and treatment.

The urinary tract undergoes many changes with age. The kidneys are affected by involutional processes, and normal age-related changes occur in renal vascular anatomy and function independent of disease. The nephrons begin to degenerate and disappear by the seventh month in utero and gradually degenerate, and their number is reduced by one-third to one-half by the seventh decade.[31] In addition to the loss of nephrons, there is some degeneration of the remaining nephrons. The degeneration starts as a sclerosis or scarring of the glomeruli, followed by atrophy of the afferent arterioles. Because of the loss of nephrons or functional units of the kidneys, a decline in function is to be expected with age. The kidneys do not concentrate urine as well because of the loss of nephrons. Under normal circumstances, however, the kidneys are capable of maintaining acid–base balance.

FACTORS THAT COMPROMISE RENAL FUNCTION

Renal function in the elderly may be compromised by one or more of the following: inadequate fluid intake, fluid loss from vomiting or diarrhea, shock due to hemorrhage, acute or chronic cardiac failure, septicemia caused by gram-negative bacteria, and injudicious use of diuretics.[15] Any one of these may result in renal ischemia and acute renal shutdown if not promptly corrected.

The minimum urinary output is about 400 mL daily. Output of 20 mL/h or less may herald acute renal failure. Acute renal failure frequently arises in the elderly and carries a mortality rate of 80% in persons 70 years of age and older. The dangers of acute renal failure include fluid overloading, which leads to congestive heart failure and pulmonary edema, and rising serum potassium level, which may cause cardiac arrest.

Diseases of the kidneys, regardless of the cause, create long-term problems. In addition to the various pathologic events associated with such diseases, the elderly person also must adapt to the normal changes of aging. The most frequent chronic kidney disease in the elderly is pyelonephritis. Other physiologic conditions that can lead to kidney dysfunction include hypertension, sodium and water retention, marked sodium or water loss, retention of potassium, and loss of serum protein. The greatest concern is inability of the kidneys to handle changing concentrations of hydrogen ion. The responses to increased hydrogen ion concentration are slowed and diminished, leading to metabolic acidosis.

Several antibiotics often used to treat infections in elderly persons are nephrotoxic, including tetracycline, cephaloridine, and gentamycin. Occasionally, penicillin also has this effect. It is not uncommon for an elderly person who has sepsis from an infection to develop acute renal failure after treatment with one of these antibiotics. It is difficult to ascertain under such circumstances whether renal failure is caused by the antibiotic or by the shock associated with the infection.

PROBLEMS WITH MICTURITION

Two of the most common and bothersome problems elderly persons encounter are nocturnal frequency of micturition and urinary incontinence. Among changes that contribute to these problems are loss of muscle tone, which results in relaxation of the perineal muscles in the female, prostatic hypertrophy in the male, bladder diverticula, sphincter relaxation, and altered bladder reflexes (Fig. 4-11). Frequently, bladder capacity is reduced.

Incomplete emptying of the bladder predisposes the elderly person to residual urine and infection. *Escherichia coli* is the most frequent cause of bladder infection in women, whereas *Proteus* species are the most common in men.[19]

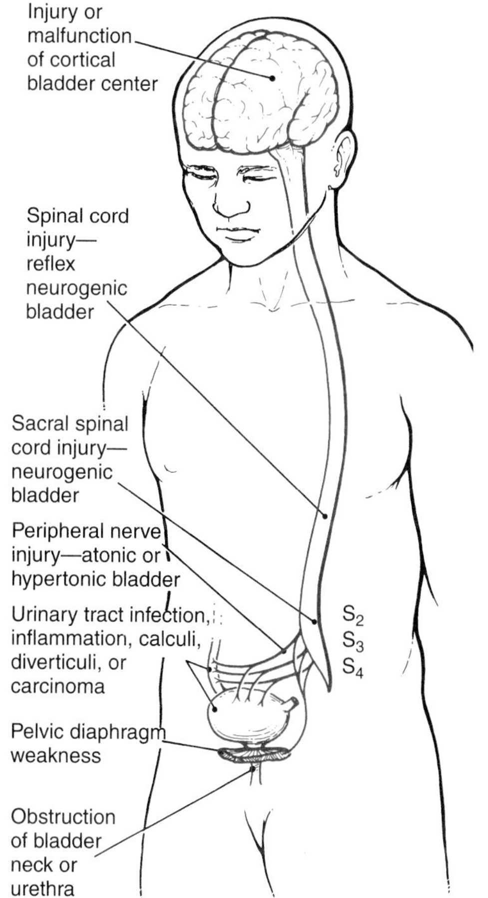

FIGURE 4-11. Stresses that contribute to urinary incontinence.

Gynecologic Changes in the Elderly Woman

In the elderly woman, objective gynecologic findings are directly related to the effects of estrogen deprivation. General atrophy occurs in the reproductive system, causing a reduction in the size of the uterus and cervix, thinning of the vaginal walls, changes in mucous secretions, and greater friability and susceptibility of vaginal tissue to irritation and infection. Because of diminished secretions, the vagina loses the normal flora that create its protective acid environment. Atrophic changes result in a vulva that is pallid and has a loss of subcutaneous fat accompanied by a flattening and folding of the labia. Breast tissue thins and sags as a result of replacement of atrophying glandular tissue with fat.

Reproductive Changes in the Elderly Man

Physiologic changes in the elderly man are also caused by lowered hormone production but occur much more gradually than in the woman. The testes undergo cellular change with no significant change in size. Fat content increases in testicular cells, and the number of cells decreases. The number of sperm ejaculated decreases by up to 50% by 90 years of age. Sperm change in size and shape and lose their fertilization ability.[8] Androgen production begins to decline at age 30 years and continues to decline until age 90. Most elderly men have some benign prostatic hyperplasia, which is considered to be a normal aging change. The changes result in a prostate that is more fibrous and has irregular thickening. The frequency of prostatic cancer also increases with age (see page 1083).

Gastrointestinal System

The gastrointestinal system is the site of many diseases in the elderly, ranging from simple dyspepsia to carcinoma. Contributing to the prevalence of these conditions are many normal features of aging.

THE MOUTH AND ESOPHAGUS

The grinding surfaces of the molars have worn down, and many elderly persons have lost most or all of their teeth. With the loss of chewing ability, they may eat only soft food, thereby developing gum and digestive problems. Altered taste sensation, caused by a decline in the number of taste buds, fosters a poor appetite, and this can result in malnutrition.

Changes in esophageal motility begin to occur with aging. Degenerative changes in the smooth muscle that lines the lower two-thirds of the esophagus result in delayed esophageal emptying, dilatation of the esophagus, and an increase in nonpropulsive contractions.[1,34] The risk of hiatal hernia in persons older than age 50 may be as high as 40% to 60%. Difficulty in swallowing is one of the primary symptoms. Hiatal hernias can mimic pulmonary distress and angina; therefore, radiography should be performed to verify the diagnosis.

THE STOMACH AND INTESTINES

It is thought that the stomach mucosa becomes thinner; however, some studies have indicated that gastric mucosa remains normal in individuals up to 80 or 90 years of age.[1] It is generally thought that gastric acid secretion is decreased with age. Pernicious anemia is common in the elderly because vitamin B_{12} is dependent on the gastric intrinsic factor for its absorption (see page 741). Gastric motility and gastric emptying appear to decrease with age.

Constipation is one of the most frequent complaints of the elderly population. In a large percentage, constipation is caused by cultural eating patterns, decreased exercise, decreased gastric motility, low fluid intake, and the ingestion of drugs such as antihypertensives and sedatives. Constipation in elderly persons is compounded by the abuse of purgatives, laxatives, and enemas, which are used to resolve constipation—thus creating a vicious cycle.

Diseases of the colon that are common in the elderly include diverticulosis, diverticulitis, polyposis, and cancer of the colon (see page 759). Diverticulosis is considered to be a disease of aging, with the majority of diverticula arising in the sigmoid colon. Most of these diseases are asymptomatic, but occult blood in the stool is common, especially with colon cancer.

THE PANCREAS AND HEPATOBILIARY SYSTEM

The changes in the pancreas with age are associated with pancreatic ductal epithelial hyperplasia and intralobular fibrosis.[1] On rare occasions, this fibrosis may lead to atrophy. The volume of pancreatic secretions declines and enzyme output diminishes with advanced age. However, the importance of these changes in causing dysfunction or nutritional impairment has not been thoroughly researched.[1]

Liver size and hepatic blood flow decrease with advancing age. Hepatocytes tend to be larger and have increased nuclear DNA. A brown, atrophied appearance of the liver is seen in older persons as a result of deposited lipofuscin granules in hepatocytes. However, this trait has also been found in younger individuals who have cachexia or malnutrition.[1] Hepatic parenchymal fibrosis may be present, but it has no apparent functional significance.

Aging and Cancer

Cancer is a serious problem, regardless of age. Because cancers are multifaceted diseases whose prevalence often increases with age, a brief discussion of cancer and aging is presented here. Even though the prevalence of cancer is higher in older persons, certain types are diagnosed less frequently in this age group, including cervical cancer and sarcoma.

FACTORS ASSOCIATED WITH CANCER IN THE AGING

Several factors are associated with cancer, although the exact cause is unknown. Constant irritation from smoking a pipe can cause oral cancers, chewing tobacco can result in cancer of the mouth, and smoking cigarettes can lead to carcinoma of the lung. The percentage of lung cancer was once highest in men, but the disease is increasing in women because of the increased number of women who smoke.

Environmental factors such as air pollution, food additives, asbestos, and certain chemicals are carcinogenic. According to the National Research Council, evidence indicates that most common cancers are influenced by diet, although there are no precise estimations of the impact of foods on cancer. Chemical carcinogens produce different effects at different periods of life. Chemical carcinogenesis occurs most readily in the aged. The assumption is that there is either an accumulated effect on the DNA of the cell or an accumulated risk for a cell to become malignant.

PREVALENT CANCERS IN THE AGING

The majority of persons with carcinoma of the colon are in the older age group. This cancer is usually very slow-growing and remains localized for a long time. Early surgical removal is beneficial.

Cancer of the prostate is the most common tumor of men older than 85 years of age.[22] The disease is known to metastasize to the pelvis, vertebrae, and other bony sites, as well as to the brain. Breast cancer is common in elderly women and is often discovered during examination for other conditions.

Chronic lymphocytic leukemia, lymphosarcoma, and myeloma are malignancies with a high incidence in the elderly population. Hodgkin's disease tends to run a rapid course in the aged, but malignancies of the lung, oral cavity, larynx, and gastrointestinal tract seem to have a similar prognosis in young and old.

Aging and Infections

Both nosocomial and community-acquired infections are more common in the elderly. Predisposing factors include a decline in immune competence, chronic illness, diminished organ reserves, development of resistant organisms, alteration in natural barriers, inadequate nutrition, and diminished sensory perception. In the immune system, T lymphocytes are reduced and neutrophils become less efficient with advanced age, thereby decreasing the elderly person's ability to fight infectious diseases. Also, the fever response to infectious disease may be blunted or absent; this factor increases the morbidity and mortality associated with infections in the elderly population.[27]

Elderly persons are especially susceptible to respiratory, urinary tract, and skin infections because of the systemic changes discussed previously. Also, the presentation of infections in the elderly may be somewhat atypical, compared with those in younger adults.[37] A summary of atypical presentations of pneumonia, tuberculosis, UTIs, and skin infections is presented in Table 4-17.

TABLE 4-17

ATYPICAL PRESENTATIONS OF COMMON INFECTIONS IN ELDERLY PERSONS

Pneumonia	Blunted fever response; decreased evidence of consolidation in 30% of patients; confusion, disorientation, and changes in behavior are common presenting signs and symptoms.
Tuberculosis	Cough, weight loss, and weakness may be subtle symptoms and may be attributed to other chronic diseases; chest pain, hemoptysis, and night sweats are seen in later stages of disease.
Skin infections	Decreased inflammatory response may delay diagnosis; peripheral vascular disease will decrease erythema, warmth, and swelling, which are commonly used to determine infection.
Urinary tract infections	Blunted fever response; anorexia, nausea, vomiting, and abdominal pain; confusion and change in behavior; increased incidence of asymptomatic bacteriuria.

(Adapted from Fraser, D. [1993]. Patient assessment: Infection in the elderly. *Journal of Gerontologic Nursing, 19*, 5.)

Pharmacology and the Elderly

Aged persons use one-third of all prescribed drugs in this country. Most take several drugs and also use over-the-counter agents frequently. All drugs can pose risks to elderly persons and can decrease their mental, physical, and functional status.[32] Nutritional status may be impaired by long-term use of certain drugs.

The elderly are the least able to tolerate injudicious use of drugs because many physiologic changes make them respond to medication in more variable ways than do younger adults. These physiologic changes result in a system that is less able to distribute, metabolize, and excrete drugs. The liver, kidneys, and heart are most involved with drug excretion and metabolism. Because they have lost some of their efficiency, compounds may accumulate and cause toxicity. The cumulative effects of trauma, prior illnesses, accidents, and disabilities further reduce the aging person's ability to handle drugs.

PHARMACOKINETIC FACTORS

Pharmacokinetic factors (those related to drug disposition in the body) have been studied in relation to absorption in the gastrointestinal tract, which would theoretically be reduced in elderly as a result of changes in intestinal mucosa, blood flow, and motility. However, there is not yet convincing evidence that alterations in absorption actually occur.[34] With age, the total body composition changes, resulting in a higher percentage of fat tissue and less lean tissue and water. The disposition of drugs that are selectively used in different tissues is affected. Also, body size decreases, so the concentration of a drug in the body is higher with standard dosages. Plasma binding by albumin in the elderly decreases 20%. Drugs that are normally plasma focused are therefore increased in concentration in the tissues.

Metabolism of drugs by the liver is diminished in the elderly by poor circulation to the liver, by a reduction in the hepatic mass, and by the possible decrease in hepatic enzymes. Any disease of the liver aggravates this situation considerably. Some of the most common drugs metabolized by the liver that have increased half-life in the elderly are the antidepressants diazepam (Valium) and chlordiazepoxide (Librium).

Another problem is reduced excretion caused by diminished renal function. Renal reserve is markedly reduced as people age, and the ability to excrete drugs is also markedly reduced. Drug action in the elderly is also altered by changes in tissue responses. There may be an increased threshold to a drug's actions. There may be a decrease in the number of receptive sites for the drug, coupled with a decrease in the necessary enzymes. A summary of alterations in the pharmacokinetic variables in the elderly is presented in Table 4-18.

TABLE 4-18

ALTERATION OF PHARMACOKINETIC VALUES IN THE ELDERLY

FACTOR	ALTERED PHYSIOLOGY	CLINICAL IMPORTANCE
Absorption	Elevated gastric pH Reduced gastrointestinal blood flow Possible changed number of absorbing cells Possible altered gastrointestinal motility	Studies have not supported any loss of absorptive ability
Distribution	Decreased total body water Decreased lean body tissue mass per kg body weight Increased body fat	Higher concentration of drugs distributed in body fluids Possible longer duration of action of fat-soluble drugs
Protein binding	Decreased serum albumin concentrations	Increased unbound plasma concentrations of highly protein-bound drugs
Metabolism	Decreased hepatic blood flow; decreased hepatic mass; possible decreased enzyme activity	Decreased hepatic clearance
Elimination	Decreased glomerular filtration rate Decreased renal plasma flow Altered tubular function	Decreased renal clearance of drugs and metabolites

SELECTED HIGH-RISK DRUGS

Listed high among drugs that can be dangerous to the elderly are antibiotics, such as tetracyclines and gentamycin. Antibiotics are excreted by the kidneys, and reduced kidney function can lead to toxic accumulation of the agents. Mental disturbances, gastrointestinal side effects, and rashes are some toxic effects.[34]

If diuretics, which cause potassium loss, are given in combination with digoxin, the danger of dysrhythmias is greatly increased. The effect of digitalis on the conduction system is enhanced by low serum potassium levels. The elderly person does not display the toxic effects of digoxin, such as gastrointestinal and ocular symptoms, that usually arise in younger adults. This makes digoxin one of the drugs that places the older individual at grave risk. Digoxin blood levels are not always a good guide to toxicity; the elderly person more commonly exhibits electrocardiographic changes and confusion. Toxic blood levels may not be seen, but the effects may be present.

Many of the antihypertensive agents have diverse side effects, but they all possess the ability to cause hypotension. Orthostatic hypotension can lead to falls and fractures. Elderly persons should be warned of this possibility, and if they are taking antihypertensives they should be cautioned not to rise too rapidly from a supine or sitting position.

Many elderly persons develop nutritional problems from long-term use of medications such as laxatives. Mineral oil can interfere with absorption of nutrients and vitamins in the intestinal tract, and its use should be discouraged.

REFERENCES

1. Altman, D. F. (1990). Changes in gastrointestinal, pancreatic, biliary, and hepatic function with aging. *Gastroenterology Clinics of North America, 19,* 227.
2. American College of Obstetricians and Gynecologists. (1996, January). Hypertension in pregnancy. *ACOG Technical Bulletin No. 219.* Washington, DC: Author.
3. American Lung Association, *Lung Disease Data 1998–1999.* www.LungDisease.org.
4. Andresen, G. P. (1998). As America ages: Assessing the older patient. *RN, 61*(3), 46–55.
5. Ashburn, S. S. (1992). Biophysical development during middlescence. In C. S. Schuster & S. S. Ashburn (Eds.), *The process of human development* (3rd ed.). Philadelphia: Lippincott.
6. Bellantoni, M. (1995). Osteoporosis and other metabolic disorders of the skeleton in aging. In W. Reichel (Ed.), *Care of the elderly: Clinical aspects of aging* (4th ed.). Baltimore: Williams & Wilkins.
7. Betz, C. L., Hunsberger, M. M., & Wright, S. (1994). *Family centered nursing care of children* (2nd ed.). Philadelphia: Saunders.
8. Birren, J. E., & Schaie, K. W. (Eds.). (1990). *Handbook of the psychology of aging* (3rd ed.). San Diego: Academic Press.
9. Bottoms, S. F. Smoking. (1996). *Contemporary OB/GYN, 41*(12), 13–14.
10. Brehm, B. (1993). *Essays on wellness.* New York: HarperCollins.
11. Bush, B. T. (1998). Substance abuse. In J. Stein (Ed.), *Internal medicine* (5th ed.). St. Louis: Mosby.
12. Carnevali, D. L., & Patrick, M. (1993). *Nursing management for the elderly* (3rd ed.). Philadelphia: Lippincott.
13. Centers for Disease Control. (1989). Progress toward achieving the 1990 national objectives for physical fitness and exercise. *Morbidity and Mortality Weekly Report, 38,* 449.
14. Charlton, A. (1994). Children and passive smoking: A review. *Journal of Family Practice, 38,* 267.
15. Clauw, D. J. (1998). Chronic fatigue syndrome. In J. Stein (Ed.), *Internal medicine* (5th ed.) St. Louis: Mosby.
16. Cotran, R. S., Kumar, V., and Robbins, S.L. (1999). *Robbins' pathologic basis of disease* (5th ed.). Philadelphia: Saunders.

17. Coustan, D. R. Gestational diabetes. (1996). *Contemporary OB/GYN, 41*(7), 18–22.
18. Dacey, J., & Traver, J. (1991). *Human development across the lifespan*. Dubuque, IA: Brown.
19. Davies, I. (1992). Biology of aging—Theories of aging. In J. C. Brockehurst (Ed.), *Textbook of geriatric medicine and gerontology* (4th ed.). New York: Churchill Livingstone.
20. Dawes, B. (1996). Neurologic and cognitive function. In A. G. Lueckenotte (Ed.), *Gerontologic nursing*. St. Louis: Mosby.
21. Dunn, P. A., & Feinberg, R. F. (1996). Oncofetal fibronectin: New insight into the physiology of implantation and labor. *Journal of. Obstetric Gynecologic and Neonatal Nursing, 25,* 753–757.
22. Ebersole, P., & Hess, P. (1998). *Toward healthy aging: Human needs and nursing response* (5th ed.). St. Louis: Mosby.
23. Egerman, R. S., & Sibai, B. M. (1997). Recognizing and managing HELLP syndrome and its imitators. *Contemporary OB/GYN, 42*(10), 129–149.
24. Eliopoulos, C. (1997). *Gerontological nursing* (4th ed.). Philadelphia: Lippincott.
25. Fairholt, F. (1859). *Tobacco: Its history and associations*. London: Chapman and Hall.
26. Frantz, R., & Ferrell-Torry, A. (1993). Physical impairments in the elderly populations. *Nursing Clinics of North America, 28,* 363.
27. Fraser, D. (1993). Patient assessment: Infection in the elderly. *Journal of Gerontologic Nursing, 19,* 5.
28. Fukuda, K. (1994). Chronic fatigue syndrome: A comprehensive approach to its definition and study. *Annals of Internal Medicine, 121,* 953–959.
29. Gabbe, S. G. (1996). Diabetes mellitus. *Contemporary OB/GYN, 41*(7), 13–14.
30. Garite, T. J., & Lockwood, C. J. (1996). A new test for diagnosis and prediction of preterm delivery. *Contemporary OB/GYN, 41*(1), 77–93.
31. Guyton, A. C., & Hall, J. E. (1996). *Textbook of medical physiology* (9th ed.). Philadelphia: Saunders.
32. Hayflick, L. *How and why we age*. (1994). New York: Ballantine.
33. Hensel, S. (1996). Sensory function. In A. G. Lueckenotte (Ed.), *Gerontologic nursing*. St. Louis: Mosby.
34. Hume, A., & Owens, N. (1995). Drugs and the elderly. In W. Reichel (Ed.), *Care of the elderly: Clinical aspects of aging* (4th ed.). Baltimore: Williams & Wilkins.
35. Lydyard, P., & Grossi, C. (1998). Development of the immune system. In I. Roitt, J. Brostoff, & D. Male (Eds.), *Immunology* (5th ed.). St. Louis: Mosby.
36. Malseed, R., & Harrigan, G. (1989). *Textbook of pharmacology and nursing care*. Philadelphia: Lippincott.
37. Matteson, M., McConnell, E., & Linton, A. (1997). *Gerontological nursing: Concepts and practice* (2nd ed.). Philadelphia: Saunders.
38. May, K. A., & Mahlmeister, L. R. (1994). *Maternal and neonatal nursing: Family-centered care* (3rd ed.). Philadelphia: Lippincott.
39. Moss, A. (1995). Diagnosis and management of heart disease. In W. Reichel (Ed.), *Care of the elderly: Clinical aspects of aging* (4th ed.). Baltimore: Williams & Wilkins.
40. Murray, R. B., & Zentner, J. P. (1997). *Health assessment and promotion through the life span*. Stamford, CT: Appleton & Lange.
41. O'Brien, C. (1997). Approach to the problem of alcohol abuse and dependence. In W. N. Kelley (Ed.), *Textbook of internal medicine* (3rd ed.). Philadelphia: Lippincott-Raven.
42. O'Brien, C. P. (1997). Approach to the problem of substance abuse. In W. N. Kelley (Ed.), *Textbook of internal medicine* (3rd ed.). Philadelphia: Lippincott-Raven.
43. Rubin, E., & Farber, J. L. (1994). *Pathology* (2nd ed.) Philadelphia: Lippincott-Raven.
44. Santrock, J. W. (1997). *Life span development*. Dubuque, IA: Brown.
45. Sauer, G. C. (1997). *Manual of skin diseases* (7th ed.). Philadelphia: Lippincott, 1997.
46. Scheibmeir, M., & O'Connell, K. A. (1997). In harm's way: Childbearing women and nicotine. *Journal of Obstetric, Gynecologic and Neonatal Nursing, 26,* 477–484.
47. Schiller, A. L. (1994). Bones and joints. In E. Rubin & J. L. Farber (Eds.). *Pathology* (2nd ed.). Philadelphia: Lippincott.
48. Schneider, E., & Rowe, J. (1996). *Handbook of the biology of aging* (4th ed.). San Diego: Academic Press.
49. Shafran, S. D. (1991). The chronic fatigue syndrome. *American Journal of Medicine, 90*(6): 730–739.
50. Shuster, C. S., & Ashburn, S. S. (1992). *The process of human development* (3rd ed.). Philadelphia: Lippincott.
51. Sibai, B. M., & Usta, I. M. (1997). Preeclampsia. *Contemporary OB/GYN, 42*(7), 15–26.
52. Simpson, K. R., Moore, K. S., & LaMartina, M. H. (1993). Acute fatty liver of pregnancy. *Journal of Obstetric, Gynecologic and Neonatal Nursing, 22,* 213–219.
53. Smolak, L. (1993). *Adult development*. Englewood Cliffs, NJ: Prentice Hall.
54. Sokol, R. J., & Martier, S. (1996). Alcohol. *Contemporary OB/GYN, 41*(12), 19–23.
55. Strong, T. H. (1997). Factors that provide optimal umbilical protection during gestation. *Contemporary OB/GYN, 42*(3), 82–105.
56. Stunkard, A. J., & Wadden, T. A. (1997). Obesity. In W. N. Kelley (Ed.), *Textbook of internal medicine* (3rd ed.). Philadelphia: Lippincott-Raven.
57. Svikis, D., & Huggins, G. (1997). Substance abuse in pregnancy: Screening and intervention. *Contemporary OB/GYN, 41*(4), 32–52.
58. Tucker, L., & Friedman, G. (1989). Television viewing and obesity in adult males. *American Journal of Public Health, 79*(4), 516.
59. Vesely, D. L. (1998). Weakness. In J. Stein (Ed.), *Internal medicine* (5th ed.). St. Louis: Mosby.
60. Walker, M. (1992). The physiology of normal aging: Implications for nursing management of critically compromised adults. In T. Fulmer & M. Walker (Eds.), *Critical care nursing of the elderly*. New York: Springer.
61. Walsh, S. W. (1997). The role of oxidative stress and antioxidants in preeclampsia. *Contemporary OB/GYN, 42*(5), 113–124.
62. Wong, D. L. (1997). *Essentials of pediatric nursing* (5th ed.) St. Louis: Mosby.
63. Wong, D. L., & Perry, S. E. (1997). *Maternal child nursing care*. St. Louis: Mosby.
64. Youngbluth, M. (1996) Viral infections of the lower respiratory tract. In S. T. Shulman, J. P. McPhair, & L. R. Peterson (Eds.), *The biology and clinical basis of infectious diseases* (5th ed.). Philadelphia: Saunders.
65. Zuspan, F. P. (1997). Chronic hypertension. *Contemporary OB/GYN, 42*(5), 15–22.

Chapter

5

Concepts of Stress, Exercise, and Sleep

Barbara L. Bullock / Patricia Vidmar

KEY TERMS

adaptation
aerobic capacity
aerobic exercise
basal metabolic rate (BMR)
circadian rhythm or pattern
dyssomnias
fast-twitch fibers
feedback—negative and positive
homeostasis
maladaptation
maximal oxygen uptake (VO_2)
melatonin
MET
myoglobin
nonrapid eye movement sleep (NREM)
oxidative phosphorylation
parasomnias
rapid eye movement sleep (REM)
reticular activating system (RAS)
slow-twitch fiber
slow wave sleep
stress
stressors
systems theory

Physiologic functions that promote health are influenced by various changes in life-style. Stress, both physiologic and psychological, and the adaptations of the body to stressors are part of normal daily living. Exercise essential to health and the adjustments of the body to exercise activities promote adaptations by the cardiovascular and other body systems. Sleep is the integral component in maintaining the physiologic balance for all humans. The effect of stress and the restorative values of exercise and sleep are part of a large number of factors involved in the maintenance of homeostasis. Physiologic and psychological adaptation to multiple internal and external changes affects how the body reacts to stressors. Changes in stressors, exercise, and sleep are factors that can cause an alteration to health and may promote a disease state or, conversely, may promote a state of wellness.

HOMEOSTASIS AND ADAPTATION

Homeostasis is defined as the maintenance of static or constant conditions in the internal environment of the body.[17] It requires constant adjustments by the organs and tissues of the body to maintain an optimal functioning environment. Homeostasis is challenged by external and internal stressors; these are stimuli that constantly confront the body. Discussions throughout the text indicate how specific organs and tissues accomplish the balancing act to maintain the constant environment that is optimal for body functioning.

Adaptation is defined as adjustment of an organism to a changing environment. It refers to adjustments that are made as a result of stimulation or change, with the end result of modifying the original situation. An adaptive response is a type of negative feedback that maintains the organism in the steady state (see below). Physiologic adaptation refers to the adjustments made by the organs and systems to stress or physiologic disruption. This response is often called compensation for abnormal stimuli. **Maladaptation** is disruptive, a disordering of the physiologic response. This positive feedback can be considered a vicious cycle—if not interrupted, it can cause illness and death.

Systems Theory

Systems theory is one of the older models for organizing and examining relationships among units. It describes *closed systems* as those that do not interact or exchange energy with their environments. The sciences of physics and physical chemistry are limited to the examination of closed systems. Conversely, *open systems* do exchange matter, energy, and information with their environments.[40] A relative state of balance, or dynamic equilibrium, called the *steady state* is achieved. Man, as an open physiologic organism, uses relationships among his component parts to achieve this state. The steady state is said to exist when the composition of the system is constant despite continuous exchange of components of the system. The three fundamental qualities of open systems are structure, process, and function. *Structure* refers to the arrangement of all defined elements at a given time. *Process* is the transformation of matter, energy, and information between the system and the environment. *Function* is related to the unique manner that each open system uses to achieve its required end.

FEEDBACK SYSTEMS

A feedback scheme describes the fundamental qualities of open systems. In the human, this means that if a factor becomes excessive or inadequate in the body, alterations in function will be initiated to decrease or increase that factor in an attempt to bring it into normal range. **Feedback** is the process of self-regulation by which open systems determine and control the amount of input and output of the system. The two types of feedback in the human body are negative and positive feedback. **Negative feedback** refers to a process of returning to a state of equilibrium; **positive feedback** indicates movement away from equilibrium. Negative feedback causes a function to increase when it falls below a set point or decrease if it rises above a set point. Positive feedback leads to a continuation of the process and moves it away from homeostasis. Unchecked, it will produce illness and finally death. In the human body, negative feedback can be readily illustrated by many functions. Flowchart 5-1 illustrates the feedback system used to maintain the balance of thyroid hormones. Loss of hormonal control, for example, causes disease states because the body can either produce too many hormones or not enough and the metabolic processes are altered.

FLOWCHART 5-1 **Feedback System**

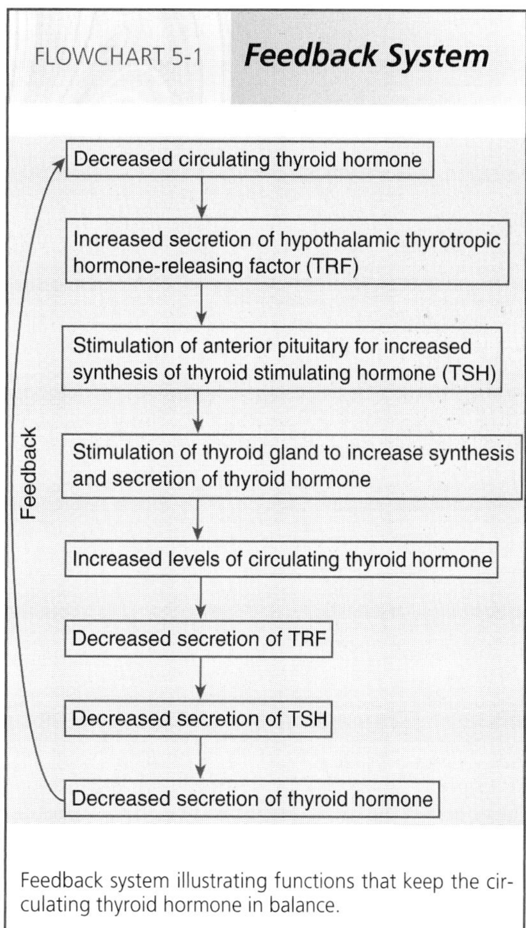

Feedback system illustrating functions that keep the circulating thyroid hormone in balance.

STRESS

All persons experience certain amounts of stress during each stage of the development process, which may relate to physiologic changes or to environmental influences. **Stress** has been defined as the nonspecific response of the body to any demand placed on it.[34] Stress-producing factors are called **stressors**; these may be physiologic or psychological, or both. The stressors may be pleasant or unpleasant and may evoke many different emotional or psychological responses while eliciting similar physiologic reactions. Reactions to stressors may be adaptive or maladaptive.

Closely associated with stress is the concept of *emotions*. This concept includes a wide range of behaviors, expressed feelings, and changes in body states.[31] Emotions often elicit the stress response, which can be viewed as a physiologic response to the emotion that encompasses the reported feelings. Stressors may be actual physical threats or perceived threats. They also may be the emotional side of joys or sorrows that elicit a physiologic reaction.

The Stress Response

The individual, as a system, has physiologic, psychosocial, environmental, and other stressors (Flowchart 5-2). These stressors may produce adaptive coping response, or they may result in physical changes that become pathologic.

Hans Selye pioneered the study of the effects of stress on the human body. He studied the nonspecific

FLOWCHART 5-2 **Examples of Stressors**

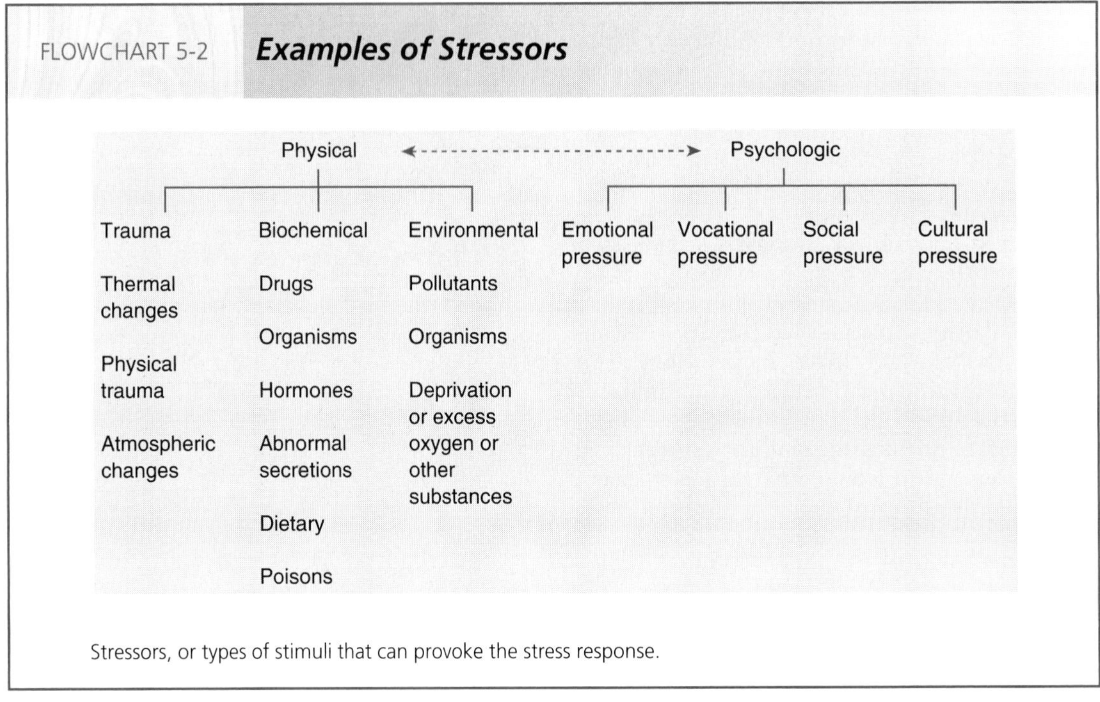

Stressors, or types of stimuli that can provoke the stress response.

response of the body to a demand and noted differences in individual abilities to withstand the same demands. He defined stress as a specific syndrome that is nonspecifically induced. He also defined stressors as tension-producing stimuli that potentially could cause disequilibrium.[34] This perception of the significance of the stressor is important and varies among individuals. Individuals differ in what produces stress and in their reactions to stressors. The response to the same stressor can vary from one day to the next. In this way, the Selye model, which was due to his use of animal models, differs from humans whose response is variable.[1]

Some types of stress are positive and these are called *eustress*. The sources are associated with some sort of control over the outcome and include such stressors as getting married, buying a house, and travel. Negative stress is termed *distress* and reflects situations over which persons have little control, including such conditions as sickness, death, and divorce.[34] The perception of stress has important implications for health and it has been shown that the hormonal changes in response to eustress are less harmful than those of distress.[10] The emotions of anger, hostility, and distrust are particularly damaging to health (see page 146).

Psychological and physiologic stressors both elicit a response that includes enlargement of the adrenal cortex, atrophy of the thymus gland, and sympathetic nervous system activation. A pattern including fatigue, loss of appetite, joint pains, gastric upset, and other nonspecific complaints comprised the syndrome that Selye called "the syndrome of just being sick." Later, he termed this conditions the general adaptation syndrome (GAS).[4]

STAGES OF THE GENERAL ADAPTATION SYNDROME

The GAS may be elicited by a variety of stimuli or stressors and may be physiologic, psychogenic, sociocultural, or environmental in nature. GAS is described in the following three stages: (1) alarm stage, (2) stage of resistance, and (3) stage of exhaustion (Flowchart 5-3).

Alarm Stage

In the alarm stage, a stressor causes an initial activation of the defensive abilities of the body. The hypothalamus is activated, releasing corticotropin-releasing hormone, which stimulates the adenohypophysis to release adrenocorticotropic hormone (ACTH). Glucocorticoids from the adrenal cortex are then released (see page 660). The so-called *fight-or-flight* mechanism is activated mainly through the sympathetic nervous system (SNS), which releases two catecholamines, *norepinephrine and epinephrine*. These hormones (see page 662) cause vasoconstriction in the skin, viscera, and kidneys and vasodilation in the vessels of the heart and skeletal muscles. They produce an increased rate and force of cardiac contractions and increase in the systemic blood pressure. These physiologic actions prepare the body for an assault.

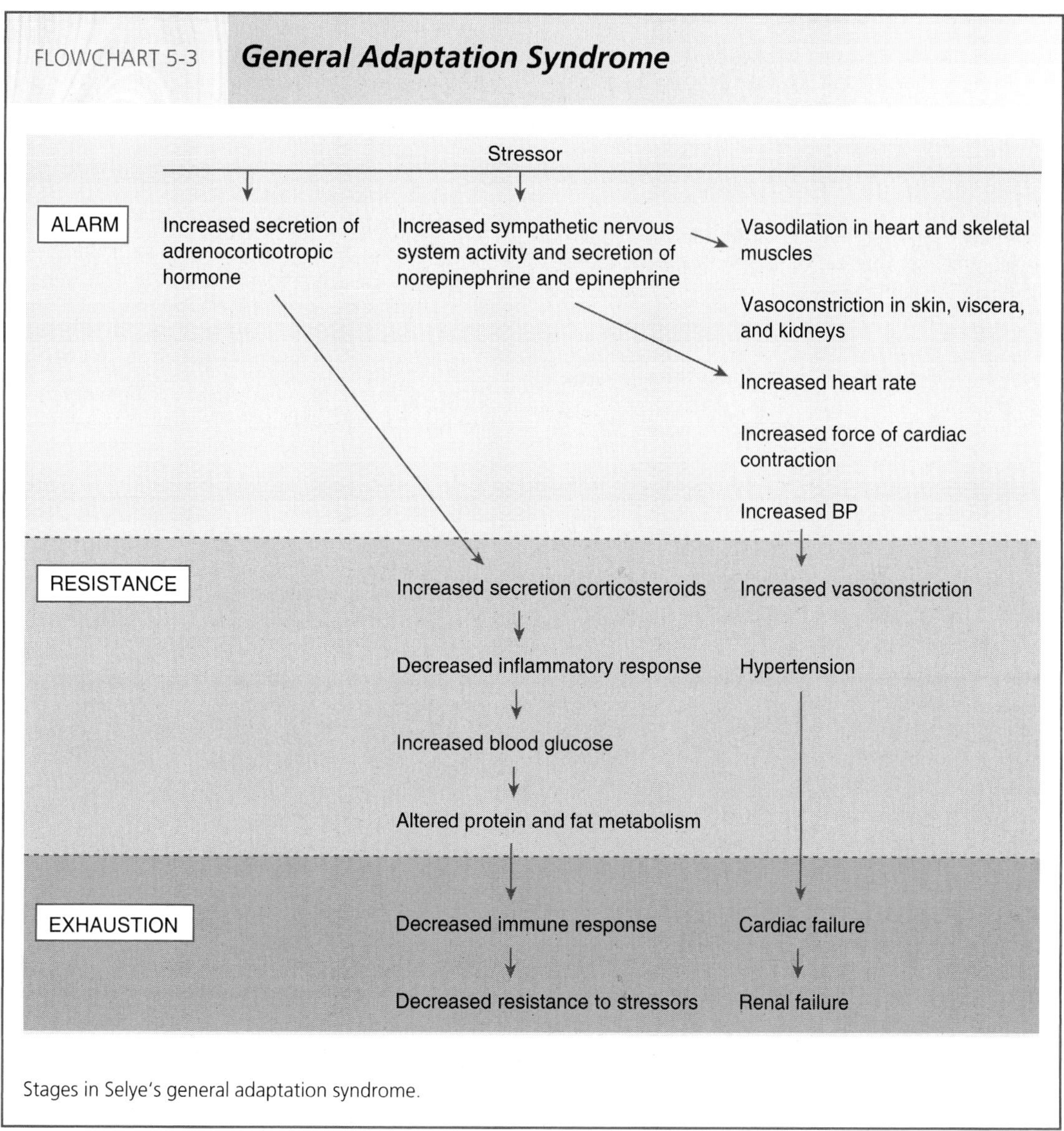

Stages in Selye's general adaptation syndrome.

Stage of Resistance

In the stage of resistance, levels of corticosteroids, thyroid hormones, glucagon, and aldosterone are increased. The adrenal cortex enlarges and secretes corticosteroids. This increases blood sugar for available energy and stabilizes the inflammatory response. Immune suppression due to excess circulating corticosteroids causes decreased lymphocyte reproduction and a marked decline is seen in the T lymphocytes.[17] This leads to a depression of the primary antigen–antibody response (see page 296). If infection is present, this suppression causes delayed clearing of the organisms and delayed healing, which is detrimental if it persists.

Stage of Exhaustion

If stage 3 or exhaustion occurs, resistance to the stressor is depleted and death ultimately occurs. Exhaustion is frequently caused by the lack of immunologic defense and is considered to be immunodeficiency secondary to stress.

LOCAL ADAPTATION SYNDROME

Localized reaction to stressors is called the local adaptation syndrome (LAS), which is illustrated by the process of inflammation. The usual outcome of inflammation is localization and destruction of the foreign substance that triggered the process.[32] The LAS assumes the same general pattern as the GAS with an acute phase followed by a resistance phase, and finally, exhaustion. Exhaustion of the LAS causes breakdown of the localizing mechanism and spreading of the process, ultimately leading to a generalized response.

Physiologic Responses to Stress

Physiologic response to stress stimuli (stressors) fall into separate, yet interactive, mechanisms including neurologic and endocrine effects on the immunologic system. These mechanisms may promote adaptation to the stressor, but long-term application of stressors ultimately causes end-organ dysfunction through these same mechanisms.[26]

NEUROLOGIC MECHANISMS

Both the voluntary and autonomic divisions of the nervous system are reactive to stress. The voluntary system is mediated through the cerebral cortex, which reacts to the stressor. The cerebral cortex directs the muscles to move to avoid danger and this movement effects the flight response. The combination of vasodilation in the skeletal muscle and the voluntary flight response are sometimes termed the *musculoskeletal response* to a stressor.[9]

The involuntary autonomic nervous system (ANS) is regulated through input from the hypothalamus. In the stress response, stimulation of the SNS occurs. Two hormones, epinephrine and norepinephrine, which are classified as *catecholamines*, are important factors in the stress response. Both are synthesized in the adrenal medulla and are released when the SNS is activated. Norepinephrine is also synthesized and secreted at adrenergic (sympathetic) nerve terminals throughout the body and is directly released when the SNS is stimulated. Epinephrine is excreted rapidly in the urine after being biotransformed in the liver. Norepinephrine, liberated at the axon endings, is actively taken up and may be restored to the nerve terminals. Some norepinephrine may be biotransformed in the liver and excreted.

The primary action of epinephrine is to increase the rate and force of cardiac contraction. It can elevate the basal metabolic rate (BMR) by 7% to 15%.[5] This hormone is a potent stimulus for glycogenolysis in the liver, which leads to an increased blood glucose level.[17] Epinephrine also diverts blood from the viscera to the skeletal muscles, so that it provides fuel and circulation for the increased need.

Norepinephrine secretion is increased in the flight-or-fight response and in persons suffering acute physical or mental stress. Studies have shown a constant increase in norepinephrine levels in individuals under chronic, unremitting stress.[11] Norepinephrine exerts its primary control over the arterioles, leading to intense vasoconstriction and increased systemic vascular resistance, causing increased blood pressure and increased cardiac workload (see page 449). The vasoconstriction to the gut is implicated in the development of stress ulcers.

Flowchart 5-4 illustrates the sympathetic response to stress as it is mediated through epinephrine and norepinephrine. Table 5-1 details the actions of the catecholamines in terms of their effects on various membrane receptors.

ENDOCRINE MECHANISMS

Effects of Glucocorticoids

Almost any type of stress causes a significant increased in ACTH secretion by the anterior pituitary. Within minutes, ACTH causes an increased synthesis and release of glucocorticoids from the adrenal cortex.[17] These hormones, mainly in the form of cortisol, increase serum glucose and alter the metabolism of carbohydrates, fat,

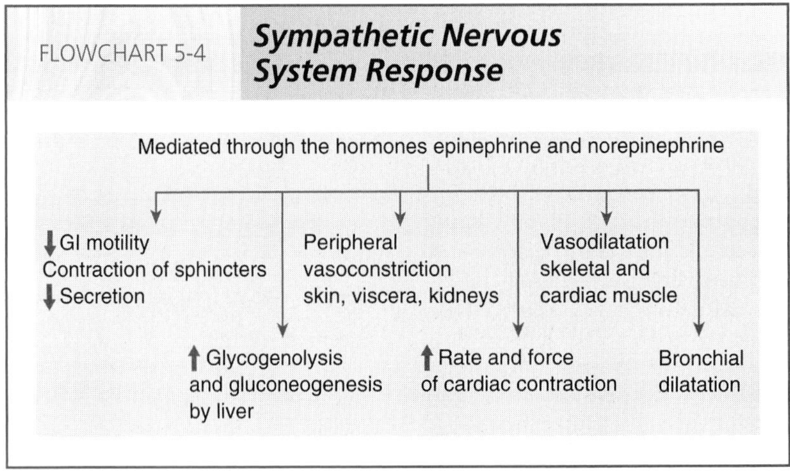

TABLE 5-1

SOME ACTIONS OF CATECHOLAMINE HORMONES

β EPINEPHRINE > NOREPINEPHRINE	α NOREPINEPHRINE > EPINEPHRINE
$\uparrow$Glycogenolysis	$\uparrow$Gluconeogenesis (α_1)
$\uparrow$Gluconeogenesis (β_2)	$\uparrow$Glycogenolysis (α_1)
$\uparrow$Lipolysis (β_3) (β_2)	
$\uparrow$Calorigenesis (β_1)	
$\downarrow$Glucose utilization	
$\uparrow$Insulin secretion (β_2)	$\downarrow$Insulin secretion (α_2)
$\uparrow$Glucagon secretion (β_2)	
$\uparrow$Muscle K+ uptake (β_2)	$\uparrow$Cardiac contractility (α_1)
$\uparrow$Cardiac contractility (β_1)	
$\uparrow$Heart rate (β_1)	
$\uparrow$Conduction velocity (β_1)	
$\uparrow$Arteriolar dilation: $\downarrow$ BP (β_2) (muscle)	$\uparrow$Arteriolar vasoconstriction; $\uparrow$ BP (α_1) (splanchnic, renal, cutaneous, genital)
$\uparrow$Muscle relaxation (β_2)	$\uparrow$Sphincter contraction (α_1)
Gastrointestinal	Gastrointestinal
Urinary	Urinary
Bronchial	Platelet aggregation (α_2)
	Sweating ("adrenergic")
	Dilation of pupils (α_1)

BP, blood pressure.
Note: α_1 and α_2 receptors are responsible for vasoconstriction and other effects and are mainly mediated by norepinephrine. β_1 and β_2 receptors are mainly mediated by epinephrine. (From Berne, R. M., & Levy, M. H. [1998]. *Physiology* [4th ed.]. St. Louis: Mosby.)

and protein. Gluconeogenesis, glycogenolysis, protein catabolism, and lipolysis are increased. The result is that more fuel is made available for energy. Cortisol may make amino acids available to damaged tissues for the synthesis of essential intracellular substances such as purines, pyrimidines, and creatine phosphate.[17]

Cortisol suppresses almost every step of the inflammatory response. It has the following effects in inflammation:

1. Stabilizes lysosomal membranes so release of proteolytic enzymes is decreased
2. Decreases the permeability of capillaries, which prevents loss of plasma into the tissues
3. Decreases movement of white blood cells into the inflamed area
4. Suppresses the immune system (see below)
5. Lowers fever due to blocking release of interleukin-1 from white blood cells[1,17]

See Chapters 9, 10, 23 and 24 for further information.

CIRCADIAN SECRETION OF GLUCOCORTICOIDS. In individuals with a day-wake/night-sleep cycle, the glucocorticoids are thought to be synchronized by light. Their concentration in blood and urine decreases during sleep and rises to its highest levels in the early morning.[17] This pattern of glucocorticoid secretion follows a particular rhythm called the **circadian rhythm or pattern**. The early morning level elevates to its daily high about 6 to 8 AM and begins to drop at about 10 AM, increasing slightly around 2 PM, and gradually declining until 10 PM (Fig. 5-1).

Disruptions in circadian rhythms are often produced by stress, which especially disturbs the rhythmic

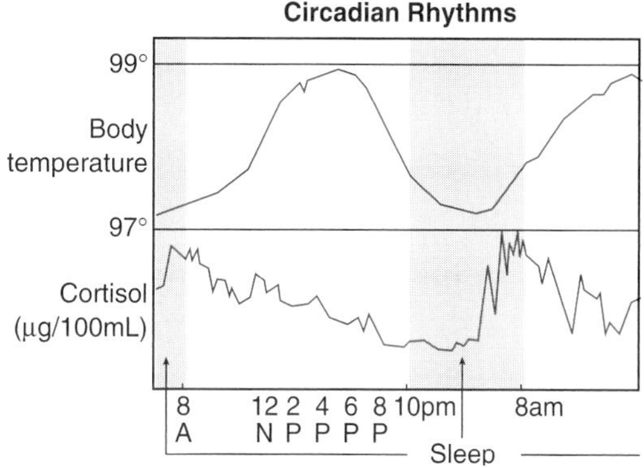

FIGURE 5-1. Circadian rhythms showing correlation of cortisol secretion and temperature changes in a 24-hour period.

patterns of blood glucose, white blood cells, and temperature regulation.[18] These alterations increase with the duration of the stress.[16] Changes in circadian rhythm may relate to illness in that phase relationships seem to be consistent in particular maladies. For example, persons with peptic ulcer disease frequently have increased gastric acid secretion causing pain in the late night or early morning hours.

EFFECTS ON THE IMMUNE SYSTEM. Stress, especially when it is chronic and unremitting, apparently lowers the body's defense, a response at least partly due to increased production of glucocorticoids (Flowchart 5-5). Glucocorticoids suppress the inflammatory response, as described above. The excessive glucocorticoid secretion causes acceleration of normal thymic atrophy and reduces T-cell responses during periods of stress.[20] When T cells are depleted there is noted a decrease in resistance to disease (see page 293). Various forms of stress, such as death of a spouse, excessive exercise, and taking exams have resulted in immune suppression and even the onset of illness.[30]

The immune suppression after overwhelming insult to the body may be lifesaving in preventing a bodywide, inflammatory response such as septicemia. The end result of this suppression may cause delayed healing and decreased resistance to infection (see page 268). Multiple organ dysfunction syndrome (MODS) is thought to be a result of exhaustion of immune defense (see page 517).

OTHER ENDOCRINE EFFECTS

The endocrine hormones are increased in the stress response through hypothalamic stimulation of the pituitary, leading to stimulation of target organ secretion. This relationship is illustrated in Flowchart 5-6. Stimulation of the pituitary can increase secretion of ACTH, antidiuretic hormone (ADH), thyroid-stimulating hormone (TSH), and others. Secretion of aldosterone is also increased from the adrenal cortex, mainly due to the effect of renin.

The increased secretion of TSH leads to increased synthesis and secretion of the thyroid hormones. This causes a small increase in BMR, which is not always coordinated with other effects of stress.[19] The thyroid hormone, thyroxine, apparently makes the body more responsive to the effects of epinephrine and may be a major effector in prolonged stress.[42]

Variable secretion of ADH from the posterior pituitary occurs in stressful situations. Certain types of stress and stress behaviors, such as alcohol ingestion, hypothermia, and certain drugs, decrease the production of ADH resulting in diuresis. Other types of stress, such as hypovolemia, anesthesia, and postsurgical stress, increase ADH production, which promotes water retention.[19]

Stress usually causes an increased level of aldosterone due to associated renin release. Aldosterone functions in sodium and water retention along with potassium excretion (see page 450).

FLOWCHART 5-5 **Immune Effects of Stress**

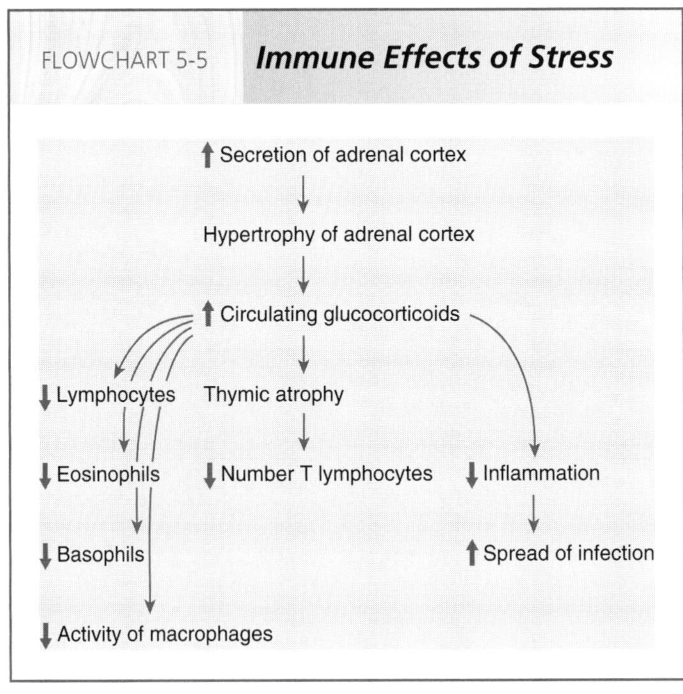

FLOWCHART 5-6 **Hormone Effects of Stress**

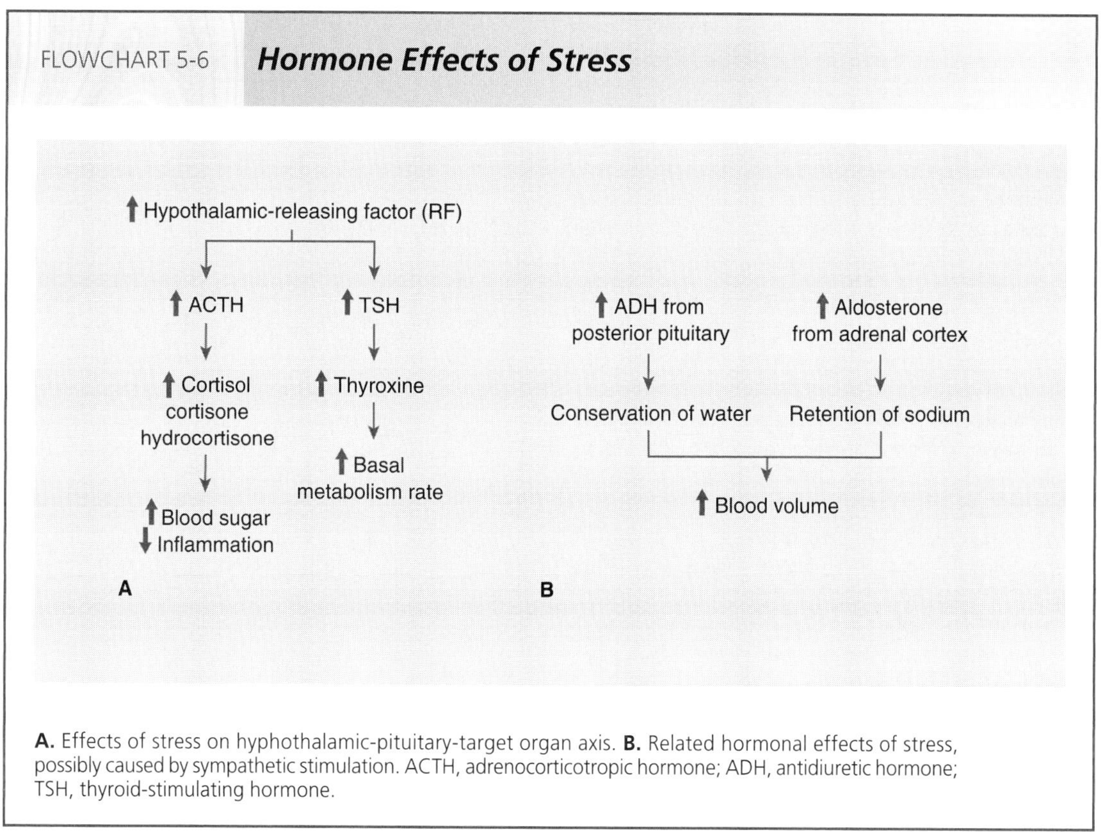

A. Effects of stress on hyphothalamic-pituitary-target organ axis. **B.** Related hormonal effects of stress, possibly caused by sympathetic stimulation. ACTH, adrenocorticotropic hormone; ADH, antidiuretic hormone; TSH, thyroid-stimulating hormone.

Stress has variable effects on growth hormone. Hypoglycemia, for example, is a potent stimulus for the release of the hormone. In the elderly, growth hormone is normally decreased and this is exacerbated by stressful life events.

Stress Effects and Disease

Many studies have been conducted to relate stress effects with actual disease development. Psychological and physical stressors have been studied correlating personality traits, genetic predisposition, and environmental, emotional, occupational, and social factors with specific disease (see below).[10] Ill health is manifested by the bodily symptoms of hyperventilation, functional bowel and musculoskeletal syndromes, along with sleep disturbances. These syndromes are strongly associated with anxiety, distress, and depressed moods and are closely linked to stressful experiences.[33] Ill health syndromes may also terminate in disease, but the exact link is not totally understood. The disease relationships are explored in the following section. The ill health is linked closely with the life situation, especially uncontrollable and undesirable life experiences.[13]

A maladaptive response of the body to stressors increases the risk of disease development. It is commonly accepted that psychophysiologic arousal can cause specific end-organ pathology in certain individuals. The chronicity of the arousal state and hyperstimulation of the end organ are necessary factors in the production of pathology.[9] Genetic predisposition to a certain disease and organ susceptibility can be influenced by physical stress, emotional stress, or both. Maladaptation is promoted when there are underlying health problems such as malnutrition or chronic diseases; these problems are often seen with the aged population.

GENETIC PREDISPOSITION

Stressors of sufficient strength or intensity can cause an alteration in normal functioning of the body. If one has a genetic or hereditary susceptibility to the stressors, the alteration may be manifested as disease.

Genetic susceptibility refers to a myriad of conditions that "run in the family" and seem to make the individual react in a particular way to certain stressors. A common example is an exaggerated allergic response that predisposes members of families to specific pollens. When the pollen count is seasonally high, these persons suffer different types of allergic responses. In this example, the stressor is the pollen count, but the response is heightened by a hyperactive, hereditary, immune reaction (see page 311).

Many other diseases seem to be familial, but the development of actual disease may require additional stressors to trigger the process. One example is the onset of a stroke (cerebrovascular accident) in the individual with a strong family history who is also obese, has high cholesterol levels, and smokes cigarettes.

ORGAN SUSCEPTIBILITY

In different individuals, all organs are not equally resistant to stressors. Some persons under equal stress conditions develop cardiovascular disorders, others develop peptic ulcers, and still others may suffer migraine headaches or other maladies. The "weak organ theory" suggests that certain organs have increased susceptibility in certain individuals.[33] Many times this susceptibility is increased when there is a genetic predisposition but in many cases, no link can be found.

Stress-Induced Disease

Selye referred to the production of disease as maladaptation and categorized stress-induced disease as indicated in Box 5-1. The stress connection of cardiovascular, immune deficiency, and digestive diseases as well as cancer and effects on other systems is explored in the following section.

CARDIOVASCULAR DISEASE

For many years it has been recognized that stress in the form of emotional, occupational, societal, cultural, hereditary, and physical stressors is important in the etiology of coronary artery disease. Major studies of the relationship of high-fat diets, stressful living situations, and personality have led to some theories concerning coronary artery disease. Individuals who have hypercholesterolemia have a greater risk of developing atherosclerotic heart disease than those with normal cholesterol levels (see page 434). In some cases, hypercholesterolemias "run in the family," in some cases they are induced by diet, and in some cases their cause is a mystery. During stressful periods, the serum cholesterol has been shown to rise, perhaps due to lipolysis induced by the increased levels of circulating catecholamines. Studies also link serum lipid levels and personality patterns.[11] Stress-induced hyperlipidemia is considered to be the principal mechanism for stress-related atherosclerosis. Stress may also induce coronary artery vasospasm, which may cause myocardial injury.[33]

Emotional stress, especially anger, can precipitate anginal pain and aggravate heart failure. Life stressors, such as bereavement and loss of employment, are significant risk factors for myocardial ischemia and infarction.[41]

Research has identified a behavior pattern consistent with hypertension and heart attack. The type A behavior pattern includes competitiveness in work, fast work pace, time pressure, inability to relax at work or play, and hostility. This personality pattern apparently offers the greatest risk for the development of symptomatic coronary artery disease even when the other risk factors are considered.[35]

BOX 5-1

SELYE'S CLASSIFICATION OF STRESS-INDUCED DISEASES

1. Hypertension
2. Heart and blood vessel disease
3. Kidney disease
4. Eclampsia
5. Arthritis
6. Skin and eye inflammation
7. Infections
8. Allergic and hypersensitivity diseases
9. Nervous and mental diseases
10. Sexual derangements
11. Digestive diseases
12. Metabolic diseases
13. Cancer
14. Immune deficiency

IMMUNE DEFICIENCY

The decreased immune response after stressful situations appears to be due to excessive glucocorticoid secretion. Physiologically or psychologically stressful events precipitate a decrease in lymphocytes and other leukocytes.

The stress-induced response of decreased immunity can be detrimental in certain conditions, such as cancer. It is often seen that an individual who was declared "cured" of cancer undergoes relapse after an acute stressful situation, such as the death of a loved one.[23] The stress-induced depression of immune system surveillance may allow for an increased rate of malignant growth.

DIGESTIVE DISEASES

The relationship of stress and peptic ulcers has been studied for years. Stress-induced ulcer disease is discussed in more detail on page 732. Duodenal ulcerations are often due to infection of the pyloric antrum with *Helicobacter pylori* bacteria that may proliferate when the immune response to the organism is decreased.[9] Overwhelming stress frequently leads to the development of stress ulcers. These may be related to gastric mucosal ischemia and gastric acid secretion. The ischemia is a result of vasoconstriction by the circulating catecholamines. The mechanism for the related gastric acid secretion is not entirely understood, but it may be due to cerebral stimulation of the vagal nerves. Hypersecretion has been demonstrated clearly in the development of Cushing's ulcers, which are associated with brain lesions. Stress ulcers are frequent in untreated individuals who experience overwhelming conditions such as shock due to trauma, surgery, burns, or infections.

Stress has been indicated in many diverse digestive conditions, such as constipation, diarrhea, ulcerative colitis, and Crohn's disease. Personality and stress factors with ulcerative colitis and regional enteritis include reports of precipitation of attacks and exacerbation of the disease with anger and anxiety.[33]

CANCER

Specific agents (stressors) are linked with cancer causation. These carcinogens are discussed on page 70. Numerous studies have linked psychosocial attitudes with development and progression of cancer. The findings vary, but depression, isolation, introverted personality, and feelings of hopelessness tend to support development of the disease.[9,23]

The relationship of stress to cancer may be that depression of the immunologic response by the stress allows cancer to be initiated.[11] Local exposure to carcinogen stressors may result in tumorigenesis. Stress can be viewed as having a twofold influence on malignancy: (1) it increases the production of abnormal cells and (2) it decreases the capability of the body to destroy these cells. This influence is mainly due to decreased surveillance by the immune system. All individuals are exposed daily to a host of potential carcinogens and resistance is multifactorial, including physiologic and behavioral responses and attitudes.[23]

OTHER SYSTEM EFFECTS OF STRESS

The skin is a target organ for stress reactivity, and when stress occurs, the vessels constrict and peripheral blood flow decreases. Some of the vasospastic conditions such as Raynaud's phenomenon are partly stress induced (see page 448). Other stress-related disorders include eczema, urticaria, psoriasis, and acne (see page 946).[33]

The musculoskeletal system exhibits stress effects by chronically tense muscles, producing the common syndromes of backache and headache.[41] Arthritis, especially rheumatoid arthritis, is aggravated by high degrees of stress and this may exacerbate symptoms.

The respiratory system participates in the acute stress reaction by hyperventilation, which may produce respiratory alkalosis (see page 183). Stress may provoke heightened allergic sinusitis and episodes of bronchial asthma (see page 311). Onset of acute asthmatic attacks often occur following periods of sleeplessness, worry, and grief.[20]

EXERCISE

Physical exercise is essential to health. It promotes cardiovascular and body system adaptation to maintain bones, muscles, hormones, and other physiologic functioning. Exercise is a type of physiologic stress that requires changes in all major systems for the body to be able to continue its motion for even short periods. Short- and long-term adaptations are discussed below in terms of effects on the body systems and energy use.

Effects on the Cardiovascular System

The cardiovascular system responds to a single bout of exercise by making multiple adaptations. The sheer anticipation of exercise causes a slight increase in heart rate. As exercise begins, heart rate, stroke volume, cardiac output, blood pressure, and blood flow all increase.[22]

HEART RATE

Heart rate increases with activity through both extrinsic and intrinsic factors. The extrinsic factors originate in the cardiovascular center of the medulla and are then transmitted through the SNS and parasympathetic nervous system of the ANS. When the cardioaccelerator nerves of the SNS are stimulated, the catecholamines (epinephrine and norepinephrine) are released. These neural hormones accelerate the depolarization of the sinus node, which causes the heart to beat faster. This acceleration can increase to the *maximal heart rate*. The factors that influence maximal heart include age, gender, level of fitness, presence of cardiovascular disease, altitude, type of exercise, and true maximal exertion.[15] The normal resting heart rate is about 70 to 80 beats/min. During a maximal exercise session that is maintained for several minutes, the heart rate may rise to a peak value of 220 beats/min minus the person's age in years.[37]

STROKE VOLUME

Stroke volume is defined as the amount of blood ejected from each ventricle per heartbeat. The factors responsible for stroke volume include venous return, ventricular distensibility, ventricular contractility, and systemic and pulmonary vascular resistance (see page 422). The principal factor with regard to exercise is *venous return*. Influence of the SNS on the heart increases heart rate and contractility. Exercise performed in the vertical position as opposed to the horizontal position results in a greater increase in stroke volume. Resting stroke volume may range from 60 to 100 mL, although maximum stroke volume in a marathon runner may reach as high as 162 mL.

CARDIAC OUTPUT

Cardiac output is amount of blood pumped by the heart per minute and is the product of heart rate times stroke volume (see page 422). Cardiac output increases during exercise to provide the exercising muscles with nutrients and oxygen necessary to continue working. At rest, the cardiac output is about 4 to 8 L/min. It may increase to as much as 20 L/min with exercise depending on age, gender, size, and physical condition.[36] This *cardiac reserve* (ability to increase cardiac output when needed) is increased as much as 50% in the athletically fit older person over the nonfit person of the same age.[17]

BLOOD PRESSURE

Blood pressure is the product of cardiac output times total peripheral resistance (see page 424). Therefore, the blood pressure changes seen during physical activity are a direct result of changes in cardiac output and peripheral resistance. The vascular bed of active muscles vasodilates, leading to decreased peripheral resistance to blood flow during exercise. The increase in cardiac output outweighs the decrease in peripheral resistance, resulting an increased mean arterial pressure.[32] The increase in mean arterial blood pressure that is seen during exercise is primarily due to increases in systolic blood pressure. It has been determined that the change in diastolic blood pressure is minimal.[37] The amount of systolic increase can range from 20 to 80 mm Hg, depending on the conditions under which the exercise is performed. The values for blood pressure are higher when exercise is performed with the arms rather than with the legs. The SNS-induced vasoconstriction in certain tissues (kidney and gut, especially) is important for the maintenance of the blood pressure.[5] Normotensive persons may experience peak exercise values in systolic blood pressure of 200 to 240 mm Hg.

BLOOD FLOW

During exercise, active muscles receive increased amounts of blood while those at rest receive less. The active muscles receive an increase in total blood flow with added blood flow being shunted from the inactive muscles. The amount of the increase in blood flow through active muscles varies with the type and intensity of the exercise and with the proportion of the total musculature involved. At rest approximately 0.8 liter of blood per minute goes to the skeletal muscles. It has been estimated that as much as 16 L/min goes to these muscles during exercise. Figure 5-2 summarizes the blood flow changes experienced during exercise. The inactive muscles of the kidneys, stomach, and intestines, particularly, receive a much decreased blood flow due to the SNS response in exercise.

As body temperature increases with exercise, more blood is sent to the skin. The thermoregulatory system responds in this way to dissipate the excessive heat production generated by working muscles and environmental temperatures.[39]

Effects on the Respiratory System

Pulmonary ventilation increases with physical activity, although the exact mechanism is unknown. It is hypothesized that afferent impulses from working of the muscles or from the central nervous system (CNS) increase activity in the motor neurons of the respiratory muscles through the spinal and supraspinal reflex centers. The result is an increase in frequency and depth of respirations.[3]

Respiratory volume is regulated through a negative feedback system, determined by carbon dioxide production in relation to carbon dioxide elimination during expiration. As a result, the carbon dioxide levels in the arterial blood probably determine the magnitude of the ventilatory response.[3]

Respiratory reserve increases when the individual is physically fit. This is especially true in the athletically fit older person. For example, in an 80-year-old nonfit person, there is an average respiratory reserve of no more than three or four times tidal volume, whereas in the athletically fit older person, it may be twice this amount.[17]

Effects on the Endocrine System

The endocrine system plays an important role during exercise. Its primary purpose is to maintain homeostatic conditions. The release of hormones from specialized glands throughout the body is controlled by the neuroendocrine system. The hormones exert their actions on target organs and cells. Table 5-2 summarizes hormone involvement during exercise.

Hormonal changes in the physically fit individual include increases in growth hormone, testosterone, estrogen, catecholamines, cortisol, and thyroid hormone. These hormones show a more marked change in early training and tend to increase less in the trained individual. Insulin levels decrease during exercise, but levels show a less marked change in the fit individual. The significance of other hormonal changes is being studied, especially in relation to sex and age differences.[42]

Effects on the Immune System

The immune system influences the body's overall response to exercise through its interaction with neural and endocrine factors.[32] The incidence of some infections

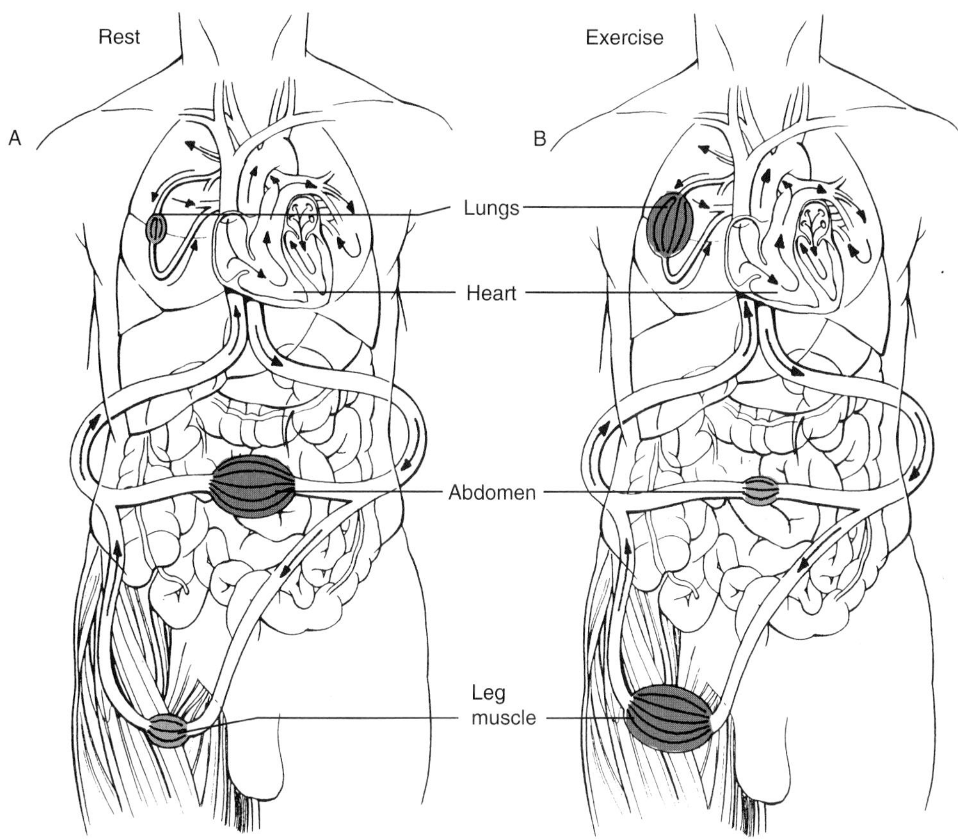

FIGURE 5-2. **A.** Schematic representation of the cardiopulmonary system of a sedentary man during standing rest. Blood flow to the heart, lungs, abdomen, and leg muscles is illustrated. **B.** The same man during exercise at maximal oxygen uptake. Blood flow to the heart, lungs, and leg muscles is increased and is markedly decreased to the abdomen.

and possibly certain types of cancer is decreased as a result of the exercise-induced bolstered function of natural killer cells, circulating T and B lymphocytes as well as cells of the monocyte/macrophage type.[32] Moderate exercise appears to bolster immune function, but a single epidose of high-intensity exercise appears to cause a dramatic decrease in the functioning of all major cells of the immune system.[28] This also has been shown to occur with overtraining.[28]

Effects on the Muscular System

Exercise increases contractile force of muscle. As is discussed below, the type and condition of the muscle fibers determines the performance that can be achieved in exercise. The *strength* of a muscle is determined mainly by the size of the muscle, whereas the *power* of muscle contraction is determined by strength, distance of contraction, and the number times that it contracts each minute.[17] The *endurance* of muscle performance depends on nutritive support, especially from glycogen.[17]

To contract, muscles must be supplied with energy through adenosine triphosphate (ATP). The generation of ATP is discussed in detail on pages 20–23. A brief review is provided below.

ENERGY PRODUCTION IN THE MUSCLE CELL

Adenosine triphosphate is generated by three basic energy systems: (1) oxidative phosphorylation, (2) glycolysis, and (3) creatine phosphate (CP). In addition, a limited supply of ATP is stored within the cell.[37]

Oxidative phosphorylation occurs within the cellular mitochondria. This aerobic reaction provides the major supply of body energy. The major metabolic substrates are fatty acids (at rest and at low exercise levels) and glucose (at high exercise intensities). Hydrogen atoms are produced during beta oxidation and the Krebs cycle. The complete oxidation of one molecule

TABLE 5-2

A SUMMARY OF HORMONAL CHANGES DURING AN EPISODE OF EXERCISE

HORMONE	EXERCISE RESPONSE	SPECIAL RELATIONSHIPS	PROBABLE IMPORTANCE
Catecholamines	Increases	Greater increase with intense exercise; norepinephrine > epinephrine; increases less after training	Increased blood glucose; increased skeletal muscle and liver glycogenolysis; increased lipolysis
Growth hormone (GH)	Increases	Increases more in untrained persons; declines faster in trained persons	Unknown
Adrenocorticotropic hormone (ACTH)-cortisol	Increases	Greater increase with intense exercise; increases less after training with submaximal exercise	Increased gluconeogenesis in liver; increased mobilization of fatty acids
Thyroid-stimulating hormone (TSH)-thyroxine	Increases	Increased thyroxine turnover with training but no toxic effects are evident	Unknown
Luteinizing hormone (LH)	No change	None	None
Testosterone	Increases	None	Unknown
Estradiol-progesterone	Increases	Increases during luteal phase of the menstrual cycle	Unknown
Insulin	Decreases	Decreases less after training	Decreased stimulus to use blood glucose
Glucagon	Increases	Increases less after training	Increased blood glucose via glycogenolysis and gluconeogenesis
Renin-angiotensin-aldosterone	Increases	Same increase after training in rats	Sodium retention to maintain plasma volume
Antidiuretic hormone (ADH)	Expected increase	None	Water retention to maintain plasma volume
Parathormone (PTH)-calcitonin	Unknown	None	Needed to establish proper bone development
Erythropoietin	Unknown	None	Would be important to increase erythropoiesis
Prostaglandins	May increase	May increase in response to sustained isometric contractions; may need ischemic stress	May be local vasodilators

(Adapted from Wilmore, J. H., & Costill, D. L. [1994]. *Physiology of sport and exercise* [p. 136]. Champaign, IL: Human Kinetics.)

of glucose produces 38 molecules of ATP, while the oxidation of one molecule of fatty acid yields 129 molecules of ATP.

Glycolysis is an anaerobic way through which muscles can acquire ATP. The generation of ATP from glycolysis occurs quickly and results in an end-product of lactate. This process of glycolysis produces only three molecules of ATP. As lactate accumulates in the muscle fiber, the cellular environment becomes more acidic. Eventually, the glycolytic enzymes cease to function optimally.

Creatine phosphate is an anaerobic pathway that provides the donation of a high-energy phosphate to adenosine diphosphate (ADP) to synthesize ATP. This process provides enough energy for about 8 seconds of exercise. When sufficient ATP is present in the mitochondria, an enzyme promotes the synthesis of CP, which stores the energy and can then transfer the energy back to the ADP when needed. This process is not adequate to support maximal muscle activity so that in active muscles dependence is greatest on the oxidative pathway.

TYPES OF MUSCLE FIBERS

Two types of muscle fibers are identified in exercising muscles—slow-twitch and fast-twitch muscles. An individual's predominant type of muscle fiber is largely the result of genetics. A direct relationship has been identified between predominant fibers type and performance in certain sports. Slow-twitch muscle fibers, for example, account for more than 90% of the total fibers in the leg muscles of marathon runners. Conversely, fast-twitch muscle fibers account for more than 80% of the total fibers in the leg muscles of sprinters.

Slow-Twitch Fibers

Slow-twitch fibers typically are aerobic, which gives them steady power and greater endurance. They tire only when their fuel supply is gone. Slow-twitch fibers (called *red muscle*) have many mitochondria, are surrounded by dense capillary beds, and contain myoglobin.[24] **Myoglobin** is an iron-containing protein similar to hemoglobin in red blood cells. It combines with oxygen and stores it until it is needed by the mitochondria. Slow-twitch fibers, therefore, are able to draw more blood and oxygen than fast-twitch fibers. Slow-twitch fibers are essential for endurance sports such as biking, long-distance running, jogging, and swimming.

Fast-Twitch Fibers

Fast-twitch fibers tend to be anaerobic. As a result, they exhibit explosive power and tend to fatigue easily. These fibers (called *white muscle*) have fewer mitochondria and fewer blood vessels than those of the slow-twitch type.[24] They do not contain myoglobin. Because fast-twitch fibers rely on anaerobic energy, they are vulnerable to an accumulation of lactic acid and rapid fatigue. The explosions of energy they provide, however, are used in sports such as sprinting, weight lifting, and swinging a golf club.

Effects on Metabolic Rate

Metabolic rate is the rate at which the body uses energy. The resting metabolic rate represents the rate of energy expenditure that is necessary to maintain basic body functions (**basal metabolic rate-BMR**) and is approximately 3.5 mL oxygen/kg per minute. This is equal to 1 **MET** (metabolic equivalent unit used to determine the amount of energy expended during activity). For an average individual, I MET burns about 1 kcal/min or 1 kcal/kg of body weight per hour.[6] Examples of energy expenditure for common physical activities are shown in Table 5-3.

TABLE 5-3

METABOLIC RATE FOR VARIOUS ACTIVITIES

ENERGY EXPENDITURE	PHYSICAL ACTIVITIES
1.5–2 METs	Standing, desk work, walking at 1–2 mph, driving a car
2–3 METs	Bowling, fishing, ironing, car washing, shopping
3–4 METs	Cycling at 6 mph, walking at 3–3.5 mph, raking leaves, window washing, janitorial work
4–5 METs	Light swimming, moderate calisthenics, hoeing a garden, painting, pushing a power mower
5–6 METs	Walking at 4 mph, cycling at 8–8.5 mph, stair climbing, garden digging
6–7 METs	Moderate swimming, backpacking, heavy calisthenics, snow shoveling, carrying or lifting 50–60 lb, hand lawn mowing
7–8 METs	Mountain climbing, walking at 6 mph, jogging at 5 mph, hand sawing, ditch digging, carrying 20 lb up stairs
8–9 METs	Competitive soccer, cycling at 13 mph, heavy weight training, climbing a ladder, moving desk or file cabinets
10+ METs	Competitive basketball, running at 6 mph, cycling at 14 mph, handball, heavy labor, heavy shoveling

Long-Term Adaptations to Exercise

Aerobic exercise is a type of exercise that improves the efficiency of the aerobic energy-producing systems. Aerobic exercise typically involves the use of large muscle groups with slow-twitch fibers. Regular aerobic exercise leads to significant long-term changes in the major systems of the body. The resting heart rate is frequently decreased as the heart beats more efficiently. Stroke volume is increased at rest and during exercise. The result of the decreased resting heart rate and the increased stroke volume is that it will provide an increase in cardiac output, especially during maximal work efforts.

Cardiac muscle fibers may hypertrophy slightly as a result of endurance training. This allows for greater force being exerted with each beat of the heart. The number of capillaries and small vessels in trained skeletal muscle is increased, which allows greater capacity for blood flow in active muscle.

Mean arterial blood pressure decreases slightly at rest in trained individuals. Long-term adjustments to maximal exercise show less increase in the blood pressure. This phenomenon is more dramatic in hypertensive individuals. Resting blood pressure is markedly decreased in hypertensives and systolic and diastolic may decrease more than 10 mm Hg.[14]

Metabolic adaptations occur in the muscular system as a result of endurance training. The mitochondria increase in size and number. The activity of oxidative enzymes increases and, along with myoglobin content increase, the amount of oxygen that is stored in individual muscle fibers also increases. The outcome of these increases is the enhancement of the oxidative capacity of the endurance-trained muscle. The capacity of skeletal muscle to store glycogen also increases. Trained muscles are better able to use fat as an energy source, which spares glycogen stores.

Maximal oxygen uptake (VO_2 max) increases in the fit individual. This measure refers to the largest amount of oxygen that can be consumed per minute. The maximal value is sometimes called **aerobic capacity** and is a functional measure of a person's physical fitness.[39] The average aerobic capacity for an untrained college man is between 42 and 46 mL oxygen/kg per minute. The untrained college woman will have an average aerobic capacity of 30 to 39 mL/kg per minute. The VO_2 max of marathoners is about 45% greater than that of the untrained person.[17]

SLEEP

Sleep is an essential component in maintaining the physiologic balance for all humans. Sleep is a basic human need on which the physical and emotional health of an individual depends. Each person needs a different amount of sleep and sleep patterns vary among individuals and societies.

Functions of Sleep

The purpose of sleep is unknown, but it probably allows the body to restore itself and prepare for daily activities. The heart and respiratory rate decrease during sleep, thus preserving respiratory and cardiac function. During sleep the body conserves energy by lowering the BMR. Epithelial and specialized cells are also repaired and revitalized during sleep.

The function of dreaming is unknown, but it is thought that some memory and problem-solving aspects are related to this function. Studies of dream content suggest that in the early stage dreams are oriented toward reality, but later in the second half of sleep the sequence of events and content becomes more emotionally intense and bizarre.[31]

Physiology of Sleep

The physiology of sleep and wakefulness is a complex phenomenon associated with many neurochemical transmitters and various areas of the brain. The coordinating mechanisms either activate or suppress the center in the brain that controls sleep. The **reticular activating system** (**RAS**) located in the upper area of the brain stem contains certain cells that maintain a person's state of being awake and alert (see page 888). The catecholamine-releasing neurons that release dopamine may be the cause of wakefulness. The spontaneous activity in the RAS excites the cerebral cortex and the peripheral nervous system. The feedback from these areas to the RAS tends to sustain the wakefulness state.[17] Neurons in the RAS probably fatigue and are susceptible to inhibition by sleep-producing chemicals. During sleep the feedback system is tremendously slowed or inhibited and activity in the RAS is very low.[38]

Sleep occurs when the wakefulness mechanism tires and the sleep-promoting neurons become active.[12] These neurons are mainly found in brain stem structures and promote deeper stages of sleep. Cortical arousal to produce wakefulness is prevented by blockage of synaptic transmission through the thalamus.[12]

Sleep may be the result of the release of serotonin or other mediators from special cells in the raphe nuclei of the pons and medulla. Serotonin may play a role in synthesis of a hypnogenic factor that directly causes sleep. Several blood-borne factors produce slow wave sleep including insulin, cholecystokinin (CCK), bombesin, and interleukin-1. CCK and bombesin are increased after food ingestion, which may be responsible for postprandial sleepiness.[12]

Sleep is composed of a set of physiologic processes involving a sequence of states within the CNS. Each sequence can be readily identified with an electroencephalogram (EEG), electromyogram, and electrooculogram by the various levels of activity that are measured. Two distinct phases of sleep have been identified by these instruments. They are REM (active sleep) and NREM (quiet sleep).[8]

As the individual falls asleep, he or she enters **nonrapid eye movement** (**NREM**) sleep, which is characterized by four progressive stages. NREM sleep is recognized by snoring, slow regular respiration, absence of body movement, and slow regular brain activity. Each stage of NREM sleep is progressively deeper. During stages III and IV of NREM sleep, slow waves are typically produced on the EEG. This is referred to as **slow wave sleep** (**SWS**) (Fig. 5-3). At the end of stage IV, individuals reenter stage III, then stage II, then finally they enter into REM sleep (Table 5-4).

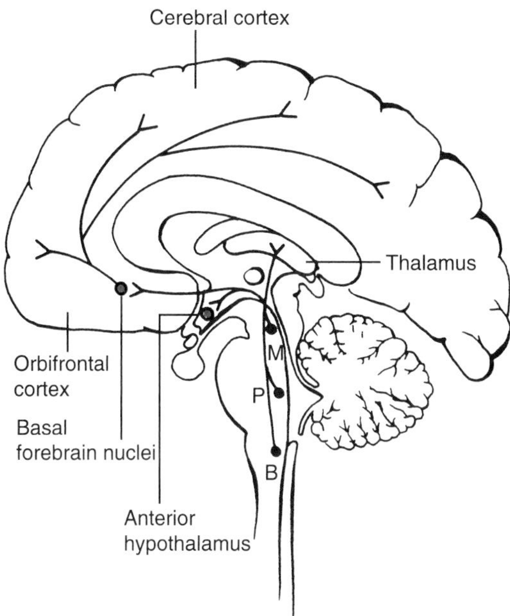

FIGURE 5-3. Generators of slow wave sleep. Slow wave sleep facilitatory stimuli originate in raphe nuclei that project rostrally to the anterior hyphothalamus, thalamus, and basal forebrain nuclei. From these centers projections reach the cortical mantle. (B, P, M = raphe nuclei; B = medulla; P = pons; M = midbrain; AH = anterior hyphothalamus; BF = basal forebrain; S = septal nuclei; CP = caudate, putamen; T = thalamus; HIP = hippocampus; PO = preoptic area.) (Culebras, A. [1996]. *Clinical handbook of sleep disorders.* Boston: Butterworth-Heineman.)

TABLE 5-4

CHARACTERISTICS OF NREM SLEEP

STAGE	CHARACTERISTICS
I	Is transitional stage between wakefulness and sleep The person is in a relaxed state but still somewhat aware of the surroundings. Involuntary muscle jerking may occur and waken the person. The stage normally lasts only for minutes. The person can be aroused easily. Constitutes only about 5% of total sleep.
II	The person falls into a stage of sleep. The person can be aroused with relative ease. Constitutes 50–55% of sleep.
III	The depth of sleep increases and arousal becomes increasingly difficult. Composes about 10% of sleep.
IV	The person reaches the greatest depth of sleep, which is called *delta sleep.* Arousal from sleep is difficult. Physiologic changes in the body include the following: Slow brain waves are recorded on an EEG. Pulse and respiratory rates decrease. Blood pressure decreases. Muscles are relaxed. Metabolism slows and the body temperature is low. Constitutes about 10% of sleep.

(Taylor, C., Lillis, C., & LeMone, P. [1997]. *Fundamentals of nursing* [3rd ed.] Philadelphia: Lippincott-Raven.)

Rapid eye movement (**REM**, desynchronized, or active) sleep is characterized by irregular respirations, absence of snoring, rapid eye movement, and twitching of the face and fingers. It usually takes about 90 minutes of sleep for an individual to reach REM sleep. Waking during REM sleep usually results in reports of dream generation and these dreams may be visual and auditory in nature.[12] Each person is different, but a typical night's sleep consists of four to six sleep cycles beginning with stage I and progressing through REM sleep (Flowchart 5-7).

Sleep Patterns

The normal human sleep–wake cycle is over a 25-hour period. Normally its onset occurs with a decrease in activity and lasts from 7 to 9 hours.[7] There is a variability of sleep needs with some individuals requiring only 4 to 5 hours a night, whereas other require 11 to 12 hours.

Sleep patterns are usually circadian with the sleep–wake cycle following the dark–light pattern of the 2-hour day. The pacemaker in the brain for this patterning is the suprachiasmatic nucleus (SCN) in the anterior hypothalamus.[27] It is stimulated by receptors in the retina. The main elements in determining wakefulness include light intensity, duration, spectrum, and time of exposure.[29]

Melatonin (secreted by the pineal gland) has potent regulatory effects on the SCN. Its secretion is stimulated by dark and is suppressed by light. Melatonin promotes sleep and its deficiency in the elderly may promote insomnia.[12]

Factors Affecting Sleep

Several factors can alter the quantity and quality of an individual's sleep in various ways throughout the lifetime. These include physical illness, sleep schedule variations, emotional stress, exercise and fatigue, weight

FLOWCHART 5-7 **A Single Normal Sleep Cycle**

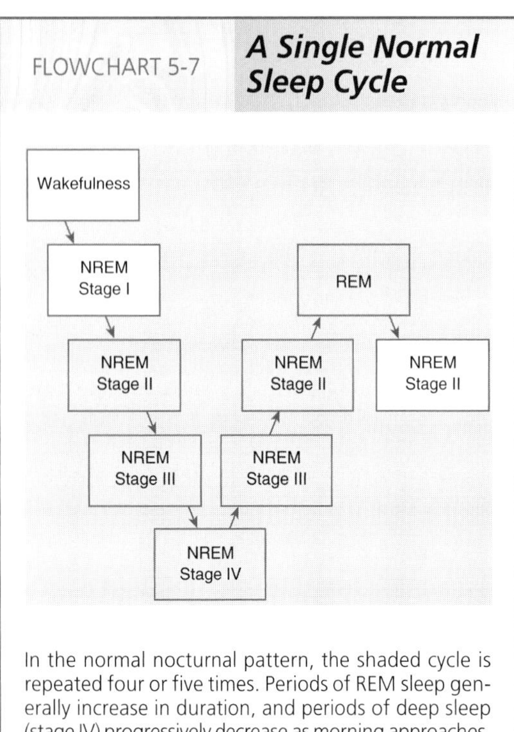

In the normal nocturnal pattern, the shaded cycle is repeated four or five times. Periods of REM sleep generally increase in duration, and periods of deep sleep (stage IV) progressively decrease as morning approaches. (Taylor, C., Lillis, C., LeMone, P. [1997]. *Fundamentals of nursing: The art and science of nursing care* [3rd ed.] Philadelphia: J. B. Lippincott.)

loss and gain patterns, environmental factors, a person's life-style and age, and various drugs and substances. Nearly every person at some time or another has had difficulty in some part of the sleep cycle.

AGING

The characteristics of sleep–wake cycles and the percentage of time spent in the various stages of sleep change over the life cycle.[31] Infants apparently have the highest amount of REM sleep, while young adults (20–40 years of age) spend 50% of their sleep time in stage II, 25% in REM, 10% in stage III, 10% in stage IV, and 5% in stage I.[12] Elderly persons spend a greater amount of time in bed than their younger counterparts but the amount of actual sleep is apparently decreased. Stage IV sleep is markedly decreased and may be absent.

Total sleep time and the total nightly amounts of sleep are age dependent, and generally sleep time is greatest in infancy and gradually decreases in childhood. The total sleep time stabilizes in adulthood until it starts to decrease with old age. In addition, the number of awakenings that occur during sleep tends to increase after age 40 years. Most of these awakenings occur during REM sleep.[12] Figure 5-4 illustrates typical patterns of sleep at different ages.

LIFE-STYLE

Many life events disrupt sleep patterns and these are not considered sleep disorders until they cause continual sleep disruption or excessive daytime sleepiness. Examples include excessive ingestion of alcohol, tobacco, or caffeine before bedtime. Intense exercise before retiring or emotionally upsetting events can disturb sleep induction. Environmental factors such as noise, too warm or cold surroundings, or unfamiliar locations all can be disturbing. Often, especially in elderly individuals, daytime naps interfere with nighttime sleep and the routine of sleeping in the daytime can become a habit.[25]

DEPRESSION

Clinical depression causes a variety of sleep disorders, from difficulty falling asleep to extended sleep periods.

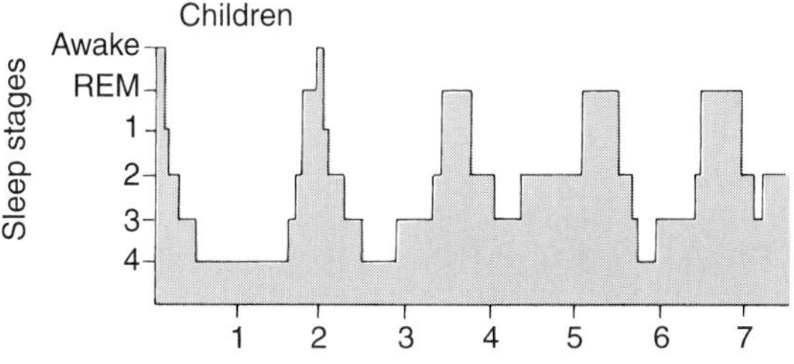

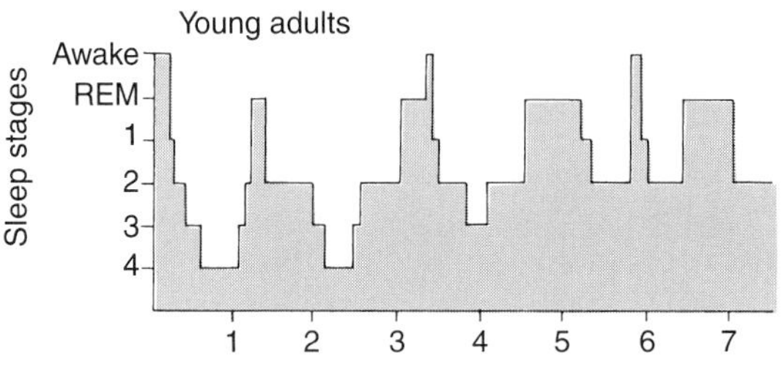

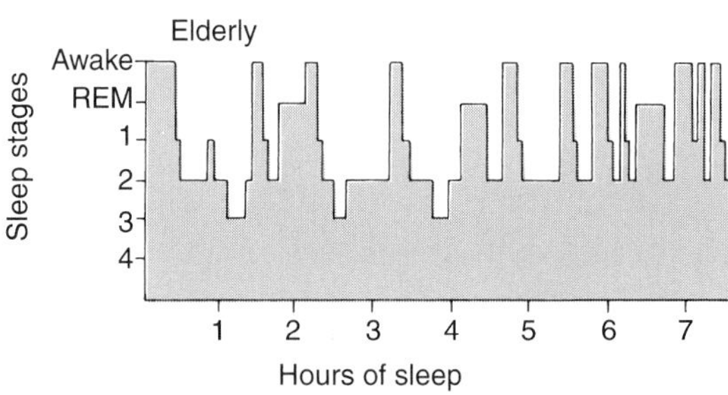

FIGURE 5-4. A comparison of developmental differences in NREM and REM cycles during nocturnal sleep for children, young adults, and elderly people. (Taylor, C., Lillis, C., & LeMone, P., [1997]. *Fundamentals of nursing: The art and science of nursing care* [3rd ed.]. Philadelphia: J. B. Lippincott.)

Analysis of sleep character shows a marked decrease in stages III and IV sleep, with increase in stages I and II and frequent, vigorous REM sleep. Sleep disruptions may be caused by neurotransmitter imbalance and measures of sleep are being used to help determine treatment approaches for depression.[12]

Sleep Pattern Disturbances

In 1972, the Association of Sleep Disorders Centers established a classification of sleep and arousal disorders based on the presenting complaint. This grouping was helpful in diagnosing sleep disorders. The disorders are classified in four basic groups: (1) disorders of initiating and maintaining sleep; (2) disorders of excessive somnolence; (3) disorders of sleeping-waking schedule; (1), (2), and (3) are classified as **dyssomnias**; and (4) dysfunctions associated with sleep, sleep stages, or partial arousals, called **parasomnias**. The classification was revised in 1990 as the International Classification of Sleep Disorders (ICSD), which is summarized in Box 5-2. For clarity, the initial classification is used in this discussion.

DISORDERS OF INITIATING AND MAINTAINING SLEEP

Disorders of initiating and maintaining sleep (DIMS) can be caused by multiple factors, both internal and external. Several aspects of an individual's sleep environment can alter sleep patterns. Examples of these aspects are noise, uncomfortable beds, and sick children. Internal factors such as stress, pain, and ingested chemicals can alter sleep patterns. These disorders are usually not diagnosed unless they chronically interrupt sleep.

Inability to sleep, or *insomnia*, may be exhibited by difficulty falling asleep, recurrent awakenings, or early morning awakening without being able to return to sleep.[25] It causes a high level of frustration in the affected individual and is described as the feeling of being tired from not getting enough sleep. It may indicate a pathologic disorder or it may be psychological in origin. Examples of pathologic disorders are pain, obstructive uropathy, hyperthyroidism, and congestive heart failure. Musculoskeletal disorders, such as arthritis, often interfere with sleep patterns. Psycho-

BOX 5-2

CLASSIFICATION OF SELECTED SLEEP DISORDERS

Dyssomnias

Intrinsic sleep disorders
- Psychophysiological insomnia
- Narcolepsy-cataplexy syndrome*
- Idiopathic and symptomatic hypersomnias*
- Sleep apnea syndromes (obstructive, central)*
- Periodic limb movement disorder

Extrinsic sleep disorders
- Inadequate sleep hygiene
- Environmental sleep disorder
- Sleep onset insomnia disorder
- Substance-dependent sleep disorders
- Nocturnal eating (drinking) syndrome

Circadian rhythm sleep disorders
- Time zone change (jet lag) syndrome
- Shift work sleep disorder
- Irregular sleep–wake pattern
- Delayed sleep phase syndrome
- Advanced sleep phase syndrome

Sleep Disorders Associated with Medical/Psychiatric Disorders

Associated with mental disorders
- (eg, psychoses, anxiety, alcoholism)

Associated with neurologic disorders*
- eg, degeneration, epilepsy, headache)

Associated with other medical disorders
- (eg. chronic obstructive pulmonary disease, asthma, gastroesophageal reflux)

Parasomnias

Arousal disorders
- Sleepwalking
- Sleep terrors

Sleep-wake transition disorders
- Rhythmic movement disorder (jactatio capitis)
- Sleep starts

Parasomnias usually associated with REM sleep
- Nightmares
- Sleep paralysis* (familial, isolated)
- REM sleep behavior disorder

Other parasomnias
- Sleep bruxism
- Sleep enuresis

* These conditions are all of central nervous system origin. *REM,* rapid eye movement. Derived from the International Classification of Sleep Disorders. (From Kelley, W. N. [1997]. *Textbook of internal medicine* [3rd ed.]. Philadelphia: Lippincott-Raven.)

logical disorders include anxiety, obsessive worrying, and depression.[2] A sleep log helps to document factors that may be causing the problem and it is critical to assess life situations, the taking of lengthy daytime naps, and drug use, especially the use of caffeine or alcohol.[25]

DISORDERS OF EXCESSIVE SOMNOLENCE

Disorders of excessive somnolence (DOES) are defined as the tendency to fall asleep when the individual becomes sedentary.[25] Excessive daytime sleepiness may indicate sleep apnea, central apnea, narcolepsy, or depression.

Sleep apnea may result from obstruction of the airway or changes in the pacemaker respiratory neurons in the brain stem.[12] There may be chronically reduced performance and inattention to the task. Individuals may cite blackouts, forgetfulness, poor concentration, and amnesia. *Obstructive apnea* occurs with progressive relaxation of the muscles of the chest, diaphragm, and throat causing airway obstruction for as long as 30 seconds.[43] The individual still attempts to breathe as the chest and abdomen continue to move. Each breath gets stronger until the obstruction is relieved. This condition most frequently occurs in the morbidly obese individual (see page 570). Defects in the brain's respiratory center that paces respiration are involved in *central apnea*. The impulse to breathe temporarily fails and air flow and chest wall movement cease. Central apnea may be the cause of crib death (sudden infant death syndrome or SIDS) in infants due to immaturity of the respiratory neurons. DOES may also be associated with head injury or brain tumors or lesions.

Narcolepsy is a condition in which the individual complains of excessive daytime sleepiness. There is also an abnormality in REM sleep.[31] During the day, the individual may suddenly fall asleep and REM sleep can occur within 15 minutes. Sleep attacks can occur at any time and may be due to brain stem dysfunction that involves failure of a waking mechanism to suppress the brain stem centers controlling REM sleep.

DISORDERS OF THE SLEEP–WAKE CYCLE

When people work the evening or night shift or travel by air across numerous times zones, the sleep–wake cycles are disrupted. Irregular patterns characterize the sleep, and frequently the sleep cycles are shortened. The inconsistent schedules result in "desynchronization" of body rhythms due to body rhythms adjusting at different rates to schedule changes. Internally it disrupts the timing of metabolic and behavioral activity in the body. Concentration is impaired, digestion is altered, and sleeping is difficult.[21] The problem then becomes chronic fatigue that occurs gradually and may result in feeling run down, depressed, and generally lacking in energy.

When the individual works the night shift, sleeping must be done during the daylight hours and the sleep pattern is disrupted. Due to days off, the circadian rhythms are almost never totally adapted to the new schedule. Individuals then become chronically sleep deprived. Sleep deprivation, like stressful events, has been linked with many diseases such as peptic ulcer disease, infections, allergies, and cancer.[12]

Jet lag syndrome results when several time zones are crossed while flying. The sleep fragmentation is due to disruption of internal circadian rhythms. The effect varies in different individuals. Research has shown that traveling west is better tolerated than eastward travel because the body adjusts more readily to lengthening its 24-hour period than to shortening it.[12]

DYSFUNCTIONS ASSOCIATED WITH SLEEP, SLEEP STAGES, OR PARTIAL AROUSALS

These dysfunctions are grouped under the term **parasomnias** and indicate a diverse group of sleep disturbances such as sleepwalking (somnambulism), night terrors, and bedwetting.[7] These conditions are occasional problems in adults and seem to occur mainly in stage II and IV sleep. Certain illness such as peptic ulcer disease and cardiovascular disease seem to be aggravated during the normal intense REM sleep periods. In these situations symptoms may occur during this time and arousal from sleep may result from chest pain or epigastric distress.[2]

FOCUS ON THE PERSON WITH A SLEEP DISORDER

J. L. is a 43-year-old former football player who has gained 150 lb since college football days. He comes to the clinic with a complaint of constant sleepiness and "nodding off" during any sedentary periods such as watching television or even at his desk at work. He weighs 385 lb with a large, protuberant abdomen. Vital signs are within normal limits, except that it is noted that accessory muscles are used in the breathing process. Mr. L.'s wife complains that he snores loudly, especially at night in bed, and awakens her with his restlessness.

Questions

1. What type of sleep disorder is probably occurring with Mr. L.? What clinical manifestations lead you to this diagnosis?
2. What are methods that could be used to diagnose this condition?
3. Explain the pathophysiology of the sleep disorder described. What alterations in the REM/non-REM pattern might be seen?
4. Compare this sleep disorder with others in the sleep disorder classification.

FOCUS ON THE PERSON WITH EXERCISE GOALS

J. J. is a healthy 22-year-old African-American woman who is just beginning an aerobic exercise program. She is 5′4″ tall and weighs 122 lb. Her exercise history is intermittent running and playing basketball. She states that she really wants to get serious because she hopes to become a world-class sprinter.

Questions

1. What changes within her body can Ms. J. expect in the initial stages of her exercise program?
2. What muscular factors must be present for the achievement of a goal of sprinting?
3. Outline the energy requirements for aerobic and anaerobic training.
4. Describe the adaptations that will occur with regular exercise.

REFERENCES

1. Adler, C., & Hillhouse, J. J. (1996). Stress, health, and immunity: A review of the literature. In T. W. Miller (Ed.), *Theory and assessment of stressful life events.* Madison, CT: International Universities Press.
2. Aldrich, M. S. (1994). Cardinal manifestations of sleep disorders. In M. H. Kryger, T. Roth, & W. C. Dement (Eds.), *Principles and practice of sleep medicine* (2nd ed.). Philadelphia: Saunders.
3. Astrand, P., & Rodahl, K. (1986). *Textbook of work physiology.* (3rd. ed.). New York: McGraw-Hill.
4. Berczi, I. (1997). The stress concept: An historical perspective of Hans Selye's contributions. In J. C. Buckingham, G. E. Gilles, & A. M. Cowell (Eds.), *Stress, stress hormones, and the immune system.* New York: Wiley.
5. Berne, R. M., & Levy, M. N. (1998). *Physiology* (4th ed.), St. Louis: Mosby.
6. Birrer, R. B. (Ed). (1994). *Sports medicine for the primary care physician* (2nd ed.). Boca Raton, FL: CRC Press.
7. Broughton, R. J. (1997). Approach to the patient with a sleep disorder. In W. N. Kelley (Ed.), *Textbook of internal medicine* (3rd ed.). Philadelphia: Lippincott-Raven.
8. Carskadon, M. A., & Dement, W. C. (1994). Normal human sleep: An overview. In M. H. Kryger, T. Roth, & W. C. Dement. *Principles and practice of sleep medicine* (2nd ed.). Philadelphia: Saunders.
9. Cooper, C. L. (1996). *Handbook of stress medicine and health.* Boca Raton, FL: CRC Press.
10. Cooper, C. L., & Payne, R. (1991). *Personality and stress: Individuals differences in the stress process.* New York: Wiley.
11. Cooper, C. L., & Watson, M. (1991). *Cancer and stress: Psychological, biological, and coping studies.* New York: Wiley.
12. Culebras, A. (1996). *Clinical handbook of sleep disorders.* Boston: Butterworth-Heineman.
13. De La Torre, B. (1994). Psychoendocrinologic mechanisms of life stress. *Stress Medicine, 10,* 107–114.
14. Fagard, R. H., & Tipton, C. M. (1994). Physical activity, fitness, and hypertension. In C. Bouchard, R. J. Shephard, & T. Stephens (Eds.), *Physical activity, fitness, and health: International proceedings and concensus statement.* Champaign, IL: Human Kinetics.
15. Froelicher, V. F. (1993). *Exercise and the heart* (3rd ed.). St. Louis: Mosby.
16. Glaser, R., & Kiecold-Glaser, J. (1994). *Handbook of stress and immunity.* San Diego: Academia Press.
17. Guyton, A. C., & Hall, J. E. (1996). *Textbook of medical physiology* (9th ed.). Philadelphia: Saunders.
18. Hafen, B. Q. (1996). *Mind/body health: The effects of attitudes, emotions, and relationships.* Boston: Allyn & Bacon.
19. Hubbard, J. R. (1992). *Behavior and immunity.* Boca Raton, FL: CRC Press.
20. Hubbard, J. R., & Workman, E. A. (1998). *Handbook of stress medicine: An organ system approach.* Boca Raton, FL: CRC Press.
21. Klein, M. (1991). *The shift worker's handbook.* Lincoln, NE: SynchroTech.
22. Lee, I, Rippe, J. M., & Wilkinson, W. J. (1995). How much exercise is enough? *Patient Care, 15,* 118–131.
23. Lewis, C. E. O'Sullivan, C., & Barraclough, B. (1994). *The psychoimmunology of cancer: Mind and body in the fight for survival.* New York: Oxford University Press.
24. Mader, S. L. (1998). *Human biology* (5th ed.). Boston: WCB McGraw-Hill.
25. Matheson, J. K. (1998). Sleep and its disorders. In J. Stein (Ed.), *Internal medicine* (5th ed.) St. Louis: Mosby.
26. Miller, T. W. (1997). *Clinical disorders and stressful life events.* Madison, CT: International Universities Press.
27. Montplaisir, J., & Godbout, R. (1990). *Sleep and biological rhythms: Basic mechanisms and applications to psychiatry.* New York: Oxford University Press.
28. Newsholme, E. A., & Parry-Billings, M. (1994). Effects of exercise on the immune system. In C. Bouchard, R. J. Shephard, & T. Stephens (Eds.), *Physical activity, fitness, and health: International proceedings and concensus statement.* Champaign, IL: Human Kinetics.
29. Rae, S. (1994). Bright light, big therapy. *Modern Maturity, 37,* 1.
30. Roitt, I., Brostoff, J., & Male, D. (1998). *Immunology* (5th ed.). St. Louis: Mosby.
31. Rozenzweig, M. R., & Leiman, A. I. (1989). *Physiological psychology* (2nd ed.) New York: Random House.
32. Rowell, L. B, & Dempsy, J. A. (1996). *Exercise regulation and integration of multiple systems.* New York: American Physiology Society by Oxford University Press.
33. Schneiderman, N., McCabe, P., & Baum, A. *Stress and disease processes.* Hillsdale, NJ: L. Erlbaum Associates.
34. Selye, H. (1956). *The stress of life.* New York: McGraw-Hill.
35. Shapiro, A. P. (1996). *Hypertension and stress.* Mahwah, NJ: Lawrence Erlbaum Associates.
36. Shephard, R. J., & Shek, D. N. (1995). Cancer, immune function, and physical activity. *Canadian Journal of Applied Physiology, 20*(3), 1–25.
37. Steele, K. D. (1994). Exercise physiology. In R. B. Birrer (Ed.), *Sports medicine for the primary care physician* (2nd ed.). Boca Raton, FL: CRC Press.
38. Tortora, G., & Grabowski, S. (1997). *Principles of anatomy and physiology* (8th ed.). New York: Harper Collins.
39. U.S. Department of Health and Human Services. (1996). *Physical activity and health: A report of the Surgeon General.* Atlanta, GA: U.S. Department of Health and Human Services, Centers for Disease Control and Prevention, National Center for Chronic Disease Prevention and Health Promotion.
40. von Bertalanffy, I. (1968). *General systems theory: Foundations, development and applications.* New York: Brazillier.
41. Weiner, H. (1992). *Perturbing the organism.* Chicago: University of Chicago Press.
42. Wilson, J. D. (1996). *Williams textbook of endocrinology* (9th ed.). Philadelphia: Saunders.
43. Zwillich, C. W. (1997). Diseases of ventilatory control. In W. N. Kelley (Ed.), *Textbook of internal medicine* (3rd. ed.). Philadelphia: Lippincott-Raven.

Chapter 6

Fluid, Electrolyte, and Acid–Base Balance

Martha Mulvey / Barbara L. Bullock

KEY TERMS

acid
acidosis
acidemia
alkalemia
alkalosis
anion gap acidosis
base
brawny edema
buffer
carbon dioxide narcosis
carpopedal spasm
hypercapnia
hypervolemia
hypocapnia
hypovolemia
Kussmaul's breathing
lymph
osmolality
osmotic pressure
paresthesias
pH
stasis dermatitis

Fluid, electrolyte, and acid–base balance is achieved through the complex cooperation of various systems of the body. Continual movement and exchange of water results in a regulated balance between plasma, interstitial fluid, and intracellular fluid. This chapter summarizes fluid, electrolyte, and acid–base balances that undergo many alterations in disease states. The basis provided here is further explored in the specific systems of the body.

NORMAL AND ALTERED FLUID BALANCE

Body fluids contain electrolytes and various amounts of protein in a large volume of water. Water, the main solvent of body fluids, is used in many metabolic processes of the body and carries waste products for excretion through the urine, skin, lungs, and feces. Water cushions, protects, lubricates, insulates, and provides structure for and resilience to the skin. An **electrolyte** is a substance that dissociates and forms ions when mixed with water; the process is called ionization. These ions are cations (positively charged electrolytes, such as sodium) and anions (negatively charged electrolytes, such as chloride). Ionic solutions readily conduct electric current, hence the term electrolyte.

The total input of water and electrolytes must be equal to the output to maintain proper balance. Water balance refers to an equilibrium maintained between intake and output of the solute.

Body Fluid Compartments

Total body fluid accounts for about 60% of body weight in the adult. This amount normally decreases with age and is affected by other components of body composition. The lean individual has a greater percentage of body water than the obese person because fat cells contain less water than muscle cells. Capillary and cell membranes separate total body fluids into two main compartments: the extracellular and intracellular. The intracellular fluid (ICF) contains different electrolytes than those present in the extracellular fluids (ECF). Approximately two-thirds of total body water is within cells of the ICF and one-third in the ECF (Fig. 6-1). The ECF is further divided into: (1) interstitial fluid (15%)—fluid located in the extravascular spaces between the cell tissues; (2) intravascular (5%)—plasma located within the vessels of the body; (3) transcellular fluid—cerebrospinal, intraocular, and gastrointestinal fluids that represent a small portion of the ECF; and (4) **lymph**—an alkaline fluid found in lymphatic vessels.

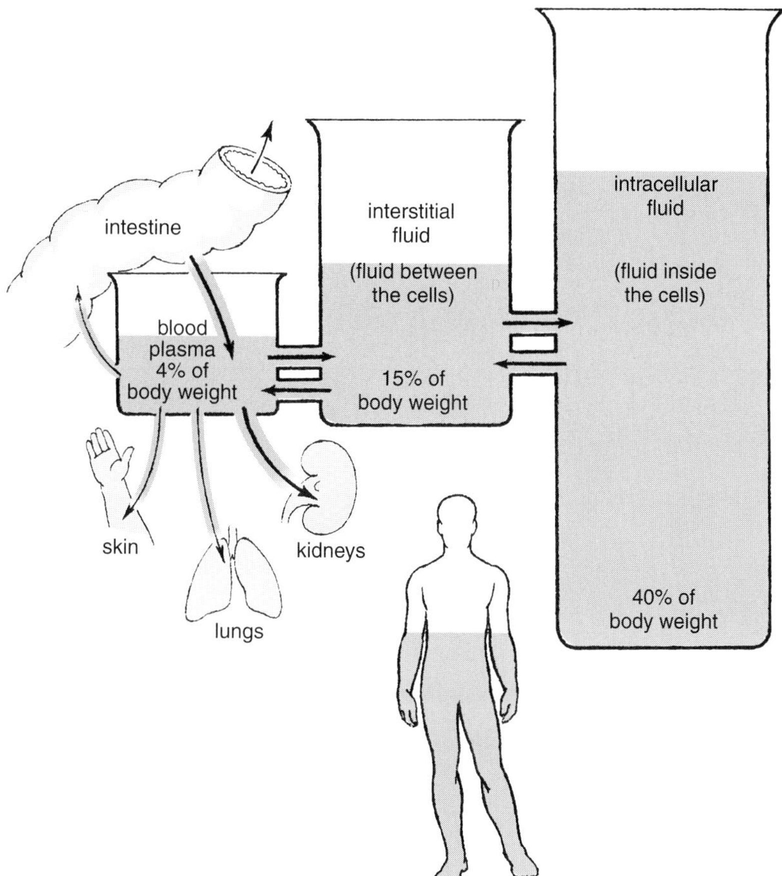

FIGURE 6-1. Main fluid compartments showing the relative percentage of body fluid in each.

Regulation of Body Fluid Balance

The volume and composition of body fluids must remain constant to support life. Water balance is maintained in equilibrium with electrolytes. The body regulates continual movement and exchange of water and electrolytes to compensate for wide variations in intake and output. Table 6-1 lists the normal laboratory values for the electrolytes and water. Unit 1, Appendix A lists laboratory values and their significance.

The amount of water intake necessary to maintain life in the adult is about 1,500 mL/m^2 of body surface area per day. Water intake, although intermittent, is usually higher than necessary, with an average total of 2,000 mL/day. Water is ingested in liquids and in foods and is also produced by oxidation of foodstuffs. It is directly conserved by the antidiuretic hormone (ADH) and indirectly conserved by aldosterone (see page 652). The kidneys, gastrointestinal tract, nervous system, and lungs, with input from the heart and glands, regulate the composition of the body fluids.

Intake of water must be balanced by output. The kidneys rid the body of excess water. Minimal renal function is 300 to 500 mL/24 h and is directly related to solute excretion of mostly urea, potassium, and sodium. The volume of urinary excretion can be increased tremendously, and usually totals approximately 1,500 mL/24 h. Water is also lost through the lungs (300 mL/24 h), skin (500 mL/24 h), and feces (200 mL/24 h). In the adult, body water gains and losses are balanced at a total of approximately 2,600 mL/24 h.

OSMOTIC FORCES IN WATER DISTRIBUTION

Osmotic forces are the principal determinant of water distribution in the body. Water accounts for the **osmotic pressure** in the tissues and cells of the body. Osmotic pressure is actually determined by the movement or draw of water through a selectively permeable membrane toward an area of greater solute concentration. To determine the osmotic pressure of a solute, the os-

TABLE 6-1

NORMAL LABORATORY VALUES FOR ELECTROLYTES AND WATER

WATER	
Serum osmolality	285–295 mOsm/kg of water 285–295 mmol/kg (SI units)
Urine osmolality	50–1,200 mOsm/kg of water 50–1,200 mmol/kg (SI units)
SODIUM	
Serum sodium	136–145 mEq/L 136–145 mmol/L (SI units)
Urine sodium	40–220 mEq/L/24 h 40–220 mmol/L/24 h (SI units)
POTASSIUM	
Serum Potassium	3.5–5.0 mEq/L 3.5–5.0 mmol/L (SI units)
Urine Potassium	25–120 mEq/L/24 h 25–120 mmol/L/24 h (SI units)
CALCIUM	
Serum Calcium	Total: 8.5–10.5 mg/dL 2.25–2.75 mmol/L (SI units) Ionized: 4.4–5.0 mg/dL 1.05–1.30 mmol/L (SI units)
Urine Calcium	100–300 mg/24 h 2.5–7.5 mmol/24 h (SI units)
PHOSPHATE	
Serum Phosphate	2.5–4.5 mg/dL, 1.7–2.6 mEq/L 0.78–1.52 mmol/L (SI units)
Urine Phosphate	0.9–1.3 g, 0.2–0.6 mEq/L
CHLORIDE	
Serum Chloride	95–108 mEq/L 98–106 mmol/L (SI units)
Urine Chloride	110–250 mEq/L 110–250 mmol/d (SI units)
MAGNESIUM	
Serum Magnesium	1.8–3.0 mg/dL, 1.5–2.5 mEq/L 0.65–1.05 mmol/L (SI units)
Urine Magnesium	6.0–10.0 mEq/24 h 3.0–5.0 mmol/24 h

molality of the solution must be determined. **Osmolality** is defined as the number of osmoles (Osm) of a substance contained within a kilogram of water; an osmole is the number of molecules in 1 g molecular weight of undissociated solute.[8] A solution with 1 Osm in each kilogram of water has an osmolality of 1 Osm/kg, and a solution with an osmolality of 1 milliosmole (mOsm) per kilogram contains 0.001 Osm/kg of solute.[8] Normal serum osmolality is 285 to 295 mOsm/kg (Box 6-1).

MOVEMENT OF FLUIDS AT THE CAPILLARY MEMBRANE

The capillaries are formed of endothelium, which is permeable to all of the solutes and water of the plasma. The endothelial layer is impermeable to the large molecules and cells in the plasma. Substances move through the gaps or spaces in the endothelial cells, and some substances, such as carbon dioxide, oxygen, and small solutes, move through the endothelial membrane as well. The process occurs by diffusion, so that near equilibrium exists at the capillary line: the amount of fluid leaving the capillary nearly equals the amount reabsorbed. This dynamic equilibrium is called *Starling's law of the capillaries* and it occurs mostly through a balance achieved between the hydrostatic pressure of the blood and the colloid osmotic pressure within the capillaries.[19]

Blood entering the capillary comes in at a *hydrostatic pressure* that is generated by the heart. This hydrostatic pressure varies in the different systemic arterioles, but it is always higher at the arteriolar end of the capillary than at the venous end (Fig. 6-2). As fluid filters out of the capillary into the tissue spaces, the hydrostatic pressure decreases. The high pressure exerted at the arteriolar end of the capillary is a simple *outward force*, or pushing force, which moves fluid from the vessel to the interstitial spaces. The hydrostatic pressure at the arteriolar end of the capillary averages 30 to 40 mm Hg, but drops to approximately 10 to 15 mm Hg at the venous end.[8] This hydrostatic pressure provides an outward force, enhanced by a negative interstitial pressure and the interstitial fluid colloid osmotic pressure (ISCOP), as shown in Figure 6-2. The ISCOP is minimal and is

BOX 6-1

SERUM OSMOLALITY

Serum Osmolality: The number of osmoles of a substance contained within a kilogram of water.
Normal value: 285–295 mOsm/kg
Calculated by the following formula:

$$\text{p Osm} = 2(\text{Na}) + \frac{\text{G}}{18} + \frac{\text{BUN}}{2.4}$$

$$(\text{serum osmolarity}) = 2 \times \text{serum sodium} + \frac{\text{serum glucose}}{18} + \frac{\text{serum urea nitrogen (BUN)}}{2.4}$$

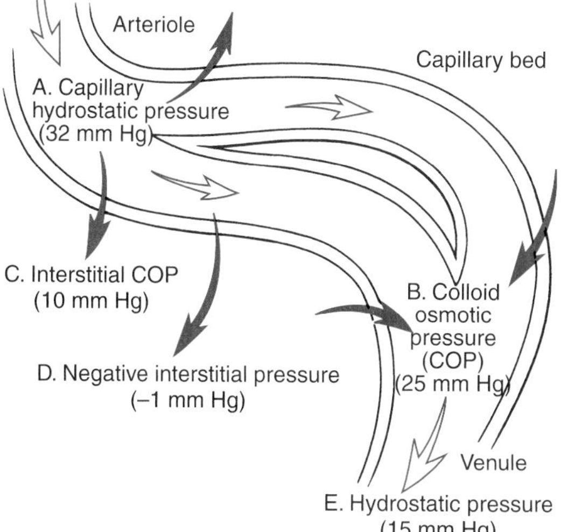

FIGURE 6-2. Fluid dynamics at the capillary line. **A.** Capillary hydrostatic pressure is higher at the arteriolar and tends to push fluid out. **B.** Colloid osmotic pressure (COP) generated by the plasma proteins maintains a constant inward pull or force. COP does not change across capillary. **C.** Interstitial COP is an outward force. **D.** Negative interstitial pressure is an outward force. **E.** Venular hydrostatic pressure is lower than the COP that is maintained in the vessel, which provides an inward force.

produced by a few plasma proteins that have escaped into the interstitial space.

The pressure exerted by the plasma proteins in the vessels, the *colloid osmotic* or *oncotic pressure* (*COP*), is an osmotic pulling or *inward force* that draws water toward it. Plasma proteins primarily exert their colloidal effect by drawing water back into the vessel. They remain in the vessel due to their larger size, which prohibits easy movement out of the vessel. The average COP is 28 mm Hg, a pressure that remains constant across the capillary. Although the amount of fluid filtered out of the vessel almost equals that reabsorbed, a larger amount is filtered into the tissue spaces than is reabsorbed. The small amounts of protein that escape into the tissue spaces during the process of fluid movement cannot be reabsorbed by the blood vessels. These excesses of fluid and protein are absorbed by the *lymphatic system* and returned through lymphatic channels to the blood. The lymphatic system carries away proteins and large matter from the tissue spaces directly into the blood capillaries.

The COP in the capillaries is mainly generated by albumin because it is the most abundant of the plasma proteins. Table 6-2 describes the concentrations and functions of major plasma proteins.

FLUID BALANCE IN BODY COMPARTMENTS

Fluids are maintained in strict volume and concentration in each of the three compartments: (1) extracellular intravascular (plasma); (2) extracellular extravascular (interstitial fluids); and (3) ICF. The relations of cations, anions, and volumes must be maintained rigidly to preserve life (Fig. 6-3). The composition of intracellular electrolytes is quite different from that of extracellular electrolytes, but the number of charges (cations and anions) is basically equal in the compartments (see page 5). The volume of fluid in the compartments is regulated by thirst, renal, and hormonal mechanisms.

Thirst

Thirst is regulated centrally but sensed peripherally as a dry mouth. It provides the primary protection against hyperosmolality. It is usually first expressed when the osmolality of plasma reaches about 295 mOsm/kg.[12] Osmoreceptors located in the thirst center in the hypothalamus are sensitive to changes in the osmolality of ECFs. As plasma osmolality increases,

TABLE 6-2

CONCENTRATION AND FUNCTION OF MAJOR PLASMA PROTEINS

PROTEINS	CONCENTRATION	FUNCTIONS
TOTAL PLASMA PROTEINS	6.0–8.0 g/dL	Synthesized by liver; maintain blood osmotic pressure; function in acid–base balance and coagulation; provide substrate for structure and energy and for transport of drugs and hormones.
ALBUMIN	3.2–4.5 g/dL (50–65% of total)	Most abundant; main protein in production of osmotic pressure; maintains blood volume; transports stored hormones; participates in binding drugs and in acid–base balance.
GLOBULIN	2.3–3.5 g/dL (30–45% of total)	Antibodies in form of immunoglobulins; provide for humoral immunity; transport iron, fats, and other substances.
FIBRINOGEN	150–400 mg/dL	Essential function in blood coagulation.

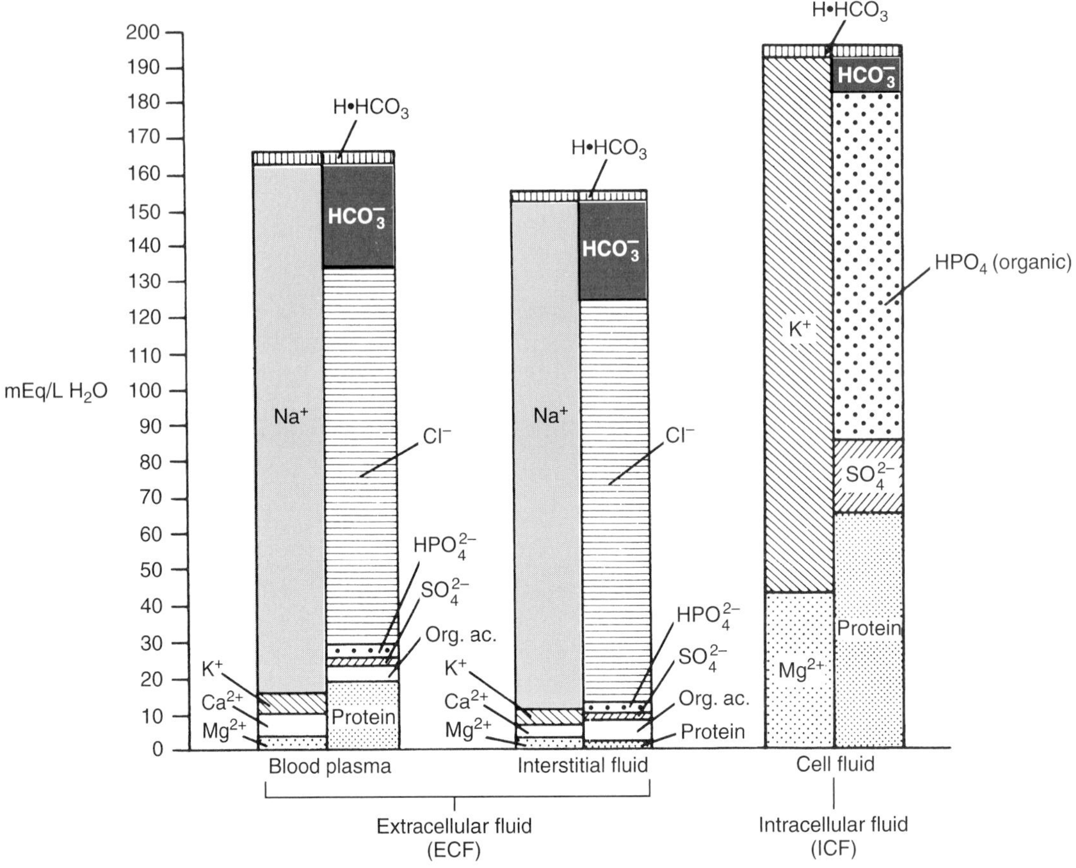

FIGURE 6-3. **Electrolyte composition of the body fluid compartments.**

the cells shrink and the sensation of thirst is experienced as a result of dehydration. This stimulates thirst through the following mechanisms:

1. Decreased renal perfusion stimulates the release of renin, which eventually leads to the production of angiotensin II (see page 450). Angiotensin II stimulates the hypothalamus to release neural substrates that are responsible for generating the sensation of thirst.[9]
2. Osmoreceptors in the hypothalamus detect elevations in osmotic pressure and activate nervous pathways that result in the thirst sensation.
3. Thirst may be induced by local dryness of the mouth in true hyperosmolar states, or it may occur to relieve the unpleasant dry sensation that results from reduced salivation.

Thirst sensation may be diminished or unrecognized in elderly and confused individuals and in individuals with decreased levels of consciousness, resulting in inadequate fluid consumption and dehydration. Generally, the thirst sensation prompts the individual to consume water, thereby correcting the hypovolemia or state of increased osmolality. After the thirst sensation has been satisfied, intake of fluid ceases.

Excessive intake of water that is unrelated to thirst usually has a psychogenic basis. Obsessive preoccupation with and indulgence in excessive water intake can lead to fluid volume overload, decreased serum osmolality, and decreased serum osmotic pressure.

Renal Regulation

The kidneys regulate the volume and electrolyte concentration of body fluids. ECF is filtered through the renal glomeruli. Selective reabsorption and excretion of water and solutes occurs in the renal tubules (see page 596). Glomerular filtration rate and renal perfusion, reflective of cardiac output, determine the rate of this process.

Hormone Regulation

Through highly complex interactions, a group of hormones regulate the fluid balance in the body. The functions of some of these hormones are described below but further detail is referred to other sections of the text.

ANTIDIURETIC HORMONE. Vasopressin or antidiuretic hormone (ADH) is formed in the hypothalamus and stored in the neurohypophysis of the posterior pituitary (see page 652). The area of ADH storage and release may overlap with the thirst center, which accounts for the integration of thirst and ADH release.[23] The major stimulus for ADH secretion is a change in sodium concentration. A few mOsm/L change of sodium will cause ADH to be released. Secretion may also occur with the stress of trauma, surgery, nausea, pain, and narcotics. The hormone increases reabsorption of water at the collecting ducts, collecting tubules, and distal tubules, thereby conserving water to correct the osmolality and restore the volume of ECF, forming a highly concentrated urine. ADH has a minor vasoconstrictive effect on the arterioles that can increase blood pressure.

ADRENOCORTICAL HORMONES. The adrenocortical hormones include aldosterone, the glucocorticoids, and a small amount of androgen hormone. Aldosterone and the glucocorticoids are active in maintaining fluid balance.

Aldosterone, a hormone secreted by the adrenal cortex, acts on the renal tubules to increase the sodium uptake. The increased sodium retention causes water retention. Aldosterone release is stimulated by changes in potassium concentration, by serum sodium concentrations, and by the renin–angiotensin system (see page 450). Normally, the rate or amount of aldosterone secretion is closely regulated by the potassium concentration, and the hormone is very effective in controlling hyperkalemia.[9]

The glucocorticoids, secreted by the adrenal cortex, exert a weak activity that promotes the reabsorption of sodium and water, which increases blood volume and causes sodium retention. This action accounts for some of the blood volume changes related to the glucocorticoids.

PROSTAGLANDINS. The prostaglandins are naturally occurring fatty acids present in many of the tissues of the body and function in the inflammatory response, blood pressure control, uterine contractions, and gastrointestinal motility. Prostaglandins antagonize ADH action by inhibiting the formation of cyclic adenosine monophosphate (AMP). Synthesis of prostaglandin, stimulated by ADH, decreases the ADH-induced cyclic AMP increase. The vasodilator action of prostaglandins increases medullary flow and thus decreases medullary hyperosmolality. These actions promote the excretion of less concentrated urine. In the kidneys, renal prostaglandins cause vasodilation and, in most cases, promote sodium excretion by inhibiting the response of the renal distal tubules to ADH. Prostaglandin-mediated renal vasodilation helps to protect the kidneys from ischemia when levels of vasoconstrictors, such as angiotensin II and norepinephrine, increase.[16] Sodium retention may result when endogenous prostaglandin production is decreased.

ATRIAL NATRIURETIC PEPTIDE. Atrial natriuretic peptide (ANP), also known as atrial natriuretic factor (ANF), was first identified in 1981. It is a peptide released from myocytes of the atria in response to increased atrial stretch. Although ANP is released on a continual basis in healthy persons, its release is accelerated by any condition that results in increased atrial stretch, especially fluid volume excess. ANP has been shown in laboratory studies to have the following effects:

1. Facilitates vasodilation and renal elimination of both water and sodium, which decreases blood volume
2. Improves glomerular filtration rate and hence increases sodium filtration by dilatation of the afferent and efferent arterioles[5,20]
3. Inhibits the reabsorption of sodium by the collecting ducts
4. Inhibits renin secretion by the juxtaglomerular apparatus, thereby preventing release of aldosterone from the adrenal cortex
5. Inhibits release of ADH[5,19]

Circulating levels of ANP have been shown to be elevated in congestive heart failure and in renal insufficiency.[19]

Edema

Edema is defined as a palpable swelling produced by expansion of the interstitial fluid volume. It may be localized or generalized, pitting or nonpitting, depending on its cause. Edema is usually thought of as accumulation of excess fluid in the skin; however, the mechanism causing skin edema also can cause fluid shifts in other vulnerable areas of the body. These fluid shifts are sometimes termed *third-space shifts* and include fluid shifts into the peritoneal area (ascites), pleural or pericardial effusions, and pulmonary edema.[13]

Table 6-3 summarizes the etiologic mechanisms that may lead to the formation of edema and fluid shifts. Essentially, the following two steps are involved in edema formation: (1) altered capillary hemodynamics that cause the movement of fluid from the vascular space into the interstitium; and (2) dietary sodium and water that are retained by the kidney. Edema cannot be clinically seen until the interstitial volume has increased to approximately 2 to 3 liters above normal.[1] The condition of edema requires a change in one or several of Starling's forces that features an increase in net filtration. The net rate of filtration out of the capillary is determined by the balance of capillary hydrostatic pressure, interstitial fluid hydrostatic pressure, plasma colloid osmotic pressure, and interstitial fluid colloid osmotic pressure.[1]

Four interrelated mechanisms are major causes of edematous states:

1. Decreased colloid osmotic pressure in the capillary
2. Increased capillary hydrostatic pressure
3. Increased capillary permeability
4. Lymphatic obstruction or increased interstitial colloid osmotic pressure

TABLE 6-3

ETIOLOGIC MECHANISMS FOR THE FORMATION OF EDEMA

ETIOLOGIC MECHANISMS	CAUSATIVE CONDITION
Increased capillary pressure	Congestive heart failure • Cor pulmonale • Right heart failure Local venous obstruction • Phlebothrombosis Pregnancy or premenstrual edema Drugs • Calcium channel blockers • Estrogens • Nonsteroidal anti-inflammatories • Fludrocortisone • Minoxidil Portal hypertension Renal failure Cushing's syndrome
Decreased colloid osmotic pressure	Liver failure Protein malnutrition Nephrosis Burns
Increased capillary permeability	Burns Allergic reactions Inflammation, sepsis Hypothyroidism Interleukin-2 therapy
Lymphatic obstruction	Surgical removal of lymph structures Inflammation or malignant involvement of lymph nodes and vessels. Filariasis

Some forms of edema result from more than one mechanism (Flowchart 6-1).

DECREASED COLLOID OSMOTIC PRESSURE

A decrease in plasma COP will increase the net filtration force and the net filtration rate of fluid into the tissues. If the plasma proteins are depleted in the blood, the inward forces are decreased, allowing the filtration effect to favor movement into the tissues. This leads to accumulation of fluid in the tissues with a decreased central volume of plasma. The kidneys respond to the decreased circulating volume by activating the renin–angiotensin system, which results in additional reabsorption of sodium and water. Intravascular volume increases temporarily. However, because the plasma protein deficit has not been corrected, the COP (the inward force) remains low in proportion to capillary hydrostatic pressure. Consequently, intravascular fluid moves into the tissues, worsening the edema and the circulatory status.

Hypoproteinemia causes decreased COP and may result from malnutrition, neoplastic wasting, liver failure, or protein loss through burns, kidneys, or the gastrointestinal tract. Albumin is the primary protein affected because it is the most abundant and also because its molecules are rather small and can pass through damaged capillary endothelium or glomeruli. When plasma protein levels are restored to normal, resolution of the edematous state will occur.

INCREASED CAPILLARY HYDROSTATIC PRESSURE

Increased capillary hydrostatic pressure changes the balance of forces toward the outward and promotes fluid remaining in the tissues. The most common cause of increased capillary pressure is congestive heart failure in which elevated systemic venous pressure is combined with increased blood volume.[20] The sodium and water retention of heart failure increases blood volume (see page 476).

Other causes of increased hydrostatic pressure include renal failure with increased total blood volume,

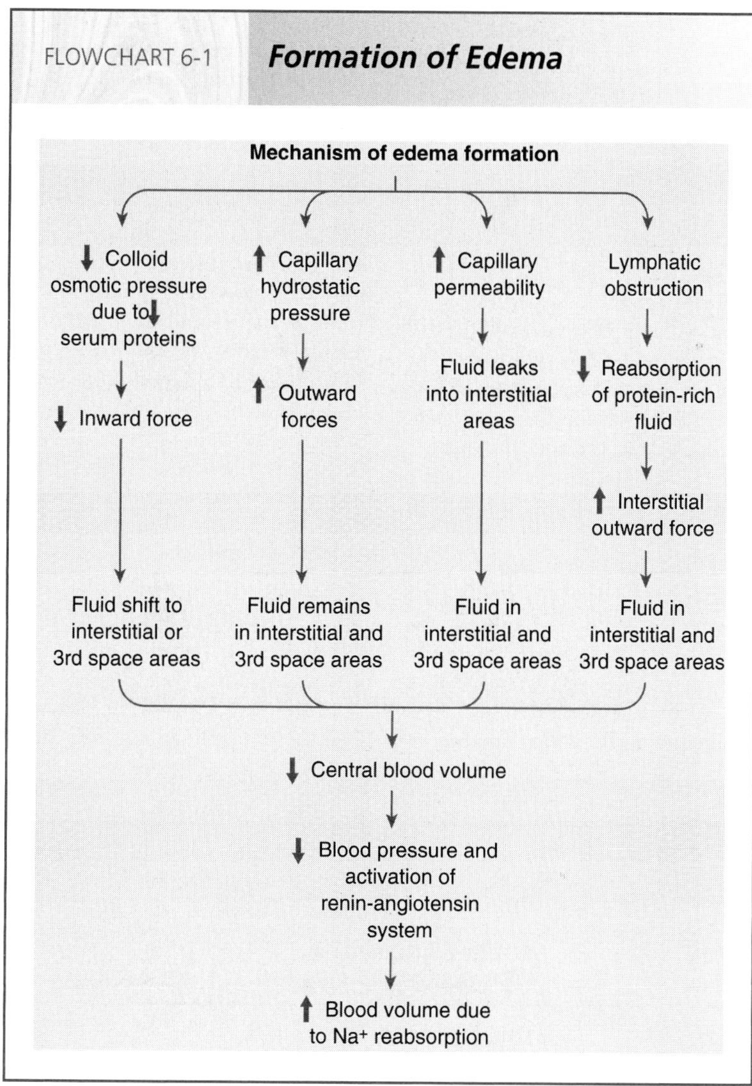

increased gravitational forces from standing for long periods of time, impaired venous circulation, and hepatic obstruction. Venous obstruction usually produces localized rather than generalized edema because only one vein or group of veins is affected.

INCREASED CAPILLARY PERMEABILITY

Direct damage to blood vessels, such as with trauma and burns, may cause increased permeability of the endothelial junctions. Localized edema may occur in response to an allergen, such as a bee sting. In certain individuals, this allergen may precipitate an anaphylactic response with widespread edema initiated by a histamine type of reaction. Inflammation causes hyperemia and vasodilatation, which lead to accumulation of fluids, proteins, and cells in an affected area (see page 254).

OBSTRUCTION OF THE LYMPHATICS

Lymphatic obstruction restricts the normal activity of the lymphatic system from removing the excess plasma proteins from the tissues and promotes the retention of fluid in the tissues. As proteins accumulate in the interstitial spaces, more water moves into the area. The most common cause of lymphatic obstruction is the surgical removal of a group of lymph nodes and vessels to prevent the spread of malignancy. Radiation therapy, trauma, malignant metastasis, and inflammation may also lead to localized lymphatic obstruction. *Filariasis*, a rare parasitic infection of the lymph vessels, can cause widespread obstruction of the vessels. The edema is usually localized.

MANIFESTATIONS OF EDEMA

The distribution of edema can give clues as to its cause. Venous or lymphatic obstruction is often localized in one extremity. Edema resulting from hypoproteinemia is generalized but is especially pronounced in the eyelids and face in the morning, due to the recumbent position assumed at night and the aid of gravitational forces. The edema of heart failure is usually greatest in the legs of an ambulatory individual, and it tends to accumulate throughout the day.[20]

Pitting edema refers to the displacement of interstitial water by finger pressure on the skin, which leaves a pitted depression. After the pressure is removed, it may take several minutes for the depression to be resolved. Pitting edema often appears in dependent sites, such as the sacrum of a bedridden individual. Similarly, gravitational hydrostatic pressure increases the accumulation of fluid in the legs and feet of an upright individual.

Nonpitting edema may be seen in areas of loose skin folds such as the periorbital spaces of the face. Nonpitting edema may occur after venous thrombosis, especially of the superficial veins. Persistent edema leads to trophic changes in the skin. These changes may progress to **stasis dermatitis** and ulcers that heal very slowly (see page 445). Nonpitting, **brawny edema** is also associated with thick, hardened skin and color changes that occur when serum proteins become trapped and coagulated in the tissue spaces.

Water Deficits and Excesses

Water and sodium imbalances usually occur together and are categorized as volume or osmolar imbalances. Volume, or isotonic, imbalances occur when sodium and water increase or decrease together in the same ratio that is normally found in the ECF spaces. Osmolar imbalances result when there is an alteration in the normal relation of water to solutes in the ECF space. The serum sodium level is the best indicator of the osmolality of blood because it is the most abundant solute in the vascular space.[15] When these imbalances occur, the manifested clinical picture is one of hypovolemia or hypervolemia.

HYPOVOLEMIA

Hypovolemia, or extracellular volume depletion, is an isotonic imbalance in which water and electrolytes are lost together in the same proportion as exists normally. The serum sodium level remains normal. Hypovolemia occurs if there is an abrupt decrease in intake of fluids or if the extracellular volume is decreased (Table 6-4).

TABLE 6-4

WATER IMBALANCES

NORMAL FUNCTION AND VALUE	SOURCE AND CAUSE OF IMBALANCE	CLINICAL MANIFESTATIONS
NORMAL FUNCTION • Removes waste products • Fluid medium for blood and tissues • Lubricate, insulates cushions, protects • Composes about 60% of body weight • Average intake 2,000 mL/d • Regulated by hormones, renal excretion, and intake.	HYPOVOLEMIA Extracellular fluid and volume depletion, may lead to intracellular loss *Etiologic factors* Dehydration, burns, hemorrhage, diarrhea, diaphoresis, vomiting, diabetes mellitus, ascites, draining wounds.	• Weight loss, tachycardia, • Thirst, dry mucous membranes • Poor skin turgor • Orthostatic hypotension • Hemoconcentration; increased hematocrit, altered BUN/serum creatinine • Increased urine specific gravity • Altered level of consciousness • Jugular veins flat, decreased CVP
NORMAL VALUE 285–295 mOm/kg Gain and loss usually equal due to thirst and replenishment and renal excretion. Increased intake leads to decreased thirst and increased urine output; decreased intake leads to thirst, decreased urine output, activation of compensatory mechanisms	HYPERVOLEMIA Extracellular fluid volume excess *Etiologic factors* May be iatrogenic (excess administration of isotonic solutions), hyperaldosteronism, congestive heart failure, renal and liver failure.	• Rapid weight gain • Ascites • Urine osmolality and decreased urine sodium • Increased CVP • Decreased hematocrit and serum proteins • Dyspnea • Hypertension

BUN, blood urea nitrogen; CVP, central venous pressure

Hypovolemia results in a decrease in the size of the extracellular space and circulatory collapse, which eventually depletes cellular fluid. Signs and symptoms of hypovolemia are related to the cause of the imbalance. In gradual fluid volume loss, the volume depletion is quite advanced by the time symptoms are manifest, owing to the fact that interstitial fluid moves to the intravascular spaces to maintain circulation. Mechanisms to compensate for hypovolemia include increased sympathetic nervous system stimulation, thirst, and release of ADH and aldosterone.

HYPERVOLEMIA

Hypervolemia, or extracellular volume excess, is an isotonic imbalance in which water and electrolytes are gained together in the same proportion as exists normally in the ECF. The serum sodium level remains normal. Hypervolemia may result from any condition that can cause excess ECF volume (see Table 6-4). Hypervolemia results in expansion of the extracellular space and circulatory overload. Signs and symptoms reflect the overload. To compensate for hypervolemia, ANP is released to promote diuresis and release of aldosterone and ADH is suppressed.

NORMAL AND ALTERED ELECTROLYTE BALANCE

The serum electrolytes are intricately involved with the body fluid balance as well as many electrical and chemical reactions of the body. The major electrolytes are presented in this section as to normal function and effect of alterations of balance.

Sodium

Sodium is the major osmotically active cation of the ECF. It regulates the osmotic pressure of the ECF and markedly affects the osmotic pressure of ICF. Sodium intake comes from the diet; requirements for body needs vary according to age and size with younger and larger individuals requiring a greater intake (from 500–2,700 mg/day). The average daily intake in the United States is 2.3 to 6.9 g.[25] Table 6-5 lists normal

TABLE 6-5

SODIUM IMBALANCES

NORMAL FUNCTION AND VALUES	SOURCE AND CAUSE OF IMBALANCE	CLINICAL MANIFESTATIONS
NORMAL FUNCTION • Regulates serum osmolality, by maintaining osmotic pressure • Close interaction between sodium and water balances • Essential in neuromuscular excitability • Regulates aspects of acid–base balance • Absorption regulated partly by aldosterone NORMAL VALUE 135–145 mEq/L Intake in diet, excess excreted in body fluids.	HYPONATREMIA* <130 m Eq/L *Etiologic factors* • Congestive heart failure • Excess hypotonic fluid administration. • syndrome of inappropriate ADH (may be due to drug therapy) • Diuretic therapy • Burns • Psychogenic polydypsia • Diaphoresis with water replacement • Adrenal insufficiency	• Causes cell swelling from decreased ECF osmolality • Cerebral edema leads to headache, stupor, coma • Peripheral and pulmonary edema • Decreased thirst • Nausea and vomiting • Muscular weakness
	HYPERNATREMIA >145 mEq /L *Etiologic factors* • Decreased ADH secretion • Excess Na^+ administration • Increased aldosterone • Impaired thirst, profuse diaphoresis • Water deprivation	• Thirst, nausea and vomiting • Cell shrinking from increased ECF osmolality leads to central nervous system irritability • Hypotension, oliguria, anuria

*Underlying mechanisms for hyponatremia and hypernatremia vary. It is important to diagnose the cause before administering treatment.

functions of sodium, as well as causes and clinical manifestations of imbalances.

HYPONATREMIA

Deficits of serum sodium are caused either from actual loss of sodium from body fluids or from excessive gains in extracellular water. The cells become swollen as water moves from ECF to ICF to compensate for the solute deficit (Fig. 6-4). Hyponatremic disorders are commonly classified as *isotonic, hypertonic,* and *hypotonic* states, depending on the serum osmolality. Normal serum osmolality is measured at 285 to 295 mOsm/L and reflects the ionic concentration of substances in the plasma. It especially reflects concentrations of sodium but can indicate increased amounts of glucose or other solutes. In hyponatremia, it is essential to recognize whether the problem is hypovolemic or hypervolemic because the treatment could be lifesaving or life threatening to the affected individual.

Isotonic Hyponatremia

This imbalance occurs with the infusion of isotonic solutions (such as dextrose 5% in water and mannitol) that are sodium free causing a decreased Na^+ in the ECF. The hyponatremia is gradually transformed from isotonic to hypotonic hyponatremia as the glucose in the isotonic solutions is oxidized and the glucose concentration decreases.[5,16]

Hypertonic Hyponatremia

The hypertonic form occurs with very high glucose states or administration of high doses of mannitol, which pull water from the cells. High glucose states are seen in diabetes mellitus. If the initial volume is normal, each 100 mg/dL increase of blood glucose decreases the serum sodium by 1.6 mEq/L.[15,19] Hypertonicity due to mannitol may occur when the drug is being administered for increased intracranial pressure.

Hypotonic Hyponatremia

The term hypotonic hyponatremia refers to a hypo-osmolar plasma associated with decreased serum sodium. The degree of hyponatremia may not reflect total body sodium. An example is hypervolemic hypotonic hyponatremia, which, as its name implies, refers to water intoxication such as can occur with an excess secretion of ADH (the syndrome of inappropriate ADH secretion). This hyponatremic individual has clinical manifestations of weight gain, edema, hypoalbuminemia, hypertension, and, sometimes, increased intracranial pressure.[16] The hypervolemic individual may have *dilutional hyponatremia,* which means that water has been reabsorbed in excess proportion to sodium.

Hypovolemic Hyponatremia

In this condition, blood volume is lost through external loss of sodium and water. The person with hypovolemic hyponatremic clinical syndrome may show signs of dehydration with a decreased urine output and signs of vascular collapse. This clinical condition may be treated with intravenous saline to correct the sodium deficit.

HYPERNATREMIA

Serum sodium excess results from decreased intake or increased output of water. Hypernatremia causes intracellular dehydration (because the fluid shifts to the serum to dilute the excess sodium) and extracellular dehydration occurs due to water loss. High osmolality is a result of hypernatremia and water moves from the ICF to the ECF to compensate for the solute excess (see Fig. 6-4). As hypernatremia develops, thirst and release of ADH are stimulated.[15] As serum sodium levels increase, water is drawn from the cells into the plasma, causing cerebral dehydration. Clinically, this leads to irritability, lethargy, weakness, convulsions, coma, and death. The clinical manifestations of the underlying condition are also manifested.

As with hyponatremic states, the underlying mechanism for the disorder may vary. Because volume and sodium are highly interactive, the classifications include hypervolemia, hypovolemia, and isovolemic hypernatremias.

FOCUS ON CELLULAR PATHOPHYSIOLOGY

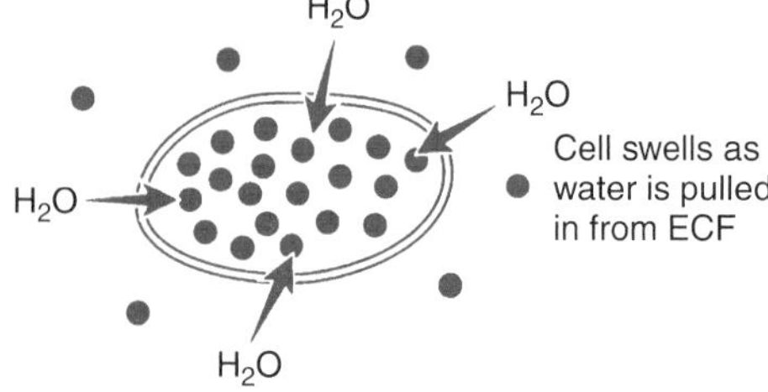

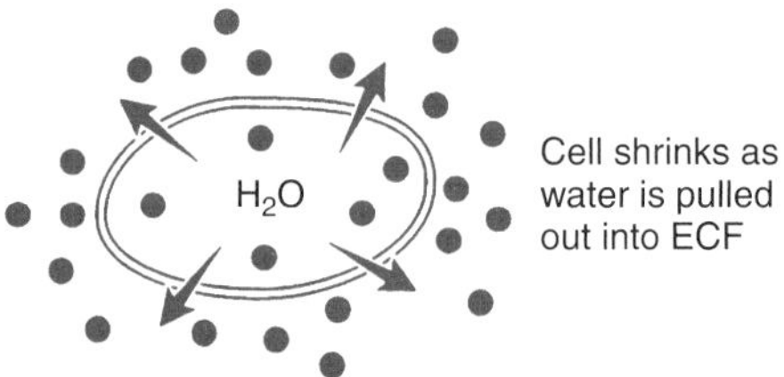

FIGURE 6-4. Effect of extracellular sodium level on cell size. (Metheny, N. M. [1996]. *Fluid and electrolyte balance* [3rd ed.] Philadelphia: Lippincott.)

Hypervolemic Hypernatremia

This type of hypernatremia is often iatrogenic, resulting from use of intravenous sodium bicarbonate or giving isotonic saline without free water to replace hypotonic insensible loss.[15] Diuretic therapy without fluid replacement also may cause edematous hypernatremia.

Hypovolemic Hypernatremia

Loss of hypotonic solutions through the kidney, skin, gastrointestinal, and respiratory tracts may lead to hypovolemic hypernatremia. Peritoneal dialysis may increase the serum sodium by removing hypotonic fluid.

Isovolemic Hypernatremia

Loss of water through the kidney or skin may be caused by failure to synthesize ADH or from failure of the kidney to respond to ADH. The isovolemia is due to increased thirst and volume intake. Failure to synthesize ADH by the hypothalamus is termed *central diabetes insipidus* and causes massive amounts of dilute urine output (see page 677). The nephrogenic type may be acquired structural renal damage or congenital disorders of renal responsiveness to ADH.[15]

Potassium

Potassium is the primary intracellular cation. It directly affects the excitability of nerves and muscles and contributes to the intracellular osmotic pressure (Table 6-6). Secretions and excretions contain large amounts of potassium. The source of potassium is the diet, which normally provides much more than is needed by the body. Urine potassium concentration varies, providing an efficient mechanism for the excretion of excess potassium to maintain the narrow range of normal serum concentrations.

Potassium moves into the cell during the formation of new tissues, the anabolic phase. During tissue breakdown, the catabolic phase, potassium leaves the cell. Potassium does not move into cells if there is a deficit of oxygen, glucose, or insulin.

The human body very effectively excretes potassium but has little mechanism for renal conservation. Potassium deficit occurs in 2 to 3 days if there is no intake.[22] The major route for the loss of potassium is the kidneys, but some loss can occur through gastrointestinal secretions or the skin. In the kidneys, the excretion of potas-

TABLE 6-6

POTASSIUM IMBALANCES

NORMAL FUNCTION AND VALUES	SOURCE AND CAUSE OF IMBALANCE	CLINICAL MANIFESTATIONS
NORMAL FUNCTION • Major intracellular cation; 98% in ICF • Influences skeletal and cardiac muscle activity; neuromuscular excitability • Important in acid–base balances, especially in ICF NORMAL VALUE • 3.5–5mEq/L • Supplied by diet. Average 50–100 mEq/d • Excreted mainly by kidney about 40 mEq/day; lost also in sweat and stool • Regulated by aldosterone; altered by acid–base imbalances.	HYPOKALEMIA <3.5 mEq/L *Etiologic factors* • Renal wasting (nephrosis) • Gastrointestinal loss • Metabolic alkalosis, • K^+ depleting diuretics, other drugs, (eg, amphotericin) • Profuse diaphoresis • Elevated glucocorticoid levels (Cushing's disease) • Laxative abuse • Lack of intake • Hyperaldosteronism	• Muscle cramping • Fatigue, weakness • Cardiac irritability, dysrhythmias • Paralytic ileus • Vomiting • Decreased concentration of urine • Respiratory muscle weakness • Increased sensitivity to digitalis • Hypotension
	HYPERKALEMIA >5mEq/L *Etiologic factors* • Renal failure • Excessive administration of K^+-conserving diuretics • Hypoaldosteronism • Metabolic acidosis • Hemolysis of red blood cells • Drugs (ie, β-adrenergic blockers, digitalis toxicity)	• Cardiac depression, dysrhythmias, cardiac arrest • Muscle weakness, paralysis • Paresthesias of face, feet, and hands • No central nervous system effects • Rarely occurs without renal dysfunction • Nausea, intestinal colic, diarrhea

sium is under the control of aldosterone at the distal tubules. At this point, hydrogen, potassium, and sodium tend to compete with each other for excretion. Sodium is usually preferred for absorption in the presence of aldosterone. If the plasma hydrogen ion concentration is elevated above normal, the tubules preferentially tend to excrete hydrogen and conserve potassium, which leads to the hyperkalemia often seen in association with acidosis. The reverse is true in alkalosis: If the hydrogen concentration is low, potassium is preferentially excreted and hydrogen is conserved, thus causing the hypokalemia associated with alkalosis (see page 181).

HYPOKALEMIA

A serum deficit of potassium affects every system (see Table 6-6). In the gastrointestinal system, anorexia, nausea, vomiting, and paralytic ileus may occur. In the muscles, flaccidity and weakness may be exhibited and may lead to respiratory muscle weakness and arrest. Cardiac dysrhythmias are common due to membrane excitability and the electrocardiogram (ECG) may show conduction blocks, paroxysmal atrial tachycardia, and increased the amplitude of the U wave (Fig. 6-5). Ventricular tachycardia and ventricular fibrillation (due to enhanced automaticity) may occur if the levels are very

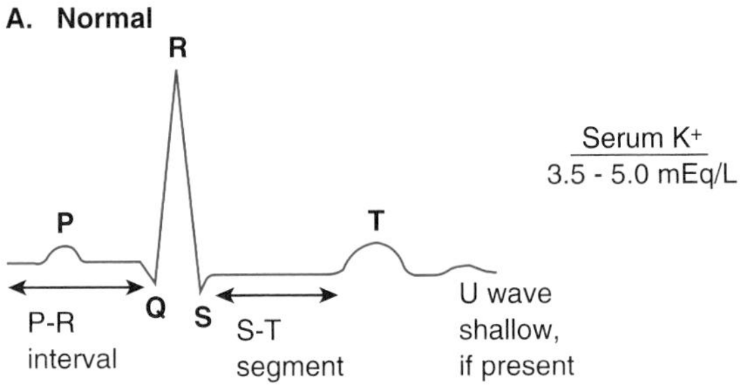

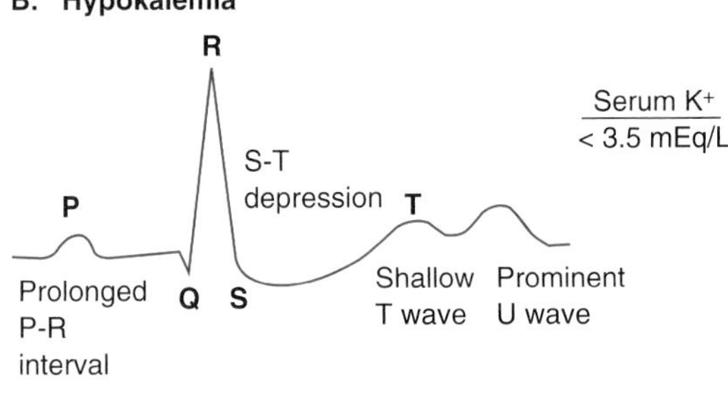

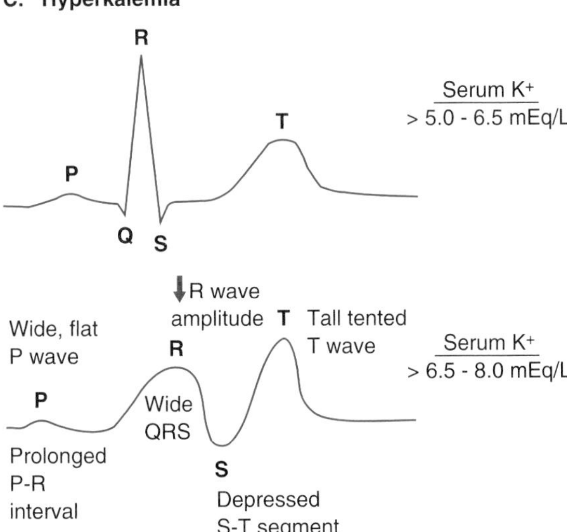

FIGURE 6-5. ECG changes with potassium imbalance. **A.** Normal ECG for Lead II. **B.** ECG for hypokalemia. **C.** ECG for hyperkalemia. At levels of 5.0 to 6.5 mEq/L; T wave increases in amplitude; P wave flattens. At levels of >6.5 mEq/L: P wave flattened; QRS wide; T wave, tall tented.

low. Central nervous system (CNS) depression and decreased deep tendon reflexes also may be noted. Hypokalemia causes decreased ability of renal tubules to concentrate waste, leading to increased water loss.

HYPERKALEMIA

Excess potassium is usually secondary to temporary or permanent kidney dysfunction (see Table 6-6). Hyperkalemia mainly affects the cardiovascular system. A decreased membrane potential causes a decrease in the intensity of the action potential, resulting in a dilated, flaccid heart. Various kinds of conduction defects may be noted together with ectopic dysrhythmia. The ECG shows a shortened PR interval, tall peaked T waves, a short QT interval, and widening of the QRS complex (see Fig. 6-5). In the gastrointestinal system, nausea, vomiting, and diarrhea are common. Initial irritability of the skeletal muscles gives way to weakness and flaccid paralysis. Digital numbness and tingling may be described.

Calcium

Calcium is combined with phosphorus to form mineral salts of bones and teeth. Ninety-nine percent is in the bones and teeth in the crystalline form, which gives hardness to these structures. Of the 1% that is circulating, approximately 45% is bound to plasma proteins, especially albumin. If its value is normal, 50% of the calcium is in the free ionized form and 5% is complexed to ions such as citrate and sulfate.[1] The ionized form of calcium is active calcium, which functions in membrane integrity, coagulation, and muscle contraction, and in the electrophysiology of the excitable cells (Table 6-7). Calcium stabilizes the cell membrane and blocks sodium transport into the cell. Its function is critical in cell excitability. Ionized calcium can be released from its bound form or bound from its ionized

TABLE 6-7

CALCIUM IMBALANCES

NORMAL FUNCTION AND VALUES	SOURCE AND CAUSE OF IMBALANCE	CLINICAL MANIFESTATIONS
NORMAL FUNCTION • Calcium, combined with phosphate, is stored in skeleton and teeth (99%). • Of 1% in blood and tissues, 50% is *ionized* and controls muscular contraction, cardiac function, nerve impulses and blood clotting; 5% is complexed to citrate and sulfate; 45% is *nonionized,* bound to serum proteins • Regulated by parathyroid hormone, calcitonin, and activated vitamin D • Absorbed mainly from small intestine and excreted in urine and feces	HYPOCALCEMIA <8.5 mg/dL *Etiologic factors* • Hypoparathyroidism • Acute pancreatitis • Inadequate vitamin D or calcium in diet • Hypoalbuminemia • Transfusion of citrated blood • Hyperphosphatemia, hypomagnesemia • Malabsorption syndrome • Alcohol abuse • Septicemia • Drugs; loop diuretics, anticonvulsants, calcitonin, gentamycin	• Increased neuromuscular excitability. • Trousseau and Chvostek signs, tetany, laryngospasm • Skeletal muscle cramps, seizures, intestinal cramping, diarrhea • Cardiac changes—ECG prolonged ST and QT intervals; congestive heart failure • Dry skin, brittle nails, dry hair • Cataracts
NORMAL VALUE • 9.0–10 mg/dL • In acidosis, ionized Ca^{++} rises due to loss from protein. • In alkalosis, levels are lowered due to protein gain.	HYPERCALCEMIA >10.5 mg/dL • Immobility • Hyperparathyroidism • Blood or bone malignancies • Renal insufficiency • Drugs: diuretics, chemotherapy, androgens, estrogen, lithium, theophylline	• Decreased neuromuscular excitability; muscle weakness, flaccidity • Renal failure, stones • CNS depression, stupor, coma • Constipation, anorexia, nausea and vomiting • Peptic ulcer disease with increased gastric acid secretion • Bone loss—may increase fracture risk • Cardiac changes—ECG short QT, bradycardia, heart block

form, depending on the serum pH. The reaction, simply stated, is a reversible equation:

$$Ca^{++} (\text{protein-bound} + H^{+}) \leftrightarrow Ca^{++} (\text{ionized}) + H^{++} (\text{protein complex})$$

The reaction is driven toward the right in acidosis, causing an increase in ionized serum calcium. In alkalosis, the reaction is driven more toward the left, which can cause hypocalcemia.[1] This is the method used by the body plasma proteins to buffer hydrogen ion (see page 181).

Calcium concentration in the blood is under the influence of *parathyroid hormone* (PTH) and *calcitonin.* PTH is released by the parathyroid glands when the extracellular level of ionized calcium is decreased. Calcitonin is released by the thyroid gland when serum calcium levels are increased and this inhibits calcium release from bone.

Vitamin D affects calcium absorption as well as bone deposition and reabsorption. Vitamin D is produced in the skin through the action of ultraviolet light and is present also in most American diets. It is changed by the liver to 25-hydroxycholecalciferol by hydroxylation and is further metabolized by the kidneys with the aid of PTH to form the most active type, 1,25-dihydroxycholecalciferol (see page 657). This substance is important in enhancing calcium uptake from the gastrointestinal tract and stimulating osteoclast activity in bone reabsorption.[8,14]

Phosphate is an anion that is also regulated by PTH and activated vitamin D. Normally, the aggregate concentration of calcium and phosphate is constant; if the calcium level increases, the phosphate level decreases. Calcium joins with phosphate to form calcium phosphate ($CaHPO_4$). If an excessive amount of $CaHPO_4$ is formed, it is not ionizable, and clinical hypocalcemia results.

Serum calcium values are affected by the serum albumin level and must be corrected when the level is abnormal. Box 6-2 shows the formula used to calculate the corrected serum calcium.

HYPOCALCEMIA

If calcium levels decrease, the blocking effect of calcium on sodium also decreases. As a result, depolarization of excitable cells occurs more readily as sodium moves in. Therefore, if the calcium levels are low, increased CNS excitability and muscle spasms occur (see Table 6-7). The results of hypocalcemia are spasms and tetany, seizures, increased gastrointestinal motility, cardiovascular problems, and osteoporosis. Muscle tetany is both common and dangerous, especially if it involves laryngeal spasm.[2] The Trousseau sign and Chvostek sign, illustrated in Figure 6-6, are clinical signs. Cardiac problems include decreased cardiac contractility and, occasionally, symptoms of heart failure. The cardiac action potential changes are seen on the ECG by prolongation of the ST segment and resultant QT interval prolongation (Fig. 6-7).[20]

HYPERCALCEMIA

Excessive levels of calcium increase the blocking effect on sodium in the skeletal muscles. This leads to decreased excitability of both muscles and nerves, eventually contributing to flaccidity (see Table 6-7). Cardiac effects include shortening of the QT interval on the ECG with virtually no ST segment (see Fig. 6-7).[17]

Phosphate

Phosphate functions with calcium to support bone formation. Most phosphate comes from dietary intake of dairy products, meat, and eggs.[26] Phosphate is the primary intracellular anion. It assists with energy transfer within the cells.[13] It is integral to the function of muscle and red blood cells (RBCs), the formation of ATP and 2,3-diphosphoglycerate (2,3-DPG), and the maintenance of acid–base balance. About 85% of body phosphate is found in the bones, and the remaining 15% is intracellular.[26] Phosphate balance is achieved by renal excretion; this process is influenced by PTH, which decreases absorption of phosphate. About 10% of plasma phosphate is protein bound. Plasma phosphate promotes acid–base balance of the

BOX 6-2

CALCULATING THE CORRECTED SERUM CALCIUM

The total serum calcium level (mg/dL) + 0.8 × (4.0 – measured albumin level in g/dL) = corrected total calcium concentration (mg/dL)

EXAMPLE: Serum albumin of 2.0 g/dL and the reported serum calcium level is 10 mg/dL.

1. The decrease in serum albumin level from normal level (difference from normal albumin of 4 g/dL) is calculated. 4 g/dL – 2 g/dL = 2 g/dL
2. The following ratio is calculated:
   0.8 mg/dL: 1 g/dL = ? mg/dL: 0.8 mg × 2
3. Calculated answer is 1.6 mg/dL
4. Corrected total serum calcium level is 10 mg/dL + 1.6 mg/dL = 11.6 mg/dL

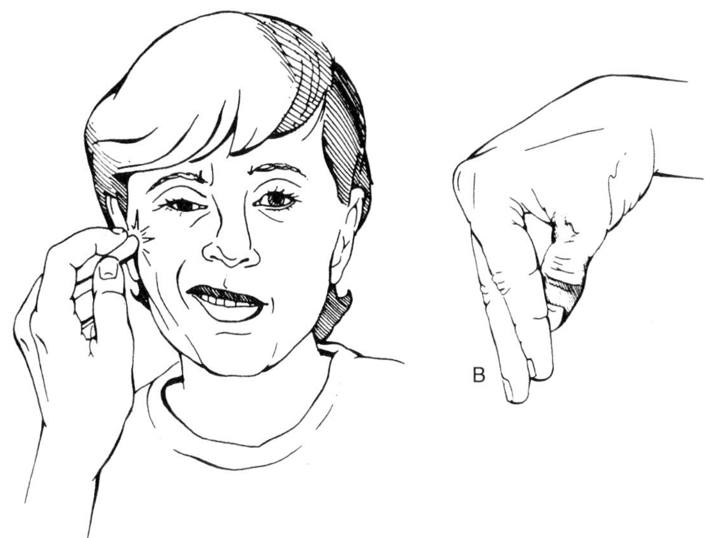

FIGURE 6-6. **A.** Chvostek's sign: a contraction of facial muscles elicited in response to a light tap over facial nerve in front of ear. **B.** Trousseau's sign: a carpopedal spasm induced by inflating a blood pressure cuff above systolic pressure.

body by acting as a buffer in the ECF. Phosphate also participates in the metabolism of glucose, fats, and proteins (Table 6-8).

HYPOPHOSPHATEMIA

Hypophosphatemia occurs through three mechanisms: decreased intestinal absorption, enhanced urinary excretion, and enhanced uptake to bone (see Table 6-8). Severe depletion can lead to abnormal formation of bone, along with skeletal, cardiac, and respiratory muscle weakness. Depletion of phosphate reduces levels of 2,3-DPG and ATP in the RBC resulting in tissue hypoxia.[1,16]

HYPERPHOSPHATEMIA

Hyperphosphatemia is often followed by a fall in plasma calcium with precipitation of calcium into the soft tissues when the plasma phosphate increases to 6 mg/dL or higher. An increased formation of $CaHPO_4$ complexes causes the clinical manifestations of hypocalcemia. It rarely occurs in the presence of normal renal function but has been described in other conditions (see Table 6-8).

Chloride

The chloride ion is the major anion of ECF (Table 6-9). The amount of chloride in the fluid closely parallels the sodium content and together they determine osmotic pressure. Bicarbonate has an inverse relationship to chloride so that when chloride moves from plasma into the RBC, bicarbonate will move back into plasma. Hydrogen ions are then formed to help release oxygen from hemoglobin (see page 344).

Chloride is a component of hydrochloric acid in the stomach. It also serves an essential role in the transport of excess carbon dioxide by RBCs (see page 346). Chloride moves into the cells by passive transport.

HYPOCHLOREMIA

Chloride depletion is seen with a variety of conditions (see Table 6-9). Metabolic alkalosis results as bicarbonate is conserved to maintain cation–anion balance. The clinical manifestations of hypochloremia are usually related to the associated metabolic alkalosis (see page 185). They also may reflect signs of hyponatremia.

HYPERCHLOREMIA

Excess serum chloride is often associated with hypernatremia, but may result from certain medications and metabolic acidosis (see Table 6-9). Hyperchloremic metabolic acidosis is common in dehydration and can lead to weakness, lethargy, and Kussmaul breathing (see page 183).

Magnesium

Magnesium is found mostly within the cells and in the bones (Table 6-10). This cation activates a number of intracellular enzyme systems and is required for protein and nucleic acid synthesis. All ATPases require magnesium for activation. Magnesium affects muscle directly by decreasing acetylcholine release at the neuromuscular junction and sympathetic ganglia, eliciting a curare-like effect. This effect can be augmented by hypercalcemia or concurrent administration of potassium. Magnesium is particularly essential in promoting neuromuscular integrity and cardiovascular function.[7] About one-third of magnesium is bound to protein and levels should be evaluated in combination with albumin levels. Magnesium is mainly regulated by renal excretion. Most magnesium is reabsorbed, but

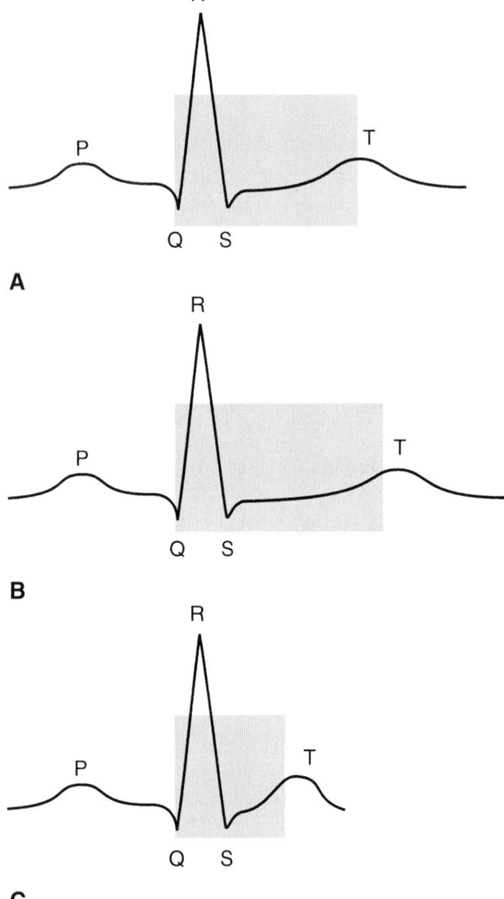

FIGURE 6-7. **A.** Normal electrocardiogram tracing. **B.** Prolongation of the QT interval in hypocalcemia may increase risk of dysrhythmias or heart block and may be associated with poor contractility. **C.** Shortening of QT in hypercalcemia may cause severe dysrhythmias that may result from increased cardiac irritability.

hypernatremia and hypercalcemia can decrease its reabsorption.[21]

HYPOMAGNESEMIA

Causes of decreased serum magnesium are listed in Table 6-10. The clinical manifestations include life-threatening cardiovascular dysrhythmias (ventricular fibrillation), increased neuromuscular irritability, paresthesias, tetany, and convulsions. The clinical signs and symptoms may be caused by refractory hypocalcemia or hypokalemia, and they respond only to magnesium therapy.[11] Hypokalemia is common in association with hypomagnesemia owing to increased renal excretion of potassium when the magnesium level is low.

HYPERMAGNESEMIA

This condition is rare but may be seen in renal failure or administration of toxic doses of magnesium (see Table 6-10). Clinical manifestations begin at a level of 4 mEq/L or greater and include lethargy, coma, cardiac dysrhythmias (sinoatrial and atrioventricular heart block), respiratory failure, and death. Because dialysis in persons with chronic renal failure does not remove magnesium well, these individuals should be restricted from ingesting magnesium-containing medications.

NORMAL ACID–BASE BALANCE

The chemical composition of the ECF is regulated within narrow limits that provide an optimal environment for maintaining normal cell function. The most precisely regulated ion concentration in ECF is that of the hydrogen ion, averaging only 0.00000004 Eq/L (40 nEq/L) with a variation of 3 to 5 nEq/L. The ionic concentration can also be expressed as nmol/L, which has the same meaning.

The regulation of the hydrogen concentration at this low level is integral to normal cellular function because of the high reactivity of hydrogen ions, especially with proteins. Deviation from normal hydrogen ion concentration can upset normal reactions of cellular metabolism by altering the effectiveness of enzymes, hormones, and other chemical regulators of cell function. Hydrogen ions can also affect the normal distribution of other ions (such as sodium and potassium) between the intracellular fluids and the ECFs, thereby disturbing a variety of cell and tissue ion-dependent functions, such as conduction, contraction, and secretion. Therefore, normal ECF hydrogen ion concentration is essential for normal body functions. The concentration is determined by the types and amounts of acids and bases present, and its regulation is commonly called acid–base balance. Some hydrogen ions are ingested in foods, but most are produced as a result of metabolism of glucose, fatty acids, and amino acids.

An **acid** is any electrolyte that ionizes in water and forms hydrogen ions and anions. An acid is a hydrogen ion donor and thus elevates the hydrogen ion concentration of the solution to which it is added. The strength of an acid is determined by its degree of ionization in water. Strong acids completely ionize in water and readily liberate hydrogen ions. Hydrochloric acid (HCl), for example, is a strong acid because 99.9% of the HCl molecules ionize in pure water. Weak acids partly ionize in water and therefore do not liberate hydrogen ions as readily as strong acids. The acidity of the solution depends on how much the acid dissociates.

A **base** is any substance that can bind hydrogen ions. An alkali is a substance that contains a base. A strong base binds hydrogen ions readily. *Hydroxides* contain a hydroxyl (OH) group and form strong bases, such as sodium hydroxide (NaOH). A weak base binds hydrogen ions less readily. Sodium bicarbonate is a

(text continues on page 176)

TABLE 6-8

PHOSPHATE IMBALANCES

NORMAL FUNCTION AND VALUES	SOURCE AND CAUSE OF IMBALANCE	CLINICAL MANIFESTATIONS
NORMAL FUNCTION Essential anion for generation of bony tissue, essential to muscle, red blood cell, and nervous system function. NORMAL VALUE 2.5–4.5 mg/dL • 85% stored in bones • Supplied in diet in red meat, fish, poultry, eggs, and milk	HYPOPHOSPHATEMIA <2.5 mg/dL *Etiologic factors* • Antacid abuse (phosphate binding) • Diabetic ketoacidosis • Alcohol withdrawal • Hyperalimentation • Respiratory alkalosis • Burn injury • Hyperparathyroidism	• Anorexia, weakness, bone pain • Muscle weakness, rhabdomyolysis • Osteomalacia • Decreased cardiac output, hypoxia, metabolic acidosis, cardiomyopathy • CNS effects: tremors, hyporeflexia, confusion, seizures, coma
	HYPERPHOSPHATEMIA >4.5 mg/dL *Etiologic factors* • Renal failure • Hypoparathyroidism • Hyperthyroidism • Vitamin D intoxication • Chemotherapeutic agents • Phosphate containing laxatives • Tuberculosis • Sarcoidosis	• Elevation of serum phosphate results in fall of serum calcium, leads to manifestations of hypocalcemia • Precipitation of calcium phosphate in tissues: renal stones, metastatic calcifications • Cardiac dysrhythmia • Tingling mouth, fingers, and toes

TABLE 6-9

CHLORIDE IMBALANCES

NORMAL FUNCTION AND VALUES	SOURCE AND CAUSE OF IMBALANCE	CLINICAL MANIFESTATIONS
NORMAL FUNCTION • Predominant anion in ECF; mainly exists with sodium or hydrogen. • Follows Na+ loss and gain. Has inverse relationship to bicarbonate. NORMAL VALUE • 98–106 mEq/L • Mainly ingested as salt. Chloride often rises in acidosis as bicarbonate drops. It decreases in alkalosis as bicarbonate increases. • Lost in urine and body secretions	HYPOCHLOREMIA <80 mEq/L *Etiologic factors* • loss of gastrointestinal secretions such as vomiting, nasogastric suction, excessive diarrhea • Burns • Diabetic ketoacidosis • Diuretics • Fever, acute infections	• CNS hyperexcitability: tremors • Metabolic alkalosis • Manifestations of hyponatremia
	HYPERCHLOREMIA >110 mEq/L *Etiologic factors* • Dehydration • Cardiac failure • Cushing syndrome • Drugs, salicylates, ion exchange resins	• Weakness • Lethargy • Kussmaul (deep, rapid) respirations

TABLE 6-10

MAGNESIUM IMBALANCES

NORMAL FUNCTION AND VALUES	SOURCE AND CAUSE OF IMBALANCE	CLINICAL MANIFESTATIONS
NORMAL FUNCTION • Mainly found in ICF and in bones • Cation that activates a number of intracellular enzyme systems • Required for protein and nucleic acid synthesis • Decreased acetylcholine release at neuromuscular junction • Promotes cardiovascular function NORMAL VALUE 1.5–2.5 mEq/L • Closely related to calcium and potassium levels	HYPOMAGNESEMIA <1.5 mEq/L *Etiologic factors* • Malabsorption, alcoholism, protein-calorie malnutrition • Diarrhea • Acute renal failure • Citrated blood • Drugs: diuretics, aminoglycosides, amphoter; and cyclosporins, treatment of hyperglycemia, citrated blood • Liver failure	• Muscle tremors, tetany • Hyperactive reflexes, confusion. • Anorexia, nausea, vomiting • Dysphagia • Cardiac dysrhythmias—ventricular fibrillation, torsades de pointes (fast ventricular tachycardia) • Paresthesias • Convulsions • Often associated with hypokalemia and hypocalcemia
	HYPERMAGNESEMIA <2.5 mEq/L *Etiologic factors* • Renal failure • Severe dehydration • Leukemia • Excessive ingestion of magnesium containing drugs • Therapy for toxemia of pregnancy or premature labor	• Sedative effect, drowsiness, lethargy • Flushing, respiratory depression. • Hypotension • Nausea, vomiting • Bradycardia, conduction system blocks • Slurred speech

weak alkali containing the bicarbonate ion, a weak base. When sodium bicarbonate ($NaHCO_3$) is added to water, it completely dissociates. A small percentage of the resulting bicarbonate ions binds hydrogen ions and forms carbonic acid ($HCO_3^- + H^+ \leftrightarrow H_2CO_3$). Because a base is a hydrogen ion acceptor, the addition of a base to a solution containing hydrogen ions lowers the hydrogen ion concentration; the opposite occurs when an acid is added.

pH and Hydrogen Ion

The **pH** is the logarithm of the reciprocal of the hydrogen ion (H^+) concentration, which means that it measures the acidity or alkalinity of a solution. One liter of water contains 0.0000001 g of hydrogen ions. For any given solution, the numeric value of pH decreases as the hydrogen ion concentration increases. Therefore, because water is neutral at a pH of 7, when hydrogen ions are added to it, the solution becomes more acidic. The greater the hydrogen ion concentration, the more acidic the solution and the more the pH number falls. Acidic solutions range in pH between 0 and 7. Alkalotic or basic solutions, conversely, have less hydrogen ion concentration and range in pH between 7 and 14. The smaller the hydrogen ion concentration, the more alkaline the solution. Box 6-3 shows the pH values of various body fluids. In the plasma and interstitial fluids, the acceptable pH range is 7.35 to 7.45.

Normal blood gas values are indicated in Table 6-11. Levels below 7.35 indicate a state of acidosis, whereas levels above 7.45 indicate alkalosis. When the hydrogen ion concentration is in the normal range of 40 nEq (nmol)/L, the pH is 7.40. Cells of the human body usually function normally when the pH of ECF (interstitial fluids and plasma) remains constant at about 7.40. Alterations in plasma H^+ concentration alter the

BOX 6-3

pH VALUES OF CERTAIN BODY FLUIDS

Gastric juice	1.2–3.0
Vaginal fluid	3.5–4.5
Urine	4.6–8.0
Saliva	6.4–6.9
Blood (arterial)	7.35–7.45
Semen	7.20–7.60
Cerebrospinal fluid	7.4
Pancreatic juice	7.1–8.2
Bile	7.6–8.6

TABLE 6-11

ARTERIAL AND MIXED VENOUS BLOOD GASES

TERM	NORMAL VALUES	IMPLICATIONS
pH	Arterial: 7.35–7.45 Venous: 7.33–7.43	• Measures H^+ concentration; acidity increases as H^+ concentration increases (pH value decreases) • Venous blood carries slightly more H^+ as a product of metabolism
Pco_2	Arterial ($Paco_2$) 35–45 mmHg Venous ($Pvco_2$) 41–51 mmHg	• Measures CO_2 partial pressure in arterial blood • Increased amount of CO_2 in venous blood • Increased $PaCO_2$ decreases blood pH • Under respiratory control
Po_2	Arterial (Pao_2) 80–100 mmHg Venous (Pvo_2) 35–49 mmHg	• Measures partial pressure of O_2 in arterial blood • Significantly less O_2 remains in venous blood
O_2 saturation	Arterial 95–99% Venous 70–75%	• Measures degree to which hemoglobin is saturated by oxygen; much greater in arterial than in venous blood
HCO_3^- Base excess	Arterial 22–26 mEq/L Venous 24–28 mEq/L $-2 \rightarrow +2$ mEq/L	• Amount of buffer present using bicarbonate; metabolic buffer • Measures difference from 24 mEq/L − 2 = 22 mEq/L of HCO_3^- + 2 = 26 mEq/L Normal ranges

functioning of the enzyme, hormones, and organs of the body.

Metabolism: Volatile and Nonvolatile Acids

In the processes of cellular metabolism, acid is continually being formed, which must be eliminated from the body. The acids formed are often described as (1) volatile acids that are excretable by the lungs, and (2) nonvolatile acids that are excreted by the kidney.

VOLATILE ACIDS

A *volatile acid* is defined as an acid that can be excreted from the body as a gas. Either the acid itself or a chemical product of the acid can be converted to a gas and excreted. Carbonic acid (H_2CO_3), produced by the hydration of carbon dioxide in body fluids, is the only volatile acid in the body. A normal adult produces 200 mL/min of carbon dioxide, which translates to about 288 L/day from metabolic reactions.[1] This results in the production of a large amount of carbonic acid. Normally, the lungs excrete carbon dioxide as rapidly as cell metabolism produces it by increasing the rate and depth of breathing. In this way, carbonic acid is not allowed to accumulate in the body and alter the pH of the ECF.

NONVOLATILE ACIDS

A *nonvolatile acid,* also called a *fixed acid,* cannot be eliminated by the lungs and must be excreted by the kidneys. All metabolic acids present in body fluids except carbonic acid are classified as nonvolatile and include sulfuric acid, phosphoric acid, lactic acid, ketoacids (acetoacetic acid, β-hydroxybutyric acid), and smaller amounts of other inorganic and organic acids. To some extent, fixed acids are neutralized by dietary fixed bases. Fruits and vegetables contain such alkaline substances as potassium citrate. In a typical American diet, however, metabolic breakdown of foodstuffs, especially proteins, leads to an excess of fixed acids and these acids must be eliminated by the kidneys to maintain a normal pH of the ECF.

Regulation of Body Fluid pH

The ECF pH is normally maintained between 7.35 and 7.45 through three main mechanisms: (1) buffer systems, (2) exhalation of carbon dioxide, and (3) kidney excretion of hydrogen.[23]

BUFFER SYSTEMS

A **buffer** is any substance that prevents major changes in the pH of body fluids by reversibly binding hydrogen. The most important buffers in the body fluids consist of weak acids (such as carbonic acid, H_2CO_3) and bases (such as $NaHCO_3^-$), together referred to as acid–base buffer pairs. In ECF fluids, the salts are primarily sodium salts, and in the intracellular fluids they are primarily potassium salts. They act within a fraction of a second for immediate defense against either increases or decreases in hydrogen ion concentration.

Buffers minimize changes in pH by taking up hydrogen ions when acids are added to body fluids or by releasing hydrogen ions when the pH of body fluids becomes too high. The function of buffers is to convert strong acids, which would strongly decrease overall pH, into weak acids, which have a minimal effect on pH. Buffers also convert strong bases, which strongly increase overall pH, into weak bases, which have a minimal effect on pH. When acid or base is added to ECF, approximately half of the added ions eventually diffuse into cells, where they are buffered. These ions or others that affect acid–base balance are exchanged across the cell membrane for intracellular ions or are accompanied into cells by ions of opposite charge. For example, if an acid is added to ECF, some of the hydrogen is buffered chemically within the ECF and some is diffused across cell membranes into cells. Because the hydrogen ion is positively charged, it must either be exchanged across the cell membrane for another cation, such as Na^+ or K^+, or be accompanied into the cell by an anion, such as Cl^-. Although both processes occur, the movement of cations out of the cell is quantitatively more important.

The pK value, described in Box 6-4, represents the pH at which a buffer pair is half dissociated. It gives a constant rate for the chemical reaction. The buffer system is most productive when the pK for the buffer is close to the pH of the fluid in which the buffer is acting. The pK is 6:1 in the bicarbonate carbonic acid buffer system as described in Box 6-4 and this value is used to determine pH by the Henderson-Hasselbalch equation.

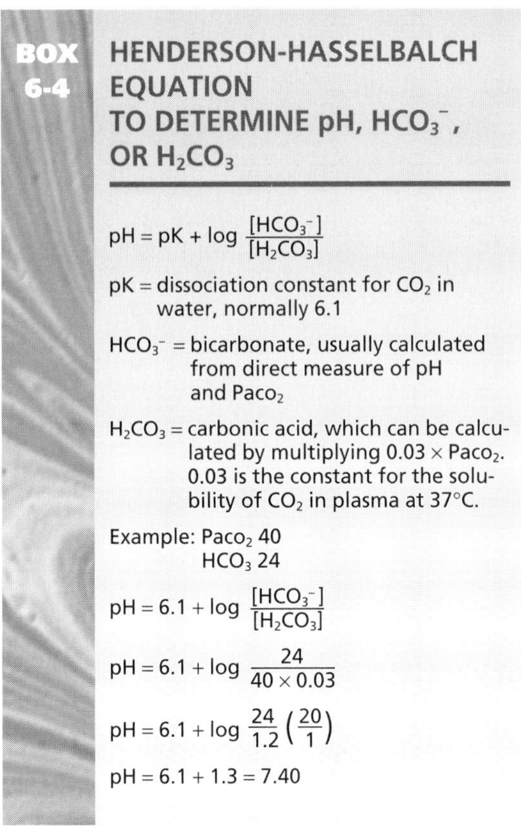

BOX 6-4 HENDERSON-HASSELBALCH EQUATION TO DETERMINE pH, HCO_3^-, OR H_2CO_3

$$pH = pK + \log \frac{[HCO_3^-]}{[H_2CO_3]}$$

pK = dissociation constant for CO_2 in water, normally 6.1

HCO_3^- = bicarbonate, usually calculated from direct measure of pH and $Paco_2$

H_2CO_3 = carbonic acid, which can be calculated by multiplying $0.03 \times Paco_2$. 0.03 is the constant for the solubility of CO_2 in plasma at 37°C.

Example: $Paco_2$ 40
HCO_3 24

$$pH = 6.1 + \log \frac{[HCO_3^-]}{[H_2CO_3]}$$

$$pH = 6.1 + \log \frac{24}{40 \times 0.03}$$

$$pH = 6.1 + \log \frac{24}{1.2} \left(\frac{20}{1}\right)$$

$$pH = 6.1 + 1.3 = 7.40$$

Carbonic Acid–Bicarbonate System

This system buffers volatile and nonvolatile acids in the interstitial fluid and in plasma. Carbonic acid–bicarbonate system is the optimum buffer system for analysis because it is the largest in the ECF and it is the easiest to measure. The following equation explains the components of the carbonic acid–bicarbonate buffer system and how each affects the other:

$$CO_2 + H_2O \leftrightarrow H_2CO_3 \leftrightarrow H + HCO_3$$

This reaction occurs in either direction and is sped up by the presence of the enzyme carbonic anhydrase. This enzyme is present in RBCs and in the renal tubular cells. The left side of the equation represents the respiratory component and the right side depicts the renal-metabolic component. When the rate that carbon dioxide is eliminated by the lungs equals the rate at which carbon dioxide is produced, hydrogen ion concentration will not change. An increase in carbon dioxide content (pressure or tension) results in the liberation of hydrogen ions; thus, the pH decreases. If alveolar ventilation is decreased, metabolically produced carbon dioxide accumulates in the blood, carbonic acid concentration rises, and blood pH falls.

A decrease in carbon dioxide tension results in fewer free hydrogen ions and, consequently, a more alkaline pH. If ventilation is stimulated so that elimination of carbon dioxide temporarily exceeds its production, the blood Pco_2 moves to a lower level and alkaline blood pH results. Thus, changes in alveolar ventilation profoundly influence blood pH. The bicarbonate ion can act as a weak base and the carbonic acid can act as a weak acid, so the system can compensate for either excess or deficit hydrogen ion.[4]

The carbonic acid–bicarbonate system is the most important extracellular buffer because it can be regulated by both the lungs and the kidneys. Normally, the carbonic acid (H_2CO_3)/bicarbonate (HCO_3^-) ratio is maintained at approximately 1:20 when the pH is 7.40. The actual content required to maintain this balance is 1.2 mEq/L of H_2CO_3 to 24 mEq/L of HCO_3^-. As long as the ratio of 1:20 is maintained, the pH will be stabilized (Fig. 6-8). If, for example, a retention of carbon dioxide and a reciprocal compensatory retention of bicarbonate occurs, the amounts might be 2.0 mEq/L of H_2CO_3 and 40 mEq/L of HCO_3^-, which would still maintain the ratio (2:40 instead of 1:20), and the pH would remain 7.40.[19,21] The respiratory system works very rapidly in the excretion or retention of carbon dioxide, whereas the renal system functions much more slowly to retain or excrete HCO_3^-.

Phosphate Buffer System

This system acts in almost the same way as the carbonic acid–bicarbonate system except that sodium salts of dihydrogen phosphate ($H_2PO_4^-$) and sodium monohydrogen phosphate (HPO_4^-) ions are used. The dihydrogen phosphate acts as a weak acid and can buffer strong bases, whereas the monohydrogen phosphate ions act as the weak base and can buffer strong acids.[19] Phosphate is highest in the ICF, so this buffer system is most active in the ICF. Phosphate also acts to buffer acids in the urine by combining Na_2HPO_4 with a strong acid such as HCl to form sodium chloride (NaCl) and sodium dihydrogen phosphate (NaH_2PO_4), a weak acid.[23] This buffering provides a mechanism for acidification of the urine and decreasing plasma acidity.

Protein Buffer System

The most plentiful buffer in body cells and plasma is the protein buffer system. All proteins can act as acidic and basic buffers by binding or donating hydrogen ion.

Hemoglobin buffers carbonic acid by causing the carbonic acid to dissociate into hydrogen ions and bicarbonate ions. At the time that carbon dioxide is moving into the cell, the oxygen from the hemoglobin is released to the tissue. This release results in reduced hemoglobin, which can combine with the hydrogen ion and provide a mechanism for carrying the acid back to the lungs. Once in the lungs, hydrogen again attaches to the bicarbonate ions and dissociates into carbon dioxide and water. The carbon dioxide gas readily diffuses out through the alveoli as new oxygen is being picked up. Their activity may be seen in both acidosis and alkalosis by releasing hydrogen or binding it when necessary.

Production of HCO_3^- by the kidney is partially dependent on ammonium (NH_4^+) production, which can produce HCO_3^-, as illustrated in Figure 6-9. This process is dependent on extraction of glutamine to

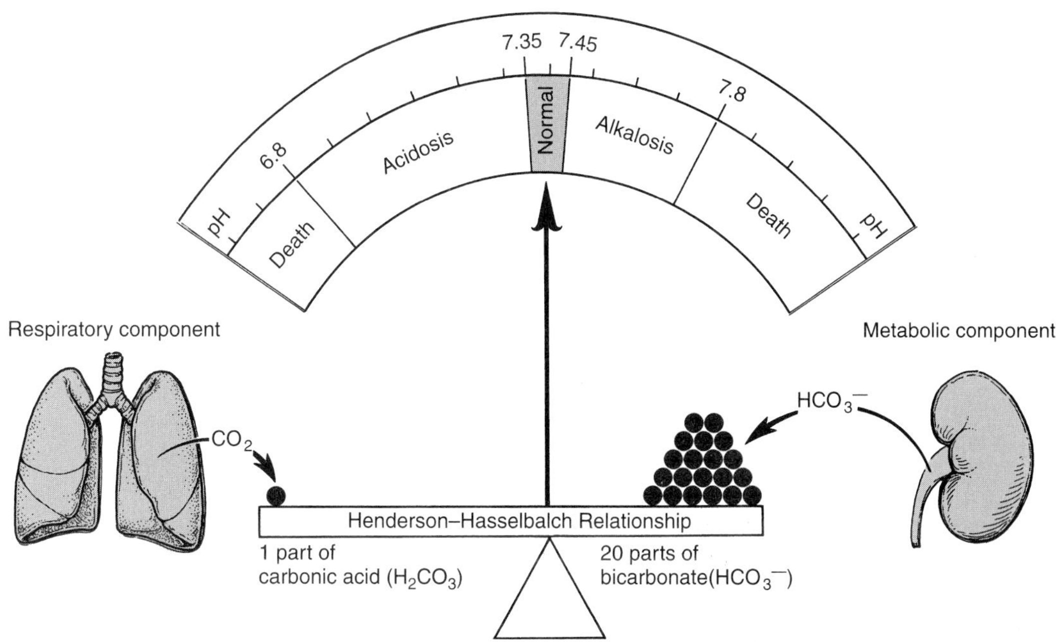

FIGURE 6-8. **Mechanisms for the defense against changes in body fluid pH.**

FOCUS ON CELLULAR PHYSIOLOGY

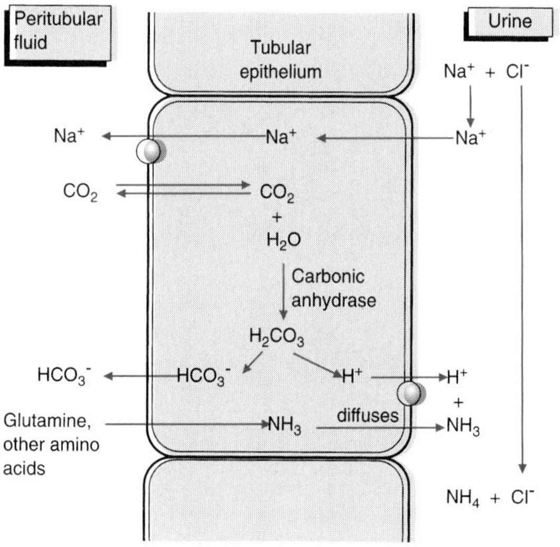

FIGURE 6-9. **Excretion of ammonia.**

liberate NH_4^+, which is actively secreted into the lumen and excreted while the HCO_3 is reabsorbed.[1,24]

RESPIRATORY REGULATION OF CARBON DIOXIDE

The respiratory system plays an important role in acid–base balance by controlling the partial pressure of carbon dioxide (P_{CO_2}) in arterial blood. As excess carbon dioxide is formed during cellular processes, most of it is picked up by the RBCs and carried to the lungs.

Alveolar ventilation is normally adjusted so that pH changes in the arterial blood are kept to a minimum. Increases of hydrogen ion concentration in body fluid (decreased pH), specifically in arterial blood and cerebrospinal fluid, result in a reflex increase in respiratory rate and depth. This respiratory response acts to blow off more carbon dioxide. The result is that the hydrogen ion concentration is decreased toward normal. Excess carbonic acid in the blood (due to failure to eliminate carbon dioxide adequately) is a powerful stimulus to ventilation. The increase in ventilation diminishes the retention of carbon dioxide and thereby minimizes the accumulation of carbonic acid in the blood. The ventilatory response also is reactive to acidosis from other acids. Fixed, nonvolatile acids cause a marked increase in ventilation rate and depth.

The respiratory system normally changes its activity to minimize shifts in pH. Respiratory activity responds rapidly to acid–base stresses and shifts blood pH toward normal in minutes. A person who is hypoventilating begins to accumulate carbon dioxide rapidly and, as a reflex, increases the rate and depth of breathing to restore the blood pH. Conversely, respiratory rate is slowed when the pH elevates, which causes the pH to approach normal. An increase in alveolar ventilation of two times normal can increase the pH of blood 0.23 pH units. Conversely, depressing ventilation to one-fourth of normal decreases the pH by 0.4 pH units.[8]

KIDNEY REGULATION OF HYDROGEN

The major role of the kidneys in maintaining acid–base balance is to conserve circulating stores of bicarbonate and to excrete hydrogen ions. The kidneys maintain ECF pH by (1) increasing urinary excretion of hydrogen ions and conserving plasma bicarbonate when the blood is too acidic and (2) increasing urinary excretion of bicarbonate and decreasing urinary excretion of hydrogen ions when the blood is too alkaline. Renal mechanisms for hydrogen ion regulation are slower (taking hours or days) than are chemical buffers or respiratory mechanisms. Renal compensation for acid–base disturbances is effective because the kidneys actually excrete hydrogen ions and eliminate them from body fluids.[6] The respiratory mechanisms described above cannot eliminate tissue-generated metabolic hydrogen ions from the body.

Renal control of acid–base balance involves three processes that occur simultaneously along the length of the nephron: (1) reabsorption of filtered bicarbonate, (2) excretion of titratable acid, and (3) excretion of ammonia. All three mechanisms involve secretion of hydrogen ions into the urine and return of bicarbonate to the plasma.

Quantitatively, the reabsorption of filtered bicarbonate is the most important process in renal acid–base regulation. Approximately 4,500 mEq $NaHCO_3$ is filtered each day. Normally, all but 1 or 2 mEq $NaHCO_3$ is reabsorbed into the plasma. Figure 6-10 illustrates the cellular mechanisms involved in the reabsorption of filtered bicarbonate.

The kidneys also excrete hydrogen ions in the form of *titratable acids,* which are the urinary buffers. These buffers consist mostly of dihydrogen phosphate ($H_2PO_4^-$) formed when hydrogen in the tubular fluid combines with monohydrogen phosphate (HPO_4^-). For each hydrogen ion excreted in the form of titratable acid, an equivalent quantity of $NaHCO_3$ is added to the blood (Fig. 6-11).

Adults normally produce 1 to 2 mEq/kg per day of fixed, nonvolatile acid, probably due to the high-protein diet consumed by meat-eating people.[3,18] If a chronic acid load is imposed on the body, the production and excretion of ammonia may increase more than 10-fold over several days. The cellular mechanisms of ammonia excretion are illustrated in Figure 6-9. Ammonia is

FOCUS ON CELLULAR PHYSIOLOGY

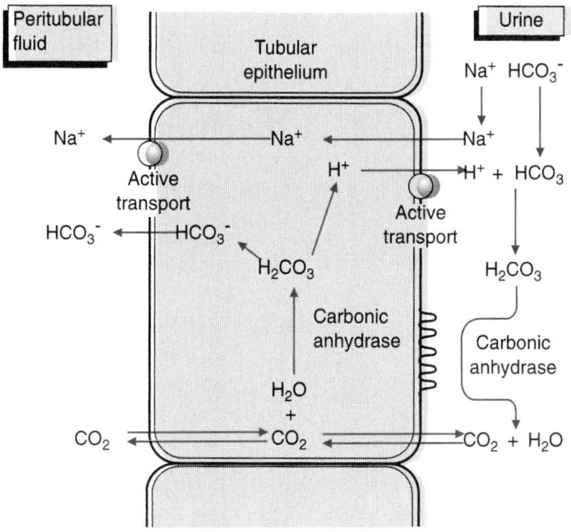

FIGURE 6-10. Reabsorption of filtered bicarbonate.

produced in the tubular cells from amino acid (glutamine) metabolism. This complex is lipid soluble and can cross the cell membrane. Ammonia, readily soluble in the luminal membrane, diffuses out of the tubular cell into the urine, where it combines with hydrogen ions to form ammonium (NH_4^+) ions. Ammonium ions penetrate cell membranes poorly, so they are effectively trapped in urine and excreted in combination with chloride.[3] For each hydrogen ion excreted with ammonia, an equivalent quantity of $NaHCO_3$ is added to the blood. Normally, the kidneys produce up to 40 mEq HCO_3^-/day from NH_4 formation.[10]

FOCUS ON CELLULAR PHYSIOLOGY

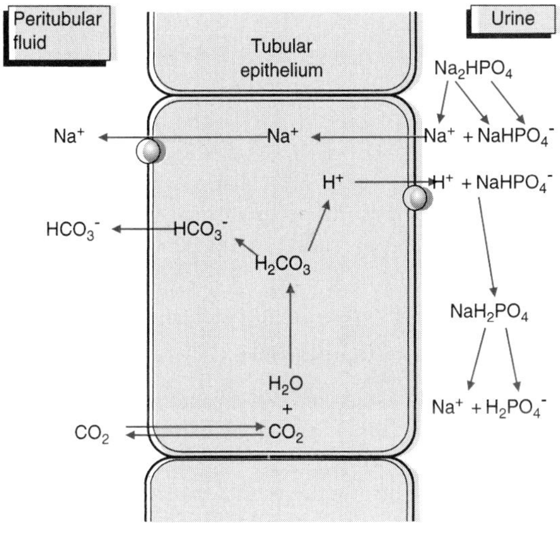

FIGURE 6-11. Production of titratable acid.

ALTERED ACID–BASE BALANCE

Alteration of the normal acid–base balance occurs when there is an accumulation of hydrogen or a loss of hydrogen due to some disruptive process and the routine compensatory mechanisms cannot overcome the disruption. The pH change itself is often more damaging than the underlying mechanism causing it.

Acidosis and Alkalosis

Arterial blood is used for assessing acid–base balance because blood is accessible and because the hydrogen ion concentration of blood affects the hydrogen ion concentration of all body fluids. Clinical evaluation of the acid–base status of a patient involves the determination of arterial pH, $PaCO_2$ and HCO_3 (see Table 6-11).

Acidosis in the body fluids refers to an elevation of the H^+ concentration above normal or a decrease in the HCO_3^- below normal, resulting in a decrease in the pH of the body fluids to below 7.35. The source of the excess hydrogen ion or altered H_2CO_3/HCO_3^- ratio can be respiratory (volatile) or metabolic (nonrespiratory or nonvolatile). **Acidemia** is defined as an acidic condition of the blood signified by an arterial pH value less than 7.35. The physiologic processes causing the acidemia are defined as acidosis (a condition of becoming acidic).

Alkalosis refers to a decrease in the H^+ concentration of the body fluids or an excess of the HCO_3^-, thus increasing pH of the body fluids to above 7.45. The source of the depletion of hydrogen ion is either elimination of carbon dioxide (hyperventilation) or a metabolic excess of primary base bicarbonate. **Alkalemia** is defined as an alkaline condition of the blood signified by arterial pH greater than 7.45. The physiologic processes causing the alkalemia define the term alkalosis (a condition of becoming alkalotic). Table 6-12 summarizes some factors that may cause acidosis and alkalosis. Table 6-13 details the physiologic effects of the pH change that occur regardless of whether the change has resulted from respiratory or metabolic alterations.

Effects of pH Changes on Potassium, Calcium, and Magnesium Balance

Integrated into the direct effects of acidosis and alkalosis on the physiologic process are their compounding effects on potassium and calcium balance. Other electrolytes, such as magnesium and phosphate, are also affected, but the systemic effects of potassium and calcium imbalances can be life threatening.

Hydrogen is preferentially excreted or retained over other cations by the renal system to maintain the blood pH. When the arterial pH falls, the excess H^+ is excreted through the kidneys. Hydrogen cannot be ex-

TABLE 6-12

DISTURBANCES OF ACID–BASE BALANCE

ARTERIAL BLOOD PH	INDICATOR OF PRIMARY ABNORMALITY	EXAMPLES OF CAUSATIVE FACTORS	COMPENSATORY MECHANISMS
Alkalemia pH > 7.45	Respiratory alkalosis $\downarrow Pco_2$ <35 mm Hg	• Hyperventilation • Anxiety • Fever, sepsis • Pain. • Aspirin poisoning • Pulmonary embolus • Pneumonia	• Kidneys retain hydrogen ions and excrete bicarbonate. • Potassium moves into cell.
	Metabolic alkalosis $\uparrow HCO_3^-$ >26 mEq/L	• Excessive ingestion of alkali (baking soda for heartburn, indigestion) • Vomiting, nasogastric suctioning • Diuretic therapy • Cushing's disease • Hyperaldosteronism.	• Alveolar ventilation decreases to retain carbon dioxide. • Kidneys increase hydrogen ion retention and excrete bicarbonate. • Potassium moves into cell.
Acidemia pH < 7.35	Respiratory acidosis $\uparrow Pco_2$ >45mm Hg	• Depression of respiratory center by drugs or disease • Obstructive lung disease • Respiratory failure from any cause • Restriction of lung movement	• Kidneys increase hydrogen ion excretion and bicarbonate retention • Potassium moves out of cell • Increased ammonia formation
	Metabolic acidosis $\downarrow HCO_3^-$ <22mEq/L	• Diabetic ketoacidosis • Lactic acidosis • Renal failure • Aspirin poisoning • Severe diarrhea • Renal tubular acidosis	• Increased alveolar ventilation • Kidneys increase hydrogen excretion and bicarbonate retention. • Increased ammonia formation • Potassium moves out of cell.

creted unless a cation is retained. Potassium is the cation usually retained; thus, hyperkalemia develops in acidosis. Potassium may also shift out of ICF because more than 50% of the excess H^+ is buffered intracellularly. The K^+ and small amounts of Na^+ leave the cell to maintain a balance with the ECF.[3] The reverse is true with alkalosis. The kidney retains H^+ to normalize the blood pH, and K^+ is wasted. The intracellular hydrogen is donated to the ECF, and K^+ is retained intracellularly. Therefore, hyperkalemia is associated with acidosis, and hypokalemia is associated with alkalosis.

Changes in the arterial pH affect the ionized calcium levels in blood. Ionized calcium in an alkalotic serum binds with serum proteins and produces the clinical effect of hypocalcemia.[2] In an acidic environment, more calcium may be released from the plasma proteins, and ionized calcium levels may rise transiently.

Serum magnesium levels also may change in response to the pH levels. Hypomagnesemia is often seen in acidosis. Symptoms include weakness, mental depression, and tetany similar to that of hypocalcemia.

Etiology and Clinical Manifestations of Acidosis and Alkalosis

Disturbances of acid–base balance may arise from respiratory or metabolic causes. The four primary types of acid–base disturbances are respiratory acidosis, respiratory alkalosis, metabolic acidosis, and metabolic alkalosis. The clinical manifestations may reflect the

TABLE 6-13

PHYSIOLOGIC EFFECTS OF ALKALEMIA AND ACIDEMIA

SYSTEM AFFECTED	ALKALEMIA	ACIDEMIA
Cardiovascular	• Palpitations due to atrial or ventricular mechanisms. • Cerebral vasoconstriction	• Dysrhythmias—ventricular fibrillation, conduction defects • Systemic vasodilation—warm, flushed skin • Myocardial depression decreased cardiac output • Pulmonary vasoconstriction
Respiratory system	• Depressed respirations • Decreased oxygen delivery to tissues	• Stimulation of respirations • Increased oxygen delivery to tissues
Central nervous system	• Light-headedness due to decreased cerebral blood flow. • Paresthesias—numbness and tingling	• Headache • Dizziness, mental cloudiness • CNS depression and coma • Convulsions
Musculoskeletal system	• Hypertonic muscles • Carpopedal spasms	• Muscle twitching to flaccid muscles • Loss of muscle protein
Metabolic effects	• Decreased serum potassium, calcium, phosphate • Increased glycolysis	• Increased serum potassium calcium, phosphate • Increased production of lactic acid • Bone loss due to buffering

underlying cause of the disturbance or those of the acidic or alkalotic condition.

RESPIRATORY ACIDOSIS

Respiratory acidosis is caused by failure of the respiratory system to remove carbon dioxide from body fluids as rapidly as it is produced in the tissues. A decrease in the pulmonary ventilation rate will increase the Pa_{CO_2} of the ECF, causing an increase in H_2CO_3. Any condition that impairs or interferes with breathing can result in respiratory acidosis (see Table 6-12). Impairment of breathing leads to an increase in Pa_{CO_2} above 45 mm Hg (**hypercapnia**), with a corresponding decrease in pH value to 7.35 or less. The pathophysiology of respiratory acidosis is summarized in Flowchart 6-2.

Severe respiratory acidosis usually is evident with the following signs and symptoms of respiratory insufficiency: cyanosis, rapid and shallow breathing, diaphoresis, and disorientation. Acute respiratory acidosis can produce **carbon dioxide narcosis**, with symptoms of headache, blurred vision, fatigue, and weakness. Prolonged acidosis may produce severe CNS symptoms, including increased intracranial pressure and permanent damage.[24] When the pH falls below 7.10, dysrhythmias, peripheral vasodilatation with dilated conjunctival and facial blood vessels, and increased intracranial pressure with papilledema may occur.

RESPIRATORY ALKALOSIS

Respiratory alkalosis is caused by the loss of carbon dioxide from the lungs at a faster rate than it is produced in the tissues (see Table 6-12). This leads to a decrease in arterial Pa_{CO_2} below 35 mm Hg (**hypocapnia**), with a pH greater than 7.45. The pathophysiology of respiratory alkalosis is summarized in Flowchart 6-3.

Symptoms of respiratory alkalosis are related to CNS irritability and include light-headedness, circumoral numbness, **paresthesias** (numbness, prickling, tingling), altered consciousness, cramps, and **carpopedal spasm** (wrist or foot) from clinical hypocalcemia (see page 172).

METABOLIC ACIDOSIS

Metabolic acidosis results from either an abnormal accumulation of fixed acids or loss of base (see Table 6-12). The arterial blood pH falls below 7.35, and the plasma bicarbonate is usually decreased below 22 mEq/L. The pathophysiology is summarized in Flowchart 6-4.

Symptoms of severe metabolic acidosis include deep, rapid respiration (**Kussmaul's breathing**), disorientation, and coma. Clinical manifestations of metabolic acidosis depend on the pH level. Arterial pH of less than 7.10 can produce severe ventricular dysrhythmias and reduction of cardiac contractility. Production of lactic acidosis may occur with associated hypotension.[2] The

FLOWCHART 6-2 **Respiratory Acidosis**

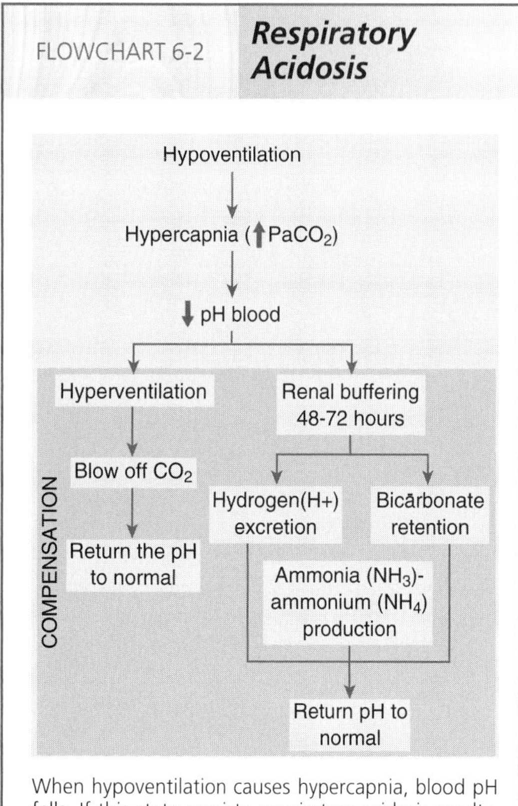

When hypoventilation causes hypercapnia, blood pH falls. If this state persists, respiratory acidosis results. Renal compensatory mechanisms can be initiated to return the pH to normal over 48–72 hours.

FLOWCHART 6-3 **Respiratory Alkalosis**

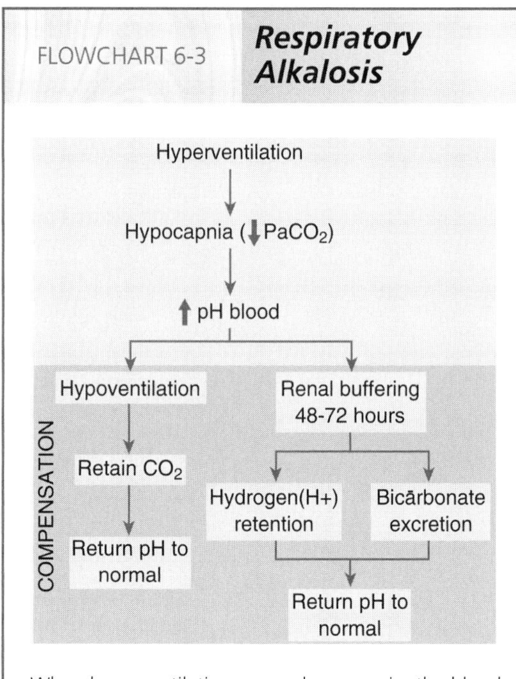

When hyperventilation causes hypocapnia, the blood pH elevates. If this state persists, respiratory alkalosis results. Compensation by the lungs usually is initiated to return the pH to normal. Renal compensation is rare since the condition usually resolves in minutes to hours.

chronic acidosis of renal failure retards bone growth and causes a variety of bone disturbances, probably due to buffering of acidosis by bone calcium.[19]

Anion Gap in Metabolic Acidosis

Evaluation of the **anion gap** is commonly used in the differential diagnosis of metabolic acidosis or in defining metabolic acidosis within mixed acid–base disorders (Table 6-14). In the ECF the sum of the concentrations of cations must equal anions. The primary ECF cation is sodium and the primary ECF anions are chloride and bicarbonate. The number of sodium ions usually exceeds the number of chloride and bicarbonate ions. The anion gap is the difference between the number of sodium ions and the number of chloride and bicarbonate ions. The anion gap identifies negative ions not measured (sulfate, phosphate, lactate, ketoacids, and albumin). The formula to compute the anion gap is: $Na^+ - (HCO_3^- + Cl^-)$. The anion gap is normally 9 to 16 mEq/L (Box 6-5).

Hyperchloremic acidosis (*normal anion gap acidosis*) is commonly due to a loss of bicarbonate ions by gastrointestinal or renal routes, with a parallel increase

FLOWCHART 6-4 **Metabolic Acidosis**

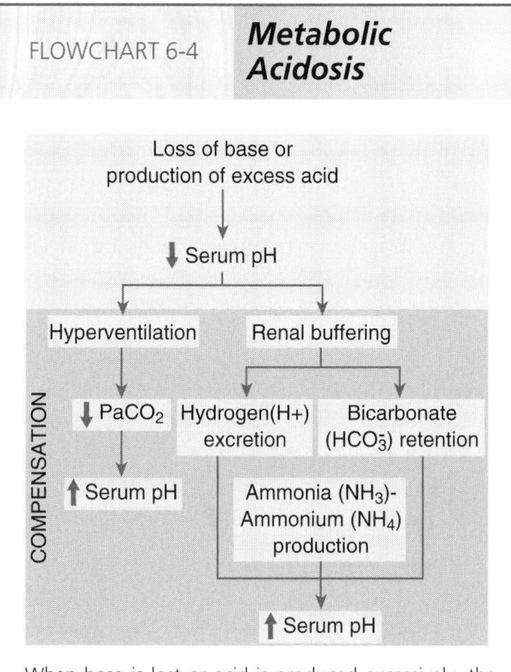

When base is lost or acid is produced excessively, the serum pH falls. If this state persists, metabolic acidosis results. Respiratory compensatory mechanisms are usually initiated quickly to attempt to return the serum pH toward normal.

TABLE 6-14

CAUSES OF METABOLIC ACIDOSIS

HIGH ANION GAP	NORMAL ANION GAP	DECREASED ANION GAP*

• Diabetic ketoacidosis
• Starvation ketoacidosis
• Alcoholic ketoacidosis
• Lactic acidosis
• Renal failure
• Salicylate poisoning
• Methyl alcohol or ethylene glycol poisonings
	• Diarrhea
	• Biliary or pancreatic fistulas
	• Excessive administration of isotonic saline or ammonium chloride
	• Renal insufficiency
	• Diuretics: aldactone, acetazolamide
	• Hyperalimentation fluid with no lactate or acetate
		• Hypermagnesemia
		• Paraproteinemic states
		  • Multiple myeloma
		  • Waldenströms macroglobulinemia

*Decreased anion gap is rare.

in chloride ions. It can also occur from an accumulation of chloride ions (acidifying salts) with a decrease in bicarbonate ions.

When hydrogen ion is added with an unmeasured anion to the ECF, it is buffered by HCO_3^- and so the HCO_3^- concentration decreases, and the unmeasured anions increase. This is called *high anion gap acidosis.* An increased anion gap is caused by conditions such as lactic acidosis, uremia, diabetic ketoacidosis, and salicylate or methanol toxicity.

METABOLIC ALKALOSIS

Metabolic alkalosis results from either a loss of hydrogen and chloride ions or addition of base to body fluids. The plasma bicarbonate increases to above 26 mEq/L, and the arterial blood pH increases above 7.45 (see Table 6-12). Secondary increase in plasma HCO_3^- is often seen with chronic respiratory acidosis as a compensation to keep the pH at or about normal levels. The pathophysiology of metabolic alkalosis is summarized in Flowchart 6-5.

Clinical manifestations of metabolic alkalosis include apathy, mental confusion, shallow breathing, polyuria and polydipsia secondary to hypokalemia, signs of volume depletion, spastic muscles, weakness, muscle cramps, dizziness, and dysrhythmias. Some of

BOX 6-5 CALCULATING THE ANION GAP IN METABOLIC ACIDOSIS

A. Na^+: 130 mEq/L
HCO_3^-: 10 mEq/L
Cl^-: 90 mEq/L
$Na^+ - (HCO_3^- + Cl^-)$
$130 - (10 + 90) = 30$ mEq/L

Gap is increased over 16.
Diagnosis is high anion gap metabolic acidosis.

B. Na^+: 136 mEq/L
HCO_3^-: 14 mEq/L
Cl^-: 112 mEq/L
$Na^+ - (HCO_3^- + Cl^-)$
$136 - (14 + 112) = 10$ mEq/L

Gap is normal.
Diagnosis is normal anion gap metabolic acidosis.

FLOWCHART 6-5 **Metabolic Alkalosis**

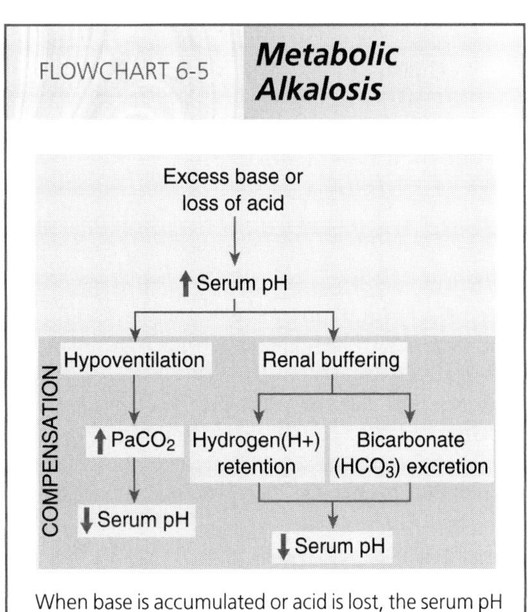

When base is accumulated or acid is lost, the serum pH elevates. If this state persists, metabolic alkalosis results. Respiratory depression is the compensation that is initiated to attempt to return the pH toward normal.

the clinical features are associated with hypokalemia or hypocalcemia. Neurologic symptoms include paresthesias and light-headedness.[3]

MIXED ACID–BASE DISORDERS

Mixed or complex acid–base disorders occur when there are two or more independent acid–base conditions that happen jointly. Some of the mixed disorders and their causes are listed below.

Respiratory and Metabolic Acidosis. This condition is manifested by an elevated PCO_2 along with a decreased HCO_3^- causing the pH to be extremely low. It may occur in such conditions as cardiopulmonary arrest, chronic renal failure with a fluid volume excess, or diabetic ketoacidosis with respiratory depression.[4]

Respiratory and Metabolic Alkalosis. This abnormality occurs when there is an increase in the pH, a decrease in the PCO_2 and an increase in the HCO_3^-. Persons with conditions such as congestive heart failure with hyperventilation and treatment with diuretics can develop metabolic alkalosis and respiratory alkalosis. Each alkalotic response blocks the compensation of the other when these disturbances are combined.

Respiratory Alkalosis and Metabolic Acidosis. This combination causes a drop in the PCO_2 far greater than would be expected as compensation for primary metabolic acidosis and the decrease in HCO_3^- is greater than necessary as compensation for primary respiratory alkalosis occurs.[24] This abnormality may be seen in salicylate intoxication.

Metabolic Alkalosis and Respiratory Acidosis. The combination of an elevated HCO_3^- and $PaCO_2$ brings the pH to near normal.[13] This may be seen in conditions such as chronic obstructive pulmonary disease being with treated with diuretics,

CORRECTION AND COMPENSATION

The two ways for an abnormal pH of arterial plasma to be returned toward normal are correction and compensation. In correction, the primary cause of the acid–base disturbance is repaired. For example, if respiratory acidosis is caused by partial blockage of the respiratory tree, removal or reduction of the obstruction improves ventilation and allows blood pH to return toward normal.

In compensation, the system or systems not responsible for causing the acid–base disturbance make physiologic adjustments to return blood pH toward normal. For example, in respiratory acidosis (high $PaCO_2$), the kidneys compensate by increasing the return of bicarbonate to the blood to return the HCO_3^-/H_2CO_3 ratio to normal. All processes of compensation are directed at returning the bicarbonate/carbonic acid ratio to 20 : 1 and restoring the normal pH of arterial plasma. The kidneys compensate for respiratory acidosis (high $PaCO_2$) by elevating the plasma bicarbonate above 26 mEq/L. The kidneys compensate for respiratory alkalosis (low PCO_2) by lowering the plasma bicarbonate below 22 mEq/L. Similar compensations are made by the kidneys in nonrenal causes of metabolic acidosis and alkalosis.[19]

The respiratory system attempts to compensate for metabolic acidosis (low HCO_3^-) by lowering the arterial PCO_2 below 35 mm Hg through hyperventilation. It attempts to compensate for metabolic alkalosis by elevating the arterial PCO_2 above 45 mm Hg through hypoventilation.

The effectiveness of the compensations depends on the amount of disruption occurring from the underlying disorder and the body's ability to make changes. Life-threatening disorders are not effectively compensated for by the slow responding renal mechanisms, but they may respond quickly to the rapid respiratory compensations.

Major disturbances of acid–base balance are rarely completely compensated. Arterial pH is returned toward normal during compensation, but rarely to normal. Therefore, the arterial pH indicates whether a process of acidosis or alkalosis is present. The arterial blood PCO_2 and the plasma bicarbonate concentration indicate which process, respiratory or metabolic, is responsible for the abnormal pH and which process is compensatory.

For example, the following blood gas data indicate an acid–base abnormality: pH = 7.22; PCO_2 = 30 mm Hg; HCO_3^- = 12 mEq/L. To interpret the data, one must look at the pH to see if there is acidemia or alkalemia. In this case, the arterial pH is below normal range (7.35–7.45) and indicates acidemia. The plasma $PaCO_2$ and bicarbonate are then examined for indications of acidosis and alkalosis. Here, the bicarbonate concentration is below normal range (22–28 mEq/L) and indicates metabolic acidosis. The arterial PCO_2 is below normal range (35–45 mm Hg) and indicates respiratory alkalosis. Because there is acidemia, the primary disturbance is one of metabolic acidosis, whereas the compensatory process is respiratory. Therefore, the data suggest partially compensated metabolic acidosis.

Examples of acid–base disturbances and blood values are shown in Box 6-6. Table 6-15 presents blood gases in such a way as to determine the type of acid–base abnormality that is occurring and where there is compensation for the abnormality. Note that the pH and HCO_3^- changes in metabolic abnormalities go in the same direction, whereas the pH and $PaCO_2$ changes go in the opposite directions in respiratory abnormalities.

BOX 6-6 EXAMPLES OF ACID–BASE ABNORMALITIES

1. Metabolic acidosis, with partial respiratory compensation
   pH 7.24 ↓
   $Paco_2$ 28 ↓
   HCO_3^- 12 ↓
2. Metabolic alkalosis with partial respiratory compensation.
   pH 7.58 ↑
   $Paco_2$ 50 ↑
   HCO_3^- 37 ↑
3. Respiratory acidosis, uncompensated.
   pH 7.22 ↓
   $Paco_2$ 56 ↑
   HCO_3^- 26 N
4. Respiratory alkalosis, uncompensated.
   pH 7.5 ↑
   $Paco_2$ 28 ↓
   HCO_3^- 22 N

N, normal

FOCUS ON THE PERSON WITH FLUID AND ELECTROLYTE IMBALANCE

A 60-year-old alcoholic woman has had nausea and vomiting for the past 5 days. She is complaining of abdominal pain after 2 weeks of drinking. She is unable to take anything by mouth. Her mucous membranes are dry. She is presenting with a blood pressure decrease on standing with a rise in pulse. Her electrolytes are as follows:

Na	134 mEq/L
K	3.1 mEq/L
HCO_3	20 mEq/L
Cl	80 mEq/L
Glucose	86 mg/dL
BUN	52 mg/dL
Cr	1.4 mg/dL

Urine and serum ketones are elevated.

Questions

1. What fluid and electrolyte imbalance is being exhibited?
2. List some contributing factors for the condition.
3. Identify reasons for laboratory changes.
4. What clinical manifestations are directly related to the condition being manifested?

See Appendix A for discussion.

TABLE 6-15

DIRECTIONS OF ACID–BASE ABNORMALITIES AND COMPENSATIONS

IMBALANCE	pH	HCO_3^-	PA_{CO_2}	BASE EXCESS
METABOLIC ACIDOSIS				
Uncompensated	↓	↓	N	↓
Partially compensated	↓	↓	↓	↓
Fully compensated	N	↓	↓	↓
METABOLIC ALKALOSIS				
Uncompensated	↑	↑	N	↑
Partially compensated	↑	↑	↑	↑
Fully compensated	N	↑	↑	↑
RESPIRATORY ACIDOSIS				
Uncompensated	↓	N	↑	N
Partially compensated	↓	↑	↑	↑
Fully compensated	N	↑	↑	↑
RESPIRATORY ALKALOSIS				
Uncompensated	↑	N	↓	N
Partially compensated	↑	↓	↓	↓
Fully compensated	N	↓	↓	↓

N, normal

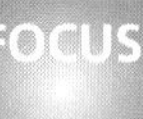

FOCUS ON THE PERSON WITH ACID-BASE IMBALANCE

A 35-year-old man suffered a generalized seizure (grand mal, tonic-clonic) 1 hour after an Achilles tendon repair.

Pre-admission Labs

Na	124 mEq/L
K	5.0 mEq/L
Cl	90 mEq/L
HCO_3	24 mEq/L
Anion gap	10
Postop Labs	
Na	112 mEq/L
K	5.0 mEq/L
Cl	74 mEq/L
HCO_3	16 mEq/L
pH	7.32
Pco_2	32

Questions

Urine ketones—normal

1. What are the abnormalities seen in electrolytes and acid-base balance?
2. What is the disorder that is presented?
3. What caused the seizure activity?
4. What clinical manifestations may be exhibited with the laboratory picture exhibited?
5. Calculate the anion gap.

See Appendix A for discussion.

REFERENCES

1. Berne, R. M., & Levy, M. N. (1998). *Physiology* (4th ed.). St. Louis: Mosby.
2. Bilezikjian, J. P. (1998). Hypercalcemia and hypocalcemia. In J. H. Stein (Ed.), *Internal medicine* (5th ed.). St. Louis: Mosby.
3. DiGiovanni, S. R., & Feldman, G. M. (1998). Disorders of acid-base balance. In J. H. Stein (Ed.), *Internal medicine* (5th ed.), St. Louis: Mosby.
4. Dubose, T. D. (1997) Approach to the patient with acid-base abnormalities. In W. N. Kelley (Ed.), *Textbook of internal medicine* (3rd ed.). Philadelphia: Lippincott-Raven.
5. Epstein, M. (1998). Disorders of sodium balance. In J. H. Stein (Ed.), *Internal medicine* (5th ed.). St. Louis: Mosby.
6. *Fluid and electrolyte disorders.* (1994). Nursing Timesavers. Springhouse, PA: Springhouse Corporation.
7. Goldhill, D. R. (1997, May/June). Calcium and magnesium. *Care of the Critically Ill, 13*(3), 112–115.
8. Guyton, A., & Hall, J. (1998). *Pocket companion to textbook of medical physiology*. Philadelphia: Saunders.
9. Halperin, M. L., & Goldstein, M. B. (1994). *Fluid, electrolyte, and acid-base physiology. A problem-based approach.* Philadelphia: Saunders.
10. Horne, M. M., Easterday-Heitz, U., & Swearingen, P. L. (1997). *Pocket guide to fluid, electrolyte, and acid-base balance* (3rd ed.). St. Louis: Mosby.
11. Humes, H. D. (1997). Approach to the patient with renal disease. In W. N. Kelley (Ed.), *Textbook of internal medicine* (3rd ed.). Philadelphia: Lippincott-Raven.
12. Kokko, J. P., & Tannen, R. L. (1996). *Fluids and electrolytes* (3rd ed.). Philadelphia: Saunders.
13. Metheny, N. M. (1996). *Fluid and electrolyte balance* (3rd ed.). Philadelphia: Lippincott-Raven.
14. Mundy, G. R., & Reasner, C. A. (1998). Physiology of bone and mineral homeostasis. In J. H. Stein (Ed.), *Internal medicine* (5th ed.). St. Louis: Mosby.
15. Narins, R. G., Faber, M. D., & Krishna, G. G. (1998). Disorders of water balance. In J. H. Stein (Ed.), *Internal medicine* (5th ed.) St. Louis: Mosby.
16. Narins, R. G. (Ed.). (1994). *Maxwell and Kleeman's clinical disorders of fluid and electrolyte metabolism* (5th ed.). New York: McGraw-Hill.
17. Poston, S. O., & Mitch, W. E. (1998). The heart and kidney disease. In R. C. Schlant, R. W. Alexander, & V. Fuster (Eds.), *The heart, arteries and veins* (9th ed.). New York: McGraw-Hill.
18. Preston, R. A. (1997). *Acid-base, fluids, and electrolytes made ridiculously simple.* Philadelphia: MedMaster.
19. Rose, B. D. (1994). *Clinical physiology of acid-base and electrolyte disorders* (4th ed.). New York: McGraw-Hill.
20. Schlant, R. C., & Sonnenblick, E. H. (1998). Normal physiology of the cardiovascular system and pathophysiology of heart failure. In R. C. Schlant, R. W. Alexander, & V. Fuster, *The heart, arteries and veins* (9th ed.). New York: McGraw-Hill.
21. Shoemaker, W. C. (1994). Fluids and electrolytes in the acutely ill adult. In W. C. Shoemaker (Ed.), *Textbook of critical care* (3rd ed.). Philadelphia: Saunders.
22. Sterns, R. H., & Narins, R. G. (1998). Disorders of potassium balance. In J. H. Stein (Ed.), *Internal medicine* (5th. ed.). St. Louis: Mosby.
23. Tortora, G., & Grabowski, S. R. (1997). *Principles of anatomy and physiology* (8th ed.). New York: HarperCollins.
24. Vander, A. (1995). *Renal physiology* (5th ed.). New York: McGraw-Hill.
25. Whitney, E. N., Cataldo, C. B., & Rolfes, S. R. (1994). *Understanding normal and clinical nutrition* (4th ed.). St. Paul, MN: West.
26. Ziyadeh, F. N. (1998). Disorders of phosphate homeostasis. In J. H. Stein (Ed.), *Internal medicine* (5th. ed.) St. Louis: Mosby.

Chapter 7

Normal and Altered Nutritional Balance

Roberta Anding

KEY TERMS

anabolic
basal metabolic rate (BMR)
catabolic
chylomicron
cortisol
deamination
essential amino acids
gluconeogenesis
glyconeolysis
insulin resistance
ketosis
linoleic acid
negative nitrogen balance
serotonin
transamination
triglyceride

Nutritional balance is a major factor in promoting health and preventing disease. Balance can be altered by increased or decreased need and excessive or deficient quantities of macro- or micronutrients. The macronutrients—carbohydrates, proteins, and fats—provide calories and other essential materials. The micronutrients—vitamins, minerals, and ultratrace minerals—provide cofactors required for metabolism. Electrolytes and water balance, central to nutritional balance, are discussed in Chapter 6. Water is essential for the absorption of nutrients, elimination of metabolic waste products, and hydration. Absorption and nutrient metabolism are also discussed in Chapters 25 and 26.

Alterations of nutritional balance affect all of the body processes and are discussed throughout the text. The nutritional problems associated with malnutrition and obesity are included in this chapter because they affect functioning of all body systems.

MACRONUTRIENTS

Macronutrients include carbohydrates, proteins, and fats. These essential nutrients are found in dietary intake and provide the substrates for metabolism for essential body processes.

Carbohydrates

Carbohydrates are the principle sources for energy in the body. They are composed of carbon, hydrogen, and oxygen. Although a minimum recommended dietary allowance (RDA) for carbohydrates has not been established (because the body synthesizes glucose from amino acid and the glycerol component of fat), leading governmental and health agencies recommend an intake of up to 60% of total calories.[2,22] Dietary carbohydrate yields 4 calories per gram (kcal/g). Dextrose administered intravenously in its liquid form yields 3 to 4 kcal/g.[78] Box 7-1 provides an application of this principle.

CLASSIFICATION

The simpler forms of carbohydrates, called simple sugars, are the mono- and disaccharides. *Monosaccharides* have one sugar unit and include glucose, fructose, and galactose. *Disaccharides* are composed of two sugar units and include sucrose, lactose, and maltose. The more complex carbohydrates are classified as *polysaccharides,* which by definition contain 10 or more monosaccharide units. They are classified as starches and dietary fiber (see below). *Oligosaccharides* are intermediate carbohydrates containing 3 to 10 sugar units. Oligosaccharides are significant in clinical nutrition because they are found in many tube feedings or enteral products.[48] Carbohydrate

CLINICAL CORRELATION

Calculation of Carbohydrate Calories in Intravenous Solutions

1,000 mL of 5% dextrose and water solution yields:

$$\frac{5\text{ g}}{100\text{ mL}} \qquad \frac{50\text{ g}}{1{,}000\text{ mL}}$$

50 g dextrose/1,000 mL × 3.4 kcal/g = 170 kcal/1,000 mL

is stored in the liver and muscle as glycogen, which is also referred to as animal starch. Table 7-1 lists the forms of carbohydrate and food sources.

DIGESTION, METABOLISM, AND FUNCTION

The digestion of carbohydrates is illustrated in Figure 7-1. They are digested more quickly than the other macro-nutrients and more than 90% of dietary intake is digested.[20]

The metabolism of carbohydrate for the most part depends on insulin (a pancreatic hormone) transporting glucose into the cells. Much of the glucose is oxidized to provide energy for all the tissues. Some glucose is converted to other carbohydrates and as a skeleton for nonessential amino acids, or protein building blocks. Excess glucose can be converted to fatty acids (for storage) or to glycogen.

The primary function of carbohydrates is to provide energy for body processes. Certain tissues of the body, particularly the brain and red blood cells, rely on glucose as a preferred energy source. In the absence of adequate carbohydrate, **gluconeogenesis** ensues to synthesize glucose from noncarbohydrate sources, primarily protein. Most gluconeogenesis occurs in the liver. Gluconeogenesis maintains blood sugar within normal limits. To prevent protein from being a substrate for gluconeogenesis the daily consumption of approximately of 100 g carbohydrate is necessary. The provision of adequate carbohydrate in the diet will also prevent **ketosis**, which can result from the rapid metabolism of fat.

DIETARY FIBER

Dietary fiber can be defined as the nonstarch polysaccharides that remain undigested or partially digested as they enter the large intestine. Fiber includes cellulose, hemicellulose, gums, pectin, and mucilages. Current estimates of adult intake of fiber in the United States indicate a consumption of about 13 g/day with recommended goals for adults being between 25 and 30 g.[2] The recommended amounts for children range from their current age plus 5 g/day to their age plus 10 g/day.[80]

The classification of fiber can be based on its physiologic function. There are two distinct types: water insoluble and water soluble. *Water-insoluble fibers* include cellulose and hemicellulose and are hydrophilic (attracting water) in nature. With sufficient fluid, insoluble fiber contributes to fecal bulking and prevents constipation. *Water-soluble fibers* include pectin, gums, and mucilages. They have the ability to form gels and serve as substrate for fermentation by intestinal bacteria. Pectin increases the viscosity of chyme (form of food that has been pulverized and mixed with stomach acid and enzymes), delaying gastric emptying time and glucose absorption. Water-soluble fiber also exerts a hypocholesterolemic effect through the adsorption of bile. Bile from the liver is composed of 70% cholesterol and is normally recycled via enterohepatic circulation. Enhanced excretion of bile may reduce serum choles-

TABLE 7-1

FOOD SOURCES FOR CARBOHYDRATES

TYPE OF CARBOHYDRATE	FOOD SOURCES
Monosaccharides	
Glucose	Breakdown of product (complex carbohydrates)
Fructose	Fruits, honey, corn syrup
Disaccharides	
Maltose	Grains
Lactose	Milk, milk products, filler in nondairy products
Sucrose	Sugar, honey, maple syrup
Oligosaccharides	Dried beans, peas (carbohydrate used in enteral medical nutrition products)
Polysaccharides	Breads, grains, starches

FOCUS ON CELLULAR PHYSIOLOGY

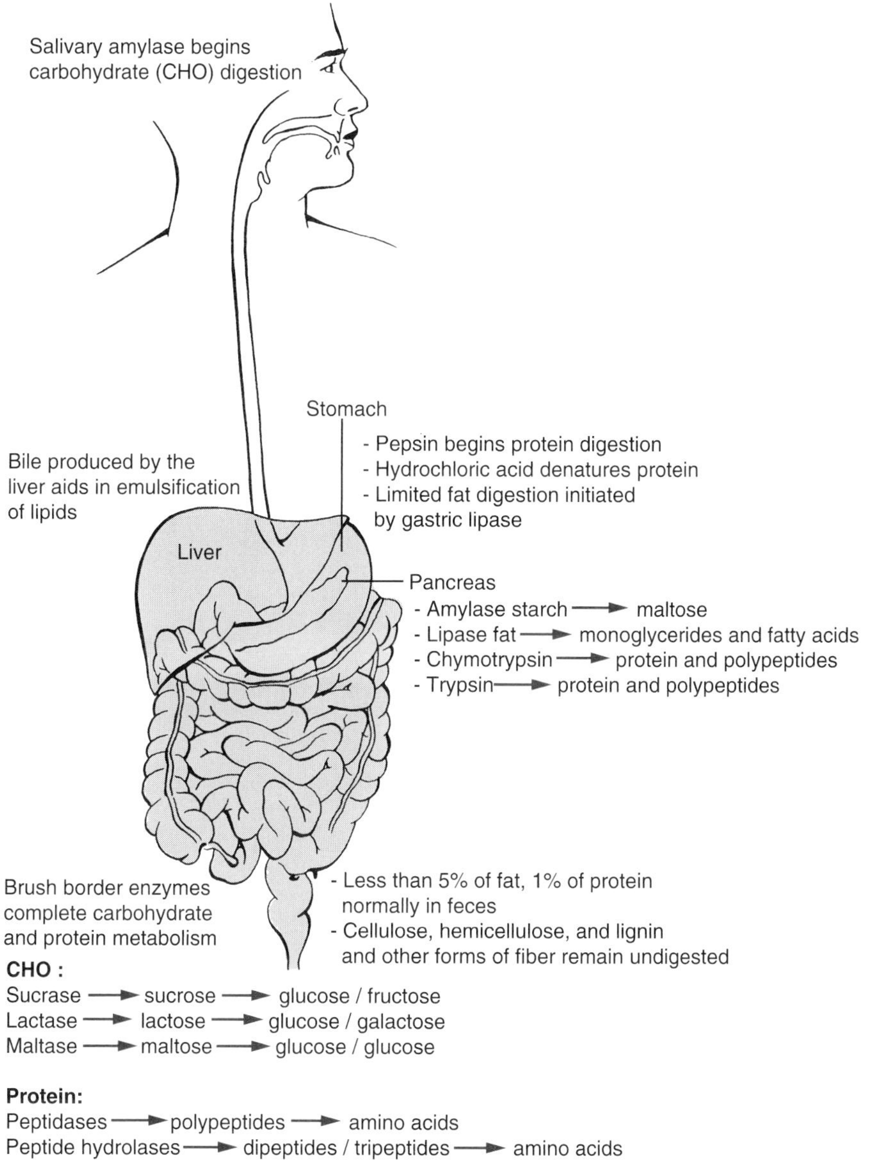
Salivary amylase begins
carbohydrate (CHO) digestion
Stomach
- Pepsin begins protein digestion
- Hydrochloric acid denatures protein
- Limited fat digestion initiated
by gastric lipase
Bile produced by the
liver aids in emulsification
of lipids
Liver
Pancreas
- Amylase starch → maltose
- Lipase fat → monoglycerides and fatty acids
- Chymotrypsin → protein and polypeptides
- Trypsin → protein and polypeptides
Brush border enzymes
complete carbohydrate
and protein metabolism
- Less than 5% of fat, 1% of protein
normally in feces
- Cellulose, hemicellulose, and lignin
and other forms of fiber remain undigested
CHO :
Sucrase → sucrose → glucose / fructose
Lactase → lactose → glucose / galactose
Maltase → maltose → glucose / glucose
Protein:
Peptidases → polypeptides → amino acids
Peptide hydrolases → dipeptides / tripeptides → amino acids

FIGURE 7-1. Summary of macronutrient digestion.

terol.[5] Table 7-2 lists the type, function, and representative food sources of both types of dietary fiber.

The proposed benefits of an adequate fiber intake include a decreased risk of constipation, diverticular disease, colon cancer, and cardiovascular disease. Increased fiber may also be used as an adjunct in the treatment of gastrointestinal disorders and diabetes. However, a sudden increase in dietary fiber may cause hyperstimulation of the bowel. Adaptation to a high-fiber diet occurs gradually and can be facilitated by increasing fluid intake. Large amounts of fiber, particularly with inadequate hydration, may cause *bezoars* (the accumulation of fiber in the stomach), intestinal obstruction, and the malabsorption of divalent cations, particularly calcium and zinc.

Proteins

The RDA for protein is 0.8 g/kg ideal body weight for healthy adults.[61] Protein requirements increase during periods of rapid growth and development such as infancy, pregnancy, and adolescence. The average intake

TABLE 7-2

MAJOR TYPES OF FIBER: THEIR SOURCES AND PHYSIOLOGIC EFFECTS

WATER-SOLUBLE FIBERS

	SOURCES
Gums	Oat bran and oatmeal Dried peas and beans
Pectin	Apples, citrus fruit, strawberries Dried peas Squash, cauliflower, cabbage, carrots, potatoes

PHYSIOLOGIC EFFECTS

Slow gastric emptying and intestinal transit time
Lower serum cholesterol levels
Delay glucose absorption, which helps improve glucose tolerance in diabetics

WATER-INSOLUBLE FIBERS

	SOURCES
Hemicellulose Cellulose	Wheat bran and whole grains and cereals Whole-wheat flour and wheat bran Vegetables: cabbage, peas, green beans, wax beans, broccoli, brussel sprouts, root vegetables Apples
Lignin	Cereals and wheat bran Mature vegetables Pears, strawberries Eggplant, green beans

PHYSIOLOGIC EFFECTS

Absorbs water to increase fecal bulk
Reduces pressure within the colon
Decreases intestinal transit time
Little effect on serum cholesterol or glucose

(Dudek, S. G. [1997]. *Nutrition handbook for nursing practice* [3rd ed.]. Philadelphia: Lippincott-Raven.)

of protein in the United States is 70 to 110 g, or about 1.5 times the needed amount. Protein must be consumed daily because there is no storage or reserve of protein in the body.

Proteins are composed or built from amino acids, which contain carbon, hydrogen, and oxygen atoms as well as nitrogen. The nitrogen fraction of the protein molecule is the amine group. Protein is the only macronutrient that contains nitrogen. Twenty amino acids are required by the body. Nine are dietary essentials because they cannot be synthesized in the body and are thus called essential amino acids. These **essential amino acids** (EAAs) must be ingested through the diet. If one EAA is lacking in the diet, nitrogen excretion exceeds nitrogen intake, causing a **negative nitrogen balance**. Eleven amino acids can be synthesized by the liver and are termed nonessential amino acids (Table 7-3).

CLASSIFICATION

Dietary protein can be classified as complete (high biologic value) or incomplete (low biologic value). *Complete proteins* contain all the EAAs in their proper proportion, indicating the ability to perform physiologically the functions of protein. *Incomplete proteins* (those lacking one or more EAA) will have their amino acids deaminated or used in transamination (see below). *Complimentary proteins*, or mutual supplementation, result from combining two incomplete proteins that are deficient in one or more EAA, thereby improving over-

TABLE 7-3

AMINO ACIDS

ESSENTIAL	NONESSENTIAL
Histidine	Alanine
Isoleucine	Arginine
Leucine	Asparagine
Lysine	Aspartic acid
Methionine	Cystine (cysteine)
Phenylalanine	Glutamic acid
Threonine	Glutamine
Tryptophan	Glycine
Valine	Hydroxyproline
	Hydroxylysine
	Proline
	Serine
	Tyrosine

(Dudek, S. G. [1997]. *Nutrition handbook for nursing practice* [3rd ed.]. Philadelphia: Lippincott-Raven.)

all protein quality. Box 7-2 lists examples of complementary proteins.

DIGESTION, METABOLISM, AND FUNCTION

The digestion of protein begins in the stomach; however, pancreatic and small intestinal proteases hydrolyze intact proteins into tripeptides, dipeptides, and free amino acids for absorption. This process is outlined in Figure 7-1. The metabolism of protein is controlled predominantly by the liver. Two significant reactions occur. **Deamination** is the process by which the amine group is removed from the amino acid molecule. The carbon skeleton that remains can be converted to some of the same intermediates formed during glucose and fatty acid metabolism. Deamination is the first step in the process of gluconeogenesis. Approximately 58% of the amino acids can be converted to glucose if the need arises. **Transamination** is the process by which nonessential amino acids are synthesized. The amine group is transferred from one amino acid to a suitable carbon skeleton.

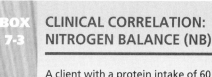

BOX 7-2 EXAMPLES OF COMPLEMENTARY PROTEINS

Rice and beans
Croutons and split pea soup
Tortilla and beans
Corn bread and chili beans
Chick peas and tahini (sesame seed)
Tofu and sesame seeds

The end-products of protein metabolism therefore depend on the process of deamination or transamination. Through deamination the amine group is converted from ammonia to urea for ultimate excretion by the kidney. The end-product of transamination is the synthesis of new amino acids.

All protein is functional. Any loss of protein represents loss of function. The primary function of protein is to build and repair tissue. Protein also:

- Provides energy at 4/kcal/g
- Forms enzymes, hormones, cells, and antibodies
- Transports lipids, vitamins, drugs, and other substances
- Maintains normal osmotic forces in the blood

When the body becomes depleted of protein, the magnitude of the loss is manifested by increasing degrees of loss of function.

Nitrogen Balance

Nitrogen balance (NB) is the amount of protein required to allow for normal physiologic functioning. NB studies are useful in determining the amount of protein required to remain in nitrogen homeostasis (ie, to achieve or maintain a positive NB). NB, which measures intake minus excretion, can be calculated by the following formula:

Intake: protein intake in grams = g nitrogen
6.25 (protein is 16% nitrogen)
Output: urinary urea nitrogen + 4g (losses through lungs, hair, skin, nails, and feces)
NB = intake − output

The clinical correlation in Box 7-3 illustrates this calculation. Figure 7-2 summarizes the concept of nitrogen equilibrium and those factors that can produce a positive or negative balance. Certain disease states alter protein requirements needed to maintain NB. These diseases and their protein requirements are summarized in Table 7-4.

BOX 7-3 CLINICAL CORRELATION: NITROGEN BALANCE (NB)

A client with a protein intake of 60 g in 24 hours has a urinary urea nitrogen loss of 10 g/24 h.
NB = 60 g protein
6.25 g (16% of protein is nitrogen)
NB = 9.6–(10 g + 4 g in skin, feces)–4.4
This client is in negative nitrogen balance.

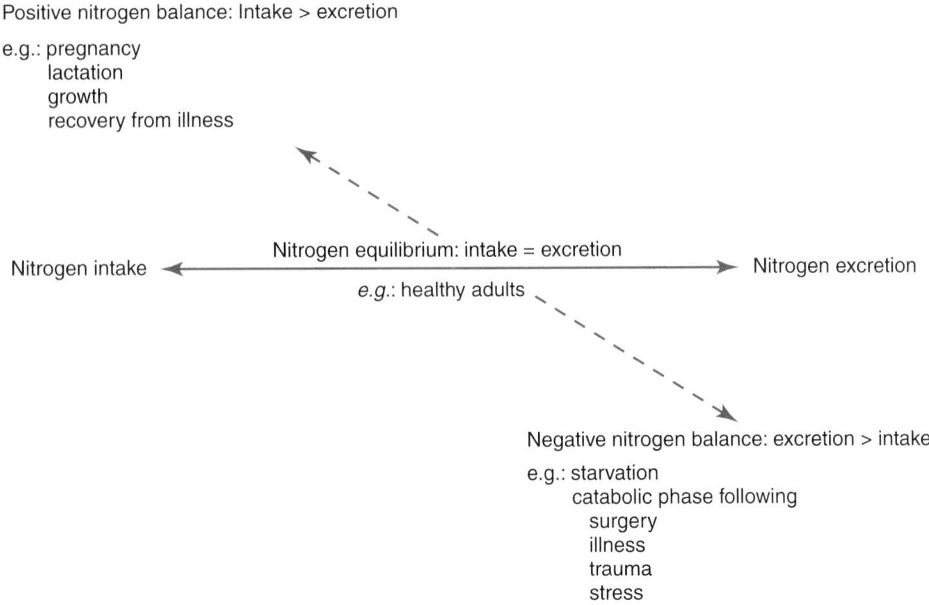

FIGURE 7-2. **States of nitrogen balance.**

Lipids

In the United States the current intake of lipid or fat for adults is approximately 34% of total calories. A national dietary goal is to decrease total fat consumption to less than 30% of total calories.[46] Although total fat intake remains above the national goal, physiologic requirements for essential fatty acids (those that must be consumed in the diet) is quite low, approximately 4% of total calories.

FATTY ACIDS

Fat is composed mostly of fatty acid, which is a substance made up of a chain of carbon atoms, hydrogen atoms, and some oxygen atoms. Fatty acids are grouped into saturated, monounsaturated, and polyunsaturated fats based on the degree to which hydrogen saturates the molecule. Trans fatty acids are a special group formed by the partial hydrogenation of a polyunsaturated vegetable oil, which change the shape of the fatty acid.

TABLE 7-4

ALTERATIONS IN PROTEIN REQUIREMENTS IN SELECT DISEASE STATES

DISEASE	PROTEIN REQUIREMENTS
Renal disease	
Early renal failure (serum creatinine 2–6 mg/mL)	0.6 g/kg (75% human biologic value—HBV)
Advanced renal failure	0.3 g/kg
Dialysis—hemo	1.0–1.2
peritoneal	1.2–1.5
Nephrotic syndrome	0.6 g plus urinary losses
Neoplastic disease	1.5–2.5 g/kg
Liver disease	
Hepatic encephalopathy	50 g/d with increased amounts of branched-chain amino acids
Cirrhosis with encephalopathy	Decreased amino acids 0.8g–1.0 g/kg
Trauma	1.0–1.5 g/kg
Sepsis	1.5–2.0 g/kg

Saturated Fatty Acids

Saturated fats or fatty acids are those that solidify at room temperature. These fatty acids can be of plant and animal origin. The molecules have no double bonds. Dietary sources include coconut oil, palm oil, and animal fats. A national goal for saturated fatty acids is to limit consumption to less than 10% of total energy intake. Saturated fats are the most atherogenic (atherosclerosis-causing) family of fatty acids. The Lipid Research Coronary Primary Prevention Trial, a classic study, demonstrated that decreasing saturated fat has a direct impact on reducing serum cholesterol values.[26]

Monosaturated Fatty Acids

Monounsaturated fats contain a single double bond. Dietary sources include olive oil, peanut oil, and canola (rapeseed) oil. Monounsaturated fats can lower serum cholesterol, although the exact mechanism is not known.[25]

Polyunsaturated Fatty Acids

Polyunsaturated fats are long-chain fatty acids with two or more double bonds. These fatty acids are liquid at room temperature and are found in vegetable oils and cold water fish. This family of fatty acids includes the essential fatty acids; linoleic (ω-6 fatty acid) and α-linolenic (ω-3 fatty acid), which must be consumed in the diet. The physiologic function of these essential fatty acids is structurally in the phospholipid layer in the cell wall and as precursors to prostaglandins, thromboxane, and prostacyclins (a group of hormone-like compounds involved in immune function, the inflammatory response, blood pressure regulation, the onset of labor, and blood clotting). There are two major classifications of polyunsaturated fats: the ω-6 and ω-3 whose functions are summarized in Table 7-5.

Trans Fatty Acids

Trans fatty acids are formed by the partial hydrogenation of a polyunsaturated vegetable oil. Hydrogenation solidifies the oil and increases shelf-life of the food. However, during this process the double bonds change from the normal *cis* configuration to the *trans* isomer. Data are emerging that trans fatty acids are associated with an increase in serum cholesterol and triglyceride concentrations thereby increasing the risk of coronary artery disease.[47] Trans fatty acids have also been implicated in other disease processes including preeclampsia.[81]

CLASSIFICATION OF FAT

Important forms of lipids include triglycerides, phospholipids, cholesterol, and lipoproteins. These can be ingested in the diet or synthesized by body processes.

Triglycerides

Triglyceride molecules have three fatty acids attached to a glycerol molecule and compose most of the lipids in food.[20] They are stored in adipose tissue to be available for energy supply.

Phospholipids

These lipids are composed of two fatty acid molecules and a phosphate group bound to a glycerol molecule. They are used as cellular structural components and in the liver and nervous system. They are found in most foods and are soluble in fat and somewhat soluble in water. This allows their use as emulsifiers in different food products.

Cholesterol

Cholesterol is a lipid in sterol form (part of a family that includes bile acids, sex hormones, and adrenocortical hormones) that is found in animal products only. There is no requirement for dietary cholesterol as humans synthesize cholesterol when dietary supply is inadequate. The most concentrated sources of cholesterol include liver, egg yolk, whole milk dairy products, beef, and pork. The physiologic functions of cholesterol include its presence as a structural component of the cell membrane and utilization as a precursor sub-

TABLE 7-5

EFFECTS OF PRODUCTS MADE FROM OMEGA-3 (ω-3) AND OMEGA-6 (ω-6) FATTY ACIDS IN MAN

SITE OF SYNTHESIS	ω-6 (LINOLEIC ACID)	ω-3 (EPA, DHA)
Cells lining blood vessels	Form prostaglandin I_2, which inhibits blood clotting	Form prostaglandin I_3, which inhibits blood clotting
Platelets* in the blood	Form thromboxane A_2, which is a strong promoter of blood clotting	Form thromboxane A_3, which is a very weak promoter of blood clotting

The net result is that ω-3 fatty acids reduce the tendency for blood to clot.
*Plate-like fragments in the bloodstream that contribute to blood clotting.
(Source: Wardlaw G. M., & Insel, P. M. [1990]. *Perspectives in nutrition.* St. Louis, Toronto, Boston: Times Mirror/Mosby.)

stance for estrogen, androgens, progesterone, cortisol, aldosterone, and vitamin D synthesis. Excess cholesterol is an important factor in the development of atherosclerosis (see page 433). Its regulation is usually very dependent on dietary intake of fats.

Lipoproteins

These molecules are compound lipids that contain both protein and various types and amounts of lipids. They are synthesized mostly in the liver and can transport insoluble lipids in the blood.[20] The lipoproteins are classified based on density into **chylomicrons**, very low-density lipoproteins, low-density lipoproteins (LDL), and high-density lipoproteins (see page 433).

DIGESTION OF FATS

Digestion of fat (mainly triglycerides) requires many steps and depends on the length of the carbon chain of the molecule. Short-chain fatty acids are those with six or fewer carbons in the chain. Medium-chain fatty acids have between 8 and 14 chains. Long-chain fatty acids have between 16 and 27 carbons. Short- and medium-chain fatty acids are water soluble and absorbed directly into the portal blood, thereby bypassing the digestion needed for the water-insoluble long-chain fats. Box 7-4 provides insight into the use of medium-chain fatty acids in clinical nutrition.

The digestion of long-chain fatty acids requires:

- Bile: to mix or emulsify the insoluble fats with the aqueous contents of the intestinal tract
- Micelle formation: the complex formed in the combining of fatty acids with bile
- Lipase: to cleave or shorten the molecules into smaller components
- Chylomicron formation or the transport vehicle that delivers the fatty acid complex to the lymphatic system

Figure 7-1 provides a summary of fat digestion. The liver is the principal organ for regulation of fat metabolism and synthesis of the transport vehicle for fatty acids, which are the lipoproteins. In the liver, fatty acids can be shortened or lengthened before they are released into circulation. As with carbohydrate, insulin is a major mediator of fat oxidation and storage. However, only 10% of the triglyceride molecule is available to be converted to glucose via gluconeogenesis.

FUNCTION

Calorically, fats are the most concentrated form of energy, supplying 9 kcal/g. In addition to providing calories, lipids also:

- Are sources of the essential fatty acids, **linoleic acid** and linolenic acid
- Contribute to satiety or a feeling of fullness
- Protect internal organs
- Contribute to the flavor and palatability of food
- Facilitate the absorption of fat-soluble vitamins
- Serve as precursors to the *eicosanoids*, a group of biologically active 20-carbon hormone-like compounds
- Provide a substrate for hormones, especially the steroid hormones
- Provide insulation of the body from excessive heat and cold
- Serve as an energy reserve

MICRONUTRIENTS

The micronutrients include the water-soluble and fat-soluble vitamins as well as the minerals. Vitamins are organic substances that help regulate thousands of body processes by assisting synthesis of various compounds. Minerals are inorganic elements and function as structural components in the body and help to regulate body processes. As opposed to the macronutrients, the micronutrients yield no energy but rather act as cofactors in metabolism.

Water-Soluble Vitamins

Water-soluble vitamins are those that are not stored in the body in appreciable amounts. Excesses are excreted readily in the urine. Due to their limited storage, daily or regular intake is necessary. Water-soluble vitamins include the B vitamins and vitamin C.

Disease states can significantly alter the need for water-soluble vitamins. Although excesses are excreted

BOX 7-4 CLINICAL USES OF MEDIUM-CHAIN FATTY ACIDS

Medium-chain fatty acids, also known as medium-chain triglycerides (MCTs), are useful in fat malabsorption syndromes. These oils do not require bile or lipase for digestion and can be used for extra calories when needed. MCTs do not contain essential fatty acids.

Diseases in which administration of MCT oils may be used for extra calories include:

- Pancreatitis
- Cirrhosis of the liver
- Inflammatory bowel disease
- Acquired immunodeficiency syndrome

in the urine, large amounts or megadoses can contribute to toxicity. A megadose is defined as 10 times the RDA. Table 7-6 summarizes the RDAs, function, food sources, deficiency disease or condition, signs and symptoms of the deficiency, factors altering requirements, and toxicity manifestations of water-soluble vitamins.

Fat-Soluble Vitamins

Fat-soluble vitamins are those vitamins absorbed along with the fats in food and stored in fatty tissues of the body. Fat-soluble vitamins are A, D, E, and K. Because these vitamins are stored in the body, short-term deficiencies have little effect on health and the development of deficiency symptoms occurs over time. Deficiency states may occur more rapidly in persons with steatorrhea (fat malabsorption). Toxicity symptoms may occur at levels as low as 10 times the RDA. Table 7-7 lists the fat-soluble vitamins, chemical name, RDAs, function, food sources, deficiency diseases, factors influencing regulation, signs and symptoms of the deficiency, and toxicity.

Minerals

Minerals are inorganic compounds that are vital in human nutrition and cell function. Minerals have many physiologic roles; some, such as calcium, serve structural roles, whereas others, such as magnesium, are involved in muscular contraction and nerve excitability. As a group, minerals also function:

- As cofactors in enzymatic reactions
- To maintain acid–base balance
- To maintain osmotic pressure
- To transfer essential compounds across cell membranes

Mineral balance is affected by interactions of minerals with other dietary components and by the presence of other minerals. For example, large doses of iron can reduce zinc absorption and supplemental doses of zinc can reduce copper absorption.

Minerals can be classified by the amount required by the body. Macrominerals are those with essential intake needs of greater than 100 mg/day. Microminerals are those required in small amounts and are also termed trace or ultratrace minerals. The macro- and microminerals are listed in Table 7-8. The functions, RDAs, food sources, deficiency states, factors influencing requirements, signs and symptoms of deficiency, and toxicity of specific minerals are presented in Table 7-9. The activities of other minerals are covered in detail in other areas of the text.

Antioxidants

Antioxidants are a select group of vitamins and minerals that protect the cell membrane from damage. The antioxidants include vitamin E, vitamin C, β-carotene (precursor to vitamin A), and selenium.

Proposed benefits of antioxidants include retardation of the aging process, cancer prevention, immune enhancement, and reduction of cardiovascular disease. The strongest evidence for antioxidants and disease prevention is reduction of coronary artery disease and cancer incidence. Epidemiologic studies have demonstrated a reduction of morbidity and mortality from coronary artery disease with supplemental vitamins E and C. The proposed mechanism of action is that potent antioxidants prevent the oxidation of LDL cholesterol, the most atherogenic of the cholesterol carrying proteins. Oxidized LDL becomes converted to foam cells and stimulates the binding of monocytes to the endothelial wall[17] (see page 434).

Antioxidants have a significant role in the prevention of cancer, but this role is site specific. Additionally, high doses of β-carotene may actually increase the risk of lung cancer in high-risk individuals.[73]

Examples of site-specific prevention include:

- Selenium and prostate cancer[11]
- Vitamin C and oral cancer[10]
- Vitamin E and colon cancer[67]

SIGNS OF NUTRITIONAL BALANCE

Nutritional balance promotes health and prevents disease. Good nutritional status is manifested through various physical and emotional signs, as shown in Box 7-5. An alteration in any of the physical and emotional signs of good nutrition may indicate systemic disorders, food allergies, malnutrition, or obesity. Specific measurements of nutritional status are discussed within the appropriate alterations section and throughout the text.

MALNUTRITION

Malnutrition is defined as an inadequate intake of macronutrients or micronutrients that causes impairment of the physiologic function of the body. It may be the result of inadequate intake, excessive losses, or increased requirements. The incidence of malnutrition has been estimated to affect 50% of hospitalized patients.[78]

Protein-calorie malnutrition (PCM) is a continuum with *marasmus* (starvation or semistarvation) at one end and *kwashiorkor* (protein deficiency, also known as hypoalbuminemic malnutrition) at the other (Fig. 7-3). PCM, as seen in the hospitalized patient, is generally classified into three categories:

(text continues on page 201)

TABLE 7-6

FUNCTIONS AND ALTERATIONS IN WATER-SOLUBLE VITAMINS

VITAMIN	RDA	FUNCTION	FOOD SOURCES	DEFICIENCY	FACTORS INFLUENCING REQUIREMENTS	SIGNS AND SYMPTOMS	TOXICITY
Vitamin B Thiamine	1.0–1.5 mg	Metabolism through oxidative reaction	Pork, whole grains, organ meats	Beriberi, chronic alcoholism	Alcoholism, fever, infection, hyperthyroidism, burns, trauma, chronic antacid use	Anorexia, fatigue, peripheral neuropathy, footdrop, cardiomegaly, depression	Nausea and vomiting
Riboflavin	1.2–1.7 mg	Coenzyme flavin, mononucleotide, citric acid, beta-oxidation	Milk, dairy products	Cheilosis, ariboflavinosis	Thyroid dysfunction, burns, trauma, diabetes, alcoholism, oral contraceptives, tricyclic antidepressants	Seborrheic dermatitis, scrotal dermatitis, growth failure, photophobia	None known
Niacin	13–19 mg	Coenzyme NAD, NADP, formation of ATP, oxidation/ reduction, reactions, immune competence	Mushrooms, enriched grain products, tuna, chicken, can be synthesized from dietary tryptophan	Pellegra	Alcohol, thyroid disorders, neoplasia, isoniazid for tuberculosis burns	Diarrhea, dermatitis, dementia, weakness, fatigue	In large amounts, nicotinic acid functions as a vasodilator; nausea, vomiting, hypocholesterolemic effect
Pyridoxine (B_6)	1.6–2.0 mg	Coenzyme form, pyridoxical phosphate, transamination of amino acids, synthesis of hemoglobin, neurotransmitter synthesis	Meat, fish, poultry, bananas, cantaloupe, broccoli	Irritability, depression	Uremia, burns, advancing age, neoplastic disease, liver disease medication, uremia, isoniazid, hydralazine, high protein diets, asthma, degenerative diseases	Stomatitis, glossitis, cheilosis, anemia (after prolonged deficiency)	Irreversible nerve damage, ataxia

Folic acid	180–200μg	One carbon transfer reaction, synthesis of RBC, nucleotides, RNA, DNA, proteins	Orange juice, liver, green leafy vegetables	Megaloblastic anemia/macrocytic anemia	Fevers, burns, alcoholism, ileal disease, inflammatory bowel disease, gluten-induced enteropathy, gastrectomies, periods of increased growth, medications, methotrexates, common deficiency in elderly, adolescent females	Smooth, sore tongue; dementia; diarrhea; weight loss	May mask B_{12} deficiency
B_{12}	2μg	Coenzyme transfer of methyl (CH_3) groups, synthesis of nucleic acids and choline, RBC formation	Animal protein	Megaloblastic anemia, pernicious anemia	Vegetarian, gastrectomy patients, ileal resection, gastric bypass surgery, intestinal parasites, medications such as neomycin, potassium chloride	Loss of appetite, weight loss, glossites, leukopenia, thrombocytopenia, tingling in extremities, dementia	None known
Vitamin C (ascorbic acid)	60 mg	Collagen formation, cartilage formation, synthesis of bile, acts as a reducing agent, wound healing	Green peppers, citrus fruit, strawberries, broccoli, cabbage	Scurvy	Cigarette smoking, alcoholic, oral contraceptive users, cancer, surgical patients, burns	Capillary fragility, hemorrhagic disorders, fatigue, anorexia, muscle pain, gingivitis	Diarrhea, nausea, excess converted to oxalate and form kidney stones, interfere with urine glucose tests, rebound scurvy

ATP, adenosine triphosphate; NAD, nicotinamide adenine dinucleotide; NADP, nicotinamide adenine dinucleotide phosphate; RBC, red blood cell.

TABLE 7-7

FUNCTIONS AND ALTERATIONS IN FAT-SOLUBLE VITAMINS

VITAMIN	RDA	FUNCTION	FOOD SOURCES	DEFICIENCY	FACTORS INFLUENCING REQUIREMENTS	SIGNS AND SYMPTOMS	TOXICITY
Vitamin A (retinoids) beta carotene (precursor)	800–1000 µg	Visual adaptation adrenal hormone biosynthesis, mucopolysaccharide and glycoprotein synthesis, maintenance of epithelial structure, wound healing, immunocompetence	Whole milk, butter, carrots	Xerophthalmia	Preterm infants, gastrointestinal dysfunction, respiratory ailments, burns, trauma	Night blindness, keratinization of epithelial cells, diarrhea	Nausea, vomiting, alopecia, hypercalcemia, long bone tenderness, pregnant women and persons with chronic renal disease may be more susceptible
Vitamin D cholecalciferol, synthesized via ultraviolet light	5–10µg	Absorption of calcium and phosphorus, calcium reabsorption from kidney, removal of calcium and phosphorus from bone, immunoregulatory	Milk, dairy products	Rickets, osteomalacia	Tropical sprue, regional enteritis, pancreatic insufficiency, gastric resection, jejunoileal bypass, chronic renal failure, hypoparathyroidism, medications (anticonvulsants, cimetidine, isoniazid), total parenteral nutrition	Bone pain, increased serum alkaline phosphatase, decreased serum calcium, levels, bone demineralization	Nausea, vomiting, anorexia, headache, diarrhea, conclusion, calcification of soft tissue
Vitamin E (tocopherols)	8–10 mg	Antioxidant, cell membrane integrity, immunoregulatory	Vegetable oil	Hemolytic anemia	Increased intake of polyunsaturated fats, steatorrhea, protein calorie malnutrition, infancy, cystic fibrosis, short bowel syndrome, respiratory distress syndrome, retrolental fibroplasia, bronchopulmonary dysplasia, smoking	Increased platelet aggregation, neurological abnormalities, decreased serum creatinine, excessive creatinuria	Nausea, headache, antagonist to vitamin K
Vitamin K (phylloquinone) diet (menoquinone) gut flora	65–80 µg	Clotting factors	Greens, broccoli, cauliflower	Hemorrhagic disease	Stage of life cycle (newborn, elderly), renal failure, ulcerative colitis, chronic pancreatitis, biliary dysfunction, medications (antibiotics, coumadin, cholestyramine)	Prolonged bleeding times	With prescription menadione, jaundice, anemia

MARASMUS. This is semistarvation caused by poor intake, where fat and muscle via gluconeogenesis provide most of the calories for survival. It is characterized by a reduction of body weight but a preservation of serum proteins and immune competence unless it is very severe. The maintenance of serum proteins is at the expense of somatic (muscle) and visceral (organ) protein. Figure 7-4 illustrates the presence of severe marasmus.

KWASHIORKOR. Kwashiorkor means "the disease that the first child gets when the second one comes" and is typically seen in underdeveloped countries where children are weaned from the breast to a protein-poor gruel[65] (Fig. 7-5). The pathophysiology of kwashiorkor is evidenced by a low ratio of protein to calories. Clinically, a "flaky paint" dermatitis, hair changes, and systemic edema are seen (see Fig. 7-5). Hypoalbuminemic malnutrition, or hospital-based kwashiorkor, develops in persons who have the stress of injury or infection with poor intake or inappropriate nutritional support. There is a generalized protein loss with increasing impairment of visceral function, evidenced by a decrease in immunocompetence and hypoalbuminemia. This condition is also known as stressed starvation.

COMBINED MALNUTRITION. Combined marasmus and kwashiorkor is commonly seen in the elderly or in persons with chronic disease. The stress of illness or trauma with protein depletion is superimposed on a marasmic individual. Survival rates are poor without early nutritional intervention.

Calorie Reserves in Starvation

During starvation, physiologic sources of calories include glycogen (stored carbohydrate), somatic and visceral protein, and fat. In the early hours of a fast, glycogen serves as the primary energy source. Metabolism favors glucose homeostasis to support tissues dependent on glucose as a sole energy source, which include the brain, nerves, red blood cells, and renal medulla. During the initial stage of starvation, a fall in arterial blood glucose levels causes a decrease in insulin, which is a major **anabolic** hormone. As insulin levels fall, the levels of the counterregulatory or **catabolic** hormones increase. The major catabolic hormone involved in the process is glucagon (see page 663). The decrease in the insulin/glucagon ratio stimulates **glycogenolysis** and the release of hepatic glucose. The process of glycogenolysis is the major source of glucose for approximately 24 hours. Gluconeogenesis from protein serves as the major source of glucose after the initial stage of starvation. Urinary excretion of nitrogen (from protein catabolism) increases as daily losses of 12 g nitrogen become common. As the fast continues, the decreased level of insulin allows lipolysis, the release and oxidation of free fatty acids, and synthesis of ketones. The brain cannot use free fatty acids because fatty acids do not cross the blood–brain barrier. Ketones and ketoacids, released in fat oxidation, can cross the blood–brain barrier and serve as alternative energy sources for the brain, a major consumer of glucose. This process is known as *ketoadaptation*.[82] The rate of protein breakdown is slowed, and urinary nitrogen losses become approximately 3 to 5 g/day. Serum proteins, such as albumin (also known as the proteins of homeostasis), are preserved until the individual is close to death and fat reserves are exhausted. At this point, gluconeogenesis increases, nitrogen excretion increases, and death is likely.[80]

TABLE 7-8

MINERALS

MACROMINERALS (RDA >100 MG/D)	MICROMINERALS (RDA <100 MG/D)
Calcium	Iron
Phosphorus	Copper
Sodium	Zinc
Potassium	Manganese
Magnesium	Iodine
Chlorine	Molybdenum
Sulfur	Fluorine
	Selenium
	Cobalt

Losses of skeletal lean body mass as well as from metabolically active tissue such as the gut and pancreas reduces caloric need and slows the rate of deterioration. Fatigue is common and reduces the level of voluntary movement, again reducing caloric need. A decrease in cardiac workload and bradycardia contribute to the overall decrease in **basal metabolic rate (BMR)**.

Nutritional / Metabolic Consequences of Stress

Hypoalbuminemic malnutrition, or stressed starvation, has a profound effect on body composition, protein use, and organ function. Neuroendocrine control mechanisms are altered and mediate changes in nutritional status. Increases in catecholamines as well as increased levels of glucagon increase the blood glucose level. Hyperglycemia in stress is often referred to as "stress diabetes." The hyperglycemia does stimulate insulin release, but **insulin resistance** coupled with increases in glucagon levels, allows hyperglycemia to persist. Gluconeogenesis is accentuated, and losses of protein continue at a greater rate than with simple starvation alone.

TABLE 7-9

FUNCTIONS AND ALTERATIONS IN SELECTED MINERALS

MINERAL	RDA	FUNCTION	FOOD SOURCES	DEFICIENCY	FACTORS INFLUENCING REQUIREMENTS	SIGNS AND SYMPTOMS	TOXICITY
Zinc	12–15 mg	Ligand in albumin, nucleotides, thymus integrity, cellular immunity, sexual maturation	Oysters, wheat germ, crab, shrimp, red meat	Growth retardation, delayed secondary sex characteristics	Trauma, burns, surgery, inflammatory bowel, short bowel syndrome, increased intake of fiber, recovery from malnutrition, total parenteral nutrition	Hair loss, inflammation of skin, poor wound healing, decreased taste	Decreased use of copper, iron decrease in HDL cholesterol; diarrhea; nausea and vomiting; immunosuppression
Copper	1.5–3 mg	Component of enzymes of iron metabolism, cross-binding of collagen, myelination of nerves	Meat, liver, cocoa, legumes, nuts, affected by soil conditions	Rare, induced by copper; free total parenteral nutrition; microcytic hypochromic anemia; increased serum cholesterol levels	Short bowel, chronic diarrhea, Crohn's disease, celiac disease, burns, antacids, high zinc intake	Skeletal demineralization, impaired glucose tolerance, depigmentation of hair	Vomiting
Selenium	55–70 μg	Antioxidant, glutathione, peroxidase	Fish, organ meats, eggs, shellfish	Muscle pain, muscle wasting, heart disease	AIDS, cystic fibrosis, cancer	Growth retardation, muscle pain/weakness, cardiomyopathy	Narrow range of essentiality to toxicity; nausea, vomiting; death
Iron	10–15 mg	Essential component of hemoglobin, respiratory oxidation, enzyme cofactor, hydroxylation of lysine and proline	Heme: liver, lean red meat, oysters; non-heme: green leafy vegetables	Hypochromic, microcytic anemia	Vegetarians, runners, periods of rapid growth, bioavailability decreased with tannins, calcium carbonate, magnesium oxide, zinc/copper, oxalate	Shortness of breath, impaired motor development[137] spoon-shaped nails (koilonychia), increased susceptibility to infection	Excess unbound iron, promotes bacterial/fungal growth hemochromatosis

AIDS, acquired immunodeficiency syndrome; HDL, high-density lipoprotein.

BOX 7-5

SIGNS OF GOOD NUTRITION

Growth, body size	Normal rate of growth in children Normal weight for height, frame size, age in adults Body mass index (BMI) between 19 and 25 Maintenance of usual body weight within 10% Average skinfold thickness measurements for age and weight Normal fat distribution
Muscular and skeletal systems	Good muscle tone; can walk or run without pain
Hair	Shiny, firm, not easily plucked
Skin	Clear, slightly moist; pink mucous membranes
Lips	Smooth, not chapped or swollen
Nails	Firm, pink, smooth
Face	Skin color uniform; smooth, not swollen
Mouth	Pink tongue with surface papillae (small projections from the mucous membrane that covers the tongue); not swollen Pink, firm, nonbleeding, nonswollen gums Bright teeth, no pain, no cavities
Eyes	Bright, clear, shiny; no sores at corners of eyelids; no prominent blood vessels
Glands	Face, neck not swollen
Behavior	Alert, energetic, good attention span, cheerful, productive
Cardiovascular system	Normal heart rate and rhythm, normal blood pressure
Gastrointestinal system	No palpable organs or masses (in children liver edge may be felt); normal digestion and elimination; good appetite
Nervous system	Normal reflexes and vibratory sense; good coordination, psychological stability
Immune system	Resistant to infection
Laboratory studies	Normal blood, urine, and stool laboratory studies Normal serum albumin levels, serum transferrin levels, creatinine levels, and total lymphocyte count

(Adapted From Eschelman, M. M. [1996]. *Introduction to nutrition and diet therapy* [3rd ed.] Philadelphia: Lippincott-Raven.)

In this hypermetabolic state, there is an increase in lipolysis, but there is a marked decline in ketone production, possibly due to adequate levels of circulating insulin. This failure to ketoadapt has the greatest clinical implications for the obese individual. Often viewed as having ample calorie reserves, the major calorie source in stressed starvation is protein, not fat. Therefore, an obese person may not be perceived at nutritional risk based on physical size rather than on the degree of stress. In clinical nutrition, the provision of intravenous dextrose prevents ketoadaptation. Therefore, nutritional support with adequate protein, should begin as soon as possible.

Skeletal muscle is catabolized to gain access to the *branched-chain amino acids*, which serve as energy substrates through gluconeogenesis. Hepatic protein synthesis shifts from the production of the proteins of homeostasis(albumin, transferrin, prealbumin, and retinol-binding protein) to the production of acute-phase reactants, such as interleukin-1, ceruloplasmin, and clotting factors, thereby contributing to hypoalbuminemia. Alterations in the serum levels of the proteins of homeostasis can be used to assess the degree of nutritional depletion (Table 7-10). Stress can decrease the serum albumin level as much as 0.5 g/dL, even in the absence of systemic pathology.[78] Hypoalbumin-

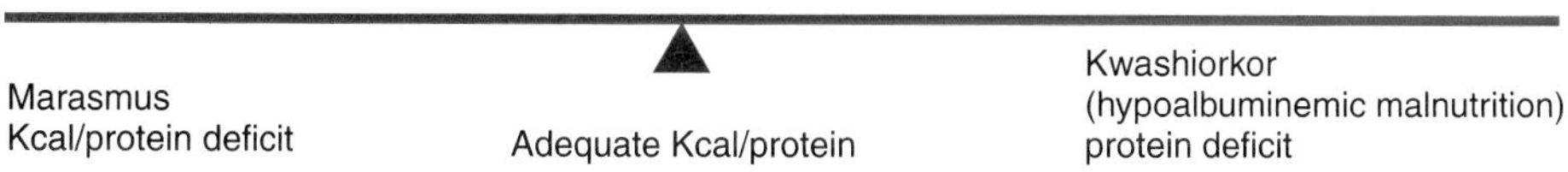

FIGURE 7-3. The continuum of marasmus and kwashiorkor. Balance requires adequate Kcal and protein. Alteration in either will tip the delicate balance.

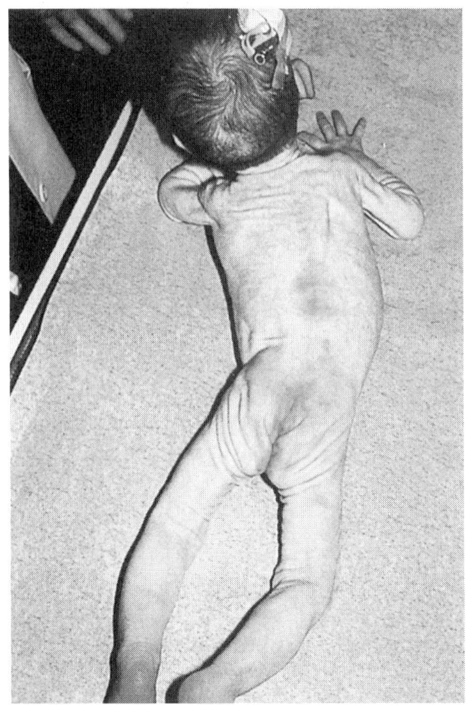

FIGURE 7-4. The child with nutritional marasmus experiences a loss of subcutaneous fat, extreme muscle wasting, and skin breakdown. (Zitelli, B. J. & Davis, H. W. [1997]. *Atlas of pediatric physical diagnosis* [3rd ed.]. Chicago: Mosby–Year Book.)

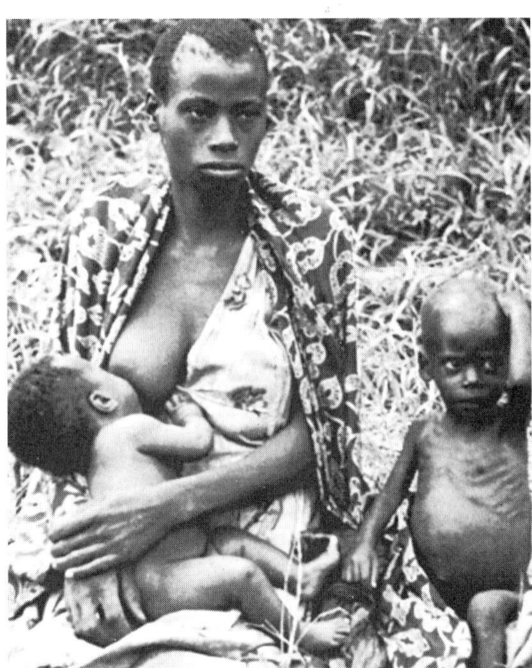

FIGURE 7-5. The older child in this picture shows the protein-calorie deprivation and the malnutrition that occurred when he was dispossessed or replaced at his mother's breast by the new baby.

emia has deleterious effects on wound healing and makes nutritional repletion difficult.

Hypermetabolism is a hallmark of stress, and this causes caloric and protein requirements to increase. Factors influencing caloric and protein requirements include the type of stress and age of the affected person. Examples of stressors that increase calorie and protein requirements are infection, fractures, trauma, fever, and metabolic diseases.

Eating Disorders

Eating disorders represent disorders of weight management ranging from anorexia nervosa (self-starvation) to bulimia nervosa (binge/purge syndrome). Risk factors for eating disorders include female gender, family history of eating disorders, affective disorders such as depression, substance abuse, obesity, history of sexual or physical abuse, and character traits of perfectionism, low self-esteem, and excessive compliance.[30]

ANOREXIA NERVOSA

Anorexia nervosa (AN) is considered to be a psychological disorder with physiologic manifestations. The diagnostic criteria are presented in Box 7-6. Nutritionally, AN is the classic example of marasmus. Although AN has been recognized since the Middle Ages, the psychogenesis of the disorder has changed during modern times. It is commonly believed that dieting and societal pressures toward thinness contribute to the development of this eating disorder and indeed, AN can be considered a diet that never ends.[8] The physical and emotional/behavioral signs and symptoms associated with AN are summarized in Box 7-7. In the United States, the incidence of AN is about 0.5% to 1%.[3]

Although all adolescents and women are exposed to cultural values that encourage slimness, only a small percentage of women become emaciated. Current research focuses on the biologic vulnerability that increases the risk of AN. Increased levels of **serotonin**, a neurotransmitter that may contribute to satiety, may be contributory to certain characteristics exhibited by anorectics including rigidity, anxiety, and obsessive behaviors.[43] Other biophysical alterations include an elevation in **cortisol** levels. Excess cortisol adversely affects appetite control mechanisms in the hypothalamus causing a decrease in hunger. Excess cortisol production may also be linked to depression, which, in turn, can affect appetite.[55]

Although biologic vulnerability exists, psychosocial factors are involved. Young women with AN are usually from enmeshed, overly close families. Separation from the family is often difficult and a sense of ineffective-

TABLE 7-10

RELATIONSHIP BETWEEN NUTRITIONAL DEPLETION AND SERUM PROTEINS

		DEGREE OF DEPLETION		
INDICATOR	**NORMAL**	**Mild**	**Moderate**	**Severe**
Albumin (g/dL)	3.5–5.5	2.8–3.4	2.1–2.7	< 2.1
Transferrin (mg/dL)	180–260	150–200	100–149	< 100
Prealbumin (mcg/dL)	200–300	10–15	5–9	< 5
Retinol-binding protein* (mcg/dL)	40–50	—	—	—

Note: To convert albumin (g/100 mL) to international standard units (nmol/L), multiply by 37.06. To convert transferrin (mg/100 mL) to standard international units (g/L), multiply by 0.01.

*Levels of < 3 mg/100 mL suggest compromised protein status. The actual degree of depletion (mild, moderate, and severe) has not been defined.

(Adapted from: Whitney, E. N., Cataldo, C. B., and Rolfes, S. R. [1994]. *Understanding normal and clinical nutrition* [4th ed.]. St Paul, MN: West.)

ness, lack of personal fulfillment, interpersonal distress, and fear of maturity may all be contributing factors.[36]

Behavioral disturbances seen in anorectics mimic those exhibited in persons undergoing simple starvation. In landmark research, Keys described a "starvation syndrome" in which healthy young male volunteers were put on restrictive diets for several months. Subjects in this study developed a preoccupation with food and food preparation as well as elaborate food rituals. Cognitively, the men exhibited difficulty with decision-making and decreased alertness. Socially, subjects withdrew from group activities, became isolated and depressed, and experienced a decrease in sex drive.[44] These biologic effects of starvation are also seen in anorectics. This underscores the importance of weight loss in the development of the symptoms seen in AN.

Medical Complications

The medical complications associated with AN depend on the variant form of the disease, whether it is a restricting type or binge-eating type (see Box 7-6). An estimated 30% to 50% of anorectics use various purging behaviors.[74] Medical complications are most severe in bulimic anorectics.[34]

Figure 7-6 illustrates the complications associated with both types of AN.

BOX 7-6

DIAGNOSTIC CRITERIA FOR ANOREXIA NERVOSA

A. Refusal to maintain body weight at or above a minimally normal weight for age and height (eg, weight loss leading to maintenance of body weight less than 85% of that expected; or failure to make expected weight gain during period of growth, leading to body weight less than 85% of that expected).
B. Intense fear of gaining weight or becoming fat, even though underweight.
C. Disturbance in the way in which one's body weight or shape is experienced, undue influence of body weight or shape on self-evaluation or denial of the seriousness of the current low body weight.
D. In postmenarcheal females, amenorrhea, ie, the absence of at least three consecutive menstrual cycles. (A woman is considered to have amenorrhea if her periods occur only following hormone, eg, estrogen, administration.)

Specific type:

Restricting type: during the current episode of anorexia nervosa, the person has not regularly engaged in binge-eating or purging behavior (ie, self-induced vomiting or the misuse of laxative, diuretics, or enemas)

Binge-eating/purging type: during the current episode of anorexia nervosa, the person has regularly engaged in binge-eating or purging behavior (ie, self-induced vomiting or the misuse of laxatives, diuretics, or enemas)

(Source: American Psychiatric Association. [1994]. *Diagnostic and statistical manual of mental disorders* [4th ed.]. Washington, DC: Author.)

BOX 7-7 PHYSICAL, MENTAL, AND BEHAVIORAL SIGNS AND SYMPTOMS OF ANOREXIA

Physical Symptoms

- Extreme weight loss and muscle wasting (anorectics may lose 25% of their body weight over a period of months); bulimics experience weight fluctuations, but may appear normal weight
- Arrested sexual development, amenorrhea
- Dry, yellow skin related to the release of carotenes as fat stores are burned for energy
- Loss of hair or change in hair texture
- Pain on touch
- Hypotension, bradycardia
- Anemia
- Constipation
- Severe sleep disturbances, insomnia
- Dental caries and periodontal disease

Mental and Behavioral Symptoms

- Bizarre eating habits, refusal to eat
- Feelings of failure, low self-esteem, social isolation
- Perfectionist, overachiever
- Preoccupation with food, dieting, and death
- Intense fear of becoming fat that does not lessen with weight loss
- Distorted body image and denial of eating disorder
- Frantic pursuit of exercise
- Frequent weighing
- Use of laxatives, diuretics, emetics, and diet pills
- Manipulative behavior

(From Dudek, S. G. [1997]. *Nutrition handbook for nursing practice* [3rd ed.] Philadelphia: Lippincott-Raven.)

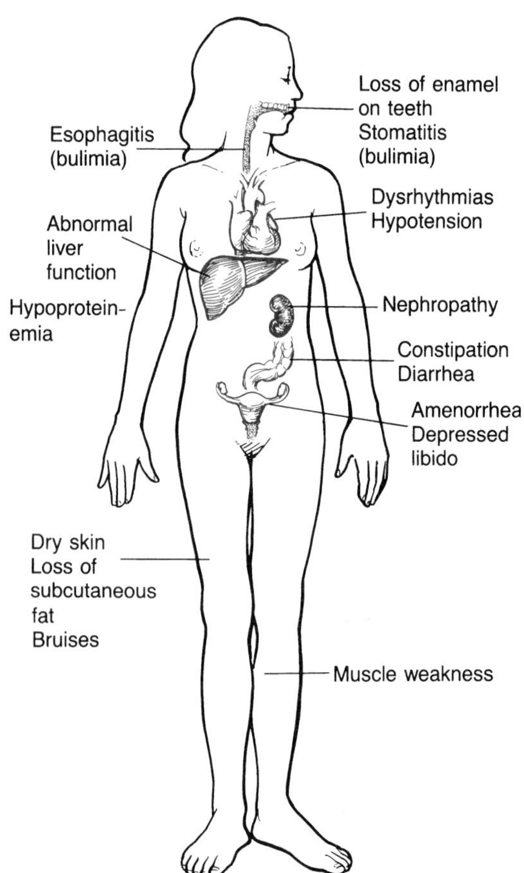

FIGURE 7-6. Complications associated with both types of anorexia nervosa.

CARDIOVASCULAR COMPLICATIONS. Cardiac abnormalities account for the majority of deaths associated with AN. It has long been documented that reductions in cardiac muscle mass, decreases in cardiac chamber size, and alterations in myocardial contractility exist in individuals with AN.[29] Clinical presentation includes hypotension, sinus bradycardia, and abnormal exercise tolerance.[66] Overzealous nutritional repletion may precipitate refeeding syndrome and congestive heart failure. This syndrome results when nutrition is introduced in quantities greater than the body can tolerate. Refeeding edema is associated with an increase in intracellular and extracellular volume and heart failure.

Decreased BMR and subnormal body temperature are associated features of starvation. Consequently, resting caloric expenditure can decrease to approximately half normal.[74] This compensatory mechanism preserves physiologic functioning, although at a lowered rate.

METABOLIC AND ENDOCRINE COMPLICATIONS. Metabolic findings in anorexia are similar to those seen in starvation (see Box 7-7). Restrictors normally experience a "fixed hypoglycemia" secondary to ketoadaptation and adequate glucogenic substrates. As weight loss progresses to a critical point, fat reserves are exhausted and gluconeogenic precursors are diminished. Profound hypoglycemia and hypoglycemic coma may develop. Hence, severe hypoglycemia represents a grave prognosis, and prompt medical treatment is warranted.[62]

Elevation in uric acid may be present and also can serve as an index of severity. Strenuous exercise, starvation, alcohol consumption, and thiazide diuretics contribute to hyperuricemia.[32] Hypogonadism is a characteristic feature of AN, and loss of needed body fat contributes to amenorrhea.

Alterations in electrolyte balance may result from refeeding. Clinicians faced with a cachectic (muscle-wasted) client often begin parenteral dextrose solutions either alone or as part of a total parenteral nutrition program. These solutions cause an increase in insulin production. Increasing levels of insulin force phosphate into the cell, resulting in hypophosphatemia. Phosphate participates in many enzymatic reactions as either adenosine triphosphate (ATP) or 2,3-diphosphoglycerate. Profound muscular weakness and progressive encephalopathy, coma, and death may develop. Hematologic disturbances associated with hypophosphatemia include hemolytic anemia and impaired leukocyte and thrombocyte function. Therefore, although the ideal form of nutritional repletion needs to be delineated for anorectics, care should be given to not increase feeding too rapidly and to monitor electrolyte disturbances. Recommended weight gain per day should not exceed 0.25 to 0.5 lb.[12]

SKELETAL COMPLICATIONS. Lack of estrogen, cortisol excess, and malnutrition are central to the pathophysiology of the bone disease exhibited in women with the disorder. In most women, the onset of the disorder occurs before peak bone mass is achieved at approximately age 24. Osteoporosis is present in over half of persons with AN and may persist after recovery, predisposing individuals to spinal vertebral crush fractures. The pathophysiology of the bone loss includes estrogen deficiency, inadequate vitamins and minerals, and a decrease in insulin-like growth factor, a potent bone trophic hormone.[31] Increased exercise may also contribute to pathologic fractures. Osteonecrosis and femoral head collapse have also been reported.[77]

GASTROINTESTINAL DISORDERS. These disorders are common in AN; the disorders can be perceived or have a true physiologic origin. Gastrointestinal distress is often presented as a reason to limit or restrict food choices. Nausea, epigastric pain, flatus, and early satiety are also common and may be related to delayed gastric emptying time, a consequence of malnutrition. This condition resolves with appropriate nutrition and weight gain.[70] Although the abdominal pain is usually benign, it may be indicative of gastric dilatation or superior mesenteric artery spasm.[58]

BULIMIA NERVOSA

Bulimia nervosa, meaning "ox hunger," is a disorder of weight maintenance characterized by preoccupation with weight and dieting and weight control through caloric restriction alternating with binge/purge behavior. The diagnostic criteria are highlighted in Box 7-8. The actual incidence of bulimia is controversial, but estimates are that 1% to 3% of adolescents and young women are affected.[3] This disorder is almost exclusively confined to women. Affected men are often those who pursue interests or

BOX 7-8 DIAGNOSTIC CRITERIA FOR BULIMIA NERVOSA

A. Recurrent episodes of binge eating. An episode of binge eating is characterized by both of the following:
   (1) Eating, in a discrete period of time (eg, within any 2-hour period) an amount of food that is definitely larger than most people would eat during a similar period of time.
   (2) A sense of lack of control over eating during the episode (eg, a feeling that one cannot stop eating or control what or how much one is eating).
B. Recurrent inappropriate compensatory behavior to prevent weight gain, such as self-induced vomiting; misuse of laxatives, diuretics, enemas or other medications; fasting; or excessive exercise.
C. The binge eating and inappropriate compensatory behaviors both occur, on average, at least twice a week for 3 months.
D. Self-evaluation is unduly influenced by body shape and weight.
E. The disturbance does not occur exclusively during episodes of anorexia nervosa.

Specify type:

Purging type: during the current episode of bulimia nervosa, the person has regularly engaged in self-induced vomiting or the misuse of laxatives, diuretics, or enemas. Nonpurging type: during the current episode of bulimia nervosa, the person has used other inappropriate compensatory behaviors, such as fasting or excessive exercise, but has not regularly engaged in self-induced vomiting or the misuse of laxatives, diuretics, or enemas.

(Source: American Psychiatric Association. [1994]. *Diagnostic and statistical manual of mental disorders* [4th ed.]. Washington, DC: Author.)

careers in which body image and weight are of paramount importance, including wrestlers and jockeys. The age of onset is usually late teens and most affected women are from the middle to upper socioeconomic classes.

A binge is defined as a larger than normal amount of food eaten within a time frame of less than 2 hours.[3] The bulimic episode is considered by the individuals as an "out of control" experience. Foods chosen are high calorie, nondietetic, and easily consumed. Purging follows the binge episode. Purging is most often accomplished by vomiting, laxative/diuretic abuse, or use of enemas. Purgatives include syrup of ipecac and various over-the-counter laxatives and caffeine-based diuretics.[56] White adolescents most commonly purge through self-induced vomiting, whereas African American adolescents most frequently purge through laxative/diuretic abuse.[21]

Unlike anorectics, affected persons are aware that the eating habits are abnormal but are unable to stop. Shame and secrecy accompany this disorder and prevent appropriate diagnosis and treatment. A guide to physical signs and symptoms is given in Box 7-9.

Pathophysiology

As with AN, dysregulation of serotonin function in the central nervous system may contribute to the symptoms exhibited in bulimic individuals. Diminished responses to satiety are common in bulimia and serotonin is a key neurochemical signal for satiety.[69]

The psychogenesis of bulimia is complex. Dieting often precipitates the disorder, with the first binge occurring while on a diet.[76] Although dieting initiates the disorder, the maintenance of the disorder is attributed to the new role binging and purging takes on. The rapid consumption of large amounts of food is followed by purging to reduce anxiety. Therefore, anxiety reduction contributes to the continuance of bulimic behavior.[76]

Medical Complications

Medical complications are common and the severity of these complications depends on the person's nutritional status and type and extent of purging behaviors. Many commonalities with AN exist if the behavior involves restriction of intake.

ELECTROLYTE AND ACID–BASE COMPLICATIONS. Electrolyte disturbances are common manifestations in binging and purging. Hypokalemia is a common and dangerous

BOX 7-9 PHYSICAL SYMPTOMS AND SIGNS IN BULIMIA NERVOSA

Presenting Physical Symptoms

Weight may be normal, overweight, or underweight
Complaints of bloating, diarrhea, swelling
Hyperactivity (mental and motor); exceptions common
Constant or extreme thirst and increased urination (hypokalemic nephropathy-hypovolemia)
May present with depression, anxiety, despair, and suicidal ideation

Physical Signs

Usually well groomed and good hygiene; definite exceptions, especially patients with a severe character disorder or chronic addictive conditions
Usually normal weight or mild to moderate obesity (exception: food restrictors or anorexia nervosa patients with associated bulimia, vomiting, purging)
Generalized or localized edema at lower extremities (compensatory renal retention of sodium and water, ie, hypovolemia with secondary hyperadosteronism or pseudo-Bartter's syndrome)
Physical findings of extreme weight loss (self-starvation) if bulimia, vomiting, and purging are complications of anorexia nervosa or food restriction
Loss of scalp hair, skin changes of anorexia nervosa
Amennorhea, effects of estrogen deficiency
Hypothermia
Swelling of parotid and other salivary glands, hyperamylasemia
Dental enamel dysplasia and discoloration due to gastric juices (vomiting)
Bruises and lacerations of palate and posterior pharynx; lesions of fingernails, fingers, and dorsum of hand(s) (due to self-induced vomiting)
Pyorrhea and other gum disorders
Diminished reflexes, muscle weakness, paralysis, and infrequently, peripheral neuropathy with muscle weakness and paralysis
Muscle cramping (with induced hypoxia or positive Trousseau's sign)
Signs of hypokalemia (cardiac dysrhythmias, hypotension, decreased cardiac output, weak pulse, poor quality heart sounds, abdominal distention, ileus, acute gastric dilatation, myopathy, shortness of breath, depression, and mental clouding)
Cardiomyopathy secondary to ipecac poisoning

(Modified from Comerci, G. D. [1997]. Medical complications at anorexia nervosa and bulimia nervosa. *Medical Clinics of North America, 74* [5], 1293.)

electrolyte disturbance (see page 170). Continual vomiting and laxative and diuretic abuse precipitate hypokalemia because 80% of body potassium is excreted in the urine and 20% in the feces.[78] Other causative factors in the development of hypokalemia include decreased plasma volume, metabolic alkalosis, and coexisting magnesium deficiency.[35] Chronic laxative abuse may produce nephropathy and a urine concentration deficit. The resultant polyuria and hypovolemia result in hyperaldosteronism and the development of edema.[83] Chronic and severe dehydration stimulate the renin–aldosterone system, which promotes the retention of sodium and water along with loss of potassium.

Renal dysfunctions secondary to electrolyte abnormalities include dehydration and sodium loss. Hyponatremia stimulates the renin–aldosterone system with effects as described above. Abrupt cessation of laxative use promotes secondary hyperaldosteronism and peripheral edema results. Weaning from laxatives prevents rapid weight gain, reduces anxiety, and decreases the likelihood of return to laxatives.[79] Diarrhea from laxative abuse causes electrolyte abnormalities but does not cause a significant malabsorption of calories. Ingestion of 50 laxative tablets results in a calorie loss of only 12%, indicating that 88% of the calories from the binge have been absorbed. Therefore, laxative abuse is an ineffective method of weight control.[6,38]

Acid–base disturbances occur in bulimia secondary to the purgative method used. Metabolic alkalosis is the most common. Loss of hydrogen ions in vomiting and in diuretic abuse leads to an increase in plasma bicarbonate contributing to alkalosis (see page 192). Metabolic acidosis can occur during the starvation or restricting phase in which ketoacids are being used as a primary energy source. Laxative abuse causes a profound bicarbonate loss and leads to metabolic acidosis. Flowchart 7-1 illustrates the electrolyte/acid–base abnormalities seen in eating disorders.

FLOWCHART 7-1 **Fluid, Electrolyte, and Acid–Base Imbalances**

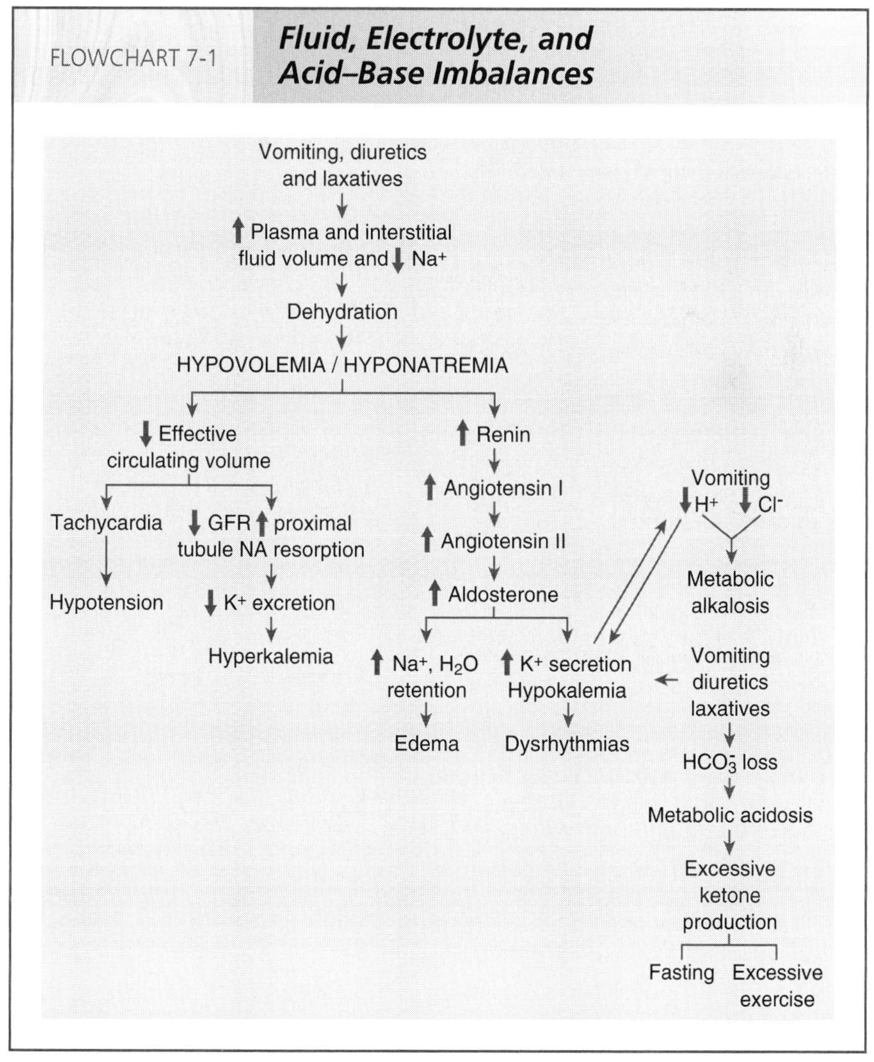

ENDOCRINE ABNORMALITIES. The endocrine disturbances in bulimia are not clearly defined or understood. Endocrine dysfunction exists and may be related to poor nutritional intake or starvation during the restricting phase.[54] Menstrual and ovulatory disturbances occur in normal-weight bulimics, but the etiology is unknown.[9]

GASTROINTESTINAL DISORDERS. Dysphagia may develop in bulimics secondary to a poor or absent pharyngeal gag reflex and increased duration of "dry" swallow. The defect in swallowing may be attributed to desensitization from prolonged vomiting as well as being a learned response.[63] Gastric rupture and esophageal tears are the most severe form of upper gastrointestinal disorders. Other effects include atrophy of smooth muscle, progressive loss of innervation, and decrease in colonic neurons. Cathartic colon, a permanent alteration in bowel function, may result in severe constipation as well as gastrointestinal bleeding. Anemia, steatorrhea, and protein-losing enteropathy may be present.

ORAL DISORDERS. In bulimic anorectics and bulimics who vomit, enamel erosion is the most common oral disorder. Other oral abnormalities include dentin hypersensitivity, caries, xerostomia (dryness of the mouth), parotid gland enlargement, and periodontal disease. The low pH of vomitus is the major cause. Postvomiting rinsing with tap water may contribute to oral disease because it reduces the buffering capacity of saliva.[1] Due to the secretive nature of bulimia, oral disorders may provide the first diagnostic clue to health professionals, particularly the dental hygienist and dentist.

DERMATOLOGIC COMPLAINTS. Bulimics often exhibit a fine dry rash on the hands secondary to dehydration. Calluses on the knuckles may be present when the fingers are used for vomiting.

NUTRITIONAL DEFICIENCIES OF ANOREXIA NERVOSA AND BULIMIA

The nutritional deficiencies exhibited in persons with eating disorders are many and varied. Chronic protein deficiency, hypoalbuminemia, and negative nitrogen balance are seen in anorectics and bulimics.[38] Vitamin deficiencies, especially water-soluble vitamins, can be evidenced by angular stomatitis, mucosal ulcers, and hair loss.[34] Zinc and copper deficiency is commonly seen in restrictors (AN) and bulimics and may impair appetite regulation. Deficiency of zinc results in altered taste acuity, altered taste sensitivity, and impairment in the sense of smell. Zinc deficiency may contribute to the chronicity of eating disorders.[40] It develops secondary to poor intake, impaired absorption, and the consumption of foods low in zinc content during a binge.

LACTOSE INTOLERANCE

The digestion and absorption of disaccharides depends on the enzyme lactase, which splits lactose into glucose and galactose for easy absorption. In some cases, lactase deficiency occurs from birth but more frequently it develops as a consequence of another disease, certain medications, or simply the process of aging.[78] Lactase deficiency is present in 2% to 8% of adults of Scandinavian or Western European extraction, but in 70% to 100% of adult Native Americans, African Americans, African Bantus, Eskimos, and descendants of peoples who live near the Mediterrainean Sea.[22].

When lactose is not rapidly hydrolyzed it attracts water, causing fullness, discomfort, cramping, nausea, and diarrhea.[78] The lactose may become food for the intestinal bacteria, which may produce irritating acid and gas.[78] The onset of the milk intolerance varies according to the degree of intolerance. Cases of absolute lactase deficiency are rare. Some adults develop symptoms after drinking milk on an empty stomach but can tolerate milk in cooking or with cereal. Often, fermented dairy products such as yogurt are better tolerated and lactose-hyrolyzed milk and lactase pills are available commercially. Lactase deficiency may develop in individuals who have diseases that produce diffuse intestinal mucosal damage or from surgery, chemotherapy, or colitis.

OBESITY

Obesity is the most common nutritional disorder in the United States and a major public health problem. Currently, obesity affects 33% of the population over the age of 20, 35% of women and 31% of men.[45] Health care costs associated with obesity are approximately $68 billion annually.[53]

Body mass index (BMI) or the Quetelet index is the preferred method of defining obesity and correlates well with more direct measures of body fatness, such as underwater weighing.[7] BMI can be calculated by the following formula:

$$\text{BMI} = \text{W}/\text{H}^2$$
$$(\text{W} = \text{weight in kilograms},\ \text{H} = \text{height in meters})$$

Obesity is defined as a BMI of 25 for ages 19 to 34 and 27 or greater after age 34.[52] A BMI of 28 is associated with a three to four times increased risk of morbidity, such as stroke, heart disease, and type 2 diabetes.[75] Figure 7-7 illustrates mortality risk associated with increasing BMI.

Types of Cellular Obesity

The number and size of adipocytes or fat cells can be used to classify the type of obesity present. *Hyperplastic obesity* is defined as an increase in the number of

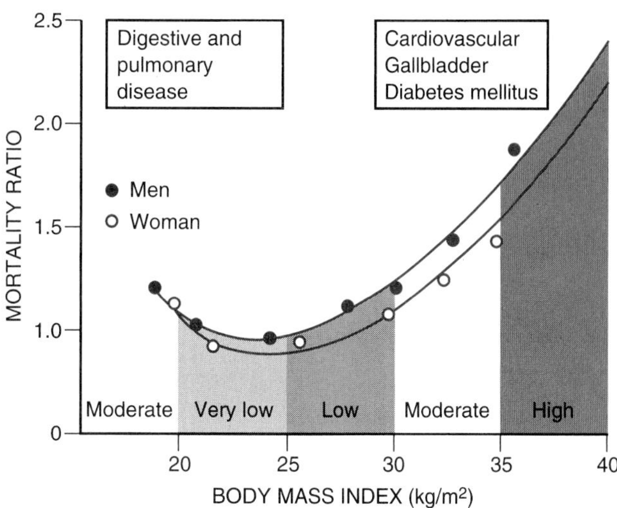

FIGURE 7-7. Body mass index and mortality risk. Data from the American Cancer Society study have been plotted for men and women to show the relationship of body mass index to overall mortality risk. At a body mass index below 20 kg/m^2 and above 30 kg/m^2, there is an increase in relative mortality. The major causes for this increased mortality are listed, along with a division of body mass index groupings into various levels of risk. (Redrawn from Bray, G. A. & Gray, D. S. [1988]. Obesity. Part I: Pathogenesis. *Western Journal of Medicine, 149*, 429.)

adipocytes present. It develops during peak periods of cell multiplication; early childhood, adolescence, and pregnancy. This type of obesity appears to be the most difficult to treat and appears to increase the risk of subsequent morbidity independent of eventual adult body weight.[51]

Hypertrophic obesity is characterized by an increase in the size of the adipocyte. This increased size is present in all obesity and 80% to 90% of adult-onset obesity is hypertrophic.

Factors Affecting Regulation of Body Weight

Regulation of body weight is a complex integration over time through short- and long-term regulation. Most individuals are predisposed to weight gain over time. Short-term regulation refers to the onset of eating on a meal-to-meal basis and is largely dependent on appetite. The social stimulus to eat and psychological factors, such as depression and anxiety, can influence appetite. Long-term regulation refers to the modulation of intake and output so that body weight is maintained within a range. The average weight gain between ages 25 and 55 is 20 lb. Although in absolute terms this gain can be viewed as weight regulation dysfunction, it represents a chronic imbalance between energy intake and expenditure of 0.3% excess intake of calories.[4]

Regulation of body weight is a multifaceted process influenced by appetite, hormones, genetics, and activity level. Obesity may result from alterations in one or a combination of any of these factors.

APPETITE CONTROL

Appetite control is regulated internally by the hypothalamus. The lateral hypothalamus, or hunger center, initiates food consumption after receiving stimuli, such as hypoglycemia. The ventromedial hypothalamus or satiety center monitors rising nutrient levels and signals the termination of hunger (satiety).[33] Other factors that signal satiety include gastrointestinal filling (causing stretch inhibitory signals to suppress the feeding center) and humoral factors through the gastrointestinal hormone, cholecystokinin, as well as the hormones, glucagon and insulin, which suppress neurogenic feeding signals from the brain.[24,33]

Appetite is also regulated by emotional factors (cerebral cortically induced) and may have little relationship to actual hunger. Many obese individuals eat as an emotional crutch, to relieve depression or anxiety, or they have a compulsive desire to eat.[20] Weight gain often increases frustration and intake of food increases in response.

ALTERATIONS OF HORMONAL REGULATION

Many physiologic cues are directed to the hypothalamus, including hormones and peptides. Some hor-

TABLE 7-11

TERMS FOR THE TWO DIFFERENT DISTRIBUTIONS OF BODY FAT

ANDROID	GYNOID
Upper body	Lower body
Apple	Pear
Abdominal	Visceral, gluteal, femoral
Central	Peripheral
Subscapular skinfold thickness > 25	Subscapular skinfold thickness < 25
Waist/hip girth ratio > 0.85	Waist/hip girth ratio < 0.85

mones are stimulated by changes in blood concentrations of macro- and micronutrients, and many affect the regulation of obesity, including the following examples:

- Thyroid hormones: a deficiency of thyroid hormone lowers BMR, whereas an excess raises it.
- Leptin: a peptide, synthesized and secreted from adipose tissue; reduces food intake and increases energy expenditure. Resistance to leptin increases with increasing body weight suggesting that obesity is linked with leptin resistance.[13]
- Insulin: obesity is often accompanied by an increase in beta-cell secretion, peripheral resistance to insulin, and the resultant hyperinsulinemia, discussed below.

The Unique Role of Insulin in Obesity

Insulin, a major anabolic (building) hormone, has a central role in the development of the major diseases associated with obesity.[15] It is especially associated with the distribution of body fat. For many years, only excess body weight (increasing BMI) was considered in determining health risk from obesity. Body fat distribution has been found equally important in predicting chronic disease risk.[41] Two major body fat distributions exist: android and gynoid obesity. Table 7-11 highlights each type.

ANDROID OBESITY. Android obesity is predominantly the result of hyperinsulinemia. Hyperinsulinemia may precede the development of obesity and be considered a cause of the obesity rather than a result. Indeed, insulin resistance and hyperinsulinemia is present in 20% to 25% of healthy, normal, glucose-tolerant individuals.[37]

Hyperinsulinemia is responsible for the "deadly quartet": upper body obesity, glucose intolerance, dyslipidemia, and hypertension.[42] Elevated serum insulin levels have been identified as an independent risk factor for coronary artery disease, which is more prevalent in obese individuals.[16] Insulin resistance is present in almost all individuals with Type 2 diabetes and is in part responsible for the increase in macrovascular disease seen in these individuals.[50] An interesting study showed that increasing sensitivity to insulin is associated with a decrease in atherosclerosis in Hispanics, non-Hispanic whites, but not in African Americans.[39]

Abdominal fat is more metabolically active than peripheral or gluteal fat. Increase in adenyl cyclase in the cell and lipoprotein lipase in the blood allows an increase in free fatty acid clearance, which decrease hepatic clearance of insulin. Rising insulin levels, a positive energy balance, and increasing plasma-free testosterone (android) yields a cascade with hyperinsulinemia as the end result. Flowchart 7-2 illustrates the metabolic derangements associated with hyperinsulinemia. Due to the ac-

FLOWCHART 7-2 **Insulin Resistance**

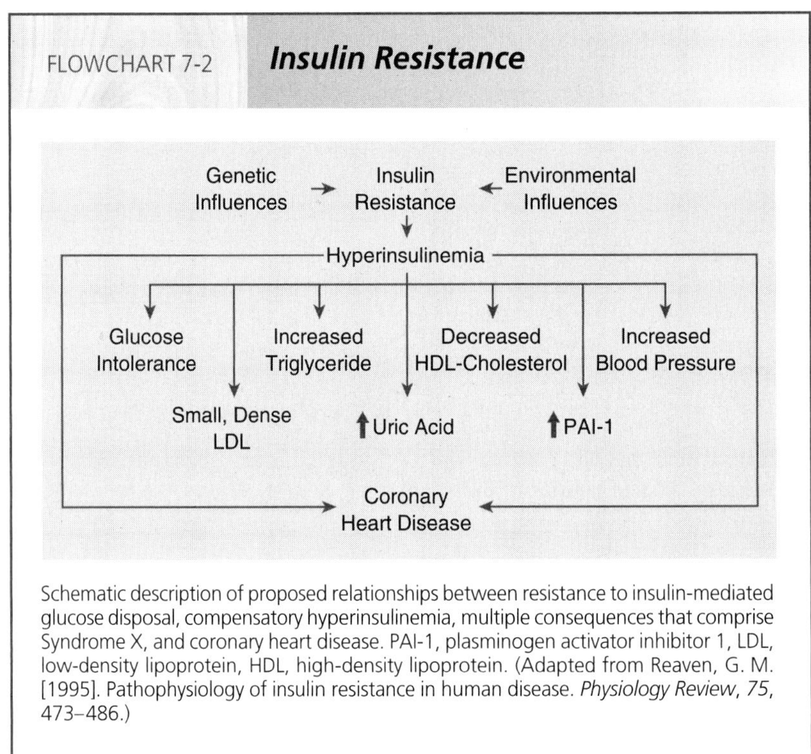

Schematic description of proposed relationships between resistance to insulin-mediated glucose disposal, compensatory hyperinsulinemia, multiple consequences that comprise Syndrome X, and coronary heart disease. PAI-1, plasminogen activator inhibitor 1, LDL, low-density lipoprotein, HDL, high-density lipoprotein. (Adapted from Reaven, G. M. [1995]. Pathophysiology of insulin resistance in human disease. *Physiology Review*, *75*, 473–486.)

cumulation of body fat in the abdominal region individuals with android obesity have an increased waist/hip ratio. A waist/hip ratio of greater than 1 in men and 0.8 in women increases the risk of the "deadly quartet." A nomogram for estimating waist/hip ratio is found in Figure 7-8.

GYNOID OBESITY. The fat distribution of the individual with gynoid obesity gives the person the typical "pear" shape, which is more commonly seen in women. The waist/hip ratio is less than 0.8. This type of obesity is less commonly associated with hyperinsulinemia than the android type.

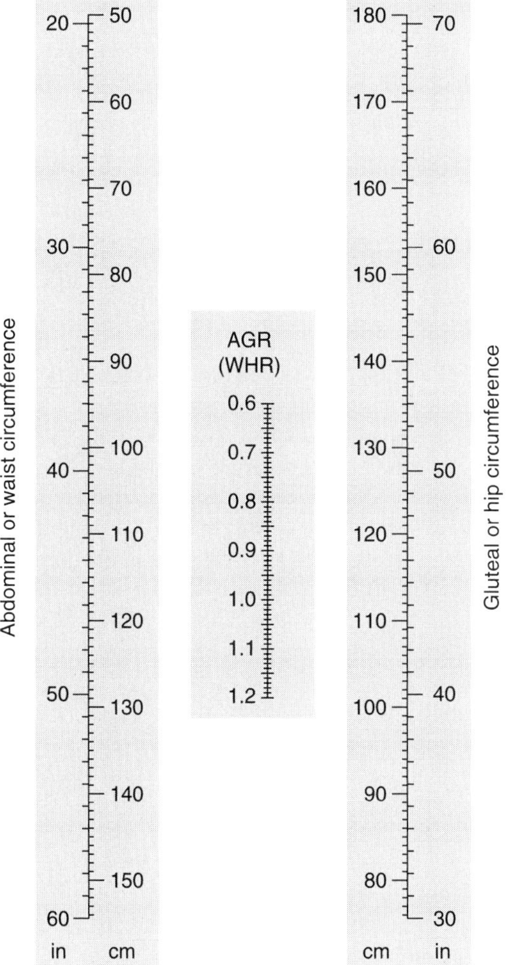

FIGURE 7-8. The abdominal (waist) and gluteal (hips) ratio (AGR) can be determined by placing a straight edge between the column for waist circumference and reading the ratio from the point where this straight edge crosses the AGR or waist–hips ratio (WHR) line. The waist or abdominal circumference is the smallest circumference below the rib cage and above the umbilicus, and the hips or gluteal circumference is the largest circumference at the posterior extension of the buttocks. (Bray, G. A. & Gray, D. S. [1988]. Obesity. Part I: Pathogenesis. *Western Journal of Medicine, 149,* 429.)

GENETIC INFLUENCES

Obesity is highly familial and may explain the poor results of obesity prevention efforts.[7] Based on twin studies, heritability is estimated to be 30% to 40% for body fat distribution, resting energy expenditure, food preference, rates of lipolysis, and physical activity.[64]

A "thrifty gene" theory has been proposed as one possible genetic expression of obesity. A thrifty metabolism is described as having a high metabolic efficiency, meaning a higher proportion of excess calories is stored as fat, equipping the individual to withstand starvation or dieting.[23] Although a single gene theory is attractive, obesity is most likely an interaction between genetic factors and the environment. Genetic influences determine whether it is possible to become obese and the environmental influences determine if the client becomes obese and to what extent.[49] The 30% increase in obesity during the past decade and the universal relationships between social class and education suggest that environmental factors such as high-fat, high-calorie diet and inactivity are potent influences.[59]

INACTIVITY

Inactivity, or lack of physical activity, contributes to the development and maintenance of obesity. Currently, 25% of men and women in the United States are inactive. These individuals have sedentary jobs, have no recreational pursuits, and avoid physical activity throughout the course of the day by taking elevators and so forth. Conversely, only 20% of the population can be considered physically active.[14]

Physical activity reduces insulin resistance, may reduce desire for foods high in fat, and burns a moderate amount of calories.[72] Other benefits of exercise include improved blood lipids, decreased risk of morbidity and mortality, increases in BMR, increases in fat oxidation, and increased sense of well-being.[71]

Although most obese individuals use more calories per any given activity, they often choose to be less active compared with their lean counterparts. Television viewing is one example of the contribution of inactivity to obesity, particularly in children. Indeed, television viewing often combines inactivity with overconsumption of high-calorie snack foods. The average child spends more time watching television than attending school.[19] Television viewing therefore displaces optional physical activities and exposes children to hundreds of food-related commercials, providing an environmental cue to eat.[60] The prevalence of obesity increases 2% for each hour of routine television viewing.[18] Restriction of television viewing has been suggested as a strategy to prevent obesity.[27]

Complications of Obesity

The complications of obesity can be categorized into two distinct risk categories: physical and psychological. Physical risk or diseases associated with obesity include[57]:

- Hypertension
- Cardiovascular and cerebrovascular disease
- Type 2 diabetes
- Gallstones (cholelithiasis)
- Osteoarthritis
- Sleep apnea
- Breast, endometrial, and ovarian cancers
- Infertility
- Birth defects

Figure 7-9 illustrates these complications. The psychological risk of obesity cannot be underestimated. Many health care providers do not understand the metabolic sequelae that contribute to obesity and view it as poor self-control.[68] Obese individuals can suffer discrimination from those who view them as lazy or lacking in willpower. Compared with normal weight women, obese women are less likely to be married, have lower incomes, and attain a lower level of education.[28]

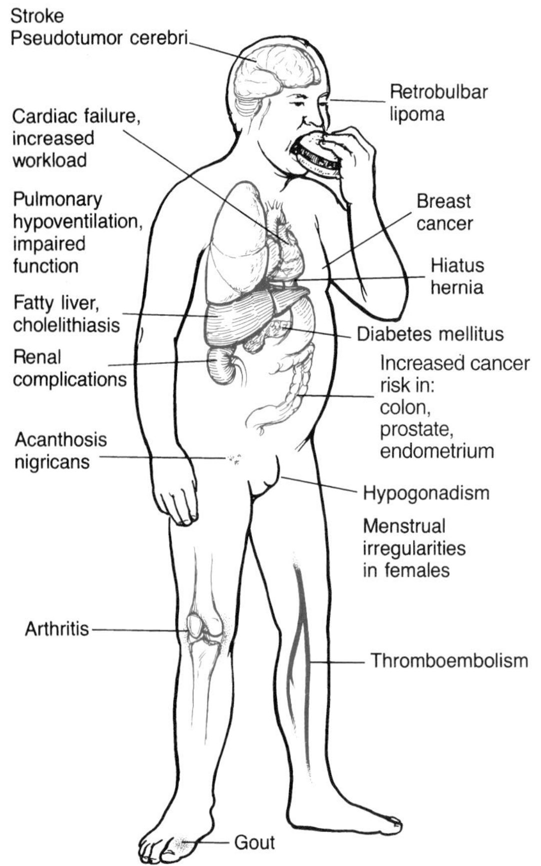

FIGURE 7-9. Complications associated with obesity.

FOCUS ON THE PERSON WITH MALNUTRITION

Mr. W. is a 5′10″ 185-lb. construction worker. He was admitted to the hospital after a fall from a scaffolding. He sustained a broken femur, radius, and two broken ribs and has internal bleeding. On day 10 of a complicated hospitalization, his albumin level is 2.0 g/dL and his weight is 162 lb. He has been maintained on D_5W as his only caloric source, and he has received only clear liquids orally.

Questions

1. What form of malnutrition does Mr. W have?
2. Describe the pathophysiologic consequences of this form of malnutrition.
3. What degree of protein depletion is indicated in the above data?
4. Compare the clinical manifestations of this form of malnutrition with other forms of malnutrition.
5. When nutritional support is initiated, what serum protein is the most sensitive marker of repletion? What nutritional support should be used to restore Mr. W's nutritional status?

See Appendix A for discussion.

REFERENCES

1. Altshulter, B. D., Dechow, P. C., Waller, P. A., & Hardy, B. W. (1996). An investigation of the oral pathologies occurring in bulimia nervosa. *International Journal of Eating Disorders, 9,* 191.
2. American Diabetes Association Position Statement. (1996). Nutrition recommendation and principles for people with diabetes. *Diabetes Care, 20,* 514–517.
3. American Psychiatric Association (1994). *Diagnostic and statistical manual of mental disorders* (4th ed.). Washington, DC: Author.
4. Belanger, B., Cupples, L., & D'Agostino, R. (1988). The Framingham Study: An epidemiological study investigating cardiovascular disease (Publication No. 88-2970). Washington, DC: U.S. Government Printing Office.
5. Bell, L. P. (1991). Cholesterol lowering effects of soluble fiber cereals as part of a prudent diet for patients with mild to moderate hypercholesterolemia. *American Journal Clinical Nutrition, 52*(6), 1020–1026.
6. Bo-Linn, G. W., et al. (1983). Purging and caloric absorption in bulimic patients and normal women. *Annals of Internal Medicine, 99,* 14.
7. Bouchard, C. (Ed.). (1994). *The genetics of obesity.* Boca Raton, FL: CRC Press.
8. Brownell, K. D. (1991). Personal responsibility and control over our bodies: When expectations exceed reality. *Health Psychology, 10,* 303–310.

9. Cantopher, T., Evans, C., Lacey, J. H., & Pearch, J. M. (1988). Menstrual and ovulatory disturbances in bulimia. *BMJ British Medical Journal, 297,* 836.
10. Chan, S. W., & Reade, P. C. (1998). The role of ascorbic acid in oral cancer and carcinogenesis. *Oral Diseases, 4*(2), 120–129.
11. Clark, L. C., Dalkin, B., Krongard, A., et al. (1998). Decreased incidence of prostate cancer with selenium supplementation: Results of a double blind cancer prevention trial. *British Journal of Urology, 81*(5), 730–734.
12. Comerci, G. D. (1990). Medical complications of anorexia nervosa and bulimia. *Medical Clinics of North America, 74*(5), 1293.
13. Considine, R. V., Madhur, K. S., & Heiman, M. L. (1996). Serum immunoreactive-leptin concentrations in normal weight and obese humans. *New England Journal of Medicine, 334,* 292–296.
14. Department of Health and Human Services. (1991). *Healthy people 2000: National health promotion and disease prevention objectives* (DHHS Publication No. 91-50212). Washington, DC: U.S. Government Printing Office.
15. DeFronzo, R. A., & Ferrannini, E. (1991). Insulin resistance: A multifaceted syndrome responsible for NIDDM, obesity, hypertension, dyslipidemia, and atherosclerotic cardiovascular disease. *Diabetes Care, 14,* 173–194.
16. Despres, J. P., Lamarche, B., Mauriege, P., et al. (1996). Hyperinsulinemia as an independent risk factor for ischemia heart disease. *New England Journal of Medicine, 334,* 952–957.
17. Diaz, M. N., Frei, B. Vita, J. A., & Keaney, J. F. (1997). Antioxidants and atherosclerotic heart disease. *New England Journal of Medicine, 337,* 408–416.
18. Dietz, L., & Gortmaker, S. L. (1985). Do we fatten our children at the television set? Obesity and television in children and adolescents. *Pediatrics, 75,* 807.
19. Dorr, A. (1986). *Television and children: A special medium for a special audience.* Beverly Hills, CA: Sage.
20. Dudek, S. G. (1997). *Nutrition handbook for nursing practice* (3rd ed.). Philadelphia: Lippincott-Raven.
21. Emmons, L. (1992). Dieting and purging behavior in black and white high school students. *Journal of the American Dietetic Association, 92,* 306–311.
22. Eschelman, M. M. (1996). *Introduction to nutrition and diet therapy* (3rd ed.). Philadelphia: Lippincott-Raven.
23. Forbes, G. B. (199). Do obese individuals gain weight more easily than nonobese individuals? *American Journal of Clinical Nutrition, 52,* 224.
24. Geary, N. (1996). Role of gut peptides in meal regulation. In L. A. Weston, & L. M. Savage (Eds.), *Obesity: Advances in understanding and treatment.* Southborough, MA: International Business Communication.
25. Ginsberg, H. N. (1998). Reduction of plasma cholesterol levels in normal men on an American Heart Association step 1 diet or a step 2 diet with added monounsaturated fat. *New England Journal of Medicine, 322,* 574–579.
26. Gordon, D. J., Salz, K. J., Roggenkamp, K. J., & Frankin, K. A. (1982). Dietary determinants of plasma cholesterol change in the recruitment phase of the Lipid Research Coronary Primary Prevention Trial. *Arteriosclerosis, 2,* 537–548.
27. Gortmaker, S. L., Dietz, W. H., & Cheung, L. W. (1990). Inactivity, diet, and the fattening of America. *Journal of the American Dietetic Association, 90,* 1247–1252.
28. Gortmaker, S. L., Must, A., Perrin, J. M., Sobel, A. M., & Dietz, W. H. (1993). Social and economic consequences of overweight in normal weight and obese humans. *New England Journal of Medicine, 329,* 1008–1012.
29. Gottdiener, J. S., Gross, H. A., Henry, W. L., Borer, J. S., & Ebert, M. H. (1978). Effects of self induced starvation on cardiac size and function in anorexia nervosa. *Circulation, 58,* 425.
30. Grilo, C. M., Devlin, M. J., Cachelin, F. M., & Yanovski, S. Z. (1997). Report of the National Institutes of Health (NIH) workshop on the development of research priorities in eating disorders. *Psychopharmacology Bulletin, 33*(3), 321–333.
31. Grinspoon, S., Herzog, D., & Klibanski, J. (1997). Mechanisms and treatment options for bone loss in anorexia nervosa. *Psychopharmacology Bulletin, 33,* 399–404.
32. Gupta, M. A., & Kavanaugh-Danelon, D. (1989). Elevated serum uric acid in eating disordered: A possible index of strenuous physical activity and starvation. *International Journal of Eating Disorders, 8,* 463.
33. Guyton, A. C., & Hall, J. E. (1996). *Textbook of medical physiology* (9th ed.). Philadelphia: Saunders.
34. Hall, R. C. W., & Beresford, T. P. (1989). Medical complications of anorexia and bulimia. *Psychological Medicine, 7,* 165.
35. Hall, R. C., et al. (1988). Refractory hypokalemia secondary to hypomagnesemia in eating disorder patients. *Psychosomatics, 29*(4), 435.
36. Herzog, D. B., & Copeland, P. M. (1985). Eating disorders. *New England Journal of Medicine, 315,* 295.
37. Hollenbeck, C. B., & Reaven, G. M. (1987). Variations in insulin stimulated glucose uptake in healthy individuals with normal glucose tolerance. *Journal of Clinical Endocrinology and Metabolism, 64,* 1169–1173.
38. Hooker, C., & Hall, R. C. W. (1989). Nutritional assessment of patients with anorexia and bulimia: Clinical and laboratory findings. *Psychological Medicine, 7*(3), 27.
39. Howard, G., O'Leary, D. H., & Zaccaro, D., et al. (1996). Insulin sensitivity and atherosclerosis. *Circulation, 93,* 1809–1817.
40. Humphries, L., Vivvian, B., Stuart, M., & McClain, C. J. (1989). Zinc deficiency and eating disorders. *Journal of Clinical Psychology, 50,* 456.
41. Jointhorp, B. (199). Obesity and adipose distribution as risk factors for the development of disease: A review. *Infusionstherapie, 17,* 24.
42. Kaplan, N. M. (1989). The deadly quartet: Upper body obesity, glucose intolerance, hypertriglyceridemia, and hypertension. *Archives of Internal Medicine, 149,* 1514.
43. Kay, H. (1997). Anorexia, obsessional behavior, and serotonin. *Psychopharmacology Bulletin, 33*(3), 335–344.
44. Keys, A., et al. (1950). *The biology of human starvation.* Minneapolis: University of Minnesota Press.
45. Kuczmarski, R. S., Flegal, S. M., Campbell, S. M., & Johnson, C. L. (1994). Increasing prevalence of overweight among US adults: The National Health and Nutrition Examination Surveys 1960–1991. *Journal of the American Medical Association, 272,* 205–211.
46. Lenfant, C., & Ernst, N. (1994). Daily dietary fat and total food energy intakes—Third national health and nutrition examination survey, phase I. *Morbidity and Mortality Weekly Report, 43*(7), 116–120.
47. Lichtenstein, A. H., Kennedy, E., Barrier, P., et al. (1998). Dietary fat consumption and health. *Nutrition Reviews, 56,* S3-S19.
48. Mahan, L. K., & Arlin, M. (1992). *Krauses' food, nutrition, and diet therapy.* Philadelphia: Saunders.
49. Meyer, J. M., & Stunkard, A. J. (1993). Genetics and human obesity. In A. J. Stunkard & T. A. Wadden (Eds.), *Obesity: Theory and therapy* (2nd ed.). New York: Raven.
50. Moller, D. E., & Flier, J. S. (1991). Insulin resistance—Mechanism, syndrome, and implications. *New England Journal of Medicine, 325,* 938–948.
51. Must, A. Jacques, P. F. Dalla, G. E., Bajema, C. J., & Dietz, W. H. (1992). Long term morbidity and mortality of overweight adolescents; A follow up of the Harvard Growth Study of 1922 to 1935. *New England Journal of Medicine, 327,* 1350–1355.

52. National Institutes of Diabetes and Digestive and Kidney Diseases. (1993). *Understanding adult obesity*. (NIH Publication No. 94-3680). Rockville, MD: National Institutes of Health.
53. National Task Force on the Prevention and Treatment of Obesity. (1996). Long term pharmacotherapy in the management of obesity. *Journal of the American Medical Association, 276,* 1907–1915.
54. Newman, M. M., & Halmi, K. A. (1988). The endocrinology of anorexia nervosa and bulimia nervosa. *Endocrinology and Metabolism Clinics of North America, 17*(1), 195.
55. Palmer, T. A. (199). Anorexia nrvosa and bulimia: Causal theories and treatment. *Nurse Practitioner, 15,* 12–21.
56. Peveler, R. C., Fairburn, C. G., Boller, I., & Dunger, P. (1992). Eating disorders in adolescents with IDDM: A controlled study *Diabetes Care, 15,* 1356.
57. Pi-Sunyer, F. X. (1993). Medical hazards of obesity. *Annals of Internal Medicine, 119,* 655–660.
58. Pomeroy, C., & Mitchell, J. E. (1989). Medical complications and management of eating disorders. *Psychiatric Annals, 19,* 488–493.
59. Prevalence of overweight among adolescents—United States 1988–1991. (1994). *Morbidity and Mortality Weekly Report, 14,* 818–821.
60. Ray, J. W., & Kleges, R. C. (1993). Influences on the eating behavior of children. In C. L. Williams & S. Y. S. Kimm (Eds.), *Prevention and treatment of childhood obesity. Annals of the New York Academy of Sciences, 699.*
61. National Academy of Sciences. (1989). *Recommended dietary allowances* (10th ed.). Washington, DC: National Academy Press.
62. Rich, L. M., Caine, M. R., Findling, J. W., & Shaker, J. L. (1990). Hypoglycemic coma in anorexia nervosa: Case report and review of the literature. *Archives of Internal Medicine, 150*(4), 894.
63. Roberts, M. W., et al. (1989). Dysphagia in bulimia nervosa. *Dysphagia, 4*(2), 106.
64. Rosenbaum, M. Leibel, R. L., & Hirsch, J. (1997). Obesity. *New England Journal of Medicine, 337,* 396–407.
65. Rossow, J. E. (1989). Kwashiorkor in North America. *American Journal of Nutrition, 49,* 58.
66. Schochen, D. D., Holloway, J. D., & Powers, P. (1989). Weight loss and the heart: Effects of anorexia nervosa and starvation. *Archives of Internal Medicine, 149,* 877.
67. Slattery, M. L. Edwards, S. L., Anderson, K., & Caan, B. (1998). Vitamin E and colon cancer. *Nutrition and Cancer, 30,* 201–206.
68. Stunkard, A. J., & Sorenson, T. I. (1993). Obesity and socioeconomic status: A complex relation (Editorial). *Mew England Journal of Medicine, 329,* 1036–1037.
69. Sunday, S. R., & Halmi, K. A. (1996). Micro and macroanalysis of patterns within a meal in anorexia and bulimia nervosa. *Appetite, 26,* 21–36.
70. Szmukler, G. I., Young, G. P., Lichtenstein, M., & Andrew, J. T. (1990). A serial study of gastric emptying time in anorexia nervosa and bulimia. *Australian and New Zealand Journal of Medicine, 20*(3), 220.
71. Thomas, P. (Ed.). (1995). *Weighing the options: Criteria for evaluating weight management programs.* Washington, DC: National Academy Press.
72. Tremblay, A., & Buemann, B. (1995). Exercise training, macronutrient balance, and bodyweight control. *International Journal of Obesity and Related Metabolic Disorders, 19,* 79–86.
73. Vaino, H., & Rautalahti, M. (1998). An international evaluation of the cancer preventive potential of caro-tenoids. *Cancer Epidemiology Biomarkers Prevention, 7,* 725–728.
74. Vaisman, N., et al. (1988). Energy expenditure and body composition in patients with anorexia nervosa. *Journal of Pediatrics, 113*(5), 919.
75. Van Itallie, T. (1985). Health implications of overweight and obesity in the United States. *Annals of Internal Medicine, 103,* 983–988.
76. Wadden, T. A., & Stunkard, A. J. (1993). Psychosocial consequences of obesity and dieting: Research and clinical findings. In T. A. Wadden & A. J. Stunkard (Eds.), *Obesity: Theory and therapy* (2nd ed.). New York: Raven.
77. Warren, M. P. (1990). Femoral head collapse associated with anorexia nervosa in a 20 year old ballet dancer. *Clinical Orthopaedics and Related Research, 251,* 171.
78. Whitney, E. N., Cataldo, C. B., & Rolfes, S. R. (1994). *Understanding normal and clinical nutrition* (4th ed.). St. Paul, MN: West.
79. Willard, S. G., Winstead, D. K, Anding, R., & Dudley, P. (1989). Laxative detoxification in bulimia nervosa. In W. G. Johnson (Ed.), *Advances in eating disorders* (Vol. 2). Greenwich, CT: JAI Press.
80. William, C. L. Bollella, M., & Wynder, E. L. (1995). Recommended goals for fiber for children. *Pediatrics, 92,* 985–988.
81. Williams, M. A., King, I. B., Sorenson, T. K., et al. (1998). Risk of preeclampsia in relation to elaidic acid (trans fatty acid) in maternal erythrocytes. *Gynecologic and Obstetric Investigation, 46*(2), 84–87.
82. Williamson, J. (1992). Physiologic stress: Trauma, sepsis, burns, and surgery. In L. K. Krause & M. A. Mahan (Eds.), *Krause's food, nutrition, and diet therapy.* Philadelphia: Saunders.
83. Wolff, H. P., Vecsei, P., & Kruch, R. (1968). Psychiatric disturbance leading to potassium depletion, sodium depletion, raised plasma renin concentration and secondary hyperaldosteronism. *Lancet, 1,* 257.

UNIT 1 APPENDIX A

PRENATAL DIAGNOSTIC TESTS

TEST	PROCEDURE	SIGNIFICANCE
I. Ultrasonography	Noninvasive procedure that uses high-frequency sound waves to provide images of fetus, placenta, and uterus. Can be done as early as 4 to 5 weeks after last menstrual period (LMP).	Determines gestational age by measuring crown–rump in 1st trimester and biparietal and femur length after 13 weeks gestation. Identifies congenital anomalies, especially of head and trunk. Cranial, spinal, thoracic, gastrointestinal, genitourinary, abdominal wall, extremity, and cardiovascular defects may be identified.
Real-time ultrasound	Adds continual cross-sectional pictures of internal structures and the motions within them.	Assessment of placental condition and location; especially important if there is vaginal bleeding. Determines presence of a pregnancy; can rule out ectopic pregnancy. Combined with other tests, can determine fetal–pelvic disproportion.
II. Doppler ultrasound	Diagnostic test for assessing the movement of blood in blood vessels and body organs. Can be used as early as 15 weeks gestation.	Detects blood flow abnormalities. Normal ratio of systolic to diastolic is 3:1 at 28 to 30 weeks gestation. Ratio normally decreases as pregnancy advances.
III. Chorionic villus sampling (CVS)	Invasive test, using ultrasound for direction, a plastic catheter is placed in the chorion and a specimen of chorionic villi is studied in a cytogenic laboratory. Usually performed between 9 and 12 weeks gestation.	Diagnoses chromosomal and metabolic disorders. May cause complications: amniotic fluid leakage, infection, intrauterine growth retardation (IUGR) or fetal death, spontaneous abortion, septic shock, and damage to placental membrane. Contraindicated in vaginal or cervical herpes infection, uterine fibroids, cervical stenosis, and RH blood incompatibilities.
IV. Amniocentesis	Invasive procedure that involves aspiration of amniotic fluid through an abdominal puncture. May be done in any trimester with adequate amniotic fluid. Ultrasound done first to confirm fetal viability, gestational age, location of placenta, and pockets of amniotic fluid.	Performed in first trimester for genetic studies such as x-linked recessive and single gene disorders. Performed in second trimester for Rh isoimmunization studies. Rh-negative mothers should have procedure at 24 to 25 weeks gestation to indicate fetal RBC hemolysis and possibly intrauterine fetal blood transfusion. Performed in third trimester to assess fetal lung maturity. Measurement of lecithin (L) and sphingomyelin (S)—two phospholipids that are normally produced by the fetus in the third trimester. They have detergent-like effect on alveoli and prevent collapse. L and S are expressed as a ratio; and a ratio of 2:1 is an acceptable measure of lung maturity. Measure of phosphatidyl glycerol also used. A positive level may indicate adequate lung maturity. Can identify missing enzymes that indicate fetal biochemical abnormalities: (1) lipid, amino acid and mucopolysaccharide abnormalities; (2) neural tube defects; (3) trisomy 21; (4) hemophilia; (5) muscular dystrophy.
V. Alpha (α) fetoprotein (AFP)	AFP is measured from amniotic fluid samples and maternal serum. AFP is produced by yolk sac and increases in the fetus at about 13 weeks gestation. Crosses the placenta to the maternal circulation.	Increased in the presence of a neural tube defect. Increased in the presence of hemorrhage or multiple pregnancy.

(continued)

UNIT 1 APPENDIX A

PRENATAL DIAGNOSTIC TESTS (Continued)

TEST	PROCEDURE	SIGNIFICANCE
VI. Acetylcholinesterase	Produced by fetal central nervous system and is more specific than AFP. Measured in amniocentesis fluid.	Increased levels indicate a neural tube defect. Decreased levels indicate fetal demise.
VII. Fetoscopy	Invasive procedure used in combination with ultrasound to diagnose and treat the fetus in utero. A needlescope (a flexible needle and endoscope) is inserted into the uterus through the abdomen. Fetal skin tissue and blood are collected.	Used to diagnose various types of genetic abnormalities. Used to diagnose blood incompatibilities, and intra uterine transfusion may be given. High risk for bleeding, infection, fetal injury, amniotic fluid leakage, and premature birth.
VIII. Percutaneous umbilical blood sampling (PUBS)	Invasive procedure that allows direct entry into fetal circulation to produce a pure specimen of fetal blood.	Used: (1) to determine fetal karyotype, (2) blood typing, (3) antibody testing, (4) acid-base evaluation, (5) assessment of hemolytic anemia, (6) to give intrauterine fetal blood transfusion. Potential complications are chorioamnionitis, premature labor, rupture of amniotic membranes, bleeding, and injury to umbilical cord.
IX. Fetal fibronectin (fFN)	Protein normally found in cervicovaginal secretions in pregnant woman approaching labor and in fetal tissue throughout pregnancy.	Normal function includes: (1) Early embryo–uterine implantation; (2) placental–uterine attachment; (3) maintenance of fetal membrane structural integrity; (4) adhesion associated with anchoring trophoblasts. Altered levels are associated with preterm labor, preeclampsia, postterm pregnancy, IUGR, and abruptio placentae.
X. Fetal biophysical profile	Test involves using a real-time ultrasound and the nonstress test to measure fetal movement, fetal breathing movements, fetal tone, amniotic fluid volume, and fetal heart rate reactivity.	High scores indicate fetal well-being with 10 of 10 being normal. (1) Normal score 2 for each variable. (2) Specific criteria for fetal movement, extension/flexion movements, acceleration of fetal heart rate, amniotic fluid volume of at least 1 cm. in two perpendicular planes, at least 30 seconds of breathing movements in 30 minutes of observation. Low scores may indicate fetal distress. (1) Results of 8 of 10 indicate possible fetal asphyxia. (2) 6 of 10 or below requires delivery for probable to certain fetal asphyxia. Indications for test include PIH, diabetes, post mature pregnancy, and suspected IUGR.

UNIT 1 APPENDIX B

LABORATORY VALUES

TEST	NORMAL VALUE	SIGNIFICANCE
Albumin	3.2–4.5 G/dL	Main plasma protein; maintains osmotic pressure; functions in binding drugs and in acid-base balance.
Aldosterone	2–9 ng/dL	Hormone responsible for sodium retention and potassium excretion.
Ammonia	12–48 mol/L	Breakdown product of protein that normally is synthesized to urea by liver to be excreted by the kidney.
Bicarbonate (HCO_3^-)	22–26 m Eq/L Arterial blood	Base buffer critical in regulating acid-base balance.
Bilirubin	0.0–1.0 mg/dL (total) 0.0–0.4 mg/dL (direct)	Substance that makes up bile pigments; most is formed from breakdown of heme from hemoglobin.
Calcium	8.5–10.5 mg/dL (total) 4.4–5 mg/dL (ionized)	Serum calcium necessary for nerve impulse transmission and muscle contraction; ionized calcium is active portion, nonionized is bound to plasma proteins.
Carbon dioxide content	24–30 mmol/L	Measured in venous blood and acts as a determinant of bicarbonate (HCO_3^-)
Carbon dioxide, partial pressure	35–45 mm Hg	Measured in arterial blood, measures pressure of carbon dioxide (CO_2) and reflects respiratory acid-base balance.
Chloride	95–108 m Eq/L	Most abundant extracellular anion; usually reflects sodium concentrations.
Creatinine	0.5–1.5 mg/dL	Byproduct of muscle catabolism from breakdown of creatine phosphokinase: all formed creatinine is excreted in urine.
Glucose	70–110 mg/dL fasting	Formed from dietary carbohydrates; essential in energy production.
Ketone (acetone)	Negative in serum and urine	Formed from fat breakdown to free fatty acids and then to ketone bodies; when formed, are excreted in urine.
Magnesium	1.5–2.5 m Eq/L	Cation concentrated in intracellular fluid; in extracellular fluid essential for neuromuscular & cardiac activity.
Osmolality	285–295 mOsm/Kg of water	Measure of the number of dissolved particles in serum; most osmolality is determined by sodium concentration.
Oxygen, partial pressure	80–100 mg Hg	Measured in arterial blood; measure pressure of oxygen (O_2) available to saturate hemoglobin.
Oxygen saturation	95–99%	Percentage of hemoglobin that is saturated with oxygen in arterial blood.
pH	7.35–7.45	Measure of hydrogen ion concentration in arterial blood; narrow range acceptable for acid-base balance.
Phosphate (Inorganic Phosphorus)	2.5–4.5 mg/dL	Principal intracellular anion; most in teeth and bones; significant relationship with calcium balance.
Potassium	3.5–5.0 mEq/L	Most abundant intracellular cation; essential in neuromuscular, cardiac and skeletal muscle Contraction.
Renin	1.6–4.3 ng/mL	Enzyme secreted by kidneys that activates angiotensinogen, which leads to vasoconstriction and water retention through aldosterone.
Sodium	136–145 mEq/L	Major cation in extracellular fluid; functions to retain water, conduction of neuromuscular impulses, regulation of acid-base balance, and close functioning with enzyme systems.
Urea nitrogen (blood urea nitrogen [BUN])	5–25 mg/dL	End product of protein metabolism; excreted by kidneys.
Uric acid	Male: 3.5–8.0 mg/dL Female: 2.8–6.8 mg/dL	By product of purine metabolism from purine foods; excess amounts are excreted in urine.

UNIT BIBLIOGRAPHY

American Psychiatric Association (1997). *Understanding sleep: The evaluation and treatment of sleep disorders.* Washington, DC: American Psychiatric Association.

Berne, R. M. & Levy, M. N. (1998). *Physiology* (4th ed.). St. Louis: Mosby.

Bijlsma, R. & Loescheke, V. (1997). *Environmental stress, adaptation and evaluation.* Boston: Birkhauser.

Buckingham, J. Gilles, G. E. & Cowell, A. M. (1997). *Stress, stress hormones and the immune system.* New York: Wiley.

Clarke, A. (Ed.) (1994). *Genetic counselling practice and principles.* New York: Rutledge.

Clarke, J. T. R. (1996). *A clinical guide to inherited metabolic diseases.* New York: Cambridge University Press.

Connor, J. M. & Ferguson-Smith, M. A. (1997). *Essential medical genetics* (5th ed.). Boston: Blackwell Scientific.

Cooper, C. L., & Watson, M., (1991). *Cancer and stress: Psychological, biological and coping studies.* New York: Wiley.

Cooper, C. L. (1996). *Handbook of stress medicine and health.* Boca Raton, FL: CRC Press.

Cooper, G. M. (1997). *The cell: A molecular approach.* Washington, DC: ASM Press.

Cox, T. M. & Sinclair, J. (Eds.) (1997). *Molecular biology in medicine.* Boston: Blackwell Scientific.

Culebras A. (1996). *Clinical handbook of sleep disorders.* Boston: Butterworth-Heineman.

Drilica, K. (1997). *Understanding DNA and gene cloning: A guide for the curious* (3rd ed.). New York: John Wiley and Sons.

Dudek, S. G. (1997). *Nutrition handbook for nursing practice* (3rd ed.). Philadelphia: Lippincott.

Eschelman, M. M. (1996). *Introduction to nutrition and diet therapy* (3rd ed.). Philadelphia: Lippincott.

Friedman, H., Klein, T. W. & Friedman, A. L. (1995). *Psychoneuroimmunology, stress and infection.* Boca Raton, FL: CRC Press.

Fuller, G. M. & Shields, D. (1998). *Molecular basis of medical cell biology.* Stamford, CT: Appleton & Lange.

Gelehrter, T. D., Collins, F. S. & Ginsburg, D. (1998). *Principles of medical genetics* (2nd ed.). Baltimore: Williams & Wilkins.

Glaser, R. & Kiecold-Glaser, J. (1994). *Handbook of stress and immunity.* San Diego: Academic Press.

Hafer, B. Q. (1997). *Mind/body health: The effects of attitudes, emotions & relationships.* Boston: Allyn and Bacon.

Holland, J. F. (Ed.)(1997). *Cancer medicine.* Baltimore: Williams & Wilkins.

Hubbard, J. R. & Workman, E. A. (1998). *Handbook of stress medicine: An organ system approach.* Boca Raton, FL.: CRC Press.

Jones, K. L. (1997). *Smith's recognizable patterns of human malformation* (5th ed.). Philadelphia: Saunders.

Jorde, L. B., Carey, J. C. & White, R. L. (1995). *Medical genetics.* St. Louis: Mosby.

Lewis, C. E., O'Sullivan, C. & Baraclough, C. (1994). *The psychoimmunology of cancer: Mind and body in the fight for survival.* New York: Oxford University Press.

King, R. A., Rotter, J. I., & Motulsky, A. G. (Eds.) (1992). *The Genetic basis of common disease.* New York: Oxford University Press.

King, R. C., & Stansfield, W. D. (1997). *A dictionary of genetics* (5th ed.). New York: Oxford University Press.

Korf, B. R.(1996). *Human genetics: A problem-based approach.* Cambridge, MA: Blackwell Science.

Lueckenotte, A. G. (Ed.) (1996). *Gerontologic nursing.* St. Louis: Mosby.

Miller, T. W. (1997). *Clinical disorders and stressful life events.* Madison, CN: International Universities Press.

Narins, R. G. (Ed) (199??521035??). *Maxwell and Kleeman's clinical disorders of fluid and electrolyte metabolism* (5th ed.). New York: McGraw-Hill.

Pawlowitzki, I. H., Edwards, J. H. & Thompson, E. A. (Eds.) (1997). *Genetic mapping of disease genes.* New York: Academic Press.

Pronsky, Z. M., et al. (1997). *Food medication interactions handbook* (10th ed.). New York: Food Interactions Co.

Robertson, J. A. (1994). *Children of choice: Freedom and the new reproductive technologies.* Princeton: Princeton University Press.

Rowell, L. B. & Dempsy, J. A. (1996). *Exercise regulation and integration of multiple systems.* New York: American Physiologic Society by Oxford University Press.

Schardein, J. L. (1993). *Chemically induced birth defects* (2nd ed.). New York: Marcel Dekker.

Scriver, A. L. Beaudet, A. L., Sly, W. S., & Valle, D. (Eds.) (1995). *The metabolic basis of inherited human diseases* (7th ed.). New York: McGraw-Hill.

Seashore, M. R. & Wappner, R. S. (1996). *Genetics in primary care and clinical medicine.* Stamford, CT: Appleton & Lange.

Simpson, J. L. & Elias, S. (1993). *Essentials of prenatal diagnosis.* New York: Churchill Livingstone.

Simpson, J. L. & Golbus, M. S. (1998). *Genetics in obstetrics and gynecology* (3rd ed.). Philadelphia: Saunders.

Snustad, D. P., Simmons, M. J. & Jenkins, J. B. (1997). *Principles of genetics.* New York: John Wiley & Sons.

Strachan, T. & Read, A. P. (1996). *Human molecular genetics.* New York: John Wiley & Sons.

Stunkard, A. J. & Watten, T. A. (Eds.) (1994). *Obesity: Theory and therapy* (2nd ed.). New York: Raven Press.

Trent, R. J. (1997). *Molecular medicine: An introductory text.* New York: Churchill Livingstone.

Vogelstein, B. & Kinzler, K. W. (1998). *The genetic basis of human cancer.* New York: McGraw-Hill.

ON-LINE REFERENCES

Access Excellence—Genetics Websites (Public Broadcasting System, PBS): *http;//outcast.gene.com/ae/RC/genetics.html*

American Journal of Human Genetics: *http://www.journals.uchicago.edu/AJHG/*

American Journal of Human Genetics—Various Human Genome Databases: *http://www.interscience.wiley.corn/jpages/0148-7299/sites.html*

American Nurses Foundation—Preparing Nurses for the Future: *http://www.ana.org/anf/hrethics.html*

Cancer Genetics Working Group—Overview: *http://www.dceg.ims.nci.nih.gov/workgrp/overview.html*

Council of Medical Genetics Organizations: *http://www.faseb.org/genetics/ashg/comgo.html*

Fragile X Bibliography: *http://www.mcet.edu/humangenome/resources/bibliography/fragilexbib.html*

Genetic Databases with emphasis on human diseases by chromosomes: *http://www.owu.edu/~jmfreed/wedgene.html*

Genetic Resources—Biological Scientific Organizations. Professional Societies. American Association for the Advancement of Science, American Board of Genetic Cournseling. The American Cancer Society: *http://www.uic.edu/depts/mcgn/genres.html*

Human Genome Project Publications: *http://www.ornl.gov/TechResources/Human Genome/publicat/publications.Html*

Internet Resources—Genetics: *http://www.auhs.edu/library/resource/genetics.html*

National Institutes of Health Gene Sequencing Databases: *http://www. ncbi.nlm.nih.gov/BLAST/*

Selected Internet Resources in Biomedicine: *http://www.med.yale.edu/library/sir/*

Unit **2**

Infections, Inflammation, and Immunity

FOCUS ON Immunologic Changes Through the Life Span

INFANT (1–12 MONTHS):

The thymus gland (for T lymphocyte maturation) weighs approximately 22 g at birth. It begins to develop mature T lymphocytes in early infancy. The phagocytosis process is mature, but the inflammatory response is slow to localize infections. Antibody production from B lymphocytes is delayed for 3 to 6 months, and much of the antibody protection is acquired from the mother's IgG. Specific immunity is developed due to infectious agent exposure and vaccinations.

TODDLER AND PRESCHOOL AGE (1–5 YEARS):

The defense mechanisms of phagocytosis are much more efficient than in infancy. The thymus continues to develop and mature T lymphocytes. Specific T and B lymphocytes are established to most organisms. IgM reaches adult levels by late infancy. IgG levels reach adult values by the age of 2, and IgA, IgD, and IgE gradually increase. Lymphoid tissues enlarge and may become sites for infections, especially the tonsils and adenoids.

SCHOOL AGE (6–12 YEARS):

The immune system becomes functionally mature by the age of 12. The phagocytic abilities are mature, and the ability to localize infection improves. The thymus gland continues to enlarge and is very active in T lymphocyte maturation. Lymphoid tissue enlarges to exceed adult size. This is associated with increased vulnerability of the tissues and mucous membranes to infection. Infections gradually decrease throughout the period.

ADOLESCENCE (13–19 YEARS):

The thymus gland attains its greatest size of about 35 g. The ability to mount immune reactions is at a peak with adult levels of T lymphocytes and all of the immunoglobulins. The immune system is highly affected by emotional and physical stress especially noted at this stage; therefore, infections (such as colds) may be seen. Nutritional alterations also may depress immune system functioning.

YOUNG ADULT AND ADULT (20–45 YEARS):

The immune system usually functions efficiently, even though there is beginning involution of the thymus gland. T lymphocytes and all of the immunoglobulins are at peak levels. During this period, many of the autoimmune diseases are diagnosed. The immune system is affected by stress, which may cause immune depression.

MIDDLE-AGED ADULT (46–64 YEARS):

Most lymphoid tissue begins a process of involution during this period, with tonsils becoming atrophied. The thymus gland continues its process of involution and is replaced by fatty connective tissue. It usually weighs less than 6 g at this time. Immune function usually is efficient unless there are intervening diseases such as cancer. Stressful lifestyles continue to affect immune functioning.

LATE ADULTHOOD (65–100+ YEARS):

The thymus gland continues to degenerate, and the total number of circulating T lymphocytes declines. B lymphocytes also decrease. The antigen–antibody responses decrease, and total immune responses—cell-mediated and humoral—decline. There are increases in the rates of different types of infections as well as increased malignancy rates. Autoimmune processes such as rheumatoid arthritis may also increase.

Chapter

8

Infectious Agents

Carol Ann Barnett Lammon

KEY TERMS

adherins
capsid
capsomere
carrier state
cestodes
Ciliata
endemic
endotoxins
eosinophilia
epidemic
epidemiology
facultative intracellular parasites
flagellates
host
iatrogenic infection
interferon
latent infection
leukocidins
leukocytosis
lymphocytosis
monocytosis
mycosis (mycoses)
nematodes
neutrophilia
nosocomial infection
oncogenic virus
pandemic
parasitism
pathogen
pleomorphic
pyrogenic
Sarcodina
Sporozoa
tissue tropism
trematodes
virions
virulence

Pathogens are microorganisms or proteinaceous substances capable of producing disease. Pathogenic agents include bacteria, viruses, prions, fungi, protozoa, and helminths. Infectious diseases are the most common cause of death worldwide.[29] In developed countries, good nutrition, insect control, immunization, sanitation, and antimicrobial chemotherapy have reduced the mortality and morbidity of infectious disease; however, microbial infections have not been eliminated. Pneumonia/influenza and the human immunodeficiency virus (HIV) are the sixth and eighth leading causes of death, respectively, in the United States.[2] The emergence of antibiotic-resistant strains of bacteria as well as previously unknown infectious agents such as prions and hantavirus have increased morbidity and mortality of infectious disease even in developed countries. Deaths due to infectious disease most commonly occur in very young, elderly, debilitated, poorly nourished, and immunosuppressed individuals.

EPIDEMIOLOGY OF INFECTIOUS DISEASE

Epidemiology is the study of how disease is produced in a population. It describes both infectious and noninfectious causes of diseases. In infectious disease, the mode of transmission, susceptibilities of populations, and ultimate outcome of the infection are studied. The interaction of the host with the causative agent in a disease-producing environment is a main factor in causation of disease.[10] An **epidemic** investigation is undertaken when there is a significant increase in the number of cases of a particular infection, greatly increased over what is considered to be the norm. An **endemic** infectious disease is one that is routinely found among certain populations. A **pandemic** is a worldwide epidemic, such as that seen with acquired immune deficiency syndrome (AIDS) or certain flu outbreaks.

PATHOPHYSIOLOGY OF INFECTIOUS DISEASE

An organism is termed a pathogen when, under certain circumstances, it can produce a disease state in the host. The readiness or ability to accomplish this state is termed the **virulence** of the organism. The terms pathogenicity and virulence are often treated as synonymous, indicating that the organism is more or less pathogenic or virulent in certain circumstances.[28]

A pathogenic microorganism typically attaches itself to a larger organism, or **host.** The relationship between the host and a pathogenic microorganism then becomes one of **parasitism**. A larger organism, the host, is damaged by coexistence with a smaller organism, the parasite. Infection is the establishment of such a host–parasite interaction. Infectious disease results when clinically observable signs and symptoms from the interaction indicate that injury to the host has occurred.[9,21]

Infectious organisms characteristically cause infection in one organ system. This propensity is called **tissue tropism** and is determined by specific biochemical substances on the surface of the organism complemented by receptors on the target organ.[26] Figure 8-1 illustrates examples of tissue tropism of common bacterial pathogens.

Each microorganism is distinct and has its own means of invasion and reproduction. All infectious organisms are communicable (transmissible) from one

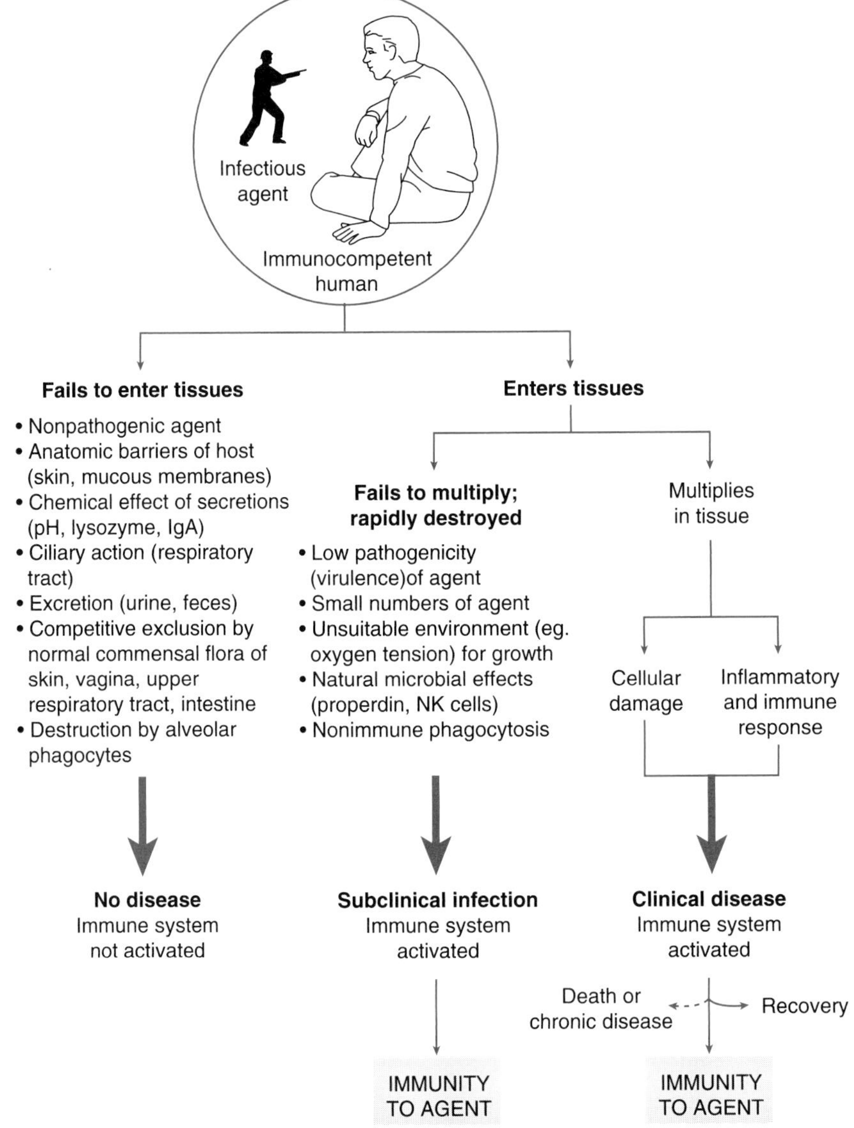

FIGURE 8-1. Possible results of an encounter with an infectious agent. (Chandrasoma, P. & Taylor, C. R. [1998]. *Concise pathology* [3rd ed.]. Stamford, CT: Appleton and Lange.)

member of the same species to another. The modes of transmission vary and depend on the source, quantity of organisms, transit survival, and a susceptible new host.[7] The process of pathogenic invasion and the development of infectious disease is summarized in Box 8-1.

Factors That Promote Infectious Disease

The occurrence of infectious diseases depends on many factors, including the virulence of the organism, the number of invading organisms, the defense mechanisms of the body, and the relationship with the normal human flora. Theobald Smith first summarized the interaction of these variables in the equation

$$P = \frac{N \times V}{R}$$

where P = probability of infection, N = number of infecting organisms, V = virulence of the infecting organism, and R = resistance of the host.[25]

THE VIRULENCE OF THE PARASITE

Some organisms are highly virulent in normal hosts, which means that in most individuals they will cause disease.[26] The mechanism of disease causation depends on the specific organism and the ability of the host to resist the onslaught of invasion. The number of invading organisms must be sufficient to overwhelm the defenses of the host (see below). Infection, then, results from the interaction of highly virulent microorganisms with an immunologically intact host or less virulent microbes interacting with a host who has some degree of impairment of host defense.[24]

Opportunistic pathogens are less virulent and only cause disease when the host's defense mechanisms are impaired.[28] The importance of opportunistic infections has been underscored by the emergence of many unusual infections in people infected with HIV, which causes AIDS. The emergence of opportunistic infections has also resulted from the administration of immunosuppressive drugs to combat disease or discourage transplant rejection. These treatment measures can impair the ability of the host to withstand infection, allowing organisms that normally reside on the surfaces of the body to gain access and cause disease. The degree of immune compromise and the elements of the immune system that are compromised are key factors in the severity of the disease manifestations. Many disease conditions and even emotional stress can also suppress the immune response and leave the individual vulnerable to disease (see p. 296).

BOX 8-1

STAGES OF PRODUCTION OF INFECTION

Virulent microorganisms must pass through the following four stages in order to cause disease:

1. The microorganism must encounter a receptive host, one whose defense mechanisms are impaired.
2. The organism must then gain entry into the host. Means of entry include inhalation, ingestion, attachment and penetration of mucous membranes, direct entry due to vector bite or trauma, and transmission across the placenta.
3. After gaining entry into the host, the organism must multiply and spread from the site of entry. Many pathogens produce enzymes and toxins that facilitate invasion and spread throughout the host.
4. Finally, the microorganism must cause host tissue injury. Pathogens can cause damage to tissues through inflammatory mobilization of phagocytic cells and cytokines. Some pathogens produce a variety of toxins that can damage host cells. Pathogens also can induce hypersensitive immune responses that damage the host's tissues.

DEFENSE MECHANISMS OF THE BODY

The defense mechanisms of the human organism are responsible for preventing multiple environmental pathogens from causing disease. These mechanisms reside on the external and internal surfaces and include physical, chemical, and immune barriers (Table 8-1). Whether the organism can cause disease largely depends on the success or failure of these mechanisms and barriers to provide adequate defense.

The main physical external barrier to infection is the skin, an intact epidermis being almost impervious to infection. The mucous membranes lining various organs also remove organisms by secreting mucus, which provides a washing effect and prevents organisms from adhering to membranes. Chemical secretions, such as hydrochloric acid in the stomach and the normally acidic pH urine, contribute to the sterile environment in the organs.

The immune system targets pathogens for destruction. When organisms gain access to the body, lymphocytes selectively recognize and destroy them, often without producing disease manifestations. The competence of the immune system, therefore, plays a major role in the outcome of infectious disease (see Chapter 10). Age, genetic factors, psychological factors, and environmental and nutritional factors affect immune competence. Clinically apparent infections occur when the defense mechanisms have not been sufficient to hold the growth of the organism in check. The pathogenesis of infection

TABLE 8-1

DEFENSE MECHANISMS OF THE BODY

MECHANISM	CHARACTERISTICS OF DEFENSE
Physical	Intact epidermis Mucus-secreting membranes Mucus blanket movement in respiratory tract Connective tissue
Chemical	Hydrochloric acid in stomach Acid pH of urine Lysozyme enzyme present in many secretions Resident flora in mouth, on skin, in large intestine
Immune	Specific antigen–antibody reactions Immunoglobin A Inflammatory response
Host factors	Age Sex Genetic susceptibilities Nutritional balance Stress—physiologic or emotional Presence of other diseases

depends on the capability of the specific organism and its ability to bypass or inactivate the defense mechanisms of the body.

NORMAL HUMAN FLORA

The human body normally harbors many thousands of different types of bacteria, with smaller numbers of other organisms.[7] The normal flora (resident bacteria) are essential in the production of vitamin K in the colon. They also produce members of the vitamin B family, but this function is not necessary with a well-balanced diet. The flora in the vaginal mucosa are protective against other bacteria. There appears to be a varying relationship at different chronological ages with different types of bacteria, which are considered to be residents or transients depending upon how long they remain without causing disease. There is a fine line between these residents and **carrier states**, which may produce disease in others exposed to the organism.

Many infections arise from normal flora of the host due to a change in organism virulence or decrease in host resistance. When the normal barriers to infections are broken, such as in hospital settings with invasive procedures, there is a much greater risk of normal flora causing infection. Infections that are caused by exposure in a hospital or other medical setting are called **nosocomial infections**. These infections would not occur if the individual had not been placed in the environment or been subjected to a particular procedure. An infection that is caused by medical personnel is termed an **iatrogenic infection.** When host resistance decreases, such as with the stress of surgery or as a reaction to antibiotic therapy, organisms normally under control will proliferate rapidly and become pathologic. If the normal microbes in an area are known, the source and significance of microorganisms isolated from a clinical infection also become known.[12] The organisms that are indigenous to specific areas vary. Table 8-2 categorizes the sites and the organisms that normally reside in those sites.

BACTERIA

Bacteria do not require living cells for growth. They are free-living organisms that use the body as a source of nutrients and as a favorable environment for growth. Bacteria can attach to epithelial tissue and, like many other types of organisms, exhibit tissue tropism.

Classification

Bacteria are classified according to their shape, staining properties, oxidative natures, and how they produce disease. Medically interesting bacteria belong to one of two categories: "typical" and "atypical."[23]

TYPICAL BACTERIA

The typical bacteria include rods and the spherical cocci according to their shape (morphology). They may be gram positive or gram negative, depending on the chemical composition of their cell walls and their absorption of staining dye. Gram-positive bacteria stain purple because their cell walls resist decolorization by acetone alcohol. Gram-negative bacteria are first decolorized and then stained with a red dye to make them stand out.[5] Within each group, the organism may be classified as pyogenic (pus producing), aerobic, or anaerobic, according to its oxidative capacities and mechanisms of disease causation.

Modes of Infection

Bacterial infection typically occurs when the bacteria overcome the host's defense mechanisms. The organism is then able to invade, multiply, and spread through the host. Bacterial pathogens have developed many ways to accomplish these goals.

Some extracellular bacteria, such as *Streptococcus salivarius*, produce **adherins,** allowing them to strongly attach to structures and penetrate to underlying tissues.[28] Other extracellular bacteria, such as the pneumococcus and streptococcus organisms, develop thick capsules of carbohydrate or protein that enables them

TABLE 8-2

NORMAL FLORA FOUND IN THE BODY

SITE AFFECTED	ORGANISM
Skin	*Staphylococcus epidermidis*
	Staphylococcus aureus
	Propionibacterium acnes (anaerobic corynebacteria)
	Lactobacilli
	Clostridium perfringens
	Acinetobacter calcoaceticus
	Aerobic corynebacteria
Nose/Nasopharynx	*Haemophilus parainfluenzae*
	Staphylococcus aureus
	Staphylococcus epidermidis
	Aerobic corynebacteria
Mouth/Oropharynx	*Staphylococcus aureus*
	Staphylococcus epidermidis
	Aerobic corynebacteria
	Alpha- and nonhemolytic streptococci
	Streptococcus mutans
	S. milleri
	S. mitis
	S. sanguis
	S. salivarius
	Branhamella catarrhalis
	Anaerobic micrococci
	Veillonella alcalescens
	Enterobacteriaceae
Small intestine	*Candida albicans*
Large intestine	Gram-negative bacilli
	Escherichia coli
	Enterobacteriaceae
	Klebsiella sp.
	Enterobacter sp.
	Candida albicans
	Bacteroides fragilis
	B. melaninogenicus
	B. oralis
	Fusobacterium nucleatum
	F. necrophorum
	Gram-positive bacilli
	Lactobacilli
	Eubacterium limosum
	Bifidobacterium bifidum
	Gram-positive cocci
	Staphylococcus aureus
	Enterococci
	Peptostreptococci
Genitourinary tract	*Lactobacillus*
Vagina	*Bacteroides*
	Peptostreptococci
	Aerobic corynebacteria
	Staphylococcus epidermidis
	Enterococci
	Candida albicans
	Trichomonas vaginalis

Note: Not all organisms are found in every individual. These organisms are common in sites listed. Other sites are usually sterile.

to escape phagocytosis.[9] Bacteria such as *Staphylococcus aureus* and *Staphylococcus pyogenes* actively secrete antiphagocytic substances known as **leukocidins** that destroy phagocytes. Table 8-3 describes some of the bacterial substances that facilitate invasion and spread of infection.

A common bacterial defense mechanism is rapid growth. Some bacteria such as *cholera* and *group A streptococcus* have such short incubation periods that they produce illness long before the primary immune response can occur.

The production of toxins also enables bacteria to grow and create illness in the host. Two hundred and twenty bacterial toxins have been specifically identified, 105 from gram-positive bacteria and 115 from gram-negative bacteria, but there probably are many more.[9] *Exotoxins* are proteins that are secreted from living cells into the surrounding medium. They are highly antigenic with variable specificity; some act on certain cell types, whereas others affect a large group of cells and tissues.[23,28] Very small quantities of exotoxin can be fatal. Exotoxins usually have a specific site of action in the body, and therefore each toxin produces specific effects. Table 8-4 describes three types of exotoxins. **Endotoxins** are lipopolysaccarides that are a component of the cell wall of gram-negative bacteria. They are released during cell division or cell destruction.[28] Endotoxin-producing bacteria are **pyrogenic**, producing fever and inflammation in the host. Endotoxins invoke the production of cytokines and activate both complement and coagulation cascades (see p. 259). They also cause the release of vasoactive peptides leading to vasodilation, hypotension, and poor organ perfusion, a condition called endotoxic or septic shock (see p. 511).

Clinical Manifestations

All bacteria are capable of localizing in specific organs and often produce an acute inflammatory reaction. The degree of tissue damage depends on the number of bacteria present, the virulence of the organism, the site of infection, and the resistance of the host to the organism.

Table 8-5 presents a classification of some of the more common gram-negative and gram-positive bacteria that affect humans, including the variable clinical pictures seen with different organisms. The list is necessarily incomplete because there are thousands of bacterial organisms.

ATYPICAL BACTERIA

The atypical group of organisms have special characteristics with regard to shape, size, or staining properties.[23] This group includes the following organisms, which have little relationship with each other except that they can cause human disease: (1) acid-fast bacilli,

TABLE 8-3

BACTERIAL SUBSTANCES THAT ENHANCE INVASION AND SPREAD OF INFECTION

SUBSTANCE	MECHANISM OF ACTION	EXAMPLE
Coagulase	Causes clotting of plasma. Enables bacteria to form a sticky fibrin layer around themselves, providing protection from host defenses.	Staphylococci
Streptokinase	Dissolves fibrin clots, allowing organism to spread through host tissues.	Streptococci
Hyaluronidase	Breaks down connective tissue and increases tissue permeability, allowing organism to spread through host tissues.	Streptococci Pneumococci Clostridia
Collagenase	Degrades collagen to facilitate deep invasion of pathogens into tendon, cartilage, and bone.	Clostridia
Elastase	Degrades and damages the elastin of blood vessel walls.	Pseudomonas
Phospholipase	Causes necrosis of muscle cell membranes, endothelial cell membranes, and RBC membranes.	Clostridia
Leukocidin	Antiphagocytic action enables bacteria to escape host defense mechanisms.	*S. Aureus* *S. pyogenes*
Adherins	Allow attachment to host cell surfaces.	*E. coli* *S. pyogenes* *T. mutans*
Slime layers and polysaccharide capsules	Allow bacteria to escape phagocytosis.	*S. pneumonia* *N. meningitidis* *H. influenza*
Waxy capsule	Allows bacteria to escape phagocytosis.	*M. tuberculosis*

especially characterized by the tubercle bacillus, *Mycobacterium tuberculosis*; (2) spirochetes, such as *Treponema pallidum*; (3) chlamydiae; (4) rickettsia; and (5) mycoplasma. Table 8-6 summarizes features of these bacteria or bacteria-like organisms.

TABLE 8-4

THREE TYPES OF EXOTOXINS

MECHANISM OF ACTION	EXAMPLES
Toxins bind to host cellular receptors, causing changes in cellular processes.	Enterotoxins (secretory diarrhea, nausea) Toxic shock syndrome
Toxins lyse erythrocytes.	Hemolysins (83 types)
Toxins consist of two parts, a vector or binding portion and an enzymatic or toxic portion that invades the cytosol of the host cell,causing damage to host cellular processes.	Diphtheria toxin (pseudomembrane) Clostridia toxin (paralysis) Cholera toxin (secretory diarrhea) Shiga toxin (hemorrhagic colitis) Verotoxins of *E. coli* O:157 H:7 (hemorrhagic colitis and hemolytic uremic syndrome)

Acid-Fast Infections

The acid-fast bacteria mainly consist of *M. tuberculosis* and *Mycobacterium leprae*. These organisms will not pick up many chemicals since they are surrounded by a waxy envelope that can only be traversed by special procedures. The name of the genus contains the root word for fungus since the organisms may form branches that suggest a fungal organism.[23] Recently, several species of *Mycobacteria* have been found to cause opportunistic infections, especially in the HIV-positive population. These species are often termed atypical acid-fast bacilli, such as *Mycobacterium avium-intracellulare*. *M. tuberculosis* organisms are common **facultative intracellular parasites**, which are able to survive and grow within macrophages and emerge to infect the host.[12,22] The organisms can also proliferate in the extracellular spaces. Humans are the only natural reservoir for *M. tuberculosis*.[28] These bacteria induce hypersensitive immune reactions to their cell wall components. Cellular responses include tissue damage resulting from chronic inflammation; the granulomatous lesion of tuberculosis is an example of such a reaction (see p. 556).[9,10]

M. leprae (Hansen's bacillus) produces a chronic infection of the skin, mucous membranes, and peripheral nerves. It results from direct and prolonged contact with an individual with active infection. Its incidence is increasing in the U.S. due to increased immigration from certain third world countries.[28]

(text continues on page 235)

TABLE 8-5

TYPICAL BACTERIA THAT CAUSE PATHOLOGIC EFFECTS IN HUMANS

BACTERIA	GRAM STAIN	MORPHOLOGY	EPIDEMIOLOGY	CLINICAL EFFECTS
Pseudomonas aeruginosa	Gram-negative	Motile rod; greenish yellow pigment formed; saprophytic but can establish infection and invade when host resistance is decreased	Commonly present on skin and mucous membranes; often attacks debilitated, immunosuppressed, burned, premature, or elderly people; transmitted by contact, especially to urinary tract, lungs, or damaged skin	Purulent drainage from wounds; characteristic greenish mucus from site of infection; bacteremia carries a 75% mortality; high fever, confusion, chills followed by circulatory collapse and sometimes leukopenia
Proteus	Gram-negative	Active motile rod; hydrolyzes urea; actively decomposes protein	Commonly present in decaying matter, soil, water, and human intestine; affects skin, urinary tract, ears, and other areas secondarily in susceptible people	Localized purulent infections may spread and cause bacteremia, symptoms of bacteremia; usually sensitive to penicillin therapy
Enterobacter, Klebsiella	Gram-negative	Short, plump, nonmotile rods; type-specific capsular antigens	Urinary tract and respiratory infections; especially pneumonia; often found in immunosuppressed, alcoholics, or people with diabetes mellitus	Symptoms of pneumonitis; productive cough, weakness, anemia; may resemble TB; responds well to aminoglycoside therapy
Shigella	Gram-negative	Nonmotile rods; aerobic or nearly anaerobic	GI tract resident; transmitted through fecal-oral route, or through contaminated food, water, swimming pools; common in countries where sanitation is poor; incubation usually less than 48 h	Fever, colicky abdominal pain, diarrhea; liquid, greenish stools may contain various amounts of blood; dehydration may result
Escherichia coli	Gram-negative	Non–spore-forming rods; different strains characterized by their antigens	Normal inhabitant of colon; may spread to urinary tract directly or through bloodstream; opportunistic organism in debilitated people	Accounts for more than 75% of urinary tract infections; abscesses may form on any area; bacteremia characterized by fever, chills, dyspnea; may develop endotoxic shock
Salmonella				
S. typhi (typhoid fever)	Gram-negative	Motile; type identified by specific antigens	Ingestion of contaminated foods, water, or milk; transmitted through fecal contamination of foodstuffs; totally transmitted by human carriers; incubation period about 10 days	Rare in U.S.; onset of fever, chills, abdominal pain, and distention; rash of small macules on upper abdomen and thorax; without treatment often causes intestinal bleeding and perforation
Other *Salmonella* organisms	Gram-negative	Varies with type	Food contamination; disease onset within hours of food ingestion	Enteritis, massive vomiting, diarrhea, dehydration, fever; antibiotic treatment normally not helpful
Haemophilus				
H. influenzae	Gram-negative	Small, pleomorphic nonmotile, aerobic non–spore-forming	Respiratory transmission, especially to very young and aged	Nasopharyngitis may be epidemic, especially in impoverished and rural populations; often outbreaks during winter months may develop into pneumonia, ear infections, rarely meningitis

(continued)

TABLE 8-5

TYPICAL BACTERIA THAT CAUSE PATHOLOGIC EFFECTS IN HUMANS (Continued)

BACTERIA	GRAM STAIN	MORPHOLOGY	EPIDEMIOLOGY	CLINICAL EFFECTS
H. ducreyi (Chancroid)	Gram-negative	Small, anaerobic, slow-growing	Sexual contact; increased incidence in males	Chancroid, painful genital ulcer, diagnosed by Gram's stain
Bordetella (*B. pertussis*)	Gram-negative	Small, aerobic, slow-growing	Respiratory droplets; very contagious; incubation about 1 wk	"Whooping cough"; characterized by catarrhal stage followed by paroxysmal cough and laryngeal stridor; without immunization, epidemics occur; immunization or disease does not provide lifelong immunity
Staphylococcus	Gram-positive	Spherical, grapelike clusters or organisms on solid media		
S. aureus	Gram-positive	Coagulase positive; remains viable on surfaces of furniture or clothing	Commonly resides on skin and mucosal surfaces; invades skin through hair follicles, thence to bloodstream; occasionally through urinary or respiratory tract	Causes: (1) *skin infections,* furuncles, boils, and carbuncles; may have localized lymphadenopathy; (2) impetigo results from exfoliative toxin from a form of *S. aureus;* (3) *pneumonia* more common in hospitalized patients; causes fever, tachycardia with localized areas of pneumonia; (4) empyema; (5) *bacteremia* may produce fever, tachycardia with abscess throughout the body, often fatal, nearly 50% mortality; (6) *acute osteomyelitis* from skin or bloodborne infection or from open or closed trauma of affected bone; high fever and bone pain; may cause much osseous destruction; (7) urinary tract infections most frequently result from contamination of indwelling catheter, ascends to kidneys from bladder; (8) toxic shock syndrome
Streptococci	Gram-positive	Spherical, anaerobe non-motile, non–spore-forming		Streptococcal *pharyngitis* very common in crowded living situations, greatest frequency ages 5–15 yr; fever, extremely painful and inflamed pharynx, tonsils, uvula; *scarlet fever* may result when a specific strain of *Streptococcus* A produces a toxin causing rash, diffuse erythema, with petechiae on soft palate, scarlet "strawberry" tongue in early stages; later tongue becomes beefy in appearance, called
Group A, *S. pyogenes* (at least 60 subtypes), B hemolytic	Gram-positive		Respiratory droplet	

				"raspberry" tongue; desquamation of skin occurs up to 3–4 wk after the disease; may occur before rheumatic fever; *rheumatic fever* may follow acute streptococcal infection and apparently is immune reaction to organism; acute *glomerulonephritis* also may follow streptococcal infection; *erysipelas,* an acute infection of the skin and subcutaneous tissue from *S. pyogenes,* causes malaise, itching, erythema that spreads rapidly with edema and encrustation; localized skin lesions, cellulitis, and pneumonia may also result
Group B, *S. agalactiae*	Gram-positive		Frequently colonize in the female genital tract, throat, and rectum; may be transmitted to susceptible person directly or by respiratory contact	May occur in puerperium to cause septicemia, pulmonary involvement, and meningitis in newborns
S. pneumoniae (pneumococcus)	Gram-positive	Diplococcal form, lancet-shaped	Transmitted by respiratory tract droplet; rapidly progressive once established	Preceded by "cold" or "sinus" complaints; fever, chills, pleuritic pain, cough productive of rusty sputum; hypoxia occurs with infiltration of lung tissue; progresses to atelectasis in one or more lobes; responds well to antibiotic therapy
Neisseria				
N. meningitides	Gram-negative	Single cocci, grows well in media with small amount of oxygen	Resides in nasopharynx of carriers, spreads through respiratory droplets; transmitted by bloodstream to meninges	*Meningococcemia* begins with cough, headache, sore throat followed by high fever and sometimes manifestations of endotoxic shock; *meningitis* evidenced by presence of meningococcus in cerebrospinal fluid and neurologic symptoms
N. gonorrhoeae (gonorrhea)	Gram-negative	Diplococcus	Humans only natural hosts; transmitted almost solely through sexual intercourse; incubation period usually less than 1 wk	Men develop dysuria, urethral discharge; because of penicillin treatment, complications are rare; women have dysuria, vaginal discharge, abnormal menstrual bleeding, Bartholin's gland may be involved; pelvic inflammatory disease may result
Corynebacterium diphtheriae (diphtheria)	Gram-positive	Nonmotile rod, club-shaped; elaborates exotoxin	Most frequently transmitted through respiratory tract but may be transmitted by skin, genitalia; incubation 1 day to 1 wk	Respiratory effect on pharynx, larynx, and trachea; formation of thick, leathery membrane on these structures, causing respiratory obstruction; exotoxin effects: heart, causing myocarditis; nervous system, causing peripheral neuritis, motor denervation; peripheral vascular collapse occurs in late stages; without antitoxin protection, mortality about 35% with 90% of those having laryngeal involvement

(continued)

TABLE 8-5

TYPICAL BACTERIA THAT CAUSE PATHOLOGIC EFFECTS IN HUMANS (Continued)

BACTERIA	GRAM STAIN	MORPHOLOGY	EPIDEMIOLOGY	CLINICAL EFFECTS
Clostridium tetani (tetanus)	Gram-positive	Anaerobic, motile rod, spore-bearing; exotoxin production	Found in soil and intestinal tract of humans and some animals; puncture or laceration of skin usual mode of entry; incubation variable, usually about 14 days	Exotoxin attacks CNS, causing muscle rigidity and spasms; pain and stiffness of jaw early symptoms; *lockjaw* refers to inability to open jaw; laryngospasm may lead to hypoxia; overall mortality 40%–60%
Clostridium difficile	Gram-positive	Obligate anaerobe spore-forming toxin-producing coccobacilli, motile due to flagella	Associated with antibiotic use	Pseudomembranous colitis: abdominal pain, leukocytosis, fever, profuse diarrhea
L. monocytogenes (listeria)	Gram-positive	Aerobic to microaerophilic, facultative intracellular organism	Food transmission, found in soil and animal feces, transmitted transplacentally during birth	Neonatal infection during birth, mother is asymptomatic or has mild flulike symptoms Meningitis —especially in cancer patients and those with renal transplants
Vibrio cholerae	Gram-negative	Motile short rods, comma-shaped flagellum	Organisms are shed in carrier's feces, which contaminates food and water supplies Two kinds of carriers: convalescent carrier sheds organism for 1 year; chronic carrier harbors organism in gallbladder and sheds organism periodically	Severe diarrhea and vomiting with fluid losses of up to 15–20 L/day Hypovolemic shock and metabolic acidosis result
V. parahaemolyticus	Gram-negative	Similar appearance; salt-loving organism	Marine organism that contaminates seafood; ingestion of undercooked or raw seafood	Explosive watery diarrhea, headache, fever, vomiting may persist for 10 days
Helicobacter pylori (Helicobacter)	Gram-negative; silver stain shows best	Pleomorphic tuft of polar flagella corkscrew motility smooth cell wall microaerophilic	Infection of GI tract; infection may also follow endoscopic exam	Gastric ulcers
Legionella pneumophila (Legionella)	Gram-negative; silver stain	Rod-shaped, motile by flagella; pili present	Airborne exposure; organism grows in air conditioning cooling towers and condensers	Causes: 1. Legionnaires disease: a pneumonia that may be mild to very severe 2. Pontiac fever (abrupt onset of fever, chills, headache, myalgias)

TABLE 8-6

ATYPICAL BACTERIA THAT CAUSE PATHOLOGICAL EFFECTS IN HUMANS

BACTERIA	MORPHOLOGY	EPIDEMIOLOGY	CLINICAL EFFECTS
MYCOBACTERIUM			
M. tuberculosis (tuberculosis)	Aerobic acid-fast; resists decolorization with acid or acid alcohol; curved spindle-shaped	Respiratory droplet; reinfection or activation of dormant infection; incubation variable, 4 to 8 weeks if not walled off	*Primary TB:* usually lung involvement, macrophages wall off viable organisms; these may be seen on radiograph as rims of calcification; *clinical TB:* fever, pleurisy, night sweats, cough, weight loss; can spread to bone or cause liquefaction and cavitation of lung
M. leprae (leprosy)	Hansen's bacillus; acid-fast rod	Prolonged exposure, especially in close contact; skin or nasal mucosa may be portal of entrance; incubation 3 to 5 years with little immunity demonstrated; endemic regions are tropical countries and some U.S. states	Destructive lesions of skin, peripheral nerves, upper respiratory passages, testes, hands, and feet; treatment may be curative
M. avium-intracellulare	Acid-fast rod	Respiratory transmission from soil, water, dairy products, birds and mammals	Chronic pulmonary disease, especially in immune-compromised individuals, especially HIV population
SPIROCHETES			
Treponema pallidum (syphilis)	Spiraled organism with helical shape resembling a spring; have flagella for organism motility	Mainly sexually transmitted with incubation about 3 weeks	Organism can penetrate any mucous membrane, enters blood and lymphatics; primary lesion of site of infection heals; secondary effects are lymphadenopathy, rash, arterial inflammation; tertiary syphilis involves CNS changes, dementia, inflammatory changes of aorta, etc.
Borrelia burgdorferi (Lyme disease)	Contain flagella longer than other spirochetes, supercoiled plasmids	Transmitted by tick bites of *Ixodes ricinus* type that feed on mice and deer; may spread locally on human skin or may disseminate by blood or lymph; localized for 1–4 weeks, disseminated 1 week to 6 months; may persist 6 months to 30 years	Skin lesions variable; neurological effects of changes in memory, mood, sleep patterns, peripheral sensory symptoms may appear like multiple sclerosis; arthritis especially in knee, often becomes chronic; vascular lesions from vascular damage
Borrelia recurrentis (relapsing fever)		Transmitted by body louse or ticks	Recurrent high fever
Leptospirosis (Leptospira)		Contact with urine of infected animals	Renal dysfunctions to renal failure; hepatic dysfunction and jaundice; headaches, myalgias, malaise, meningitis
CHLAMYDIA			
C. trachomatis	Round, non-motile gram-negative	Sexually transmitted, incubation 5–10 days Eye-to-eye transmission by droplets, hands, and contaminated clothing May also be transmitted during the birth process	Urogenital infections; lymphogranuloma-venereum Chronic keratoconjunctivitis that may lead to blindness if untreated Neonatal pneumonia and conjunctivitis Reiter's syndrome: conjunctivitis, polyarthritis, and genital inflammation
C. psittaci	Same as above	Inhalation of organism from infected birds and droppings; person-to-person transmission also occurs	Fever, myalgia, headache, pneumonia, toxic encephalitis, carditis, hepatitis; ⅓ of all patients have a false-positive test for syphilis
C. pneumoniae	Same as above; pear-shaped	Human-to-human respiratory transmission	Mild respiratory infection to pneumonia

(continued)

TABLE 8-6

ATYPICAL BACTERIA THAT CAUSE PATHOLOGICAL EFFECTS IN HUMANS (Continued)

BACTERIA	MORPHOLOGY	EPIDEMIOLOGY	CLINICAL EFFECTS
RICKETTSIA			
Rickettsia rickettsii (Rocky Mountain spotted fever)	Small organism, stains purple; usually gram-negative cell wall antigen; elaborates endotoxinlike substance	Multiply in nucleus and cytoplasm of infected cells of ticks and mammals; commonly occurs in Western hemisphere; transmitted by bite of infected tick or through skin abrasions contacting tick feces or tissue juices; incubation 3–12 days	Swelling and degeneration of endothelial cells, vascular damage, myocarditis, pneumonitis; peripheral vascular collapse may cause death; impairment of hepatic function and consumption coagulopathy may occur; severe headache, muscle pain, fever for 15–20 days; characteristic rash begins as small discrete, nonfixed pink lesions on wrists, ankles, forearms, etc., becomes petechial; mortality 7%–10%
R. prowazekii (epidemic typhus)	Small, gram-negative organism; always multiplies within cytoplasm of cells	Inhalation of dried louse feces; louse feces often rubbed into broken skin as with scratching of bite; incubation approximately 1 wk	Intense headache; continuous pyrexia for 2 wk; macular rash in axilla spreads to extremities, becomes petechial; peripheral vascular collapse as with Rocky Mountain spotted fever
R. typhi (endemic typhus)	Similar to *R. prowazekii*	Transmitted by fleas, widespread in U.S., especially southeastern and Gulf Coast states	Headache, fever, chills; fever up to 12 days; rash generalized, dull red macular, over thorax and abdomen; prognosis good with or without treatment
Coxiella burnetti (Q fever)	Appearance similar to other rickettsiae	Inhalation of infected dust, of ticks on body and lice feces; sheep, goats, cows often affected; incubation 2–4 wk; present throughout the world	Fever, headache, weakness, interstitial pneumonitis, dry cough, chest pain; hepatitis and endocarditis may follow; rash not characteristic
R. quintana (Trench fever)	Appearance like other rickettsiae	Transmitted by body louse feces into broken skin; found in Europe, Africa, North America; incubation usually 1–4 wk	Headache, fever, malaise, pain, tenderness, splenomegaly, macular rash common; recovery usually rapid
R. tsutsugamushi (Scrub typhus)	Appearance like other rickettsiae	Transmitted by chigger bite, especially in Asia, northern Australia	Fever, usually undiagnosed. Rash and eschar rarely seen
R. akari (rickettsial pox)	Small gram-negative organism	Mite vector; transmits disease to mouse or human if mouse is unavailable; disease most common in densely populated urban areas; unknown incubation period	Vesicular rash with local eschar and regional lymphadenopathy, chills, fever, headache, myalgia appear 3–7 days after initial vesicle appears
MYCOPLASMA			
M. pneumoniae	Small coccoidal to short branched filamentous cells; bulbous enlargement with a differentiated tip structure that allows organism to have a gliding movement; no cell wall	Slowly spreading, requires close contact; children affected most, then disease spreads to others in family	Rhinitis, wheezing pneumonia
Ureplasma urealyticum	Tiny; metabolize urea to ammonia; no cell wall	Isolated from GU tract as an opportunist	Nongonococcal urethritis; may play a role in perinatal mortality
M. hominis	Large colonies form "fried egg" appearance; no cell wall	Isolated from GU tract as an opportunist	Implicated in post-partum fever, post-abortal fever, pelvic inflammatory disease and pyelonephritis

Spirochetes

These bacteria are named for their helical shape, which resembles a spring. The most common spirochete is *Treponema pallidum*, which causes syphilis, a sexually transmitted infection (see p. 248). Others in this category include *Leptospira, Borrelia recurrentis,* and *Borrelia burgdorferi.* The latter is the causative organism of Lyme disease. Lyme disease is transmitted by tick bites from *Ixodes* ticks that mate on deer in fall and winter. Usually occurring from May to September, infection is most common in children. It does not occur in areas not inhabited by deer.[4]

Chlamydia

Chlamydia are a unique class of bacteria closely related to each other but only distantly related to other eubacteria.[13] They are obligate intracellular parasites that cannot be cultured on artificial media. Chlamydia possess a tropism for columnar epithelial cells of mucous membranes.[12]

Mode of Infection. Chlamydia exhibits a unique biphasic life cycle, existing in two forms in the body. The infectious form of chlamydia is the elementary body. In this form chlamydia can exist outside the cell. The elementary body attaches to microvilli of mucous membranes and penetrates the clathrin-coated pits at the bottom of the microvilli. The elemental bodies transform into the metabolically active reticulate bodies inside endosomes in the cell. Host mitochondria become associated with the endosome and are used by the organism to make energy. Chlamydia divide to form microcolonies called inclusion bodies, which can be identified by Giemsa staining. The reticulate bodies eventually mature into elementary bodies and are released from the cell by exocytosis (*C. trachomatis*) or by cell destruction (*C. Psittaci*).[12] Chlamydial infections are susceptible to erythromycin and tetracycline.[3,6,19]

Rickettsia

Rickettsia, once thought to be related to viruses because of their small size, are obligate, parasitic organisms. They possess all of the features of bacteria except that they can multiply only within certain cells of susceptible hosts.[12] The classification of rickettsia is based on the clinical features and epidemiologic aspects of the diseases they cause. The organisms are classified into three groups: (1) spotted fever group, (2) typhus group, and (3) others, including Q fever.

Mode of Infection. The normal reservoir for rickettsia most often is the arthropods, especially ticks, mites, lice, and fleas, in which they multiply without causing disease. Most rickettsial diseases are transmitted to humans through the bite or feces of the infected arthropod. An exception to this is Q fever, which is spread from person to person by airborne transmission.

Clinical Manifestations. All rickettsial diseases cause fever, and most cause a rash that is the result of rickettsial multiplication in the endothelial cells of the small blood vessels. The cells become swollen and necrotic, leading to the vascular lesions noted on or through the skin. Aggregations of lymphocytes, granulocytes, and macrophages accumulate in the small vessels of the brain, heart, and other organs.

Laboratory tests demonstrate the presence of rickettsial antigens and antibodies. Broad-spectrum antibiotics such as tetracycline suppress the growth of rickettsia, but full recovery requires an intact immune system that can develop antibodies against the organism.[19] The most common diseases resulting from rickettsial infection include Rocky Mountain spotted fever and the typhus fevers.

Mycoplasma

Mycoplasma are small microorganisms usually classified with bacteria even though they are distinctly different. They lack a cell wall and assume **pleomorphic** shapes, including spherical, pear-shaped, or filamentous cells with branching.[13] Many antibiotics are ineffective in treating mycoplasma infections.

Mode of Infection. The P1 protein is a major adherin of mycoplasma, allowing it to attach to specific tissues in the respiratory and genitourinary tract.[12] Mycoplasma infections commonly occur in the upper respiratory tract of children and young adults and in the genital and urinary tracts of young adults. Animal models implicate mycoplasma as an etiologic agent of arthritis; however, there is no convincing evidence at this time that they are an etiologic agent in humans.[12]

VIRUSES

Viruses are small obligate intracellular organisms. They are not complete cells in themselves and essentially exist as parasites on living cells. These organisms use the biochemical products and machinery of the host to replicate. Viruses vary in size, appearance, and behavior. They are classified as either DNA or RNA viruses, according to their genetic material.

The structure of the virus has been studied with the electron microscope and is described according to its appearance. Many contain nucleic acid, which is protected by a closed protein shell called the **capsid**. The capsid is made up of protein subunits called **capsomeres**. The viral nucleic acid and the capsid together are called the nucleocapsid.[8,12] Mature infective virus particles are called **virions** and contain a core of nucleic acid of either DNA or RNA. Complex virions may contain additional layers, or lipid envelopes. Figure 8-2 illustrates the different forms of viruses and their component parts.

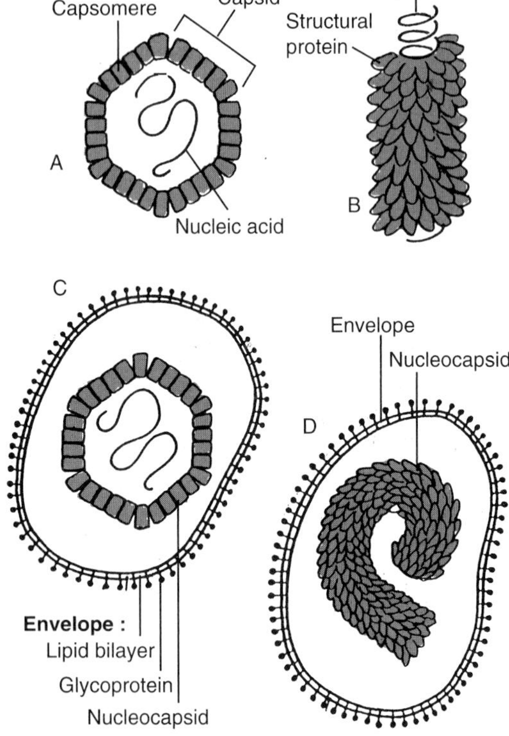

FIGURE 8-2. **Structures of viruses. The morphology varies by shape and presence or absence of an envelope. A and B represent two forms of naked or nonenveloped viruses. C and D represent two types of enveloped viruses that are highly variable in shape (pleomorphic) because the membrane is not rigid. These are more complex viruses.**

Classification

Although there are multitudes of types of viruses, most of them can be classified structurally as DNA or RNA viruses. Table 8-7 presents this classification, listing the common disease-producing groups, their modes of transmission, and the resulting symptomatology.

Mode of Infection

The protein covering of the virus is type specific. The surface structure is responsible for attachment to particular cell receptors. Infection depends on the compatibility of the viral surface with the host cell receptors and the ability of viral nucleic acid to use the host cell to manufacture viral products. All viruses are similar in their method of attachment to the specific receptors on the host cell membrane—the so-called lock-and-key attachment. Some have amino acids that are similar to the actively transported substances in the cell membrane of the host. Viruses can fool the cell, attach themselves to receptor sites on the host cell, and block the movement of normally transported materials.

Viruses appear to be species- and organ-specific and can replicate only in permissive or receptive cells. Some B lymphocytes, for example, carry receptors for the Epstein-Barr virus, whereas cells in the tracheal lining have receptors for the influenza virus. Viruses produce specific diseases that involve specific tissues, but their modes of transmission and diseases produced are numerous.

Although no one virus is typical, the replication and transmission of these organisms have been assessed extensively by studying the bacteriophage (virus that attacks bacteria). The genetic material of the bacteriophage is enclosed in an angular head or protein-containing capsid. The hollow head contains the viral genetic material and connects with a hollow cylinder of protein surrounded by protein contractile fibers. The contractile fibers coil around the cylinder like a spring. At the end of the tail, the fibers and an enzyme are important in attaching the virion to the host cell (Fig. 8-3).

Viral multiplication usually occurs in several steps (Fig. 8-4). The first step is recognition and attachment (adsorption) of the virus to the host cell. The second step is penetration or injection of viral DNA into the cell. Some viruses enter a receptive cell by endocytosis, and some fuse with the cellular membrane (see p. 15).[8,12] Replication follows through nucleic acid synthesis and assembly into new virus particles. At a certain point, these virus particles are released from the cell into the extracellular environment.[8] The formed particles can survive outside the host cell for variable periods of time, often until a new susceptible host cell can be found.

Viral infections stimulate the immune system's antibody production. Neutralizing antibodies are formed during viremia, but the main host defense is through cell-mediated immunity (see p. 285).[22] The initial response to viral infestation usually is by the mononuclear cells, the monocytes and lymphocytes. At the site of entry of viruses into the body, the immunocompetent (antigen-specific) cells accumulate and initiate the inflammatory process. Macrophages often attach to the virus and enhance T- and B-cell interaction. Exposure to viral agents initially causes the synthesis of specific IgM antibodies, followed after about 10 days by the synthesis of IgG antibodies. When the virion is sufficiently coated with antibody, it is rendered noninfectious. The specific T lymphocytes provide for long-term immunity. Viruses and other substances stimulate the production of **interferon,** a family of antiviral proteins that inhibits viral spread from cell to cell.[8]

After attachment, an eclipse stage may be entered, during which viral DNA becomes part of the host chromo-

(text continues on page 240)

TABLE 8-7

CLASSIFICATION OF VIRUSES

TYPE	NUCLEIC ACID PRESENT	EPIDEMIOLOGY/ INCUBATION PERIOD	CLINICAL MANIFESTATIONS
HERPES VIRUSES			
Varicella-zoster virus (varicella, chickenpox)	DNA	Highly contagious through respiratory droplets and contact with lesions Incubation period: 10–21 days	Fever, disseminated vesicular eruption profuse on trunk and on oral mucosa; increased risk in immunosuppressed people
Varicella zoster virus (zoster-shingles)	DNA	Reactivation of chickenpox Incubation period: variable	Follows chickenpox—may occur years after a primary attack; spreads down peripheral nerves of skin; active ganglionitis causes burning or dull pain; vesicles follow nerve fibers
Herpes simplex type 1	DNA	Skin contact (oral) Incubation period: 2–12 days	Fever, vesicular eruption of mucous membranes, conjunctivitis, oral lesions (fever blisters); encephalitis occasionally results when virus ascends to central nervous system; manifestations more severe in immunosuppressed people
Herpes simplex type 2	DNA	Skin contact (genital); attack rate with sexual contact 1:3; through small mucosal cracks Incubation period: 5–14 days	Genital vesicles, fever, burning, urinary urgency in males; dysuria, vulvar burning, dyspareunia in females
Epstein-Barr	DNA	Respiratory droplet, transfusion Incubation period: 30–50 days	Sore throat, lymphadenopathy, splenomegaly, supraorbital edema; causative agent of infectious mononucleosis; virus has been isolated from Burkitt's lymphoma
Cytomegalovirus (CMV)	DNA	Saliva, urine, feces, semen, transplacental, transfusion Incubation period: 28–49 days	Vary with age of onset: *congenital:* failure to thrive, jaundice, respiratory distress; may be fatal; *postnatal:* infection may cause anemia, hepatomegaly, lymphocytosis; *adult form:* fever, lymphocytosis, Guillain-Barré syndrome *Immunosuppressed people:* interstitial pneumonia, hepatitis, increased frequency of rejection of transplanted organs, retinitis
POXVIRUSES			
Vaccinia	DNA	Inoculation for smallpox; also used as a vector for expression of foreign genes in vaccine production Incubation period: about 2 weeks after vaccination	Probably hybrid of variola or cowpox virus; may cause widespread eczematous reaction or encephalomyelitis that causes death in 30%–40% of patients
Molluscum contagiosum	DNA	Sexual/nonsexual skin contact Incubation period: 14–50 days	3- to 5-mm, firm, smooth lesions, usually on genitalia; asymptomatic
PARVOVIRUS			
(*Erythema infectiosum or Fifth disease*)	DNA	Respiratory secretions; maternal–fetal transmission may also occur Incubation period: 10 days	10 days after mild illness, facial redness with absence of circumoral redness; rash on extremities and trunk

(continued)

TABLE 8-7

CLASSIFICATION OF VIRUSES (Continued)

TYPE	NUCLEIC ACID PRESENT	EPIDEMIOLOGY/ INCUBATION PERIOD	CLINICAL MANIFESTATIONS
ADENOVIRUS (many strains identified)	DNA	High frequency in children and military recruits; respiratory aerosol or droplet Incubation period: 7–14 days	Febrile pharyngitis; headache, regional lymphadenopathy, nasal obstruction and discharge, conjunctivitis, pneumonia
PAPOVAVIRUS			
Papillomavirus	DNA	Skin contact, contact with contaminated secretions; sexually transmitted Incubation period: 1–20 months	Solid, rounded tumors with horny projections 1–2 cm in size; often asymptomatic unless located on area of irritation; often found on hands, neck, shins, forearms, genital area
PICORNAVIRUS (Coxsackie virus A and BC many strains)	RNA	Fecal–oral contact; insects may be passive vectors Incubation period: 2–5 days	Depend on type; acute myocarditis, fever, muscle and pleuritic pain, vesicular lesions on soft plate and tonsils, pharyngitis; associated with many systemic problems
Poliovirus	RNA	Fecal–oral contact Incubation period: 2–5 days	Undifferentiated febrile illness may spread to involve anterior horn cells of spinal cord and motor nuclei of cranial nerves; causes various muscle paralyses, hemiplegia, paraplegia; bladder and respiratory muscle dysfunction; poliovaccines can prevent disease
Rhinovirus	RNA	Respiratory droplet Incubation period: 1–2 days	Common cold; fever, cough, croup, and pneumonia may develop in children; sore throat, nasal congestion, and nasal discharge without fever common in adults
CORONAVIRUS	RNA	Respiratory droplet Incubation period: 3 days	Common cold, rhinitis, pneumonia, bronchitis
PARAMYXO-VIRUSES			
Morbillivirus	RNA	Respiratory droplet Incubation period: 3–5 days	Measles rash follows exposure usually associated with rhinorrhea, rash disseminates bodywide
Paramyxovirus	RNA	Very communicable in crowded conditions; transmitted by upper respiratory tract secretions Incubation period: 15–21 days	Painful enlargement of salivary glands; orchitis occurs in 20%–35% postpubertal males; small percentage develop meningitis; or may affect other glands
ORTHOMYXO-VIRUS (influenza A, B, and C)	RNA	Epidemic, new strains evolve frequently; transmitted by infected respiratory secretions Incubation period: 18–36 hours, up to 7 days	Respiratory symptoms, cough, headache, muscle pain, fever, chills, sneezing, nasal discharge, prostration common; symptoms among strains similar

(continued)

TABLE 8-7

CLASSIFICATION OF VIRUSES (Continued)

TYPE	NUCLEIC ACID PRESENT	EPIDEMIOLOGY/ INCUBATION PERIOD	CLINICAL MANIFESTATIONS
TOGAVIRUSES (alphaviruses)	RNA	Transmitted by arthropod vectors; occur especially in summer and fall Incubation period: variable with strain	Encephalitis
FILOVIRUSES			
Ebola virus	RNA	Transmitted via contact with blood or body fluids Incubation period: 5–10 days	Hemorrhagic fever
BUNYAVIRUS			
Hantavirus	RNA	Ingestion or contact with urine or feces of rodent, rodent bites, inhalation of airborne virus from rodents' living quarters Incubation period: up to 6 weeks	Hemorrhagic fever with renal syndrome, pulmonary syndrome resembling ARDS
ARENAVIRUSES			
Lassavirus	RNA	Rat reservoir (*Mastomys nalalensis*) found in Africa; blood and body fluids precautions Incubation period: 10 days	Hemorrhagic fever
NORWALK-LIKE VIRUSES	RNA	Responsible for over ⅓ of cases of gastroenteritis; ingestion of contaminated food and water and person-to-person spread Incubation period: 48 hours	Nausea, vomiting, abdominal cramps, diarrhea, fever, chills
RHABDOVIRUS (rabies)	RNA	Animal bite of nonimmunized domestic dogs or cats or of wild animals such as skunks, foxes, raccoons, bats, wolves Incubation period: variable; average 2–6 weeks in humans	Virus introduced through mucous membranes or epidermis; replicates in striated muscle and then spreads up peripheral nerve bundles to central nervous system; passes to all organs but major effects on CNS include acute encephalitis, brain stem dysfunction and death; rapidly fatal if not treated; hydrophobia (excessive salivation) characteristic
ARBORVIRUS (four groups cause CNS disease)	RNA	Mosquito bite transmits to humans; can multiply in horses, birds, bats, snakes, insects Incubation period: 4–14 days	Age related; younger people often have high fever and convulsions; headache, fever, drowsiness, confusion, disorientation; some manifest mainly by lethargy, "sleeping sickness"; muscle weakness; residual effects range from none to convulsion; speech difficulties
HEPATITIS A	RNA	Fecal–oral enhanced by poor hygiene, overcrowding, contaminated food, water; sexual; percutaneous (uncommon) Incubation period: 15–45 days	Onset acute, most frequent in young people; causes anorexia, malaise, and other symptoms followed by jaundice; dark urine, clay-colored stools; recovery usually complete

(continued)

TABLE 8-7

CLASSIFICATION OF VIRUSES (Continued)

TYPE	NUCLEIC ACID PRESENT	EPIDEMIOLOGY/ INCUBATION PERIOD	CLINICAL MANIFESTATIONS
HEPATITIS C	RNA	Parenteral; possible fecal–oral Incubation period: 60–160 days	Clinical course variable; debilitation and liver dysfunction not infrequent, chronic hepatitis
HEPATITIS B	DNA-type	Percutaneous, sexual, maternal–infant, fecal–oral (uncommon) Incubation period: 45–160 days	Chronic active hepatitis may occur; jaundice, liver dysfunction may progress to liver failure; recovery slow
DELTA VIRUS	RNA	Blood, homosexual contact Incubation period: 28–180 days	People susceptible to hepatitis B or HBV carriers can be infected; clinical picture like HBV; may progress to chronic hepatitis
HEPATITIS E	RNA	Fecal–oral contaminated water Incubation period: 14–56 days	Chronic active hepatitis, cirrhosis, chronic carrier, like hepatitis B
RETROVIRUSES			
human immunodeficiency virus (HIV)	RNA retrovirus	Homosexual or heterosexual contact; parenteral transmission; perinatal transmission Incubation period: variable: 5–10 years in adults, more rapid onset in children	May be dormant; may cause clinical AIDS; immunodeficiency affects resistance to cytomegalovirus and Epstein-Barr virus with high percentage affected; pneumonia caused by *Pneumocystis carinii:* series of opportunistic infections; Kaposi's sarcoma; swollen lymph glands, fatigue, weight loss; clinical AIDS usually results in death

some and remains latent. The greater the capability to initiate a rapid reproductive cycle, the more virulent the virus. Activation or induction causes the latent viruses to become active and reprograms the cell for viral reproduction. Activation of latent viruses may be initiated by cold temperatures, carcinogens, or materials in food, air, or water. Each virus responds to a specific induction mechanism. Sometimes a few cells with viruses within them escape induction, so that not all affected cells are lysed. In this way the host cell carries viral DNA as part of its own DNA, and the virus can remain latent in the host tissues throughout the life of the cell.[12]

Clinical Manifestations

Each type of virus infects the host cell uniquely. The resulting signs and symptoms of the viral disease reflect the manner in which the virus has affected the host. There may be no apparent cellular change, because viral DNA may adopt a symbiotic relationship with the host cell. Conversely, cellular pathologic effects, such as death or virus-induced hyperplasia, may occur. Cytopathic effects are common and include aggregation of host cells into clusters with shrinkage, lysis, and fusion of the cells. The effects differ and are influenced by the effects of the virus on cellular synthesis of macromolecules; alteration in cellular organelles, such as the lysosomes; and changes in the host cell membrane.

Viral infections produce many diseases, including hepatitis, meningoencephalitis, pneumonia, rhinitis, skin diseases, and numerous other diseases that affect almost every body system. Some viruses are thought to be cofactors in the etiology of cancer. These viruses are called **oncogenic viruses** and include papilloma viruses, Epstein-Barr viruses (EBV), human T-cell lymphotropic virus (HTLV), and hepatitis B virus (HBV).[8] Research is being conducted on many other disease conditions, such as multiple sclerosis, diabetes mellitus, and cancer, in the hopes of finding a viral connection.[22]

Some viruses are endogenous and can remain latent within the host for years, only to be later reactivated (Fig. 8-5). Examples of this type are herpes zoster and genital herpes. In most cases the disease results from exposure to an exogenous virus, either through direct contact with another infected host or through indirect transmission, such as by means of contaminated water or shellfish.[12]

Identification of viral infections is usually by clinical symptoms, but certain laboratory tests can be used.

FOCUS ON CELLULAR PATHOPHYSIOLOGY

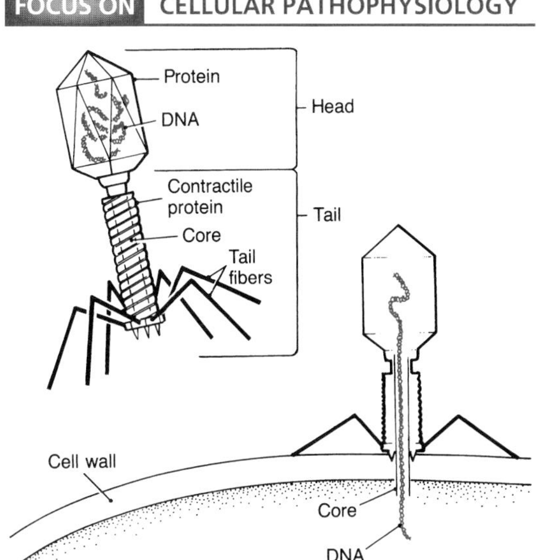
Protein
DNA
Head
Contractile protein
Tail
Core
Tail fibers
Cell wall
Core
DNA

FIGURE 8-3. A bacteriophage is a virus that attacks bacteria. It has been used to study viral activity. The bacteriophage is composed of DNA protein, a hollow core, and tail fibers. It attaches to the cell wall of an *E. coli* bacteria and injects its DNA through the bacterial cell wall.

Laboratory analysis of exposure to certain types of viruses can be made by complement-fixing antibodies, which elevate and remain elevated for a period of time following the disease. A high titer of complement-fixing antibody to a specific virus is suggestive of recent contact with that virus.[12] The polymerase chain reaction is a new test that can amplify a single DNA molecule, which yields a detectable signal, especially for viral diseases. The polymerase chain reaction technique has been used to detect hepatitis B virus in chronic hepatitis and HIV, and especially for typing of the genital human papillomavirus as well as other viruses.[5,12]

PRIONS

Prions are defined as small infectious particles that contain a protein, which is encoded by a host gene.[20] Whether or not they also contain nucleic acids is unknown; however, prions are resistant to procedures that normally would inactivate nucleic acids such as nucleases, ultraviolet light, and chemical modification by nucleophiles. Prion protein can exist in two forms: prion protein cellular (PrPc) and an abnormal form that can cause disease, prion protein scrapie (PrPsc). The normal function of the prion protein is unknown. When the

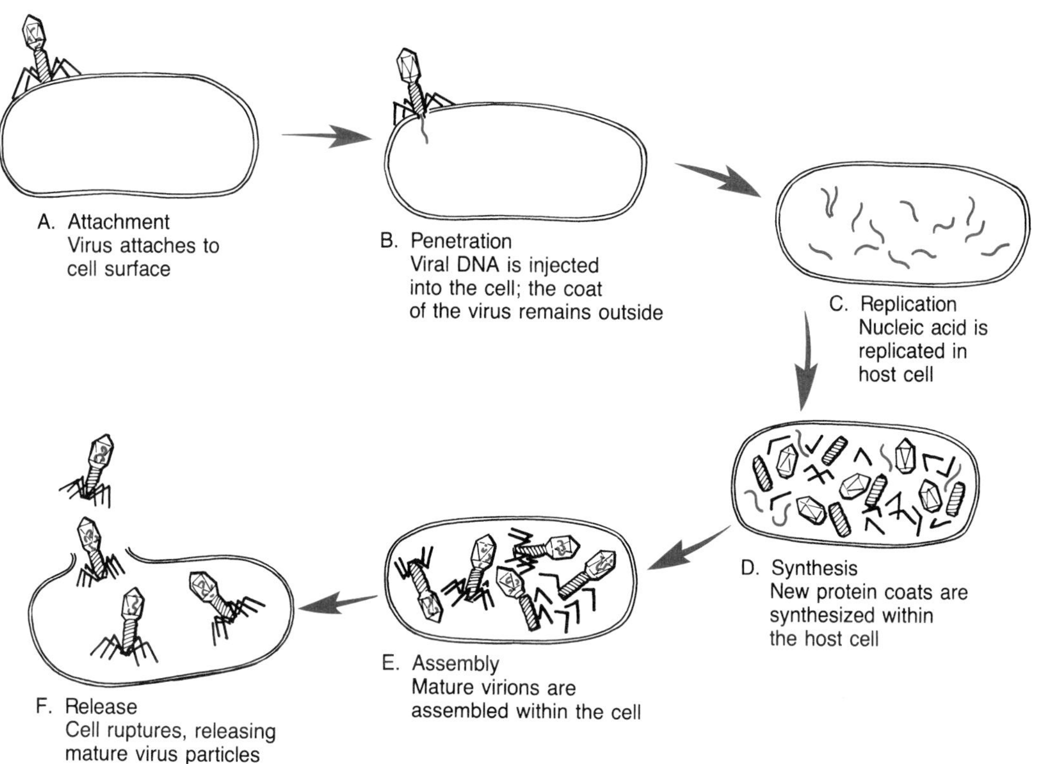
A. Attachment
Virus attaches to cell surface
B. Penetration
Viral DNA is injected into the cell; the coat of the virus remains outside
C. Replication
Nucleic acid is replicated in host cell
D. Synthesis
New protein coats are synthesized within the host cell
E. Assembly
Mature virions are assembled within the cell
F. Release
Cell ruptures, releasing mature virus particles

FIGURE 8-4. Steps in replication cycle of a virus.

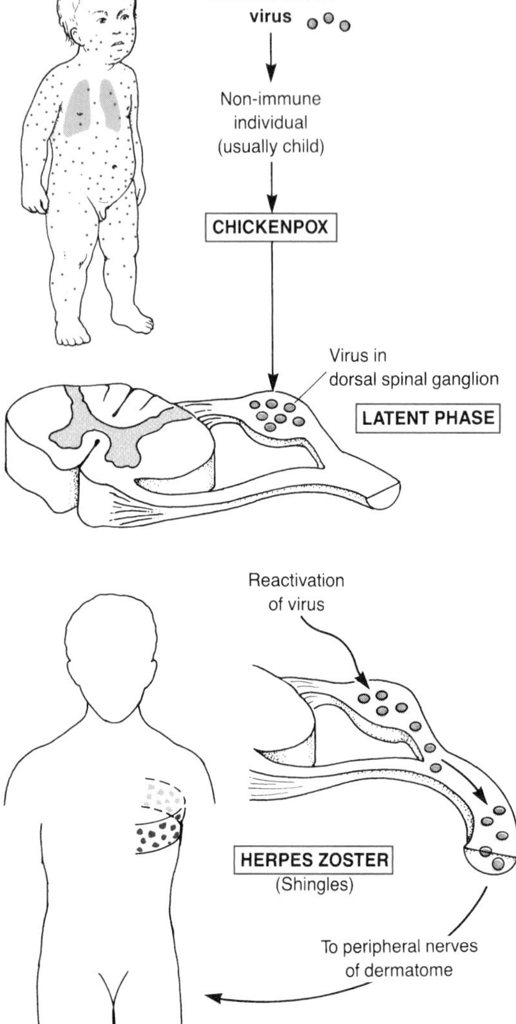

FIGURE 8-5. (*Top*) Varicella (chickenpox). Varicella-zoster virus (VZV) in droplets is inhaled by a nonimmune person (usually a child) and initially causes a "silent" infection of the nasopharynx. This progresses to viremia, seeding of fixed macrophages, and dissemination of VZV to skin and viscera. The VZV resides in a dorsal spinal ganglion, where it remains dormant for many years. (*Bottom*) Herpes zoster. Latent VZV is reactivated and spreads from ganglia along the sensory dermatomes. (Adapted from Rubin, E., & Farber, J. L. [1999]. *Pathology* [3rd ed.]. Philadelphia: Lippincott Williams & Wilkins.)

protein exists in its abnormal form it is believed to be responsible for causing a group of diseases known as transmissible neurodegenerative diseases (TNDs). Human TNDs include kuru, Creutzfeldt-Jakob disease (CJD), Gerstmann-Straussler syndrome (GSS), and fatal familial insomnia (FFI).[27] Some individuals with CJD and all persons with GSS and FFI have mutations in their prion protein gene and can pass the disease to their children.[1]

Human TNDs exibit the following four common characteristics:

1. Their major pathological manifestations occur primarily in the central nervous system.
2. The incubation times are long, ranging from 6 months for CJD to 30 years for kuru.
3. The disorders are progressive and eventually fatal.
4. Neuropathological identifying features include reactive astrocytosis with little inflammation and the presence of small vacuoles in the neurophil of the brain known as spongiform changes.[27]

There are many unanswered questions about prions. Research is ongoing to determine how an agent that may not contain nucleic acids replicates, the normal function of the PrPc protein, how the PrPc-to-PrPsc conversion causes disease, and whether prions may play a role in other chronic neurodegenerative diseases such as Alzheimer's disease.[27] Table 8-8 describes disorders associated with prions.

FUNGI

There are approximately 50,000 different species of fungi. Of these, less than a dozen cause about 90% of all fungal infections.[12] Fungi are eukaryotic organisms possessing a rigid cell wall that is chemically unlike the peptidoglycan layer of bacteria. Fungi have a cell membrane that is similar in structure to higher eukaryotes with one exception: fungal cell membranes contain ergosterol and zymosterol, whereas mammalian cell membranes contain cholesterol.[13] Antifungal medications, such as amphotericin B and ketoconazole, achieve a measure of selectivity because of this difference.[3,6,19]

Classification

Fungi grow in two forms: (1) yeasts, which reproduce by budding, and (2) molds, which grow by producing intertwined hyphae called a mycelium. Some fungi are dimorphic and, as such, can grow as either a yeast or mold depending on environmental conditions. Many pathogenic fungi, such as the organisms causing blastomycosis, histoplasmosis, and coccidiodomycosis, are dimorphic.[12]

Mode of Infection

Fungi produce disease by three mechanisms. (1) Individuals may become sensitized to specific fungous antigens, resulting in an allergic reaction. Symptoms may

TABLE 8-8

DISORDERS ASSOCIATED WITH PRIONS

DISEASE	EPIDEMIOLOGY/ INCUBATION PERIOD	CLINICAL EFFECTS
Kuru	Affects mostly adult women and children of both sexes in New Guinea; transmitted during burial ceremonies of males; family members contact the infection via ingestion of infected tissue (ritual cannibalism) or contact with infected tissue (rubbed over the survivors); the disease is declining since recognition of its cause and discontinuation of these cultural practices Incubation period: up to 30 years	Ataxia, paralysis, dementia, slurred speech, visual disturbances; death occurs within months of onset of symptoms
Creutzfeldt-Jakob disease	Transmitted by exposure to needles, instruments, electrodes used in treatment of patient with the disease, tissue transplantation (cornea), and treatment with human-derived growth hormone.* Incubation period: 6 months	Progressive dementia, dysarthria, muscle-wasting, myoclonus athetosis; death within 1 year of onset of symptoms
Gerstmann-Strausser syndrome	Inherited disorder Incubation period: unknown	Lesion in dominant parietal area of brain; unable to point, name different fingers, confuse right and left sides of body, unable to write or calculate, blindness, homonymous hemianopsia
Fatal familial insomnia	Inherited; rapidly progressive disease Incubation period: unknown but symptoms occur in middle and later life	Intractable insomnia, autonomic dysfunction, endocrine disturbances, dysarthria, myoclonus, coma; death is usual outcome

* It is recommended that individuals receiving human-derived growth hormone not serve as a blood, tissue, or organ donor.

include rhinitis, bronchial asthma, alveolitis, or generalized pneumonitis. (2) Fungi can generate toxic substances called mycotoxins that are harmful to humans. Among the most toxic are amatoxin, produced by poisonous mushrooms, and aflatoxin, which is mutagenic and a potent liver carcinogen in animals. (3) Some fungi are able to actively grow on a human host, causing an infection called a **mycosis.**[12]

Fungal organisms causing mycoses are divided into three groups, according to the part of the body they infect. **Systemic** or deep mycoses affect the internal organs or viscera. The pathogens involved can attack major systems and organs and may cause death. **Subcutaneous** mycoses infect the skin, subcutaneous tissue, fascia, and bone. Infection usually occurs from direct contamination with fungal spores or mycelia (mycelia are filamentous parts of fungi) fragments that enter wounds or broken areas of the skin. **Superficial** mycoses or dermatophytes involve only the epidermis, hair, and nails. The principal habitat of the organisms is mammalian skin.[12]

The establishment of a mycosis depends on the host defense capabilities, the route of exposure, the amount of exposure, and the virulence of the fungus. Although fungal infections do occur in otherwise healthy individuals, persons with suppressed immune systems are especially at risk. An important fungus-like organism is *Pneumocystis carinii*, which was formerly classified as a protozoan. It has been identified in immunocompromised individuals and is the most common severe, life-threatening infection among persons infected with HIV.[17] The clinical picture includes fever, cough, chest tightness, and diffuse interstitial infiltration of the lungs. It is usually fatal if not treated, and even after treatment with pentamidine, relapses are common.

Table 8-9 summarizes some of the common human fungal infections.

PROTOZOA

Protozoa are complex, unicellular organisms that may be spherical, spindle-shaped, spiral, or cup-shaped.[12] Many absorb fluids through the cell membrane, and all possess the ability to move from place to place. Pathogenesis caused by protozoa often occurs in the gastro-

TABLE 8-9

COMMON FUNGI THAT CAUSE PATHOLOGIC EFFECTS IN HUMANS

FUNGUS	MORPHOLOGY	EPIDEMIOLOGY	CLINICAL EFFECTS
Superficial dermatophytoses: tinea pedis (athlete's foot), tinea capitis (scalp ringworm), tinea corporis (body ringworm)	Branching hyphae on microscopic examination; found on keratinized portion of skin, nail plate, and hair	Contact with fungus through skin; maceration or poor hygiene favor acquisition	Fissuring of toe webs, itching, irritation, areas of alopecia, and scaling; circumscribed lesion with round borders of inflammation leads to designation of *ringworm;* treatment curative
C. albicans (systemic candidiasis)	Small, yeastlike cells; blastospores with budding; forms clusters of round growths on cornmeal agar	Contact with normal flora of mouth, stool, vagina; may be superficial or systemic in susceptible immunosuppressed people	*Oral* lesions: white plaques on mouth and tongue, may cause fissures and open sores; *urinary tract infection* after broad-spectrum antibiotic therapy or in person with diabetes mellitus; *vaginal* discharge may be profuse and irritating; *Candida* in serum may cause disseminated abscesses
C. immitis (coccidioidomycoses)	Yeastlike cells; no budding is formed; divided into multiple small cells	Soil saprophyte in southern U.S., Mexico, South America; infection occurs with inhalation of arthrospores; symptoms begin 10–14 days after inhalation	*Primary form:* respiratory infection causes flulike symptoms, sometimes pneumonia; pleural effusion may occur; *progressive form:* dissemination to regional lymph nodes, skin, meninges, etc. may occur, especially with immunosuppressed, other than Caucasian; fever, cough, chest pain, pulmonary coin lesion
H. capsulatum (histoplasmosis)	Dimorphic fungus; forms cottony white growth on glucose agar	Grows as mold, prefers moist soil; airborne exposure by cleaning chicken coops, working with soil	Cough, fever, weight loss, hilar adenopathy; progressive fibrosis of mediastinal structures; difficult to diagnose; treatment with amphotericin B may or may not be helpful; ultimate prognosis poor for disseminated type
B. dermatitidis (blastomyosis)	Dimorphic fungus; budding, round, yeastlike cells	Majority of cases in southeast, central and mid-Atlantic U.S.; infection acquired by inhalation of fungus, reservoir unknown; incubation may be about 4 wk	Fever, cough, weight loss, chest pain, pneumonia, large skin lesions; responds well to treatment with amphotericin B
C. neoformans (cryptococcosis)	Yeastlike, budding	Infection through inhalation in lungs, often opportunistic with immunosuppressed people (AIDS, lymphoma, etc.); fungus excreted in pigeon droppings	More common in males; pulmonary infection causes chest pain, cough, infiltrates; meningoencephalitis causes headache, dementia, confusion, cranial nerve palsies, cerebral edema, and death 2 wk to several years after diagnosis

(continued)

TABLE 8-9

COMMON FUNGI THAT CAUSE PATHOLOGIC EFFECTS IN HUMANS (Continued)

FUNGUS	MORPHOLOGY	EPIDEMIOLOGY	CLINICAL EFFECTS
Pneumocystis carini (PCP)	Fungus-like cysts with dark bodies	Mainly confined to immunosuppressed individuals, especially AIDS. Transmitted through respiratory droplets	Fever, nonproductive cough, shortness of breath, pneumonitis, progressive to pneumonia (PCP), often fatal
Aspergillus fumigatis (aspergillosis)	Molds, in colonies, smoky gray color	Opportunistic with immunosuppressed individuals, especially neutropenic individuals	Allergic bronchopulmonary asthmatic response, focal consolidation, lobar pneumonia

intestinal tract, genitourinary tract, and circulatory system.

Classification

The protozoa may be divided into four groups, or subphyla, which include the flagellates, sarcodina, sporozoa, and ciliata. The **flagellates** have flagella, or undulating membranes. They are considered to be some of the more primitive protozoa. This group includes members of *Giardia*, *Trichomonas*, and *Enteromonas* genera, which infect the intestinal or genitourinary tract. Other flagellates, such as *Leishmania*, tend to be localized to skin, tissue, or mucous membranes. *Trypanosoma* organisms cause a systemic disease that is often fatal. *Trichomonas vaginalis* is a common sexually transmitted protozoal infection.

Typical ameboid characteristics are seen in the subphylum **Sarcodina** (also called rhizopods or amebas). Species of the genera *Entamoeba*, *Endolimax*, and *Iodamoeba* are representative of this group.

Organisms in the **Sporozoa** subphylum have a definite life cycle that usually involves two different hosts, one of which often is an arthropod and the other a vertebrate. *Plasmodium*, a genus of the malaria parasites, is representative of this group.[18]

Organisms in the subphylum **Ciliata** are the most complex of the protozoa. These organisms have cilia distributed in rows or patches, and the shape of the organism varies according to the amount of material it has ingested. *Balantidium coli* is the only representative that is pathogenic to humans. It is a rare cause of diarrheal illness resembling amebiasis, with only a few cases having been recorded.[12]

Mode of Infection

The motility of the protozoa is accomplished by pseudopod or by the action of flagella or cilia. In *pseudopod* movement, characteristic of many ameboid cells, the projection is actively pressed forward and is rapidly followed by the rest of the organism. The movement usually is directional, toward a specific focus. *Flagella* are whiplike projections that cause rapid movement of the organism from place to place. *Cilia* are shorter and more delicate and cover the entire outer surface of the organism. The synchronous action of these structures allows the organism to move rapidly.

Reproduction may be sexual or asexual, depending on the species. The sexual cycle, when it occurs, takes place in the definitive host, whereas the asexual cycle takes place in the intermediate host. Protozoa capable of sexual reproduction are called gametes, and those capable of asexual reproduction are called zygotes. Protozoa can also form cysts, which means that they can surround themselves with a resistant membrane; this prevents destruction and allows them to live for a long time.[12] Table 8-10 summarizes several common protozoal diseases in humans.

HELMINTHS

The word *helminth* means worm and usually refers to pathogenic worms, many of which are parasitic. The common intestinal helminths are divided into three general groups: (1) **nematodes,** or roundworms; (2) **trematodes**, or flukes; and (3) **cestodes**, or tapeworms. Helminths are complex organisms in both their structure and their life cycle. Many spend part of their developmental life in several locations and in various hosts, such as fish, hogs, rats, snails, and humans. Their eggs, or larvae, often are eliminated in the feces or urine of humans and may be found in the feces on microscopic examination.[14] The mode of infection for helminths is mainly through fecal–oral transmission or through broken skin.[16]

Table 8-11 summarizes some common diseases caused by helminths. These conditions, although rarely fatal, are an important cause of disability worldwide.

TABLE 8-10

COMMON PROTOZOA THAT CAUSE PATHOLOGIC EFFECTS IN HUMANS

PROTOZOA	MORPHOLOGY	EPIDEMIOLOGY	CLINICAL EFFECTS
Entamoeba histolytica (amebiasis)	Motile trophozoite usually seen in active disease; cysts form usual means of disease transmission; anaerobic	Cysts transmitted from human feces; contaminated food, poor personal hygiene	Chronic, mild diarrhea to fulminant dysentery; stools may contain mucus and blood, may persist for months or years; numerous trophozoites found in stools; fever, abdominal cramps, and hepatomegaly common
Plasmodium vivax, Plasmodium ovale, Plasmodium malariae, Plasmodium falciparum (malaria)	Asexual phase passed in human body; multiple in liver, called *exoerythrocytic* cycle; then enter RBCs and multiply, *trophozoite* stage; as RBCs hemolyze, segments called *merozoites* released into blood	Transmitted by bite of infected female *Anopheles* mosquito; incubation period varies with type of organism from 10 days–7 wk	Anemia due to loss of RBCs; hemolyzing process with release of parasites cause chills and fever; immunologic mechanisms cause normal as well as infected RBC hemolysis; debilitation progressive; hepatitis complications may cause permanent damage
Toxoplasma gondii (toxoplasmosis)	Intracellular protozoa exist in trophozoites; cysts and oocysts form; trophozoites invade all cells; cysts often take the form of transmission; oocysts transmitted through cycle by cat; form not seen in humans	Transplacental transfusion or fecal-oral cysts; may be in lamb or pork	Focal areas of necrosis, especially of eye, but may cause CNS or disseminated effects; lymphadenopathy common in immunosuppressed people; CNS involvement leads to high mortality; may infect fetus of affected mother
Giardia lamblia (giardiasis)	Flagellated protozoan in upper small intestine; both tropozoite and cyst stages; cyst can remain viable in cold or tepid water 1–3 months	Water spread in U.S.; found in persons with achlorhydria, genetic susceptibility, Type A blood	Subtotal villous atrophy of small intestine. Inflammatory infiltrate. Incubation period 1–3 weeks, acute diarrheal period, nausea, anorexia, may last 1–2 months; chronic illness occurs rarely
T. vaginalis (trichomonas)	No cyst stage; trophozoite infects during sexual contact	Sexually transmitted	Females: watery leukorrheal vaginal discharge, pruritus and irritation of vulva; males: mild discharge

MANIFESTATIONS OF INFECTIOUS DISEASE

Early symptoms of infection are often nonspecific and include malaise, weakness, myalgias, arthralgias, headache, sleepiness, and anorexia. As infection progresses manifestations include flushed skin, chills, dehydration, lymph node enlargement (lymphadenopathy), elevation of the white blood cell count (**leukocytosis**), confusion, and delirium.[11] Fever is considered the hallmark symptom of infection. Pyrogenic agents that act on the hypothalamus to produce fever during infection include interleukin-1(IL-1), interleukin-6 (IL-6), interferon, tumor necrosis factor (TNF), and other cytokines. Weight loss may occur due to release of TNF alpha (cachectin), combined with decreased intake and increased metabolism due to the effects of fever.[11]

Infections may produce illness, as described above, or they may be inapparent or *subclinical,* in which state they are so mild that signs and symptoms are not seen. A particular form of subclinical infection is the carrier state, in which the person remains a reservoir of infection and retains the ability to infect others. Another important form of infection is **latent infection**, in which episodes of disease occur, interrupted by periods of no disease manifestation or infectivity. Herpes viral

TABLE 8-11

COMMON HELMINTHS THAT CAUSE PATHOLOGIC EFFECTS IN HUMANS

HELMINTHS	MORPHOLOGY	EPIDEMIOLOGY	CLINICAL EFFECTS
Schistosomiasis: *S. mansoni, S. haematobium, S. japonicum*	Blood flukes grow and mature in portal venous system; may attain 1–2 cm in length; life span 4–30 yr	Eggs of worm pair excreted in feces or urine of humans hatch miracidia that penetrate a specific snail host and transform into infective larvae; these penetrate human skin and are carried to rest finally in portal venous circulation; worldwide distribution	Usually asymptomatic; may cause dermatitis at focus of entry; cause mild fever and malaise; acute fever begins 1–2 mo after exposure, often associated with lymphadenopathy and hepatomegaly, eosinophil levels markedly elevated; mucosa of bowel may become ulcerative and ova may be recovered from stool specimens. *S. haematobium* causes hematuria with involvement of kidneys, ureters, bladder, and seminal vesicles
Cestodes (tapeworms; *Taenia saginata* [beef], *Taenia solium* [pork], *Hymenolepis nana* [dwarf], *Dypylidium caninum* [dog])	Segmented ribbon-shaped hermaphroditic worms; absorb food through their surface; attach to host intestinal mucosa by sucking cups; length varies with species from 1 cm–10 m	Transmitted when raw or poorly cooked beef or pork eaten; other types may be transmitted by fecal-oral route, man to man or dog to man; usually matures in adult intestines	Weight loss, hunger, epigastric discomfort; in *T. solium,* encysted larvae may deposit in muscles, eyes, and brain; leads to eosinophilia, weakness, muscle pain; anemia may result from tapeworm competition for nutrition
Nematodes	Elongated, cylindric, unsegmented organisms form a few millimeters to a meter in length; life span 1–2 mo–10 yr		
Trichinella spiralis (trichinosis)		Encysted larvae of *T. spiralis* ingested in poorly cooked pork or bear meat; larvae released in intestinal mucosa; multiply, and new larvae migrate into vascular channels throughout body; lodge in skeletal muscle, become encysted and grow for 5–10 yr	Severe inflammation of muscles in major infestation of muscle; may begin with diarrhea and fever; muscle pain, conjuctivitis, and rash may develop; eosinophilia common; neurotoxic symptoms and myocarditis may be seen
Trichuris trichiura	Embryonated eggs in soil; worms develop in small intestine; cylindrical shape	Common in southeastern U.S. and in tropical/subtropical areas	Often asymptomatic; may have abdominal pain, diarrhea, weight loss
Enterobiasis (pinworm, threadworm; *Enterobius vermicularis*)	Female 10 mm, male 3 mm; live attached to mucosa of bowel; female deposits eggs on perianal skin at night, then dies	Fecal-oral transmission, transfer of eggs from anus to mouth; contamination of bed linens, remains viable 2–3 wk; common infection in humans	Pruritus of anal and genital regions common, especially at night; bladder infection or other foci relatively rare; simultaneous treatment of entire families and group essential

(continued)

TABLE 8-11

COMMON HELMINTHS THAT CAUSE PATHOLOGIC EFFECTS IN HUMANS (Continued)

HELMINTHS	MORPHOLOGY	EPIDEMIOLOGY	CLINICAL EFFECTS
Ancylostoma duodenale, Necator americanus (hookworm)	Four prominent hooklike teeth attach worm to upper part of small intestine; adults about 1 cm in length	Affects about 700 million persons worldwide; greatest incidence in Africa, Asia, tropical Americas; transmitted by invasion of exposed skin by larvae, migrates through lungs and resides in GI tract; excretion of larvae in fecal material perpetuates cycle	Iron deficiency anemia and hyper albuminemia result from chronic intestinal blood loss; most infections asymptomatic but may have GI distress or ulcerlike pain; eosinophilia common

infections are common latent infections that can be reactivated by stress, other infections, or other factors.[7]

HEMATOLOGIC EFFECTS. Leukocytosis is an important manifestation of most infections; however, the cell type will vary depending on the nature of the infection. Acute bacterial infections typically result in **neutrophilia** or an increased neutrophil count. Accompanying neutrophilia will be eosinopenia and lymphopenia. As the infection resolves, monocytes and lymphocytes may increase. **Eosinophilia** (increased eosinophils) is typical of helminth infection. **Monocytosis** (increased monocytes) and **lymphocytosis** (increased lymphocytes) commonly accompany chronic infections such as tuberculosis.[5]

Prolonged infections also result in anemia due to decreased red blood cell (RBC) survival, compromised delivery of iron to the developing RBC, and a lack of compensatory increase in production of erythropoetin in response to the anemia.[11] The erythrocyte sedimentation rate, a nonspecific test indicating inflammation, will also increase.[5]

Changes in coagulation occur due to platelet and fibrinogen increases. A serious complication of acute infections is disseminated intravascular coagulation (DIC) (see p. 385).

CARDIOVASCULAR EFFECTS. Cardiovascular changes, which occur in response to severe infection, are mediated by interleukin-1 and TNF. Hypotension, compensatory increases in heart rate and cardiac output, and septic shock all result from the powerful vasodilatory effects of these mediators. Most cases of septic shock are due to gram-negative bacteremia, but rickettsial, chlamydial and viral infections can also cause it.[11] Activation of the complement cascade also affects the cardiovascular system. Activation of C3a and C5a of the complement cascade enhances vasodilation and hypotension (see p. 259).[15]

RENAL EFFECTS. Renal effects of infection may include proteinuria due to fever or direct infection of the renal structure itself. The stress of infection may temporarily decrease tubular reabsorption of glucose, resulting in glycosuria. Azotemia may result from the increased nitrogen load when tubular cells are destroyed by the infecting agent. Oliguria will accompany hypotension and septic shock due to decreased renal perfusion.[12]

HEPATOBILIARY EFFECTS. Jaundice, an ominous sign of liver damage, may accompany severe infections. It may result from direct damage to the hepatocytes by infecting agents, formation of infectious lesions in the liver, or overload of the liver with heme pigments due to hemolytic effects of the infection.[11]

SEXUALLY TRANSMITTED DISEASES AND INFECTIONS

Sexually transmitted diseases (STDs) or infections (STIs) may be caused by bacterial, viral, fungal, protozoal, and parasitic organisms. STDs and STIs are spread through vaginal intercourse, anal intercourse, and oral sex. The outcome of contracting an STD or STI ranges from mild irritation and discomfort to death. The number of different STDs and STIs classified by the Centers for Disease Control (CDC) has grown from only a few to over 50 disorders.[2]

Individuals who engage in unprotected sex are especially at risk of contracting these infectious diseases. Additionally, opportunistic infections may occur in individuals with immunodeficiencies. Controlling STDs and STIs offers a public health challenge of the highest magnitude. Essential components of this effort include education regarding STDs and safe sex practices to avoid them, offering clinics for diagnosis and treatment, and tracing, notification, and treatment of any contacts of an individual with a known STD. Table 8-12 describes some of the common STDs.

TABLE 8-12

SEXUALLY TRANSMITTED DISEASES AND INFECTIONS

INFECTION	INCUBATION PERIOD	CLINICAL MANIFESTATIONS
BACTERIAL		
Neisseria gonorrhoeae (gonorrhea)	Males: 3–10 days Females: 2 weeks or more Newborn conjuctivitis: 1–12 days after birth	Male: GU: yellow mucopurulent penile discharge, dysuria, frequency, malaise, 5–10% asymptomatic infection Female: 50% asymptomatic; GU: dysuria, frequency, green or yellow vaginal discharge, abnormal menses, backache, abdominal and pelvic pain, pruritus and burning of the vulva Anal infection: 50% of males and most females asymptomatic; pruritus, mucopurulent rectal discharge, rectal bleeding, rectal pain, tenesmus, constipation Pharyngeal infection: fever, lymphadenopathy, tonsillitis; 60% asymptomatic
Treponema pallidum (syphilis)	Primary stage: 10–90 days, average 21 days	Primary stage: small red papule changes to small ulcer, then to a hard chancre at site of entry; lymphadenopathy
	Secondary stage: 6 weeks after primary lesion occurs	Secondary stage: generalized maculopapular rash, especially on palms and soles; skin lesions, condylomata lata; systemic symptoms include fever, headache, anorexia, sore mouth, alopecia
	Latency: 4–12 weeks after beginning of stage 2	Asymptomatic
	Tertiary stage: 1 year to a lifetime after secondary lesions occur	Gummas, cardiovascular lesions, neurosyphilis
		Congenital syphilis: prematurity, IUGR, hepatosplenomegaly, bone marrow depression, bone and skin lesions, retinal inflammation, glaucoma, blood dyscrasias, nephrotic syndrome, CNS involvement
Haemophilus ducreyi (chancroid)	Up to 10 days	Maculopapular lesion on penis or vulva that progresses to a pustule and eventually to a painful, shallow, ragged ulcer 1–3 cm in diameter, inguinal lymphadenopathy, buboes (fluid-filled lymph nodes) develop 7–10 days after initial lesion; these lesions may rupture and further spread disease through self-inoculation
Calymmatobacterium granulomatis (granuloma inguinale)	Variable	Papule that progresses to a spreading necrotic ulcer with extensive scarring; Disease may spread to bones, joints, and liver
Chlamydia (lymphogranuloma venereum)	5–21 days	Small painless papule or vesicle that usually heals spontaneously, followed by painful lymphatic involvement and possibly scarring and obstruction, malaise, fever, headache
Chlamydia trachomatis (chlamydia)	GU symptoms: 7–21 days Newborn conjunctivitis: 4–14 days after birth Newborn pneumonia: 3–11 weeks after birth	Female: may be asymptomatic, lower abdominal pain, heavy vaginal discharge with a fishy odor, dysuria, frequency, vaginal bleeding, arthritis–dermatitis syndrome Male: may be asymptomatic, urethritis, clear penile discharge, epididimitis, Reiter's syndrome Newborn: conjunctivitis and pneumonia
Haemophilus corynebacterium or *Gardnerella vaginalis* (vaginosis)	Varies	Thin grey, heavy, malodorous vaginal discharge with little or no vaginal and cervical irritation; odor increases when secretions are in contact with alkaline secretions such as semen or menses

(continued)

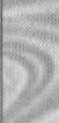

TABLE 8-12

SEXUALLY TRANSMITTED DISEASES AND INFECTIONS (Continued)

INFECTION	INCUBATION PERIOD	CLINICAL MANIFESTATIONS
Shigella (shigellosis)	24–48 hours after anal/oral contact	Fever, abdominal distress, diarrhea may progress to dysentery with severe cramping, abdominal pain, tenesmus, and bloody mucus from rectum
Campylobacter jejuni (Campylobacter enteritis)	1–7 days after anal/oral contact	Fever, abdominal pain, diarrhea, malaise, anorexia, headache, arthralgia, myalgia
VIRAL INFECTIONS		
Herpes virus hominis–type 2 (genital herpes)	3–7 days	Single or multiple vesicles >1 mm in diameter that rupture spontaneously, leaving a red, swollen, painful ulcer that scabs and heals after 24–72 hours; lesions in males are located on the glans penis, prepuce, buttocks and inner thighs; 90% of lesions in females are located on the cervix; primary infection lasts 3–4 weeks, then infection becomes latent, subsequent episodes usually last 7–10 days Neonatal infections: can occur in utero or during birth; symptoms appear during first month of life and include local infections of eyes, skin, and mucous membranes; severe disseminated infections can occur, including CNS involvement
Human papillomavirus (condylomata acuminata [genital warts])	1–3 months	Cauliflower-like lesions on penis, vulva, within vagina, cervix, and rectum; possible increased risk of cancer after infection
Human immunodeficiency virus (HIV) (acquired immunodeficiency syndrome: AIDS)		HIV infection is a complex infection affecting T4 helper cells (see Chapter 11 for more information)
Cytomegalovirus (CMV)	20–50 days	Malaise, fever, lymphadenopathy, pneumonia, hepatosplenomegaly, superinfections (especially severe in immunosuppressed persons); retinal and GI infections are common May be transmitted in utero to fetus, resulting in spontaneous abortion, fatal illness, or normal infant with no signs of infection; 10% show microcephaly, retarded growth, hepatosplenomegaly, hemolytic anemia, and pathologic fractures of long bones
Hepatitis B (Hepatitis B)	45–180 days (average 60–90 days)	Jaundice, hepatomegaly, anorexia, abnormal liver function, abdominal discomfort, clay-colored stools, tea-colored urine
FUNGAL		
Candida albicans (candidiasis)	Varies	Pruritus, white exudate on mucous membranes, irritation to mucous membranes Not always sexually transmitted
PROTOZOAN		
Trichomonas vaginalis (trichomoniasis)	4–20 days (average 7 days)	Female: itching, burning vulva and vagina; profuse, thin, frothy, greenish-yellow to greenish-white vaginal discharge with foul odor; vaginal pH > 4.2, small, deep red "strawberry spots" on cervix

(continued)

TABLE 8-12

SEXUALLY TRANSMITTED DISEASES AND INFECTIONS (Continued)

INFECTION	INCUBATION PERIOD	CLINICAL MANIFESTATIONS
		Male: may be asymptomatic, slight penile discharge, pruritus, and mild dysuria
Entamoeba histolytica (amebiasis)	Variable time period after anal/oral or anal/genital contact	May be asymptomatic, mild diarrhea to dysentery; infection may spread to other organs such as the liver
Giardia lamblia (giardiasis)	Variable time period after anal/oral or anal/genital contact	Explosive diarrhea, distension and flatulence, upper GI distress; milder symptoms may last for months with malabsorption and weight loss
PARASITIC		
Sarcoptes scabiei (scabies)	Days to weeks	Intense pruritus; burrows in skin appear as wavy short lines with a small papule or vesicle at one end; common burrow sites include finger webs, anterior surface of wrists and elbows, axillary folds, beltline, inner thighs, external genitalia (males), nipples, lower buttocks; secondary infections may occur due to scratching
Phthirius pubis (pediculosis pubis) [crabs])	1–2 weeks	Mild to severe pruritus; allergic sensitization occurs after ~5 days accompanied by itching, redness, inflammation; secondary infections may occur due to scratching

REFERENCES

1. Borman, S. Prion research accelerates. *Chemical and Engineering News,* Feb. 9, 1998. Website:http://pubs.acs.org/hotartcl/cenear/980209/cows.html.
2. Centers for Disease Control and Prevention: NCHS Website:http://www.cdc.gov/nchs www/faq/deaths1.htm 1996.
3. Clark, J., Queener, S., & Karb, V. (1997). *Pharmacologic basis of nursing practice.* St. Louis: C.V. Mosby.
4. Davis, A. T. (1997). Zoonoses. In S. Shulman, J. Phair, L. Peterson, & J. Warren (Eds.), *The biologic and clinical basis of infectious diseases* (5th ed.). Philadelphia: W. B. Saunders.
5. Gaedeke, M. (1996). *Laboratory and diagnostic test handbook.* Menlo Park: Addison Wesley.
6. Gerding, D., Shulman, S., and Phair, J. (1997). Antimicrobial therapy. In S. Shulman, J. Phair, L. Peterson, & J. Warren (Eds.), *The biologic and clinical basis of infectious diseases* (5th ed.). Philadelphia: W. B. Saunders.
7. Grimes, D. (1991). *Infectious diseases.* St. Louis: C. V. Mosby.
8. Herold, B., & Spear, P. (1997). Virus–host interactions. In S. Shulman, J. Phair, L. Peterson, & J. Warren (Eds.), *The biologic and clinical basis of infectious diseases* (5th ed.). Philadelphia: W. B. Saunders.
9. Hoeprich, P. (1997). Host–parasite relationships and the pathogenesis of infectious diseases. In P. Hoeprich, M. Jordan, & A. Ronald (Eds.), *Infectious diseases* (5th ed.). Philadelphia: J. B. Lippincott.
10. Hoeprich, P. (1994). Resistance to infection. In P. Hoeprich, M. Jordan & A. Ronald (Eds.), *Infectious diseases* (5th ed.). Philadelphia: J. B. Lippincott.
11. Hoeprich, P. & O'Grady, L. (1994). Manifestations of infectious diseases. In P. Hoeprich, M. Jordan, & A. Ronald (Eds.), *Infectious diseases* (5th ed.). Philadelphia: J. B. Lippincott.
12. Joklik, W., Willett, H., Amon, D., & Wilfert, C. (1992). *Zinserr's microbiology* (20th ed.). Norwalk, CT: Appleton and Lange.
13. Jones, R. (1995). Chlamydial diseases. In G. Mandell, J. Bennett, & R. Dolin (Eds.), *Mandell, Douglas and Bennett's principles and practices of infectious diseases* (4th ed.) New York: Churchill Livingstone.
14. Krogstad, D. J. (1998). Blood and tissue protozoa. In M. Schaechter (Ed.), *Mechanisms of microbial disease* (3rd ed.). Baltimore: Williams & Wilkins.
15. McPhee, S., Lingappa, V., Ganong, W., & Lang, J. (1995). *Pathophysiology of disease: An introduction to clinical medicine.* Stamford, CT: Appleton and Lange.
16. Merlin, T., Gibson, D., & Connor, D. (1999). Infections and parasitic diseases. In E. Rubin & J. Farber (Eds.), *Pathology* (3rd ed.). Philadelphia: Lippincott Williams & Wilkins.
17. Plorde, J. (1994). *Pneumocystis carinii.* In J. C. Sherris (Ed.), *Medical microbiology: An introduction to infectious diseases* (3rd ed.). Stamford, CT: Appleton & Lange.
18. Plorde, J. (1994). Sporazoa. In J. C. Sherris (Ed.), *Medical microbiology: An introduction to infectious diseases* (3rd ed.). Stamford, CT: Appleton and Lange.
19. Pooley, R., & Peterson, L. (1997). Mechanisms of microbial susceptibility and resistance to antimicrobial agents. In S. Shulman, J. Phair, L. Peterson & J. Warren (Eds.), *The biologic and clinical basis of infectious diseases* (5th ed.). Philadelphia: W. B. Saunders.
20. Prusiner, S. (1992). Chemistry and biology of prions. *Biochemistry, 31,* 12277–12288.
21. Relman, D. and Falkow, S. (1995). A molecular perspective of microbial pathogenicity. In G. Mandell, J. Bennett, & R. Dolin (Eds.), *Mandell, Douglas and Bennett's principles and practices of infectious diseases* (4th ed.). New York: Churchill Livingstone.
22. Samuelson, J. & von Lichtenberg, F. (1994). Infectious diseases. In R. Cotran, V. Kumar, & L. Robbins (Eds.), *Robbins' pathologic basis of disease* (5th ed.). Philadelphia: W. B. Saunders.

23. Schaecter, M. (1998). Introduction to pathogenic bacteria. In M. Schaechter, G. Medoff, & B. I. Eisenstein (Eds.), *Mechanisms of microbial disease* (3rd ed.). Baltimore: Williams & Wilkins.
24. Shulman, S. T. & Phair, J. (1997). Host–bacteria interactions. In S. T. Shulman, J. Phair, L. Peterson, & J. Warren (Eds.), *The biologic and clinical basis of infectious diseases* (5th ed.). Philadelphia: W. B. Saunders.
25. Smith, T. (1934). *Parasitism and disease.* Princeton: Princeton Press.
26. Tramont, E. & Hoover, D. (1995). General or nonspecific host defense mechanisms. In G. Mandell, J. Bennett, & R. Dolin (Eds.), *Mandell, Douglas and Bennett's principles and practices of infectious diseases* (4th ed.). New York: Churchill Livingstone.
27. Tyler, K. (1995). Prions. In In G. Mandell, J. Bennett, & R. Dolin (Eds.), *Mandell, Douglas and Bennett's principles and practices of infectious diseases* (4th ed.). New York: Churchill Livingstone.
28. Warren, J. (1997). Bacteria–host interactions. In S. Shulman, J. Phair, L. Peterson, & J. Warren (Eds.), *The biologic and clinical basis of infectious diseases* (5th ed.). Philadelphia: W. B. Saunders.
29. World Health Organization (1997). *World health report 1997.* Website: http://www.who.ch/whr/1997 fig.2e.gif.

Chapter 9

Inflammation

Judith Bryan

KEY TERMS

abscess
acute inflammation
adhesion
adhesion molecules
angiogenesis
arachidonic acid
autocoids
bradykinin
chemotaxis
chronic inflammation
cicatrix
cicatrization
complement system
C-reactive protein
cytokine
dehiscence
emigration
endogenous pyrogens
extravasation
exudates
granulomatous inflammation
granulation tissue
histamine
keloids
kinin system
labile cells
leukotrienes
lymphadenitis
lymphangitis
margination
monocyte-macrophage system (mononuclear phagocyte system [MPS])
opsonin
pavementing
permanent cells
prostaglandins
serotonin
stable cells
systemic inflammatory response syndrome
thromboxanes

Inflammation is a defensive response of vascularized living tissue to cellular injury caused by endogenous or exogenous agents. Injury normally is prevented by the body's intact skin and mucous membranes, which include both physical and chemical barriers (Box 9-1). These barriers are called the *first line of defense*. When their integrity has been breached, inflammation and the nonspecific mechanisms of immunity form the *second line of defense*. The specific immune responses constitute the *third line of defense*.[8] The process of inflammation is closely related to the process of immunity (see Chap. 10).

Inflammation can be defined as the entire complex of tissue changes in reaction to injury. These changes characteristically involve vascular and cellular responses working together in a coordinated manner to destroy substances recognized as being foreign to the body.[9]

The most common causes of inflammation include (1) infection from microorganisms in the tissues; (2) physical trauma, often with the release of free blood in the tissues; (3) chemical, irradiation, mechanical, or thermal injury, causing direct irritation to the tissues; and (4) immune reactions, causing tissue-damaging hypersensitive responses. A wound is a break or interruption of the continuity of a tissue caused by mechanical or physical means, and it commonly initiates the inflammatory response (Table 9-1). The intensity of the inflammatory process is usually proportional to the degree of tissue injury.

The causation, location, and extent of the tissue injury may vary, but the sequence of physiologic events that constitutes the inflammatory response is very similar. The inflammatory response is called a nonspecific response because the pattern of events is similar regardless of the stimulus. The goal of the inflammatory response is essentially to rid the organism of both the initial cause of injury and the consequences of the injury.[4] Whether the injury is a small surgical incision or a reaction to a bacterial invasion, the body will activate those physiologic responses designed to protect the tissue from further injury.

Acute inflammation is the immediate and early response to an injurious agent. **Chronic inflammation** is of longer duration and follows a persis-

BOX 9-1 MECHANISMS OF HOST DEFENSE

- Physical and chemical barriers
  - Morphologic integrity of skin, mucous membranes
  - Sphincters
  - Epiglottis
  - Normal secretory and excretory flow
  - Endogenous microbial flora
  - Gastric acidity
- Inflammatory response
  - Circulating phagocytes
  - Complement
  - Other humoral mediators (bradykinins, fibrinolytic systems, acid cascade)
- Reticuloendothelial system
  - Tissue phagocytes
- Immune response
  - T lymphocytes and their soluble products
  - B lymphocytes and immunoglobulins

tent, self-perpetuating course, with the source of the inflammation being unresolved. Chronic inflammation may either result in healing or develop into **granulomatous inflammation.**

The inflammatory response and the process of repair are closely intertwined. The sequence of events in the inflammatory response culminates in the healing process. For example, inflammation alleviates infection, thereby initiating wound healing.[4] Healing ideally involves the return of tissue to its previous state. Healing can range from complete regeneration of functional tissue to production of a collagenous scar that only restores the mechanical integrity of the injury site.[8]

Although the inflammatory response is usually beneficial, it can be excessive, resulting in additional cellular injury or in the **systemic inflammatory response syndrome** (SIRS), which often leads to multiple organ failure.[5] SIRS became evident in the 1970s in intensive care patients with multiple organ failure.[2] It is commonly associated with sepsis.

ACUTE INFLAMMATION

Acute inflammation is of short duration, lasting from minutes to several days, and is characterized by vascular and cellular changes (Fig. 9-1). The mediators of inflammation cause and are caused by these changes. Because of the vascular and cellular alterations, fluids, proteins, and white blood cells from the vascular system arrive into the interstitial tissue in a process called *exudation.*

TABLE 9-1

TYPES OF MECHANICAL AND PHYSICAL WOUNDS

WOUND	DEFINITION
MECHANICAL	
Incision	Caused by cutting instrument; wound edges are in close proximity, aligned
Contusion	Caused by blunt instrument, usually disrupting skin or organ surface; causes hemorrhage or ecchymosis of affected tissue
Abrasion	Caused by rubbing or scraping of epidermal layers of skin or mucous membranes
Laceration	Caused by tissue tearing, with blunt or irregular instrument; tissue nonaligned with loose flaps of tissue
Puncture	Caused by piercing of tissue or organ with a pointed instrument accidentally, such as with a nail, or intentionally, such as venipuncture
Projectile or penetrating	Caused by foreign body entering tissues at high velocity; fragments of foreign missile may scatter to various tissues and organs
Avulsion	Caused by tearing of a structure from its normal anatomic position; damage to vessels, nerves, and other structures may be associated
PHYSICAL	
Microbial agents	Living organisms may affect skin, mucous membranes, organs, and bloodstream; secrete exotoxins; or release endotoxins or affect other cells
Chemical agents	Agents toxic to specific cells include pharmaceutic agents, substances released from cellular necrosis, acids, alcohols, metals, and others
Thermal agents	High or low temperatures can produce wounds of various thicknesses; these in turn may lead to cellular necrosis
Irradiation	Ultraviolet light or radiation exposure affects epithelial or mucous membranes; large doses of whole-body radiation cause changes in CNS, blood-forming system, and GI system

FOCUS ON CELLULAR PATHOPHYSIOLOGY

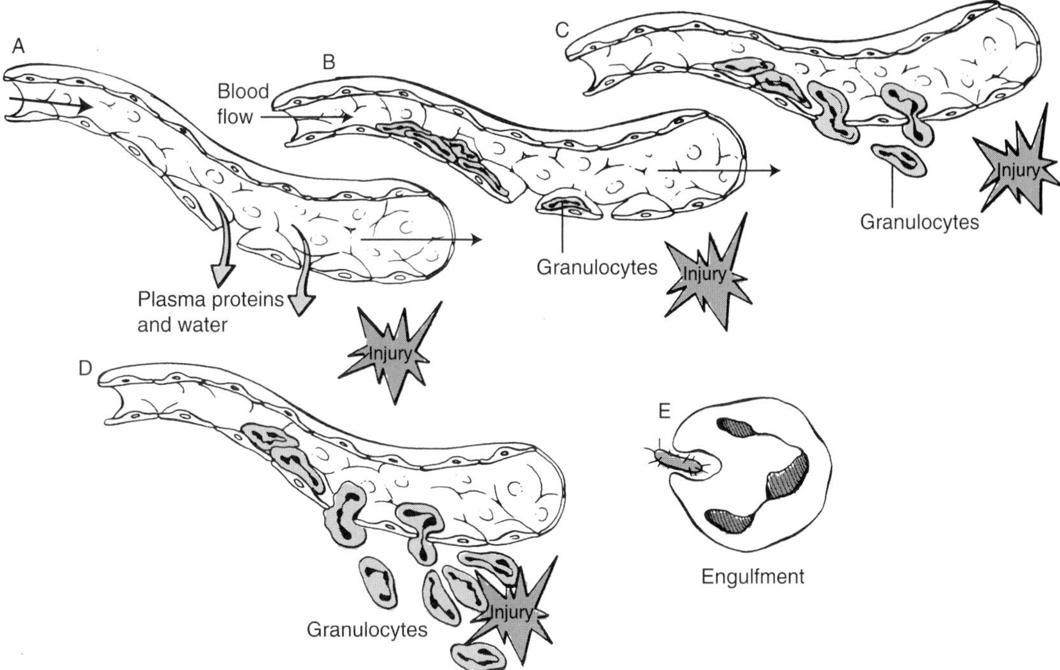

FIGURE 9-1. Phases of acute inflammation.

Vascular Phase

Acute inflammation is characterized by exudation of fluid and plasma proteins and the emigration of leukocytes, primarily neutrophils.[4] The initial response to cellular injury is a neural reflex that causes transient vasoconstriction, resulting in a decreased blood flow. The vasoconstriction is followed by vasodilatation (called the hyperemic response). Arterioles in the injured area dilate and channels in the capillary bed close, causing increased blood flow to the injured tissues (Fig. 9-2). The increased blood flow brings phagocytic cells, oxygen, and nutrients to the area of injury. The duration of vasodilatation depends on the stimulus. Dilated vessels and the increased capillary permeability lead to the loss of protein-rich fluid into the extravascular tissue. The reduced intravascular osmotic pressure and increased osmotic pressure of the interstitial fluid, combined with increased hydrostatic pressure, lead to edema. The fluid may dilute the injurious chemicals and bring complement, antibodies, and other chemotactic substances to the area (see p. 257). The plasma proteins leaked into the tissues provide an osmotic gradient, or pull, that brings more water in from the plasma. As the protein-rich fluid moves into the extravascular tissues, there is an increased concentration of red cells in the small vessels, causing an increased viscosity of blood. The resultant slowing of circulation causes stasis and heralds the beginning of the cellular phase of inflammation.[4]

Cellular Phase

The cellular phase involves the movement of neutrophils in a process called **extravasation.** Neutrophils are highly mobile cells and arrive first at the site of injury to begin phagocytosis and release inflammatory mediators capable of digesting proteins, including elastin and collagen.[8] The cells accomplish extravasation through **margination, pavementing, adhesion, emigration**, and **chemotaxis.**

MARGINATION, PAVEMENTING, AND ADHESION

Within an hour or so after the initiation of the inflammatory response, the blood becomes more viscous, due to the fluid exudation described above, and granulocytes and monocytes move toward the endothelial lining of the vessel in a process called margination. The slow movement of blood allows the polymorphonuclear leukocytes (PMNs), mostly neutrophils, to drop to the side of the capillary to form a layer closely approximated to the endothelial lining. As more leukocytes line the endothelium, the appearance of the endothelial surface is called pavementing (see Fig. 9-1). The platelets and a few red blood cells may join the PMNs on the endothelial lining.

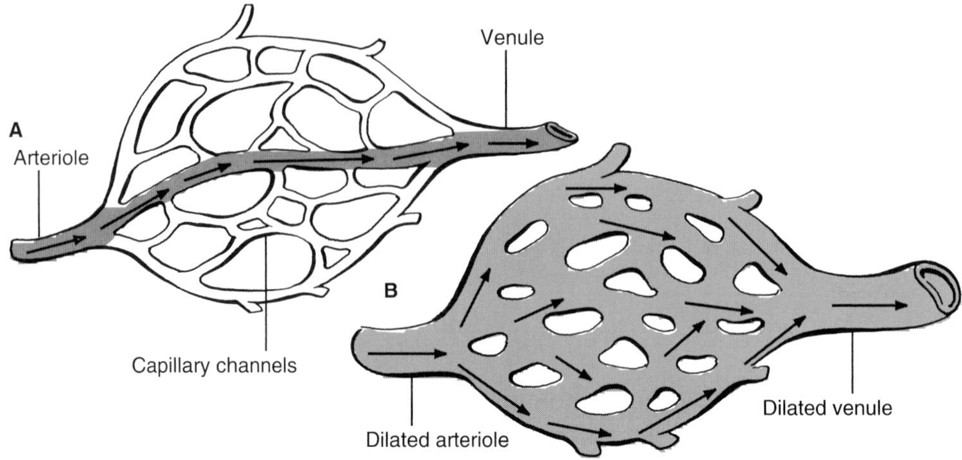

FIGURE 9-2. **A.** Normal capillary circulation. **B.** Hyperemia increases capillary flow, especially through exchange vessels around the capillary channels. Increased blood flow to the area brings cells and nutrients. The redness of an inflamed area is caused by hyperemia.

Adhesion of inflammatory cells to the endothelial lining is a critical aspect in the recruitment of these cells to the sites of tissue injury.[7] The endothelial cells normally repel passing blood cells, but the changes that occur during inflammation appear to inhibit this property. The adherence is effected by glycoproteins, called **adhesion molecules**, which are responsible for guiding inflammatory cells into extravascular sites of inflamed tissue. The adhesion receptors involved belong to the molecular families of selectins, immunoglobulins, and integrins.[13] The action of the molecules is influenced by the duration of inflammation, the type of inflammatory stimulus, and blood flow conditions. The molecules have varying functions that localize leukocytes to sites of tissue injury and participate in interactions between neutrophils, endothelial cells, and platelets.[13]

EMIGRATION

In the initial phases of the inflammatory reaction, **cytokines** such as lymphokines may be released from cells at the inflammatory site. Once lymphocytes and mononuclear cells arrive at the site, they may release additional cytokines and further enhance cellular migration by acting on the local endothelium.[12] Once the leukocytes are firmly adhered to the surface of the endothelium, they insert pseudopods into the junctions between the endothelial cells and the basement membrane. Eventually they move into the extravascular spaces. This active process is followed by the cytoplasm streaming toward the projected extension. The entire leukocyte then arrives in the tissue spaces. The first leukocytes on the scene are neutrophils. Monocytes (macrophages) and lymphocytes arrive later. Red blood cells may passively leak into the tissues along with the PMNs or because of hydrostatic pressure changes.

CHEMOTAXIS

Directional orientation for the movement of the PMNs is through chemotaxis—the movement of additional white blood cells to an area of inflammation in response to the release of chemical mediators by neutrophils, monocytes, and injured tissue. The cells move along a concentration gradient that is composed of substances such as bacterial toxins, products of tissue breakdown, and activated complement factors.

PHAGOCYTOSIS: RECOGNITION AND ATTACHMENT

Phagocytosis is a highly specific process that requires recognition of the foreign particle by the phagocyte before actual attack and engulfment can take place. The major phagocytes are PMNs and macrophages. Phagocytes have surface receptors that enable them to attach nonspecifically to bacteria and other foreign particles.[11] Phagocyte attachment is greatly enhanced in the presence of specific proteins called **opsonins**. Opsonins include immunoglobulins, especially IgG, and the opsonic fragment C3b, which bind to bacterial surfaces to form a bridge between the surfaces and the phagocytes, thereby promoting phagocytosis. When the foreign particles are recognized, their receptors are attached by the leukocyte, and phagocytosis occurs. Macrophages also may respond to opsonized or other foreign material.

Phagocytosis involves the engulfment of foreign material. The cytoplasm of the phagocyte flows around the foreign particle and ingests it. Cytoplasmic lysosomes attach to the ingested particle and release hydrolytic enzymes into it, which often kill the microorganisms or dissolve foreign proteins (Fig. 9-3). In the process, the phagocyte often dies and releases its proteolytic enzymes into the surrounding tissue, causing injury to surrounding cells and resulting in the digestion of the cell membrane of the phagocyte.

Accumulations of large numbers of phagocytes in the area of inflammation lead to pus accumulations and, eventually, the destruction and removal of foreign material. Phagocytosis localizes or walls off foreign material, preventing the spread of the process to other areas. Phagocytosis is an energy-dependent process and stimulates the production of hydrogen peroxide within the lysosomes of the phagocyte. The pH of the lysosome drops to about 4.0, which enhances the action of the hydrolytic enzymes.[3] This lowered pH is directly harmful to some pathogens, but also is the pH at which many lysosomal enzymes are most active.[9] The quantities of hydrogen peroxide produced are apparently not sufficient to induce a bactericidal effect, but they increase in the presence of myeloperoxidase (a lysosomal enzyme), which catalyzes the reaction between H_2O_2 and chloride ions to form hypochlorite, which is bactericidal.[9]

Superoxide, formed during oxidative metabolism, is a lethal oxidant that results in bacterial killing in a process called the respiratory oxidative burst.[3] During phagocytosis there is a burst of metabolic activity inside the phagocyte, resulting in increased oxygen uptake. As a result, oxygen is converted to superoxide free radical, hydrogen peroxide, and hydroxyl radical, which contribute to potent microbicidal activity in the phagolysosome.[13]

Most microorganisms ingested by phagocytes are immediately destroyed; however, some microbes survive and multiply within phagocytes. *Salmonella typhi* (cause of typhoid fever), *Mycobacterium tuberculosis* (cause of tuberculosis), and *Brucella abortus* (cause of brucellosis) are examples of bacteria that multiply intracellularly.[11]

FOCUS ON CELLULAR PATHOPHYSIOLOGY

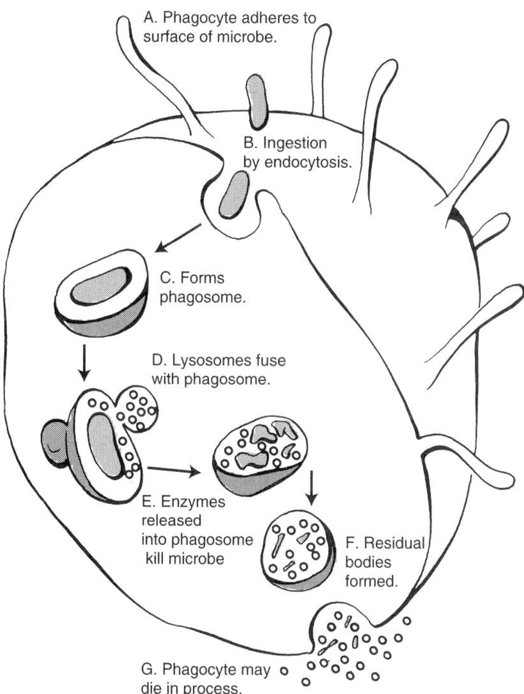
A. Phagocyte adheres to surface of microbe.
B. Ingestion by endocytosis.
C. Forms phagosome.
D. Lysosomes fuse with phagosome.
E. Enzymes released into phagosome kill microbe
F. Residual bodies formed.
G. Phagocyte may die in process.

FIGURE 9-3. Phagocytosis is a specific process in which the foreign particle is contacted and engulfed by a phagocyte. Once engulfed, the phagocytic vesicle becomes attached by lysosomes, which release proteolytic enzymes to destroy the foreign particle. Residual particles may remain within the phagocyte, or the phagocyte may be destroyed in the process.

Mediators of Inflammation

Many mediators of the inflammatory system are responsible for the effectiveness of the response to and limitations of tissue damage. General factors that promote a beneficial inflammatory reaction include adequate blood supply, nutrition, age, and general health. Some of the chemical mediators known to play an important role in promoting inflammation are discussed below. A complicated interplay among the various mediators and a cooperative system, with enhancers and depressors to the response, promote an effective response (Table 9-2).

VASOACTIVE AMINES

Histamine and **serotonin** have similar actions and are considered to be the principal mediators of the vascular phase of inflammation.[4] Basophils, mast cells, and platelets are important sources of these vasoactive mediators.

Histamine causes dilatation of the arterioles and increases vascular permeability of the venules, but constricts large arteries. It is contained mostly in mast cells, basophils, and platelets. Many agents promote the release of histamine from tissue, including mast cell and IgE reactions, C3 and C5a fragments, trauma, heat, and lysosomes of neutrophils.[4,13]

Some serotonin is present in the platelets, but the major source of this amine is the mucosal layer of the gastrointestinal tract. It is not present in mast cells of humans. Release from platelets occurs when platelet aggregation is stimulated. Figure 9-4 illustrates the cellular sources of chemical mediators.

TABLE 9-2

SUMMARY OF MEDIATORS OF ACUTE INFLAMMATION

MEDIATOR	SOURCE	ACTION: Vascular Leakage	ACTION: Chemotaxis	ACTION: Other
Histamine and serotonin	Mast cells, platelets	+	–	
Bradykinin	Plasma substrate	+	–	Pain
C3a	Plasma protein via	+	–	Opsonic fragment (C3b)
C5a	liver; macrophages	+	+	Leukocyte adhesion, activation
Prostaglandins	Mast cells, from membrane phospholipids	Potentiate other mediators	–	Vasodilation, pain, fever
Leukotriene B_4	Leukocytes	–	+	Leukocyte adhesion, activation
Leukotriene C_4, D_4, E_4	Leukocytes, mast cells	+	–	Bronchoconstriction, vasoconstriction
Oxygen metabolites	Leukocytes	+	±	Endothelial damage, tissue damage
PAF	Leukocytes; mast cells	+	+	Bronchoconstriction Leukocyte priming
IL-1 and TNF	Macrophages; other	–	+	Acute phase reactions Endothelial activation
IL-8	Macrophages Endothelium	–	+	Leukocyte activation
Nitric oxide	Macrophages Endothelium			Vasodilatation Cytotoxicity

(Cotran, R. S., Kumar, V., & Collins, T. [1999]. *Robbins' pathologic basis of disease* [6th ed.]. Philadelphia: W. B. Saunders.)

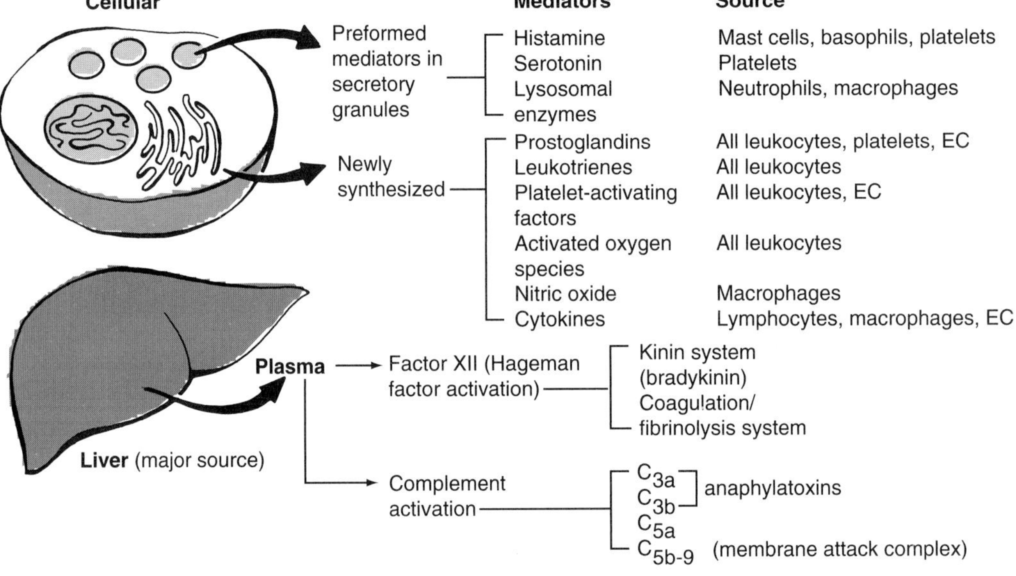

FIGURE 9-4. Chemical mediators of inflammation. (Cotran, R. S., Kumar, V., & Collins, T. [1999]. *Robbins' pathologic basis of disease* [6th ed.] Philadelphia: W. B. Saunders.)

COMPLEMENT SYSTEM

The **complement system,** a major mediator of inflammation, affects vascular responses as well as leukocyte adhesion, chemotaxis, and enhanced phagocytosis in the inflammatory response. The term "complement" was originally used to describe the activity in serum, which could complement the ability of a specific antibody to cause lysis of bacteria.[14] The system contains about 20 distinct proteins and their cleavage products. Complement components normally are present in the blood in the form of zymogens or pro-enzymes requiring proteolytic cleavage to become active.[18] These are sequentially activated, with each component activating the next in the series (Flowchart 9-1). The complement system enhances chemotaxis, increases vascular permeability and, in the final conversion, causes cell lysis. Fixation (activation) of complement at the C1q level is by antigen–antibody interaction. C1 complement consists of a single C1q molecule, two C1r molecules, and two C1s molecules.[18] This classic pathway continues a reaction pattern until the C8 and C9 enzymes are activated. The complement components, C3 and C5, are the most important inflammatory mediators. They increase vascular permeability and cause vasodilatation by assisting in the release of histamine from mast cells. C3 assists in the process of phagocytosis. C5a is a powerful chemotactic agent for neutrophils, monocytes, eosinophils, and basophils.[18] Figure 9-5 shows the modulation of the adaptive immune response through complement activity. The inflammatory process is greatly diminished in the absence of complement enzymes.

The alternative pathway is activated by the chance binding of C3b to hydroxyl groups on the surface of a microorganism.[7,18] The cascade continues from C3b to the terminus at C8 and C9, but no memory is produced.

AUTOCOIDS (ARACHIDONIC ACID METABOLITES)

Prostaglandins, thromboxanes, and **leukotrienes** belong to a group of so-called **autocoids (arachidonic acid metabolites)**, or local, short-range hormones that exert their effects locally and either decay spontaneously or are destroyed enzymatically (Fig. 9-6).[4,13] These substances can be synthesized by most connective tissue, blood, and parenchymal cells. Prostaglandins have histamine-like effects and are involved in fever and in the transmission of pain impulses. Thromboxanes are involved in the platelet response to blood vessel injury.[7,13] Leukotrienes cause vasodilatation and increased permeability.

FLOWCHART 9-1 ***The Complement Cascade***

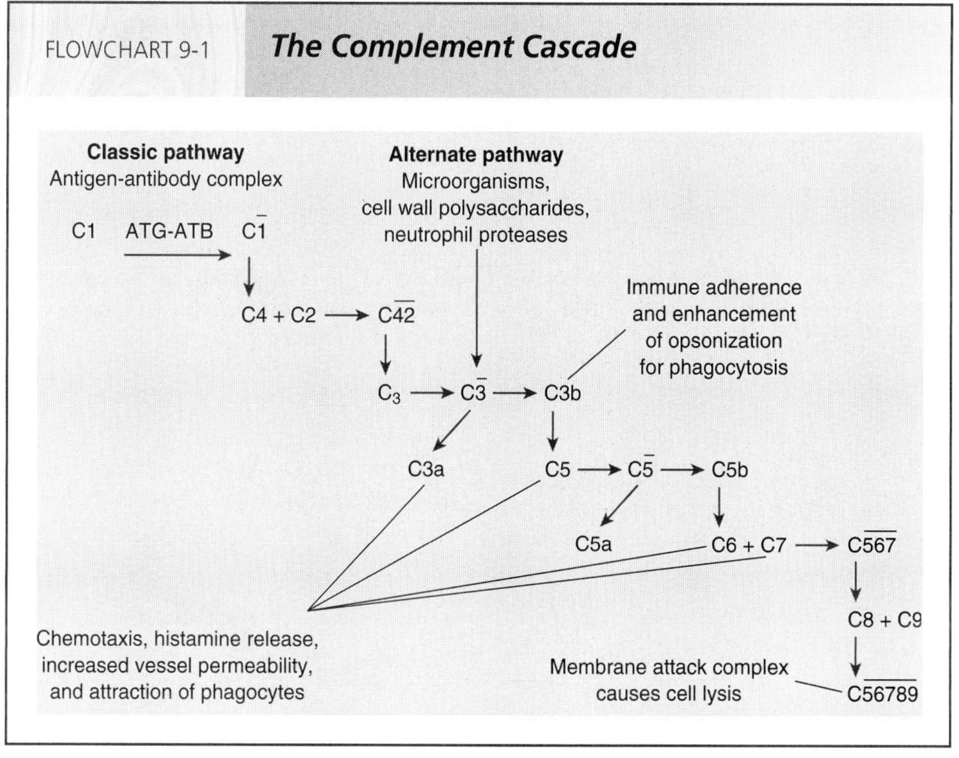

FOCUS ON CELLULAR PATHOPHYSIOLOGY

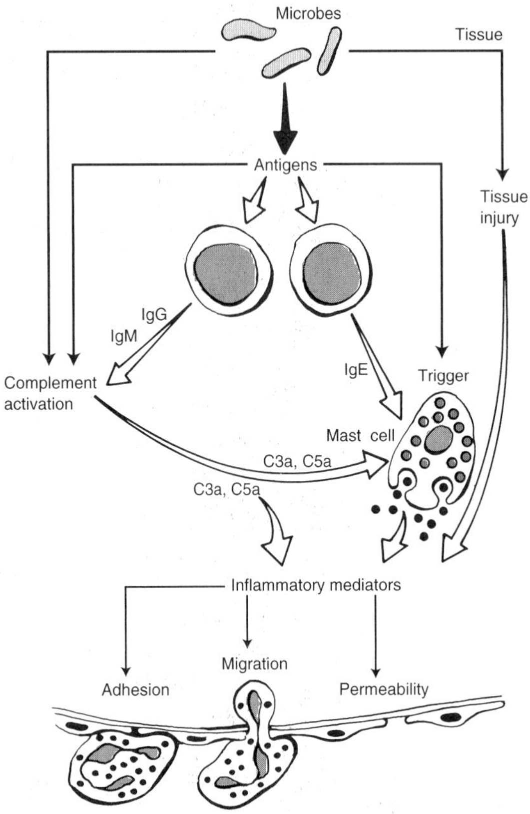

FIGURE 9-5. The adaptive immune system modulates inflammatory processes via the complement system. Antigens (e.g., from microorganisms) stimulate B cells to produce antibodies including IgE, which binds to mast cells, while IgG and IgM activate complement. Complement can also be activated directly via the alternative pathway. When triggered by antigen, the sensitized mast cells release their granule-associated mediators and eicosanoids (products of arachidonic metabolism, including prostaglandins and leukotrienes). In association with complement (which can also trigger mast cells via C3a and C5a), the mediators induce local inflammation, facilitating the arrival of leukocytes and more plasma enzyme system molecules. (Roitt, I., Brostoff, J., & Male, D. [1998]. *Immunology* [5th ed.]. Philadelphia: Mosby.)

During cell injury, phospholipids become available for conversion to prostaglandins. Other mediators of inflammation, such as **bradykinin**, also have been shown to stimulate prostaglandin synthesis. Some of the prostaglandins function as vasodilators by enhancing vascular permeability. This leads to edema, with increased concentrations of these substances in the fluids and exudates of inflammatory reactions. The mechanism by which prostaglandins increase fever is not known, but local production is thought to affect the hypothalamus, which then transmits the information to the vasomotor system, resulting in stimulation of the sympathetic nervous system.

KININS AND THE COAGULATION SYSTEM

The **kinin system** begins with activation of a plasma protein called the Hageman factor (XII), which is also a component of the clotting cascade. Factor XII is activated by surface-active agents, endotoxins, cartilage contact, and contact with basement membrane tissue. It causes the activation of coagulation proteins, conversion of prekallikrein to kallikrein, plasmin interaction with complement, and fibrinolysis (Flowchart 9-2).[7] Activated Hageman factor converts plasma prekallikrein to the enzyme kallikrein, resulting in the release of kinins.

One of the most important of the kinins is bradykinin, which mediates vasodilatation, increased vascular permeability, contraction of smooth muscle, and pain sensation.[13] The action of bradykinin is quickly inactivated by an enzyme called kininase.[4]

LYMPHOKINES

Lymphokines are protein mediators released from helper T lymphocytes during immunologic reactions and are from a group of extracellular factors called cytokines. Cytokines produced from lymphocytes are called lymphokines. This group of vasoactive substances has a major role in immunologic reactions and also induces chemotaxis for neutrophils (PMNs) and macrophages.[9]

NEUTROPHIL MEDIATORS

The lysosomes of neutrophils contain potent proteins and proteases that can activate the alternative pathway for complement and release kinin-like substances and cationic proteins, all of which increase vascular permeability.[7] As the neutrophils die and release their lysosomal products into the surrounding tissue, chemotaxis and vasodilatation are enhanced.

Exudates

In the process of inflammation, different types of exudates are formed, the analysis of which may offer clues to the nature of the process. An **exudate** is fluid or matter collecting in a cavity or tissue space. There are many types of exudates, which are described according to their constituents (Table 9-3). The following exudates are commonly seen in inflammation:

- Serous exudate—a protein-rich fluid that escapes into the tissues in the early stages of inflammation. Because of its high protein content, it draws water and thus is responsible for the edema at the site of an inflammatory reaction.

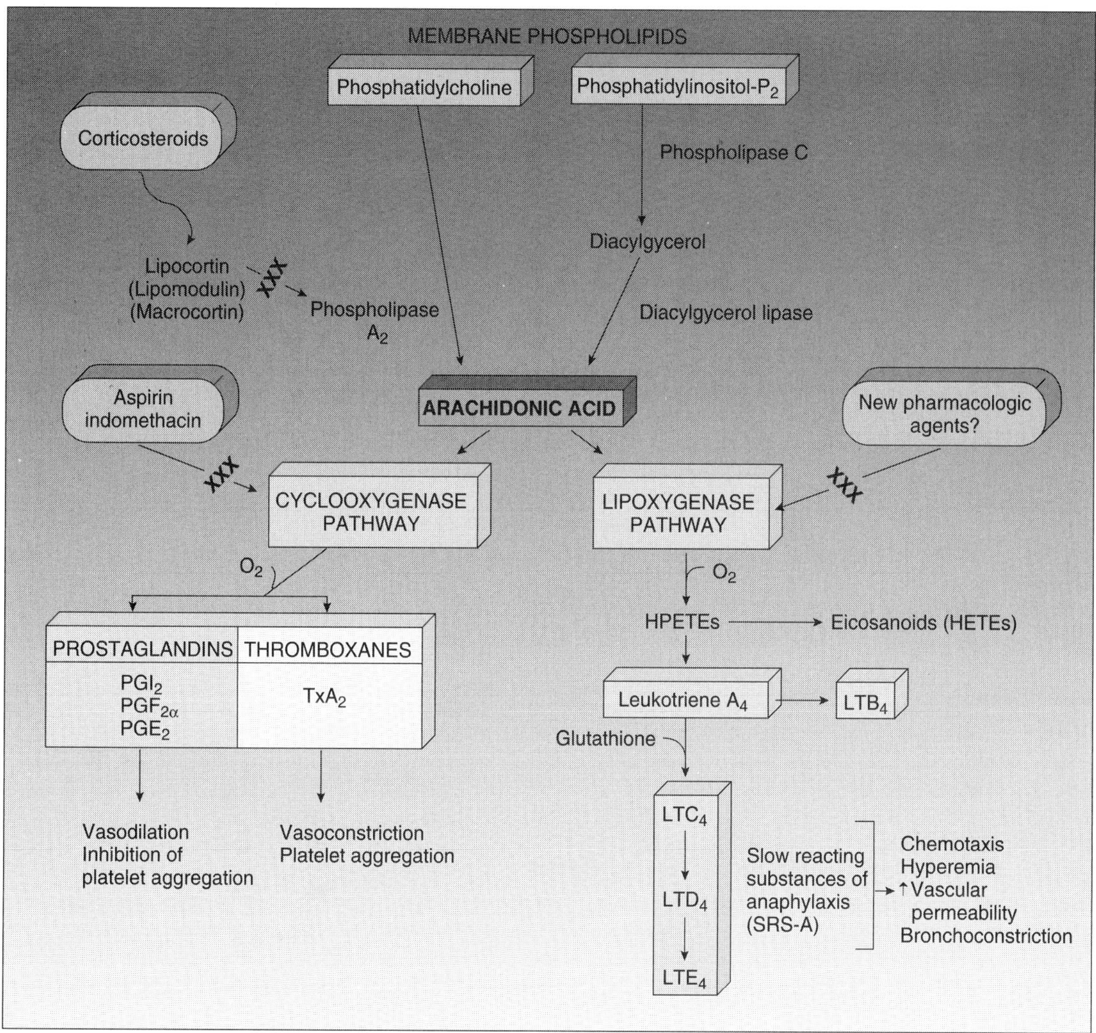

FIGURE 9-6. Arachidonic acid metabolism: Lipid mediators of inflammation cause (1) the release of cyclo-oxygenase products leading to prostaglandins and thromboxanes, and (2) the lipogenase pathway leading to the leukotrienes. (Adapted from Rubin, E. & Farber, J. L. [1999]. *Pathology* [3rd ed.] Philadelphia: Lippincott Williams & Wilkins.)

- Purulent exudates—those that contain pus, which is really a combination of phagocytic neutrophils and "pus-producing" organisms localized on a battlefield to prevent the infection from spreading system wide.

Outcomes of Acute Inflammation

The nature and intensity of the injury, the site of the injury, the tissue affected, and the responsiveness of the host impact the inflammatory process. The injury often leads to acute inflammation, which may resolve, undergo healing through regeneration or scarring, develop into a chronic inflammatory process, or result in an **abscess** (Flowchart 9-3). Chronic inflammation and abscess formation are discussed below.

The ideal outcome of acute inflammation is the complete resolution of the site of injury to normal. When the injury is of short duration and of limited scope, with minimal tissue damage, resolution is the expected outcome. Regeneration of tissue and/or scarring occur when there is more extensive tissue damage (see p. 265).

CHRONIC INFLAMMATION

Chronic inflammation is a persistence of the inflammatory process and may follow a less predictable course than acute inflammation. The chronically inflamed area usually is infiltrated by mononuclear leukocytes, mostly macrophages and lymphocytes. However, certain types of chronic inflammation, such

FLOWCHART 9-2

Hageman Factor Activation and Inflammatory Mediator Production

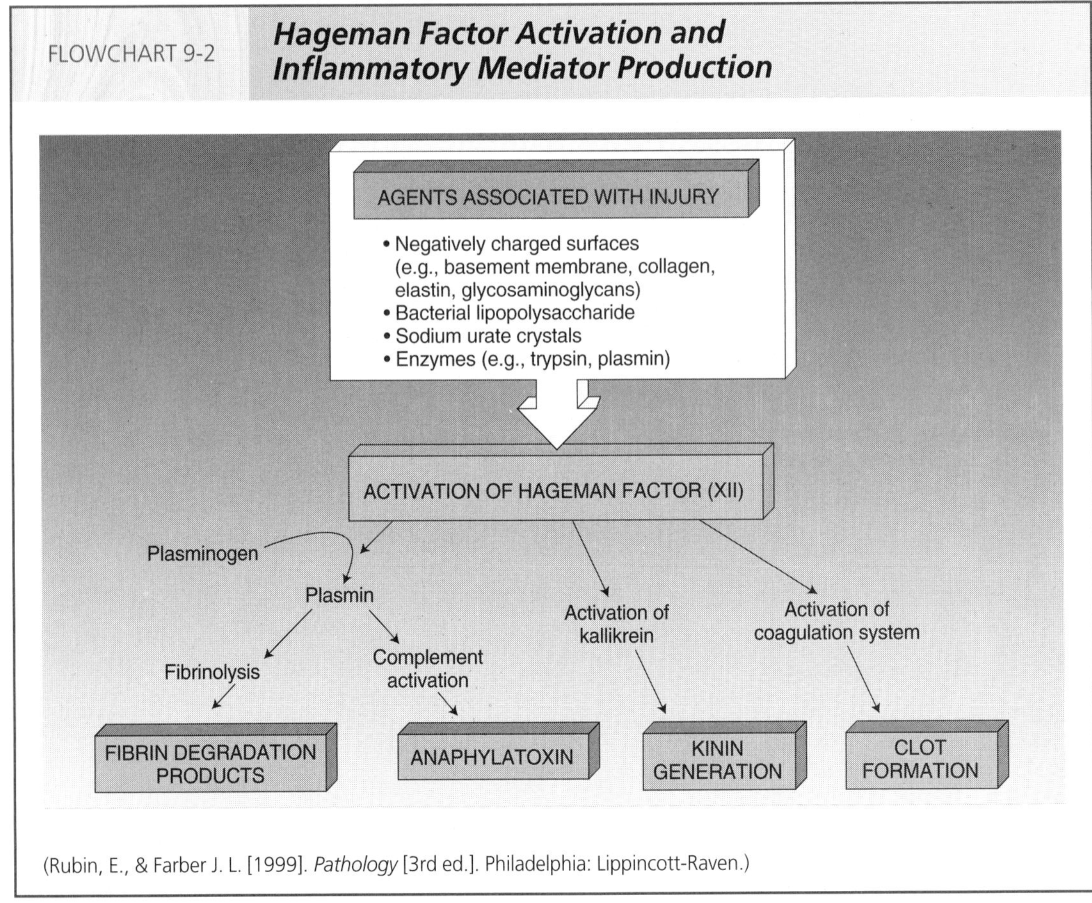

(Rubin, E., & Farber J. L. [1999]. *Pathology* [3rd ed.]. Philadelphia: Lippincott-Raven.)

as osteomyelitis, may contain neutrophils for months, and some types of acute inflammation have increased numbers of lymphocytes in the early phase.[7] When macrophages are the predominant cells, they divide and multiply and release chemotactic substances that attract more macrophages (Flowchart 9-4). The inflammatory process may begin as a low-grade, poorly cleared inflammation or as an acute inflammation that is not totally resolved by the body.

Chronic inflammation results in infiltration of the site with fibroblasts, increased amounts of collagen deposits, and varying amounts of scar tissue formation. The scar tissue and underlying inflammation often cause organ dysfunction. Chronic inflammation may begin insidiously with a low-grade fever and no other apparent symptoms.

Cells of Chronic Inflammation

The **mononuclear phagocytic system (MPS)** includes blood monocytes and tissue macrophages. Even though monocytes emigrate early toward acute inflammation, they are not the primary cell type at the site of injury until about 48 hours after the injury. The monocyte becomes a macrophage when it reaches extravascular tissue. Macrophages are not only phagocytic but have the unique capability to increase their cell size, increase levels of lysosomal enzymes, and become metabolically more active.[15] After activation, the macrophages secrete several biologically active products that serve as mediators in chronic inflammation. Macrophages eventually disappear in acute inflammation but continue to accumulate in chronic inflammation.

Granulomatous Inflammation

Granulomatous inflammation is a type of chronic inflammation characterized by the accumulation of modified macrophages and initiated by either infectious or noninfectious agents. The most predominant example of granulomatous inflammation is tuberculosis.

LOCAL AND SYSTEMIC EFFECTS OF INFLAMMATION

The local effects of inflammation are found in the area of injury. All types of inflammation have in common the following five cardinal signs: calor (heat), dolor

TABLE 9-3

CHARACTERISTICS OF EXUDATES IN INFLAMMATORY PROCESSES

TYPES	COMPONENTS	EFFECTS
Serous	Plasma-like effusion with no cells	Characteristic of early inflammation; also seen in other conditions such as heart failure and pleural effusions
Purulent or suppurative	Effusion contains white blood cells, bacteria, proteins and tissue debris; caused by pyogenic bacteria	May cause surrounding tissue damage; may localize in abscess formations, usually walled off from systemic circulation
Fibrinous	Exudate contains large amounts of fibrinogen	Forms thick, sticky meshwork that may cause areas to stick together
Membranous	Exudate contains fibrinous or fibrinopurulent material with necrotic cells	Often found on mucous membranes; characteristic of certain microorganism infection
Serosanguinous	Contains both serous and hemorrhagic material	Caused from bleeding as well as serous exudation, as in injury or burns
Hemorrhagic	Contains large numbers of red blood cells and usually other cells	Caused when blood vessels are damaged or permeable to red blood cells
Mucinous	Contains large amounts of mucous and epithelial cells	Caused by inflammatory conditions such as allergic rhinitis or the common cold

(pain), rubor (redness), tumor (swelling), and loss of normal function. These manifestations result from vasodilatation, exudation, and irritation of nerve endings. The vasodilatation is associated with the release of chemical mediators. Exudation results from fluid and white blood cell movement into the affected area. Nerve endings are irritated by chemical mediators, causing pain and sometimes loss of functioning.

The systemic manifestations of acute inflammation are known as the acute-phase reactions. These indicate the reaction of the body to the inflammatory process and include fever, leukocytosis, decreased appetite, altered sleep patterns, and changes in plasma levels of the acute phase proteins, especially C-reactive protein, antibody, and complement. Changes in the levels of these proteins are mediated by interleukin-6, a cytokine syn-

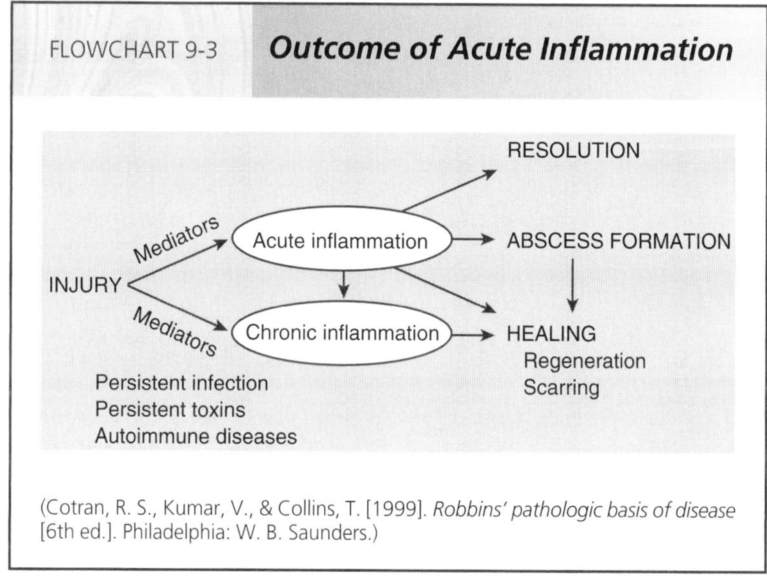

(Cotran, R. S., Kumar, V., & Collins, T. [1999]. *Robbins' pathologic basis of disease* [6th ed.]. Philadelphia: W. B. Saunders.)

FLOWCHART 9-4 **The Accumulation of Macrophages in Chronic Inflammation**

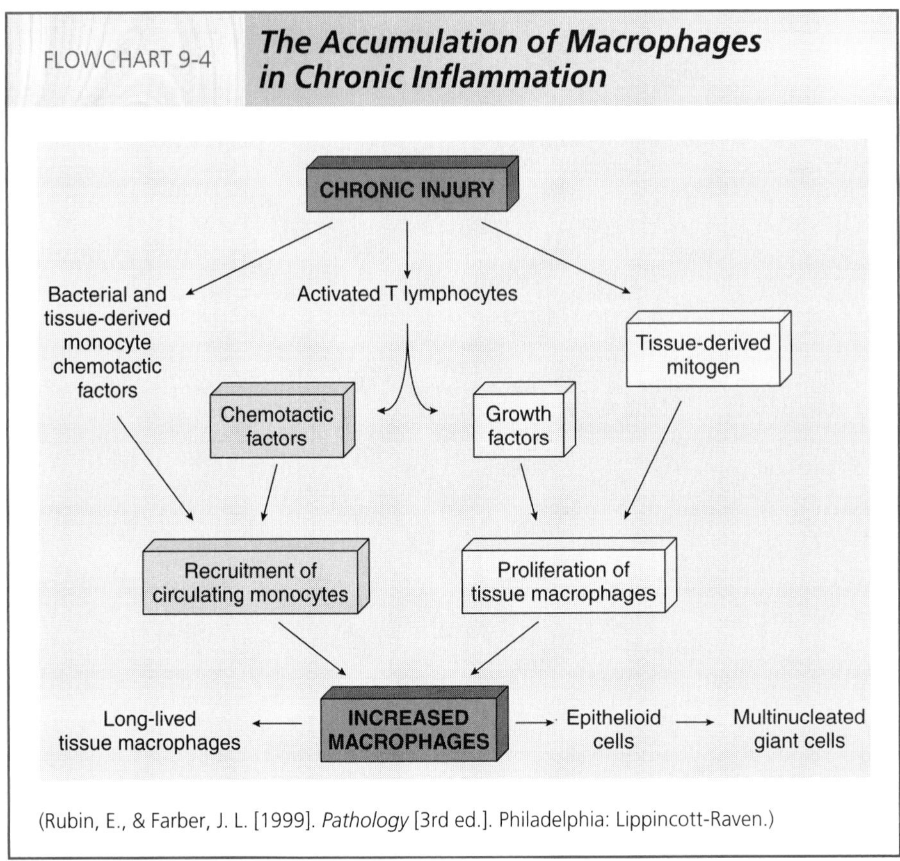

(Rubin, E., & Farber, J. L. [1999]. *Pathology* [3rd ed.]. Philadelphia: Lippincott-Raven.)

thesized at sites of inflammation by various cell types.[13] **C-reactive protein** is an acute phase reactant that has opsonic properties as well as having a modulating effect on inflammatory and immune responses.[13]

Lymphadenopathy

Lymphadenopathy is a sign of a severe, localized infection. It results when the local lymph nodes and vessels drain the infected material, which becomes enmeshed in the follicular tissue of the nodes. Increased lymphatic flow is characteristic of localized inflammation. If an inflammation of the lymphatic vessel occurs, it is termed **lymphangitis.** If it affects the lymph nodes, it is termed **lymphadenitis**. The lymph system serves to localize and isolate infections and prevent their entrance into the bloodstream.

Fever

Fever is an almost universal phenomenon of illness, particularly of inflammation. Its purpose is unknown, but up to a certain point it is considered a defense against disease. High body temperatures intensify the effect of interferons. A high body temperature speeds up the body's reactions and may help the body tissue repair themselves more quickly.[7] It is thought to be caused by the release of **endogenous pyrogens** from macrophages and possibly from eosinophils, which are activated by phagocytosis, endotoxins, immune complexes, and other products. These pyrogens act on the temperature-regulating centers in the hypothalamus to elevate the thermostat set-point. It has been suggested that interleukin-1 (formerly called endogenous pyrogen) causes fever by inducing the hypothalamus to release prostaglandin E2, which acts on the hypothalamus to evoke the fever response.[9,15] When the set-point becomes increased to a higher than normal level, mechanisms for raising the body temperature are activated.[8] The body initiates heat-conservation measures, including vasoconstriction, piloerection (gooseflesh), and shivering, to drive the body temperature up to a new level. These mechanisms, along with conscious heat-conservation measures, such as covering with blankets, aid the body in attaining the new set-point. Therefore, the new set-point may be 38° to 40°C. Above 40°C the temperature control regulation can become seriously impaired, causing central nervous system damage. When the set-point is reached or the stimulus is removed, the body initiates cooling measures, including vasodilatation (flush) and sweating, to maintain the set-point. If the set-point returns to normal, the fever rapidly dissipates. This rapid resolution has been termed "breaking of the fever," and it may signify that the causative agent has been destroyed. Effective antibiotic therapy can rapidly destroy the bacteria that produce pyrogens and cause a rapid recovery of the temperature control mechanism. Also, antipyretic agents, such as aspirin and acetaminophen, can impede the formation of prostaglandins from arachidonic acid and reduce fever.[7]

Leukocytosis and Leukopenia

Leukocytosis refers to an elevation in the white blood cell count. The rise in the number of cells is selective, according to the causative agent. For example, pyogenic bacteria often cause an increase in the neutrophil count, whereas helminthic infections may cause eosinophilia (see p. 246).

In advanced or overwhelming infections, leukopenia may occur. The onset of a depletion of neutrophils indicates that the system is unable to mount an adequate defense.

RESOLUTION OF INFLAMMATION: HEALING

For the body to maintain normal structure and function, foreign material must be removed or isolated to prevent deleterious effects. Ideally, this occurs with a process called healing. Wound healing begins with inflammation. There is no distinct line between the time when inflammation ends and healing begins. Healing follows several typical steps or stages. The first stage requires a cleanup of cellular debris, organisms, or clot, which is carried out mostly by macrophages and a few neutrophils. The reparative process follows and is accomplished through: (1) simple resolution, (2) regeneration, or (3) replacement by a connective tissue scar. Flowchart 9-5 indicates the possible pathways of the reparative responses.

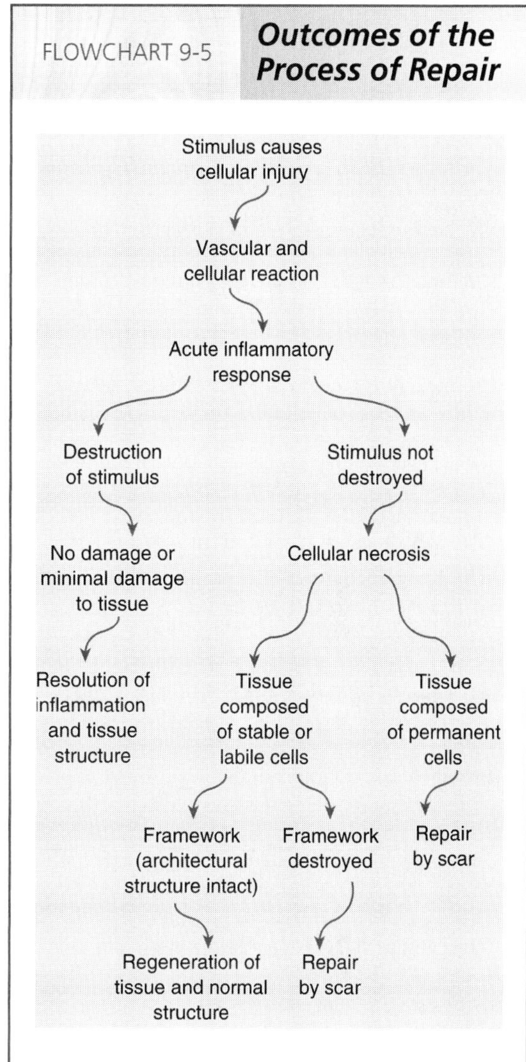

Simple Resolution

Simple resolution involves no destruction of normal tissue and probably goes on continuously in the human body. The offending agent is neutralized and destroyed. The vessels return to their normal permeability, and excess fluid exudation is reabsorbed. Any defensive cells in the area are either reabsorbed or cleared by tissue macrophages.

Regeneration

Regeneration refers to the replacement of lost or necrotic tissue with tissue that is structurally and functionally identical.[7] It is part of the reparative process to heal and reconstitute damaged tissue. The intact, healthy neighbor cells surrounding the dead cells undergo mitosis and proliferate to replace the cells lost in the tissue. This process usually occurs to the greatest degree in epithelial tissue. Certain glands and organs can regenerate functional parenchymal cells if the architectural support structure remains intact.

In the healthy human body, the process by which cell growth and reproduction occurs is still essentially unknown. Certain cell types have different patterns of reproduction (see below). Control substances are probably secreted by cells that act as a feedback mechanism to stop or slow growth when an adequate number of cells is produced.[9] Certain types of cells removed from the body can be grown in a laboratory culture if the medium is suitable. These cells stop growing when small amounts of their own secretions are allowed to collect in the culture medium. Thus, the secretions are probably the control substances that limit cell growth and reproduction.

Cells may be classified according to reproductive capability. Regenerative capacity varies among tissues, but generally the more specialized the tissue, the less capable it is of regeneration. The general pattern of reproduction of cell types follows:

- All **labile cells** undergo complete regeneration by the proliferation of reserve cells. Labile cells reproduce continually since they are constantly being depleted through daily processes. Examples of labile cells include the epithelial cells of the skin and mucous membranes.
- **Stable cells** regenerate if they are stimulated to do so. For example, bone injury causes fibroblasts to differentiate into osteoblasts and osteocytes. Muscle, bone, liver, kidney, and lung tissues are moderately regenerative, and synovial cells in the tendons may be reformed under optimal healing conditions.
- **Permanent cells** such as heart muscle and nerve cell bodies are generally incapable of mitosis in adults. Death of these cells requires replacement by scar tissue.

Repair by Scar

Repair by scar occurs when dead tissue cells are replaced by viable cells of a different type than the original cells. The new cells form **granulation tissue**, which later matures to fibrous scar tissue. Granulation tissue is proliferative connective tissue that is highly vascularized. The gradual laying down of collagen by these connective tissue cells eventually causes a dense fibrous scar to form.[7] Collagen is the main component that provides strength to healing wounds.[4] The scar begins as collagen bridges the defect and provides the initial strength to a wound.

As granulation tissue forms, it is very vascular and bleeds readily. As the scar forms, it tends to mold to the shape of the surrounding tissue and increases in tensile strength by compressing the collagen. In the early weeks, the scar is red because of the many blood vessels infiltrating it. The new vessels originate by a budding or sprouting from vessels adjacent to the wound in a process called **angiogenesis**, or neovascularization. The new vessels are leaky and allow fluid and protein to pass through them into the extravascular spaces. This leakiness accounts for edema that remains after the acute inflammation has subsided. The red scar begins to fade as healing becomes complete and less blood is needed. The vessels become smaller and the scar assumes a white, fibrous appearance.

Wound remodeling occurs throughout healing. Contraction, or shortening, of the scar is effective in pulling the wound edges closer together in the early stages of scar formation. **Cicatrization** denotes formation of mature scar tissue with less elasticity than most normal tissue. The **cicatrix** has been described as less vascular, pale, and contracting scar tissue. The pale appearance is due to lack of pigmentation of connective (scar) tissue.[7]

Epithelialization also occurs from the wound margins across the surface of the wound. This process is important to reestablish a protective covering of the surface of the healed wound. The epithelial cells at the wound margins begin active mitosis and cell migration on the surface of the granulation tissue that has formed (Fig. 9-7).

HEALING BY FIRST INTENTION

First-intention healing refers to scar tissue that is laid down across a clean wound with edges in close approximation. The edges are sealed together by a blood clot, which dries to protect and seal the wound. The best example is a clean surgical wound closed by sutures (Fig. 9-8). An acute inflammatory reaction occurs within the first 24 hours, with neutrophilic infiltration of the area. By the third day, macrophages have largely replaced the neutrophils and have removed the cellular debris. Collagen fibers are lined up vertically but do not bridge the incision.[4] By the fifth day, the collagen fibrils begin to bridge the defect. Maximum vascularization occurs at this time. Collagen continues to accumulate to form a firm, tough scar, progressively increasing in strength until about the end of the first month. Epithelialization across the superficial layers restores a smooth contour.

FOCUS ON CELLULAR PATHOPHYSIOLOGY

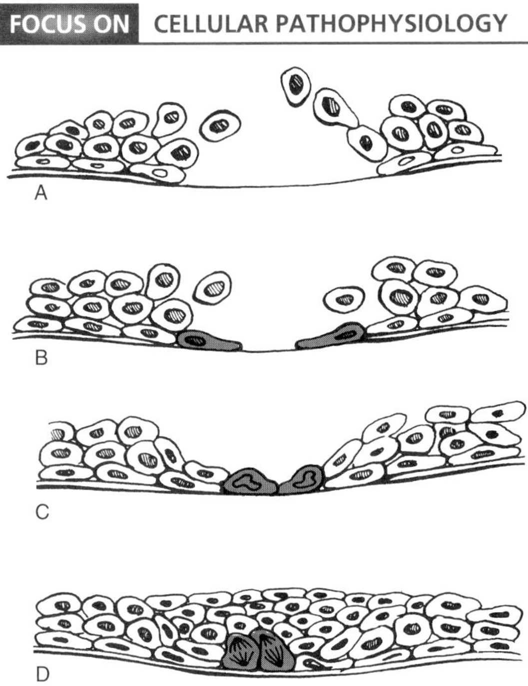

FIGURE 9-7. Reepithelialization of a wound. **A.** With injury, epidermal cells detach from basement membrane and enlarge. **B.** Undifferentiated basal cells migrate toward center of wound defect. **C.** Contact inhibition occurs when migrating cells meet in the center and touch. **D.** Basal cells proliferate to restore epidermis.

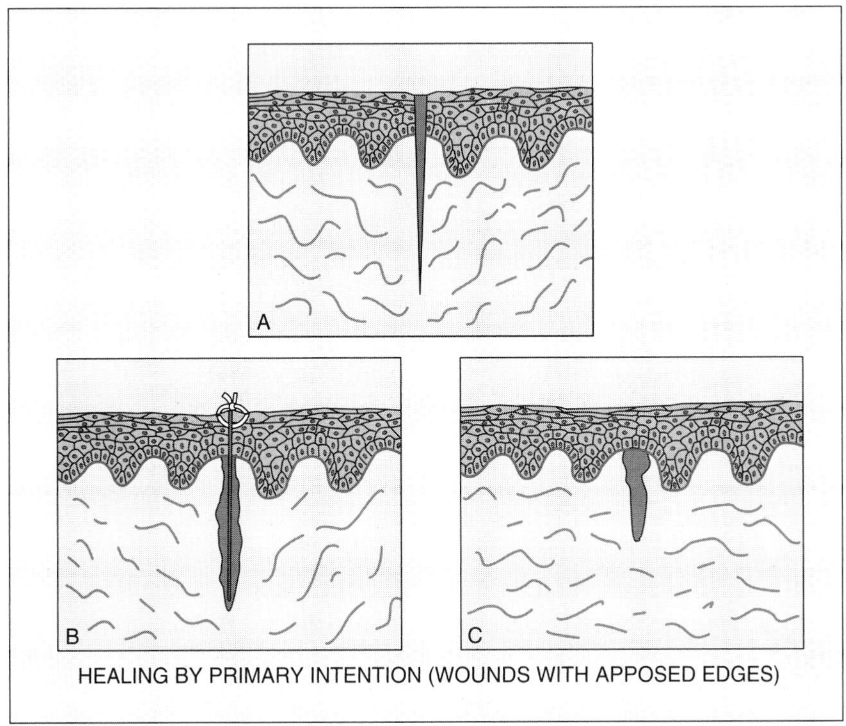

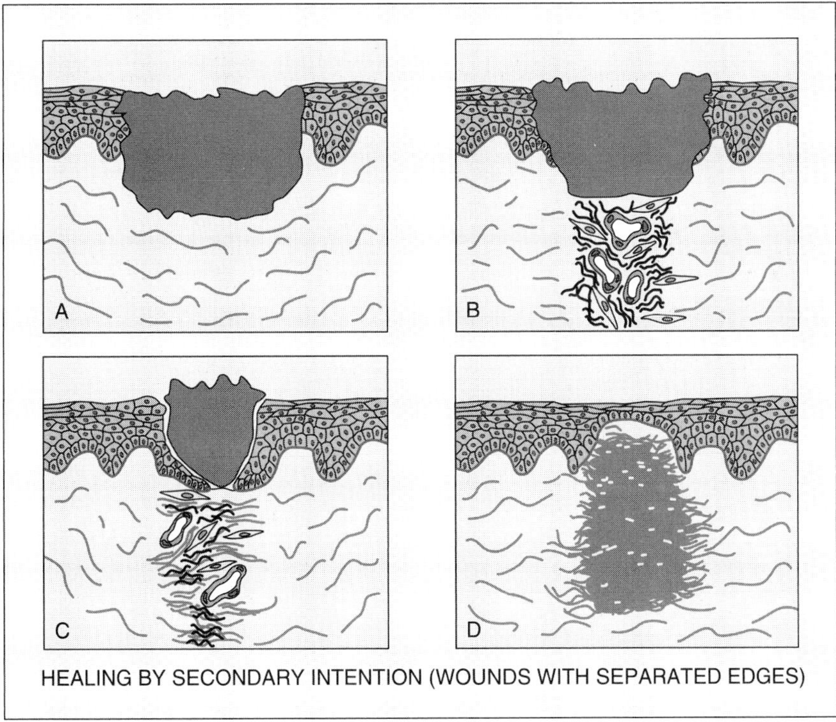

FIGURE 9-8. **Top.** Healing by primary intention. **A.** A wound with closely apposed edges and minimal tissue loss. **B.** Such a wound requires only minimal cell proliferation and neovascularization to heal. **C.** The result is a small scar. **Bottom.** Healing by secondary intention. **A.** A gouged wound, in which the edges are far apart and in which there is substantial tissue loss. **B.** This wound requires wound contraction, extensive cell proliferation, and neovascularization (granulation tissue) to heal. **C.** The wound is reepithelialized from the margins, and collagen fibers are deposited in the granulation tissue. **D.** Granulation tissue is eventually reabsorbed and replaced by a large scar that is functionally and cosmetically unsatisfactory. (Rubin, E., & Farber, J. [1999]. *Pathology* [3rd ed.]. Philadelphia: Lippincott Williams & Wilkins).

The scar initially is bright red from the extensive vascularization, but it decreases in size and changes to a thin white line as vascularity decreases. For the first month, tensile strength closely parallels the collagen content of the wound.[7]

HEALING BY SECOND INTENTION

Second-intention healing parallels first-intention healing except that it occurs in wounds in which large sections of tissue have been lost or in wounds complicated by infection. More time is necessary to remove the necrotic debris and infection from this type of wound. The inflammatory reaction is more extensive across the larger wound surface, and the wound remains inflamed for a longer period. These wounds often become contaminated and heal over the surface only to open up again due to infectious processes smoldering below the surface.

Large amounts of granulation tissue must be formed. The wound must granulate from its margins and base, with collagen gradually filling the defect. Wound contraction is mostly caused by myofibroblast contraction that tends to pull the wound edges into closer proximity. Myofibroblasts anchor themselves to the wound margins and begin the process of contraction that pulls the edges together (see Fig. 9-8).

Surface reepithelialization over the large surface begins and eventually restores a multilayered epithelium. The underlying scar is large and deforming due to the large amount of granulation that is formed.

Second-intention healing is required in third-degree burns, deep skin ulcerations, infected wounds, and other large wounds. Structures normally found in the scarred area cannot be replaced, so hair follicles, sweat glands, and melanin-producing cells are lost.

Factors That Delay Wound Healing

Both local and systemic factors affect the body's ability to heal a wound. Oxygen deficiencies, malnutrition, and electrolyte imbalances are examples of conditions that can markedly affect the efficiency of the normal defense mechanisms. Immune suppression and clotting deficiencies also can disturb the primary closure of a wound surface. The effects of systemic bodily stress from injury or illness produce immune suppression, resulting in delayed healing. Box 9-2 describes local and general factors that can delay wound healing.

Aberrant Healing

Aberrant means deviating from the normal, typical, or usual. In healing wounds, deviations from the normal may cause complications, deformity, and decreased function of the injured tissue. The results of aberrant healing depend on where the wound is located, the degree of deviation, and the modifying factors present in the patient. Aberrant healing results from abnormalities in healing mechanisms that lead to formation of excess scar tissue, contractures, constrictions, or adhesions.

EXUBERANT GRANULATION AND KELOIDS

Exuberant granulations, or "proud flesh," occur when there is an excessive accumulation of scar tissue. They may vary in size from small to very large protrusions of granulation tissue that block the epithelialization of the wound.[16] Once removed, they do not return.

BOX 9-2 FACTORS THAT DELAY WOUND HEALING

Local Factors

- Excessive accumulation of necrotic tissue and debris: difficult to clear and heal
- Large areas of injury: extend the amount of inflammation
- Infections: must be cleared before healing can begin
- Failure to close a dead space: allows for fluid and debris to collect
- Wound dehiscence or eviceration: requires clearance of infection and reclosure
- Retained foreign body: inflammation continues to remove agent
- Hematoma: blood must be removed before inflammation is effective

Systemic Factors

- Age: Cell replacement is slower in aged individuals, epithelialization is impaired.
- Systemic diseases or immune deficiency: Decreased inflammatory cells are available to mount the response.
- Diseases that decrease systemic circulation: Decreased blood flow does not allow the delivery of mediators and cells to the area. Conditions such as atherosclerosis and diabetes affect healing.
- Malnutrition: Inadequate stores of proteins, fats, vitamins, and carbohydrates slow and sometimes interrupt the healing process.
- Drug-induced immune suppression: Decreases inflammatory cells.
- Edema of tissues: Slows the clearing of inflammatory debris.

An excessive deposition of collagen at the wound site results in a **keloid**.[1] The main defect in the production of a keloid may be inadequate lysis of excess collagen by collagenase. Elevated levels of propylhydroxylase, an enzyme necessary for collagen formation, may contribute to the excess scar formation. Research has demonstrated that in contrast to normal fibroblasts, keloid fibroblasts synthesize collagen at a rapid rate, possibly because of excessive histamine in the area.[6,10,17] Keloid formation tends to be more common among dark-skinned people and is characterized by abundant, broad, and irregular collagen bundles, with more capillaries and fibroblasts than expected for a scar of the same age.[17] Persons under the age of 30 also have a propensity for development of these abnormalities. Keloids tend to recur after removal. They can result with any wound but occur most often around the face, neck, and shoulders (Fig. 9-9).

EXCESSIVE CONTRACTURE

Wound contracture is a normal part of healing and involves migration of wound margins toward the center due to myofibroblasts. Some wounds continue to contract after closure, and a disfiguring scar or disability results. The ability of a wound to close depends in part on the flexibility of the surrounding skin. Skin on the scalp and tibial area has limited flexibility, especially if little subcutaneous tissue is present. Contractures over joints may interfere with joint mobility. They can occur in any area, skin, and subcutaneous tissue, as well as after bone fractures and tendon, muscle, or nerve injuries.

DEHISCENCE AND EVISCERATION

Dehiscence is the surface disruption that results in the bursting open of a previously closed wound. This can occur as a result of interruption of primary or secondary healing. Dehiscence occurs when the strength of the collagen framework is not adequate to resist the forces imposed on the wound. Poor collagen synthesis often is related to poor circulation.

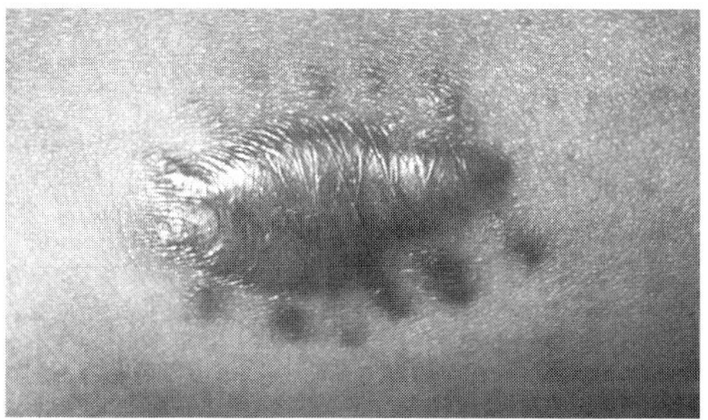

FIGURE 9-9. Close-up of a keloid that has developed at the site of prior surgery. Keloids are raised, hard, irregular, itchy scars on the skin. They consist of a mass of collagen. (© Photo Researchers.)

Evisceration refers to the internal organs moving through a dehiscence. This most frequently occurs with the abdominal organs and is a life-threatening situation. Common activities contributing to dehiscence are vomiting, coughing, and ileus.[5]

STENOSIS AND CONSTRICTION

If scar tissue forms in and around tubular areas, such as the ureter or esophagus, a stricture may develop, leading to narrowing or obstruction of an opening. Because scar tissue normally contracts, tubular structures are vulnerable to stricture development. Excessive scarring may occur around an incision line as a consequence of inflammation.

ADHESIONS

When serous or mucous membrane surfaces are inflamed, the exudate may cause scar tissue to bind or adhere to adjacent surfaces. Adhesions commonly occur in the peritoneal cavity between loops of bowel or abdominal viscera, especially after abdominal surgical procedures. Partial or complete intestinal obstruction can result from the fibrinous bands extending from organ to organ or from organ to peritoneal wall. Adhesions also frequently develop after pleuritis, causing dense, fibrous pleural adhesions that obliterate the pleural space and restrict respiratory excursion.

FOCUS ON THE PERSON WITH A COMPLICATED WOUND

Mr. J. is an obese, white, 45-year-old male who sustained a deep lacerating wound to his left thigh 4 days ago. Mr. J. was trimming a large tree with a chainsaw when he lost his balance on the ladder and dropped the saw onto his leg. He was taken to the emergency room immediately after the accident. The wound was cleansed and sutured in the operating room because of the extensive injury. He was given prophylactic antibiotics and pain medication and sent home. He is now complaining of increasing pain and an elevated temperature. The 7-inch-long wound is deep red and warm to the touch, with a purulent discharge coming from the base of the wound.

Questions

1. Describe the phases of wound healing.
2. What is the stage of healing?
3. What factors are necessary, in this case, to promote healing?
4. What are the factors, in this case, that may delay wound healing ?
5. What wound care teaching would you provide for Mr. J.?

FOCUS ON THE PERSON WITH A COMPLICATED WOUND

Mrs. G. is an obese, black, diabetic female, age 65, who underwent surgery for an abdominal tumor 6 days ago. She has a large, raised scar on her neck from a previous surgery. The pathology report was positive for a malignancy. She had a transverse incision that measured 4 inches and was secured with staples. Every other staple was removed on the 6th day and replaced with butterfly strips.

She was to wear an abdominal binder. While assisting with her morning care, Mrs. G. coughed and stated she felt something draining on her abdomen. Serous drainage was noted on the binder.

Questions

1. What are the factors listed in the case study that alert you to a wound complication?
2. What caused the drainage on the binder?
3. What is the explanation for the thick, raised scar on the neck ?
4. When Mrs. G. is to be discharged, what information should you give her regarding her wound care?

REFERENCES

1. Alster, T. S. & West, T. B. (1997). Treatment of scars: A review. *Annals of Plastic Surgery, 39*(4), 418–432.
2. Baue, A. E. (1997). Multiple organ failure, multiple organ dysfunction syndrome, and systemic inflammatory response syndrome. Why no magic bullets? *Archives of Surgery, 132,* 7.
3. Cohn, R. M. & Roth, K. S. (1996). *Biochemistry and disease: Bridging basic science and clinical practice.* Philadelphia: Williams & Wilkins.
4. Cotran, R. S., Kumar, V., and Collins, T. (1999). *Robbins' pathologic basis of disease* (6th ed.). Philadelphia: W. B. Saunders.
5. Davis, M. G., & Hagen, P. O. (1997). Systemic inflammatory response syndrome. *British Journal of Surgery, 84,* 7.
6. Ehrlich, H. P., Cremona, O. & Gabbiani, G. (1998). The expression of alpha 2, beta 1 integrin and alpha smooth muscle actin in fibroblaststs grown on collagen. *Cell Biochemistry, 16*(2), 129–137.
7. Fantone, J. C. & Ward, P. A. (1999). Inflammation. In E. Rubin & J. L. Farber, *Pathology* (3rd ed.). Philadelphia: Lippincott.
8. Gallin, J. I., Goldstein, I. M., & Snyderman, R. (1992). *Inflammation: Basic principles and clinical correlates* (2nd ed.). New York: Raven Press.
9. Guyton, A. C., & Hall, J. E. (1996). *Textbook of medical physiology* (9th ed.). Philadelphia: W. B. Saunders.
10. Kishi, N. H., Tsuchiya, Y., Yamada, H., & Tajima, S. (1997). Exposure of fibroblasts derived from keloid patients to low-energy electromagnetic fields: Preferential inhibition of cell proliferation, collagen synthesis, and transforming growth factor beta expression in keloid fibroblasts in vitro. *Annals of Plastic Surgery, 5,* 536–541.
11. Lim, D. (1998). *Microbiology* (2nd ed.). Boston: WCB McGraw-Hill.
12. Lydyard, P., & Grossi, C. (1998). Cell involved in the immune response. In I. Roitt, J. Brostoff, & D. Male, *Immunology* (5th ed.). St. Louis: Mosby.
13. Male, D. (1998). Cell migration and inflammation. In I. Roitt, J. Brostoff, & D. Male, *Immunology* (5th ed.). St. Louis: Mosby.
14. Morello, J. A., Mizer, H. E., Wilson, M. E., & Granato, P. A. (1998). *Microbiology in patient care* (6th ed.). Boston: WCB McGraw-Hill.
15. Tortora, G. J., Funke, B. R., & Case, C. L. (1998). *Microbiology: An introduction* (6th ed.). Menlo Park: Addison Wesley Longman.
16. Tredget, E. E., Nedelec, B., Scott, P. G., & Ghahary, A. (1997). Hypertrophic scars, keloids, and contractures: The cellular and molecular basis for therapy. *Surgical Clinics of North America, 77*(3), 701–730.
17. Tuan, T. L. & Nichter, L. S. (1998). The molecular basis of keloid and hypertrophic scar formation. *Molecular Medicine Today, 4*(1), 19–24.
18. Walport, M. (1998). Complement. In I. Roitt, J. Brostoff, & D. Male, *Immunology* (5th ed.). St. Louis: Mosby.

Chapter

10

Normal Immunology

Robert L. Ismeurt / Barbara Bullock

KEY TERMS

antibody
antigens
antigenic determinants
autoimmunity
chemotaxis
complement
hapten
immunity
immunocompetent cells
immunogenicity
lymphocytes
major histocompatability complex (the human leukocyte antigens)
opsonization
phagocytes
psychoneuroimmunology
recognition
specificity

The immune system consists of cells and organs that defend the body against invasion by microorganisms, damage by foreign substances, and damage and disease within cells of the body. On a discrete level, the immune system functions to protect the human body from the damages of physical injury and microbial invasion. On a more general level, however, the immune system plays a critical role in the overall maintenance of basic cellular integrity. The organs, cells, and chemicals of the immune system are intricately organized to maintain health at a cellular level and to identify and respond appropriately to threats to that health. Knowledge of the organs, immune cells, and the chemicals utilized by the immune system for communication are an essential basis for understanding human health and disease.

The immune response is induced by the introduction of a foreign particle or organism at the cellular level, and involves a variety of organs, cells, and chemicals in a complex process aimed at removing or destroying the foreign particles. The inherent capacities of the immune system to distinguish what is foreign from what belongs to the body, to self-regulate a response pattern, to have very specific responses to each pathogen, and to maintain a record of immunologic activity for future responses provide protection from foreign intrusion.

Knowledge in the area of immunology and the immune response is rapidly expanding through both basic research and from observations during many clinical situations. Most scientific knowledge of immune cells, chemicals, and functions has been gained in the 20th century with description of the primary cells of the specific immune response (two types of **lymphocytes** known as B-cells and T-cells) in 1966.[24] Knowledge of the basic chemicals of immune cell communication (immunotransmitters called cytokines) has blossomed in the past 20 years. Additionally, knowledge of the interactions between the brain and the immune system is undergoing a revolutionary expansion within the field of psychoneuroimmunology (see p. 290).

OVERALL CHARACTERISTICS OF THE SPECIFIC IMMUNE SYSTEM RESPONSE

Even though the immune system is described by its discrete cellular and chemical components, it is essential to acknowledge and comprehend its overall characteristics, which form the patterns of immunologic self. The specifics of the processes are discussed throughout the chapter.

Historically, the immune system has been described as having five cardinal features.

SELF/NOT SELF TOLERANCE. Discrimination of self from not-self (called *self/not-self tolerance*, or threat/non-threat identification) is the recursive ability of the immune cells to engage in the process of exploring the cellular environment. Healthy self cells are left alone, and the immune cells identify and mount responses against foreign cells as well as cancerous or infected self-cells. Much of the maturation process of T cells, for example, involves just the process of repetitive error-free self identification that leads to self tolerance. When self destruction occurs it is called **autoimmunity**. T cells that fail these trials in the thymus are destroyed prior to maturation (by cells in the thymus called *nurse cells)* and not allowed to enter the circulation. The ability of the immune cells to carry out this process, time after time, without failure is a unique feature of the immune system.

SELF-REGULATION. Self-regulation is the ability of the immune system to initiate, maintain, and down-regulate immune activity independent of the nervous system or other controls. Thus, the immune system can carry out its functions, if needed, without direct input from other systems in the body.

SPECIFICITY. **Specificity** is the ability of the immune system to design and implement an immune response that is targeted only to a single, specific antigen or foreign cell. The generalized inflammatory response, a first-line defense against cellular invasion, responds equally to any and all antigen that is encountered. The specific response that is developed provides cells and chemicals targeted to each individual antigen.

DIVERSITY. The body has the ability to develop a specific response to an indefinite number of different antigens. Current opinion in immunology suggests that the human genetic repertoire provides us with an ability to mount a specific response to about 100,000 different antigens.[11] Yet the human body can, over time, generate immune responses to even synthetic antigens, and it is now demonstrated that it can create new cellular receptor sites in immature immune cells based on information provided by other, nonspecific immune cells, and that upon maturation the newly created cells can bind with and provide for a specific response to a nearly endless number of antigens over the course of the life span.[11,20]

MEMORY. Once the immune system identifies antigen and mounts an immune response, it can store a memory of the antigen and keep memory cells available throughout the life span to provide for a prompter response to secondary exposure. Only the immune system and central nervous system share these unique characteristics.

Antigen and Hapten Recognition

An **antigen** is a molecule that is capable of inducing a detectable immune response when introduced into the body. When an antigen stimulates an immune response, it is said to have **immunogenicity**.[20] It stimulates the immune response, denoting an active production of **antibodies** or sensitized cells. Most antigens and *immunogens* (an antigen with immunogenicity) are proteins, but other large molecules, such as polysaccharides, nucleoproteins, and protein fragments, may also function in this way.

Several characteristics appear to determine whether a molecule can stimulate an immune response, including such aspects as size, foreignness, shape, and solubility. Some molecules become antigenic only when they are combined with a carrier. Called **haptens,** these substances when uncombined fail to elicit an immune response because they are small. These molecules cannot serve as complete antigens until they are combined with protein carriers. An example is the contact allergens, which probably attach to proteins of the skin and stimulate the proliferation of a subpopulation of T-cells sensitized to the substance. Later exposure to the allergen leads to a more rapid reaction (see p. 288). Examples of haptens include poison ivy, some drugs, dust particles, dandruff, industrial chemicals, and poisons.

Major Histocompatability Complex (The Human Leukocyte Antigens)

The genetic information of any individual is somewhat unique from all other individuals of the same species, and cells and tissues of that individual are marked with cell-surface proteins to identify them as belonging to that individual. The **major histocompatability complex** (MHC) is the region of the genetic information that codes for this identifying information.[4] In humans this information is coded on a short arm of chromosome 6, and is often called the Human Leukocyte Antigen (HLA). Many possible allele combinations can occur from this genetic information—so many that no two individuals have an exact match. The proteins produced by the MHC are used for a variety of immunologic activities. MHC Class I molecules (proteins) normally are on the surface membrane of most of the cells in the body to help identify those cells as self. MHC-II molecules (and to a lesser extent MHC-I molecules) are used by the immune system to help label and identify foreign antigen. MHC-II, for example, is necessary for the presentation of foreign antigen to certain lymphocytes (T helper cells) that identify pathogens and activate the specific immune responses (see p. 283). MHC-III coding is less well understood at present, but seems to code for **complement** system chemicals and activation.[11]

The MHC molecules play an essential role in the immune system's ability to identify self (and not activate a response) and non-self (and to then activate an appropriate immune response). **Phagocytes** search for cells that are foreign antigens (not MHC-self-marked), and mature T-helper lymphocytes have the ability to recognize and respond only to MHC-coupled messages. It is during T lymphocyte maturation in the thymus gland that these lymphocytes undergo a series of tests of self/not-self recognition based upon MHC classification. Only those T lymphocytes that successfully pass these tests are the mature, immune-competent cells that enter circulation.

LYMPHOID ORGANS AND TISSUES

The lymphoid organs include the bone marrow, thymus, lymph nodes, associated lymphoid tissues, and spleen (Fig. 10-1). The bone marrow and thymus are the primary central lymphoid organs that serve as the location for most new lymphocyte creation and differentiation into type and function. The tissues play a role in the chemical control of the immune system. The peripheral lymphoid organs (such as the lymph nodes, associated lymphoid tissues, and spleen) function to assist the various cells of the immune system to efficiently carry out their role in defense of cellular integrity. Many of the cells of the immune system are found within the lymphatic organs, in addition to the blood stream and interstitial fluids. Some immune cells travel throughout the lymphoid tissues and organs, entering and leaving most tissue spaces with ease.

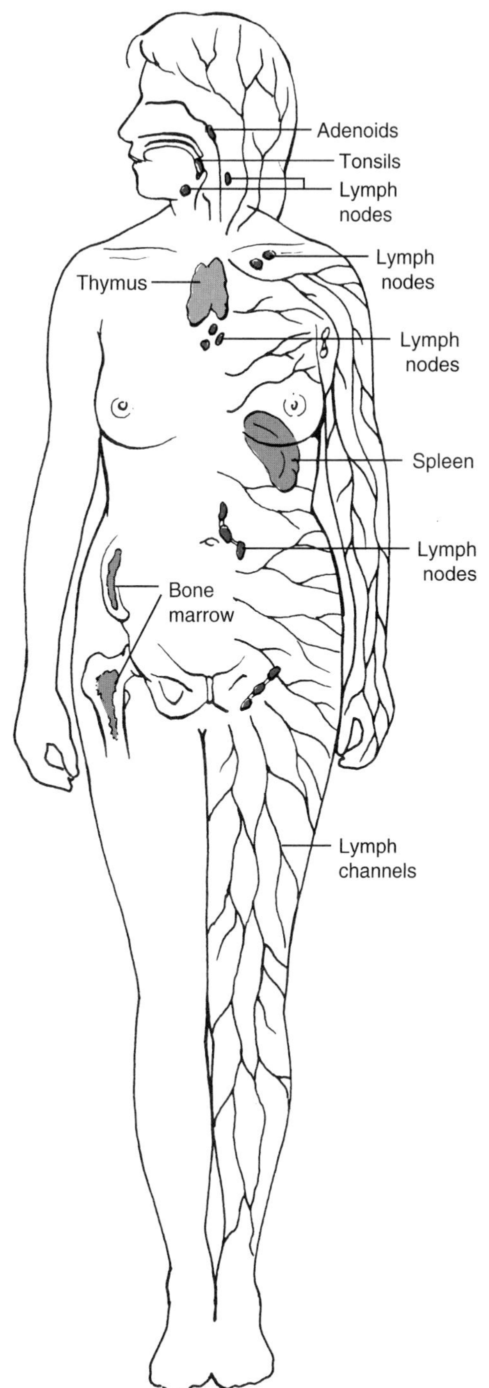

FIGURE 10-1. Illustration of major lymphoid organs and tissues. The bone marrow produces and matures B lymphocytes, and the thymus gland processes and matures T lymphocytes from immature cells produced in the bone marrow. The lymph nodes and tissues drain and filter much of the tissue spaces. The lymphoid cells in the spleen and other organs trap antigens. The lymph channels provides a system to circulate lymph fluid, which contains large numbers of lymphoid cells.

Central Lymphoid Organs

The bone marrow and the thymus gland are the central lymphoid organs. They function in forming and maturing lymphocytes.

BONE MARROW

The marrow compartments of the bones of the human body contain the parent or stem cells from which lymphoid cells are derived. These compartments, described on p. 338, contain red and yellow marrow. The red marrow provides all of the blood cells of the body. Yellow marrow stores lipids, serving as an energy reserve. The immature T lymphocytes are formed in the bone marrow, but these cells must travel to the thymus gland to mature into immunocompetent cells. The originating cells, called pluripotent hematopoietic stem cells, produce all of the circulating blood cells; thus, in addition to lymphoid and myeloid cells (white blood cells [WBCs]), they produce the erythrocytes (red blood cells [RBCs]) and thrombocytes (platelets) (see p. 338).

Billions of WBCs are found in interstitial fluids, lymph channels, and lymphoid organs and tissues. The total number of lymphocytes, alone, in adults is about 10^{12} cells, with about 1% in the blood and the remaining 99% within tissue spaces.[19,21] The bone marrow is capable of producing billions of WBCs per day if needed. The production, storage, and maturation of WBCs is an ongoing process, and also can be stimulated by immune activation. Most WBCs mature in the bone marrow, but some lymphocytes travel to other sites for specialized maturation.

THYMUS

The thymus gland, a primary lymphoid organ, is located in the mediastinal area of the chest (see Fig. 10-1). The thymus and other lymphatic tissues undergo marked changes in size in relation to age (Fig. 10-2). The thymus weighs about 20 gm. at birth, grows rapidly in children, and reaches maximum size at puberty (about 35 gm), after which it gradually begins the process of involution. Involution progresses from the cortical zone to the medullary area.[19] The gland never completely disappears, but in elderly people it becomes a collection of reticular fibers, some lymphocytes, and connective tissue.

The thymus processes and matures lymphocytes in large numbers from the early years of life until puberty and at diminishing rates throughout adult life. Lymphocyte maturation is the process of transformation of lymphocyte precursor cells into antigen-specific lymphocytes regulated only to respond to specific antigens under proper conditions of antigen **recognition** (see p. 282). Immature immune cells travel via the blood stream from the bone marrow to the cortex of the thymus for maturation and development. In the medullary area of the thymus, lymphocytes appear to become more differentiated and to undergo a series of steps that allows them to discriminate between self and non-self tissue. They thus become **immunocompetent cells**. They leave the thymus and enter the circulation able to recognize self tissues and to identify and react to foreign (nonself) tissues. Many of the cells developing in the thymus (called thymocytes) die in the gland, as they are unable to mature successfully.[19]

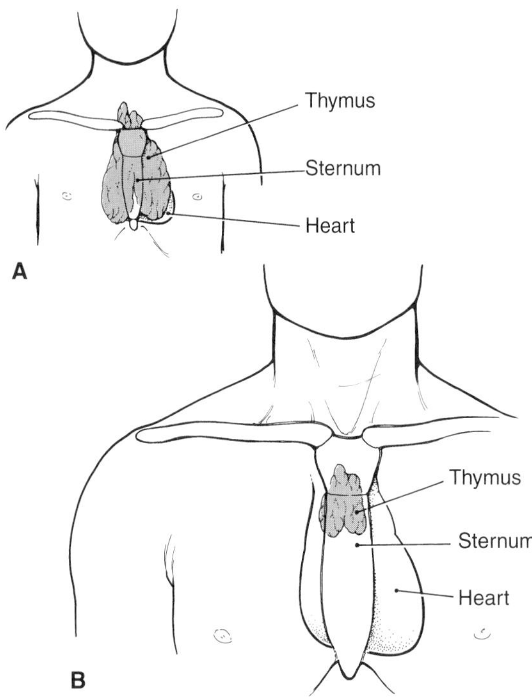

FIGURE 10-2. **A.** Large, active thymus gland in childhood. **B.** Atrophy and fat infiltration in adulthood.

The process of lymphocyte maturation occurs in the cortical and medullary areas under the influence of the thymic hormones. The thymic hormones are a group of hormones that have been proposed to play a role in attracting T lymphocyte precursors and promoting their maturation in the thymus.[17]

Peripheral Lymphoid Organs and Tissues

The peripheral or secondary lymphoid organs and tissues include the lymph nodes, the mucosa-associated lymphoid tissue, and the spleen.

LYMPH NODES

Lymph nodes are encapsulated secondary lymphoid organs that are systematically distributed throughout the body to receive and process the lymph circulation. Human lymph nodes are 1 to 25 mm in diameter and are round or kidney-shaped. They often are seen at branches of the lymphatic vessels and are found in clusters at strategic locations, such as the neck, axillae, and groin, where large amounts of lymph drainage occurs.[9] A lymph node consists of an outer portion, called the *cortex*, and an inner portion, called the *medulla* (Fig. 10-3). The cortex is further broken down into smaller compartments, including the outer cortex and the paracortex. The outer cortex is organized into lymphoid follicles, some of which contain germinal centers. The lymphoid follicles and germinal centers contain mostly B lymphocytes but may contain a few T lymphocytes and macrophages. Some lymphocytes reproduce in the germinal centers, through a clonal process. They may then be retained in the node or seeded into the bloodstream. The paracortex includes the thymus-dependent zone, which is believed to contain chiefly T lymphocytes. Different types of free cells are held in place in the node by reticular and collagen fibers. The lymph sinusoid is a thin-walled vessel through which lymph flows. The lymph sinus in the subcapsular space is like a hollow space that conducts the lymphatic flow.

Lymph circulation serves to return interstitial fluids to the circulatory system, as well as to provide immune

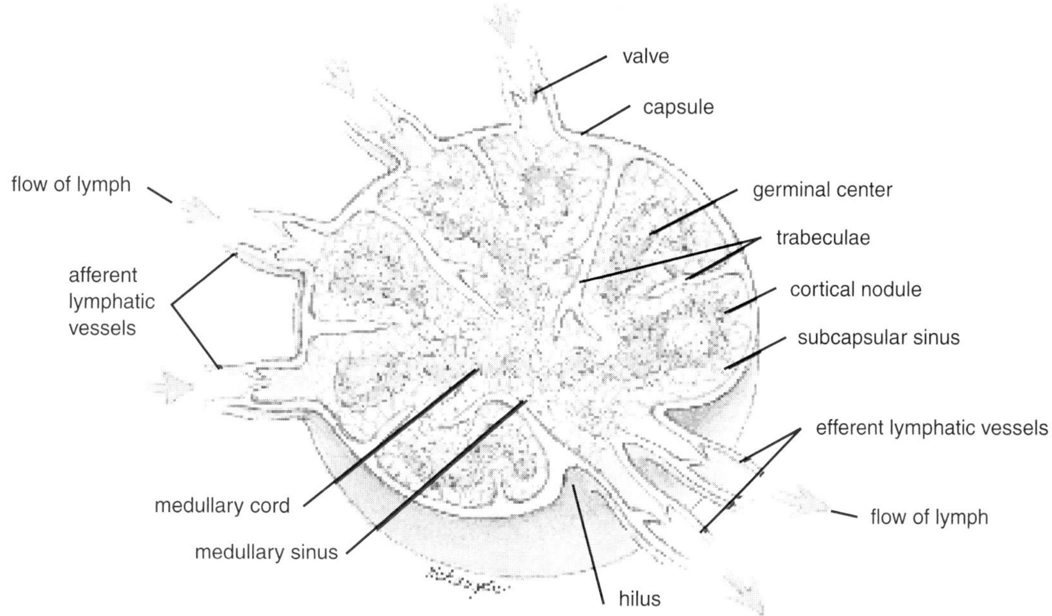

FIGURE 10-3. **Basic organization of a lymph node.**

system access to interstitial drainage. Basically, lymph nodes serve as a series of in-line filters, so that all lymph in the lymph vessels is filtered by at least one node and is thus exposed to large numbers of immunocompetent cells. Lymph flows into the cortex from afferent channels, which are lined with lymphocytes. The lymph then passes through the cortical, paracortical, and medullary regions. Lymph leaves the medulla through efferent lymphatic channels, which are also lined with lymphocytes, and drains into the venous channels for return to the blood stream. Many immunocompetent cells and macrophages circulate from the blood stream to lymph nodes continuously throughout their life spans.

MUCOSA-ASSOCIATED LYMPHOID TISSUE (MALT)

In addition to the lymph channels and peripheral lymph nodes in the interstitial spaces, aggregates of lymphoid tissue are found in many organs, especially those of the gastrointestinal and respiratory tracts.[19] These aggregates are called mucosa-associated lymphoid tissue (MALT) and are further identified by their specific locations. The presence of lymphoid tissue in these locations can, through secretory IgA and other immune factors, prevent successful entry of microorganisms into the body.

The gut-associated lymphoid tissues (GALT) are lymph node–like tissues in the gastrointestinal tract that collect antigen from the epithelial surfaces in the lumen of the bowel. The lymphocytes in GALT, both B lymphocytes and T lymphocytes, form a follicle that protrudes within the lumen to enhance potential contact with antigen entering the GI tract. These specialized protruding tissues include the tonsils, adenoids, the vermiform appendix, and specialized structures in the small intestines called Peyer's patches (see Fig. 10-1). Aggregates of lymphocytes on the epithelial mucosa of the respiratory airways are known as bronchial-associated lymphoid tissues (BALT). Generally, the lymphocytes in BALT aggregates are those with specificity for airborne pathogens, whereas the lymphocytes in the GALT aggregates are those specific for enteric pathogens. These specific lymphocytes, aggregating and protruding into the lumen of the airway or bowel, increase the ability of the immune system to come into contact with pathogens upon their arrival and to capture and/or destroy the pathogens before they colonize or penetrate the cellular layer. The work of the BALT is facilitated by the flow of mucus out of the lungs through the ciliary action of the columnar epithelial cells and by the cough reflex.

SPLEEN

The spleen is the largest internal lymphatic organ, weighing about 180 to 240 g. It is surrounded by a capsule of fibers that penetrate into the organ, and the variety of cells within the organ are supported with a reticular framework (Fig. 10-4). It can function as a reservoir for blood in its venous sinuses and pulp. As the spleen

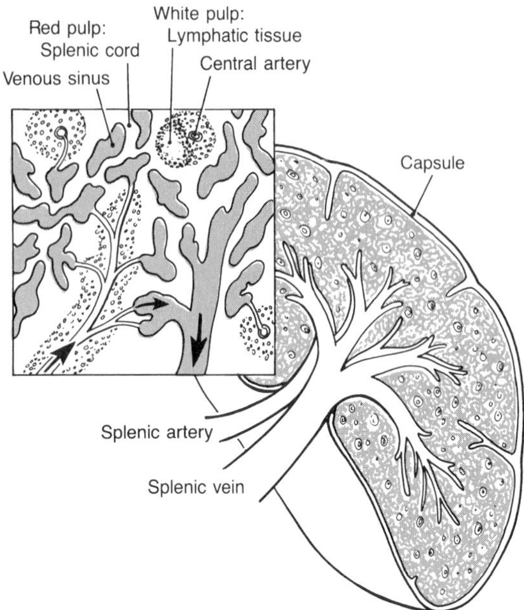

FIGURE 10-4. **Organization of lymphoid tissue in spleen. Note venous sinuses in red pulp. This tissue is innervated by post-ganglionic sympathetic nerve fibers.**

enlarges, the quantity of red blood cells within its *red pulp* also can increase. Another of the main functions of the spleen is to process the red blood cells that squeeze through its pores. Red cells that are nearing the end of their life span often break down here. Specialized macrophages in splenic tissue clear cellular debris and process hemoglobin.

Many phagocytic cells, especially macrophages, line the pulp and sinuses of the spleen. Groups of lymphocytes and plasma cells throughout the parenchyma of the spleen are called the *white pulp.* These cells function in the process of immunity to clear blood-borne pathogens. Interestingly, selective white blood cell aggregates in the spleen are directly innervated with sympathetic nerve fibers, and so are influenced by and influence central nervous system functioning.

STRUCTURAL AND PHYSIOLOGIC BARRIERS IN BODILY DEFENSE

In addition to the lymphoid organs and tissues themselves, other organs can serve immune functions. Table 10-1 indicates immune defenses as first-line, second-line, and third-line defenses.

Physical barriers tend to prevent entry of pathogens or foreign particles and serve an immune defense function. The skin is the primary barrier to entry into the body. The tight junctions of cells in the skin, the presence of antibacterial peptides, and the shedding property of surface cells in the skin make it difficult for pathogens to colonize or to enter. The mucous membranes are also physical barriers to invasion at the cellular level because of cellular alignment, ciliated epithelial functions, longitudinal flow over their surfaces, the movement of mucus, the presence of microbe-active enzymes, various pH levels, and fatty acids. Saliva, tears, and mucus all serve to carry away potential cellular threats. Urine flow in the urinary tract serves a similar protective function. These anatomic barriers serve to stop pathogens or foreign substances from entering the body and allow for rapid clearance from the body of those entering the pulmonary, GI, and GU systems.

Physiologic barriers to infection include pH, soluble factors in tissue and tissue secretions, temperature, and to some degree the presence of commensal organisms. Acidic pH, in particular, is a barrier to pH-sensitive pathogens. Many chemicals released by cells in the mucous membranes are known to be bacterially active and function through enzymatic reactions. High tissue or body temperature may be a defensive mechanism against temperature-sensitive pathogens. Commensal organisms in the GI tract serve to regulate

TABLE 10-1

IMMUNE DEFENSES

FIRST-LINE DEFENSES	SECOND-LINE DEFENSES	THIRD-LINE DEFENSES
BARRIERS TO ENTRY	NONSPECIFIC IMMUNITY	SPECIFIC IMMUNITY
Intact skin	Antimicrobial substances (HCL in stomach, etc.)	T lymphocytes
Commensal organisms	Phagocytic white blood cells—neutrophils, macrophages	B lymphocytes
Saliva	Inflammatory process	Antibodies
Mucus	Natural killer cells	Memory cells
Tears		
Chemical substances		

pH, available pathogen food supply, and available binding sites and access points for microbial invasion. The competitive nature of commensal organisms, when altered by administration of antibiotics (for example), can result in overgrowth of even the normally benign commensal microbes; generally, however, they serve to limit colonization by pathogenic microbes.

CELLS OF THE IMMUNE SYSTEM

The cells that make the immune system include cells of nonspecific immunity and those of adaptive, specific immunity. The cells are derived from stem cells of the bone marrow, which produce two lineages of WBCs (see p. 338).

The cells of the myelocytic (monocyte/macrophage and granulocytes) lineage function in various ways to trap and destroy antigen. They may process and destroy the antigen by phagocytosis or chemical mediators.

The B lymphocytes and T lymphocytes, and apparently the natural killer (NK) cells, are classified within the lymphocytic lineage. T lymphocytes and B lymphocytes are activated for processes of immune response that are each time specific to a particular antigen. Lymphocytic cells are capable of recognizing antigen, or foreign particles, through the use of MHC recognition and other chemical pathways. Unit 2, Appendix A describes cells and other immune studies.

Cells of Innate, Non-specific Immunity

Innate immunity includes the interaction of phagocytes with antigen as well as chemical mediators from other WBCs. The functions of these cells are detailed in Chapter 13.

MACROPHAGES

One type of phagocyte in the immune system is the macrophage. Derived from monocytes, macrophages are the mature cells of the mononuclear phagocyte system (or monocyte-macrophage system). Macrophages function in phagocytosis of antigen and in processing and presenting antigen to specific lymphocytes.[19] Tissue macrophages make up a network of phagocytic cells throughout the body. These have special names in different areas: Kupffer cells in the liver, alveolar macrophages in the lungs, peritoneal macrophages in the peritoneal cavity, histiocytes in the connective tissue, and others. In the central nervous system, the special cells of the neuroglia classification called *microglia* have the ability to undergo changes and develop the property of phagocytosis during pathologic states. Fig. 10-5 shows these different monocytes and macrophages.

Macrophages serve an essential function in removing foreign and devitalized material from the body (see p. 265). Macrophages also have an important cooperative role in the immune response, but how they function is not entirely understood. These cells trap and process antigens to present them to specialized lymphocytes. They may play a secondary or accessory role in promoting lymphocyte activity and may function as an intermediary between specific T cells and specific B cells.

The macrophage moves by ameboid motion toward a chemical concentration of soluble substances released into its environment by antigens or by lymphocytes. This is called movement toward a *chemotactic gradient*, or signal, that is elicited by soluble substances such as cytokines (see p. 285). The *monocyte migration inhibition factor* and the *macrophage-activating factor*, which, respectively, tend to retain the macrophage in an area and increase its phagocytic activity, are especially important cytokines. The release of these cytokines results from activation of the macrophage by organisms and in association with lymphocytes and/or NK cells.[21]

NEUTROPHILS

Neutrophils are the most numerous and the most important cellular component of the innate, non-specific immune response. They serve, along with macrophages, to complete the phagocytic family of cells and are a first-line defender in the body against bacterial invasion, colonization, and infection (see p. 360).

EOSINOPHILS AND BASOPHILS

Eosinophils are believed to play a pivotal role in defense against parasitic infections (see p. 362). They are components of innate immunity but can be activated by lymphocytes, and serve a role in adaptive immunity involving both antibody responses (humoral immunity) and NK cell responses (cell-mediated immunity). They particularly target antibody-coated parasites.

Basophils are believed to play a role in protecting mucosal surfaces throughout the body, and, like mast cells, they release substances that assist other cells in the inflammatory response.

MAST CELLS

Mast cells are derived from bone marrow cells that are distinct from basophils (see p. 362). They are believed to migrate as immature cells to the tissues, where they mature (rarely are they seen in circulation when mature).[11] Membrane-bound granules that contain proteoglycans such as chondroitin sulfate (in GI mucosal mast cells) and heparin (such as in pulmonary mucosal mast cells) are contained within the mast cell cytoplasm. Histamine content depends on whether the mast cell is based in connective tissue or mucosal tissue. Mast cells serve to provide substances that are supportive and enhancing of immune responses. Basophils are able to produce and secrete many of the

FOCUS ON CELLULAR PHYSIOLOGY

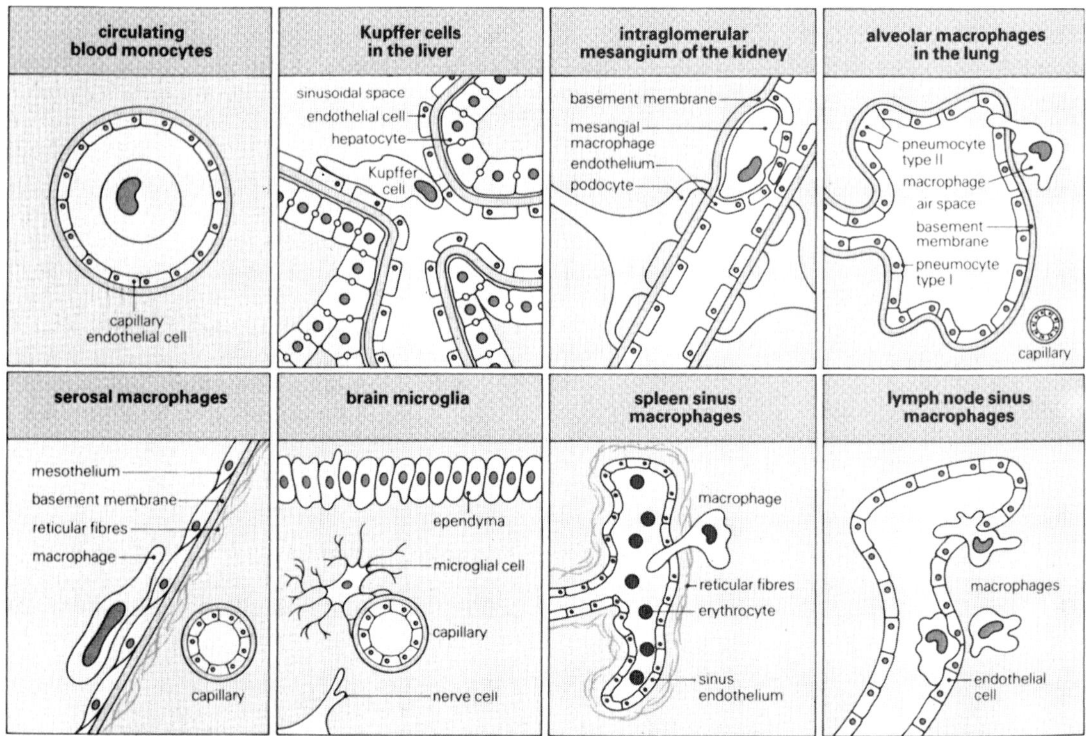

FIGURE 10-5. Mononuclear phagocyte system. The mononuclear phagocyte system includes blood monocytes and phagocytes resident in tissues or fixed to the endothelial layer of blood capillaries. In the liver the resident macrophages are known as Kupffer cells, whereas in the kidneys they are called the intraglomerular mesangial cells. Alveolar and serosal (e.g., peritoneal) macrophages are "wander" macrophages. Brain microglia are cells that enter the brain around the time of birth and differentiate into fixed cells. (From I. Roitt, J. Brostoff, & D. Male [1998]. *Immunology* [5th ed.]. St. Louis: C. V. Mosby).

same chemicals as mast cells and share similar triggering mechanisms for activation (such as IgE binding).[1]

Cells of Adaptive, Specific Immunity

The two groups of cells responsible for adaptive, specific immunity are the B and T lymphocytes. They are essential for producing immunity to diseases and protection from other foreign agents.

B LYMPHOCYTES

The B lymphocytes are responsible for *humoral immunity*, or *immunoglobulin-mediated immunity*, which is specific immunity for antigens that are found outside of the host cells. Typically humoral immunity is activated in bacterial infection. Most humoral immunity requires the T lymphocyte interaction described on page 288.

B lymphocytes originate in the bone marrow and mature either there or in some other site. The maturing site is clearly identified in birds as the bursal sac. In humans, where no equivalent bursa area occurs, the cells are said to mature in the "bursa-equivalent" tissues and are thus called B cells. They are capable of proliferating and differentiating into *plasma cells* and *memory cells* when exposed to their specific antigen (Fig. 10-6). Plasma cells are capable of secreting large quantities of specific immunoglobulin, the immune active portion of humoral immunity. Immunoglobulin secreted by plasma cells is called *antibody*. B lymphocytes do not need to directly contact foreign antigens but serve to release antibodies that contact and attach to foreign antigens, and thus generate an immune response.

Memory cells serve the purpose of stockpiling a specific clone of B cells, so that immediate production of large quantities of the specific immunoglobulins results when the cells are next exposed to a particular antigen. Thus, plasma cells activate and secrete antibody, whereas memory cells stand by for future activation.

Immunoglobulins

Antibody has exquisite specificity for particularly targeted antigen, so that within the many classes of antibody are molecules that recognize only their specific

FOCUS ON CELLULAR PHYSIOLOGY

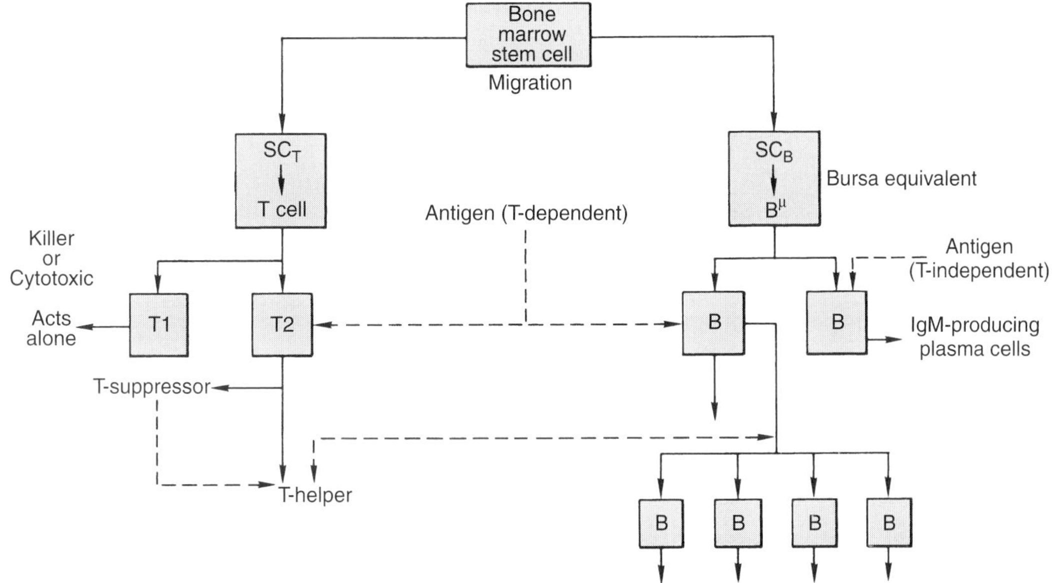

FIGURE 10-6. Schematic appearance of T and B lymphocyte maturation. Both T and B lymphocytes arise from the bone marrow stem cell (SC) and migrate to the thymus gland (T cell) or to an unknown area (B cell), where they mature to immunocompetent cells. The T cells may act in cooperation with B cells or alone. Some antigens can stimulate B cells.

antigen.[21] The specificity resides in a portion of the molecule that has binding affinity for antigen.

The basic unit of every immunoglobulin molecule is a symmetric arrangement of four polypeptide chains. Two of the polypeptide chains, called *heavy chains (H)*, are identical and have a greater molecular weight than the two *light chains (L)*. These heavy and light chains are kept together as a symmetric four-chain molecule (H_2L_2).[18] The chains are held together by disulfide bonds and remain viable across a wide range of conditions (heat stability, for instance).

Figure 10-7 shows a representative model of an immunoglobulin. The Fab (fragment, antigen-binding) portion is the *variable* portion, and the Fc (fragment, crystallizable) portion is the *constant* portion of the immunoglobulin class. The constant portion almost certainly directs the biologic activity of the antibody and perhaps the distribution or location of the immunoglobulin within the body.[21] The variable portion provides individual specificity for binding antigen and varies among immunoglobulin molecules. To be specific in response, an antigen and an antibody must chemically fit together precisely, the way the right key fits into a lock (Fig. 10-8). The antigen-binding, or variable, region of the antibody binds only similar structures on antigen. The variable binding sites are referred to as **antigenic determinants**.

Several theories have been proposed to explain immunoglobulin specificity. One of these, the *clonal-*

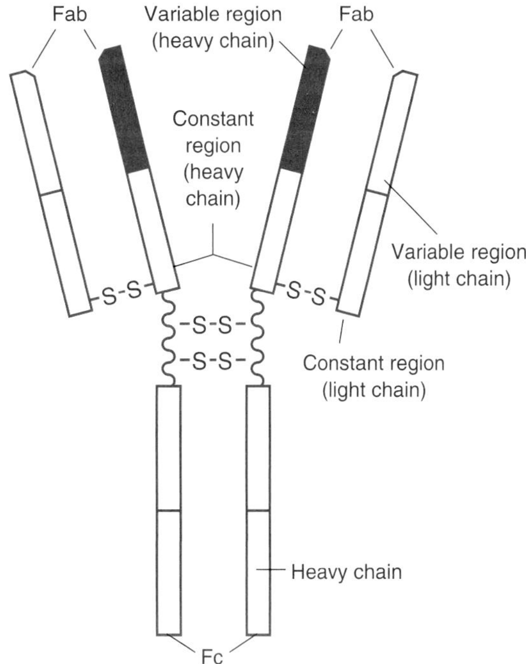

FIGURE 10-7. Schematic appearance of an immunoglobulin molecule showing two light and two heavy polypeptide chains. The constant portion, or Fc, accounts for the biologic activity, and the variable portion, or Fab, provides for the binding of specific antigen. (S-S = disulfide bonds.)

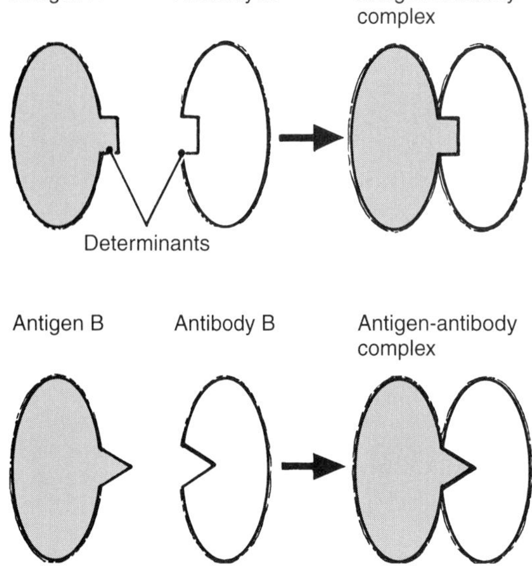

FIGURE 10-8. **Highly schematic appearance of specificity of antibody for antigen, the so-called lock-and-key response.**

selection theory, proposes that each B lymphocyte contains all the genetic information necessary to produce all possible specific antibodies.[11] Thus, the gene for specific antibody is activated by contact with the antigen, and large amounts of the antibody are formed.[18] The binding of antigen stimulates the available number of B cells that recognize it to proliferate, producing sufficient cells to mount an immune response.[18] The clonal-selection model assumes that large amounts of antigenic stimulation trigger the immunocompetent lymphocyte to clonally reproduce and for those new cells to make large amounts of specific antibody.[18]

Five major classes of immunoglobulins have been identified: IgG, IgM, IgA, IgE, and IgD. The classification depends on the structure of the heavy-chain portion of the molecule (the molecular weight of the immunoglobulins), but the size and shape of the molecule also seem to influence characteristics of the immunoglobulin, such as whether it is most specific for airborne or enteric or secretory pathogens. Table 10-2 lists the main properties of each major classification.

TABLE 10-2

IMMUNOGLOBULIN CLASSIFICATION

	IMMUNOGLOBULIN				
CHARACTERISTIC	**IgG**	**IgA**	**IgM**	**IgD**	**IgE**
Serum concentration (mg/dL)	1000	200	120	3	0.05
Molecular weight	150,000	160,000 (serum) 400,000 (secretory)	900,000	180,000	190,000
Serum half-life (days)	23	6	5	3	2
Binds to mast cells	–	–	–	–	+
Fixes complement	+ +	–	+ + +	–	–
Antiviral activity	+	+ + +	+	?	?
Antibacterial lysis	+	+	+ + +	?	?
Total (%)	75–80	10–15	6	1	0.002
Crosses placenta	+	–	–	–	–
Function	Major antibody formed in secondary response; most common antibody in response to infection; long-lived	External secretions and surfaces, saliva, tears, mucus, bile, colostrum; protective function in preventing entry of microorganisms through portals of entry	First antibody formed in primary response; mediates cytotoxic responses; can produce antigen-antibody complexes that precipitate	Not known; found with IgM on surface of B cells	Reaginic antibody binds to mast cells and basophils; causes allergic symptoms through attaching to mast cells and release of histamine and other substances

–: negative; +: positive; + +: active; + + +: highly active.

IgG. IgG makes up about 75% of the antibodies normally circulating in plasma. Various subtypes of IgG exist, each with slightly different biologic characteristics.[18] IgG antibody freely diffuses into the extravascular spaces to interact with antigen. The amount of IgG synthesized is closely related to the amount of *antigenic* stimulation presented to the host. In prenatal life, it diffuses across the placental barrier to provide the fetus with passive immune protection until the infant can produce an adequate immune defense.

IgG has been shown to carry the major burden in neutralizing bacterial toxins, which result partly because of its ability to fix complement (see p. 290). This function is essential in accelerating the process of phagocytosis.

IgA. Most IgA is in the form of *secretory* IgA in the external body secretions, such as saliva, sweat, tears, mucus, bile, and colostrum. It provides a defense against pathogens on exposed surfaces of the body, especially those entering the respiratory and gastrointestinal tracts. More than 85% of plasma cells in the intestinal area produce IgA. Secretory IgA is derived from specific plasma cells.

IgA is associated in seromucous secretions with another protein known as the *secretory component.* IgA and secretory component interact to form a specific defense against bacterial and viral antigens. The first exposure causes increased amounts of secretory IgA and secretory component to be formed, so that on second exposure the body surfaces are defended by specific antibody when exposed to that specific antigen. IgA antibodies also may function to inhibit the adherence of pathogens to mucosal cells.

IgM. Often called the macroglobulin (because it is the largest), IgM is the first immunoglobulin produced in quantity during an immune response, and so levels rise early in the course of an infection. IgM (in association with IgD) is efficient in agglutinating antigen, fixing complement, and lysing cell walls. It is present in high concentrations in the bloodstream and can react efficiently with bacteria and viruses that are bloodborne. The levels of IgM normally decrease after the first week of antigen exposure, and the IgG response increases.[18]

IgD. IgD is present in plasma in very low concentrations and is readily broken down (half-life in plasma is 2 to 8 days). Its exact function is not well understood, but its presence on lymphocyte surfaces together with IgM suggests that it may be a receptor that helps bind antigens to the cell surfaces.[21] Its levels are elevated in chronic infections.

IgE. IgE serves, apparently, to activate mast cells. Concentrations of IgE are low in the serum, because the antibody normally remains firmly fixed on tissue surfaces. It is found on surface membranes of basophils and mast cells and also on mucosal surfaces, such as conjunctival, nasal, and bronchial mucosa.[18] IgE contact with a specific antigen triggers the release of the mast cell granules.

Many parasitic infectious agents (protozoa and helminths [worms] in particular) are resistant to phagocytic killing by neutrophils or macrophages. IgE antibodies bind to helminth surfaces and activate mast cells and eosinophils, causing them to secrete their granular contents. The released proteins serve to lyse the parasite and, additionally, may mediate the release of other chemicals involved in the immunologic response to parasitic infections.

IgE is also called the reaginic antibody because it is involved in immediate hypersensitivity reactions (Type I; allergy). The released vasoactive amines, when widespread, cause the signs and symptoms of allergy and anaphylaxis (see p. 311). Higher serum levels of IgE occur in allergy-prone people and in those infected with certain parasites, especially helminths.[18]

T LYMPHOCYTES

The long-lived T lymphocytes account for about 75% of the serum lymphocytes. Their life span ranges from a few months to nearly the duration of a person's life, and they account for many aspects of long-term immunity. The T lymphocytes originate from stem cells in the bone marrow but are matured in the thymus gland; thus, they are known as T lymphocytes and are sometimes called *thymocytes.* These cells develop distinctive receptors on their cell surfaces as they mature, which allows them to bind to specific proteins found in circulation on the surface of other cells, and makes their functions different from those of B cells. The T lymphocytes can proliferate rapidly in the thymus and lymph nodes and clonally produce large numbers of antigen-specific cells.

The T lymphocytes leave the thymus to enter special regions called thymus-dependent zones, mainly in the paracortical region of the lymph nodes and part of the white pulp of the spleen. They may remain in the lymphoid tissue, enter the blood circulation, or enter the extravascular spaces to encounter antigens that correspond to the membrane receptors on their surfaces. This movement is in part controlled by thymic hormones, and certainly by a large number of other immunotransmitters, the cytokines (see p. 285).

T lymphocytes often circulate via the blood stream in a fixed pattern, between specific lymph node groups and specific tissues, to increase the likelihood of contact with the antigens for which they have specific binding sites. If a T cell encounters its specific antigen, it activates, and it can divide and proliferate to form a clone of T cells that can destroy the antigen or that can orchestrate the actions of other cells in the immune system to mount an immune response. The T lymphocyte family can be functionally divided into three subgroups: *helper, killer,* and *suppressor cells*. These various T lymphocytes have different functions within the immune system attained during maturation in the thymus. They are further distinguished by the presence of different cell-surface proteins, called clusters of differentiation, on their outer surfaces (Fig. 10-9).

Clusters of Differentiation (CDs)

The CD surface proteins serve the immune system as binding sites that allow immune cells to bind, or attach, to specific types of circulating chemical messengers or to other cellular membrane proteins. CD molecules are expressed on the surface of a lymphocyte during the maturation process. They serve as markers to chemically identify the different types of T lymphocytes, as different function in immune cells is in part related to different, specific types of surface protein markers.

Clusters of differentiation appear to distinguish cells according to their lineage and type of differentiation, and are clearly identifiable in the laboratory using specific, known monoclonal antibodies for attachment and labeling. There are many different CD molecules, and often an immune cell has many CD markers on its surface; their CD designations are based on which is the predominant marker on a cell.

Most blood T lymphocytes are classified as those that express CD4 (Th) and CD8 (Tc) markers. The lymphocytes with CD4 markers mainly help or induce an immune response, whereas those with CD8 markers are mainly cytotoxic. Suppressor T cells (T_s) have been functionally identified and often are classified as CD8, but both CD4 and CD8 T cells have been shown to suppress the immune response.[14] Several hundred CD proteins are now known, and an individual immune cell may be covered with scores of different CD markers, and with scores of the same marker over and over. A systemic nomenclature has been developed to identify the CD subsets. Some of the specific markers are described in Unit 2, Appendix B.

T Lymphocyte–Antigen Recognition

T lymphocytes recognize antigen in the form of peptide fragments that are bound to the surface of antigen-

FOCUS ON CELLULAR PHYSIOLOGY

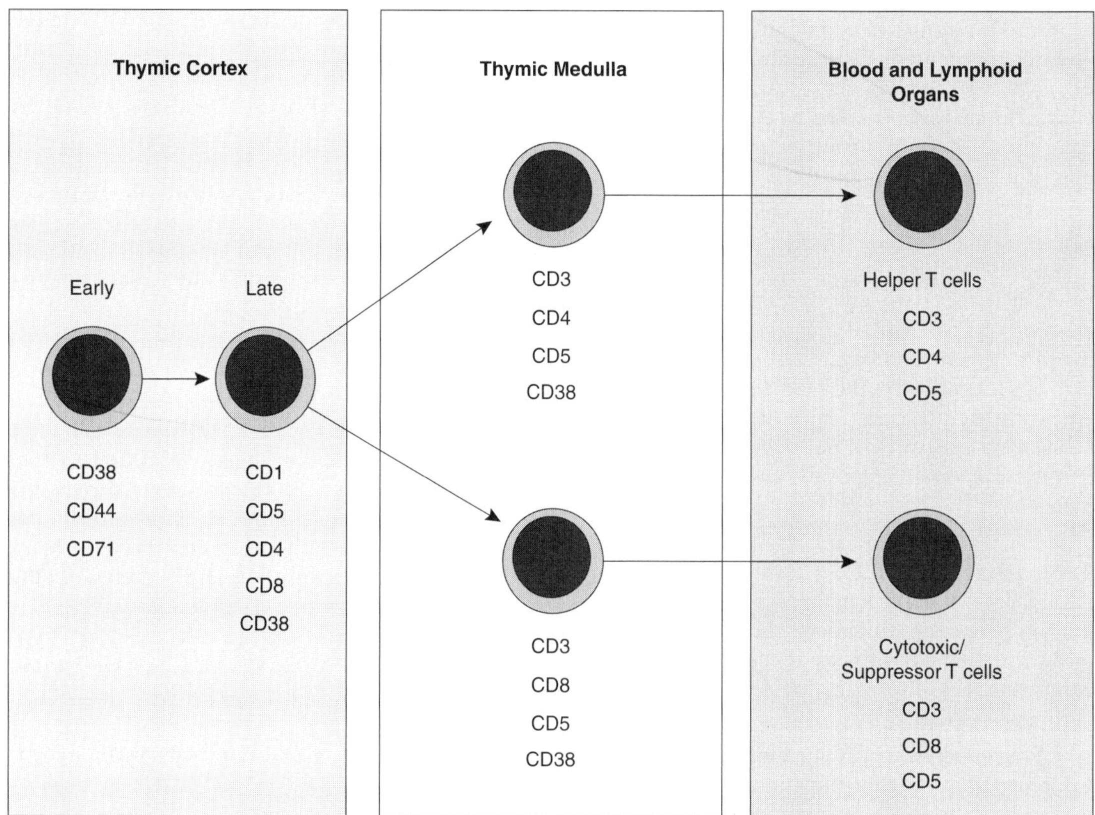

FIGURE 10-9. Membrane marker changes during thymic T-cell maturation. (Rubin, E., & Farber, J. L. [1999]. *Pathology* [3rd ed.]. Philadelphia: Lippincott Williams & Wilkins.)

presenting cells (APCs, such as macrophages) at the site of the major histocompatability complex (MHC) molecules on the APCs.[10] The T lymphocyte marker is called the T cell antigen receptor (TCR); it recognizes only these antigenic peptides that are bound to MHC molecules.[10] The result is that individual T lymphocytes respond only to a specific combination of antigen and MHC. This combination of presented MHC self-molecule with a foreign antigen fragment prior to activation of T cells is necessary as a protection against an autoimmune response: if the T lymphocyte reacted to all antigen fragments it encountered, it might begin to attack healthy cells as well as infected cells.

Helper T Cells

Helper T (Th) cells stimulate B lymphocytes to differentiate into antibody producers and serve to activate cytotoxic T lymphocytes and other T cell responses; they are therefore responsible for activating the specific immune response. To this degree, Th cells are often described as being the key to activation of a specific immune response. Th cells also activate and recruit macrophages. A chemical message from an antigen-sensitized T lymphocyte induces sensitized B cells to divide and mature into plasma cells, which begin to synthesize and secrete immunoglobulins. The synthesis of IgM antibody seems to be the least dependent on T cell activity, whereas the IgA response is usually dependent on this T cell activity. Another group of Th cells interacts with the macrophages, with the result of enhancing their destruction of pathogens.[11]

Helper T (Th) lymphocytes are designated CD-4 cells since that marker predominates on their surface membrane. The CD-4 surface protein, additionally, serves as the site where antigen, in the presence of an MHC molecule, is presented to the Th cell (attached) so that recognition of antigen and immune activation can be initiated (see p. 272). Helper T 1 cells (T_h1) and helper T 2 cells (T_h2) are subsets of Th cells that, although similar in CD-4 classification, are distinct in the types and quantities of cytokines (immune-based chemical messengers) that they release. Through their differing cytokine profiles, the T_h1 and T_h2 CD-4 cells regulate different aspects of immune activation and orchestration (Fig. 10-10).[21] Recently identified T_h0 cells have cytokine patterns overlapping T_h1 and T_h2 cells, and share functions as well.[7]

Killer (Cytotoxic) T Lymphocytes

Some CD-8 T lymphocytes become cytotoxic T lymphocytes (CTLs). These cells develop in the thymus, are activated in the periphery by Th cells, undergo transformation, and then engage in direct lysis of infected cells (see Fig. 10-10). CTLs contain granules that can form openings in cell membranes and produce and secrete proteolytic enzymes and other chemical toxins into the infected cells. They also can lyse an infected cell, and they demonstrate direct antiviral activity toward the infecting virus.

CTLs thus bind to the surface of the infected cell, disrupt its membrane, and kill it by altering its intracellular environment. CTLs secrete cytotoxic proteins onto the target, or foreign, cell and kill it.[10] The toxic proteins, often called *lymphotoxins* (chemotactic substances), include perforin (cytolysin) and granzymes (complement-like proteases).[10] The substances may be *chemotactic*, establishing a chemical gradient that helps to bring leukocytes and other substances into the area. The cytotoxic cells can stimulate the target cell to commit suicide, a mechanism called *apoptosis*. The mechanisms used by the cells are not well understood but involve fragmentation of the DNA and disintegration of the cell.[11] After killing, the activated cytotoxic T cell moves on with the ability to kill again.[10]

In addition to directly lysing virally infected cells, CTLs are also active in the destruction of some of the parasitic organisms. The recognition mechanism of the T cells must be tightly controlled to discriminate between self and nonself because they recognize the membrane proteins of the host cell rather than free antigen. Therefore, CTLs are the chief mechanisms to react to and reject foreign tissue.[17,21] The lymphokines secreted draw macrophages to the area and stimulate the production of interferon, which may function to suppress the spread of viruses from cell to cell.

Suppressor T Cells

Suppressor T cells reduce the humoral response. The production of immunoglobulins against a particular antigen can be reduced or abolished in the presence of these cells. The mechanism of action may be to control the production of immunoglobulins, either by regulating the proliferation of B cells or by inhibiting the activity of helper T cells. Suppressor T cells are among those T lymphocytes that have as their principal cell surface marker the CD-8 molecule.

NATURAL KILLER (NK) CELLS

Some lymphocytes cannot be classified as T or B lymphocytes because they lack the surface markers that are characteristic of these cells. Morphologically, these cells are mainly large granular lymphocytes (LGLs) and account for up to 15% of blood lymphocytes. They are generally considered a third member of the lymphocyte family and may be derived from uncommitted T cells (as they seem to mature in the thymus, but without T cell surface characteristics). Unlike B and T cells, NK cells can spontaneously react to antigen without prior sensitization or activation being demonstrated; thus they are said to be natural killers. Uniquely, NK cells can lyse targets not expressing any self MHC molecules. NK cells are functionally identified through their abilities to kill virus-infected cells, tumor cells, and targets coated with IgG antibody (due to CD 16 surface protein that is on IgG surface receptors).[11] The

FOCUS ON CELLULAR PHYSIOLOGY

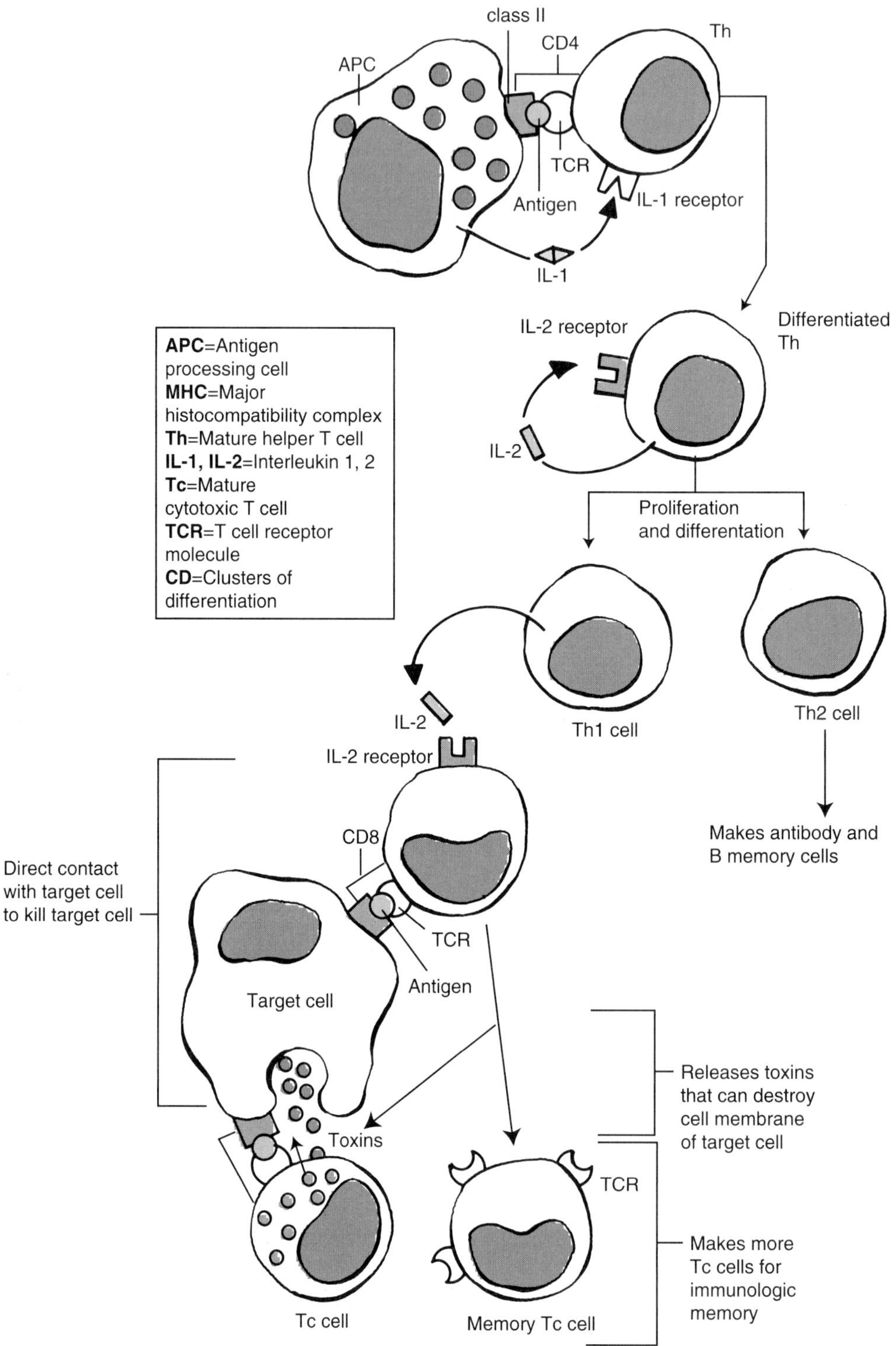

FIGURE 10-10. Cell mediated response. The T helper cell and specific cytokines serve a critical function in activating the cytotoxic T cell.

ability to kill (lyse) target cells is called *natural killer activity* or *antibody-dependent cellular cytotoxicity*, depending on the specific activity of the cell. NK cells also may release interferon or other cytokines and may be important in the regulation of immune response and production of granulocytes (neutrophils, basophils, or eosinophils) and macrophages.[11]

CYTOKINES: CHEMICAL MESSENGERS OF THE IMMUNE SYSTEM

To carry out the many complex activities and processes of the immune response (both nonspecific and specific), the immune system is diffused with a large family of chemicals. First discovered in lymphocytes and thus originally referred to as *lymphokines*, these immunotransmitters are generally called *cytokines*.[11] They are small-molecular-weight soluble proteins. Scores of cytokines have been discovered within the past two generations, and they have been classified into four major groups: the interleukins (IL), interferons (IFN), tumor necrosis factors (TNF), and transformation growth factors (Table 10-3).

Properties of Cytokines

In addition to apparently specific, discrete messages that can be carried by cytokines, they have the characteristic of pleiotropism, meaning that they appear to deliver different messages under differing cellular/chemical conditions. Their unique nature as pleiotropic agents suggests that cytokines individually contribute part of a larger, orchestrated message within the immune system; many chemicals, mixed carefully by the cells of the immune system, are necessary to deliver the complex messages necessary for integrated and coordinated function of the immune system's many components. Further, it is now clearly demonstrated that not only do immune cells have the capability to produce large numbers of different cytokines and to express cell surface receptor sites for the cascade of cytokines, but these chemicals also are produced in nonimmune cells (such as cells in the hypothalamus) and that there are receptor sites within numerous central nervous system locations for cytokines.[16]

TYPES OF IMMUNITY

As previously described, the term **immunity** refers to all of the mechanisms used by the body to prevent foreign material from causing harm to the body. The agents may be microorganisms or other environmental factors. The various types of immunity include innate and acquired (passive and adaptive).

Innate Versus Acquired Immunity

Innate immunity refers to those factors a person is born with to prevent disease. These factors, broadly speaking, can be physical barriers, such as skin, the ability to cough, or mucous membranes. Chemical barriers also work cooperatively to decrease microorganism invasion. The internal factors include mononuclear phagocytes and leukocytes.

Acquired immunity refers to passive and active immune processes. *Passive acquired immunity* occurs in early neonatal life, when some of the mother's immunity, which was passed through the placenta prenatally, continues to protect the infant from disease. This immunity protects only for the first few months of life. *Acquired active immunity* involves the response mounted by the person's own immune system. It requires all of the factors described earlier. Scientists have discovered the process of inducing acquired immunity through vaccination. The resultant individual response can be induced against microorganisms and their products as well as against thousands of natural and synthetic compounds. The vaccine prepared uses the least amount of antigenic material to provide the maximum human response and, thus, protection from disease.

Innate Immunity

A particular type of innate immunity is species specificity of infectious organisms. This refers to the natural immunity that humans have to infectious agents that cause disease in other animal species.

Barrier protections and the nonspecific inflammatory response are described in Chapter 9 (see also Table 10-1). These forms of protection against bodily harm are the initial lines of defense in the immune system, yet they are nonspecific in nature. They function in conjunction with the specific immune response in most situations.

Adaptive Immunity

The specific, adaptive immune response is responsible for the protection of the human body from disease. It requires a cellular and/or humoral response to an antigen. This type of immunity is an active process of specific recognition of antigen and the production of a bank of cells that "remember" the antigen and quickly respond to repeat antigen introduction. When the immune system cannot overwhelm the antigen, disease or death may occur.

Cell-Mediated Immunity

Cell-mediated immunity, caused by T-lymphocyte activity, is mediated through contact between T cells and antigen and by cytokines.[22] The interaction sets off a complex series of steps leading to subsequent destruction of the antigen.

TABLE 10-3

REPRESENTATIVE CYTOKINES

FAMILY	ALTERNATIVE NAMES	PRODUCER CELLS	ACTIONS
Interleukins (hematopoietins)	IL-2 (T cell growth factor)	T cells	T cell proliferation
	IL-3 (multicolony colony stimulating factor)	T cells, thymic epithelial cells	Synergistic action in early cell formation
	IL-4	T cells, mast cells	B cell activation, IgE
	IL-5	T cells, mast cells	Eosinophil growth, differentiation
	IL-6	T cells, macrophages	T and B cell growth and differentiation
	IL-7	Bone marrow cells	Growth of pre-B and pre-T, cells
	IL-9	T cells	Mast cell–enhancing activity
	IL-11	Fibroblasts in bone marrow stroma	Synergistic action with IL 3 and IL 4
	IL-13	T cells	B cell growth and differentiation; inhibits macrophage cytokine production
	IL-15	T cells	IL 2–like
	IL-1 α	Macrophages, epithelial cells	Fever, T cell activation, macrophage activation
Unassigned	IL-1 β	Macrophages, epithelial cells	Fever, T-cell activation, macrophage activation
	IL-1 RA	Macrophages	Binds IL 1 receptor as natural antagonist of IL 1
	IL-10	T cells, macrophage, Epstein-Barr virus	Potent suppressor of macrophage functions
	IL-12 (NK cell stimulatory factor)	B cells, macrophages	Activates NK cells, induce CD4 T-cell differentiation to TH 1–like cells
	MIF (macrophage inhibitory factor)	T cells, others chondrocytes, monocytes	Inhibits macrophage migration
	TGF β	T cells	Inhibits cell growth; anti-inflammatory
Interferons	IFN-γ	T cells, NK cells	Macrophage activation, increased MHC expression
	IFN-α	Leukocytes	Antiviral, increased MHCI expression
	IFN-β	Fibroblasts	Antiviral, increased MHCI expression
Tumor necrosis factor family (TNF)	TNF α (cachectin)	Macrophages, NK cells	Local inflammation, endothelial activation
	TNF β (lymphotoxin)	T cells, B cells	Killing, endothelial activation
	CD 40 ligand	T cells, mast cells	B cell activation, class switching
TNF Family	CD 27 Ligand	T cells	Stimulates T cell proliferation
	CD 30 Ligand	T cells	Stimulates T and B cell proliferation
Chemokines	IL-8 (NAP-1)	Macrophages, others	Chemotactic for neutrophils, T cells
	MCP-1 (membrane co-factor protein)	Macrophages, others	Chemotactic for monocytes

(Summarized from Janeway C., & Travers, P. [1997]. *Immunobiology* [3rd ed.]. New York: Current Biology Ltd., Garland Publishing.)

Cell-mediated reactions mainly involve T lymphocyte, macrophage, and cytokines, but antibody from B lymphocytes can act as an essential link in some cell-mediated reactions.[22] The reactions invariably produce memory, and subsequent exposure to the specific antigen results in an active response.

The T lymphocyte recognizes antigen by receptors on the surface of the T cell, called T-cell receptor molecules (TCRs), with the CD-4 or CD-8 molecules acting as co-receptors. After antigen recognition, Th cells activate and orchestrate a variety of specific responses that may also involve NK cells, activated macrophages, and, if needed, B cell production of antibodies (see Fig. 10-10). Destruction of the antigen may occur through the release of soluble chemical compounds directly into the target cell membrane or through the secretion of cytokines (Flow Chart 10-1).

Direct contact with an antigen frequently is called *killer activity*, and some T lymphocytes are directly cytotoxic in function. Killer activity is mediated through a group of cytotoxic T cells that function in the destruction of cells with the identified surface antigens. The specific recognition is through a lock-and-key type approach (see Fig. 10-8). To protect healthy self-cells from being attacked by the cell-mediated response, the Th cells recognize and respond only to specific surface molecules.

THE ROLE OF Th CELLS

The Th cells (CD-4+ T lymphocytes) recognize only antigen fragments that attach to their TCRs and CD-4 molecules in the presence of the MHC-II molecules on the surface of the antigen presenting (processing) cell (APC). APCs are a variety of cell types, mainly macrophages, that have ingested antigen, broken it down into fragments, and expressed these fragments on their cell surface, where they may be encountered by T cells. Basically, a macrophage encounters, engulfs, and lyses the antigen in circulation (see Fig. 10-10). After lysis, the macrophage expresses on its own cell surface antigen fragments (essentially proteins) that indicate that it has contacted foreign antigen. It attaches the foreign antigen on its own surface in juncture with its own MHC-II molecules. Upon contact with a CD-4 Th cell, the antigen/MHC-II complex binds to the TCR/CD-4 molecules on the surface of the Th cell and a complex is formed that tells the Th cell the chemical nature of

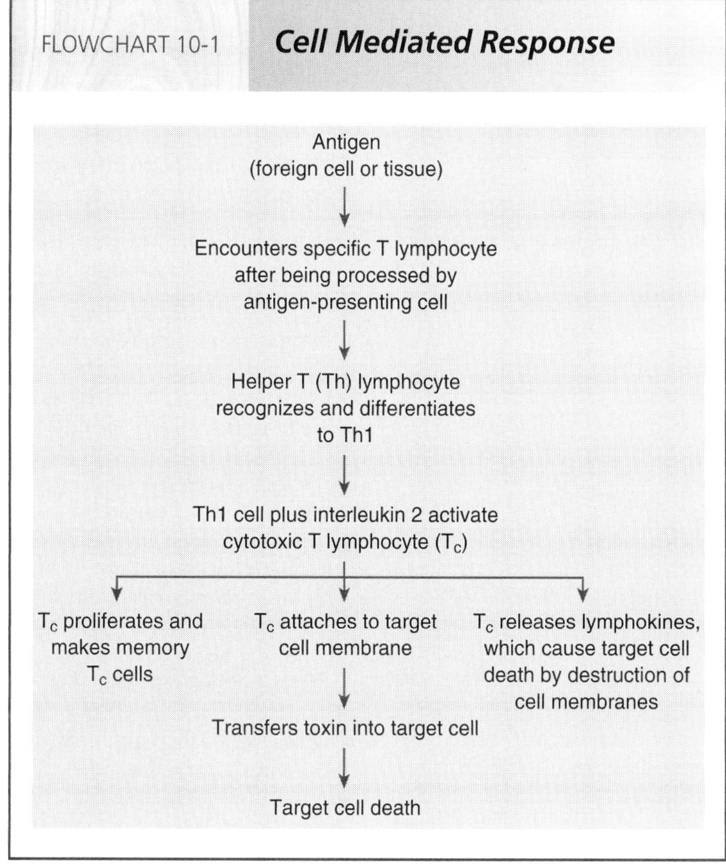
FLOWCHART 10-1 Cell Mediated Response
Antigen
(foreign cell or tissue)
Encounters specific T lymphocyte
after being processed by
antigen-presenting cell
Helper T (Th) lymphocyte
recognizes and differentiates
to Th1
Th1 cell plus interleukin 2 activate
cytotoxic T lymphocyte (T_C)
T_C proliferates and
makes memory
T_C cells
T_C attaches to target
cell membrane
T_C releases lymphokines,
which cause target cell
death by destruction of
cell membranes
Transfers toxin into target cell
Target cell death

..ntigen. The APC then secretes a chemical messenger (the cytokine Interleukin I) that binds to the Th cell surface to confirm the message and allows for activation of the Th cell for immune response to the antigen (the cytokine is called the "second messenger").

Only the linking of the APC with the Th cell, followed by the second messenger cytokine, can trigger the T cell response and thus initiate a full specific immune response. Coupling and binding of the APC with the Th cell is further assisted by the presence on the surface of those cells of other proteins called *fusion molecules*, which hold the two cells together tightly while message delivery is ongoing. Once the message is delivered and confirmed, the Th cell is activated into two subsets (Th1 and Th2). It can then use its genetic information to initiate cascades of other specific immune response, including both B cell activation leading to antibody secretion in the humoral response and activation of CTLs and NK cells as the cell-mediated response.[22] Thus, a pathogen that has penetrated the external barriers and survived the nonspecific inflammatory response is then challenged with the specific response of Th cells. These cells find and destroy the pathogen in the serum, interstitial spaces, and lymph, and even within infected host cells.

ROLE OF Tc LYMPHOCYTES AND NK CELLS

The CD8 lymphocyte may become activated when it contacts its specific antigen. As shown in Figure 10-10, it divides and differentiates into a clone of cytotoxic T lymphocytes, which can directly destroy the antigen (tumors cells and virally infected cells, especially). The cytotoxic T lymphocytes and NK cells may directly destroy the antigen by binding to the cell and producing a break in its membrane. This results in disruption of the intracellular osmotic environment and the death of the cell. The activated killer cell also may release cytotoxic substances directly into the target cell.

The NK cells (described on p. 283) function in host defense in the early phases of infection with several intracellular pathogens, especially herpes virus. They also can kill certain lymphoid tumor cells.[11] The mechanism of recognition of affected and unaffected cells is not entirely known, but altered MHCI or changes in cell surface glycoproteins by virus or bacteria may be the signal.[11]

The activated T lymphocytes release cytokines, which affect other lymphocytes by enhancing or suppressing their activity. These cells also may create a chemotactic gradient that causes macrophages to accumulate in the area. The activation of a very few antigen-specific T cells leads to a reaction that involves a large number of macrophages that destroy the antigen.[1] The specific antigen involved may be foreign tissue (transplant reactions), intracellular parasites (such as viruses or mycobacteria), soluble protein, or penetrating chemicals. The chemotactic gradient also attracts eosinophils, basophils, and neutrophils to the area.

The T cells function in immunosurveillance to detect cells in the host that have foreign antigens on their surface. The T cells can be thought of as defensive cells that patrol the blood and tissue spaces. This self-protective function is what prevents the transplantation of tissue from one person to another unless the antigens on the surface of the cells in the tissue are similar enough for the host tissue to accept the transplanted tissue as self.

Humoral Immunity

Humoral immunity refers to immunity effected by antibodies (specific immunoglobulins) that serve to coat the surface of an antigen and thus target it for destruction by polymorphonuclear neutrophils and macrophages. The interaction of antigen with antibody activates the classic pathway of the complement system (see p. 290).

Most antigens are recognized by T helper cells through the process of antigen presentation, which promotes the activation of B cells with specificity for the antigen. These B cells are believed to be activated, or made ready for immune activity, by direct T-cell interaction or by T-cell-secreted chemicals, or they can be directly activated by antigen. In some cases, a macrophage serves as an intermediary between the T and B cells. Activation causes the B cell to divide and differentiate into an active B cell called a *plasma cell*, which secretes specific immunoglobulin to target the antigen for destruction (Fig. 10-11).

Primary and Secondary Immune Response

The immune response is divided into two phases: primary and secondary. These are determined by the pattern of exposure to antigen.

Primary Immune Response

The first time a particular antigen enters the body, a characteristic pattern (called the primary immune response) of antibody production is induced. As the antigen binds to specific B cells and T cells, chemical induction takes place causing activation. The B cells proliferate and differentiate into specialized antibody-producing plasma cells. After about 6 days, antibodies specific to the antigen can be measured in the blood. This *lag* or *latent* phase is the time during which activation of T and B lymphocytes is taking place.[20] The first antibodies or immunoglobulins to be produced in measurable quantities usually are IgM. These are produced in large quantities, with levels increasing up to 14 days and then gradually declining to little IgM production after a few weeks.[3,13] After the initial IgM elevation, IgG immunoglobulins appear at about day 10, peak at several weeks, and maintain high levels much longer. Some antigens create more difficulty for the

FOCUS ON CELLULAR PHYSIOLOGY

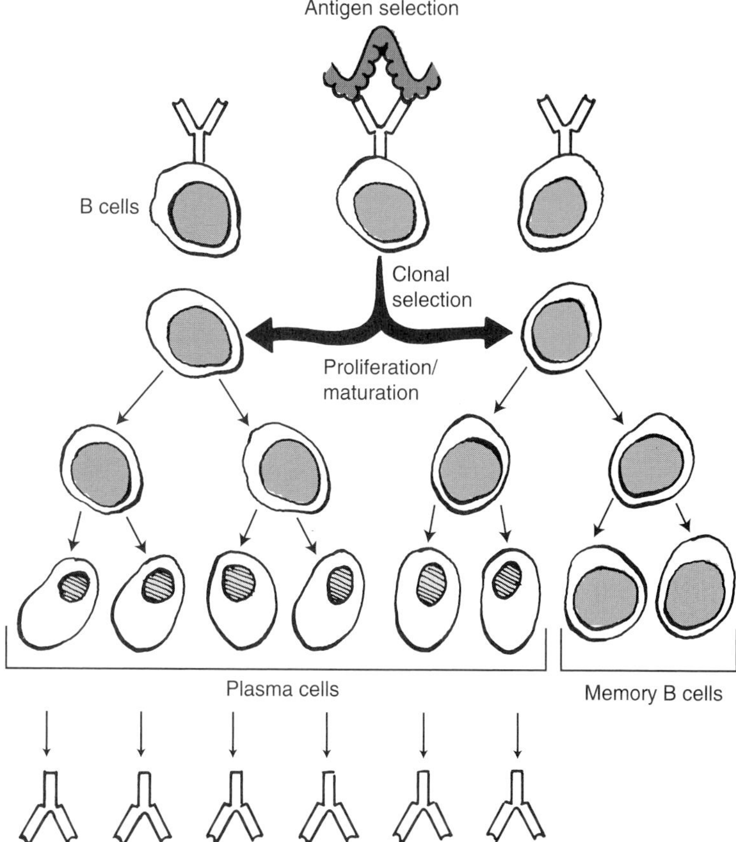

FIGURE 10-11. Once the B cell has been activated (usually by the helper T cell), it divides and differentiates into plasma cells and memory cells. The plasma cells make and release immunoglobulins that cover the antigen through opsonization. This targets the antigen for destruction by phagocytes.

immune cells to recognize, and the specific response may take months to generate.

During the course of the primary immune response, the immunoglobulins improve in their ability to bind the inducing antigen. The mechanisms responsible for this change are not known, but probably firmer binding occurs because of greater precision in matching surface receptors. IgG is considered the highest-affinity antibody that binds antigenic groupings firmly. After a time, a *steady-state phase* is reached in the specific immune response, during which antibody synthesis and degradation are about equal. Then a *declining phase* occurs, when the synthesis of new antibody decreases, in response to declining stimulation from antigen. Figure 10-12 shows primary and secondary immune responses to the same antigen.

Secondary Immune Response

The secondary response differs from the primary response in that the production of specific antibodies for the antigen begins almost immediately. Specific im-

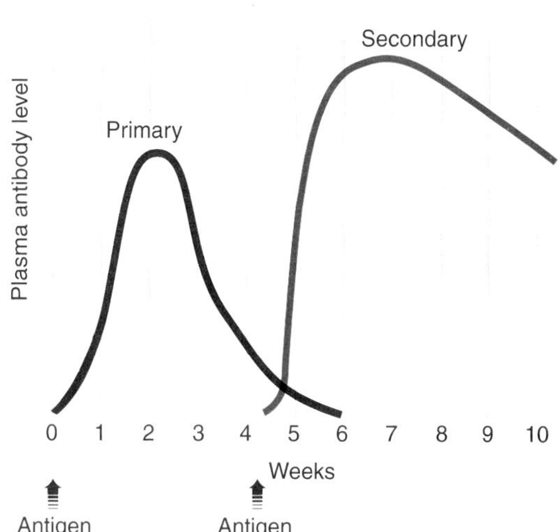

FIGURE 10-12. Primary and secondary immune response by antibody to the same antigen.

munoglobulin is produced early and in large amounts, and more antibody may be produced overall. The secondary response is called the *memory response* because the immune system responds much faster to a second exposure to a particular antigen.

Both T and B memory cells are involved in the secondary response because of T and B memory cells that were produced in the primary reponse. As the antigen is reintroduced into the host, the cells begin immediate production of specific antibodies that bind antigen quickly. Small amounts of antigen stimulate a highly specific response with the antibody.[20]

Complement Activation

Complement is a system of functionally linked proteins and their fragments that circulate in the serum as inactive molecules. Complement system components are normally activated only at localized sites as needed. More than two dozen complement proteins have now been identified. They are capable of interacting with one another in a sequential activation cascade that is designated by the letter C and by numbers (such as C3), with nine numbers indicating the major molecules and symbols or names indicating the components of those molecules (see p. 259).

The *classic pathway* for the activation (fixation) of complement involves binding the first component, C1, with a portion of the immunoglobulin molecule that begins the cascade of complement activation, essential in promoting the inflammatory process and the specific response. In most cases, an antigen–antibody (ATG–ATB) reaction is required for the activation of complement along the classical pathway. The system promotes inflammation by chemically increasing vascular permeability, by **chemotaxis**, and by phagocytosis. It finally causes lysis of the foreign cell. Activation of complement also promotes **opsonization** of target material. Opsonization occurs when the complement proteins attach to antigen particles, setting the stage for phagocytosis by neutrophils or macrophages.

Complement fixation is the result of complement-fixing antibody, especially IgG. The results of the components of the cascade may cause some damage to normal tissue around the foreign tissue, and in some cases, this process can be damaging to the host.

The *alternate complement activation* described on page 259 results in no immunologic memory because there is no ATG–ATB reaction. The complement factors participate in the inflammatory reaction, which may cause normal tissue damage.

Thymus-Independent B-Cell Response

Certain non-self antigens, designated as thymus-independent antigens, elicit strong B-cell responses without T-cell interaction. Examples include *Escherichia coli*, pneumococcal polysaccharide, dextrans, and other large polymers.[17] Antibody responses to T-independent antigens are usually weaker than those requiring a T-cell interaction. They tend to generate mainly IgM responses, and the secondary response is much less active on repeat exposure to antigen. This would indicate that the memory factor in this type of response is poor.[7]

PSYCHONEUROIMMUNOLOGY AND NORMAL IMMUNITY

As modern research expands our knowledge of immune function in relationship to health and disease, it becomes increasingly clear that the immune system plays a role not only in infectious diseases but also in many (perhaps most) disease conditions, acts of health restoration, and processes of health maintenance. Immune mediation of coronary artery disease, diabetes, chronic demyelinating nervous disorders, and even various mental illnesses is now well documented.[2] The collective belief that such immunologically mediated diseases can be influenced by cognitive thoughts and affective feelings is well documented as well.[15] The traditions of psychosomatic medicine, behavioral medicine, and holistic medicine probably predate recorded history. It has only been within the past 30 or 40 years that the research support and theoretical understanding of brain-immune interactions has matured to a level that brings comprehension and the promise of uniform clinical applications.[12]

It is within the field of **psychoneuroimmunology** (PNI) that we now have emerging a solid physiologic, empirical, and theoretical understanding of how the mind influences immunologically mediated diseases.

The term psychoimmunology was first used in 1964, and the term psychoneuroimmunology was first used in 1981.[23] Psychoneuroimmunology is a multidisciplinary field of study that proposes a model of bidirectional interactions between the central nervous (CNS), endocrine, and immune systems such that all are modulated by and influence the subjective experiences and psychological state of an individual.[2,15] Thus, the patterns of biological functioning and psychosocial functioning may be reflections of shared processes.[12] Of importance to a general discussion of immunology are the following two central features of PNI: (1) chemical pathways used for shared communication and (2) shared patterns of organismic response to issues of self/not self and threat/not threat.

There are chemical pathways used for shared communication between CNS cells and immunologically competent cells. The thymus, spleen, GALT, and many other immune tissues are innervated by postganglionic autonomic nervous system fibers, and, indeed, the synaptic connections are between nerve cells and immune cells (individually and in clumps). Additionally, we now know that immunotransmitters are produced in the specific cells in the CNS and in immune cells, as are neurotransmitters and endocrine hormones and a variety of other chemical messengers. Further, there are receptor sites for cytokines not only on immune cells but also in the CNS, and there are receptor sites for neurotransmitters not only on brain cell membranes but also on the cell membranes of a wide variety of immunocompetent cells. The emerging model is of networks within the brain and immune systems that communicate locally and globally to one another, to other organ systems, and to the body as a whole. It has been postulated that there are no organ-specific chemical messengers, only the messengers of the organism as a whole, which can be used in system-wide communication as well as in subsystem communications.[3]

In addition to the brain–immune system communications taking place using shared pathways and chemical messengers, the communication is about shared patterns of organismic response to issues of self/not-self and issues of threat/not-threat. The immune patterns historically identified as being unique to the immune system may, thus, reflect organismic patterns of self: the concepts of stored memory from prior mastered experience; of general inflammatory and also specific, discreet responses to not-self; the recursive nature of self/not-self validation; the ability to adapt to a diverse environment; and the ability to self-regulate may be shared along the common communication pathways for the purpose of holistic integration of immune and CNS functions for overall health. Acute stress responses, such as the sympathetic-adrenal medullary response (SAM activation with catecholamine release), generally have an immune-enhancing effect, and chronic activation of the hypothalamic-pituitary adrenal cortical responses most often has a immune-suppressive effect.[2] Further, survey and experimental research documents a relationship between perceptions of stress, predicted immunologic response, and morbidity and mortality in immunologically mediated diseases.[5,6,12] The field of PNI is relatively new, and our knowledge, as exciting as it is, only gives preliminary glimpses of how immune and neural systems communicate and influence one another. It is clear, however, that immune function is influenced by cognitive and affective experiences in the CNS, with predictable outcomes in terms of immune enhancement and immune suppression.

REFERENCES

1. Abbas, A., Lichtman, A., & Pober, J. (1991). *Cellular and molecular immunology*. Philadelphia: W. B. Saunders.
2. Ader, R., Madden, K., Felten, D., Bellinger, D., & Schiffer, R. (1996). Psychoneuroimmunology: Interactions between the brain and immune system. In B. Fogel, R. Schiffer, & S. Rao (Eds.), *Neuropsychiatry* (pp. 193–215). Baltimore: Williams & Wilkins.
3. Breard, J., Costa, O., & Kordon, C. (1995). Organization and functional relevance of neuroimmune networks. In B. Leonard & K. Miller (Eds.) *Stress, the immune system and psychiatry* (pp. 17–45). Chichester, UK: John Wiley & Sons.
4. Brodsky, F. M. (1997). Antigen presentation and the major histocompatability complex. In D. P. Stites, A. I. Terr, & T. G. Parslow (Eds.), *Medical immunology* (9th ed.). Stamford, CT: Appleton & Lange.
5. Cohen, S. & Herbert, T. (1996). Health psychology: Psychological factors and physical disease from the perspective of human psychoneuroimmunology. *Annual Review of Psychology, 47,* 113–142.
6. Fawzy, F., Fawzy, N., Arndt, L., & Pasnau, R. (1995). Critical review of psychosocial interventions in cancer care. *Archives of General Psychiatry, 52,* 100–113.
7. Feldmann, M. (1998). Cell cooperation in the antibody response. In I. Roitt, J. Brostoff, & D. Male, *Immunology* (5th ed.). St. Louis: Mosby.
8. Greenberg, P. D. (1997). Mechanisms of tumor immunology. In D. P. Stites, A. I. Terr, & T. G. Parslow (Eds.), *Medical immunology* (9th ed.). Stamford, CT: Appleton & Lange.
9. Guyton, A. C., & Hall, J. E. (1997). *Human physiology and mechanisms of disease* (6th ed.). Philadelphia: W. B. Saunders.
10. Imboden, J. B. (1997). T lymphocytes & natural killer cells. In D. P. Stites, A. I. Terr, & T. G. Parslow (Eds.), *Medical immunology* (9th ed.). Stamford, CT: Appleton & Lange.
11. Janeway, C. & Travers, P. (1997). *Immunobiology: The immune system in health and disease.* New York: Garland Publishing.
12. Kiecolt-Glaser, J., & Glaser, R. (1995). Psychoneuroimmunology and health consequences: Data and shared mechanisms. *Psychosomatic Medicine, 57*(3), 269–276.
13. Kuby, J. (1992). *Immunology.* New York: W. H. Freeman.
14. Lydyard, P. & Grossi, C. (1998). The lymphoid system. In I. Roitt, J. Brostoff, & D. Male, *Immunology* (5th ed.), St. Louis: Mosby.
15. Maier, S., Watkins, L., & Fleshner, M. (1994). Psychoneuroimmunology: The interface between behavior, brain, and immunity. *American Psychologist, 49*(12), 1004–1017.
16. Oppenheim, J. J. & Ruscetti, F. (1997). Cytokines. In D. P. Stites, A. I. Terr, & T. G. Parslow (Eds.), *Medical immunology* (9th ed.). Stamford, CT: Appleton & Lange.
17. Parslow, T. G. (1997). Immunogens, antigens, and vaccines. In D. P. Stites, A. I. Terr, & T. G. Parslow (Eds.), *Medical immunology* (9th ed.). Stamford, CT: Appleton & Lange.
18. Parslow, T. G. (1997). Immunoglobulins and immunoglobulin genes. In D. P. Stites, A. I. Terr, & T. G. Parslow (Eds.), *Medical immunology* (9th ed.). Stamford, CT: Appleton & Lange.
19. Parslow, T. G. (1997). Lymphocytes and lymphoid tissue. In D. P. Stites, A. I. Terr, & T. G. Parslow (Eds.), *Medical immunology* (9th ed.). Stamford, CT: Appleton & Lange.
20. Parslow, T. G. (1997). The immune response. In D. P. Stites, A. I. Terr, & T. G. Parslow (Eds.), *Medical immunology* (9th ed.). Stamford, CT: Appleton & Lange.
21. Peakman, M., & Vergani, D. (1997). *Basic and clinical immunology.* New York: Churchill Livingstone.
22. Rook, G. & Balkwill, F. (1998). Cell-mediated immune reactions. In I. Roitt, J. Brostoff, & D. Male, *Immunology* (5th ed.) St. Louis: Mosby.
23. Solomon, G. (1987). Psychoneuroimmunology: Interactions between central nervous system and immune system. *Journal of Neuroscience Research, 18,* 1–9.
24. Talmage, D. (1997). History of immunology. In D. P. Stites, A. I. Terr, & T. G. Parslow (Eds.), *Medical immunology* (9th ed.). Stamford, CT: Appleton & Lange.

Chapter 11

Altered Immunity

Miguel da Cunha / Barbara L. Bullock

KEY TERMS

allergen
allergies
anaphylaxis
angioedema
antigen-presenting cell (APC)
apoptosis (programmed cell death)
atopy
autoantibodies
chemotaxis
complement system
cytokine
ELISA (enzyme-linked immunosorbent assay)
erythroblastosis fetalis
granulomatous hypersensitivity response
hapten
helper T-cell (Th, T4, CD4$^+$ T-cells)
HIV (human immune deficiency virus)
histocompatibility antigens
hypersensitivity reactions
interleukins (IL)
kernicterus
natural killer (NK) cells
opportunistic infections
opsonins
pannus
rheumatoid factor
suppressor T-cells (T8, CD4$^-$ T-cells)
syncytia
thymosins
urticaria
Western blot

An intact immune system helps maintain the body's ability to defend itself against foreign invasion from microorganisms and other foreign materials. A myriad of alterations can occur that prevent or exaggerate this defensive function. These alterations have been classified as immune deficiency syndromes on one extreme and hypersensitive immune responses on the other. There are multiple alterations that may result in disease states; only a small, representative group are presented in this chapter.

IMMUNE DEFICIENCY SYNDROMES

Immune deficiency syndromes (IDSs) may be classified as primary and secondary. Primary IDSs are rare, usually congenital in nature and caused by heritable defects of specific genes (e.g., X-linked severe combined immunodeficiency syndrome, or SCID). Most IDSs are secondary, or acquired; as the term implies, they represent a loss of a previously effective immune response. That loss can be a result of a single insult (e.g., infection with the human immunodeficiency virus), or it can be due to multiple insults, as in the case of malnutrition, stress, aging, or iatrogenic conditions, such as those resulting from cancer, immune suppressive (e.g., anti-rejection drugs), and long-term steroid therapies.

Regardless of type or etiology, the fundamental consequence of IDSs is an increased vulnerability to opportunistic diseases, such as infections and malignancies.

Examples of opportunistic diseases and their relationship to immune dysfunctions are given in Table 11-1. T-lymphocyte defects often result in opportunistic infections that are aggressive and persistent. Those caused by B-lymphocyte defects are usually chronic and recurrent.

Primary Immune Deficiency Syndromes

As hereditary and sometimes congenital disorders, primary IDSs result in failure of development of specific components of the immune system and may involve a variety of cells and non-specific defense mechanisms.[29] The three major cells of the immune system are T and B lymphocytes and phagocytic cells (see p. 277). In addition, adequate functioning of the **complement system** is essential for immune defense. It is therefore conve-

TABLE 11-1

SELECTED OPPORTUNISTIC DISEASES AND IMMUNE DYSFUNCTION

OPPORTUNISTIC DISEASES	IMMUNE DYSFUNCTION
BACTERIAL INFECTIONS	
Bacterial sepsis, *Salmonella* sp., *Legionella* sp.	T-cell defect
Streptococci, Staphylococci, *Haemophilus* sp.	B-cell defect
Pseudomonas aeruginosa, Staphylococci	Phagocyte defect
Neisseria sp., other pyogenic bacteria	Complement defect
VIRAL INFECTIONS	
Enteroviral encephalitis	B-cell defect
Cytomegalovirus (CMV), Epstein-Barr virus (EBV), chronic infections with respiratory and intestinal viruses	T-cell defect
Hepatitis viruses	B-cell defect
FUNGAL, PROTOZOAL INFECTIONS	
Candida sp., *Pneumocystis carinii, Toxoplasma* sp.	T-cell defect
Severe intestinal giardiasis (*Giardia lamblia*)	B-cell defect
Candida sp., *Nocardia* sp., *Aspergillus* sp.	Phagocyte defect
MALIGNANCIES	
Kaposi sarcoma (KS), non-Hodgkin's lymphoma, primary brain lymphoma	Combined T- and B-cell defects Complement defect Phagocyte defect

nient to classify primary IDSs according to the specific causative cellular or immune dysfunction: T-cell disorders, B-cell disorders and antibody deficiencies, phagocyte disorders, and complement disorders. Since T-cells are directly involved in regulation of B-cells, deficiencies caused by these lymphocytes are often classified as combined lymphocyte defects. One disorder, Louis-Barr syndrome or *ataxia telangiectasia,* does not fall under the classification above, but represents an important group of IDSs of variable etiology: a defect in DNA repair. Table 11-2 presents selected examples of primary IDSs, their immune dysfunctions, genetics, and clinical manifestations with age of onset.

T-CELL AND COMBINED T- AND B-CELL DISORDERS

Primary, isolated T-cell disorders are rare and often result from T-cell maturation defects. In *DiGeorge syndrome,* for example, an embryogenic error in thymus development causes impairment of T-cells, in the presence of adequate B-cell function. Another rare disorder involves selective absence of **suppressor T-cells (T8)** with impairment of natural killer (NK) cells and has been identified only in Mennonite groups in the eastern United States.[9,16] Partial T-cell losses have also been identified and are associated with disorders such as chronic mucocutaneous candidiasis with extensive infection of the mouth and esophagus, skin, and nails.

In most instances, however, since proper T-cell activity is essential for T-cell to B-cell interaction, primary T-cell dysfunctions will secondarily affect B-cell function and antibody production. As a result, children with primary T-cell dysfunctions often present with fulminating infections by a variety of bacteria, fungi, and viruses. Common viral diseases of childhood often result in fatal outcomes. In the case of *severe combined immune deficiency (SCID) syndromes,* failure of cell-mediated and humoral immunities results in complete loss of immune response and a high mortality rate. In one case with worldwide recognition, a Texan boy with SCID (known only as David, the Bubble Boy) was able to survive approximately 12 years secluded within a plastic, pathogen-free environment. Combined lymphocyte deficiencies account for approximately 25% of all primary IDSs.

ANTIBODY DEFICIENCIES

As previously mentioned, many B-cell deficiencies are secondary to T-cell dysfunction. Typically, patients with B-cell defects and their resulting antibody deficiencies present with recurrent pyogenic infections, including pneumonia, otitis media, and sinusitis. Antibody disorders may occur in the form of isolated deficiencies (e.g, selective IgA deficiency) or may involve several immunoglobulins. One characteristic example of the latter category is *X-linked agammaglobulinemia,*

(text continues on page 295)

TABLE 11-2

SELECTED EXAMPLES OF PRIMARY IMMUNE DEFICIENCY SYNDROMES

DISORDER	IMMUNE DYSFUNCTION	GENETICS	CLINICAL MANIFESTATIONS
Agammaglobulinemia (Bruton type)	Antibody deficiency Failure in B-cell development from pre-B-cells	X-linked recessive Location: Xq, 22 **Age of onset:** early infancy	Absence of serum immunoglobulins Severe recurrent infections: Conjunctivitis Pharyngitis Otitis media Bronchitis Pneumonias Skin infections Persistent intestinal giardiasis Increased risk for: Vaccine-associated poliomyelitis Fatal echovirus encephalitis *Pneumocystis carinii* pneumonia Autoimmune diseases
Ataxia telangiectasia (Louis-Barr syndrome)	DNA repair defect Cell cycle abnormalities Impaired lymphocyte development	Autosomal recessive Chromosome fragility Location: 11q, 22–23 **Age of onset:** early childhood	Cerebellar ataxia Multiple, progressive telangiectases (eye, face, hands, neck, knees) Cancer susceptibility: lymphomas Recurrent infections Radiation hypersensitivity Progressive neurologic degeneration Absence of thymus Hypoplastic gonads
Chédiak-Higashi syndrome	Phagocyte disorder Leukocyte motility and intracellular defects NK cells defect	Autosomal recessive Location: 1q, 42–44 **Age of onset:** childhood	Neutropenia Abnormal neutrophils with reduced bactericidal activity Recurrent infections Acute episodes of fever Decreased pigmentation of hair and skin Photophobia Nystagmus Cancer susceptibility: lymphomas Hepatosplenomegaly Generalized lymphadenopathy
Common variable immune deficiency	Antibody deficiency, varying from hypogammaglobulinemia to agammaglobulinemia Presence of autoantibodies, which disrupt immune system homeostasis Probable T-cell mediation	Probably polygenic **Age of onset:** adolescence to adulthood	Susceptibility to autoimmune diseases: Pernicious anemia Hemolytic anemia Rheumatoid arthritis
DiGeorge syndrome (thymic hypoplasia)	Primary T-cell disorder Variable degrees of T-cell dysfunction, from mild to complete deficiency; B-cell function can be affected	Autosomal dominant Location: 22q, 11–12 **Age of onset:** early infancy	Absence of thymus and parathyroids Total absence of cell-mediated immunity Hypocalcemia and tetany Congenital heart/great vessels defects Abnormal mouth, ears, facies Persistent fungal and viral infections
Isolated IgA deficiency	Antibody deficiency Occasionally, presence of *anti-IgA* antibodies.	"Familial" Autosomal dominant(?) **Age of onset:** childhood	Most persons are asymptomatic In some, recurrent infections: Respiratory (sinopulmonary) Gastrointestinal (diarrhea) Urogenital
Leukocyte adhesion disease, type 1 (LADS-1)	Phagocyte disorder Decreased motility, adherence (reduced integrins), endocytosis	Autosomal recessive Location: 21q, 21–22 **Age of onset:** early childhood	Delayed separation of umbilical cord Recurrent infections: Severe, scarring skin infections Gingivitis Systemic bacterial infections

(continued)

TABLE 11-2

SELECTED EXAMPLES OF PRIMARY IMMUNE DEFICIENCY SYNDROMES (Continued)

DISORDER	IMMUNE DYSFUNCTION	GENETICS	CLINICAL MANIFESTATIONS
Severe combined immune deficiency syndrome (SCID)	Primary combined T- and B-cell deficiency or primary T-cell dysfunc-ion, which blocks T-cell to B-cell interaction Decreased total lymphocyte count	X-linked recessive Location; Xq, 13 **Age of onset:** early childhood	Failure to thrive and diarrhea in early infancy Recurrent, severe infections: *Candida albicans* *Pneumocystis carinii* *Pseudomonas* sp. Cytomegalovirus Varicella Various other bacteria "Graft-versus-host" reaction (from transplacental transfer or maternal T-cells)
Complement disorders	Complement system deficiencies	Autosomal recessive (various genes) **Age of onset:** variable	C1, C2 deficiency: hereditary angioedema (recurrent episodes of localized edema of skin and mucous membranes) C3 deficiency: recurrent infections by pyogenic bacteria C1, C2, C4 deficiency: increased risk of immune complex–mediated diseases and systemic lupus erythematosus (SLE) C5 to C8 deficiencies: recurrent neisserial (gonococcal, meningo-coccal) infections

often termed Bruton disease, which results from B-cell maturation arrest in early stages of development, so that affected persons have few or no B-cells. Consequently, they lack serum immunoglobulins of all types, with the occasional exception of small amounts of IgG. This disorder is predominantly expressed in males because it is X-linked. Protected by maternal antibodies, young boys affected with this disorder usually remain healthy for the first 6 to 12 months of life. After that age, they are continuously vulnerable to infections, especially upper respiratory and ear infections (during cold episodes). These often progress to pneumonia, which, if untreated, leads to the development of bronchiectasis. Most skin and nail infections are caused by streptococci, staphylococci, *Haemophilus influenzae*, gram-negative bacteria, and various species of mycoplasma and ureaplasma.[32]

PHAGOCYTE DISORDERS

Inflammatory cells whose primary function is phagocytosis include cells of the monocyte-macrophage system and polymorphonuclear leukocytes. These cells emigrate from the vascular compartment by means of complex mechanisms involving chemotaxis and cellular motility. Phagocyte disorders result from impairments of these functions, causing decreased availability of protective cells at the sites of inflammation. In addition, their bactericidal activity is often impaired, contributing to the host's increased susceptibility to infections by pyogenic bacteria.

Chédiak-Higashi syndrome (CHS), an example of this category of primary IDSs, is an autosomal recessive disorder that results in defective neutrophils with intracellular inclusions, deficient microtubular structures, and decreased **chemotaxis**. As a result of these abnormalities, leukocyte motility is severely impaired and bactericidal activity is significantly reduced. In addition, **natural killer (NK) cell** function is also impaired, causing failure of cancer immunosurveillance and resulting in increased susceptibility to malignancies. Children with CHS are often pale, with slate-grey skin and light-colored hair, who typically present with a history of repeated infections and acute episodes of fever. Hepatosplenomegaly and hypersplenism predisposes them to thrombocytopenia, and intracranial bleeding is not uncommon. Many of these children develop hematologic malignancies, especially lymphomas and acute lymphoblastic leukemia, which, together with intracranial hemorrhages, account for a high number of deaths.

COMPLEMENT DEFICIENCIES

Genetic deficiencies of various proteins of the complement system have been identified. According to the function of each protein, or group of proteins, complement deficiencies have multiple consequences (see Table 11-2). A complement disorder involving protein C_1 is the cause of an autosomal dominant condition termed *hereditary angioneurotic edema* (HAE). The pathogenesis of HAE is a deficiency of an inhibiting factor involved in the activation of the complement cascade's classical pathway. The disease is characterized by recurrent episodes of angioedema of various body parts, responsible for various pathologies including abdominal pain, cramping, vomiting (due to edema of the intestines), and possible asphyxiation (due to edema of the upper respiratory passages). Other complement deficiencies may affect phagocyte activity (especially due to the **opsonins** of the C_3 to C_5 group) or may predispose to autoimmune disease (due to the C_2 and C_4 proteins).[1]

Secondary Immune Deficiency Syndromes

Secondary immune deficiency syndromes represent damage to an originally competent immune system. They can be caused by various environmental stressors, such as aging, stress, nutritional deficiencies, disease processes, chemical, physical and biological insults (Box 11-1). Since integrity of T-cell function, from maturation to immune competent responses, is essential to the regulation of most of the immune system, any condition that impedes adequate T-cell activity will secondarily affect other immune components. For example, T-cell impairment will impact cytolytic T-cell activity (due to interleukin-2 deficiency), antibody production (defective T-cell to B-cell interaction), macrophage function (lack of macrophage-directed lymphokines), NK cell activity (decreased interleukin-2 stimulation), and various other combined deficiencies. Thus, it is expected that an initial T-cell failure will result in increased susceptibility to infections (decreased cell-mediated and humoral immunity) and to malignancies (impaired cancer immunosurveillance due to deficient macrophage and NK cell function). A classic example of T-cell depletion that impacts immune function as a whole is HIV infection, in which the virus has a preference for the ultimate regulatory cell, the helper T-cell (see p. 287).

DETERMINANTS OF SECONDARY IMMUNE DEFICIENCY SYNDROMES

Whether caused by biologic, environmental, or iatrogenic events, conditions that affect the normal functioning of the immune system may precipitate a secondary immune deficiency syndrome.

BOX 11-1 CAUSES OF SECONDARY IMMUNE DEFICIENCY

Biologic Determinants
Aging
Stress

Nutritional Deficiencies
Proteins, carbohydrates, lipids
Vitamins: A, B complex
Trace elements: iron, zinc

Malignant Disease

Infections
Postviral infection
Chronic infection

Iatrogenic
Radiation therapy
Cancer chemotherapy
Immunosuppressive therapy
Multiple transfusions
Certain medications

Miscellaneous
Recreational drug abuse
Maternal alcoholism

Aging

The concept that aging results from a "wearing out" of the immune system has been extensively studied, and progressive declines in immune function in the aged individual are usually seen. These declines include the interrelated factors of decreased availability of thymosin and impaired T-cell function.[13] **Thymosin** is the thymus hormone necessary for full maturation of T-cells whose pure reduction can be initiated at about age 40. Pure T-cell dysfunction does not appear to be significant until after age 60. The increased incidence of cancer among the elderly is probable evidence of age-related immune deficiency. The increased prevalence of autoimmune disease in the elderly parallels an increased production of autoantibodies.

Stress

An exciting discovery of recent times is the interaction among immune, endocrine, and neurologic mechanisms. The field of *psychoneuroimmunology* is rapidly developing and has began to clarify many of the influences of *stress* on immune response. It has been demonstrated that immune system cells express receptors to norepinephrine, enkephalins and endorphins, corticotropin-releasing factor (CRF, a hypothalamic hormone), adrenocorticotropin (ACTH, released by the pituitary), and glucocorticoids, which allows them to be modulated by many of the molecules of the neuro-endocrine-immune regulatory loops.[11] As a result of these interactions, the initiation of an immune reaction may trigger the release of CRF by the hypothalamus and/or activation of the sympathetic nervous system. In the first pathway, pituitary stimulation by CRF results in the production of ACTH or the neuropeptide α-endorphin. ACTH induces adrenal production of corticosteroids. The subsequent modulation of immune system cells will depend on the concentration of CRF, ACTH, and beta-endorphin, and can result in increased or decreased immune function. The release of many of these endocrine hormones can be triggered by stress. A stressful situation that occurs prior to an immune response may leave immune system cells suppressed by corticosteroids and unable to respond to antigenic stimulation. The level of circulating corticosteroids will determine the duration of immune suppression, so that the higher the stress, the greater the likelihood of a prolonged immune suppression. In many instances, the immune system does not distinguish between "good" and "bad" stress; it simply registers alterations in homeostasis, so one's immune response may be identical no matter what the stressor (see p. 140).

Nutritional Deficiencies

Worldwide, nutritional deficiencies (and in developing countries, HIV infection) are the most common causes of secondary immune deficiency. It has been estimated that 400 million people are affected.[36] However, even in developed countries, malnutrition continues to present a threat to the various segments of the population, not so much in terms of generalized malnutrition but of specific nutritional deficiencies that impair immune function. In addition to decreased availability of food products, other factors that influence adequate nutrition include: (1) conditions that affect intestinal absorption of necessary substances, such as parasitic infections, celiac disease, or gastric achlorhydria; (2) the uncontrolled use of pesticides, which are transferred to food and result in impairment of cellular metabolism necessary for immune response; and (3) various socioeconomic factors such as poverty, poor sanitation, and reduced access to health care.

Nutritional deficiencies affect most areas of immune response, including cell-mediated immunity, phagocyte activity, complement activation, and **cytokine** production. Various dietary elements are essential for the differentiation and maturation of immune system cells, including vitamins (e.g., A, B_{12}, folic acid) and trace metals (e.g., zinc. iron, selenium, chromium, copper), in addition to adequate amounts of carbohydrate, lipid, and protein substrates. Reduced dietary intake as a result of poor availability of food will impact all these needs, even if above the levels of malnutrition or starvation.

Protein-energy malnutrition (PEM) is of significant importance as a cause of immune deficiency, especially if present during fetal life. Immune responses significantly affected by PEM include cell-mediated immunity (indicated by decreased helper T-cell count and lower helper/suppressor ratio), phagocytosis, chemotaxis, complement activation, and especially, bactericidal activity by phagocytes.[32] In addition, immunization-induced antibody production is markedly reduced in the presence of PEM. Better response to immunization can be achieved even if short-term nutritional supplementation is given prior to and after immunization.

Iatrogenic Causes

The treatment of several disorders (e.g., cancer) with immunosuppressive therapies is a common cause of secondary immune deficiencies in the modern world. Malignant disease often causes malnutrition as a result of protein wasting, with consequent immune suppression. It is ironic that in addition to cancer itself, many, if not most, cancer chemotherapeutic agents are also immunosuppressive, so that the treatment compounds the effects of the disease. Especially immunosuppressive are the alkylating agents, such as the nitrogen mustards (e.g., mechlorethamine, chlorambucil, cyclophosphamide); the nitrosoureas (e.g., carmustine, lomustine, semustine); and the triazines (e.g., dacarbazine), among many others. The other major cancer treatment modality, radiotherapy, also causes significant myelosuppression and immune deficiency. A total radiation dose of 2.5 to 4.5 grey (gy; 1 gy = 100 rad) to the whole bone marrow causes aplasia (lack of blood cell production) and pancytopenia (decrease in all blood cells), as does segmental (partial) treatment with doses between 30 and 40 gy. For comparison, the total dose given to the cervical, axillary, and mediastinal nodes for Hodgkin disease is 40 gy, and myelosuppression (albeit a temporary one) is an expected adverse event in the treatment of this form of lymphoma.

Human Immunodeficiency Virus (HIV) Disease

Although HIV disease is a secondary immunodeficiency syndrome, it is discussed as a separate entity since it has had devastating socioeconomic ramifications and has caused historic changes in the field of immunology. Significant discoveries have been made recently about the pathophysiology of human immunodeficiency virus (HIV) infection, including the viral structure and the natural history of the disease. These new developments have greatly contributed to a better understanding of mechanisms of viral attachment, with potential impact on future disease control and treatment.[4]

HIV disease was first reported in the United States in 1981, and at the end of that year the number of reported cases for the whole country was 257. In 1983 HIV disease was declared epidemic, and the figures continued to steadily increase. By the end of the millennium, the number of reported cases in the U.S. will probably have reached the 1,000,000 mark. Such reported numbers represent total cumulative counts of all cases of acquired immune deficiency syndrome (AIDS–Category C disease) reported to the Centers for Disease Control and Prevention (CDC) since 1981, and includes persons who are still alive and those who have already died (approximately 60% at any point in time). These figures indicate a progressing epidemic, albeit a heterogeneous one; although some groups (male homosexuals) have shown a slight decline in new infections, among others (heterosexual females and adolescents) the rate of spread is steadily increasing. The modes of HIV transmission have been well identified and have remained unchanged throughout the history of this disease (Fig. 11-1).

The link between immune deficiency and AIDS became apparent early in the epidemic, since many of the opportunistic diseases observed (e.g., *Pneumocystis carinii* pneumonia and Kaposi sarcoma) had been previously reported among other groups of immune-suppressed persons. More detailed research and observation of greater numbers of infected individuals revealed that **helper T-cells** are the preferred host cells for this virus. HIV-induced helper T-cell death accounted for the progressive loss of both cell-mediated and humoral immune function. Other cell types have also been shown to be susceptible to HIV infection (Box 11-2).

THE VIRUS

Human immune deficiency virus, type I (HIV-1) is a non-oncogenic, cytopathic retrovirus (RNA-containing) belonging to the subfamily *lentivirus* ("slow virus"). Other lentiviruses found in non-human animals share some morphologic and pathogenic properties with HIV. They all cause slow, progressive wasting disorders, including neurologic degeneration, that are often fatal.

The HIV virion, or free viral particle, is approximately 100 to 120 nm (1 nm = one billionth of a meter) in diameter and consists of a central core surrounded by a lipid envelope (Fig. 11-2). Immediately inside the lipid membrane, a protein layer, p17, lines the inner surface of the virus. The inner cone-shaped core consists of a major capsid protein layer, p24, which surrounds the viral genome and several protein molecules, including protease, integrase, and reverse transcriptase. The viral genome consists of two copies of an RNA molecule bound to a nucleic acid–binding protein, p9, and capped on both ends by long terminal repeat (LTR) sequences. The RNA genome is approximately

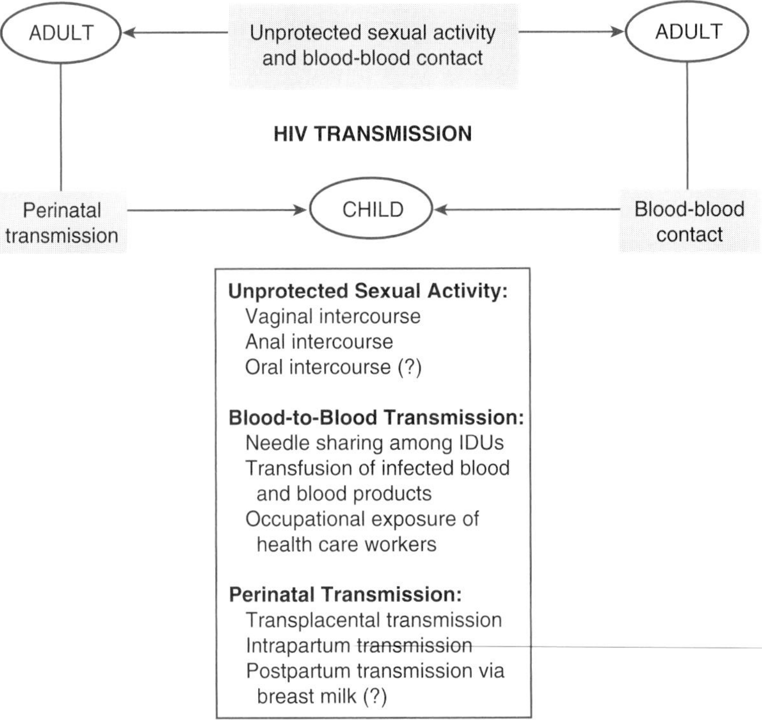

FIGURE 11-1. Conceptual model of HIV transmission. The three known modes of transmission are integrated with adult and children populations and individually characterized.

> **BOX 11-2**
> ## CELLS SUSCEPTIBLE TO HIV INFECTION
>
> ### Infection Observed in Vitro
> CD4+ lymphocytes
> Monocyte/macrophages
> Microglia
> Bone marrow CD34+ precursor cells
> Monocytic T-cell lines
> Glioma and neuroblastoma cell lines
> Tumor cell lines from colon and liver
>
> ### Infection Observed in Vivo
> CD4+ lymphocytes
> Monocyte/macrophages
> Epithelial Langerhans cells
> Follicular dendritic cells
> Brain endothelial cells
> Microglia, astroglia, oligodendroglia
> Undefined cells in the retina, cervix, and colon
>
> (DeVita, V. T., Hellman, S., & Rosenberg, S. A. [Eds.] [1997]. *AIDS: Etiology, diagnosis, treatment and prevention* [4th ed.]. Philadelphia: Lippincott-Raven.)

10 kilo-bases long and includes three major genes: *gag*, which encodes structural (core) proteins; *pol*, whose proteins reverse transcriptase, protease, polymerase, and endonuclease are directly involved in viral replication; and *env*, which codes for envelope glycoproteins. The gene *pol* also regulates ribonuclease H activity. The remaining genes, including *tat, rev,* and *nef*, are involved in the regulation of viral replication.[30] There are approximately 1,200 molecules of p24 and 80 molecules of reverse transcriptase in each HIV particle.[19]

The envelope consists of a lipid bilayer that has molecules of glycoproteins (gp41 is a transmembrane molecule, and gp120 units caps each gp 41 molecule) which loosely bind to CD4 receptors.[32] Both glycoproteins play important roles in the recognition of host cells' receptors. There are up to 280 molecules of gp120 in each HIV particle.[19]

HIV LIFE CYCLE

Like all viruses, HIV is an essential parasite and must infect target cells in order to replicate. Initial attachment requires recognition of a cellular receptor, CD4, although direct infection of $CD4^+$ cells has been reported. Many of the cell lines that are susceptible to HIV infection are **antigen-presenting cells (APC)**, and their eventual death further contributes to failure of immune response (see Box 11-2).[37] In addition, the ubiquitous distribution of many of these cells is responsible for the wide dissemination of HIV infection.

Figure 11-3 illustrates the various phases of the viral life cycle. The early events in the cycle (attachment, internalization, reverse transcription, and DNA duplication) constitute the afferent functions. The later events of the cycle (the efferent) include integration, transcription, and translation of viral proteins.

Viral Attachment: The Chemokine Connection

Following entry of HIV into the blood stream, specialized macrophages phagocytize the viral particles and transport them to lymph nodes, where they encounter

FOCUS ON CELLULAR PATHOPHYSIOLOGY

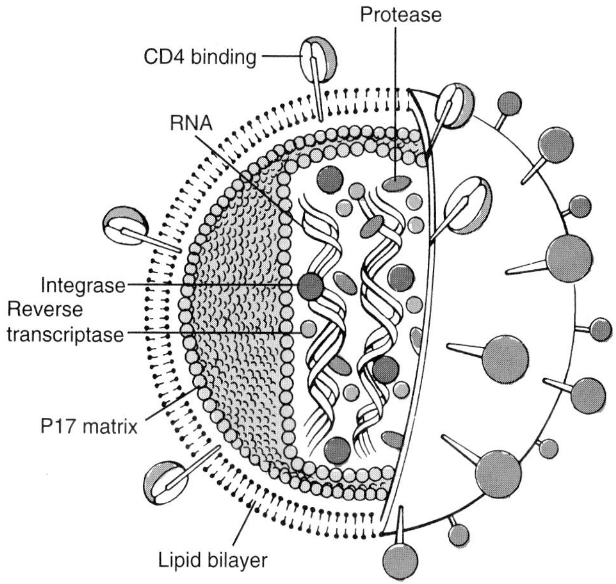

FIGURE 11-2. Structure of the human immunodeficiency virus (HIV). The envelope consists of a phospholipid bilayer studded with transmembrane glycoprotein gp41 to which attach molecules of glycoprotein gp120 (CD4 binding site). The internal layer consists of a protein p17 matrix. The conical core is formed by protein p24 and encloses the two copies of the RNA genome, and viral-encoded reverse transcriptase, integrase, and protease enzyme molecules.

FOCUS ON CELLULAR PATHOPHYSIOLOGY

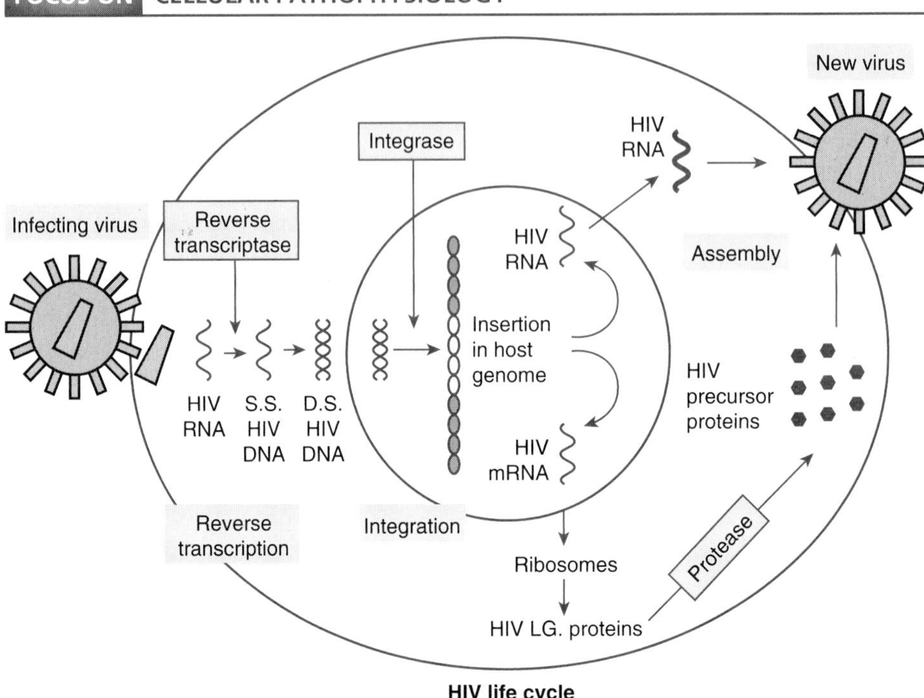

FIGURE 11-3. Life cycle of the human immunodeficiency virus (HIV), illustrating the sequence of events from attachment of an infecting viral particle to the budding of new viruses. Highlighted are the key enzymes in viral replication—reverse transcriptase, integrase, and protease—with the areas where they impact replication, reverse transcription, integration, and viral assembly highlighted in white. (S.S. HIV DNA = single-stranded HIV DNA; D.S. HIV DNA = double-stranded HIV DNA.)

an abundance of CD4$^+$ T-cells. Viral gp120 initiates the attachment process by binding to the host cell's CD4 receptor, but final fusion with the host cell requires viral interaction (via gp41) with another cellular co-receptor. The cooperation of another co-receptor in the binding process was first suggested by unsuccessful attempts at infecting HIV onto mouse cells engineered to express CD4.[37] In mid-1996, several research papers in *Science, Nature,* and *Cell* were published identifying HIV co-receptors.[40] The key element in this discovery is a group of chemoattractant cytokines secreted by CD8$^+$ T-cells, termed *chemokines.* Human chemokines (more than 25 chemokines and 11 receptors are known) belong to either the alpha family (or CXC), which act primarily on neutrophils, or the beta family (or CC), which act on lymphocytes, monocytes, mast cells, and eosinophils.[27] Some cytokines (including the types Rantes, MIP-1alpha, and MIP-1beta) bind and block specific receptors, which are also used by HIV for attaching to host cells. Primary HIV strains (i.e., those entering the body, prior to replication) use a beta-chemokine receptor, CKR-5 (chemokine receptor 5), on the surface of macrophages, and beta-chemokines can inhibit HIV attachment by blocking that receptor. Figure 11-4 presents a conceptual model to illustrate the relationship between CD4 and CKR-5 receptors. Subsequent generations of viruses (those that emerged from infected cells) bind to another receptor, CXCR4 (CX chemokine receptor 4), which is not bound by primary viruses. This discovery suggests that important functional differences exist between primary and secondary viruses.

By blocking HIV receptors, chemokines may represent an important weapon against viral attachment. It was suggested that elevated levels of beta-chemokine control HIV load and replication in individuals who do not progress to AIDS after infection with HIV (termed non-progressors, or long-term survivors). High levels of beta-chemokines also explain the fact that some individuals appear to have increased resistance to infection, such as the sexual partners of HIV-infected persons who never become infected.[27] One intervention possibility would be to develop vaccines aimed at increasing levels of chemokines, or to decrease (down-regulate) the number of receptors to chemokines. In addition, the fact that beta-chemokines, as proteins, are under genetic control opens new doors to the possibility of future genetic intervention towards HIV resistance.

FOCUS ON CELLULAR PATHOPHYSIOLOGY

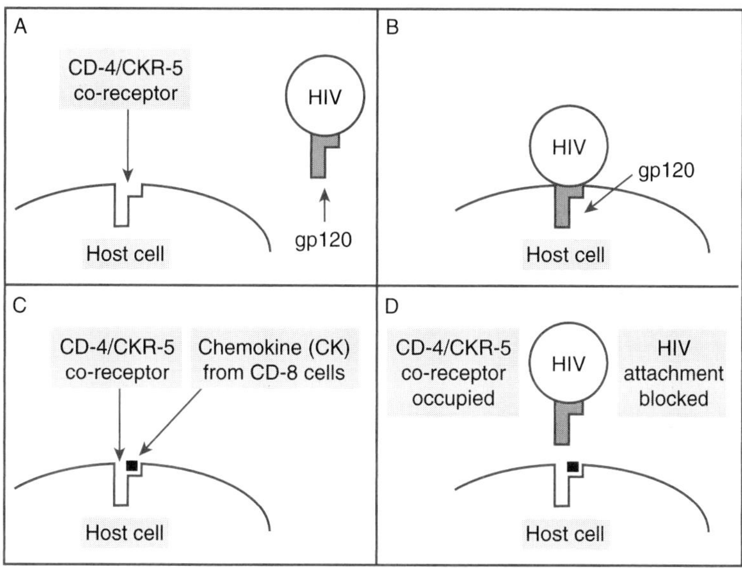

FIGURE 11-4. HIV attachment: The chemokine connection. **A.** CD4/CKR-5 co-receptors and viral gp120 are the recognition sites for HIV attachment. **B.** If the host cell CD4/CKR-5 co-receptor is unoccupied, HIV attaches and initiates the replication cycle. **C.** Chemokines (CK) secreted by CD8 cells bind to the CKR-5 portion of the co-receptor. **D.** With the host cell co-receptor partially occupied by a chemokine molecule, the HIV particle is unable to attach, preventing further viral replication.

Internalization and Integration

Recognition and attachment are followed by fusion of the viral envelope with the host cell membrane, which has a similar lipid constitution. The virus core enters the host cell (internalization) and is then uncoated to reveal its RNA genome and its *gag* and *pol* proteins. Reverse transcriptase, a *pol*-encoded enzyme, then mediates the process of reverse transcription of the viral genetic information from RNA to single-stranded DNA.

Because of the high rate of replication error, reverse transcription is the phase of the viral cycle that generates most of the viral genomic variability that allows HIV to escape immune surveillance and to develop resistance to antiretroviral therapy. The single-stranded viral DNA molecule then undergoes duplication and emerges as a double-stranded DNA molecule capable of penetrating into the nucleus and competent for integration into the host cell's genome. The integration process is mediated by another viral-encoded enzyme, integrase. Integration of the viral genome into the host cell's genetic material appears to be essential for viral replication, and integration occurs at a fixed position in the genome of the cell.

Activation and Virus Assembly

Integration results in an infected host cell that has acquired the genomic complement of HIV as a provirion, and the cluster of viral genes replicates as original cellular genes, so that upon cell division, the resulting daughter cells also carry copies of the provirion. This state of permanent infection is maintained in approximately 1% of all infected cells. Activation of infected cells is necessary for the completion of viral replication. T-lymphocyte activation results from exogenous influences, such as cytokines, and other physiologic stimuli. Under these influences, the remaining 99% of infected cells will undergo activation and initiate transcription and translation of viral proteins. The first products are large protein molecules (Gag-Pol protein) of high molecular weight. The viral-encoded protease then cleaves these large molecules into smaller units, amenable to being assembled with other viral components (including RNA molecules) into new viruses. The assembly process is completed near the host cell membrane, and the emerging viruses are released by budding out of the host cell, utilizing cell membrane components to form its own lipid envelope.

A thorough understanding of the HIV life cycle is essential for the development of antiviral strategies. Currently, the only antiretroviral agents available are reverse transcriptase inhibitors and protease inhibitors. Given the complexity of viral replication, many points in the HIV life cycle, for which antiretroviral intervention will be eventually developed, remain to be ex-

TABLE 11-3

T4 CELL COUNTS AND T4/T8 CELL RATIOS IN HIV DISEASE

IMMUNE STATUS	T4 COUNT (CELLS/MM^3)	T4/T8 CELL RATIO
Competent immune system	650–1,200	2:1
"Suppressed" immune system	500–200	1:1
AIDS-indicator values	<200	0.5:1

plored. Potential cellular targets include mechanisms to block viral attachment and post-infection cellular activation. Viral targets appear to be more promising and include inhibition of integrase and various other replication-related enzymes.

Consequences of Viral Replication

HIV infection results in two major consequences—the number of viruses in plasma increases, and infected cells progressively die. Until recently, helper T-cell (T4) counts and the helper-to-suppressor (T4/T8) ratio were standard methods of assessing disease progression, since they are cost effective and easily available procedures. Table 11-3 illustrates the relationship among immune status, T4 cell count, and T4/T8 cell ratio. Currently, T4 cell counts alone are still useful in determining initiation of prophylaxis against opportunistic infections. A T4 cell count of 200 or fewer cells/mm^3 is an AIDS-defining value and signals the possibility of impending diseases such as *Pneumocystis carinii* pneumonia, the most prevalent opportunistic infection in HIV disease (see p. 307). At these T4 cell values, treatment with medications such as trimethoprim-sulfamethoxazole or pentamidine isethionate is usually initiated. However, the exclusive use of T-cell counts as predictors of disease outcome has many disadvantages: T4 counts fluctuate from count to count and show significant circadian variations. Also, a large number of HIV-infected individuals exists who remain asymptomatic in spite of markedly decreased T-cell counts. Ratios between helper and suppressor T-cells (T4/T8 ratios) have also proved ineffective as predictors of disease progression, as they involve two cell populations with double variability. These deficiencies led to searches for better disease progression markers.

Recent studies indicate plasma viral load (number of circulating HIV particles per milliliter) is a strong, independent predictor of clinical outcome.[25] Viral load determination became possible after the development of polymerase chain reaction (PCR), a technique that allows minute amounts of genetic material to be serially replicated until a concentration adequate for testing is reached.[22] The correlation between viral load and disease progression is shown in Table 11-4. Currently, a combination of viral load determination and T4 cell counts is used as criteria for initiation of antiretroviral therapy (Table 11-5).[8]

Various models to explain T-cell loss have been proposed (Box 11-3). The possibility that HIV infection might trigger autoimmune destruction of T-cells is remote, as is cytotoxicity caused by viral replication (new viruses emerge by budding, with major cell disruption). HIV particles have been observed within bone marrow stem cells, indicating that the progenies of such cells would be born already infected. The models best supported by research evidence are **apoptosis** and **syncytia** formation. Apoptosis is a form of genetically-induced cell death that occurs in physiologic and pathologic conditions.[2,3,18,28] In HIV infection, the binding of viral gp120 to cellular receptors activates the caspase enzyme cycle, with the consequent destruction of the host cell.[13] Compounding the damage by individual infected cells is the fact that infected and uninfected cells cluster together in syncytia. This is a term used to designate fusion of cells resulting in large masses of cytoplasm with multiple nuclei. The resulting loss of normal tissue architecture causes the death of infected and healthy cells. The combination of apoptosis and syncytia formation accounts for the excessively high rate of cell death observed in HIV disease.

Given the two major consequences of HIV infection—viral increase and host cell death—it is of paramount importance that treatment approaches for HIV disease include antiretroviral agents and some

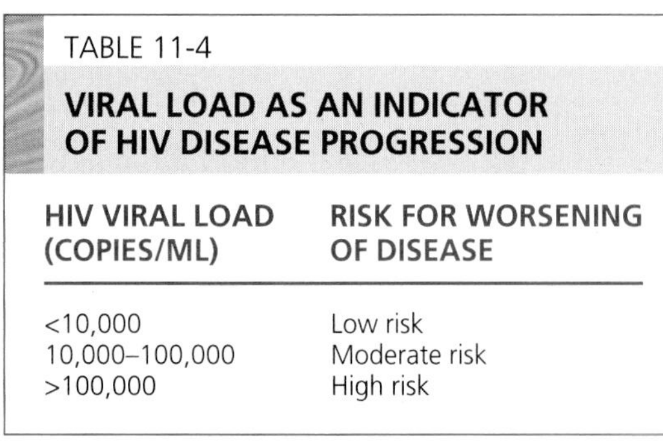

TABLE 11-4

VIRAL LOAD AS AN INDICATOR OF HIV DISEASE PROGRESSION

HIV VIRAL LOAD (COPIES/ML)	RISK FOR WORSENING OF DISEASE
<10,000	Low risk
10,000–100,000	Moderate risk
>100,000	High risk

TABLE 11-5

INDICATIONS FOR INITIATION OF ANTIRETROVIRAL TREATMENT IN THE CHRONICALLY HIV-INFECTED ADULT/ADOLESCENT PATIENT

STATUS	RECOMMENDATION
Symptomatic (including Category B symptoms) T-cell count: any value Viral load: any value	Treat all
Asymptomatic T-cell count <500/mm^3 *or* viral load >20,000/mL (RT-PCR)	Treatment should be offered, based on disease-free survival and patient's willingness to accept treatment
Asymptomatic T-cell count >500/mm^3 *and* viral load <20,000/mL (RT-PCR)	Some experts recommend treatment; others prefer to delay treatment and observe

(Centers for Disease Control and Prevention. [1998]. Report of the NIH Panel to Define Principles of Therapy of HIV Infection and Guidelines for the Use of Antiretroviral Agents in HIV-Infected Adults and Adolescents. *Morbidity and Mortality Weekly Report (MMWR); 47*(RR-05), 43–82.)

modality of T-cell replenishment, perhaps with the use of biologic response modifiers. Currently the only successful weapons are antiretroviral therapies, but intensive research is being conducted on vaccine development and biologic response modifiers.

CLINICAL SPECTRUM OF HIV DISEASE

HIV disease has been classified by the CDC for both adult/adolescent and pediatric populations.[6,7] These definitions should be considered as reference parameters for classification purposes only.

Adult HIV Disease

The CDC classification of adult HIV disease is based on clinical findings (Clinical Categories A, B, and C) and on T4 cell counts (Categories 1, 2, and 3). The parameters for this classification are summarized in Table 11-6.

An appropriate exposure is a contact with a pathogen that results in infection. Following such an exposure, HIV gains access to the host's circulation and initiates replication. Recent research data indicate that the virus immediately starts its replication cycle, without a latent period. This has two significant implications: an infected person may be able to transmit HIV soon after infection, and therapy planning and initiation should be considered as soon as possible. The sequence of events that follows represents a continuum of disease progression, with asymptomatic and symptomatic periods. The disease course is highly variable with respect to disease events and time frame. The time line represented in Figure 11-5 summarizes this progression, and the question marks (?) along the line reflect the variability in time frame.

CATEGORY A DISEASE. This disease is represented by a heterogeneous group of events (Box 11-4). It includes newly infected symptomatic persons who may or may not be aware of their infection status. Approximately 2 to 4 weeks after infection, 90% of all infected persons develop a transient influenza- or mononucleosis-like symptomatology termed *acute retroviral syndrome (ARS)*, or *primary HIV infection*. The most common symptoms of ARS include fever, pharyngitis, headache, malaise, and, at times, a diffuse skin rash, a roseola-like eruption occurring mainly on the trunk and limbs. Other symptoms may include arthralgias, lymphadenopathy, gastrointestinal findings, and photophobia. This temporary and self-limiting illness usually subsides within a few days, and the infected person returns to an asymptomatic status.

Acute retroviral syndrome probably represents an attempt by the immune system to control the infection in its early stages. With virus multiplication progressing unopposed, seroconversion usually occurs within 6 to

BOX 11-3

MODELS OF T-CELL LOSS

HIV (gp 120)–induced apoptosis
Formation of syncytia
Infection of stem cells
Replication-induced cytotoxicity
Autoimmune mechanisms

TABLE 11-6

1993 REVISED CLASSIFICATION SYSTEM FOR HIV INFECTION AND EXPANDED AIDS SURVEILLANCE CASE DEFINITION FOR ADOLESCENTS AND ADULTS*

	CLINICAL CATEGORIES		
CD4⁺ T-CELL CATEGORIES	(A) Asymptomatic, Acute (Primary) HIV or PGL†	(B) Symptomatic, Not (A) or (C) Conditions†	(C) AIDS-Indicator Conditions†
(1) ≥500/mm^3	A1	B1	C1
(2) 200–499/mm^3	A2	B2	C2
(3) <200/mm^3 AIDS-indicator T-cell count	A3	B3	C3

HIV: human immunodeficiency virus; AIDS: acquired immunodeficiency syndrome; PDL: persistent generalized lymphadenopathy.
* The shaded cells illustrate the expanded AIDS surveillance case definition. Persons with AIDS-indicator conditions (Category C) as well as those with CD4⁺ T-lymphocyte counts <200/mm^3 (Category A3 or B3) are reportable as AIDS cases in the United States and Territories, effective January 1, 1993.
† See text for discussion.
(From the U.S. Centers for Disease Control and Prevention. [1992]. 1993 revised classification system for HIV infection and expanded surveillance case definition for AIDS among adolescents and adults. *MMWR, 41* [No. RR-17], 1.)

12 weeks after infection. This seroconversion time represents the time it takes for HIV-infected asymptomatic persons to yield positive results on antibody tests such as the **ELISA** (enzyme-linked immunosorbent assay) and the **Western blot**. Once seroconversion occurs, most persons will continue to test HIV antibody–positive. The lack of detectable antibodies may occur during a time called the "seroconversion window" during which a virally infected individual will have a negative result on an antibody test. For this reason, it is imperative that tests with negative results be repeated at determined intervals to confirm the absence

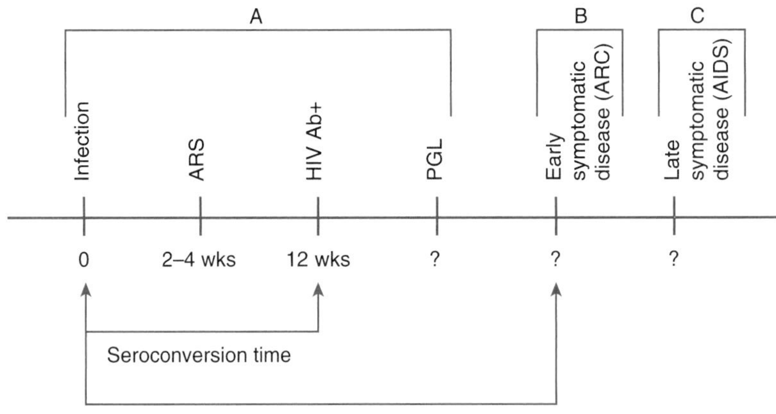

FIGURE 11-5. Timeline model of HIV disease, from infection (time 0) to the development of late symptomatic disease (Category C, or AIDS). Illustrated here are the highlights of HIV disease C. ARS = acute retroviral syndrome; HIV Ab⁺ = HIV antibody positive, the marker for seroconversion; PGL = persistent generalized lymphadenopathy; ARC = AIDS-related complex, a term no longer used. Seroconversion time, expressed in weeks, marks the individual's conversion to HIV-antibody positivity, signaling infection. Incubation time, measured in years (median time above 13 years), expresses the length of the asymptomatic phase, with the development of early symptomatic disease (Category B). Refer to text for further details.

BOX 11-4

CATEGORY A ADULT HIV DISEASE

Acute Retroviral Syndrome (ARS), or Primary HIV infection

Negative HIV antibody test
Acute, self-limiting, influenza-like symptomatology occurring 2–4 weeks after infection; rash may occur
Most symptoms subside after a few days

Asymptomatic Infection

Positive antibody test (2 ELISAs + 1 WB)
No disease process

Persistent Generalized Lymphadenopathy (PGL)

Positive antibody test (2 ELISAs + 1 WB)
Lymphadenopathy (>1 cm diameter at two or more extra-inguinal sites for more than 3 months)

(Centers for Disease Control and Prevention. [1992]. 1993 revised classification system for HIV infection and expanded surveillance case definition for AIDS among adolescents and adults. *Morbidity and Mortality Weekly Report (MMWR), 41*[RR-17], 1.)

of HIV infection. After the resolution of acute retroviral syndrome, infected persons regain an asymptomatic state and may remain relatively healthy for a long time.

The term *asymptomatic infection* refers to the absence of clinical manifestations that can be directly attributed to the HIV infection. In some cases, a few nonspecific manifestations, such as headache and lymphadenopathy, may be seen in this otherwise asymptomatic phase. The next significant landmark, which occurs at variable periods of time, is the development of *persistent generalized lymphadenopathy (PGL)*, lymph node enlargement to diameters greater than 1 cm and occurring at two or more extra-inguinal sites for longer than 3 months. Despite the absence of clinical findings in the majority of cases, occasional non-specific manifestations such as anemia, neutropenia, and thrombocytopenia may occur. The most HIV-specific change seen during this phase is a steady decline in helper T-cells, corresponding at times to annual losses of 40 to 80 cells/mm^3 in untreated individuals. The median duration of the asymptomatic phase, often termed incubation time, as limited by the diagnosis of HIV-related disease processes (Category B disease) has been reported to be as long as 12 years.

CATEGORY B DISEASE. Formerly termed AIDS-related complex, this condition represents early symptomatic disease (non-Category A, non-Category C symptoms), usually precipitated by a progressive loss of helper T-cells and resulting from long-standing infection with HIV. The depression of immune function facilitates the development of conditions that are relatively rare among immunocompetent persons (Box 11-5). These include **opportunistic infections** caused by various microorganisms, such as viruses (e.g., varicella-zoster virus), fungi (e.g., *Candida albicans*), and protozoa (e.g., *Toxoplasma sp.*), as well as a variety of conditions such as fever, night sweats, chronic diarrhea, fatigue, headache, hairy leukoplakia, idiopathic thrombocytopenic purpura, pelvic inflammatory disease, peripheral neuropathy, and cervical dysplasia. The severity of the manifestations of the infections ranges from minor to life-threatening.

BOX 11-5

CATEGORY B ADULT HIV DISEASE

(Former Terminology: AIDS-Related Complex, or ARC)

"Symptomatic conditions in an HIV-infected adolescent/adult that are not *included among conditions listed in clinical Categories A or C. For classification purposes, Category B conditions take precedence over those in Category A" [CDC definition, from MMWR 1992, 41 (RR-17)].*

- Usually a positive antibody test (2 ELISAs + 1 WB)
- *Examples* of conditions include, but are not limited to:
  - Oropharyngeal candidiasis (oral thrush)
  - Vulvovaginal candidiasis persistent, frequent, or poorly responsive to treatment
  - Cervical dysplasia (moderate to severe), or cervical carcinoma in situ
  - Constitutional symptoms, such as fever (38.5°C or diarrhea lasting >1 month
  - Oral hairy leukoplakia
  - Herpes zoster (shingles) involving at least two distinct episodes or more than one dermatome
  - Pelvic inflammatory disease (PID), particularly if complicated by tubo-ovarian abscess
  - Peripheral neuropathy

(Centers for Disease Control and Prevention. [1992]. 1993 revised classification system for HIV infection and expanded surveillance case definition for AIDS among adolescents and adults. *Morbidity and Mortality Weekly Report (MMWR), 41*[RR-17], 1.)

CATEGORY C DISEASE. This represents a series of more severe disease processes and opportunistic diseases that are AIDS defining and result from severely depressed T4 cell counts below 200 cells/mm^3 (Box 11-6). These include opportunistic infections caused by protozoa, viruses, bacteria and fungi; malignancies; neurologic disorders; and HIV wasting syndrome. Although some of the opportunistic infections can be avoided or managed with adequate prophylactic or therapeutic intervention, their underlying cause is the host's severe immune dysfunction. Even if controlling *Pneumocystis* pneumonia spares many lives, a T4 cell count below 50 cells/mm^3 greatly increases the risk of recurring opportunistic diseases and death. However, the use of antiretroviral therapy, especially with multiple drug protocols, has significantly reduced the incidence of AIDS-related morbidity and mortality, and many clinicians have been following patients with counts below 10 cells/mm^3 for as long as 5 to 7 years.[34]

Pediatric HIV Disease

Most children with HIV disease acquired the virus from their HIV-infected mothers (87%); of the remaining, 9% were infected by transfusion of contaminated blood and blood products (including hemophiliacs treated with clotting factors), and 4% are still under investigation. There are three outcomes for children born to HIV-infected mothers:

- 10% to 15% develop AIDS in the first few months of life and die soon after.
- 15% to 20% are relatively well during infancy, but gradually become chronically ill and die in childhood.
- 65% to 75% will thrive. They are not infected.

BOX 11-6

CATEGORY C HIV ADULT DISEASE (AIDS-DEFINING)

(Synonym: AIDS)

"Category C includes the clinical conditions below. For classification purposes, once a Category C condition has occurred, the person will remain in Category C" [CDC definition, from MMWR 1992, 41(RR-17)].

- Usually positive antibody tests (2 ELISAs + 1 WB)
- AIDS-defining conditions (*complete list*):

Opportunistic Infections

Pneumocystis carinii pneumonia (PCP)
Candidiasis of bronchi, trachea, or lungs
Esophageal candidiasis
Cytomegalovirus (CMV) disease (other than liver, spleen, or nodes)
CMV retinitis (with loss of vision)
Herpes simplex: chronic ulcers (>1 month), herpetic bronchitis, pneumonitis, esophagitis
Mycobacterium avium complex (MAC) or *M. kansaii,* disseminated or extrapulmonary
Mycobacterium tuberculosis infection, any site
Mycobacterium sp. infection, any site
Recurrent pneumonia
Toxoplasmosis of the brain
Salmonella septicemia
Coccidioidomycosis, disseminated or extrapulmonary
Cryptococcosis, extrapulmonary
Cryptosporidiosis, chronic intestinal (>1 month)
Histoplasmosis, disseminated or extrapulmonary
Isosporiasis, chronic intestinal (>1 month)

Malignancies

Kaposi sarcoma (KS)
Invasive cervical cancer
Lymphomas: primary lymphoma of brain, Burkitt's lymphoma, immunoblastic lymphoma

Neurologic manifestations

HIV-related encephalopathy (including AIDS dementia complex)
Progressive multifocal leukoencephalopathy (PML)

HIV wasting syndrome

Unintentional weight loss of 10% or more of body weight, within a 6-month period

(Centers for Disease Control and Prevention. [1992]. 1993 revised classification system for HIV infection and expanded surveillance case definition for AIDS among adolescents and adults. *Morbidity and Mortality Weekly Report (MMWR), 41*[RR-17], 1.)

This indicates that a child born to an infected mother has only a 25% to 30% chance of being infected. The chances of infection are a function of maternal viral load. Therefore, reducing the number of maternal circulating viruses is of paramount importance in reducing the rate of infection. A study, conducted by the AIDS Clinical Trials Group 076 (ACTG 076), treated HIV-infected pregnant women with antiretrovirals, which resulted in a decrease in the rate of transmission by two-thirds (to 8%).[12] A recent study reported a significantly lower rate of transmission (to 1%) by combining zidovudine (AZT) treatment with Cesarean delivery.[22]

Pediatric HIV disease is classified according to clinical parameters into Categories N, A, B, and C, and according to immunologic categories by correlation of immunologic dysfunction with T4 lymphocyte count and percentage of total lymphocytes (Tables 11-7 and 11-8). As in adult disease, these classifications are meant to serve as guidelines to clinicians and are subject to periodic change.

Clinical category N represents no detectable symptoms of HIV disease, and Category A reflects a mild disease pattern (Box 11-7). The signs and symptoms of the disease become increasingly severe in categories B and C (Boxes 11-8 and 11-9). As with adults, *P. carinii* pneumonia is the most common opportunistic disease in children with HIV. Another major cause of morbidity and mortality is lymphoid interstitial pneumonitis (LIP), a chronic, progressive lung interstitial disease that presents often without cough and fever and with an unremarkable chest examination. LIP may accompany lymphadenopathy, enlarged parotid glands (parotitis), and digital clubbing. In the case of either disease, children who develop pulmonary disease have a poor prognosis. The most common opportunistic diseases in pediatric HIV infection are listed in Table 11-9.

SELECTED OPPORTUNISTIC DISEASES IN HIV DISEASE

Pneumocystis carinii Pneumonia (PCP)

This pulmonary infection is a relatively rare disease outside the group of severely immune-suppressed persons. Among HIV-infected individuals, PCP is the presenting disease in 65% of all cases and accounts for approximately 75% of all deaths in HIV disease. PCP is caused by a fungus-like organism, formerly classified as a protozoan, which results in a pattern of interstitial pulmonary consolidation similar to that seen in fungal pneumonias. Research supports the belief that infection with P. carinii occurs during early life, and the microorganism is kept in check by an intact immune system until immunosuppression occurs. In this sense, PCP as seen in HIV-infected adults represents a reactivation of a preexisting infection. HIV-infected persons at highest risk for developing PCP include those with a baseline T4 cell count of 200 or fewer cells/mm3, those with thrush and fever, and those who have previously had an episode of PCP. Manifestations of PCP include a persistent, nonproductive cough; progressive shortness of breath; tachypnea; and fever.

Toxoplasmosis

This infection is the second most common neurologic disease in AIDS and is caused by a protozoan, *Toxoplasma gondii*, whose definitive host is the domestic cat. Humans usually acquire the microorganism by

TABLE 11-7

PEDIATRIC HIV DISEASE CLASSIFICATION*

IMMUNOLOGIC CATEGORIES	CLINICAL CATEGORIES: N: No Signs/ Symptoms	A: Mild Signs/ Symptoms	B: Moderate Signs/ Symptoms†	C: Severe Signs/ Symptoms†
1: No evidence of suppression	N1	A1	B1	C1
2: Evidence of moderate suppression	N2	A2	B2	C2
3: Severe suppression	N3	A3	B3	C3

*Children whose HIV infection status is not confirmed are classified by using the above grid with a letter E (for perinatally exposed) placed before classification code (e.g., EN2).

† Both Category C and lymphoid interstitial pneumonitis in Category B are reportable to state and local health departments as acquired immunodeficiency syndrome (AIDS).

(Centers for Disease Control and Prevention. [1994]. 1994 Revised classification system for human immunodeficiency virus infection in children less than 13 years of age. *Morbidity and Mortality Weekly Report (MMWR), 30*(RR-12), 1–11.)

TABLE 11-8

PEDIATRIC HIV DISEASE IMMUNOLOGIC CATEGORIES BASED ON AGE-SPECIFIC T4 LYMPHOCYTE COUNTS AND PERCENT OF TOTAL LYMPHOCYTES

	AGE OF CHILD					
	< 12 Months		1–5 Years		6–12 Years	
IMMUNOLOGIC CATEGORY*	μL	%	μL	%	μL	%
1	≥1,500	≥25	≥1,000	≥25	≥500	≥25
2	750–1,499	15–24	500–999	15–24	200–499	15–24
3	≤750	<15	<500	<15	<200	<15

* Category 1: No evidence of suppression; Category 2: Evidence of moderate suppression; Category 3: Severe suppression. (Centers for Disease Control and Prevention. [1994]. 1994 Revised classification system for human immunodeficiency virus infection in children less than 13 years of age. *Morbidity and Mortality Weekly Report [MMWR], 30*[RR-12], 1–11.)

ingesting its oocysts (ova) excreted in cat feces or in cysts present in inadequately cooked meats. Infection with *T. gondii* is the most common cause of focal encephalitis in HIV-infected persons. Immunologic evidence for the presence of *T. gondii* can be found in a least 50% of the adult U.S. population, which again suggests that the disease seen in HIV-infected persons is a reactivation of previous infection. Clinical manifestations of toxoplasmosis include headache, fever, hemiparesis, seizures, ataxia, aphasia, altered mental states, confusion, dizziness, and coma.

BOX 11-7 CATEGORIES N AND A PEDIATRIC HIV DISEASE

Category N: Non-symptomatic

- No signs and symptoms of HIV-related disease
- One of the conditions listed in category A (below)

Category A: Mildly Symptomatic

- Two or more of the following, but none of the conditions listed in categories B and C:
  - Lymphadenopathy (≥0.5 cm at more than two sites. Bilateral = one site)
  - Hepatomegaly
  - Splenomegaly
  - Dermatitis
  - Parotitis
  - Recurrent or persistent upper respiratory infection, sinusitis, or otitis media

(Centers for Disease Control and Prevention. [1994]. 1994 revised classification system for human immunodeficiency virus infection in children less than 13 years of age. *Morbidity and Mortality Weekly Report [MMWR], 30*[RR-12] 1–11.)

Chronic Cryptosporidiosis

This common debilitating disease is caused by a variety of species of the genus Cryptosporidium, a coccidian protozoan commonly found in farm animals and recently reported in humans. Sources of infection include infected humans and contaminated food or water. Fecal–oral transmission is the presumed mode of transmission. In persons with AIDS, this infection causes a persistent, voluminous, watery diarrhea, resulting in massive fluid loss and weight loss. Spread to other organs, such as the lung and gallbladder, has been reported.

Isosporiasis

This enteric infection is caused by the coccidian protozoan *Isospora belli* and produces symptoms similar to those of cryptosporidiosis. Although rare in the United States, it has been reported in increasing numbers among immigrants from the Caribbean and Africa.

Recurrent Pneumonias

Pneumonias of varying etiology were included for the first time in the AIDS-defining diseases category in 1993. The term recurrent pneumonia is defined by the CDC as bacterial or viral pneumonias occurring at the rate of two or more episodes per year.

Tuberculosis (TB)

Mycobacterium tuberculosis at pulmonary or extrapulmonary sites was also included among Category C diseases in the 1993 classification revision. Mycobacterial tuberculosis may be the presenting illness in HIV-infected individuals, especially among injecting-drug users. TB has been an increasing concern due to its

(text continues on page 310)

BOX 11-8

CATEGORY B PEDIATRIC HIV DISEASE: MODERATELY SYMPTOMATIC

- HIV-related symptoms other than those in Categories A or C
- *Examples* of conditions include, but are not limited to:
  - Anemia, neutropenia, or thrombocytopenia persisting for ≥30 days
  - Bacterial meningitis, pneumonia, or sepsis (single episode)
  - Candidiasis, oropharyngeal, persisting >2 months in children older than 6 months
  - Cardiomyopathy
  - CMV infection, onset before 1 month of age
  - Diarrhea, recurrent or chronic
  - Hepatitis
  - Herpes simplex virus (HSV) stomatitis, recurrent
  - HSV bronchitis, pneumonitis, or esophagitis, onset <age 1 month
  - Herpes zoster (shingles) in two distinct episodes or in more than one dermatome
  - Leiomyosarcoma
  - Lymphoid interstitial pneumonitis (LIP) or pulmonary hyperplasia complex
  - Nephropathy
  - Nocardiosis
  - Persistent fever, lasting >1 month
  - Toxoplasmosis, onset <age 1 month
  - Varicella, disseminated (complicated chickenpox)

(Centers for Disease Control and Prevention. [1994]. 1994 revised classification system for human immunodeficiency virus infection in children less than 13 years of age. *Morbidity and Mortality Weekly Report [MMWR], 30*[RR-12], 1–11.)

BOX 11-9

CATEGORY C PEDIATRIC HIV DISEASE: SEVERELY SYMPTOMATIC

Any condition listed in 1987 classification (*MMWR* 1987, *36,* 225–230) (except LIP), including:

- Serious bacterial infections, multiple or recurrent (2-year period), *including* septicemia, pneumonia, meningitis, bone or joint infection, abscess of internal organ or body cavity, and *excluding* otitis media, superficial abscesses, indwelling catheter-related infections
- Candidiasis, esophageal or pulmonary (bronchi, trachea, lungs)
- Coccidioidomycosis, disseminated
- Cryptococcosis, extrapulmonary
- Cryptosporidiosis or isosporidiosis with diarrhea persisting >1 month
- CMV disease, onset >age 1 month
- Encephalopathy
- Herpes simplex virus (HSV) mucocutaneous ulcer persisting >1 month, or HSV bronchitis, pneumonitis, or esophagitis in child > age 1 month
- Histoplasmosis, disseminated
- Kaposi sarcoma
- Lymphomas: primary, of the brain; Burkitt lymphoma; immunoblastic or large cell lymphoma
- *Mycobacterium* tuberculosis, disseminated or extrapulmonary, or other mycobacterium species, disseminated
- *Mycobacterium avium* complex (MAC) or *M. kansaii,* disseminated
- *Pneumocystis carinii* pneumonia (PCP)
- Progressive multifocal leukoencephalopathy (PML)
- *Salmonella* (non-typhoid) septicemia, recurrent
- Toxoplasmosis of the brain, onset >age 1 month
- Wasting syndrome

(Centers for Disease Control and Prevention. [1994]. 1994 revised classification system for human immunodeficiency virus infection in children less than 13 years of age. *Morbidity and Mortality Weekly Report [MMWR], 30*[RR-12], 1–11.)

TABLE 11-9

MOST FREQUENT OPPORTUNISTIC DISEASES IN PEDIATRIC HIV DISEASE

DIAGNOSIS	FREQUENCY (%)
Pneumocystis carinii pneumonia	36
Lymphoid interstitial pneumonitis	24
Recurrent bacterial infections	20
HIV wasting syndrome	15
Candida esophagitis	15
HIV encephalopathy	14
Cytomegalovirus disease	8
Mycobacterium avium infection	6
Pulmonary candidiasis	4
Herpes simplex disease	4
Cryptosporidiosis	4
Other opportunistic infections	6
Malignancies	2

communicability and increased prevalence. In addition, some strains of *M. tuberculosis* have become resistant to traditionally efficient therapeutic agents. Clinical manifestations include persistent cough, fever, night sweats, fatigue, and weight loss.

Mycobacterium avium Complex (MAC)

This rare type of tuberculosis is found in 20% to 40% of persons with advanced HIV disease, resulting from infection with *Mycobacterium avium*, or *M. kansasii.* The hallmark of this infection is extensive extrapulmonary involvement. The gastrointestinal tract is usually the site of entry, and dissemination to the bone marrow, lymph nodes, and liver is common. Clinical manifestations include fever, anorexia, night sweats, malaise, weight loss, and weakness. Cough, headache, diarrhea, and abdominal pain are other symptoms of this infection.

Malignancies

Various types of malignancies are considered to be AIDS-defining diseases among HIV-infected persons and are included in Category C disease.

Kaposi sarcoma (KS), an angiosarcoma, is significantly prevalent (26%) among HIV-infected gay and bisexual men, but has remained rare in other HIV-infected groups. Susceptibility to KS is increased by infection with a sexually transmitted type of herpes virus termed KSHV (Kaposi sarcoma herpes virus), in the same manner that infection with human papilloma virus increases the risk of cervical cancer in infected women.[13] This epidemic form of KS is more aggressive and has a higher metastatic potential than the other major KS type found in elderly men of Mediterranean ancestry. Although not clearly defined, it appears that the two variants may be separate disease entities. The AIDS-associated KS is generally quite aggressive and causes purple, raised lesions that affect the skin, mucous membranes, gastrointestinal tract, lymph nodes, and lungs.[13]

Invasive cervical carcinoma in HIV infection and in the presence of a positive HIV test is an AIDS-defining condition. Other gynecologic manifestations, such as abnormal vaginal cytology, can also occur in early symptomatic HIV disease. By including these disorders of the female reproductive system, this classification emphasizes the risk of AIDS to women.

AIDS-related lymphomas are common, with approximately 6% of all persons with AIDS developing a lymphoma during their lifetime.[13] Immune deficiency is a definite predisposing factor, so that those persons with CD4 counts below 50/mm^3 are at high risk. The majority of the lymphomas are aggressive B-cell tumors that present in an advanced stage.[13] The location of the lymphomas varies and can involve lymph nodes as well as extranodal sites. Central nervous system lymphomas are 1000 times more common in the person with AIDS than in the general population.[13] The pathogenesis of lymphoma is discussed in Chapter 13.

Neurologic Diseases

Various neurologic diseases become more frequent as HIV disease advances and T4 cell counts decline. The most common examples of HIV infection on cells of the nervous system are *progressive multifocal leukoencephalopathy* (PML) and *AIDS dementia complex* (ADC). PML, like other opportunistic diseases, is caused by the JC virus, a human papovavirus that results in selective areas of demyelination. Approximately 4% of AIDS patient are affected. PML causes a progressive loss of mental acuity and motor functioning within weeks to months of onset. ADC is a subcortical dementia with cognitive, behavioral, and motor deficits and is one of the most common CNS complications of untreated HIV disease. The precise etiology of ADC is still questionable, although most evidence points to direct consequences of HIV infection of brain cells, such as the microglial cells and neurons. Clinical features of ADC include impaired concentration, forgetfulness and mental slowing (cognition); apathy, confusion, hallucinations, personality changes (behavioral); and unsteady gait, leg tremors, and impaired handwriting (motor).

Other infections that affect the central nervous system include cryptococcal meningitis, cytomegalovirus (CMV) infection, cerebral toxoplasmosis, mycobacterial infections, and herpes infections.

HIV Wasting Syndrome

This syndrome was first identified in sub-Saharan African countries and described under the term "slim disease." It was later associated with HIV infection. HIV wasting syndrome is defined as unintentional weight loss of more than 10% of a person's body mass within 6 months. The precise etiology or pathogenesis of this syndrome is unknown, but it probably represents an entity similar to the anorexia/cachexia syndrome seen in cancer patients, which is refractory to weight-gaining measures. It is often associated with massive and persistent diarrhea.

HYPERSENSITIVITY AND AUTOIMMUNE REACTIONS

When an adaptive immune response becomes inappropriately exaggerated, it is termed a hypersensitive response.[32] The classic term for an immunologic, tissue-damaging reaction is **hypersensitivity reaction,** which refers to an exaggerated response of the immune system to an antigen. The antigen that elicits the response produces different responses, depending on a person's genetic predisposition for an exaggerated response. In some cases, the antigen that produces the response is unknown. Four types of hypersensitivity reactions were described by Coombs and Gell in 1975, but these four types may have overlapping features.[32]

Classifications of Tissue Injury Caused by Hypersensitivity

Type I to Type IV hypersensitivity reactions are described in this section according to their underlying pathophysiologic mechanisms and how they manifest themselves in different diseases (Table 11-10). Figure 11-6 shows a summary diagram of the four types of hypersensitivity reactions.

TYPE I: IMMEDIATE HYPERSENSITIVITY: ATOPY AND ANAPHYLAXIS

Immediate hypersensitivity reactions are IgE-mediated reactions that may manifest as atopic or, in the extreme, anaphylaxis. These reactions, commonly called **allergies**, occur in organs that are exposed to environmental antigens. Many types of antigens (**allergens**) can initiate the hypersensitivity state in susceptible people. The most common of these are environmental

TABLE 11-10

CLASSIFICATION OF HYPERSENSITIVITY STATES

TYPE	CAUSE	RESPONSIBLE CELL OR ANTIBODY	IMMUNE MECHANISM	EXAMPLES OF DISEASE STATES
I—Immediate hypersensitivity (anaphylaxis, atopy)	Foreign protein (antigen)	IgE	IgE attaches to surface of mast cell and specific antigen, triggers release of intracellular granules from mast cells	Hay fever, allergies, hives, anaphylactic shock
II—Cytotoxic hypersensitivity	Foreign protein (antigen)	IgG or IgM	Antibody reacts with antigen, activates complement, causes cytolysis or phagocytosis	Transfusion, hemolytic drug reactions, erythroblastosis fetalis, hemolytic anemia, vascular purpura, Goodpasture's syndrome
III—Immune complex disease	Foreign protein (antigen) Endogenous antigens	IgG, IgM, IgA	Antigen-antibody complexes precipitate in tissue, activate complement, cause inflammatory reaction	Rheumatoid arthritis, systemic lupus erythematosus, serum sickness, glomerulonephritis
IV—Delayed/cell-mediated	Foreign protein, cell, or tissue	T lymphocytes	Sensitized T cell reacts with specific antigen to induce inflammatory process by direct cell action or by activity of lymphokines	Contact dermatitis, transplant graft reaction, granulomatous diseases

FOCUS ON CELLULAR PATHOPHYSIOLOGY

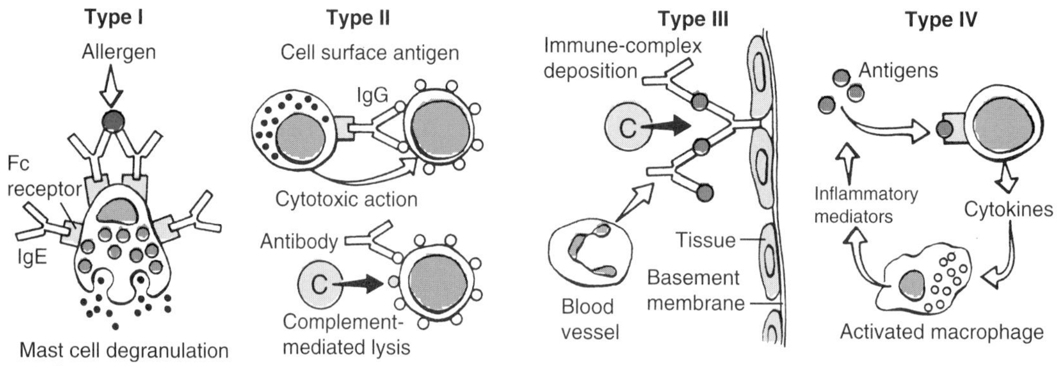

FIGURE 11-6. Four types of hypersensitivity reactions. Type I: Mast cells bind IgE via their Fc receptors. On encountering allergen the IgE becomes cross-linked, inducing degranulation and release of mediators that produce allergic reactions. Type II: Antibody is directed against antigen on an individual's own cells (target cell) or foreign antigen, such as transfused red blood cells. This may lead to cytotoxic action by K cells, or complement-mediated lysis. Type III: Immune complexes are deposited in the tissue. Complement is activated and polymorphs are attracted to the site of deposition, causing local tissue damage and inflammation. Type IV: Antigen-sensitized T cells release lymphokines following a secondary contact with the same antigen. Cytokines induce inflammatory reactions and activate and attract macrophages, which release inflammatory mediators. (Roitt, I., Brostoff, D., & Male, D. [1998]. *Immunology* [5th ed.] St. Louis: Mosby.)

allergens, such as pollens, dander, foods, insect bites, and certain household cleaning agents. Drug sensitivity reactions can effect the same response. The allergic reactions include such conditions as hay fever, asthma, atopic eczema, drug allergies, and anaphylactic shock. Susceptibility to allergy is determined by genetic factors and by other factors that allow for exposure to the allergen.[5]

Atopy is the most common of the immediate hypersensitivity reactions. The skin, respiratory tract, and gastrointestinal system are especially affected. Anaphylaxis is an acute response that involves cardiovascular, respiratory, cutaneous, and gastrointestinal reactions.

Pathophysiology of the Type I Response

Pathophysiologically, the immune response is activated when antigen binds to IgE antibodies attached to the surface of mast cells. Mast cells are present in profusion in connective tissue, skin, and mucous membranes. The reaction proceeds when the IgE molecule specific for a particular antigen becomes cross-linked on the surface of the mast cell and triggers the release of intracellular granules. This granule exocytosis releases stored mediators and causes synthesis of leukotrienes and cytokines. Most of the stored mediators are composed of histamine, which induces the acute inflammatory events. The leukotrienes and cytokines induce a late-phase chronic inflammatory response that involves T lymphocytes, monocytes, eosinophils, and neutrophils.[20]

Histamine is probably the most potent mediator in the Type I response. It constricts smooth muscle and causes microvascular peripheral vasodilatation along with an increase in vascular permeability, resulting in local vascular congestion and edema.[38] The constriction of smooth muscle in the bronchioles accounts for the bronchiolar constriction often associated with the allergic reaction (Fig. 11-7).

The late-phase reaction, caused by the synthesis of potent mediators, is associated with smooth muscle contraction and sustained edema.[20] The mediators, especially leukotrienes and prostaglandins, are apparently very important in long-term reactions such as chronic asthma.

Allergic Rhinitis

This common condition occurs in 10% to 12% of the U.S. population. It is also known as hay fever and represents an atopic reaction to inhaled allergens, such as pollens, dust, and animal danders. The effects are localized in the nasal mucosa and the conjunctiva of the eye. The clinical manifestations include paroxysmal sneezing, watery drainage from the nose, drainage to the back of the throat, cough, and itching of the nose and conjunctivae.[38] Fever is not present unless there is a secondary bacterial infection.

Bronchial Asthma

Atopic allergy may cause bronchial asthma, frequently induced by the inhalation of environmental

FOCUS ON CELLULAR PATHOPHYSIOLOGY

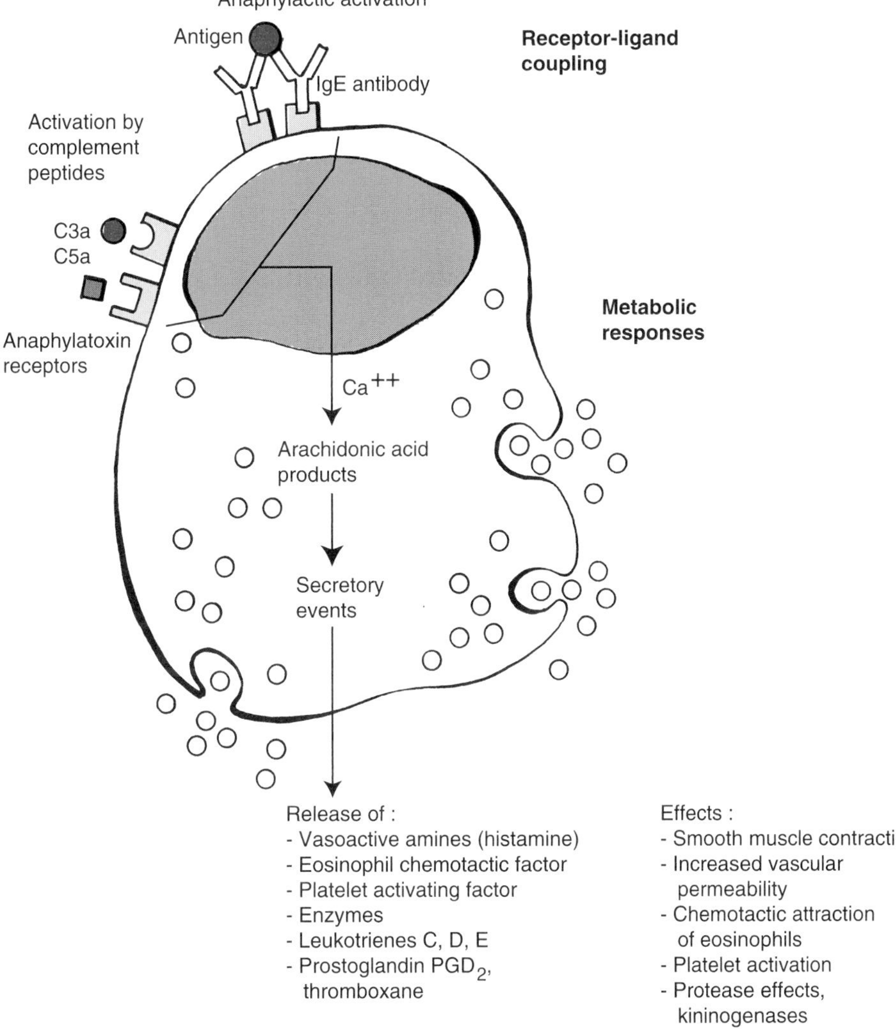

FIGURE 11-7. Type I hypersensitivity. Activation of the mast cell and the potent inflammatory mediators released or synthesized by the cell. (Adapted from Rubin, E. & Farber, J. L. [1999]. *Pathology* [3rd ed.]. Philadelphia: Lippincott Williams & Wilkins.)

antigens (see p. 558). The mechanism for bronchial asthma may result from the interaction of antigen with specific IgE antibodies; the inflammation produces mucosal edema, increased secretion of mucus, and bronchospasm, all of which cause narrowing of the airways and increased airway resistance. The early signs and symptoms of asthma are dyspnea and wheezing. Repeated attacks result in hypertrophy of the bronchial muscle, which can exaggerate bronchoconstriction and increase the severity of each subsequent attack. Bacterial or viral infections may precipitate asthmatic attacks.

Atopic Eczema

Atopic eczema (dermatitis) is an acute or chronic, noncontagious, inflammatory condition that may occur after contact with irritants to which a person has a specific sensitivity. In some cases, it results from a cell-mediated reaction (see p. 318); in others, it is mediated by IgE, with liberation of chemotactic mediators into dermal areas. It often is associated with respiratory allergy.[5]

Atopic eczema causes urticaria and angioedema. The typical wheal-and-flare reaction is seen almost immediately after the allergen penetrates the skin (such as by an insect sting). **Urticaria** involves the superficial capillaries, and **angioedema** involves the capillaries of the deeper skin layers. The wheals of urticaria have well-defined margins, erythema, and vesicles filled with clear fluid. Pruritus frequently is severe. Angioedema causes nonpitting swelling of localized areas of the skin.[13] This skin reaction to an allergen frequently is associated with respiratory hypersensitivity, especially hay fever or another type of allergy. Drug reactions may result in the same dermatologic manifestations, probably caused by the same mechanisms.

Late-phase reactions may also be seen in the skin and may have the appearance of a lump in the skin, which is painful rather than pruritic. A more widespread edematous response may appear about 8 hours after the initial acute reaction in some individuals.[20]

Anaphylaxis and Anaphylactic Shock

Anaphylaxis is defined as an antigen-specific allergic hypersensitivity reaction of the body to a foreign protein or a drug. It is mediated primarily by IgE interaction with mast cells, but non-IgE reactions may occur. Anaphylactic shock occurs when the reaction becomes systemic and thus a life-threatening event (see p. 512). The reaction results when a person has been previously sensitized to the antigen and may occur in a matter of minutes. The antigen–antibody reaction occurs on the mast cells in the connective tissue and around small blood vessels. It causes the mast cells to release histamine and other mediators, which results in contraction of smooth muscle and increased vascular permeability.

The clinical manifestations of anaphylaxis include respiratory, cardiovascular, cutaneous, or gastrointestinal tract manifestations (Box 11-10).[23] The respiratory obstruction, manifested by hoarseness, inspiratory stridor, chest tightness, or wheezing, is the cause of fatalities in 70% of deaths due to anaphylaxis.[23] Dermatologic symptoms, such as wheal-and-flare skin reactions, are usually present and precede the more severe events. Cardiovascular collapse, seen by the presence of hypotension, shock, and dysrhythmias, complicates the anaphylactic picture.

BOX 11-10 CLINICAL MANIFESTATIONS OF ANAPHYLAXIS

Respiratory
Bronchospasm
Laryngeal edema
Inspiratory stridor
Wheezing

Cardiovascular
Hypotension/circulatory shock
Dysrhythmias
Syncope

Dermatologic
"Wheal and flare" reactors
Urticaria
Angioedema
Flushing
Pruritus

Gastrointestinal
Nausea, vomiting
Diarrhea
Abdominal cramping

TYPE II: CYTOTOXIC HYPERSENSITIVITY

In type II hypersensitivity response, a circulating antibody, usually IgG or IgM, reacts with an antigen on the surface of a cell. Because people normally have antibodies to antigen of the ABO blood group not present on their own membranes, the antigen may be a normal component of the membrane. It also may be a foreign antigen, such as a pharmacologic agent, that adheres to the surface of the host's own cells. Antibodies produced to self red blood cells may produce an autoimmune hemolytic anemia. The effect on the host depends on the numbers and types of cells destroyed.

Examples of the Type II hypersensitivity response include (1) antigens on erythrocytes, (2) antigens on neutrophils, (3) antigens on platelets, (4) antigens on basement membrane, and (5) stimulation and inhibition of cellular function.[10] These are briefly discussed following a review of some of the general pathophysiologic features of the Type II response.

Pathophysiology of Type II Hypersensitivity

The pathophysiology of Type II hypersensitivity usually involves the activation of complement and resultant destruction of red blood cells or specific target cells. Opsonic coating of target cells with IgG antibody sets the stage for effector cells to destroy the target cells.[21] Specific IgG or IgM activation of complement results in the complement effects of chemotaxis and cell lysis (Fig. 11-8). Red cell destruction may be triggered by IgG opsonization and the attachment of lymphocytes or macrophages to the cell surface.[13,21]

Antigens on Erythrocytes

Examples of reactions that destroy red blood cells are transfusion reactions, erythroblastosis fetalis, autoimmune hemolytic anemia, and drug-induced hemolysis.

Transfusion Reactions. These reactions may result when antibodies in the recipient's serum react against antigens in the donor's red blood cells. It causes hemolysis of donor red blood cells with the liberation of large

FOCUS ON CELLULAR PATHOPHYSIOLOGY

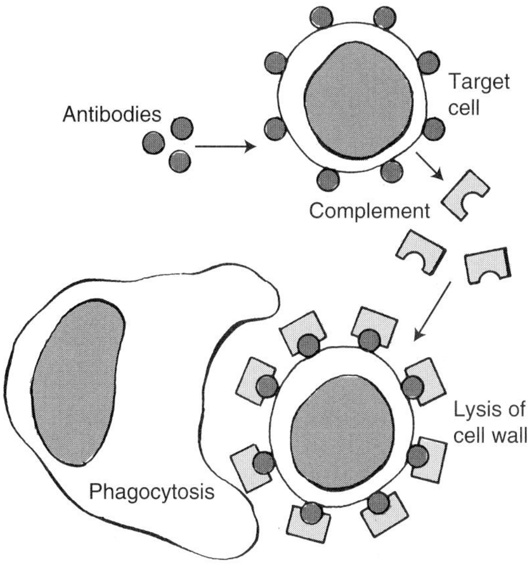

FIGURE 11-8. Type II hypersensitivity response. The target cell is covered with antibody that activates complement and sets the stage for phagocytosis.

quantities of hemoglobin into the plasma. Some of the hemoglobin is broken down into unconjugated bilirubin. If the amount of free hemoglobin is greater than the ability of the liver to conjugate and excrete, the excess diffuses into the tissue or through the renal glomeruli into the renal tubules. Precipitation of large amounts of hemoglobin in the renal tubular fluid forms sharp needles in the acid urine, which can cause tubular damage and obstruction.[15] Precipitation in the tubules of the shells of red blood cells also frequently contributes to tubular damage and renal failure. Transfusion reactions may also increase the risk of renal failure by causing circulatory shock, renal vasoconstriction, and decreased renal blood flow.

The antigenic nature of mismatched blood transfusions depends on the type and Rh factor of the donor blood (see p. 341). For example, people with type A blood possess anti-B antibodies. Therefore, the incompatible blood is coated with antibodies, usually of the IgM class. This causes agglutination of the donor cells, and lysis rapidly follows.[21]

Signs and symptoms of a transfusion reaction include chills, fever, low back pain, hypotension, tachycardia, anxiety, hyperkalemia, nausea and vomiting, red or port wine–colored urine, and occasionally urticaria. These may progress to shock and irreversible renal failure. Hemolytic reactions are fatal in 10% of ABO-incompatible transfusions, which occur when large amounts of incompatible blood are transfused, usually as a result of human error.[15]

Erythroblastosis Fetalis. **Erythroblastosis fetalis** may result if a mother without Rh antigens carries a child with Rh antigens or if mother and fetus have ABO incompatibility. A mother who lacks Rh antigens on her red blood cells (Rh-negative) can be sensitized to the Rh antigen carried on the cells of the fetus by mixing her red blood cells with fetal red blood cells. If the woman again becomes pregnant with a fetus that has Rh antigens, her anti-Rh antibodies may cross the placenta and enter the fetal circulation. The result is destruction of fetal red blood cells through a hemolytic reaction. More commonly, ABO blood group incompatibility causes the free passage of antibodies from the mother through the placenta to the fetus.[13,38] Blood types interact in different ways, but the result is attachment and hemolysis of fetal red blood cells by maternal antibodies. Hemolysis of fetal red blood cells results in severe anemia, which may lead to heart failure. Also, the release of high concentrations of bilirubin from hemoglobin may cause fetal brain damage, called **kernicterus,** as unconjugated bilirubin passes across the blood–brain barrier, with the result of edematous swelling of brain parenchyma. The mechanism by which unconjugated bilirubin crosses the blood–brain barrier is not clearly understood, but the barrier apparently is more permeable in neonates and premature infants.[13] Hyperbilirubinemia is common in an affected infant who survives for more than several days. This increased bilirubin level usually is manifested as jaundice and is termed *icterus gravis.* The red cell activity in bone marrow increases, and extramedullary hematopoiesis begins in the liver, spleen, and perhaps other organs to compensate for lost red blood cells. The risk of erythroblastosis fetalis in subsequent pregnancies can be reduced by administering anti-Rh antibodies to the mother within 72 hours after the birth of the first Rh-positive infant. More difficult to predict is ABO erythroblastosis, but the condition can be monitored if both parents are aware of their blood incompatibility.

Autoimmune Hemolytic Anemia. Two types of hemolytic anemias with a probable autoimmune basis are *warm antibody disease* and *cold antibody disease.* Warm antibody disease is termed autoimmune hemolytic anemia and usually is due to IgG antibody that attacks the host's own red blood cells. The disease can be life-threatening, depending on the amount of hemolysis. The red blood cells develop a limited life span, and the resulting anemia can be severe. Autoimmune hemolytic disease may develop for no known reason, or it may be associated with other autoimmune diseases, cancer, or systemic infection.[13]

Cold antibody disease results when an autoantibody, usually IgM, binds to erythrocytes at temperatures below 31°C. These temperatures may be reached in the fingers or toes during very cold weather. The red blood cells thus coated with cold antibodies reenter the general circulation, activate complement, and hemolyze the red blood cells. These hemolytic attacks occur only after exposure to cold and tend to be self-limiting. The major diagnostic criterion for hemolytic anemia is the Coombs' antiglobulin test. In this test, agglutination of red blood cells occurs when immunoglobulins are attached to the red blood cell membranes.[31]

Drug-Induced Hemolysis. This may result from drug-antibody complexes that bind passively to red blood cells and initiate the complement reaction. Other drugs may act as **haptens** and bind to a red blood cell carrier. Antibody is formed and induces hemolysis of the red blood cells. Some drugs produce changes in the surface antigens of the red blood cells, resulting in antibody production against the host's own erythrocytes. Most drug-induced hemolytic reactions stop once use of the drug is discontinued. Box 11-11 lists some drugs that have been implicated in producing immune hemolytic anemias.

Antigens on Neutrophils

Blood transfusion reactions may be caused by nonerythrocyte antigen incompatibilities. These may be due to neutrophil antigens. Maternal antibodies to the fetal neutrophil antigens may cause neonatal leukopenia, and antibodies against donor leukocytes may cause destruction of the neutrophils, with fever, chills and hypotension.[10]

Antigens on Platelets

Neonatal thrombocytopenia and post-transfusion febrile reactions may occur as a result of destruction of platelets. Idiopathic thrombocytopenic purpura results when a person develops antibodies against self platelet membrane antigens. These antiself antibodies may cause a destruction of platelets with resultant thrombocytopenia and bleeding.[10]

Antigens on Basement Membrane

The best illustration of a specific target cell hypersensitivity reaction is *Goodpasture's syndrome,* which is a rapidly occurring condition characterized by the development of antiglomerular basement membrane antibodies (anti-GBM). These antibodies are directed at the glomerular basement membrane of the kidneys as well as the basement membrane of the pulmonary alveoli. The initiator is unknown, but the condition is associated with the flu, or it may follow the inhalation of hydrocarbons, especially cigarette smoke.[20]

The disease is diagnosed by the presence of hemoptysis, iron-deficiency anemia, and rapidly progressing glomerulonephritis. It may rapidly progress to death with the destruction of the basement membranes, leading to hemoptysis and renal failure. Goodpasture's disease is primarily a disease of young white males (the male/female ratio is 6 : 1).[14] Both pulmonary and glomerular improvement have been seen as a result of plasmapheresis and steroid therapy.

Stimulation and Inhibition of Cellular Function

These reactions are often classified as a Type V hypersensitivity because the antibodies that interact with antigens on cells cause either stimulation or inhibition of the cellular function rather than cell death.[10]

Examples of this type of hypersensitivity include Graves' disease, myasthenia gravis, and pernicious anemia. *Graves' disease* is caused by IgG antibodies that bind to the TSH receptor on the follicular cells of the thyroid gland.[10] This binding leads to stimulation of enzyme systems that stimulate the secretion of thyroid hormone (see p. 686). *Myasthenia gravis* is an autoimmune disease that results when IgG antibody is directed against acetylcholine receptors at the motor end plate. The end result is a failure of neuromuscular transmission (see p. 1010).[10] *Pernicious anemia* may be caused by antibodies that bind to intrinsic factor, thus inhibiting the absorption of vitamin B_{12} (see p. 355). Figure 11-9 illustrates how the anti-receptor antibodies function to cause the effects of Graves' and myasthenia gravis.

BOX 11-11 DRUG-INDUCED IMMUNE HEMOLYTIC ANEMIAS

1. Drug absorption mechanism
2. Membrane modification mechanism
3. Immune complex mechanism

Partial List of Drugs

Aminosalicylic acid (PAS)
Antihistamines
Cephalothin
Chlorinated hydrocarbons
Chlorpromazine
Dipyrone
Insulin
Isoniazid
Levodopa
Mefenamic acid
Melphalan
Methyldopa
Penicillin
Pyramidon
Quinidine
Quinine
Rifampin
Stibophen
Sulfonamides
Sulfonylureas
Tetracyclines

(Adapted from Stites, D. P, Terr., A. J., & Parslow, T. G. [1998]. *Basic and clinical immunology* [9th ed.]. Norwalk, CT: Appleton & Lange.)

FOCUS ON CELLULAR PATHOPHYSIOLOGY

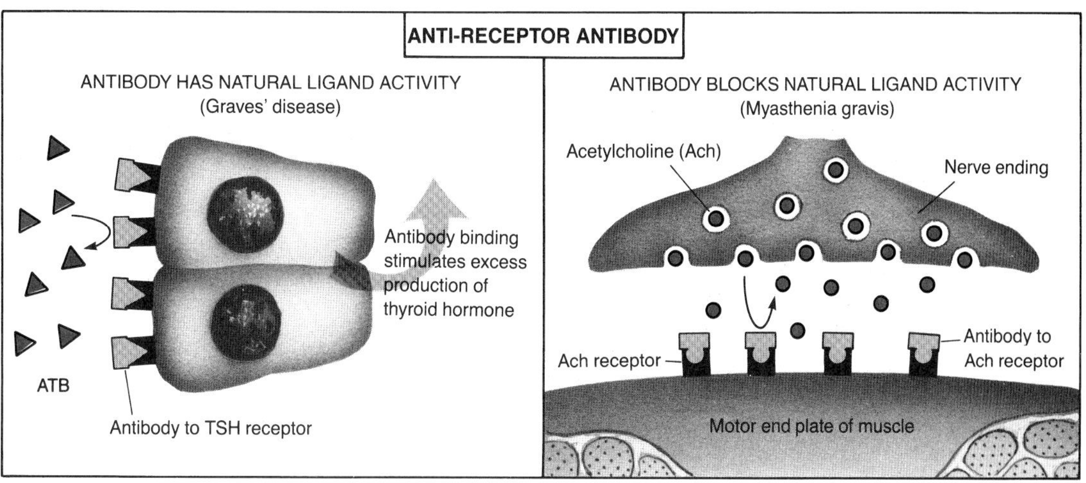

FIGURE 11-9. Type II hypersensitivity. Noncytotoxic antireceptor antibodies in Graves' disease and myasthenia gravis. The binding of the antibody to the TSH receptor in Graves' disease results in hyperthyroidism, whereas the inhibition of synaptic transmission in myasthenia gravis leads to profound muscle weakness. (Rubin, E. & Farber, J. L. [1999]. *Pathology* [3rd ed.]. Philadelphia: Lippincott-Raven.)

TYPE III: IMMUNE COMPLEX DISEASE

Immune complex disease results in the formation of antigen-antibody complexes that activate a variety of serum factors, especially complement.[13] This results in precipitation of complexes in vulnerable areas, leading to inflammation as a consequence of complement activation. The end result is an intravascular, synovial, endocardial, or other membrane inflammatory process that affects the vulnerable organs (Fig. 11-10). Each person apparently has some unique vulnerability in target organs.

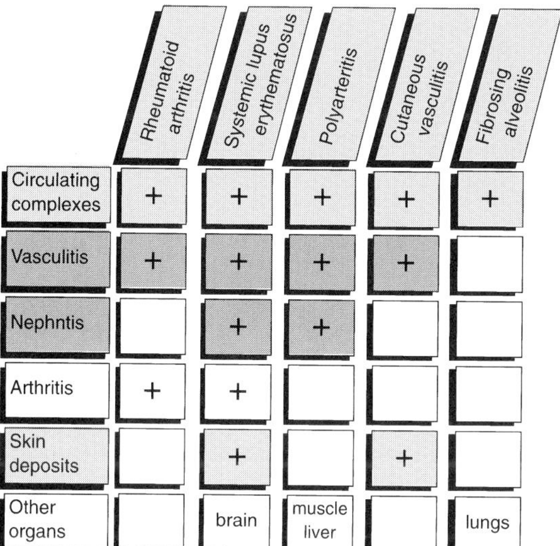

	Rheumatoid arthritis	Systemic lupus erythematosus	Polyarteritis	Cutaneous vasculitis	Fibrosing alveolitis
Circulating complexes	+	+	+	+	+
Vasculitis	+	+	+	+	
Nephritis		+	+		
Arthritis	+	+			
Skin deposits		+		+	
Other organs		brain	muscle liver		lungs

FIGURE 11-10. Immune complex deposits and their clinical effects.

Antigen-antibody complexes may be present in the plasma but may not cause disease manifestations. If the complexes are not removed by the mononuclear phagocyte system, they may lodge in the tissue, where they initiate an inflammatory reaction that leads to tissue destruction. The complexes frequently are small, and their size seems to determine whether they will be cleared and whether they can lodge at a place where significant damage can occur. The antigen-antibody complexes that remain in solution cause reactions when they circulate through the body and lodge in the tissue and small vessels.[39] Increased vascular permeability allows the complexes to be deposited in the extravascular spaces. Deposition also appears to be greater at points of high pressure, high flow, and turbulence.[32] Once precipitated, the immune complexes initiate the inflammatory process by activating complement and releasing vasoactive substances from the defense cells (Flowchart 11-1). Box 11-12 summarizes the pathogenesis of inflammatory lesions in type III reactions.

Serum sickness and Arthus reactions are classic examples of the Type III reactions. More usual, however, are the common, systemic autoimmune conditions, most of which are classified as Type III reactions.

Serum Sickness

Serum sickness results from injection of large doses of foreign material and can cause various types of

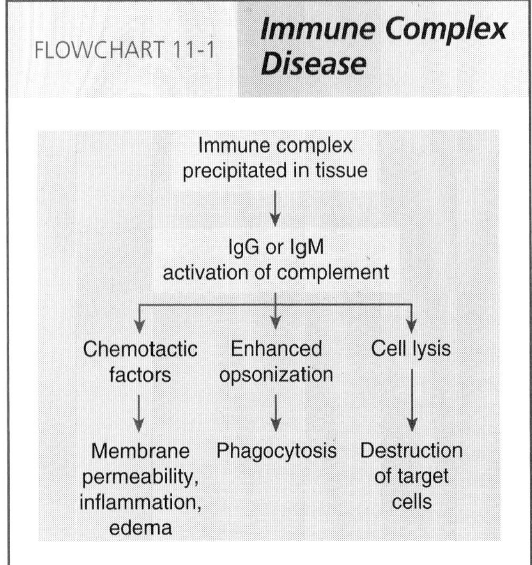

FLOWCHART 11-1 **Immune Complex Disease**

arthritis, glomerulonephritis, and vasculitis. Antigen-antibody complexes form in the bloodstream and precipitate into vulnerable areas. Serum sickness was first reported after passive immunization with horse serum (equine tetanus antitoxin), which contains at least 30 antigens. It can cause an acute reaction or a chronic condition. Vaccines, protein-based drugs, and bee stings may cause this condition, and in rare cases it may occur as an allergic reaction to penicillins, sulfonamides, and cephalosporins.[39]

If the antigen concentration is greater than the antibody concentrations, the resulting antigen-antibody complexes tend to be small and remain in solution for as long as 8 to 15 days after initial injection. Immune complexes are deposited throughout the vasculature of the body; complement is activated, and neutrophils and macrophages move into the area in response to chemotactic signals. Phagocytosis of the immune complexes begins with the release of lysosomal enzymes into the area, and this causes acute vasculitis with destruction of the elastic lamina of the arteries. Once phagocytosis of the immune complexes is complete, the inflammatory process decreases, leaving some scarring of the blood vessel walls.[10,13]

Renal glomerular deposits of complexes occur even when the immune complex concentrations are not high, probably because of the efficient filtering action of the kidneys. The complexes form characteristic deposits in the glomerular walls that activate complement and lead to destruction of glomerular tissue. Increased permeability of the glomerular basement membrane often produces hematuria and proteinuria. Figure 11-11 shows the process of vasculitis and glomerulonephritis that can result.

Arthus Reaction

Another Type III disorder, the Arthus reaction, involves inflammation and cellular death at the site of injection of antigen into a previously sensitized person. Pathologically, it causes acute, localized edema with tissue inflammation and little vasculitis.[33] Antibody precipitation and complement activation cause all of the effects of inflammation, with activation of the complement fragments through C89, which destroys antigen and surrounding tissue (see p. 259).

Hypersensitive pneumonitis may be an Arthus reaction from the inhalation of antigenic materials from molds, plants, or animals.[32] This reaction is due to primarily IgG response, but some relationship with the Type I and IV hypersensitivity reactions has been described.[10,13,33]

Other Type III Conditions

Many of the common autoimmune conditions are classified as immune complex disorders. The mechanism for inflammation and damage is the precipitation of immune complexes into vulnerable areas. Immune complex disorders are dynamic, constantly changing processes that are manifested in the tissues in which they become lodged. Systemic lupus erythematosus (SLE), rheumatoid arthritis, and some types of glomerulonephritis are examples. SLE and rheumatoid arthritis are discussed more fully on pages 323 to 324. Glomerulonephritis is described in detail on pages 624 to 627.

TYPE IV: CELL-MEDIATED HYPERSENSITIVITY

Type IV response is the result of specifically sensitized T lymphocytes without the participation of antibodies. Type IV reactions typically occur 24 to 72 hours after exposure of a susceptible individual to an of-

BOX 11-12 PATHOGENESIS OF TYPE III REACTIONS

1. Antigen (endogenous or exogenous)–antibody complexes form
2. Localization of complexes in vessels, often in joint areas
3. Activation of complement inflammatory pathway
4. Chemotaxis for cells and exudate
5. Inflammation with swelling, heat, and pain in joints and tissues
6. Infiltration of area with polymorphonuclear leukocytes and macrophages
7. Tissue damage and destruction
8. Continuing inflammation and fibrin deposition
9. Scarring and collagen deposition; may cause joint or tissue deformity

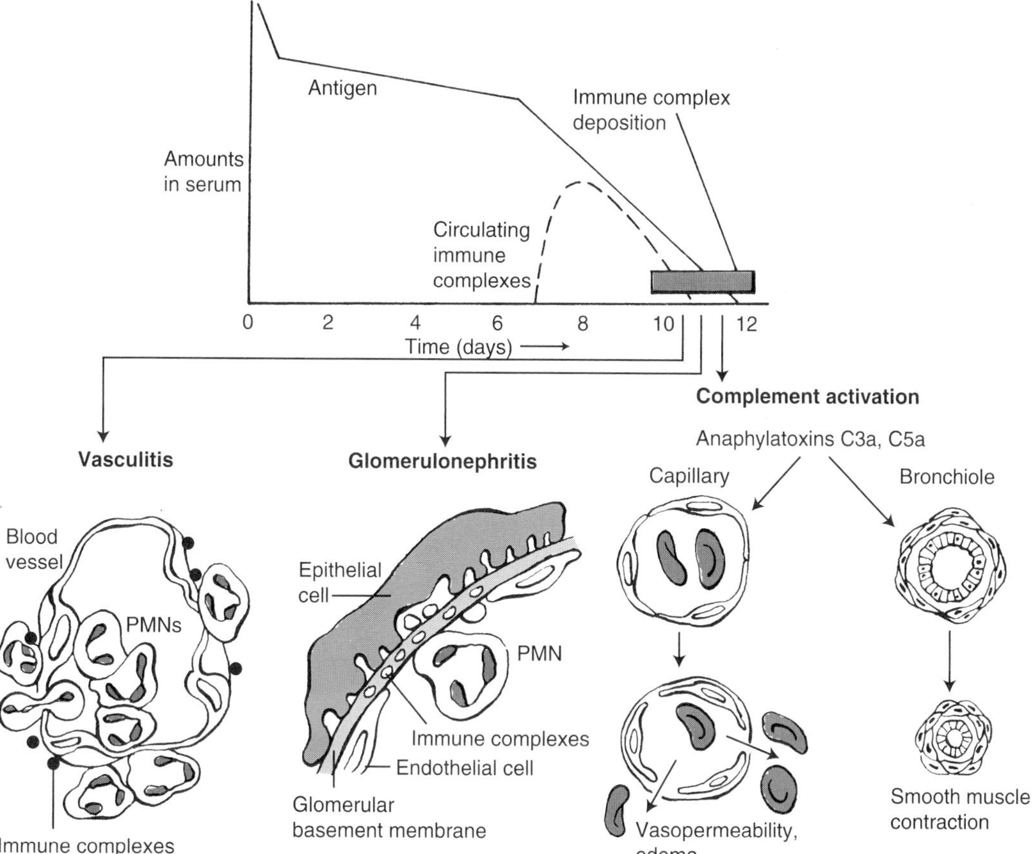

FIGURE 11-11. Type III hypersensitivity. In the serum sickness model of immune complex tissue injury, antibody is produced against a circulating antigen and immune complexes form in the blood. These complexes deposit in tissues such as blood vessels and glomeruli and, augmented by complement activation, induce tissue injury or dysfunction responses. (Rubin, E., & Farber, J. L. [1999]. *Pathology* [3rd ed.]. Philadelphia: Lippincott-Raven.)

fending antigen, which is why they are called delayed reactions. Delayed hypersensitivity responses are due to the specific interaction of T cells with antigen. The T cells react with the antigen and release lymphokines that draw macrophages into the area. Macrophages release monokines. These substances enhance the inflammatory response that destroys the foreign material (Figure 11-12).

Direct T cell–mediated cytotoxicity is causative in many of the following conditions: (1) contact dermatitis, (2) infections, (3) granulomatous inflammation, (4) certain autoimmune diseases, and (5) transplant or graft rejection.[10] The phenomenon of transplant and graft rejection has greatly enlarged the understanding of the immune system and is discussed in a separate section below.

Contact Dermatitis

A common allergic skin reaction, contact dermatitis seems to be a T-cell response with a delayed reaction. It occurs on contact with certain common household chemicals, cosmetics, and plant toxins. Common antigens are leather, drugs, dyes in clothing, poison ivy, and poison oak.[10] These may alter the normal skin protein so that it becomes antigenic, or they may act as haptens that combine with proteins in the skin.[32]

The area of contact becomes red and indurated with well-circumscribed lesions. Vesicles begin to appear that are mainly confined to the epidermis. Lymphocytes and macrophages infiltrate the area and react against the epidermal cells. Sterile, protein-rich fluid fills the blebs. If the blebs are opened, the antigen may be spread to a new area. The affected cells are destroyed, slough off, and are replaced by regenerating new cells. Exposure to the chemicals in poison ivy is an example of contact dermatitis that causes a reaction even though the chemicals are not proteins. The chemicals have the ability to bind to cell membrane proteins and are recognized by antigen-specific lymphocytes.[33] The effect reaches its greatest intensity 24 to 48 hours after exposure.

FOCUS ON CELLULAR PATHOPHYSIOLOGY

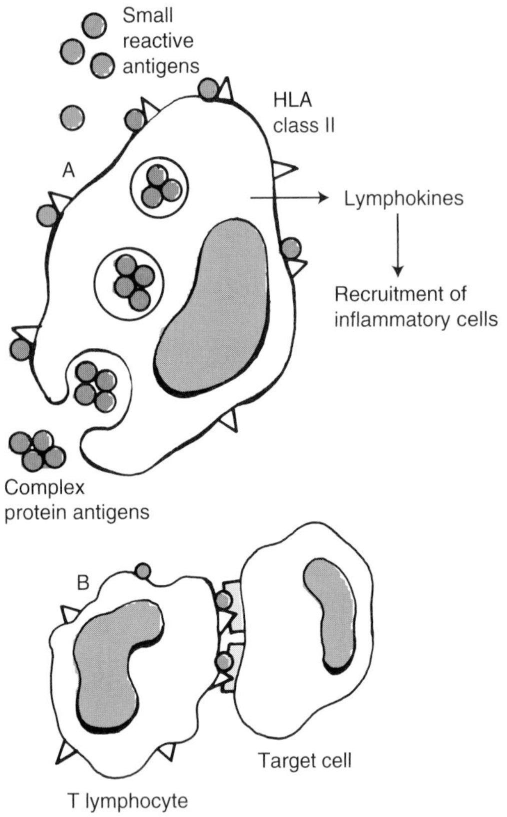

FIGURE 11-12. Type IV cell-mediated hypersensitivity. The response in **A** is the delayed type with macrophage processing of the antigen for the sensitized T lymphocyte. The result is the release of lymphokines and recruitment of inflammatory cells. In **B** the T lymphocyte recognizes a foreign cell such as a virally infected cell, a histoincompatible cell, or a tumor cell, and targets it for destruction through direct interaction or release of lymphokines.

Infections

Delayed hypersensitivity responses often are caused by infectious agents, such as mycobacteria, protozoa, and fungi. These organisms present a chronic antigenic stimulus, and the T lymphocytes and macrophages react, sometimes conferring protective immunity against later exposure.

The tuberculin response is the best example of the delayed hypersensitivity response as a result of infection with mycobacteria. It is used to determine whether a person has been sensitized to the disease. Reddening and induration of the site begin within 12 hours of injection of tuberculin and reach a peak in 24 to 72 hours.[32] It is mainly a dermal reaction. The positive response occurs because of the presence of antigen-specific T cells that are activated to secrete cytokines and lymphotoxin. They react due to the presence of mycobacterium organisms that the macrophages are unable to destroy.

Granulomatous Hypersensitivity Response

Granulomatous hypersensitivity response is the most important form of delayed hypersensitivity because it results in the formation of granulomas in different areas of the body. It usually results from microorganisms being present within macrophages or other substances that the cell is unable to destroy.[32] The epithelioid cell is the characteristic morphologic feature and appears as a large, flattened cell that may be derived from activated macrophages. Sometimes the formation of multinucleated giant cells surrounded by T lymphocytes occurs.[32] The granuloma may be surrounded by fibrosis, with contained necrotic material.

Precise classification of diseases that manifest delayed hypersensitivity with or without granuloma formation is difficult. A wide variety of chronic diseases are included, most of which are related to infectious agents. Table 11-11 lists examples of granulomatous inflammation with etiology and tissue reaction.

Autoimmune Diseases

Certain conditions involve direct T-cell reactivity against normal host antigens and lead to progressive destruction of these cells. Examples of T cell–mediated autoimmunity include insulin-dependent diabetes mellitus, Hashimoto's thyroiditis, and probably rheumatoid arthritis and multiple sclerosis. Rheumatoid arthritis is a complex disease that also involves antibodies, including IgM anti-IgG autoantibody, called rheumatoid factor).[20]

Transplant or Graft Rejection

When tissues containing nucleated cells are transplanted from one person to another, T-cell responses almost always trigger a response against the transplanted organ.[20] Rejection of tissue and transplanted organs involves several of the hypersensitivity responses, which essentially leads to destruction of the transplanted tissue. Targeting of transplanted organs depends on whether the **histocompatibility antigens** are similar enough between the donor and the recipient to prevent activation of the rejection phenomenon. These surface antigens on cells distinguish them from other people and from other organs. These are the *self-proteins* to which a person develops tolerance. Identical twins have identical histocompatibility antigens, so that organs or tissue can be transplanted from one to the other with ease. Since it is rare to have identical twins, donor and recipient tissues are matched from families or donor banks; the closer the match, the more likely the transplantation will be successful.[32] Various forms of rejection are common, and prevention is essential in securing a functioning transplanted organ.

TABLE 11-11

EXAMPLES OF GRANULOMATOUS INFLAMMATIONS

DISEASE	CAUSE	TISSUE REACTION
Tuberculosis	*Mycobacterium tuberculosis*	*Noncaseating tubercle (granuloma prototype)*: a focus of epithelioid cells, rimmed by fibroblasts, lymphocytes, histiocytes, occasional Langhans' giant cell; *caseating tubercle:* central amorphous granular debris, loss of all cellular detail; acid-fast bacilli
Leprosy	*Mycobacterium leprae*	Acid-fast bacilli in macrophages; granulomas and epithelioid types
Syphilis	*Treponema pallidum*	*Gumma:* Microscopic to grossly visible lesion, enclosing wall of histiocytes; plasma cell infiltrate; center cells are necrotic without loss of cellular outline
Cat-scratch disease	*Gram-negative bacillus*	Rounded or stellate granuloma containing central granular debris and recognizable neutrophils; giant cells uncommon

(Cotran, R., Kumar V., & Collins, T. [1999]. *Robbins' pathologic basis of disease* [6th ed.]. Philadelphia: W. B. Saunders.)

FIRST-SET, SECOND-SET, AND HYPERACUTE REJECTION

First-set rejection usually occurs 11 to 15 days after grafting. The initial graft is accepted but is rejected due to T-cell response.[20] This delayed response reflects the time necessary for the T lymphocyte to become sensitized to the transplanted antigens. There is cell injury through secretion of lymphokines and direct cytotoxicity.[10] If the recipient is regrafted with tissue from the previous donor, there will be a much more rapid rejection process. This is called second-set rejection. The reaction does not occur if the recipient is grafted with tissue from another donor. Hyperacute rejection is a fulminant reaction that occurs within minutes after transplantation and is characterized by severe necrotizing vasculitis (due to damage to the vasculature of the graft).[10] It is due to the presence in the recipient's blood of high levels of preformed antibodies against antigens on the transplanted cells.

ACUTE REJECTION

Acute rejection is a complex reaction that involves both cell-mediated and humoral responses. It may occur days to months after transplantation and is called acute because it progresses rapidly once it has begun.[10] It is the process by which the immune system of the host recognizes, develops sensitivity to, and attempts to eliminate the antigenic differences of the donor organ. It causes cellular destruction and failure of the grafted organ or tissue. Cytolytic T lymphocytes may either attack grafted tissue directly or secrete chemotactic lymphokines that enhance the activity of macrophages in tissue destruction. Humoral responses may be due to circulating antibodies that were formed during previous exposure to the antigen.

After transplantation, the lymphocytes become sensitized as they pass through the donor site. There is parenchymal cell necrosis and infiltration of the tissue with lymphocytes. The humoral component causes the deposition of immune complexes in the small vessels of the graft, acute vasculitis, and ischemic changes.

CHRONIC REJECTION

Progressive rejection is common in most transplanted tissue, and there is a slow deterioration of organ function over a period of time, usually months to years. The T lymphocyte (Type IV reaction) causes a relentless destruction of parenchymal cells. The cardinal features of chronic rejection are obliteration of the lumen of the blood vessels by proliferating smooth muscle cells and interstitial fibrosis. Grafts may be damaged by the recurrence of the original disease process that produced a need for the transplant in the first place.[32]

Autoimmunity

Autoimmune disease results when a specific adaptive immune response occurs against self antigen instead of a foreign antigen. The result is a tissue-damaging response that causes chronic inflammatory injury and may eventually be lethal.[20] The response may be cell mediated, through the T lymphocytes, or it may involve immune complexes being deposited into tissues. A wide spectrum of autoimmune responses has been divided clinically into non–organ-specific and organ-specific diseases. Figure 11-13 indicates the

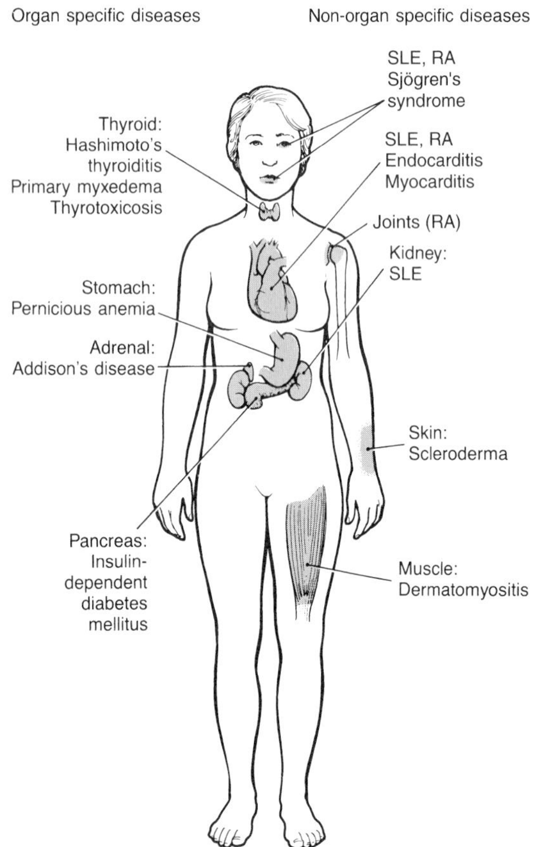

FIGURE 11-13. **Autoimmune diseases have been classified as organ specific and non–organ specific. Organ-specific diseases only affect certain organs. Non–organ specific diseases can target multiple organs and have system-wide effects. SLE: systemic lupus erythematosus; RA: rheumatoid arthritis.**

spectrum of common organ-specific and non–organ-specific diseases. Unit 2, Appendix A lists many diagnostic tests used for autoimmunity. Many of these are described in other sections of the book. The relationships of destructive autoimmune reactions are clearly demonstrated in myasthenia gravis, Graves' disease, rheumatoid arthritis, systemic lupus erythematosus (SLE), and others (Table 11-12). SLE, rheumatoid arthritis, and scleroderma are considered in further detail in the section below. The possibility of autoimmunity as a causative factor has been proposed in conditions as diverse as multiple sclerosis, hepatitis, and cancer.

PATHOPHYSIOLOGY OF TISSUE INJURY

The manifestations of autoimmune disease are based on the cells or tissues that are targeted for attack and destruction by the immune system. It may include humoral mechanisms, cell-mediated mechanisms, or a combination of both.[20]

Autoantibodies are antibodies that are produced against the body's own cells or tissue components, and include rheumatoid factor (RH factor), antinuclear antibody (ANA), and others. They may be demonstrated by presence in the blood stream or in tissue samples. The problem with the demonstration of these autoantibodies is that they may be present in individuals who have no indication of autoimmune disease.

There is strong evidence for the presence of *autoimmune human T cells* in certain diseases, such as insulin-dependent diabetes mellitus in which the beta cells of the islets of Langerhans are selectively destroyed by specific T cells.[20] These cells are not easily identified, but the outcome of their effects appear to be autoimmune in nature. A major challenge in the study of autoimmune disease is to identify the autoantigens recognized by T cells and to use this information to control the activity of these T cells.[20]

The mechanisms of autoimmune disease production may be seen as in the Type II, Type III, and Type IV hypersensitivity reactions. In these, injury may be

TABLE 11-12

AUTOIMMUNE DISEASES

SINGLE ORGAN OR CELL TYPE	SYSTEMIC
PROBABLE	PROBABLE
Hashimoto's thyroiditis	Systemic lupus erythematosus
Autoimmune hemolytic anemia	Rheumatoid arthritis
Autoimmune atrophic gastritis of pernicious anemia	Sjögren's syndrome
Autoimmune encephalomyelitis	Reiter's syndrome
Autoimmune orchitis	POSSIBLE
Goodpasture's syndrome*	Inflammatory myopathies
Autoimmune thrombocytopenia	Systemic sclerosis (scleroderma)
Insulin-dependent diabetes mellitus	Polyarteritis nodosa
Myasthenia gravis	
Graves' disease	
POSSIBLE	
Primary biliary cirrhosis	
Chronic active hepatitis	
Ulcerative colitis	
Membranous glomerulonephritis	

* Target is basement membrane of glomeruli and alveolar walls. (From Cotran, R., Kumar, V., & Collins, T. [1999]. *Robbins' pathologic basis of disease* [6th ed.]. Philadelphia: W. B. Saunders.)

produced when (1) antibody becomes attached to the cell membrane of target cells, activates complement, and with the help of macrophages caused destruction of the target tissue (Type II); (2) antigen and antibody form immune complexes that are deposited in tissues, inducing a complement-mediated reaction (Type III); or (3) cell-mediated destruction of target tissues results from sensitized T lymphocytes destroying target tissue through lymphokines and/or macrophage assistance (Type IV).[32]

EPIDEMIOLOGY OF AUTOIMMUNE DISEASE

Observations of autoimmune phenomena have resulted in the following generalizations:[13,32]

- Specific autoimmune phenomena occur with greater frequency in certain families, which suggests a genetic disorder related to a fundamental disorder of thymic immune control.
- Autoimmune diseases are more common in females than in males, which indicates a relation between the sex hormones and the immune response.
- Elderly people have a greater prevalence of autoantibodies, which may be the result of genetic errors because of the wearing out of the immune system through the aging process.
- Viruses may play a role in the occurrence of autoimmunity because of their ability to disrupt the immune system at any one of several levels.
- Sequestered tissue (tissue and protein not normally in contact with T and B cells) may be exposed to these cells through disease or disruption.
- Tissue self-antigen is altered by disease or injury so that the host no longer recognizes it as self.

SYSTEMIC LUPUS ERYTHEMATOSUS (SLE)

SLE is a multisystem, chronic, remitting and relapsing, rheumatic disease that may assume several forms. The greatest frequency of the disease is found in women 20 to 40 years of age. It is much more common and more severe in African-American women, with a reported incidence of 1 in 245.[13]

Antinuclear antibodies (ANAs) are demonstrated in the serum of more than 95% of persons with SLE. They may represent antibodies to DNA, to nucleoproteins, or to other nuclear components. The presence of antibodies against double-stranded DNA is highly specific for SLE.[10]

Pathology

Pathologically, immune complexes are formed between antinuclear antibodies and nuclear antigens and are found in the serum, small blood vessels, skin, and glomerular basement membrane.[10] The immune complexes initiate the complement reaction, and serum complement levels are frequently decreased during active attacks of SLE. This causes widespread degeneration of connective tissue, especially in the heart, glomeruli, blood vessels, skin, spleen, and retroperitoneal tissue. Skin changes include atrophy, dermal edema, and fibrinoid infiltration. The renal glomeruli characteristically demonstrate fibrinoid changes, necrosis with scarring, and deposits of immunoglobulin and complement in the basement membrane.[10]

Clinical Manifestations

Stiffness and pain in the hands, feet, or large joints are common complaints. The joints appear red, warm, and tender but do not exhibit the deformities of rheumatoid arthritis. The exposed skin shows signs of a patchy atrophy. An erythematous rash frequently occurs in a butterfly pattern over the nose and cheeks. The dermis becomes edematous, and discoid lesions are found on the face, neck, and scalp, beginning as localized erythematous plaques. Alopecia is common.[24]

Renal involvement, a serious complication, results from the precipitation of immune complexes in the renal glomeruli. The course of renal involvement is characterized by remissions and exacerbations ranging in severity from mild proteinuria to massive hematuria and proteinuria, finally resulting in total renal failure.[24]

Systemic problems, including fever, fatigue, anorexia, and weight loss, are common. Cardiopulmonary effects include pericarditis, pleural effusions, and pneumonitis. Raynaud's phenomenon is observed in approximately one-third of affected persons (see p. 442). Neurologic manifestations are often nonspecific and include headaches, organic brain syndrome, and seizures. Besides antibody demonstration, hematologic abnormalities include hemolytic anemia, thrombocytopenia, and leukopenia.

The prognosis for SLE depends upon the degree of effect on target organs. The 10-year survival has improved from 50% to 90% with the advent of dialysis, the use of glucocorticoids, and renal transplantation.[24]

RHEUMATOID ARTHRITIS

Rheumatoid arthritis(RA) is a chronic, systemic, inflammatory disease that specifically affects the small joints of the hands and feet in its early stages and involves the larger joints in later stages. It occurs throughout the world and affects 1% to 2% of the population, with a more common incidence in women.[42]

Pathology

RA is nonsuppurative but finally results in the destruction of cartilage and joints. It has many extraarticular manifestations, including neurologic, hematologic, cardiac, pulmonary, and ocular conditions (Box 11-13).

The pathophysiologic manifestations of rheumatoid arthritis appear to result from T lymphocytes

BOX 11-13

ARTICULAR AND EXTRA-ARTICULAR MANIFESTATIONS OF RHEUMATOID ARTHRITIS

- **Subcutaneous nodules:** Firm, freely movable rubbery or granular nodules caused by deposition of extra-articular granulation tissue. Usually found at joint points such as knuckles and elbows.
- **Synovial cysts:** Called Baker's cysts in popliteal fossa; filled with synovial fluid that may be found in periarticular areas in elbow, shoulder, or small joints.
- **Arthritis:** Bilateral involvement of the small joints and later the large joints; hands joints are usually swollen and may be red. Inflammation leads to disability from destruction of cartilage, bone, and tendons. Flexion contractures are common. Osteoporosis, vertebral compression fractures, and avascular necrosis of the femoral head are common and may relate to treatment with corticosteroids. Usually at least three joint areas are involved.
- **Systemic rheumatoid vasculitis:** Immune complex–mediated inflammation in small and medium-sized arteries. It may be life-threatening if in a critical area. Causes pericardial, cardiac, pulmonary, and other types of lesions. Digital necrosis is common.
- **Compression neuropathy:** Mainly causes peripheral nerve entrapment with carpal tunnel syndrome. Paresthesias, pain, burning, muscle wasting, and weakness are common symptoms.
- **Cardiac disease:** Pericardial lesions and effusions are common and may or may not be symptomatic. Conduction system abnormalities from blockages due to rheumatic nodules around the atrioventricular node may cause heart block.
- **Pleuropulmonary disease:** Pleural effusions or pleuritic chest pain are relatively common. Pulmonary fibrosis or progressive interstitial lung disease may be seen with or without rheumatoid nodules in the lung parenchyma.
- **Episcleritis and scleritis:** Episcleritis is an inflammatory condition of the connective tissue between the sclera and conjunctiva. Scleritis is of the sclera and can cause scleral perforation.
- **Sicca syndrome:** A condition of dry eyes and dry mouth that can result from infiltration of the lacrimal and salivary glands with lymphocytes.

specific for an antigen in the joints, and they release lymphokines. The disease also involves antibodies, especially an IgM anti-IgG called **rheumatoid factor (RF)**.[20] RF is present in 85% to 90% of persons with rheumatoid arthritis and may be stimulated by a self-antigen, an antigen in the synovial cavity, or an infectious antigen. The RF-IgG complexes are present in the rheumatoid lesions and apparently activate complement to promote the inflammatory response.

Acute attacks of rheumatoid arthritis occur as the RF-IgG complexes precipitate in the synovial fluid. Complement is activated that attracts polymorphonuclear leukocytes, whose main function appears to be phagocytosis of the complexes. The lysosomal enzymes released by these cells intensify the inflammatory reaction and increase destruction of the articular cartilage. Granulation tissue and inflammatory cells form a mass of tissue called **pannus** that erodes the articular cartilage.[10] The joint space is destroyed, and the resultant scarring may completely immobilize the joint or cause bleeding and thrombosis in the area.

Rheumatoid subcutaneous nodules often are seen and are described as firm, non-tender, oval masses up to 2 cm in diameter. They are present on the forearms and sometimes the Achilles tendons, or attached to underlying periosteum or tendons.

Other systems also are affected. A necrotizing arteritis may lead to thrombosis of small arteries. Fibrinous pericarditis, cardiomyopathy, and valvular lesions may affect the heart. Pleuritis and interstitial fibrosis may affect the lungs.[13]

Clinical Manifestations

The signs and symptoms of rheumatoid arthritis are due to both systemic and local inflammatory lesions. Fatigue, weakness, joint stiffness, and vague arthralgias are early symptoms. The individual complains of morning stiffness, which gradually improves after rising. Joints in the hands or feet may be inflamed and swollen; these symptoms tend to spread symmetrically, so that the corresponding joints on the contralateral extremity become involved. Systemic symptoms are variable and rarely cause significant problems.[42]

Laboratory values, besides the positive RF, include a normochromic or hypochromic anemia, mild leukocytosis with eosinophilia, and elevated erythrocyte sedimentation rate. Synovial fluid shows exudation with polymorphonuclear leukocytes, and the fluid has a turbid appearance.[17]

The course of rheumatoid arthritis is variable, with remissions and exacerbations. Some people have a relatively benign disease, whereas in others it progresses to severe deformity and total disability.

SCLERODERMA

Scleroderma, also called systemic sclerosis, is a relatively uncommon condition that involves thickening and fibrosis of the skin together with vascular, organ, and

FOCUS ON THE PERSON WITH HIV

C. H. is a 28-year-old divorced female with an 8-year-old daughter. Since her divorce 5 years ago, she has dated casually but has not been sexually active. Ms. H. reported that her husband was her only sex partner. She is now a graduate student who presented to the Student Health Service with a severe vaginal yeast infection, which has been refractory to short-term treatment with antifungal vaginal treatment. Physician examination revealed mild lymphadenopathy of the cervical chains, and pelvic examination was positive for a whitish discharge and vaginal and vulvar inflammation consistent with yeast infection. *Candida sp.* was confirmed by wet mount preparation and blood was drawn for HIV screening. During a follow-up visit, Ms. H. was informed that her HIV antibody tests (2 ELISAs and a confirmatory Western Blot) were positive. When questioned about any other HIV-related manifestations, Ms. H. was unsure about having experienced acute retroviral syndrome symptoms, but acknowledged an episode of "sore throat with swollen lymph nodes in her neck sometime in the past." Ms. H. believes that she acquired the virus from her husband, who reportedly had had various sexual relationships during the times they were separated. Laboratory tests indicate a T4 cell count of 360/mm^3. A repeat count showed 300 cells/mm^3. Ms. H.'s daughter was tested for HIV and the results were negative. Treatment with zidovudine (AZT) was initiated and psychosocial intervention with counseling was begun.

Questions

1. Why did Ms. H.'s persistent yeast infection alert the medical team to the possibility of HIV infection?
2. If Ms. H. was infected by her husband several years ago, how did she remain healthy for such a long time?
3. If Ms. H. was a blood donor and had been routinely tested for HIV antibody, how long after infection would she become positive?
4. What is the significance of acute retroviral syndrome (ARS)?
5. Considering the modes of transmission of HIV, why is Ms. H.'s disease probably caused by her ex-husband?
6. What is the significance of the T4 count?
7. What is the mode of action of antiretrovirals such as zidovudine (AZT)? What are its limitations and side effects?
8. Considering the prognosis of HIV infection, what psychosocial interventions would be recommended?

See Appendix A for discussion.

FOCUS ON THE PERSON WITH HYPERSENSITIVITY RESPONSE

J. E., a 37-year-old woman, was working in her yard when she received a sting on the right wrist from a yellow-jacket wasp. Several minutes later she complained of a itching sensation and cramping abdominal pain. She then became acutely short of breath with wheezing. A patchy erythema radiating from the area of the sting was noted along with swollen eyelids and lips. A neighbor took her to an emergency center where she became very faint. Vital signs were: blood pressure, 60/34; pulse, 156; respirations, 40. Epinephrine 1/1000 was immediately administered intravenously along with 100 mg of hydrocortisone. Withing minutes, an improvement in the respiratory rate was noted and blood pressure increased to 100/70 with a pulse rate of 112.

Questions

1. What type of hypersensitivity response is described above?
2. Explain the pathophysiologic mechanism involved in producing the clinical picture.
3. What is the rationale for the treatment given?
4. How could this reaction be prevented? What should Mrs. E. be taught to prevent this occurrence?

See Appendix A for discussion.

immunologic derangements. It affects about four times as many women as men, with the highest on-set between ages 50 to 60 years. The disease appears to follow a more severe course in African-American women.[13] Different forms of the disease exist, but the initial onset usually is marked by Raynaud's phenomenon (see p. 442). The condition may be more prevalent than is thought because of missed diagnoses.

The initial skin changes of edema may be accompanied by arthralgia or morning stiffness. This is followed by skin thickening that results from accumulation of collagen in the dermis.[35] The skin changes are continuous, causing taut restrictions over joints, the thoracic cavity, and even the face. The serum ANA is positive in 90% of persons with systemic sclerosis, and other antibodies may be demonstrated. As the disease progresses, organ changes occur. Patchy fibrosis of the myocardium may result from intermittent myocardial ischemia produced from decreased circulation. Pulmonary changes are varied and may include interstitial inflammatory fibrosis and vascular injury.[13] Progressive renal insufficiency and marked hypertension result from renovascular changes. The gastrointestinal changes are varied and include esoph-

ageal reflux, malabsorption, intussusception, and volvulus. Endocrine changes include hypothyroidism and reproductive disorders.[35] In some cases affected persons are said to have the CREST syndrome, which is a more limited form of scleroderma that may develop visceral changes much later in the course of the disease, if at all. The CREST syndrome refers to the manifestations of calcinosis (calcium deposits in various body tissues), Raynaud's phenomenon, esophageal dysmotility, sclerodactyly (fixed semi-flexed fingers with tightened skin), and telangiectasia (permanent dilatation of the capillaries in various areas of the body).[13]

Morbidity and mortality depend on the degree of organ involvement, and a 60% overall 5-year survival rate is reported in systemic scleroderma.[35]

REFERENCES

1. Abbas, A. K., Lichtman, A. H., & Pober, J. S. (1997). *Cellular and Molecular Immunology* (3rd ed.). Philadelphia: W. B. Saunders.
2. Ameisen, J. C. (1995). HIV infection and T-cell death. In C. Gregory (Ed.), *Apoptosis and the immune system* (pp. 115–142). New York: Wiley-Liss.
3. Barinaga, M. (1996). Forging a path to cell death [research news]. *Science, 273,* 735–737.
4. Broder, S., Merigan Jr., T. C., & Bolognesi, D. (Eds.). (1994). *Textbook of AIDS medicine.* Baltimore: Williams & Wilkins.
5. Brostoff, J. & Hall, T. (1998). Hypersensitivity type I. In I. Roitt, J. Brostoff, & D. Male, *Immunology* (5th ed.). St. Louis: C. V. Mosby.
6. Centers for Disease Control and Prevention. (1992). 1993 revised classification system for HIV infection and expanded surveillance case definition for AIDS among adolescents and adults. *Morbidity and Mortality Weekly Report (MMWR), 41*(RR-17), 1.
7. Centers for Disease Control and Prevention. (1994). 1994 revised classification system for human immunodeficiency virus infection in children less than 13 years of age. *Morbidity and Mortality Weekly Report (MMWR), 30*(RR-12), 1–11.
8. Centers for Disease Control and Prevention. (1998). Report of the NIH Panel to Define Principles of Therapy of HIV Infection and Guidelines for the Use of Antiretroviral Agents in HIV-Infected Adults and Adolescents. *Morbidity and Mortality Weekly Report (MMWR), 47*(RR-05), 43–82.
9. Chan, A. C., Kadlacek, T. A., Elder, M. E. et al. (1994). ZAP-70 deficiency in an autosomal recessive form of severe combined immunodeficiency. *Science, 264,* 1599–1601.
10. Chandrasoma, P. & Taylor, C. R. (1998). *Concise pathology* (3rd ed.). Stamford, C. T.: Appleton & Lange.
11. Clancy, J. Jr. (1998). *Basic concepts in immunology: A student's survival guide.* New York: McGraw-Hill.
12. Connor, E. M., Sperling, R. S., Gelber, R. et al. (1994). Reduction of maternal–infant transmission of imunodeficiency virus type 1 with zidovudine treatment. *New England Journal of Medicine, 331,* 1173–1180.
13. Cotran, R. S., Kumar, V., & Robbins, S. L. (1999). *Robbins' pathologic basis of disease* (6th ed.). Philadelphia: W. B. Saunders.
14. Couser, W. G. (1998). Glomerular diseases. In J. Stein (Ed.), *Internal medicine* (5th ed.) St. Louis: Mosby.
15. Donegan, E. & Bossom, E. L. (1997). Blood banking and immunohematology. In D. P. Stites, A. I. Terr, & T. G. Parslow (Eds.), *Medical immunology* (9th ed.). Stamford, CT: Appleton & Lange.
16. Elder, M. E., Lin, D., Clever, J., et al. (1994). Human severe combined immunodeficiency syndrome due to a defect in ZAP-70, a T-cell tyrosine kinase. *Science, 264,* 1596–1599.
17. Firestein, G. S. (1997). Rheumatoid arthritis. In W. N. Kelley (Ed.), *Textbook of internal medicine* (3rd ed.). Philadelphia: Lippincott-Raven.
18. Gougeon, M. L. & Montagnier, L. (1993). Apoptosis in AIDS. *Science, 260,* 1269–1270.
19. Hahn, B. H. (1994). Viral genes and their products. In S. Broder, T. C. Merigan Jr., & D. Bolognesi (Eds.), *Textbook of AIDS medicine* (pp. 21–43). Baltimore: Williams & Wilkins.
20. Janeway, C. A. & Travers, P. (1997). *Immunobiology: The immune system in health and disease* (3rd ed.). New York: Current Biology/Garland.
21. Male, D. (1998). Hypersensitivity—Type II. In I. Roitt, J. Brostoff, & D. Male, *Immunology* (5th ed.). St. Louis: C. V. Mosby.
22. Mandelbrot, L., LeChenadec, J., Berrebi, A., et al. (1998). Perinatal HIV-1 transmission: Interaction between zidovudine prophylaxis and mode of delivery in the French Perinatal Cohort. *Journal of the American Medical Association, 280,* 55–60.
23. Marquardt, D. L. (1998). Anaphylaxis. In J. H. Stein, *Internal medicine* (5th ed.). St. Louis: Mosby.
24. McGuire, J. L. & Lambert, R. E. (1997). Systemic lupus erythematosus and overlap syndromes. In W. N. Kelley (Ed.), *Textbook of internal medicine* (3rd ed.). Philadelphia: Lippincott-Raven.
25. Mellors, J. W., Munoz, A. M., Giorgi, J. V. et al. (1997). Plasma viral load and $CD4^+$ lymphocytes as prognostic markers of HIV-1 infection. *Annals of Internal Medicine, 126,* 946–954.
26. Melroe, N. H., Stawarz, K. E., Simpson, J., & Henry, W. K. (1997). HIV RNA quantitation: Marker of HIV infection. *Journal of the Association of Nurses in AIDS Care, 8,* 31–38.
27. O'Brien, T. R., & Goedert, J. J. (1998). Chemokine receptors and genetic variability: Another leap in HIV research [editorial]. *Science, 279,* 317–318.
28. Oyaizu, N. & Pahwa, S. (1995). Role of apoptosis in HIV disease pathogenesis. *Journal of Clinical Immunology, 15*(5), 217–227.
29. Puck, J. M. (1997). Primary immunodeficiency diseases. *Science, 278,* 1835–1841.
30. Ratner, L. (1996). Genetic organization of HIV. In S. Gupta (Ed.), *Immunology of HIV infection* (pp. 3–22). New York: Plenum Medical Books.
31. Rodgers, R. P. C. (1997). Clinical laboratory methods for detection of antigens and antibodies. In D. P. Stities, A. I. Terr, & T. G. Parslow, *Basic and clinical immunology* (9th ed.). Stamford, CT: Appleton & Lange.
32. Roitt, I., Brostoff, J., & Male, D. (1998). *Immunology* (5th ed.). Philadelphia: Mosby.
33. Rubin, E. & Farber, J. L. (1999). *Pathology* (3rd ed.). Philadelphia: Lippincott.
34. Saag, M. S. (1997). Clinical spectrum of human immunodeficiency virus diseases. In V. T. DeVita, S. Hellman, & S. A. Rosenberg (Eds.), *AIDS: Etiology, diagnosis, treatment and prevention* (4th ed.) (pp. 203–213). Philadelphia: Lippincott-Raven.
35. Seibold, J. R. (1997). Scleroderma and Raynaud's syndrome. In W. N. Kelley (Ed.), *Textbook of internal medicine* (3rd ed.). Philadelphia: Lippincott-Raven.
36. Staines, N., Brostoff, J., & James, K. (1994). *Introducing immunology* (2nd ed.). St. Louis: Mosby.

37. Staprans, S. I., & Feinberg, M. B. (1997). Natural history and immunopathogenesis of HIV-1 disease. In M. A. Sande & P. A. Volberding (Eds.), *The medical management of AIDS* (5th ed.) (pp. 29–55). Philadelphia: W. B. Saunders.
38. Stites, D. P., Terr, A. I., & Parslow, T. G. (1997). *Basic and clinical immunology* (9th ed.). Stamford, CT: Appleton & Lange.
39. Terr, A. I. (1997). Immune complex allergic disease. In D. P. Stites, A. I. Terr, & T. G. Parslow, *Basic and clinical imunology* (9th ed.). Stamford, CT: Appleton & Lange.
40. Weiss, R. A. (1996). HIV receptors and the pathogenesis of AIDS. *Science, 272,* 1885–1886.
41. Young, J. A. T. (1994). The replication cycle of HIV. In P. T. Cohen, M. A. Sande, & P. A. Volberding (Eds.), *The AIDS knowledge base: A textbook on HIV disease from the University of California, San Francisco, and the San Francisco General Hospital* (2nd ed.). Boston: Little, Brown.
42. Zvaifler, N. J. (1998). Rheumatoid arthritis. In J. Stein (Ed.), *Internal medicine* (5th ed.). St. Louis: Mosby.

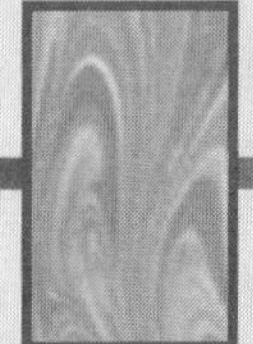

UNIT 2: CASE STUDY

Systemic Lupus Erythematosus

Introduction to the Patient

L. L. is a 41-year-old Asian-American female who is being seen in the clinic with vague complaints of fever, fatigue, weight loss, and arthralgias in all of the joints. The onset of this condition has been insidious over perhaps 6 months to a year.

Present Illness

Ms. L. has noticed pronounced fatigue, weight loss, loss of hair, an erythematous rash over the cheeks and bridge of the nose, and migratory, transient arthralgias of the knees and hands. She made the clinic appointment a month ago and has felt worse while waiting to be seen.

Social History

Ms. L. works as a seamstress in a dry cleaning establishment close to her home. She often works 12 hours or more in her job. She is married and has one child, a boy, aged 9. Her husband is an engineer working for an architectural design firm. Ms. L. does not drink alcohol or smoke cigarettes.

Past Medical History

Ms. L. states that her health has been good, with only a few episodes of flu and a cold or two per year. She denies significant menstrual problems or urinary tract infections.

Family History

Ms. L.'s parents immigrated to the U.S. when she was a child. Both parents are living. Her father suffered a stroke 10 years previously and has residual paralysis of the left arm and weakness of the left leg. Her mother cares for her father, and both parents live in Ms. L.'s home. The mother has diagnosed pernicious anemia and is treated with monthly injections of vitamin B12. Ms. L. has an identical twin sister who lives on the East Coast. Her brother lives in Houston close by her home. Both siblings are alive and apparently well. Ms. L.'s husband and son are in good health.

Physical Examination

Ms. L. is a thin Asian woman who is very pale and anxious appearing. She is 5 ft. tall and weighs 90 lbs. Her temperature is 100°F, blood pressure is 110/70, and pulse is 90. Examination indicates normal cardiac and respiratory sounds. She complains of tenderness on mobilization of wrist joints, but no apparent deformity is present. A malar rash over the cheeks and bridge of the nose is present. Hair is very thin and lacks luster. She states that she has had some pleuritic type chest pain, which is not present currently. Lymphadenopathy is present in the cervical and axillary areas.

Diagnostic Tests

Chest x-ray is essentially normal.

Lab values indicate Hgb 10, Hct. 28, platelets 100,000/µL, WBC 4000/µL, + ANA, + VDRL, BUN 35, creatinine 1.8.

CRITICAL THINKING QUESTIONS

1. What features in the above case support the diagnosis of systemic lupus erythematosus (SLE)?
2. Discuss the pathophysiology of SLE, including its various presentations.
3. What etiologic factors influence the onset of this disease? How is it related to drug therapies?
4. Discuss the diagnostic tests performed on Ms. L. and their significance.
5. What genetic and familial factors are especially important in planning for effective care of this patient?
6. Construct a plan of care for the management of this patient through drug therapy, prevention of complications, and long-term management.

Besides your pathophysiology text, you will need a good pharmacology textbook, a medical immunology text, a pathology text, and current research articles to complete this case study. Suggested references follow:

Karch, A. (2000). *Focus on nursing pharmacology.* Philadelphia: Lippincott Williams & Wilkins.

Roitt, I., Brostoff, J., & Male, D. (1998). *Immunology* (5th ed.). St. Louis: Mosby.

Rubin, E. & Farber, J. L. (1999) *Pathology* (3rd ed.). Philadelphia: Lippincott-Raven.

UNIT 2 APPENDIX A

IMMUNOLOGIC DIAGNOSTIC TESTS

TEST	NORMAL VALUE	SIGNIFICANCE
Alpha$_1$ antitrypsin	76–189 mL/dL	Serine protease inhibitor, synthesized by liver; binds with elastases and proteases to inhibit their damage to lung tissues. Deficiency of substance associated with early-onset emphysema, liver disease, glomerulonephritis and connective tissue disease.
Anti-glomerular basement membrane antibodies (anti-GBM)	Negative	Detects circulating anti-GBM antibodies that damage GBM in glomeruli, may cause severe glomerulo nephritis and damage to pulmonary capillary basement membranes (as in Goodpasture's syndrome).
Antimyocardial antibodies	Negative	Auto-antibodies that reacted against cardiac muscle that can damage the heart; may be present after myocardial infarction, rheumatic fever, or cardiac surgery.
Antinuclear antibodies (ANA)	Negative	Screening test for diagnosing autoimmune diseases, especially systematic lupus erythematosus (SLE). Also may be positive with scleroderma, rheumatoid arthritis, cirrhosis of the liver, infectious mononucleosis, and malignancy.
Antistreptolysin O (ASO)	< 100 IU/mL	Antibodies developed to beta-hemolytic *Streptococcus* organism. Antibodies appear 1–2 weeks after an acute streptococcal infection and may remain elevated for months.
Bence-Jones protein	None detected in serum or urine	Free light chains of immunoglobulin molecules, seen in about half of all patients with multiple myeloma.
C-reactive protein (CRP)	Usually not present	Acute-phase protein seen 6–10 hours after acute inflammatory processes; a non-specific test helpful in monitoring phases of rheumatic fever and rheumatoid arthritis.
Cold agglutinins	1:8 antibody titer	Autoantibodies of the IgM class that agglutinate human erythrocytes at temperatures <37°C. Elevated levels often found in persons with primary atypical pneumonias, influenza, cirrhosis of the liver, and other clinical problems.
Complement		
Total	75–160 μ/mL	Complements make up about 10% of serum globulins; which function in inflammatory response.
C3	86–184 mg/dL	Most abundant component, essential to carry out cascade of activated complement proteins; may be decreased in immundeficiency and in SLE.
C4	20–58 mg/dL	Second most abundant complement component; increased in acute inflammation and decreased in SLE, primary immune deficiency, and other conditions.
Coombs' test		
Direct	Negative	Detects antibodies attached to red blood cells that may cause cellular damage; positive in erythroblastosis fetalis, autoimmune hemolytic anemia, hemolytic transfusion reactions, and some drug reactions.
Indirect	Negative	Detects free circulating antibodies; positive in incompatible cross-matched blood, acquired hemolytic anemia anti-Rh antibodies.
Cryoglobulins (cryoproteins)	Up to 6 mg/dL	Serum globulins of IgG or IgM classification, elevated with autoimmune conditions, such as SLE, and other conditions such as lymphocytic leukemia and acquired hemolytic anemias.
Erythrocyte sedimentation rate (ESR)	Depends on method, usually: Female: 1–25 mm/hr Male: 0–17 mm/hr	Measures rate at which red blood cells settle in mm/hour. Rate is increased in inflammatory conditions such as infections and collagen diseases.

UNIT 2 APPENDIX A (Continued)

TEST	NORMAL VALUE	SIGNIFICANCE
Haptoglobulins	16–199 mg/dL	Globulins that combine with free hemoglobin during hemolytic reactions; may be elevated in certain inflammatory conditions and cancers, and decreased in hemolytic anemias, severe liver diseases, and certain other conditions.
Immunoglobulins		
IgG	614–1295 mg/dL	Major immunoglobulin, has antibacterial and antiviral activity; decreased in primary deficiency, bone marrow suppression, leukemia; increased in infections and autoimmune disorders.
IgA	60–309 mg/dL	Found in secretions (respiratory, gastrointestinal, etc.). Decreased in primary deficiency, malignancies; increased in autoimmune disorders and chronic infections. Found
IgM	53–334 mg/dL	mainly in blood. Decreased in lymphocytic leukemia, primary deficiency; increased in lymphosarcoma, infections mononucleosis, skin reactions, certain infections.
IgE	10–179 IU/mL	Located in tissues and blood; increases during allergic reactions and anaphylaxis.
Lupus erythematosus cell test (LE cell)	Negative	Nonspecific screening test for SLE. Test rarely done since ANA and anti-DNA tests are more sensitive; also may be positive with rheumatoid arthritis, scleroderma, and drug-induced lupus.
Lymphocytes		
T lymphocytes	60–80% 600–2400 cells/μL	Cellular immunity and directing humoral immunity; decreased in immunodeficiency diseases (both primary and secondary), acute viral infections, increased in certain autoimmune diseases.
B lymphocytes	4–16% 50–250 cells/μL	Humoral immunity through specific antigens. Decreased in immunodeficiency (both primary and secondary); increased in acute and chronic lymphocytic leukemias, multiple myeloma, auto immune conditions.
Protein Total	6–8 g/dL	Total protein composed of albumin and globulins.
Albumin	3.5–5 g/dL	Mainly responsible for maintaining serum colloid osmotic pressure, affecting acid-base balance; and drug carrying. Decreased in malnutrition, liver disease, many systemic conditions; increased in dehydration and exercise.
Globulin	1.5–3.5 g/dL	Major globulins are alpha 1, alpha 2, beta, and gamma globulins. May be decreased in deficiency states, liver disease, hypocholesterolemia, nephrotic syndromes, lymphocytic leukemia. May be elevated in collagen diseases, certain neoplasms, infections, trauma, and obstructive jaundice depending on the type of globulin affected.
Rheumatoid factor (RF)	<30 IU/mL	Screening test for antibodies (IgM, IgG, or IgA) found in sera of persons with rheumatoid arthritis. Also elevated in SLE, scleroderma, infectious mononucleosis, tuberculosis, leukemia, old age, and other conditions.
Thyroid antibodies (thyroglobulin antibodies)	Negative	Antibodies to self thyroid; combine with thyroglobulin and cause inflammatory lesions of the gland.

UNIT 2 APPENDIX B

COMMON CD MARKERS

MARKER	CELL AFFECTED	SIGNIFICANCE
CD 4	T-helper	Co-receptor for MHC class II molecules. Helps or induces immune responses. Has receptor for HIV-1 and HIV-2 gp120.
CD 5	B cell T cells	Co-stimulator in both T and B cells; may be physiologic ligand in B cells.
CD 8	T-cytotoxic	Co-receptor for MHC class I molecules. Predominantly cytotoxic; biased towards certain bacterial and viral antigens.
CD 16	NK cell/neutrophils, macrophages	Reliable marker for presence of NK cells, which recognize and kill certain tumor and virus-infected cells.
T_s	T suppressor	May be function of CD 4 and CD 8 T cells, but function with negative regulation of signal transduction to limit immune reactivity.

UNIT BIBLIOGRAPHY

Abbas, A. K., Lichtman, A. H., & Pober, J. S. (1997). *Cellular and molecular immunology* (3rd ed.). Philadelphia: W. B. Saunders.

Bach, F. H. & Auchincloss Jr., H. (Eds.) (1995). *Transplantation immunology.* New York: John Wiley.

Benjamini, E., Sunshine, G., & Leskowitz, S. (1996). *Immunology: A short course* (3rd ed.). New York: Wiley-Liss.

Brent, L. (1997). *A history of transplantation immunology.* New York: Academic Press.

Brostoff, J., Gray, A., Male, D., & Roitt, I. (1998). *Case studies in immunology.* Philadelphia: Mosby.

Charlesworth, E. N. (Ed.) (1996). *Cutaneous allergy.* Cambridge, MA: Blackwell Science.

Clancy, J. (1998). *Basic concepts in immunology: A student's survival guide.* New York: McGraw-Hill.

Davies, H. (1997). *Introductory immunobiology.* New York: Chapman & Hall.

Elgert, K. D. (1996). *Immunology: Understanding the immune system.* New York: Wiley-Liss.

Frank, M. M., Austen, K. F., Claman, H. N., & Unanue, E. R. (1995). *Samter's immunologic diseases,* Vols. I and II (5th ed.). New York: Little, Brown.

Glaser, R. & Kiecolt-Glaser, J. (Eds.) (1994). *Handbook of human stress and immunology.* New York: Academic Press.

Herbert, W. J., Wilkinson, P., & Stott, D. I. (1995). *The dictionary of immunology* (4th ed.). New York: Academic Press.

Janeway, C. A., & Travers, J. (1997). *Immunobiology: The immune System in health and disease* (3rd ed.). New York: Garland Publishing.

Kaplan, A. P. (Ed.) (1997). *Allergy* (2nd ed.). Philadelphia: W. B. Saunders.

Kuby, J. (1997). *Immunology* (3rd ed.). New York: W. H. Freeman.

Male, D., Cooke, Owen, M. A., Trowsdalde, J., & Champion, B. (1996). *Advanced immunology* (3rd ed.). Philadelphia: Mosby.

Mandel, G., Bennett, J. & Dolin, R. (Eds.)(1995). *Mandell, Douglas, and Bennett's principles and practices of infectious diseases* (4th ed.). New York: Churchill Livingstone (1997).

Peakman, M. & Vergani, D. (1997). *Basic and clinical immunology.* New York: Churchill Livingstone.

Playfair, J. H. L. (1996). *Immunology at a glance* (6th ed.). Cambridge, MA: Blackwell Science.

Roitt, I., Brostoff, J., & Male, D. (1998). *Immunology* (5th ed.). Philadelphia: Mosby.

Schaechter, M., Medoff, G. & Eisenstein, B. I. (1998). *Mechanisms of microbial disease* (3rd ed.). Baltimore: Williams & Wilkins (1996).

Sell, S. (1996). *Immunology, immunopathology, and immunity* (5th ed.). Stamford, CT: Appleton & Lange.

Sheehan, C. (1997). *Clinical immunology: Principles and laboratory diagnosis* (2nd ed.). Philadelphia: Lippincott.

Shulman, S., Phair, J., Peterson, L. & Warren, J. (1997). *The biologic and clinical basis of infectious diseases* (5th ed.). Philadelphia: W. B. Saunders (1996).

Stevens, C. D. (1996). *Clinical immunology and serology: A laboratory perspective.* Philadelphia: F.A. Davis.

Stiehm, E. R. (Ed.) (1996). *Immunologic disorders in infants and children* (4th ed.). Philadelphia: W. B. Saunders.

Stites, D. P., Terr, A. I., & Parslow, T. G. (Eds.) (1997). *Medical immunology* (9th ed.). Stamford, CT: Appleton & Lange.

Tizard, I. R. (1995). *Immunology: An introduction* (4th ed.). Philadelphia: Saunders College Publishing.

Widmann, F. K. (1998). *An introduction to clinical immunology* (2nd ed.). Philadelphia: F. A. Davis.

BIBLIOGRAPHY—HIV DISEASE

Adam, B. D. & Sears, A. (1996). *Experiencing HIV: Personal, family, and work relationships.* New York: Columbia University Press.

Berger, J. R. & Levy, R. M. (Eds.) (1997). *AIDS and the nervous system* (2nd ed.). Philadelphia: Lippincott-Raven.

Bartlett, J. G. & Finkbeiner, A. K. (1996). *The guide to living with HIV infection* (Johns Hopkins AIDS Clinic) (3rd ed.). Baltimore: Johns Hopkins Press.

Broder, S., Merigan Jr., T. C., & Bolognesi, D. (Eds.) (1994). *Textbook of AIDS medicine.* Baltimore: Williams & Wilkins.

Catalán, J., Sherr, L., & Hedge, B. (Eds.) (1997). *The impact of AIDS: Psychological and social aspects of HIV infection.* Amsterdam: Harwood Academic Publishers.

Cohen, P. T., Sande, M. A., & Volberding, P. A. (Eds.) (1994). *The AIDS knowledge base: A textbook on HIV disease from the University of California, San Francisco, and the San Francisco General Hospital* (2nd ed.). Boston: Little, Brown.

Cotton, D. R. & Watts, D. H. (Eds.) (1997). *The medical management of AIDS in women.* New York: John Wiley & Son.

DeVita, V. T., Hellmann, S., & Rosenberg, S. A. (Eds.) (1997). *AIDS: Etiology, diagnosis, treatment, and prevention* (4th ed.). Philadelphia: Lippincott.

Faden, R. & Kass, N. E. (Eds.) (1996). *HIV, AIDS, and childbearing: public policy, private lives.* New York: Oxford Press.

Fahey, J. L. & Flemming, D. S. (Eds.) (1996). *AIDS/HIV: Reference guide for medical professionals* (4th ed.). Baltimore: Williams & Wilkins.

Friedman-Kien, A. E. & Cockerell, C. J. (1996). *Color atlas of AIDS* (2nd ed.). Philadelphia: Saunders.

Gendelman, H. E., Lipton, S. A., Epstein, L., & Swindells, S. (Eds.) (1998). *The neurology of AIDS.* New York: Chapman & Hall.

Golematis, B. C. & DeVita Jr, V. T. (Eds.) (1996). *AIDS and malignancies: Current concepts and perspectives.* New York: John Wiley.

Green, J. & McCreaner, A. (Eds.) (1996). *Counselling in HIV infection and AIDS* (2nd ed.). Cambridge, MA: Blackwell Science.

Gupta, S. (Ed.) (1996). *Immunology of HIV infection.* New York: Plenum Medical Books.

Harrison, M. J. G. & McArthur, J. C. (1995). *AIDS and neurology* (Clinical Neurology and Neuroscience Monographs). New York: Churchill Livingstone.

Huber, J. T. (1996). *HIV/AIDS community information services: Experiences in serving both at-risk and HIV-infected populations.* New York: Haworth Press.

Huber, J. T. & Gillaspy, M. L. (1996), *HIV/AIDS and HIV-related terminology: A means of organizing the body of knowledge.* New York: Haworth Press.

Levy, J. A. (1994) *HIV and the pathogenesis of AIDS.* Washington, DC: ASM Press.

Mann, J. & Tarantola, D. (Eds.) (1996). *AIDS in the world II: Global dimensions, social roots, and responses.* The Global AIDS Policy Coalition. New York: Oxford University Press.

Morrow, W. J. W., & Haigwood, N. L. (Eds.) (1993). *HIV: Molecular organization, pathogenicity, and treatment.* New York: Elsevier.

Muma, R. D., Lyons, B. A., Borucki, M. J., & Pollard, R. B. (1997). *HIV manual for health care professionals* (2nd ed.). Norwalk: Appleton & Lange.

Nokes, K. M. (Ed.) (1996). *HIV/AIDS and the older adult.* Washington, DC: Taylor and Francis.

O'Donnell, M. (1996). *HIV/AIDS: Loss, grief, challenge, and hope.* Washington, DC: Taylor and Francis.

Pizzo, P. A. & Wilfert, C. M. (Eds.) (1994). *Pediatric AIDS: The challenge of HIV infection in infants, children, and adolescents* (2nd ed.). Baltimore: Williams & Wilkins.

Powell, J. (1996). *AIDS and HIV-related diseases: An educational guide for professionals and the public.* New York: Plenum (Insight Books).

Sande, M. A., & Volberding, P. A. (Eds.) (1997). *The medical management of AIDS* (5th ed.). Philadelphia: W. B. Saunders.

Schochetman, G. & George, J. R. (Eds.) (1994). *AIDS testing: A comprehensive guide to technical, medical, social, legal, and management issues* (2nd ed.). New York: Springer-Verlag.

Stine, G. J. (1996). *AIDS: Biological, medical, social, and legal issues* (2nd ed.). Englewood Cliffs, NJ: Prentice Hall.

Webber, D. W. (Ed.) (1997). *AIDS and the law* (3rd ed.). New York: John Wiley & Sons (Wiley Law Publications).

Wormser, G. P. (Ed.) (1996). *A clinical guide to AIDS and HIV.* Philadelphia: Lippincott-Raven.

Wormser, G. P. (Ed.) (1998). *AIDS and other manifestations of HIV infection* (3rd ed.). Philadelphia: Lippincott-Raven.

CLASSIC BIBLIOGRAPHY—HIV/AIDS

AIDS: Epidemiologic and clinical studies (Vol. 2). (1989). Reprints from The New England Journal of Medicine. Waltham, MA: NEJM Books.

Clinical Studies, (1987). *AIDS: Epidemiological and clinical studies.* Reprints from *The New England Journal of Medicine.* Waltham, MA: Massachusetts Medical Society.

Cole, H. M., & Lundberg, G. D. (Eds.)(1986). *AIDS: From the beginning.* Chicago: American Medical Society.

Kulstad, R. (Ed.) (1988). *AIDS 1988: AAAS symposia papers.* Washington, DC: American Association for the Advancement of Science.

Kulstad, R. (Ed.) (1986). *AIDS: Papers from Science, 1982–1985.* Washington, DC: The American Association for the Advancement of Science.

Shilts, R. (1987). *And the band played on: Politics, people, and the AIDS epidemic.* New York: St. Martin's Press.

Sontag, S. (1989). *AIDS and its metaphors.* New York: Farrar, Strauss and Giroux.

USEFUL WEBSITES—HIV/AIDS

AIDS Education and Training Centers (ETC) for Texas and Oklahoma (The University of Texas—Houston Health Science Center School of Public Health): http://www.sph.uth.tmc.edu/www/utsph/jmeyer/aidsetc.htm

Centers for Disease Control and Prevention (CDC) homepage: http://www.cdc.gov/

Centers for Disease Control and Prevention (CDC), Morbidity and Mortality Weekly Report (MMWR): http://www.cdc.gov/epo/mmwr/mmwr.html

Internet HIV/AIDS resources: http://www.sph.uth.tmc.edu/www/utsph/jmeyer/info.htm

Journal of the American Medical Association (JAMA) AIDS Website: http://WWW.AMA-ASSN.ORG/special/hiv/hivhome.htm

National Pediatric and Family HIV Resource Center (University of Medicine and Dentistry of New Jersey): http://www.pedhivaids.org/

Unit
3

Hematology

FOCUS ON Hematologic Changes Through The Life Span

INFANT (1–12 MONTHS):

Physiologic anemia is common with production of more and more mature erythrocytes. Lymphoid tissue grows rapidly during infancy and begins to provide for immunity after the first few months. Early immunity is provided by fetal transfer of antibodies from placental blood. Gradual development of immune competence occurs.

TODDLER AND PRESCHOOL AGE (1–5 YEARS):

The phagocytic system and the immune system are much more efficient than in infancy. Lifetime immunity to specific diseases is often gained by immunizations or exposure to diseases. Immunoglobulin levels gradually increase to adult levels. Red blood cell formation is normally induced, but dietary deficiencies of iron and proteins may produce anemias.

SCHOOL AGE (6–12 YEARS):

The immune system becomes functionally mature. Enlargement of the lymphoid tissues, especially the tonsils and adenoids, is common. Thymic function is very active in the production of lymphocytes. Erythrocyte formation is normal, but anemias are common due to diet and growth factors.

ADOLESCENCE (13–19 YEARS):

Thymic function remains maximal to provide for lifetime immunity and disease protection. All cellular components are usually normal unless there is intervening disease, malnutrition, or trauma. Dietary habits are often poor, and anemias related to diet are common. Eating disorders are at their peak, especially in females, and nutritional imbalances may affect all of the hematologic system.

YOUNG ADULT AND ADULT (20–45 YEARS):

Normal blood cell counts are usual in the presence of health. These provide for maximal oxygenation and protection from disease. Red marrow is found in the ribs, sternum, pelvis, vertebrae, and a few other bones and is responsible for making all of the blood cells. By age 20, most people have become immune to many of the infectious agents in the environment. The immune system functions maximally in the absence of stress and disease. Anemias are common in women, especially in the childbearing ages.

MIDDLE-AGED ADULT (46–64 YEARS):

In the healthy individual, there are no major changes in the values of blood cells. Immunity remains intact even though there is gradual thymic involution and decrease in the production of lymphocytes. Stress, illness, and trauma may markedly affect the production of blood cells and the ability to resist infection.

LATE ADULTHOOD (65–100+ YEARS):

Blood production is not usually altered in the healthy elderly person, but it may be altered by diseases, nutritional deficiencies, and trauma. Hemoglobin and hematocrit levels often decline slightly and often are related to diet. Immune response is slower, and T-lymphocytes levels may decline. Older adults are more susceptible to infectious complications, and response to therapy may be less effective than in younger persons. Leukocytes and platelets may be decreased, and depleted levels are regenerated much more slowly than in the younger individual. There is an increase in some of the autoantibodies.

Chapter

12

Normal and Altered Erythrocyte Function

Brenda K. Shelton

KEY TERMS

agglutinogens
agglutinins
apoferritin
blood group
blood type
carbaminohemoglobin (CO_2Hgb)
colony-forming units (CFUs)
2,3 diphosphoglycerate (2,3 DPG)
erythropoietin hormone
ferritin
haptoglobin
hemachromatosis
hematopoiesis
intrinsic factor
koilonychia
methemoglobin
oxyhemoglobin
pluripotential stem cells
polycythemia
porphyrin structure (heme)
red blood cell aplasia
splenomegaly
stem cell theory
thrombocytosis
transferrin

All living cells require materials to survive and to perform homeostatic functions. Blood, in conjunction with interstitial fluid, provides a means for delivery and removal of essential substances and waste products to the cells. Transportation of cellular and humoral messages by the blood helps to integrate physiologic processes, enabling the body to function as a unified whole.

The primary roles of blood are to integrate body functions and to meet the needs of specific tissues. This is accomplished through transportation, regulation, and protection mechanisms. Blood transports oxygen, nutrients, waste products, and hormones from one place to another. Regulation is accomplished through buffers in the blood (see p. 178), plasma proteins, and heat transport, such as muscle-generated temperature. The protective function of the blood includes activities by antibodies and phagocytes to protect against disease and coagulation factors that participate in hemostasis.

BLOOD COMPONENTS

Blood consists of a clear yellow fluid called *plasma*, in which cells and other substances are suspended. Ninety-nine percent of the cells are red blood cells (RBCs), also known as erythrocytes. Other cells in the plasma include the white blood cells (WBCs) and the platelets, which are discussed in Chapters 13 and 14.

Although plasma is intravascular and interstitial fluid is extravascular, they both have a similar composition, except that plasma contains a high protein concentration. Proteins are the major solutes in plasma and consist primarily of albumins, globulins, and fibrinogen. High blood concentration of proteins maintains the intravascular volume by colloid oncotic (osmotic) pressure (see p. 159). In addition to holding water in the intravascular spaces, plasma proteins bind with substances such as lipids and metals, such as iron, that contribute to blood viscosity. Plasma proteins also participate in the coagulation of blood and regulation of acid-base balance.

The blood volume is the sum of volumes of plasma and cells of blood in the vascular system. It can be calculated from either plasma volume or cell volume. Although numerous factors affect blood volume, compensatory mechanisms enable total blood volume to remain relatively stable in the healthy person. For example, clinical conditions decreasing RBC volume (e.g., anemia) are balanced by increased plasma volume, establishing a consistent blood volume despite changes in the plasma-to-cell ratio. Capillary dynamics and renal mechanisms play major roles in maintaining plasma volume. The constituency of blood rapidly and continuously changes, but the general characteristics remain relatively constant. General physical characteristics of the blood and causes of variations are summarized in Table 12-1. Unit 3, Appendix A provides detailed information on hematologic values and diagnostic tests used in specific blood disorders.

Formation of Blood Cells

Hematopoiesis is a term used to describe the normal formation of blood cells in the bone marrow. It is a dynamic process, with rapid turnover of blood cells. There are greater reserves of white blood cells, and the normal ratio of white blood cell precursors to RBC precursors is between 2 : 1 and 4.5 : 1.[17] However, RBC formation is the best understood of hematopoietic cell formation and differentiation.

BONE MARROW

Bone marrow meets the body's changing demands for cells by maintaining a reserve supply of cells. In the adult, the bone marrow produces all hematopoietic cells. At birth and throughout early childhood, red marrow is present in all bone marrow cavities, and blood cells are formed in the red marrow, liver, and spleen.[17] By age 20 to 25 years, red marrow is present in the cranial bones, vertebrae, sternum, ribs, clavicles, scapulae, pelvis, and proximal ends of the femur and humeri. Other marrow areas become inactive, infiltrated with fat, and are called yellow marrow. In the aged person, red marrow no longer fills the cranial bones and lower vertebrae.[6] The blood supply to the marrow comes from thin-walled arteries with large lumens that branch into a network of capillaries to become a bed of sinusoids. Between the sinuses lies the hematopoietic tissue in which blood cells are formed. At a predestined maturation point, blood cells gain access through small openings in the walls of the sinusoids, and maturation is completed in the circulatory system and tissues.[21] Loss of integrity of the sinus walls or increased need may allow the release of immature cells into the circulation.

STEM CELLS

The **stem cell theory** currently explains how specific hematopoietic cells are created and supplied when needed (Fig. 12-1). Stem cells have the morphologic appearance of small mononuclear cells that resemble

TABLE 12-1

CHARACTERISTICS OF BLOOD

CHARACTERISTIC	NORMAL	ALTERATIONS
Color	Arterial: bright red Venous: dark red or crimson	Hypochromic (light color) in anemia Lighter color in dilution
pH	Arterial: 7.35–7.45	Decreases in systemic acidosis such as renal failure, diabetic crisis, infection
	Venous: 7.31–7.41	Increases in alkalosis such as vomiting, diuretic use, or hyperventilation
Specific gravity	Plasma: 1.026 RBC: 1.093	—
Viscosity	3.5–4.5 times that of water	Loss of plasma volume such as dehydration Increased cell production such as polycythemia Abnormal immunoglobulin such as multiple myeloma
Volume	Plasma volume 45 mL/kg Cell volume 30 mL/kg Average male is about 5000 mL	Fat tissue contains little water, so total blood volume best correlates to lean body mass Women have more fat, and therefore blood volume is usually lower than men Plasma volume rises with progression of pregnancy Volume increased with immobility and decreases with prolonged standing. May be due to changes in pressure on glomerulus and glomerular filtration rate. Blood volume highest in neonate and lowest in elderly Lack of nutrients causes decreased RBC and plasma formation Increased environmental temperature increases blood volume

FOCUS ON CELLULAR PHYSIOLOGY

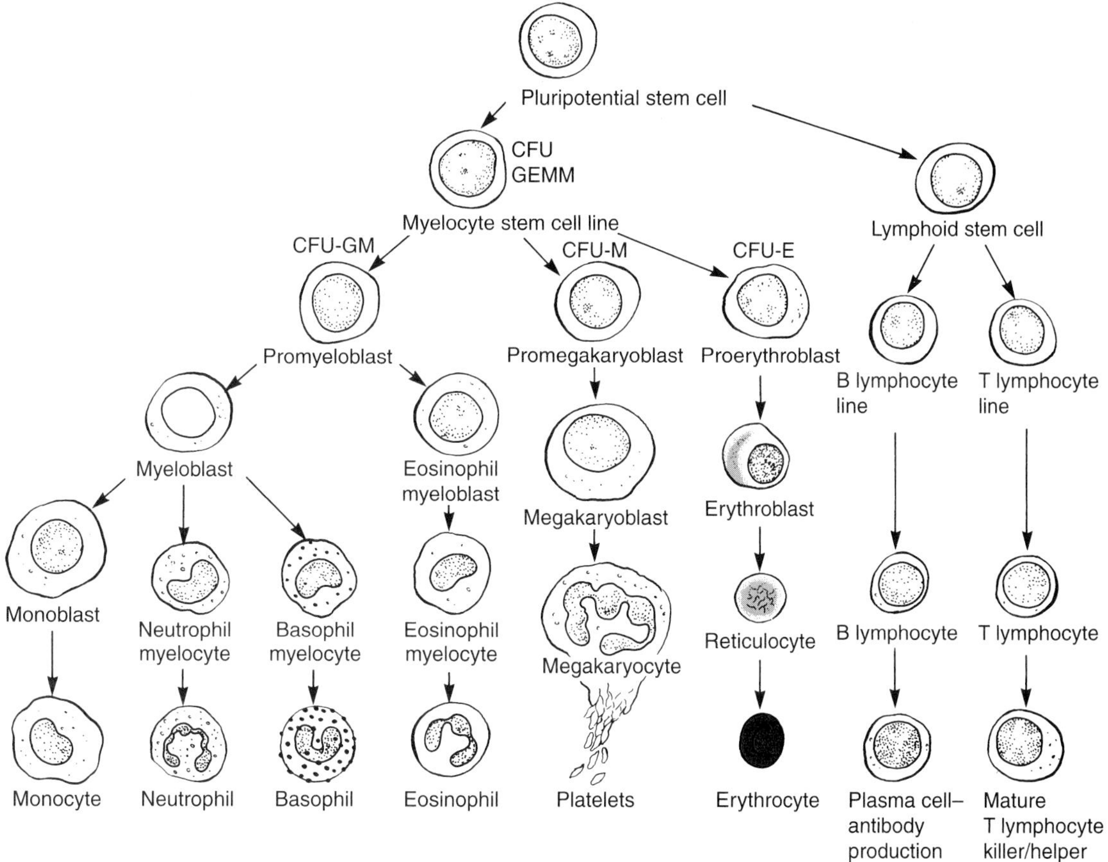

FIGURE 12-1. Differentiation of hematopoietic blood cells. Colony-forming units (CFUs) are groups of cells that can become committed to a specific blood line. CFU-GEMM has the potential to form any cell line except lymphocytes. CFU-GM forms granulocytes and monocytes, CFU-M forms megakaryocytes, and CFU-E forms erythrocytes.

lymphocytes. These cells apparently have the ability to divide and differentiate into a specific cell line when stimulated, and are thus called **pluripotential stem cells.** These pluripotential stem cells transform to committed precursor (early) cells, then finally differentiate (mature) into recognizable hematopoietic cells.[6] They become grouped in pools or compartments called **colony-forming units (CFUs)**. These units can maintain themselves and produce cells that become committed to a certain line of blood cells.[21] Colony-forming units that are designated to form erythrocytes are termed CFUE, those that form granulocytes and monocytes have the designation CFUGM, and those forming megakaryocytes are termed CFUM.[6,21]

Complex feedback loops of humoral regulation involve colony-stimulating and inhibiting factors. These factors regulate the proliferation and differentiation of blood cells into mature cells.[17] As noted in Figure 12-1, the stem cell becomes committed to the lymphoid or trilineage myeloid stem cell lines, but it maintains the property of self-renewal.[2] Pools of pluripotent or uncommitted stem cells must be present, because once the cell line becomes differentiated (e.g., proerythroblast), the cells are in active cell division and cannot initiate other cells.[21] The pool of stem cells can recover if injured but not lethally damaged, which works in favor of chemotherapeutic agents that damage differentiated cells but may not affect the stem cells.[2]

SPLEEN

The spleen is a large, highly vascular organ with elements of the lymphoid and mononuclear phagocyte systems. It is located in the left upper abdominal cavity, directly beneath the diaphragm, above the left kidney, and behind the fundus of the stomach. It has a connective tissue capsule from which trabeculae (supporting strands) extend inside the organ and form a framework with small spaces that contain splenic pulp.

The major areas of the spleen are the red pulp, the white pulp, and the venous sinuses. As can be seen in Figure 12-2, a small splenic artery, which divides into several branches before entering the concave side of the spleen, penetrates into the splenic pulp and terminates in highly porous capillaries. Blood moves from these capillaries into the red pulp and then gradually squeezes through the trabecular network, eventually ending up in the venous sinuses.[31] The white pulp and venous sinuses contain large numbers of phagocytic and immunocompetent cells that cleanse the blood of old RBCs or platelets and many pathogens. The destruction of old or imperfect RBCs is sometimes referred to as "culling." Approximately half of the cells located within the splenic sinuses are phagocytic, and the others are lymphocytes. The exposure of cells in the blood to phagocytic cells in the venous sinuses gives a large surface area for removal of unwanted debris in the blood. After passing through the spleen as described, the capillaries empty into thin-walled veins that terminate in the splenic veins, which itself terminates in the portal vein.

Although the spleen is not necessary for survival, it is involved in four important functions: (1) production of lymphocytes in the white pulp; (2) destruction of erythrocytes in the red pulp; (3) filtration and trapping of foreign particles in both areas, providing a surface for destroying bacteria and viruses; and (4) storage of blood.[21] The normal adult spleen holds about 150 to 200 mL of blood, but because of its structure, it has the capacity to enlarge when the blood volume is increased.[16] In fetal life, the spleen is active in hematopoiesis, a function that mostly ends at or before birth.[14]

Splenic Enlargement and Infarction

Splenic enlargement (**splenomegaly**) is seen in some infectious conditions in the same manner as is seen with lymph node enlargement. It may also be enlarged with hemolyzed RBCs or platelets, in conditions of hemolytic anemia or immune thrombocytopenia purpura (ITP) (see p. 383). It may accompany hyperviscosity syndromes, such as multiple myeloma.[17] Congestive splenomegaly may result from chronic venous congestion and commonly is found with alcoholic cirrhosis of the liver (see p. 762). Occasionally, splenomegaly results from venous congestion in severe right heart failure. Whatever the cause, a dragging sensation in the left upper quadrant is often described. If massive splenomegaly exists, rupture of the spleen may result from trauma to the abdomen. Rupture causes massive intraperitoneal hemorrhage and, frequently, hemorrhagic shock.

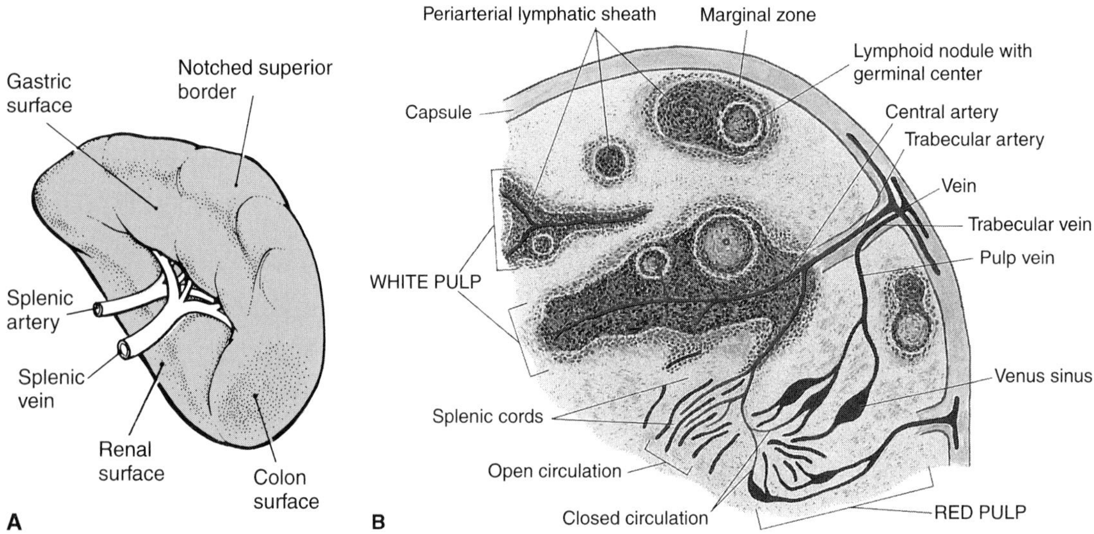

FIGURE 12-2. Anatomy of the spleen. **A.** Appearance of the spleen. **B.** Red and white pulp in splenic structure. (**B** from Rubin, E., & Farber, J. [1999]. *Pathology* [3rd ed.]. Philadelphia: Lippincott.)

Splenic infarction occurs when there is occlusion of the major splenic artery or its branches. It may result from systemic emboli localizing in the spleen.[16] Splenic infarction may present with sudden and severe left upper quadrant abdominal pain.

NORMAL ERYTHROCYTE STRUCTURE

Erythrocytes (RBCs) are nonnucleated, biconcave disks. This shape provides a large surface–volume ratio that permits distortion of the cells without stretching their membrane. Thus, RBCs can traverse very small capillaries, and normal RBCs adapt to the sinusoids of the spleen, escaping without being trapped and destroyed. The unique shape of erythrocytes also is conducive to gas exchange. The membrane of the RBC is made of lipids and proteins, making the cell resilient, flexible, and water-insoluble. Erythrocytes contain hemoglobin, which binds loosely with oxygen and carbon dioxide to carry essential gases to and away from the tissues.

Hemoglobin

The protein hemoglobin is a conjugated, oxygen-carrying red pigment formed throughout the life span of the erythrocyte (Fig. 12-3). Two molecular components are produced during hemoglobin synthesis: (1) the **porphyrin structure (heme)** that contains iron and (2) the polypeptide chains that make up globin. Heme is a large disk that contains iron and porphyrin, a nitrogen-containing organic compound.[21] The adult hemoglobin molecule (HbA) is composed of a globin (made of two alpha and two beta large polypeptide chains) with four heme (iron porphyrin) complexes.[21] The structure of hemoglobin changes in the last 3 months of gestation from primarily fetal hemoglobin (HbF) to HbA. In certain congenital hemolytic anemias the HbF persists, which, along with globin chain synthesis imbalance, provides the basis for the pathophysiology of these disorders (see p. 350).

One iron atom is present for each heme molecule. Each of the four iron atoms of the molecule combines reversibly with an atom of oxygen, forming **oxyhemoglobin**. The high density of hemoglobin in each RBC allows a large amount of oxygen to be transported. The disk shape of the erythrocytes provides a large surface area per unit mass of hemoglobin, enhancing gas exchange in both the pulmonary and systemic capillary system.

Red Blood Cell Antigens

More than 300 RBC antigens have been identified, the molecular structure of which is determined by genes at various chromosomal loci.[14] Because distinct RBC antigenic properties are genetically determined, they are almost never precisely the same among individuals. The antigens in the blood of one person may react with plasma or cells of another, especially during or after a blood transfusion. The antibody to the RBC antigen attaches to the antigenic sites and may cause hemolysis or agglutination of the RBCs.[17]

BLOOD CLASSIFICATION

Blood is classified into different groups and typed according to the antigens present on the red cell membrane. The term **blood group** refers to any well-defined system of RBC antigens in which 21 systems are recognized.[17] The term **blood type** refers to identification of

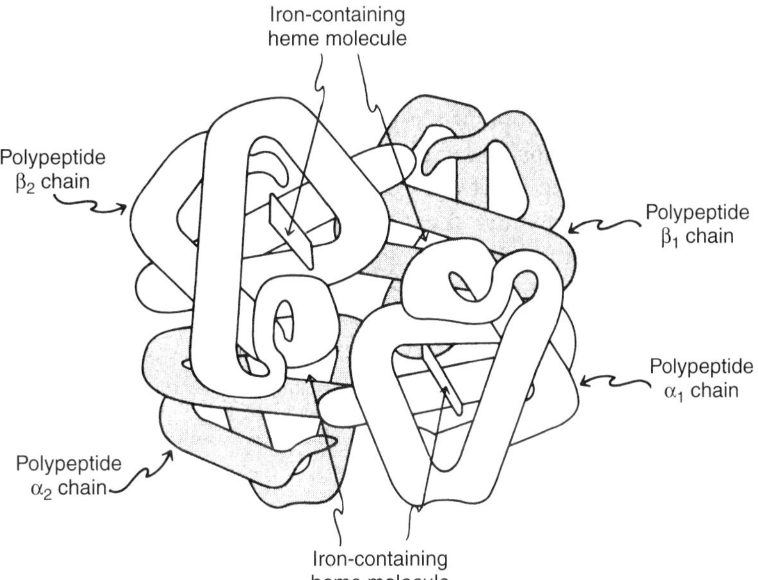

FIGURE 12-3. **Structure of the hemoglobin molecule. Note the alpha and beta chains and the iron-containing heme molecules.**

the antigens to determine a person's blood group.[19] These antigens, carried on the RBC surface, and antibodies, carried in the circulating plasma, are used for typing of blood so that it can be used for transfusion. Characteristics of blood types, their incidence, and transfusion compatibilities are found in Table 12-2. The antigens most commonly present on RBC membranes are antigens A, B, and Rh. These make up the ABO system of antigens and the Rh system.

ABO System

Type A and B surface antigens are called **agglutinogens,** and plasma antibodies that can cause agglutination are called **agglutinins**. Antibodies to the agglutinogens are almost always present if the agglutinogens are not present on a person's RBCs.[20] For example, anti-A agglutinins are present in the plasma of someone who does not have a type A agglutinogen. A person may inherit neither of these antigens (type O), or one (A or B), or both (A and B). Type O blood is referred to as the universal donor because it lacks A or B antigens. Type AB is the universal recipient because it contains neither anti-A nor anti-B antibodies. Either may contain other antigens that can account for a blood transfusion reaction.[19]

Rh System

The Rh type is determined by the presence or absence of particular antigens on the RBC. Type Rh negative refers to the absence of these antigens, and Rh positive refers to the presence of these antigens. There are six types of Rh factors: C, D, E, c, d, and e.[19] The most common is D, which, when present, accounts for the Rh+ (positive) designation. Eighty-five percent of whites and 95% of African Americans in the United States are Rh+.[7,8] Blood that does not have the D antigen is called Rh– (negative).

NORMAL DEVELOPMENT AND FUNCTION OF ERYTHROCYTES

The normal life span of adult RBCs is 120 days. Old RBCs are continuously destroyed, and new ones are regenerated for replacement. The total RBC mass remains constant, with a balance being maintained between destruction and replacement. The main function of RBCs is to carry oxygen to the tissues and transport carbon dioxide back to the lungs for elimination.

Erythropoiesis

The process of RBC formation is called erythropoiesis. It is an orderly process of maturation of RBCs for their maximum function in binding with oxygen and carbon dioxide. Erythrocytes are formed in the blood islands of the yolk sacs during the first several weeks of gestation.[21] During the second trimester of pregnancy, fetal RBCs are produced in the liver, spleen, and lymph nodes. After birth, the bone marrow becomes the principal site

TABLE 12-2

BLOOD TYPES AND TRANSFUSION COMPATIBILITY

BLOOD TYPE	% OF POPULATION	CHARACTERISTICS	RBCs CAN TRANSFUSE	PLASMA OR PLATELETS CAN TRANSFUSE
O	44%	Neither antigen A or B	O	O A B AB
A	43%	Antigen A on RBC No anti-A antibodies Contains anti-B antibodies	A O	A AB
B	9%	Antigen B on RBC No anti-B antibodies Contains anti-A antibodies	B O	B AB
AB	4%	Both antigen A and antigen B on RBC No anti-A and no anti-B antibodies in plasma	AB A B O	AB
D	85%	RH+	RH+ RH–	RH+ RH–
No D	15%	RH–	RH–	RH+ RH–

of RBC production.[14] After adolescence, the red marrow takes over the major erythropoietic function. This marrow cell pool and splenic reserve of stored cells provide a constant supply of peripheral RBCs.

The mature RBC is the end result of several divisions and differentiations before reaching the final stage of maturity. During maturation, the nucleus decreases in size until it disappears, the total size of the cell shrinks, the amount of ribonucleic acid lessens, and hemoglobin synthesis increases. Figure 12-4 illustrates the cellular stages from the proerythroblast through the formation of the mature erythrocyte. Hemoglobin reaches a concentration of 34% of cell volume. The reticulocyte is the final stage before the mature erythrocyte is formed. It normally remains in the marrow about 1 day and then in the bloodstream 1 day before becoming a mature erythrocyte.[16] Normally, only 1% to 2% of the erythrocytes in the blood are in the form of reticulocytes, but this proportion increases when there is rapid RBC turnover, such as with hemolysis and sudden blood loss.[6,7]

FOCUS ON CELLULAR PHYSIOLOGY

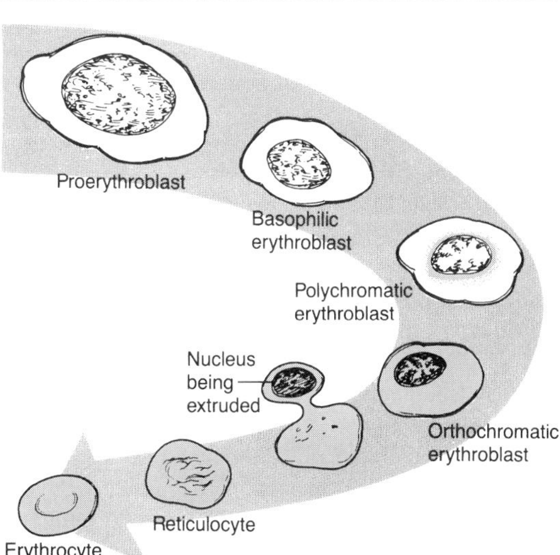

FIGURE 12-4. Development of red blood cell. Proerythroblast stage is the first stage following the erythroid colony-forming unit (CFU-E), which is a cell with a very large nucleus. The basophilic erythroblast stage is when hemoglobin synthesis begins. The polychromatic erythroblast, or normoblast stage, is the last stage of DNA synthesis and cell division. Hemoglobin synthesis continues. The orthochromatic erythroblast stage shows the shrinking and autolysis of the nucleus. The remains of the nucleus are extruded from the cell. In the reticulocyte stage, the cell does not have a nucleus and enters the circulation, where it becomes a mature erythrocyte. The erythrocyte is a disk-shaped, pliable cell that can move in tight spaces to pick up or release oxygen.

SUBSTANCES NEEDED FOR ERYTHROPOIESIS

Substances essential for the proper formation of hemoglobin and RBCs include iron, vitamin B_{12}, copper, cobalt, pyridoxine, and folic acid.

Iron

Iron is essential for the production of heme, and about 65% of body iron is present in hemoglobin.[14] The total amount of iron in the body equals about 4 g, with 15% to 30% of this amount being stored as **ferritin**, primarily in the liver. Ferritin (storage iron) is formed from a combination of iron with a protein called **apoferritin**.[17] It is readily available for hemoglobin synthesis when needed through the aid of a beta-globulin called **transferrin**. Transferrin has specific binding capabilities that facilitate the transfer of iron across the membranes of immature erythrocytes. Transferrin also carries the iron released from worn-out erythrocytes to the bone marrow, where it is reused for hemoglobin synthesis.[21] The presence of nonoxidized iron in these alternate forms allows the formation of hemoglobin, which is capable of binding and releasing oxygen normally. Oxidized ferric iron, however, results in the formation of **methemoglobin**, which cannot carry oxygen.[3] Certain drugs, such as nitrates, phenacetin, sulfonamides, and lidocaine, may cause the production of excess ferric iron.[21]

Daily losses of iron are replaced by dietary intake or transferred to apoferritin to make ferritin. Iron is absorbed mostly in the duodenum by an active process that apparently continues until all of the transferrin is saturated.[3] When transferrin can accept no more iron, absorption of iron almost entirely ceases; conversely, if the stores are depleted, larger amounts of iron are absorbed.[14] The result is a feedback mechanism that keeps a stable level of iron for hemoglobin synthesis. Inadequate dietary intake or absorption of iron leads to iron deficiency anemia (see p. 356).

Vitamin B_{12}

Vitamin B_{12} is essential for the synthesis of deoxyribonucleic acid (DNA) molecules within the RBCs. This large molecule does not easily penetrate the mucosa of the gastrointestinal tract, but must be bound to a glycoprotein known as the **intrinsic factor** for its absorption. The intrinsic factor is secreted by the parietal cells of the gastric mucosa and binds to vitamin B_{12} to protect it from the digestive enzymes.[3] After absorption from the lower gastrointestinal tract, vitamin B_{12} is stored in the liver and is available for the production of new erythrocytes. Longstanding lack of B_{12} leads to macrocytic anemia (pernicious anemia) (see. p. 355).

Copper and Cobalt

Copper is a catalyst in the formation of hemoglobin and in this way helps to make RBCs.[17] Cobalt is a mineral in the vitamin B_{12} molecule, so that its deficiency will lead to the same type of macrocytic anemia as that seen with lack of the intrinsic factor.

Folic Acid

Folic acid (pteroylglutamic acid) is necessary for the synthesis of RBC DNA and its maturation. Lack of folic acid causes folic acid anemia, a type of macrocytic anemia that readily responds to dietary replacement (see p. 355).[11]

Pyridoxine

Pyridoxine (vitamin B_6) is involved with absorption of amino acids and the synthesis of heme precursors. Anemia resulting from pyridoxine deficiency occurs more frequently as a result of a hereditary or acquired defect than as a consequence of malnutrition.

FACTORS THAT INFLUENCE ERYTHROPOIESIS

Erythropoiesis is stimulated by a decrease in the partial pressure of oxygen in the arterial blood. The regulation of RBC mass is through the **erythropoietin hormone**, which is released when there is a sensed hypoxemia. The regulation is very sensitive to minor changes of oxygen consumption by tissues, and this maintains the normal production of RBCs. The resulting hypoxemia stimulates erythropoietin release from the kidneys and bone marrow production of more RBCs. Partial pressure of oxygen may also decrease due to pathologic conditions such as anemia, chronic obstructive lung disease, poor blood flow, and heart failure. Chronic hypoxemia produces constant erythropoiesis stimulus and erythrocytosis (see p. 345).

Erythropoietin hormone stimulates erythropoietin-responsive pluripotent stem cells in the bone marrow to produce increased numbers of RBCs through conversion of certain stem cells to proerythroblasts. These cells are part of a fast cycling system for RBC production that matures them faster than other precursor cells.[21] Erythropoietin principally comes from renal glomerular epithelial cells, but some may be released from liver epithelium. Normal kidneys produce 85 to 90% of erythropoietin.[17] The usual stimulus for erythropoietin secretion is hypoxia, but androgens and possibly other hormones have an effect on its secretion. The androgen connection accounts for the higher RBC count in men than in women.[21] A negative feedback system is established, with hypoxemia being a stimulus for erythropoietin and resulting in increased production of RBCs (Flowchart 12-1).

FLOWCHART 12-1 **Feedback Mechanism For Maintaining Red Blood Cells**

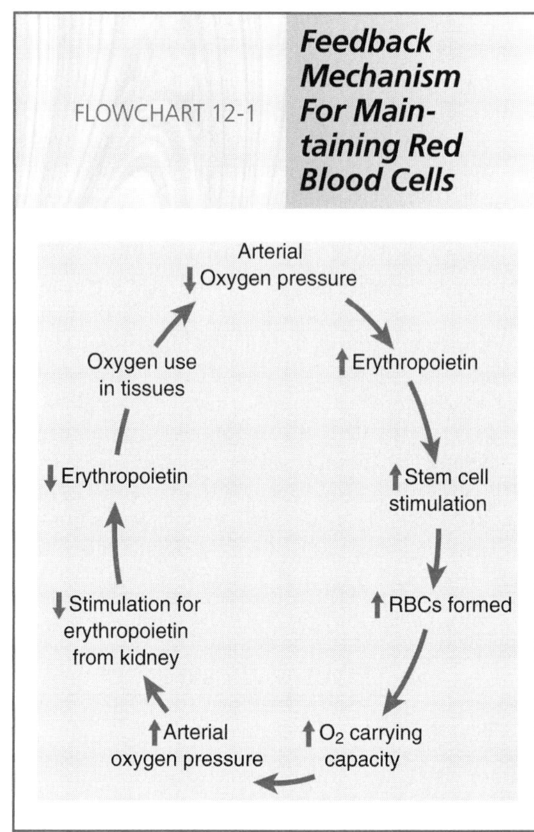

Energy Production in Erythrocytes

Mature erythrocytes cannot synthesize nucleic acids, complex carbohydrates, lipids, or proteins because they do not have a nucleus or other intracellular organelles. Because there are no mitochondria for oxidative metabolism, the energy of mature RBCs is generated from the metabolism of glucose by the anaerobic pathway (glycolysis). Because their energy is produced anaerobically, RBCs do not use any of the oxygen that they transport.[21] RBCs are uniquely rich in **2,3 diphosphoglycerate (2,3 DPG)**, which is a low-energy side product of glycolysis.[17] 2,3 DPG functions as a prime regulator for hemoglobin's ability to unload oxygen to the tissues. The RBCs apparently generate 2,3 DPG whenever there is hypoxia of the tissues, and the effect may be seen on the oxyhemoglobin dissociation curve (see p. 542).

Even without a nucleus, the RBC is metabolically active and requires energy to provide the following functions: (1) maintenance of osmotic stability through intact membrane pumps and active transport of sodium and potassium; (2) maintenance of iron in the reduced ferrous state; and (3) modulation of hemoglobin function by generating 2,3 DPG.[17]

Oxygen and Carbon Dioxide Transport

Most of the oxygen that crosses the alveolocapillary membrane in the lungs combines with the heme portion of hemoglobin into a loose bond called oxyhemoglobin. Hemoglobin saturation with oxygen usually is approximately 95% in arterial blood, and oxygen is rapidly released when it reaches the tissues. Normal venous blood and the tissues both demonstrate a partial pressure of oxygen at about 40 mm Hg, with a hemoglobin saturation of about 70%.[14] Fully saturated hemoglobin from the lungs transports and releases oxygen at the tissue level to meet cellular needs. The affinity of hemoglobin for oxygen is affected by hydrogen ion concentration, carbon dioxide levels, the amounts of 2,3 DPG, and body temperature. Increases in any of these factors cause a decreased affinity for oxygen and hemoglobin and more effective oxygen unloading to the tissues. This could be viewed as a compensatory mechanism for improved tissue oxygenation. The presence of excess 2,3 DPG may hinder oxygen loading in the lungs, but this is counterbalanced by an increased tendency to unload oxygen at the tissue level.[14]

Transport of carbon dioxide from the tissues to RBCs occurs in two major ways:

1. It directly combines with hemoglobin amine radicals to form **carbaminohemoglobin (CO_2Hgb)**. This reversible reaction is a loose bond, allowing CO_2 to be easily released into the alveoli by diffusion from higher to lower gaseous pressure.[14] About 20 to 25% of CO_2 is carried in this manner.
2. About 70% of the CO_2 is carried in the dissolved form of bicarbonate.[3] When CO_2 is released from the tissue cell, it diffuses into the RBC and combines with water, with carbonic anhydrase as the catalyst, and forms carbonic acid. Carbonic acid (H_2CO_3) almost immediately dissociates into free hydrogen and bicarbonate ions. Free hydrogen attaches to hemoglobin because it is a powerful acid-base buffer, and bicarbonate is free to diffuse into the plasma or attach to a positive ion within the RBC. When bicarbonate diffuses into the plasma, it usually is replaced by chloride in the chloride shift (Fig. 12-5).[31] This is made possible by a bicarbonate-chloride carrier protein that rapidly moves these ions in opposite directions. The end result is a greater amount of chloride in venous RBCs than in arterial cells, and CO_2 is carried from the tissue cells as bicarbonate ions in the plasma.[14]

Destruction of Erythrocytes

When RBCs reach their life span at about 120 days after release into the circulation, breakdown of the cells occurs. Failing glucose metabolism in aging erythrocytes causes a gradual decrease in the amount of adenosine triphosphate (ATP). Without an adequate supply of ATP, cells are no longer able to maintain normal function. RBCs are normally removed from circulation and lysed by the spleen or liver. After lysis of the RBC, iron is recycled by transferrin, and the heme molecule is converted to bilirubin that is conjugated and excreted as bile by the liver and in the urine as urobilinogen (Fig. 12-6).[14] A small percentage of RBCs undergo intravascular destruction. When the RBC membrane lyses, hemoglobin moves out of the cells and becomes bound with a plasma globulin called **haptoglobin**.[21] The resulting complex prevents renal excretion of hemoglobin. The complex is then taken up by phagocytic cells in the liver and processed. When the amount of hemoglobin presented for uptake exceeds renal absorptive capacity, free hemoglobin and methemoglobin appear in the urine.[17] The membranous remains of RBCs are called "ghosts" when they are present in blood samples.[25]

FOCUS ON CELLULAR PHYSIOLOGY

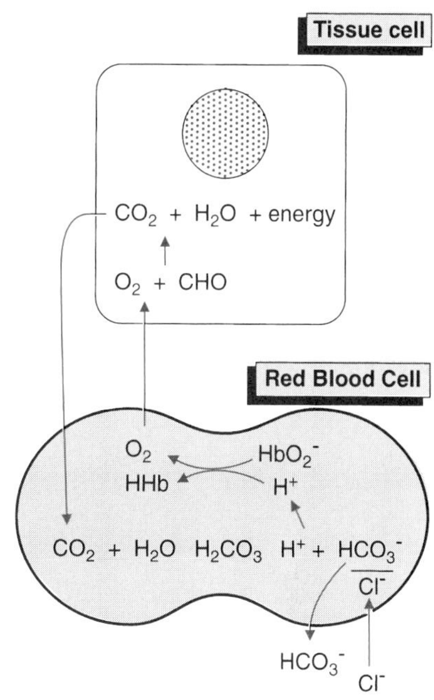

FIGURE 12-5. In the process of gas exchange with the tissue cell, the red blood cell picks up carbon dioxide (CO_2), which becomes carbonic acid (H_2CO_3) and dissociates into hydrogen (H^+) and bicarbonate (HCO_3^-). It can then donate a bicarbonate (HCO_3^-) to the plasma, which is exchanged for a chloride ion (Cl^-). This method for donating a buffer to the extracellular fluid is called the "chloride shift."

DISORDERS OF ERYTHROCYTES

Erythrocyte diseases are mainly classified into those that cause an excessive number of RBCs and those that cause a decreased number of RBCs. An increased number of RBCs may be termed erythrocytosis or polycythemia, whereas a decreased number is termed anemia.

Erythrocytosis

The term erythrocytosis, often termed **polycythemia**, encompasses a group of conditions characterized by an increase in the hematocrit.[4] The hematocrit is normally greater in men than in women, but if this value is above 50%, the viscosity of the blood increases significantly. Table 12-3 lists the causes of erythrocytosis along with pertinent clinical features.

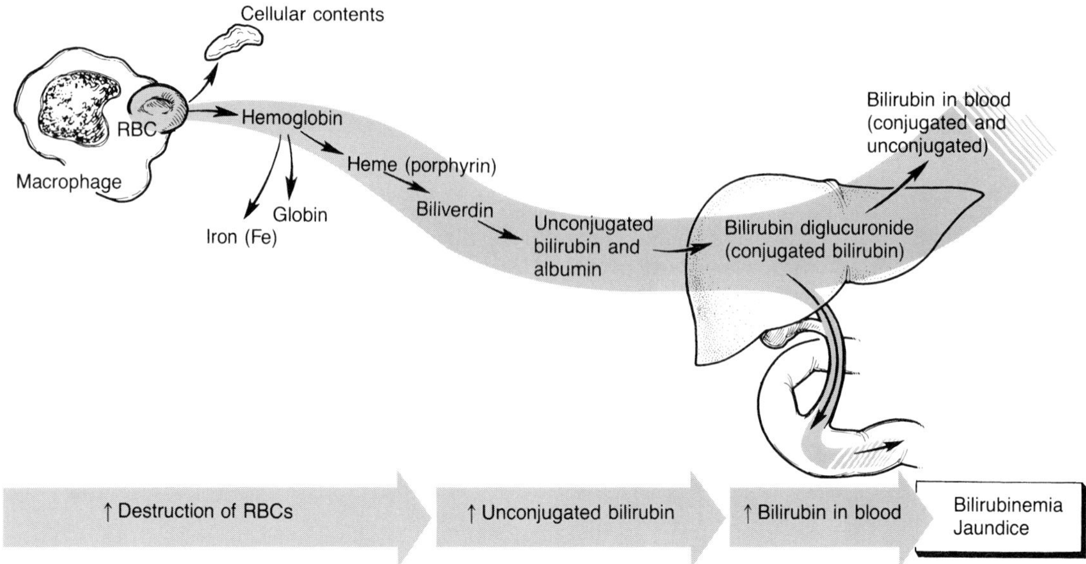

FIGURE 12-6. **Hemolysis of RBCs causes the release of heme, which becomes unconjugated bilirubin and must be conjugated in the liver for excretion into the bile. Increased amounts of bilirubin lead to bilirubinemia and jaundice.**

TABLE 12-3

CAUSES OF ERYTHROCYTOSIS

CAUSATIVE FACTORS	RESULTS
I. Relative erythrocytosis—caused by hemoconcentration due to dehydration or plasma loss	I. No actual increase in RBC mass occurs, but hematocrit increases due to loss of plasma volume.
II. Increased RBC mass—erythropoietin-induced	II. Increased hematocrit is due to stimulation of bone marrow from erythropoietin.
Altered hemoglobin structure and function	Oxygen-carrying capacity altered, causing hypoxic stimulation of renal erythropoietin-producing cells.
Aberrant erythropoietin production	Some tumors, e.g., renal cell carcinomas, produce erythropoietin-like substances that cause erythrocytosis.
High altitudes	When oxygen levels are decreased in areas of high altitude, a hypoxic stimulus for RBC production occurs.
Chronic obstructive lung diseases (COPD)	Severe COPD causes decreased arterial oxygen and erythropoietin stimulation.
Cyanotic congenital heart diseases	Due to intracardiac shunting, arterial oxygen levels are decreased, providing a renal erythropoietin stimulation.
III. Physiologic erythrocytosis—seen in newborn	III. At birth, the hematocrit ranges from 45–65%. It gradually decreases to normal levels during infancy.
IV. Blood transfusion	IV. Excessive administration of RBCs, as in "blood doping," may increase the hematocrit.
V. Polycythemia vera	V. A neoplastic condition of production of RBCs and other blood cells may lead to splenomegaly and increased viscosity.

SECONDARY ABSOLUTE ERYTHROCYTOSIS

The most commonly recognized causes of secondary erythrocytosis are hypoxemia and overproduction of erythropoietin.[15] Hypoxemia causes decreased tissue oxygenation, which in turn stimulates an increase in blood levels of erythropoietin. Elevated erythropoietin levels stimulate the bone marrow to produce more RBCs.[9]

In the process of acclimatization to high altitudes, which have a low atmospheric oxygen level, the RBC volume slowly rises. This appropriate response makes more RBCs and hemoglobin available for oxygenation.

Many persons who have chronic pulmonary disease or who are heavy smokers are hypoxemic and subsequently develop an increased hematocrit level. The possible mechanism for hypoxemia in cigarette smokers is that carbon monoxide from the smoke displaces oxygen from the hemoglobin.[15]

Overproduction of erythrocytes results when there is inappropriate, excessive production of erythropoietin. This condition has been associated with renal disease, malignant tumors, or conditions in which there is a disturbance of renal blood flow.[15]

Secondary erythrocytosis is always related to elevated levels of circulating erythropoietin, and the bone marrow remains normal without increased proliferation of leukocytes. This proliferation of erythropoietin may represent a normal renal response to tissue hypoxemia, or it may result from production of erythropoietin from an outside or uncontrolled source.[15]

RELATIVE (SPURIOUS) ERYTHROCYTOSIS

Characterized by a normal erythrocyte count and a reduced plasma volume, this condition is mainly caused by dehydration. The pathogenesis of the condition when it becomes chronic is not known, but a condition of chronic plasma depletion is usually present.[15] The chronic type has been seen in hypertensive individuals and is often related to smoking.

POLYCYTHEMIA VERA

Polycythemia vera is a myeloproliferative disorder in which there is increased production of all the formed elements (RBCs, granulocytes, and platelets) of blood. The condition is relatively rare, occurring slightly more frequently in men than in women and between ages 50 and 70, but the cause is unknown.[15,16]

Pathophysiology

Abnormal bone marrow proliferation initially involves white and red cell elements and later also causes **thrombocytosis.**[16] There is evidence that the disease is a neoplastic disorder that stimulates abnormal erythropoietin-hypersensitive stem cells while suppressing normal stem cells.[15,16] Proliferation of hematopoietic cells results in an increase in blood counts, blood viscosity, and blood volume. The liver and spleen become congested and packed with RBCs that cause stasis and thrombosis and may lead to infarction. Vascular thrombosis is more often the result of thrombocytosis.[16] The course of the disease may change, resulting in aplastic, fibrotic, or even leukemic bone marrow, or polycythemia may be gradually replaced by anemia. Acute myeloblastic leukemia is a common consequence in persons treated with chlorambucil or marrow irradiation. This transformation may occur in the natural progression of the disease or, possibly, may be the result of therapy.[9,16]

Clinical Manifestations

The clinical onset of polycythemia vera is insidious. Most symptoms appear to be related to the increased blood volume, increased blood viscosity, and changes in cerebral blood flow. Lightheadedness, visual disturbances, headaches, and vertigo may be described. Ruddy cyanosis of the face usually is apparent. Pruritus is a common complaint, possibly caused by histamine release from the basophils.[16] Increased cardiac work may be manifested by eventual congestive heart failure. Thrombophlebitis and thrombosis of digital arteries, accompanied by gangrene, may occur.

Polycythemia vera is differentiated from secondary polycythemia by the appearance of abnormalities of other hematopoietic cells and the normal or lower-than-normal levels of serum and excreted erythropoietin. Laboratory studies may show increased hematocrit, hemoglobin, RBC mass, basophils, eosinophils, neutrophils, thrombocytes, leukocyte alkaline phosphatase, serum B_{12} and B_{12}-binding protein, and uric acid. The RBC count may be 7 to 9 million/L or higher, and the total blood volume is elevated.[4]

Anemias

The term anemia refers to a condition in which there is a decrease in hemoglobin concentration, the number of circulating RBCs, or the volume of packed cells (hematocrit) compared with normal values. Anemias usually are categorized according to cause or morphology (Table 12-4). The type of anemia present is diagnosed by the underlying mechanism of the disease. Almost all anemias can be divided into two kinds: (1) those caused by impaired RBC formation and (2) those caused by excessive loss or destruction of RBCs. The reticulocyte count is of primary importance in diagnosis, as it reflects the early release of immature erythrocytes commonly seen in acute blood loss or hemolysis. It is also important to ascertain the size, shape, color, and hemoglobin content of RBCs by blood smear. Morphologic characteristics of RBCs usually are

TABLE 12-4

CLASSIFICATION OF ANEMIAS

TYPE	MORPHOLOGIC CHARACTERISTICS	CAUSES
Aplastic	Normocytic, normochromic RBCs, depletion of leukocytes and platelets	Drug toxicity Genetic failure Radiation Chemicals Infections
Hemolytic	Normocytic, normochromic, increased number of reticulocytes	Mechanical injury RBC antigen–antibody reaction Complement binding Chemical reactions Hereditary membrane defects
Macrocytic or megaloblastic; pernicious or folic acid	Macrocytic with variation in size (anisocytosis), shape (poikilocytosis) of RBCs	Inadequate diet Lack of intrinsic factor for pernicious anemia Impaired absorption
Microcytic; iron deficiency; chronic blood loss	Microcytic; hypochromic	Inadequate diet Blood loss, chronic Increased need
Posthemorrhagic; acute hemorrhage	Normocytic, normochromic, increased number of reticulocytes within 48–72 h	Loss of blood leading to hemodilution from interstitial fluid within 48–72 h Internal or external hemorrhage, leading to blood volume depletion

used in the classification of anemias. The morphologic features and their significance are found in Table 12-5.

Anemias each have unique clinical manifestations that correlate to the specific malfunction; however, some common manifestations are found regardless of the underlying disorder. Signs and symptoms of anemia relate to inadequate RBC volume, lack of RBCs to carry out normal functioning, or mechanisms used by the body to compensate for loss of RBC function. Those signs and symptoms are summarized in Figure 12-7.

APLASTIC ANEMIA

Aplastic anemia occurs as a result of reduced bone marrow function and causes a drop in levels of all blood elements. The number of pluripotent stem cells appears to decrease, and the blood-forming cells are not formed or matured.[13,16] A severe anemia results, with the formed RBCs sometimes appearing morphologically immature.[12] The cells may be macrocytic or normocytic and are usually normochromic. The prognosis of aplastic anemia is variable, dependent upon the causative agent and reversibility.[5] The cause of aplastic anemia is poorly understood, and in more than one-half of cases it is unknown.[12,23] Genetic failure of bone marrow development (e.g., Fanconi's syndrome) or injury to stem cells (e.g., whole-body irradiation) may prohibit the cells' reproduction and differentiation. Physical, chemical, infectious, and pharmacologic agents have all been implicated in the etiology of aplastic anemia. These factors are summarized in Table 12-6.

A routine blood examination and marrow aspiration with biopsy provide essential information regarding bone marrow function. The marrow is usually hypocellular, and biopsy may reveal large areas of fat with clusters of lymphocytes, reticular cells, and plasma cells.[5,12] Uptake of iron by the marrow is decreased, and serum iron is increased (termed **hemachromatosis**).[12] Smears most frequently show normocytic, normochromic RBCs that are profoundly decreased in number.[5,12] The onset of symptoms is usually gradual, reflecting progressive loss of cell function. Oxygen transport problems with anemia may be present, but due to a shortened life span of platelets and WBCs, patients more often first present with bleeding or infection.[32] Weakness, dyspnea, headaches, and syncope are common. The most common causes of death are severe hemorrhage, such as intracranial hemorrhage, or overwhelming infection and septic shock.[5,13]

Pure **red blood cell aplasia** is associated with, but much less common than, aplastic anemia. It may be congenital, immunologically mediated, drug-induced, or preleukemic, or it may follow a viral infection.[13] RBC aplasia frequently occurs as a secondary response to end-stage renal failure (see p. 623). It is characterized by severe normocytic, normochromic anemia with no reticulocyte response.[11]

TABLE 12-5

MORPHOLOGIC ALTERATIONS OF RED BLOOD CELLS

CELL CHANGES	DESCRIPTION	FIGURE
Normocytic/ normochromic	Normal size of cell Normal hemoglobin concentration/ normal color	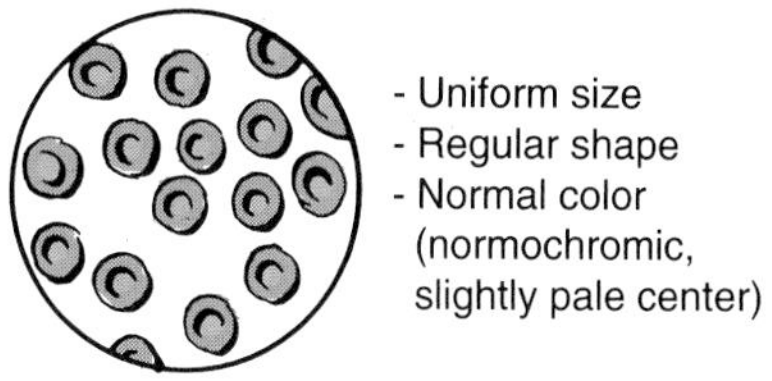 - Uniform size - Regular shape - Normal color (normochromic, slightly pale center)
Microcytic/ hypochromic	Cell < 7μ in diameter Decreased hemoglobin/ decreased color Caused by impaired hemoglobin synthesis	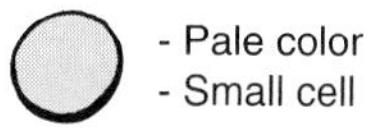 - Pale color - Small cell
Macrocytic	9μ in diameter Caused by impaired DNA synthesis	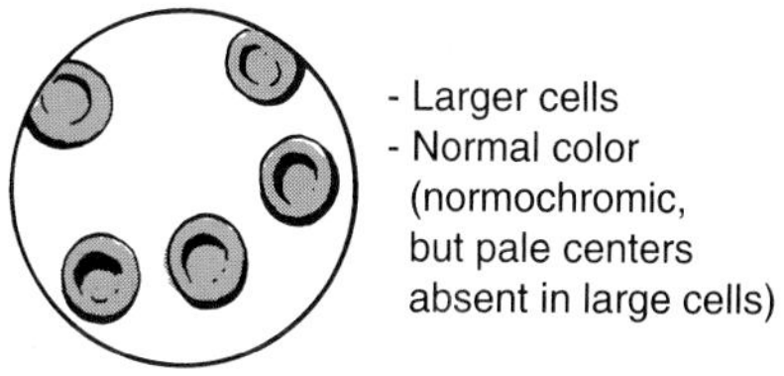 - Larger cells - Normal color (normochromic, but pale centers absent in large cells)
Ansiocytosis	Variations in RBC size; cells may be macrocytic or microcytic May be seen with many anemias	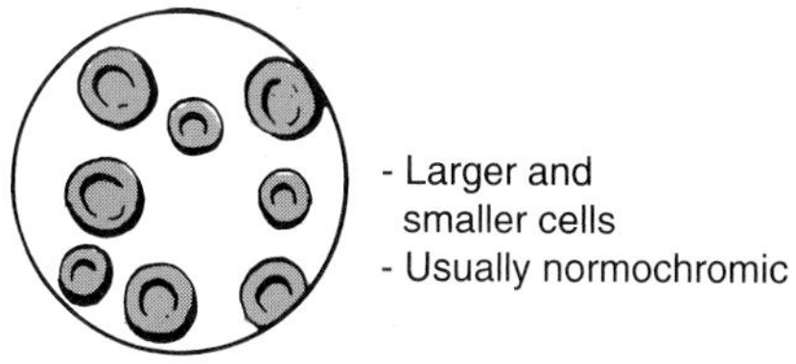 - Larger and smaller cells - Usually normochromic
Poikilocytosis	Variations in shape of RBC May be seen with many anemias	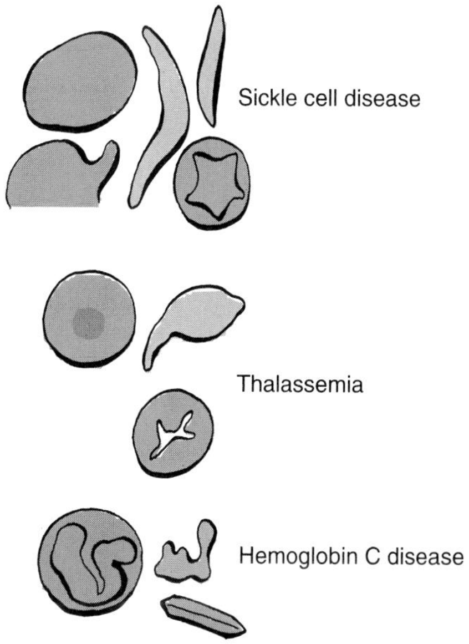 Sickle cell disease Thalassemia Hemoglobin C disease

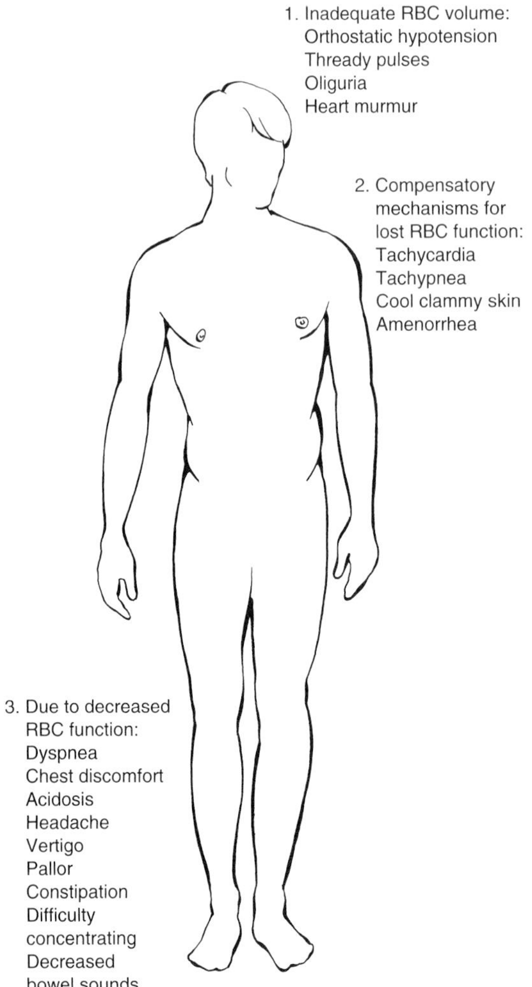

FIGURE 12-7. Clinical manifestations of anemia.

TABLE 12-6

ETIOLOGIES OF APLASTIC ANEMIA

RISK GROUP	EXAMPLES
Diseases/ disorders	Immune suppression Post-orthoptic liver transplant Pregnancy Vitamin B_{12} deficiency
Infections	Cytomegalovirus Epstein-Barr virus Hepatitis
Medications	Anticonvulsants—felbamate, phenytoin, trimethadione Anti-dysrhythmics—quinidine, norpace, procainamide, ticlodipine Anti-inflammatory—gold, indomethacin, phenylbutazone Anti-microbials—sulfonylureas (e.g., methimazole, albendazole), chloramphenicol Antineoplastic agents—many may cause, but most commonly associated with alkylating agents Quinines
Toxins	Arsenic Benzene Herbicides Insecticides Lacquers Paint thinner Radiation Toluene (glue) and trinitrotoluene

HEMOLYTIC ANEMIA

In the hemolytic anemias, the life span of the RBC may be shortened by a diverse group of intrinsic or extrinsic factors that can adversely affect the cell. Shortened RBC life span may be compensated for by an increase in erythrocyte production, which results in an increase in circulating reticulocytes. Hemolytic anemias are classified by mechanisms of RBC injury, although categories often overlap (Table 12-7). The more common diseases are discussed in greater detail below.

Red Cell Membrane Defects

Inherited and acquired disorders of the RBC membrane include conditions such as hereditary spherocytosis, acquired immune hemolytic anemia, blood transfusion reactions, and glucose-6-phosphate dehydrogenase deficiency.

HEREDITARY SPHEROCYTOSIS. Hereditary spherocytosis refers to a group of inherited hemolytic anemias that are mainly due to inherited autosomal dominant conditions that result in a molecular defect of the RBC membrane.[25,33] RBCs are spherical in shape and are prematurely destroyed by the spleen. The cells rapidly hemolyze in a hypotonic solution. Hereditary spherocytosis is suspected in hemolytic disease of the neonate when there is a change in the shape of the RBC to a spherical shape. It may present with severe hemolysis in childhood, or it may be less severe and first manifested in early adulthood. Clinical signs depend on the amount of hemolysis present and can include jaundice, splenomegaly, and signs of anemia. The splenic enlargement is characteristic and is a key determinant in clinical expression.[11] Crises in hereditary spherocytosis are related to associated problems, such as infections, especially parvovirus, and gallstones.[30]

An associated hemolytic anemia is hereditary elliptocytosis, which resembles hereditary spherocytosis except that the RBCs have an oval appearance. The disease usually is less severe and is associated with splenomegaly.[6]

ACQUIRED IMMUNE HEMOLYTIC ANEMIAS. Acquired immune hemolytic anemias result from premature destruction of the RBCs by autoantibodies in the im-

TABLE 12-7

ETIOLOGIES OF HEMOLYTIC ANEMIA

RISK GROUP	EXAMPLES
Abnormalities of membrane or shape of cell	Hereditary
	Elliptocytosis
	Spherocytosis
	Stomatocytosis
	Acquired
	Anemia of liver disease (stomatocytes, acanthocytes, target cells)
	Anemia of uremia (echinocytes)
	Chronic lymphocytic leukemia
	Exotoxemia (spherocytes)
	Immune hemolytic anemia (spherocytes)
	Membrane sensitivity to complement—paroxysmal nocturnal hemoglobinuria
Metabolic abnormalities	Glycolytic pathway enzyme deficiencies
	Hexose-monophosphate shunt enzyme deficiencies
	Purine and pyrimidine pathway enzyme deficiencies
	Pyruvate kinase deficiency
Hemoglobinopathies	Disorders of Hemoglobin Structure
	Hemoglobin C, D, and E disorders
	Porphyria
	Sickle cell anemia
	Disorders of Hemoglobin Synthesis
	Glucose-6-phosphate dehydrogenase (6-GPD) deficiency
	Thalassemias (alpha and beta)
Physical damage to the RBC	Blunt trauma injury
	Chemical hemolysis
	Microangiopathic—hemolytic transfusion reactions
	RBC fragmentation due to turbulent flow—artificial heart valves, endocarditis, extracorporeal bypass, continuous veno-venous hemofiltration (CVVH), exercise
	Red blood cell parasitization—malaria, babesiosis
	Thermal injury
Unknown mechanism	Autoimmune disease—C_1 inhibitor deficiency, scleroderma, systemic lupus erythematosus (SLE), Wilson's disease, Wiscott-Aldrich's disease
	Diabetes mellitus
	Fludarabine phosphate
	IgA deficiency
	Illicit drugs—cocaine, PCP
	Infections—Brucella, HIV
	Medications—carboplatin, cisplatin, cyclosporine, dapsone, interferon (alpha and beta), lovastatin, mefloquine, methyldopa, mitomycin, penicillin, phenazopyridine, quinidine, quinine, rifampicin, rifampin, tacrolimus
	Naphthalene
	Ovarian cyst
	Snake bites
	Spider bites
	Ulcerative colitis

mune system that have specificity against blood group antigens.[25] It is diagnosed by the Coombs' test. A positive direct Coombs' test means that a plasma protein, usually IgG or complement, has become fixed to the surface of a RBC. The type involving IgG is associated with lymphoma, systemic lupus erythematosus, and drug reactions, or it may be idiopathic.[30] Some people with this type of disease have an antibody against a specific antigen on their own RBCs.[33] The indirect Coombs' test induces agglutination of RBCs if antiRBC antibodies are present in the suspected serum (see Unit 3, Appendix A). Both direct and indirect Coombs' tests may be positive in hemolysis, especially in drug-induced hemolytic disease.[4,33]

HEMOLYTIC BLOOD TRANSFUSION REACTIONS. Hemolytic blood transfusion reactions are good examples of secondary defects of the red cell membrane. The antigens in the blood of one person may react with plasma or cells of another, especially during or after a blood transfusion. The antibody to the RBC antigen attaches to the antigenic sites and may cause hemolysis or agglutination of the RBCs.[17] When incompatible blood is transfused, the antigen-antibody reactions within the recipient of transfusion cause systemic reactions. The four types of transfusion reactions are febrile, allergic, acute hemolytic, and delayed hemolytic. A summary of the defining features for these reactions is included in Table 12-8.

These reactions are immunologically mediated and directed at the antigens in the transfused blood that are deemed foreign. Major hemolysis usually results from incompatibilities of the ABO system or, occasionally, the Rh factor.[31] Other hemolytic reactions may be directed toward any of the other RBC antigens. Hemolysis usually occurs intravascularly, but it also may occur in extravascular spaces. Laboratory tests show hemoglobinemia, elevated bilirubin, and often a positive direct Coombs' test.[25] Symptoms of the reaction usually involve the sudden onset of restlessness, anxiety, fever, chills, flushing, chest or back pain, nausea, and vomiting, and then early onset of disseminated intravascular coagulation, renal failure, and shock.

GLUCOSE-6-PHOSPHATE DEHYDROGENASE (G6PD) DEFICIENCY. G6PD deficiency is a deficiency of an X-linked RBC enzyme. It occurs in 13% of African American males, and 25% of African American females are carriers.[17] Levels of the enzyme usually decrease as the cell ages, so that older cells are more susceptible to hemolysis. One in four carriers is subject to hemolysis. Such factors as oxidant drugs (e.g., sulfonamides), viral or bacterial infections, and diabetic ketoacidosis may precipitate hemolysis in susceptible people.[4] Once the triggering event is discontinued, recovery usually occurs.[4,17] Profound hemolytic anemia, due to G6PD deficiency in red blood cells of all ages, may occur in affected African blacks and people of Mediterranean descent.[6]

HEMOGLOBINOPATHIES. Hemoglobinopathies are inherited disorders characterized by structural changes in hemoglobin. The broad types of diseases manifesting abnormalities of hemoglobin synthesis are described as qualitative or structural (e.g., sickle cell disease) and quantitative (e.g., thalassemias).[6]

Sickle Cell Trait and Sickle Cell Anemia

Sickle cell trait and sickle cell anemia are two related genetic disorders of hemoglobin. Sickle cell is an autosomal recessive disease in which the normal amino acid, glutamic acid, is replaced by valine; the hemoglobin molecule synthesized from the altered globin chain is termed HbS. Sickle cell trait is carried by heterozygous individuals; sickle cell anemia occurs when an individual is homozygous.[18,27] These syndromes occur almost exclusively in African-Americans, with about 10% of these individuals carrying HbS on the hemoglobin molecule (sickle cell trait). About 0.2% of African-Americans exhibit the actual disease.[9] Due to improved diagnosis and more effective immediate treatment for crises, the prognosis for sickle cell anemia is improving, and more persons are surviving to adulthood.[18]

Because the sickle cell trait is heterozygous, RBCs require very low oxygen tension to precipitate the characteristic sickling effect, and overall RBC life span usually is not affected.[18] Therefore, most people with the sickle cell trait have no symptoms unless they suffer a severe hypoxic episode.

In sickle cell anemia, the abnormal amino acid sequence alters the solubility of hemoglobin. At low blood pH and with decreased oxygen tension, the HbS precipitates out of solution, and the cells become sickle-shaped and then obstruct small vessels.[18] The characteristic shape usually returns to normal when oxygen again becomes available, but irreversible ischemia and infarction of tissues may have occurred by that time. After vascular obstruction, RBC hemolysis occurs, shortening the RBC life span from a normal of 120 days to about 10 to 15 days. Bilirubin is released from the hemoglobin during hemolysis, and increased conjugated and unconjugated bilirubin accumulates in the plasma.[18] Hemolyzed RBC fragments are trapped in the spleen, and the entire organ eventually may become infarcted. Infection or hyperviscosity of the blood increases the chances of sickling.[1,24] Flowchart 12-2 summarizes the pathophysiology of sickle cell anemia.

Sickle cell anemia is diagnosed by electrophoresis of the hemoglobin molecule. Abnormal hemoglobin will provide a different electrophoresis pattern (see Unit 3, Appendix A). The disease is also recognizable by decreased hematocrit and hemoglobin and elevated reticulocytes, bilirubin, and uric acid. The bone marrow often becomes hyperplastic, with evidence of increased erythropoiesis.[26] Reticulocytes and even normoblasts may be released into the circulating blood.[18]

Sickle cell anemia causes symptoms beginning at about 6 months of age. Signs and symptoms of sickle cell anemia vary in severity but may include jaundice. The symptoms depend upon the number of sickled and hemolyzed cells, although the most common cause of death is intracranial hemorrhage.[1] Sickle cell crises are described by their pathophysiologic mechanism. A summary of these crises and key clinical features is included in Table 12-9.

Thalassemias

Thalassemias are intrinsic, congenital disorders that result from defects in the synthesis of hemoglobin and cause a hypochromic, microcytic anemia. They are classified as major and minor, according to the features of the disease, which include stillbirth, severe hemolytic anemia, and mild to moderate anemia.[28] Many different defects involving beta, alpha, or delta-beta hemo-

TABLE 12-8

SUMMARY OF TRANSFUSION REACTIONS

TRANSFUSION REACTION	FREQUENCY OF REACTION	POTENTIAL CAUSES	SYMPTOMS
Febrile non-hemolytic transfusion reaction	1:5 platelets 1:100 red blood cells (RBCs)	Recipient antibodies to donor leukocytes Bacterial contamination Inflammatory cytokine release	Rise in temperature 1°C (1.8 F) or greater within two hours after transfusion Chills
Delayed hemolytic transfusion reaction	1:2,500 RBCs	Extravascular hemolysis of RBCs	May be clinically occult Fatigue Pallor Anemia Dyspnea Mild jaundice Unexpected drop in hemoglobin New (+) Coombs test
Bacterial contamination	1:350 platelets 1:2,500,000 RBCs	Contamination of the blood product, occurring during procurement, storage, preparation, or administration of product.	Fever Chills Sepsis
Transfusion-related acute lung injury	1:10,000 RBCs also with cryoprecipitate	Activation of complement and histamine release, resulting in increased pulmonary capillary permeability	Respiratory distress, which may be accompanied by: Fever Chills Cyanosis Hypotension
Acute hemolytic reaction	1:25,000 RBCs	Administration of incompatible blood Preexisting antibodies against transfused RBCs, resulting in massive hemolysis Improper administration (i.e., with dextrose solution)	Fever Chills Nausea Dyspnea Low back pain Hemoglobinurea Pain at infusion site Tachycardia Hypotension Cardiovascular collapse Renal failure Disseminated intravascular coagulopathy
Urticarial reaction (plasma allergy)	1:1,000 blood products	Recipient responds to donor proteins	Flushing Hives Itching
Anaphylaxis	1:150,000 blood products	Severe immune response to a foreign substance	Generalized flushing Dyspnea Stridor Chest pain Hypotension Nausea Abdominal cramps Loss of consciousness
Transfusion associated graft-versus-host disease	Rare, true incidence unknown	Allogenic lymphocytes in the transfused blood engraft in the patient who is profoundly immunodeficient.	Fever Rash Hepatitis Diarrhea Bone marrow suppression Infection

(Adapted from Labovich, T. M. [1997]. Transfusion therapy: Nursing implications. *Clinical Journal of Oncology Nursing, 1*[3], 61–72.)

FLOWCHART 12-2 **Pathophysiology of Sickle Cell Anemia**

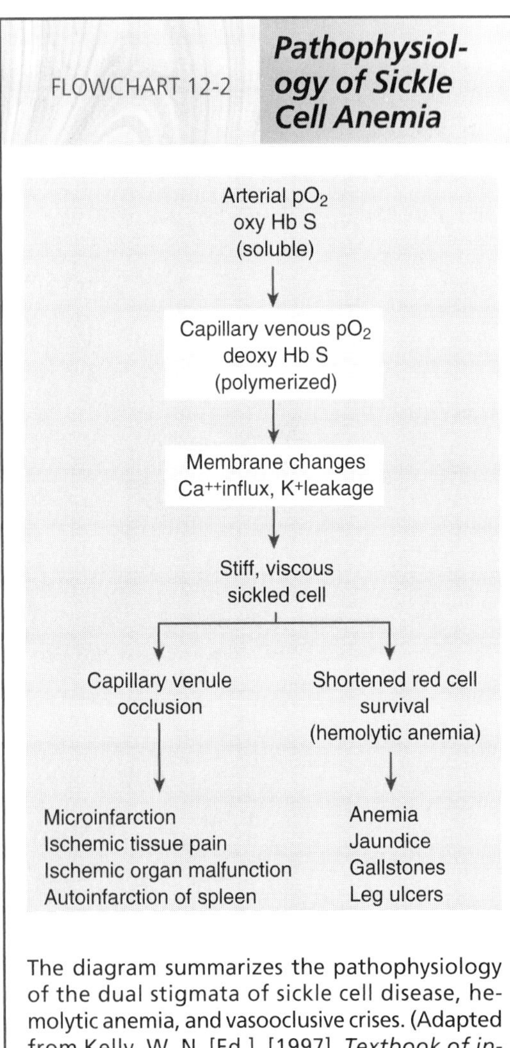

The diagram summarizes the pathophysiology of the dual stigmata of sickle cell disease, hemolytic anemia, and vasooclusive crises. (Adapted from Kelly, W. N. [Ed.], [1997]. *Textbook of internal medicine* [3rd ed.] Philadelphia: J. B. Lippincott.)

TABLE 12-9

CRISES OF SICKLE CELL ANEMIA

TYPE OF CRISIS	CLINICAL FEATURES
Vaso-occlusive crisis	This is the most common form of crisis This crisis causes severe pain for the patient Microvasculature is obstructed by large amounts of sickle cells
Anemic crisis	Red cells are depleted due to hemolysis and splenic sequestration Folate deficiency due to hemolysis exacerbates problem
Aplastic crisis	Bone marrow production of RBCs is suppressed Usually due to infection (especially viral) Rapid RBC turnover exacerbates problem
Acute sequestration crisis	Occurs in age 8 mo–2 y Sudden enlargement of spleen or liver occurs Splenic and hepatic discomfort is severe Acute abdominal symptoms are present May lead to intra-abdominal sepsis and death
Hemolytic crisis	Rare type of crisis May be due to precipitating factor such as infection rather than sickle cell disease Hemolysis continues even after hypoxia is corrected

(Adapted from Shelton, B. K. [1996]. Hematologic disorders. In J. Hebra, & M. M. Kuhn (Eds.); *Manual of critical care nursing*. Boston: Little, Brown.)

globin chains are known, and many forms of these diseases have been diagnosed. Disease involving defects of beta-chain synthesis occurs most frequently in inhabitants of the Mediterranean areas, Central Africa, Asia, the South Pacific, and parts of India.[28] Defects in alpha-chain synthesis are most frequent among southern Asians. Delta-beta thalassemias are very rare. The effects vary markedly, depending on whether the disorders are heterozygous or homozygous.[4]

Thalassemia major is homozygous and exhibits ineffective erythropoiesis and peripheral hemolysis, which stimulates enlargement of the red marrow to increase RBC formation.[28] Typical expansion of the bone marrow leads to thin cortical bone, causing enlargement of the bones of the face and jaws. The long bones become vulnerable to fracture. Sometimes the liver also becomes involved in erythropoiesis, resulting in hepatomegaly. The condition manifests with severe hemolytic anemia along with hypochromic, microcytic RBCs.[17] Death may occur early in fetal life, although a less severe form of the disease may permit the homozygote to survive to adulthood. Transfusion therapy has diminished some of the effects of the disease.[26] Growth retardation is common, as are marked splenomegaly and hepatomegaly. Clinical manifestations include profound anemia, wasting, jaundice, hepatomegaly, and a characteristic "chipmunk" face.[28]

Thalassemia minor is a heterozygous disorder that may be a chronic, asymptomatic, mild anemia. It is diagnosed by blood smear (hypochromic, microcytic

RBCs) and must be differentiated from iron deficiency anemia by electrophoresis, which shows that most of the hemoglobin is HbA due to deficient HbB (beta).[4,17]

MACROCYTIC ANEMIA: MEGALOBLASTIC ANEMIA

Megaloblastic anemias refer to those disorders that demonstrate large, immature, poorly functional erythrocytes.[10,11] These are also called macrocytic or megaloblastic anemias. The two most common causes are vitamin B_{12} deficiency (pernicious anemia) and folate (folic acid) deficiency. Other conditions, such as drug-induced suppression and inborn errors, also may produce this type of anemia.

Vitamin B_{12} deficiency is a common form of megaloblastic anemia, usually called pernicious anemia. It affects up to 1% of elderly adults in the United States, especially those of Northern European descent.[6] It is an autoimmune disease leading to progressive loss of parietal cells in the stomach, causing failure of secretion of hydrochloric acid and the intrinsic factor. The intrinsic factor is a glycoprotein that is essential to bind vitamin B_{12} and protect it from degradation by intestinal enzymes.[4] The body readily stores vitamin B_{12} so that development of this type of anemia requires years of utilization of bodily stores. The clinical features include chronic anemia and neurologic defects from lesions in the spinal cord with symptoms such as ataxia and a burning sensation in the soles of the feet.

TABLE 12-10

MACROCYTIC ANEMIA

	VITAMIN B_{12} DEFICIENCY	FOLIC ACID (FOLATE) DEFICIENCY
Pathophysiology	Pernicious anemia is decreased serum vitamin B_{12} due to decreased absorption. Bound by intrinsic factor (IF) secreted by parietal cells of stomach, to protect from destruction until absorbed in the ileum	Malabsorption of dietary folic acid due to lack of intake or absorption
Etiology	Familial incidence, fair complexion Related to autoimmune diseases associated with gastric mucosal atrophy Higher incidence in autoimmune disorders: SLE, myxedema, Graves' disease Common in Northern Europeans; rare in children, Blacks, and Asians Occurs postoperatively with gastric or small bowel surgery Parasites that compete for nutrient (e.g.; fish, tapeworm) Increased requirement—pregnancy	Immature GI tract—infants Poor dietary intake—adolescents, pregnant and lactating women, alcoholics, elderly, cancer, excessive cooking of foods Poor GI absorption—intestinal disease (jejunitis, small bowel resection, sprue), prolonged anticonvulsants and estrogens Folate antagonists—anti-metabolite antineoplastics, alkylating agents, nitrous oxide Inborn errors of metabolism—defective folate metabolism Increased requirement—pregnancy, hemolytic anemia, myeloproliferative disease
Clinical presentation	Inhibited growth of all cells—anemia, leukopenia, thrombocytopenia Demyelination of peripheral nerves to spinal cord (occurs in approximately 10%) Triad: weakness, sore tongue, paresthesias	Similar to B_{12} deficiency but without neurologic symptoms Signs of poor oxygenation: dizziness, irritability, dyspnea, pallor, headache, oral ulcers, tachycardia
Diagnostic tests	Schilling test + – failure to secrete HCl even after histamine administration ↓Hgb and RBC Macrocytosis ↑ MCV and ↓ MCHC ↓ WBC and Plts ↑ LDH	Macrocytosis ↑ MCV and ↓ MCHC Serum folate < 4 mg/dL Abnormal platelet appearance ↑ Reticulocyte count
Management	Parenteral vitamin B_{12} Iron replacement for life	Folic acid supplements Foods high in folic acid: beef liver, peanut butter, red beans, oatmeal, asparagus, broccoli

(Shelton, B. K. [1998]. Anemia. In C. R. Ziegfeld, B. G. Lubejko, & B. K. Shelton [Eds.], *Oncology fact finder: Manual of oncology nursing*. Philadelphia: Lippincott.)

Folic acid anemia results from a lack of folic acid in the diet, malnutrition, chronic alcoholism, increased need (pregnancy and infancy), and antagonistic drugs (chemotherapeutic and anticonvulsant drugs).[6] It causes impaired DNA synthesis and megaloblastic transformation of RBCs.[4] The clinical manifestations include severe anemia with evidence of megaloblastic RBCs, which can be readily treated with dietary supplementation. A summary of macrocytic anemias is included in Table 12-10.

MICROCYTIC ANEMIA: IRON DEFICIENCY ANEMIA

Iron deficiency anemia is characterized by deficient hemoglobin synthesis caused by a lack of iron.[22] With severe deficiency, the RBCs become microcytic and hypochromic because of low concentrations of hemoglobin. This is the most common type of anemia, and it occurs in all geographic locations and in all age groups.[22] The main causes of iron deficiency are increased loss, as in chronic or acute bleeding, and decreased dietary intake. Iron deficiency is common among preschool children, presumably because of increased dietary need and poor dietary supply.[9] It also occurs in the elderly, adolescents, and the indigent, possibly due to poor dietary intake.[22] Because iron is absorbed mostly in the duodenum and its ionization and absorption are enhanced by gastric hydrochloric acid, iron deficiency anemia may accompany pernicious anemia or gastrectomy.[22] Also, malabsorption syndromes impair absorption of iron along with other nutrients.[22]

Laboratory diagnosis includes evidence of decreased levels of serum iron, transferrin (stored iron), and apoferritin (iron-binding protein produced by the liver) in the early stages (see Unit 3, Appendix A). Anemia, characterized by microcytic and variably sized hypochromic RBCs, is a relatively late manifestation.[21]

Clinical manifestations of iron deficiency are nonspecific, and their onset is insidious; as many as 20% of affected adults have normal iron indices.[22] Fatigue, tachycardia, irritability, and pallor with epithelial abnormalities, such as sore tongue, cracks in the corners of the mouth, or stomatitis, are present. Thinning or spooning of the nails (**koilonychia**) occasionally is encountered. Pica, or the craving for non-food substances, may be striking. Affected people may crave dirt, starch, or ice.[22] Late manifestations may include cardiac murmurs, congestive heart failure, loss of hair, and pearly sclera.[9]

POSTHEMORRHAGIC ANEMIA

Posthemorrhagic anemia occurs after acute or chronic blood loss, although chronic blood loss usually results in iron deficiency anemia. Both plasma and RBCs are lost during a hemorrhage, so hemoglobin level and RBC count are normal immediately after a hemorrhage.[10] The dominant clinical picture is usually that of hypovolemia and shock.

Blood volume is restored by the movement of fluid from the interstitial spaces into the capillaries, causing dilution of the remaining RBCs (dilutional anemia) with a maximum effect in 48 to 72 hours.[8] This dilute blood carries too few RBCs to efficiently oxygenate the tissues. Normocytic, normochromic anemia is accompanied by reticulocytosis up to 15%.[17] In acute massive bleeding, this compensatory effect requires up to 1 week and may not occur in time to be life saving without transfusions of whole blood.

CHRONIC DISEASE ANEMIAS

Anemias of chronic disease are those that exhibit a mild-to-moderate decrease in hemoglobin concentration. There is a decrease in the proliferation of RBCs and a shortened RBC survival.[22] This very common anemia is associated with various types of infections, autoimmune diseases, neoplastic diseases, and inflammatory disorders (Box 12-1).[11,29] The reticulocyte count is less than 2%, and the RBC morphology is usually normochromic and normocytic but may be hypochromic.[11] The anemia is caused by failure of transport of storage iron into the plasma, leading to failure of hemoglobinization. The diagnosis is made by finding increased iron stores in the bone marrow and by elevated plasma ferritin levels.[6] This condition has an insidious onset; the symptoms are vague, with pallor and fatigue, and they must be differentiated from iron deficiency anemia.[22]

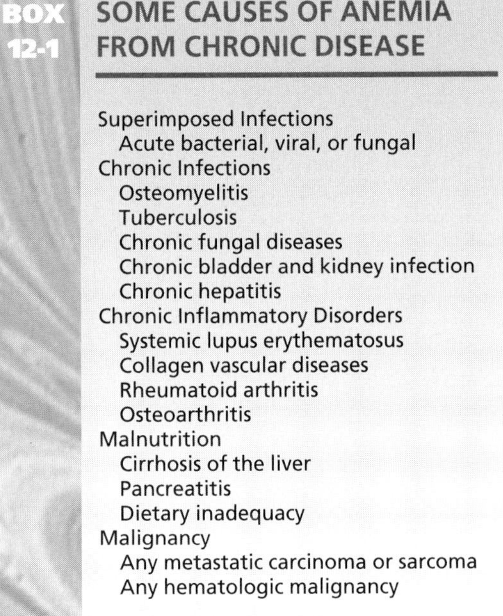

BOX 12-1 SOME CAUSES OF ANEMIA FROM CHRONIC DISEASE

- Superimposed Infections
  - Acute bacterial, viral, or fungal
- Chronic Infections
  - Osteomyelitis
  - Tuberculosis
  - Chronic fungal diseases
  - Chronic bladder and kidney infection
  - Chronic hepatitis
- Chronic Inflammatory Disorders
  - Systemic lupus erythematosus
  - Collagen vascular diseases
  - Rheumatoid arthritis
  - Osteoarthritis
- Malnutrition
  - Cirrhosis of the liver
  - Pancreatitis
  - Dietary inadequacy
- Malignancy
  - Any metastatic carcinoma or sarcoma
  - Any hematologic malignancy

FOCUS ON THE PERSON WITH ANEMIA

M. P., 44-year-old woman, was seen by her family physician because she was feeling worn-out and unable to carry out activities of daily living. She indicated that her menstrual periods were very heavy, lasting 8 to 9 days and occurring every 21 days. She also reported that she had been dieting to lose 20 pounds. Examination revealed a thin, pale woman with spooning of the nails and thin, lifeless hair.

Questions

1. What is the most probable diagnosis for this woman? What laboratory test would be used and what would confirm the diagnosis suspected?
2. Compare the pathophysiology, clinical picture, and laboratory features of the different types of anemias.
3. What treatment would be effective in this form of anemia? What teaching should be used to prevent recurrence of this clinical picture?

See Appendix A for discussion.

REFERENCES

1. Adams, R. J., McKie, V. C., Brambilla, D., et al. (1996). Stroke prevention trial in sickle cell anemia. *Controlled Clinical Trials, 19*(1), 110–129.
2. Baserga, R. (1998). Principles of molecular cell biology of cancer: The cell cycle. In V. T. DeVita, S. Hellman, and S. A. Rosenberg (Eds.), *Cancer: Principles and practice of oncology* (5th ed.). Philadelphia: Lippincott.
3. Berne, R. M. & Levy, M. N. (1998). *Physiology* (4th ed.). St. Louis: Mosby.
4. Bonner, H. & Erslew, A. J. (1999). The blood and lymphoid organs. In E. Rubin and J. L. Farber, *Pathology* (3rd ed.). Philadelphia: Lippincott.
5. Brodsky, R. A. (1998). Biology and management of acquired severe aplastic anemia, *Current Opinion in Oncology, 10*(2), 95–99.
6. Chandrasoma, P. & Taylor, C. R. (1998). *Concise pathology* (3rd ed.). Stamford, CT: Appleton & Lange.
7. Chernecky, C. C., & Berger, B. J. (1997). *Laboratory tests and diagnostic procedures* (2nd ed.). Philadelphia: Saunders.
8. Coffland, F. I., & Shelton, D. M. (1995). Blood component replacement therapy, *Critical Care Nursing Clinics of North America, 5*(1), 543–556.
9. Cotran, R. S., Kumar, V., & Collins, T. (1999). *Robbins' pathologic basis of disease* (6th ed.). Philadelphia: W.B. Saunders.
10. Erickson, J. M. (1996). Anemia. *Seminars in Oncology Nursing, 12*(1), 2–14.
11. Fairbanks, V. F., Hines, J. D., Mazza, J. J., & Hocking, W. G. (1995). The anemias. In J. J. Mazza (Ed.), *Manual of clinical hematology* (2nd ed.). Boston: Little, Brown.
12. Fonseca, R., & Tefferi, A. (1997). Practical aspects in the diagnosis and management of aplastic anemia. *American Journal of the Medical Sciences, 313*(3), 159–169.
13. Guinan, E. C. (1997). Clinical aspects of aplastic anemia. *Hematology-Oncology Clinics of North America, 11*(6), 1025–1044.
14. Guyton, A. & Hall, J. E. (1996). *Textbook of medical physiology* (9th ed.). Philadelphia: Saunders.
15. Hocking, W. G. (1995). Primary and secondary erythrocytosis. In Mazza, J. J. (Ed.), *Manual of clinical hematology* (2nd ed.). Boston: Little, Brown.
16. Hutton, J. L. (1998). The leukemias and polycythemia vera. In J. H. Stein (Ed.), *Internal medicine* (5th ed.). St. Louis: Mosby.
17. Jandl, J. H. (1996). *Blood: Textbook of hematology* (2nd ed.). Boston: Little, Brown.
18. Jones, L. (1998). Sickle cell anemia: Avoiding crises, organ damage. *Annals of Internal Medicine, 128*(12 pt 1), 1055–1056.
19. Labovich, T. M. (1997). Transfusion therapy: Nursing implications. *Clinical Journal of Oncology Nursing, 1*(3), 61–72.
20. Male, D. (1998). Hypersensitivity—Type II. In I. Roitt, J. Brostoff, & D. Male. *Immunology* (5th ed.). St. Louis: Mosby.
21. Mazza, J. J. (1995). Hematopoiesis and hematopietic growth factors. In J. J. Mazza (Ed,), *Manual of clinical hematology* (2nd ed.). Boston: Little, Brown.
22. Means, R. T. (1998). Iron deficiency anemia, anemia of chronic disease, sideroblastic anemia, and iron overload. In J. Stein (Ed.), *Internal medicine* (5th ed.). St. Louis: Mosby.
23. Nakao, S. (1997). Immune mechanisms of aplastic anemia. *International Journal of Hematology, 66*(2), 127–134.
24. Ohene-Frempong, K. Weiner, S. J., & Sleeper, L. A. (1998). Cerebrovascular accidents in sickle cell disease: Rates and risk factors. *Blood, 91*(1), 288–294.
25. Petz, L. D., Allen, D. W., & Kaplan, M. E. (1995). Hemolytic anemia: Congenital and acquired. In J. J. Mazza (Ed.), *Manual of clinical hematology* (2nd ed.). Boston: Little, Brown.
26. Petz, L. D., Calhoun, L., Shulman, I. A., et al. (1997). The sickle cell hemolytic transfusion reaction syndrome. *Transfusion, 37*(4), 382–392.
27. Rodgers, G. P. (1997). Overview of pathophysiology and rationale for treatment of sickle cell anemia. *Seminars in Hematology, 34*(3 Suppl 3), 2–7.
28. Schnall, S. F., & Benz Jr., E. J. (1995). Abnormalities of hemoglobin. In J. J. Mazza (Ed.), *Manual of clinical hematology* (2nd ed.). Boston: Little, Brown.
29. Shelton, B. K. (1998). Anemia. In C. R. Ziegfeld, B. G. Lubejko, & B. K. Shelton (Eds.), *Oncology fact finder: Manual of oncology nursing*. Philadelphia: Lippincott.
30. Shelton, B. K. (1996). Hematologic disorders. In J. Hebra, & M. M. Kuhn (Eds,), *Manual of critical care nursing*. Boston: Little, Brown.
31. Shier, D., Butler, J. & Lewis, R. (1996). *Hole's anatomy and physiology* (7th ed.). Dubuque, IA: Wm. C. Brown.
32. Storb, R. (1997). Aplastic anemia. *Journal of Intravenous Nursing, 20*(6), 317–322.
33. Winkelmann, J. C. (1998). Hemolytic anemia. In J. Stein (Ed.), *Internal medicine* (5th ed.). St. Louis: Mosby.

Chapter

13

Normal and Altered Leukocyte Function

Brenda K. Shelton / Amy Beth Soloman

KEY TERMS

agranulocytes
Bence-Jones protein
dysmyelopoiesis
giant cells
granulocytes
granulomatous disease
immunocytes
leukemoid reaction
lymphadenopathy
mononuclear phagocyte system
myeloproliferative disorders
pancytopenia
phagocytes
preleukemic syndrome
Reed-Sternberg cells

Leukocytes, the white blood cells or WBCs, are larger and less numerous than erythrocytes, and play a key role in the defense mechanisms of the body. As the name implies, leukocytes are almost white (the Greek *leukos* means "white").

The two important functions of the leukocytes are (1) to defend the body against invasion by foreign organisms, and (2) to produce, transport, and distribute defensive elements (e.g., antibodies) that are necessary for the immune response. The subtypes of leukocytes each have different functions that work together to produce a total integrated and effective defensive response to perceived injury or invasion by pathogens.

NORMAL LEUKOCYTE STRUCTURES

There are normally about 5,000 to 10,000 leukocytes per microliter, or 5 to 10^9 per liter of adult human blood.[11] **Granulocytes** (polymorphonuclear leukocytes, or polys) make up the largest portion of the total number of leukocytes, and **agranulocytes** constitute the remainder. The three types of granulocytes are neutrophils, eosinophils, and basophils. Lymphocytes and monocytes are the two types of agranulocytes. Specific cellular characteristics and their staining features are described in Table 13-1. The proportions of different types of WBCs are determined by counting cells in a diluted blood sample; the results are called the *differential white blood cell count.* This count varies with age, and the significance of alterations is important in identifying infectious disorders and leukocyte diseases (see Unit 3, Appendix B).

Granulocytes

Granulocytes have large granules and horseshoe-shaped nuclei. Their background cytoplasm stains blue to pink with Wright's stain, which enhances their morphologic identification (see Table 13-1). The specific features of each of the granulocytes follow:

NEUTROPHILS. These granulocytes are the most numerous, making up 35% to 65% of the total WBC count. This count varies with age. These cells are often called polymorphonuclear leukocytes (polymorphs or PMNs). These PMNs are called segmented *(segs)* neutrophils when they are mature and *bands* (stabs) when they are immature. The nucleus of the immature cell looks like a thick, curved band; normally, less than 5% of the WBC count will be in this form. The neutrophil has special organelles called peroxisomes that contain several powerful oxidizing agents, including hydrogen peroxide, superoxide, and hydroxyl ions.[33] Neutrophils are active phagocytes and their purpose is to kill bacteria.

TABLE 13-1

OVERVIEW OF LEUKOCYTES

CELL TYPE	CHARACTERISTICS	WRIGHT'S STAINING CYTOPLASM	WRIGHT'S STAINING CYTOPLASMIC GRANULES	WRIGHT'S STAINING NUCLEUS	DIAGRAM
GRANULOCYTES (POLYMORPHONUCLEAR LEUKOCYTES, POLYS)					
Neutrophils	Have small; fine, light pink or lilac acidophilic granules when stained and a segmented, irregularly lobed, purple nucleus	Blue to pink	Lilac	Purple-blue	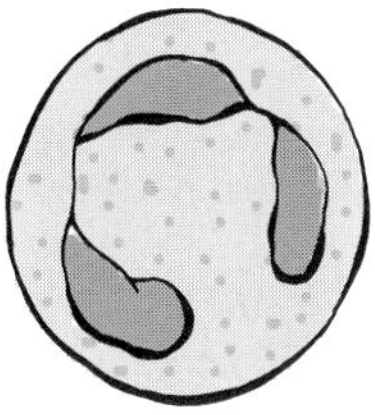 Neutrophil
Eosinophils	Have large round granules that contain red-staining basic mucopolysaccharides and multilobed purple-blue nuclei	Blue to pink	Red	Purple-blue	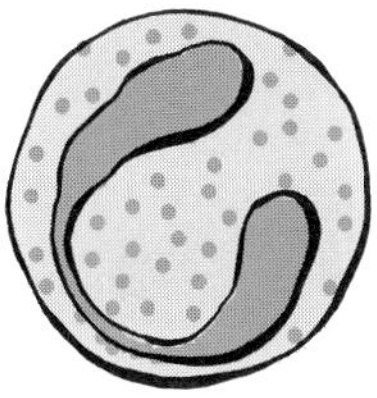 Eosinophil
Basophils	Coarse blue granules conceal the segmented nucleus. Granules contain histamine, heparin, and acid mucopolysaccharides.	Blue to pink	Blue-black	Purple-blue	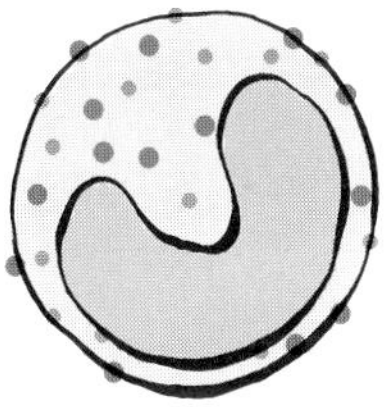 Basophil
AGRANULOCYTES					
Lymphocytes	Small cell with a large, round, deep-staining, single-lobed nucleus and very little cytoplasm. The cytoplasm is slightly basophilic and stains pale blue	Pale blue	—	Dark blue	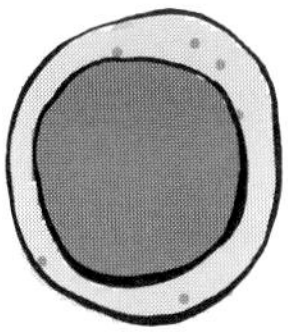 Lymphocyte
Monocytes	Large cell with a prominent, multi-shaped nucleus that sometimes is kidney-shaped. Chromatin in the nucleus looks like lace, with small particles linked together like strands. The gray-blue cytoplasm is filled with many fine lysozymes that stain pink with Wright's stain.	Gray-blue	Pink	Blue lighter than lymphocytes	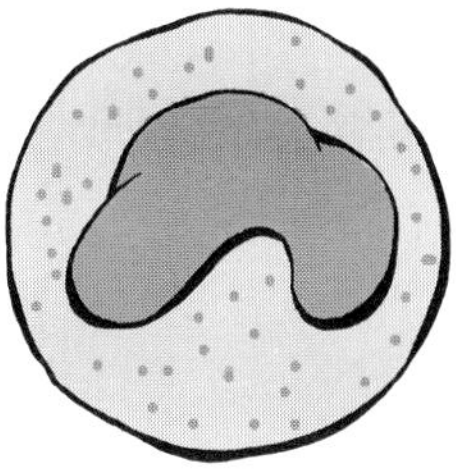 Monocyte

Eosinophils. These constitute about 0.5% to 5% of the normal WBC count, which varies with age, but larger numbers are found in the mucosa of the intestinal tract and of the lung. They contain hydrolytic enzymes in their granules and also release highly reactive forms of oxygen.[21] They increase in number in allergic reactions and with parasitic infestation.

Basophils. These normally constitute less than 1% of the normal WBC count in all age groups, but they are found in larger numbers in the connective tissue and pericapillary area. They contain histamine, heparin, and small quantities of bradykinin and serotonin.[21] They increase in number during inflammatory and allergic reactions.

Agranulocytes

The agranulocytes are so named because the granules in their cytoplasm are not readily visible (see Table 13-1). They have a large, deep-staining nucleus. The features of the monocytes and lymphocytes (both called mononuclear leukocytes) follow:

Monocytes. These normally constitute 3% to 8% of the normal WBC count. Organelles within the monocyte, especially lysosomes and peroxisomes, contain powerful bactericidal agents and proteolytic enzymes.[33] These cells are immature macrophages. Macrophages have multiple functions in disposing of foreign material and ridding the body of waste material, especially following an inflammatory process.

Lymphocytes. These compose 25% to 38% of the normal WBC count and consist of two types: T lymphocytes and B lymphocytes. These cells, also called *immunocytes,* are the cells responsible for the specific immune response (see Chap. 10).

NORMAL LEUKOCYTE DEVELOPMENT AND FUNCTION

Multipotential or uncommitted stem cells in bone marrow differentiate into unipotential, or committed, stem cells that ultimately become leukocytes, erythrocytes, or platelets (see Figure 12-1). The two major functional groups of leukocytes are **phagocytes** and **immunocytes**. Phagocytes, including neutrophils and monocytes, function in the ingestion and destruction of antigens and in cellular waste removal. Immunocytes are the lymphocytes and function in the specific immune response.

Genesis and Life Span of Leukocytes

The multipotential, or uncommitted, stem cells in bone marrow differentiate into the specific WBC line and mature through several morphologic stages. Granulocytes and monocytes are apparently derived from a common committed stem cell. Neutrophils, basophils, and eosinophils are formed in the bone marrow and can be stored there until needed. A precursor to the monocyte called the promonocyte is also formed and differentiated in bone marrow, then released into the circulation as a monocyte. The monocyte can leave the blood for the tissues, where it enlarges and is transformed or matured into a lysosome-filled macrophage. The macrophage is much larger than the monocyte, which is essential for the phagocytosis of large particles and debris (see p. 362).

Lymphocytes are formed from a pluripotent, or uncommitted, stem cell that becomes committed to the lymphocyte line (see p. 338). T lymphocytes travel to the thymus gland, where they mature into antigen specific cells. B lymphocytes develop and mature in the bone marrow.[21]

The life span of circulating WBCs is short, often only hours. The average life span of a neutrophil is about 6 hours, but during serious infections it may be only about 2 hours.[16] A summary of the normal circulating and tissue life span of specific WBCs is shown in Table 13-2.

Functions of Neutrophils

The main function of the neutrophils is to defend the body from infection through the process of phagocytosis, a defensive activity also performed by macrophages. The process involves antigen ingestion and destruction, followed by cellular waste removal (Table 13-3). For neutrophils to accomplish their defensive purpose, they must perform the following: (1) accumulate in sufficient numbers at the right place; (2) attach to the foreign material or agent; (3) envelop or engulf the agent; and (4) dispose of the debris (Fig. 13-1).[12] Alterations in any of these functions result in defective phagocytosis and a defective defensive response.[6]

The stimulation of tissue injury or the presence of a pathogen (antigen) that has breached the barrier defenses stimulates the inflammatory-immune response and initiates a WBC (both neutrophil and monocyte-macrophage) response. The complement system, which is activated in the immune response, provides a chemical wall (chemotaxis) that causes WBCs to move toward the source of the injury. WBCs migrate to the affected area, wall it off, and prevent the spread of injury or infection (see p. 256). This process ensures that adequate numbers of WBCs are present to perform activities required for phagocytosis. Tightly packed WBCs in the area can then rapidly destroy the antigen.

Phagocytosis is promoted by physical factors such as heat, an antigen-induced positive electrical charge,

TABLE 13-2

LIFE CYCLE OF WHITE BLOOD CELLS

CELL TYPE	DEVELOPMENT AND MIGRATION	LIFE SPAN
GRANULOCYTES		
Neutrophils Eosinophils Basophils	Mature in the bone marrow. Maturing granulocytes that are no longer dividing accumulate as a reserve in the bone marrow. Normally about a 5-day supply in the bone marrow.	Average of 12 hours in the circulation. About 2 to 3 days in the tissues.
AGRANULOCYTES		
Lymphocytes	T lymphocytes are constantly circulating, following a path from the blood to the lymphatic tissue, through the lymphatic channels, and back to the blood through the thoracic duct. B lymphocytes are largely noncirculating. They remain mainly in the lymphoid tissue and may differentiate into plasma cells.	Life span varies. Small population of memory lymphocytes survives for many years. Most T lymphocytes of the peripheral lymphatic tissue recirculate about every 10 hours.[19] Mature plasma cells have a survival rate of about 2 to 3 days.
Monocytes	Monocytes spend less time in the bone marrow pool than granulocytes.	Circulation is about 36 hours.[3] After the monocyte has been transformed into a mobile or fixed macrophage in the tissues, its life ranges from months to years.

TABLE 13-3

FUNCTIONAL ACTIVITY OF PHAGOCYTIC CELLS

FUNCTIONAL PROCESS	DESCRIPTION OF ACTIVITY
Phagocytosis	Process similar to how ameba ingests its nutrients. The phagocyte changes its shape and opens up one side of its protoplasm, creating a vacuole (also called phagosome) that engulfs and fuses the protoplasm of the two cells. Microorganisms, old cells, and foreign particles are destroyed by phagocytosis.
Degranulation	After foreign material is engulfed in a phagosome, degranulation occurs. This process involves lysosomes (granules) fusing with the internal membrane of the phagosome and emptying their contents into its vacuole. The granules contain hydrolytic enzymes that cause the dissolution of the phagosome contents and, eventually, lysis of the phagocyte itself.
Killing	Killing is the process by which the microorganism contained within the membrane-bound phagosome dies. Most hydrolytic enzymes contained in the granules serve a digestive function and are not directly involved in killing. What actually kills the microorganism is peroxidation of hydrogen peroxide, which, in the presence of iodide, destroys the microbial membrane. Only a few organisms (e.g., acid-fast bacilli causing tuberculosis and leprosy) survive inside a phagocyte.
Diapedesis	The ability of cells to "slide" in an ameba-like action through the capillary vessel walls. This activity involves development of a pseudopod-like projection that is projected through the wall, and permits incremental movement until the entire cell passes through and is then able to accumulate at the site of injury or pathogenic invasion.
Chemotaxis	Chemical substances, called chemotactic agents or mediators, are released from the infected or necrotic tissues and provide a signal for the leukocytes to move toward the source of the bacterial invasion. Chemotactic agents include the complement system, plasminogen, the fibrinolytic system, kallikrein (the kinin system), and substances released from the phagocytes. This process, called chemotaxis, is dependent on a concentration gradient. A greater concentration of the chemotactin causes more leukocytes to move toward the source.
Pinocytosis	Process meaning "cell drinking"; cellular engulfment of tiny particles suspended in a droplet of fluid.
Opsonization	Opsonization is defined as alteration to the antigenic surface of a pathogen that renders it accessible to the phagocyte. Opsonization is mediated by activation of the complement protein system or by specific antibodies. Activation of complement results in attachment of C3b to the surface of the particle, which, with specific antibody, allows it to be recognized and phagocytosed by the leukocyte.

FOCUS ON CELLULAR PHYSIOLOGY

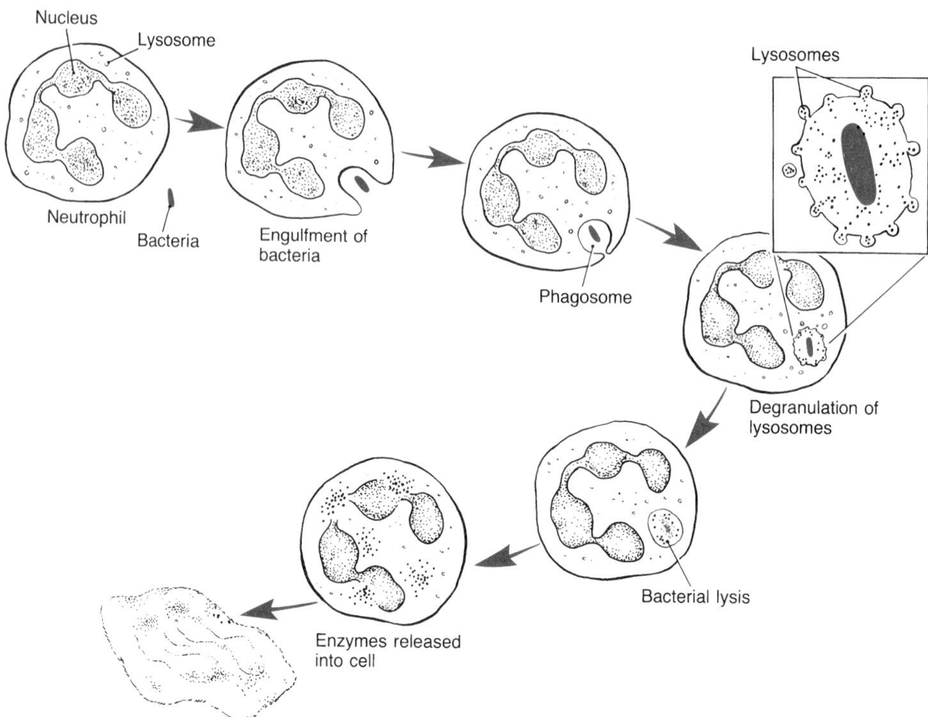

FIGURE 13-1. Phagocytosis of bacteria by neutrophils.

or specific antigenic surface properties.[22] In infections, the fever that is produced may serve as a protective mechanism that enhances phagocytosis and hastens removal of pathogenic material (see p. 256).

Monocyte-Macrophage Functions

The **mononuclear phagocyte system** (occasionally referred to as the reticuloendothelial system) is a large system of stationary and mobile macrophages. It includes all the fixed and mobile phagocytic cells in the liver, spleen, lymph nodes, and gastrointestinal tract. Fixed macrophages in these organs exist in equilibrium with mobile macrophages. All tissue macrophages, including the Kupffer cells of the liver and alveolar macrophages in the lungs, originate from the mobile circulating macrophages, which have as their source blood monocytes.[33]

Macrophages ingest large particles, large amounts of debris, and inert materials. If a particle is a very large, multinucleated foreign body, **giant cells** may be produced from fusion of several macrophages.[5] This ability is important to prevent the spread of infection, particularly with encapsulated organisms (e.g., pneumococcus, streptococcus, or mycobacterium). Macrophages are responsible for removing the debris that accumulates in infectious process as well as necrotic debris. If a foreign agent is introduced to the body, the macrophages will surround it and wall it off from the rest of the body.

Macrophages also clear aged and damaged cells. Certain tissue macrophages break down and recycle RBCs by binding with globin and transporting heme to be recycled into new hemoglobin. Macrophages of the liver, spleen, and bone marrow can bind free iron to apotransferrin, forming transferrin (see p. 753).[22]

Basophil and Eosinophil Function

The precise functions of eosinophils and basophils are not well understood, but these cells are known to participate in inflammatory and allergic reactions. They cause some of the signs and symptoms of allergic reactions.[21] People with allergies often have elevated levels of immunoglobulin E (IgE). When basophilic receptor sites for IgE are attached, histamine and other substances are released that increase chemotaxis and enhance the allergic response (see p. 312). The number of basophils increases in some of the **myeloproliferative disorders**, such as polycythemia vera.

Eosinophils weakly exhibit phagocytosis and chemotaxis, but their primary function is probably to detoxify foreign proteins.[26] Because of their location in the mucosa of the intestinal tract and the lungs, they probably detoxify foreign proteins through the production of toxic reactive oxygen intermediates.[26] The circulating level of eosinophils is increased (eosinophilia) as a result of worm infestation and parasitic infections. In trichinosis, the numbers of eosinophils can increase 25% to 50%.

Functions of Lymphocytes

Lymphocytes demonstrate immunocytic functions both in lymphoid tissue and in circulation (see Chap. 10). They do not possess phagocytic capabilities, but function to protect the body against specific antigens. This specific immunity is integrated with other general immune responses. The lymphocytes move freely from the blood to the lymphoid tissues, patrolling the tissue spaces for recognizable foreign material, which when encountered is targeted for destruction.[5]

NONMALIGNANT WHITE BLOOD CELL DISORDERS

Because each leukocyte subtype has a defined function, attacks by a particular foreign agent elicit the response of a specific type of leukocyte. Significant increases or decreases in the numbers of any type of leukocyte are known as quantitative alterations. Significant functional abnormalities of the cells are called qualitative alterations. Nonmalignant white blood cell disorders are conventionally divided into quantitative and qualitative disorders according to whether they are characterized by an increase in the numbers of leukocytes or by an impairment in the functional competence of the leukocytes.

Quantitative Leukocyte Alterations

Alterations in the number of specific WBC subtypes can be influenced by a wide variety of diseases and exposures. Elevations of specific cell lines are identifiable by the suffixes *-philia* or *-cytosis*, as indicated by neutrophilia or monocytosis. Deficiencies of specific cell subtypes are recognizable by the suffix *-penia*. If the entire WBC count is decreased due to bone marrow suppression, it is termed **pancytopenia.** Specific WBC count decrease is often associated with one or more factors suppressing the WBC production in the bone marrow, and the clinical manifestations reflect increased susceptibility to infection. Common key quantitative WBC disorders addressed below include neutrophil, eosinophil, basophil, monocyte, and lymphocyte alterations, as well as myelodysplastic syndrome.

NEUTROPHILIA

Neutrophilic leukocytosis (neutrophilia) is defined as an absolute neutrophil count greater than 7,500/L of blood.[11] Acute bacterial infections often cause increases in the number of immature, nonsegmented neutrophils (also called stabs or bands) in the peripheral blood.[42] This increase is called a "shift to the left," which refers to writing bands or stabs on the left-hand side of the page (a procedure no longer done, but the expression remains). As the differential count returns to a normal balance of all the different white blood cells, the infection is likely to be subsiding. Chronic inflammation or infection and chronic blood loss stimulate increased levels of granulocytes, and a mild neutrophilia also may be seen in the third trimester of pregnancy.[8]

The term **leukemoid reaction** refers to persistent neutrophilia of 30,000 to 50,000/L, which usually results from an acute infection (e.g., malaria) but may be mistakenly diagnosed as a leukemia.[16] The neutrophils in this reaction resemble those of leukemic origin, but leukemoid reactions lack the number of immature cells, WBC alkaline phosphatase, thrombocytopenia, or WBC clonal changes in the bone marrow that are seen with leukemia.

The clinical manifestations of neutrophilia relate to the underlying causative factors and may include fever and other signs of infection or inflammation. In many cases, the neutrophilia is an incidental finding on routine WBC counts.

NEUTROPENIA

Neutropenia is defined as a decreased level of the absolute neutrophil count. It may be characterized as mild, moderate, or severe based on the neutrophil count. Individuals with mild neutropenia have cell counts of 1000 to 1500 cells/mm^3; those with moderate neutropenia have 500 to 1000 cells/mm^3; and those with severe neutropenia have counts below 500 cells/mm^3.[9] Neutrophils are decreased in diseases involving bone marrow production (e.g., agranulocytosis, aplastic anemia) or when excess destruction occurs. The specific cause of neutropenia may be determined by diagnostic tests such as bone marrow aspiration with biopsy, antinuclear antibody (ANA), serum immunoglobulin electrophoresis, folate, B_{12}, and antineutrophil antibody tests.[16]

A diminished number of neutrophils alters the body's defenses against bacterial invaders. In the first week of neutropenia, those pathogens most likely to cause infection are bacterial; however, there is an increased risk of fungal infection after 7 to 10 days, and a risk of infection with opportunistic organisms (organisms capable of causing disease in the host with impaired immune defenses) beyond 21 to 30 days.[29] Without the phagocytic WBC response, neutropenic individuals are also unable to localize or contain an infection, so early and rapid infection dissemination is common.

The neutropenic person not only has less of a defense against invading pathogens but also displays fewer signs and symptoms. He or she exhibits few local symptoms such as pain, erythema, or exudates (e.g., pus) (see p. 262). Fever, malaise, and nonspecific aches (myalgias or arthralgias) may be the only symptoms of infection in the affected individual.

EOSINOPHIL, BASOPHIL, AND MONOCYTE ALTERATIONS

When the differential counts for eosinophils, basophils, and monocytes are elevated or decreased, the cause and clinical manifestations are specific to the underlying causative conditions.

Eosinophilia is defined as an absolute eosinophil count that exceeds 500/mm^3. It is often associated with allergy and parasitic infections. It also can be caused by a large number of unusual systemic diseases such as sarcoidosis, pernicious anemia, polycythemia vera, and Addison's disease.[14] *Eosinopenia* occurs when the absolute eosinophil count is less than 50/mm^3. The decrease may be due to severe infection, shock, or adrenocortical stimulation.[42] It may also be associated with pancytopenia.

Basophilia is defined as an absolute basophil count exceeding 50 to 100/mm^3 of blood. It is often associated with myeloproliferative disorders, chronic granulocytic leukemia, and polycythemia vera.[14] *Basopenia* occurs when the absolute basophil count is less than 20/mm^3 of blood. It is often associated with suppression of other granulocytes in drug-induced or other causes of bone marrow suppression.[42]

Monocytosis refers to an absolute monocyte count greater than 600/mm^3 in adults. It may occur in nonpyogenic bacterial infections, such as active tuberculosis. Monocyte counts also are seen to be elevated in chronic inflammatory disorders such as ulcerative colitis, as well as viral infections.[31] *Monocytopenia* is defined as an absolute monocyte count less than 100/mm^3 in adults. It may be seen with administration of immunosuppressive agents or in other conditions that cause pancytopenia.

LYMPHOCYTE ALTERATIONS

Lymphocytosis is an increase in the number of lymphocytes above 4000/mm^3 in adults. It often occurs in viral diseases and in lymphocytic leukemia. *Lymphopenia* results from a suppression of lymphocyte production in the bone marrow and is seen in association with any factor that can cause bone marrow suppression.

Infectious Mononucleosis

Infectious mononucleosis (IM) is primarily a disease of adolescents and young adults in the United States.[32] The causative agent is the Epstein-Barr virus (EBV), which is transmitted mainly through oral secretions. EBV subclinically infects from 90% to 100% of the world's population by age 5.[13] Infections from cytomegalovirus (CMV) and hepatitis A, as well as Hodgkin's disease and drug reactions from diphenylhydantoin, hydralazine, and other drugs, can mimic IM.[40]

The active disease is associated with the brief appearance of IgM antibodies against EBV. Hematologic changes are characteristic, with an initial mild leukopenia leading to an elevation to 15,000 to 30,000 by the second week. Atypical lymphocytes are seen in the peripheral blood in the second through fourth weeks. This disease is characterized by cervical **lymphadenopathy**, fever, sore throat, and splenomegaly. Profound fatigue, malaise, and weakness are also commonly described. Neurologic manifestations occur in approximately 1% of affected persons; these may include Guillain-Barré syndrome, Bell's and other cranial nerve palsies, and transverse myelitis.[13]

MYELODYSPLASTIC SYNDROME

Myelodysplastic syndrome (MDS) is a hematologic disorder of the bone marrow characterized by abnormal hematologic cell production (**dysmyelopoiesis**) and low peripheral blood counts.[20,43] MDS is also referred to as **preleukemic syndrome**, or a subacute myeloid leukemia that may progress to an acute leukemic state (see p. 365).[16] It is most common in adults over 60 years of age but has affected every age group, including infants.[3] The etiology of this disease is unknown, but some affected individuals have been exposed to toxic chemicals, especially benzene.[8]. Most affected individuals have a mean survival of 2 to 4 years, either from progressive pancytopenia or leukemic transformation.[1,16]

Stem cell cloning of cells is dysfunctional, leading to production of fewer hematopoietic cells or abnormal, short-lived cells. The bone marrow displays both normal stem cells and clone cells. Initially, clone cells of MDS are pluripotent and capable of differentiation (e.g., giving rise to all bone marrow cell lines). Over time, those same clone cells lose the ability to differentiate along multiple cell lines and can no longer mature the granulocyte cell line. At this stage, the bone marrow produces mostly immature myeloblasts, with increased size.[16,41] Bone marrow is suppressed and fails to produce adequate numbers of hematopoietic cells. Progression from MDS to an acute myelogenous leukemia occurs in 20% to 40% of patients.[8] The greater the number of blasts in the bone marrow of the MDS patient at diagnosis, the higher the chance of conversion of MDS to acute leukemia.[16] It is now known that as many as 50% of people with acute leukemia had previous bone marrow changes indicative of MDS.[17]

The most common clinical findings in MDS are anemia, neutropenia, and thrombocytopenia. Infections and bleeding are common presenting symptoms.

Qualitative Leukocyte Alterations

Defective leukocyte quality is less common than quantitative disorders and much more difficult to identify.

The qualitative abnormalities of granulocytes result in defective physical and chemical functions. Neonates are particularly prone to qualitative alterations due to complement deficiencies and immature adhesion properties of the neutrophil.[21] Most of these disorders involve defects in the phagocyte or its locomotion. One such disorder is *lazy leukocyte syndrome*, seen with intrinsically abnormal leukocytes. Complement disorders that alter the phagocytic and chemotactic responses of granulocytes are associated with collagen vascular disorders (e.g., systemic lupus erythematosus) or bacterial infections. Drugs such as aspirin, corticosteroids, colchicine, paclitaxol, and phenylbutazone can also cause dysfunction of the phagocyte.[21] Ethanol causes a significant decrease in leukocyte migration and chemotaxis during acute intoxication.[16]

Several qualitative abnormalities of the granulocytes are inherited. Altered nuclear structure and appearance, excessive granulation of the cytoplasm, and hypersegmentation of neutrophils occur. These alterations may affect phagocytosis or may have no clinical implications. **Granulomatous diseases** are rare qualitative defects of the granulocytes, especially neutrophils, that result in defective bactericidal activity. In chronic granulomatous disease, there is an inherited X-linked absence of neutrophil and monocyte oxidative metabolism that is necessary for the killing of bacteria.[39] The disease results in severe recurrent infections of the skin, lymph nodes, lungs, liver, and bones with catalase-positive microorganisms (those that destroy their own hydrogen peroxide).[8,10]

MALIGNANT WHITE BLOOD CELL DISORDERS

Malignant white blood cell disorders include: (1) leukemias, progressive proliferations of abnormal leukocytes; (2) lymphomas, neoplasms of the lymphoreticular organs that present as solid tumors; and (3) plasma cell myelomas, malignant neoplasms of plasma cells.

Leukemias

Leukemias are malignant proliferations of WBCs that are classified by the dominant cell type. This group of malignancies constitutes about 7% to 8% of all cancers and has no specific gender or ethnic distribution.[24] Leukemias are the most common malignancies in children.[34] In general, the prognosis in children is better than that for adults, but each leukemia subtype has specific prognostic implications.

The abnormal overproduction of malignant cells is initially confined to the bone marrow, but the cells later invade other organs of the body and tissue, causing anemia, infection, and thrombocytopenia. If untreated, leukemic cells will replace all normal hematopoietic cells and lead to death.

CLASSIFICATION

Leukemia is classified according to the onset and duration of the disease and the type of abnormal cells present in the bone marrow. *Acute leukemia* is characterized by large numbers of immature leukocytes that cause a rapid onset and disease progression. *Chronic leukemia* is identified by the excessive numbers of mature leukocytes found in the bone marrow and periphery and has a more gradual onset and progression. If abnormal proliferation of granulocytic leukocytes or their precursors is found in the blood or bone marrow, the leukemia may be called *granulocytic, myelogenous*, or, most commonly, *myelocytic*. If abnormal proliferation of lymphocytes or monocytes is seen, the leukemia is called *lymphocytic* or *monocytic*, respectively. Leukemias are named with either *acute or chronic* preceding the cell type involved (e.g., acute myelocytic leukemia [AML] or chronic lymphocytic leukemia [CLL]). The French-American-British (FAB) classification system further differentiates acute leukemia subtypes based upon abnormal cell types. The FAB classifications for acute leukemias are included in Table 13-4.

ETIOLOGY

To date, no definitive cause of leukemia has been identified, but genetic, environmental, and disease factors are thought to predispose an individual to leukemia. There is a concordance in identical twins of approximately one in four when one develops leukemia.[36] The congenital chromosomal abnormality of Down syndrome (trisomy of chromosome 21) increases the risk of developing leukemia by 20-fold.[23,36] Acquisition of the Philadelphia chromosome (a translocation between chromosomes 22 and 9) is characteristic of chronic myelogenous leukemia. Exposure to ionizing radiation and chemicals,including benzene, arsenic, pesticides, chloramphenicol, phenylbutazone, and antineoplastic agents (especially alkylating agents), is also known to cause leukemia.[36] The development of leukemia after treatment with alkylating agents for other cancers is called *secondary leukemia*. Diseases such as MDS, myelofibrosis, polycythemia vera, and refractory anemia increase one's risk of leukemia.[17,20] Support for a viral causation has resulted from study of the human T-cell leukemia virus (HTLV-1), which has been shown to induce acute leukemia in animals.[6,36]

PATHOPHYSIOLOGY

The abnormal functions of leukemia are the result of malignant WBCs suppressing normal bone marrow function or are related to leukemic cell invasion of other body tissues. Leukemic cells inhibit normal bone marrow production of erythrocytes, platelets, and immune function. Histopathologic and prognostic features of acute leukemias are described in Table 13-5.

TABLE 13-4

FAB CLASSIFICATION OF ACUTE LEUKEMIA

CLASS	CELLULAR FINDINGS	%	PROGNOSIS	HISTO-CHEMISTRY	DIAGRAM
M_0	Acute undifferentiated (not classifiable)	?	Poor	—	
M_1	Acute myeloblastic leukemia without maturation and <3% promyelocytes	20%	Complete response in 65–80%; quick relapse after post-remission therapy	Sudan black and peroxidase negative Peroxidase identified by monoclonal antibody	
M_2	Acute myeloblastic leukemia with some maturation, >3% promyelocytes	20–30%	Complete response in 65–80%; quick relapse after post-remission therapy	Strongly peroxidase positive	
M_3	Acute promyelocytic leukemia (APHL) with >30% promyelocytes	5–7%	Good for 2 to 7-year remission	Strongly peroxidase positive	
M_4	Acute myelomonocytic leukemia containing myelocytes and monocytes with > 20% peripheral blood evidence, with or without bone marrow evidence	22–30%	Best in adults	Strongly peroxidase positive May have prictate (PAS) positive cells	
M_5	A. Acute monocytic leukemia, poorly differentiated B. Acute monocytic leukemia well differentiated	10–19%	Worst in adults	May be peroxidase and PAS positive Nonspecific esterase stains are strongly positive	
M_6	Erythroleukemia has a predominance of erythroblasts and severe erythropoiesis	1–5%	Poor	RBC precursors are positive Ringed sideroblasts are seen with iron stains	
M_7	Megakaryocytic leukemia	2–5%	Variable	Variable Platelet peroxidase can be demonstrated by electron microscope	
L_1	Childhood (pre-B and T cell) lymphoblastic predominance		Best in children >90% remission	PAS positive Peroxidase negative	

(continued)

TABLE 13-4

FAB CLASSIFICATION OF ACUTE LEUKEMIA (Continued)

CLASS	CELLULAR FINDINGS	%	PROGNOSIS	HISTO-CHEMISTRY	DIAGRAM
	Homogeneous small blasts with scant cytoplasm and little variation from cell to cell Round nucleus with a single small nucleolus			Acid phosphatase positive Naphthyl esterase positive if T-ALL	
L_2	Adult (pre B and T cell) lymphoblastic predominant Heterogeneous large cells with more abundant cytoplasm than L_1 Variation from cell to cell Irregularly shaped nucleus, often with multiple nucleoli		2 to 10-year remission Often relapse from first remission in <2 years	Same as L_1	

(Summarized from Rubin, E., & Farber, J. [1999]. *Pathology* [3rd ed.]. Philadelphia: Lippincott Williams & Wilkins.)

CLINICAL MANIFESTATIONS

The following clinical manifestations may be seen in leukemia:

- Anemia with a hematocrit between 20% and 30% and a hemoglobin of 8 to 10 gm/dL causes fatigue, shortness of breath, pallor, and malaise secondary to decreased oxygen carrying capacity.
- Thrombocytopenia, with platelet counts as low as 20,000, causes petechiae, bruising, bleeding, and, infrequently, hemorrhage.
- Leukopenia or neutropenia increases the risk for infection and life-threatening sepsis.
- Other manifestations of leukemia such as neurologic dysfunction result from immune dysfunctional cells infiltrating organs and tissue, such as the central nervous system.
- Chloromas are skin infiltrations near bony prominences that are often seen with myelocytic leukemia.
- Gum infiltration is typical of acute monocytic leukemia, and central nervous system leukemia is most likely to occur with acute lymphocytic leukemia.

Key clinical features of the acute leukemias are described in Table 13-5. Comparisons of chronic forms of myelogenous and lymphocytic leukemia are found in Table 13-6.

Malignant Lymphomas

Malignant lymphomas are cancers involving only lymphocytes during their maturation or storage in the bone marrow. Lymphomas are classified by their cellular characteristics into Hodgkin's lymphoma and non-Hodgkin's lymphomas. Malignant lymphomas constitute about 5.5% of all malignancies in Western countries; however, for unknown reasons the incidence has been increasing over the past decade.[1,34] The prognosis for patients with lymphoma depends upon the cellular subtype, stage of disease at diagnosis, and specific genetic and phenotypic markers. Lymphoma is the third most common malignancy in children.[27,38] Lymphoma in children has unique clinical features and a better overall prognosis than lymphoma in adults.[27,38]

HODGKIN'S LYMPHOMA

Also known as Hodgkin's disease (HD), this lymphoma constitutes less than 1% of all cancers and only 15% of lymphomas.[2,18] Hodgkin's disease has a bimodal incidence pattern, prevailing in young adults (16 to 30 years of age) and also in the fifth decade.[8] It is slightly more common in men than women.[28] It is considered to be curable in up to 80% of affected persons who receive immediate and aggressive treatment.[28]

TABLE 13-5

FEATURES OF ACUTE LEUKEMIAS

FEATURE	ACUTE MYELOCYTIC LEUKEMIA (AML)	ACUTE LYMPHOCYTIC LEUKEMIA (ALL)
Age of incidence	Adult years—peak incidence 60 years 10% of all diagnosed in childhood	Highest incidence in 3 to 4-year-olds Often < 15 years Adults of any age
Gender	M > F 3:2	M > F 5:4
Biggest risk factors	Ionizing radiation Chemical exposure Genetic abnormalities	Ionizing radiation Anti-neoplastic chemotherapy Virus Genetic abnormalities
Survival	1–3 years with treatment; 3–6 months with some long-term survivors	2–5 years depending upon clinical features and histopathology
Peripheral blood	Variable WBC count with myeloblasts, decreased absolute neutrophil count, thrombocytopenia, and anemia	Increased, decreased, or normal WBC count, lymphocytosis (usually > 25,000 or >40%), thrombocytopenia, and anemia
Bone marrow	Hypercellular (> 50% myeloblasts) Auer rods (red-staining rods in the cytoplasm of myeloblasts characteristic of AML)	Hypercellular with infiltrating lymphoblasts
Cytogenetics	Chromosomal aberrations—trisomy 21, Bloom syndrome, trisomy 8, and deletions of the long arm of chromosomes 5 and 7	Variable chromosome number or structure: t(8;14) (q 24; q 32) t(2;8) or t(8;22) trisomy 21.
Immunologic identification	Not identified due to lack of cALLa antigen Lack of T and B cell determination	85% have cALLa antigen Lack B or T cell characteristics
Treatment	Combination chemotherapy with cytosine arabinoside and daunorubicin, idarubicin, or mitoxantrone Blood products Bone marrow transplant	Combination chemotherapy with vincristine, prednisone, methotrexate, l-asparaginase Blood products Bone marrow transplant
Common signs and symptoms	Gum, skin, soft tissue infiltration Oral infection Gingival hyperplasia Small vascular occlusions Disseminated intravascular coagulation Bleeding—epistaxis, petechiae	Meningeal, CNS involvement Chills Hepatosplenomegaly Bone/joint pain

Etiology

The bimodal age distribution of HD suggests more than one possible etiologic factor. An infectious source for HD has been validated by research findings linking HD to Epstein-Barr virus in as many as 20% of cases.[13,21] Clusters of disease within families or geographic regions also suggest an infectious source.[13] Exposure to carcinogens such as ionizing radiation and antineoplastic chemotherapy has also been associated with HD.[8] Both non-Hodgkin's lymphoma and HD have an increased incidence in persons who are immune compromised, especially those infected with the human immunodeficiency virus (HIV).[28]

Pathophysiology

Hodgkin's disease is characterized by proliferation of a tumor in which only a small proportion of the cells are malignant and the majority are normal reactive lymphocytes, plasma cells. The characteristic malignant cells, called **Reed-Sternberg cells**, are probably multinucleated, giant cell mutations of the T-lymphocyte and are always present in the lymph node at the time of diagnosis with HD. The size and prominent nucleolus of this cell make it unmistakable on pathologic examination.[8,10] Infiltration of the nodes with eosinophils and plasma cells occurs and is associated with lymph node necrosis and fibrosis.[10]

Hodgkin's disease may involve a defect in the B or T lymphocytes, although T-lymphocytic abnormalities are more common. Lymph nodes affected by HD show obliteration of the normal lymph node structure and its replacement with cells characteristic of the disease.

Clinical Manifestations

Laboratory findings of HD include normocytic, normochromic anemia, even when there is no bone marrow involvement.[30] Affected persons will also have neutrophilia, monocytophilia, lymphopenia, and normal or increased platelet counts. In late stages of the disease, bone marrow infiltration can occur, produc-

TABLE 13-6

FEATURES OF CHRONIC LEUKEMIAS

FEATURE	CHRONIC MYELOCYTIC LEUKEMIA (CML)	CHRONIC LYMPHOCYTIC LEUKEMIA (CLL)
Age	20- to 60-year-old; peak age 40 Infrequent in children	Greatest incidence at 60 years and older
Gender	Slightly higher in males over females	2 : 1 incidence in males over females
Biggest risk factors	Ionizing radiation Chemical exposure	Unknown
Survival	1 to 10 years; mean 3 years	2–25 years
Peripheral blood	Increased WBC with mature granulocytes but all developmental stages present Early thrombocytosis, late thrombocytopenia and anemia	Some elevation of small lymphocytes Thrombocytopenia with anemia in late stages
Bone marrow	Hyper cellular (< 50% blasts) Megakaryocytosis	> 30% lymphocytes
Cytogenetics	85% have aberration of Philadelphia chromosome	Random unconfirmed chromosomal aberrations
Immunologic identification	Not identified	Majority have B cell markers 1–3% have T cell markers
Common signs and symptoms	Splenomegaly, bone tenderness, pallor, hypermetabolic symptoms, diaphoresis, weight loss, anorexia, weakness	Painless lymphadenopathy, hepatosplenomegaly, fatigue, hypersensitivity to insect bites

ing worsening anemia, thrombocytopenia, and generalized leukopenia.[30]

The most common clinical manifestation of HD is an enlarged, non-tender lymph node. The most common sites are high cervical (29%), and supraclavicular (41%).[28] Lymph nodes often fluctuate in size, but remain firm and movable. Fevers without chills are common, although no specific pattern of occurrence is typical. Pruritus without rash is a common complaint, although the precise incidence and prognostic significance of its presence are unknown.[28] Night sweats, abdominal pain, and weight loss of more than 10% are constitutional symptoms that portend a worse prognosis.[30] Other signs and symptoms that occur due to disease infiltration of visceral organs include chest discomfort, dyspnea, bone pain, abdominal distention, and an enlarged spleen.

The severity of HD is established by clinical and histopathologic staging. The Ann Arbor staging system for HD considers lymph node involvement, extranodal disease, and constitutional symptoms (Table 13-7).

TABLE 13-7

ANN ARBOR STAGING* CLASSIFICATION OF HODGKIN'S DISEASE

STAGE	CLASSIFICATION
I	Involvement of a single lymph node region (I) or single extralymphatic site (I_E)
II	Involvement of two or more lymph node regions on the same side of the diaphragm (II), which may also include the spleen (II_S), localized extralymphatic involvement (II_E), or both (II_{SE}), if confined to the same side of the diaphragm
III	Involvement of lymph node regions on both sides of the diaphragm (III), which may also include the spleen (III_S), localized extralymphatic involvement (III_E), or both (III_{SE})
IV	Diffuse or disseminated involvement of extralymphatic sites (e.g., bone marrow, liver, or multiple pulmonary metastases), with or without lymph node involvement

*The presence of fever, night sweats, or unexplained weight loss of 10% or more of body weight over 6 months is designated by the letter *B*. The letter *A* indicates absence of these symptoms.
Clinical staging (CS) refers to the use of noninvasive tests; pathologic staging (PS) refers to staging based on invasive or surgical procedures (e.g., laparoscopy or laparotomy with splenectomy). Thus a patient with CSIIA Hodgkin's disease may prove to have $PSIV_{S+He+}$ on the basis of positive liver and splenic biopsies.
(Stein, J. (Ed.), [1998] *Internal medicine* (5th ed.). St. Louis: Mosby.)

NON-HODGKIN'S LYMPHOMA

Non-Hodgkin's lymphoma (NHL) is the most common type of malignant lymphoma, constituting 85% of all cases.[18,24] Unlike HD, this disease most often affects adults, particularly between the ages of 50 to 70 years of age.[15] NHL also is more common in men than women and in whites than African-Americans.[21] NHL may involve B or T lymphocytes and more often involves extranodal sites than does HD.[44]

Etiology

Non-Hodgkin's lymphoma probably arises from combinations of environmental and genetic factors. As with other hematologic malignancies, viruses, herbicides, organic solvents, and ionizing radiation are known risk factors for NHL.[10,18] The high incidence of NHL seen with HIV disease and the link between Epstein-Barr virus and Burkitt's lymphoma (a type of NHL) also validate the potential for an infectious etiology.[13] Gastric lymphoma has been positively identified with *Helicobacter pylori* infection, warranting antimicrobial therapy even in asymptomatic patients.[25]

Pathophysiology

Non-Hogkin's lymphoma is pathophysiologically similar to HD, but there are no Reed-Sternberg cells and the specific mechanism of lymph node destruction is different. The abnormal lymph node tissue is identified by changes in tissue architecture and patterns of infiltration. The distribution of malignant cells within specific regions of the lymph node further defines the lymphoma as follicular (germinal), interfollicular, mantle, or medullary. The tissue is then described by the pattern of infiltration as nodular or diffuse.[8]

Various staging systems exist using histopathologic characteristics. Although many differences exist, grouping as low grade, intermediate grade, or high grade based on the cell maturity and growth pattern is standard. Low-grade lymphomas are slow growing and have well differentiated cells, whereas high-grade lymphomas are rapidly growing and have poorly differentiated cells (Table 13-8).[16,37]

Clinical Manifestations

Hematologic profiles show only lymphocytopenia unless the bone marrow is involved. Non-Hogkin's lymphoma usually first presents with enlarged, non-tender lymph nodes, although there is no typical location such as seen with HD. In fact, 15% to 25% of patients also present with extranodal disease, most commonly in the gastrointestinal tract or nasopharynx.[19] Other reported sites include skin, bone, thyroid, breast, lung, testis, and brain.[19] The incidence of multisystem disease is high. A summary of potential signs and symptoms and tumor locations is shown in Table 13-9. Non-Hodgkin's lymphoma in children is significantly different than in adults. The key differences in the two presentations are described in Table 13-10.[28]

TABLE 13-8

WORKING FORMULATION OF NON-HODGKIN'S LYMPHOMA

LOW GRADE

A. Small lymphocytic
  Consistent with CLL
  Plasmacytoid
B. Follicular, predominately small cleaved cell
C. Follicular, mixed small cleaved and large cell

INTERMEDIATE GRADE

D. Follicular, large cell
E. Diffuse, small cleaved cell
F. Diffuse, mixed small and large cell
G. Diffuse, large cell

HIGH GRADE

H. Large cell immunoblastic
I. Lymphoblastic
J. Small noncleaved cell
  Burkitt
  Non-Burkitt

MISCELLANEOUS CATEGORIES

K. Cutaneous T cell
L. Adult T-cell leukemia/lymphoma

(Rubin, E. & Farber, J. [1999]. *Pathology* [3rd ed.]. Philadelphia: Lippincott Williams & Wilkins.)

Plasma Cell Neoplasms

Plasma cell neoplasms or multiple myeloma are a group of related disorders, which are associated with proliferation and accumulation of immunoglobulin-secreting cells (plasma cells). They account for 1.1% of all cancers.[35] The disease occurs slightly more frequently in men than women and is the most common lymphoid malignancy in African-Americans.[24] The mean age at diagnosis is 68 to 70 years, although it has been reported in adults of all ages.[35] Despite effective initial responses to therapy, only 10% of patients survive for 5 years or more, with an average survival of only 24 to 36 months after diagnosis.[4,7]

ETIOLOGY

The etiology of plasma cell neoplasms is unknown, but there is a connection with chromosomal translocations involving chromosome 14 and with conditions of sustained immune stimulation (such as autoimmune diseases or allergies). Exposure to chemicals, food processing, and agricultural products has been linked with the disease.[35]

TABLE 13-9

SIGNS AND SYMPTOMS OF NON-HODGKIN'S LYMPHOMA

SYMPTOM	CAUSE
Lymphadenopathy and leukemia-like symptoms	Tumor growth in the lymph nodes or bone marrow
Gastrointestinal disturbance: pain, nausea, vomiting, malabsorption, or bleeding	Abdominal or pelvic mass; obstruction or erosion of the GI tract
Recurrent renal infections, pain, bleeding	Renal mass or obstruction
Peripheral neuropathy, cranial nerve palsies, headaches, visual disturbance, seizures, mental status changes or other CNS symptoms	Meningeal/intracranial/ocular tumor and pressure
Thyroid and other endocrine abnormalities	Thyroid/adrenal mass
Pulmonary symptoms: SOB, cough, chest pain, pulmonary infiltrates, etc.	Pulmonary mass
Systemic symptoms: weight loss, fatigue, night sweats	More extensive disease and tumor growth, high rate of cell necrosis, paraneoplastic hormone, and electrolyte abnormalities

(Ziegfeld, C. R. & Shelton, B. K. [1998]. Malignant lymphomas. In C. R. Ziegfeld & B. G. Lubejko [Eds.], *Oncology fact finder: Manual of cancer care.* Philadelphia: Lippincott.)

PATHOPHYSIOLOGY

When plasma cells become malignant, they proliferate uncontrollably and create excessive abnormal immunoglobulins.[2] In this proliferation process, they infiltrate the bone marrow, then the bone matrix, causing osteolytic bone lesions. Myeloma cells then proliferate outside the bone marrow in all lymphoid tissues where plasma cells normally reside. Since plasma cells are located in virtually all organs of the body, excess cell proliferation and abnormal immunoglobulin production affect almost all organ systems of the body.

Malignant plasma cells create a homogeneous antibody termed *monoclonal gammopathy*, determined by the specific malignant cell's characteristics. Excessive and abnormal immunoglobulins (antibodies) are one of the defining features of this disease. Based on the immunoglobulin created, multiple myeloma can be categorized as IgG, IgA, IgD, and IgM, in order of incidence. IgE multiple myeloma is very rare.[10] The type of immunoglobulin present often determines the aggressiveness of the disease and the prognosis for the affected individual. For example, IgG myeloma is progressive with a mean survival of 3 to 4 years, whereas IgD meyloma is an aggressive disorder with a mean survival of about 1 year.[8]

Production of excess immunoglobulin produces high plasma viscosity, and the excreted light chains are

TABLE 13-10

CLINICAL PRESENTATION OF NON-HODGKIN'S LYMPHOMA (NHL) IN CHILDREN AND ADULTS

PARAMETER	CHILDREN	ADULTS
Incidence	Rare	Common
Median age at presentation	10–15 years	55–70 years
Clinical presentation	Extranodal	Nodal
Histology	Diffuse pattern Undifferentiated cells Blastic appearance of cells Arise from early precursor cells and are antigen independent	Frequently nodular pattern Differentiated, frequently cleaved cells Small dormant lymphocytes Arise from fully differentiated cells and are antigen dependent
Growth rate	High mitotic rate	Low mitotic rate
Immunophenotype	50–70% are B-cell	70–90% are B-cell
Paraproteins	None	Rare (5%)
Clinical course	Rapidly proliferative	Variable—often indolent
Curability	60–80%	< 30% (except 40–70% in intermediate NHL, particularly noncleaved cell of follicular origin)

thought to be toxic to the renal tubules.[4] The laminated, crystalline casts in the distal tubules damage and obstruct the tubules.

CLINICAL MANIFESTATIONS

The clinical presentation of multiple myeloma is caused by abnormal plasma cell function, excess and abnormal immunoglobulin, and infiltration of the organs of the mononuclear phagocyte system with the malignant plasma cells. The major clinical findings are detectable in bone and bone marrow function, immune competence, and renal function. There is frequently associated normocytic, normochromic anemia, hypercalcemia, and hyperuricemia, along with an elevated erythrocyte sedimentation rate.[8]

Bone or back pain is the most common symptom.[35] Malignant plasma cells erode the matrix of the bone, causing lytic lesions seen radiographically as punched-out holes within the bone (Fig. 13-2). Although the lesions may occur anywhere in the skeleton, they are most frequently noted in the vertebral column, ribs, skull, pelvis, femurs, clavicles, and scapulae.[35] The bones may have so many holes that simple movements cause pathologic fractures, particularly of the weight-bearing bones such as in the pelvis or the femur. If untreated, pathologic fractures alter mobility and may cause collapse of vertebrae with subsequent spinal cord compression. Invasion of the bone marrow is evidenced by pallor and weakness caused by secondary anemia and by bleeding indicative of concomitant thrombocytopenia. Despite these other debilitating symptoms, the most common cause of death is infection.

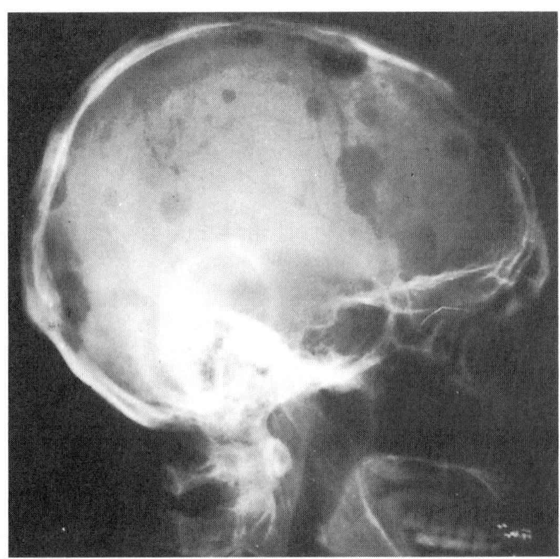

FIGURE 13-2. **Multiple myeloma. A radiograph of the skull shows numerous "punched-out" radiolucent areas. (Rubin, E., & Farber, J. L. [1999] *Pathology* [3rd ed.]. Philadelphia: Lippincott.)**

High plasma viscosity results in a high risk of thrombotic disorders such as deep vein thrombosis, pulmonary embolism, and thrombotic or embolic stroke.[4,7] Hyperviscosity may initially present as Raynaud's phenomenon, intermittent claudication, or unexplained cool extremities. Occlusions of venous and arterial vessels are found with equal frequency.

TABLE 13-11

CLINICOPATHOLOGIC CORRELATES IN MYELOMA

CLINICAL FEATURES	UNDERLYING PATHOLOGY
Anemia (usually normochromic, occasionally macrocytic or leukoerythroblastic)	Due to combination of accelerated red cell destruction, nutritional factors, and replacement of marrow by tumor.
Bone pain	Lytic lesions weaken bone, causing compression with or without collapse; may compress nerve roots in spine. Release of osteoclast-activating factor (OAF) contributes to lysis.
Renal disease	Due to combination of light chain deposition in tubules, hypercalcemia, amyloid, and renal infection.
Hypercalcemia symptoms	Due to lytic lesions and effects of OAF.
Infections	Due to decreased ability to produce specific antibody (especially bacteria such as pneumococcus).
Hyperviscosity syndrome	Due to high levels of Ig, producing microcirculatory impairment; typically seen in plasmacytoid lymphoma producing IgM (macroglobulinemia) but may occur with myeloma producing IgG or IgM.
Bleeding diathesis	Due to combination of thrombocytopenia, hyperviscosity, and amyloid.
Arthritis	Due to amyloid deposits or rarely uric acid (secondary gout, especially following treatment).
Neuropathy	Due to root compression or amyloidosis.

(Chandrasoma, P. & Taylor; C. R. [1998]. *Concise pathology* [3rd ed.]. Stamford, CT: Appleton & Lange.)

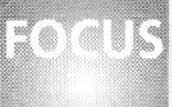

FOCUS ON THE PERSON WITH CHRONIC MYELOGENOUS LEUKEMIA

Mr. G. J., a 65-year-old man, was admitted for chemotherapy following the diagnosis of chronic myelogenous leukemia. He had a white blood cell count of 250,000/mm^3 with most of the cells being mature granulocytes. Examination revealed marked splenomegaly, anemia, and temperature of 100.8°F. Mr. J. reported a weight loss of 32 pounds during the past 6 months and upper abdominal tenderness along with nonspecific arthralgias.

Questions

1. Describe the pathophysiology of chronic myelogenous leukemia (CML). Compare it with the other forms of leukemia.
2. What is the clinical marker that is characteristic of CML?
3. Why do anemia, bleeding, and opportunistic infections occur with CML? What types of infections might be seen in this individual?
4. Describe the clinical picture that results from the accelerated phase of the disease.
5. What is the purpose of chemotherapy in CML? What is a common side effect of this therapy?

The incidence and severity of renal failure also correlates to the amount of immunoglobulin protein found in the urine.[4] Myeloma nephrosis occurs because of infiltration and precipitation of the light chains (**Bence-Jones protein**) in the distal tubules as the urine is concentrated. Pathologic interstitial inflammation and fibrosis further impair kidney function, leading to uremia. Table 13-11 describes the clinicopathologic correlates in myeloma.

REFERENCES

1. American Joint Committee on Cancer. (1998). *AJCC cancer staging handbook* (5th ed.). Philadelphia: Lippincott-Raven.
2. Anderson, K. C. (1997). Plasma cell tumors. In J. F. Holland, et al. (Eds.), *Cancer medicine* (4th ed.). Baltimore: Williams & Wilkins.
3. Applebaum, F. R. (1998). Bone marrow failure and myelodysplasia. In J. Stein (Ed.), *Internal medicine* (5th ed.). St. Louis: Mosby.
4. Barlogie, B., Jagannath, S., Epstein, J., et al. (1997). Biology and therapy of multiple myeloma in 1996. *Seminars in Hematology, 34*(1 suppl 1), 67–72.
5. Barnetson, R., Gawkrodger, D., & Britton, W. (1998). Hypersensitivity—Type IV. In I. Roitt, J. Brostoff, & D. Male, *Immunology* (5th ed.). St. Louis: Mosby.
6. Beverley, P. (1998). Tumour immunology. In I. Roitt, J. Brostoff, & D. Male, *Immunology* (5th ed.). St. Louis: Mosby.
7. Boccadoro, M., & Pileri, A. (1997). Diagnosis, prognosis, and standard treatment of multiple myeloma. *Hematology-Oncology Clinics of North America, 11*(1), 111–131.
8. Bonner, H., Bagg, A., & Cossman, J. (1999). The blood and the lymphoid organs. In E. Rubin & J. L. Farber, *Pathology* (3rd ed.). Philadelphia: Lippincott.
9. Boxer, L. A. (1997). Approach to the patient with leukopenia. In W. N. Kelley (Ed.), *Textbook of internal medicine* (3rd ed.). Philadelphia: Lippincott-Raven.
10. Chandrasoma, P. & Taylor, C. R. (1998). *Concise pathology* (3rd ed.). Stamford, CT: Appleton & Lange.
11. Chernecky, C. C., & Berger, B. J. (1997). *Laboratory tests and diagnostic procedures* (2nd ed.). Philadelphia: W. B. Saunders.
12. Cotran, R. S., Kumar, V., and Collins, T. *Robbins' Pathologic Basis of Disease* (6th ed.). Philadelphia: W.B. Saunders, 1999.
13. Crowe, S. (1994). Virus infections of the immune system. In D. P. Stites, A. I. Terr, & T. G. Parslow (Eds.), *Basic and clinical immunology* (8th ed.). Norwalk, CT.: Appleton & Lange.
14. Emerson, S. G. (1997). Approach to the patient with leukocytosis. In W. N. Kelley (Ed.), *Textbook of internal medicine* (3rd ed.). Philadelphia: Lippincott-Raven.
15. Freedman, A. S. & Nadler, L. M. (1997). Non-Hodgkin's lymphoma. In J. F. Holland, et al. (Eds.), *Cancer medicine* (4th ed.). Baltimore: Williams & Wilkins.
16. Friedenberg, W. R. (1995). Disorders of granulocytes: Qualitative and quantitative. In Mazza, J. J. (Ed.), *Manual of clinical hematology* (2nd ed.). Boston: Little, Brown.
17. Giles, F. J., & Koeffler, H. P. (1994). Secondary myelodysplastic syndromes and leukemias. *Current Opinion in Hematology, 1*(4), 256–260.
18. Glass, A. G., Karnell, L. H., & Menck, H. R. (1997). The National Cancer Data base report on non-Hodgkin's lymphoma. *Cancer, 80*(12), 2311–2320.
19. Greer, J. P., Macon, W. R., List, A. F., et al. (1993). Non-Hodgkin's lymphoma. In G. R. Lee, T. C. Bithell, J. Foerstler, J. W. Athens, & J. N. Lukens (Eds.), *Wintrobe's clinical hematology* (9th ed.). Malvern, PA: Lea and Febiger.
20. Jacobs, P. (1997). Myelodysplasia and the leukemias. *Disease-A-Month, 43*(8), 505–597.
21. Jandl, J. H. (1996). *Blood: Textbook of hematology* (2nd ed.). Boston: Little, Brown.
22. Janeway, C. A. & Travers, P. (1997). *Immunobiology: The immune system in health and disease* (3rd ed.). New York: Garland Publishing.
23. Jorde, L. B., Carrey, J. C., & White, R. L. (1995). *Medical genetics.* St. Louis: Mosby.
24. Landis, S. H., Murray, T., Bolden, S., & Wingo, P. A. (1998). Cancer statistics, 1998. *CA: A Cancer Journal for Clinicians, 48*(1), 6–11.
25. Lee, J., & O'Morain, C. (1997). Who should be treated for *Helicobacter pylori* infection? A review of consensus conferences and guidelines. *Gastroenterology, 113*(6 suppl), S99–106.
26. Lydyard, P. & Grossi, C. (1998). Cells involved in the immune response. In I. Roitt, J. Brostoff, & D. Male, *Immunology* (5th ed.). St. Louis: Mosby.
27. Magrath, I. T. (1997). The treatment of pediatric lymphomas: Paradigms to plagiarize? *Annals of Oncology, 8*(suppl.). 7–14.
28. Mauch, P. M. & Bonadonna, G. (1997). Hodgkin's disease. In J. F. Holland, et al. (Eds.), *Cancer medicine* (4th ed.). Baltimore: Williams & Wilkins.
29. Merlin, T. L., Gibson, D. W., & Connor, D. H. (1994). Infections and parasitic diseases. In E. Rubin & J. L. Farber, *Pathology* (2nd ed.). Philadelphia: Lippincott.
30. Miller, T. P. & Grogan, T. M. (1998). Hodgkin's disease and non-Hodgkin's lymphoma. In J. Stein (Ed.), *Internal medicine* (5th ed.). St. Louis: Mosby.
31. Pagana, K. D., & Pagana, T. J. (1998). *Mosby's diagnostic and laboratory text reference* (3rd ed.). St. Louis: Mosby.
32. Pagano, J. S. (1997). Epstein-Barr virus infections and the infectious mononucleosis syndrome. In W. N. Kelley (Ed.),

Textbook of internal medicine (3rd ed.). Philadelphia: Lippincott-Raven.

33. Parslow, T. G. (1994). The phagocytes: Neutrophils and macrophages. In D.P. Stites, A.I. Terr, & T.G. Parslow (Eds.), *Basic and clinical immunology* (8th ed.). Norwalk, CT: Appleton & Lange.
34. Pui, C. H. (1996). Acute leukemia in childhood. *Current Opinion in Hematology, 3*(4), 249–258.
35. Salmon, S. E. & Cassady, J. R. (1997). Plasma cell neoplasms. In V. T. DeVita, S. Hellman, & S. A. Rosenberg, *Cancer: Principles and practice of oncology* (5th ed.). Philadelphia: Lippincott-Raven.
36. Scheinberg, D. A., Maslak, P. & Weiss, M. Acute leukemias. In V. T. DeVita, S. Hellman, & S. A. Rosenberg, *Cancer: Principles and practice of oncology* (5th ed.). Philadelphia: Lippincott-Raven.
37. Schipp, M. A., Mauch, P. M., & Harris, N. L. Non-Hodgkin's lymphoma. In V. T. DeVita, S. Hellman, & S. A. Rosenberg, *Cancer: Principles and practice of oncology* (5th ed.). Philadelphia: Lippincott-Raven.
38. Shad, A. & Magrath, I. (1997). Non-Hodgkin's lymphoma. *Pediatric Clinics of North America, 44*(4), 863–890.
39. Spitznagel, J. K. (1997). Constitutive defenses of the body. In M. Schaechter, G. Medoff, & B. I. Eisenstein, *Mechanisms of microbial disease* (3rd ed.). Baltimore: Williams & Wilkins.
40. Straus, S. E. (1997). Herpes simplex virus and its relatives. In M. Schaechter, G. Medoff, & B. I. Eisenstein, *Mechanisms of microbial disease* (3rd ed.). Baltimore: Williams & Wilkins.
41. Tien, H. F., Wang, C. H., Chuang, S. M., et al. (1995). Acute leuekmic transformation of myelodysplastic syndrome—immunophenotypic, genotypic, and cytogenetic studies. *Leukemia Research, 19*(9), 595–603.
42. Treseler, K. M. (1995). *Clinical laboratory and diagnostic tests* (3rd ed.). Stamford, CT: Appleton & Lange.
43. Utley, S. M. (1996). Myelodysplastic syndromes. *Seminars in Oncology Nursing, 12*(1), 51–58.
44. Veronese, M. L., Schichman, S. A., & Croce, C. M. (1996). Molecular diagnosis of lymphoma. *Current Opinion in Oncology, 8*(5), 346–352.

Chapter 14

Normal and Altered Hemostasis

Theresa Pluth Yeo

KEY TERMS

alpha 2 antiplasmin
anticoagulants
antithrombin III
coagulopathy
degranulation
ecchymoses
fibrin degradation products
heparin cofactor II
homocysteine
hyaline
megakaryocytes
melena
methionine
paraproteinemias
plasminogen activator inhibitor-1
prostacyclin (PGI2)
protein C
protein S
prothrominase
serine proteases
thrombocythemia
thrombocytopenia
thrombophillia
thromboxane A2
tissue factor
tissue thromboplastin
von Willebrand factor (vWF)
zymogens

Hemostasis is a complex and highly evolved process that maintains blood fluidity under normal conditions but rapidly responds to vascular injury, arresting bleeding and then allowing blood to clot quickly to prevent hemorrhage. Platelets play an essential role in hemostasis. The process of coagulation (clotting) is a part of the process of hemostasis, which finally terminates in fibrinolysin. Alterations in blood coagulation may be caused by many factors and may result in coagulation deficiencies or thrombosis (the formation of a blood clot in the vascular system).

STRUCTURE AND FUNCTION OF PLATELETS

Platelets (also called thrombocytes) are anucleate fragments of **megakaryocytes**, which are formed in the bone marrow and released into the circulation. The normal platelet concentration in the blood is about 150,000 to 400,000.[15] Platelets have an inner zone that contains a large contingent of organelles, including contractile microfilaments, along with a variety of granules that secrete specific substances (Fig. 14-1).

Platelets are continually being formed by the bone marrow to maintain normal levels in the body. They are functionally active in the circulation for 8 to 12 days, then are eliminated from circulating blood mainly by the macrophages in the spleen. At any given time only two thirds of the total available platelets are circulating. The remaining platelets congregate in the red pulp of the spleen. Besides their function in hemostasis, which is the formation of the platelet plug, platelets also participate in inflammation and fibroblast proliferation.[10]

NORMAL HEMOSTASIS

Normal hemostasis involves interactions among blood vessel endothelium, the platelets, and the plasma coagulation factors. It will cause the arrest of bleeding through injury-induced vascular constriction and the activation of endothelial factors, platelets, and coagulation factors. Once a clot is formed, activation of the fibrinolytic system breaks down the formed clot and promotes healing. There is a delicate balance between

FOCUS ON CELLULAR PHYSIOLOGY

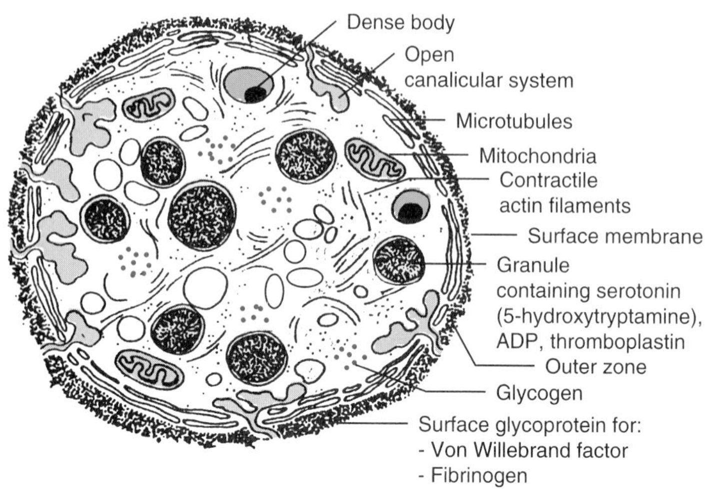

FIGURE 14-1. Structure of the platelet.

the coagulation and fibrinolytic systems (Fig. 14-2). A disturbance at either end disrupts the hemostatic balance and affects both systems.

Vascular Endothelium

Vascular endothelial cells line the walls of the blood vessels and normally inhibit coagulation and platelet aggregation while encouraging clot breakdown through fibrinolysis (see p. 381). Inhibition of coagulation is accomplished in several ways: (1) normal endothelial tissue has a smooth texture that does not allow platelet adherence; (2) the endothelial cells contain negatively charged proteins, which repel the clotting factors and platelets; and (3) circulating anticoagulant proteins suppress the formation of blood clots.[7]

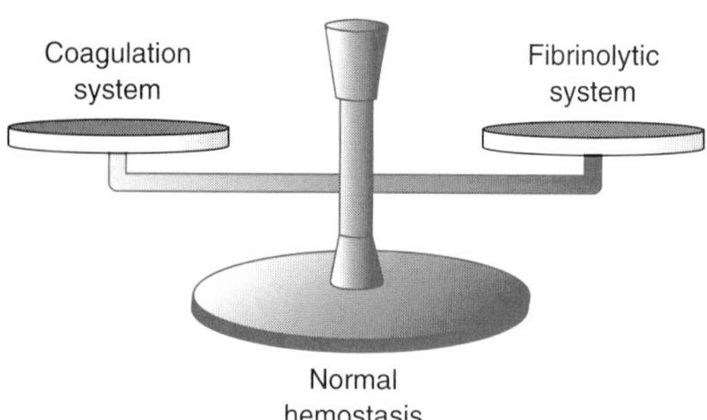

FIGURE 14-2. Balance between the coagulation and fibrinolytic systems.

Normal endothelial cells synthesize and secrete basement membrane and extracellular matrix containing the proteins collagen, fibronectin, and von Willebrand factor.[7] These adhesive and highly reactive proteins are deep in the subendothelium and are separated from blood cells, platelets, and plasma factors.

When the endothelium is injured, the normal conditions are altered and the reactive elements are stimulated, promoting platelet adhesion. This is often considered to be the first step in the process of hemostasis.

Events of Hemostasis

Hemostasis is divided into four main events: (1) vasoconstriction, (2) platelet plug formation, (3) blood coagulation, and (4) fibrin clot formation. The coordination of all four events is essential for normal hemostasis, as illustrated in Flowchart 14-1.

VASOCONSTRICTION

Vasoconstriction occurs immediately after the wall of a vessel is injured, diminishing blood flow into and out of the vessel. This constriction is initiated by local nervous reflexes and sustained through the biochemical mediators, serotonin and histamine, which are released from platelets in the damaged subendothelial wall. **Thromboxane A2** (TXA2), a fatty acid synthesized and released from the activated platelets, causes smooth muscle contraction and prolonged vasoconstriction.[4]

FLOWCHART 14-1 **Hemostatic Mechanisms**

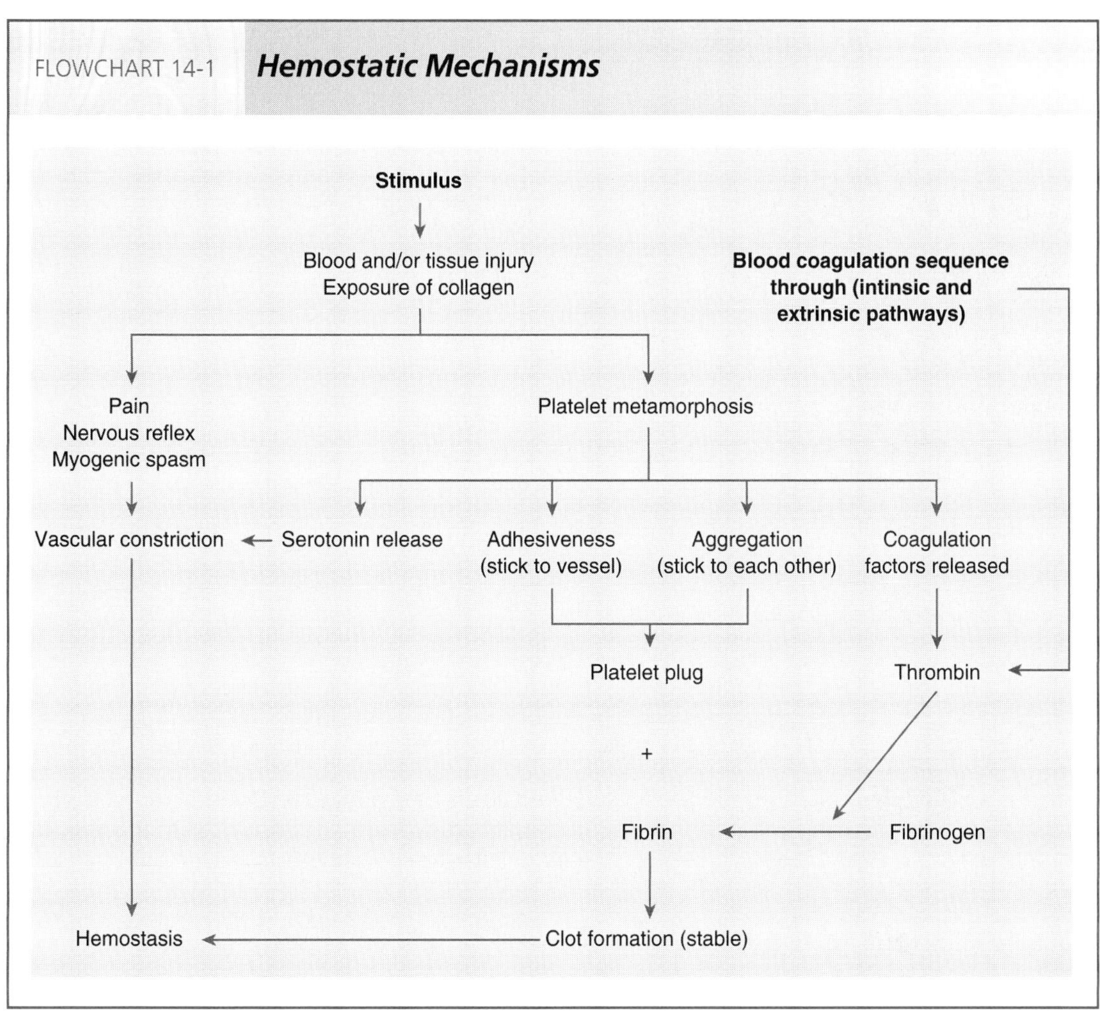

The greater the portion of vessel traumatized, the greater the degree of spasm. A sharply cut vessel, such as one clean cut by a sharp razor blade, undergoes less spasm and thus bleeds longer than a crushed vessel.[10]

PLATELET PLUG FORMATION

The surface of the endothelial cell membrane provides binding sites for adhesive proteins when subendothelial collagen is exposed through injury.[6] Within seconds of blood vessel damage, *primary hemostasis*, or formation of a platelet plug, occurs as platelets aggregate to control blood loss from capillaries, small arterioles, and venules (Fig. 14-3). If the damage is small, the platelet plug can arrest bleeding completely; thus, it closes minute ruptures in vessels that occur hundreds of times per day.[10] When exposed to collagen and other foreign substances (such as antigen-antibody complexes, thrombin, proteolytic enzymes, endotoxins, and viruses), platelets undergo a dynamic change in appearance and begin the process of adhesion and activation. In platelet *adhesion*, the platelets swell, become sticky, and adhere to the collagen fibril on the basement membrane at the site of injury. Platelet adhesion requires **von Willebrand factor (vWF)**, a large plasma protein that binds receptors on the platelet membrane, building a bridge between the activated platelets and the subendothelium.[11]

Platelet activation is stimulated by thrombin, adenosine diphosphate (ADP), thromboxane A2, or epinephrine, triggering further morphologic and biochemical changes in the platelets.[20] The activated platelets release the contents of their granules (also called **degranulation**). The granules contain many substances such as fibrinogen, vWF, factor V (proaccelerin or labile factor), platelet-derived growth factor, heparin-neutralizing protein, and ADP (which is also released from disrupted red blood cells and damaged tissue). Release of ADP attracts other platelets and further aids in platelet adhesion and aggregation, thereby creating a cycle of platelet activation. The effects of ADP are counteracted by two prostaglandin derivatives, TXA2 and **prostacyclin (PGI2)**.[19] TXA2, which produces vaso-

FOCUS ON CELLULAR PATHOPHYSIOLOGY

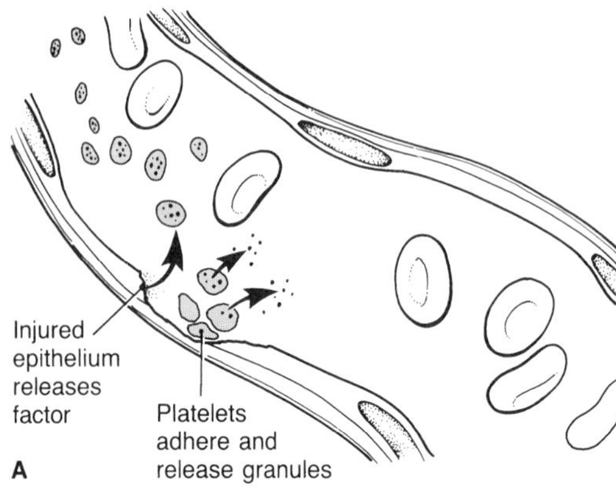

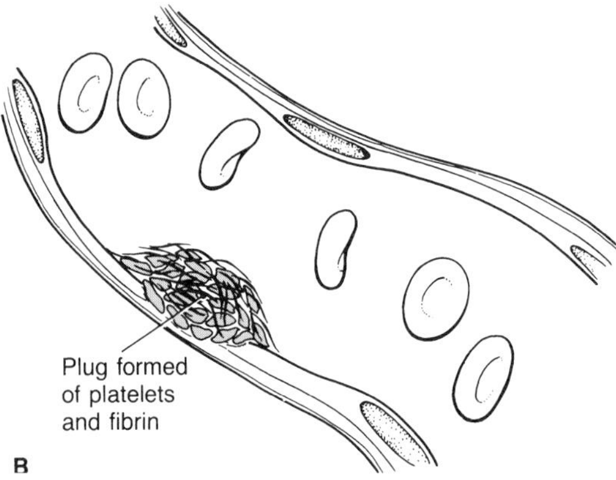

FIGURE 14-3. **A.** Damaged vessel endothelium is a stimulus to circulating platelets, causing platelet adhesion. Platelets release mediators. **B.** Platelet aggregation results.

constriction after initial injury, also promotes platelet degranulation, releasing more ADP. Conversely, prostacyclin inhibits TXA2, causing vasodilatation and inhibiting platelet degranulation. The effect is to promote platelet aggregation at the site of injury but prevent adherence to normal endothelium.[10]

BLOOD COAGULATION

Blood coagulation, or *secondary hemostasis*, is an essential host defense system that prevents blood loss, particularly from larger vessels, in order to maintain the integrity of the closed circulatory system. Secondary hemostasis normally takes several minutes to occur. It consists of the formation of a solid fibrin clot through sequential activation of the plasma proenzymes or clotting factors in the plasma coagulation system through the intrinsic or extrinsic pathways (see below).

The three basic reactions that constitute the sequential process of blood coagulation include: (1) forming prothrombin activator in response to tissue or endothelial damage, (2) catalyzing the conversion of prothrombin to thrombin, and (3) converting soluble fibrinogen to solid fibrin polymer threads.

Blood coagulation occurs through two delineated pathways: the intrinsic pathway and the extrinsic pathway. These pathways converge with the activation of factor X, which causes the conversion of prothrombin to thrombin, at which point the system is called the common pathway for blood coagulation (Flowchart 14-2).

Coagulation Factors

The coagulation (clotting) factors are glycoproteins that are plasma proenzymes (**zymogens**) and belong to a group of proteolytic enzymes called **serine proteases.** Table 14-1 summarizes these factors and indicates the international nomenclature used for each. All of the clotting factors are essential to the normal coagulation sequence. Without the sequential activation, clotting will not occur.

The liver is essential for the synthesis of most of the coagulation factors and for removal of activated coagulation products. Vitamin K is required for the synthesis of factors II, VII, IX, and X in the liver. Vitamin K occurs in two forms; K1 is found in vegetable oils and leafy plants, and K2 is synthesized by bacteria in the colon. K1 and K2 are both fat-soluble and are absorbed

FLOWCHART 14-2 **Pathways of Blood Coagulation**

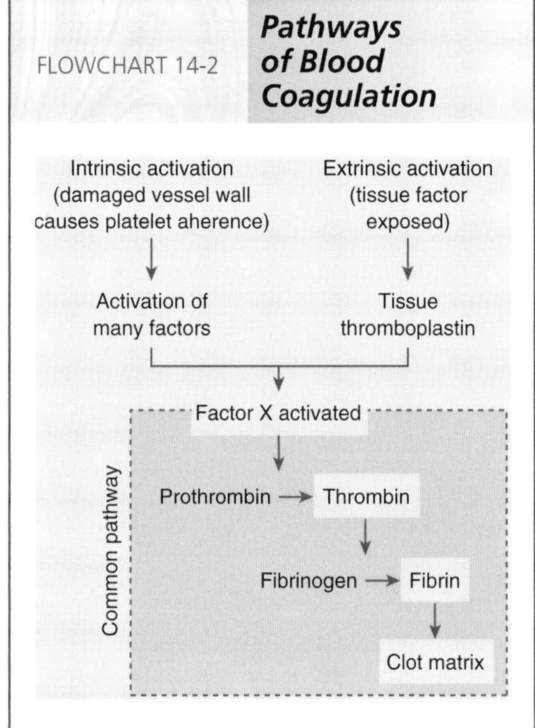

TABLE 14-1

BLOOD COAGULATION FACTORS

FACTOR (INTERNATIONAL NOMENCLATURE)	COMMON SYNONYMS	REMARKS
I	Fibrinogen	Soluble macromolecule, synthesized in liver, fibrin precursor
II	Prothrombin	Synthesized in liver, vitamin K required for formation
III	Tissue thromboplastin; thrombokinase	Phospholipid; involved in activation of extrinsic pathway
IV	Calcium	Involved in several complexes of coagulation process
V	Proaccelerin; labile factor; Ac-globulin; Ac-G	Synthesized in liver; modifier protein, not enzyme; required in prothrombin activator complex
(VI)	Obsolete term	Same as factor V
VII	Proconvertin; stable factor; serum prothrombin conversion accelerator	Part of enzyme complex in extrinsic pathway; synthesized in the liver; vitamin K required for formation
VIII	Antihemophilic globulin (AHG); antihemophilic factor (AHF); antihemophilic factor A	Required for intrinsic pathway function; possibly synthesized in liver, spleen, RES, or kidneys
IX	Plasma thromboplastin component (PTC); Christmas factor; antihemophilic factor B	Synthesized in liver; requires vitamin K; needed for intrinsic pathway function
X	Stuart-Prower factor; Stuart factor	Synthesized in the liver; requires vitamin K, needed for both intrinsic and extrinsic pathways
XI	Plasma thromboplastin antecedent (PTA); antihemophilic factor C	Substrate in intrinsic activator enzymatic complex; needed for intrinsic system activation, area of synthesis unknown
XII	Hageman factor; contact factor; antihemophilic factor D	Involved in first step of activation of intrinsic system; area of synthesis unknown
XIII	Fibrin stabilizing factor (FSF); fibrinase	Causes amide cross-linkage fibrin; stabilizes clot formation, synthesized by platelets and possibly other proteins, may be activated by liver

only in the presence of bile salts. Vitamin K catalyzes the last of several steps leading to the production of many coagulation factors.

The clotting factors are effective only when present on membrane surfaces with protein co-factors, such as factor VII and V. Calcium ions play a critical role in coagulation, as most of the reactions in the coagulation cascade are calcium dependent or require calcium in order for the proteins to interact with the cell membrane surface.

When activated, proteolytic enzymes cause a series of successive reactions in a cascading sequence. The sequentially derived product of one reaction supplies the protease essential for the next reaction.

Fibrinogen (factor I), prothrombin (factor II), and factors XII, IX, and X are essential procoagulation factors. Fibrinogen is synthesized in the liver at a rate that usually corresponds to the rate of use or need. Vitamin K–dependent factors, II, VII, XII, IX, and X, and proteins C and S are also synthesized exclusively by the liver.

Intrinsic Pathway

The intrinsic pathway of coagulation is activated through components already present in the blood. The mechanism for initiating clotting begins within the vessel (it usually requires several minutes).[20] When the blood comes into contact with collagen or damaged endothelium, an intrinsic activator-enzyme complex is formed. The Hageman factor (activated factor XII), a proteolytic enzyme, activates the conversion of factor XII to factor XIIa in the presence of calcium. Factor XIIa converts XI to XIa. Factor XIa then activates the conversion of factor IX to IXa. Factor IXa and factor VIIIa, on membrane surfaces, form *factor Xa activation complex*, which consists of activated factor IX, factor VIII, calcium (factor IV), and phospholipids. Activated factor X then combines with factor V, calcium, and phospholipids to form prothrombin activator or **prothrombinase**. Within seconds, prothrombin activator initiates the proteolytic cleavage of two prothrombin peptide bonds to form thrombin. The amount of thrombin formed is closely related to the amount of prothrombin activator present. Once thrombin is formed, the final clotting pathway is set in motion, and fibrinogen is converted to fibrin by cleavage of two peptide bonds (Flowchart 14-3).

Extrinsic Pathway

Whereas the intrinsic pathway plays an important role in the growth and eventual maintenance of the fibrin clot, the extrinsic pathway is critical in the initiation of fibrin development. The extrinsic pathway for co-

FLOWCHART 14-3 **Blood Coagulation Sequence**

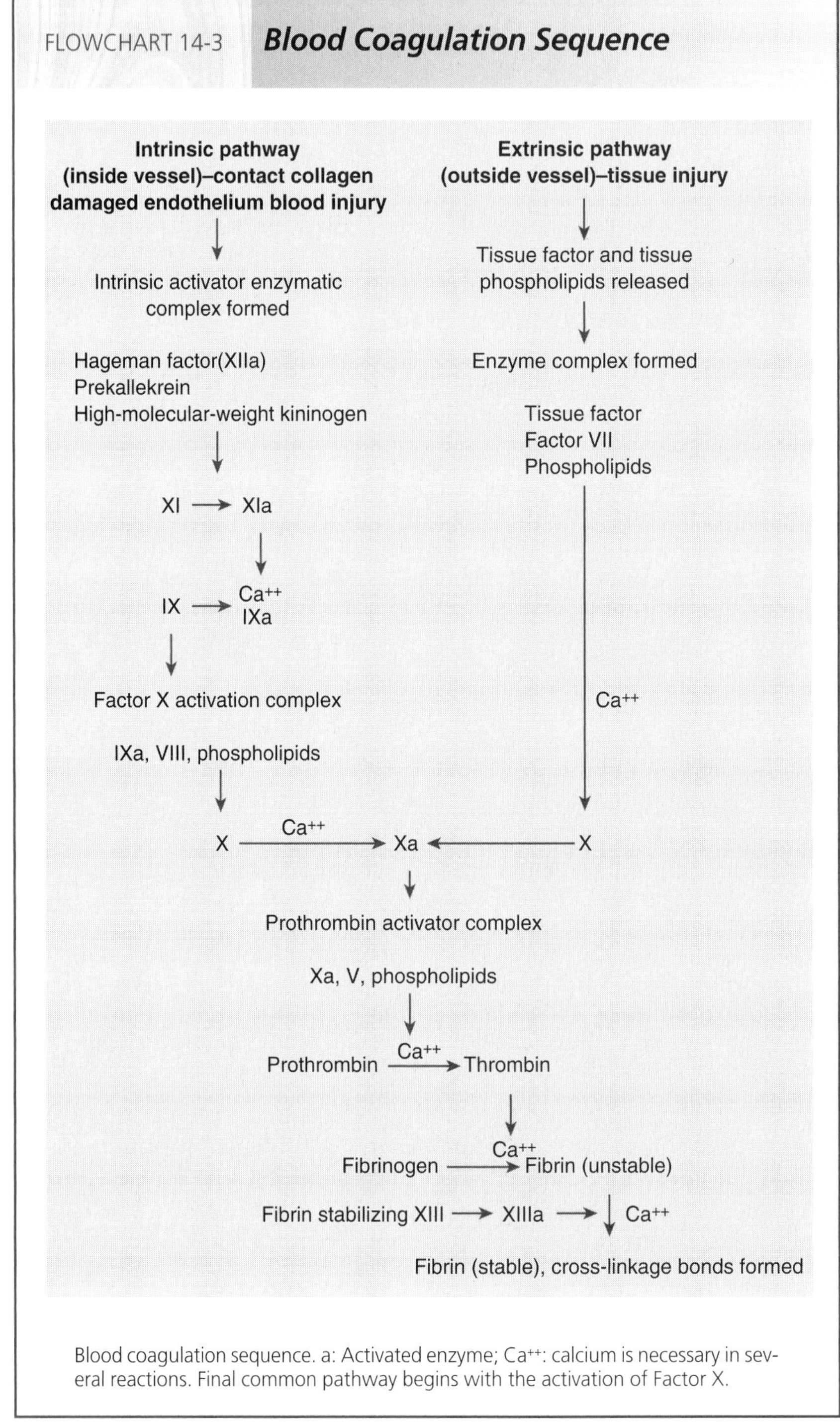

Blood coagulation sequence. a: Activated enzyme; Ca^{++}: calcium is necessary in several reactions. Final common pathway begins with the activation of Factor X.

agulation is triggered by factors not normally present in the blood but found in the tissues. Specifically, the extrinsic pathway requires **tissue factor** and factor VII. Because there are fewer steps in the extrinsic pathway than in the intrinsic, it occurs rapidly, often within seconds.[20] When blood comes in contact with a traumatized vascular wall or extravascular tissue, tissue factor, a proteolytic enzyme, and phospholipids from the cell membrane are released. Tissue factor initiates the extrinsic pathway as a cofactor in a complex composed of factor VII, calcium, and phospholipids. This complex activates the conversion of factor VII to factor VIIa (**tissue thromboplastin**), catalyzed by factor X. Factor X forms factor Xa to become part of the prothrombin activator complex, which then converts prothrombin to thrombin. Thrombin, in turn, converts fibrinogen to fibrin and a clot is formed. Thrombin accelerates the fibrin clot formation process by its ability to activate factors V and VIII. (see Flowchart 14-3).

Final Common Pathway

The intrinsic and extrinsic pathways merge into the common pathway with the activation of factor X and formation of the prothrombin activator complex (see Flowchart 14-3). The main event of the final common pathway is the conversion of prothrombin to thrombin, which in turn enzymatically converts fibrinogen to fibrin, forming the clot matrix. The rate of the blood coagulation reaction is generally related to the amount of prothrombin activator formed and the degree of activation of factor X. If either is inhibited or stopped because of the absence of a clotting factor, the coagulation process becomes altered and excess bleeding results.

Thrombin plays a central role in hemostasis in general. It acts on fibrinogen, factors V, VIII, XIII, platelet membrane glycoprotein, and proteins C and S. Thrombin also recruits platelets into the hemostatic plug, thereby controlling the rate of plug formation. It acts more slowly on the intrinsic, or platelet-altered side, than on the extrinsic, or tissue factor–exposed, side.[4]

FIBRIN CLOT FORMATION AND CLOT COMPOSITION

Clot formation occurs when fibrinogen is converted by the action of thrombin to fibrin. Fibrin is the structural protein that forms into the fibrin polymer. The blood clot is composed of a meshwork of polymerized fibrin threads that have become attached to blood cells, platelets, and plasma products. The fibrin threads adhere to the damaged vessel surface, holding the clot in place and preventing blood loss. The meshwork is produced by spontaneous aggregation of fibrin monomer to form polymer threads. Fibrin-stabilizing factor (XIII), which is released from platelets entrapped in the clot and is activated by thrombin, acts on the fibrin to form covalent cross-links that stabilize the clot and make it resistant to dissolution.[10,20]

Blood coagulation occurs faster with severe trauma to the vascular wall than with minor trauma. The sequence of physical events takes place in a comparatively short time. After a vessel is severed, platelets aggregate, and the fibrin polymer develops into a clot in as little as 15 seconds and up to 6 minutes. The fibrin clot mechanically blocks blood flow and prevents blood loss. Clot retraction follows and may take 30 to 60 minutes.

Clot Retraction

Clot retraction is a platelet-dependent process that begins a few minutes after the clot has formed. Platelets entrapped in the clot continue to release fibrin-stabilizing factor, causing the fibrin threads to shorten and create a stronger, denser bond. Clot retraction pulls the edges of the broken vessel closer together, which allows the vascular wall to mend. Fibrin-thread contraction causes plasma and clotting factors to be expressed from the clot. Failure of a clot to retract often indicates a decreased number of platelets.[11]

Fibrinolysis

Fibrinolysis, or lysis of blood clots, is the final event of hemostasis. It is a mechanism for limiting clot formation and facilitating endothelial cell regrowth and vessel recanalization.

Fibrinolysis is mediated by plasmin (Flowchart 14-4). Plasmin is formed from inactive circulating plasminogen by the action of several plasminogen activators. During the initial phase of hemostatic platelet plug formation, the platelets and endothelial cells release tissue plasminogen activators, which convert plasminogen to plasmin. There are several naturally occurring plasminogen activators, including tissue-type plasminogen activator (t-PA) and urokinase-type plasminogen activator (u-PA). T-PA type is fibrin selective, and its catalytic activity is enhanced several hundred-fold when it binds to fibrin. U-PA is less fibrin selective than t-PA.[16] The plasminogen activators are stimulated by thrombin to convert plasminogen to plasmin. After plasmin is formed, it degrades fibrin into **fibrin degradation products** (FDPs). FDPs have anti-thrombotic capabilities and block fibrin-binding sites and platelet surface glycoprotein binding sites, thereby dissolving the clot.

Macrophages can also activate t-PA and u-PA and facilitate degradation of the fibrin clot from the endothelial and platelet surfaces, providing another pathway for fibrin degradation. Macrophage-mediated fibrinolysis may occur during the recanalization of the vessel.[16]

To maintain a balance between coagulation and fibrinolysis, plasminogen activation and plasmin activity are regulated by two inhibitors: **alpha-2 antiplasmin** and **plasminogen activator inhibitor-1**, which bind the active enzymes and prevent excessive

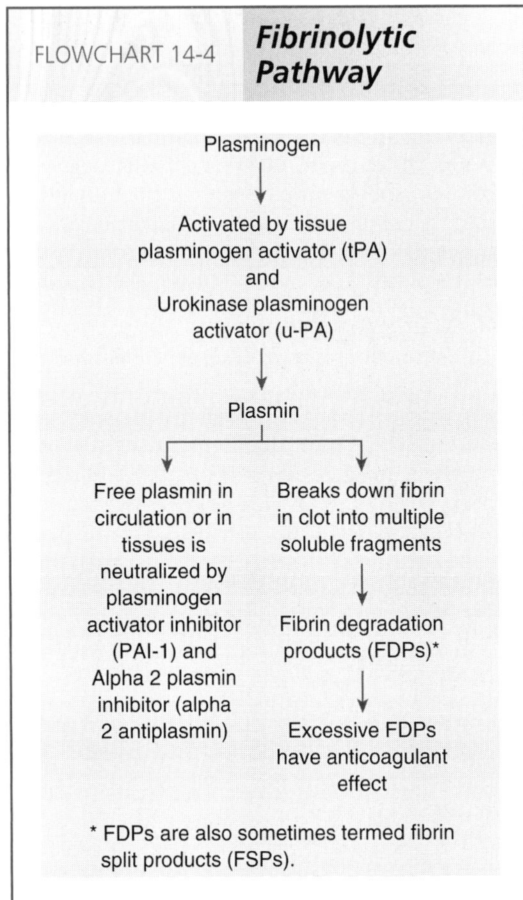

tion. A small amount of free thrombin is released from the surface of the clot into the circulation when the clot is dissolved. Free thrombin is neutralized by antithrombin III, preventing coagulation from occurring in the bloodstream. Thrombotic tendencies develop when plasminogen is deficient or defective. Hemorrhagic disorders result when alpha-2 antiplasmin or plasminogen activator inhibitor-1 is defective.

FLOWCHART 14-4 Fibrinolytic Pathway
Plasminogen
Activated by tissue plasminogen activator (tPA) and Urokinase plasminogen activator (u-PA)
Plasmin
Free plasmin in circulation or in tissues is neutralized by plasminogen activator inhibitor (PAI-1) and Alpha 2 plasmin inhibitor (alpha 2 antiplasmin)
Breaks down fibrin in clot into multiple soluble fragments
Fibrin degradation products (FDPs)*
Excessive FDPs have anticoagulant effect
* FDPs are also sometimes termed fibrin split products (FSPs).

Natural Anticoagulants

Natural **anticoagulants** produced in the coagulation and fibrinolytic systems retard the coagulation process and prevent excessive clot formation.[8] **Protein C** and **protein S** are vitamin K–dependent, proteolytic plasma proteins that have an anticoagulant function. Protein C inactivates factors V and VIII and enhances fibrinolysis at the endothelium-plasma interphase. Protein S serves as a cofactor in the inactivation of factors V and VIII. Other circulating anticoagulants include C-1 inhibitor, which neutralizes factor XIIa, and tissue factor pathway inhibitor, which blocks factor VIIa/TF. **Antithrombin III (ATIII)** is a plasma protein that inhibits several serine proteases in the coagulation cascade. ATIII blocks factors IXa, Xa, and thrombin. Most thrombin (85% to 90%) is absorbed into the fibrin strands. As a control mechanism, the remaining thrombin combines with ATIII, blocking the effect of thrombin on fibrinogen and inactivating thrombin. **Heparin cofactor II (HCFII)** is an enzyme inhibitor that resembles ATIII.

Intrinsic heparin is produced and secreted by circulating basophils and tissue mast cells. Heparin stops the coagulation cascade by inhibiting factors IX and X and thrombin, acting in both the intrinsic and extrinsic pathways. Intrinsic heparin greatly accelerates the effects of ATIII.

DISORDERS OF HEMOSTASIS

Disorders of platelet function and platelet plug formation and deficiencies of any of the clotting factors produce patterns of coagulation disruptions with varying clinical manifestations. The impairments may result from genetic deficiencies, defects in the clotting factors, or suppression of clotting components.

Laboratory tests that are helpful in diagnosing disorders of hemostasis are summarized in Appendix C. These tests are effective in confirming the presence of a clinical bleeding problem, the pathway involved, and often, the components that are defective.[21]

The Hemophilias

Low levels, or lack, of even one of the coagulation factors can lead to abnormal bleeding problems. The term *hemophilia* loosely defines several different hereditary coagulation deficiencies of the intrinsic pathway. The types of hemophilia include deficiencies of any of the following:

- Factor VIII (lack of vWF), causing von Willebrand disease
- Factor VIII from a different mode of inheritance than von Willebrand (hemophilia A)
- Factor IX (hemophilia B or Christmas disease)
- Factor XI (hemophilia C or Rosenthal's disease)

More than 90% of the hemophilias are caused by deficiencies of factors VIII, IX, and X.[7]

VON WILLEBRAND DISEASE

Von Willebrand disease is the most common hereditary bleeding disorder, usually resulting from an inherited autosomal dominant trait. Approximately 20 variants of the disease have been identified, with the most common being Type 1, which results in a reduced quantity of circulating vWF. Von Willebrand disease has been shown to be associated with autoimmune and lymphoproliferative conditions, such as systemic lupus erythematosus (SLE) and Bernard-Soulier syndrome (an autosomal recessive disorder in which a platelet glycoprotein is absent or dysfunctional and unable to bind with von Willebrand factor).[5,13]

Von Willebrand disease is characterized by a qualitative platelet abnormality caused by deficiency of vWF, which in turn gives rise to a secondary decrease in levels of factor VIII.[6,8] Because of this deficiency, both the adhesion of platelets to the injury-exposed endothelial collagen and coagulation are impaired.

Von Willebrand disease produces a prolonged bleeding time with mild to moderate bleeding disorder.[11] Epistaxis, gastrointestinal bleeding, and menorrhagia are common manifestations.

HEMOPHILIA A

Hemophilia A (factor VIII deficiency) is the most common type, accounting for 85% of all cases and occurring at a rate of 1 in 10,000 births.[8,12] This disease is genetically transmitted through a sex-linked recessive gene that is located on the X chromosome and therefore affects males almost exclusively. Females are usually asymptomatic carriers, but in rare cases may manifest the disease. There is a high mutation rate for this disease, such that one-third of these hemophiliacs will have no family member with the disease.[8,12]

In this condition factor VIII is produced, but it has a molecular defect and does not promote coagulation. Several genetic deletions, nonsense mutations, and splicing errors have been documented. The majority of severely affected persons have DNA mutations that prevent any synthesis of factor VIII.[8]

Hemophilia A is considered to be the classic hemophilic disorder and is characterized by spontaneous or traumatic subcutaneous and intramuscular hemorrhages. The severity of the hemorrhage depends on the coagulation factor levels. In mild hemophilia, factor VIII levels are borderline at 0.05 U/mL (normal range is 0.5 to 2.0 U/mL). Generally, this level of deficiency causes problems only with post-traumatic or post-surgical bleeding. Factor VIII levels below 0.02 U/mL result in spontaneous bleeding episodes. Hematuria and bleeding from the mouth, gums, lips, and tongue are common. The joint hemarthralgias cause extreme pain and deformity of the joint over time.[11]

HEMOPHILIA B

Hemophilia B, also called Christmas disease, is a factor IX deficiency. It is an X-linked autosomal recessive defect that accounts for 10% to 15% of all cases of hemophilia. The defect results from point mutations or deletions within the gene causing either the inability to form or to activate factor IX. Clinically it is indistinguishable from hemophilia A, but plasma assays show a decreased level of factor IX. Bleeding tends to be less severe than in hemophilia A, although the disease can occur with varying degrees of severity.

HEMOPHILIA C

Hemophilia C, or Rosenthal's disease, is a deficiency of factor XI. It is transmitted as an autosomal recessive trait and accounts for 2% of all hemophilia cases. It is a mild bleeding disorder manifested by bruising, epistaxis, and menorrhagia.

Antibody-Mediated Alterations in Coagulation

Some coagulation abnormalities result from the presence of antibodies against coagulation factors. These abnormalities may disrupt coagulation as a consequence of other disease states.

IMMUNE THROMBOCYTOPENIA PURPURA (ITP)

Immune thrombocytopenia purpura (ITP), previously called idiopathic thrombocytopenia purpura, is the most common autoimmune disorder of platelet consumption. The two types of ITP are acute and chronic. Acute ITP occurs exclusively in children and is often preceded by an acute viral infection. Chronic ITP occurs in adults; unlike acute ITP in children, there is often no identifiable secondary disease or preceding illness.

In all forms of ITP, antiplatelet antibodies bind to normal platelet membrane, resulting in phagocytosis by the splenic macrophages.[5] Platelet survival is impaired and the platelet count becomes markedly decreased.[6,14]

In acute ITP, bruises are found on the legs and hemorrhagic bullae on the gums and lips. Epistaxis is common. Spontaneous recovery is seen in 80% of children within 6 months, and normal platelet levels usually return 9 to 12 months after the onset of illness.[5] Chronic ITP, in contrast, becomes a life-long condition. Other diseases may be associated with ITP, including conditions such as sarcoidosis, SLE, thyrotoxicosis, carcinomatosis, tuberculosis, lymphoproliferative disorders, and drug hypersensitivity.[11]

LUPUS ANTICOAGULANT

Lupus anticoagulant is an antibody (IGG or IGM) against a phospholipid glycoprotein complex that causes hypercoagulability through platelet activation. The antibody was called "lupus anticoagulant" because it was often found in persons having SLE. The term is now recognized to be a misnomer because lupus anticoagulant occurs more frequently in persons without SLE than those with SLE. Lupus anticoagulant often is associated with thrombosis, fetal loss, and thrombocytopenia with or without autoimmune disease.[5,14] Clotting factor deficiencies often are associated, but lupus anticoagulant is generally associated with thrombosis rather than with abnormal bleeding. Clinical manifestations may be absent, and the presence of lupus anticoagulant frequently is discovered incidentally. The procoagulant state is often indicated by venous and arterial thromboses, which may be associated with cerebral and ocular ischemia or spontaneous miscarriages.[8]

CIRCULATING ANTIBODIES TO COAGULATION FACTORS

Circulating antibodies to coagulation factors are usually specific inhibitors, which means that they inhibit only a single factor. The development of antibodies to coagulation factors results in an increased risk of hemorrhage. This phenomenon has been observed in many disease states. For example, 5% to 20% of persons treated for hemophilia A develop an antibody to factor VIII. The bleeding tendencies from the factor VIII antibody are identical to those of hemophilia A disease and may account for reports of hemophilia in females.

Circulating antibody anticoagulants have also been documented as a cause of bleeding in other conditions, including multiple myeloma and other **paraproteinemias,** SLE, hemophilia B, inhibition of the thrombin-fibrinogen reaction, Down syndrome, and after massive blood transfusions. The clinical and laboratory presentation resembles that of an inherited factor deficiency.

Acquired Alterations in Coagulation

A large group of coagulation disorders is secondary to other medical conditions and involve factors necessary in the production of the coagulation factors. Vitamin K deficiency, liver disease, and massive transfusion syndrome are among those most frequently seen.

VITAMIN K DEFICIENCY

Deficiency of vitamin K may result from several conditions. A newborn infant normally is deficient in vitamin K due to an immature liver and lack of intestinal bacteria that are needed to synthesize vitamin K. Newborn infants are often given injections of vitamin K to prevent any bleeding. Obstructive liver disease and malabsorption disorders can also cause a vitamin K deficiency. Obstructive liver disease blocks the flow of bile necessary for the absorption of fat and fat-soluble vitamin K. Inadequate dietary intake of vitamin K also may result in deficiency. Vitamin K deficiency may be induced by coumarin-derivative anticoagulants given therapeutically. Coumadin (warfarin) competes for vitamin K receptors and therefore blocks binding of vitamin K.

The major consequence of vitamin K deficiency is the development of a bleeding diathesis due to a deficiency of clotting factors VII, IX, X, and prothrombin. This condition is characterized by development of hematomas, hematuria, **melena, ecchymoses**, and bleeding from the gums.[8]

LIVER DISEASE

Liver disease can lead to **coagulopathy** and platelet dysfunction with **thrombocytopenia**, if hypersplenism or bone marrow suppression is present. Alterations in liver function, caused by conditions such as hepatitis, disseminated intravascular coagulation (DIC), shock, acute poisoning, acute alcohol-induced liver dysfunction, and hepatic failure, can cause bleeding due to lack of coagulation factors. Reduced coagulation factor synthesis, failure to remove activated products, impaired clearance of fibrolytic enzymes, and accompanying DIC all may contribute to the bleeding problems.

MASSIVE TRANSFUSION SYNDROME

Abnormal bleeding may develop in persons who receive a large volume of transfused blood over a short period of time. This may occur for the following reasons:

- Banked blood is usually deficient in factors V and VIII and platelets. It is also collected into bags that contain citric acid, which prevents clotting.
- Shock, hypothermia, and organ failure often accompany massive transfusion and probably cause more ongoing bleeding than the transfusion products themselves. Shock leads to tissue ischemia and release of cellular products that induce DIC. Liver failure augments bleeding through decreased production of clotting factors and decreased clearance of fibrinogen-fibrin degradation products. Hypothermia (<33°C) is a major cause of bleeding in surgical patients, especially trauma victims, and results in decreased function of coagulation factors and altered endothelial function.

DRUG-INDUCED COAGULATION ABNORMALITIES

Certain drugs—notably the cephalosporin drugs, beta-lactam antibiotics, mithramycin, adriamycin, and bicarbonate and magnesium ions—may produce abnormalities in coagulation.[11,13] The cephalosporins antagonize vitamin K, thus causing bleeding due to lack of prothrombin. Mithramycin and adriamycin activate the fibrinolytic system. When given in high doses, the cephalosporins and the beta-lactams can impair platelet function. Drug-induced coagulation abnormalities may be the cause of altered coagulation or platelet abnormalities in a person who has no other conditions that might cause bleeding.

Deficiencies of Circulating Anticoagulation Proteins

A congenital or acquired absence of specific circulating proteins can cause clotting abnormalities. The more common abnormalities include deficiencies of protein C and protein S, ATIII, and heparin cofactor II.

PROTEIN C AND PROTEIN S DEFICIENCIES

Individuals congenitally deficient in protein C or protein S demonstrate a predisposition to recurrent venous thrombosis (pulmonary embolism and deep vein thrombosis). Autosomal dominant inherited deficiency of protein C was first described in 1981.[13] Deficiencies of protein C and S can be acquired through vitamin K deficiency, liver disease, or with administration of coumarin drugs. Acquired deficiencies have been found with DIC, renal failure, and preeclampsia and in women taking oral contraceptives.

Low plasma levels are associated with an increased risk of thrombotic events, but many affected persons are asymptomatic. Several cases of arterial thrombosis have recently been reported involving myocardial infarction and femoral, renal, radial, and ulnar arterial thromboses in patients with documented protein C or S deficiency.[2,19]

ANTITHROMBIN III DEFICIENCY

Autosomal dominant hereditary deficiency of ATIII is mainly associated with venous thrombosis. ATIII deficiency can be acquired in much the same manner as the protein C and S deficiencies. It has been observed in women taking oral contraceptives; in patients with liver disease, massive obesity, thrombosis, and eclampsia; and in premature infants.[3]

Thrombosis of the legs and pulmonary embolus are common. Coagulation tests are usually normal, although FDPs may be elevated. This disorder is often unrecognized clinically, but thrombotic events increase with age as the result of a combination of ATIII deficiency and other risk factors for thrombotic disease.

HEPARIN COFACTOR II DEFICIENCY

Heparin cofactor II deficiency is inherited as an autosomal dominant trait, but can be acquired in liver disease, DIC, and preeclampsia and by patients on prolonged hemodialysis. It is activated by heparin sulfate and neutralizes thrombin, without affecting factor Xa. It is manifested clinically as deep vein thrombosis, transient ischemic attacks, and stroke.[3]

Disseminated Intravascular Coagulopathy (DIC)

Disseminated intravascular coagulopathy (formerly called disseminated intravascular coagulation) is a common, acquired disorder of coagulation. DIC results from activation of hemostasis by simultaneous disturbances in the coagulation and fibrinolytic systems, causing a cycle of concurrent thrombosis and hemorrhage. It is not a primary entity but rather occurs secondarily to another disorder, such as shock or septicemia. DIC is often a life-threatening medical emergency and the mortality rate is high—50% to 90% depending on the precipitating event.[11] The reported incidence varies greatly, probably reflecting the degree to which the diagnosis is pursued. Known etiologies of DIC include sepsis and infection, malignant neoplasms, complications of obstetric and gynecologic conditions, liver disease, metabolic disturbances, circulatory disorders, brain injury, crush injury, transfusion reactions, congenital defects, immune disorders, and hematologic disease (Box 14-1). Venomous snakebite is the most common cause of DIC worldwide.

PATHOPHYSIOLOGY

The pathophysiology of DIC is complex and not completely understood. The mechanisms of DIC are multiple and interrelated, causing overlap of certain processes and creating a self-perpetuating vicious circle of pathologic processes. The process begins with endothelial damage, release of tissue thromboplastin (TTP), and activation of factor X. Damage to the endothelium, which occurs in endotoxic and other types of septic shock, hypoxia, and low cardiac output states, activates the intrinsic clotting pathway. In septic shock, endotoxins can activate platelets, causing platelet adhesion and formation of tissue thromboplastin in both the intrinsic and extrinsic pathways. TTP is released from endothelial cells as a result of burns, brain injury, MI, surgical injury, cancers, and obstetric accidents (Flowchart 14-5).

Factor X can be activated by these same mechanisms, directly by excessive release of pancreatic and hepatic enzymes, or by venomous snake bites. Activation of factor X causes increased amounts of thrombin to be produced, leading to fibrin formation. Widespread coagulation occurs intravascularly in the small vessels. The ensuing coagulopathy activates the fibrinolytic system. Large amounts of circulating plasminogen are converted to plasmin, and prothrombin is converted to thrombin. Thrombin is deposited intravascularly, causing vessel obstruction. Plasmin degrades fibrin into FDPs, which are anticoagulants and inhibitors of platelet function. Bleeding worsens (Flowchart 14-6). The clotting factors are depleted and hemorrhage occurs, creating a paradoxical condition of thrombosis in the presence of hemorrhage.[11,13] Natural anticoagulants, proteins C and S,

BOX 14-1 CAUSES OF DISSEMINATED INTRAVASCULAR COAGULATION (DIC)

Obstetric Complications and Accidents

Abruptio placentae
Septic abortion
Hydatidiform mole
Puerperal sepsis
Intrauterine fetal death
Eclampsia
Toxemia
Retained dead fetus syndrome
Amniotic fluid embolism
Saline abortion

Infections

Bacterial (gram-negative and -positive septicemia, meningococcemia)
Viral (herpes, rubella, hepatitis, cytomegalovirus, Reye's)
Rickettsial (Rocky Mountain spotted fever)
Protozoal (*Falciparum malariae,* trypanosomiasis)
Mycoses (Histoplasmosis, aspergillosis)

Neoplasms: Solid Tumors

Carcinomas (prostate, pancreas, lung, breast, others)
Metastatic disease

Hematopoietic Disorders

Acute promyelocytic leukemias
Hemolytic transfusion reaction
Sickle cell anemia
Rhabdomyolysis
Anaphylaxis
Deficiency of proteins C or S

Vascular Disorders

Giant hemangiomas
Purpura fulminans
Aneurysms
Coarctation of aorta and other large vessels
Takayasu's aortitis
Prosthetic arterial grafts
Collagen vascular disease (acute vasculitis, glomerulonephritis, ployarteritis, SLE, amyloidosis)
Congestive heart failure with pulmonary embolus
Hemolytic uremia syndrome
Myocardial infarction
Cardiac arrest
Shock
Hypothermia

Renal Disorders

Renal graft rejection
Nephrotic syndrome
Proliferative glomerulonephritis
Renal allograft rejection

Massive Tissue Damage

Massive traumatic injury (head trauma, gunshot wounds, stab wounds)
Trauma requiring extensive surgical intervention
Extensive burns
Major vessel thrombosis
Extracorporeal circulation
Fat embolism
Heat stroke
Frostbite

Gastrointestinal Disorders

Acute and chronic liver disease
Acute pancreatitis
Liver transplantation
Cirrhosis

Endocrine

Diabetic ketoacidosis
Lactic acidosis
Cushing's syndrome

Other

Snakebite
Drug reactions (any drug, any duration of treatment)
Graft-versus-host disease
ARDS
Status epilepticus

and ATIII are overwhelmed and are not able to regulate the abundance of thrombin.

CLINICAL MANIFESTATIONS

Diagnosis of DIC is made on the basis of clinical presentation and laboratory test results, which are reported in a DIC screen (see Appendix C). Clinical manifestations vary from mild ecchymosis and oozing to severe bleeding from any opening in the skin. Acrocyanosis often occurs in the digits and is manifested as cold, mottled fingers and toes. Hypoxemia may cause dyspnea, cyanosis, and air hunger. Neurologic or renal symptoms may result from microthrombi that occlude the small vessels. The onset of DIC may be acute, as seen in acute obstetric emergencies, or may develop more gradually, as with metastatic cancers.

Altered Fibrinolysis

Thrombotic tendencies develop when plasminogen is deficient or defective (see p. 390). Hemorrhagic disorders result when alpha-2 antiplasmin or plasminogen activator inhibitor-1 (PAI-1) are defective, which is usually a congenital condition. Normally, alpha 2-antiplasmin functions to neutralize any plasmin that escapes the fibrin clot, while PAI-1 complexes with tissue plasminogen activator probably to prevent premature dissolving of the fibrin clot.[9]

Primary fibrinolysis results when massive amounts of plasminogen activator are released into the system.

FLOWCHART 14-5 **The Pathophysiology of Disseminated Intravascular Coagulation (DIC)**

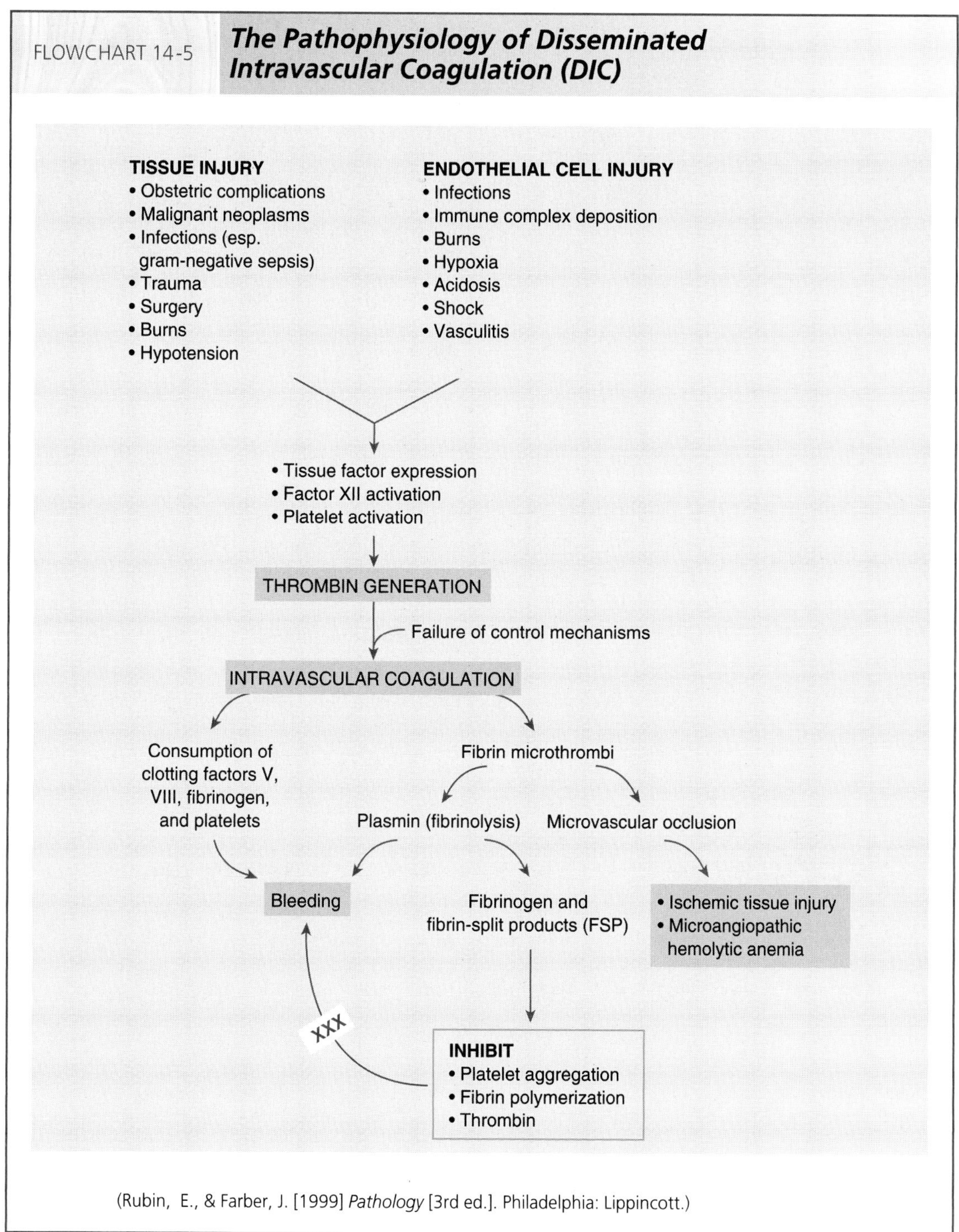

(Rubin, E., & Farber, J. [1999] *Pathology* [3rd ed.]. Philadelphia: Lippincott.)

Plasminogen activators can be released by activator-rich neoplastic tissue such as prostatic carcinoma. Severe anoxia, shock, or surgical procedures may also precipitate release of the plasminogen activators, in which case the condition may actually be secondary to DIC. Primary fibrinolysis reactions and DIC are similar conditions. Both are associated with increased fibrinolytic activity, but through different mechanisms. Primary fibrinolysis results from excessive activation of plasminogen, resulting in a marked increase in bleeding potential at any vulnerable sites, such as the mucous membranes, gastrointestinal system, and intracerebral areas. In DIC, the fibrinolysis occurs as a secondary response to a hypercoagulable state.

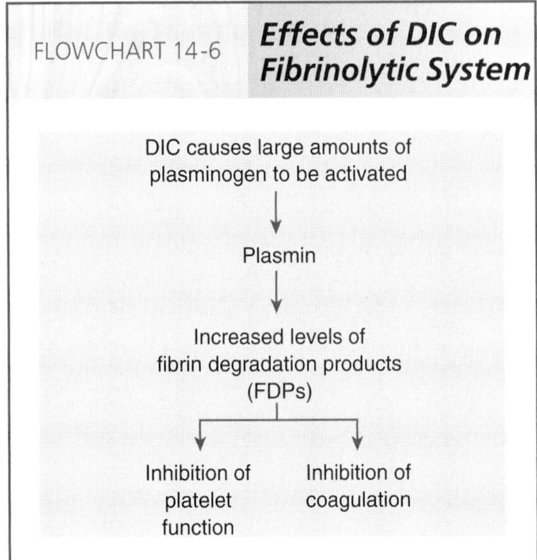

Altered Platelet Quantity and Function

Platelet disorders can include deficiency (thrombocytopenia), excess (thrombocytosis) or functional disorders. They may be acquired or may result from biochemical abnormalities in the blood.

THROMBOCYTOPENIA

Thrombocytopenia is a quantitative platelet disorder defined as a platelet count below 100,000 platelets/mm^3 of blood.[15] Thrombocytopenia may be primary or secondary. Primary immune/idiopathic thrombocytopenia purpura (ITP) is described on page 383. Secondary thrombocytopenia is often associated with drug hypersensitivities, viral infections, and some of the autoimmune conditions. Some drugs that may induce secondary thrombocytopenia are chlorothiazide derivatives, gold thiomalate, diphenylhydantoin, acetaminophen, quinidine, heparin, sulfonamides, chloramphenacol, antimetabolites, and antihistamines.[5] Platelet destruction results from antibodies that target the platelets for destruction. Table 14-2 classifies causes of thrombocytopenia by mechanism.

When the platelet count falls below 50,000, there is an increased potential for hemorrhage associated with trauma such as surgery or accidents. A platelet count between 10,000 to 20,000 is associated with petechiae, ecchymosis, purpura, and bleeding from mucous membranes. When the platelet count is below 5,000, the risk of fatal hemorrhage through the gastrointestinal tract, respiratory system, or central nervous system is great. Failure of a clot to retract often indicates a decreased number of platelets.[10]

Heparin-Induced Thrombocytopenia

Heparin-induced thrombocytopenia (HIT) has been found to occur in approximately 5% of all individuals treated with heparin and may be mild or severe.[22] The etiology of HIT is probably an antibody-mediated reaction directed against heparin and platelet factor 4. The antibodies deplete platelets, but they also activate them and promote thrombosis.[1,8,17]

The thrombi noted in HIT are aggregates of platelets that precipitate in small vessels; thus the condition is often called *white clot syndrome.*[1] Unrecognized HIT can cause the rapid development of arterial, venous, cerebral, coronary, and pulmonary thromboses. Any loss of circulating platelets also increases the risk of minor or major bleeding.

THROMBOCYTOSIS

Thrombocytosis (**thrombocythemia**) is a quantitative abnormality in which there is an increased number of platelets in the peripheral blood. In general, an increased number of platelets is not problematic. Transient thrombocytosis is a normal physiologic response to infection, stress, trauma, exercise, and ovulation. Counts of 400,000 to 1,000,000/mm^3 of blood usually have little or no pathyphysiologic effect, but counts greater than 1,000,000 may result in thrombosis or in bleeding if the excessive numbers of platelets are dysfunctional.[15]

Primary thrombocytosis is a myeloproliferative disorder in which the megakaryocytes in the bone marrow overproliferate. It is associated with chronic nonlymphoblastic leukemia, polycythemia vera, and myelofibrosis. Clinical manifestations include splenomegaly, increased bruisability, and microthromboemboli in the fingers or toes.

ALTERATIONS IN PLATELET FUNCTION

Platelet function disorders include alterations in platelet adherence, which cause prolonged bleeding times despite a normal platelet count. These disorders arise from a variety of platelet function defects and can be inherited, as in von Willebrand disease, or acquired.

The inherited platelet problems are quite rare and include lack of cell membrane glycoprotein, reduced or absent cytoplasmic storage granules, platelet enzyme deficiency, or von Willebrand plasma factor deficiency.[8] These affect platelet adhesion, aggregation, and subsequent secretion, depending on the defect manifested.

Acquired platelet function disorders are more common and are caused by drugs, systemic reactions, and hematologic alterations.[5] Examples of drugs known to affect platelet function include anti-inflammatory agents (especially aspirin), antimicrobials, antidepressants, and adrenergic blocking agents. Systemic disorders include chronic renal disease and autoimmune diseases. Hematologic disorders include chronic myeloproliferative diseases, leukemias, myelodysplastic syndromes, and those of altered protein function.[8]

TABLE 14-2
CLASSIFICATION OF THE THROMBOCYTOPENIAS

TYPE OF DISORDER	ETIOLOGY
DECREASED PRODUCTION	
Hypoproliferation	Toxic agents, especially drug toxicity; radiation, infection; constitutional factors (Fanconi's anemia, etc.); idiopathic aplastic anemia; paroxysmal nocturnal hemoglobinuria; myelophthisis (tumor, fibrosis, etc.)
Infective thrombopoiesis	Megaloblastic anemia; Di Guglielmo's syndrome; familial thrombocytopenia
ABNORMAL DISTRIBUTION	Congestive splenomegaly; myeloid metaplasia, lymphoma
DILUTIONAL LOSS	Massive blood transfusion
DYSFUNCTION	
Drug-induced	Drugs that cause platelet dysfunction include aspirin, nonsteroidal anti-inflammatory drugs, alcohol, antihistamines, tricyclic antidepressants, phenothiazines
Systemic disease	Renal disease; liver disease; myeloproliferative diseases; hereditary protein disorders; leukemia and myelodysplasia, multiple myeloma
ABNORMAL DESTRUCTION	
Consumption	Disseminated intravascular coagulation, vasculitis; thrombotic thrombocytopenia (TTP)
Immune mechanism	Idiopathic thrombocytopenic purpura (ITP); drug-induced thrombocytopenia; chronic lymphocytic leukemia, lymphoma, lupus erythematosus, neonatal thrombocytopenia; posttransfusion purpura
Direct trauma	Cardiopulmonary bypass, hemodialysis, continuous arteriovenous or veno-venous hemofiltration (CAVH, CVVH)

(Adapted from Beck, W. S. [1985]. *Hematology* [4th ed.]. Cambridge, MA: MIT Press, and Barnard, D. L. [1989]. *Clinical hematology*. Oxford: Heinemann Medical.)

Thrombosis

Thrombosis is defined as the presence of blood clot in the vascular circuit (see p. 444). The pathophysiology of thrombosis, first described by Rudolf Virchow, is commonly referred to as Virchow's triad and includes (1) changes in the vessel wall, (2) changes in blood flow, and (3) changes in the coagulability of blood.

VASCULAR INJURY

Thrombosis of the vessels, both arterial and venous, is usually initiated by adherence of the platelets to the injured endothelial lining. Arterial thrombosis is related to direct alterations of the arterial endothelium, whereas venous thrombosis is seen in vessels with poor vessel tone and decreased blood flow. Both arterial and venous thrombosis may be seen in association with endothelial dysfunction caused by elevated plasma **homocysteine**. Arterial thrombosis is often the result of atherosclerotic damage to the vessel wall. The thrombotic process is initiated by chemical mediators that trigger platelet adhesion and aggregation, in much the same manner as in normal hemostasis. Synthesis of TXA2 recruits more platelets into the thrombus.

Venous thrombosis occurs in blood vessel walls that appear histologically normal. It seems that a generalized reduction in vessel tone and low blood flow are important pathophysiologic factors. Hyperhomocystenemia occurs in 5% to 7% of the general population.[23] Homocysteine is an amino acid produced from the catabolism of **methionine**, which is another amino acid. Elevated homocysteine levels can cause endothelial dysfunction by depressing protein C and enhancing the activity of factors XII and V. There is epidemiologic evidence that even mild hyperhomocysteinemia is an independent risk factor for atherosclerosis and atherothrombosis, including premature coronary artery disease, and recurrent arterial thrombi.[23] It has also been implicated in venous thrombosis.[8]

Vitamins B_{12}, B_6, and folate are essential for methionine synthesis. Nutritional deficiencies of the vitamin cofactors may lead to hyperhomocysteinemia. Several disease states—chronic renal failure, hypothyroidism, pernicious anemia, and carcinoma of the breast, ovary, and pancreas—have been associated with elevations of plasma homocysteine.[23]

HYPERCOAGULABILITY STATES

Hypercoagulability can be defined as the risk of venous and arterial thrombosis in circumstances that would not cause thrombotic conditions in a normal individual. There is an inherited tendency towards thrombosis, which has been referred to as **thrombophilia.**[17] Persons with thrombophilia are at life-long risk of thrombosis. Specific hypercoagulable conditions include thrombotic thrombocytopenia purpura (TTP), ATIII deficiency, heparin cofactor II deficiency, protein C and S deficiencies, and several other rare diseases. TTP is discussed in this section; other conditions are discussed elsewhere in this chapter. Deficiencies in anticoagulant proteins ATIII, proteins C and S, and tissue factor pathway inhibitor predispose affected individuals to thromboembolic events. Initial episodes usually occur in early adulthood. The most common manifestations are deep vein thrombosis and pulmonary embolism, but arterial thrombosis also can occur (Box 14-2).

Primary or Inherited Hypercoagulable States

A specific primary or inherited hypercoagulable state is identifiable in over 50% of patients with thrombophilia. Although the prevalence of prothrombotic mutations in the general population is high, most affected individuals do not have any clinically apparent thrombotic complications, which indicates that most episodes of thrombosis are probably precipitated by acquired prothrombotic insults in these patients (Box 14-3). ATIII deficiency is the most common coagulation defect associated with thrombophilia. Resistance to activated proteins C and S, tissue factor pathway inhibitor, and components of the fibrinolytic system are involved less often.

Certain clinical indicators may suggest hypercoagulable states, including a family history of thrombosis, recurrent spontaneous thrombosis, unusual sites of clot formation, thrombosis at a young age, resistance to anticoagulant therapy, recurrent spontaneous abortion, and thrombosis during pregnancy.[12]

BOX 14-2 MANIFESTATIONS OF HYPERCOAGULABLE STATES

- Deep vein thrombosis
- Pulmonary embolus
- Axillary, femoral, subclavian thrombosis
- Superficial phlebitis
- Stroke
- Myocardial infarction
- Warfarin-induced skin necrosis
- Gangrene
- Recurrent fetal loss
- Thrombocytopenia

BOX 14-3 CAUSES OF HYPERCOAGULABLE STATES

Primary or Inherited Disorders

- Protein S deficiency
- Protein C deficiency
- Antithrombin III deficiency
- Heparin cofactor II deficiency
- Resistance to activated protein C
- Hypoplasminogenemia
- Dysplasminogenemia
- Plasminogen activator deficiency
- Decreased tissue plasminogen activator
- Increased plasminogen activator inhibitor
- Increased histidine-rich glycoprotein
- Dysfibrinogenemia
- Factor V deficiency
- Homocysteine deficiency

Secondary or Acquired Disorders

- Increased levels of plasminogen activator inhibitor-1
- Polycythemia vera
- Antiphospholipid antibody syndrome
- Cancer
- Nephrotic syndrome
- Estrogen therapy
- Obesity
- Immobilization
- Sepsis
- Advanced age
- Trauma
- Venous stasis
- Mechanical devices (intra-aortic balloon pump or vascular catheters)

Secondary or Acquired Hypercoagulability States

Secondary or acquired hypercoagulability states are thought to be caused by increased venous stasis, activation of the coagulation system, platelet activation, vascular disorders, prolonged immobilization, obesity, congestive heart failure, and post-surgical stasis (see Box 14-3). The coagulation system is tenuous, and its delicate balance is frequently upset in critically ill patients.

Thrombotic Thrombocytopenia Purpura

Thrombotic thrombocytopenia purpura (TTP) is a rare, often fatal hypercoagulable disorder characterized by severe thrombocytopenia, hemolytic anemia, neurologic deficits, renal failure, and fever. The incidence of TTP is increasing due to its association with HIV infection.

The etiology of TTP is poorly understood, but the prodromal symptoms, which resemble influenza, suggest a viral causation.[8] Endothelial cell damage activates vWF and other procoagulant factors, causing an immune vasculitis. The megakaryocytes multiply and

FOCUS ON THE PERSON WITH A COAGULOPATHY

Ms. I. P., a 35-year-old female, was brought to the emergency ward of a large metropolitan hospital, complaining of excessive bleeding following a therapeutic abortion performed 5 days earlier. She appeared to be in acute distress, with cold, mottled fingers and toes along with severe vaginal bleeding and evidence of nasal and oral bleeding. She was examined and taken to the operating room, where a large segment of retained placenta was removed. Laboratory tests included abnormal coagulation studies, especially partial thromboplastin times (67 seconds for aPTT) and a decreased fibrinogen count (105 mg/dL). An increased titer of fibrin degradation products (35 μg/mL) was found.

Questions

1. What is the coagulopathy described?
2. What risk factors did Ms. P. exhibit?
3. Describe the pathophysiology of the disorder and explain the reasons for the symptoms she experienced.
4. Why was the surgical procedure performed on a critically ill patient? What other treatment measures might be effective?

intimal hyperplasia occurs. **Hyaline** thrombi, composed of dense aggregates of platelets surrounded by fibrin, occlude the arterioles, capillaries, and venules.[5] Platelet adhesion and aggregation leads to obstruction of the vessel and ischemia to the surrounding tissue.

Platelet counts are 2,000 to 10,000/mm^3, with decreased hemoglobin and elevated lactic dehydrogenase (LDH). Other coagulation studies are also abnormal.

Ten percent of patients with TTP will die if not treated within 3 months of onset. Death usually results from renal failure, stroke, or MI.

REFERENCES

1. Aster, R. H. (1995). Heparin-induced thrombocytopenia and thrombosis. *New England Journal of Medicine, 332*, 1374.
2. Beattie, S., Norton, M. & Doll, D. (1997). Coronary thrombosis associated with inherited protein S deficiency: A case report. *Heart & Lung, 26*(1), 118.
3. Bennett, J. S. (1997). Thrombotic disorders. In W. N. Kelley (Ed.), *Textbook of internal medicine* (3rd ed.). Philadelphia: Lippincott-Raven.
4. Berne, R. M. & Levy, M. N. (1998). *Physiology* (4th ed.). St. Louis: Mosby.
5. Bonner, H., Bogg, H. & Cossman, J. (1999). The blood and the lymphoid organs. In E. Rubin & J. L. Farber, *Pathology* (3rd ed.). Philadelphia: Lippincott.
6. Chandrasoma, P. & Taylor, C. R. (1998). *Concise pathology* (3rd ed.). Stamford, CT: Appleton & Lange.
7. Colman, R., Hirsh, J., Marder, V., & Salzman, E. (1994). *Hemostasis and thrombosis: Basic priniciples and practice* (3rd ed.). Philadelphia: J. B. Lippincott.
8. Cotran, R. S., Kumar, V., & Collins, T. (1999). *Robbins' pathologic basis of disease* (6th ed.). Philadelphia: W.B. Saunders.
9. George, J. N. (1998). Hemostasis and fibrinolysis. In J. H. Stein (Ed.), *Internal medicine* (5th ed.). St. Louis: Mosby.
10. Guyton, A. C. & Hall, J. E. (1996). *Textbook of medical physiology* (9th ed.). Philadelphia: W. B. Saunders.
11. Jandl, J. H. (1996). *Blood: Textbook of hematology* (2nd ed.). Boston: Little, Brown.
12. Jorde, L. B., Carey, J. C., & White, R. L. (1995). *Medical genetics.* St. Louis: Mosby.
13. Lee, G. R., Bithell, T. C., Foerster, J., Athens, J. W., & Lukens, J. N. (1993). *Wintrobe's clinical hematology* (9th ed.). Philadelphia: Lea & Febiger
14. Male, D. (1998). Hypersensitivity—Type II. In I. Roitt, J. Brostoff, & D. Male, *Immunology* (5th ed.). St. Louis: Mosby.
15. Pagana, K. D. & Pagana, T. J. (1998). *Mosby's diagnostic and laboratory text reference* (3rd ed.). St. Louis: Mosby.
16. Sasahara, A., & Loscalzo, J. (1997). *New therapeutic agents in thrombosis and thrombolysis.* New York: Marcel Dekker.
17. Schafer, A. (1994). Hypercoagulable states: Molecular genetics to clinical practice. *Lancet, 344*(12), 1739.
18. Schafer, A. (1998). Thrombocytopenia and disorders of platelet function. In J. Stein (Ed.), *Internal medicine* (5th ed.). St. Louis: Mosby.
19. Svensson, P. & Dahlback, B. (1994). Resistance to activated protein C as a basis for venous thrombosis. *New England Journal of Medicine, 330*(8), 517.
20. Tortora, G. J. & Grabowski, S. R. (1997). *Principles of anatomy and physiology* (8th ed.). New York: Harper-Collins.
21. Treseler, K. M. (1995). *Clinical laboratory and diagnostic tests* (3rd ed.). Stamford, CT: Appleton & Lange.
22. Warkentin, T. E., & Kelton, J. G. (1996). A 14-year study of heparin-induced thrombocytopenia. *American Journal of Medicine, 101*, 502.
23. Welch, G. & Loscalzo, J. (1998). Homocysteine and atherothrombosis. *New England Journal of Medicine, 338*(15), 1035.

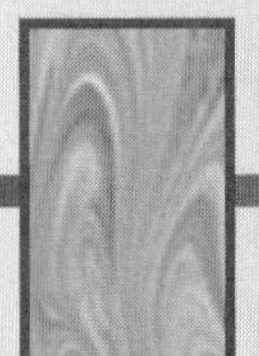

UNIT 3: CASE STUDY

Hematology

Introduction to the Patient

J. G., a 32-year-old Mexican-American male, presented to a local emergency department with substernal chest pain, diaphoresis, shortness of breath, nausea, and right leg pain. An electrocardiogram revealed an acute MI. The patient underwent coronary artery bypass surgery and right femoral-popliteal bypass graft placement after angiographic documentation of coronary and right femoral artery obstructions. Intravenous heparin therapy, followed by oral warfarin anticoagulation therapy, was started prior to discharge.

Social History

The psychosocial history revealed that the patient did not smoke cigarettes or drink alcohol on a regular basis. He worked at a construction site and was the sole support for a wife and three children under the ages of 6.

Past Medical History

The patient's past medical history was significant for two episodes of deep vein thrombosis between the ages of 18 and 23. At age 28, he developed left radial and ulnar artery occlusions, treated with heparin. He was followed for 2 years while taking warfarin sodium (Coumadin) but subsequently was lost to follow-up until this admission.

Family History

There was a family history of early heart disease in an uncle who succumbed to an MI at age 41. The family history also included hyperlipidemia but no hypertension, stroke, or diabetes mellitus. His younger sister had suffered a deep vein thrombosis while pregnant.

Physical Examination

Mr. G. was in obvious distress. He was 5 ft. 10 in. tall and weighed 167 lb. He was alert and oriented but very anxious. Blood pressure on admission was 155/88, and pulse was 132. No pulmonary rales were present, and heart sounds indicated no gallop rhythms. He was complaining of substernal chest pain, radiating to the left arm and jaw. The right foot was pale and mottled in appearance; no pulses were found by palpation or Doppler examination.

Diagnostic Tests

Routine cardiac workup indicated elevated CPK-MB enzymes (865 IU/L) and an acute anterior myocardial infarction by 12-lead electrocardiogram. Blood gases indicated hypoxemia and respiratory alkalosis.

Angiography of the right leg demonstrated a right calf embolus. Subsequent cardiac catheterization revealed an occluded left anterior descending coronary artery but no evidence of coronary artery atherosclerosis.

The complete blood count and platelet counts were normal on two separate occasions. Protein S, antithrombin III, and plasminogen levels were within normal levels. The PTT taken before heparin therapy was initiated was within normal limits. The patient's protein C level while on Coumadin was markedly reduced at 31% (the normal range is 48% to 152%). A sample taken from the patient's mother was 50% functionally and 55% immunologically, confirming the suspected diagnosis of inherited protein C deficiency.

CRITICAL THINKING QUESTIONS

1. Which risk factors suggest an inherited anticoagulant deficiency?
2. Which screening tests should be performed in young persons with recurrent thrombosis? Discuss the implications of the diagnostic tests performed.
3. Describe the importance of patient compliance and medical follow-up as it relates to the outcome of this case.
4. Discuss the pathophysiology evident in the case presented.
5. Considering the multiple factors leading to the patient's diagnosis, construct a plan of care for acute management and then consider the long-term teaching and care of this patient.

Besides your pathophysiology text you will need a good pharmacology textbook, a medical hematology textbook, a pathology text, and current research articles to complete this case study. Suggested references follow:

Karch, A. (2000). *Focus on nursing pharmacology*. Philadelphia: Lippincott Williams & Wilkins.

Jandl, J. H. (1996). *Blood: Textbook of hematology* (2nd ed.). Boston: Little, Brown.

Rubin, E. & Farber, J. L. (1999). *Pathology* (3rd ed.). Philadelphia: Lippincott-Raven.

UNIT 3 APPENDIX A

LABORATORY TESTS OF RED BLOOD CELL FUNCTION

TEST	NORMAL VALUES	CLINICAL IMPLICATIONS OF ABNORMAL VALUES
Hemoglobin (HgB)	• Infant, first day: 14–20 g/dL • Child l yr: 10–14 g/dL • Child 6–10 yr: 11–15 g/dL • Adult female: 12–16 g/dL • Adult male: 13.5–17.5 g/dL • Adult > 65 yr: 11.7–17 g/dL	Levels decreased with reduced RBC production, blood loss, and hemolysis. Levels may appear decreased when hemoglobin is abnormal (e.g., sickle cell anemia). The hemoglobin level is usually approximately one third of the hematocrit; variations in this relationship may indicate intervening variables affecting the accuracy of one test or the other.
Hematocrit (H)	• Infant, first day: 50–62% • Child 1 yr: 32–40% • Child 6–10 yr: 33–43% • Adult female: 37–47% • Adult male: 40–54% • Adult > 65 yr: 35–50%	Decreased with reduced RBC production, blood loss, and hemolysis. Levels are easily influenced by fluid volume status; hypervolemia leads to lower hematocrit without actual decreased RBCs, and hypovolemia and hemoconcentration reflects a higher hematocrit than actually exists. Immature RBCs (e.g., reticulocytes) that have a large mass will make the hematocrit appear higher.
Erythrocyte count	• Infant, first day:3.3–5.3 mL/mm³ • Child 1 yr: 3.8–4.8 mL/mm³ • Child 6–10 yr: 4.1–5.2 mL/mm³ • Adult female: 3.8–5.1 mL/mm³ • Adult male: 4.3–5.7 mL/mm³ • Adult > 65 yr: 3.8–5.8 mL/mm³	Levels decreased with reduced RBC production, blood loss, and hemolysis. Abnormally shaped RBCs (e.g., sickled cells, schistocytes, helmet cells, target cells) will not be counted in the RBC level.
RBC smear	Normocytic, normochromic cells	Evidence of schistocytes (fragmented RBCs) on RBC smear is a sign of sheared and damaged RBCs, which occurs during the hemolysis process. Other abnormalities occur with liver disease, renal failure, hypertension, and artificial heart valves.
Reticulocyte count	• Female: 0.5–2.5% of RBC count • Male: 0.5–1.5% of RBC count	Increased reticulocyte (immature RBCs) count occurs in response to blood loss. As the RBC mass decreases, the body's compensatory response is to release immature RBCS (called reticulocytes) to replace RBCs until stabilization occurs. Small elevations (2–4%) of reticulocytes occur with recent blood loss, but levels exceeding 4 % of the total RBC mass indicate hemolysis.
Mean corpuscular volume (MCV)	87–103 nm³	This test of the average size of each RBC reflects the maturity level and degree of hemoglobin content. Large immature cells such as reticulocytes increase the MCV; inadequate hemoglobin content causes microcytosis and decreases MCV.
Mean corpuscular hemoglobin (MCH)	26–34 pg/cell	This test of the average amount of to hemoglobin in each RBC reflects the amount of active and functional hemoglobin. Disorders of hemoglobin production (e.g., iron deficiency, sickle cell anemia) cause decreased MCH.
Mean corpuscular hemoglobin concentration (MCHC)	31–37 g/dL	This test of the average saturation of oxygen to hemoglobin in each RBC reflects the amount of functional hemoglobin. The MCHC is reduced when oxygen saturation is inadequate due to abnormal hemoglobin (e.g., sickle

(continued)

UNIT 3 APPENDIX A

LABORATORY TESTS OF RED BLOOD CELL FUNCTION (Continued)

TEST	NORMAL VALUES	CLINICAL IMPLICATIONS OF ABNORMAL VALUES
		cell anemia) or when another gas has replaced oxygen in the hemoglobin molecule (e.g., carbon monoxide poisoning).
Platelets	150,000–400,000 cells/mm^3	Platelet production by bone marrow is reduced when marrow is exposed to radiation, toxic chemicals, and certain medications. Decreased platelets also occur as platelets are trapped in small clots of hemolyzed RBCs and because of excessive sensitivity of the spleen to remove cells. When large foreign bodies are in the bloodstream (e.g., intravenous catheters, heart valves, pacemakers), platelets adhere to the foreign object and cause decreased platelet counts, at least temporarily. Inflammatory processes stimulate platelet aggregation and may cause initial decreases in platelet count, but the body usually compensates by accelerating production.
WBC	5.0–10.0 × 10^6/mm^3	Inflammatory processes result in leukocytosis, occurring secondary to the other bleeding disorder.
BUN	2–20 mg/dL	Increased creatinine and BUN occur when the level of hemolysis is so significant that intravascular heme, globin, iron, and waste products cause toxic damage to the kidneys and induce renal dysfunction.
Creatinine	0.2–1.0 mg/dL	See above.
Bilirubin (Total)	0.2–1.2 mg/dL	When the demands for conjugation of RBC breakdown products exceeds the body's ability to maintain a constant removal, hyperbilirubinemia results. More rapid onset of hemolysis is likely to produce higher levels of bilirubin. The bilirubin level correlates to the degree of jaundice; higher levels produce more jaundice.
Erythrocyte sedimentation rate (ESR)	0–20 mm/h	RBCs usually quickly settle and stack in a straight column within a capillary tube when they are the usual tiny biconcave discs; with inflammation, this process requires more time. The ESR is prolonged with inflammatory disorders such as autoimmune disease; it may be used to monitor response to treatment, although it is not diagnostic of any disorder.
Serum folate	1.5–15 ng/mL	Serum folate reflects the amount of available vitamin building blocks for creation of normal RBCs. Folate is low in folate/folic acid deficiency.
Serum iron level	50–170 mg	Iron stores in the body are usually constant through means of normal intake and recirculation from hemolyzed RBCs, but levels are decreased in iron-deficient anemia, pregnancy, or certain gastrointestinal diseases. Peptic acid of the stomach aids absorption of iron, and iron-deficient anemia can occur when the stomach is diseased or resected.

UNIT 3 APPENDIX A

LABORATORY TESTS OF RED BLOOD CELL FUNCTION (Continued)

TEST	NORMAL VALUES	CLINICAL IMPLICATIONS OF ABNORMAL VALUES
Total iron binding capacity (TIBC)	20–45%	Iron is bound to hemoglobin approximately one third of the time, but may be decreased if iron stores are inadequate. Iron-deficient anemia usually requires low serum iron levels and poor binding capacity.
Ferritin level	100–200 ng/mL	Ferritin is a precursor to iron and is reflective of the body's ability to create new iron stores. Ferritin may be low in iron-deficient anemia related to nutritional deficit, and must be present for the body to accelerate RBC production in times of blood loss.
Transferrin level	200–400 mg/dL	Transferrin is used to bind and recirculate iron from hemolyzed cells. Transferrin may be low when hemolysis has occurred and large amounts of iron are bound to transferrin.
Haptoglobin level	60–270 mg/dL (fasting)	Since haptoglobin normally binds with heme to facilitate removal from the circulation, free levels of serum values decrease when extra-splenic hemolysis is occurring since more heme needs to transport back to the liver prior to removal or recirculation.
Hemoglobin electrophoresis	Normal A and S	The proteins involved in hemoglobin demonstrate a specific pattern when separated, but abnormal hemoglobin S is present with sickle cell anemia.
Schilling test	8–40% excretion in 24 hr.	Measure absorption of vitamin B_{12}. Radioactive B_{12} is administered and amount in a 24 hour urine collection is measured used to diagnose pernicious anemia
Coomb's test (direct/indirect)	Negative	The presence of minor RBC antigens (not usual A or B antigens) can be detected through-this agglutination test. Some minor antigens detected through this means are Kell, E, and cold.
A positive indirect Coombs' indicates the presence of antibody to specific antigen and can identify specific red cell antigens used to identify blood system antibodies.		A positive direct Coombs' indicates that antibody (usually IgG) is present on washed RBCs. Will be positive in immune hemolytic anemias and hemolytic transfusion reactions.

WHITE BLOOD CELL DIFFERENTIAL AND CLINICAL IMPLICATIONS TOTAL WHITE BLOOD CELL (WBC) COUNT: CHILD < 2 YRS: 6,200–17,000/mm³: CHILD > 2 YRS/ADULT: 5,000–10,000/mm³

CELL TYPE	CHILD < 2 YRS % OF WBC	CHILD > 2 YRS/ ADULT % OF WBC	CELL FUNCTIONS	ELEVATED	DECREASED
GRANULOCYTES					
Neutrophils	Segments (mature): 2,400–4000/mm³ 25–35% of total	3,000–7,000/mm³ 50–70% of total	• Recognize, ingest, and kill pyogenic bacteria	• Acute pyogenic infections • Anti-dysrhythmic agents • Cancer • Emotional stress • Exercise • Fever • Hemorrhage • Hemolysis • Inflammation (e.g, gout, arthritis) • Lithium carbonate • Metabolic/chemical poisoning • Pregnancy, delivery • Thyrotoxicosis • Tissue necrosis	• Allopurinol • Amphotericin • Anaphylaxis • Anticonvulsants • Antithyroid drugs • Bactrim • Captopril • Chemotherapy agents • Folic acid deficiency • Hypersplenism • Infection—especially severe or chronic • Increased age • Ionizing radiation exposure • Loop diuretics • Malnutrition • Methyldopa • Nonsteroidal anti-inflammatory drugs (NSAIDs) • Phenothiazines • Psychiatric drugs—haloperidol • Rickettsial infection • Systemic lupus erythematosus (SLE) • Thiazide diuretics • Viral infection
Neutrophil bands	Bands (immature): 800 ± 200/mm³ < 8.5% of total	500 + 100/mm³ < 8% of total	• Same as neutrophils		
Eosinophils	200 ± 50/mm³ 2–4% of total	50–250/mm³ 1–4% of total	• Weakly exhibit phagocytosis and chemotaxis.[23] • Present in large numbers in the intestinal tract and lungs; thought to help to detoxify foreign proteins	• Allergy/asthma • Cancer • Dermatologic conditions (e.g., eczema, psoriasis) • Exercise • Parasitic infection	• Adrenocortical stimulation (e.g., corticosteroid treatment) • Cushing's disease • Severe infection • Stress • Shock

				• Penicillin • Pernicious anemia • Pulmonary disorders • Serum sickness • Worm infestation	
Basophils	50 ± 10/mm³ 0.5–1% of total	40 + 10/mm³ 0.5–1% of total	• Contain histamine, heparin, bradykinin, and serotonin • Present in small numbers in the blood and in larger numbers in the connective tissue and pericapillary areas • Prevent clotting in the microcirculation and cause some of the signs and symptoms of allergic reactions	• Chronic hypersensitivity reactions • Myeloproliferative disorders (chronic leukemia) • Myxedema/hypothyroidism • Ulcerative colitis	Adrenocortical stimulation (e.g., corticosteroid treatment) • Cushing's disease • Severe infection • Stress • Shock
AGRANULOCYTES					
Lymphocytes	7,000 ± 2,000/mm³ 60 + 15%	1,000–4,000/mm³ 20–40% of total	• Antigen presentation to granulocytes and macrophages • Activation of antigen-antibody reactions • Recognition of cell mutations (malignant cells) and presenting them to granulocytes and macrophages • Cytokine production and activation	• Chronic lymphocytic leukemia • Viral illness—mumps, rubella, rubeola, hepatitis, varicella, cytomegalovirus (CMV), mononucleosis (EB virus) • Toxoplasmosis	• Acute tuberculosis • Adrenocortical stimulation (e.g., administration of corticosteroids) • Alkylating agents and antimetabolites • HIV disease • Ionizing radiation exposure • Lymphoid malignancies (e.g., lymphoma, leukemia) • Terminal uremia
Monocytes	700 ± 200 mm³ 3.5–8% of total	100–600/mm³ 2–6% of total	• Most enter tissues and differentiate into macrophages • Phagocytose large particles and inert materials (e.g., wood, metal) • Fuse several macrophages into a giant cell to remove very large particles • Clean debris left after granulocytes perform phagocytosis • Return released iron to transferrin for transportation back to the bone marrow	• Chronic inflammatory conditions • Chronic ulcerative colitis • Nonpyogenic bacterial infections (e.g., tuberculosis, subacute bacterial endocarditis, syphilis, brucellosis) • Viral infection	• Adrenocortical stimulation (e.g., corticosteroid administration) • Administration of immunosuppressive agents • Overwhelming infections • Stress

UNIT 3 APPENDIX C

NORMAL BLOOD COAGULATION VALUES

TEST	NORMAL VALUES	SIGNIFICANCE OF ALTERED VALUES
Clotting or coagulation time	6–17 min (glass tube) 19–60 min (siliconized tube)	Prolonged in deficiency of all clotting factors except VIII and VII; rarely used
Partial Thromboplastin, time (PTT)—activated PTT most commonly done	PTT 60–90 sec. aPTT 30–45 sec.	Screening test used to detect abnormalities of the intrinsic clotting pathway Prolongation indicates deficiencies in either the intrinsic or common pathway
Prothrombin time (PT)	PT 12–15 sec. measured against a control.	Measures the extrinsic and common pathways and reflects vitamin K–dependent factors Prolongation may be secondary to deficiencies of proteins of extrinsic and common pathways
International Normalized Ratio (INR)	Used in anticoagulation therapy. Normal 1.0 Anticoagulation: Thrombosis 2.0 Artificial Valves 3.0–4.0	Method to standardize prothrombin time reporting. It is based on the PT ratio if a standard reference thromboplastin was used. Thromboplastin sensitivity is determined by the manufacturer and is called the International Sensitivity Index (ISI). PT determinations are converted to INR by dividing PT patient by PT reference lab.
Bleeding time	Normal: 2–10 minutes	Gross test of primary hemostasis and platelet function; earlobe or arm surface used, clean superficial wound time to stop bleeding Screens for von Willebrand's disease and platelet disorders
Thrombin time (TT)	24–35 seconds	Measures thrombin-induced conversion of fibrinogen to fibrin Prolonged with hypofibrinogenemia but normal in the hemophilias
Platelet count	150,000–400,000 μL	Electronically counted. Increased levels (thrombocytosis) occur with malignancies, myeloproliferative diseases, polycythemia vera, and others. Thrombocytopenia occurs secondary to decreased production and survival of platelets.
Clot retraction time	Begins in 30 minutes Complete in 12–24 hours	Time for a clot to retract and express serum and degree of retraction; decreased with decreased platelet count
Coagulation factor assays Factors V, VIII Fibrinogen Plasminogen Protein C Protein S Antithrombin III Factor IX antigen	Results expressed as a percent of normal	Used to assess for absence of specific clotting factors when inherited disorders are suspected
Disseminated intravascular coagulopathy (DIC) screen	Prothrombin time: 11–15 sec. Fibrin degradation products (FDP) < 10 μg/mL. aPTT. 25–40 sec. Fibrinogen titer: 200–400 mg/100 mL Platelet count: 150,000–400,000/mm³	PT and PTT prolonged FDPs increased Fibrinogen decreased Platelets' decreased Indicative of onset of DIC
Heparin antibody test	Negative	Used when PTT is abnormally prolonged in a patient receiving heparin; also used with decreased platelet levels or if patient fails to respond to heparin
Fibrinogen	200–400 mg/dL	Plasma protein synthesized by the liver; activated by thrombin to produce fibrin strands for clot formation. Increased levels may be seen with oral contraceptive use, collagen diseases, acute infections, hepatitis. Deficiency results from DIC, severe liver disease, and other systemic condition.

UNIT BIBLIOGRAPHY

American Joint Committee on Cancer. (1998). *AJCC cancer staging handbook* (5th ed.). Philadelphia: Lippincott-Raven.

Beattie, S., Norton, M. & Doll, D. (1997). Coronary thrombosis associated with inherited protein S deficiency: A case report. *Heart & Lung, 26*(1), 118.

Beutler, E. (Ed.) (1995). *William's hematology* (5th ed.). New York: McGraw-Hill.

Chandrasoma, P. & Taylor, C. R. (1998). *Concise pathology* (3rd ed.). Stamford, CT: Appleton & Lange.

Chernecky, C. C. & Berger, B. J. (1997). *Laboratory tests and diagnostic procedures* (2nd ed.). Philadelphia: W.B. Saunders.

Coller, B., Owen, J., & Jesty, J. (1987). Deficiency of plasma protein S, protein C or antithrombin III and arterial thrombosis. *Arteriosclerosis, 17*(5), 1148.

Colman, R., Hirsh, J., Marder, V. & Salzman, E. (1994). *Hemostasis and thrombosis: Basic principles and clinical practice* (3rd ed.). Philadelphia: J.B. Lippincott.

Cotran, K. S., Kumar, V. & Collins, T. (1999). *Robbins' pathologic basis of disease* (6th ed.). Philadelphia: W. B. Saunders.

Davie, E., Fujikawa, K., & Kisiel, W. (1991). The coagulation cascade: Initiation, maintenance, and regulation. *Biochemistry, 30*(43), 10363.

Detmer, W. M., McPhee, S., Nicoll, D., & Chou, T. (1992). *Pocket guide to diagnostic tests.* Norwalk, CT: Appleton & Lange.

DeVita, V. T., Hellman, S., & Rosenberg, S. A. (1997). *Cancer: Principles and practice of oncology* (5th ed.). Philadelphia: J. B. Lippincott.

Esmon, C. (1989). The roles of protein C and thrombomodulin in the regulation of blood coagulation. *Journal of Biological Chemistry, 264*(9), 56.

Fahs, S. & Friedland, M. (1996). Evaluation of the bleeding patient. *Clinician Reviews, 1996.*

Formstone, C., Hallam, P., & Tuddenham, E. (1996). Severe perinatal thrombosis in double and triple heterozygous offspring in a family segregating two independent protein S mutations and a protein C mutation. *Blood, 87*(9), 922.

Furie, B. & Furie, B. (1988). The molecular basis of blood coagulation. *Cell, 53*(5), 505.

Hoffman, R. (Ed.) (1995). *Hematology: Basic principles and practice* (2nd ed.). New York: Churchill Livingstone.

Holland, J. F. (Ed.) (1997). *Cancer medicine* (4th ed.). Baltimore: Williams & Wilkins.

Jandl, J. H. (1996). *Blood: Textbook of hematology* (2nd ed.). Boston: Little, Brown.

Janeway, C. A. & Travers, P. (1997). *Immunobiology: The immune system in health and disease* (3rd ed.). New York: Current Biology Ltd./Garland Publishing.

Lee, G. R., Bithell, T. C., Foerster, J., Athens, J. W., & Lukens, J. N. (1993). *Wintrobe's clinical hematology* (9th ed.). Philadelphia: Lea & Febiger.

Mazza, J. J. (Ed.) (1995). *Manual of clinical hematology* (2nd ed.). Boston: Little, Brown.

McBrien, N. (1997). Thrombotic thrombocytopenia purpura. *American Journal of Nursing, 97*(2), 322.

Miller, D. R., Baehner, R. L., & Miller, L. P. (Eds.) (1995). *Blood diseases of infancy and childhood* (7th ed.). St. Louis: Mosby.

Nordfang, O., Bjorn, S., Valentin, S., Nielson, L. Wildgoose, P., Beck, T. & Hedner, U. (1991). *Biochemistry, 30,* 224.

Pizzo, P. A. & Poplack, D. G. (Eds.) (1993). *Principles and practices of pediatric oncology* (2nd ed.). Philadelphia: Lippincott.

Roitt, I, Brostoff, J. & Male, D. (1998). *Immunology* (5th ed.). St. Louis: Mosby.

Rubin, E. & Farber, J. L. (1999). *Pathology* (3rd ed.). Philadelphia: Lippincott.

Schafer, A. (1994). Hypercoaguable states: Molecular genetics to clinical practice. *Lancet, 344*(12), 1886.

Schaechter, M., Medoff, G., & Eisenstein, B. I. (1997). *Mechanisms of microbial disease* (3rd ed.). Baltimore: Williams & Wilkins.

Stein, J. H. (Ed.) (1998) *Internal medicine* (5th ed.). St. Louis: Mosby.

Stites, D. P., Terr, A. I. & Parslow, T. G. (1997). *Medical immunology* (9th ed.). Stamford, CT: Appleton & Lange.

Treseler, K. M. (1995). *Clinical laboratory and diagnostic tests* (3rd ed.). Stamford, CT: Appleton & Lange.

Welch, G. & Loscalzo, J. (1998). Homocysteine and atherothrombosis. *New England Journal of Medicine, 338*(15), 2022.

SELECTED ON-LINE REFERENCES

Blood: Journal of the American Society of Hematology. *http://www.bloodjournal.org/*

Yale Library: Selected Internet resources. *http://www.med.yale.edu.library/sir*

Hematology resources. *http://www.cc.emory.edu/*

Blood Cells, Molecules, and Diseases (journal). *http://seconde.scripps.edu/Welcome.html*

Diseases and Common Conditions Health Links University of Washington. *http://www.hslib.washington.edu/conditions/*

Dr. Deloughery's Famous Handouts, Oregon Health Sciences University. *http://www.ohsu.edu/cliniweb/handouts/list.html*

Cells of the Blood: Department of Microbiology and Immunology. *http://www.micro.msb.le.ac.uk/MBChB/bloodmap/Blood.html*

Vanderbilt Histology and Blood. *Webmaster@www.mc.vanderbilt.edu*

Aplastic Anemia Answer Book. http://medic.med.UTH.TMC.edu

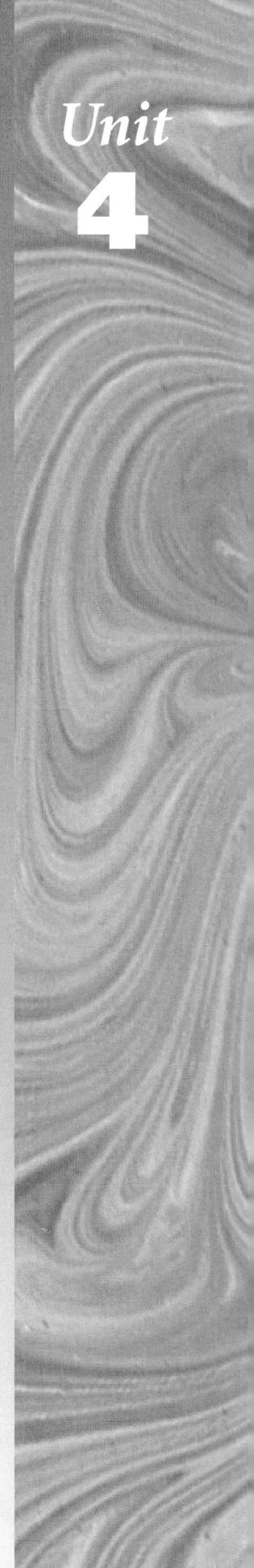

Circulation

FOCUS ON Circulatory Changes Through The Life Span

INFANT (1–12 MONTHS):

The heart doubles its weight and gradually shifts from the horizontal to a more vertical position. At birth, ventricles are equal in size, but left ventricular muscle mass increases as systemic blood pressure increases from approximately 80/50 to 90–100/50–60. Average pulse declines from approximately 150 bpm to 110 bpm. Gradual development of vasoconstriction and vasodilatation properties of arteries occurs.

TODDLER AND PRESCHOOL AGE (1–5 YEARS):

Heart weight increases fourfold from birth due to increased muscle mass, mainly in left ventricle. Heart rate gradually declines to about 90 to 100 bpm. Blood pressure is approximately 90–100/50–60. Vessels grow to supply the growing child.

SCHOOL AGE (6–12 YEARS):

By age 12, heart muscle mass is almost 10 times heavier than at birth. It assumes the normal vertical position of adulthood. Heart rate averages 70–80 bpm and blood pressure is approximately 100–110/60–70. Blood vessels grow and thicken to accommodate increased pressure.

ADOLESCENCE (13–19 YEARS):

Age of onset of adolescence variable with sexual changes. Heart size doubles in this period, increasing its pumping capacity, and it may outstrip that of the vessels supplying the tissues, accounting for some complaints of muscle aches and chest pains. Vessels increase in length and thickness. Cardiac output increases according to the physical size of the individual, which increases the blood pressure to an average of 110–120/60–70. Pulse averages 60–70 bpm, with females often having a higher rate (70–80 bpm).

YOUNG ADULT AND ADULT (20–45 YEARS):

Adult cardiac size with establishment of normal rhythm is attained. Maximum cardiac output of 70–85 mL/kg of body weight is attained at about age 30. Blood pressure increases to 100–120/60–80 with average heart rate of 72 bpm. Arteries have decreased elasticity, and varicose veins may be seen with increased abdominal pressure such as pregnancy. Alcohol, drug, or nicotine abuse can weaken the myocardium. Early atherosclerotic changes may be seen, which may progress as age increases.

MIDDLE-AGED ADULT (46–64 YEARS):

Heart efficiency may decrease to 80% or less as aging occurs. Decline in cardiac output is 1% per year. Cardiac reserve declines and maximum heart rate decreases, so that exercise tolerance may decrease. Blood pressure is 120–130/70–80 with pulse of 60–80 bpm. Decreased elasticity of arteries and increased incidence of atherosclerosis lead to development of coronary artery disease or peripheral vascular disease, with an increased incidence in males versus females. Varicose veins are common in both sexes.

LATE ADULTHOOD (65–100+ YEARS):

Left ventricular hypertrophy with atrial and valvular thickening and calcification of cardiac valves is common. Decline in myocardial contractility causes decreased cardiac output to 70% of that at age 30; this decreases progressively as age increases. Decreased elasticity and thickening of all peripheral vessels cause an increase in the systemic vascular resistance. There is increased incidence of atherosclerosis of arteries, which increases the risk of coronary artery disease. Varicose veins are common.

Chapter

15

Normal Circulatory Dynamics

Barbara L. Bullock

KEY TERMS

action potential
afterload
automaticity
autoregulation
capacitance vessels
catecholamines
chordae tendineae
conductivity
contractility
distensibility/compliance
ejection fraction
exchange vessels
excitability
inotropic state
intercalated disks
myocardial oxygen consumption
myocardial work
preload
pulse pressure
refractory period
rhythmicity
systemic vascular resistance
total peripheral resistance
trabeculae carneae
voltage dependent calcium channels
voltage-gated sodium channels

The dynamic circulatory system supplies oxygen and nutrients to the tissues of the body and removes and transports metabolic wastes to the excretory organs. Blood acts as the carrier. The heart pumps the blood through the arteries to the arterioles, which interconnect with the capillaries, venules, and veins to return blood to the heart. The vessels carrying the blood must remain intact and the pumping mechanism must maintain a dynamic action for continual movement of blood. The basis for the pumping mechanism is the heart's cellular structure, which contracts and relaxes in a continual sequence to maintain blood flow. Two major divisions of the *circulatory system* have been identified that accomplish the purposes of circulation and oxygenation of blood. The *systemic* division supplies oxygen and nutrients to the body tissues and brings blood back to the heart. The *pulmonary* division sends blood to the lungs for carbon dioxide removal and oxygen uptake, after which the newly oxygenated blood returns to the heart.

HEART

Structure of the Heart

The heart is composed of four pumping chambers: the right and left atria and the right and left ventricles. The atrioventricular (AV) sulcus or groove separates the atria from the ventricles; the interventricular sulci or grooves separate the ventricles from one another. When viewing the heart's surface, these landmarks are often not clearly visible due to the deposition of epicardial fat. The right atrium and ventricle receive blood from the systemic veins and pump it to the lungs through the pulmonary artery. The left atrium and ventricle receive blood from the pulmonary veins and pump it to the systemic arteries through the aorta. Figure 15-1 shows the general structure of the heart and its blood vessels.

ATRIA (SING., ATRIUM)

The *right atrium* is a low-pressure, thin-walled chamber that receives blood from the superior and inferior vena cavae and from the veins that drain the heart. The *left atrium* is slightly smaller than the right and receives blood from the four pulmonary veins that return oxygenated blood from the lungs to the heart.

The atrial walls are composed of three layers: (1) *epicardium*, a thin outer layer that is continuous with the outer layer of the ventricles; (2) *myocardium*, the middle or muscular layer of the atria, discontinuous with that of the ventricles; and (3) *endocardium*, a thin, continuous, inner layer that covers the inner surface of the atria, valves, ventricles, and vessels entering and leaving the

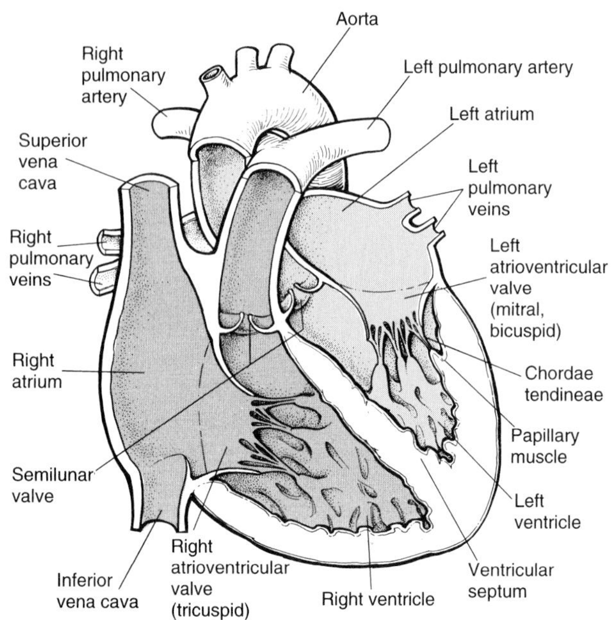

Atria: Low pressure chambers and reservoirs that serve as separate pumps from ventricles.
Ventricles: High pressure chambers; generate pressure sufficient to sustain arterial pressure of 120/80 mm Hg. Left ventricular pressure 120/0-10; right ventricular pressure 25/0-5. Aortic pressure 120/80.
Atrioventricular valves: Attached to papillary muscles by chordae tendineae, which prevent valvular eversion into the atria during ventricular contraction.
Semilunar valves: Aortic and pulmonic valves lie between the ventricles and the exiting arteries; prevent the backflow of blood from the arteries into the ventricles when the ventricles relax.
Aorta
Right pulmonary artery
Left pulmonary artery
Left atrium
Superior vena cava
Left pulmonary veins
Right pulmonary veins
Left atrioventricular valve (mitral, bicuspid)
Right atrium
Chordae tendineae
Papillary muscle
Semilunar valve
Left ventricle
Right atrioventricular valve (tricuspid)
Inferior vena cava
Right ventricle
Ventricular septum

FIGURE 15-1. **Internal anatomy of the heart.**

heart (Fig. 15-2). The myocardium of the atria is much thinner than that of the ventricles and accounts for the lower pressures that the atria maintain. The atria serve mostly as storage reservoirs and conductive passageways for blood movement to the ventricles.

Dividing the right and left atria is the *membranous atrial septum*, a structure that prevents the communication of blood between the atria. This septum houses the fossa ovalis, which originates as a fetal communication, the foramen ovale (see p. 495).

VENTRICLES

Like the walls of the atria, the ventricular walls are composed of three layers: epicardium, myocardium, and endocardium (see Fig. 15-2). The *right ventricle* has the appearance of a bellows, with a myocardial layer that is thicker than in the atrial walls but thinner than in the left ventricle. The *left ventricle* is more circular than the right. Its myocardium is much thicker than in the right ventricle, which allows the left ventricle to achieve the high pressures required for systemic arterial circulation (see Fig. 15-1).

Dividing the ventricles is the *ventricular septum*, a thick muscular structure that becomes membranous as it approaches the AV valves. This septum contains the branches of the conduction tissue for the transmission of an impulse (Fig. 15-3). It also provides an important fulcrum during contraction of the ventricles (see p. 416).

The inner surface of the ventricles contains areas of raised muscle bundles called the **trabeculae carneae** that are undercut by open spaces. The *papillary muscles* project from the trabeculated surface, giving rise to two groups of papillary muscles in the left ventricle and three groups in the right. These muscles project strong fibrous strands called **chordae tendineae**, which attach to the margins of the AV valves (see Fig. 15-1).

ATRIOVENTRICULAR VALVES

The AV valves, which separate the atria from the ventricles, include the mitral and the tricuspid valves (Fig. 15-4). The *mitral (bicuspid) valve* lies between the left atrium and the left ventricle. It is composed of two leaflets of fibroelastic tissue that slightly overlap when the valve is closed. The margins of the valve are attached to the fibrous chordae tendineae. The *tricuspid valve* is composed of three leaflets and lies between the right atrium and the right ventricle. The leaflets, also composed of fibrous tissue, are thinner than those of the mitral valve. These leaflets are attached to chordae tendineae that project from the right ventricular papillary muscles. The *annulus* (valve ring) that surrounds each valve is quite compliant and distorts its shape during ventricular contraction.

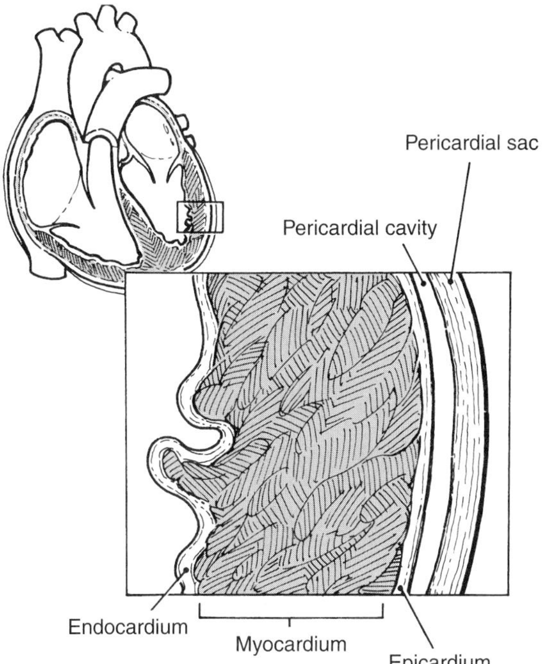

FIGURE 15-2. Cross-section showing the layers of the ventricles. Note the thin endocardial layer in relation to the thick myocardium.

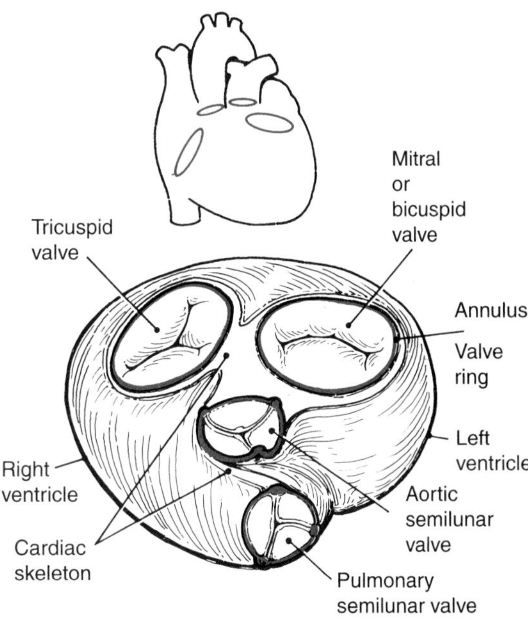

FIGURE 15-4. Fibrous rings of cardiac skeleton surround the heart valves as viewed from above. Valves are in the closed position.

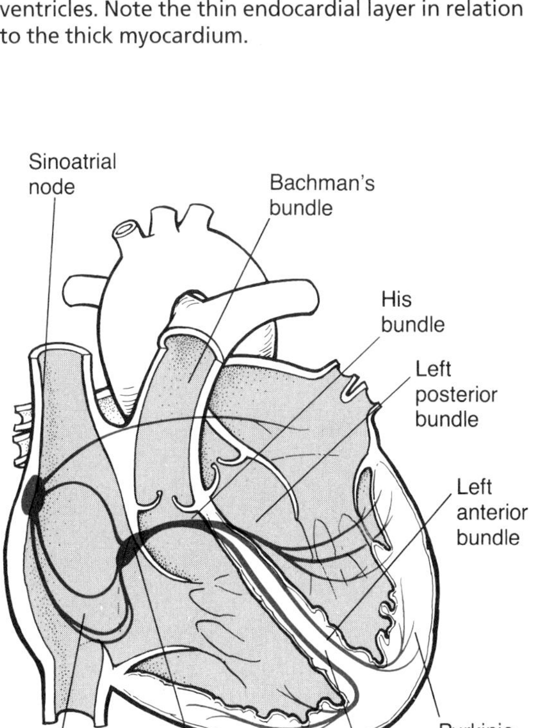

FIGURE 15-3. Location of pathways for the heart's conduction system.

SEMILUNAR VALVES

The *aortic* and *pulmonary valves* are called semilunar valves because their cusps are similar to half-moons in appearance (see Fig. 15-4). Each valve contains three cusps whose margins meet when the valves are closed. The valves close when they are filled with blood during the diastolic or resting phase of the cardiac cycle (see p. 416). The aortic and pulmonic valves are similar in structure except that the aortic valve is composed of slightly thicker fibrous cusps and gives off the coronary arteries (see below). Strong fibrous tissue or valve rings support both valves.

FIBROUS CARDIAC SKELETON

The fibrous cardiac skeleton holds together the main structures of the heart. It provides a firm anchor that attaches the atrial and ventricular muscles and the valvular tissue (see Fig. 15-4). It is composed of compact fibroelastic tissue around the valves and is continuous with the membranous portion of the ventricular septum, where it provides support for the aortic cusps, especially the right coronary and the noncoronary cusps.[17] The bundle of His, described on page 409, penetrates this fibrous area and at the crest of the muscular septum divides into the right and left bundle branches.

MAJOR ARTERIES OF THE HEART

The two major arteries leading from the heart are the *pulmonary artery* and the *aorta* (Fig. 15-5). The pulmonary artery leads from the right ventricle to the lungs and branches into smaller and smaller vessels that finally become the pulmonary capillary bed (where oxygen and carbon dioxide exchange occurs). The pulmonary capillaries then become venules and finally the four pulmonary veins described below.

The aorta is the main systemic artery and carries oxygenated blood to all body tissues. This artery has branches that become smaller and smaller, terminating finally in systemic arterioles and capillaries where exchange for oxygen and nutrition occurs.

GREAT VEINS OF THE HEART

The *superior* and *inferior venae cavae* return systemic venous blood to the heart. After blood passes through the systemic vascular (capillary) bed, it passes through venules, small veins, larger veins, and finally to the inferior and superior vena cavae (see Fig. 15-5).

The *pulmonary veins*, usually four in number, carry oxygenated blood from the lungs back to the left atrium. They bring blood pumped to the lungs by the right ventricle back to the left side of the heart to be circulated.

CORONARY ARTERIES

Two main coronary arteries arise from the sinuses of Valsalva of the aortic valve. The *right coronary artery* (*RCA*) arises from the right coronary sinus and the *left coronary artery* (*LCA*) arises from the left coronary sinus (Fig. 15-6).

The RCA usually arises as a singular vessel from the right coronary ostium, but two vessels may arise from this position. This second vessel, if present, is called the *conus artery*. When a single coronary artery arises on the right side, the conus artery is the first branch off the right main coronary artery.[17] The RCA travels in the AV

Arteries
Vasculature has thicker, more muscular walls, high pressure resistance circuit. Elastic property of the larger arteries permits distention to accommodate blood ejected from the left ventricle recoiling to propel blood forward. As blood moves to the periphery, arteries subdivide to become arterioles which can dilate or constrict in response to autonomic nervous system control. Dilation decreases resistance to flow; constriction increases resistance, thus decreasing and increasing the diastolic pressure maintained within the arterial circuit.

Capillaries
Large bed of single-layer walled vessels. Oxygen and nutrients are delivered to the tissues and carbon dioxide and wastes are picked up. Exchange is dependent on hydrostatic and oncotic pressures produced by actual generative forces from the heart and plasma proteins respectively.

Veins
Small veins called venules receive and collect blood from the capillaries and empty into veins. Veins have greater distensibility than arteries and lower pressures, thus this is called a capacitance system. Venous valves within the veins help to maintain a forward flow of blood toward the heart.

Pulmonary Circulation
The vasculature has thinner walls, greater distensibility, less resistance to blood flow. Pressure is 1/5 of systemic pressure. Primary function: takes up oxygen and gives off carbon dioxide.

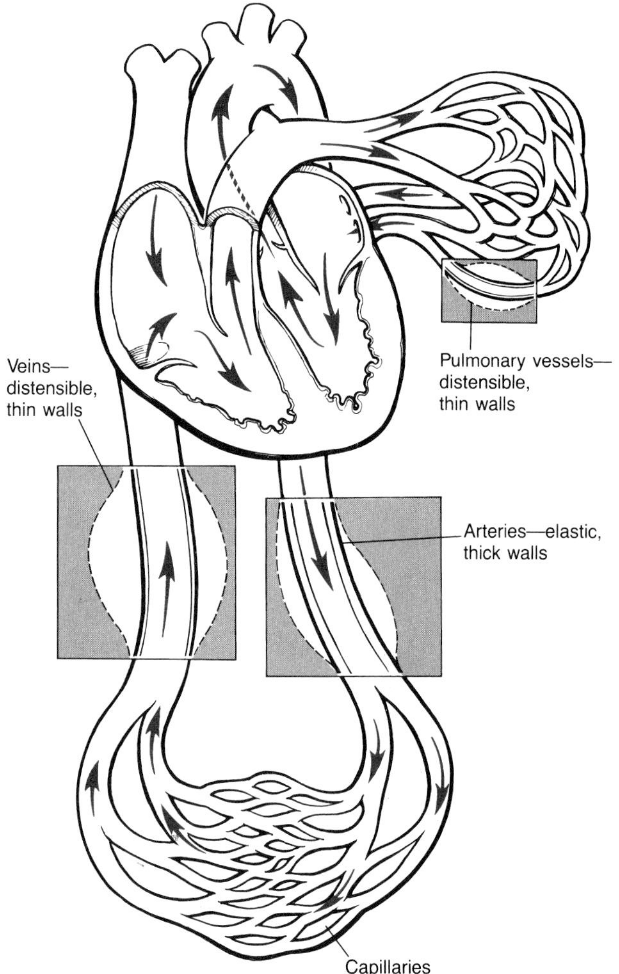

FIGURE 15-5. **Blood flow through the systemic and pulmonary vasculature circuit.**

Coronary arteries arise from 2 of the pouchlike dilations at the base of the aorta called the sinuses of Valsalva.

Right coronary artery (RCA): most frequently supplies the sinoatrial (55% of hearts) and atrioventricular (90%) nodes, right ventricle (RV), posterior septum and posterior left ventricle (LV). It turns downward in the posterior interventricular groove and is called the posterior descending coronary artery.

Left coronary artery (LCA): divides into the left anterior descending (LAD) and circumflex arteries. The LAD gives off 1-4 diagonal arteries which supply the LV wall. The LAD supplies the anterior LV and the apex of the heart. The circumflex artery supplies part of the anterior and lateral LV.

Veins of the heart: blood is returned from the heart muscle through the thebesian veins (which drain the septa and ventricular walls directly into the heart chambers) the small cardiac vein, middle cardiac vein, and great cardiac vein which drain into the coronary sinus and thence into the right atrium. Anterior cardiac veins enter the right atrium directly.

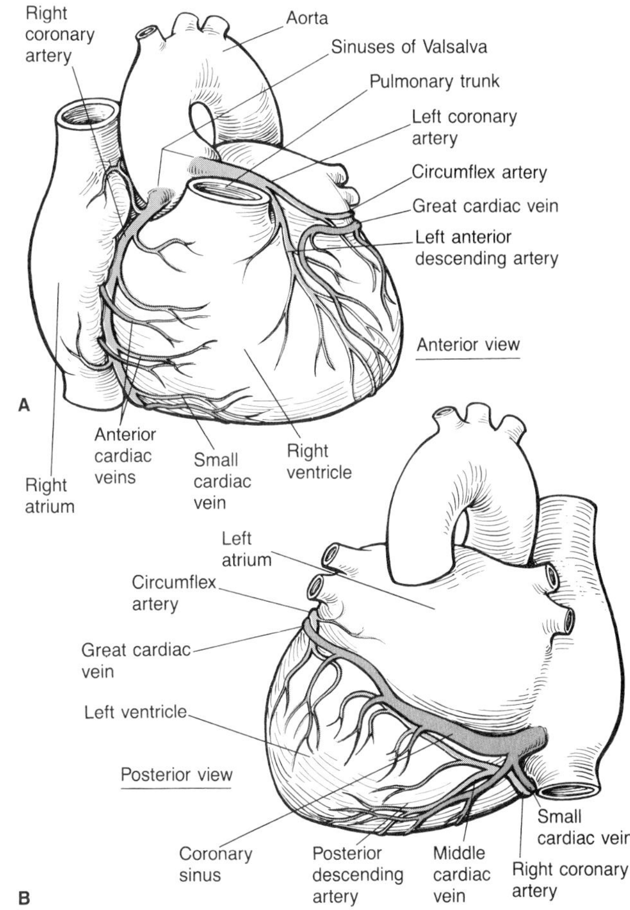

FIGURE 15-6. **Coronary arteries and veins. A. Anterior view. B. Posterior view.**

groove (sulcus) and turns downward in the posterior interventricular sulcus where it is called the *posterior descending coronary artery*. In about 55% of human hearts, the RCA supplies blood to the sinoatrial (SA) node through a branch called the sinus node artery. In about 90% of hearts it supplies the AV node through the AV nodal artery.[17] In most hearts, the RCA supplies the posterior surface of the right and left ventricles and the posterior interventricular septum. In a few hearts, it may extend to supply part of the lateral and apical surfaces. In these cases it is called a dominant RCA.

The *left main coronary artery* (*LMCA*) arises from a single ostium in the left coronary sinus. It travels in the AV sulcus for a short distance and then divides (bifurcates) into the *left anterior descending* (*LAD*) and the *left circumflex* coronary arteries. Other branches, called *diagonal arteries*, may stem from the bifurcation. These arteries, two to six in number, provide blood to the anterior surface of the left ventricle. The LAD descends in the anterior interventricular sulcus and supplies blood to the anterior left ventricle, the anterior interventricular septum, and the apex of the heart. Septal branches of the LAD supply the septum. The circumflex artery branches off the LMCA at a sharp angle and its branches supply blood to the lateral left ventricle and various portions of the posterior wall. It supplies the SA node in approximately 45% of hearts and usually supplies the left atrium. In a small percentage of persons the circumflex supplies the posterior left ventricle and interventricular septum, and thus is called a dominant circumflex artery.

Table 15-1 summarizes the normal blood supply to the myocardium and variations that may occur. Both coronary arteries receive their blood when the aortic valve closes during the diastolic or resting phase of the heart.

The coronary arteries divide into smaller and smaller branches that penetrate deeply into the myocardial muscle. They form a network of capillaries that supply the myocardial cells. Numerous functional and nonfunctional anastomoses exist between the coronary vessels, which can enlarge when the flow in one arterial branch

TABLE 15-1

NORMAL BLOOD SUPPLY TO MYOCARDIUM

CORONARY ARTERY	AREA SUPPLIED	VARIATIONS
Right coronary artery (RCA)	SA node in 55% of hearts; AV node in 90% of hearts; posterior surface of right and left ventricles; posterior interventricular system	Dominant when it supplies lateral and apical left ventricle
Left main coronary artery		
Left anterior descending (LAD)	Anterior left ventricle; apex of heart; anterior interventricular septum	In 5–10% of hearts supplies AV node; antero-lateral left ventricle
Circumflex (Cx)	SA node in 45% of hearts; left atrium; posterior lateral surface left ventricle	In 5–10% of hearts supplies AV node; dominant where it supplies entire left ventricle; interventricular septum

SA, sinoatrial; AV, atrioventricular.

decreases. Enlargement of anastomoses can improve blood flow to myocardial segments, thus providing *collateral circulation*. The endocardial layer is the only portion of the heart that receives oxygen and nutrients from the blood that circulates within the chambers. The rest of the heart receives its oxygen and nutrients from branches of the coronary arteries.

CORONARY VEINS

The coronary veins enable blood to drain from the myocardium and empty into the right atrium (see Fig. 15-6). They consist of the coronary sinus and its branches, the anterior right ventricular veins, and the thebesian veins. The coronary sinus and its branches receive the majority of drainage from the left ventricle. The coronary sinus is basically an extension of the great coronary vein. The anterior cardiac veins drain the right ventricle and usually empty directly into the right atrium. The remaining venous blood empties into the heart through the small thebesian veins. These tiny venous outlets drain directly into the right atrium.[17]

PERICARDIUM

A fibrous sac called the *parietal pericardium* surrounds the heart. A second, inner layer that is in contact with the outside of the heart is called the *visceral pericardium* or the *epicardium* (see Fig. 15-2). Between the parietal and visceral layers is normally about 10 to 50 mL of clear fluid, an ultrafiltrate of blood plasma, which allows for free movement of the heart within the sac.[17] Ligaments attach the fibrous layer to the sternum and the diaphragm, keeping the heart in a normal position. This fibrous layer is also attached to the great vessels at the area where they enter and leave the heart. The pericardium limits distention of the heart.

CONDUCTION SYSTEM

Normal contraction of the heart is initiated by specialized conductive tissues, which are actually myocardial muscle cells with fewer myofibrils than the other myocardial cells. Figure 15-3 shows the location of the conductive structures within the heart: the SA node, atrial internodal tracts, AV node, bundle of His, right and left bundle branches, and terminal or Purkinje network.

Sinoatrial or Sinus Node

The *sinoatrial* or *sinus (SA) node* is a small mass of cells located near the entrance of the superior vena cava into the right atrium. The SA node normally serves as the heart's pacemaker because of its ability to generate an impulse through spontaneous diastolic depolarization (see p. 419). The node receives blood from the SA node artery, which may arise from the RCA or the left circumflex. Specific cells in the SA node include nodal cells, transitional cells, and atrial muscle cells. The nodal cells are easily recognized microscopically and are thought to be the source of normal impulse formation by the SA node. The transitional cells are located at the margins of the SA node and may provide a pathway for distribution of the impulses formed in the nodal cells.[17] The atrial muscle cells are supplied with sympathetic nerve supply and the SA node is directly innervated by a branch of the vagus nerve.

Atrial Internodal Tracts

The *atrial internodal tracts* extend from the SA node and are difficult to distinguish from surrounding cardiac muscle. The pathways are designated as the *anterior, middle*, and *posterior internodal tracts*. The electrical impulse that the SA node generates travels rapidly along these tracts to merge at the AV node. Bachman's bundle (the anterior internodal tract) conducts the impulse to the left atrium. The remaining tracts travel through the right atrium.

Atrioventricular Node, Bundle of His, and Purkinje Network

The *atrioventricular (AV) node* and *bundle of His* form an interconnecting structure between the atria and ventricles that functionally joins the two units. The AV node lies in the lower portion of the right atrium at the juncture of the atrial septum. It is composed of dense fibrous tissue that continues into the bundle of His. The AV node, along with the bundle of His pathway, is the only functional connection between the atrial and ventricular muscles. The slow conduction in the AV node may be partly due to the unspecialized structure of its cells, and it allows for atrial emptying and filling of the ventricles (see p. 416). The area of the AV node and bundle of His is richly supplied with adrenergic and cholinergic fibers of the autonomic nervous system (ANS). The bundle of His directly connects with the AV node and crosses into the membranous portion of the ventricular septum. It is composed of fibrous tissue with a few myofibrils and terminates in the bifurcation of the common bundle into the right and left bundle branches.

The *right and left bundle branches* travel down the interventricular septum to terminate in the Purkinje network. The *right bundle branch* descends superficially in the endocardium of the right ventricular septum. It divides into numerous branches that penetrate the walls of the right ventricle. The *left bundle branch* fans into two main fascicles—the posterior and anterior—that travel in the left interventricular septum for varying distances. The posterior fascicle sends its branches to the left lateral and posterior walls and the papillary muscles. The anterior fascicle primarily goes to the anterior and lateral wall of the left ventricle. The fascicular branches subdivide into smaller and smaller subbranches and terminate in the Purkinje network.

The *Purkinje network* is composed primarily of Purkinje cells that have few myofibrils and are joined end-to-end by intercalated disks that aid in the property of accelerated conduction of the impulse (see below). A Purkinje fiber is composed of many Purkinje cells in a series. These fibers lie in the deepest layer of the myocardium and supply the papillary muscles and apical parts of the ventricles. Thus, the apical portion of the ventricles contracts before the basal parts, facilitating the excitation of the right and left ventricles.[2]

Myocardial Cellular Structure and Function

Cardiac muscle cells, though similar to skeletal muscle cells in many ways, have some fundamental differences. Figure 15-7 illustrates the transverse tubules (T tubules), associated sarcoplasmic reticulum (SR), and myofibrils that are common in all muscle cells. The junctions between cardiac muscle cells consist of **intercalated disks**, which form tight connections that allow impulses to pass rapidly from one cell to the next. Permeable gap junctions between the cell membranes allow free diffusion of ions so that **action potentials** (APs) travel instantaneously from one muscle cell to the next[11] (see below).

The *myofibril* is the contractile unit of the myocardial muscle cell. Its action occurs through the movement of *actin* on *myosin* in the sarcomere unit. The thin actin filament also is associated with two inhibitory proteins, *tropomyosin* and *troponin*. The activity of these proteins in muscle contraction is described in detail on page 783. The myocardial muscle cell has a poorly developed SR but a highly developed T tubule system. This tubular system probably contributes to the intracellular release of calcium.[2] The cardiac cell contains a large number of mitochondria that have been shown to store calcium along with the adenosine triphosphate (ATP) necessary for muscle contraction. Glycogen and lipid are also stored within the cells.

The major function of the myocardial cell is to contract and propel blood into the circulation. It requires a constant production of ATP, which in turn requires nutrients for energy production.

CONTRACTION OF CARDIAC MUSCLE

Cardiac muscle contraction occurs in much the same way as skeletal muscle contraction except that cardiac muscle functions as a whole unit. If one cardiac cell contracts, the impulse spreads to all the muscle cells and the entire unit contracts. The two units in the myocardium (atrial and ventricular) are functionally joined by portions of the conduction system: the AV node and the bundle of His.

The AP (see below) generated from the SA node spreads across the muscle and causes the SR to release calcium into the sarcoplasm. Calcium binds with troponin causing a conformational change in troponin, which is transmitted to tropomyosin and exposes myosin-binding sites on actin filament. Actin then slides on myosin. The calcium ion apparently has two major roles in excitation–contraction: (1) as the trigger substance or initiator and (2) as the regulator of contraction.[14] The initiation of the AP causes a rapid influx of sodium. The **voltage-gated sodium channels** are responsible for the rapid inward movement of sodium that results in the rapid upstroke of the AP.[15] This property is critical in the self-generating AP that is characteristic of cardiac muscle. This inherent "leakiness" of fibers of the conduction system is the basic cause for their self-excitation or spontaneous depolarization[11,15] (see p. 412).

As the AP travels down the extensive T tubular system, it comes close to the terminal cisternae of the SR, whereby a coupling mechanism (that remains unclear)

FOCUS ON CELLULAR PHYSIOLOGY

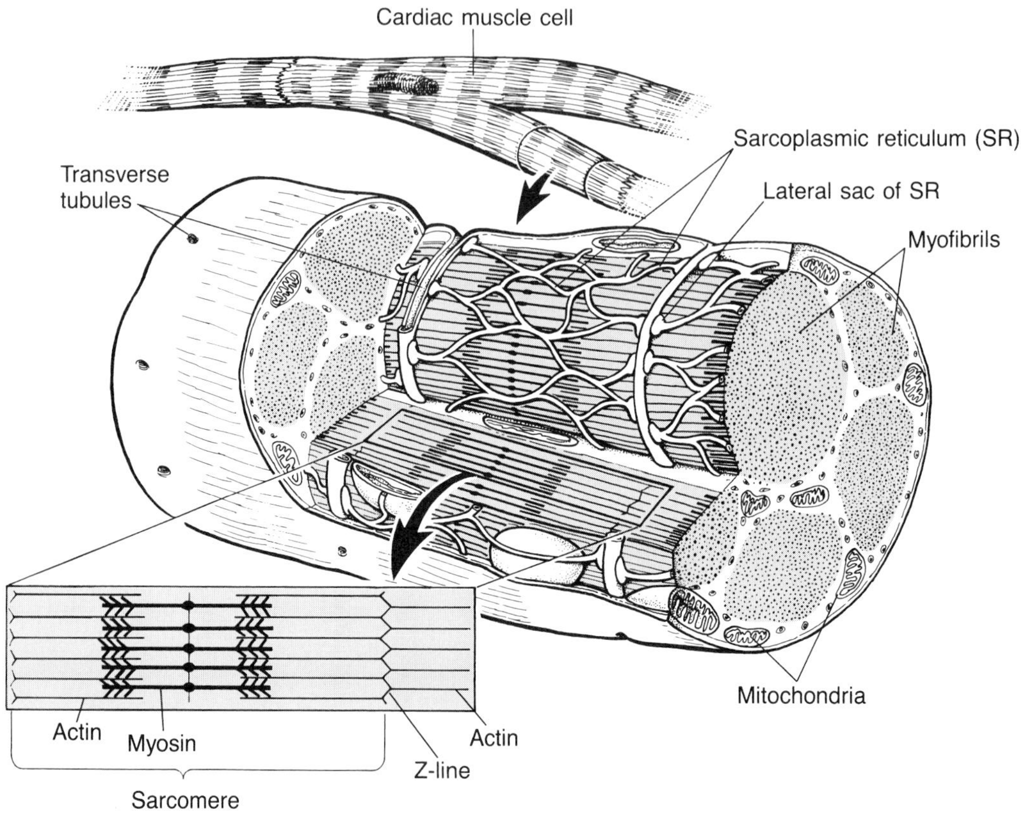

FIGURE 15-7. Structure of a cardiac muscle cell.

causes the SR to release large amounts of calcium into the sarcoplasm. This free calcium binds with troponin and, thus, inhibits both troponin and tropomyosin. Energy for the contraction is obtained from ATP, which is split by an ATPase site on the myosin filament when it interacts with actin.[14]

The rate and amount of myocardial tension that is developed directly relates to the amount of calcium available to bind with troponin.[2,16] The T tubules possess a large number of **voltage-dependent calcium channels** that open rapidly in response to the propagated AP and allow extracellular calcium to move down its concentration gradient into the cell. Calcium ions diffuse into the myofibrils to promote the reactions that cause the sliding of actin on myosin, which is an identical process to that of skeletal muscle contraction. Cardiac muscle contraction differs from that of skeletal muscle in that a large quantity of extra calcium ions diffuses into the sarcoplasm from the T tubules directly at the time of the AP. This accounts for the strength of the cardiac contraction because the poorly developed SR of the cardiac muscle does not store enough calcium to provide full contraction without this mechanism.[11]

Calcium must be returned to the SR through a continually active calcium pump that decreases the concentration of free cytosolic calcium. A decreased level of calcium in the sarcoplasmic fluid restores the inhibition of actin and myosin by the troponin–tropomyosin complex. The sarcomere unit then returns to the resting position.

Action Potential

An action potential (AP) is an electrical current generated by excitable tissue, in this case, the heart. Figure 15-8 illustrates the AP of human ventricular myocardium with the electrolyte changes that occur in the different stages. When the myocardial muscle cell is at rest, the resting membrane potential is approximately −85 to −95 mV. When an AP occurs, the membrane potential changes from a negative to a slightly positive value, a process called *depolarization*. The cardiac muscle cell remains depolarized for a longer period than do other excitable cells, which explains the plateau phase of the cardiac AP. The physiologic importance of this phase is that it allows for a longer contraction in cardiac muscle. *Contraction* begins during the plateau phase of the AP and

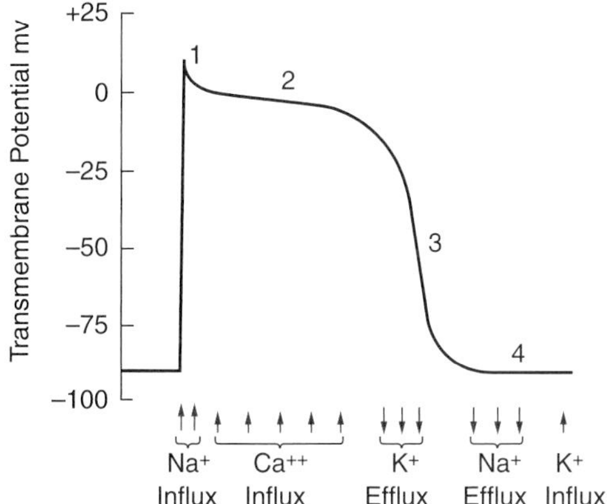

FIGURE 15-8. Schematic action potential of human ventricular myocardium together with probable electrolyte movements. The initial phase 0 spike and overshoot is related to a sudden influx of Na^+. This is followed by a slower, maintained influx of Ca^{++} during the plateau phase 2. The phase of Ca^{++} efflux is not well defined for human ventricular myocardium, but presumably it occurs during phase 4. (From R. W. Alexander, R. C. Schlant, & V. Fuster [Eds.], [1998]. *Hurst's the heart* [9th ed.]. New York: McGraw-Hill.)

reaches its peak of strength during early repolarization. Depolarization is followed by *repolarization* and a return to the resting state. As noted in Figure 15-8, these changes in potential and state of cardiac muscle can be described in terms of discrete phases: phase 0 denotes depolarization; phase 1 indicates complete depolarization and contraction; phase 2 is a plateau phase of maximum cardiac contraction; phase 3 is the period of repolarization; and phase 4 indicates the myocardium at rest. Application to the electrical events of the heart is found below.

The term **refractory period** is used to describe various actions in phase 1, 2, and 3 in both atrial and ventricular muscle. During the *absolute refractory period* (phases 1 and 2), the membrane is completely depolarized and the myocyte is contracting; no stimulus can cause it to respond or contract again. The *relative refractory period* (phase 3) occurs when the muscle membrane is repolarizing and a strong stimulus will cause it to contract again.[11]

METABOLISM OF CARDIAC MUSCLE

Cardiac muscle requires constant production of ATP. This muscle stores little ATP, so oxygen and nutrients for energy production must be constantly supplied through blood from the coronary arteries. Most ATP is produced in the numerous myocardial mitochondria using fatty acids and other nutrients, especially lactate and glucose. If one substance is not available, cardiac muscle can efficiently use another. The amount of ATP normally produced is equivalent to the work needed to pump incoming blood into the arteries with sufficient pressure to maintain vital body functions.

Function of the Heart

The function of the heart is considered in terms of the electrical and mechanical activities of the myocardial muscle. The cellular aspects provide a better understanding of the process. The electrical events precede and initiate the mechanical response and require certain properties inherent to cardiac muscle cells: **automaticity**, **rhythmicity**, **excitability**, and **conductivity**. The mechanical events of cardiac contraction are the result of four major determinants: **preload, afterload, contractility**, and **distensibility**. The heart rate, normally an extrinsic influence, helps to determine *cardiac output*.

ELECTRICAL EVENTS OF THE CARDIAC CYCLE

The cardiac cycle is initiated through specialized conduction tissue whose pacemaker cells spontaneously and rhythmically depolarize. The critical threshold is gradually reached; spontaneous depolarization occurs and is followed by repolarization (Fig. 15-9).

Spontaneous Depolarization

The SA node is the heart's pacemaker because spontaneous depolarization occurs most frequently here and supersedes the discharge of other potential pacers. This is due to a less negative resting membrane potential (−55 to −60 mV) in the SA node than in other cardiac muscle fibers and to increased membrane permeability to sodium. The depolarization of the SA node suppresses the AV node, bundle of His, and Purkinje fibers (the His–Purkinje system) by depolarizing them before they can compete as pacemakers.[11]

The conduction tissue has been called a cascade of potential pacers that fire at different rates and can take over pacemaker function if the more rapid pacemaker is not operational.[11] Figure 15-10 shows the approximate potential rates of the inherent cardiac pacemakers.

Excitation of cardiac muscle normally follows a strict sequential pattern. The excitation wave (propagated AP) begins at the SA node and is propagated through the internodal pathways, causing depolarization of the atrial muscle and excitation of the AV node.

At the AV node, the impulse slows as it passes through the dense fibrous tissue, allowing time for the atria to complete contraction before sending the depolarization wave to the ventricles. The impulse then travels down the bundle of His and the bundle branches to the Purkinje network, causing rapid depolarization and ventricular contraction.

Properties of Cardiac Muscle

For the above actions to occur, the properties of automaticity, rhythmicity, excitability, and conduc-

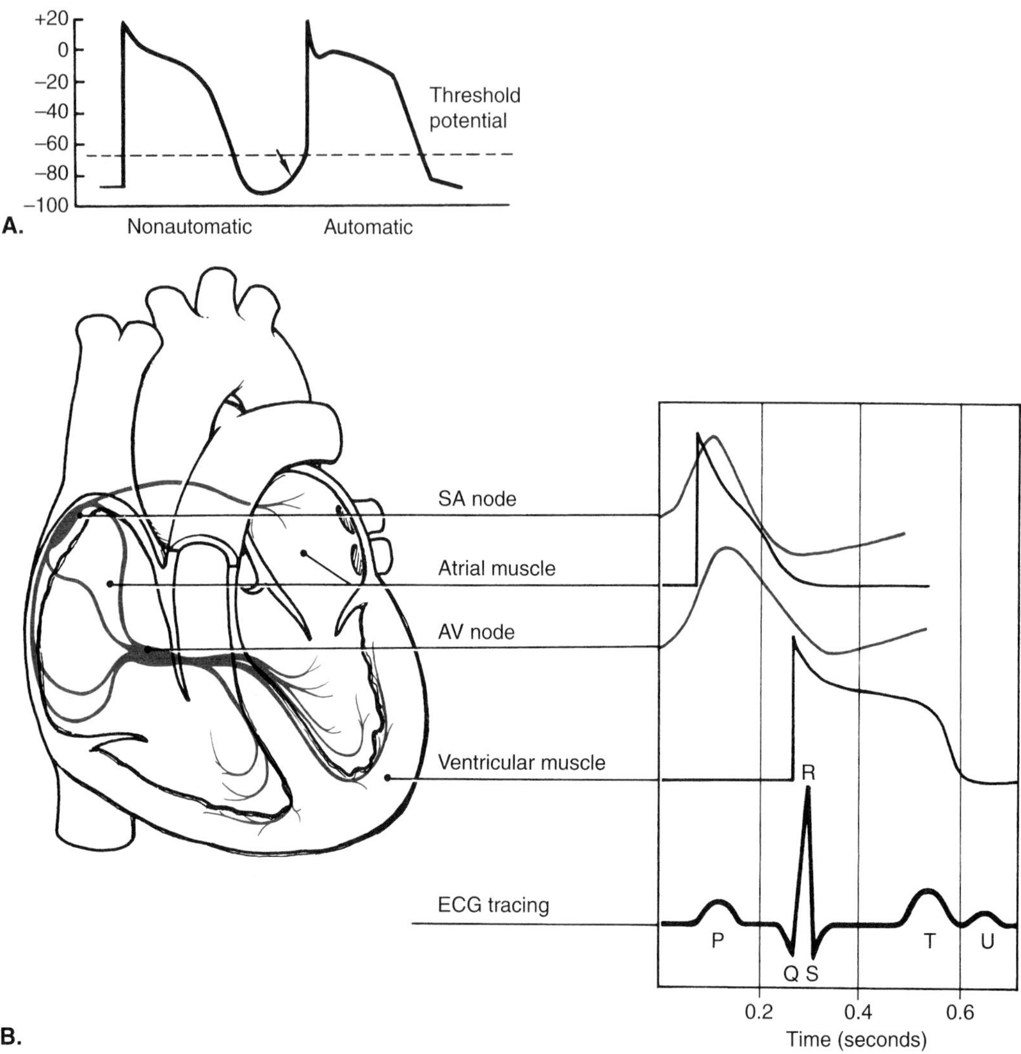

FIGURE 15-9. **A.** The nonautomatic cell depolarizes with a stimulus of adequate strength. The automatic cell depolarizes at regular intervals through increased permeability to sodium. **B.** Various areas of the conduction system depolarize through automatic and nonautomatic mechanisms.

tivity must be present. The electrocardiogram (ECG) described on pages 428 to 430 graphically depicts the electrical events of the cardiac cycle.

AUTOMATICITY. Automaticity is a property of conductive tissue in which spontaneous APs are generated within the tissue. This process occurs through slow diastolic depolarization during phase 4 of the AP. When the threshold level is reached, an AP is generated. The AP usually arises in the SA node, where an inward leakage phenomenon allows sodium to drift into the cell, thus making the resting membrane potential unstable. All parts of the conduction system retain the property of automaticity but do so at inherently different rates. The rate of this diastolic depolarization in phase 4 is more rapid in the SA node. Thus, it fires more frequently. These SA node impulses dominate other automatic regions simply because they are formed with greater frequency.

The calcium–sodium channels become inactivated and the potassium channels open, producing a hypernegativity in the fiber. Closing of the potassium channels follows, and the inward-leaking sodium ions overbalance the outward flux of potassium. The result is that the resting potential moves again toward threshold and discharge.[11] The process is a recurring self-

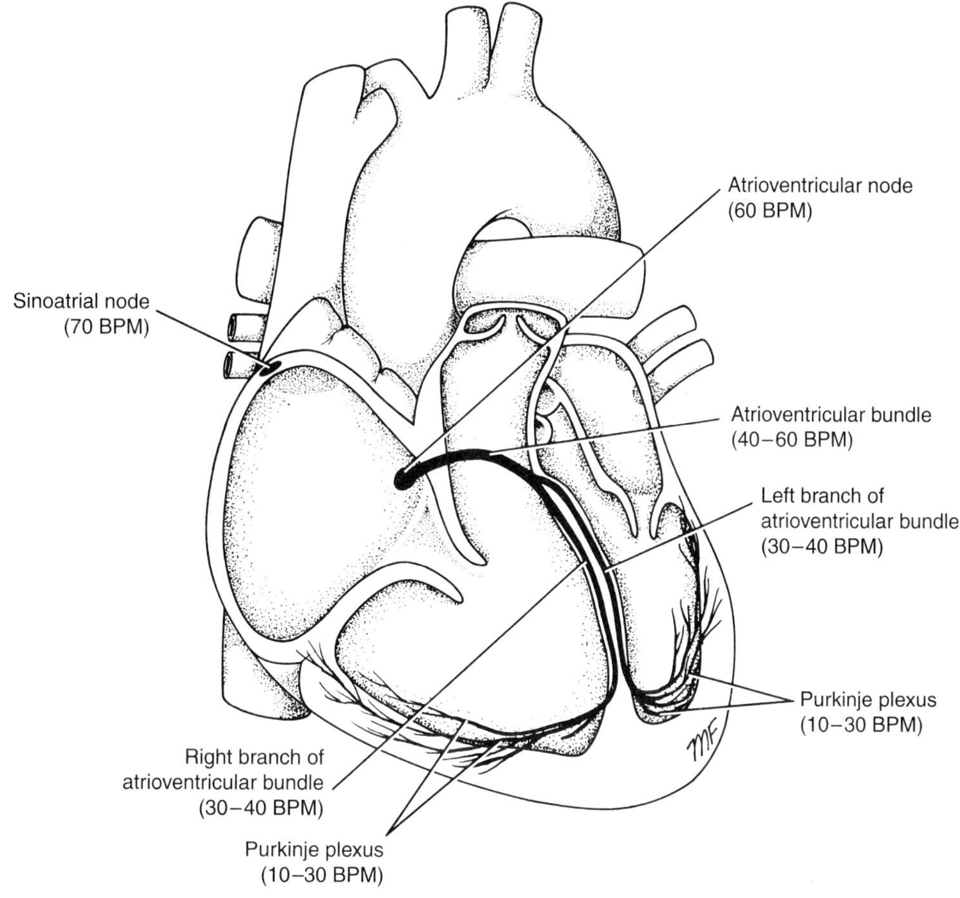

FIGURE 15-10. **Approximate rates of inherent cardiac pacemakers.**

excitation, recovery from the AP, hyperpolarization, drifting of the resting potential to threshold once again to re-excitation.[2,11] Over and over the process occurs as the heart continues to beat. Flowchart 15-1 summarizes the process of excitation–contraction and actin–myosin relaxation.

The term *abnormal automaticity* refers to abnormal changes in transmembrane potentials of cardiac cells. Abnormal automaticity can occur almost anywhere in the heart.[18] Table 15-2 describes factors that enhance and depress automaticity. Pharmaceutical agents, hypoxemia, and injury are some factors that can alter the threshold for myocardial response. Some medications raise the threshold for generation of the AP and thus decrease the rate of diastolic depolarization. This drug action is especially effective if ectopic impulses are causing ventricular dysrhythmias (see p. 455). Other medications enhance automaticity by increasing the rate of diastolic depolarization, thus increasing cardiac rate and irritability.

The body's intrinsic ANS also influences depolarization. Parasympathetic influences through the vagus nerve slow the rate of diastolic depolarization and decrease the rate of SA node automaticity. Sympathetic influences increase the automaticity and the rate of diastolic depolarization.

RHYTHMICITY. Rhythmicity is an important property of the conduction tissue that is characteristic of all potential pacemakers of the heart. This term refers to the rhythmic or regular generation of an AP. The leakage phenomenon described above remains consistent, allowing for the same amount of time from one depolarization to the next. Therefore, the AP discharges regularly.

The sympathetic nervous system (SNS) and the parasympathetic system (PSNS) may influence rhythmicity. SNS stimulation in stress may increase irritability and promote ectopic beats (see p. 421). A cyclic increase and decrease in cardiac rate due to respiratory influences on the vagus nerve of the PSNS result in an increased cardiac rate on inspiration and a decreased rate on expiration in certain persons. Influences such as electrolyte imbalances and pharmaceutical agents may also alter rhythmicity.

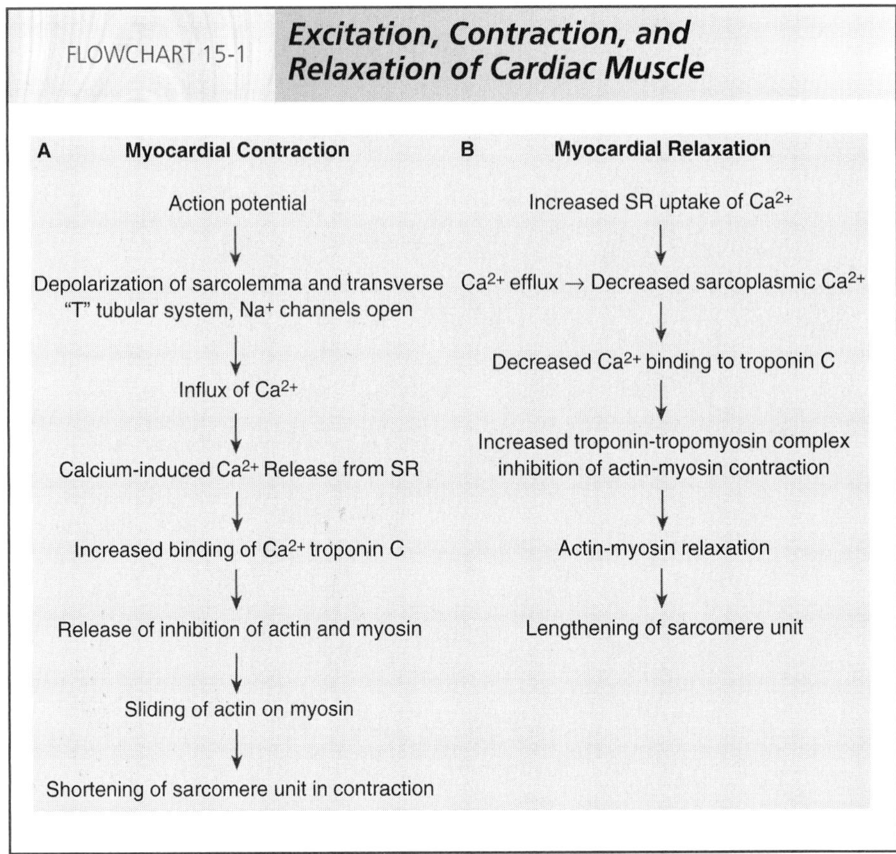

A Myocardial Contraction
Action potential
Depolarization of sarcolemma and transverse "T" tubular system, Na^+ channels open
Influx of Ca^{2+}
Calcium-induced Ca^{2+} Release from SR
Increased binding of Ca^{2+} troponin C
Release of inhibition of actin and myosin
Sliding of actin on myosin
Shortening of sarcomere unit in contraction
B Myocardial Relaxation
Increased SR uptake of Ca^{2+}
Ca^{2+} efflux → Decreased sarcoplasmic Ca^{2+}
Decreased Ca^{2+} binding to troponin C
Increased troponin-tropomyosin complex inhibition of actin-myosin contraction
Actin-myosin relaxation
Lengthening of sarcomere unit

FLOWCHART 15-1 **Excitation, Contraction, and Relaxation of Cardiac Muscle**

EXCITABILITY. Excitability refers to the ability of the cell to respond to stimulation. In the heart muscle, excitability denotes the ability of the cardiac muscle cell to respond to an impulse in an adjacent muscle cell. This property means that the threshold impulse generated in one muscle cell can be readily transmitted to the next until the entire muscle unit is depolarized and contracts. Excitability is important in normal impulse conduction as indicated and can be a basis for various alterations in the cardiac cycle, especially as seen in dysrhythmias such as ectopic beats (see p. 455).

CONDUCTIVITY. Impulse transmission in cardiac muscle is affected mostly by the structure of the intramyocardial cells, which allows the current to flow easily from one cell to the next. Therefore, threshold current from one cell rapidly passes to and depolarizes the adjacent cell. Conductivity is effected through the intercalated disks (tight junctions) between the myocardial muscle cells. It may be slowed when these junctions are altered, such as with intracellular damage from ischemia or infarction.[1] Excitability and conductivity are closely related and essential properties; excitability refers to being able to respond to a stimulus, whereas conductivity means allowing the stimulus to be passed from one cell to the next.

MECHANICAL EVENTS OF THE CARDIAC CYCLE

The mechanical events of the heart are those that result from the response to the electrical excitation and provide the cardiac output and blood pressure. Cardiac output equals the stroke volume (volume per ventricle per beat) times the heart rate and is measured in liters per minute. The arterial blood pressure reflects the pressure generated by the left ventricle on contraction and the pressure maintained in the arterial circuit on ventricular relaxation.

Factors Regulating the Mechanical Events

PRELOAD. This term refers to the degree of stretch (myocardial muscle length) before contraction. Preload is provided by venous return and refers to the volume that causes a degree of stretch in the ventricles. The response to increased preload is an inherent increase in the force of the cardiac contraction within certain limits. Starling described this phenomenon in 1918, noting that the energy of contraction is related to the length of the muscle fiber; thus, the principle is often called *Starling's law of the heart*, even though others have contributed to the study of this phenomenon.[14] In Starling's law, the increased fiber length is related to increased blood volume, which causes the initial stretch, and it responds with an increased force

TABLE 15-2

SOME FACTORS THAT ENHANCE AND DEPRESS AUTOMATICITY

FACTORS	RESULTS
ENHANCING FACTORS	
Sympathetic nervous system stimulation	Fever, pain, anxiety, trauma, illness, exercise all lead to increased pulse, blood pressure, and respiration. These increase cardiac irritability and automaticity.
High-output states	Conditions such as hyperthyroidism, anemia, and AV fistulas increase the volume that the heart must pump, increasing cardiac work and irritability.
Congestive heart failure and hypoxia	These conditions may decrease available oxygen to the myocardium and enhance the ectopic pacemakers. Stretch of the ventricular myocardium also increases irritability.
Drugs	Sympathomimetics such as epinephrine and norepinephrine directly increase normal and abnormal automaticity. Vagolytics such as atropine block parasympathetic effects and indirectly enhance automaticity. Toxic levels of digitalis can increase automaticity.
Electrolyte imbalances	Hypokalemia enhances normal automaticity.
DEPRESSING FACTORS	
Parasympathetic nervous system	Stimulation of this system causes direct depression of the heart's normal pacemakers.
Electrolyte disturbances	Hyperkalemia depresses normal and abnormal automaticity.
Acute myocardial infarction	Inferior wall MI can enhance PSNS activity and depress automaticity, especially at the AV node.
Drugs	Many antiarrhythmic drugs suppress the normal pacemakers and depress automaticity. Examples include β-adrenergic blockers and digitalis.

AV, atrioventricular; MI, myocardial infarction; PSNS, parasympathetic nervous system.

of contraction. Commonly used terms to describe the ability of the ventricle to receive blood are **distensibility** or **compliance**, both of which refer to the ratio of ventricular volume change to ventricular diastolic pressure change. *Decreased compliance* means increased ventricular stiffness, often seen in ischemia of cardiac muscle. A normally functioning ventricle can increase volume without a significant increase of pressure, such as during exercise stress. Ischemia, pericardial restriction, and hypertrophy are examples of factors that can affect compliance by limiting venous inflow or limiting the contractility that normally would occur. Increased ventricular distensibility without effective contraction may be present in heart failure.

A variety of factors can affect end-diastolic (just before ventricular contraction) volume or preload. Intravascular blood volume depletion decreases preload, whereas overload of intravascular volume increases it. Decreased efficiency of cardiac contractility, such as with heart failure, increases preload (see p. 474). Body position can greatly influence preload because blood tends to pool in dependent parts of the body due to loss of vascular resistance. Loss of effective negative intrapleural pressure, which helps to return blood to the heart, can cause a significant decrease in preload.[4]

AFTERLOAD. Afterload refers to the resistance that the aortic and pulmonary valves normally maintain, the condition and tone of the aorta, and the resistance that the systemic and pulmonary arterioles offer. Afterload is the net force per unit cross-sectional area across the myocardial wall during ejection and is estimated by using Laplace's law: *Wall stress* = PR/2h, where P = intracavitary pressure, R = radius of curvature, and h = wall thickness.[16] Afterload is determined primarily by aortic impedance, which is mainly determined by systemic vascular resistance or SVR (see p. 431). Because wall stress is difficult to measure, the mean arterial pressure (MAP) is used to approximate afterload.

The MAP is calculated by the following formula: systolic pressure + 2 × diastolic pressure ÷ 3.

Increased blood viscosity and increased preload also contribute to afterload. Pathophysiologic states, such as hypertension and aortic stenosis, significantly increase afterload. As afterload increases, so does cardiac work and oxygen consumption. Greater muscle mass is required to maintain cardiac output against chronic increased resistance. Over time, the ventricular muscle mass increases, leading to cardiac hypertrophy.

CONTRACTILITY. Contractility refers to the force of contraction that myocardial muscle generates. This property may be expressed in terms of the **inotropic state**, which is referred to as positive (+) if the force of contraction is increased and negative (−) if the force of contraction is decreased. Both preload and afterload influence contractility, but contractility may change independently. The SNS, through the influence of catecholamines, increases force of contraction[11] (see p. 421). Also, by increasing the recoil of ventricular muscle on diastole, diastolic ventricular pressure is decreased, which allows for greater filling, greater fiber stretch, and, therefore, a stronger contraction.[9] Increased contractility is termed *hyperkinesis*, while depressed contractility is called *hypokinesis*.

Recently, pharmacologic agents called *calcium channel blockers* have been developed to close or partially close calcium channels and, thus, decrease myocardial contractility. In ischemic heart disease or hypertrophic cardiomyopathy, calcium channel blockers can be used to decrease available calcium and cause a negative (−) inotropic state. The end result is decreased blood pressure and less cardiac ischemia.[5,8] Some antiarrhythmic medications block *sodium channels* with similar cardiac effects. Many antiarrhythmic medications are classified according to their membrane/channel action.[18]

HEART RATE. Stress in any form stimulates the SNS, increasing cardiac rate. This increased rate leads to increases in cardiac output and ventricular contractility. Rate changes are often called the *chronotropic effect*, with a positive effect referring to an increased rate and a negative effect referring to a decreased rate. Alteration in heart rate is a significant factor in changes of cardiac output.

Phases of the Cardiac Cycle

The cardiac cycle is defined by one complete period of contraction (systole) and relaxation (diastole). Table 15-3 describes some terms essential in understanding the cardiac cycle. The events of the cardiac cycle from the atria through the ventricles during systole and diastole follow.

ATRIAL FILLING AND CONTRACTION. As the atria receive blood from the incoming veins, blood accumulates in these structures until ventricular pressures fall below atrial pressures. As the atrial pressure rises, the flow of blood passively opens the AV valves and enters the ventricles. Approximately 70% of blood flow from the atria to the ventricles occurs passively. Atrial contraction, which follows atrial depolarization from the SA pathways, provides the "atrial kick" to move the remaining atrial blood into the ventricles.

VENTRICULAR FILLING, CONTRACTION, AND RELAXATION. Rapid ventricular filling occurs after the AV valves open. Blood moves into the ventricles passively and then actively in response to the atrial kick. Ventricular depo-

TABLE 15-3

TERMS USED TO DEFINE THE CARDIAC CYCLE

TERM	DEFINITION
Cardiac output	Amount of blood pumped from heart/ minute; cardiac output = stroke volume × heart rate; normal = 4–8 L/min
Cardiac index	Cardiac output indexed to square meters of body surface area; normal = 2.5–4.0 L/min/m^2
Stroke volume	Amount of blood ejected from each ventricle beat; this is not all of the blood in each ventricle, but about 60–75% of the volume, and is called the *ejection fraction*
End-diastolic volume	Amount of blood in the ventricle just before systole
Ejection fraction	Ratio of stroke volume to end-diastolic volume. Measure of left ventricular function; normal = 67 ± 9%
Isovolumic contraction	Period of ventricular pressure rise prior to opening of semilunar valves
Ejection	Period when ventricular pressure exceeds arterial pressure, and blood is ejected from heart
Incisura	Inscription of a pressure recording that occurs when aortic valve closes; caused by a momentary reversal of pressures between aorta and left ventricle
Isovolumic relaxation	Rapid drop of pressure in ventricles toward diastolic pressure. Occurs prior to opening of atrioventricular valves and ventricular filling
Systole	Contraction of the heart
Diastole	Relaxation of the heart

larization and contraction occur from the conduction pathways and Purkinje activation of the muscle. Ventricular systole occurs in discrete phases:

1. Ventricular pressure begins to rise, causing increased tension around the AV valve structures and closure of the mitral and tricuspid valves. This *isovolumic contraction* period occupies the time between onset of ventricular contraction and opening of the semilunar valves.[14]
2. The ventricles eject blood when the pressure in the ventricles exceeds the diastolic pressures maintained in the aorta and the pulmonary artery. This increased pressure opens the semilunar valves, allowing blood to flow into the arteries. This period is termed *rapid ventricular ejection*.
3. After ejection of the stroke volume, the pressure in the ventricles begins to fall. At a certain point, the pressure falls below the arterial diastolic pressure and the semilunar valves close. On a pressure tracing, closure of the aortic valve is indicated by the *incisura* or *aortic dicrotic notch*. The *isovolumic relaxation phase* occurs as pressure continues to descend in the ventricles toward the low diastolic pressure. This lasts until the pressure in the ventricles falls below the atrial pressure, when rapid ventricular filling begins again. Figure 15-11 summarizes the events of the cardiac cycle.

The mechanical events occur at the same time in both the right and left sides of the heart. Normally, right and left ventricular outputs are equal, even though the stroke volumes between the chambers may vary slightly. Respiratory excursion, for example, may cause a temporary increase in right ventricular output. When the left ventricle receives this increased volume, however, it increases its output to balance the minute cardiac output.

Figure 15-12 shows some significant differences between the chambers in terms of pressures and oxygen saturations. It can be readily seen that left-sided pressures exceed the right. The aortic systolic and diastolic pressures are much higher than those in the pulmonary artery. The diastolic pressure in both ventricles is normally very low, approaching zero. The oxygen saturations also show a significant change from the arterial to the venous circulations.

Heart Sounds

The normal heart produces two major distinct sounds: S_1, the first heart sound or mitral sound, and S_2, the second heart sound or aortic sound. The S_1 occurs when the ventricles begin contraction, at the beginning of cardiac systole. It has always been attributed to closure of the AV valves but that may or may not be a component of the sound. Acceleration and deceleration of blood with tensing of the valve structures and cardiac vibrations probably produces the S_1.[18] Normally, this sound is best heard in the fifth intercostal space in the midclavicular line (the apex) (Fig. 15-13).

The S_2 is mainly due to closure of the semilunar valves. It has two components: the aortic and pulmonary closure sounds. During the inspiratory phase of respiration, venous return to the right side of the heart increases, which increases the volume in the right ventricle and thereby increases right ventricular ejection time. The pulmonary valve closes slightly after the aortic valve, producing a physiologic splitting sound. This split is more obvious in young persons and during hyperventilation. This sound is best heard in the aortic and pulmonary areas at the second intercostal spaces (see Fig. 15-13).

The third heart sound, S_3 (ventricular gallop), may be normally heard in young children but is usually pathologic in adults. When heard, the S_3 occurs after the S_2. It results from tensing of the chordae and AV ring during the end of the rapid-filling phase.[13] The S_3 is most frequently heard when a dilated ventricle or volume overload is present, especially with heart failure.

The fourth heart sound, S_4 (atrial gallop), occurs with increased ventricular pressure during atrial contraction. It is heard immediately before S_1 and may be associated with hypertension or decreased ventricular compliance. Both S_3 and S_4 are heard best at the apex with the bell portion of the stethoscope.

Other sounds may be heard with pathology of the heart and its valves. Figure 15-14 phonetically illustrates the common normal and abnormal heart sounds.

Myocardial Work

Myocardial work is generated by the ventricular wall tension during systole. This wall tension creates the pressure to eject blood into the arteries. Cardiac work is often expressed in terms of **myocardial oxygen consumption**. The amount of oxygen consumed is closely related to the amount of stress developed in the ventricular wall. The major factors that affect oxygen consumption include the amount of myocardial muscle mass, the contractile or inotropic state, the heart rate, and the intramyocardial tension generated.[14] The total oxygen supply for the work of myocardial muscle is delivered by the blood from the coronary arteries. Myocardial oxygen extraction of up to 70% leaves little oxygen reserve. Increased delivery of oxygen is needed in stress situations because of enhanced contractility and tachycardia that are induced by the catecholamines, especially epinephrine. Figure 15-15 illustrates the oxygen extraction of various body organs.

Cardiac Reserve

Cardiac reserve refers to the ability of cardiac output to increase to match increases in metabolic demand. Cardiac output can increase five- to sixfold during exercise.[11] The mechanisms it uses to do so include changes in heart rate and stroke volume, increased oxygen extraction, cardiac dilatation, and hypertrophy.

Increases in heart rate enhance the cardiac output within certain physiologic limits. Increasing the rate of

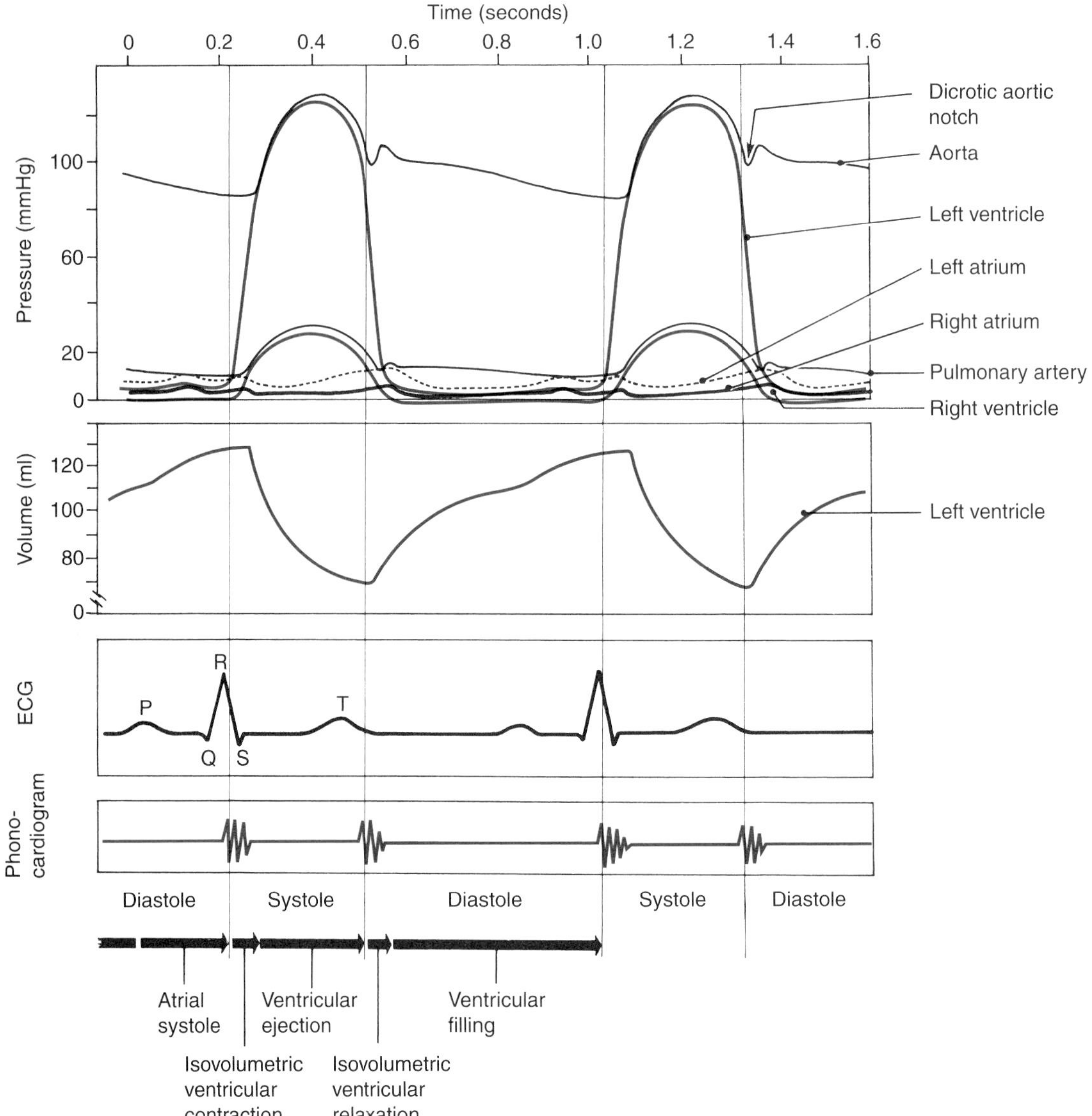

FIGURE 15-11. **Events of the cardiac cycle indicating changes in volume and pressure related to the electrocardiogram and heart sounds.**

contraction and maintaining the stroke volume will also increase the cardiac output. Increased heart rate results from increased sympathetic nervous effect (see p. 421). Heart rate is the main mechanism that changes during exercise and through tachycardia cardiac output increases two to three times.

The stroke volume is approximately 70 to 100 mL. In the normal person this amount relates to size, fitness level, and age. During exercise, venous return to the heart increases along with the stroke volume, adding to the increased cardiac output achieved by tachycardia. A good indicator of the heart's ability to maintain contractility is the relationship between the end-diastolic volume and the stroke volume. This result is called the **ejection fraction,** measured as a percentile (normally about 60–75%).[11] In other words, if the ventricle receives 100 mL of blood during a cardiac cycle, it should pump out 60 to 75 mL with each beat. In the normal heart, increased return of blood to the heart usually causes an increased ejection fraction through the Starling principle described earlier. A decrease in ejection fraction is the hallmark of ventricular failure because the ventricle is unable to pump effectively (see p. 474).

Oxygen extraction is the percent of oxygen that is extracted from the blood as it passes through the tissues. Many systemic tissues extract a greater percent of oxy-

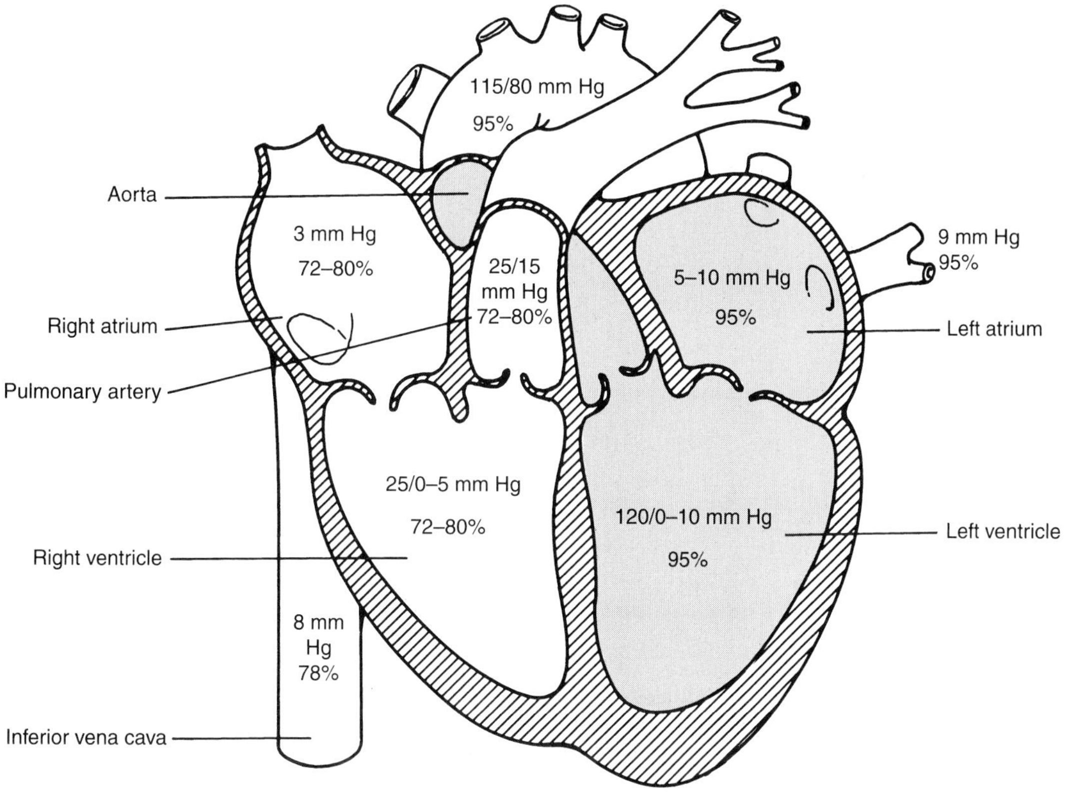

FIGURE 15-12. Normal pressures and oxygen saturated on the hemoglobin as found in the great vessels and cardiac chambers.

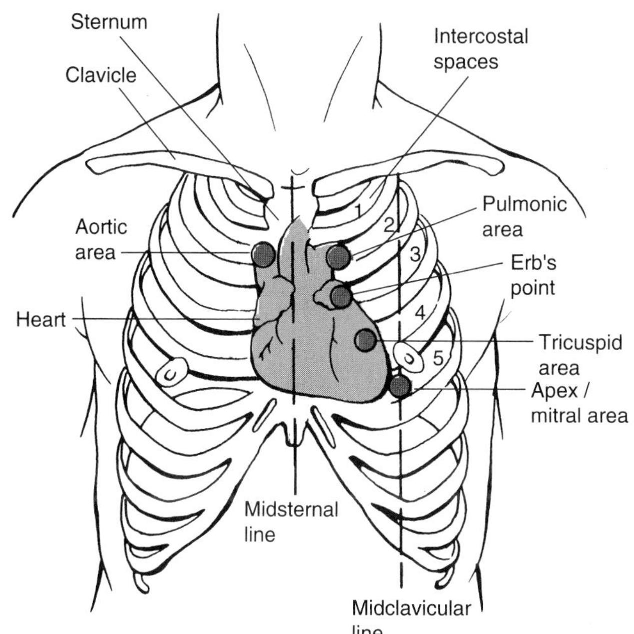

FIGURE 15-13. Locations of the auscultatory points for the various heart sounds. Note that the mitral sound is heard directly over the point of maximal impulse (PMI), which is also the apex of the heart (normally at about the midclavicular line).

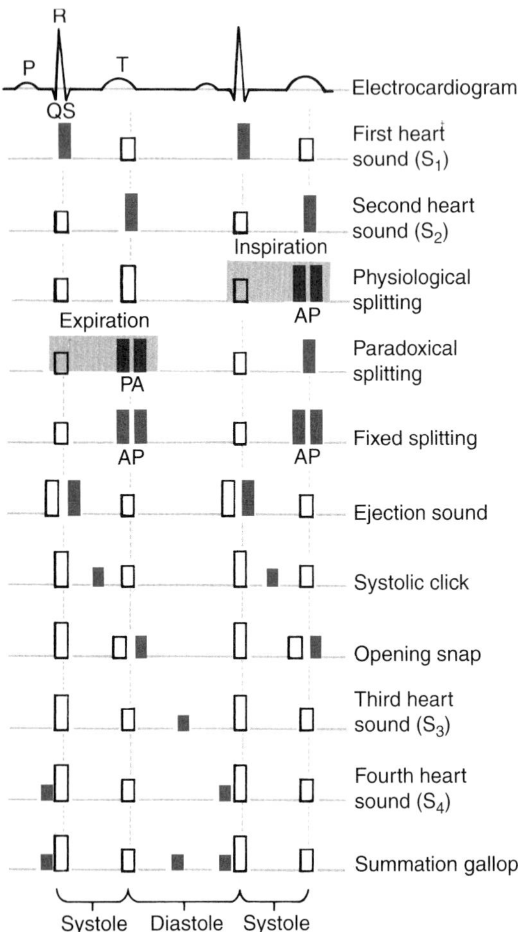

FIGURE 15-14. **Illustration of the heart sound related to the electrocardiogram. Some normal and pathologic sounds are illustrated.**

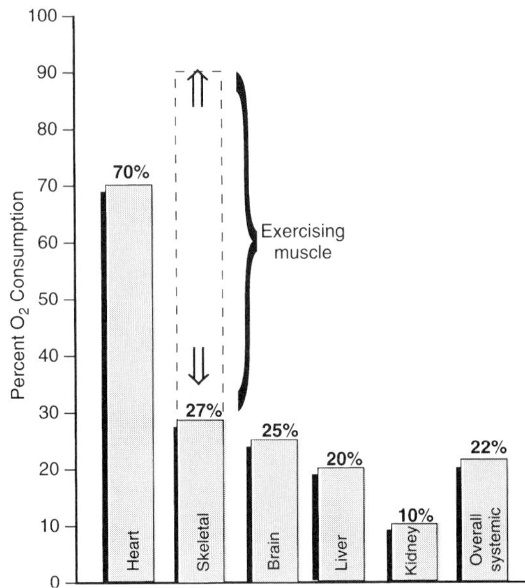

FIGURE 15-15. **Normally the brain extracts 25% of the oxygen delivered to it. The liver, kidney and systemic cells take 10–20%. The skeletal muscle oxygen extraction depends upon whether it is resting or exercising. The heart normally extracts 70–75% of oxygen delivered to it.**

gen from the blood to increase tissue oxygenation to meet metabolic demand. At rest the heart already extracts about 70% to 75% of its supplied oxygen so this mechanism is of less use to the heart during periods of increased demand than to the systemic tissues.[14]

Systemically, the *redistribution of cardiac output* helps to maintain vital tissue perfusion in increased demand situations. During such periods, maintaining blood flow to the brain, heart, and tissues that acutely require blood flow results in decreased blood flow to less essential areas.[14] The two main mechanisms for redistribution of blood flow in the heart are apparently local autoregulation and ANS control. **Autoregulation** is the mechanism by which coronary blood flow remains constant. It involves a myogenic mechanism, arteriolar vasodilatation, and local chemical regulation through vasodilator substances, especially carbon dioxide, hydrogen, potassium, and prostaglandins. The *autonomic nervous system* increases or decreases heart rate either through sympathetic or parasympathetic nervous system activation.

Cardiac dilatation and *hypertrophy* are compensatory mechanisms for overload situations. Temporary dilatation results in the Starling principle of enhanced contractility, but continued dilatation is a classic sign of heart failure. Hypertrophy results mainly when the work that the heart must perform consistently increases. Hypertension is the most frequent cause of hypertrophy (see p. 447).

Myocardial Perfusion

Changes in aortic pressure mainly regulate coronary blood flow. Filling of the coronary arteries occurs following closure of the aortic valve and filling of the sinuses of Valsalva, early in diastole. The perfusion pressure is normally maintained by an adequate mean arterial pressure of 90 to 100 mm Hg. A close parallel exists between the level of myocardial metabolic activity and coronary blood flow. A decrease in the ratio of oxygen supply to oxygen demand releases a vasodilator substance that decreases coronary arteriolar resistance.[2] The vasodilator may be adenosine, which is released with hypoxemia or increased metabolic activity of the heart. Substantial mechanical dysfunction, called myocardial stunning, may be seen after short periods of myocardial ischemia. A combination of calcium overload and generation of hydroxyl and superoxide free radicals may be the cause of the impaired myocardial contractility[6] (see p. 467).

AUTONOMIC INFLUENCES ON CARDIAC ACTIVITY

The divisions of the ANS, sympathetic and parasympathetic, exert external influences on myocardial contractility and rate. The cardiovascular center in the medulla receives input from other areas of the brain and relays messages throughout the body. In the heart, such messages include the ANS adjustment of the heart rate and contractility to the body's demands. The ANS has an enhancing or restraining effect on the inherent pacemaker system and can alter the automaticity of abnormal pacemaker systems.

Sympathetic Nervous System

The chemical mediators of the SNS are norepinephrine and epinephrine, collectively called **catecholamines**. The SNS releases these mediators during the stress reaction. These mediators stimulate α- and β-adrenergic receptors on target cells, which cause specific effects (see p. 900). Receptors from the SNS are present in the atrial wall, ventricles, and SA and AV nodes. When stimulated, these cardioaccelerator fibers release *norepinephrine*, which stimulates β_1-receptors to increase the rate of depolarization and impulse transmission through the conduction tissue.[2] Increased sympathetic tone increases cardiac rate and the contractility of myocardial muscle. The increased contractility is due to enhanced calcium entry through the myocardial muscle calcium channels.[11,14] SNS stimulation predominantly affects the SA node and causes a sinus tachycardia such as that seen in response to exercise or fear. Stimulation of the SNS also can increase the irritability of myocardial muscle cells, causing abnormal or early depolarization, such as with premature atrial or ventricular contractions. These abnormal stimuli are usually referred to as *ectopic foci* because their effects are from an AP outside the normal conduction system (see p. 455).

The effects of the SNS on the coronary arteries are somewhat more complex. Norepinephrine causes coronary artery vasoconstriction and increased oxygen extraction by the myocardial cell. Some individuals have a hyperactive response to norepinephrine and exhibit coronary artery vasospasm during stressful situations. Ischemia results and causes the liberation of metabolites that, in turn, can cause vasodilation. The reaction may lead to angina pectoris and even myocardial infarction. *Epinephrine*, which is released from the adrenal glands, has a secondary dilating action on the coronary arteries. Its main actions are to produce tachycardia and increase contractility (a positive inotropic effect).

Prostaglandins, a group of chemically related substances, may be stimulated secondarily in the sympathetic stress response. They are synthesized by the myocardial cells and arteries and usually dilate the coronary arteries.[10,11]

Normally, autoregulation of coronary blood flow appears to counteract the effects of neural stimulation. The changes of perfusion pressure are counteracted by changes in vascular resistance, so that blood flow remains rather constant. Autoregulation is probably due to the response of smooth muscle in the arterioles to stretch, so that when the local blood pressure rises the vessels constrict, and when it falls, they dilate.[11] When SNS stimulation induces coronary vasoconstriction, coronary autoregulation usually overrides the mechanism and ischemia is prevented.[6]

Parasympathetic Nervous System

The PSNS is mediated through the chemical transmitter *acetylcholine*, which is released from vagal fibers. The major effects of vagal stimulation are a restraining or slowing influence on the SA node, atrial muscle, and AV node. Vagal stimulation slows the heart rate by restraining the rate of diastolic depolarization in the conduction tissue. It causes only a slight decrease in ventricular contractility.

A balance exists between SNS and PSNS stimulation of the heart, but the predominant system appears to be the PSNS. Evidence supporting this is that resting heart rate is usually lower than the inherent automatic SA pacing rate.[4]

BARORECEPTORS

Baroreceptors are pressure-sensitive structures present mostly in the carotid sinus and the aortic arch (Fig. 15-16). Decreased systolic blood pressure causes a reflex sympathetic response with increased pulse, increased contractility, and vasoconstriction. Increased pressure stimulates stretch receptors and causes a reflex vagal response, which decreases heart rate and passive vasodilation in the systemic arterioles.[16] This explains the significant bradycardia seen during episodes of acute increase in blood pressure.

There is also a reflex, called *Bainbridge reflex*, which responds to venous pressure. The receptor for this reflex is located in the right atrium and venae cavae. When the pressure is increased, nervous impulses are sent to the medulla. The SNS is stimulated to increase the rate and force of the cardiac contraction.[12] Whether this reflex is due to blocking of the vagal impulses or atrial stretch receptors is unknown. The significance of the reflex is questionable.[10]

CHEMORECEPTORS

The body's major chemoreceptor is the *medulla oblongata*, but special receptors are also located in the *carotid* and *aortic bodies*. Chemical changes in the blood, especially in pH, carbon dioxide, and oxygen levels, alter cardiac and respiratory activity. Respiratory changes

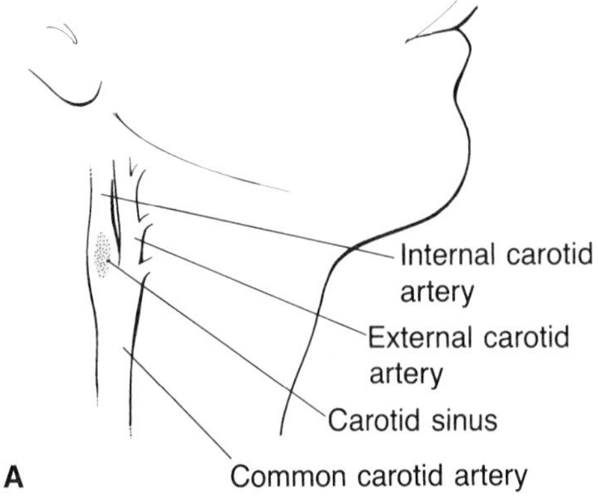

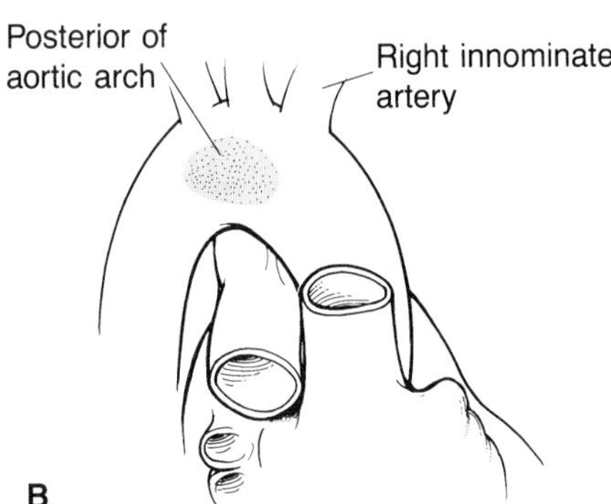

FIGURE 15-16. **Location of the baroreceptors in (A) the carotid sinus area, and (B) the aortic arch area.**

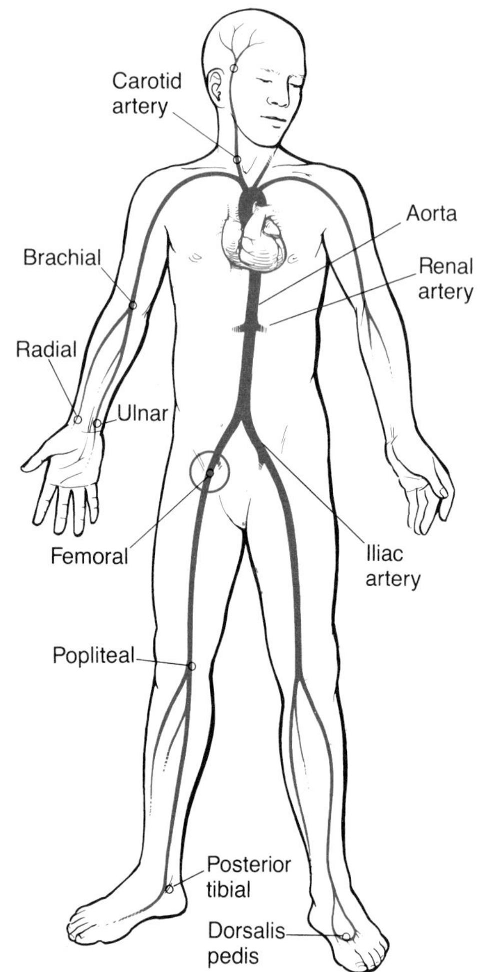

FIGURE 15-17. **Major systemic arteries of the body. The circles represent points at which the pulse can be palpated.**

are detailed on page 535. Cardiac effects result from a reflex sympathetic discharge or inhibition. Discharge occurs with increased Pa_{CO_2} levels sensed by the medulla oblongata or decreased oxygen levels sensed by the carotid and aortic bodies. Sympathetic discharge results in tachycardia, vasoconstriction, and increased myocardial contractility. Sympathetic inhibition results from decreased Pa_{CO_2} and increased pH. These serve to reduce the vasoconstrictor effect, leading to passive vasodilatation.[16]

SYSTEMIC CIRCULATION

The systemic circulation consists of the arteries and veins that circulate blood to and from the tissues. The systemic arteries supply oxygen to the cells of all of the organs, while the systemic veins carry carbon dioxide and waste products of cellular metabolism back to the lungs (see Fig. 15-5).

Structure of the Systemic Circulation

ARTERIES

Figure 15-17 shows the main arteries of the body. Arteries are less numerous and have thicker walls than veins. The largest systemic artery is the *aorta*. The aorta divides into medium-sized arteries, which then divide into smaller arteries, which finally become the smallest arteries, called *arterioles*.

The arteries are composed of three layers: *tunica intima, tunica media, and tunica externa* or *adventitia* (Fig. 15-18). The layers contain variable amounts of collagen and muscle fibers according to the type of artery. Basically, however, the outer coat supports or gives shape to the vessel, the middle or muscular coat regulates the vessel's diameter, and the inner coat provides a smooth passageway for blood flow.

The large arteries are called *elastic vessels* because they can stretch or increase their width to receive the stroke volume of the heart and then contract or resume their original shape, pushing the blood forward. The *nutrient arteries* are branches of the elastic vessels; they supply oxygen and nutrients to the organs and tissues. The ar-

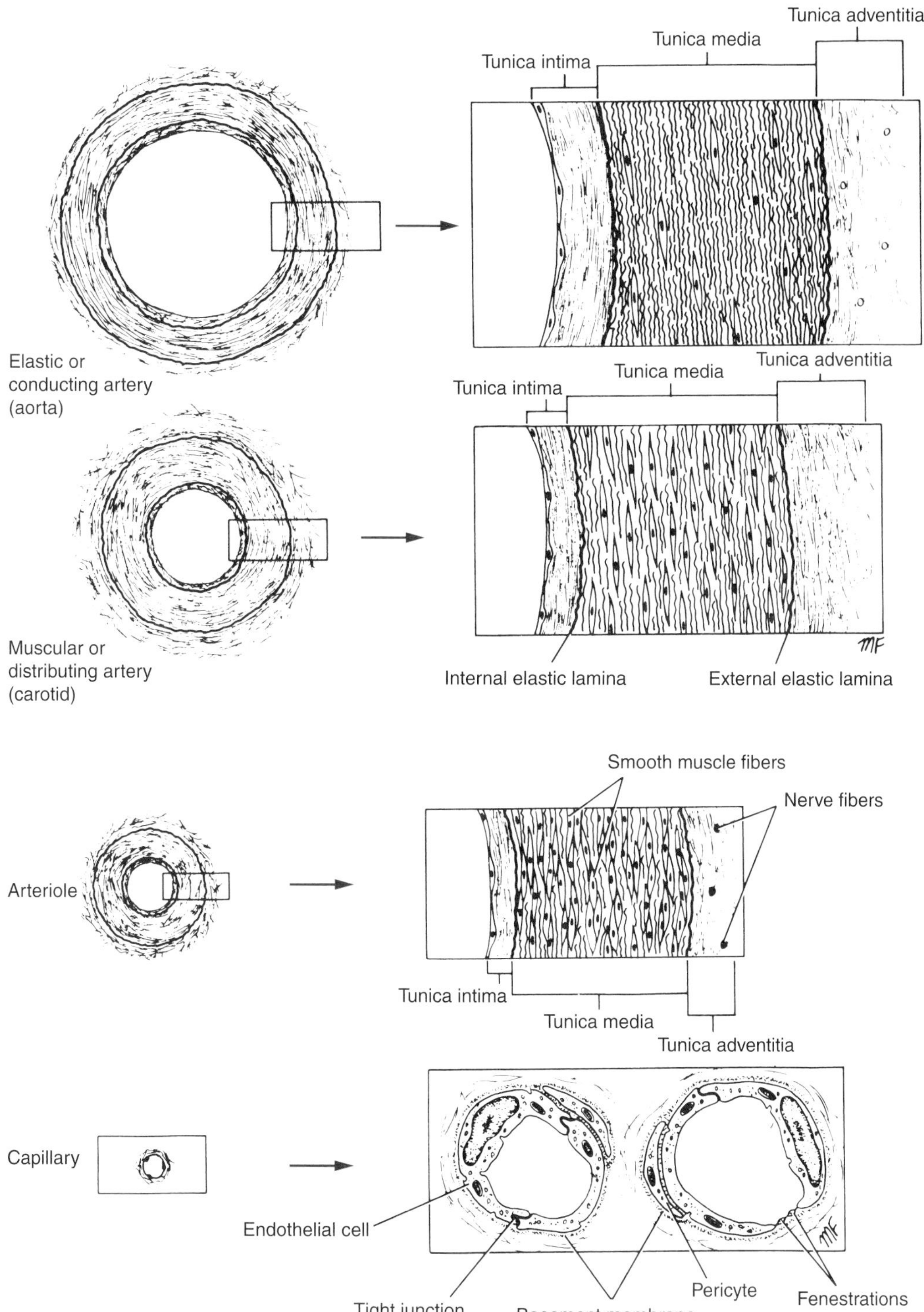

FIGURE 15-18. **Layers of the aorta, artery, arterioles, and capillary.**

terioles lead into the capillary bed. The arterioles offer varying degrees of resistance to circulating blood by constricting or dilating, which regulates the volume and pressure in the artery and the capillary bed.

CAPILLARIES

A network of tiny blood vessels provides the microcirculation through which materials enter or leave the circulating blood. A *capillary* consists of a single layer of endothelial cells that line up in such a way as to allow for exchange of fluids, dissolved gases, and small molecules. The capillaries hold back large molecules, such as the plasma proteins, to provide oncotic pressure (see p. 161). Capillary pressures differ among organs and systems.

VEINS

Figure 15-19 illustrates the major veins of the body. These veins vary in anatomic position in different persons. The smallest veins are the venules, which receive their blood from the capillaries. These vessels have very thin walls through which some nutrients and oxygen may leave and waste products may enter. Capillaries and venules are often called **exchange vessels**. Venules join together to form veins. Veins contain approximately 75% of circulating blood volume at any one time. Because they have the capability to stretch and hold blood, they are called **capacitance vessels**. The larger veins have valves, which are endothelial flaps or folds interspersed along their inner surface (Fig. 15-20). These valves prevent the backflow of blood and are numerous in the lower extremities, especially in skeletal muscle areas.

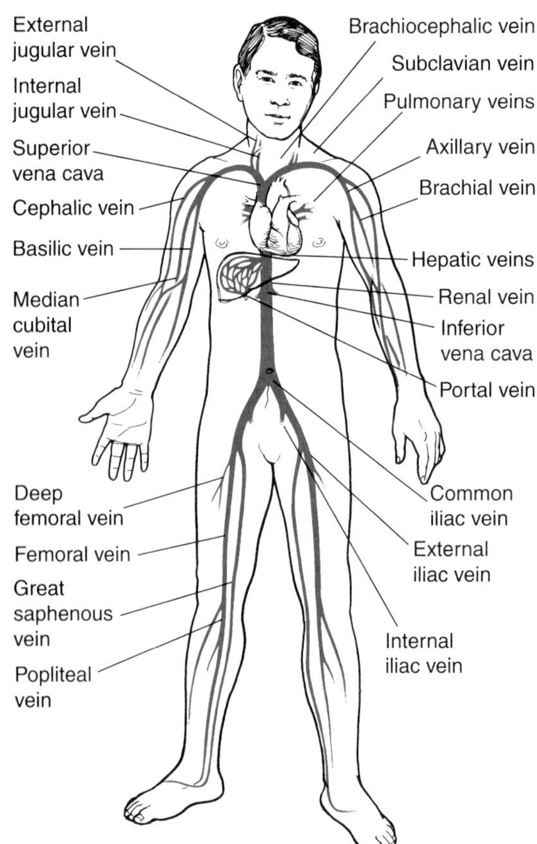

FIGURE 15-19. Some systemic veins of the body.

LYMPHATIC CIRCULATION

The lymphatic circulation is a secondary route to move fluids from tissues and into the circulation. Lymph vessels begin as blind-ended capillaries. They connect the lymph nodes and provide a secondary circulatory system. Approximately 2 liters of fluid remains in the interstitial spaces every day, which diffuses into the lymph capillaries. The lymph vessels effectively remove any excess plasma proteins that have leaked into the interstitial area.

The movement of lymph through the large lymphatic vessels occurs because of arterial pulsations and muscle movement. The lymphatic vessel valves prevent backflow. Lymph flow in the thoracic duct is approximately 1.3 mL/kg body weight per hour.[11] If the lymphatic circulation is decreased or blocked, *lymphedema* (edema of high-protein content) occurs (see page 165).

Function of the Systemic Circulation

FACTORS CONTROLLING ARTERIAL CIRCULATION

Arterial blood pressure is determined by cardiac output and resistance to blood flow. The highest pressure is the *systolic pressure*, which is achieved by the contracting left ventricle in the ejection of its stroke volume. The *diastolic pressure*, maintained or stored as potential energy in the aorta during diastole, permits a continuous forward flow of blood. The difference between the systolic and diastolic pressures is the **pulse pressure**. The *mean arterial pressure* is the average pressure maintained in the aorta (see p. 415).

Blood pressure changes as blood courses down the arteries, being highest in the aorta and lowest in the capillary system. Vasoconstriction in the arterioles increases diastolic pressure (because of increased **total peripheral** or **systemic vascular resistance**; TPR or SVR) and decreases capillary pressure (see below). Arteriolar vasodilatation causes decreased diastolic pressure (decreased TPR or SVR) and increased capillary pressure. The terminal portion of the arteriole contains precapillary sphincters that constrict and relax with autonomic stimulation or with local changes in temperature, pH, and oxygen levels.

The sounds described in auscultating blood pressure are called *Korotkoff sounds* (Fig. 15-21). They are generated after placement of a cuff around an extremity

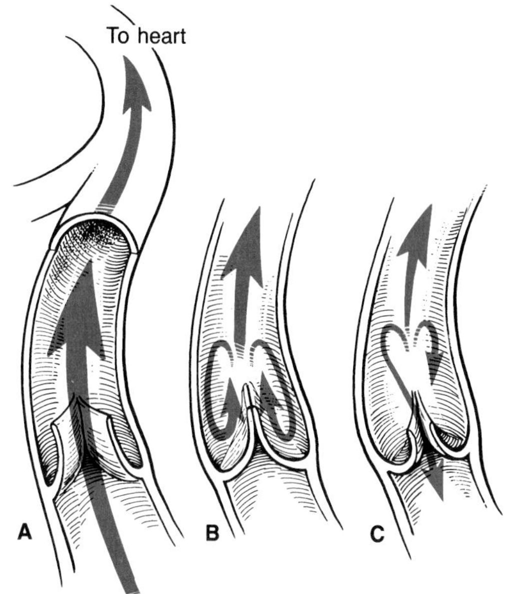
To heart
A
B
C

FIGURE 15-20. **Valves of the larger systemic veins. A. Blood can move forward through the valves to the heart. B, C. Valves distend with blood and close to prevent backflow, which causes perpetual movement of blood toward the heart. Blood moves from higher pressure to the lower pressure produced by the negative intrathoracic pressure and the low pressure in the right atrium.**

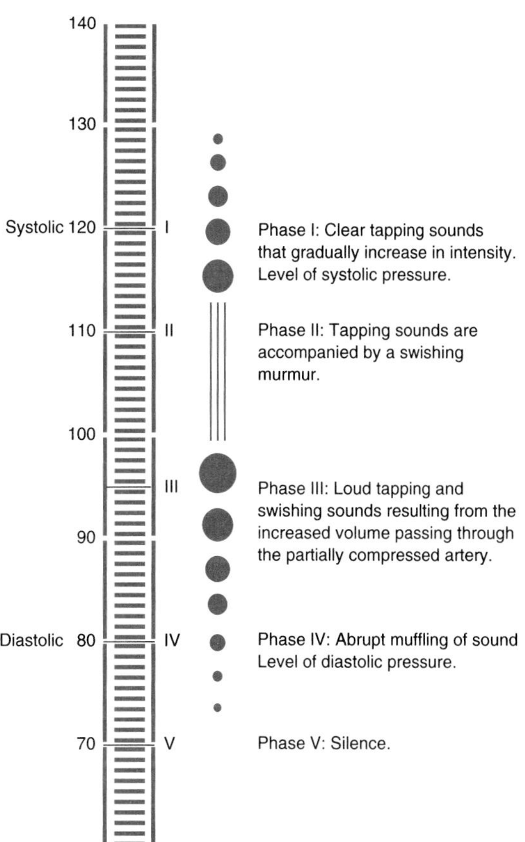
140
130
Systolic 120
110
100
90
Diastolic 80
70
I
II
III
IV
V
Phase I: Clear tapping sounds that gradually increase in intensity. Level of systolic pressure.
Phase II: Tapping sounds are accompanied by a swishing murmur.
Phase III: Loud tapping and swishing sounds resulting from the increased volume passing through the partially compressed artery.
Phase IV: Abrupt muffling of sound Level of diastolic pressure.
Phase V: Silence.

FIGURE 15-21. **Korotkoff sounds. A compression cuff is placed over a peripheral artery and the pressure is increased to the level of occlusion of the artery. As the pressure is gradually released, the typical sounds are auscultated. Phases I through V are described.**

with pressure sufficient to occlude blood flow. As the cuff pressure is released, the beating sounds begin when the pressure falls below the systolic blood pressure. As the cuff pressure is continually released, the sounds become muffled and disappear at the point of diastolic pressure. It is generally appreciated that an error of 8 to 10 mm Hg (systolic pressure underestimated by 4 to 5 mm Hg and diastolic pressure overestimated by the same amount) occurs with this indirect measurement.[10] The sounds are basically produced by turbulence of blood flow through the constricted segment. Flow of blood in an unconstricted artery is silent.

The pulse pressure normally is about 50 mm Hg. High systolic and low diastolic pressures increase or widen the pulse pressure. Low systolic and high diastolic pressures decrease or narrow the pulse pressure. Increased pulse pressure is usually the result of increased stroke volume, decreased peripheral volume, or decreased SVR. These factors might occur during exercise, fever, with aortic insufficiency, or sometimes with atherosclerosis. A narrowed pulse pressure can occur with increased SVR, decreased cardiac output, hypovolemia, or other conditions.

Determinants of Blood Pressure

Contraction of the left ventricle moves its stroke volume into the aorta. The left ventricle pumps against the elastic resistance of the aortic wall, the resistance offered by the arterioles, and the residual volume in the aorta. Therefore, direct determinants of arterial blood pressure include cardiac output, vascular resistance, aortic impedance (resistance to flow), and diastolic arterial volume.

The activity of the ANS and the renin–angiotensin–aldosterone system also influence blood pressure levels (see p. 449). Variations of blood pressure occur with normal daily activities. Body posture, muscular activity, emotions, and use of tobacco, coffee, and vasoactive drugs also influence blood pressure.

CARDIAC OUTPUT. The amount of blood ejected from the heart is partly determined by the length of end-diastolic fibers. Changes in stroke volume vary in healthy persons and increased ventricular volume at the end of diastole will, of itself, produce a stronger ventricular contraction. If an individual is hypovolemic, the decreased end-diastolic fiber length leads to a decrease in the force of ventricular contraction and, subsequently, a decrease in cardiac output and blood pressure.

VASCULAR RESISTANCE. Vascular resistance is often called systemic vascular resistance (SVR) or total peripheral resistance (TPR) and refers to the impedance that the arterioles offer to blood flow. The major factor that determines SVR from a major artery is the caliber or radius of the arteriole. Constriction of the arterioles increases resistance and raises the blood pressure. Dilatation of the arterioles decreases resistance and decreases blood pressure.[11] Stimulation of the sympathetic nerves causes vasoconstriction, a mechanism that is important in blood pressure elevations with exercise or fear. Humoral mechanisms can increase or decrease SVR. Prostaglandins, renin, kinins, and many other substances are under study in relation to their regulation of SVR.

AORTIC IMPEDANCE. Aortic impedance is offered by the elastic aortic wall and the aortic valve. The aortic valve normally remains closed until the pressure in the left ventricle exceeds the pressure maintained in the aorta. After this occurs, the valve opens and the ventricle must pump against the resistance offered by the elastic aortic wall. When elasticity increases, such as with aging, more aortic impedance is offered to the left ventricle. Also, with narrowing of the aortic valve, impedance requires an increased ventricular force to eject its contents.

DIASTOLIC ARTERIAL VOLUME. The amount of blood remaining in the aorta on diastole is related to the factors mentioned above. If cardiac output is increased and SVR is also elevated, increased amounts of blood remain in the arterial circuit during diastole. Increased amounts of blood usually increase diastolic pressure and resistance against which the ventricle has to pump. If cardiac output is increased and SVR is decreased, the "run-off" (flow of blood down a pressure gradient) decreases the diastolic volume and resistance against which the heart is pumping.

FACTORS CONTROLLING VENOUS CIRCULATION

Blood in the veins does not normally pulsate as it does in arteries. Movement of blood from the systemic veins to the heart is due to (1) pressure differences; (2) skeletal, thoracic, and visceral muscle pressures; and (3) valves that prevent the backflow of blood. Pulsations may be seen in the jugular veins, which reflect the activity of the right atrium and right ventricle. Abnormalities in venous circulation can result from many conditions, such as fluid overloading, venous insufficiency, and constrictive pericarditis.

Venous return to the heart depends on the following interrelated factors[2]:

1. *Pressure difference* from venules to the right atrium. The average pressure at the level of the systemic venules is 16 mm Hg; this decreases to about 0 mm Hg at the level of the right atrium. Blood flow then moves along its pressure differential from higher to lower.
2. *The skeletal muscle pump* moves blood back to the right atrium as the muscle movement, in an action called *milking*, opens the proximal valves and closes the distal valves. A continual forward movement of blood occurs (Fig. 15-22).
3. *Via the respiratory pump* the normal processes of inspiration and expiration generate pressure differences in the thoracic cavity. Increased negativity produced during inspiration pulls blood toward the heart.
4. *The venous valves* prevent backflow that might occur with gravitational forces and with increased thoracic pressures.

PULMONARY CIRCULATION

Structure of the Pulmonary Circulation

The pulmonary circulation is composed of the pulmonary artery, smaller pulmonary arteries, arterioles, capillaries, venules, and pulmonary veins. These vessels carry systemic or less oxygenated blood from the right

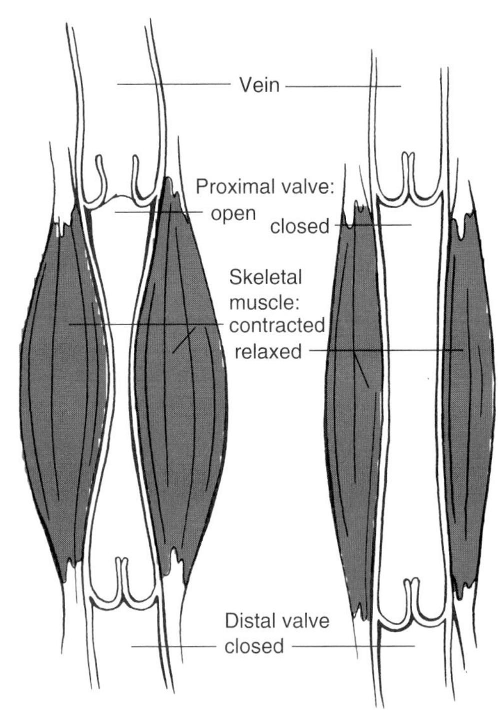

FIGURE 15-22. The skeletal muscle pump returns blood to the heart by a massaging motion that compresses the vein, opens the proximal valve, and closes the distal valve. When the muscle relaxes, both valves are closed. The net effect is a continual forward movement of blood.

side of the heart to be oxygenated in the pulmonary capillary bed. The blood then returns to the left side of the heart, where it is circulated to the body.

The pulmonary circulation depends on the pulmonary arterial circuit, which carries blood from the right ventricle to the pulmonary artery to the smaller pulmonary arteries and the pulmonary arterioles. In the extensive pulmonary capillary bed, exchange of oxygen and carbon dioxide occurs between the vessels and the alveoli. From the capillary system, pulmonary venules become pulmonary veins and finally the four pulmonary veins enter the left atrium of the heart, carrying oxygenated blood. Because pressures in the pulmonary system are low, pulmonary arteries have larger diameters, thinner walls, and less elastic tissue than do systemic arteries (see p. 422).

Function of the Pulmonary Circulation

The purpose of the pulmonary circulation is to remove carbon dioxide carried in and on the red blood cells and to saturate the hemoglobin of the red blood cells with oxygen. The carbon dioxide moves across the alveolocapillary membrane into the alveoli and is exhaled. Through a net diffusion of oxygen from the alveoli across the membrane to the pulmonary capillary system,

TABLE 15-4

TERMS RELATING TO NORMAL ELECTROPHYSIOLOGY AND CARDIAC DYSRHYTHMIAS

TERM	DEFINITION
Absolute refractory period	Period where cardiac cell cannot accept any stimulus, regardless of intensity, to initiate an impulse
Accessory pathway	An extra or analogous pathway bypassing the AV node
Action potential	A change in electrical activity along the cell membrane initiating an impulse; each cardiac cell has five phases: 0, 1, 2, 3, and 4
Automaticity	Electrical property of cardiac cells that permits spontaneous depolarization generating an electrical impulse; groups of these automatic cells make up the heart's primary pacemakers: SA node, AV node, and ventricles
Circus movement	Continuous stimulation of the myocardium through conduction pathways within the myocardium
Conduction	Flow of electrical impulses through the cardiac conduction system. Normal conduction occurs in this way from the SA node to the ventricles
Aberrant conduction	Impulses that are abnormally conducted through the ventricles due to a delay in the refractory period in the bundle branches; seen on the ECG as a change in QRS morphology
Antegrade conduction	Impulses flow forward through the conduction system
Retrograde conduction	Impulses flow backward through the conduction system
Compensatory pause	A pause that occurs after a premature complex; a premature beat that does not interrupt the cardiac cycle is a full compensatory pause and is equal to twice the R to R interval between two normal beats
Reentry	Phenomenon where an impulse returns to reexcite a previously stimulated region of the myocardium through a pathway; usually the impulse is sinus or ectopic in origin and occurs in an area of slowed conduction with unequal response time in the myocardium
Rhythm	
Active rhythm	A rhythm stimulated by a premature ectopic focus that maintains a rate faster than a normal pacemaker and assumes control of cardiac rhythm regardless of the underlying rhythm
Ectopic rhythm	Impulses that originate outside of the SA node due to the inability of the SA node to generate an impulse
Normal sinus rhythm	A series of impulses generated by the SA node and conducted through the conduction system in a normal fashion
Passive rhythm	Impulses generated by a lower pacemaker when the primary pacemakers slow or fail; also termed as escape rhythm

AV, atrioventricular; ECG, electrocardiogram; SA, sinoatrial.

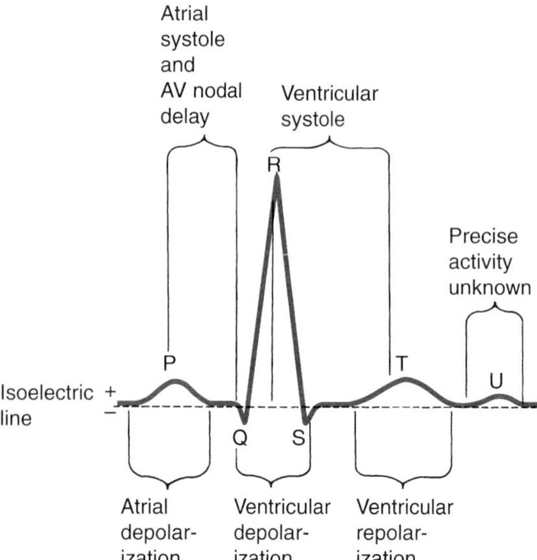

FIGURE 15-23. **Correlation of mechanical and electrical activity within the heart.**

oxygen is made available to be saturated on the hemoglobin (see page 541). The now oxygen-saturated hemoglobin is transported in the blood to the left heart where it is pumped to the systemic tissues and released.

The pressures in the pulmonary arterial circuit are much lower than in the systemic circuit, but they are maintained in much the same way as are systemic arterial pressures. Constriction of the pulmonary arterioles increases the pulmonary vascular resistance and the right ventricle increases its pressure to empty its contents. Dilatation of the vessels decreases the resistance to the right ventricle. More detail on hemoglobin saturation and pulmonary dynamics is given in Chapters 12 and 19.

CARDIOVASCULAR DIAGNOSTIC PROCEDURES

Many diagnostic procedures are used in the differential diagnosis of cardiovascular diseases. They include blood studies and noninvasive and invasive diagnostic studies (see Unit 4 Appendices A, B, and C).

Electrocardiogram

The ECG graphically depicts the electrical events of the cardiac cycle. The waveforms produced are of (1) the electrical activity (AP) generated as electrical impulses spread through the conduction system, and (2) the recovery of myocardial cells following depolarization. Table 15-4 defines terms relating to normal electrophysiology and cardiac dysrhythmias. Further discussion of dysrhythmias is found on page 455. Figure 15-23 correlates the appearance of the ECG to electrical and mechanical events in the heart.

BASICS OF THE ELECTROCARDIOGRAM

The heart's conduction system creates an electrical field that is distributed to the body surfaces and recorded as specific waveforms. SA node depolarization is inscribed as the P wave. The PR interval is the time it takes for the impulse to traverse the atria and the AV node. As the impulse travels down the bundle of His, bundle branches, and Purkinje fibers, the QRS complex is formed. Finally, the T wave represents repolarization. Figure 15-24 shows the normal appearance of a single cardiac cycle recorded in the lead II position. Illustrated are the times of the normal intervals as represented on a strip of recording paper.

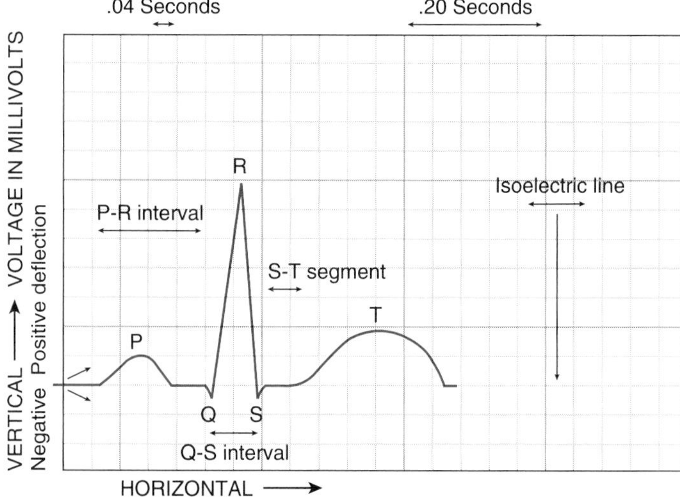

FIGURE 15-24. **One cardiac cycle from the lead II position. Components of the cardiac cycle include (1) P wave, indicating atrial depolarization; (2) P-R interval, the time it takes the impulse to traverse the AV node; (3) QRS, ventricular depolarization; (4) ST segment, the time of ventricular contraction; and (5) T wave, ventricular repolarization. Each small square is 0.04 seconds in time. The normal P-R interval is 0.12 to 0.20 seconds. The normal QRS is 0.06 to 0.10 seconds.**

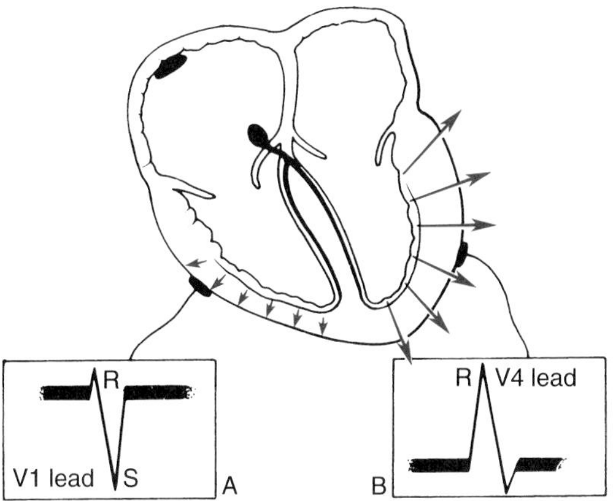

FIGURE 15-25. **A.** As the depolarization wave spreads from endocardium to epicardium in the right ventricle, the small muscle produces a small positive wave in V1. The deep S wave reflects left ventricular depolarization, which is seen as moving away from the V1 lead position. **B.** Endocardial to epicardial depolarization produces a tall R wave in V4 because of the thick muscle mass of the left ventricle.

Because the myocardium is depolarized from endocardium to epicardium, a positive electrode placed on the epicardial surface of the heart normally shows a positive inscription. If a large amount of muscle mass is depolarized, a large inscription is formed. Smaller muscle masses inscribe smaller R waves (Fig. 15-25).

Positive and negative electrodes placed in various locations on the body surface sense the electrical impulses. One positive and one negative electrode make a lead. Leads record the magnitude, direction, and surface potential of impulses generated by cardiac cells. Electrical impulses moving toward a positive electrode produce a predominantly positive deflection of the QRS complex (R wave) while impulses traveling away from a positive electrode produce predominantly negatively deflected QRS (QS) complexes (Fig. 15-26).

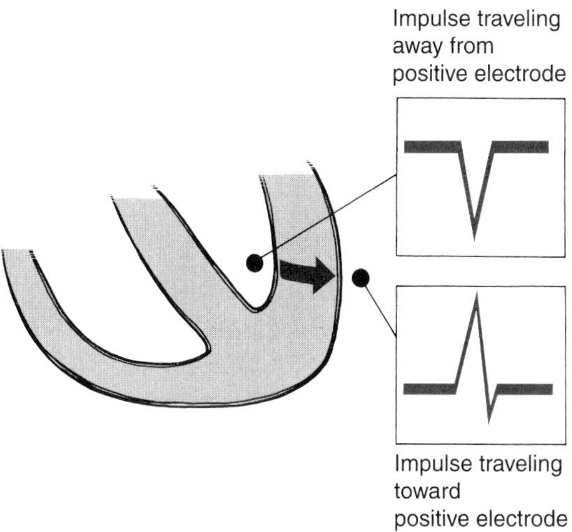

FIGURE 15-26. Appearance of QRS complex relative to cardiac placement of a positive electrode.

THE 12-LEAD ELECTROCARDIOGRAM

The 12-lead ECG is composed of six limb and six precordial leads. These leads are made up of both bipolar and unipolar leads. Bipolar leads were first identified by Einthoven as a triangular lead system composed of a positive and a negative electrode placed at equal distances from the heart (Fig. 15-27). The electrodes are placed on the left arm, right arm, and left leg and are termed limb leads. In lead I, the positive electrode is on the left arm with the negative on the right. In lead II, the negative electrode is on the right arm with the positive on the left leg. In lead III, the positive electrode is on the left leg with the negative on the left arm. The bipolar leads view the heart from the frontal plane gathering data from the superior, inferior, right, and left surfaces.

The unipolar leads consist of the augmented limb leads and the precordial chest (V) leads. The augmented limb leads are so called because the electrical voltage is so small that it must be amplified to be seen. The chest

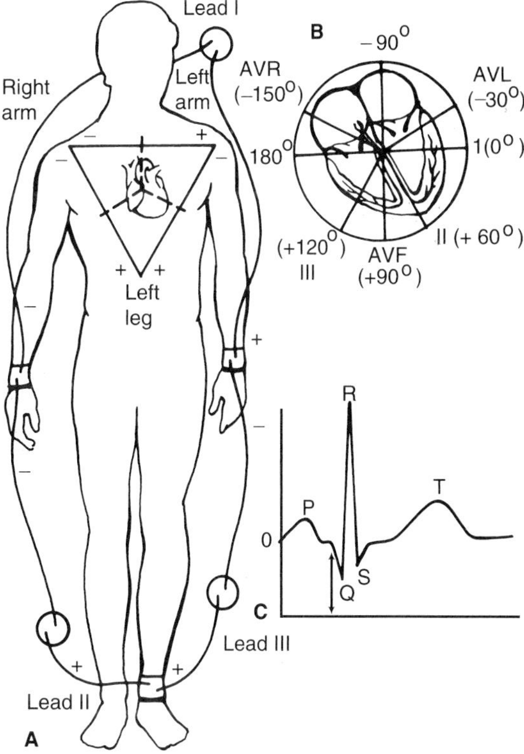

FIGURE 15-27. **A.** The standard electrocardiographic (ECG) leads with their attachments to the body. **B.** ECG tracings recorded with leads I, II, and III. **C.** The normal ECG from lead II.

leads view the horizontal plane of the heart. A positive electrode is placed on either the left arm (aVL), right arm (aVR), or left leg (aVF) (Fig. 15-28).

Precordial leads provide six views (V_1 through V_6) of electrical activity of the heart on the horizontal plane (see Fig. 15-28). Due to the position of the electrodes in the precordial area, these leads are particularly useful in detecting atrial and ventricular activity and chamber hypertrophy and in providing a mirror image of posterior heart activity.[3] The electrodes are placed in specific locations on the anterior chest wall and each gives specific important information that can be supportive of different diagnoses, particularly myocardial ischemia or infarction (see p. 465 and 469). Referring to Figure 15-29, one can note that the majority of the electrical impulses move away from the electrode in V_1, producing a small, positive R wave and a deep, negative S wave. Due to the placement of the V_2 through V_6 electrodes and the flow of the electrical forces, the R wave appears to grow, becoming more positive and reaching maximum height in V_4 to V_5. This is known as *R wave progression on the precordium* and is characteristic of normal ECGs. The R waves in V_5 and V_6 then become somewhat smaller.

Figure 15-29 illustrates a normal 12-lead ECG. The 12-lead is useful in diagnosing acute and nonacute myocardial infarction, atrial and ventricular hypertrophy, and congenital defects. It can also detect the dysrhythmias associated with acute or chronic heart disease. In the diagnosis of acute myocardial infarction, the 12-lead ECG assesses anatomic areas or surfaces of the heart perfused by the right and left coronary arteries. Patterns reflecting ischemia, injury, and necrosis can be detected by examining these areas (see p. 468).

EXERCISE ELECTROCARDIOGRAPHY

The exercise test is used to assess those persons at risk for significant coronary artery disease and dysrhythmias that may be induced in controlled exercise situations. This test may be used to determine the presence of cardiac pathology, especially coronary artery disease.[7]

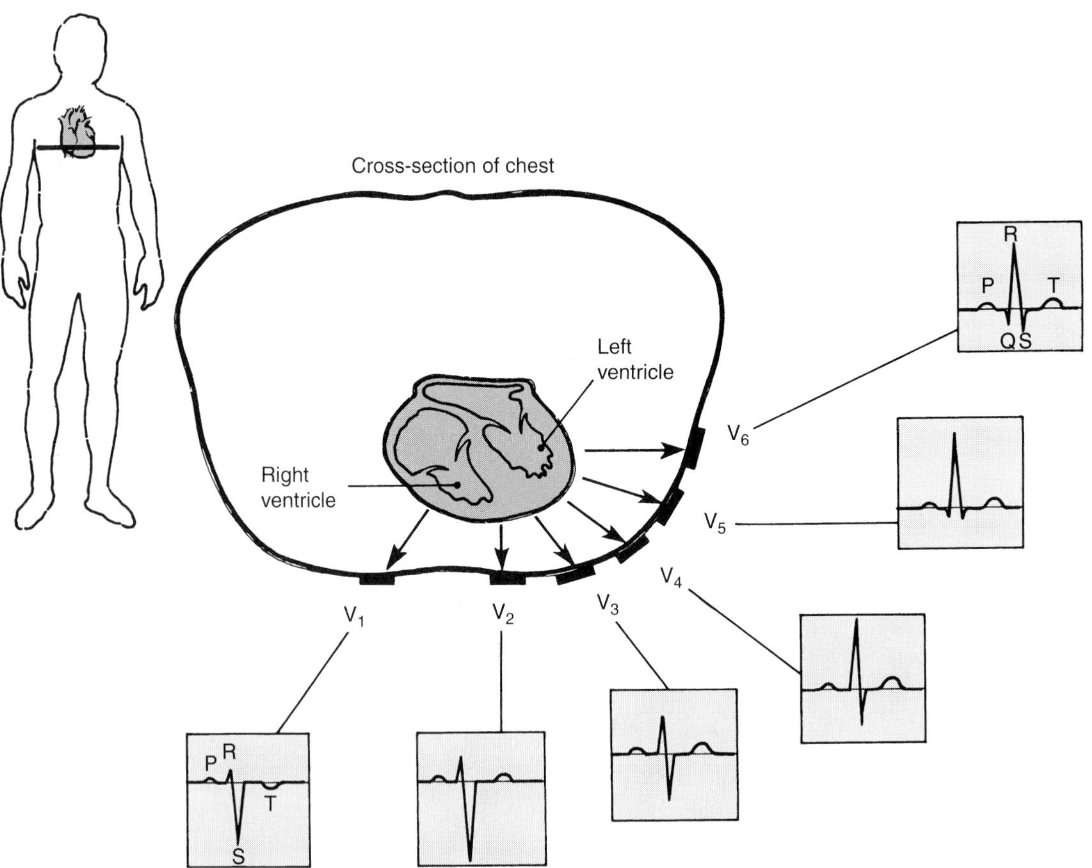

FIGURE 15-28. Appearance of QRS complexes in precordial leads of a 12-lead electrocardiogram.

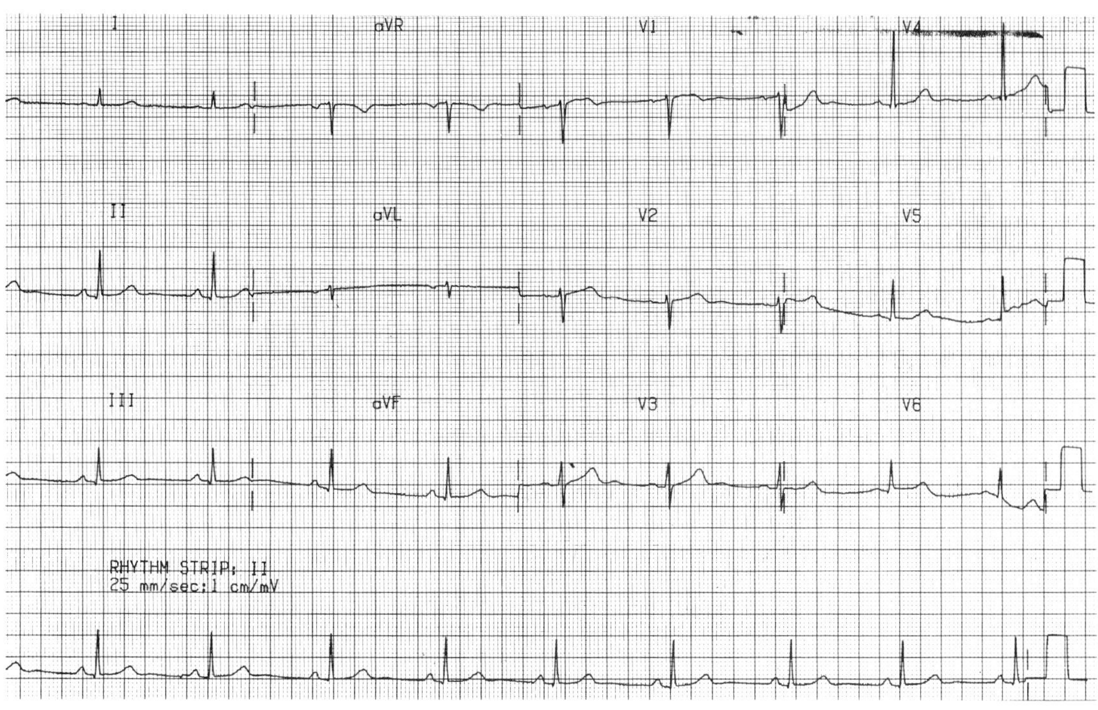

FIGURE 15-29. A normal 12-lead electrocardiogram.

REFERENCES

1. Alexander, R. W., Roberts, R., & Pratt, C. M. (1998). Diagnosis and management of patients with acute myocardial infarction. In R. W. Alexander, R. C. Schlant, & V. Fuster, et al. (Eds.), *Hurst's the heart* (9th ed.). New York: McGraw-Hill.
2. Berne, R. M., & Levy, M N. (1998). *Physiology* (4th ed.). St. Louis: Mosby.
3. Castellanos, A., Kessler, K. M., & Myerburg, R. J. (1998). The resting electrocardiogram. In R. W. Alexander, R. C. Schlant, & V. Fuster, et al. (Eds.), *Hurst's: The heart* (9th ed.). New York: McGraw-Hill.
4. Cheitlin, M. D., Sokolow, M., & McIlroy, M. B. (1997). *Clinical cardiology* (7th ed.). Norwalk, CT: Appleton & Lange.
5. Dell'Italia, L. J., & Pearce, D. J. (1998). Chest pain. In J. H. Stein (Ed.), *Internal medicine* (5th ed.). St. Louis: Mosby.
6. Factor, S. M., & Bache, R. J. (1998). Pathophysiology of myocardial ischemia. In R. W. Alexander, R. C. Schlant, & V. Fuster, et al. (Eds.), *Hurst's: The heart* (9th ed.). New York: McGraw-Hill.
7. Fisch, C. (1997). Electrocardiography, exercise stress testing, and ambulatory monitoring. In W. N. Kelley (Ed.), *Textbook of internal medicine* (4th ed.). Philadelphia: Lippincott-Raven.
8. Frishman, W. H., & Sonnenblick, E. H. (1998). Beta-adrenergic blocking drugs and calcium channel blockers. In R. W. Alexander, R. C. Schlant, & V. Fuster (Eds.), *Hurst's the heart* (9th ed.). New York: McGraw-Hill.
9. Frohlich, E. D., & Re, R. N. (1998). Pathophysiology of systemic arterial hypertension. In R. W. Alexander, R. C. Schlant, & V. Fuster, et al. (Eds.), *Hurst's: The heart* (9th ed.) New York: McGraw-Hill.
10. Ganong, W. F. (1997). *Review of medical physiology* (17th ed.). Norwalk, CT: Appleton & Lange.
11. Guyton, A. C. & Hall, J. E. (1996). *Textbook of medical physiology* (9th ed.). Philadelphia: Saunders.
12. Opie, L. H. (1998). *The heart: Physiology and metabolism* (3rd ed.) New York: Lippincott-Raven.
13. O'Rourke, R. A., Shaver, J. A., Soletti, R., Silverman, M. E., & Schlant, R. C. (1998). The history, physical examination, and cardiac auscultation. In R. W. Alexander, R. C. Schlant, & V. Fuster (Eds.), *Hurst's: The heart* (9th ed.). New York: McGraw-Hill.
14. Schlant, R. C., Sonnenblick, E. H, & Katz, A. M. (1998). Normal physiology of the cardiovascular system. In R. W. Alexander, R. C. Schlant, & V. Fuster, et al. (Eds.), *Hurst's: The heart* (9th ed.). New York: McGraw-Hill.
15. Stiles, G. L. (1998). Structure and functioning of cardiovascular membranes, channels, and receptors. In R. W. Alexander, R. C. Schlant, & V. Fuster, et al. (Eds.), *Hurst's: The heart* (9th ed.). New York: McGraw-Hill.
16. Tortora, G. J., & Grabowski, S. R. (1997). *Principles of anatomy and physiology* (8th ed.). New York: HarperCollins.
17. Waller, B. F., & Schlant, R. C. (1998). Anatomy of the heart. In R. W. Alexander, R. C. Schlant, & V. Fuster, et al. (Eds.), *Hurst's: The heart* (9th ed.) New York: McGraw-Hill.
18. Woosley, R. L. (1998). Antiarrhythmic drugs. In R. W. Alexander, R. C. Schlant, & V. Fuster, et al. (Eds.). *Hurst's: The heart* (9th ed.) New York: McGraw-Hill.

Chapter 16

Altered Circulatory Function

Barbara L. Bullock

KEY TERMS

afterload
apoptosis
atheroma
brawny edema
carotenoid pigment
cellulitis
collateral circulation
dyslipoproteinemias
endothelium
hypertrophy
intermittent claudication
ischemic neuropathy
lipoproteins
papilledema
renin
rubor
subclavian steal
tumor necrosis factor
ventricular remodeling

Alterations in circulatory function include disturbances in blood flow in the arterial, venous, and lymphatic circulations. Arterial hypertension affects circulatory function and predisposes individuals to multiple problems. *Peripheral vascular disease* is a term that in its broadest sense applies to disease of any blood vessel outside the heart and to disease of the lymph vessels. Arterial diseases are common and are closely related to the process of atherosclerosis. Venous pathology includes the common problems of varicose veins and deep vein thrombosis. Pathology of the lymphatic system is often secondary to some other problem, such as infection or malignancy. Primary or essential hypertension is the most common disease in the United States and, like arterial diseases, is closely related to atherosclerosis.

CELLULAR STRUCTURE OF THE VESSEL WALL

The structure of the vessel wall is composed of endothelial and smooth muscle cells (see p. 422). The endothelial layer is a single layer that lines the tunica intima. The **endothelium** is active in many metabolic functions (Box 16-1). Between the endothelium and the smooth muscle of the tunica media is a layer of connective tissue. The *tunica intima* consists of the endothelium and the connective tissue. The *tunica media* contains smooth muscle layers of varying thicknesses depending on the vessel's size. Blood vessels with more than 28 layers of smooth muscle cells have a vascular supply system, called the *vasa vasorum*, which penetrates the exterior of the vessel wall and supplies it with blood.[2] The *tunica adventitia* is the outer layer of the vessel and is composed of connective tissue, small vessels that produce the vasa vasorum, and nerves.

ALTERED FUNCTION OF ARTERIES

The majority of the pathologies seen in the arterial circulation are due to atherosclerosis. Other causes include congenital weakness of the arteries, inflammation, or vasospastic conditions. Atherosclerosis is discussed in some depth below because of its effect on all major arteries of the body.

BOX 16-1

FUNCTIONS OF ENDOTHELIAL CELLS OF THE BLOOD VESSELS

Permeability barrier
Vasoactive factors: nitric oxide (endothelium-derived relaxing factor), endothelin
Antithrombic agent production: prostacyclin (PGI_2), adenine metabolites
Prothrombic agent production: factor VIIIa (von Willebrand factor)
Anticoagulant production: thrombomodulin, other proteins
Fibrinolytic agent production: tissue plasminogen activator, urokinase-like factor
Procoagulant production: tissue factor, plasminogen activator/inhibitor, factor V
Inflammatory mediator production: interleukin-1, cell adhesion molecules
Receptors for factor IX, factor X, low-density lipoproteins, modified low-density lipoproteins, thrombin
Growth factor production: blood cell colony-stimulating factor, insulin-like growth factors, fibroblast growth factor, platelet-derived growth factor
Growth inhibitor: heparin
Replication

TABLE 16-1

FACTORS IMPLICATED IN THE DEVELOPMENT OF ATHEROSCLEROSIS

FACTOR	RELATIONSHIP TO DISEASE
Age	Increased frequency with advancing age
Weight	Probably related to diet; obesity correlates with increased frequency of myocardial infarction
Heredity	Increased frequency at early age within certain families points to familial predisposition that also may reflect dietary habits
Diet	Diet high in saturated fats with frequency of hyperlipidemia increases ischemic heart disease
Sex	Significantly increased in men until age 75 years or greater, when it approaches equality
Diabetes mellitus	Almost twofold increase as compared with nondiabetics; also relates to obesity
Cigarette smoking	Correlates with number of cigarettes smoked and decreases when smoking stops
Hypertension	Correlates with degree of hypertension; diastolic pressure the most important figure
Occupation or life-style	Behavior pattern (type A or B personality) inconclusive but risk appears to be twofold with type A personality

Atherosclerosis

Atherosclerosis is a common response of an artery to numerous, different forms of insult.[22] It is a disease of large and medium-sized arteries that begins as a fibrofatty plaque on the artery's intimal surface. The disease is usually asymptomatic until impeded arterial blood flow causes ischemia or infarction of the affected organ.

ETIOLOGY

Many factors have been studied in the development of atherosclerosis (Table 16-1). All the factors correlate, and two or more of them usually interact when pathology is expressed. The risk factors for atherosclerotic vascular disease are exactly the same as for coronary artery disease (CAD) and can be classified as alterable and unalterable (see p. 457).

Table 16-2 shows the proposed cellular mechanisms of the atherogenic risk factors. Complications of atherosclerosis include CAD, stroke, mesenteric occlusion, and gangrene of the extremities. These atherosclerotic diseases account for more than 50% of the annual mortality in the United States.[3] Because a significant degree of arterial occlusion must be present for the disease to become symptomatic, actual incidence of atherosclerosis, both reported and unreported, can only be surmised.

Because feeding animals a diet high in cholesterol induces atherosclerosis and because the disease process rarely occurs in humans unless their cholesterol levels are greater than 160 mg/dL, hyperlipidemia is considered a major causative factor.[22] The lipid in the atheroma is derived from serum lipoproteins, as discussed next.

Relationship of Lipid Metabolism to Atherosclerosis

The lipids of the body exist mostly in the form of **lipoprotein** particles, which have been divided into classes according to their density. The major classes are chylomicrons, very low-density lipoproteins (VLDLs),

TABLE 16-2

MECHANISMS OF ATHEROGENIC RISK FACTORS

RISK FACTOR	CELLULAR MECHANISM
Hypertension	Increased SVR, endothelial damage, increased platelet adherence, increased permeability of endothelial lining. Renin–angiotensin system may induce cellular changes.
Cigarette smoking	Endothelial damage from carbon monoxide. Platelet aggregation. Smoking-induced increased SVR leads to endothelial damage.
Elevated serum cholesterol level, especially with low HDL cholesterol levels	Increased LDL cholesterol damages endothelium and causes accumulation on endothelial lining and proliferation of smooth muscle cells.

HDL, high-density lipoprotein; LDL, low-density lipoprotein; SVR, systemic vascular resistance.

intermediate-density lipoproteins (IDLs), low-density lipoproteins (LDLs), and high-density lipoproteins (HDLs) Table 16-3 details the functions and normal values of each class. These particles have a lipid core with associated proteins, called apolipoproteins.[22] Each class contains a different amount of cholesterol, which determines its atherogenic propensity.

Two metabolic pathways for lipoprotein synthesis and release have been identified: the *exogenous* and *endogenous cholesterol transport pathways*. These pathways work together in the formation of cholesterol. Figure 16-1 illustrates their function and relationship with the end result of increasing or decreasing serum cholesterol. As Figure 16-1 shows, the liver hepatocyte is essential in the formation of LDL; this lipoprotein is the major factor in cholesterol transport in the plasma.[2] The liver clears approximately 70% of plasma LDL by binding LDL to surface receptors. LDL can also be transported through other receptor pathways in most body cells, which causes the entire lipoprotein to move inside the cell for structural purposes.[10] The cell controls its own internal cholesterol concentration by decreasing absorption of LDL when its concentration within becomes too great.

The LDL that remains in the blood has the highest concentration of cholesterol of all lipoprotein classes. Scavenger cells of the mononuclear phagocyte system degrade some LDL, which may contribute to the development of atherosclerosis by making more cholesterol available in the plasma.[4]

The HDL carries cholesterol to the liver for removal from the body. This cholesterol is principally free cholesterol that the liver rapidly degrades. Persons who have defects in this degradation process have **dyslipoproteinemias**, increased intracellular cholesteryl esters, and premature atherosclerosis. The literature has repeatedly described an inverse relationship between CAD and HDL cholesterol levels, so that this "good cholesterol" has been termed protective in preventing CAD.[23] By inference, HDL probably helps to prevent other atherosclerotic diseases because the atherogenic process is the same for all arteries.

FAMILIAL HYPERCHOLESTEROLEMIA. Familial hypercholesterolemia is a common genetic defect and in its more common heterozygous form is found in about 1/500 persons.[23] It results from a mutation in the LDL receptor gene (on the short arm of chromosome 19), causing a loss of feedback control and elevated cholesterol levels.[4] As cholesterol accumulates in the plasma and throughout the body cells and tissues, premature onset of atherosclerotic lesions begins.

The relationship between circulating cholesterol levels and the development of atherosclerosis closely relates to serum LDL levels. In other words, levels between 600 and 1,000 mg/dL lead to early onset CAD and death before the age of 20 years in individuals who are genetically homozygous (incidence about 1 per million persons) for familial hypercholesterolemia.[2] Male heterozygotes with LDL cholesterol levels from 250 to 500 mg/dL often suffer from premature myocardial infarction at about age 40 to 45.[23]

Other defects in lipoprotein and apolipoprotein synthesis may lead to changes in LDL or LDL-like serum concentrations and in early onset atherosclerosis. Identifying the genetic source of the atherogenic lesion is important because some types respond to cholesterol-lowering drugs; nicotinic acid therapy may improve others.[2]

PATHOPHYSIOLOGY

The earliest lesion of atherosclerosis is the fatty streak that often develops within the first decade of life.[4,6,22] In experimental studies, the first change seen is the adhesion of monocytes to an intact endothelial surface.[6] This adhesion initiates a self-perpetuating focus of chronic inflammation, which produces endothelial injury and depends on elevated lipid levels for its continuation.[20] The monocytes are converted to macrophages and their uptake of lipids leads to the formation of lipid droplets, called *foam cells*, that are deposited on the

TABLE 16-3

FUNCTION AND NORMAL VALUES OF LIPOPROTEIN PARTICLES

LIPOPROTEIN	VALUE	FUNCTION
Total cholesterol	<200 mg/dL	Serum lipoprotein, metabolized by the liver. Necessary for the production of steroid hormones, cellular membranes, and bile acids.
Chylomicrons		Source is dietary (exogenous). Dominant core is triglyceride, not thought to play a part in atherogenesis.
Very low-density (VLDL)		Synthesized by the liver (endogenous). Core lipoprotein is triglyceride, may play a part in HDL structure when catabolized.
Intermediate-density lipoprotein (LDL)		Catabolized by liver through interaction with LDL receptors on hepatocyte membranes. Triglyceride removed from lipoprotein until LDL particles are formed.
Low-density lipoprotein (LDL)	<160 mg/dL	LDL supplies cholesterol to cells for cell membrane and steroid hormone synthesis. Many cell membranes have receptors for LDL. High-fat diet may suppress LDL receptor activity so that particles circulating in plasma are not removed. Exposure of LDL to endothelial cells causes peroxidation and increased negative charge. This may cause chemotaxis for blood monocytes and accumulation of cholesterol esters in macrophages and smooth muscle cells, leading to atherosclerotic plaque.
High-density lipoprotein (HDL)	>35 mg/dL	In two forms. Larger HDL carries more cholesterol and returns it to liver for excretion in the bile. Larger form can be converted back to smaller form, which increases its atherogenic potential. Normally, HDL is thought to be preventive in atherosclerosis development.

tunica intima. These early fatty streaks result from macrophages taking up LDL, which only can result from chemical changes in LDL produced by the cells in the arterial wall.[6] The foam cells produce a number of inflammatory cytokines including **tumor necrosis factor** (TNF) and *procoagulant tissue factor*. LDL oxidation or **apoptosis** (cell suicide), which TNF may partially induce, may kill the lipid-filled macrophages. The resulting lipid cores and spaces fill with cellular debris and cholesterol.[6] Smooth muscle proliferates due to growth factors produced by many substances, including platelets, fibrinogen, thrombin, and even the smooth muscle cells themselves. The smooth muscle cells must migrate from their normal placement in the tunica media to the tunica intima in response to chemotactic stimuli.[25]

The actual atherosclerotic lesion is called an **atheroma** or an atheromatous plaque. Atheromas are composed of fatty and fibrofatty material white to yellow in color. An atheroma protrudes into the artery and may compromise vascular supply to the involved tissue.[22] The process exhibited represents an inflammatory response that contains large numbers of macrophages. Eventually fibroproliferation and thrombosis result.[1]

As shown in Figure 16-2, atheromas have essentially three components: (1) cells of smooth muscle, macrophages, and other leukocytes; (2) connective tissue with collagen, elastic fibers, and proteoglycans; and (3) lipid deposits both intracellularly and extracellularly.[4] The plaque's center becomes necrotic and contains cellular debris, lipid-laden foam cells, calcium, cholesterol crystals, and a mass of lipid material. The lipid core is often bright yellow due to the presence of **carotenoid pigment**.[6] The smooth muscle cells form on the surface and make a fibrous cap.

Thrombosis on the plaque is induced by erosion or disruption of the surface, which exposes the subendothelial connective tissue to platelet aggregation and gradual induction of the intrinsic coagulation system (see p. 379). The cause of the disruption is unknown, but it may be due to a destructive process that the macrophages initiate.[6]

Atherosclerotic lesions differ among body areas and individuals. Coronary artery lesions, for example, are fibrous, and in long-standing lesions, the fibrosis may convert the atheroma to a fibrous scar.[4] The lesion may exist for years as a quiescent plaque that suddenly becomes activated, causing vasoconstriction, increased inflammatory cells, and thrombus formation.[1]

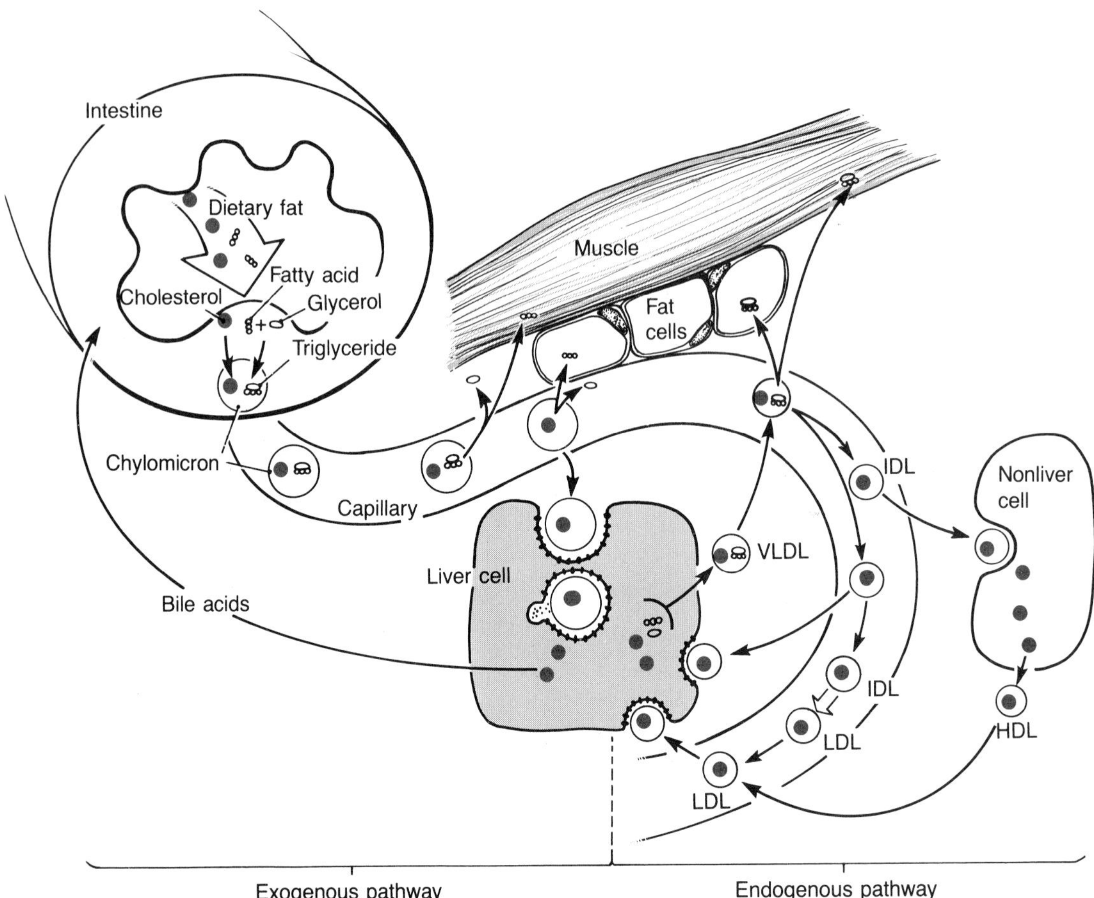

FIGURE 16-1. Exogenous and endogenous cholesterol transport pathways. In the exogenous pathway, dietary fat is absorbed as cholesterol and fatty acids from the intestinal mucosa. Triglycerides are formed from fatty acid and glycerol linkages. Both triglycerides and cholesterol are packaged into chylomicrons that are absorbed into the circulation. In the capillaries, the bonds holding the fatty acids in triglycerides are split by lipoprotein lipase. Fatty acids are removed, leaving cholesterol-rich lipoprotein. These are taken up by liver cells and either secreted into the intestine (as bile acids) or packaged as very low density lipoproteins (VLDL), which are secreted into the circulation. This first step in the endogenous cycle is followed by the removal of triglyceride from the VLDL, leaving the intermediate density lipoprotein (IDL) in the circulation. Some IDL is taken up by the liver or non-liver tissues to form low-density lipoproteins (LDL). Most of the LDL in circulation bind to hepatocytes or other cells and are removed from the circulation. High density lipoproteins (HDL) take up cholesterol from cells. This cholesterol is esterified by a specific enzyme, causing the esters to be transferred to LDL and taken up by cells. (Adapted from Rubin, E. & Farber, J. L. [1999]. *Pathology* [3rd ed.]. Philadelphia: Lippincott Williams & Wilkins.)

Plaques are labeled as *complicated plaques* when they exhibit any of the following:

- *Significant calcification*—leads to a stiff, brittle artery that does not accommodate well the dynamic flow of blood through it.
- *Ulceration* or *thrombosis*—ulceration of the surface may dislodge the debris within the plaque, causing embolization to a smaller artery. Thrombosis occurs when platelets adhere to a site of endothelial activation or injury and activation of the coagulation mechanism results in obstruction of the vessel lumen.
- *Hemorrhage*—bleeding into the plaque results from disruption of thin-walled capillaries that provide blood to the plaque; the formed hematoma may occlude the vessel lumen or be localized in the plaque.
- *Weakened medial wall*—results when the plaque extends into the wall, accounting for the association of atherosclerosis and aneurysm formation; disruption of medial blood supply or calcium infiltration may cause aneurysm formation.[4]

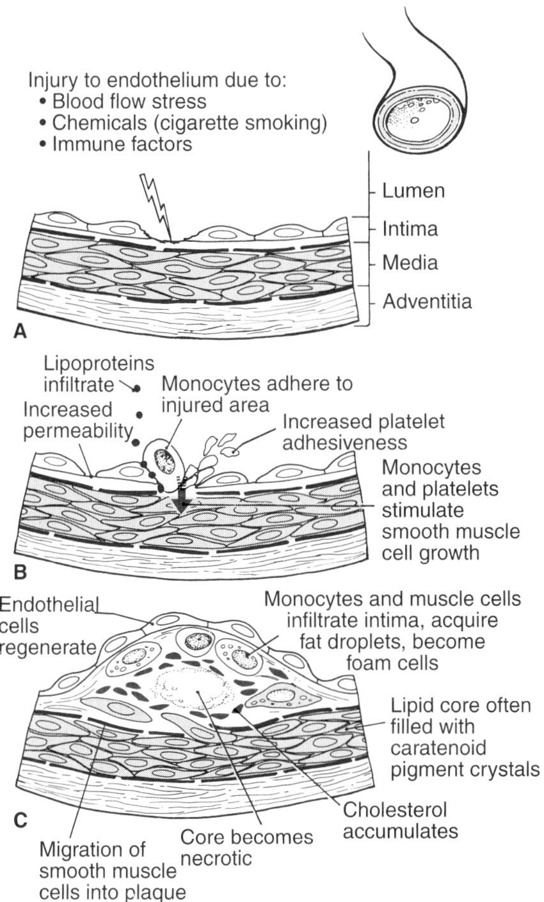

FIGURE 16-2. The process of atherogenesis and formation of an atheroma. **A.** Endothelial injury initiates process. **B.** Platelets and monocytes adhere and stimulate growth of smooth muscle. **C.** The generation and migration of smooth muscle cells add to formation of the atheroma. Lipid deposits are both intracellular and extracellular. The center of the atheroma becomes necrotic.

CLINICAL MANIFESTATIONS

Even though atherosclerosis may affect any artery, the aorta, coronary, carotid, and iliac arteries are involved with the greatest frequency. The abdominal aorta is involved more frequently than the thoracic, and the lesions tend to locate at ostia and bifurcations.[4]

A wide range of clinical effects may result from the ischemia and infarction of specific areas. Table 16-4 summarizes some of these effects.

Embolization from a thrombosed atheroma causes the characteristic signs of arterial occlusion in a distal artery:

- Diminished or absent pulses
- Skin pallor, cyanosis, or both
- Pain
- Muscle weakness

A large embolus may arise from a thrombosed atheroma in the descending aorta and may travel to the terminal aorta. If the embolus occludes both the iliac arteries and terminal aorta, it is known as a saddle embolus.

Occlusive Disease of the Lower Extremity

Occlusive disease of the terminal aorta and its branches produces ischemia in distal tissues. Most occlusive disease in this area is chronic and slowly progressive. The result is a profusion of collateral circulation that may forestall symptoms for some time.

PATHOPHYSIOLOGY

The bifurcation of the aorta to the iliacs is the most common site for the development of peripheral atherosclerosis. Most individuals who have narrowing at the femoral-popliteal area also have disease at the aorto-iliac bifurcation.[17] Men are affected more frequently than are women and the mean age for symptomatic lesions is 60 years. The prevalence and severity of occlusive disease increase if the individual suffers from concomitant diabetes mellitus. Lesions in the arteries of the legs are often associated with CAD or carotid artery disease or with abdominal aortic aneurysms.

Gradual occlusion of an atherosclerotic terminal aorta or of other large vessels can cause ischemia to the part supplied. When a large artery is obstructed, pressure in the smaller arteries distal to it decreases and blood flow declines. As the main arterial trunk progressively narrows, **collateral circulation** develops to maintain blood flow. Collateral vessels are native, undeveloped vessels that can enlarge when blood flow to them gradually decreases through the main arterial channel. Collateral circulation has been demonstrated in most of the main arteries, especially the coronary and leg arteries.[8] The process results from a complex series of inflammations and cellular proliferations that cause the rudimentary vessels to enlarge and provide blood supply to ischemic tissue (Fig. 16-3). This compensatory action may provide circulation to the limb or myocardium for an extended time. Limb-threatening arterial insufficiency may result as the lesion progresses, leading to gangrene if the cellular deprivation of oxygen is critical enough to cause cell death.

CLINICAL MANIFESTATIONS

If the terminal aorta is affected, clinical manifestations include intermittent claudication, loss of peripheral hair, shiny skin, and impotence in men. If a peripheral artery is affected, pain and color changes in the affected leg are common.

TABLE 16-4

CLINICAL AND PATHOLOGIC EFFECTS OF ATHEROSCLEROSIS IN DIFFERENT ANATOMIC SITES

SITE	CLINICAL AND PATHOLOGIC EFFECTS
Abdominal/terminal aorta	Ischemic effects in lower extremities; gangrene of toes, feet; effects of fusiform abdominal aneurysm; embolism of atherosclerotic debris to smaller arteries
Aortoiliac and femoral arteries	Intermittent claudication; gangrene of toes, feet; aneurysm formation in iliac arteries
Coronary arteries	Angina pectoris; conduction disturbances; myocardial infarction
Carotid and vertebral arteries	Transient ischemic attacks; cerebrovascular accident or stroke
Renal artery	Hypertension; renal ischemia (hematuria, proteinuria)
Mesenteric arteries	Intestinal ischemia (ileus, bowel perforation with peritonitis)

Pain

Various types of pain are described that are related to the degree of impairment of circulatory supply. **Intermittent claudication** is an aching, persistent, cramplike, squeezing pain that occurs after a certain amount of exercise of the affected extremity.[12] Rest without change of position relieves intermittent claudication, which occurs in almost all affected persons at some stage of the disease. It is frequently the first symptom an affected individual notices, often beginning in the arch of the foot or calf of the leg.

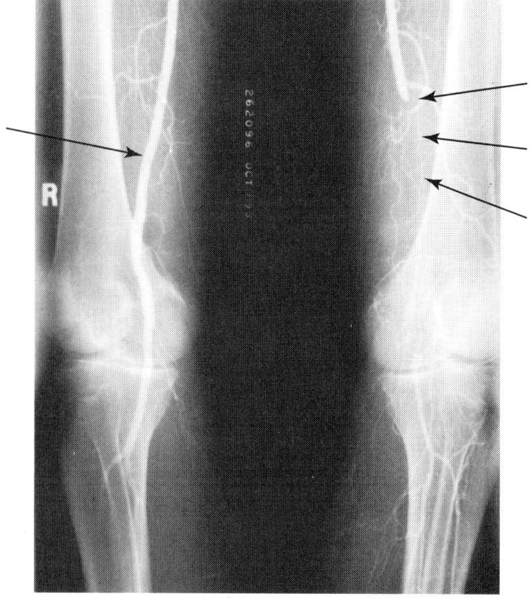

FIGURE 16-3. Arteriogram showing arterial obstruction and collateral circulation. Arrow on left shows normal right femoral artery circulation; arrows on right show complete blockage of left femoral artery and profuse collateral circulation.

Rest pain is usually localized in the digits. Affected individuals describe it as a severe ache or a gnawing pain, often occurring at night and persisting for hours at a time. Severe ischemia of tissues and sensory nerve terminals cause rest pain, which may herald the onset of gangrene.[12] Elevation of the extremity may aggravate rest pain; dependency may relieve it.

Pain of **ischemic neuropathy** usually occurs late in the disease with severe ischemia. This severe pain is often associated with various types of paresthesias. It may be described as a shocklike sensation that usually occurs in both the foot and leg and follows the distribution of the peripheral sensory nerves. The pain of ulceration and gangrene is usually localized to the areas adjacent to ulcers or gangrenous tissue. It is severe, persistent, and frequently worse at night. The pain is described as an aching sensation and sometimes may be associated with sharp, severe stabs of pain.

Coldness or Cold Sensitivity

Coldness or sensitivity to cold is a frequent symptom. Complaints of coldness in the toes on exposure to a cold environment may be associated with color changes such as blanching or cyanosis. The temperature of the feet is colder to the touch than the rest of the body; this finding may vary with a person's activity level and complaints of ischemic leg pain.

Impaired Arterial Pulsations

Pulsation in the posterior tibial and dorsalis pedis arteries is impaired or absent in the majority of lower extremity occlusions. Impairment of pulsations in the popliteal and femoral arteries is less frequent. Pulsations may improve on rest, which indicates that some alterations in blood flow may be due to arterial spasm.

Color Changes

Affected extremities may be of a normal color; however, in advanced disease, cyanosis or an abnormal red color called **rubor** may be visible, particularly when the extremity is in a dependent position. Postural color changes are often asymmetrical, and affected extremities or digits become abnormally blanched after being elevated for a few minutes. When the extremity is in a dependent position, a delay of 5 to 60 seconds may be required for color to return to the skin. The part first becomes abnormally red and then gradually the rubor decreases. Rubor is due to maximal dilatation of the arterioles and capillaries in response to inadequate flow.

Ulceration and Gangrene

Ulcerative lesions may occur spontaneously on an ischemic extremity or they may result from trauma, such as pressure on the toenails from shoes. In the absence of diabetes mellitus, gangrene is rare unless it develops after some trauma.[17] Bruises, nicks, or cuts in the skin; freezing; burning; or application of strong, irritating medicines or chemicals may cause the initial injury that does not heal, leading to ulceration and eventually gangrene. Ulceration and gangrene are usually confined to one extremity at a time. They may be manifested by small spots on a digit or involve a whole extremity.

Ulcers may develop on the tips, between, or at the base of the flexor surface of the toes. The area around the ulcer is painful and may swell or exhibit redness at the margin. Secondary infections are common and lead to abscess formation, cellulitis, and spread of infection. Gangrene and ulceration related to diabetes are discussed on page 702.

Edema

Edema of the feet and legs may occur when obstruction is severe. It is most evident when the legs are in a dependent position. The edema is not as dominant as that seen with venous occlusions (see p. 443). Associated ischemic skin lesions, capillary atony, deep venous thrombosis, and lymphangitis contribute to the edema.

Sexual Dysfunction

Occlusive disease of the terminal aorta can decrease the blood supply to the vascular tree supplying penile circulation. Affected men may report the inability to attain or maintain an erection, especially men with total occlusion of the terminal aorta.[17]

Superficial Thrombophlebitis

At some stage of the disease, superficial nonvaricose veins are involved in a type of thrombophlebitis (see p. 445). This condition occurs in about 40% of persons with atherosclerotic occlusive disease. The smaller veins are usually involved with lesions or are red, raised, indurated, tender, cordlike veins that measure approximately 0.5 to 3.0 cm long. The lesions usually cause permanent occlusion of the veins, but the redness and symptoms of thrombophlebitis subside, usually in 1 to 3 weeks after onset.[12]

Other Changes

As a result of moderate to severe chronic ischemia, small scars, depressions, or pitting may form on the tips of the toes. Nail growth is slow and nails may become thickened and deformed. They also may be paper thin. The toes or an entire foot may appear shrunken, with atrophied muscles. Therefore, the calf or thigh may decrease in size. Skin that is deprived of blood often becomes translucent and shiny.

Thromboangiitis Obliterans or Buerger's Disease

Buerger's disease affects the small and medium-sized arteries, and the medium-sized, mostly superficial, veins of the extremities. It is mainly seen in young men between ages 20 and 35 years but its frequency is increasing in women.[12] It almost invariably affects individuals who use tobacco and may represent an autoimmune reaction to it.[12] It frequently results in arterial occlusion, causing ischemia and gangrene in the extremities. The nonatherosclerotic lesion consists of microabscesses with a central focus of polymorphonuclear leukocytes usually surrounded by mononuclear cells.[4]

PATHOPHYSIOLOGY

Pathologically, the gross characteristics of vessels affected by thromboangiitis vary depending on the age of the lesions at the time of examination. The vessels appear contracted at the site of destruction. The occluded segments are indurated but not brittle. The arteries are more frequently obliterated than are their accompanying veins. In the diseased vessel, the occlusion may extend for variable lengths and then stop abruptly. Occlusions may occur at two different levels in the same vessel, and between these sites the vessel may be completely patent.[14]

CLINICAL MANIFESTATIONS

Clinical manifestations include:

- Pain (intermittent claudication or rest pain)
- Increased sensitivity to cold

- Decreased pulses in the extremities
- Color changes including rubor and cyanosis of the extremities
- Hair loss in the extremities
- Thin, shiny skin
- Coexisting migratory phlebitis
- Low serum cholesterol concentration
- Eventually, ulceration and gangrene

The most striking physiologic change is the impairment of arterial blood flow. Blood flow through peripheral arteries in the extremities is reduced, particularly in more distal portions. Arteriolar spasm contributes to the ischemia and its presence varies among individuals and perhaps with the disease's stage.

Occlusive Disease of the Upper Extremity

Just as atherosclerosis is the major cause of lower extremity occlusion, it also is the main cause of upper extremity occlusion. Lesions tend to be located at the bifurcations of the arch vessels and the common carotid arteries.[12] The proximal left subclavian artery is most frequently affected, excluding the common carotid artery occlusions, which are described in Chapter 31.

Upper extremity ischemia is very uncommon due, in part, to the **subclavian steal**. This phenomenon refers to cerebral ischemia that results from a diversion of blood from the circle of Willis back through vertebral artery on the affected side to the ischemic arm. The steal is invariably produced by exercising the arm and cerebral flow moving retrograde to the arm.[17] The syndrome usually presents with the typical picture of transient ischemic attacks or other central nervous system dysfunction. Diagnostic studies, especially using Doppler techniques, demonstrate obstruction to blood flow.

Aortic and Arterial Aneurysms

An aneurysm is a localized dilatation of the arterial wall. It develops at a site of weakness of the tunica media. Pathologically, aneurysms may be described as fusiform, aortic dissection (dissecting hematoma), or saccular on the basis of their appearance. Aneurysms may be classified as abdominal or thoracic according to their location on the aorta. Some aneurysms are found on the peripheral arteries, especially those in the cerebral circulation or at sites of surgical incisions (false aneurysms). The majority of aneurysms are related to atherosclerosis, but they may also be related to a hereditary disruption of elastin in the medial wall.[25] Some aneurysms are due to congenital defects, infections such as syphilis, and trauma.

FUSIFORM ANEURYSMS

Fusiform aneurysms produce circumferential arterial dilatation. The arterial wall balloons on all sides (Fig. 16-4). During this process, the aneurysmal sac fills with necrotic debris and thrombi. Calcium infiltrates the area. The sac dilates because of a weakened medial layer. The dangers of this type of aneurysm include rupture, embolization to a peripheral artery, pressure on surrounding structures, and obstruction of blood flow to organs supplied by the tributary arteries.

Abdominal Aortic Aneurysms

Almost all abdominal aortic aneurysms are fusiform; most arise at a level below the branchings of the renal arteries. They often extend to and include the iliac arteries (see Fig. 16-4). Significant atherosclerosis may exist elsewhere in the body.[25] These aneurysms are three to four times more common in men than women, often affect individuals with a strong family history of aneurysms, and occur in the seventh or eighth decade of life.[17]

Clinical manifestations are usually nonexistent. Occasionally, the person discovers a pulsatile abdominal mass. More frequently, a physical examination performed for some other reason, such as vague abdominal symptoms or poor peripheral circulation, reveals the aneurysm. Pain of recent onset may herald an expanding aneurysm with impending rupture.[17] Pressure from a large or enlarging abdominal aortic aneurysm on surrounding abdominal organs, together with lack of blood supply to the intestines, can precipitate ileus or intestinal obstruction.

Physical examination reveals a pulsatile abdominal mass. Due to intra-aneurysmal clot, the size of the

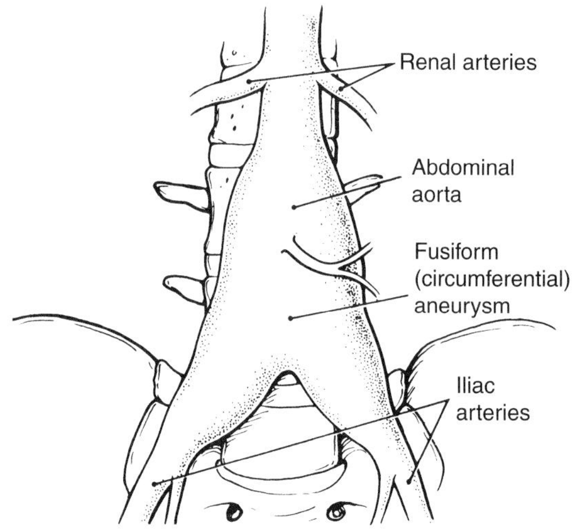

FIGURE 16-4. Fusiform aneurysm of the aorta.

aneurysm may not be appreciated on angiographic studies. A radiograph of the abdomen often confirms the aneurysm's presence due to a rim of calcification seen in the vessel wall. Rupture may be the first sign of the aneurysm with bleeding frequently occurring into the retroperitoneal space. In such instances, exsanguination is generally prevented due to the location of the hemorrhage. The initial symptoms of this type of rupture include abdominal pain and hemorrhagic shock.

Thoracic Aneurysms

Thoracic aortic aneurysms related to atherosclerosis are usually fusiform and may be located in the ascending, arch, or descending segments of the aorta. Those that result from medial necrosis are usually dissecting in nature; syphilitic aneurysms are often saccular in nature (see below).

Most thoracic aneurysms are asymptomatic and are detected incidentally on chest radiograph.[17] The most common clinical manifestation is deep, aching back pain that may be associated with erosion of the ribs or may indicate expansion of the aneurysm with impending rupture. Compression of respiratory structures and of the recurrent laryngeal nerve may cause dyspnea, hoarseness, and coughing. Rupture that is the initial manifestation of this type of aneurysm is usually fatal.

AORTIC DISSECTION

Aortic dissection, previously called dissecting aneurysm, is also termed *dissecting hematoma*. Tearing and degeneration of the medial layer allow blood to separate the artery's intimal layer from the adventitial layer (Fig. 16-5). Weakening of the medial layer appears to be essential to the process of dissection.[5] Aortic dissection most frequently occurs in the ascending aorta. Eighty percent of individuals with aortic dissection also have systemic hypertension (see p. 447).

Dissecting hematomas are also associated with the autosomal dominant disorder called *Marfan's syndrome*. Marfan's syndrome is characterized by degeneration of the elastic fibers of the aortic media, usually beginning at the aortic root and spreading segmentally throughout. Physical manifestations of this disorder include long arms and legs, thin hands and feet, lax ligaments, and deformities of the thoracic cage.[4]

Clinical manifestations of a aortic dissection often present a striking change in appearance, depending on the location of the dissection. External rupture may lead to exsanguination, but more frequently, the process involves dissection from the initial point away from the heart. As it dissects through the aortic segment, it often causes obstruction to vessels branching off the aorta. If it occurs across the arch of the aorta, color changes and cerebral ischemia may be noted suddenly. Aortic regurgitation may result if the dissection occurs retrograde through the aortic valve.

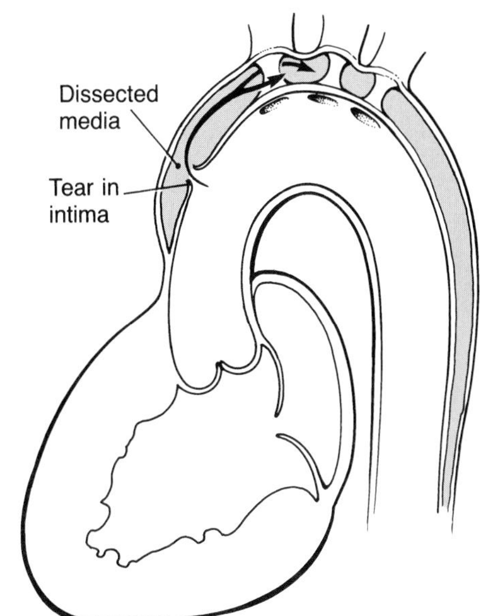

FIGURE 16-5. **Consequences of dissection from the ascending aorta across the arch of the aorta.**

The affected person usually complains of the sudden onset of severe, tearing chest pain that radiates to the back, abdomen, and hips.[5] The mortality rate with aortic dissection is very high. In the initial 24 hours after dissection, a 35% mortality rate is reported and it continues to be high in the first and second weeks.[17] Two main factors that determine the mortality are the place of origin of dissection and whether the process is self-limiting.[4]

SACCULAR ANEURYSMS

Saccular aneurysms are more frequently associated with syphilis or congenital malformations than with atherosclerosis. They are characterized by an outpouching on one side of an artery (Fig. 16-6). Common congenital saccular aneurysms are described as *berry aneurysms* when they occur on the arteries of the circle of Willis. The danger of these intracerebral aneurysms is intracranial rupture and bleeding (see p. 1010).

Saccular syphilitic aneurysms most frequently arise on the ascending and descending thoracic aorta. They can compress the mediastinal structures, place pressure on the surrounding skeletal structures, thrombose, or rupture. Syphilitic (luetic) aneurysms are rarely reported in the United States because of improved treatment and measures to control syphilis.[3] A common saccular aneurysm is the *false aneurysm* that may form at a surgical site for arterial repair. False aneurysms have been reported after revascularization surgeries, such as aortoiliac bypass of the lower extremities, and repair of arteries damaged by trauma. This aneurysm

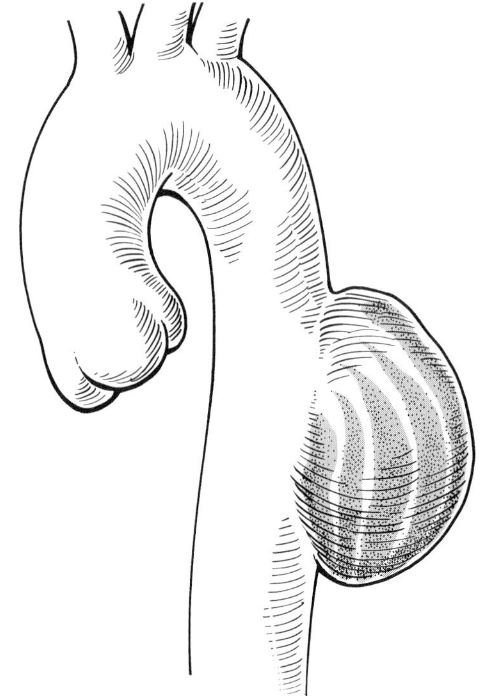

FIGURE 16-6. **Saccular aneurysm of the descending aorta.**

may erode into a surrounding structure and rupture, causing grave effects.[5]

Arteriolosclerosis

Arteriolosclerosis, as its name implies, involves degeneration of the intima and media of small arteries and arterioles. When arteriolosclerosis affects the kidney, hypertension results, but hypertension often initiates the condition. Arteriolosclerosis also may occur in the peripheral arteries and arterioles of the aged, and is often considered to be a change of normal aging.

Arteriospastic Disorders

RAYNAUD'S PHENOMENON

Raynaud's phenomenon (RP) is the clinical syndrome of episodic constriction of the small arteries or arterioles of the extremities, resulting in intermittent pallor and cyanosis of the skin of the fingers, toes, and sometimes the ears or nose. After an episode of constriction, hyperemia may produce rubor. RP is associated with several conditions and diseases. It is a vasospastic disorder that produces temporary changes in skin color and is often secondary to some underlying disorder.[21]

Primary Raynaud's Phenomenon or Raynaud's Disease

This disease occurs predominantly in women, and heredity may play a role in its development. Symptoms usually develop between ages 20 and 40 years. Because investigators rarely are able to examine sections of the blood vessels in cases of early Raynaud's disease, little is known of the pathologic changes in its initial stages. In advanced stages, the intima of the digital arteries is thickened.

The typical clinical picture of primary RP is color changes of the extremities on exposure to cold. At first, only the tips of the fingers are involved, but later, the more proximal parts also exhibit color changes. All the fingers of both hands usually undergo color changes that include pallor, cyanosis, and rubor. The sequential change from pallor to cyanosis and finally to rubor is characteristic.[26] The toes, nose, or ears may also exhibit these changes.

Pallor is caused by spasm of the arterioles and possibly the venules. During this time, blood flow into the capillaries is decreased or absent, causing the affected part to appear dead white. Cyanosis results from capillary dilatation, which occurs later in the course of the disease. Blood flow becomes sluggish with extraction of more oxygen. Rubor indicates excessive hyperemia due to reactive vasodilatation. Exposure to emotional or thermal (cold) stimuli initiate vasoconstriction with subsequent color changes in the digits. Pain characterizes advanced disease, often associated with ulceration on the tips of the digits. Paresthesias such as numbness, tingling, throbbing, and dull aching may be present. During an actual attack, coldness of the digits is evident, sensory acuity is decreased, and other vasomotor syndromes, such as migraine, may be described.

Secondary Raynaud's Phenomenon

A large group of seemingly unrelated conditions may share RP as one of their features (Box 16-2). The link with connective tissue disease, especially scleroderma, is notable in that RP may precede skin changes by months or years.[21] This type of RP, called secondary RP, necessitates the evaluation for the presence of an underlying condition. Table 16-5 compares the clinical features of primary RP with that picture associated with connective tissue disease.

Arteritis

Arteritis is a general term for inflammation an artery. This term replaces the earliest vasculitic syndrome termed *periarteritis nodosa*, named for nodules seen along the course of the small arteries.[27] The process can involve small or medium-sized arteries. It may result from infection or generalized systemic disease. Numerous conditions can be classified as arteritis; the most common are infective aortitis, Takayasu's disease, polyarteritis nodosa, and giant cell arteritis.

BOX 16-2

MECHANISTIC CLASSIFICATION OF RAYNAUD'S PHENOMENON

Vasospastic

Primary (idiopathic) Raynaud's phenomenon
Drug-induced
β-Adrenergic blockers
Ergot
Methysergide
Pheochromocytoma
Variant angina
Migraine

Structural

Vibration syndrome
Arteriosclerosis
Thromboangiitis obliterans
Cold injury (frostbite, pernio, immersion foot)
Neurovascular compression (thoracic outlet syndrome, carpal tunnel syndrome, crutch pressure)
Chemotherapy (bleomycin, vinblastine)
Polyvinyl chloride disease
Connective tissue disease
Systemic sclerosis
Systemic lupus erythematosus
Overlap syndrome
Polymyositis/dermatomyositis
Rheumatoid arthritis

Hemorrheologic

Cryoglobulinemia
Cryofibrinogenemia
Cold agglutinin disease
Paraproteinemia (plasma cell dyscrasia)
Polycythemia (essential thrombocythemia, polycythemia vera)

(Source: Kelley, W. N. [1997]. *Textbook of internal medicine* [3rd ed.]. Philadelphia: Lippincott-Raven.)

Infective aortitis mainly results from infection of the aortic wall by blood-borne pathogens. These organisms enter through the vasa vasorum and commonly lodge in a previously damaged area, such as an aneurysm, atherosclerotic area, or area of aortic trauma.[17] The clinical picture varies and may only be recognized by an unexplained persistent febrile illness in an individual with atherosclerosis, aortic valvular surgery, or a known aortic aneurysm.

Takayasu's disease causes inflammation of the aorta and upper branches. The condition primarily affects young women and is believed to have an autoimmune basis.[2] It is classified according to the amount of involvement of the aorta: (1) that restricted to the aortic arch and its branches, (2) that involving the descending thoracic aorta and the abdominal aorta, and (3) that involving both the arch and descending aorta.[2] As the arterial disease becomes established, ischemic symptoms involving the upper extremities and central nervous system are common.[17]

Polyarteritis nodosa is a vasculitis of the medium-sized arteries of middle-aged men. It tends to affect the branchings and bifurcations of arteries with an inflammatory process that may lead to weakening of the wall and development of aneurysms. This condition is often thought to be a connective tissue disorder but its etiology is unknown. Symptoms vary with the location of the lesions.

Giant cell arteritis is a special type of arteritis that is found mainly in the cerebral arteries, especially the temporal, but may involve the aorta.[17] This common form of vasculitis is seen in greatest incidence in older adults, usually at about the age of 70.[23] The affected artery is infiltrated with granulomatous inflammations that contain giant cells that vary widely in number. These areas become foci for necrosis. The affected artery then becomes swollen, irregular, and fragmented. Thrombosis may obliterate the vessel lumen.[23] Symptoms include headache and temporal pain, which may be accompanied by fever, malaise, and generalized muscular aching. If the temporal artery is affected the area over the temporal artery will be swollen, tender, and red.

ALTERED FUNCTION OF VEINS

Veins have walls that contract or relax, intact endothelium to prevent clotting, and valves that promote blood flow to the heart. Normally, the valves of larger veins and communicating veins prevent retrograde flow of blood in the superficial and deep veins, which promotes forward blood flow. The system provides a venous pump that enables individuals to maintain an upright position. When a person is standing, the pressure of blood in the feet rises to about 90 mm Hg. When standing continues, as much as 15% to 20% of the blood volume can be sequestered and effectively lost from the circulation.[5] Walking causes the muscles to contract and squeeze blood into the veins and propel it toward the heart. When the muscles relax the venous valves prevent the backflow of blood to the periphery. The structure of the veins, discussed on page 424, provides the basis for normal blood return to the heart.

Obstructive Diseases of the Veins

Obstructive lesions of the veins may be permanent or temporary, partial or complete. Obstruction to some portion of the main trunk causes the distal large veins to dilate, which results in incompetent valves.

TABLE 16-5

CLINICAL FEATURES HELPFUL IN DISTINGUISHING PRIMARY RAYNAUD'S PHENOMENON FROM RAYNAUD'S PHENOMENON OF EARLY CONNECTIVE TISSUE DISEASE

FEATURE	PRIMARY RAYNAUD'S PHENOMENON	RAYNAUD'S PHENOMENON SECONDARY TO CONNECTIVE TISSUE DISEASE
Sex	Overwhelmingly female	Male or female
Age of onset	Menarche	Mid-20s and later
Extent of involvement	Usually all digits	Frequently a single digit to start
Symptoms	Mild to moderate	Moderate to severe
Attack precipitated by emotional stress	Yes	Rarely
Ischemic injury	No	Yes
Finger edema	Rare	Common
Periungual erythema	Rare	Common
Evidence of other vasomotor syndromes (eg. migraine)	Yes	No

(Source: Kelley, W. N. [1997]. *Textbook of internal medicine* [3rd ed.]. Philadelphia: Lippincott-Raven.)

The small veins and venules may be damaged permanently as a result of pressure, stretching, hypoxemia, and malnutrition. Permanent impairment in interchange of fluid may result from disruption of small vessels. Damaged venous capillaries may function normally when the person is in a recumbent position but inadequately when the person stands. This inadequacy is due to increased hydrostatic pressure and sometimes to associated incompetent valves.

THROMBOSIS IN THE VENOUS SYSTEM

Lesions in veins may produce localized thrombi in small veins or extensive thrombi in the larger veins. Classically, thrombosis is associated with *Virchow's triad*: (1) venous stasis, (2) changes in the wall of the vein, and (3) a hypercoagulable state. Venous thrombosis may result from an inflammatory or traumatic lesion of the endothelium of the vein wall. In most cases, however, no evidence is found of either. An inflammatory reaction may develop in the vein wall as a reaction to primary thrombosis, so that phlebitis ensues several hours after the thrombus is formed. The terms *thrombophlebitis* (with inflammation) and *phlebothrombosis* (without inflammation) have been largely replaced by the term *deep vein thrombosis* (*DVT*), which mainly refers to thrombosis in the deep veins of the legs.

Pathophysiology

A thrombus develops as a result of slowed flow in the venous bloodstream and is associated with platelet aggregation. After several days and after development of a secondary reaction in the wall of the thrombosed vein, a sudden proximal extension may protrude from the end of the original organizing thrombus. Emboli may develop at this time from the proximal extension, or the new clot may stick and become organized. Emboli may be small or large; they tend to lodge in the vessels of the pulmonary circulation (see p. 575).

A thrombus organizes from its outer margins centrally. In some veins, the entire thrombus organizes with complete and permanent occlusion of the lumen (Fig. 16-7). In a large thrombus, involution usually occurs by a process of partial fibrosis and partial lysis, which is probably due to the action of naturally occurring fibrinolysins (plasmins) in the blood. In most cases, the center disappears and a varying portion of the periphery may organize on a fibrous ring.

The degree of inflammatory reaction in the different layers of the veins varies. In some persons, the thrombus causes minimal reaction; in others an intense reaction extends throughout all layers. Inflammatory cells, leukocytes, lymphocytes, and fibroblasts accumulate and cause congestion of capillaries in and around the venous wall.

Venous thrombosis obstructs venous blood flow and relates to the size and location of the involved vein. If it occurs in superficial veins and in short segments, collateral circulation will compensate. This compensation may occur in obstruction of the saphenous vein of the leg or a larger vein of the arm (eg, median basilic or cephalic) because of the numerous anastomoses that occur. Collateral channels may become evident even after obstruction of the superior or inferior vena cava.

When thrombosis occurs in the iliofemoral or axillary veins, the collateral circulation compensates only partially and venous pressure increases in the veins distal to the thrombosis. This increased pressure

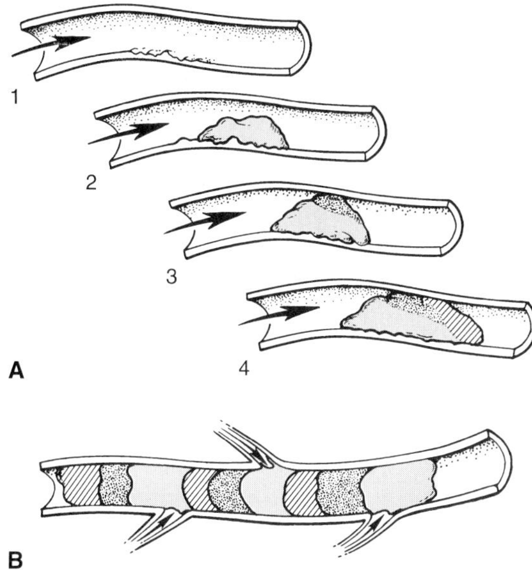

FIGURE 16-7. **A.** Stages in the development of phlebothrombosis: 1, intimal damage, sluggish circulation; 2, platelet aggregation; 3, occlusion of the lumen of the vein; 4, blood clot propagates. **B.** Clot propagates clot at each point of entry of the small veins.

results in distention of all veins and even venules of the limb. The increased pressure in the venules and capillaries causes intense congestion of these areas. Pressure changes inhibit normal reabsorption of fluid and electrolytes from the tissues in the venous end of the capillaries. Edema of the affected limb then develops.

Idiopathic thrombophlebitis is a recurrent condition that produces segmental lesions in the small and medium-sized veins. The thrombus may be recanalized and the lumen restored, but more frequently the vein becomes completely obliterated. *Suppurative thrombophlebitis* differs in that it usually results from bacterial invasion. The wall of the vein becomes markedly inflamed and leukocytes infiltrate the area. Bacteria within the thrombus and portions of the endothelium ultimately lead to abscesses. The infection may follow the course of the vein and may erode into the tissues surrounding the vein. This condition is often termed **cellulitis**, which refers to a diffuse infection of the skin or subcutaneous tissue. *Chemical thrombophlebitis* may result from venous irritation from drugs (eg, antibiotics or potassium) or other chemicals that gain access to the venous circulation. The thrombus becomes adherent and completely organized, resulting in a vein that is contracted, fibrotic, and cordlike.

Clinical Manifestations

Symptoms and signs of thrombophlebitis develop acutely and usually persist for 1 to 3 weeks. In small or medium-sized veins, acute thrombophlebitis rarely produces systemic reactions. With involvement of the larger vessels, the body temperature may rise to as high as 102°F (39°C). Thrombosis of superficial veins often involves redness, pain, tenderness, and localized edema.

Deep vein thrombosis may produce calf pain and tenderness in the calf muscles. Enlargement of the calf and a positive Homans' sign (pain in the calf muscle when the foot is dorsiflexed) may result. Thrombosis of the iliofemoral vein usually produces a typical, acute, clinical picture. Moderate to severe pain in the thigh and groin with diffuse pain throughout the limb is described. Superficial veins may be prominent and distended in the edematous limb. The skin of the leg and thigh may be slightly cyanotic. Thrombosis may be accompanied by impaired or absent pulses from associated arterial spasm. Fever and tachycardia may also be associated. Pitting edema is characteristic with onset a few days after the obstruction ensues. As the edema becomes chronic, it may be associated with skin changes and **brawny edema**. The skin becomes thick, hardened, infiltrated with plasma proteins, and often has an "orange-peel" appearance. The edema is different from cardiac edema in that it does not pit on digital pressure.

Thrombosis of the axillary and subclavian veins produces a clinical picture similar to that of iliofemoral thrombosis. The axillary vein becomes tender, prominent, and enlarged with pitting edema in the forearm and hand. Superficial veins of the entire arm are prominent and those of the pectoral region on the affected side may be distended.

Venous Insufficiency and Stasis

Chronic venous insufficiency results from stasis (stagnation) of venous blood flow, especially in the iliofemoral veins. Old iliofemoral thrombophlebitis leaves behind a thickened, inelastic vein wall, damaged venous valves, and a partially or sometimes completely obstructed lumen. In the lower extremity, the three groups of veins—deep, communicating, and superficial—normally have thin, elastic walls and segmentally spaced valves of the bicuspid type. Venous flow against gravity in the lower limbs is possible by action of the calf muscle and the competent valves. Muscular compression of the elastic veins forces blood upward and the valves prevent retrograde flow. This mechanism fails in chronic venous insufficiency, usually because of incompetent valves. The result is venous hypertension in the affected system.

Ambulatory venous pressure becomes high, which upsets the normal equilibrium of capillary fluid exchange and causes congestion and edema. Stasis also results from the high ambulatory pressures, as manifested by changes in the skin and subcutaneous tissues around the distal third of the leg and around the ankle. Changes that may occur include edema, hyperpigmentation, dermatitis, induration (a firm, hard area), stasis cellulitis, and ultimately, venostasis ulcers (Fig. 16-8). The amount of edema varies according to length of dependency of the affected limb. In chronic stasis, brawny edema and a characteristic light brown pigmentation in white skin and a darker pigmentation in black skin are visible. Pain may be present. A dull ache in the affected leg may develop after the individual has been standing for variable periods. Affected individuals usually describe the pain as more severe when standing still rather than when walking. The pain usually disappears within 5 to 30 minutes after the person assumes a recumbent position with the leg elevated. Nocturnal muscular cramps may be reported.

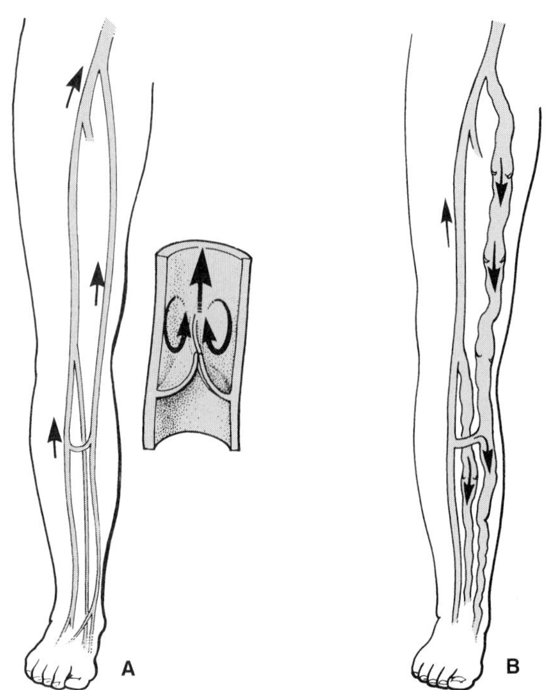

FIGURE 16-9. **Varicose veins. A. Normal vein with competent valves. B. Incompetent valves with tortuous, dilated segments promote stasis of blood in lower extremities.**

Varicose Veins

Varicose veins are dilated, elongated, and tortuous superficial veins of the lower extremities. They are produced by incompetent valves and increased intraluminal pressure (Fig. 16-9). Varicose veins vary from a small group of dilated veins to involvement of the leg's whole venous system. Varicosities probably develop because of an inherent weakness in the vein's structure. Superficial veins dilate when they lack normal resistance against pressure. Primary varicose veins may develop from hereditary predisposition, pregnancy, prolonged standing, and marked obesity. Prolonged periods of standing favor development of varicosities because of the high gravitational pressure within the veins. Obesity places external pressure on the veins, especially the iliofemoral veins. Estimates are that up to 50% of the general population over age 50 have varicose veins, with women affected four times more often than men.[4,23]

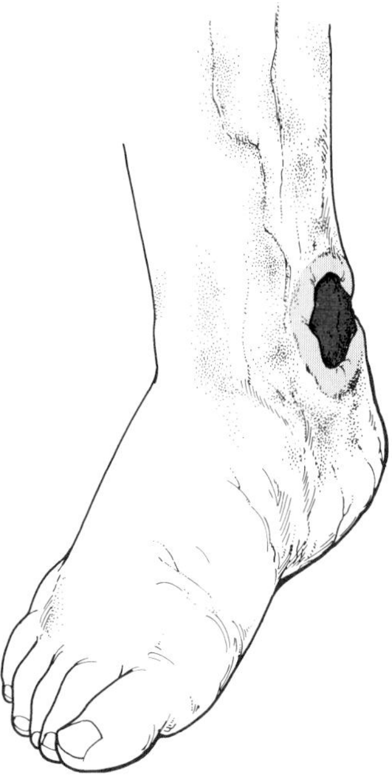
FIGURE 16-8. **Stasis dermatitis with a stasis ulcer from long-term venous stasis.**

Deep venous thrombosis often gives rise to secondary varicosities. Loss of valve sufficiency places unusual strain on the superficial veins. A frequent finding is the presence of localized dilatations just distal to the venous valves. Valve incompetency is due primarily to extreme dilatation in the affected veins, which causes separation of the valve cusps. In primary varicose veins, incompetency tends to progress downward in the saphenous main channel and its tributaries. In secondary varicose veins, which arise because of deep vein insufficiency, incompetency tends to progress upward from incompetent perforating veins in the lower third of the leg.

Varicose veins can lead to chronic venous insufficiency. In the early stages, affected individuals may notice localized pain and heat after prolonged standing. Persistent edema may develop, together with trophic skin changes and stasis ulcers (see Fig. 16-8). The stasis ulcers heal slowly due to poor blood supply and often become infected.

ALTERED FUNCTION OF THE LYMPHATIC SYSTEM

The lymphatic system serves the essential function of draining excess fluids and proteins from the interstitial space. This system provides the only means for returning plasma proteins that have leaked into the interstitial space to the general circulation. Wherever tissue fluid levels increase, lymphatic drainage also increases. When fluids continually escape into the interstitial space, such as with venous obstruction and heart failure, edema may not be noted because of increased compensatory lymphatic drainage. In this way, lymphatic flow is an essential method for control of tissue fluid volume.

Obstruction of the lymph vessels interferes with the system's control mechanism and may precipitate or contribute to edema. Numerous factors may cause *lymphedema*, which is the term for edema that results from lymphatic obstruction. Primary or idiopathic lymphedema is rare. Examples include *Milroy's disease*, a congenital lymphedema noticeable at birth (usually caused by faulty development of lymphatic channels) and *lymphedema praecox*, which affects females predominantly between ages 9 and 25 years and is characterized by swelling of the feet.

Secondary lymphedema is much more common than the primary form. Obstruction of the lymph channels may result from malignant metastatic infiltration of the lymph nodes and channels. Inflammation or infection of the channels may result in fibrosis and obstruction. A common cause of lymphedema is surgical removal or irradiation of the lymph nodes to prevent spread of malignancy.

Lymphedema essentially results from stasis. Chronic stasis often leads to brawny edema, which describes skin that appears thick, hardened, infiltrated with plasma proteins, and often like an "orange peel." This edema is differentiated from cardiac edema in that it does not pit on digital pressure.

Lymphedema can be categorized as inflammatory or noninflammatory. *Lymphangitis* is the term for inflammation of the lymph vessels, usually from bacterial organisms. *Lymphadenitis* refers to inflammation of the lymph nodes. Lymphangitis is characterized by painful red streaks following the lymph vessels, which may eventually involve the lymph nodes as well. β-Hemolytic streptococci most commonly cause lymphangitis, but any virulent pathogen may initiate it. Systemic effects include a marked temperature elevation, malaise, and chills. Localized edema occurs and may become progressive if attacks recur. Chronic lymphangitis may follow, causing fibrosis of the affected area, further brawny edema, skin changes, and sometimes ulcerations.

SYSTEMIC HYPERTENSION

Hypertension is the most common disease in the United States, affecting 20% to 35% of adults.[15] It is a direct risk factor for and contributor to heart and vascular disease, especially myocardial infarction, congestive heart failure, and cerebrovascular accident. Its etiology is poorly understood and the condition is generally asymptomatic until complications develop. The frequency of sudden death is markedly increased among hypertensive persons.

Hypertension is defined as abnormal elevation of the systolic arterial blood pressure with age-related differences (Table 16-6). Systolic levels normally fluctuate within certain limits depending on body position, age, and stress. Blood pressure varies widely during the course of the day with a surge early in the morning after rising from sleep. This finding may, in part, account for the early morning increase in sudden death, heart attacks, and strokes.[11] Variations are definitely noted with activity (such as running) when the systolic pressure elevates and diastolic pressure may fall.[10]

The Joint National Committee on Detection, Evaluation, and Treatment of High Blood Pressure describes hypertension in terms of stages (Table 16-7). Blood pressure readings (to classify the hypertensive individual) are based on three readings at each visit with at least two visits.[15] Researchers have noted that blood pressure can be markedly elevated at one time and normal at another. This phenomenon is called *labile hypertension*; this condition must be monitored for progression.

The most common feature of hypertension is mixed elevation of systolic and diastolic pressures. Occasionally, the diastolic pressure is elevated without a significant increase in systolic pressure, most commonly in persons under age 45.[15] Increase in systolic pressure

TABLE 16-6

HYPERTENSION AS IT RELATES TO DIFFERENT AGE GROUPS

AGE GROUP	NORMAL	HYPERTENSIVE
Infants	80/40	90/60
Children		
7–11 y	100/60	120/80
Teenagers		
12–17 y	115/70	130/80
Adults		
20–45 y	120–125/75–80	135/90
45–65 y	135–140/85	140/90–160/95
> 65 y	150/85	160/90 (borderline)

TABLE 16-7

STAGES OF HYPERTENSION AS DEFINED BY THE JOINT NATIONAL COMMITTEE ON DETECTION AND EVALUATION OF HYPERTENSION

CATEGORY	SYSTOLIC BLOOD PRESSURE (mm Hg)		DIASTOLIC BLOOD PRESSURE (mm Hg)
Normal	<130		<85
High normal	130–139		85–89
Hypertension			
Stage 1	140–159	*or*	90–99
Stage 2	160–179	*or*	100–109
Stage 3	180–209	*or*	110–119
Stage 4	>210	*or*	>120

without diastolic elevation may occur in elderly persons, or in persons with hyperdynamic circulation (eg, hyperthyroidism) or aortic insufficiency. This type of hypertension is called *isolated systolic hypertension.*

Hypertension is described as *essential (primary, idiopathic) hypertension,* which has no specific etiologic basis, and *secondary hypertension,* which results from a known cause. *Benign* and *malignant hypertension* refer to the course of the disease, either of which may result from essential or secondary hypertension. Benign hypertension is a misnomer because it causes permanent damage, even though its onset is gradual and begins with blood pressure levels only slightly above normal. It is chronic with secondary effects that are not clinically evident for many years. Malignant hypertension refers to rapidly progressive, uncontrollable pressure elevation that causes rapid onset of end-organ complications, including renal failure, cerebrovascular accident, retinal hemorrhages, congestive heart failure, and encephalopathy.

Etiology

The etiology of essential hypertension is unknown, but it has been associated with several risk factors, including advancing age, race, genetic predisposition, obesity, neural mechanisms, sodium intake, and renal vasopressors.

Of secondary forms of hypertension, renal parenchymal and renovascular disease are the most common causative factors.[16] Hypertensive episodes are frequent in alcoholic individuals (up to 50% in noncardiac alcoholics), especially when measurements are made close to the point of ethanol intake.[21] Endocrine hyperfunction related to cortical and medullary hypersecretion account for less than 0.5% of all cases of hypertension.[11] Pregnancy-induced hypertension occurs in approximately 10% of pregnancies and may present as a multisystem disease with cerebral, renal, and hepatic changes[18] (see p. 92). When the causative factor of secondary hypertension is treated, the blood pressure may return to normal. Table 16-8 lists the etiologies associated with essential and secondary hypertension.

TABLE 16-8

CAUSES OF HYPERTENSION

TYPES OF HYPERTENSION	CAUSES
Essential, idiopathic, or primary	• Related to obesity, hypercholesterolemia, atherosclerosis, high-sodium diet, diabetes, stress, type A personality, familial history, smoking, and lack of exercise
Secondary	• Renovascular Parenchymal disease, such as acute and chronic glomerulonephritis Narrowing, stenosis of renal artery—due to atherosclerosis or congenital fibroplasia • Cushing's disease or syndrome • Drugs Oral contraceptives Sympathomimetic drugs Alcohol • Pregnancy • Primary aldosteronism • Renin-secreting tumors • Pheochromocytoma • Coarctation of the aorta

Pathophysiology

Blood pressure is normally maintained within rather narrow limits. During sleep, it may fall to 60/40 mm Hg or less; during exercise, marked increases may be noted that often correspond to changes in heart rate and cardiac output. Total peripheral resistance (TPR) or systemic vascular resistance (SVR) is an important factor in the regulation of arterial blood pressure. It is the sum of all resistances offered by the body's vascular beds. Vascular resistances vary with different organs, but SVR has the greatest effect on the mean arterial blood pressure (see p. 424). Very small changes in arteriolar diameter, also called the precapillary sphincter diameter, significantly affect both systemic arterial pressure and blood flow. When arteriolar constriction occurs, SVR increases, which in turn increases afterload.

LEFT VENTRICULAR HYPERTROPHY AND VENTRICULAR REMODELING

In hypertension, the left ventricle must usually empty against an elevation of the **afterload** (resistance). Higher afterload requires the ventricle to develop more pressure to empty its contents. Consistent increase in workload causes the left ventricle to increase its muscle mass (**hypertrophy**) through an increase in the diameter of the individual muscle fibers. Although left ventricular hypertrophy (LVH) is a compensatory mechanism early in the disease process, it becomes an independent cardiovascular risk factor over the long term.[19] Even though the increased muscle mass allows the heart to achieve greater pressures to maintain cardiac output, the heart requires more blood flow and oxygen to drive the pump. The increased muscle mass increases the myocardial need for oxygen and usually reduces ventricular compliance. Together with a muscle mass that needs more oxygen to sustain its increased workload is an acceleration of the coronary atherosclerotic process, a phenomenon frequently noted with hypertension. Myocardial blood flow is thus reduced, increasing the risk of cardiac ischemia and infarction.[7] Eventually, the heart will be unable to keep up with the demand; heart failure or myocardial infarction may result.

The term **ventricular remodeling** refers to changes in the ventricle's contour. Macroscopically, LVH may be *concentric* with a proportional thickening of the left ventricle and the interventricular septum. *Disproportionate thickening* of the interventricular septum more than that of the left ventricular free wall may be seen in persons with borderline hypertension. An *eccentric pattern* combines some hypertrophy with left ventricular chamber enlargement[28] (Fig. 16-10).

Pathologic hypertrophy results when the remodeling causes distortion of the ratio of cardiac myocyte to collagen mass. LVH from hypertension is associated with delayed relaxation and impaired ventricular filling, apparently due to infiltration of the myocardium with fibrosis that replaces some myocytes.[28] The relative amount of collagenous tissue determines myocardial stiffness and may cause the poor compliance seen in hypertensive hearts.[28]

MECHANISMS OF INCREASED SYSTEMIC VASCULAR RESISTANCE

In most types of hypertension, the arterioles offer abnormally increased resistance to blood flow. This resistance increases SVR, decreases capillary blood flow, and results in increased resistance against which the heart must pump. The major hemodynamic alteration is a progressively increasing vascular resistance, achieved through an increase in the tone of arteriolar and venular smooth muscle.[9] Many factors can stimulate the myo-

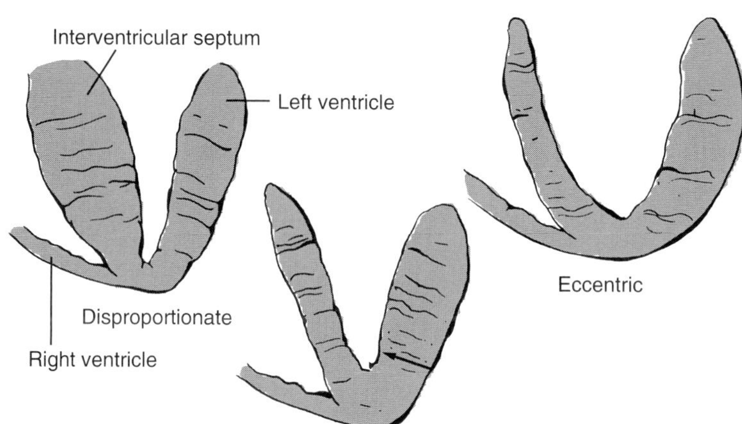

FIGURE 16-10. Remodeling of the left ventricle in relation to arterial hypertension. (1) Disproportionate thickening involves greater septal hypertrophy than LV free wall thickening. (2) Concentric hypertrophy involves main thickening of the left ventricle from endocardium to epicardium. (3) Eccentric hypertrophy involves both hypertrophy and ventricular enlargement.

cytes of the vascular smooth muscle, such as adrenergic input, catecholamines, and angiotensin II. The end result is increased availability of calcium to permit the enhanced state of contractility.[9]

The endothelium of the vessels participates in the process through endothelium-derived factors that cause constriction. These factors include endothelin, superoxide anions, endoperoxides, and thromboxane. Several enzymes inhibit the vasodilating factors of the endothelium resulting in vessel constriction. An example is the inhibition of nitric oxide, which is a potent endothelially produced relaxing substance that affects factors such as angiotensin II. Impaired nitric oxide synthesis or the vascular response to it is seen in aging, hypertensive vascular disease, and hyperlipidemia.[9]

Renin has been implicated in the causation of hypertension in the following way:

1. When blood flow to the kidneys decreases, the juxtaglomerular cells release renin (a proteolytic enzyme), which reacts with angiotensinogen (a plasma protein formed by the liver) to form angiotensin I, which an enzyme in the lungs then converts to angiotensin II. Angiotensin II is a potent vasoconstrictor.
2. The target for the angiotensin II effect is the arterioles. Circulating angiotensin II also stimulates aldosterone secretion which, in turn, increases blood volume by conserving sodium and water (Flowchart 16-1).
3. Angiotensin II can be changed to generate angiotensin III, which has many of the same physiologic effects as angiotensin II.
4. Angiotensin II also may be changed to angiotensin IV, which appears to have effects on the central nervous system and electrolyte balance.[13,24]

This renin–angiotensin–aldosterone system is a normal regulator of blood pressure and blood volume that goes awry in hypertension.

Increased serum renin levels are not present in every form of hypertension but they correlate well with some

FLOWCHART 16-1 **Renin–Angiotensin–Aldosterone System**

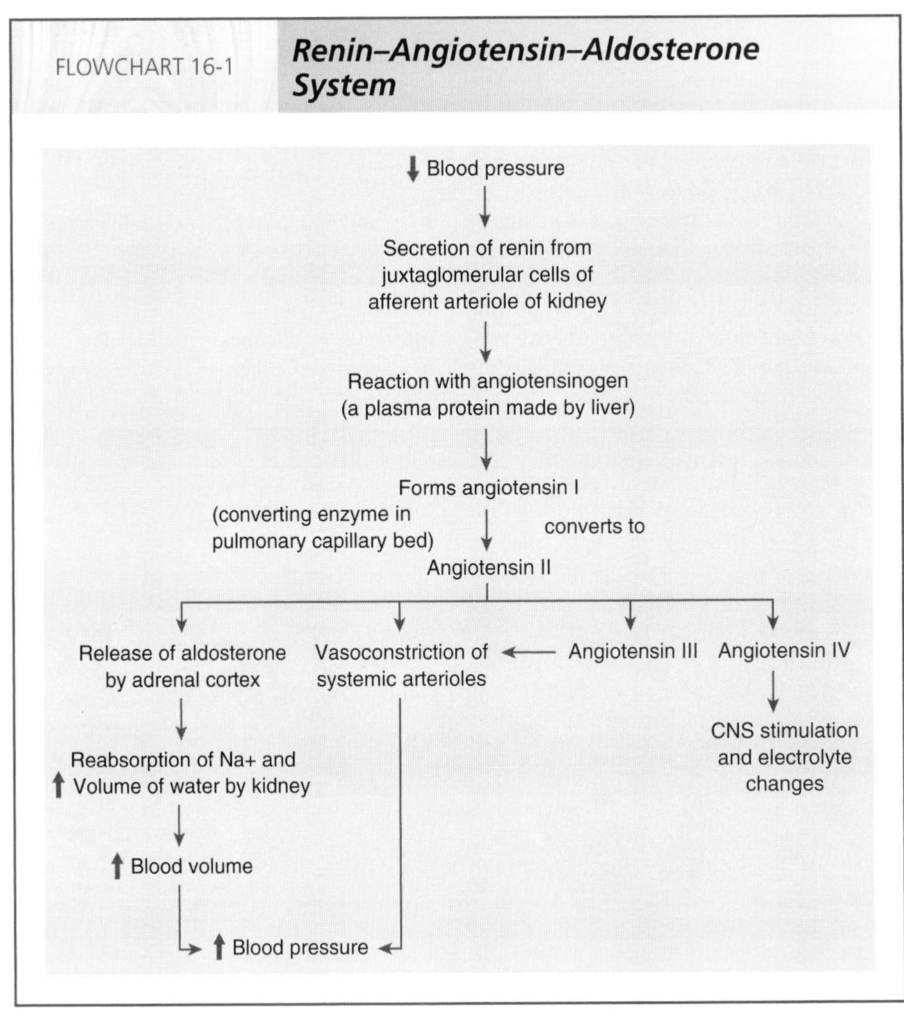

types, especially the accelerated or malignant form.[9] It is important to correlate plasma renin activity with daily sodium intake because renin is usually released with decreased levels of sodium and is suppressed by increased levels. Plasma renin activity can estimate the amount of generated angiotensin II.

Complications

The signs and symptoms that hypertensive individuals exhibit are mainly complications of sustained hypertension. Hypertension is often categorized as stage 1: mild; stage 2: moderate; stage 3: severe; or stage 4: very severe (see Table 16-7). It also may be labile or that with isolated systolic hypertension. Mild or moderate hypertension is often asymptomatic or affected individuals may describe vague symptoms such as "head stuffiness" or dizziness. It is frequently discovered on a screening blood pressure check. When mild or moderate hypertension is sustained, a great possibility exists of target organ damage (see below). Stage 3 hypertension is a blood pressure of 180 to 209 systolic and 110 to 119 diastolic and requires treatment within a few days. Very severe (accelerated, or malignant) hypertension, often seen in the emergency setting, is extremely high with a diastolic pressure of greater than 125 mm Hg in conjunction with **papilledema** (optic disk swelling).[11] Very rapid renal, cardiac, and cerebral damage may occur if the blood pressure is not controlled quickly. Labile hypertension is a common result of stress or other disease conditions. It is characterized by wide fluctuations in blood pressure and assessment for target organ damage is essential. Isolated systolic hypertension may be associated with many disease conditions and is common in elderly individuals. It carries the same risks for cardiovascular damage as mild or moderate hypertension.[11]

When symptoms do occur, hypertension is usually far advanced. The classic symptoms of headache, epistaxis, dizziness, and tinnitus thought to be associated with high blood pressure are no more common in hypertensive than in normotensive individuals. Unsteadiness, waking headache, blurred vision, depression, and nocturia have been shown to be increased in untreated hypertension.[11] The prognosis for uncontrolled hypertension is dismal. Statistics of premature death correlate with levels of blood pressure elevation. The risk of cerebrovascular accident, for example, is five times higher for hypertensive than for normotensive individuals.

Table 16-9 summarizes the end organs affected by hypertension and how these effects manifest themselves. The target organs most frequently affected are the eyes, the heart and vascular system, the brain, and the kidney.

HYPERTENSIVE RETINOPATHY

Changes in the retina (retinopathy) provide some objective clues to hypertension's clinical course. The Keith-Wagener-Barker funduscopic classification indicates a I rating for minimal arteriolar narrowing; II for more significant narrowing and arteriovenous nicking; III for flame-shaped hemorrhages and cotton wool exudates; and IV for the above changes with papilledema (Fig. 16-11). Studies have associated retinopathy with 5-year survival rates of 85% for group I, 50% for group II, 13% for group III, and 0% for group

TABLE 16-9

HYPERTENSIVE EFFECTS ON TARGET ORGANS

ORGAN	EFFECT	MANIFESTED BY
Heart	Myocardial infarction	ECG changes; enzyme elevations
	Congestive failure	Decreased cardiac output; S_3 or summation gallop auscultated: cardiomegaly on radiograph
	Myocardial hypertrophy	Increased voltage R wave in V_3–V_6; increased frequency of angina; left ventricular strain, manifested by ST- and T-wave changes
	Dysrhythmias	Usually ventricular dysrhythmias or conduction defects
Eyes	Blurred or impaired vision	Nicking arteries and veins; hemorrhages and exudates on visual examination
	Encephalopathy	Papilledema
Brain	Cerebrovascular accident	Severe occipital headache, paralysis, speech difficulties, coma
	Encephalopathy	Rapid development of confusion, agitation, convulsions, death
Kidneys	Renal insufficiency	Nocturia, proteinuria, elevated blood urea nitrogen level, creatinine
	Renal failure	Fluid overload, accumulation of metabolites, metabolic acidosis

ECG, electrocardiogram.

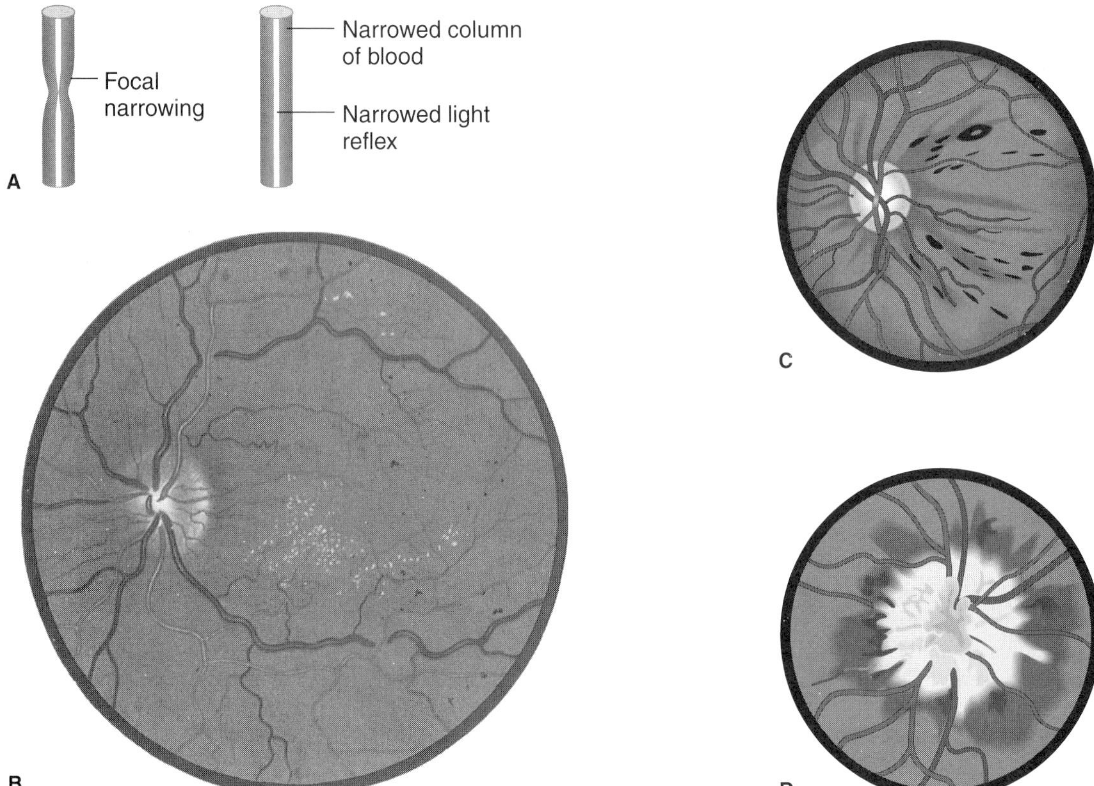

FIGURE 16-11. Hypertensive changes on the retina of the eye. **A**. Arteries show areas of focal or generalized narrowing. **B**. Venous tapering and blurring of the optic disk can be seen. **C**. Superficial retinal hemorrhages show as flame-shaped red streaks. **D**. Engorgement and swelling of disk result from severe hypertension, called papilledema. (Adapted from Bates, B. [1999]. *Guide to physical examination and history taking* [7th ed]. Philadelphia: Lippincott Williams & Wilkins.)

IV.[11] Papilledema is always associated with malignant hypertension.

HYPERTENSIVE CARDIOVASCULAR DISEASE

Hypertension increases the rate of atherosclerotic changes. This atherosclerosis may affect any major artery, including the coronaries. Manifestations of peripheral vascular disease, aneurysms, or myocardial ischemia or infarction may occur. Hypertension is the most common cause of LVH, which can increase coronary ischemia.

Myocardial ischemia may result from atherosclerosis of the coronary arteries along with associated LVH. The risk for developing a myocardial infarction is increased. Dysrhythmias are common and relate to decreased myocardial blood flow and ischemia.

Congestive heart failure frequently occurs in the uncontrolled hypertensive patient. The hypertrophied left ventricle finally cannot maintain the elevated pressures and the compensatory mechanisms of heart failure complicate the disease's course (see p. 476).

HYPERTENSIVE CEREBROVASCULAR DISEASE

The effects of hypertension on the brain are due to microhemorrhages or occlusion of cerebral vessels that produce the cerebrovascular accident or stroke.

When blood pressure rises to extremely high (accelerated or malignant) levels, hypertensive encephalopathy may occur. The effects of this condition can be readily reduced if the blood pressure is reduced before any cerebral damage occurs.

Stroke

Vascular lesions may cause either a hemorrhagic or ischemic stroke. The increasing pressures may cause dilatation of the small, sometimes nonelastic, and aged vessels. Dilatation, in turn, causes breaks in the vessel and hemorrhage into the brain parenchyma. The dilatations of the smaller intracerebral arteries are called *Charcot-Bouchard microaneurysms*. These microaneurysms may rupture and cause signs of intracerebral hemorrhage. In the process of aneurysm formation, the vessels undergo some repair, which eventually leads to thickening and tortuosity of the endothelium.[4]

Ischemic infarcts often occur from associated atherosclerosis of the extracranial vessels (carotids and vertebrals). Obstruction to blood flow is usually produced by a thrombus on an atherosclerotic plaque .

Hypertensive Encephalopathy

This ominous manifestation results from leakage of water and electrolytes from the brain capillaries into its tissues. This leakage produces cerebral edema and is often associated with papilledema (optic disk swelling). Encephalopathy is most commonly seen in malignant hypertension or when a hypertensive state assumes a malignant, uncontrolled pattern. Severe headache, confusion, or lethargy followed by agitation, convulsions, coma, and frequently death may herald the condition. Hypertensive encephalopathy must be differentiated from other neurologic conditions; a long-standing history of increased blood pressure can support its diagnosis.

HYPERTENSIVE RENAL DISEASES

Benign nephrosclerosis results from chronic hypertension and is characterized by hyaline lesions in the arterioles. Nephrosclerosis decreases blood flow to the renal parenchyma and over time may cause renal insufficiency, especially in individuals who experience trauma or hemorrhage.[4]

In malignant hypertension, nephrosclerosis may be very severe. The severe increase in blood pressure causes vascular necrosis due to endothelial injury, vascular coagulation, and fibroid necrosis. Onset of renal insufficiency and renal failure will be sudden.

Renal failure is a common outcome of diabetic changes in the nephrons that hypertension often accelerates. When essential hypertension is the cause, renal insufficiency frequently results from progressive damage to the small arteries and arterioles. Progressive hyaline sclerosis leads to ischemic death of nephrons and to fibrosis, which causes contracted kidneys. With significant loss of nephrons, renal failure ensues.

FOCUS ON THE PERSON WITH PERIPHERAL VASCULAR DISEASE

J. B. is a 60-year-old white man who sought medical attention due to increasing problems with intermittent claudication and loss of color in the left leg. He was found to have absent pulses in the left foot, even with Doppler studies. A femoral arteriogram showed complete occlusion of the femoral artery several inches above the left knee. Extensive collateral circulation could be seen; and the dorsalis pedis artery was weakly outlined. Except for a history of tobacco smoking, no other risk factors were identified. No other atherosclerotic lesions were noted. A femoral popliteal bypass was recommended to restore circulation to the left foot.

Questions

1. Describe the process of atherosclerotic occlusion of a vessel.
2. What is the basis for the development of collateral circulation?
3. Why did Mr. B. have the symptoms described?
4. What is the relationship between smoking and atherosclerotic arterial disease?
5. Describe the principle of Doppler studies and how a femoral arteriogram is done.
6. How would the surgical procedure recommended restore arterial circulation?

REFERENCES

1. Alexander, R. W., & Griendling, K. K. (1998). Coronary ischemic syndromes: Relationship to the biology of atherosclerosis. In R. W. Alexander, R. C. Schlant, & V. Fuster (Eds.), *Hurst's: The heart* (9th ed.). New York: McGraw-Hill.
2. Benditt, E. P., & Schwartz, S. M. (1994). Blood vessels. In E. Rubin & J. L. Farber (Eds.), *Pathology* (2nd ed.). Philadelphia: Lippincott.
3. Cheitlin, M. D., Sokolow, M., & McIlroy, M. B. (1994). *Clinical cardiology* (6th ed.). Norwalk, CT: Appleton & Lange.
4. Cotran, R. S., Kumar, V., & Robbins, S. L. (1994). *Robbins' pathologic basis of disease* (5th ed.). Philadelphia: Saunders.
5. Daising, M. C., Lalka, S. G., Sawchuk, A. P., & Mohler, E. R. (1997). Vascular medicine. In W. N. Kelley (Ed.), *Textbook of internal medicine* (3rd ed.). Philadelphia: Lippincott-Raven.
6. Davies, M. J. (1998). Pathology of coronary atherosclerosis. In R. W. Alexander, R. C. Schlant, & V. Fuster (Eds.), *Hurst's: The heart* (9th ed.) New York: McGraw-Hill.
7. Devereaux, R. B., & Roman, M. J. (1997). Cardiac structure and function in hypertension. In A. Zanchetti & G. Mancia (Eds.), *Handbook of hypertension, Vol. 17: Pathophysiology of hypertension*. New York: Elsevier Science.
8. Factor, S. M., & Bache, R. J. (1998). Pathophysiology of myocardial ischemia. In R. W. Alexander, R. C. Schlant, & V. Fuster (Eds.), *Hurst's: The heart* (9th ed.). New York: McGraw-Hill.
9. Frohlich, E. D. (1998). *Hypertension: Evaluation and treatment*. Baltimore: Williams & Wilkins.
10. Guyton, A. C., & Hall, J. E. (1996). *Textbook of medical physiology* (9th ed.). Philadelphia: Saunders.
11. Hall, W. D. (1998). Diagnostic evaluation of the patient with systemic arterial hypertension. In R. W. Alexander, R. C. Schlant, & V. Fuster (Eds.), *Hurst's: The heart* (9th ed.). New York: McGraw-Hill.

12. Joyce, J. W., & Rooke, T. W. (1998). Diagnosis and management of diseases of the peripheral arteries and veins. In R. W. Alexander, R. C. Schlant, & V. Fuster (Eds.), *Hurst's: The heart* (9th ed.). New York: McGraw-Hill.
13. Jeunemaitre, X., Soubrier, F., Kotelevtsev, Y. V., Lifton, R. P., Williams, C. S., & Charru, A. (1992). Molecular basis of human hypertension: Role of angiotensinogen. *Cell, 71,* 1–20.
14. Juergens, J. L., Fairbaim, J. E., & Spittell, J. A. (1986). *Peripheral vascular diseases* (5th ed.). Philadelphia: Saunders.
15. Kaplan, N. M. (1998). *Clinical hypertension* (7th ed.). Baltimore: Williams & Wilkins.
16. Klag, M. J., & Whelton, P. K. (1996). Hypertension. In J. D. Stobo, D. B. Hellmann, P. W. Ladenson, B. G. Pety, & T. A. Traill (Eds.), *The principles and practice of medicine* (23rd ed.). Stamford, CT: Appleton & Lange.
17. Lindsay, J., Beall, A. C., & DeBakey, M. E. (1998). Diagnosis and treatment of diseases of the aorta. In R. W. Alexander, R. C. Schlant, & V. Fuster (Eds.), *Hurst's: The heart* (9th ed.). New York: McGraw-Hill.
18. May, K. A., & Mahlmeister, L. R. (1998). *Maternal and neonatal nursing: Family-centered care* (3rd ed.). Philadelphia: Lippincott-Raven.
19. Motz, W., & Scheler, S. (1997). Arterial hypertension and left ventricular hypertrophy. In L. Hannson & W. H. Birkenhager (Eds.), *Handbook of hypertension, Vol. 18: Assessment of hypertensive organ damage.* New York: Elsevier Science.
20. Poston, L. (1998). Mechanisms of atherosclerosis: Part II. Relations between monocytes, macrophages, and the endothelium. In A. Halliday, B. J. Hunt, L. Poston, & M. Schachter (Eds.), *An introduction to vascular biology: From physiology to pathophysiology.* New York: Cambridge University Press.
21. Regan, T. J. (1998). Alcohol and nutrition. In R. W. Alexander, R. C. Schlant, & V. Fuster (Eds.), *Hurst's: The heart* (9th ed.). New York: McGraw-Hill.
22. Ross, R. (1998). Factors influencing atherogenesis. In R. W. Alexander, R. C. Schlant, & V. Fuster (Eds.), *Hurst's: The heart* (9th ed.). New York: McGraw-Hill.
23. Rubin, E., & Farber, J. L. (1994). *Pathology* (2nd ed.). Philadelphia: Lippincott.
24. Santos, R., Simoes, E., Silva, A. C., et al. (1996). Evidence for a physiological role of angiotensin (1–7) in the control of hydroelectrolyte balance. *Hypertension, 27,* 875–884.
25. Schachter, M. (1998). Mechanisms of atherosclerosis: Introduction and current concepts. In A. Halliday, B. Hunt, L. Poston, & M. Schachter (Eds.), *An introduction to vascular biology.* New York: Cambridge University Press.
26. Seibold, J. R. (1997). Scleroderma and Raynaud's syndrome. In W. N. Kelley (Ed.), *Textbook of internal medicine* (3rd ed.). Philadelphia: Lippincott-Raven.
27. Waller, B. F. (1998). Nonatherosclerotic coronary heart disease. In R. W. Alexander, R. C Schlant, & V. Fuster (Eds.), *Hurst's: The heart* (9th ed.). New York: McGraw-Hill.
28. Weber, K. T., Sun, Y., & Cambell, S. E. (1997). Hypertensive heart disease: Structural remodeling and the role of hormones. In A. Zanchetti & G. Mancia (Eds.). *Handbook of hypertension, Vol. 17: Pathophysiology of hypertension.* New York: Elsevier Science.

Chapter

17

Altered Cardiac Function

Barbara L. Bullock

KEY TERMS

anaerobic metabolism
antistreptolysin O titer
atheroma
collateral circulation
creatine kinase (creatinine phosphokinase)
dilatation
hypertrophy
hypokinesis
infarction
insufficiency
ischemia
juxtaglomerular cells
pulsus paradoxus
reperfusion
stenosis
troponin T and I

Cardiovascular disease (CVD) is the leading cause of death and disability in the United States and in most other industrialized nations. Ischemic heart disease accounts for almost one-fourth of deaths in persons over the age of 35.[48] Sudden, out-of-hospital deaths account for more than half of all coronary fatalities.[48] One of every three men and one of every 10 women can expect to develop CVD before the age of 60 years.[30] During the past 30 years mortality rates have declined for the various forms of cardiovascular diseases (Fig. 17-1). Improved CVD mortality figures may reflect widespread application of cardiopulmonary resuscitation, better medical control of emergencies, control of hypertension, lower cholesterol diets, and numerous other factors. Heart failure is a form of CVD that may result from cardiac, pulmonary, or renal disease. Other cardiac disabilities include valvular disease due to congenital or infective causes as well as congenital malformations of the heart.

This chapter focuses on diseases inherent to the heart and its structures. The cardiac dysrhythmias are included because they cause alterations in the cardiac output and occur in many different cardiac conditions.

CARDIAC DYSRHYTHMIAS

An alteration in the normal rhythm of the cardiac cycle is often labeled as dysrhythmia, arrhythmia, or ectopic rhythm. A widely accepted term is *dysrhythmia,* which is defined as an abnormality of the formation or conduction of an electrical impulse that causes an alteration in heart rate or regularity. A dysrhythmia occurs when some factor alters the normal action potential of the heart.

Mechanisms of Dysrhythmias

The two primary mechanisms that initiate alterations in normal cardiac rhythm are:

- *Abnormal automaticity:* Normal automaticity is that found in the normal pacemaker of the heart as described on page 412. Abnormal automaticity refers to abnormal changes in the transmembrane potentials of cardiac muscle cells.[50] It may be classified as *enhanced automaticity* (in which the rate of discharge is increased) or *depressed automaticity* (in which the rate is decreased).
- *Re-entry phenomena:* Re-entry develops when an impulse has the ability to re-excite tissue previously depolarized through anatomic or functional circuits.[53] The rate of impulse conduction and the length of the refractory period influence the presence of re-entry phenomena. Figure 17-2 illustrates how the impulses may enter the circuit and generate recurrent dysrhythmias. Continuous excitement of the myocardium by normal or abnormal paths is described as *a circus movement* or *re-entrant excitation.*[53]

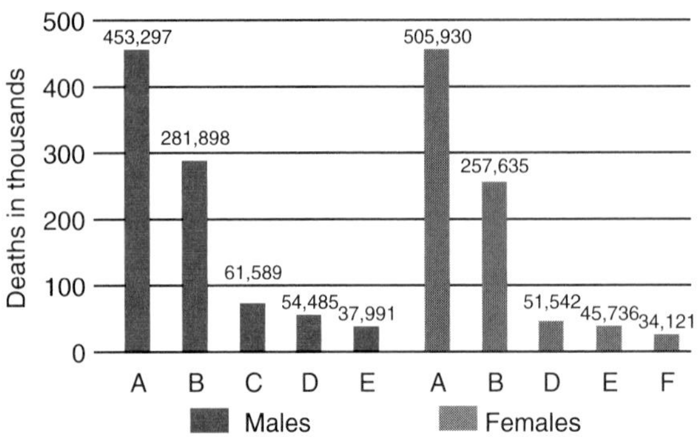

A

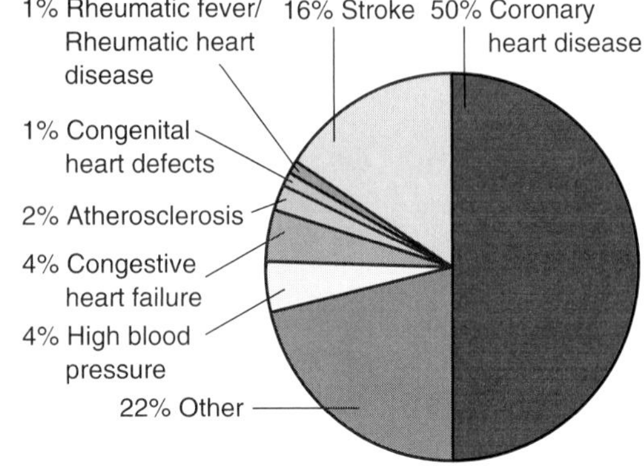

B

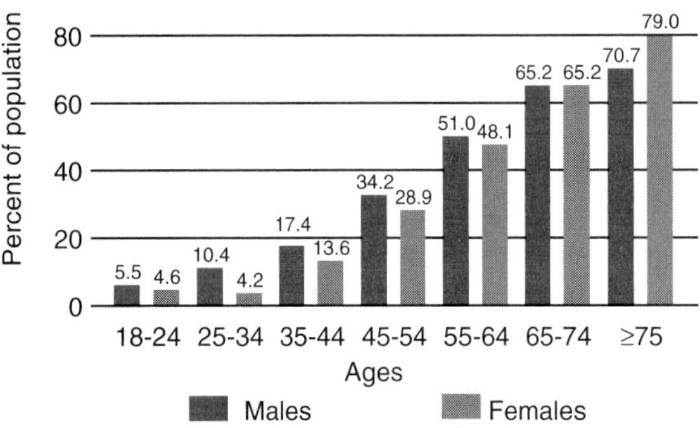

C

FIGURE 17-1. **A.** Leading causes of death for all males and females. **B.** Percentage breakdown of deaths from cardiovascular diseases. **C.** Estimated prevalence of cardiovascular diseases by age and sex. (Source: American Heart Association, Inc., Dallas, TX, 1999; http:www.amhrt.org/statistics/03cardio.html)

Alterations in cardiac rhythms can result from many etiologies (Table 17-1). The most common include disease or injury to the cardiac muscle, structures, or conduction system; systemic diseases; drug intoxication; electrolyte imbalances; and exercise.[27] Hypokalemia in association with stimulation from catecholamines is a potent cause of dysrhythmias, especially ventricular re-entry circuits.[53]

Dysrhythmias are clinically significant as indicators of underlying heart disease or they may produce life-threatening electrical events with catastrophic hemodynamic results. Dysrhythmias may be present with or without clinical signs or symptoms and in individuals with and without advanced cardiac disease. Clinical symptoms in the individual with a normal heart are usually not noted unless the heart rate exceeds 180 beats/min or slows to below 40 beats/min.[54] The hemodynamic effects of dysrhythmias vary depending on the heart rate, rhythm, and the presence of significant underlying heart disease.

Common Cardiac Dysrhythmias

It is convenient to discuss cardiac dysrhythmias according to their anatomic site of origin. The basic cardiac dysrhythmias are classified following the normal conduction pathway of the heart as sinus, atrial, junctional, and ventricular dysrhythmias, and heart blocks. Characteristics of each disturbance are summarized in Table 17-2 along with an example rhythm strip. Detailed information concerning the dysrhyth-

A

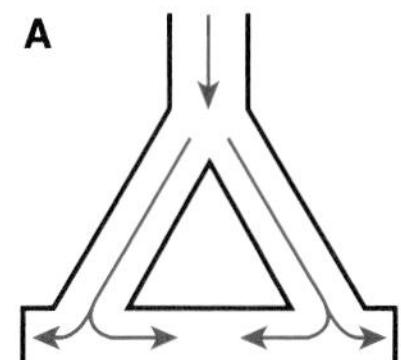

Normal propagation through the Purkinje fiber to depolarize the ventricle

B

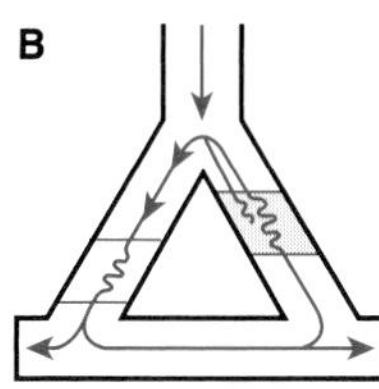

Shaded area on right indicates diseased (ischemic) myocardium. Activation is blocked in that direction and passes retrograde to the other side and reenters the proximal conducting circuit. The propagating impulse does not meet refractory myocardium and continues to activate excitable tissue.

FIGURE 17-2. A schematic reentry pathway.

mias can be found in sources indicated in the Unit bibliography.

CORONARY ARTERY DISEASE/ ISCHEMIC HEART DISEASE

Coronary heart disease (*CHD*), a term used interchangeably with the term *coronary artery disease* (*CAD*), causes about 800,000 new heart attacks and about 450,000 recurrent heart attacks each year.[26] Other terms related to CAD, such as *ischemic heart disease* (IHD) and cardiovascular disease may be used interchangeably with CAD. Men have a higher incidence than women and at an earlier age, but beyond age 65 women have a nearly equal incidence.[2]

TABLE 17-1

ETIOLOGIES OF DYSRHYTHMIAS

ETIOLOGY	EXAMPLES
Underlying cardiac disease	Coronary artery disease; cardiomyopathies; valvular lesions; congenital defects: rheumatic heart disease
Acute myocardial infarction	
Systemic/metabolic diseases	Diabetes; hypertension; pulmonary disorders; hyperthyroidism; anemia
Electrolyte imbalance	
Anesthesia	
Drug intoxication	Digitalis Other prescription and illegal drugs
Central nervous system disorders	
Psychoneurogenic disorders	
Exercise	

Coronary artery disease almost always results from atherosclerosis of the coronary arteries, a fact that has led to widespread research into the causes of atherosclerosis (see p. 433). Numerous theories exist regarding the pathophysiology of atherosclerosis, with most theorists agreeing that it begins early in life and progresses over decades. Many factors probably interact to accelerate the atherogenic process. These have been identified as risk factors in epidemiologic studies because they seem to reflect an increase in the probability of a person developing coronary atherosclerosis but do not predict the severity or extent of an atherosclerotic lesion.[24]

Risk Factors

Certain risk factors determine a person's probability for developing CAD (Table 17-3). They are divided into two categories: risk factors that can be altered by life-style changes and risk factors that cannot be altered.

ALTERABLE RISK FACTORS

Among the alterable risk factors for CAD are high-fat diet, smoking, hypertension, sedentary life-style, and diabetes mellitus. Individuals can diminish the probability of developing CAD by making certain life-style changes in these areas.

Diet

A high-fat diet is a main factor in the development of CAD. In the United States, the consumption of a high-fat, high-carbohydrate diet was standard in most households until the 1970s when education by governmental agencies and the American Heart Association began to advocate a low-fat diet. Despite educational efforts, the diet in the United States remains higher in fat than in most other nations. The liver readily uses foods high in saturated fat content to make cholesterol. Coronary risk is directly related to serum cholesterol: the higher the plasma cholesterol level, the greater the individual's risk for CAD. Those who have plasma cholesterol levels below 160 mg/dL have less than half the risk of myocardial infarction (MI) than those with levels of 250 mg/dL or greater.[24] Table 17-4 lists the various forms and risks of serum cholesterol levels.

As discussed in Chapter 16, cholesterol, when carried by low-density lipoproteins (LDLs) is associated with an increased risk of CAD, whereas cholesterol car-

(text continues on page 461)

TABLE 17-2

CHARACTERISTICS OF CARDIAC DYSRHYTHMIAS

Rhythm: Sinus bradycardia
Mechanism: PSNS (vagal) influence
Origin: Sinus node
Characteristics: Sinus rhythm < 60 bpm

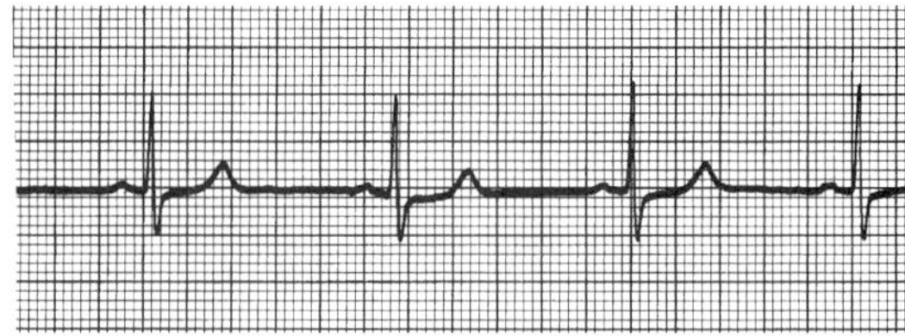

Rhythm: Sinus tachycardia
Mechanism: SNS influence
Origin: Sinus node
Characteristics: Sinus rhythm > 100 bpm

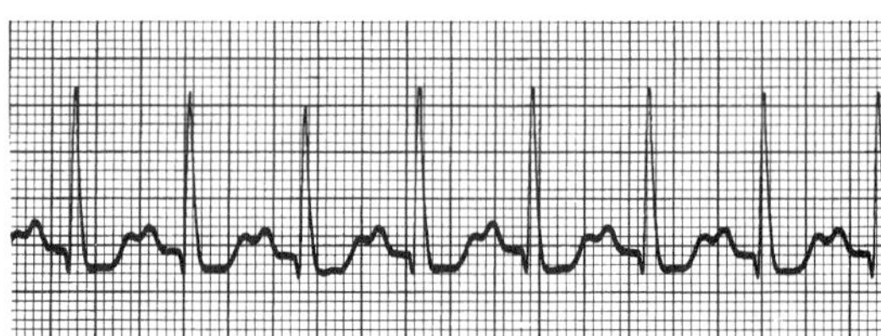

Rhythm: Sinus arrhythmia (sinus dysrhythmia)
Mechanism: Respiratory vagal influences
Origin: Sinus node
Characteristics: Sinus rhythm/irregular rhythm

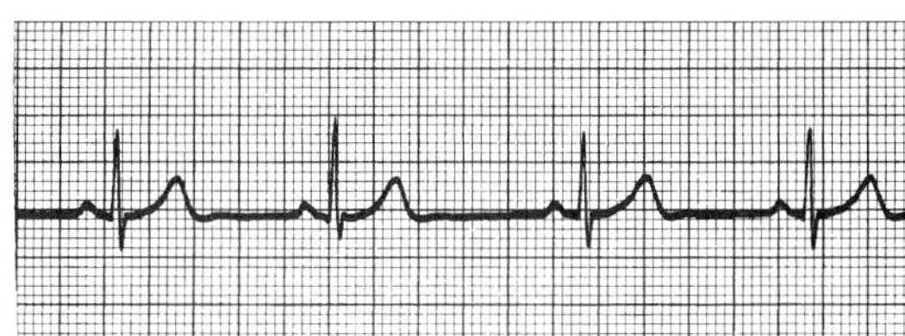

Rhythm: Sinus arrest
Mechanism: Depression of SA node due to disease or vagal influence
Origin: Sinus node
Characteristics: No P wave with no QRS or with escape junctional beat

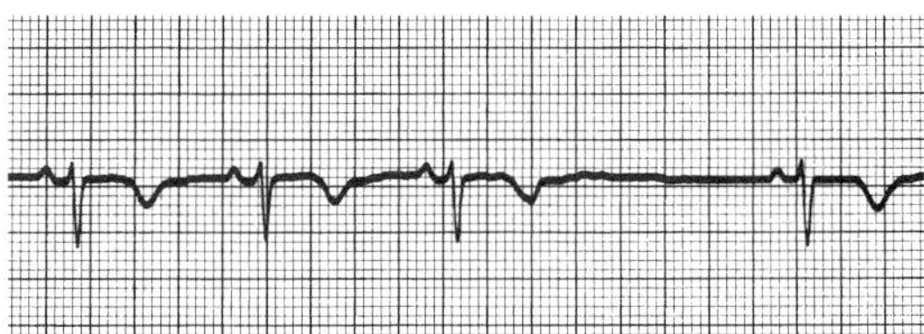

Rhythm: Premature atrial contractions (PACs)
Mechanism: Ectopic atrial impulse
Origin: Atria
Characteristics: Premature abnormal P wave followed by normal QRS and pause following

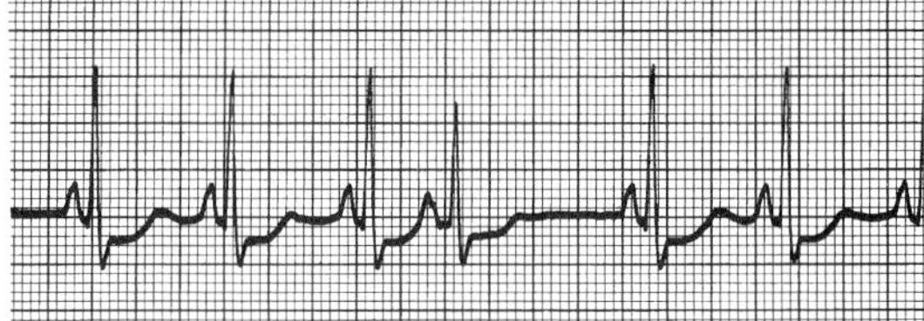

Rhythm: Atrial tachycardia (PAT or AT)
Mechanism: Reentry or automaticity increased
Origin: Atria
Characteristics: Onset of more than 6 PACs in a row; rate often > 150 bpm

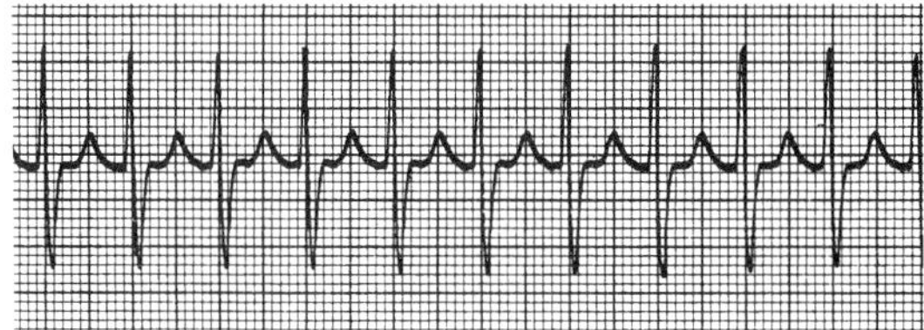

Rhythm: Atrial flutter
Mechanism: Reentry
Origin: Atria
Characteristics: Ectopic site initiates impulse at rate of 250 to 350 bpm; ventricle blocks every 2nd, 3rd, or 4th beat; "saw-toothed" appearance of P waves

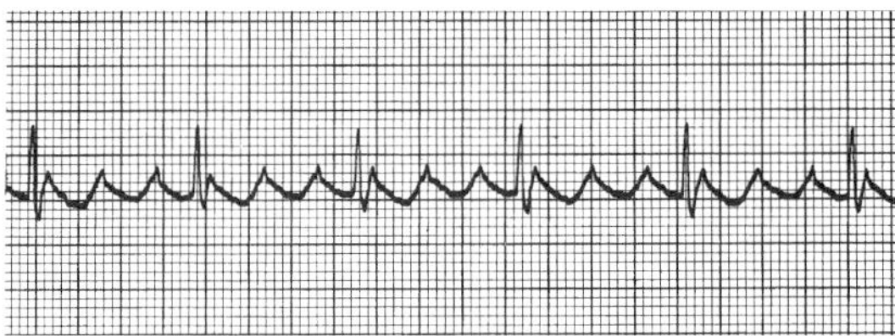

(continued)

TABLE 17-2

CHARACTERISTICS OF CARDIAC DYSRHYTHMIAS (Continued)

Rhythm: Atrial fibrillation
Mechanism: Reentry
Origin: Atria
Characteristics: Impulse formation so rapid that atria cannot contract normally; many impulses are blocked at AV node; giving irregularly irregular rhythm

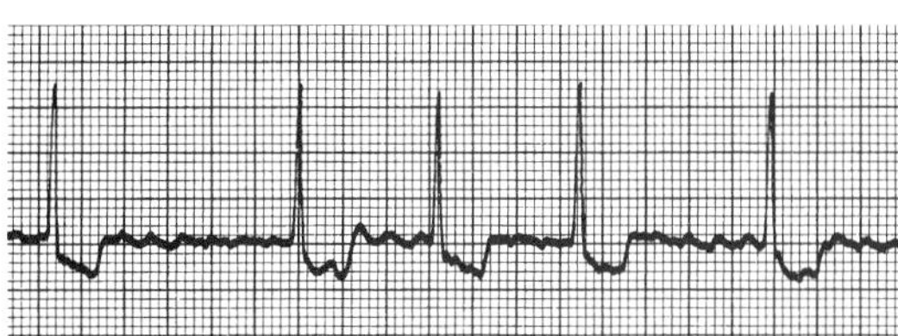

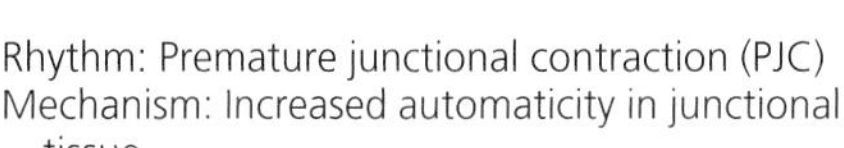

Rhythm: Premature junctional contraction (PJC)
Mechanism: Increased automaticity in junctional tissue
Origin: AV node or bundle of His
Characteristics: An inverted P wave or no P wave on premature beat, followed by pause usually interrupting an entire cycle

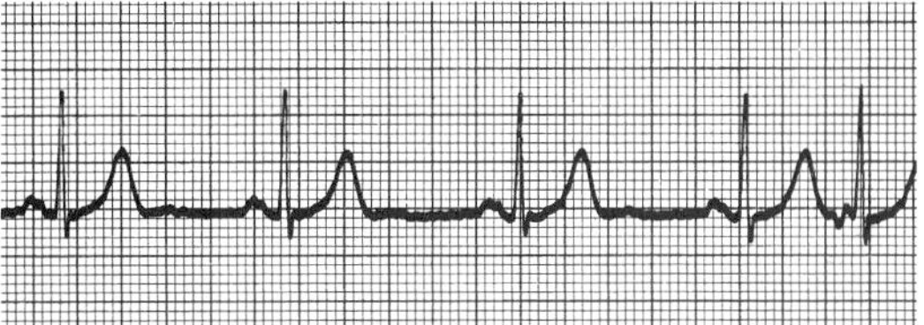

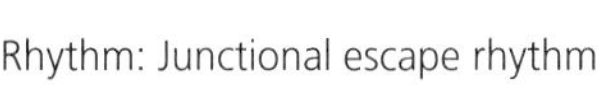

Rhythm: Junctional escape rhythm
Mechanism: Junctional tissue assumes pacemaking function when SA node fails
Origin: AV node or bundle of His
Characteristics: Rate usually 60 bpm or less; inverted P or no P; rhythm usually regular

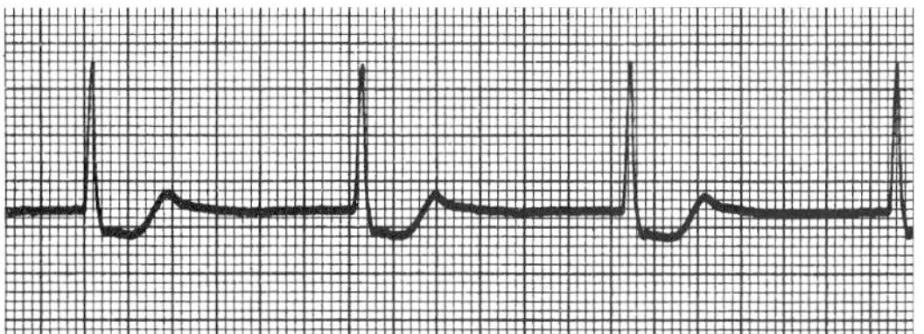

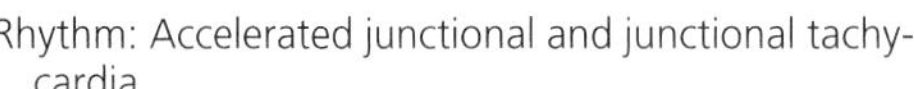

Rhythm: Accelerated junctional and junctional tachycardia
Mechanism: Increased automaticity of junctional tissue
Origin: AV node or bundle of His
Characteristics: Accelerated junctional rate of 60–100 bpm; junctional tachycardia at rate > 100 bpm

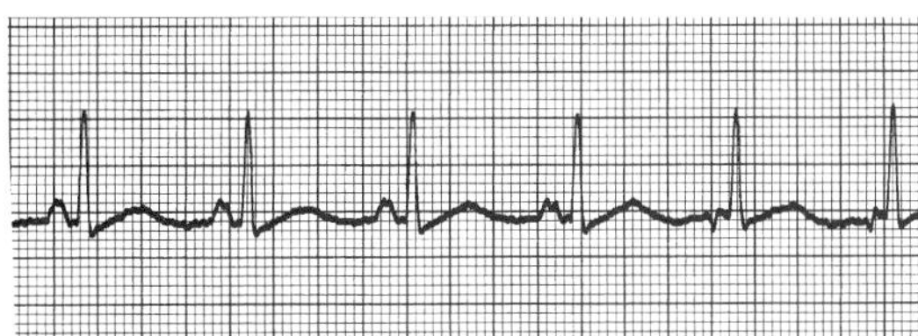

Rhythm: Premature ventricular contractions (PVCs)
Mechanism: Ectopic ventricular impulse
Origin: Ventricles
Characteristics: Wide QRS occurs prematurely and is followed by compensatory pause

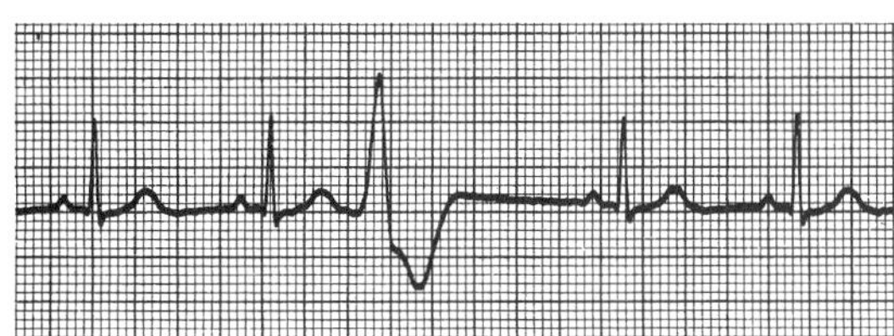

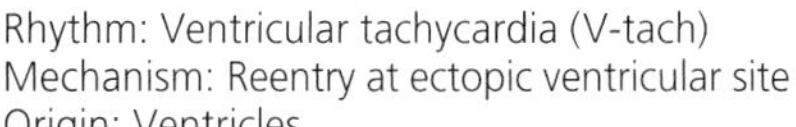

Rhythm: Ventricular tachycardia (V-tach)
Mechanism: Reentry at ectopic ventricular site
Origin: Ventricles
Characteristics: More than 3 PVCs in a row; rate in established rhythm 100 to 250 bpm

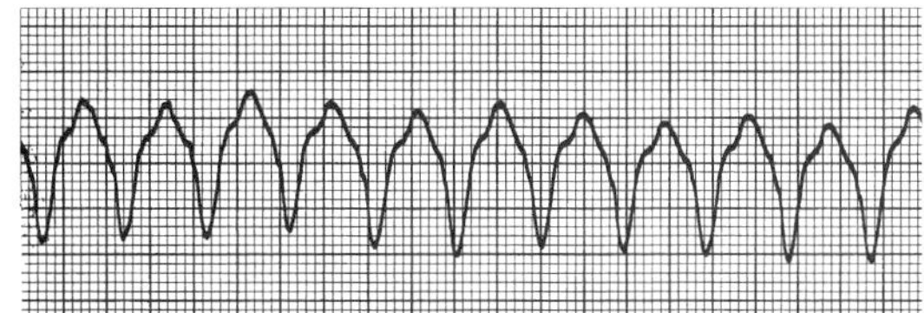

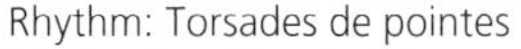

Rhythm: Torsades de pointes
Mechanism: Reentry/triggered early after depolarization
Origin: Ventricles
Characteristics: Twisting and turning motion of baseline; often related to idiosyncratic reaction to certain medicines

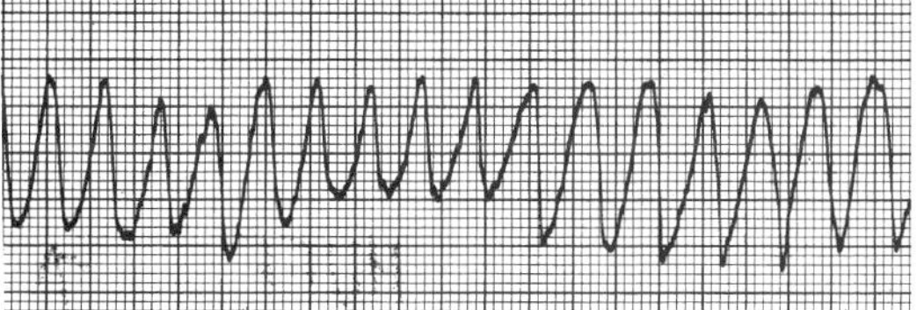

(continued)

TABLE 17-2

CHARACTERISTICS OF CARDIAC DYSRHYTHMIAS (Continued)

Rhythm: Ventricular fibrillation
Mechanism: Reentry
Origin: Ventricles
Characteristics: Multiple ectopic impulses cause the ventricles to quiver; no identifiable complexes; no cardiac output

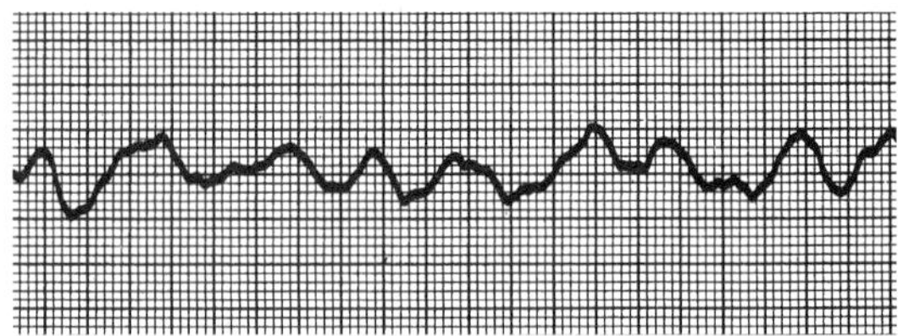

Rhythm: Idioventricular rhythm (agonal)
Mechanism: Loss of all pacemakers except Purkinje
Origin: Ventricles
Characteristics: Wide QRS complexes, slow rate, 10–40 bpm, often terminal rhythm

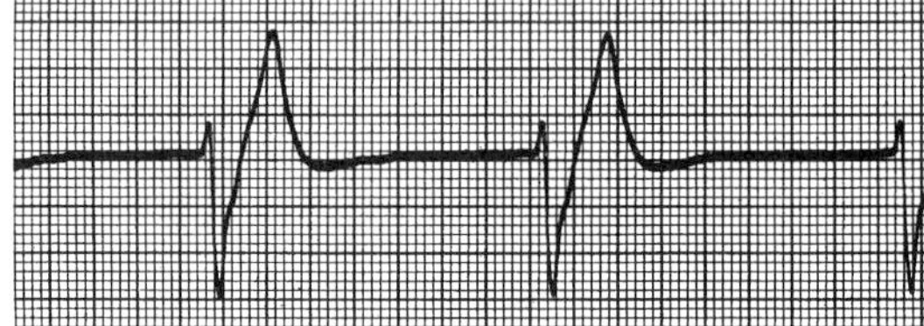

Rhythm: Asystole
Mechanism: No electrical activity in heart
Characteristics: No P waves, QRSs, or T waves; straight line on EKG

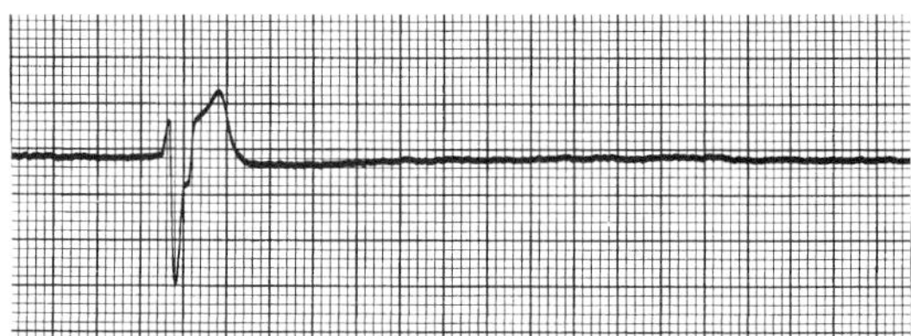

Rhythm: First degree heart block
Mechanism: Slowing of impulse at AV node
Origin: AV node
Characteristics: Sinus rhythm with prolonged P-R, >.2 seconds; regular rhythm

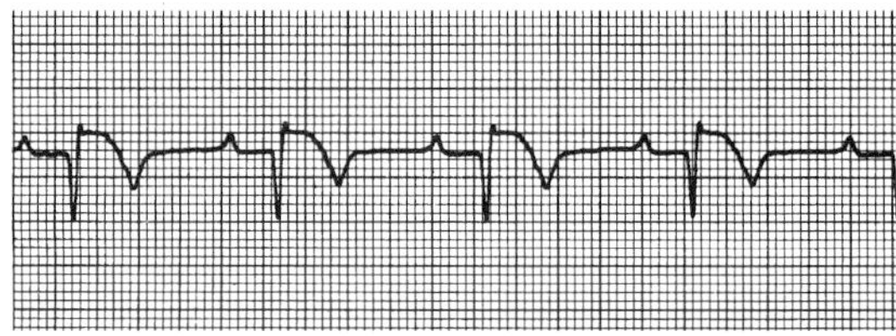

Rhythm: Mobitz I heart block (Wenckebach)
Mechanism: Progressive delay of conduction through AV node
Origin: AV node
Characteristics: Gradual lengthening of P-R interval until a QRS is dropped; produces an irregular rhythm

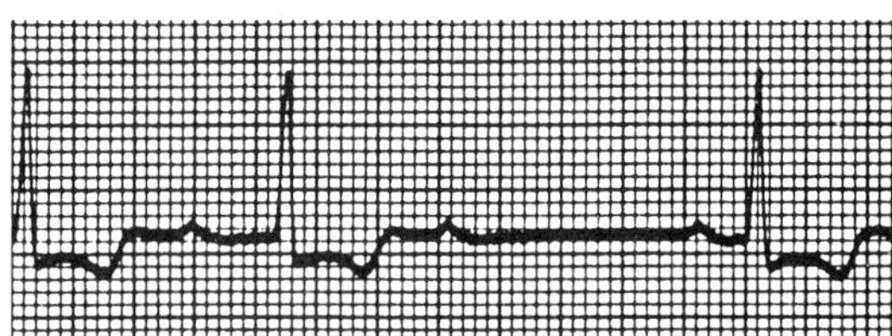

Rhythm: Mobitz II heart block
Mechanism: Block at AV node allows every 2nd, 3rd, or 4th impulse to pass
Origin: AV
Characteristics: Every 2nd, 3rd, or 4th P wave is conducted to the ventricles; P-R interval is constant in conducted beat, rhythm usually regular; rate usually < 50 bpm

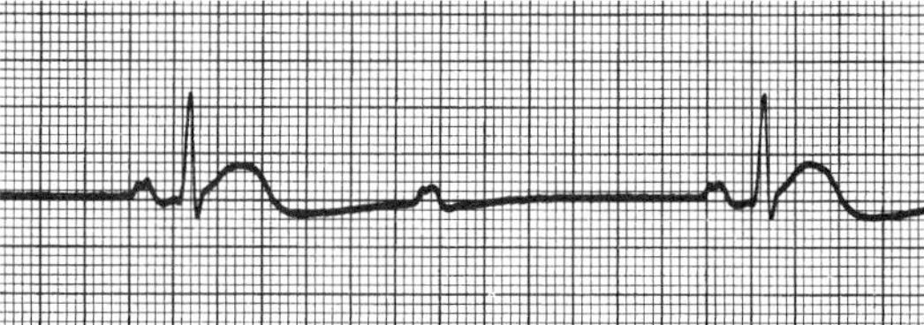

(continued)

TABLE 17-2

CHARACTERISTICS OF CARDIAC DYSRHYTHMIAS (Continued)

Rhythm: Third degree heart block (complete heart block)
Mechanism: Complete block at AV node; no impulses pass; escape pacemaker causes ventricles to beat
Origin: AV node
Characteristics: P waves are regular; QRS complexes regular and very slow; sometimes QRSs are wide; no consistent P-R interval

Rhythm: Ventricular standstill
Mechanism: No ventricular beats; SA node continues to fire
Origin: AV node
Characteristics: Outcome of complete heart block; P waves appear, but no QRS complex; no cardiac output

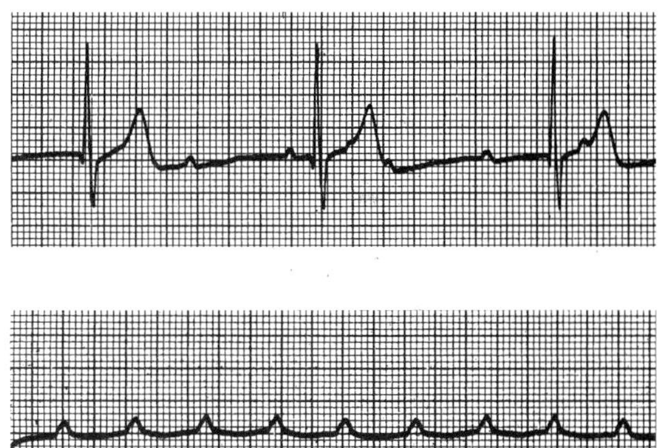

ried by the high-density lipoproteins (HDLs) tends to exert a protective effect in preventing CAD. Factors such as regular exercise, age (children and premenopausal women), and low-fat diet increase HDL levels and apparently decrease the risk of CAD.[24] The diet in the United States is gradually consisting of less saturated fats and this may be a major factor in the declining mortality figures for CAD.[24] A small percentage of cases of hyperlipidemia are due to a hereditary disorder (see p. 434).

TABLE 17-3

RISK FACTORS FOR CORONARY ARTERY DISEASE

RISK FACTOR	PATHOLOGIC BASIS FOR DISEASE
ALTERABLE	
Diet	High-fat, high-carbohydrate diet leads to high serum plasma cholesterol.
Smoking	Multiple factors lead to altered HDL/LDL ratios, altered oxygen levels in myocardium, increased risk of dysrhythmias and sudden cardiac death.
Hypertension	Mechanism not known but enhances atherogenesis and increases oxygen consumption by myocardium.
Stress	Hypothesized that type A behavior is characterized by increased risk of CAD; statistical relationship with increased incidence of CAD during or following stressful life events.
Sedentary life-style	Altered HDL/LDL relationship increases risk of significant plaque; exercise improves collateral circulation.
Diabetes mellitus	All atherosclerotic disease processes are increased due to altered carbohydrate/fat metabolism; mechanism not clear.
Alcohol	Correlation mainly through elevated blood pressure and other associated risk behaviors.
NONALTERABLE	
Age	All atherosclerotic diseases increase with increased age.
Sex	Men have increased incidence prior to age 60; after that male/female incidence is nearly equal.
Race	Equal incidence if rule out hypertension which is more common in African Americans; Orientals have a lower incidence in general, which may relate to diet.
Genetics	Early CAD is often found to run in families and may be related to genetic hyperlipidemia.

CAD, coronary artery disease; HDL, high-density lipoprotein; LDL, low-density lipoprotein.

TABLE 17-4

SERUM CHOLESTEROL AND CAD RISKS

TYPES OF LIPIDS	SOURCE	FUNCTIONS AND CAD RISKS
Chylomicron	80–95% triglyceride (TG)	Low risk, little association with CAD; largest lipoprotein, transports triglycerides to fat and muscle and liver
Very low-density lipoprotein (VLDL)	45–65% TG 25% cholesterol	Synthesized by liver, primarily transports triglycerides to tissue capillaries and fat and muscle cells
Low-density lipoprotein (LDL)	70% cholesterol	Major cholesterol transport; uptake of LDL in arteries can result in the development of atherosclerosis; high levels seen with familial hyperlipoproteinemias, smokers, diabetics; often elevated in obese individuals
High-density lipoprotein (HDL)	25% cholesterol	Carrier that removes cholesterol from tissues and transports it to the liver for catabolism and excretion; levels are increased in premenopausal women, athletes, moderate alcohol drinkers

(Source: Pagana, K. D., & Pagana, T. J. [1992]. *Mosby's diagnostic and laboratory test reference.* St. Louis: Mosby-Year Book.)

Cigarette Smoking

Smoking, especially of cigarettes, has been labeled the single most preventable cause of premature death in the United States.[30] Current evidence indicates that a person's risk of CAD decreases rapidly after quitting smoking and by 1 year later the risk is similar to that of nonsmokers.[28,30] Smoking decreases HDL cholesterol, increases LDL cholesterol, and alters oxygen transport by increasing carbon monoxide in the blood supply to the myocardium.[24] Because of the oxygen uptake problem, smokers have a greatly increased risk of cardiac dysrhythmias and sudden death. Over the past 20 years, smoking has declined from 50% to 31% among men and 32% to 27% among women, a finding that probably has contributed to the declining mortality rate from CAD.[24] Despite this encouragement, an increased incidence of smoking in young persons aged 13 to 18 may portend increased CAD in future years.[24]

Hypertension

High blood pressure, described in Chapter 16, is a significant risk factor for CAD that can be decreased with regular administration of antihypertensive drugs, proper diet, and regular exercise. The risk of CAD is related to the elevation of the systolic and diastolic pressure, especially in men over age 50 years and in the elderly population.[18] Alcohol consumption compounds the problem of hypertension although in moderation, it has been shown to increase HDLs. Drinking alcohol often is correlated with increased smoking behavior, alcoholism, cirrhosis of the liver, obesity, and other systemic problems.[6,38]

Stress

Theorists have continually posited that behavioral factors, especially environmental stress and reactions to stressors, are correlated with an increased incidence of CAD. The type A behavior pattern, characterized by competitiveness, impatience, aggressiveness, and time urgency, has yet to be convincingly documented as causative in CAD.[30] Stressful life events, job problems, limited social support, and life-style changes have all been associated with increased incidence of CAD, although the mechanisms are unknown. These psychosocial factors may also be associated with other risk factors, such as diet and smoking.

Sedentary Life-Style

Lack of exercise has been implicated as an increased risk for CAD. Decreased risk results if a person engages in regular, moderate, or vigorous physical activity over a period of months to years. Controlled studies are difficult to conduct but all of the correlates of moderate exercise with its accompanying attendant psychological and physical improvement seem to have a positive effect on decreasing CAD. Moderate exercise also affects serum cholesterol by increasing the serum HDL level.

Diabetes Mellitus (DM)

Diabetes mellitus alters carbohydrate and fat metabolism and increases the frequency of coronary and other atherosclerotic diseases. The mechanism by which DM causes atherogenesis is poorly understood, and the evidence is inconclusive as to whether elevated concentrations of serum lipoproteins occur in persons who have adequate control of their disease.[40] It is the consensus, however, that control of serum glucose slows the onset of atherosclerosis.[40]

NONALTERABLE RISK FACTORS

Among the nonalterable risk factors for CAD are age, sex, race, and genetic heritage.

Advancing Age

Advancing age is associated with an increased incidence of CAD. Because atherosclerosis is a gradual process that is well established in men by young adulthood and progresses over time, all forms of atherosclerotic disease are manifest more commonly with increased age.[24]

Sex

Gender differences favor an incidence in men approximately 10 years earlier than women. Female hormones may be protective but if the woman is diabetic, smokes cigarettes, or takes oral contraceptives, her risk often approaches that of the man. Over the age of 65, the incidence of CAD becomes nearly equal between the sexes.[24]

Genetic Predisposition

Family history of atherosclerotic disease is a strong factor in the development of CAD. History taking in the young person suffering from acute MI will often reveal a close family member with early CAD. Despite controlling the other risk factors, risk is definitely increased when heart disease "runs in the family." Persons with a family history of premature CAD (before age 55 years) in first-degree relatives have two to five times the risk of those without this history.[24] This risk is further increased when other risk factors are present in the individual and in the family.

Pathophysiology of Coronary Artery Disease

ATHEROSCLEROTIC CORONARY ARTERY DISEASE

The lesions of coronary atherosclerosis develop progressively in much the same manner as those of atherosclerosis of the other major arteries (see p. 433). The initial change occurs early in life and consists of a fatty streak that may develop into a fibrous plaque or **atheroma**. This atheromatous plaque is white, becomes elevated, and partially occludes the lumen of the artery (Fig. 17-3A). The core of the plaque becomes necrotic, and hemorrhage and calcification may result.[7] Thrombosis on or around the plaque may also occur, partially or completely occluding the lumen of the vessel (Fig. 17-3B).

Lesions are usually asymptomatic until the atherosclerotic process is well advanced, occluding 75% or more of the vascular supply to the area. Sometimes total occlusion of a vessel does not cause **ischemia** to a supplied area because of the development of **collateral circulation.** Although almost no communication exists among the larger coronary arteries, many communicating channels are present among the smaller arteries. When slowly developing lesions occur these channels dilate and provide needed blood flow to the myocardial muscle[16] (Fig. 17-4).

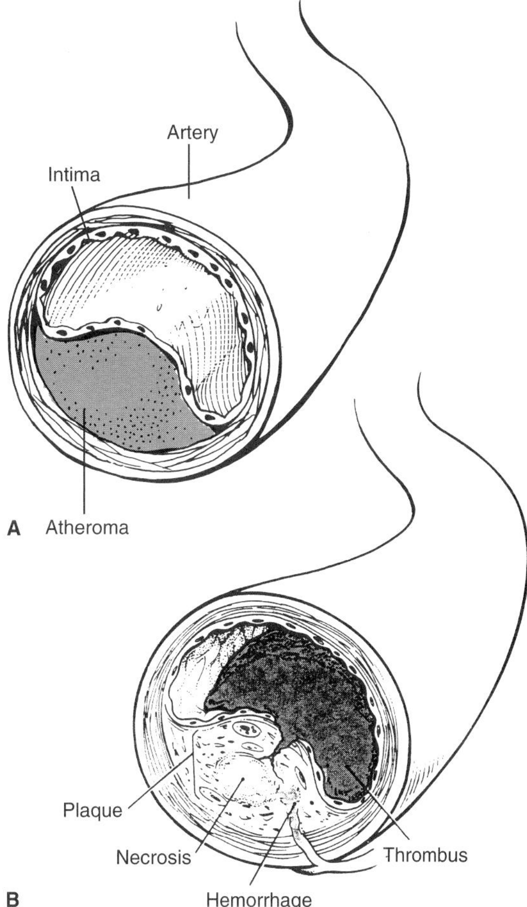

FIGURE 17-3. **A.** Illustrations of atheromatous plaque. **B.** Thrombosis of atheromatous plaque.

Atherosclerotic plaques tend to appear at bifurcations, curvatures, and taperings of arteries. The right and left main coronary arteries branch sharply off the aorta and thus become prime targets for the development of atheromas. The vessels then bifurcate and taper rapidly so that these areas also can become affected more rapidly than other vessels.

As the coronary artery lumen narrows with increasing plaque formation, resistance to blood flow increases and myocardial muscle blood supply is compromised. Normal myocardial muscle has an efficient oxygen up-

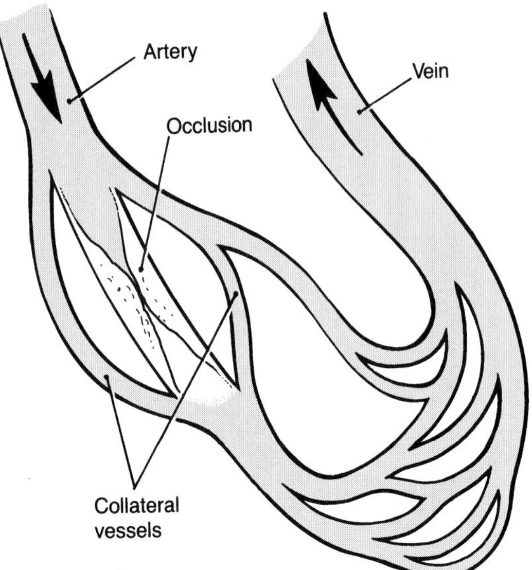

FIGURE 17-4. **Collateral channels can compensate for slowly developing lesions to provide myocardial blood flow until the atherosclerosis progresses beyond the limits of collateral supply.**

take (70–75%). As the amount of blood flow through the vessel decreases, oxygen uptake cannot increase significantly, resulting in compromise of oxygen supply to the tissues. When this compromise causes myocardial ischemia, angina pectoris (heart pain produced by ischemia) results. Further compromise or lack of blood supply may cause necrosis of the myocardial muscle, or MI.

A considerable latent period of two to four decades usually exists between the onset of arterial lumen narrowing and symptomatic disease.[41] After this amount of time symptoms may begin when the lumen is obstructed over 75%.[41] The event that produces **infarction** may be sudden and involve hemorrhage into an atherosclerotic plaque, thrombosis on an established plaque, or coronary artery spasm. Table 17-5 indicates the multiple mechanisms that can lead to IHD.

NONATHEROSCLEROTIC CORONARY ARTERY DISEASE

Although most cases of CAD result from atherosclerosis, other factors can cause significant impairment of blood flow to the heart (Box 17-1).[51] Especially important among these is cocaine abuse, the effects of which are discussed later in the section on MI.

Angina Pectoris

The term *angina pectoris* describes pain that is substernal or radiating to other areas that is caused by ischemia

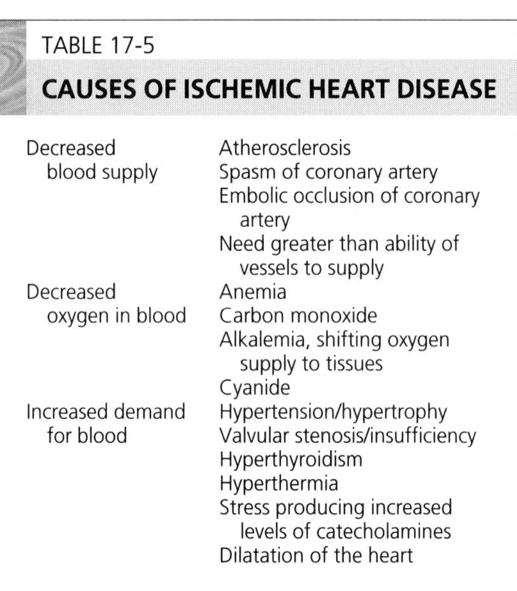

TABLE 17-5

CAUSES OF ISCHEMIC HEART DISEASE

Decreased blood supply	Atherosclerosis Spasm of coronary artery Embolic occlusion of coronary artery Need greater than ability of vessels to supply
Decreased oxygen in blood	Anemia Carbon monoxide Alkalemia, shifting oxygen supply to tissues Cyanide
Increased demand for blood	Hypertension/hypertrophy Valvular stenosis/insufficiency Hyperthyroidism Hyperthermia Stress producing increased levels of catecholamines Dilatation of the heart

of heart muscle. Its manifestations often precede the onset of MI.

PATHOPHYSIOLOGY OF MYOCARDIAL ISCHEMIA

The pain, described by an affected individual, results from an imbalance between myocardial oxygen supply and demand (Fig. 17-5). Insufficient oxygen is being supplied to the myocardial cell for it to function effectively.[39] This condition almost always relates to atherosclerotic narrowing of the coronary arteries. For a

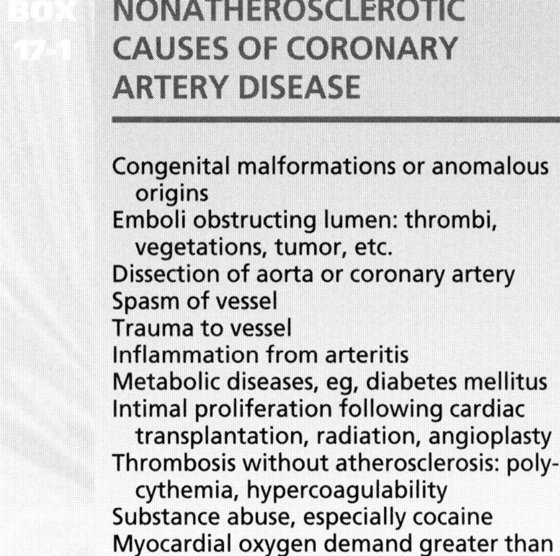

BOX 17-1

NONATHEROSCLEROTIC CAUSES OF CORONARY ARTERY DISEASE

Congenital malformations or anomalous origins
Emboli obstructing lumen: thrombi, vegetations, tumor, etc.
Dissection of aorta or coronary artery
Spasm of vessel
Trauma to vessel
Inflammation from arteritis
Metabolic diseases, eg, diabetes mellitus
Intimal proliferation following cardiac transplantation, radiation, angioplasty
Thrombosis without atherosclerosis: polycythemia, hypercoagulability
Substance abuse, especially cocaine
Myocardial oxygen demand greater than supply, eg, systemic hypertension

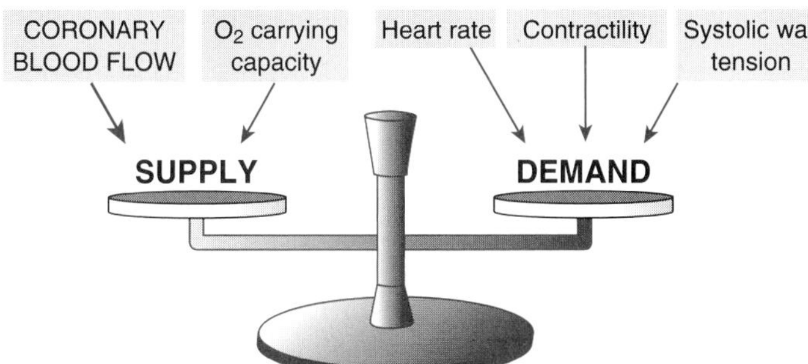

FIGURE 17-5. Myocardial oxygen supply and demand are usually in balance. In angina pectoris, either supply decreases in relation to demand or demand exceeds supply.

long time, as blood flow decreases, the myocardium avoids ischemia through autoregulation of coronary blood flow, probably as a result of smooth muscle relaxation of the arterioles in response to the release of adenosine, a powerful vasodilator of the coronary vasculature. This vasodilation decreases resistance in the coronary arteriolar bed and increases blood flow to the myocardial muscle.[13] When this mechanism fails to meet the metabolic needs of the myocardium, ischemia results, causing pain. The pain is intermittent and often is relieved by rest or taking a vasodilator, such as nitroglycerin.

Ischemia suggests that changes are reversible and cellular function can be restored with restoration of oxygen to the affected muscle. **Anaerobic metabolism** is used to produce adenosine triphosphate during oxygen insufficiency but the resulting accumulation of lactic acid impairs left ventricular function. Impaired left ventricular function results in decreased strength of cardiac contraction and impaired wall motion. The degree of impairment depends on the size of the ischemic area. Depression of left ventricular function may lead to a temporary decrease in stroke volume and to changes in systemic blood pressure.

The heart is unique in that it can be manipulated or operated on without pain; however, ischemia of cardiac muscle causes intense pain. The cause of the pain is not fully understood, but ischemic myocardial muscle releases acidic substances (lactic acid) that may then stimulate the nerve endings in the muscle, conducting pain through the sympathetic nerves to the middle cervical ganglia and through the thoracic ganglia to the spinal cord.

The referred nature of the pain (to the left or right arm or neck) probably is linked to interconnections in the sympathetic nerves. These nerve fibers enter the spinal cord all the way from C3 to T5 (Fig. 17-6).[16,42] When ischemia is very severe, an individual may describe cardiac pain as crushing in quality and substernal in location. Researchers do not entirely understand the pain's source but believe it may stem from sensory nerve endings from the heart to the pericardium that reflect pain sensation to the great vessels.[16]

The ischemic episodes causing the chest pain of angina pectoris usually subside in minutes if the imbalance is corrected. Ischemia is totally reversible, and a return to normal metabolic, functional, and hemodynamic balance usually occurs. The episodes are a warning of significant vascular occlusion and the increased risk for MI.

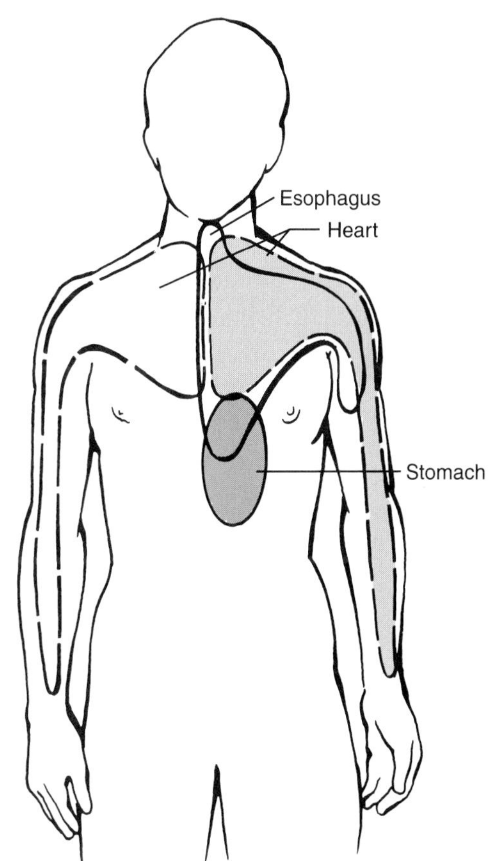

FIGURE 17-6. Referred pain from the heart extends to the dermatomes C3–T8, left arm, shoulder, back, substernal region, neck, axilla, and occasionally the stomach, with complaints of indigestion. Referred pain from the esophagus and stomach may be misinterpreted as pain from the heart.

CLINICAL MANIFESTATIONS OF ANGINA PECTORIS

The clinical features of angina pectoris relate to the pain and the person's physiologic response to it. Individuals typically describe anginal pain as substernal, a feeling of tightness or fullness, or oppression. The pain may radiate down one or both arms or into the neck and jaws.

Characteristically, the person becomes immobile and also may exhibit pallor, profuse perspiration, and dyspnea. The dyspnea may be a compensatory result of temporary cardiac failure induced by left ventricular hypokinesis (see p. 478). It also may result from anxiety causes by pain onset.

Classically, activity (physical or emotional stress) precipitates angina, which is relieved in minutes with rest or the administration of a coronary vasodilator, such as nitroglycerin. During the anginal attack, typical electrocardiographic (ECG) changes occur, including T-wave inversion, ST-segment depression, and minor ST elevation when ischemia is severe and progressive (Fig. 17-7).[47] Approximately 50% to 70% of persons with angina pectoris who have had no previous MI have a normal resting ECG. Changes, either symptomatic or asymptomatic, may be produced when the individual is placed on a treadmill and monitored during exercise stress. Levels of cardiac enzymes in blood drawn during or after an anginal attack are usually normal. This finding helps to differentiate angina from MI.

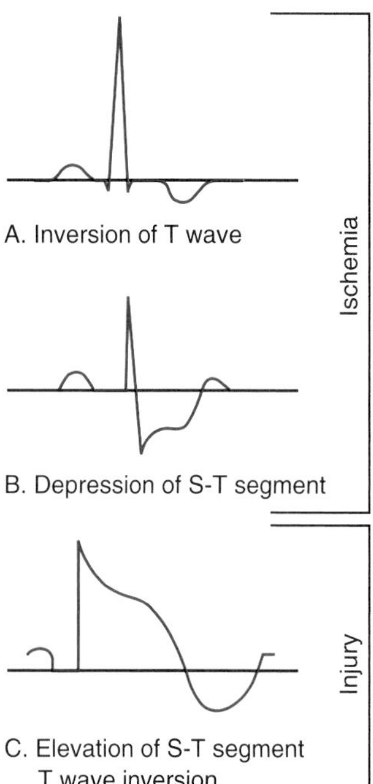

FIGURE 17-7. **ECG changes associated with ischemia and injury.**

Various descriptions of angina have to do with the clinical presentation exhibited and whether a pattern exists (Table 17-6). Box 17-2 presents the Canadian Cardiovascular Society Functional Classification of Angina Pectoris, which is widely used to classify the severity of angina pectoris.

Stable Angina

Most angina first presents as stable angina, which has a characteristic pattern of known precipitators. Onset may occur due to specific activities such as exercise, eating, sexual behavior, emotional upset, or life-changing events (see Box 17-2).

Variant or Prinzmetal's Angina

Episodes of angina that occur exclusively at rest and that exercise or emotional stress do not precipitate characterize variant (Prinzmetal's) angina. Vari-

TABLE 17-6

TYPES OF ANGINA

Stable	Symptoms predictable, onset due to certain level of activity, eating, sexual behavior, etc.
Variant or Prinzmetal's	Not precipitated by activity or stress; often occurs at night; demonstrated due to coronary vasospasm rather than atherosclerosis
Silent ischemia	Noted during exercise testing without complaint of chest pain; increased incidence of dysrhythmias
Unstable or preinfarctional	Pain becomes increasingly severe with more frequent episodes; usually seen in a person with a previously stable anginal pattern; often progresses to infarction if left untreated
Ischemic myocardial dysfunction, "stunned myocardium"	Ischemia produces significant contractility problems; may be due to decreased production of adenosine triphosphate or production of oxygen free radicals or abnormal calcium transport

BOX 17-2

CANADIAN CARDIOVASCULAR SOCIETY FUNCTIONAL CLASSIFICATION OF ANGINA PECTORIS

I. Ordinary physical activity, such as walking and climbing stairs, does not cause angina. Angina results from strenuous or rapid or prolonged exertion at work or recreation.
II. Slight limitation of ordinary activity. Walking or climbing stairs rapidly, walking uphill, walking or stair climbing after meals, in cold, in wind, or when under emotional stress, or only during the few hours after awakening. Walking more than two blocks on the level and climbing more than one flight or ordinary stairs at a normal pace and under normal conditions.
III. Marked limitations of ordinary physical activity. Walking one to two blocks on the level and climbing more than one flight under normal conditions.
IV. Inability to carry on any physical activity without discomfort—anginal syndrome may be present at rest.

(Summarized from Campeau, L. [1976]. Grading of angina pectors [letter] *Circulation, 54,* 522–523. Copyright 1976 American Heart Association, Inc.)

ant angina is thought to result from coronary artery vasospasm usually occurring on vessels that have some degree of atherosclerotic obstruction. Some affected persons have no demonstrable CAD. The triggering mechanism for the vasospasm is unknown.[47] This form of angina tends to be more common in women than in men and may be associated with other arterial vasospastic conditions.[39] ST-segment elevation in leads recording the ischemic event is characteristic and this elevation returns to normal when the pain (ischemia) is relieved.

Silent Ischemia

Ischemia is asymptomatic in many persons with significant coronary artery narrowing. The mechanism for the induction of ischemia is an imbalance between supply and demand so that the heart is receiving insufficient oxygen to meet its needs. Silent ischemia is often first noted during a stress test in which the changes are noted but the individual has no complaints of chest pain. The evidence for the ischemia is ST-segment depression and T-wave inversion. The condition may be associated with increased incidence of ventricular dysrhythmias and sudden death.[5]

Unstable or Preinfarctional Angina

As atherosclerotic disease progresses in the coronary arteries, pain may become more severe and occur more often. Pathologically, platelet emboli have been noted as well as nonocclusive thrombi localizing over a fissured plaque.[9] Clinically, the anginal episodes change in character, duration, and intensity usually in persons with a long history of stable angina. The quality of the chest pain is similar to stable angina, but the pain may occur at night or after less and less activity during the day. Each successive attack may last longer than earlier attacks. Increasing severity or frequency of anginal attacks herald an impending MI. The ECG often shows continual signs of ischemia and injury.

Ischemic Myocardial Dysfunction (Stunned Myocardium)

The term "stunned myocardium" refers to persistent mechanical dysfunction of the ventricle due to ischemia. This type of ischemic injury is not sufficient to produce an MI but the myocardium demonstrates significant **hypokinesis.**[49] This condition has been described in association with angina, post-thrombolytic therapy, after percutaneous coronary angioplasty, and after coronary artery bypass procedures. The actual pathophysiology is unknown but it may be associated with depression of adenosine triphosphate levels perhaps due to inadequate oxygen for formation. Other postulated mechanisms include damage caused by oxygen free radicals or abnormal calcium transport.[13] The oxygen free radicals are a product of **reperfusion** and induce ventricular dysfunction by an unknown mechanism, possibly peroxidation of unsaturated fatty acids of intracellular organelles[13] (see p. 38). Researchers have noted that if the "stunned heart" is allowed to rest with the use of an intra-aortic balloon pump or supported with an inotropic drug (one that increases contractility), it often will regain contractility and be able to support an adequate blood pressure in a period of several days.[49]

Myocardial Infarction

Myocardial ischemia is differentiated from MI on the basis of the pathologic results of the process. The pathology occurs on a continuum in which the myocardium is first temporarily deprived of adequate oxygen for function and then the deprivation causes cell death. Cell death manifests as infarction (myocardial death). Infarction in myocardial muscle is permanent and the infarcted area must be repaired by scar.

Myocardial infarction is the single most common cause of death in the United States. Most MIs are due to thrombosis that has developed on an atherosclerotic plaque effectively occluding a coronary artery. An increasing incidence of MI has been reported in individuals who use cocaine.[46] MIs related to cocaine abuse are often seen in younger men rather than middle-aged or older adults who have primarily atherosclerotic disease of the coronary arteries.[17,46]

PATHOPHYSIOLOGY

Ischemic necrosis of the myocardium, or MI, results from prolonged ischemia to the myocardium, which causes irreversible cell damage and muscle death. The time between onset of ischemia and myocardial muscle death occurs with irreversible injury to myocytes in the subendocardium and the wavefront of cell death moves to include more of the myocardium. In experimental models the onset of irreversible cell injury is 20 to 40 minutes with the extent of necrosis largely complete within 3 to 6 hours.[7] The resulting size of the infarct depends on the following factors:

- The extent, severity, and duration of the ischemic episode
- The amount of collateral circulation
- The metabolic needs of the myocardium at the time of the event[7]

When cocaine is involved, the MI may be due to sympathomimetic effects (tachycardia, hypertension, and vascular constriction), increased thrombogenicity due to platelet aggregation, constriction of the coronary arteries, direct myocardial muscle damage, and premature atherosclerosis.[46]

Functionally, MI causes the following:

- Reduced contractility with abnormal wall motion
- Altered left ventricular compliance
- Reduced stroke volume
- Reduced ejection fraction
- Elevated left ventricular end-diastolic pressure[6,42]

Alterations in function depend not only on the size but also the location of an infarct. Anterior left ventricular infarcts often result from occlusion of the left anterior descending coronary artery. Posterior left ventricular infarcts often arise from right coronary artery obstruction, whereas lateral wall infarcts usually arise from circumflex artery obstruction. Table 17-7 lists affected coronary arteries, the areas of resulting infarction, and the percentage of infarcts that result from the lesions. This distribution varies because of individual differences in coronary artery supply.[4]

The infarct is also described in terms of where it occurs on the myocardial surface. The *transmural infarct* extends from endocardium to epicardium. The *subendocardial* type is located on the endocardial surface extending varying distances into the myocardial muscle. *Intramural infarction* is often seen in patchy areas of the myocardium and is usually associated with long-standing angina pectoris. For the most part, these descriptive terms have been replaced by the terms *Q-wave infarction* and *non–Q-wave infarction*, which reflect the ECG appearance of Q waves in association with the clinical picture of MI (see p. 472). The initiating events of infarction are coronary occlusion but Q-wave infarction usually results from sustained coronary occlusion and extensive necrosis, whereas non–Q-wave may have early spontaneous or thrombolytic therapy-induced reperfusion for at least a part of the affected area.[1]

Acute MIs are often described as having a central area of necrosis (infarction) that is surrounded by an area of injury; the area of injury is surrounded by a ring of ischemia (Fig. 17-8). The amount of myocardial dysfunction that results depends not only on the size of the necrotic lesion but also on the amount of injury and ischemia in the area. Each area emits characteristic ECG

TABLE 17-7

CORONARY ARTERY LESIONS AND AREAS OF INFARCTION

CORONARY ARTERY AFFECTED	PERCENTAGE OF CASES	AREAS OF INFARCTION
Left anterior descending	40–50	Anterior left ventricle; apex; anterior interventricular septum
Right coronary artery	30–40	Inferior/posterior wall of left ventricle; posterior interventricular septum; right ventricle
Left circumflex	15–20	Lateral wall of left ventricle

(Summarized from Cotran, R. S., Kumar, V., & Collins, T. [1999]. *Robbins' pathologic basis of disease* [6th ed.]. Philadelphia: Saunders.)

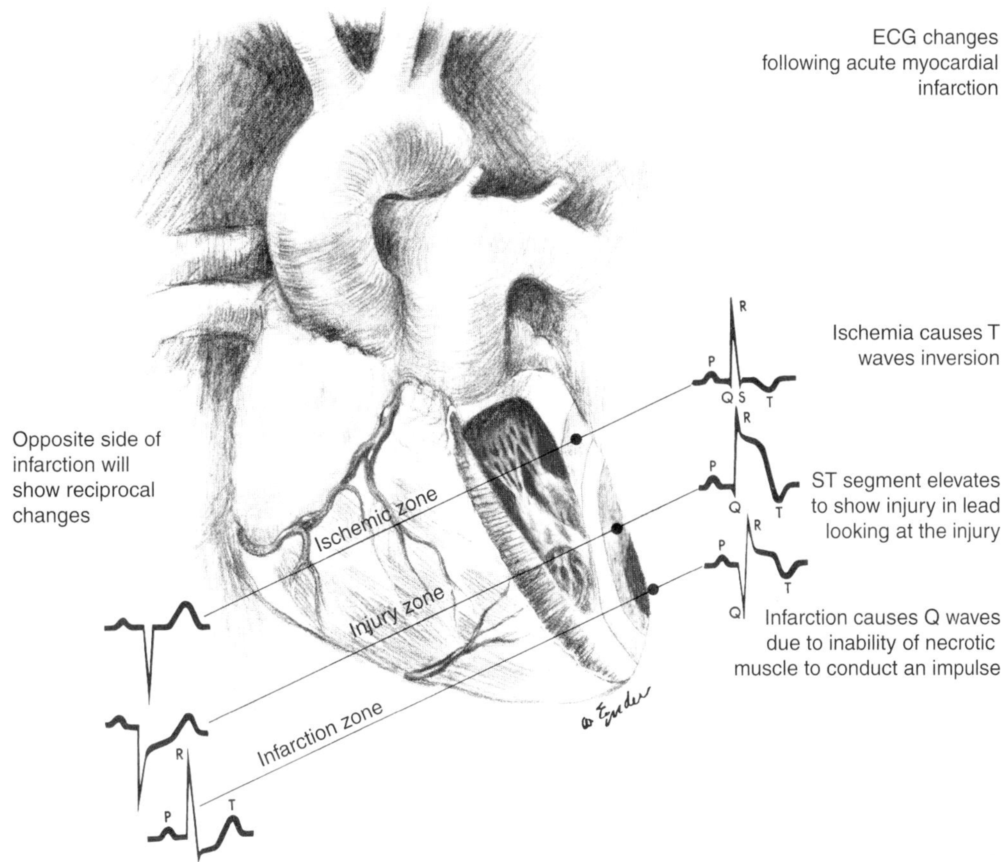
ECG changes following acute myocardial infarction
Ischemia causes T waves inversion
ST segment elevates to show injury in lead looking at the injury
Infarction causes Q waves due to inability of necrotic muscle to conduct an impulse
Opposite side of infarction will show reciprocal changes
Ischemic zone
Injury zone
Infarction zone
P
Q
R
S
T

FIGURE 17-8. **Most acute MIs have a central area of necrosis surrounded by an area of injury and an area of ischemia.**

patterns that help to localize and determine the extent of the infarct on a 12-lead ECG (Table 17-8).

When myocardial muscle cells die, they liberate their intramyocardial cellular enzymes. These enzymes can be used to date an infarct and partially to judge its severity.[1] Table 17-9 summarizes the importance and reliability of the specific plasma markers.

Because the affected myocardial muscle does not regenerate after an infarction, healing requires the formation of scar tissue that replaces the necrotic myocardial muscle. A series of morphologic changes range from no apparent cellular change in the first 6 hours to total replacement by scar tissue. Figure 17-9 illustrates these changes.

Scar tissue inhibits contractility; its significance depends on the amount of scar tissue formed. As contractility falls, heart failure may ensue and the body may begin to use the compensatory mechanisms described on page 476 in an attempt to maintain cardiac output. Ventricular dilatation is common. If a large amount of ventricular myocardium is lost, contractility may be greatly compromised and cardiogenic shock may ensue.

Right ventricular infarction may occur with occlusion of the right coronary artery and the resulting inferior wall infarction. When infarcts affect the posterior wall of the left ventricle and the posterior interventricular septum, they extend to the right ventricular wall in 15% to 30% of cases.[7] The central venous pressure may be elevated markedly if acute right ventricular failure develops (see p. 479). Low right ventricular output may cause cardiogenic shock[1] (see p. 482). The diagnosis of right ventricular infarction is difficult but may be established by right-sided ECG leads and echocardiographic studies.

CLINICAL MANIFESTATIONS

The clinical manifestations of MI depend on the infarct's severity, the individual's previous physical condition, and whether earlier infarcts have occurred. They may reflect changes in the autonomic nervous system. The location of the infarct may affect symptoms, including magnitude and location of pain. Manifestations can range from sudden death due to dysrhythmias or

TABLE 17-8

LOCATION OF INFARCT BY ELECTROCARDIOGRAM

SITE	LEADS OF ECG	CHANGES NOTED
Inferior	II, III, aVF	ST-segment elevation—acute; abnormal Q waves—the depth represents the extent of infarction; Q-wave change usually persists and is diagnostic of old MI
Inferolateral	II, II, aVF, V_4–V_6	ST-segment elevation—acute; abnormal Q waves develop and persist
True posterior	V_1	Tall R wave, called a reciprocal change
Anterior/apical	V_2–V_4	ST-segment elevation—acute; development of abnormal Q waves
Anterior (extensive)	I, aVL, V_1–V_6	ST-segment elevation—acute; development of abnormal Q waves
Anterolateral (extensive)	I, II, aVL, V_4–V_6	ST-segment elevation—acute; development of abnormal Q waves
Anterolateral	I, aVL	ST-segment elevation—acute; development of abnormal Q waves
Right ventricular	V_4R–V_6R, V_1–V_3	ST-segment elevation—acute; development of abnormal Q waves

* Conditions such as bundle branch block and ventricular hypertrophy may alter the appearance for the diagnosis of MI.

ventricular rupture to no symptoms whatsoever. Typical symptoms include:

- Acute, substernal, radiating chest pain with areas of radiation following nerve channels as described on page 465
- Diaphoresis
- Dyspnea
- Nausea and vomiting
- Extreme anxiety
- Any type of dysrhythmia
- Fever

TABLE 17-9

SPECIFIC PLASMA MARKERS IN MYOCARDIAL INFARCTION

PLASMA MARKER	ELEVATES	PEAKS	PERIOD OF ELEVATION	SIGNIFICANCE
I. Creatinine phosphokinase (CPK)	4–8 h	12–36 h	72 h	Enzyme released with myocardial muscle damage, also elevates with brain and skeletal muscle damage
Isoenzymes				
CPK I (BB)	0	0	0	Produced mostly by brain
CPK II (mB)	4–8 h	12–36 h	72 h	Produced by heart Released with myocardial damage
CPK III (mm)	0	0	0	Produced mostly by skeletal muscle. May elevate with trauma, invasive procedures, or surgery.
II. Troponin T	12–16 h	24–36 h	10–12 d	Part of sarcomere complex of myocardial muscle cell, may be increased with skeletal injury, but levels much higher with cardiac injury
Troponin I	12–16 h	24–36 h	10–12 d	Part of sarcomere complex of myocardial muscle cell; not present in skeletal muscle; specific marker for myocardial injury
III. Myoglobin	2 h	7–12 h	Up to 20 d	Part of sarcomere unit in skeletal and myocardial muscle In absence of skeletal trauma, early indicator of MI

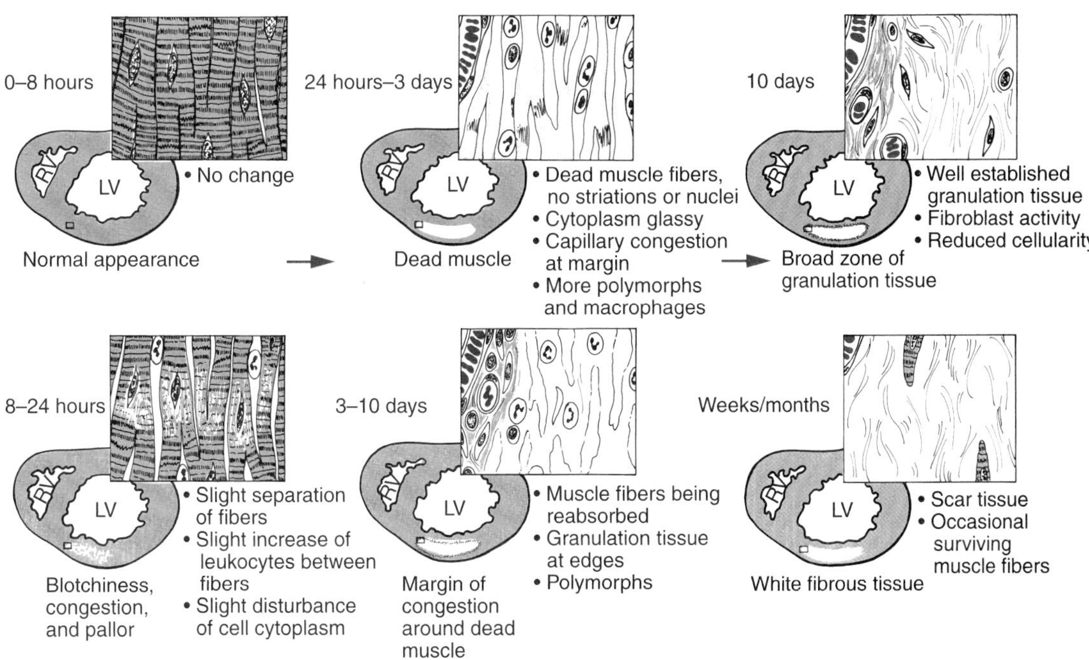

FIGURE 17-9. Pathologic appearance of myocardial infarction over time.

Figure 17-10 illustrates the clinical picture of MI. Often the clinical features reveal associated complications.

DIAGNOSIS

Diagnosis of MI is made on physical examination as well as specific diagnostic tests. Absence of typical symptoms cause approximately 23% of MIs to go unrecognized.[1] Of these atypical symptoms, respiratory difficulties, nausea, vomiting, and epigastric pain are common. The response of most individuals is to deny the possibility that an MI is occurring so that atypical symptoms are either ignored or attributed to another cause.

Laboratory Studies

Laboratory studies are very helpful in the diagnosis of acute MI (see Unit Appendices A and B). The complete blood count often reveals an elevated leukocyte count, which rises with the fever that occurs with the onset of myocardial necrosis. The erythrocyte sedimentation rate increases in the early period after MI.

Cardiac enzyme and other plasma marker levels elevate because of cellular damage. Their values elevate and return to normal in a characteristic pattern after an MI (see Table 17-9). Because the factors are present in other tissues, coexisting disease can produce misleading elevations. Isoenzymes provide more specific accuracy. The isoenzyme **creatinine phosphokinase**-MB (CK-MB) is usually considered diagnostic of MI, espe-

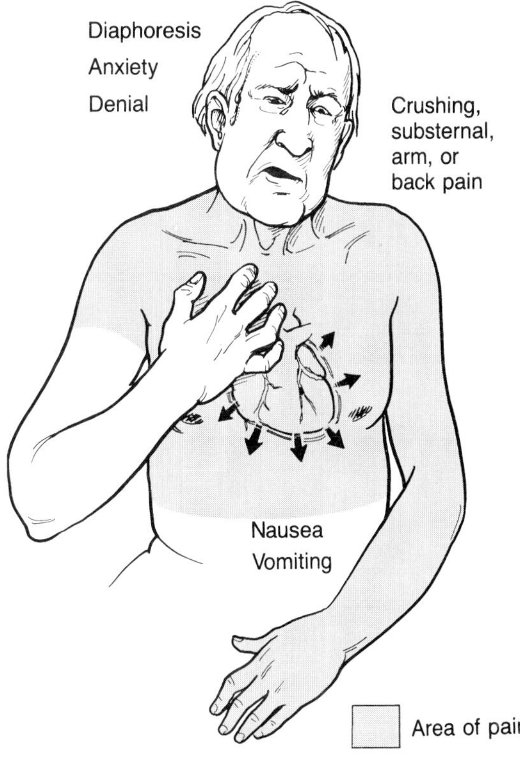

FIGURE 17-10. Clinical picture of myocardial infarction. Some or all of the signs and symptoms may be present.

cially in the presence of increased levels of **troponin T** and **I.**[1] Myoglobin elevation is an early indicator of myocardial damage in the absence of skeletal muscle damage but its sensitivity may not be reliable after 10 to 12 hours because of rapid renal clearance.[1]

Myocardial Imaging

Myocardial infarction imaging has proved to be a sensitive indicator of acute myocardial damage (see Unit Appendix C). The technetium pyrophosphate combines with calcium in the damaged myocardial cells and shows up on a scan as a "hot spot." Also, the multigated blood pool scan is used to calculate end-diastolic volume, end-systolic volume, ejection fraction, and stroke volume. These values are beneficial in evaluating the effects of infarction on myocardial function.

Electrocardiographic Changes

The ECG changes of acute MI consist of pronounced Q waves and ST elevation. These changes are reflected in the leads overlying the area of injury, so that the infarction can be generally localized by the ECG (see Table 17-8). In the acute phase, only ST-segment and T-wave changes are seen. Over the following 36 to 48 hours, Q-wave changes develop. In the early phase, the ECG diagnosis is "probable" acute MI, which changes to acute MI when Q waves are added to the ST- and T-wave changes. Over time, the ST-segment and T-wave changes return to normal but the Q wave persists as evidence of an old infarction and can be used to localize the defect throughout the person's life. Figure 17-11 shows a 12-lead ECG with characteristic changes of an acute inferior MI.

COMPLICATIONS

Complications of MI are related to the size of the infarct itself, the location of the injury, and the changes that have occurred within the infarcted area.

Dysrhythmias

The most common complication of acute MI is a disturbance in cardiac rhythm. Seen in 90% of MIs, dysrhythmias result from numerous predisposing factors, including: (1) tissue ischemia, (2) hypoxemia, (3) sympathetic and parasympathetic nervous system influences, (4) lactic acidosis, (5) hemodynamic abnormalities, (6) drug toxicity, and (7) electrolyte imbalance.[1] The basic mechanisms for cardiac rhythm abnormalities are abnormal *automaticity* and *re-entry*, or both together (see p. 455). The most common dysrhythmias associated with MI are listed in Table 17-10. Dysrhythmias may cause a decline in cardiac output and an increase in cardiac irritability, which further compromise myocardial perfusion. The most common cause of death outside of the hospital in individuals with MI is probably ventricular fibrillation.

Congestive Heart Failure and Cardiogenic Shock

Congestive heart failure (CHF), discussed on page 474, is a state of circulatory congestion produced by myocardial dysfunction. MI compromises myocardial function by reducing contractility and producing ab-

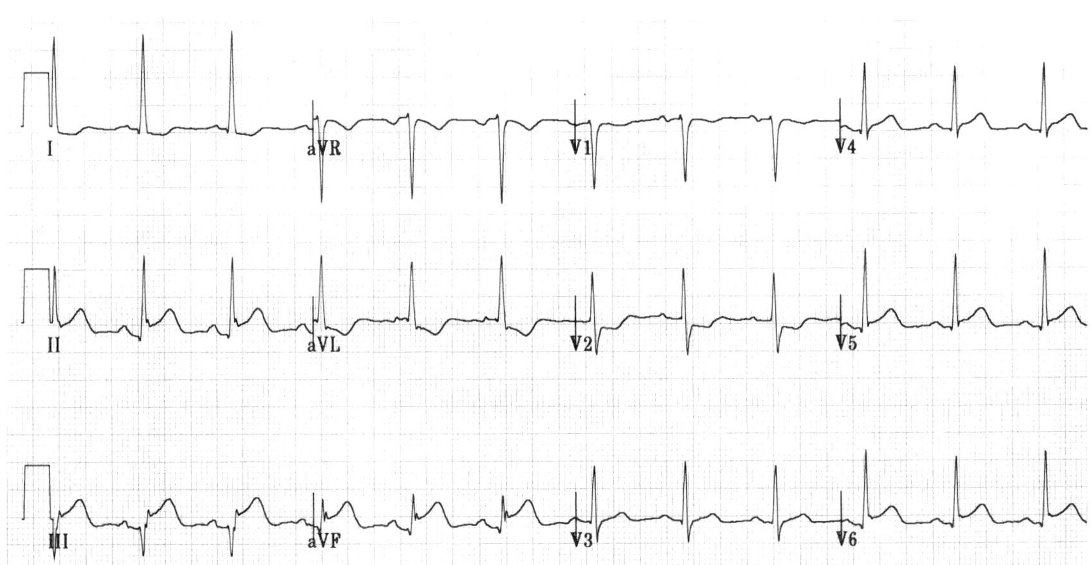

FIGURE 17-11. Acute changes seen in inferior myocardial infarction. Note S-T segment elevation in leads II, III, and aVF. Deep Q wave is evident in lead III.

TABLE 17-10

COMMON DYSRHYTHMIAS AFTER MYOCARDIAL INFARCTION

TYPE OF DYSRHYTHMIA	EXAMPLES
Ventricular	Premature ventricular contractions Ventricular tachycardia Ventricular fibrillation
Atrial	Premature atrial contractions Atrial flutter Atrial fibrillation
Conduction defects	Bundle branch block, right or left Second-degree heart block Third-degree or complete heart block
Sinus	Sinus tachycardia Sinus bradycardia Sinus arrhythmia (dysrhythmia)

normal wall motion. As the ability of the ventricle to empty becomes less effective, stroke volume falls and residual volume increases, which may lead to pulmonary edema. The fall in stroke volume elicits compensatory mechanisms to maintain cardiac output. The classic picture of left heart failure then may result (see p. 478).

Cardiogenic shock results from profound left ventricular failure, usually from a massive MI. This pump failure shock follows MI in 10% to 15% of cases; mortality is approximately 80%.[1]

Thromboembolism

Mural thrombi are common in postmortem examinations of individuals who die of MI. In a study of 924 fatalities due to acute MI, 44% had mural thrombi attached to the endocardium.[7] These thrombi are usually associated with large infarcts and, therefore, probably occur more frequently in nonsurvivors than survivors. Mural thrombi adhere to the endocardium and overlie an infarcted area. Fragments, however, can produce systemic arterial embolization. Autopsy studies reveal that 10% of individuals who die of MI also have arterial emboli to the brain, kidneys, spleen, or mesentery.[7,41]

Almost all pulmonary emboli originate in the veins of the lower extremities. Bed rest and heart failure predispose an individual to venous thrombosis and pulmonary embolism. Both occur in those with acute MI.

Pericarditis

This syndrome associated with MI was first described by Dressler and is often called Dressler's syndrome. It usually occurs after a transmural infarction; a pericardial friction rub occurs in about 10% to 20% of affected individuals.[44] Pericarditis is usually transient, appearing in the first week after infarction (see p. 494).

Myocardial Rupture

Rupture of the free wall of the left ventricle accounts for 10% of in-hospital deaths due to acute MI.[41] Rupture causes immediate cardiac tamponade and death. Cardiac tamponade restricts filling of the heart and causes an immediate decline in the blood pressure (Fig. 17-12). Rupture of the interventricular septum is less common, occurs with extensive myocardial damage, and produces an interventricular septal defect.[1] Rupture of the papillary muscle is an uncommon complication of MI and is more common with right coronary artery occlusions.[1] It results when necrosis and rupture of the papillary muscle cause the release of the chordae tendenae and immediate onset of mitral regurgitation (Fig. 17-13). Symptoms of heart failure usually follow the sudden, severe onset of mitral regurgitation (see p. 485).

Ventricular Aneurysm

This event is a late complication of MI that involves thinning, ballooning, and hypokinesis of the left ventricular wall after a transmural infarction. The aneurysm often creates a paroxysmal motion of the ventricular wall with ballooning out of the aneurysmal segment on ventricular contraction (Fig. 17-14). The dysfunctional area often fills with necrotic debris and clot, and some-

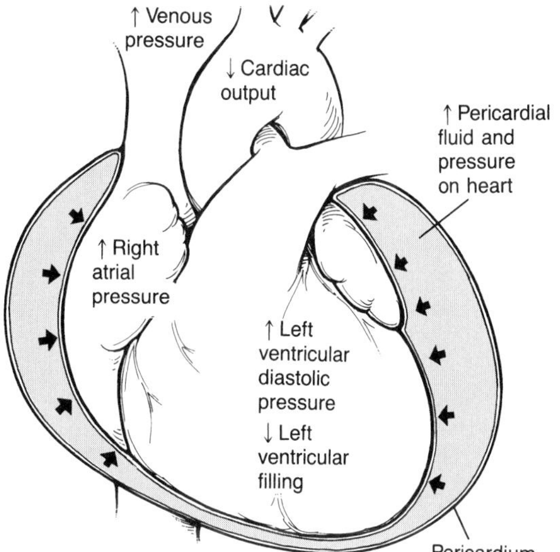

FIGURE 17-12. Cardiac tamponade. This condition may be due to rupture of the myocardium after infarction or it may be seen with trauma to the heart or hemorrhagic pericarditis.

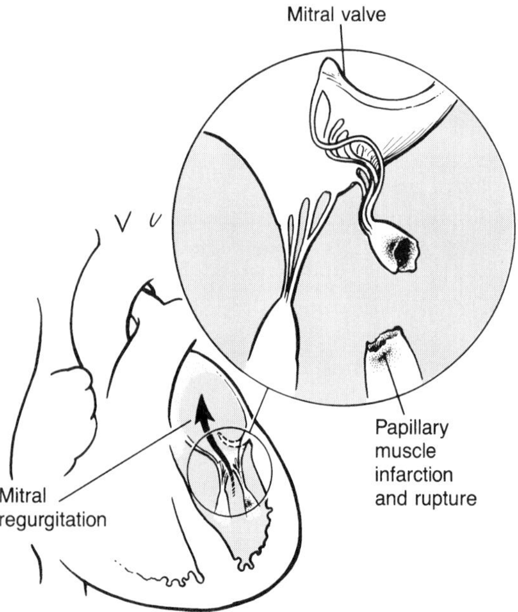

FIGURE 17-13. **Production of acute picture of mitral regurgitation due to papillary muscle infarction and rupture.**

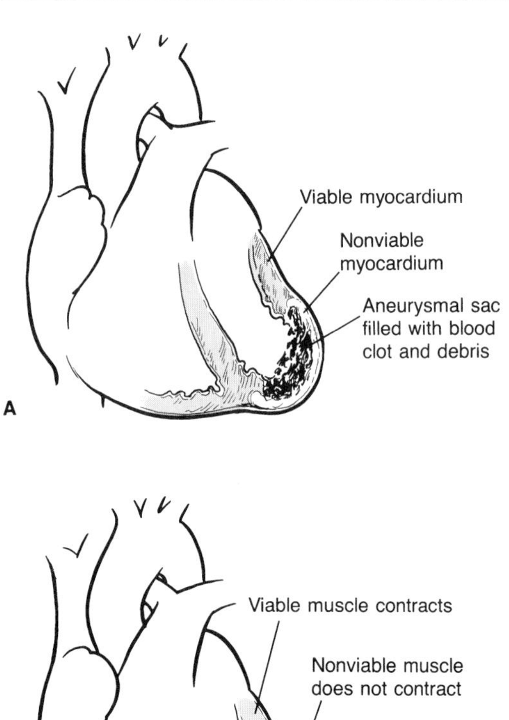

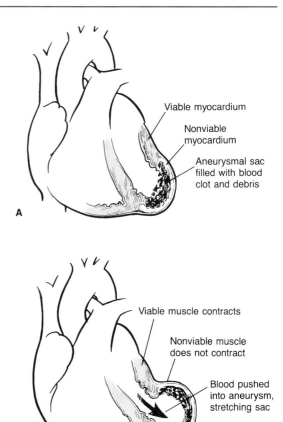

FIGURE 17-14. **Appearance of the ventricular aneurysm. A. When the myocardium is relaxed, the aneurysm remains as an aneurysmal sac, usually located at the apex of the heart. B. When the myocardium contracts, blood is pushed into the sac, causing it to bulge. This also decreases cardiac output.**

times is rimmed by a calcium ring. The debris or clot may fragment and travel into the systemic arterial circulation.[1] Occasionally, these aneurysms rupture, causing tamponade and death, but usually the problems that result are due to declining ventricular contractility or embolization.

HEART FAILURE

Heart or cardiac failure refers to a constellation of signs and symptoms that result from the heart's inability to pump enough blood to meet the body's metabolic demands. The pump, itself, is impaired and unable to supply adequate blood to meet the cellular needs. Cardiac failure is one type of *circulatory failure*, a term that also includes hypoperfusion resulting from extracardiac conditions, such as hypovolemia, peripheral vasodilatation, and inadequate oxygenation of hemoglobin. *Circulatory congestion* may result from cardiac or noncardiac causes. Cardiac causes are called *congestive heart failure*; noncardiac causes include conditions of increased blood volume such as those resulting from salt retention and those primarily resulting from decreased peripheral resistance.[43]

An old, but useful, classification of heart failure is *left-sided* and *right-sided* on the basis of clinical manifestations. It has further been divided into *forward* and *backward effects* to explain its low-output and venous congestion components. Forward and backward failure are related to *systolic* and *diastolic dysfunction*, which are the current clinical classifications in use for heart failure.[43] In some cases, the forward (systolic dysfunction) or low-output syndrome dominates, whereas in others, the congestive (diastolic dysfunction) phenomenon is the major manifestation. These concepts are discussed in detail in the section below.

The causes and mechanisms for heart failure vary and include intrinsic myocardial disease, malformation or injury, and secondary abnormalities. Table 17-11 describes the intrinsic and extrinsic causes of heart failure. Myocardial failure is often the cause of death in terminal illness of noncardiac etiology. Box 17-3 lists the functional classification of heart failure corresponding to degree of disability resulting from the cardiac dysfunction.

TABLE 17-11

CAUSES OF HEART FAILURE

CAUSES	MECHANISMS
INTRINSIC	
Myocardial infarction	Loss of myocardial muscle leads to hypokinesis or akinesis of muscle
Cardiomyopathy/myocarditis	Disease of myocardium cause impairment of contractility
Congenital heart disease	Shunts cause increased preload; hypoxia causes decreased contractility
Valvular heart defects	May cause increased preload or afterload, eventually leading to inability to compensate
Pericarditis/cardiac tamponade	Impair filling of heart, decrease cardiac output
EXTRINSIC	
Systemic hypertension	Chronic increase in afterload, leads to left ventricular hypertrophy and finally inability to maintain compensation
Chronic obstructive pulmonary disease	Leads to hypoxemia and pulmonary hypertension. causes increased afterload in right ventricle
Pulmonary embolism	Increased afterload due to obstruction in pulmonary arteries, overloads right ventricle
Anemia	Due to lack of oxygen with decreased red blood cell count, increased heart rate and hypoxemia may lead to heart failure
Thyrotoxicosis	Hyperthyroidism increases metabolism with chronic increased stress on the heart
Metabolic/respiratory acidosis	Acidosis depresses contractility of the myocardium
Blood volume excess/polycythemia	Increased volume leads to increased preload; increased red blood cell count increases viscosity and thus overloads the heart
Drug toxicity	Some drugs are cardiotoxic
Cardiac dysrhythmias	Increased rate or irritability may increase stress on heart or decrease available oxygen
Metabolic diseases	Connective tissue diseases may decrease myocardial contractility; altered metabolites may be toxic to myocardium

Pathophysiology

The onset of heart failure may be acute or insidious. It is often associated with systolic or diastolic overloading and with myocardial weakness. As the physiologic stress on the heart muscle reaches a critical level, the muscle's contractility decreases and cardiac output declines, but venous input to the ventricles remains the same or increases.

NEW YORK HEART ASSOCIATION FUNCTIONAL CLASSIFICATION OF HEART FAILURE

Class I: No symptoms noted with normal daily activity.
Class II: Symptoms noted with normal daily activities but they subside with rest.
Class III: Symptoms noted with minimal activity; may or may not be symptom-free at rest.
Class IV: Symptoms usually present at rest and worsened by any type of activity.

The systemic responses to the decreasing cardiac output are predictable and include:

1. Reflex increase in sympathetic activity
2. Release of renin from the **juxtaglomerular cells** of the kidneys
3. Anaerobic metabolism by affected cells
4. Increased extraction of oxygen by the peripheral cells

The heart's responses to increased blood volume in the ventricles are also predictable and include short-term and long-term mechanisms. These include:

1. Dilatation of the heart's chambers, especially in acute CHF
2. Hypertrophy of the myocardium, especially in chronic heart failure

In *acute or short-term mechanisms*, as the end-diastolic fiber length increases, the ventricular muscle responds with dilatation and an increased force of contraction (Starling mechanism; see p. 414). In *long-term mechanisms*, ventricular hypertrophy increases the ability of the heart muscle to contract and push its volume into the circulation. The pathology of the predisposing condition determines whether heart failure is acute or insidious in onset because compensation often occurs for long periods before clinical manifestations develop.

An example of the long-term mechanisms or compensation is that resulting from the excessive workload of systemic hypertension (see p. 447). Because the ventricles must pump against increased pressure (increased afterload), the ventricular myocardium hypertrophies, the heart pumps with more force, and the heart rate is often elevated. These mechanisms may maintain normal cardiac output for years prior to the onset of failure. Symptoms of CHF signal that the pump can no longer keep up with cellular demands.

An example of acute onset of heart failure is an extensive MI that causes direct impairment of cardiac contractility, a sudden decrease in cardiac output, and insufficient available time for the development of hypertrophy. The end result may be cardiogenic shock or pulmonary edema or both (see p. 482).

SYSTEMIC RESPONSES OR "COMPENSATIONS" IN HEART FAILURE

Systemic responses or "compensations" in heart failure may preserve the individual's life, but they usually aggravate the underlying condition. The major responses are presented below, but a large number of neurohormonal factors are being investigated for their role in compensation, which may eventually lead to progression of heart failure.[34] Some of these factors include eicosanoids, cytokines, endothelial derived factors, neuropeptide Y, and arginine vasopressin (AVP). The maladaptation that eventually results may be caused by apoptosis (cell suicide) signalled by some factor that goes awry.[32]

Sympathetic Response to Heart Failure

A decrease in cardiac output results in decreased blood pressure, which causes a reflex stimulation of the sympathetic nervous system (SNS). The SNS causes an increase in the rate and force of contraction of the ventricles through the conduction system and through an increase in ventricular irritability. It also results in vasoconstriction of the arterioles throughout the body. SNS activity is sustained inappropriately for unknown reasons and it causes a degeneration of the previously compensated heart by continual increase in ventricular workload. The intense vasoconstriction contributes to increased afterload.[26]

The SNS activity is mediated through the hormones, epinephrine and norepinephrine (see p. 421). These hormones increase the rate and force of cardiac contractions and function in systemic arteriolar vasoconstriction.[43]

Renin–Angiotensin–Aldosterone System

When blood pressure decreases, the renal juxtaglomerular cells release renin. Renin acts on angiotensinogen, a plasma protein the liver produces, to form angiotensin I. An enzyme present mostly in the lungs converts angiotensin I to angiotensin II (Fig. 17-15). Angiotensin II is a potent vasoconstrictor that constricts renal arterioles, stimulates the brain's thirst center, and stimulates the secretion of aldosterone by the adrenal glands.[16] These actions cause vasoconstriction, which leads to increased blood pressure and expansion of the blood volume through the aldosterone effect of sodium preservation. In persons with heart failure this system increases cardiac preload and afterload through fluid volume retention (aldosterone effect) and vasoconstriction (angiotensin II effect). Increasing the workload on a heart that is already failing is a temporary mechanism to improve the stroke volume but it is at the ultimate expense of the ability of the heart to compensate.

Myocardial Oxygen Needs and Supply

Myocardial oxygen needs in heart failure may increase due to increased stress on the myocardial muscle (as with hypertension), increased heart rate, or ventricular enlargement.[43] The available oxygen and oxygen needs partially determine the heart's ability to compensate for the problem producing the heart failure.

Oxygen extraction from the red blood cells to the tissues increases when the circulation is inadequate and perfusion is diminished. Normally, peripheral tissue extracts about 30% of oxygen from red blood cells but it can extract greater amounts during periods of poor perfusion. This mechanism is not very useful to the myocardial tissue because it already extracts most of the available oxygen (see p. 418).

Atrial and Ventricular Natriuretic Peptides or Factors

Atrial natriuretic peptide (ANP) is mainly produced by specialized atrial cells; brain natriuretic peptides (BNPs) are released mainly by ventricular myocytes. The concentration of these substances is increased in heart failure and the action is to promote diuresis through a direct renal action. ANP also suppresses aldosterone, renin, and AVP. ANP is released with atrial distention. The purpose of these substances in heart failure is not clear and the action is probably overwhelmed by the other factors that tend to promote sodium and water retention and vasoconstriction.[43]

Starling's Law of the Heart

When the heart is not pumping all its contents, increased amounts of blood remain within. This residual

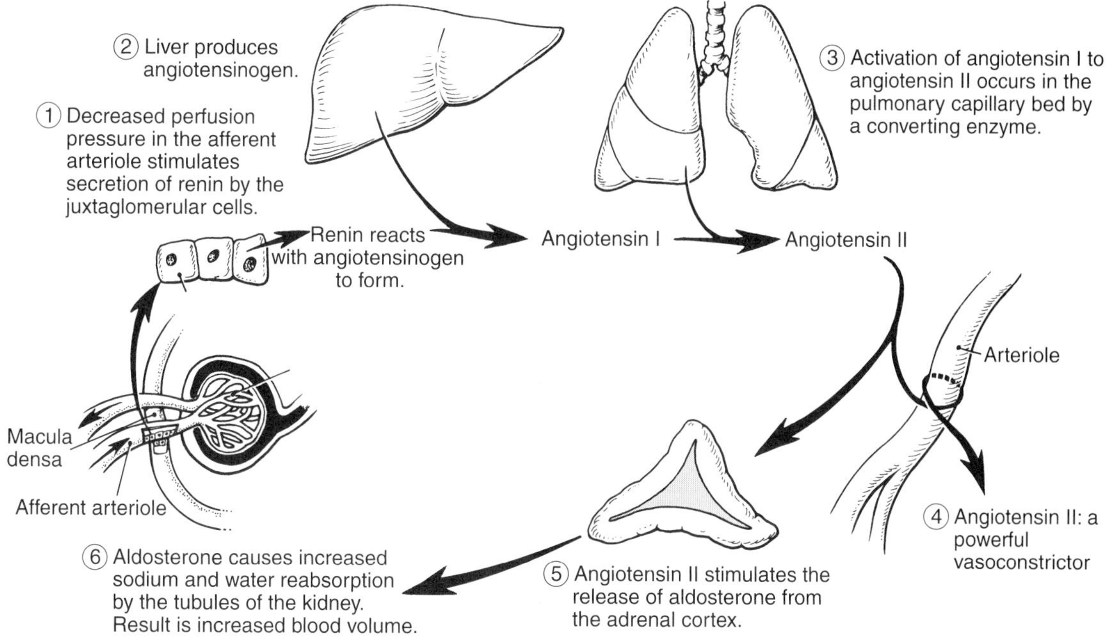

(2) Liver produces angiotensinogen.
(1) Decreased perfusion pressure in the afferent arteriole stimulates secretion of renin by the juxtaglomerular cells.
Renin reacts with angiotensinogen to form.
Angiotensin I
Angiotensin II
(3) Activation of angiotensin I to angiotensin II occurs in the pulmonary capillary bed by a converting enzyme.
Arteriole
Macula densa
Afferent arteriole
(4) Angiotensin II: a powerful vasoconstrictor
(5) Angiotensin II stimulates the release of aldosterone from the adrenal cortex.
(6) Aldosterone causes increased sodium and water reabsorption by the tubules of the kidney. Result is increased blood volume.

FIGURE 17-15. The renin-angiotensin-aldosterone system.

volume increases diastolic fiber length. The inherent compensatory mechanism is an increase in the force of recoil so that the heart responds with increased stroke work and volume[16] (see p. 414). Over time, a nearly normal stroke volume may be sustained due to increased end-diastolic fiber length.[43] As the diastolic fiber length is continually increased, the Starling mechanism becomes less effective in maintaining stroke volume. The increased end-diastolic fiber length increases the energy requirements on the already overworked myocardium and often the overburdened heart cannot supply those requirements. Increased blood volume from renal conservation adds to the diastolic volume overloading.

Hypertrophy of the Myocardium

When increased stress is placed on any chamber of the heart, hypertrophy can result. This physiologic myocardial response is due to chronically increased workload. The individual myocardial muscle cells increase in size but not in number. Hypertrophy probably results when the wall tension of the chamber must continuously increase on systole to eject the contents of the chamber, such as with systemic hypertension (see p. 447). Ventricular hypertrophy is more common than atrial hypertrophy and provides for compensatory adaptation to a chronically increased workload. Hypertrophy increases the myocardial requirement for oxygen. Oxygen is supplied by the coronary arteries, and energy is produced by an increasing number of mitochondria, which proliferate early in the process of developing hypertrophy.[16] As long as the oxygen supply from the coronary arteries and the mitochondrial production of adenosine triphosphate keeps up with the enlarging muscle, the ventricle will pump very efficiently. When an imbalance between oxygen supply and demand occurs, ischemia and cardiac dysfunction result. Capillary supply to the hypertrophied myocardium does not increase adequately to supply the increased muscle mass and ischemia, even in the absence of CAD may occur.[26] The deterioration of cardiac function in hypertrophy has led to the hypothesis that the heart is "energy starved" and this contributes to cardiac failure by promoting myocardial cell death.[20]

Dilatation of the Heart

Dilatation refers to enlargement of cardiac chambers. It often occurs because of increased volume of blood that enters the heart. The ventricles are always dilated in acute CHF. Dilatation often coincides with hypertrophy, especially if the stressful event causing the failure is chronic, such as chronic systemic hypertension.

Radiographic enlargement of the cardiac shadow characterizes heart failure. In the normal heart, increased input to the ventricle results in increased ventricular force of contraction but no permanent enlargement occurs. As the cardiac reserve fails, the ventricle is unable to pump out all of its contents and thus enlarges.

Dilatation imposes a mechanical disadvantage on the ventricles. As ventricular volume increases, a large portion of the mechanical energy of contraction is expended in imparting tension to the fibers and a smaller portion for fiber recoil or shortening. Usually, the greater the dilatation, the more ineffective the cardiac contraction. Ineffective ventricular contraction is called ventricular **hypokinesis** and may affect the left or right ventricle.

A heart that is greatly dilated also works at a metabolic disadvantage because its need for oxygen is increased. More blood to the myocardium is required, which may not be supplied by the coronary arteries.

Left Heart Failure

Left heart failure (LHF) occurs when left side of the heart is unable to pump the total volume of blood it receives from the right side of the heart. As a result, the pulmonary circuit becomes congested with blood (backward effects) that cannot be moved forward and the systemic blood pressure falls (forward effects). The most common cause of left heart failure is MI. Other causes include systemic hypertension, valvular stenosis or insufficiency, and cardiomyopathy.

PATHOPHYSIOLOGY

The diastolic dysfunction (*backward effects*) of LHF results from the volume overload of the left ventricle or in some cases the left atrium. Because the left heart cannot discharge its normal ejection fraction, increased end-diastolic volume causes blood to accumulate in the left atrium, into the four pulmonary veins, and the pulmonary capillary bed (PCB). As the volume of blood in the lungs increases, the pulmonary vessels enlarge. The pressure of blood in the PCB increases. When it reaches a certain critical point (about 25–28 mm Hg), fluid passes across the pulmonary capillary membrane into the interstitial spaces around the alveoli and finally into the alveoli (Flowchart 17-1). Actual alveolar pulmonary edema occurs when the rate of fluid transudation exceeds the ability of the plentiful lymphatic drainage to remove it from the interstitial spaces. Acute pulmonary edema (APE) results as the alveoli fill with fluid; this impairs gas exchange, which can be life-threatening (Fig. 17-16). Higher PCB pressures may cause microhemorrhages in the sacs or rust-colored sputum due to the presence of hemosiderin-laden alveolar macrophages.[7] The presence of large amounts of these hemosiderin-laden macrophages (heart failure cells) is often indicative of long-standing cases of pulmonary congestion, as may be seen with mitral stenosis[7] (see p. 485). The congestive phenomena of LHF result from the overloading of the left ventricle.

The systolic dysfunction (*forward effects*) of LHF results from the inability of the left heart to pump its contents into the circulation. The left heart cannot pump its normal stroke volume out to the aorta. Thus, the systemic blood pressure decreases. This decrease is sensed by the baro-receptors and a reflex stimulation of the SNS causes increased heart rate and peripheral vasoconstriction. The renin–angiotensin–aldosterone system is stimulated, leading to further vasoconstriction, together with sodium and water retention. The inherent compensatory mechanisms of the body are to preserve blood volume and pressure even at the expense of organs and tissues (see Flowchart 17-1). The end result is to increase the preload and afterload, which then contributes to the workload on the already overburdened heart.

Chronic LHF often occurs in mitral valve disease and it may progressively occur in cardiomyopathy and post-MI. In the last two conditions, pulmonary congestion may be evidenced but APE does not occur unless additional stress increases the cardiac demand. Gradual onset, such as with mitral stenosis, may cause pulmonic pressures greater than 30 mm Hg without symptoms of APE. In conditions of sudden onset, such as acute MI, this level would cause APE.

FLOWCHART 17-1 ***Left Heart Failure***

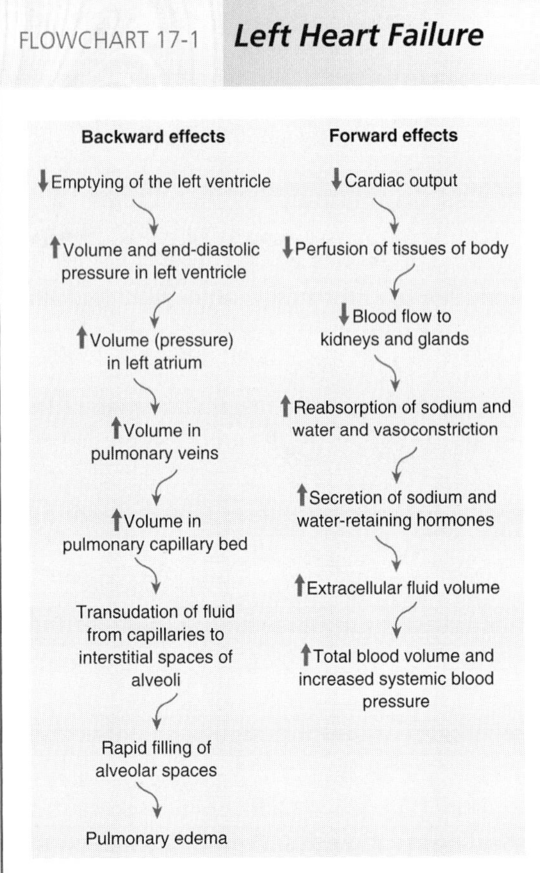

Highly schematic representation of the pathophysiology of left heart failure.

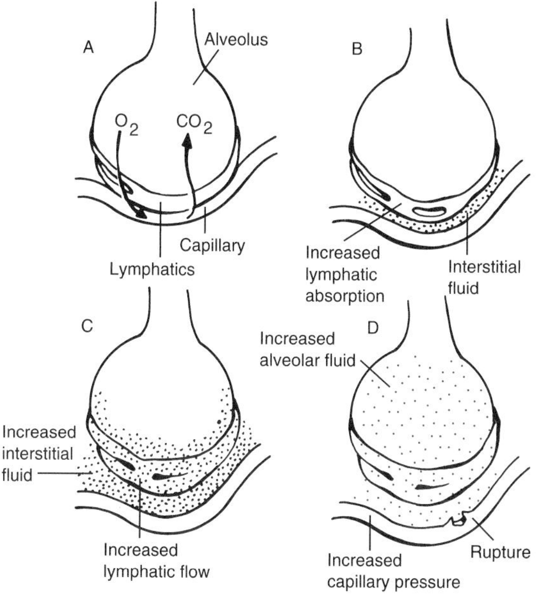

FIGURE 17-16. **A–D. Stages in the progression of pulmonary edema due to left heart failure.**

CLINICAL MANIFESTATIONS

Clinical manifestations of LHF are as follows:

- Affected individuals exhibit dyspnea in the early stages of LHF, when fluid begins to accumulate in the PCB and the formation of interstitial edema causes a defect in oxygenation.[41] The oxygen saturation of blood decreases, causing the chemoreceptors to stimulate the respiratory center. The respiratory rate increases at first during exercise and later even at rest. Shortness of breath on exertion (dyspnea on exertion, DOE) is a common and relatively early symptom. The person may complain of breathlessness when walking or after eating a heavy meal.
- Easy fatigue, weakness, and dizziness result when hypoxia of the body tissues occurs because of decreased cardiac output and decreased oxygen saturation of the blood. Dizziness is the result of hypoxia to the brain. As failure and hypoxia worsen, disorientation, confusion, and ultimately unconsciousness can occur. Loss of potassium induced by increased levels of aldosterone also causes muscle weakness.
- *Orthopnea* is a term that indicates the inability to breathe in a supine position. In chronic LHF, interstitial and alveolar pulmonary edema may be present all of the time; the affected individual assumes an upright position so fluid gravitates to the bases of the lungs, making breathing easier. As fluid begins to collect in the pulmonary capillaries, the person assumes an upright position so that fluid collects in the bases of the lung fields and pulmonary blood flow increases in the apices.[43]
- Auscultation of the heart reveals an S_3 gallop and a paradoxical split of the second sound on expiration (see p. 417). A *pulsus alternans*, characterized by alternating weaker and stronger pulsations in the peripheral arteries, often occurs and indicates a poorly functioning ventricle.
- Paroxysmal nocturnal dyspnea (PND) refers to the onset of acute episodes of dyspnea at night. The cause is unknown but it may result from improved cardiac performance at night during recumbence. This causes increased reabsorption of fluid that has accumulated in the lower half of the body into the systemic veins, where it is returned to the heart. The increased fluid returns to and overloads the left ventricle, causing acute pulmonary congestion until the individual assumes the orthopneic position. Affected individuals describe acute breathlessness and a feeling of smothering.[49] This particular breathing difficulty is considered to be a very specific symptom of LHF.[49]
- *Cardiac asthma* is an old term for wheezing due to bronchospasm induced by heart failure. The bronchioles may react to the increased fluid in the alveoli, constrict, and produce the characteristic wheezing.[6,49]
- Acute pulmonary edema is always a life-threatening condition characterized by dyspnea of sudden onset, basal rales, gasping respirations, extreme anxiety, rapid weak pulse, increased venous pressure, and decreased urinary output. The skin is cool and moist to the touch, ashen gray, or cyanotic. A cough accompanied by expectoration of frothy white, pink-tinged, or bloody sputum may be present (Fig. 17-17). Most attacks gradually subside in 1 to 3 hours, usually with treatment, but they may progress rapidly to shock and death.[43]

Right Heart Failure

Right heart failure (RHF) occurs when the output of the right ventricle is less than the input from the systemic venous circuit. As a result, the systemic venous circuit is congested (backward effects) and output to the lungs decreases (forward effects). The major cause of RHF is LHF; the right ventricle fails because of the excessive pulmonary pressures generated by failure of the left heart. Other causes include chronic obstructive lung disease, pulmonary embolus, right ventricular infarction, and congenital heart defects, especially those that involve pulmonary overloading and pulmonary hypertension. *Cor pulmonale* is RHF that results from lung disease and over 50% of cases in the United States are caused by emphysema and chronic bronchitis.[29]

PATHOPHYSIOLOGY

The diastolic dysfunction (backward or congestive effects) of RHF occurs due to the right ventricle being unable to pump all of its contents forward. Therefore, the end-diastolic volume of the right ventricle increases and causes excessive volume in the right

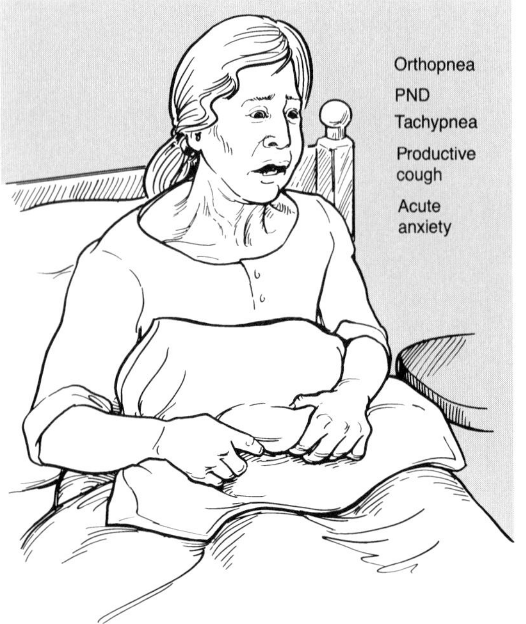

FIGURE 17-17. **Pulmonary signs and symptoms of left heart failure.**

atrium, which leads to increased volume and pressure in the systemic venous circuit. The increased volume and pressure are transmitted to distensible organs, such as the liver and spleen. Increased pressure in the peritoneal vessels leads to transudation of fluid into the peritoneal cavity. Increased pressure at the capillary line causes fluid to move into the interstitial space and systemic peripheral edema results (Flowchart 17-2).

The systolic dysfunction (forward or low output effects) of RHF occurs due the inability of the right ventricle to maintain its output to the lungs. This results in a decreased pulmonary circulation and decreased return to the left side of the heart. These forward effects of RHF cause all of the forward effects of LHF (see Flowchart 17-2).

CLINICAL MANIFESTATIONS

The clinical manifestations of RHF reflect both forward and backward effects.

- Dependent, pitting edema may be noted in the sternum or sacrum of a bedridden person, as well as in the feet and legs of a person in the sitting position.
- Enlargement of the spleen and liver can cause pressure on surrounding organs, respiratory impingement, and organ dysfunction. Inadequate deactivation of aldosterone by the liver may lead to additional fluid retention. Jaundice and coagulation problems may result with severe, long-standing, decompensated RHF. Ascites also occurs when RHF is severe and may cause respiratory distress and abdominal pressure. Pleural effusions may appear due to the increased capillary pressure.
- Jugular venous distention is common and the level of the distention provides an index of decompensation.
- With pure RHF (that not precipitated by LHF), the pulmonary symptoms are minimal to absent, whereas engorgement of the venous and portal systems is significant.[7] The peripheral edema may be massive. When RHF is due to lung disease, the underlying lung problem will present its symptoms, as well as the cardiac dysfunction.

Diagnosis of Congestive Heart Failure

Diagnostic methods in heart failure include radiology studies, hemodynamic monitoring, and clinical examination. These support the evidence of the underlying clinical disorder.

FLOWCHART 17-2 ***Right Heart Failure***

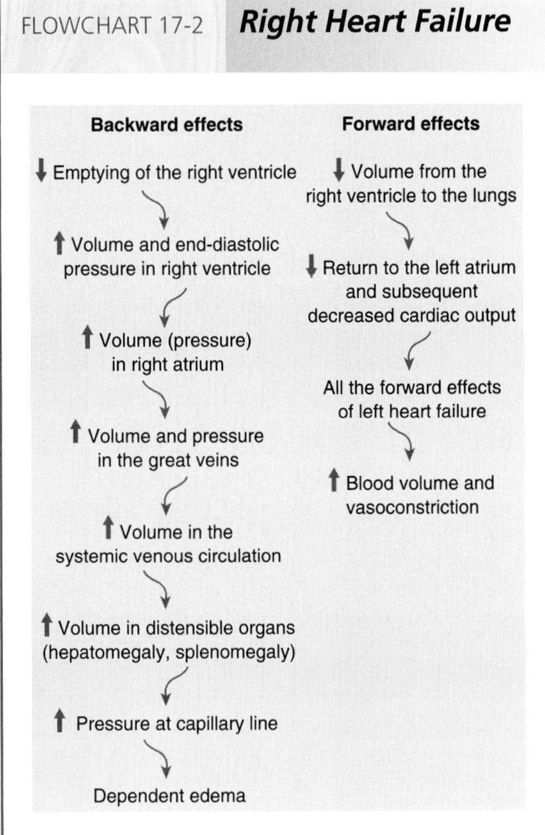

Highly schematic representation of the pathophysiology of right heart failure.

RADIOLOGIC CHANGES

In LHF, radiologic evidence of cardiac enlargement is noted by an increased size of the left ventricular shadow. The left ventricle extends past the midclavicular line and fluid effusion may be present throughout the lung fields (Fig. 17-18). In RHF, the right ventricular shadow can be seen extending out from the right sternal border. Pulmonary markings may be decreased due to decreased pulmonary circulation (Fig. 17-19).

HEMODYNAMIC MONITORING

The balloon-tipped flow-directed catheter (pulmonary artery catheter) is an effective monitoring system for assessing pulmonary and systemic circulations. The pulmonary artery catheter is threaded into the pulmonary artery where it finally halts in a vessel slightly smaller than the inflated balloon tip, blocking the flow of blood from the right ventricle.[8] A pressure reading at this time reflects the diastolic pressures of the left ventricle if there is no concomitant mitral valve disease. This pulmonary artery wedge pressure (PAWP) reflects its pressures because of the continuous circuit to the left heart. Thus pressure measurements reflect the left ventricular end-diastolic pressure. Figure 17-20 illustrates the pressures measured by the pulmonary artery catheter.

The end-diastolic volume is elevated in the failing heart. Because an increase in end-diastolic volume is often associated with an increase in end-diastolic pressure, the end-diastolic pressure can be used as an indicator of ventricular function.[43] The pulmonary artery catheter also measures central venous pressure (right atrial pressure). This catheter also can be used to measure cardiac output by the thermodilution method, in which a computer analyzes a temperature differential between two points on the catheter. The normal cardiac output is approximately 4 to 8 L/min. The level of decreased cardiac output in persons with CHF helps to determine the necessary treatment. Table 17-12 describes the normal values of data that can be derived from hemodynamic monitoring.

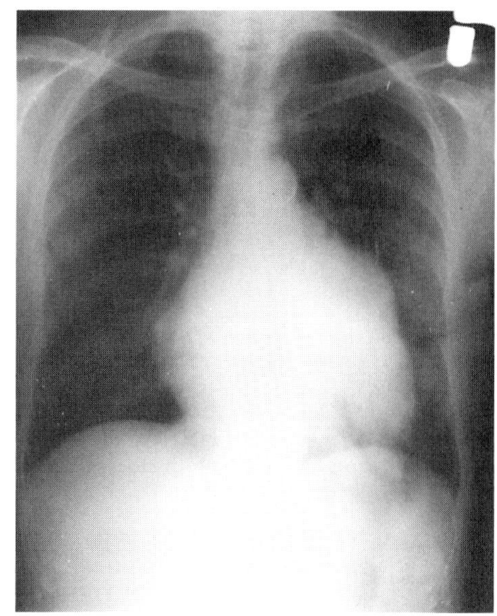

FIGURE 17-19. Radiologic changes in right heart failure. Note right ventricular shadow extending from the right sternal border.

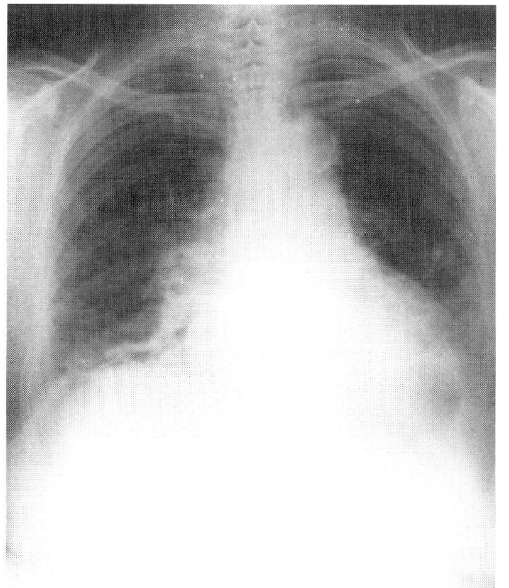

FIGURE 17-18. Radiologic changes in left heart failure. Note left ventricular enlargement and fluid effusion in lung fields.

CLINICAL EXAMINATION

The patient with heart failure presents with a variety of signs and symptoms that often indicate the underlying cause of the cardiac dysfunction. The history may indicate shortness of breath, fatigability, and peripheral edema. Pallor, tachycardia, pulmonary rales, and venous congestion are common findings. Gallop sounds, the S_3 or S_4 or a combination of the two, may be heard (see p. 417). Diagnostic echocardiography often shows a hypokinetic ventricle and nuclear imaging techniques may assess ventricular volume, shape, and motion[22] (see Appendix Table C).

Arterial and venous blood gases often show hypoxemia (decreased partial pressure of oxygen or PaO_2). Oxygen saturation often remains normal until decompensation is severe. The partial pressure of carbon dioxide ($PaCO_2$) may be low early in CHF due to hyperventilation but in late-stage CHF, the $PaCO_2$ may become elevated (see Table 6-11).

A. Catheter advanced to right atrium, balloon is inflated. Pressure is low, usually 2–5 mm Hg.

B. Catheter is floated to right ventricle with the balloon inflated. Wave-forms indicate a systolic pressure of 25–30 mm Hg and a diastolic pressure of 0–5 mm Hg.

C. As the catheter moves into the pulmonary artery, the systolic pressure remains the same but the diastolic pressure elevates to 10–15 mm Hg.

D. The balloon in deflated and the catheter is moved until it can be wedged in a smaller vessel when the balloon is inflated. The pressure recorded is that pressure in front of the catheter. It is an approximate measure of the left ventricular end diastolic pressure.

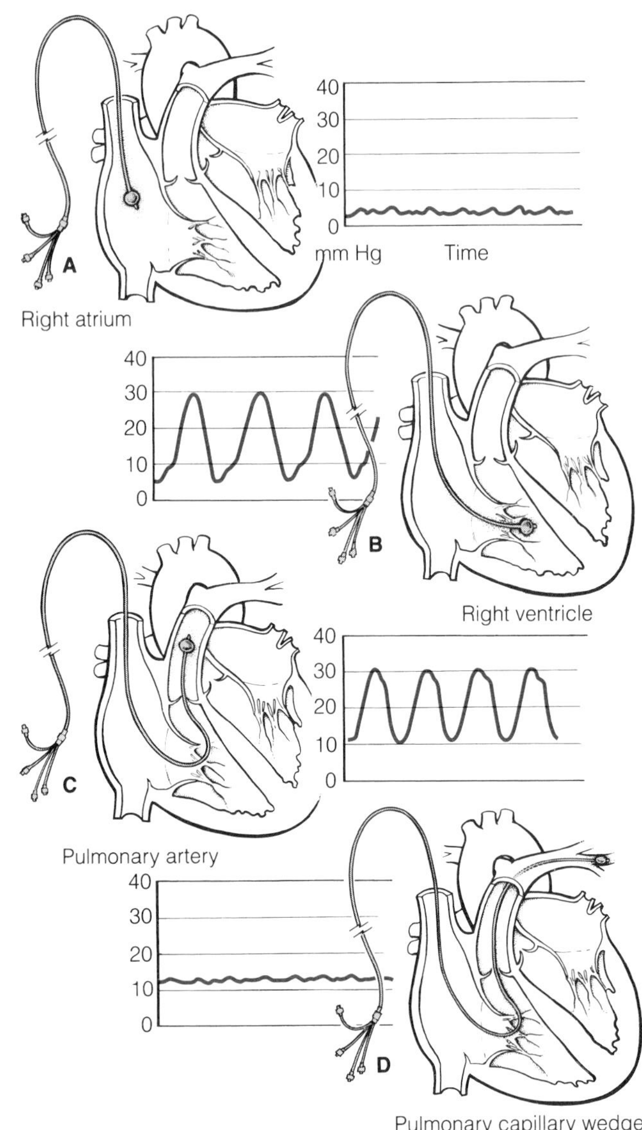

FIGURE 17-20. Insertion of a flow-directed cardiac catheter.

Other helpful laboratory tests include the serum sodium and potassium. Serum sodium levels are often low in CHF even though body sodium levels are almost always elevated. This laboratory picture results from the retention of sodium and water and is called *dilutional hyponatremia*. Serum potassium may be decreased due to the aldosterone effect and the administration of potassium-depleting diuretics. Other laboratory values may be altered depending on the underlying cause of the CHF (see Appendix Table A).

Cardiogenic Shock

Heart failure may lead to cardiogenic shock with a low-output component, the congestive phenomena, or both. Cardiogenic shock often occurs when more than 40% of the left ventricle is nonfunctional. It always carries a grave prognosis with a mortality rate of over 80%.[1] The most common cause of cardiogenic shock is MI; however, cardiomyopathy, dysrhythmias, cardiac tamponade, pulmonary embolism, or any factor that can depress myocardial function may precipitate this syndrome.

PATHOPHYSIOLOGY

Cardiogenic shock results from decreased ability of the left or right ventricle to maintain minimally adequate cardiac output. The result is decreased systolic

TABLE 17-12

NORMAL VALUES OF HEMODYNAMIC DATA

DATA	NORMAL VALUES	SIGNIFICANCE
Central venous pressure (CVP)/ right atrial pressure (RAP)	1–5 mm Hg	Reflects volume of blood returning to the right atrium from the systemic venous circulation
Pulmonary artery pressure (PAP)	17–32/4–13 mm Hg	Reflects pressure generated by right ventricle to eject its stroke volume; affected by preload and pulmonary vascular resistance (afterload)
Pulmonary artery wedge pressure (PAWP)	12–15 mm Hg	Reflects left ventricular end-diastolic pressure, a measure of preload; influenced by left ventricular contractility in absence of mitral valve disease
Cardiac output (CO) (stroke volume × heart rate)	4–8 L/min	Total volume pumped by the heart per minute
Cardiac index (CI)	2.8–4.2 L/min/m^2	Cardiac output indexed to body surface area
Systemic blood pressure	100–140/60–80	Reflects pressure required to eject blood from the left ventricle and pressure maintained in the arterial circuit
Mean arterial pressure (Systolic BP + 2 × Diastolic BP ÷ 3)	70–100	Reflects the average pressure maintained in the arterial circuit
Systemic vascular resistance	1,100–1,400 dynes/sec/HRU	Good measure of the resistance afforded by the arterioles, which is a significant determinant of afterload

blood pressure with reduced peripheral perfusion resulting in intense SNS stimulation. This increases vasoconstriction and markedly increases the heart rate causing further taxation on an already overtaxed heart. SNS stimulation markedly decreases renal perfusion and increases the risk for acute renal failure (see p. 613).

Anaerobic metabolism begins in peripheral cells as vital oxygen deprivation occurs. The effect of this energy production is to keep cells viable, but the production of lactic acid as a by-product leads to metabolic acidosis (see p. 514). Acidosis depresses cardiac function. Further depression of cardiac function may result from a *myocardial depressant factor* released from cells in shock situations.[7,14] Comprehensive coverage of the shock state is found on page 503.

CLINICAL MANIFESTATIONS

Diagnosis of cardiogenic shock is often one of exclusion. Sometimes hypovolemic or even septic shock must be ruled out. The symptoms and signs that the affected individual presents are analyzed. The blood pressure is very low and the individual exhibits cold, clammy skin, diaphoresis, tachycardia, mental confusion, and decreased urinary output. Physical examination reveals *gallop rhythms*, sometimes venous engorgement, and the effects of acute hypotension. The ECG often shows cardiac dysrhythmias and evidence of MI. The chest x-ray usually shows a dilated or enlarged heart, which may be accompanied by the pulmonary infiltrates of APE. The pulmonary artery catheter usually reveals elevated pulmonary wedge pressures and decreased cardiac output.[14]

VALVULAR DISEASE

Valvular disease refers to a condition, such as **stenosis** or insufficiency, that may interfere with valve functions and blood flow through the heart. The main etiologic factor, worldwide, is rheumatic fever, but it may also be caused by bacterial endocarditis or congenital valvular problems.[19]

In *valvular stenosis*, the valve orifice (opening) narrows and the valve leaflets (cusps) fuse together in such a way that the valve cannot open freely. This narrowing of the opening obstructs of blood flow. As a result, the chamber behind the affected valve must build up more pressure to overcome resistance. The muscle fibers in that chamber must thicken to do more work to push the blood through the narrowed opening. Gradually, the myocardial muscle hypertrophies in response to the added workload.

With *valvular insufficiency* (regurgitation), the valve cannot close completely. The incomplete closure usually results from scarring and retraction of the valve leaflets. As a result, blood is permitted to flow backward (retrograde) through the opening. The heart chamber, which receives the additional retrograde flow, is then forced to pump the added regurgitant volume together with the volume being received. As a response to the increased volume present in the chamber behind the regurgitant valve, the muscle fibers lengthen or stretch. This dilatation of muscle fibers increases the surface area to accommodate the additional volume. Both hypertrophy and dilatation are compensatory mechanisms that occur in the presence of specific valvular defects.

When stenosis and regurgitation occur simultaneously, the defect is called a *mixed lesion*, and usually is a feature of advanced disease. In the clinical setting, lesions are classified in terms of the predominant mechanical load that is placed on the heart leading also to the classification of valvular defects. Stenosis can be predominant or "pure," as can regurgitation, or the lesions can be mixed. In addition to having a mixed lesion on one valve, disease may be on another valve at the same time. This finding is called combined valvular disease, which may present a rather complex clinical picture depending on the number of valves involved and the types of lesions.

Rheumatic Fever

Rheumatic fever is an inflammatory disease that occurs in susceptible persons after untreated pharyngeal infection with group A β-hemolytic streptococci. It appears to be an individual immune reaction to the streptococcal organism and affects 1% to 3% of individuals with untreated streptococcal sore throat.[19] The production of streptococcal antigenic response may activate cytotoxic T cells that may then cross-react with certain cardiac structures and cause acute inflammation of the heart[41] (Fig. 17-21). The disease causes inflammation of the joints, heart, skin, and nervous system. The most common age of onset is 9 to 11 years, and frequency is greatest in areas of crowded, substandard living conditions.[19,41] Recurrent attacks of rheumatic fever are common in susceptible, untreated individuals and carry a greater risk of valvular disease or rheumatic heart disease with each recurrence.

PATHOPHYSIOLOGY

The joints are affected with an exudative synovitis with associated subcutaneous nodules. A characteristic pancarditis (endocarditis, myocarditis, and pericarditis) is present, with endocarditis usually being the most severe. *Aschoff bodies* are the diagnostic lesions of rheumatic fever and consist of granular fibrinoid material surrounded by histiocytes that are found in the connective tissue of the heart.[4] *Verrucae*, which are small, warty vegetations produced by fibrin or ground substance, appear

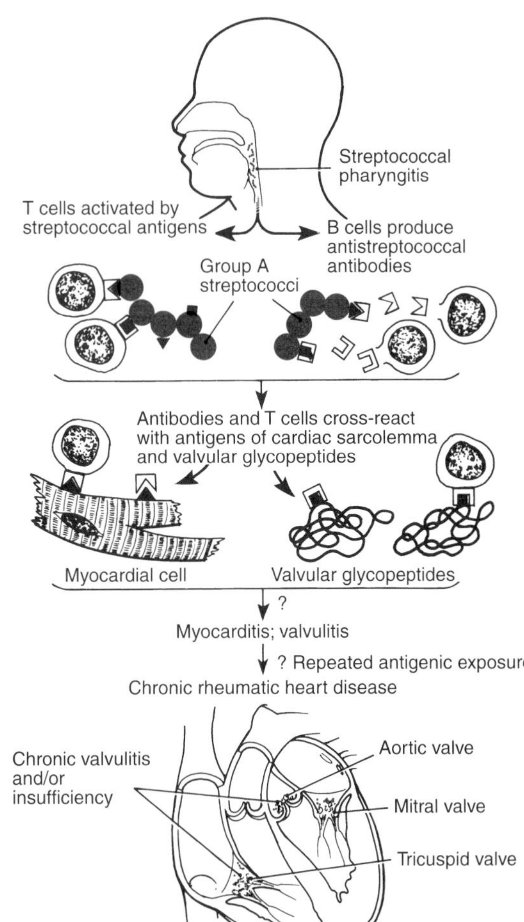

FIGURE 17-21. **Pathophysiology of rheumatic heart disease. (Modified from Rubin, E. & Farber, J. L. *Pathology* [2nd ed.]. Philadelphia: J. B. Lippincott, 1994).**

on the valve leaflets. They apparently cause inflammation and exudation, leading to interadherence of the leaflets. They also may develop in a line on the chordae tendineae and produce scarring and shortening of these structures over time.[7] During the acute phase of rheumatic fever, the valves and endocardial surface are inflamed and edematous. Nervous system involvement is manifested by Sydenham's chorea (rapid, jerky, involuntary movements of the arms and legs), and emotional instability.[19] No diagnostic central nervous system lesion has been found to explain this manifestation.

CLINICAL MANIFESTATIONS

Onset of the disease may be acute or subacute. The acute form causes any or all of the following:

- Migratory polyarthritis, which refers to inflammation that moves from joint to joint

- Subcutaneous nodules that appear over the extensor surfaces of joints, such as the wrist or elbows[19]
- Characteristic low-grade and intermittent fever that may be as high as 102°F (39°C) in severe pericarditis or myocarditis[19]
- Tachycardia out of proportion to the level of the fever that may be associated with mitral or aortic murmurs, cardiac enlargement, and congestive heart failure
- Sydenham's chorea, which may begin up to 3 months after the streptococcal infection
- Erythema marginatum, a pink, erythematous rash on the trunk and extremities that often appears in concentric circles that fade and enlarge in minutes to hours
- Rheumatic arteritis, pneumonitis, and pleuritis (relatively rare)
- Chronic rheumatic carditis that may run a fatal course over a few months; rheumatic carditis is rare and cardiac involvement is subsequently expressed through valvular defects, often years after the initial disease.[6]

Most cases of rheumatic fever last less than 12 weeks. The onset in later years of valvular dysfunction usually can be prevented by treatment of later streptococcal infections.

The subacute form of rheumatic fever may be not diagnosed or may be described as a flulike episode with or without recurrences. This form accounts for the many persons who have no history of rheumatic fever when they are diagnosed with valvular disease in later life.

Laboratory tests are not diagnostic, but the erythrocyte sedimentation rate (ESR) and the **antistreptolysin O** (ASO) titers are increased after streptococcal infection. Blood cultures do not show evidence of streptococcal organisms.

Mitral Stenosis

Stenosis of the mitral valve impairs blood flow from the left atrium to the left ventricle (Fig. 17-22*A*). The impairment is due to an abnormality in the structure of the valve leaflets that prevents the valve from opening completely in diastole. The most common cause of mitral stenosis is scarring after rheumatic endocarditis, but other conditions are also implicated. Table 17-13 presents the etiology, pathophysiology, clinical manifestations, and diagnostic tests that are helpful in understanding mitral stenosis. Heart sounds are characteristics and are illustrated in Figure 17-22*B*. The uninterrupted course of mitral stenosis is long and progresses toward total disability and death. The onset of the dysrhythmia, atrial fibrillation, adds an additional burden to the already compromised hemodynamics and may predispose to systemic emboli.[36] Pulmonary hypertension develops after long exposure to high pulmonary pressures and may cause permanent vascular changes along with the development of RHF.[37]

Mitral Regurgitation or Insufficiency

Mitral regurgitation is described as the backflow of blood from the left ventricle across the mitral valve to the left atrium during ventricular systole. Regurgitation occurs when the mitral valve fails to close completely. The most common causes of mitral regurgita-

(text continues on page 488)

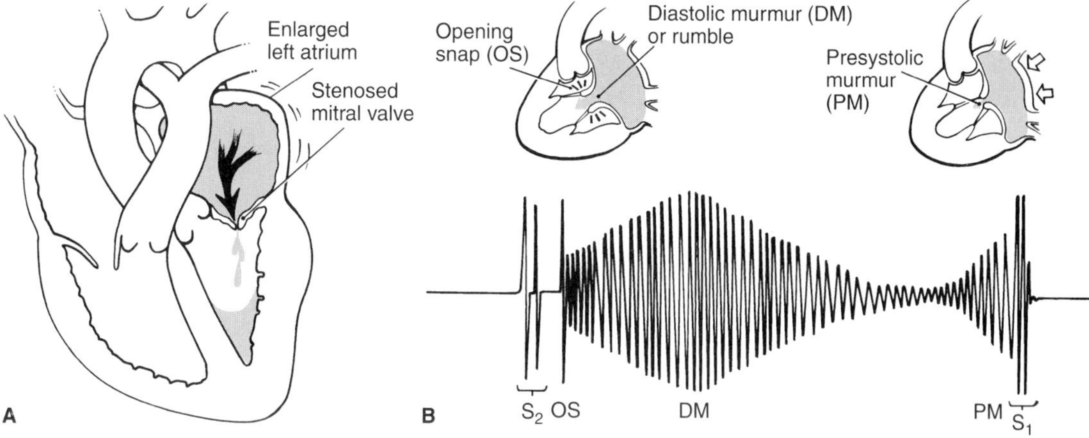

FIGURE 17-22. **A.** Mitral stenosis as viewed during atrial contraction. **B.** The diastolic rumble is produced due to obstruction of blood flow from left atrium to left ventricle. The stiff valve produces an opening snap (OS). The murmur intensity decreases in mid-diastole. Atrial contraction increases flow across the stiff valve, causing a presystolic increase in the murmur intensity.

TABLE 17-13

VALVULAR DISEASE

ETIOLOGY	PATHOPHYSIOLOGY	CLINICAL MANIFESTATION	DIAGNOSTIC TESTS
MITRAL STENOSIS			
Rheumatic endocarditis Congenital Neoplasm Atrial Thrombi Connective tissue disease Acute/subacute bacterial endocarditis. (ABE/SBE)	Valve leaflets thicken, calcify, commisures become fused, chordae tendinea shorten When mitral valve orifice decreases from 4–6 cm. normal to 1.0–2.0 cm. Produces gradient across the valve; Left atrial (LA) pressure rises, LA dilates, hypertrophies Decreased flow from LA to left ventricle (LV) leads to decreased cardiac output Increased LA volume/pressure reflected to lungs Pulmonary congestion and edema Chronic increased LA pressure leads to Pulmonary hypertension Right heart failure (RHF) results	Onset of symptoms with decrease orifice size to 1/3 to 1/2 normal Early symptoms: fatigue, dyspnea on exertion Progressive fatigue and dyspnea Palpitations from atrial dysrhythmias, especially atrial fibrillation (AF) Decreased blood pressure especially with onset of AF Pulmonary congestion and pulmonary edema as stenosis is severe Hemoptysis with pulmonary hypertension Signs and symptoms of RHF	*Heart Sounds* Loud first heart sound (S_1) Opening snap Diastolic rumble *Radiology* Chest film shows straightening of left ventricular shaw, enlargement of pulmonary artery Kerley's B. lines represent pulmonary edema *ECG* Broad notched P wave in lead II (P mitrale) Right ventricular hypertrophy Atrial dysrhythmias if present *Echocardiogram* LA enlargement Loss of posterior leaflet motion
MITRAL REGURGITATION OR INSUFFICIENCY			
Rheumatic endocarditis Mitral valve prolapse ABE/SBE Ruptured papillary muscle after myocardial infarction (MI) Extreme cardiac dilatation	Mitral valve remains open in ventricular systole; results in regurgitant and systemic blood flow *Acute* Sudden onset regurgitation of blood into LA on Ventricular systole Decreased cardiac output (CO) and increased volume and pressure in pulmonary capillary bed. Acute pulmonary edema (APE) *Chronic* Gradual dilatation LA, may become aneurysmal Decreased CO Increased pulmonary congestion and APE Increased pulmonary pressure/pulmonary hypertension RHF and left heart failure (LHF)	*Acute* Sudden onset respiratory distress, cough, white or pink frothy sputum Orthopnea Decreased blood pressure *Chronic* Exercise intolerance Fatigue Dyspnea Palpitations due to atrial dysrhythmias, especially atrial fibrillation (in 75% cases) Signs and symptoms of RHF	*Heart Sounds* Loud systolic murmur high pitched at apex Irregular heart rhythm due to AF *Radiology* LA and LV enlargement Pulmonary venous changes *ECG* Enlarged P wave in lead II Right ventricular hypertrophy Atrial dysrhythmias, if present *Echocardiogram* Estimates severity of regurgitation Shows wall motion abnormalities
MITRAL VALVE PROLAPSE			
Congenital displacement of posterior leaflet of mitral valve	Mostly asymptomatic May cause mitral regurgitation (MR), which de-	Nonexertional chest pain Palpitations, due to atrial and ventricular dysrhythmias	*Heart Sounds* Systolic murmur may be crescendo in nature

(continued)

TABLE 17-13

VALVULAR DISEASE (Continued)

ETIOLOGY	PATHOPHYSIOLOGY	CLINICAL MANIFESTATION	DIAGNOSTIC TESTS
Autosomal dominant condition in Marfan's syndrome Greatest incidence in females; symptomatic in 2nd to 4th decades of life	termines hemodynamic alterations May be vulnerable to SBE, could lead to increased MR	If MR present, may have pulmonary symptoms	Various clicks *Radiology* Normal cardiac shadow *ECG* Normal except for frequent dysrhythmias; atrial tachycardia, atrial fibrillation, premature ventricular contractions, ventricular tachycardia *Echocardiogram* Determines degree of insufficiency
AORTIC STENOSIS			
Rheumatic endocarditis Congenital, bicuspid valve, hypertrophic cardiomyopathy Degenerative calcific valve (seen mainly in elderly persons) SBE on previously damaged valve	Onset of gradient when valve decreases from 2.6–3.5 cm. to ⅓ normal Amount of gradient indicates severity Increased workload leads to hypertrophy of LV. Hypertrophy compensatory to maintain CO Over time, LHF may result Decreased blood flow to hypertrophical myocardium leads to ischemia	Blood pressure decreases slightly, pulse pressure narrows Chest pain on exertion and later at rest Syncope, "gray-outs"; when cerebral circulation is inadequate Symptoms of LHF in late stages	*Heart Sounds* Systolic ejection murmur Loud, best heard in aortic area *Radiology* Cardiac shadow may be normal until LHF occurs; then dilatation of LV Apical bulging may be seen; Calcification of valve ring may be noted *ECG* LV hypertrophy *Echocardiogram* Valve structure and motion defects Ventricular function
AORTIC INSUFFICIENCY OR REGURGITATION (AR)			
Rheumatic endocarditis Syphilis ABE Dissecting hematoma ascending aorta	*Acute* ABE causes perforation and destruction of valve Dissecting hematoma causes dilatation of valve ring Acute AR leads to sudden increase in end-diastolic volume (EDV) marked LV dilatation, sudden onset LHF *Chronic* Rheumatic endocarditis leads to fibrosis and retraction of valve Syphilis causes dilatation of ascending aorta Increased EDV leads to increased contraction; constant load causes hypertrophy/dilatation of LV LHF results	*Acute* Signs & symptoms LHF and APE Cardiogenic shock and death *Chronic* Asymptomatic for years Fatigue Dyspnea Exercise intolerance Chest pain Signs and symptoms of LHF Blood pressure increased systolic/ low diastolic Corrigan's pulse (water hammer)—Intense upstroke with quick downstroke	*Heart Sounds* Diastolic murmur begins shortly after S_2 and ends before S_1 Austin Flint with severe AR, diastolic rumble at apex *Radiology* Cardiac shadow enlarged LV *ECG* LV hypertrophy Increased incidence of ventricular dysrhythmias *Echocardiogram* Increased chamber size Wall motion abnormalities

tion are mitral valve prolapse and rheumatic valve disease. Table 17-13 summarizes the etiology, hemodynamics, clinical manifestations, and diagnostic tests useful in understanding MR.

In mitral regurgitation, cardiac output is divided into regurgitant and systemic flows (Fig. 17-23*A*). The amount of regurgitant flow is determined by the degree of mitral valve incompetence and the resistance to flow through the aortic valve. Regurgitant flow increases proportionately to mitral valve orifice size. Characteristic heart sounds are illustrated in Figure 17-23*B*. The course of mitral regurgitation depends on the causative factor. It may be slowly progressive, leading to pulmonary congestion and hypertension, or it may cause the sudden onset of APE (such as with rupture of the papillary muscle).

Mixed Mitral Stenosis and Regurgitation

A mitral valve that has both fused commissures and structures that fail to close properly exhibits a mixture of mitral stenosis and regurgitation. Most mixed mitral lesions result from rheumatic heart disease. The course of these mixed lesions depends on which one is predominant. If the degree of stenosis is greater than the degree of incompetence, there is a smaller amount of backflow of blood across the mitral valve during systole and a smaller amount of forward flow of blood across the valve in diastole. If incompetence is greater than stenosis, there is more backflow of blood across the valve in systole and more forward flow of blood across the valve in diastole.[52] The clinical manifestations depend on the degree or obstruction and backflow.

Mitral Valve Prolapse

Mitral valve prolapse, also called floppy mitral valve syndrome, billowing mitral leaflet syndrome, and systolic click-murmur syndrome, is a common condition, occurring in 3% to 8% of adults.[33] It is caused by posterior displacement of the posterior cusp of the mitral valve and is probably a congenital abnormality of the valve tissues in which the large posterior leaflet bulges back into the left atrium during systole. The etiology, hemodynamics, clinical manifestations, and diagnostic tests are summarized in Table 17-13.

Aortic Stenosis

Aortic stenosis involves obstruction to outflow of blood from the left ventricle to the aorta and the obstruction may lie at the level of the valve, above the valve, or below the valve.

Significant narrowing of the valve orifice leads to a decrease in blood flow from the left ventricle to the aorta.

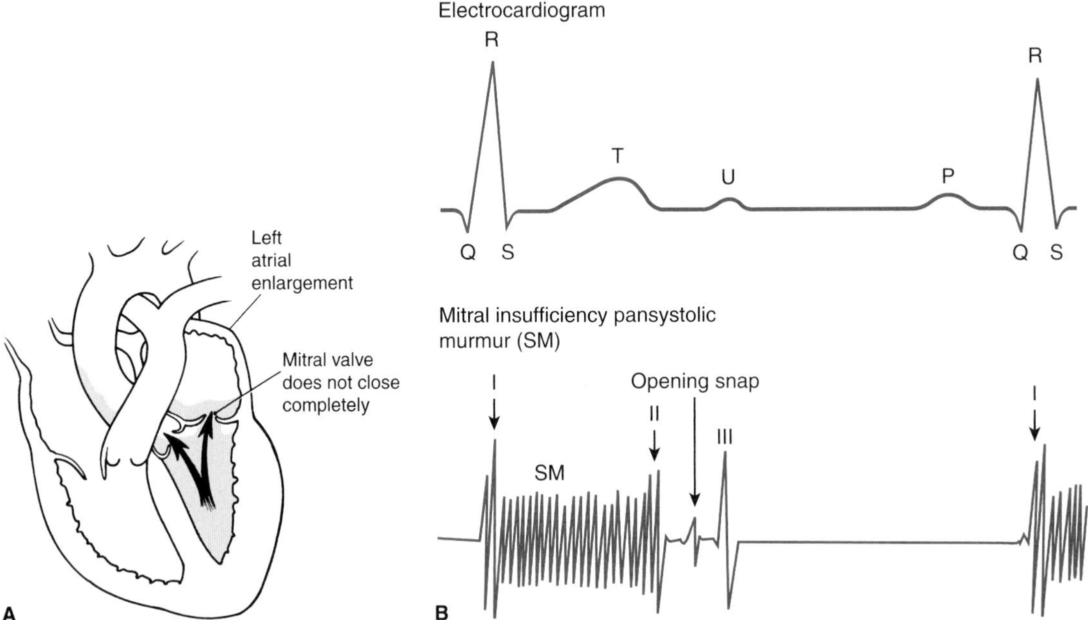

FIGURE 17-23. **A.** Stroke volume in mitral insufficiency is divided into regurgitant and systemic flows. The greater the degree of mitral insufficiency, the more regurgitance there will be. The left atrium gradually dilates unless the onset of insufficiency is sudden when rapid dilatation is seen. **B.** A pansystolic murmur of high intensity is usual with little or no opening snap. The S3 is frequently present.

The obstruction of outflow from the left ventricle leads also to strain or pressure load on the left ventricle that occurs as the left ventricle tries to push blood through the narrowed opening (Fig. 17-24*A*). This resistance to ejection is reflected by an increase in pressure in the left ventricle to force more blood through the stenotic valve during systole. Characteristic heart sounds are illustrated in Figure 17-24*B*. Table 17-13 presents etiology, hemodynamics, clinical manifestations, and diagnostic tests that are useful in understanding aortic stenosis.

Aortic Regurgitation or Insufficiency

Aortic regurgitation is incomplete closure of the aortic valve. It can occur as a chronic or acute lesion. During systole, blood is ejected out of the left ventricle through the aortic valve and into the aorta, but some of it flows back into the ventricle during diastole when the pressure in the aorta exceeds that in the left ventricle. The left ventricle also receives blood from the left atrium during diastole and left ventricular end-diastolic volume increases[35] (Fig. 17-25*A*). Characteristic heart sounds are illustrated in Figure 17-25*B*. Table 17-13 presents etiology, hemodynamics, clinical manifestations, and diagnostic tests that are useful in understanding aortic regurgitation.

Mixed Aortic Stenosis and Regurgitation

When aortic stenosis and regurgitation are both present, the condition is referred to as a mixed lesion. The majority of individuals with aortic valve disease have mixed lesions.[36] Both myocardial hypertrophy and dilatation are present and the clinical features of both conditions may be present. Either stenosis or regurgitation usually predominates over the other hemodynamically.

ALTERATIONS IN LAYERS OF THE HEART

Diseases of any of the three layers of the heart may result from various causes. The most common of these diseases are infective endocarditis, cardiomyopathy, and pericarditis.

Infective Endocarditis

Infective endocarditis affects the lining of the heart and is caused by an invading microorganism. Causative agents include bacteria, fungi, rickettsiae, and, rarely, viruses and parasites. The disease has been described by a variety of terms: (1) subacute bacterial endocarditis (SBE); (2) acute bacterial endocarditis (ABE); (3) prosthetic valve endocarditis; (4) native valve endocarditis; and (5) nonbacterial thrombotic endocarditis.[12] Although considerable overlap among the clinical pictures of endocarditis exists, the terms SBE and ABE have descriptive value in presenting the course of the disease. Table 17-14 compares acute and subacute bacterial endocarditis.

The epidemiology of SBE and ABE includes congenital heart disease, rheumatic fever, mitral valve prolapse, prosthetic valves, bacteremia or sepsis from other types of organisms, intravenous drug abuse, and degenerative changes in the cardiac valves.

PATHOPHYSIOLOGY

The invading organism of SBE is usually of low virulence and the process can develop gradually over weeks or months.[12] The disease usually affects an already damaged heart, such as one with congenital or rheumatic heart disease. The most common causative organism is α-streptococcus or *Streptococcus viridans*.

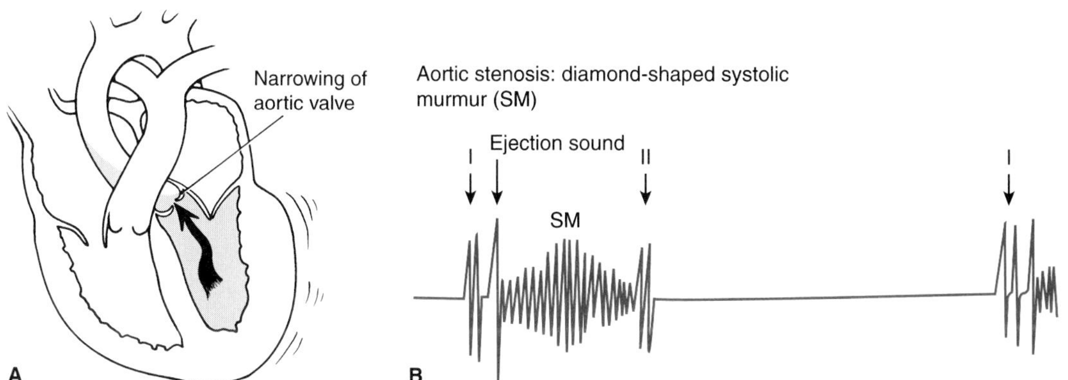

FIGURE 17-24. **A.** View of aortic stenosis during systole. **B.** Murmur for aortic stenosis often includes an ejection sound with a diamond-shaped murmur (crescendo-descrescendo sound) of high frequency.

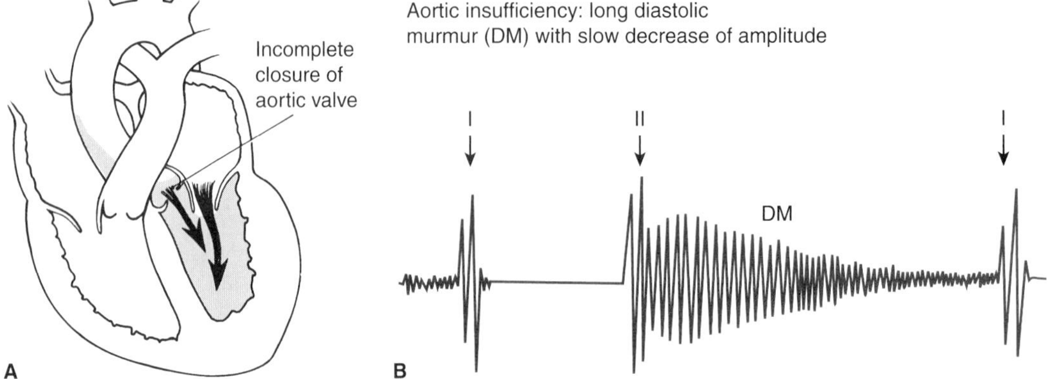

FIGURE 17-25. **A.** View of aortic insufficiency during early ventricular diastole. **B.** Murmur of mild aortic insufficiency includes a long diastolic murmur of decreasing amplitude of high frequency.

Acute bacterial endocarditis often occurs in persons with normal hearts but can affect those who have damaged hearts. Because the organism is of high virulence, the process usually progresses very rapidly and causes significant valvular damage. The most common causative organism is *Staphylococcus aureus.* The tricuspid or pulmonary valves are affected in over 50% of cases of ABE in intravenous (IV) drug abusers but the aortic and mitral valves may also be affected.

The organisms traveling in the bloodstream attach to the endocardial lining of a normal heart or to the area of defect of an abnormal heart.[4] After attaching themselves, the organisms become enmeshed in deposits of fibrin and platelets, with vegetations occurring on the leaflets of the valves.[4,7] These vegetations vary in size, shape, and color and may become quite friable depending on the invading organisms[41] (Fig. 17-26). ABE often produces large friable vegetations that embolize and produce embolic abscesses; SBE produces smaller vegetations that also embolize and lodge in the microcirculation and spleen. The vegetations produced by the infectious process settle on the cardiac valves and invade the leaflets. These vegetations prevent normal alignment of the cusps and may, therefore, cause incomplete closure or regurgitation, leading to cardiac murmurs. The murmurs produced correspond to the affected valve.

If the vegetations grow and infiltrate the downstream side of the valve, small fragments may break off as blood is pushed through the valve orifice. These fragments from left heart valves may embolize to the cerebral and systemic circulations. If they embolize from the valves on the right side of the heart, pulmonary emboli result.

TABLE 17-14

COMPARISON OF ACUTE AND SUBACUTE BACTERIAL ENDOCARDITIS

CHARACTERISTIC	ACUTE	SUBACUTE
Duration of clinical symptoms	< 6wk	> 6wk
Causative organisms	*Staphylococcus aureus,* β-streptococci	α-streptococci
Virulence of organism	Highly virulent	Less virulent
Condition of valves	Previously normal Valve perforations common	Previously damaged Valve perforations rare
Population affected (Persons with)	Drug abusers Prosthetic valves Septic conditions	Congenital heart conditions Prosthetic valves Rheumatic heart disease

(Adapted from E. Rubin, E., & Farber, J. L. [1999]. *Pathology* [3rd ed.]. Philadelphia: Lippincott-Raven.)

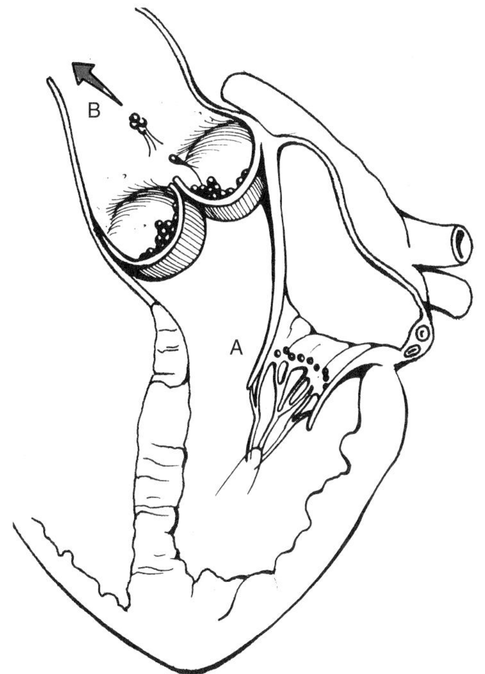

FIGURE 17-26. **A.** Subacute bacterial endocarditis usually localizes on an already diseased or damaged valve. Small vegetations may embolize into the arterial circuit if they form on the mitral or aortic valves. **B.** Acute bacterial endocarditis produces large friable vegetations on a normal valve.

CLINICAL MANIFESTATIONS

The clinical manifestations of infective endocarditis include fever, hematuria, splenomegaly, petechiae, Osler's nodes, and anemia. Cardiac murmurs are common. The fever and its related symptomatology depend on the type of infection.

With ABE, the fever has a rapid onset with spikes to high elevations that are accompanied by shaking chills.[12] In SBE, the fever is usually low grade, intermittent with elevations, and without chills. In addition, complaints of weakness, fatigue, night sweats, anorexia, and arthralgias, and exhibition of splenomegaly are common.

In both types of infective endocarditis, there may be *Osler's nodes*, which are painful, tender, red, subcutaneous nodules in the pads of the fingers; *Janeway's lesions*, which are flat, small, irregular, nontender, red spots on the palms and soles; and *Roth's spots*, which are retinal hemorrhages that have a white or yellow center surrounded by a red, irregular halo.[7,12]

The diagnosis of infective endocarditis is based on positive blood cultures, which are present in the majority of cases. The positive blood cultures and the cardiac valvular disruption confirm the diagnosis. Also, a normocytic, normochromic anemia and an elevated sedimentation rate may be noted. Many cases of SBE are probably not diagnosed at the time of infection. If ABE is not treated, the clinical course is rapid and often fatal. The prognosis depends on the offending organism and the stage at which it is treated.[35] Table 17-15 summarizes the major clinical manifestations of bacterial endocarditis.

Diseases of the Myocardium

The term cardiomyopathy refers to a group of myocardial diseases that primarily affect the heart's pumping ability but are not due to disease or dysfunction of other cardiac structures (eg, valves, CAD).[25] *Primary or idiopathic myocardial disease* refers to conditions affecting the ventricular muscle that have an unknown origin. *Secondary cardiomyopathy* designates conditions in which the causative factors are known. The cardiomyopathies have been classified as congestive, restrictive, and hyper-trophic. *Myocarditis* is a term used for inflammation of the myocardium, which may be due to infection, chemical agents, or hypersensitivity responses.

CONGESTIVE OR DILATED CARDIOMYOPATHY

Congestive or dilated cardiomyopathy, also called *idiopathic dilated cardiomyopathy*, is usually of unknown etiology but may be associated with ischemic cardiac disease, beriberi, thyrotoxicosis, alcoholism, childbirth or the postpartum period, diabetes mellitus, drug toxicity (especially from daunorubicin), cobalt therapy, and certain neuromuscular disorders (Box 17-4). This type of cardiomyopathy is the most common of the various forms and the incidence appears to be increasing worldwide.[3] The striking effect of congestive cardiomyopathy is immense cardiomegaly with the activation of compensatory mechanisms leading to remodeling of the ventricular shape, which leads to further myocardial dysfunction.[3] The enlargement is a combination of dilatation and hypertrophy of the heart (Fig. 17-27) that leads to a hypokinetic myocardium with the usual onset of biventricular CHF.[3]

Symptoms include exertional dyspnea, fatigue, paroxysmal nocturnal dyspnea, and pulmonary edema with symptoms of RHF late in the disease's course. Atrial and ventricular gallops may be noted on auscultation. Peripheral edema and hepatomegaly are signs of RHF. The prognosis depends on the underlying cause, with ischemic cardiomyopathy exhibiting a poorer prognosis than nonischemic forms.[3]

TABLE 17-15

SUMMARY OF THE MAJOR CLINICAL MANIFESTATIONS OF INFECTIVE ENDOCARDITIS

MANIFESTATION	HISTORY	EXAMINATION	INVESTIGATIONS
Systemic infection	Fever, chills, rigors, sweats, malaise, weakness, lethargy, delirium, headache, anorexia, weight loss, backache, arthralgia, myalgia Portal of entry: oropharynx, skin, urinary tract, drug addiction, nosocomial bacteremia	Fever, pallor, weight loss, asthenia, splenomegaly	Anemia, leukocytosis (variable), raised erythrocyte sedimentation rate, blood culture, results positive, abnormal cerebrospinal fluid
Intravascular lesion	Dyspnea, chest pain, focal weakness, stroke, abdominal pain, cold and painful extremities	Murmurs, signs of cardiac failure, petechiae (skin, eye, mucosae), Roth's spots, Osler's nodes, Janeway lesions, splinter hemorrhages, stroke, mycotic aneurysm, ischemia or infarction of viscera or extremities	Blood in urine, chest roentgenogram, echocardiography, arteriography, liver-spleen scan, lung scan, brain scan, CT scan, histology, culture of emboli
Immunologic reactions	Arthralgia, myalgia, tenosynovitis	Arthritis, signs of uremia, vascular phenomena, finger clubbing	Proteinuria, hematuria, casts, uremia, acidosis, polyclonal increases in gamma globulins, rheumatoid factor, decreased complement, immune complexes in serum, antistaphylococcal teichoic acid antibodies

CT: computed tomography.
(From Alexander, R. W., Schlant, R. C., & Fuster, V. [Eds.] [1998]. *Hurst's the heart* [9th ed.]. New York: McGraw-Hill.)

CAUSES OF DILATED CARDIOMYOPATHY

- Ischemic cardiomyopathy
- Valvular disease
- Idiopathic cardiomyopathy (often familial)
- Toxic cardiomyopathy (including alcohol, chemotherapeutic agents, cocaine, lead, carbon monoxide, other drugs)
- Infections (including viral, bacterial, fungal)
- Systemic disorders (eg, systemic lupus erythematosis, scleroderma, sarcoidosis)
- Postpartum cardiomyopathy
- Metabolic abnormalities (including nutritional, endocrine, electrolyte abnormalities)
- Other rare causes (eg, Duchenne muscular dystrophy, myotonic dystrophy, Friedreich's ataxia)

RESTRICTIVE CARDIOMYOPATHY

Restrictive cardiomyopathy describes the clinical picture of constrictive pericarditis, the underlying cause of which is actually myocardial.[45] The etiology is generally unknown, but it has been described in association with such diverse conditions as amyloidosis, hemosiderosis, and glycogen storage disease. In the systemic myocardial disorders, abnormal substances infiltrate the myocardial muscle apparently causing dysfunction of the ventricle. In the idiopathic form extensive fibrosis is evident but no pathologic substrate can be identified.[45] Symptoms of biventricular failure are common. Ventricular filling is impeded and the end-diastolic pressure of the ventricles usually becomes exceedingly high. The prognosis for survival is poor and death often results from CHF. Congestive and restrictive cardiomyopathies are mostly differentiated on the basis of the presence or absence of cardiomegaly.

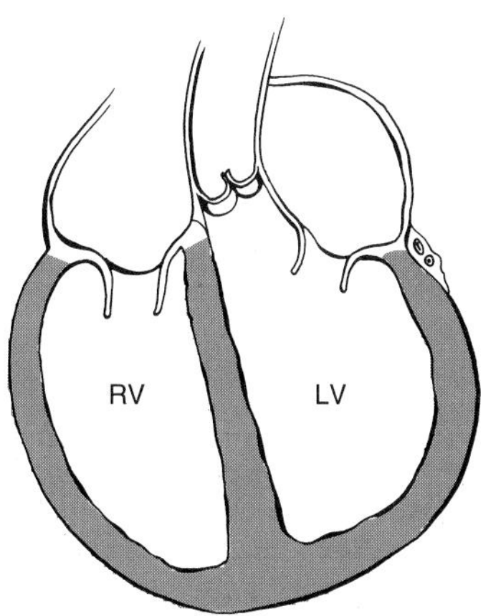
Biventricular dilatation leads to hypokinetic heart with marked decrease in cardiac output and congestive heart failure. May have "usual" associated mitral or tricuspid insufficiency.
RV
LV

FIGURE 17-27. **Congestive or dilated cardiomyopathy.**

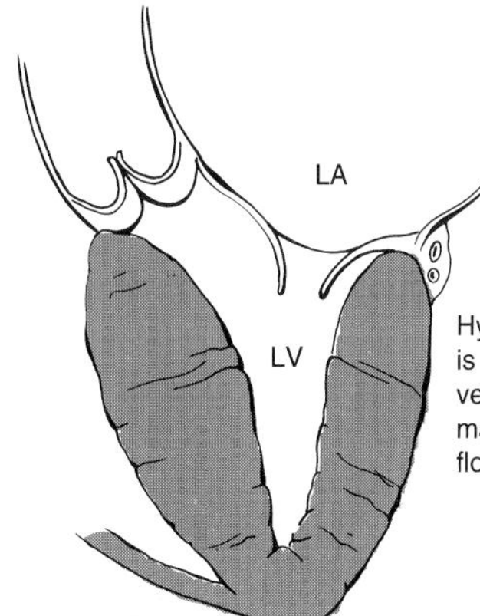
LA
LV
Hypertrophic cardiomyopathy is an asymmetric increase in ventricular muscle mass that may cause obstruction to blood flow during ventricular contraction.

FIGURE 17-28. **Hypertrophic cardiomyopathy.**

HYPERTROPHIC CARDIOMYOPATHY

Hypertrophic cardiomyopathy usually refers to an asymmetrical increase in ventricular muscle mass. It has received many labels, including *idiopathic hypertrophic subaortic stenosis* and *hypertrophic obstructive cardiomyopathy*.[23]

The etiology of this condition is unknown. Familial occurrence is noted with no predominance for either sex. Certain studies support a mutation in protein synthesis in the genes that encode for the myocardial sarcomere.[23]

Pathologic features include an asymmetrical hypertrophy of the left ventricular myocardium with usually greater hypertrophy in the ventricular septum than in other ventricular areas.[23] Small or normal ventricular chamber size and disorganization of myocardial muscle cells, especially of the myofibrils, may occur. Because of the septal hypertrophy, the left ventricular cavity is misshapen and, on contraction, the hypertrophied septum may cause obstruction to the flow of blood from the ventricle (Fig. 17-28). Any condition that enhances contractility increases the degree of obstruction. The associated left ventricular hypertrophy causes impairment of ventricular filling during diastole and reduced ventricular compliance. The heart often shows enlargement of the atria, fibrosis in the left ventricular wall, and enlargement of the leaflets of the mitral valve.[23]

The clinical manifestations vary and may be due to (1) left ventricular outflow obstruction, (2) diastolic dysfunction, (3) myocardial ischemia, and (4) dysrhythmias.[23] These dysfunctions may cause symptoms of LHF, including exertional dyspnea, angina, periods of syncope, and orthopnea. Obstruction of ventricular outflow is more severe under stress and may be reduced or abolished with β-blocking drugs. The diastolic dysfunction results from abnormalities in relaxation and filling that cause a prolongation in the rapid filling phase of diastole. Myocardial ischemia is indicated by the ECG changes of decreased blood flow. Various forms of rhythm alterations may result and are related to myocardial ischemia or conduction system effects or both. Sudden cardiac death may occur during or just after vigorous physical activity, notably in young athletes with no reported prior symptoms.[23] The prognosis is variable due to the complexity of the disease expression with some individuals exhibiting no symptoms throughout life while others progress to end-stage heart failure.[23]

MYOCARDITIS

Inflammation of the myocardium may result from an infectious process, chemical agents such as chemotherapeutic drugs, or hypersensitivity responses. Viruses, especially the coxsackieviruses, bacteria, protozoa, metazoa, and fungal infections have all been implicated in its causation. Myocarditis is often a self-limiting condition that is manifested by tachycardia, symptoms of heart failure, and gallop rhythm on auscultation. Flulike symptoms occur in approximately 60% of persons diagnosed with myocarditis usually before the onset of the cardiac symptoms.[31] Many types of myocarditis resolve with bed rest, fluid restriction, and limited drug therapy. In a small percentage of affected persons, the disease is progressive and leads to all of the manifestations of dilated, congestive myocardiopathy.

Pericarditis

Pericarditis is an inflammation of the pericardium that may be secondary to many conditions including open heart surgery (the leading cause), MI, viral or bacterial infections, anticoagulants, or trauma.[44] Generalized conditions such as uremia, systemic lupus erythematosus, rheumatoid arthritis, or malignancies such as lung or breast cancer or lymphoma also may involve the pericardium.

ACUTE PERICARDITIS

In acute pericarditis, serous, serofibrinous, or purulent exudates form on the epicardial and pericardial surfaces.[7] The nature of the exudates depends on the underlying cause. The volume of the exudates also varies. Small volumes usually do not encroach on cardiac function but larger volumes restrict cardiac input and produce a cardiac tamponade (see p. 473).

Clinical Manifestations

Some of the clinical features of acute pericarditis include fever, pain, pericardial friction rub, ECG changes, pericardial effusion with cardiac tamponade, and a paradoxic pulse.

Individuals may describe the pain as severe, sharp, and aching. It is usually precordial or substernal, and it may radiate to the left or right shoulder, arms, and elbows. On occasion, pain may spread to the jaw, throat, and ears. Deep breathing, sneezing, coughing, moving, or changing position may intensify the pain. The pain may be relieved when the person sits up and leans forward. Acute pericarditis is often confused with the pain of myocardial ischemia, which may lead to misdiagnosis.[6]

In addition to pain, one of the most important physical signs of pericarditis is a *friction rub* that is heard best at the apex and at the lower left sternal border. It is an intermittent, transitory sound that imitates the sound of sandpaper rubbing together. This loud, "to and fro," leathery sound may disappear on one day and reappear on the next.

Acute pericarditis can produce the following changes on ECG: (1) ST elevation in two or three standard limb leads and precordial leads V_2 through V_6; (2) reciprocal depressions occur in AVR and V_1; (3) low R-wave voltage is characteristic without Q waves; and (4) following the acute stage, the ST segments return to normal and T waves invert.[44]

Pericardial Effusion

Pericardial effusion refers to a collection of noninflammatory fluid that accumulates in the pericardial sac. This fluid may be serous, serosanguineous, chylous, or, rarely, of other compositions, such as cholesterol.[6] *Serous effusions* are seen in CHF and in hypoproteinemia, such as that due to liver failure. *Serosanguineous effusions* result from blunt chest trauma, especially postcardiopulmonary resuscitation. Chylous effusions contain lipid droplets, being seen especially with conditions causing lymphatic obstruction. Hemopericardium refers to accumulation of blood in the pericardial sac.

Purulent pericarditis with pus or inflammatory exudate is not considered to be an effusion but large volumes of bacterial, mycotic, or parasite-laden fluid can accumulate and produce a reddened, granular, inflammatory reaction. If the fluid accumulates rapidly, it can cause cardiac compression.

With pericardial effusion, the heart sounds are faint and the apical impulse may disappear. The chest film shows enlargement of the cardiac silhouette. The heart may appear as a "water bottle" configuration. The echocardiogram detects the presence of pericardial fluid.

When fluid accumulates rapidly or in an amount large enough to impair cardiac function, the condition is referred to as *cardiac tamponade* (see Fig. 17-12). The amount of fluid that can cause tamponade varies according to the rate of fluid accumulation. In rapid accumulation of fluid, 250 mL may produce significant obstruction. When an effusion develops slowly, 1,000 mL or more may accumulate before significant symptoms develop. As fluid collects in the pericardial sac, the pressure rises in the pericardial cavity to a level equal to the pressures in the heart during diastole. The first structures to be compressed are the right atrium and ventricle because they have the lowest diastolic pressures. This compression causes increased venous pressure with decreased right atrial filling. Jugular venous distention and systemic venous congestion with edema and hepatomegaly result. There is also a decrease in diastolic filling of the ventricles, which leads to decreases in stroke volume and cardiac output. A characteristic sign of cardiac tamponade is **pulsus paradoxus**. This is a large inspiratory reduction in arterial pressure that can be heard with a stethoscope. In pulsus paradoxus, the systolic blood pressure drops more than 10 mm Hg during inspiration. If the tamponade is severe, pulsus paradoxus may be palpated as a weakness or disappearance in the arterial pressure during inspiration.

CHRONIC CONSTRICTIVE PERICARDITIS

Chronic constrictive pericarditis results from the healing of acute pericarditis and formation of granular tissue that gradually contracts to form a firm scar surrounding the heart. This scar causes constriction of the heart and, therefore, interferes with filling of the ventricles. This complication is similar to the physiologic abnormality that results from pericardial effusion except that it develops slowly over weeks to months.

Clinical manifestations of chronic constrictive pericarditis are weakness, fatigue, weight loss, anorexia, and edema. Individuals may complain of abdominal discomfort due to systemic venous congestion. This discomfort is due to hepatic congestion and swelling of the abdomen. A characteristic sign of constrictive pericarditis is jugular neck vein distention, which is indicative of elevated venous pressure.

The echocardiogram may show pericardial thickening and paradoxic septal motion in constrictive pericarditis. Also noted on the echocardiogram is that the left ventricular wall moves distinctly outward in early diastole, after which there is little or no change.[11,44] The chest film may be diagnostic when calcification appears in the pericardium.

CONGENITAL CARDIOVASCULAR DISEASE

Congenital cardiovascular disease is an abnormality of structure or function of the heart, circulatory system, or both usually resulting from an alteration in or failure of development. The condition may cause a cardiovascular shunting defect, which refers to blood flow through an abnormal communication between the heart chambers or between the pulmonary and systemic circulations. It may also cause an obstructive defect that results in increased intraventricular or intra-atrial pressures.

The frequency of congenital cardiovascular malformations is difficult to determine because many are asymptomatic and not diagnosed in infancy. A bicuspid aortic valve and mitral valve prolapse are common asymptomatic congenital defects. Researchers estimate that a cardiovascular malformation complicates about 8/1,000 live births.[15]

The causes of congenital heart disease vary and appear to result from multifactorial interactions between genetic and environmental systems. A specific causative factor usually cannot be identified. Some environmental insults include viral infection (especially rubella) in the first 8 weeks of pregnancy and maternal drug and alcohol abuse. Hereditary factors may be involved in such conditions as atrial septal defect (ASD), patent ductus arteriosus (PDA), and coarctation of the aorta. Evidence has shown that a significant number of defects may be produced by single-gene defects and that the same defect may be produced by mutant genes at different loci[21] (see p. 56). Some lesions are more prevalent in females, some in males, and some have equal frequencies. Extracardiac anomalies occur in approximately 25% of infants with significant cardiac anomalies.[15] Preterm infants often have persistence of the ductus arteriosus, a structure that normally closes at birth. Stillborn infants have a very high frequency of complex cardiac anomalies.

Abnormalities of the formation of the heart or great vessels causes pathophysiologic problems that affect the blood flow to the lungs or the body. Alterations to the oxygenation of the blood also may occur. These alterations often lead to heart failure in the infant or adult, depending on the nature of the congenital defect.

Embryology of the Heart

Cardiovascular embryology involves the development of the heart and vasculature at specific times in fetal development. Understanding congenital heart defects requires a basic understanding of when and how these structures develop.

DEVELOPMENT OF THE HEART

The heart begins to develop in the embryo from day 18 and is complete by day 56.[21] A *primitive straight cardiac tube* composed of an outer myocardium and an inner endocardium loops to form a primitive atrium and ventricle, followed rapidly by a large *truncus arteriosus*. The tube doubles over on itself during the second month of gestation to form *two parallel pumping systems*, each having two chambers and a great artery (the truncus arteriosus). As a consequence of this doubling, the heart begins to situate in the left side of the chest. An endocardial cushion develops within the common chamber and is the first of the structures to divide the chambers of the heart. From the endocardial cushion, the mitral and tricuspid orifices develop (Fig. 17-29). The large truncus divides into the *aorta* and *pulmonary arteries*. Rotation of the truncus coils the aortopulmonary septum and creates the normal spiral relationship between the aorta and pulmonary artery. The truncus arteriosus is connected to the dorsal aorta by six pairs of *aortic arches* that appear and disappear at different times during the formation of the heart and vessels. Abnormalities of the regression of the arch system in a number of sites can produce a wide variety of arch abnormalities. Partitioning of the heart is accomplished by *septa* that form actively and passively. The major septa of the heart are formed between the 27th and 37th days of development.[21]

FETAL CIRCULATION

In addition to formation of heart and vessel structures, changes occur in the fetal circulation that will enable the newborn to survive in the extrauterine environment. During fetal growth, the placenta performs the duties of respiration, excretion, and nourishment for the fetus. The three essential structures are the *ductus venosus*, a vessel that connects the umbilical vein to the inferior vena cava; the *foramen ovale*, an opening in the interatrial septum; and the *ductus arteriosus*, a vessel that joins the main pulmonary artery and the distal aortic arch.

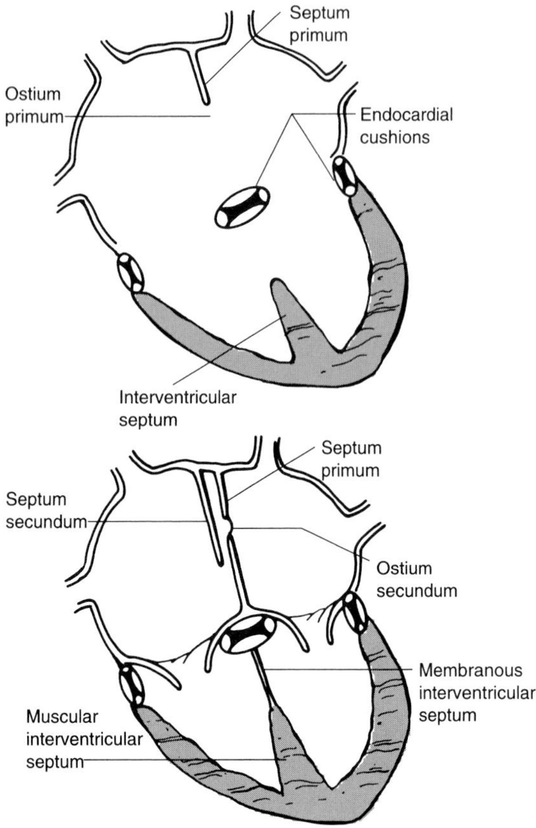

FIGURE 17-29. **Schematic appearance of the process of formation of septi and valves in early cardiac development.**

During fetal life, blood passes from the placenta along the umbilical vein through the ductus venosus and into the inferior vena cava, where it is mixed with venous return from the lower extremities. It enters the right atrium and is mainly channeled through the foramen ovale, a one-way valve, into the left atrium where it is channeled to the rest of the body to provide oxygen and nutrients to all of the tissues. Blood flow from the head and upper extremities returns to the superior vena cava, is channeled into the right ventricle, and is pumped out the pulmonary artery. Because of the nonfunctioning, nonexpanded lungs, the resistance to blood flow into the lungs is higher and blood shunts through the ductus arteriosus into the descending aorta (Fig. 17-30). Because of the resistance of the lungs, the pressures in the right ventricle and those in the right atrium are elevated, causing a right-to-left shunt of blood across the foramen ovale into the left atrium.

CHANGES AT BIRTH

Birth changes are as follows: the newborn cries and expands its lungs, the resistance in the pulmonary circulation decreases, and the pressure lowers in the right side of the heart. With dilatation of the pulmonary vessels and lowered pulmonary arterial pressure, the flow is diminished through the ductus arteriosus and it gradually closes, usually becoming a thin ligament-like structure within 6 to 8 weeks after birth. Clamping the umbilical cord leads to clotting of blood in the umbilical vein and ductus venosus; the latter occludes within 1 to 5 days to become a ligament also. The increased systemic resistance created with clamping of the umbilical arteries is transmitted to the left atrium. This, in conjunction with increased venous return from the lungs, causes the pressure in that chamber to exceed right atrial pressure, thus tending to create a left-to-right flow through the foramen ovale. The foramen ovale acts as a one-way valve, and the tendency toward reversal of flow causes the flap of the valve to close. Closure is followed by gradual, permanent obliteration of the opening by fibrous adherence of the flap to the interatrial septum within 6 to 8 months.

Shunts

Because blood flows along the path of least resistance from higher to lower pressures, most congenital defects having an abnormal communication between chambers or vessels end up with a *left-to-right shunt.* A portion of blood returned to the left heart is diverted back into the pulmonary circuit before it can reach the systemic capillaries. This often causes increased volume in the right heart and subsequently, in the pulmonary circuit. Most ASDs and ventricular septal defects (VSDs) as well as PDA result in a left-to-right shunt. The result is pulmonary overloading and eventually, pulmonary hypertension and congestion.

Pulmonary hypertension results from increased pressures in the pulmonary vascular bed usually produced by a large left-to-right shunt. The pulmonary vasculature begins to undergo changes that eventually destroy the ability of the pulmonary arterioles to deliver blood to the pulmonary capillaries.[15] The amount of pulmonary resistance can be estimated from data obtained at cardiac catheterization. Significant pulmonary hypertension may indicate permanent damage and a poor prognosis. The systemic circulation also may become impaired if the shunt is large. The result may be right ventricular failure due to the continual volume and pressure that the right ventricle is required to pump.

Right-to-left shunts occur when desaturated, systemic, venous blood is diverted to the left side of the heart without passing through the capillaries of the lungs. For this condition to occur, there must be a communication from the right heart to the left heart,

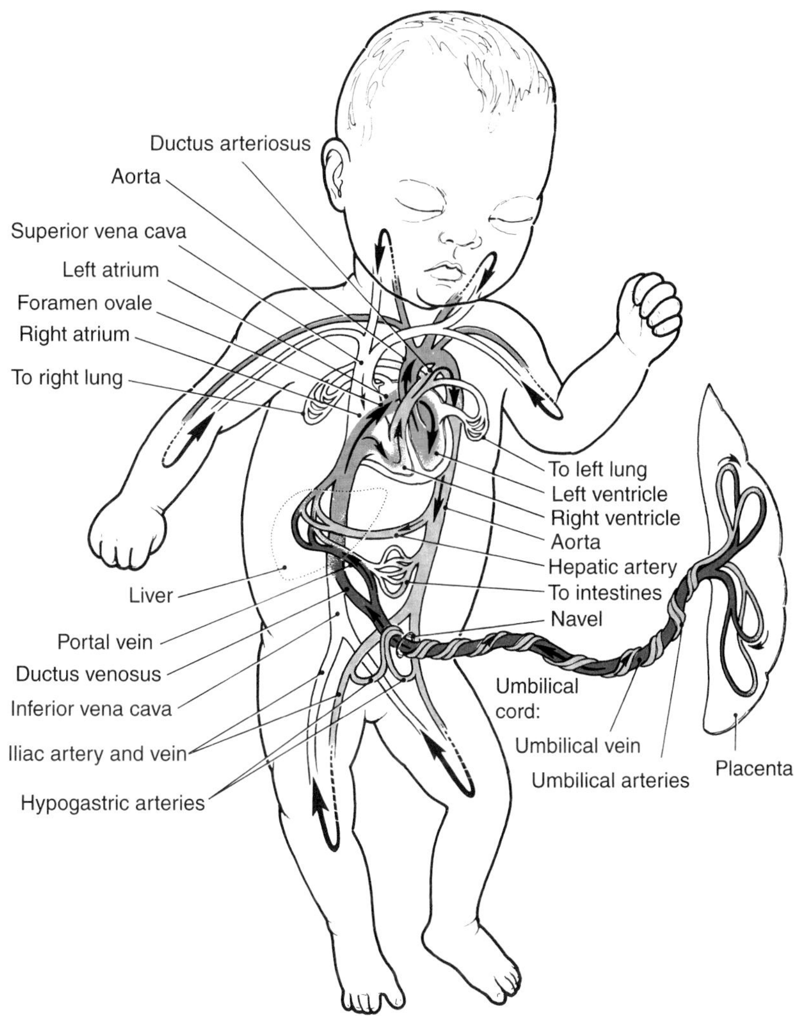

FIGURE 17-30. **Diagrammatic illustration of fetal circulation. Arrows show the direction of blood flow.**

and the pressures in the right heart must exceed those of the left. The common signs and symptoms include cyanosis, polycythemia, clubbing, squatting, and failure to thrive. When cyanosis is present, the shunt is large, with about one-third of the arterial hemoglobin being unsaturated. Polycythemia is the normal reaction of the body to the lack of oxygen. The kidneys release erythropoietin, which stimulates the release of more red blood cells. The increased numbers of erythrocytes increase blood viscosity. Clubbing also occurs with long-term polycythemia and cyanosis. The ends of the phalanges become bulbous and the nails curved (Fig. 17-31). The cause of clubbing may be dilatation and engorgement of the local capillaries in an attempt to gain oxygen. The condition is usually seen in children who may assume a squatting position, which may be a way of centralizing the available oxygen. Failure to thrive and growth retardation may be related to tissue hypoxia and poor nutrient absorption.

Congestive Heart Failure

One child in five with any type of congenital heart defect will develop CHF.[13] It often develops early in life in the severe defects with significant shunting. In small ASDs or VSDs, CHF, if seen, develops after years of pulmonary hypertension from the left-to-right shunt. In infants, CHF may be fulminant or insidious and may be associated with respiratory tract infections. It is manifested by difficulty breathing and rapid grunting respirations.[15] Symptoms of right heart failure are less common and usually seen in association with pulmonary hypertension or cyanosis.

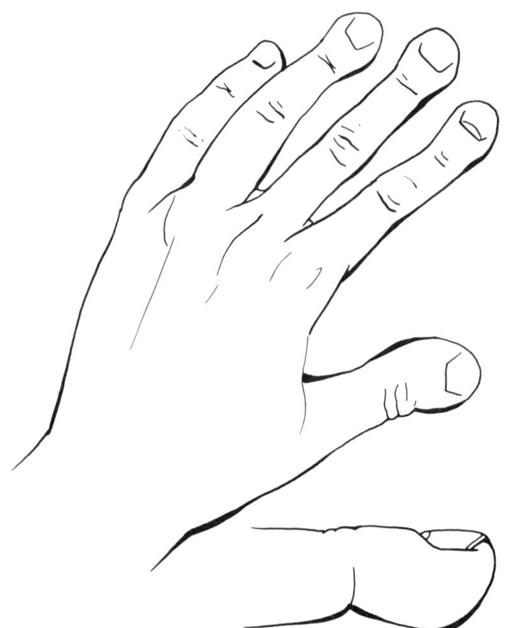

FIGURE 17-31. Clubbing of the fingers from chronic hypoxemia.

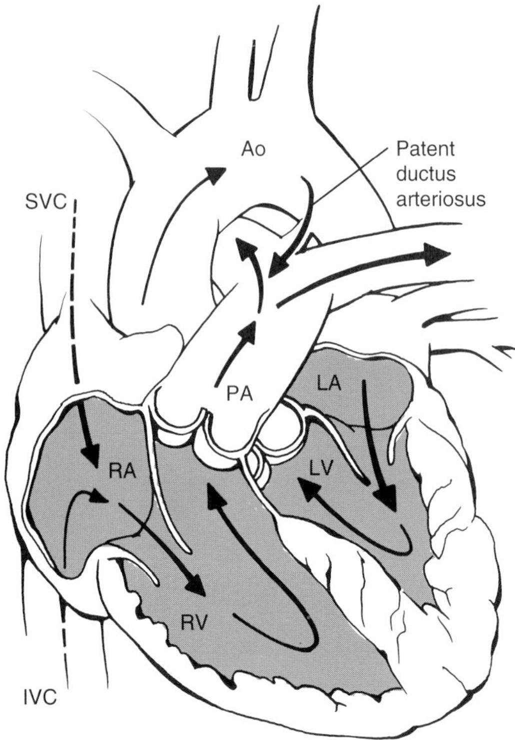

FIGURE 17-32. Blood flow in patent ductus arteriosus.

Common Congenital Cardiovascular Defects

Although multiple defects can occur during gestation, several defects are more common than others. These defects can cause shunting, obstruction to blood flow, and heart failure.

PATENT DUCTUS ARTERIOSUS

When the embryonic ductus arteriosus fails to close after birth, it persists as a shunt between the pulmonary artery and the aorta (Fig. 17-32). It often occurs as an isolated defect and is the second most common congenital defect in infants and children.[13] The patent ductus often does not manifest in the early postnatal days, but within about 2 weeks the blood flow through the ductus from the aorta to the pulmonary artery first produces a systolic and then a continuous machinery-like murmur, indicating a constant flow of blood through the shunt. The result of this condition is increased volume and pressure in the pulmonary system, basically short-circuiting one-fourth to three-fourths of left ventricular output. The signs and symptoms depend on the volume of the shunt; often the child is asymptomatic. The condition is usually discovered on routine physical examination when the murmur is detected. Other symptoms include pulmonary congestion and manifestations of heart failure.

ATRIAL SEPTAL DEFECTS

Congenital ASDs are very common and result from failure of the atrial septum to close. There are various forms: *ostium primum, persistent atrioventricular communis*, and *ostium secundum*. Figure 17-33 shows the location of the common types of ASDs.

Clinical manifestations depend on the size of the defect and the volume of shunted blood. The majority of ASDs are asymptomatic but right ventricular hypertrophy, frequent respiratory infections, feeding difficulties, dyspnea, fatigability, and growth retardation may develop with larger defects.

VENTRICULAR SEPTAL DEFECTS

Considered to be the most common congenital heart lesions, VSDs account for 8% to 20% of congenital heart disease. During fetal development, the ventricular septum grows in a cephalad (headward) fashion and fuses at the endocardial cushion. It begins as a muscular septum with a membranous portion at the point of closure.[21] The shunt of blood in a VSD is almost always left-to-right from the high pressure in the left ventricle to the lower pressure in the right ventricle (Fig. 17-34). The shunt produces a holosystolic murmur of a high grade, often creating a palpable

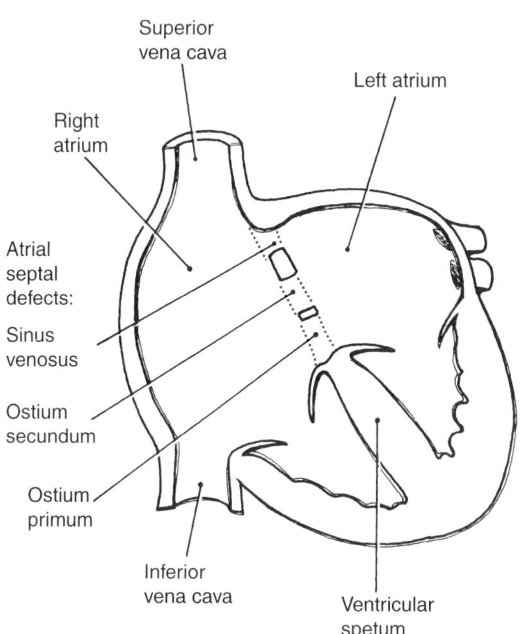

FIGURE 17-33. **Location of the common types of atrial septal defects.**

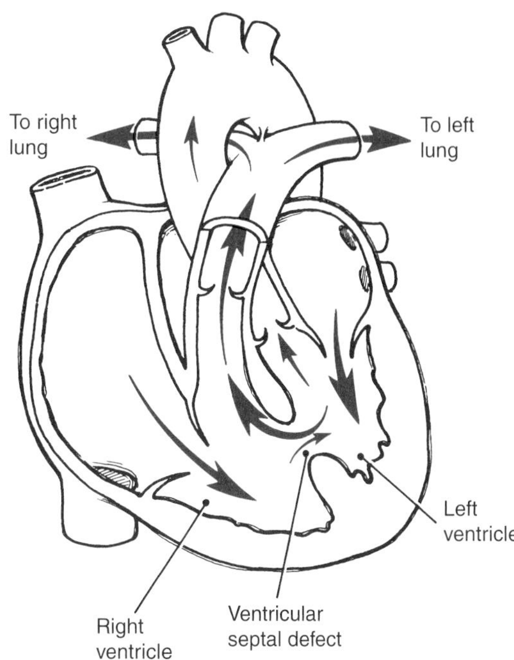

FIGURE 17-34. **Blood flow in ventricular septal defect.**

thrill on the chest wall. In a large shunt, there is significant overloading of the right ventricle and pulmonary circulation. In the small defect, the shunt of blood is much smaller and may be occluded during part of ventricular systole by the contraction of the muscular septum.

Clinical manifestations of VSDs depend on the amount of pulmonary overloading and right ventricular strain. In some cases (as many as 10–30%), the defect apparently closes spontaneously and a preexisting murmur then disappears.[15] Pulmonary hypertension and right ventricular failure are signs of poor prognosis and the defect may progress to a cyanotic condition if the right ventricular pressures become high enough to reverse the shunt to right-to-left.

The term Eisenmenger's syndrome is used to describe pulmonary hypertension that results in a reversed shunt. It accounts for about 7% of adult congenital heart disease more commonly in women than in men.[10] It can be seen in any of the defects where there is a reversal of shunt to a bidirectional or right to left shunt but it most commonly is seen with VSD.[10]

TETRALOGY OF FALLOT

This condition was first described by Fallot in 1888. It is the primary cause of cyanotic heart disease and is more common in boys than girls. It involves the combination of pulmonary stenosis, VSD, dextroposition of the aortic root, and **hypertrophy** of the right ventricle (Fig. 17-35). The degree of pulmonary stenosis is responsible for the volume and direction of the shunt. It increases right ventricular pressure, causing shunting of blood from the right ventricle to the left through the VSD. Pulmonary stenosis also decreases pulmonary blood flow and the available blood for oxygenation. Direct pumping of blood to the aorta from the right ventricle causes direct access of venous blood to the systemic circulation.

Clinical manifestations include cyanosis, clubbing, hypoxia, polycythemia, and susceptibility to infections. *Cyanosis* may be severe and deepens during exertion, pulmonary infection, and dyspnea. *Clubbing* of the fingers also depends on the degree of cyanosis. The *oxygen saturation* in the arterial system may be 80% (normal, 95–98%) or lower, while venous oxygen saturation may be below 60% (normal, 75–80%). *Polycythemia* is compensatory and causes increased blood volume and elevated hematocrit. *Dizziness and convulsions* may be caused by periods of cerebral anoxia. *Squatting* is often a habitual response that may relieve the dizziness by supplying more blood to the brain. *Stunting of growth* from the continual hypoxia is characteristic when there is severe cyanosis. Complications of the condition include pulmonary infections, heart failure, cerebral embolism, subacute bacterial endocarditis, and brain damage from hypoxia.

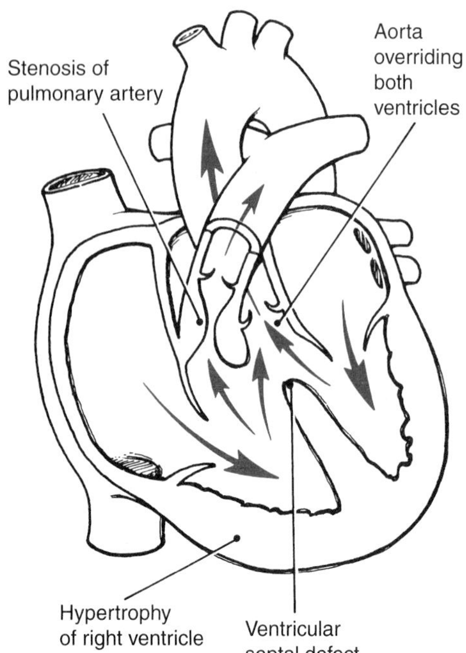

FIGURE 17-35. **Blood flow in tetralogy of Fallot.**

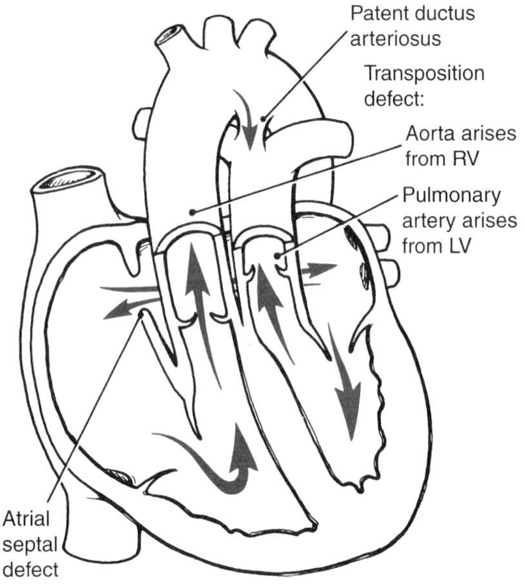

FIGURE 17-36. **Blood flow in transposition of the great vessels.**

TRANSPOSITION OF THE GREAT VESSELS

In the fourth week of gestation, the common truncus arteriosus is divided into the pulmonary artery and the aorta. The two vessels rotate so that the pulmonary artery lies anterior and in the right ventricle and the aorta arises posterior and in the left ventricle, thus providing for normal blood flow. In transposition, this rotation does not occur and the aorta arises anteriorly from the right ventricle and the pulmonary artery arises posteriorly from the left ventricle. Blood is pumped from the right ventricle through the aorta to the systemic system, and returns through the cavae to the right atrium. Blood from the left ventricle passes through the pulmonary artery to the lungs and returns through the pulmonary veins to the left atrium (Fig. 17-36). These two closed circuits are obviously incompatible with life.

Other defects usually associated with this condition include ASDs, VSDs, and enlarged bronchial arteries to carry blood from the aorta to the lungs. In some cases, the ductus arteriosus remains patent and the foramen ovale remains open due to the increase in right atrial pressure.

The clinical manifestations depend on the amount of intermixing of blood from the associated life-sustaining defects. *Cyanosis* may be severe or minimal to absent; it is intensified with exertion. *Dyspnea* is common, and *CHF* frequently occurs in early infancy. Death within the first year is common.

COARCTATION OF THE AORTA

The aortic arch develops between the fifth and seventh weeks of gestation.[21] The area of the aorta near the ductus arteriosus may develop improperly, leaving a restricted lumen proximal to, at, or distal to the insertion of the ductus.[15] Postductal coarctation obstructs blood flow beyond the left subclavian artery so the blood pressure in the upper extremities is much higher than in the lower extremities (Fig. 17-37). No cyanosis is evident because the ductus closes at birth.

The clinical manifestations result from high blood pressure and decreased circulation to the lower extremities. Headaches, dizziness, epistaxis, and intermittent claudication, coolness, or pallor in the lower extremities may be noted. Preductal or ductal coarctation usually results in persistent patency of the ductus with blood shunting from the pulmonary artery to the aorta. The result is cyanosis of the lower extremities. In either case, CHF may result, especially after 5 years of age.[15]

OTHER DEFECTS

Some of the other congenital heart defects include:

- *Total anomalous pulmonary venous connection*, in which the pulmonary veins are connected to the right atrium
- *Truncus arteriosus*, in which the embryonic truncus fails to divide into the aorta and pulmonary arteries
- The *endocardial cushion defect*, in which the valves and septi fail to form adequately and may result in a one-chambered heart
- *Ebstein's malformation*, in which the basic abnormality is downward displacement of the tricuspid

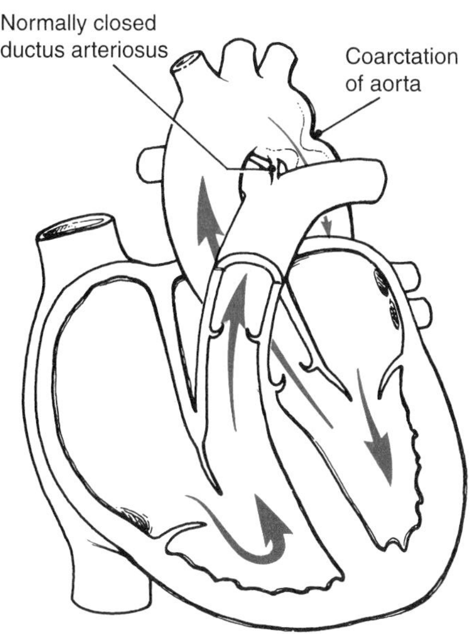

FIGURE 17-37. **Postductal coarctation of the aorta.**

FOCUS ON THE PERSON WITH CARDIAC PROBLEMS RELATED TO IV DRUG ABUSE

J.J. is an 18-year-old white woman who has been living "on the streets" with friends for the past 8 months. She is a known IV drug abuser who is brought into the emergency room with sudden onset of high fever, shaking chills, and complaints of difficulty breathing. Examination shows a thin-to-emaciated young woman with splenomegaly, petechiae all over the skin surfaces, and loud systolic and diastolic murmurs with a gallop rhythm. There are rales in the bases of the lungs, and her pulse is 146 with a respiratory rate of 32.

Questions

1. What is the probable diagnosis for Ms. J.?
2. Describe clearly the basis on which you made the diagnosis. What definitive laboratory analysis is used to determine the diagnosis? Include risk factors and clinical manifestations in your assessment.
3. Outline the pathophysiology of the condition, including causative organisms and the target structures of these organisms.
4. Considering the clinical manifestations, what is the prognosis?
5. What is the appropriate treatment for this condition? What are preventative steps to avoid recurrence of this condition?

valve, making part of the right ventricle a part of the right atrium. This decreases output to the lungs and increases right atrial pressures. If there is an associated ASD, a right-to-left shunt causes a cyanotic clinical picture.[9]

- *Tricuspid atresia*, in which the tricuspid valve does not form or there is no right ventricle. A hypoplastic pulmonary artery may be present and a PDA must be present to sustain life. The right atrium is enlarged and the left ventricle is hypertrophied.
- *Isolated pulmonic stenosis*, a relatively common congenital anomaly that produces symptoms when it is severe
- *Bicuspid aortic valve* refers to development of the aortic valve with only two cusps. This defect is common and usually asymptomatic.
- *Mitral valve prolapse*, discussed on page 488

REFERENCES

1. Alexander, R. W., Roberts, R., & Pratt, C. M. (1998). Diagnosis and management of patients with myocardial infarction. In R. W. Alexander, R. C. Schlant, & V. Fuster (Eds.), *Hurst's: The heart* (9th ed). New York: McGraw-Hill.
2. American Heart Association. (1998). *Facts and figures.* Dallas, TX: Author.
3. Bristow, M. R., Bohlmeyer, T. J., & Gilbert, E. M. (1998). Dilated cardiomyopathy. In R. W. Alexander, R. C. Schlant, & V. Fuster (Eds.), *Hurst's: The heart* (9th ed.). New York: McGraw-Hill.
4. Chandrasoma, P., & Taylor, C. R. (1998). *Concise pathology* (3rd ed.), Stamford, CT: Appleton & Lange.
5. Chattergee, K. (1998). Ischemic heart disease. In J. H. Stein (Ed.), *Internal medicine* (5th ed.). St. Louis: Mosby.
6. Cheitlin, M. D., Sokolow, M., & McIlroy, M. B. (1994). *Clinical cardiology* (6th ed.). Norwalk, CT: Appleton & Lange.
7. Cotran, R. S., Kumar, V., & Collins, T. (1999). *Robbins' pathologic basis of disease* (6th ed.). Philadelphia: Saunders.
8. Daily, E. K., & Schroeder, J. S. (1994). *Techniques in bedside hemodynamic monitoring* (5th ed.). St. Louis: Mosby.
9. Davies, M. J. (1998). Pathology of coronary athrosclerosis. In R. W. Alexander, R. C. Schlant, & V. Fuster (Eds.), *Hurst's: The heart* (9th ed.). New York: McGraw-Hill.
10. Deanfield, J. E., Gersh, B. J., Warnes, C. A., & Mair, D. D. (1998). Congenital heart disease in adults. In R. W. Alexander, R. C. Schlant, & V. Fuster (Eds.), *Hurst's: The heart* (9th ed). New York: McGraw-Hill.
11. DeMaria, A. N., & Blanchard, D. G. (1998). The echocardiogram. In R. W. Alexander, R. C. Schlant, & V. Fuster (Eds.), *Hurst's: The heart* (9th ed.). New York: McGraw-Hill.
12. Durack, D. T. (1998). Infective endocarditis. In R. W. Alexander, R. C. Schlant, & V. Fuster (Eds.), *Hurst's: The heart* (9th ed.). New York: McGraw-Hill.
13. Factor, S. M., & Bache, R. J. (1998). Pathophysiology of myocardial ischemia. In R. W. Alexander, R. C. Schlant, & V. Fuster (Eds.), *Hurst's: The heart* (9th ed.). New York: McGraw-Hill.
14. Francis, G. S. (1998). Congestive heart failure. In J. H. Stein (Ed.), *Internal medicine* (5th ed.). St. Louis: Mosby.
15. Freed, M. D., & Plauth, W. H. (1998). The pathology, pathophysiology, recognition, and treatment of congenital heart disease. In R. W. Alexander, R. C. Schlant, & V. Fuster (Eds.), *Hurst's: The heart* (9th ed.). New York: McGraw-Hill.
16. Guyton, A. C., & Hall, J. E. (1996). *Textbook of medical physiology* (9th ed.). Philadelphia: Saunders.

17. Hollander, J. E., Hoffman, R. S., Burnstein, J. L., Shih, J. D., & Thode, H. C. (1996). Cocaine associated myocardial infarction: Mortality and complications. *Archives of Internal Medicine, 155,* 1081–1086.
18. Kannel, W. B. (1996). Blood pressure as a cardiovascular risk factor: Prevention and treatment. *Journal of the American Medical Association, 275,* 1571–1576.
19. Kaplan, E. L. (1998). Acute rheumatic fever. In R. W. Alexander, R. C. Schlant, & V. Fuster (Eds.), *Hurst's: The heart* (9th ed.). New York: McGraw-Hill.
20. Katz, A. M. (1996). Is the failing heart an energy-starved organ? *Journal of Cardiac Failure, 2,* 267–272.
21. Keller, B. B., & Markwald, R. R. (1998). Embryology of the heart. In R. W. Alexander, R. C. Schlant, & V. Fuster (Eds.), *Hurst's: The heart* (9th ed.). New York: McGraw-Hill.
22. LeJemtel, T. H., Sonnenblick, E. H., & Frishman, W. H. (1998). Diagnosis and management of heart failure. In R. W. Alexander, R. C. Schlant, & V. Fuster (Eds.), *Hurst's: The heart* (9th ed.). New York: McGraw-Hill.
23. Maron, B. J. (1998). Hypertrophic cardiomyopathy. In R. W. Alexander, R. C. Schlant, & V. Fuster (Eds.), *Hurst's: The heart* (9th ed.). New York: McGraw-Hill.
24. Maron, D. J., Ridker, P. M., & Pearson, T. A. (1998). Risk factors and the prevention of coronary heart disease. In R. W. Alexander, R. C. Schlant, & V. Fuster (Eds.), *Hurst's: The heart* (9th ed.). New York: McGraw-Hill.
25. Mason, J. W. (1998). Classification of cardiomyopathies. In R. W. Alexander, R. C. Schlant, & V. Fuster (Eds.), *Hurst's: The heart* (9th ed). New York: McGraw-Hill.
26. Moser, D. K. (1998). Pathophysiology of heart failures update: The role of neurohumor activation in the progression of heart failure. *AACN Clinical Issues, 9*(2), 157–171.
27. Myerberg, R. J., Kessler, K. M., & Castellanos, A. (1998). Recognition, clinical assessment, and management of arrhythmias and conduction disturbances. In R. W. Alexander, R. C. Schlant, & V. Fuster (Eds.), *Hurst's: The heart* (9th ed.). New York: McGraw-Hill.
28. National Center for Health Statistics. (1996). *Health, United States, 1995.* (DHHS Publication No. 96-1232). Washington, DC: US Government Printing Office.
29. Newman, J. H., & Ross, J. C. (1998). Chronic cor pulmonale. In R. W. Alexander, R. C. Schlant, & V. Fuster (Eds.), *Hurst's: The heart* (9th ed.). New York: McGraw-Hill.
30. Oberman, A. (1997). Epidemiology and Prevention of Cardiovascular Diseases. In W. N. Kelley (Ed.), *Textbook of internal medicine* (3rd ed.). Philadelphia: Lippincott-Raven.
31. O'Connell, J. B., & Renlund, D. G. (1998). Myocarditis and cardiomyopathies. In R. W. Alexander, R. C. Schlant, & V. Fuster (Eds.), *Hurst's: The heart* (9th ed). New York: McGraw-Hill.
32. Olvetti, G., Abbi, R., & Quaini, F. (1997). Apoptosis in the failing human heart. *New England Journal of Medicine, 336,* 1131–1141.
33. O'Rourke, R. A. (1998). Mitral valve prolapse syndrome, In R. W. Alexander, R. C. Schlant, & V. Fuster (Eds.), *Hurst's: The heart* (9th ed.). New York: McGraw-Hill.
34. Packer, M. (1992). The neurohomonal hypothesis: A theory to explain the mechanism of disease progression in heart failure. *Journal of American College of Cardiology, 20,* 248–254.
35. Rahimtoola, S. H. (1998). Aortic valve disease. In R. W. Alexander, R. C. Schlant, & V. Fuster (Eds.), *Hurst's: The heart* (9th ed.). New York: McGraw-Hill.
36. Rahimtoola, S. H., Enriquez-Sarano, M., Schaff, H. V., & Frye, R. L. (1998). Mitral valve disease, In R. W. Alexander, R. C. Schlant, & V. Fuster (Eds.), *Hurst's: The heart* (9th ed.). New York: McGraw-Hill.
37. Rahimtoola, S. H. (1998). Valvular heart disease. In J. Stein (Ed.), *Internal medicine* (5th ed.). St. Louis: Mosby.
38. Regan, T. J. (1998). Alcohol and nutrition. In R. W. Alexander, R. C. Schlant, & V. Fuster (Eds.), *Hurst's: The heart* (9th ed.). New York: McGraw-Hill.
39. Roberts, R. (1997). Ischemic heart disease. In W. N. Kelley (Ed.), *Textbook of internal medicine* (3rd ed.), Philadelphia: Lippincott-Raven.
40. Ross, R. (1998). Factors influencing atherogenesis. In R. W. Alexander, R. C. Schlant, & V. Fuster (Eds.), *Hurst's: The heart* (9th ed.). New York: McGraw-Hill.
41. Rubin, E., & Farber, J. L. (1998). *Pathology* (3rd ed.). Philadelphia: Lippincott-Raven.
42. Schlant, R. C., & Alexander, R. W. (1998). Diagnosis and management of patients with chronic ischemic heart disease. In R. W. Alexander, R. C. Schlant, & V. Fuster (Eds.), *Hurst's: The heart* (9th ed,). New York: McGraw-Hill.
43. Schlant, R. C., Sonnenblick, E. H., & Katz, A. M. (1998). Pathophysiology of heart failure. In R. W. Alexander, R. C. Schlant, & V. Fuster (Eds.), *Hurst's: The heart* (9th ed.). New York: McGraw-Hill.
44. Shabetai, R. (1998). Diseases of the pericardium. In R. W. Alexander, R. C. Schlant, & V. Fuster (Eds.), *Hurst's: The heart* (9th ed.). New York: McGraw-Hill.
45. Shabetai, R. (1998). Restrictive, obliterative, and infiltrative cardiomyopathies. In R. W. Alexander, R. C. Schlant, & V. Fuster (Eds.), *Hurst's: The heart* (9th ed.). New York: McGraw-Hill.
46. Smith, A. L., & Schlant, R. C. (1998). Effect of noncardiac drugs, electricity, poisons, and radiation on the Heart. In R. W. Alexander, R. C. Schlant, & V. Fuster (Eds.), *Hurst's: The heart* (9th ed.). New York: McGraw-Hill.
47. Theroux, P., & Waters, D. (1998). Diagnosis and management of patients with unstable angina. In R. W. Alexander, R. C. Schlant, & V. Fuster (Eds.), *Hurst's: The heart* (9th ed.). New York: McGraw-Hill.
48. Thom, T. J., Kannel, W. B., Silbershatz, H., & D'Agostino, R. B. (1998). Incidence, prevalence, and mortality of cardiovascular disease in the United States. In R. W. Alexander, R. C. Schlant, & V. Fuster (Eds.), *Hurst's: The heart* (9th ed.). New York: McGraw-Hill.
49. Traill, T. A. (1996). Left ventricular dysfunction: Mechanisms and symptoms. In J. D. Stobo, D. B. Hellmann, P. W. Ladenson, B. G. Petty, & T. A. Traill (Eds.), *The principles and practice of medicine* (23rd ed.). Stamford, CT: Appleton & Lange.
50. Waldo, A. L., & Wit, A. L. (1998). Mechanisms of cardiac arrhythmias and conduction disturbances. In R. W. Alexander, R. C. Schlant, & V. Fuster (Eds.), *Hurst's: The heart* (9th ed.). New York: McGraw-Hill.
51. Waller, B. F. (1998). Nonatherosclerotic coronary heart disease. In R. W. Alexander, R. C. Schlant, & V. Fuster (Eds.), *Hurst's: The heart* (9th ed.). New York: McGraw-Hill.
52. Weiss, J. L. (1997). Valvular heart disease. In W. N. Kelley (Ed.), *Textbook of internal medicine* (3rd ed.). Philadelphia: Lippincott-Raven.
53. Woosley, R. L. (1998). Antiarrhythmia drugs. In R. W. Alexander, R. C. Schlant, & V. Fuster (Eds.), *Hurst's: The heart* (9th ed.). New York: McGraw-Hill.
54. Zipes, D. P. (1997). Cardiac arrhythmias. In W. N. Kelley (Ed.), *Textbook of internal medicine* (3rd ed.). Philadelphia: Lippincott-Raven.

Chapter 18

Shock

Maria A. Smith / Barbara L. Bullock

KEY TERMS

acute lung injury
adult respiratory distress syndrome
anaerobic glycolysis
anaphylactoid reaction
anaphylaxis
catecholamines
diffuse alveolar damage
disseminated intravascular coagulation
endotoxin
enterobacteria
epinephrine
exotoxin
lactate
lactic acidosis
multiple organ dysfunction syndrome
myocardial depressant factor
norepinephrine
prostaglandins
splanchnic organ
systemic inflammatory response syndrome (SIRS)

Shock is a life-threatening disturbance of hemodynamics that results in failure to maintain adequate perfusion of vital organs. This state of hypoperfusion is not a specific disease but a clinical syndrome that involves numerous organs and systems. The occurrence of the shock state represents the most severe complication of a variety of diseases. Loss of circulating fluid volume (hypovolemic shock), an inadequate pump (cardiogenic shock), systemic infection (septic shock), and generalized arteriolar and venous dilatation (neurogenic or anaphylactic shock) are causative factors. The responses of the body, called compensatory mechanisms, cause changes in volume, flow, and oxygen transport regardless of the initiating event. These mechanisms are the main factors that lead to survival, whereas failure of adequate compensation can lead to circulatory failure and death.[15] Therapeutic intervention can alter the interactions; however, it should address not only the primary cause but also the systemic effects of the shock.

STAGES OF SHOCK

There are essentially three stages of the shock state, which lie on a continuum progressing from one stage to the next. The terms used to describe these stages vary. Compensated (nonprogressive), decompensated (progressive), and irreversible are used in this discussion. Persons experiencing shock progress through fairly distinguishable phases ranging from compensation to various degrees of decompensation to a refractory state that is irreversible (Flowchart 18-1). The clinical picture illustrates progressive deterioration in compensatory mechanisms throughout body systems and organs (Table 18-1).

Compensated (Nonprogressive) Shock

Compensated shock represents the initial or early phase during which, in response to the initial insult, certain physiologic compensatory mechanisms are activated. These mechanisms, described below, may compensate for the shock state and return the body to its normal functional state. Early intervention, such as fluid replacement, may restore the blood pressure and prevent hypoxic tissue damage that results from hypoperfusion. Any tissue damage incurred in the process is repaired through the process of inflammation and healing.

Clinical manifestations that predominate in the initial stage are directly related to the compensatory ac-

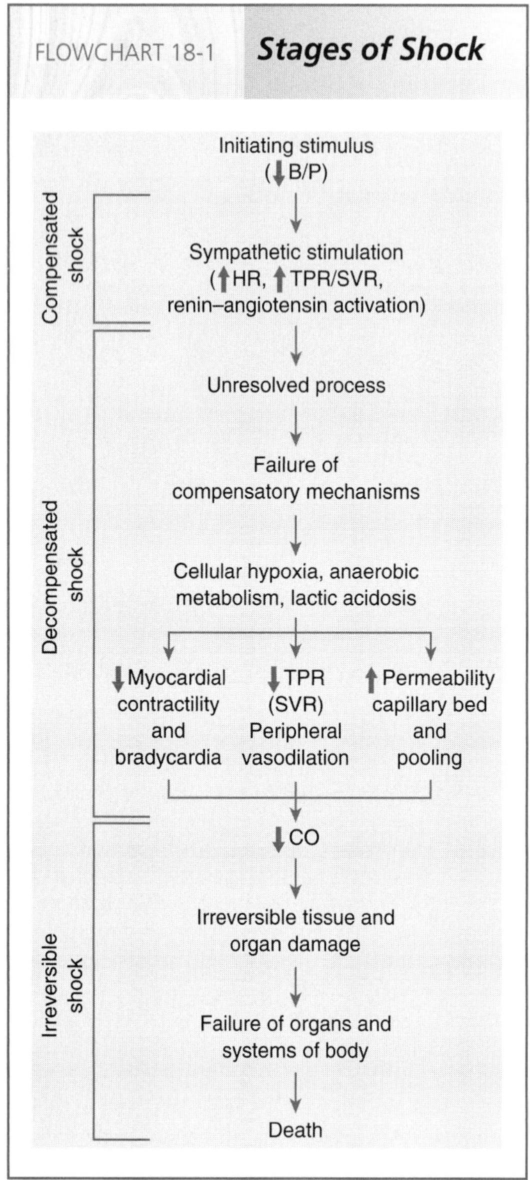

tivities of sympathetic nervous system (SNS) activation and hormonal responses. These manifestations include pallor, diaphoresis, pupillary dilatation, tachycardia, tachypnea, complaints of thirst, hypoactive bowel sounds (due to vasoconstriction of the gut), and decreased urinary output.

COMPENSATORY MECHANISMS

A sufficient blood pressure (BP) is required to maintain an adequate perfusion pressure to supply oxygen and essential nutrients to the cell. When the blood pressure is inadequate to maintain perfusion, a series of compensatory actions is initiated by the body to maintain blood flow to the heart and brain. These mechanisms involve alterations in blood volume and vascular diameters through nervous system and hormonal mechanisms. The interactive nature of these mechanisms allows for a combination of volume and vascular events. Cellular hypoxia from inadequate perfusion requires that ATP be produced through a process of **anaerobic glycolysis**, which temporarily maintains the viability of the cell.

Blood pressure is the product of cardiac output (CO) times total peripheral resistance (TPR), also called systemic vascular resistance (SVR). It is expressed by the equation BP = CO X TPR (see p. 424). In shock, a response that increases CO and TPR may raise BP and restore tissue perfusion.

Blood Volume and Vascular Response

Shock results in changes in blood volume and blood vessels. These changes cause alterations in CO, TPR (SVR), autonomic (especially SNS) responses, and intravascular fluid volume. The mechanisms of these changes are mainly through hormonal changes.

CARDIAC OUTPUT CHANGES. Cardiac output is the product of stroke volume (SV) and heart rate (HR) (see p. 414). Left ventricular ejection or SV is dependent on an adequate venous return. Many shock conditions decrease venous return, which then decreases SV and CO. Normal compensation for a decrease in venous return is an increased HR to maintain constant CO as well as hormonal interaction to retain intravascular fluid volume.

TOTAL PERIPHERAL RESISTANCE (SYSTEMIC VASCULAR RESISTANCE). Total peripheral resistance refers to the total resistance blood encounters as it flows through the systemic circulation and is determined primarily by changes in the diameter of the arterioles. Resistance to flow is inversely related to vessel radius. Systemic blood pressure is increased when vessels are constricted and decreased when vessels are dilated if fluid volume is unchanged. A small change in arteriolar diameter can have a profound effect on BP, with constriction increasing it and dilatation decreasing it. The constriction of the arterioles, in certain shock states, is a normal compensation for the low BP and helps to increase BP by centralizing blood volume.

SYMPATHETIC NERVOUS SYSTEM INTERACTION. Nervous system control of blood flow and pressure is mediated through the autonomic nervous system (ANS), the sympathetic and parasympathetic divisions (see p. 421). Sympathetic nervous system stimulation is critical in regulating blood flow and pressure through its ability to increase HR and TPR. In the shock state, the SNS reflexes are initiated, resulting in powerful responses, including: (1) arteriolar constriction in most areas of the body, thus increasing the TPR; (2) constriction of veins and venous reservoirs to maintain adequate venous return; and (3) marked increase of HR.[6] This compensation is essential to tolerate losses in blood volume. In

TABLE 18-1

CLINICAL MANIFESTATIONS RELATED TO DEGREE OF SHOCK

CLINICAL MANIFESTATION	COMPENSATED (NONPROGRESSIVE)	DECOMPENSATED (PROGRESSIVE)	IRREVERSIBLE
Sensorium	Oriented to time, place, and person	Oriented to person and possibly place	Disoriented to comatose
Communication	Speech clear	Speech slurred	Speech significantly slurred to no communication
Pulse rate/quality	Sinus tachycardia/ bounding to slightly decreased	Sinus tachycardia/ decreased to variable	<60 or >150/weak, thready, difficult to feel
Blood pressure	Slightly increased to low normal	Decreased	Systolic <80, diastolic inaudible
Urinary output	20–50 mL/hr	20–30 mL/hr	<20 mL/hr
Skin color	Slightly pale	Pale	Mottled
Acid–base balance	Normal	Slightly acidotic	Severely acidotic

the absence of the SNS response, only 15% to 20% of the blood volume can be lost before death is produced. With SNS activation, a 30% to 40% loss can be sustained before death results.[6]

HORMONAL RESPONSE. The hormones responsible for blood pressure regulation are the **catecholamines** (**epinephrine** and **norepinephrine**), the renin–angiotensin system, and antidiuretic hormone. Hormones act by altering arteriolar diameter, which increases blood flow to vital organs during stress and redistributes blood during losses in hemorrhage or shock. They also function to conserve fluid volume, which can function to increase BP. The catecholamines, epinephrine and norepinephrine, are released by the adrenal medullae and various adrenergic terminals located throughout the body.[4] They are categorized as short-term, immediate determinants of blood pressure. Epinephrine accounts for about 80% of the catecholamines released from the adrenal medullae and causes vasoconstriction in many vascular beds (excluding the liver and skeletal muscles), along with a marked cardiac stimulation (increasing HR). Norepinephrine causes vasoconstriction in essentially all of the blood vessels of the body, which greatly increases the TPR.[6] In shock, with the stimulation of the SNS, both the sympathetic nerve terminals and adrenal medullae are stimulated to secrete their catecholamines. The SNS terminals secrete norepinephrine, which accounts for the clinical effects of vasoconstriction (e.g., pallor and sweating). Epinephrine secreted from the adrenal medullae circulates to all body tissues and has a metabolic effect five to ten times greater than norepinephrine.[6] The effect of the renin–angiotensin system (sometimes called the renin–angiotensin–aldosterone system) in restoration of BP is shown in Flowchart 18-2. The system is initiated by decreased vascular tension, which reduces renal perfusion pressure and volume. The effect is to increase blood volume through aldosterone and increase TPR through angiotensin II.

Antidiuretic hormone (ADH), or vasopressin, is released by the posterior pituitary in response to an increased serum osmolality, water deficit, or low blood volume. ADH causes water reabsorption by the kidneys by increasing the permeability of the renal distal tubules and collecting ducts (see p. 598). Increased permeability results in water reabsorption into the plasma (increasing blood volume) and thus, a more concentrated urine. It also has a vasoconstrictor effect on the arterioles throughout the body (increasing TPR).[6]

Energy Production

The cellular mitochondria require oxygen for aerobic oxidation of carbohydrates, which takes place when pyruvate enters the Krebs cycle (see p. 20). When oxygen is not present in shock, pyruvate is converted to **lactate** without entering the Krebs cycle. This action results in a marked reduction of ATP molecule formation. The resulting lactate production and limited ATP generation leads to **lactic acidosis.**[13] The lactic acid is absorbed into the central circulation and metabolic acidosis results (see p. 183). This action is a temporary fix to keep cells viable since cells without adequate ATP fail to maintain their structural integrity and rapidly die.

Decompensated (Progressive) Shock

Decompensated shock represents a condition in which compensatory responses fail to restore blood pressure and tissue perfusion (see Flowchart 18-1). The complications of shock usually begin to develop during this

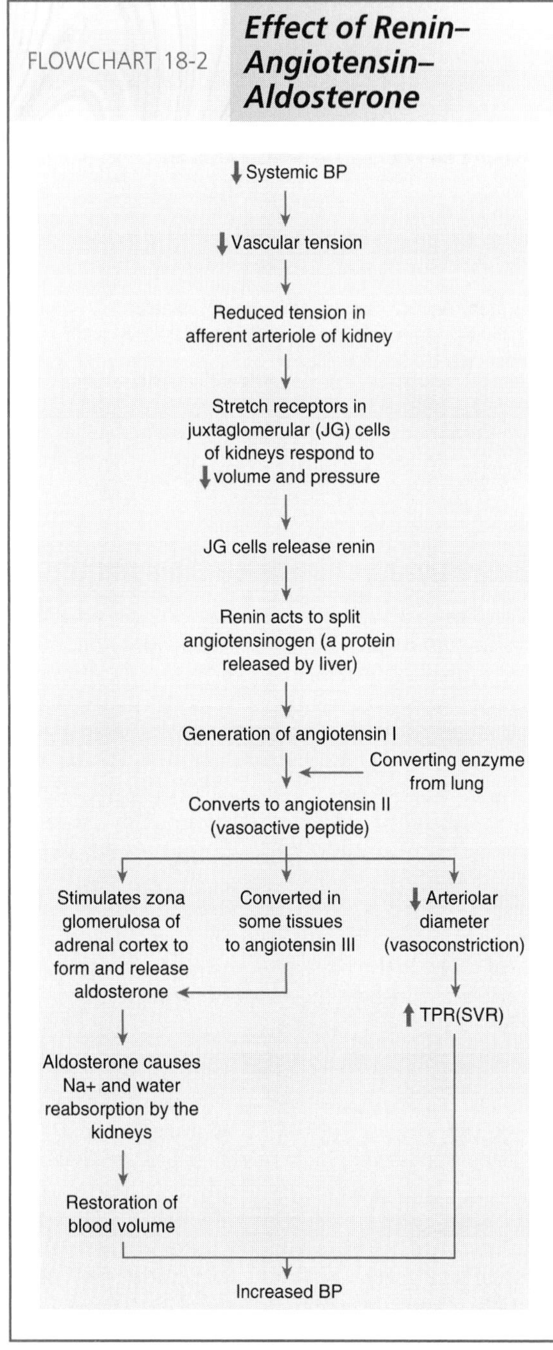

↓ Systemic BP
↓ Vascular tension
Reduced tension in afferent arteriole of kidney
Stretch receptors in juxtaglomerular (JG) cells of kidneys respond to ↓ volume and pressure
JG cells release renin
Renin acts to split angiotensinogen (a protein released by liver)
Generation of angiotensin I
Converting enzyme from lung
Converts to angiotensin II (vasoactive peptide)
Stimulates zona glomerulosa of adrenal cortex to form and release aldosterone
Converted in some tissues to angiotensin III
↓ Arteriolar diameter (vasoconstriction)
↑ TPR(SVR)
Aldosterone causes Na+ and water reabsorption by the kidneys
Restoration of blood volume
Increased BP

FLOWCHART 18-2 **Effect of Renin–Angiotensin–Aldosterone**

time (see p. 514). The BP and vascular response decline and injury to the tissues and vital organs results. Anaerobic glycolysis results from tissue hypoxia and generates lactic acid; this results in a metabolic acidosis. Poor blood flow in the tissues prevents removal of carbon dioxide; this causes the formation of high concentrations of intracellular carbonic acid.[6]

Hypoxia may lead to depression of the vasomotor center in the medulla and depression of the SNS responses. The pancreas may become ischemic, and it then releases a substance called **myocardial depressant factor**, which decreases myocardial contractility and further compromises the blood flow to the system.

Vasodilatation and pooling result from continued hypoxia, contributing to the deterioration. As the shock progresses, histamine and bradykinin are released. These activate the arachidonic acid pathway, which generates prostaglandin (PGE_2) and prostacyclin (PGI_2), both of which have vasodilating properties (see p. 257). Other factors that lead to loss of peripheral vascular tone include (1) acidemia, (2) catecholamine depletion from vascular smooth muscle nerve endings, and (3) decreased central sympathetic system activity caused by cerebral ischemia.

The clinical manifestations associated with the decompensated stage are related to organ failure and the development of complications.[7] Levels of consciousness and orientation decrease. Bradycardia from cardiac depression may ensue, causing progressive hypotension. Urine output ceases and peripheral and pulmonary edema may develop. Abdominal distention and paralytic ileus are common. The skin becomes cold, ashen, and diaphoretic. Metabolic acidosis is common due to lactic acid accumulation. Without rapid and effective intervention to treat the source of the shock, the irreversible stage will be entered.

Irreversible Shock

Irreversible shock denotes the final stage and is the point at which the person degenerates despite therapeutic intervention (see Flowchart 18-1). The line between decompensated and irreversible shock is clinically difficult to ascertain, since therapy may for a time return the BP to near normal as the circulatory system continues to deteriorate.[6] The irreversible point results from acidosis, destructive enzymes, and tissue (organ) death.[7] Ischemic cell death is manifested by renal, heart, pulmonary, and brain dysfunction.

TYPES OF SHOCK

Shock can be classified by etiology, by major pathophysiological impairment, or by clinical manifestations. For example, hypovolemic shock is caused by loss of intravascular volume; cardiogenic shock is the result of cardiac decompensation; and distributive shock results from internal fluid loss or redistribution. Table 18-2 compares the pathophysiological processes of shock by mechanisms of causation and clinical manifestations.

(text continues on page 509)

TABLE 18-2

TYPES OF SHOCK

CATEGORY	MECHANISMS	CLINICAL MANIFESTATIONS
I. Hypovolemic Shock	Results from loss of circulating fluid volume. Circulating volume deficits reduce cardiac output, lower blood pressure, and impair tissue perfusion. Compensatory mechanisms include SNS stimulation, renin–angiotensin activation, and ADH secretion.	SNS compensation produces vasoconstriction (pallor), tachycardia, diaphoresis, decreased urine output, concentrated urine, nausea, vomiting, ileus. As shock progresses, compensations fail and complications begin.
A. Hemorrhagic	A. Results from a significant loss of whole blood from trauma, gastrointestinal bleeding,coagulation defects, and other conditions.	A. Tachycardia, tachypnea, pallor, diaphoresis, anxiety, decreased urine output, and altered gastrointestinal function.
B. Dehydration	B. Results from an extensive loss of body fluid that depletes tissue fluid.	B. Usual onset rather gradual; SNS mechanisms not as dramatic as in hemorrhagic shock. Skin turgor is poor and eyeballs may be soft.
C. Burn	C. Results from loss of plasma proteins, which alters colloid osmotic pressure and leads to edema. Chemical mediators in tissues enhance fluid exudation to tissues. Central blood volume is markedly depleted.	C. SNS response not effective in increasing BP, and renal and tissue perfusion is markedly impaired. Immune response impaired with increased risk of septic shock.
II. Cardiogenic Shock	II. Impaired cardiac output due to myocardial damage (i.e., myocardial infarction), inadequate ventricular filling (i.e., cardiac tamponade), life-threatening cardiac dysrhythmias.	II. SNS stimulation and renin–angiotensin activation cause tachycardia, pallor, increased blood volume, and central venous pressure. Compensatory mechanisms quickly fail and progression to decompensation occurs.
A. Excessive preload: • Acute myocardial infarction • Myocarditis/myocardiopathy • Mitral/aortic valvular insufficiency • Ventricular septal defects, congenital conditions causing right heart failure • Chronic obstructive pulmonary disease	A. Poor cardiac contractility leads to increased end-diastolic pressure and decreased BP. SNS is activated to increase afterload; renin–angiotensin increases preload (aldosterone) and afterload (angiotensin II). Heart unable to pump under increased stress. CO decreases, BP decreases, tissue perfusion declines, and acidosis impairs cardiac functioning further.	A. B/P very low. Tachycardia, pallor, narrow pulse pressure from vasoconstriction. Central venous pressure elevates. Pulmonary or systemic edema may be seen. Urine output decreased. Cardiac murmurs of heart failure (S_3, S_4) or of underlying condition.
B. Reduced preload: • Pericardial tamponade • Right ventricular infarction (RVI) • Tension pneumothorax	B. Restriction of input to the heart occurs with tamponade and tension pneumothorax. RVI causes decreased blood flow to left ventricle due to poor contractility. Standard SNS responses occur, but increased HR does not compensate for filling defect.	B. Marked decrease in BP, increased HR. Narrow pulse pressure, elevated central venous pressure (jugular venous distention). Urine output decreased.

(continued)

TABLE 18-2

TYPES OF SHOCK (Continued)

CATEGORY	MECHANISMS	CLINICAL MANIFESTATIONS
C. Excessive afterload: • Pulmonary embolism (PE) (massive) • Systemic hypertension • Aortic stenosis	C. Gradual onset of heart failure and shock occurs when heart cannot maintain the pressures required from hypertension and aortic stenosis. The hypertrophied left ventricle decompensates, heart failure ensues, blood pressure declines. In massive pulmonary embolus, sudden right heart failure develops from obstruction to flow.	C. Pulmonary edema often occurs with a progressive decline in BP. Signs and Symptoms of left heart failure that degenerates to shock-level BP. In PE, acute symptoms of right heart failure occur, BP declines, and shock ensues.
III. Distributive Shock	III. Profound and massive vasodilatation results in inappropriate distribution of blood volume and failure to maintain an adequate BP. SNS stimulation cannot overcome underlying problem.	
A. Neurogenic (Vasogenic) • CNS damage to vasomotor center • Cerebral edema • General anesthetic medullary depression • Cervical spinal cord injury	A. SNS inhibition or PSNS stimulation causes widespread vasodilatation and peripheral pooling. In spinal cord, injury blocking SNS allows PSNS-induced bradycardia. Peripheral pooling causes decreased BP and the SNS is unable to compensate.	A. Decreased BP, may lead to mental confusion, syncope. Pulse may be decreased or increased according to the effect on the medullary and peripheral nervous system. Often self-limiting but may lead to metabolic acidosis and irreversible shock.
B. Septic Shock • Endotoxin mediated • Exotoxin mediated	B. Wide spread sepsis from gram-negative or gram-positive organisms. Toxins produce vasodilatation and peripheral pooling. Mediators of inflammation potentiate the vasodilatation. SNS response cannot overcome vasodilatation. Capillary endothelial damage, micro emboli, myocardial depression, and organ failure are common effects.	B. In early stages, tachycardia increases cardiac output, BP exhibits increased systolic and decreased diastolic pressures. Progression leads to peripheral pooling, decreased urine output, signs and symptoms of complications of shock.
C. Anaphylactic/Anaphylactoid • IgE mediated: certain drugs, foods, insect venoms, pollens • Non–IgE mediated: iodinated contrast material, dextran, opiates, mannitol, nonsteroidal anti-inflammatory drugs, polymixin B, blood transfusions to IgA-deficient patient, and local anesthetics	C. Drastic, acutely developing and progressing type of shock. • Anaphylaxis occurs with IgE-mediated reactions. Molecules of IgE bind with allergen and tissue mast cells, releasing histamine, which causes vascular permeability and smooth muscle constriction. Occurs on re-exposure to an antigen. • Non–IgE-mediated reactions can be induced on first contact. May be induced by direct mast cell activation or IgG interactions (in specific cases). • Physiologic response is vasodilatation, and peripheral edema, and bronchoconstriction. SNS cannot overcome vasodilating stimulus.	C. Signs and symptoms are exactly the same whether the mechanism is IgE- or non–IgE mediated. Tachycardia, low BP, bronchoconstriction (some cases), cardiovascular collapse. May progress to manifestations of decompensated shock if not treated. • Respiratory: hoarseness, stridor • Skin: edema of face, mouth, larynx, urticaria, pruritis, flushing • Chest tightness, wheezing • Hypotension, dysrhythmias • Nausea, vomiting, diarrhea • Disorientation to coma

Hypovolemic Shock

Hypovolemic shock is a shock state resulting from loss of circulating fluid volume. This shock results from any condition that significantly depletes normal volumes of whole blood, plasma, or water. The underlying pathology, regardless of the exact type of fluid loss, is related to actual circulatory fluid pressure/volume deficits (see Table 18-2). Decreased circulating fluid volume decreases venous return, which reduces cardiac output and, subsequently, lowers BP. Lowered BP impedes tissue and organ perfusion and impairs oxygen and nutrient delivery. This leads to ischemia and, eventually, necrosis, with resulting organ malfunction and shock (Flowchart 18-3). Compensatory mechanisms are activated to adjust for the reduced tissue and organ perfusion. These mechanisms include sympathetic nervous system stimulation to increase HR and TPR, activation of the renin–angiotensin system, and increased secretion of ADH. These mechanisms, working together, result in an increase in BP. If treatment is effective, shock remains in the nonprogressive stage and a crisis is averted or resolved. If the fluid volume loss is overwhelming or therapeutic measures are ineffective, the initial stage of shock may progress to the irreversible stage.

FLOWCHART 18-3 **Pathophysiology of Hypovolemic Shock**

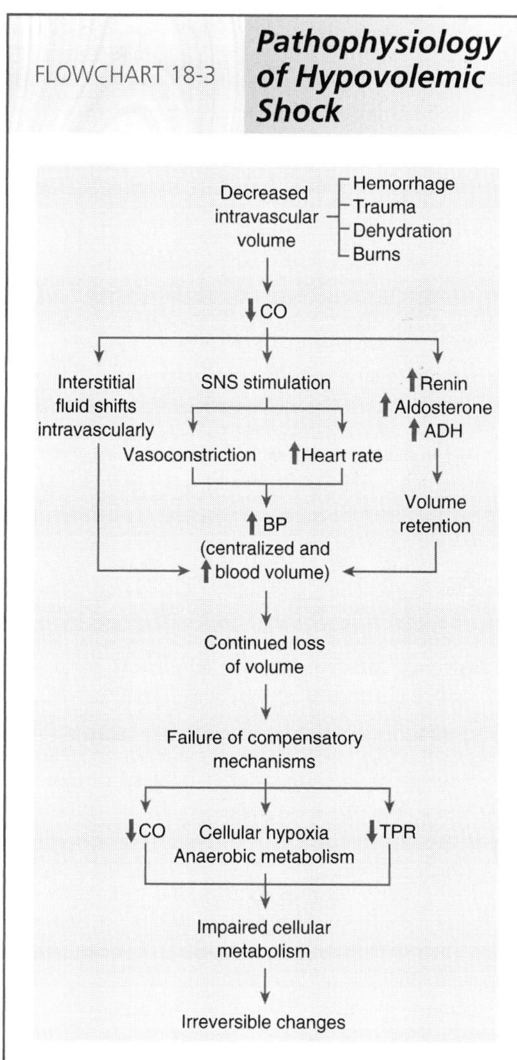

HEMORRHAGE

Hemorrhagic shock occurs as a result of massive loss of whole blood. Some conditions that can produce this loss include gastrointestinal bleeding, postoperative hemorrhage, hemophilia, childbirth, and trauma. In order for shock to occur, blood loss must be extensive and immediate. Minimal loss of blood, up to 10% of the total volume (500 cc), does not produce noticeable changes in blood pressure or cardiac output. Blood loss of 15% to 20% reduces cardiac output and average BP systolic to 90 to 100 mmHg. Blood loss of between 35% and 45% of the total blood volume reduces both cardiac output and BP to zero.[6] Mortality in hemorrhagic shock can range from 10% to 30%.[11] Blood loss results in hypoperfusion to body cells and tissues, which causes reduced oxygen to the cells and cellular components. These overall effects perpetuate the oxygen deficit cycle to cells and body organs. Clinical manifestations exhibited depend on the actual volume of blood lost and whether the loss was sudden or gradual. Compensatory mechanisms range from mild to severe tachycardia, hypotension, and vasoconstriction.

Trauma

Trauma, in the forms of crushing injuries to muscles and bones, gunshot wounds, and penetration of blood vessels, viscera, or other vital organs by knives or sharp instruments, produces the shock state primarily through extensive and sudden blood loss. An astounding amount of blood lost internally due to trauma can be concealed in tissue, organs, and "third spaces" for variable lengths of time before symptoms of shock are manifested. For example, the thigh muscle can hold up to 1,000 mL of blood resulting from a fractured femur or a tear in a femoral vessel without a noticeable increase in thigh diameter. The abdomen can hold even larger quantities of blood. Loss of 1 L of whole blood represents a significant hemorrhage, especially if it goes undetected and uncorrected.

Trauma also can produce shock related to sepsis due to the access of organisms to the blood stream from open wounds or from contamination from peritonitis. This type of shock is discussed on page 511.

DEHYDRATION

Dehydration can result in hypovolemic shock from extensive and profound loss of body fluid. The following conditions can cause dehydration:

- Profuse sweating
- Extensive gastrointestinal fluid loss related to diarrhea, vomiting, or upper gastrointestinal suctioning
- Diabetes insipidus
- Ascites
- The diuretic phase of acute renal failure
- Diabetic ketoacidosis
- Addison's disease and hypoaldosteronism
- Lack of adequate fluid volume intake
- Osmotic diuresis
- Injudicious use of diuretics

Dehydration must be severe to produce a shock state. It results from significant interstitial and intracellular fluid shifts. Simple or moderate dehydration does not produce symptomatology consistent with shock, because fluid moves along a pressure gradient from tissue spaces to the intravascular space. Fluid volume in the vascular compartment is maintained at the expense of the tissues. Once fluid volume loss becomes severe, however, the transfer of water is not sufficient to maintain intravascular volume, and the shock state ensues.

BURNS

Burns, especially third-degree burns, often cause hypovolemic shock due to loss of plasma proteins through the burn surface. Fluid loss results from an increase in capillary endothelial permeability that occurs within the initial 24 hours after the burn. Cellular metabolism disruption also occurs, which results in loss of normal electrolyte homeostasis and altered oxygen transport and uptake of nutrients by essential organs.

In burns, the chemical mediators of inflammation are released, which cause peripheral vasodilatation and increased capillary permeability and may promote local tissue ischemia at the burn site. These mediators aggravate the compensatory mechanisms for hypovolemia and make the hypotension more profound. Burn patients also are especially susceptible to infection due to (1) loss of the natural skin barriers and (2) immune system compromise due to the burn injury. Extensive burns initiate marked alterations in all body systems, and the complications of shock are frequently seen.

Cardiogenic Shock

Shock directly attributable to impaired or compromised cardiac output is referred to as cardiogenic shock. The predominant cause of cardiogenic shock is myocardial infarction. Shock develops in approximately 5% to 7% of these individuals. Cardiogenic shock does not respond well to treatment, and mortality rates are frequently greater than 80%.[1]

Three categories of conditions can induce shock of cardiac origin: those causing excessive preload, those causing reduced preload, and those causing excessive afterload (see Table 18-2). Regardless of the category, the end result is an inability of the heart to maintain CO, and the standard compensatory mechanisms are initiated. These mechanisms overload the heart's ability to respond since the underlying problem is in the heart itself.

In myocardial infarction, cardiogenic shock usually develops when the total amount of myocardium lost reaches a critical point (approximately 40% of left ventricular mass) and myocardial function begins to deteriorate (see p. 482).[5] Stroke volume and, subsequently, CO is decreased. Sympathetic compensatory mechanisms ensue with increased heart rate, but the CO falls short due to limited availability of oxygen and nutrients to the cardiac musculature. Total peripheral resistance is significantly elevated and the SNS-mediated vasoconstriction increases afterload, forcing the myocardium to work even harder in an effort to sustain adequate CO. Preload is increased due to renin–angiotensin compensation and renal conservation. Flowchart 18-4 illustrates the pathophysiologic processes.

Sustained hypotension results from decreased CO and increased SVR. It reduces blood flow to essential body organs, impeding their ability to function normally and forcing cellular anaerobic metabolism.[14]

Signs indicative of cardiogenic shock may include varying degrees of pulmonary edema, severe hypotension, oliguria/anuria, cold and diaphoretic skin with pallor, decreased or altered sensorium, tachycardia, and abdominal distention with hypoactive or absent bowel sounds.

Distributive Shock

Distributive shock develops as a consequence of profound and massive vasodilatation, resulting in inappropriate distribution of blood volume. Blood volume is shifted from central/core organs and vessels to peripheral vascular beds, especially venous beds. The net result is an increase in capacitance relative to the intravascular blood volume. In this form of shock, blood volume is not reduced; rather, there is an increase in vessel capacitance (decreased TPR) that accommodates this set volume.

Increased vessel diameter expands vascular capacity, effectively reducing venous return to the heart. The balance between volume and vascular capacity is disrupted. Sympathetic stimulation, the major compensatory mechanism in shock, may be lost or unable to overcome the vasodilatory effects of the primary defect without intervention. The clinical effects depend on the underlying mechanism causing the shock. Three forms of distributive shock are described: neurogenic, septic, and anaphylactic (see Table 18-2).

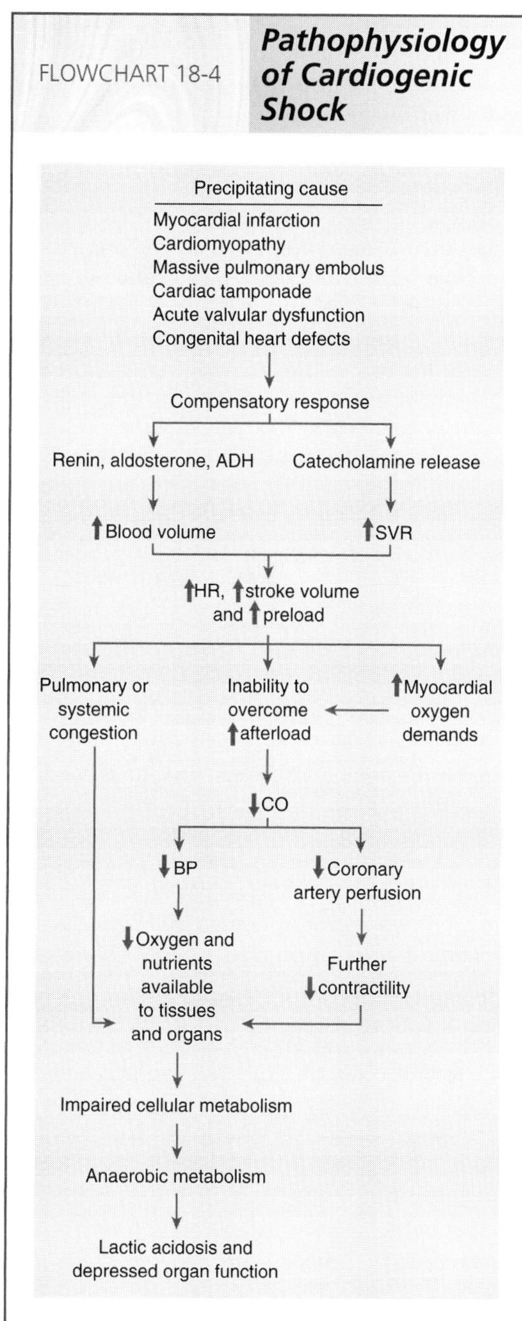

NEUROGENIC SHOCK (VASOGENIC SHOCK)

Neurogenic shock (vasogenic shock) is the result of loss of vasomotor tone that induces generalized vasodilatation. Loss of sympathetic control of blood vessel tone from central (vasomotor) or spinal cord injury results in pooling of blood in storage or capacitance vessels and **splanchnic organ** capillaries. Conditions that depress vasomotor function directly or indirectly adversely affect the vascular control. Direct injury of the vasomotor center may result from a penetrating object such as a bullet. Indirect injury results from cerebral edema, with increased intracranial pressure from head trauma or ischemia of the brain.[15] Neurogenic shock may also be caused by medullary brain stem depression from deep general anesthesia and drug overdose (especially barbiturates, opiates, and tranquilizers). Spinal cord injury and high spinal anesthesia can induce profound vasomotor failure because of interruption of sympathetic pathways to blood vessels, blocking vasoconstriction and promoting vasodilatation. Persons having acute cervical spinal cord injuries often exhibit bradycardia since there is unopposed action of the parasympathetic nervous system on the heart. Flowchart 18-5 demonstrates the consequences of neurogenic shock.

SEPTIC SHOCK

Septic shock results from widespread sepsis that causes hypotension, organ dysfunction, oliguria, lactic acidosis, and alteration in mental status.[2] This form of shock is most often initiated by gram-negative organisms that release **endotoxins**, proteases, and other products. Gram-negative septicemia carries a 60% mortality rate despite treatment. Gram-positive organisms also can precipitate septic shock by the release of **exotoxins**, polysaccharide A, capsular polysaccharides, peptidoglycans, C substance, enzymes, and hemolysins.

Septic shock is the terminal point of the **systemic inflammatory response syndrome (SIRS)**. Sepsis is defined as SIRS caused by infection.[13] Severe septic SIRS is complicated by organ dysfunction, hypoperfusion, and hypotension (see p. 254).

Causative Organisms

Enterobacteria are the micro-organisms most commonly associated with gram-negative sepsis. These include *Escherichia coli, Klebsiella, Proteus, Pseudomonas,* and others. The origin of the underlying sepsis for individuals may be in of two sources: (1) the community or (2) the hospital (nosocomial).[9,13] Most cases are nosocomially acquired as a complication of therapeutic measures such as indwelling urinary catheters.

In the majority of cases, gram-negative organisms initiate the process. Many gram-negative bacilli produce hemolysins, proteases, and elastases. These break down tissue barriers, damage the membrane of phagocytic cells, and degrade immunoglobulins. Gram-negative organisms have a unique structure that aids in their ability to survive and thrive. Endotoxin is a lipopolysaccharide (LPS) portion of the outer membrane of gram-negative bacteria. The release of LPS by the bacterial membrane initiates the clinical manifestations of sepsis. LPS binds LPS-binding protein (LBP), which attaches to monocytes and macrophages by a specific cell

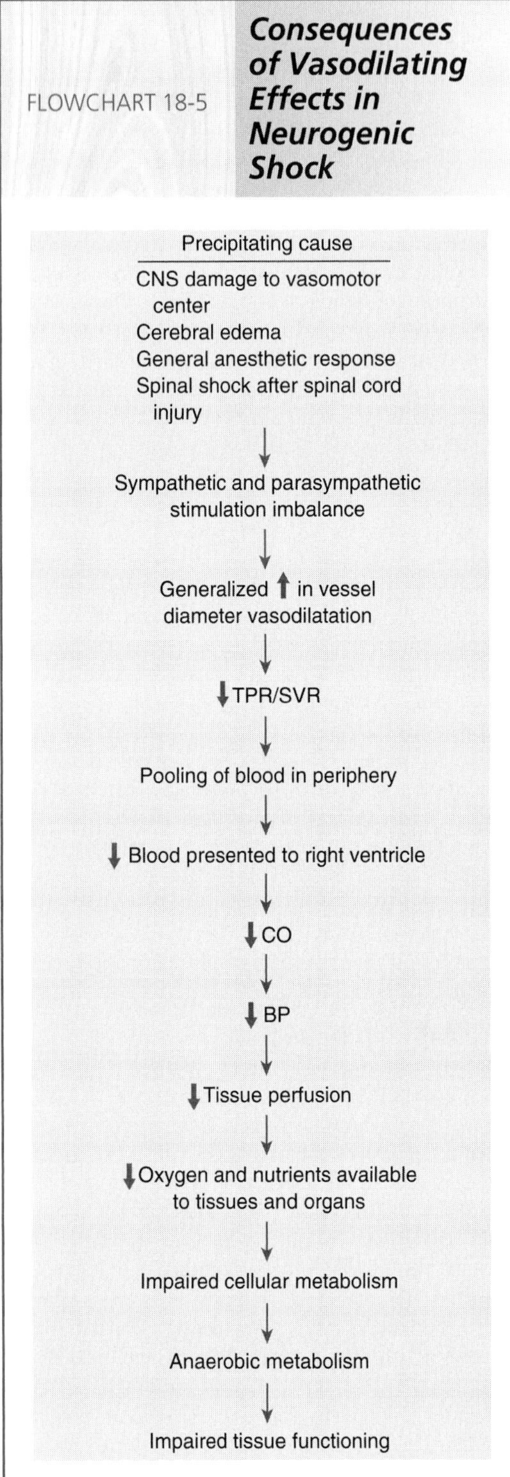

surface receptor and induces release of tumor necrosis factor (TNF) and interleukin-1 (IL-1).[9] The macrophage system also activates the release of cytokines and other substances such as complement, coagulation factors, and **prostaglandins**. Many of these factors in combination cause capillary damage, which initiates plasma leakage and fluid loss. This capillary insult is the basis for the development of **adult respiratory distress syndrome** (ARDS) (see p. 514).

FLOWCHART 18-5
Consequences of Vasodilating Effects in Neurogenic Shock
Precipitating cause
CNS damage to vasomotor center
Cerebral edema
General anesthetic response
Spinal shock after spinal cord injury
Sympathetic and parasympathetic stimulation imbalance
Generalized ↑ in vessel diameter vasodilatation
↓TPR/SVR
Pooling of blood in periphery
↓ Blood presented to right ventricle
↓CO
↓BP
↓Tissue perfusion
↓Oxygen and nutrients available to tissues and organs
Impaired cellular metabolism
Anaerobic metabolism
Impaired tissue functioning

Systemic Effects

The overall systemic effects of septic shock are shown in Flowchart 18-6. They are initiated by an infectious agent, which enters the body and overwhelms the normal defenses. As a consequence of host defense activity, mediators of shock are liberated. The collective effects of these mediators are vasodilatation, capillary endothelial cell damage, platelet aggregation with microemboli, myocardial depression, and impaired myocardial contractility. The alterations in peripheral venules and arterioles as well as those of myocardial function impair tissue and organ perfusion, resulting in lactic acidemia. Lactic acidemia further depresses myocardial contractility, TPR, and the vital organ functions. Death ensues predictably unless this chain of events is interrupted.[10]

Clinical Manifestations

Physiological signs and symptoms indicative of septic shock include elevated temperature, heart rate, and respirations; lowered BP; altered mental status; and decreased urine output. The initial symptoms are nonspecific, but sepsis can be suspected when a focal site, such as a urinary tract infection, is identified.[9] An elevated white blood cell count may not always be seen, especially in elderly or immunocompromised persons.

In the early stages of septicemia, the affected person may demonstrate a greater than normal CO, which results from a high metabolic rate induced by the bacterial toxin. The typical BP response is an elevation in the systolic and a decrease in the diastolic pressures (a reaction to the decreased TPR). The skin may be warm and flushed with a very elevated body temperature. As the compensations fail, the BP falls and the appearance of the shock state may be very much like that of hemorrhagic shock.[6]

ANAPHYLACTIC SHOCK AND ANAPHYLACTOID REACTIONS

Anaphylactic shock, or **anaphylaxis**, is the most drastic, acutely developing, and rapidly progressing of the forms of shock. This form of shock results from an explosive, widespread allergic, or hypersensitivity, reaction. Onset can occur in a matter of seconds. Profound peripheral vascular collapse may become well established in only a few minutes without intervention, and death can occur in an hour or so.

Anaphylaxis results from an IgE-mediated (allergic) reaction. A reaction that is clinically identical to anaphylaxis can occur in the absence of IgE reactions and is termed an **anaphylactoid reaction.**[18] Flowchart

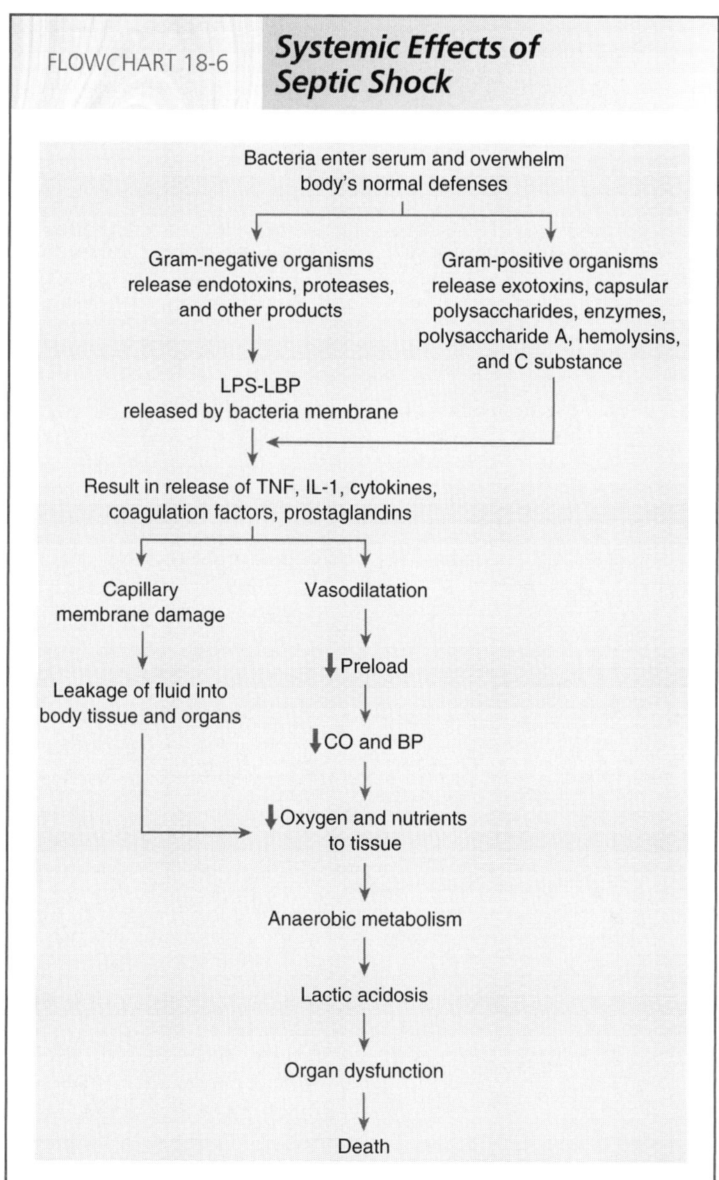
Bacteria enter serum and overwhelm body's normal defenses
Gram-negative organisms release endotoxins, proteases, and other products
Gram-positive organisms release exotoxins, capsular polysaccharides, enzymes, polysaccharide A, hemolysins, and C substance
LPS-LBP released by bacteria membrane
Result in release of TNF, IL-1, cytokines, coagulation factors, prostaglandins
Capillary membrane damage
Leakage of fluid into body tissue and organs
Vasodilatation
↓Preload
↓CO and BP
↓Oxygen and nutrients to tissue
Anaerobic metabolism
Lactic acidosis
Organ dysfunction
Death

FLOWCHART 18-6 **Systemic Effects of Septic Shock**

18-7 summarizes the pathophysiologic processes in this type of shock.

Anaphylactic Shock

In allergic mechanisms, allergens bind to and crosslink antigen-specific IgE molecules on the surface of the tissue mast cells. This initiates mast cell degranulation, resulting in the release of vasoactive, chemotactic, and enzymatic mediators (see p. 311). Measurable amounts of histamine and tryptase are detectable in the serum. Histamine induces most of the recognized manifestations of anaphylaxis. It dilates blood vessels, constricts respiratory smooth muscle, and increases vascular permeability. The clinical presentations relate to upper airway obstruction, lower airway obstruction, and cardiovascular, cutaneous, and gastrointestinal abnormalities.

Anaphylaxis rarely occurs after initial exposure, but re-exposure to an antigen may induce this hypersensitivity reaction. The mechanism by which antigen–antibody reactions induce shock is directly related to the effects of the substance liberated at the onset of the reaction.[18] Specifically, the shock state develops as a consequence of hypotension from profound vasodilatation and low CO. This reaction is from central fluid volume deficits that are caused by increased capillary permeability and peripheral pooling of blood. Compensatory mechanisms are not capable of reversing or retarding the progression of this form of shock because the initial shock-producing insult develops rapidly and

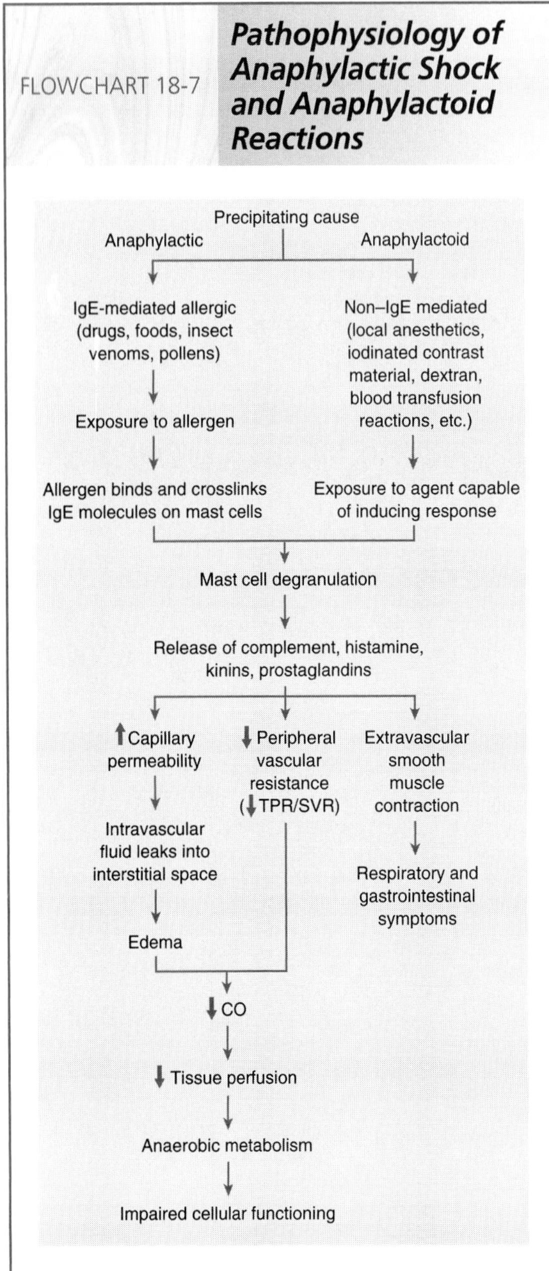

acutely. The pathologic developments of severe laryngeal spasm, edema, and bronchoconstriction compound the shock state by adding further hypoxemia to the overall pattern of response. Hypoxemia perpetuates the cycle of anaerobic metabolism and lactic acid production.

Anaphylactoid Reactions

Non-IgE–mediated reactions may cause the clinical picture of anaphylaxis. They may be due to nonimmunologic release of mediators that induce the vascular collapse.[18] The most common form of shock is induced by injection of local anesthetics, such as in dental or minor surgical procedures. Ionic compounds, such as radiographic contrast material and the antibiotic polymyxin B, also may induce the reaction. Polysaccharides such as dextrans probably cause direct mast cell activation, and certain drugs act in this same manner.[18]

COMPLICATIONS OF SHOCK

Complications that are directly caused by the shock state are devastating and often fatal. These complications stem from and are produced by the pathologic processes inherent in shock. Pathology is often seen in a number of organs (Fig. 18-1). The three most common processes that induce severe complications are vasodilatation with inadequate tissue and organ perfusion, damage to the capillary endothelial lining, and activation of clotting factors. Complications of these processes include lactic acidosis, ARDS, disseminated intravascular coagulation, and multiple organ dysfunction.

Lactic Acidosis

The basis for lactic acidosis in shock is the relentless production of lactic acid related to continual hypoxia of tissues from impaired perfusion. Hypoperfusion to tissues deprives them of oxygen. Cells are unable to metabolize nutrients appropriately without oxygen. In the absence of sufficient oxygen, cells are forced into anaerobic metabolism. In this state, pyruvate is converted to lactic acid.

Lactic acid exerts two major effects on the body. In prolonged anaerobic situations such as shock, it depresses myocardial contractility. This reduces myocardial functioning and interferes with cardiac output, thus establishing a cycle of further compromised tissue perfusion. The second adverse effect of lactic acid production is impairment of cellular metabolic function from metabolic acidosis (see p. 183).

Adult Respiratory Distress Syndrome (ARDS)

Following prolonged shock-induced hypoxia, injury to the alveolar wall causes generalized interstitial pneumonitis (shock lung) and is considered a causative agent of ARDS, a respiratory crisis. This condition also results from an acute injury to the alveolar capillary membrane from direct or indirect causes.[7] Direct causes of injury include aspiration of gastrointestinal acid or inhalation of toxic substances (such as smoke inhalation). Indirect causes include responses to systemic

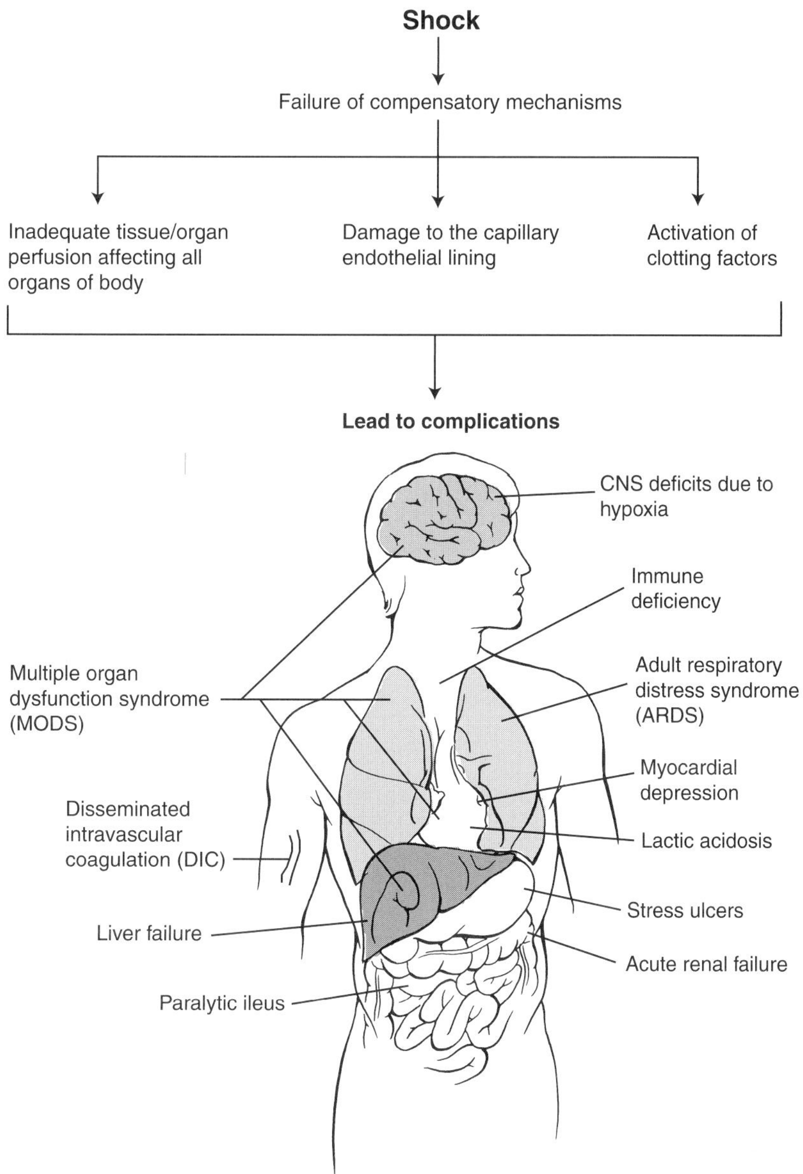

FIGURE 18-1. Complications of shock.

chemical mediators from conditions such as sepsis, trauma, and pancreatitis. Whatever the cause, a common response of **acute lung injury** (ALI) due to a massive inflammatory response by lung tissue is seen (see p. 568). Another term for ALI is **diffuse alveolar damage** (DAD), which is a precursor to the clinical syndrome of ARDS. Neutrophils are attracted and activated by various mediators released by alveolar macrophages and the endotoxic activation of complement. Neutrophils release several toxic products that cause alveolar capillary membrane damage and increase membrane permeability. These inflammatory mediators include proteolytic enzymes, oxygen free radicals, prostaglandins, leukotrienes, and platelet-activating factor.[17]

Diffuse alveolar damage increases permeability of the alveolar basement membrane, allowing interstitial and alveolar pulmonary edema through fluid, proteins, and blood cells crossing into the alveolar space. Hypoxemia is believed to be caused by intrapulmonary shunting and occurs early in the course of the condition.[17] The fluid extravasation into the pulmonary capillary membrane bed also causes protein and fibrin aggregation, which leads to hyaline membranes identical to those seen in premature infants.[17] This leads to reduced functional capacity and poor pulmonary compliance. Resulting symptomatology includes respiratory symptoms of rapid, shallow breathing; dyspnea; and pulmonary infiltrates throughout all lung fields, which produce a refractory hypoxia. Respiratory acidosis results in late stages from profound hypercapnia (see p. 183).

Disseminated Intravascular Coagulation

Disseminated intravascular coagulation (DIC) is a complex coagulopathy that occurs secondarily to a major body insult, frequently that of shock. The bases for the development of DIC are abnormal platelet aggregation and activation of factors of clotting, both of which are prominent features of shock. In response to the platelets and clotting factors, generalized coagulation occurs in the microcirculation, a condition which impedes capillary flow. In addition, the clotting process consumes fibrin, platelets, and other factors of clotting and initiates fibrinolysis. Active fibrinolysis produces and releases fibrin degradation products, which are the end products of fibrin, fibrinogen, and plasmin lysis. The presence of these fibrin degradation products, plus the consumption of platelets and other clotting factors, interrupts subsequent coagulation and leads to widespread bleeding (see p. 385).

Symptoms of microcirculation (capillary) coagulation are present, including cool skin with mottling

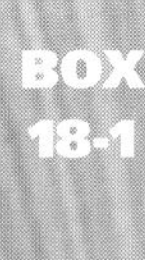

BOX 18-1 ETIOLOGY OF MULTIPLE ORGAN DYSFUNCTION SYNDROME

- Inadequate or delayed resuscitation
- Significant soft tissue injury
- Persistent hypoperfusion and shock
- Systemic infection
- Burns over 30% of body surface area
- Renal failure
- Liver failure
- Trauma
- Coma on admission
- Multiple blood transfusions
- Persistent hypoxia
- Age over 65 years

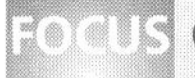

FOCUS ON THE PERSON IN SHOCK

D. M. is a 35-year-old mother of two, who was received in the emergency room following a tornado that destroyed a shopping center where she was a customer. She received a severe open pelvic fracture (she was struck by a wooden building support beam—part of the wooden beam is still protruding from the wound). The patient presents in a C-collar, on a backboard with Mast trousers and three peripheral intravenous lines.

Physical examination findings include:

General appearance: Pale, in obvious distress

Vital signs: BP 70/46, HR 148, R 38

Neuro: Glasgow Coma Scale = 14 (confused but appropriate); movement bilateral upper extremities and right lower extremity intact; no movement in left leg and questionable sensation in left lower leg

Chest: Breath sounds absent on right, multiple areas of soft tissue injury on anterior chest wall

Cardiac: Tachycardia

Abdomen: Large pelvic laceration from anus through perineum to left iliac crest with open symphysis pubis fracture with a through-and-through 4-inch wooden stake protruding from wound. Multiple bony fractures apparent with exposed left iliac vessels; bowel visible through exposed peritoneum and large amount of active bleeding.

Laboratory and radiological findings include:

Lab: Na 140, K 2.9, Cl 121, CO_2 14, BUN 9, Cr 0.8, Hgb 5.6, Hct 17.1

Chest x-ray: Right pneumothorax

Pelvic x-ray: Completely separated symphysis pubis, multiple bony defects

Questions

1. What type of shock is D. M. exhibiting?
2. From the clinical picture described, explain the source of the shock.
3. Explain the pathophysiology of this form of shock.
4. What signs and symptoms validate this type of shock?
5. What would be the expected course of treatment for this type of shock?
6. After resolution of the initial shock state, what potential complication is this patient susceptible to that may lead to a second shock episode?

and cyanotic nail beds and concomitant signs of profuse bleeding, especially from puncture sites, incisions, and the gastrointestinal tract. The overall picture of DIC is one of a vicious circle of coagulation and anticoagulation.

Multiple Organ Dysfunction Syndrome

The term multiple organ system failure, or **multiple organ dysfunction syndrome** (MODS), refers to a progressive loss of function in two or more organs following a major bodily insult. Precipitating factors include a variety of diseases and mechanisms that usually precipitate shock and cause organ hypoxia (Box 18-1). The most common cause of MODS is sepsis and/or septic shock.[3] Mortality is directly related to the number of systems that fail and is highest with failure of three or more organs, ranging from 80% to 100%.[3] With failure of two organs, mortality drops to between 45% and 55%.[16] Multiple organ dysfunction syndrome often begins with pulmonary failure and is manifested by ARDS. This may be followed rapidly by acute renal failure. Cardiovascular effects may then occur as a result of septic mediators or shock-induced myocardial depression. Gastrointestinal and liver dysfunction are common and may be manifested by paralytic ileus and altered liver function tests. Central nervous system deficits are closely related to the magnitude of the shock state. The onset of immune deficiency depletes the host's ability to withstand opportunistic organisms. The onset of the syndrome of DIC markedly decreases the chance for survival, because it further damages oxygen-depleted tissues and organs.

The clinical signs of MODS are variable, depending upon the systems primarily affected. Respiratory abnormalities associated with ARDS precipitate further tissue hypoxia.[12] Other signs of MODS include confusion, decreased urine output, evidence of gastrointestinal bleeding, thrombocytopenia, altered coagulation studies, glucose intolerance, and worsening of a previously stable shock picture. Thus, the triad of intravascular sepsis, respiratory failure, and renal dysfunction presents a poor outcome.

REFERENCES

1. Alexander, R. W., Roberts, R., & Pratt, C. M. (1998). Diagnosis and management of patients with acute myocardial infarction. In R. W. Alexander, R. C. Schlant, & V. Fuster (Eds.), *Hurst's the heart* (9th ed.). New York: McGraw-Hill.
2. American College of Chest Physicians/Society of Critical Care Medicine Consensus Committee. (1992). Definitions for sepsis and organ failure and guidelines for the use of innovative therapies in sepsis. *Critical Care Medicine, 20*(6), 864.
3. Beal, A. L., & Cerra, F. B. (1994). Multiple organ failure syndrome in the 1990s. *JAMA, 271*(3), 226.
4. Goldstein, D. S. (1995). *Stress, catecholamines and cardiovascular disease*. New York: Oxford University Press.
5. Grella, D. R., & Becker, R. C. (1994). Cardiogenic shock complicating coronary artery disease: Diagnosis, treatment and management. *Current Problems in Cardiology, 19*(12), 727.
6. Guyton, A. C. (1996). *Textbook of medical physiology* (9th ed.). Philadelphia: W. B. Saunders.
7. Leier, C. V. (1997). Approach to the patient with hypotension and shock. In W. N. Kelley (Ed.), *Textbook of internal medicine* (3rd ed.). Philadelphia: Lippincott-Raven.
8. Livingston, D. H., & Deitch, E. A. (1995). Multiple organ failure: A common problem in surgical intensive care unit patients. *Annals of Medicine, 27,* 13.
9. Noskin, G. A. & Phair, J. P. (1997). Approach to the patient with bacteremia and sepsis. In W. N. Kelley (Ed.), *Textbook of internal medicine* (3rd ed.). Philadelphia: Lippincott-Raven.
10. Parillo, J. E. (1995). Septic shock in humans: Clinical evaluation, pathogenesis, and therapeutic approach. In W. C. Shoemaker et al. (Eds.), *Textbook of critical care* (3rd ed.), Philadelphia: W. B. Saunders.
11. Peitzman, A. B., et al. (1995). Hemorrhagic shock, *Current Problems in Surgery, 32*(11), 925.
12. Rinaldo, J. E., & Clark, M. (1998). Multiple organ dysfunction in the context of ARDS. In J. H. Stein (Ed.), *Internal medicine* (5th ed.) St. Louis: Mosby.
13. Sanders, L. I. & Cobbs, C. G. (1998). Gram-negative bacteriemia and the sepsis syndrome. In J. H. Stein (Ed.), *Internal medicine* (5th ed.). St. Louis: Mosby.
14. Sharma, M. & Becker, R. C. (1998). Hypotension and cardiogenic shock. In J. H. Stein (Ed.), *Internal medicine* (5th ed.). St. Louis: Mosby.
15. Shoemaker, W. C. (1995). Shock states: Pathophysiology, monitoring, outcome prediction and therapy. In W. C. Shoemaker et al. (Eds.), *Textbook of critical care* (3rd ed.), Philadelphia: W. B. Saunders.
16. St. John, R. C., & Dorinsky, P. M. (1994). An overview of multiple organ dysfunction syndrome. *Journal of Laboratory and Clinical Medicine, 124*(4), 478.
17. Steinberg, K. P. & Hudson, L. D. (1997). Approach to the management of the patient with acute respiratory distress syndrome. In W. N. Kelley (Ed.), *Textbook of internal medicine* (3rd ed.). Philadelphia: Lippincott-Raven.
18. Terr, A. I. (1997). Anaphylaxis and urticaria. In D. P. Stites, A. I. Terr, & T. G. Parslow, *Medical immunology* (9th ed.). Stamford, CT: Appleton & Lange.

UNIT 4: CASE STUDY

Cocaine-Induced Cardiomyopathy

Introduction to the Patient

B. W. is a 34-year-old African-American male who has sought medical attention with a chief complaint of chest pain of 4 hours' duration. The pain radiates down the left arm and is associated with a feeling that the heart is "racing away." He appears to be very anxious and is perspiring profusely.

Present Illness

Mr. W. has noticed occasional chest "twinges" over the past 3 months. When pressed, he admits that they were often associated with use of cocaine. This episode was different in onset in that it began following use of cocaine and continued as unremitting, substernal, squeezing pain. It was not relieved by rest or use of antacids. Mr. W. admits to daily use of cocaine, which is administered through the nasal route. In the past few weeks he has increased his drug use and has experienced symptoms including palpitations, ringing in the ears, chest pains, and paranoia.

Social History

Mr. W. is an accounts executive for a large bank. His career is very stressful, and he began using cocaine occasionally approximately 5 years ago. The desired effect of the cocaine use was to increase energy and enhance clarity of thinking. Mr. W. is married and has two children, a boy, age 2 and a girl, age 5. He states that his wife does not use cocaine and that she doesn't know of his use of the drug.

Past Medical History

Mr. W. states that his health is excellent, and until last year he was exercising daily at the gym. He admits to smoking about a pack of cigarettes daily since he was 17 years of age. He drinks "socially," one or two mixed drinks daily. He had an appendectomy at age 22. When he was 18 he was in a serious automobile accident with fracture of the femur and a concussion. He reports no residual effects.

Family History

Mr. W.'s father died at age 54 of a myocardial infarction. His mother had a slight stroke last year at age 60 but has nearly recovered. His two brothers, ages 32 and 38, are apparently in good health. His sister, age 40, had surgery for a ruptured ovarian cyst but recovered with no further problems.

Physical Examination

Mr. W. is an ill-appearing adult who is oriented to time and place. He is perspiring profusely and appears very anxious. He states that he is 6 ft. tall and weighs 176 lbs. Initial blood pressure is 180/100 with a heart rate of 142. Heart sounds include a questionable gallop or perhaps an S4. Lung fields are clear and the rest of the examination is unremarkable.

During the initial examination, Mr. W. developed a rapid atrial rhythm on the dynamic monitor, which was diagnosed as paroxysmal atrial tachycardia. This rhythm spontaneously converted to sinus tachycardia with frequent, unifocal PVCs. During the rhythm change, the blood pressure dropped to 90/60 but returned to previous levels after conversion.

Diagnostic Tests

12-lead electrocardiogram indicates S-T elevation in V3 through V5. Chest x-ray indicates an enlarged left ventricle with no congestion in the lung fields.

Lab values are normal except for the CPK, which was elevated to 560 U/mL. The CPK-MM was 70 U/mL, the CPK-BB was 0 U/mL, and the CPK-MB was 490 U/mL.

CRITICAL THINKING QUESTIONS

1. What are the physiologic effects of cocaine on the body systems? Draw a flow chart showing the effects of cocaine use on the cardiovascular system.
2. What are the possible diagnoses suggested by the above clinical picture? How does the use of cocaine affect the clinical picture presented?
3. How do the data found in the diagnostic tests help in making a clinical diagnosis? What further diagnostic tests would be helpful in determining the diagnosis?
4. Based on known cardiac and nervous system toxicity of cocaine, what are possible effective treatment strategies?
5. What drug therapy may be effective in treating this condition? What drugs may have toxic effects on the heart affected by cocaine?
6. Considering the complexities of cocaine addiction and the psychosocial picture presented, construct a plan of care for managing this patient.

Besides your pathophysiology text, you will need a good pharmacology textbook, a medical cardiovascular textbook, a pathology text, and current research articles to complete this case study. Suggested references follow:

Alexander, R.W., Schlant, R.C., & Fuster, V. (Eds.) (1998). *Hurst's the heart* (9th ed.). New York: McGraw-Hill.

Karch, A. (2000). *Focus on nursing pharmacology.* Philadelphia: Lippincott Williams & Wilkins.

Rubin, E., & Farber, J.L. (1999). *Pathology* (3rd ed.). Philadelphia: Lippincott-Raven.

UNIT 4 APPENDIX A

Laboratory Studies Useful in Diagnosis of Cardiovascular Disease

TEST	NORMAL VALUE	SIGNIFICANCE
I. Erythrocyte sedimentation rate	NB: 0–2 mm/hr <Age 20: 3–13/mm/hr Ages 20–60: Males: 0–10 mm/hr Females: 0–20 mm/hr >Age 60: 15–30 mm/hr	Nonspecific test roughly measuring concentrations of fibrinogen and serum globulins. Rate increases in all inflammatory diseases, infectious or connective tissue, e.g., rheumatic fever, bacterial endocarditis
II. Red blood cell (RBC, erythrocyte)	NB: 4.8–7.1 mil/mm^3 Neonate: 4.1–6.4 mil/mm^3 Ages 1–60: Males: 4.4–5.7 mil/mm^3 Females: 4.0–5.3 mil/mm^3 >Age 60: 3.0–5.0 mil/mm^3	Certain anemias will show a decreased number of RBCs; cardiac workload increases due to decreased oxygen in blood and tissue deprivation. Polycythemias have increased numbers of RBCs and result from tissue hypoxia or myeloproliferative disease; cause increased blood viscosity and increased cardiac workload.
III. Hemoglobin	NB: 14–24 g/dL Infant: 10–15 g/dL <Age 20: 11–16 g/dL Ages 20–60: Males: 13–17 g/dL Females: 12–15 g/dL >Age 60: 10–17 g/dL	Value decreased due to decreased production (lack of iron, genetic abnormalities, protein depletion, loss from bleeding); cause decrease in oxygen-carrying capacity, lead to symptoms of anemia and increased cardiac workload.
IV. White blood cell	NB: 9–10 10^3/mm^3 Infant: 6–17.5 10^3/mm^3 <Age 20: 5–10 10^3/mm^3 Ages 20–60: 4–10 10^3/mm^3 >Age 60: Males: 4.25–14 10^3/mm^3 Females: 3.1–12 10^3/mm^3	May indicate cardiac or vascular infection. Increased in Myocardial infarction, burns, gangrene, and myeloproliferative disorders. Physiologic increase in exercise and pain. Decreased in bone marrow suppression.
V. Platelet count	NB: 140–300,000/mm^3 Infant: 200–473,000/mm^3 <Age 20: 150–450,000/mm^3 Ages 20–60: 250–500,000/mm^3 >Age 60: Males: 330–1,430,000/mm^3 Females: 255–1,392,000/mm^3 >Age 90: 70–175,000/mm^3	Difficult to count; best to use automated counter. Increased production in myeloproliferative diseases and thrombocytosis. Increased numbers may lead to thrombosis. Decreased production—thrombocytopenia may result from drug reaction, autoimmune conditions, bone marrow suppression. Causes bleeding, purpura, petechiae.
VI. Prothrombin time (measured against a control) • International normalized ratio (INR)	NB: 12–21 sec <Age 20: 12–20 sec Ages 20–60: 12–13.8 sec >Age 60: 12–15 sec INR: Thromboembolism 2.0–3.0. Artificial heart valves 3.0–4.0.	Decreased circulating prothrombin due to decreased production; causes bleeding. Increased circulating prothrombin may cause increased propensity to clot. INR used to monitor anticoagulation states. INR method for standardizing Protime ratio. Thromboplastin from animal source is compared with human source, giving the International Sensitivity Index (ISI). The PT ratio (measured value/control) is a match with the ISI for the reagent used. The Protime and INR are both reported so that decisions regarding anticoagulation may be made.
VII. Partial Thromboplastin time (PTT) • Reported as activated PTT	NB: <90 sec <Age 20: 39–53 sec Ages 20–60: 35–45 sec >Age 60: 35–45 sec	Screening test for coagulation factors both intrinsic and extrinsic. Prolonged in hemophilia, heparin therapy, liver disease. Shortened in increased activity of clotting factors such as in thrombosis and some malignant tumors.
VIII. Fibrinogen	NB: 150–300 mg/dL <Age 20: 200–400 mg/dL Ages 20–60: 160–300 mg/dL >Age 60: 470–485 mg/dL	Important coagulation factor. A significant decrease may be caused by disseminated intravascular coagulation, liver disease, congenital deficiencies; leads to bleeding disorders. Increased levels occur with trauma, neoplasms and infections. May increase thrombosis in vascular system.

(continued)

UNIT 4 APPENDIX A

Laboratory Studies Useful in Diagnosis of Cardiovascular Disease (Continued)

TEST	NORMAL VALUE	SIGNIFICANCE
IX. Sodium (Na^+)	NB: 126–166 mEq/L <Age 20: 138–146 mEq/L Ages 20–60: 136–145 mEq/L >Age 60: 134–147 mEq/L	Sodium is essential cation in normal cardiac function. Increased levels occur in dehydration and lead to hemoconcentration and changes on serum osmolality. Decreased levels occur in sodium loss due to diarrhea and vomiting, diuretic use endocrine disorders. Often associated with water excess such as with liver disease, congestive failure. Sodium and water overload lead to increased plasma volume and increased preload.
X. Potassium (K^+)	NB: 5.0–7.7 mEq/L <Age 10: 3.5–4.7 mEq/L Ages 10–20: 3.4–5.6 mEq/L Ages 20–60: 3.5–5.5 mEq/L >Age 60: Males: 3.5–5.6 mEq/L Females: 3.5–5.2 mEq/L	Potassium is essential in electrophysiology of the heart. Hypokalemia commonly occurs with loss of GI fluids, diuresis, ketoacidosis, and with lack of intake. Cell membrane becomes less excitable; muscle weakness results. Hyperkalemia mainly results with renal insufficiency; may be seen temporarily with excess intravenous administration of K^+ or hemolysis of RBCs. Causes increased irritability of cell membranes and significant cardiac dysrythmias.
XI. Calcium (Ca^{++}) (total serum)	NB: 6.2–11 mg/dL <12 years: 8.8–10.8 mg/dL Ages 12–60: 8.4–10.2 mg/dL >Age 60: 8.8–10 mg/dL	Calcium levels necessary for bone structure, blood coagulation, muscle contraction, nerve impulse transmission, and enzyme activation. Increased levels caused by bony destruction (invasive bone disease), disuse atrophy of bone, conditions of increased concentrations of serum proteins, and hyperparathyroidism. May cause neurologic changes, renal stones, increased fatiguability. Decreased levels occur in hypoalbuminemia, osteoblastic bone conditions, decreased ingestion, hypoparathyroidism; cause increased muscle tone and irritability, increased neuromuscular activity, bronchospasm.
XII. Magnesium	NB: 1.4–2.9 mEq/L <Age 20: 1.6–2.6 mEq/L Ages 20–60: 1.5–1.95 mEq/L >Age 60: 1.5–1.95 mEq/L	Magnesium is critical in many intracellular functions and activates many enzyme systems. Increased levels due to renal insufficiency, or with over administration of magnesium-containing substances; causes vasodilatation, drowsiness, muscle weakness. Decreased levels may be seen with cirrhosis, pancreatitis, malabsorption, diuretic therapy, alcoholism, and decreased albumin. May cause weakness, tremor, dizziness, convulsions, and confusion.
XIII. Cholesterol*	*Total* NB: 50–100 mg/dL <Age 10: 110–200 mg/dL Ages 10–30: 120–220 mg/dL Ages 30–60: 130–240 mg/dL >Age 60: 130–140 mg/dL	Cholesterol is a fat (lipid)-related fatty acid that is synthesized by the body and ingested in the diet. It cannot be used for energy but is important in maintaining cell membranes and in producing steroid hormones. Levels are decreased in malnutrition, hepatic disease, hyperthyroidism, and some cancers. Increased levels are related to diet, genetic predisposition, hypothyroidism, and possibly other hormone problems. May lead to increased atherosclerosis and arterial obstruction of coronary arteries and other major arteries.

(continued)

UNIT 4 APPENDIX A

Laboratory Studies Useful in Diagnosis of Cardiovascular Disease (Continued)

TEST	NORMAL VALUE	SIGNIFICANCE
	Low density lipoprotein (LDL) NB: 20–60 mg/dL <Age 20: 60–140 mg/dL Age 20–60: 70–200 mg/dL >Age 60: 90–200 mg/dL	LDL form carries most atherogenic cholesterol. Increased levels are directly related to onset and severity of atherosclerosis.
	High density lipoprotein (HDL) NB: 0–60 mg/dL <Age 20: 35–75 mg/dL Ages 20–60: 35–90 mg/dL >Age 60: 35–90 mg/dL	HDL form of cholesterol protects against and prevents atherosclerosis. Increased levels are induced with regular exercise.

* All values approximate and variable with diet and lifestyle changes.

UNIT 4 APPENDIX B

Serum Enzymes and Protein Markers

TEST	NORMAL VALUE	SIGNIFICANCE
I. Creatine kinase (creatinine phosphokinase, CPK) Isoenzymes: CK - BB CK - MM CK - MB	Total: NB: 65–180 IU/L Adult Males: 10–190 IU/L Females: 8–150 IU/L CK - BB 0% total CK - MM 94–100% total CK MB 0–6% total	Enzymes are found in high concentrations in skeletal, heart, and cerebral cortex. Increased levels indicate damage to one of these areas. Normal levels usually reflect only skeletal muscle. Total CPK is markedly increased by trauma, intramuscular injections, certain drugs, exercise, surgery, and pregnancy. CK - MM reflected by total CPK. CK - MB rises within 4–6 hours after acute MI,* peaks in 18–24 hours, returns to normal within 72 hours. Correlates well with extent of infarction.
II. Troponin I and Troponin T	Troponin I: negative Troponin T: negative.	Proteins are found in myofibrils; highly specific for cardiac muscle damage. They are not found in skeletal muscle. Troponin I can be detected within 4 hours after MI and may remain elevated for 1–2 weeks. Troponin T detects smaller amounts of damage and may remain elevated for up to 1 week.
III. Myoglobin	Serum, all ages: 0–90 ng/mL Urine, all ages: Negative	Levels of this globin complex (found in muscle tissue) increase with cardiac and skeletal muscle damage. May also be elevated with high fevers, diabetic ketoacidosis, and familial myoglobinuria. Excreted by urine when in excess amounts in plasma. First elevates after MI in 2–3 hours, peaks in 2–4 hours, remains elevated for 72 hours or longer.
IV. Lactic dehydrogenase (LDH)	Total: NB: 300–1500 IU/L <Age 20: 50–150 IU/L Ages 20–60: 100–190 IU/L >Age 60: 100–190 IU/L Isoenzymes LDH_1: 14–26% LDH_2: 27–37% LDH_3: 13–26% LDH_4: 8–16% LDH_5: 6–16%	Levels of LDH are elevated in cardiac, RBC pulmonary, liver, skeletal muscle, and other organ damage. The isoenzyme LD_1 is primarily found in heart and RBCs, elevates in MI and anemia, and remains elevated for 1 week or longer. This test is primarily used for noncardiac causes. LDH_1 found in heart, RBCs, kidneys, brain. LDH_2 found in heart, RBCs, kidneys, brain. LDH_3 found in lungs, spleen, pancreas, adrenals, thyroid, lymphatic, heart. LDH_4 found in liver, skeletal muscle, kidneys, brain. LDH_5 found in liver, skeletal muscle, kidneys.

* May be detected as early as 1 hour.

UNIT 4 APPENDIX C

Noninvasive and Invasive Diagnostic Tests

TEST	PURPOSE	SIGNIFICANCE
I. Chest x-ray	Noninvasive test Used to evaluate cardiac size and configuration; pleural or pericardial effusion, or intrapulmonic congestion. Pulmonary vasculature can be assessed for size, which reflects blood flow.	Right or left ventricular or atrial dilatation may indicate heart failure or other cardiac problems. Pulmonary congestion may indicate pulmonary edema or pulmonary infections. Pericardial effusion may be seen with enlargement of cardiac shadow. Pleural effusion usually seen at bases of lungs.
II. Echocardiography	Noninvasive test Ultra sound used to examine the heart with high-frequency sound that creates an image of the heart by using pulsed, reflected sound. Signal or echo locates the dynamically moving heart and produces wavy lines on recording. M-mode study, two-dimensional study and Doppler are forms.	Useful test in assessing ejection fraction, segmental wall motion, systolic and diastolic ventricular volumes, mural thrombi or atrial masses, mitral valve prolapse, pericardial effusion, congenital heart defects. M-mode evaluates motion of different parts of the heart, which can be watched or recorded on paper. Two-dimensional (2-D) produces a series of brightness dots that give a motion-picture like scan of heart valves. Doppler (Continuous wave Doppler) gives essential information about blood flow; which adds to M-mode and 2-D information about cardiac structure and movement. Direction of blood flow can be assessed by measuring echoes reflected from RBCs. Audio signals yield information about high speed jets of blood and can determine pressure gradients. Transesophageal echocardiography (TEE) views the heart through a transducer placed at the end of an endoscope in the esophagus. Especially effective in viewing left atrium, mitral valve, and aorta. Coronary arteries can be viewed to detect stenosis, atherosclerosis, and congenital abnormalities.
III. Phonocardiography	Noninvasive test Transducer is placed on various areas of chest wall to record heart sounds simultaneously with electrocardiographic tracing.	Test rarely used but allows precise timing of cardiac events and helps to visualize heart sounds heard with a stethoscope. May be used to record carotid, venous, and apical precordial pulsations.
IV. Radionuclide imaging	Noninvasive tests except for administration of radiotracers. Used to provide information about cardiac pathology.	Test results are analyzed for (1) perfusion defects—"cold spots"—or (2) localization of radiotracer in a damaged area—"hot spot" imaging.
A. Myocardial perfusion imaging (MPI)	Radioisotopes are used and the distribution is projected on a screen. Test is performed with exercise to compare uptake during exercise and at rest. A. Two basic techniques: 1. Planar imaging places camera over heart in several views. 2. Single photon emission computed tomography (SPECT) obtains data from multiple views similar to computed tomography (CT).	Perfusion defects are areas of decreased tracer uptake. If this occurs during exercise and returns to even distribution at rest, it is called a *reversible perfusion defect.* If it is a constant defect, it is called a *fixed perfusion defect.* The reversible type is found in persons with onset of ischemia (angina) during exercise. The fixed defect may be due to the presence of an existing MI. "Hot spot" imaging involves the used of a radiotracer, T_c-pyrophosphate (PYP),

(continued)

UNIT 4 APPENDIX C

Noninvasive and Invasive Diagnostic Tests (Continued)

TEST	PURPOSE	SIGNIFICANCE
	B. Two main radionuclides used: technetium – 99m (T_c) and thallium 201 (Tl).	which binds to calcium released from necrotic cells in acute MI. This imaging is done only in cases in which the serum enzymes are not diagnostic.
B. Gated blood pool imaging (GBPI)	Procedure used to assess left and right ventricular function by the change in volume of the chamber during the cardiac cycle. When a radioactive tracer is mixed in the blood, the counts from the chamber are proportional to the volume of blood in the chamber. The radionuclide used is T_c pyrophosphate.	Good procedure for assessing global left ventricular function and ejection fraction. Used for assessing persons with ischemic heart disease and intracardiac shunts in congenital heart disease.
V. Positron emission tomography (PET)	Procedure exceeds the capability of SPECT. Pharmacologic stress agents, dipyridamole and adenosine, evoke hyperemic responses. Measures regional myocardial blood flow.	Extremely accurate for detecting coronary artery disease (CAD) Can evaluate the effects of CAD on regional myocardial tissue function.
VI. Magnetic resonance imaging (MRI)	Procedure used to visualize the heart and great vessels. Acquires images noninvasively without interference from bone or soft tissues.	Used to assess cardiac anatomy and physiology, ventricular and valvular function, pericardial integrity, and for vascular imaging. Can denote wall thickness, location and extent of masses, thrombi, and congenital heart disease.
VII. Doppler studies	Use ultrasound waves to evaluate systemic flow. Can be used to determine direction and velocity of blood flow and establish patency of peripheral arteries and veins.	Useful in peripheral arterial occlusive diseases and in venous thrombosis. Can be used in congenital conditions such as arteriovenous malformation and patent ductus arteriosus.
VIII. Coronary arteriography	An invasive procedure that is performed by placing a catheter into the femoral artery and passing it retrograde to the right or left main coronary arteries. The arteries are injected with radio-opaque dye and the filling image is recorded on film.	Procedure specifically performed to evaluate CAD. It localizes lesions in specific coronary arteries and their branches. It also outlines any collateral circulation that has developed.
IX. Right and left heart catheterization	Right heart catheterization: Procedure is invasive and involves cannulating the veins leading to the right heart and injecting a dye to measure intracardiac and intravascular pressures. Cardiac output, ejection fraction, and oxygen saturations are measured. Left heart catheterization: Procedure often performed with coronary arteriography to measure left heart pressures and ejection fraction.	Right heart catheterization is useful for evaluating congenital heart diseases (location of defect and size of any shunts) and congestive heart failure. Left heart catheterization is often performed to evaluate value defects and left heart failure.
X. Angiography	General term used to refer to injection of vessels with contrast material. *Arteriography* is injection of an artery to determine patency. *Venography* is injection of any vein to determine patency.	Arteriography is used to outline atherosclerotic or other obstructive diseases of any artery. Venography is used to localize venous thrombosis.

UNIT BIBLIOGRAPHY

American Heart Association. (1998). *AHA guide to heart attack treatment, recovery, and prevention.* Dallas: AHA.

Aronow, W. S, Stemmer, E. A., Wilson, S. E. (1997). *Vascular disease of the elderly.* Armonk, NY: Futura Publishing.

Bharati, S. & Lev, M. (1996). *The pathology of congenital heart disease.* Armonk, NY: Futura Publishing.

Bloom, S., Lie, J. T. & Silver, MD. (1997). *Diagnostic criteria for cardiovascular pathology: Acquired disease.* Philadelphia: Lippincott.

Braunwald, E. (Ed.) (1997). *Heart disease: A textbook of cardiovascular medicine* (5th ed.). Philadelphia: Saunders.

Carabello, B. A. & Crowford, F. A. (1997). Valvular heart disease. *New England Journal of Medicine, 337,* 32.

Cotran, R. S., Kumar, V., & Collins, T. (1999). *Robbin's pathologic basis of disease* (6th ed.). Philadelphia: Saunders.

Damjanov, I. & Linder, J. (Eds.) (1996). *Anderson's pathology* (10th ed.). St. Louis: Mosby.

DeMello, W. C., & Janse, M. J. (1998). *Heart cell communication in health and disease.* Boston: Kluwer Academic Press.

Devereux, R. B. (1995). Recent developments in the diagnosis and management of mitral prolapse. *Current Opinion in Cardiology, 10,* 107–116.

Drzewiecki, J. K. (1998). *Analysis and assessment of cardiovascular function.* New York: Springer Verlag.

Folkman, J., & D'Amore, P. A. (1996). Blood vessel formation: what is its molecular basis? *Cell, 87,* 1153.

Froelicher, V. F. & Quagletti, S. (1997). *Handbook of ambulatory cardiology.* Philadelphia: Lippincott-Raven.

Frolich, E. D. (1998). *Hypertension: Evaluation and treatment.* Baltimore: Williams & Wilkins.

Goldstein, D. S. (1995). *Stress, catecholamines, and cardiovascular diseases.* New York: Oxford University Press.

Gotto, A. M. (1997). Cholesterol management in theory and practice. *Circulation, 96,* 4424.

Gotto, A. M. (1995). *Multiple risk factors in cardiovascular disease.* Boxton: Kluwer Academic.

Grossman, W. (1992). Diastolic dysfunction in congestive heart failure. *New England Journal of Medicine, 325,* 1552.

Halliday, A. (1998). *An introduction to vascular biology.* New York: Cambridge University Press.

Hansson, L, & Birkenhager, W. H. (1997). *Assessment of hypertensive organ damage.* New York: Elsevier.

Hollenberg, N. K. (1998). *Hypertension: Mechanisms and therapy* (2nd ed.). Philadelphia: Current Medicine.

Hu, F. B. et al. (1997). Dietary fat intake and the risk of coronary heart disease in women. *New England Journal of Medicine, 337,* 1491.

Iskandrian, A. E. & Verani, M. S. (1997). *New developments in cardiac nuclear imaging.* Armonk, NY: Futura Publishing.

Kaiser, F. E., Morley, J. E., & Coe, R. M. (1997). *Cardiovascular disease in older people.* New York: Springer.

Kaplan, N. M. (1998). *Clinical hypertension* (7th ed.). Baltimore: Williams & Wilkins.

Kushwaha, S. S., Fallon, J. T, & Fuster, V. (1997). Restrictive cardiomyopathy. *New England Journal of Medicine, 336,* 267–276.

LaBarthe, D. R. (1998). *Epidemiology and prevention of cardiovascular diseases: A global challenge.* Gaithersburg, MD: Aspen.

Marks, A. R., & Taubman, M. B. (1997). *Molecular biology of cardiovascular diseases.* New York: Marcel Dekker.

Mercuri, M. (1998). *Noninvasive imaging of atherosclerosis.* Boston: Kluwer Academic Press.

Narula, J. et al. (1996). Apoptosis in myocytes in end-stage heart failure. *New England Journal of Medicine, 335,* 1182.

Opie, L. H. (1998). *The heart: Physiology from cell to circulation* (3rd ed.). Philadelphia: Lippincott-Raven.

Richardson, D. R., Randall, D. C. & Speck, D. F. (1998). *Cardiopulmonary system.* Madison, CT: Fence Creek.

Rubin, E. & Farber, J. L. (1999). *Pathology* (3rd ed.). Philadelphia: Lippincott.

Schoen, F. J. & Gimbrone, M. A. (Eds). (1995). *Cardiovascular pathology: Clinicopathologic correlations and pathogenetic mechanisms,* Baltimore: Williams & Wilkins.

Silver, M. D. (1996). *Cardiovascular pathology* (2nd ed.). New York: Churchill Livingstone.

Steinberg, D. (1997). Oxidative modification of LDL and atherogenesis. *Circulation, 95,* 1062.

Svennsson, L. G. & Crawford, E. S. (1997). *Cardiovascular and vascular disease of the aorta.* Philadelphia: Saunders.

Thun, J. et al. (1997). Alcohol consumption and mortality among middle-aged and elderly U. S. adults. *New England Journal of Medicine, 337,* 1705.

Topol, E. (1998). *Textbook of cardiovascular medicine.* Philadelphia: Lippincott-Raven.

Zanchetti, A. (1997). *Hypertension and the heart, vol. 18.* New York: Plenum Press.

Zanchetti, A. & Mancia, G. (1997). *Pathophysiology of hypertension, vol. 17.* New York: Elsevier.

ON-LINE REFERENCES

Ask NOAH: Heart Disease and Stroke—www.noah.cuny.edu/heart disease/heartdisease.html

Congenital Heart Disease Web Ring—www.webring.org/cgi-bin/webring?ring=little hearts-&list

Heart and Stroke A–Z Guide—www.amhrt.org/Heart and Stroke A Z Guide/

Heart Failure Online—www.heartfailure.org/

Heart Information Network—www.heartinfo.org/

Live Healthier, Live Longer—rover.nhlbi.nih.gov/chd/

PediHeart—www.pediheart.org/

Yale University School of Medicine Heart Book—www.med.yale.edu/library/heartbk/

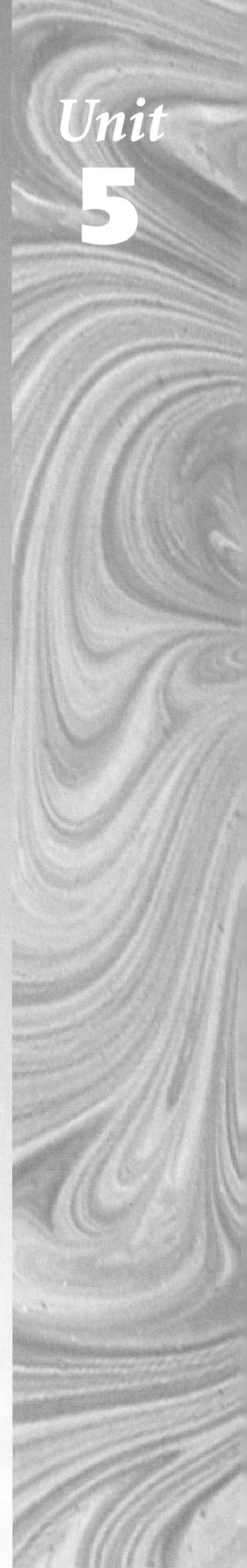

Pulmonary Function

FOCUS ON
Pulmonary Changes Through the Life Span

INFANT (1–12 MONTHS):

Chest wall is round with A-P dimensions equal. Upper respiratory tract is delicate with decreased resistance against infectious agents. Infections rapidly spread from throat and bronchi to ears. Respiratory rate is increased to increase gas exchange through developing alveolar surfaces.

TODDLER AND PRESCHOOL AGE (1–5 YEARS):

Respiratory rate declines to 20–30/minute. Lung volumes improve as lung fields mature. There is increased susceptibility to sinus and bronchial infections.

SCHOOL AGE (6–12 YEARS):

Breathing becomes deeper and slower. Chest broadens and flattens, assumes an adult-type configuration. Lung weight increases 10 times from birth.

ADOLESCENCE (13–19 YEARS):

Lungs grow slowly relative to growth of body. Respiratory rate slows to 16–20/minute. Inadequate oxygen may be available for body growth, which may contribute to "growing pains." Lungs are mature size by age 17 to 18.

YOUNG ADULT AND ADULT (20–45 YEARS):

Maximal breathing capacity exists until age 30. Breathing deeper and slower at rates of 12–20/minute. Declines in lung volumes begin to occur beyond age 30. Lung increases its weight 20 times from birth.

MIDDLE AGED ADULT (46–64 YEARS):

Lungs become less elastic and exhibit less compliance, especially after age 50. The thorax shortens, and the chest cage becomes stiffer. Exercise tolerance declines and may decrease up to 75% of normal, especially if there is associated smoking behavior.

LATE ADULTHOOD (65–100+ YEARS):

Compliance decreases significantly and the chest wall stiffens. Respiratory muscles function less effectively. Vital capacity decreases to 50–65% of age 30. Cough reflex is less effective in clearing the airway. Air trapping and alveolar size increase.

Chapter

19

Normal Pulmonary Function

Lynda Mackin / Barbara L. Bullock

KEY TERMS

acinus
airway resistance
alpha 1-antitrypsin
alveolar-capillary membrane
alveolar dead space
alveolar ventilation
anatomic dead space
bronchoconstriction
Brownian movement
carbaminohemoglobin
chemoreceptors
collateral ventilation
compliance
conducting airways
critical oxygen tension
elastance
hemoglobin
Hering-Breuer reflex
hydrogen hemoglobin
intrapleural pressure
intrapulmonic pressure
laminar flow
mediastinum
mucociliary escalator system
net bacterial lung clearance
oxyhemoglobin
oxyhemoglobin dissociation curve
perfusion
pores of Kohn
respiratory acidosis
respiratory alkalosis
respiratory zone
shunting
surface tension
surfactant
Starling forces
tidal volume
tissue hypoxia
tissue resistance
turbulent flow
ventilation-perfusion mismatching

To understand the pathophysiologic mechanisms of pulmonary disease, an understanding of normal pulmonary structure and function is needed. This chapter provides an overview of key concepts. The pulmonary system provides for gas exchange through oxygen intake and elimination of carbon dioxide. Multiple complex structures must function in harmony to accomplish this task.

NORMAL STRUCTURE OF THE PULMONARY SYSTEM

The pulmonary system is composed of upper and lower airways surrounded by a protective thoracic cage. The airways serve as a conduit for air transport that terminates in the alveoli, the parenchymal unit of the lungs, across which gas exchange occurs (Fig. 19-1).

Upper Airway

The upper airway is composed of the nose, oral cavity, and pharynx. As inhaled air passes through the nose and mouth and into the pharynx, it is filtered, warmed, and humidified.

NOSE AND PARANASAL SINUSES

The outer parts of the nose are composed of cartilage and bone. Air enters the nose through openings called *nares* or *nostrils.* The nasal septum separates the nose into the right and left sections. Inside the nose, hair follicles called *vibrissae* act as filters for the inspired air. These filters are effective only for large particles; the smaller particles are inhaled more deeply into the lower respiratory structures. Nonciliated stratified squamous epithelium lines the outer one-third of the nasal cavity. The posterior portions are lined with pseudostratified ciliated columnar epithelium. The *turbinates* are bony protrusions in the superior portion of the nasal cavity that serve to separate inhaled air into different air streams and warm and humidify it. There are three turbinates on each side of the nose: the inferior, middle, and superior. Posterior to the turbinates are the *paranasal sinuses.* These air-filled cavities provide mucus for the nose and a site for sound and spoken voice resonance. The paranasal sinuses include the

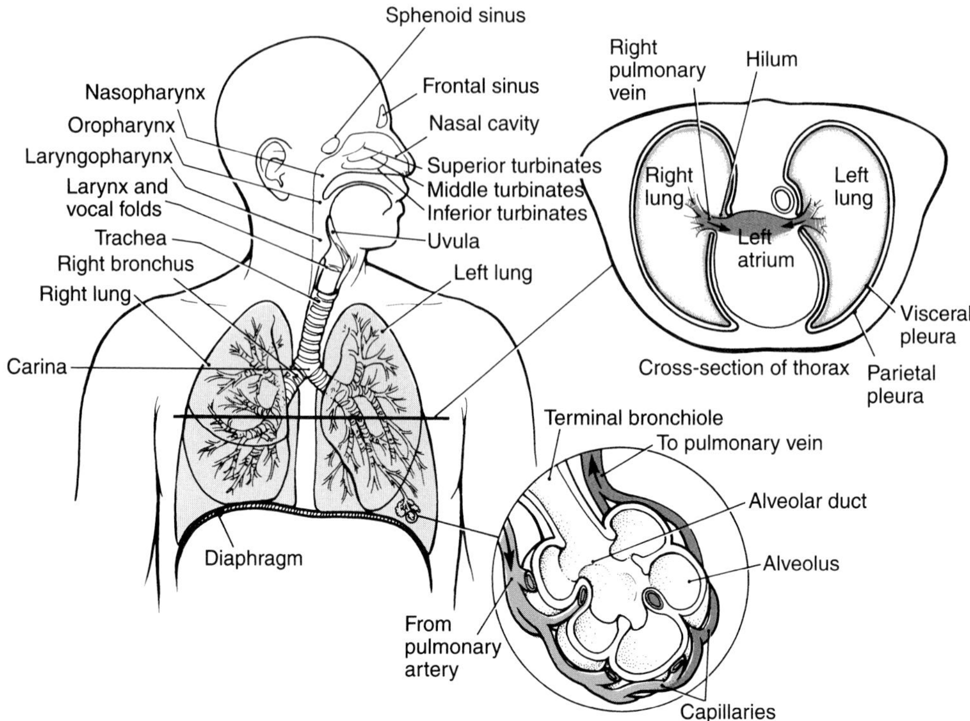

FIGURE 19-1. **The respiratory system.**

maxillary, ethmoid, sphenoid, and frontal sinus cavities. The *olfactory region,* which contains receptors responsible for the sense of smell, is located near the middle and superior turbinates. Figure 19-1 illustrates the location of these upper airway structures.

ORAL CAVITY

The oral cavity is an alternative portal of entry for air into the respiratory tract. It is lined by stratified squamous epithelium with glands that secrete saliva. The outer portion of the oral cavity is called the *vestibule* and consists of the lips, gums, and teeth. The roof of the mouth is composed of the *hard palate* (anterior) and *soft palate* (posterior). The main function of these structures is to move food from the mouth into the esophagus in the process of swallowing. The posterior portion of the oral cavity is bordered by the *palatopharyngeal arch,* the *palatoglossal arch,* and the *palatine tonsil.* The tonsilar structures are composed of lymphoid tissue and play a role in immune defense and protection from foreign matter. The fleshy appendage that hangs down from the soft palate is called the *uvula.*

PHARYNX

The pharynx is composed of the *nasopharynx,* the *oropharynx,* and the *laryngopharynx* (see Fig. 19-1). The entire pharynx serves as a conduit to the lower airways. The nasopharynx is lined with pseudostratified ciliated columnar epithelium. Lymphoid tissues of the nasopharynx include the *pharyngeal tonsils,* or *adenoids,* which are found in the posterior portion of the nasopharynx.

The oropharynx is inferior to the nasopharynx. On the lateral portions of the nasopharynx, bilateral *eustachian tubes* (auditory tubes) are found. The eustachian tubes connect the nasopharynx to the middle ear and allow for pressure equalization between the two areas. The *lingual tonsil* is part of the oropharynx and is located at the base of the tongue. The laryngopharynx is the lower portion of the pharynx near the opening of the larynx. It is superior to the esophagus. Both the oropharynx and laryngopharynx are lined with stratified squamous epithelium.

Lower Airway and Lungs

The lower airway is composed of the larynx, trachea, bronchi, bronchioles, and alveoli (see Fig. 19-1). The branches of the bronchi, bronchioles, and alveoli make up the lungs. The lungs lie in the thoracic cavity, separated from each other by the **mediastinum**. The central portion of the mediastinum where the lung "roots" are found is referred to as the *hili* (or *hilum*). Each lung is a cone-shaped, spongy structure with a narrow end at the top and wide bases at the bottom. The top of the lung is referred to as the *apex* (plural, *apices*) and the bottom of the lung is the *base*. Each lung is composed of lobes: three on the right and two on the left.

Bronchopulmonary segments are structural and functional subdividions of lung lobes. The right and left lung each contain 10 bronchopulmonary segments (Fig. 19-2). The segments are divided into smaller segments and eventually terminate in the alveolar sacs. Gas exchange takes place at the terminal portion of the lower airway.

LARYNX

The larynx, or voice box, is inferior to the base of the tongue and superior to the trachea. It is composed of nine cartilages: thyroid, cricoid, epiglottis (all single cartilages) and arytenoid, corniculate, and cuneiform (all paired cartilages). These cartilages are supported by ligaments, membranes, and extrinsic and intrinsic muscles. The inner surfaces of the larynx are lined with mucous membranes. The *vocal cords* are located in the larynx. The three primary functions of the larynx are to provide a pathway for airflow from the upper airways into the lowers airways; to separate air from food or liquids, thus preventing aspiration; and to serve as a site for resonance of spoken voice.

TRACHEA, BRONCHI, AND BRONCHIOLES

Inhaled air passes through the larynx and into the trachea. The trachea is composed of C-shaped cartilaginous rings that provide firm support. The trachea subdivides at the *carina* into *right* and *left main stem bronchi.*

The bronchi are large, cartilage-containing airways that serve as the central passageway to the right and left lungs, respectively. The right main stem bronchus is shorter and wider than the left, projecting off the trachea more vertically than the left. This explains why aspiration tends to occur more frequently in the right lung.

The right and left main stem bronchi divide into the *lobar bronchi*, which further divide into the *segmental bronchi*. The segmental bronchi then divide into the subsegmental bronchi or *bronchioles*. The bronchioles are further subdivided into *terminal* (non-respiratory) *bronchioles* and subdivide again into *respiratory bronchioles*, which lead to *alveolar ducts* and finally terminate in the *alveolar sacs* (*alveoli*) (Fig. 19-3). The proximal segments, such as the terminal bronchiole, do not participate in gas exchange and are referred to as **conducting airways**. The distal portions of the airway, such as the respiratory bronchioles and alveoli, are where actual gas exchange occurs, so these segments are called the **respiratory zone**.

The diameter of each of these successive segments is smaller than the last, but the number of airways that branch out from each successive segment is greater than that of the previous one. This series of anatomic divisions is called the *generations of bronchi*. By the time the segments have reached the respiratory bronchiole level, there have been 24 generations or subdivisions.

ALVEOLI

The majority of the lung itself is composed of tiny grapelike sacs called alveoli (alveolus, singular). The surfaces of the alveoli are covered with a rich network of pulmonary capillaries and therefore serve as the functional units where gases are exchanged. The *alveolar-capillary interspace* separates the alveolus from the pulmonary capillary (Fig. 19-4).

The alveoli have a volume of about 2500 mL in the adult. There are approximately 300 million alveoli in the lung, thus accounting for a surface area about the size of a tennis court (approximately 70–100 m^2). These alveoli do not have separate connections with the terminal bronchiole but are of various shapes and

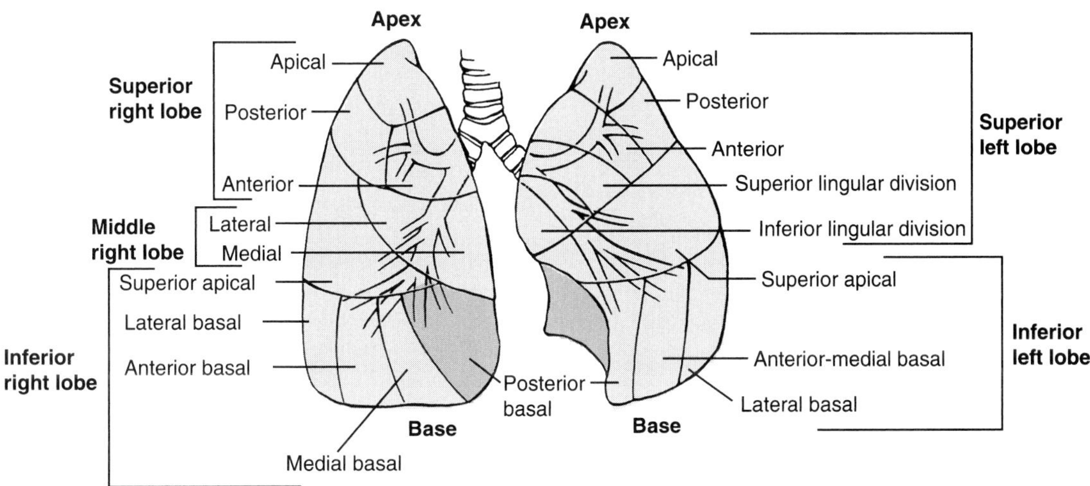

FIGURE 19-2. Bronchopulmonary segments and lobes of the lung.

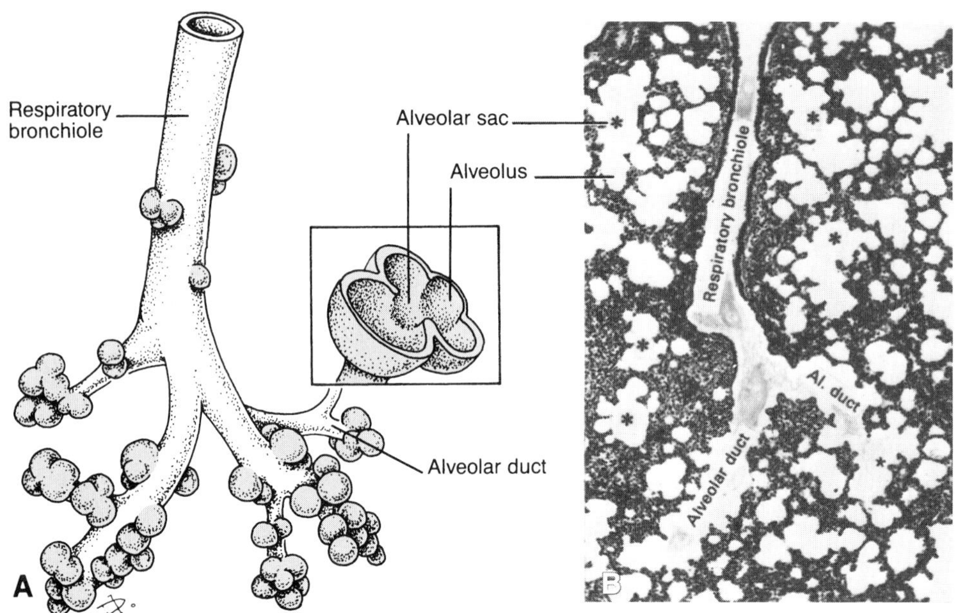

FIGURE 19-3. Schematic diagram **(A)** and low-power view **(B)** of the respiratory bronchiole leading into alveolar ducts (child's lung). *Asterisks* in **B** indicate alveolar sacs. (Cormack, D. H. [1993]. *Essential histology.* Philadelphia: J. B. Lippincott.)

are interconnected, resembling a long corridor with adjacent rooms. Each group of respiratory bronchioles, alveolar ducts, and alveoli is referred to as a *primary lobule* or **acinus.** Each primary lobule is approximately 3.5 cm in size and contains about 2000 alveoli.[2]

FOCUS ON CELLULAR PHYSIOLOGY

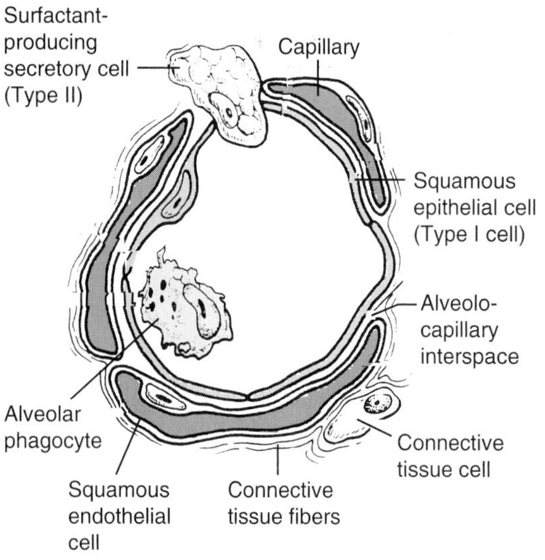

Surfactant-producing secretory cell (Type II)
Capillary
Squamous epithelial cell (Type I cell)
Alveolo-capillary interspace
Alveolar phagocyte
Connective tissue cell
Squamous endothelial cell
Connective tissue fibers

FIGURE 19-4. Representation of a single alveolar-capillary interspace. Note Type I and Type II cells and supporting connective tissue cells and fibers.

Several different cell types compose the alveolar walls. These include squamous epithelial cells (also called Type I cells or *Type I pneumocytes*), surfactant producing secretory cells (Type II cells or *Type II pneumocytes*), and squamous endothelial cells (see Fig. 19-4). Type I cells compose most of the alveolar surface area. The alveolus contains alveolar macrophages. These macrophages play a role in defense against foreign particles or microorganisms.

The connective tissue fibers and cells and gel-like hyaluronic acid molecules that surround and support the alveolar structures are called the *interstitium.* The interstitium also contains neural fibers, lymphatic structures, and water. If necessary, the water-containing capacity can be increased by more than 30% without effecting pressure changes in the lungs.[2]

Small openings between the alveoli are called the **pores of Kohn** (Fig. 19-5). These openings range from 3 to 13 microns in size and allow air to move between adjacent alveoli.[2] Within a second after gas is taken in, all alveoli in an acinus have the same gas concentration. In young children, the pores of Kohn are not as well developed as those of adults. The pores of Kohn provide an alternative ventilatory pathway called **collateral ventilation** when there is obstruction in the small airways.

Substances Important in Maintaining Alveolar Integrity

Two substances are essential for the maintenance of alveolar expansion and integrity of the alveolar mem-

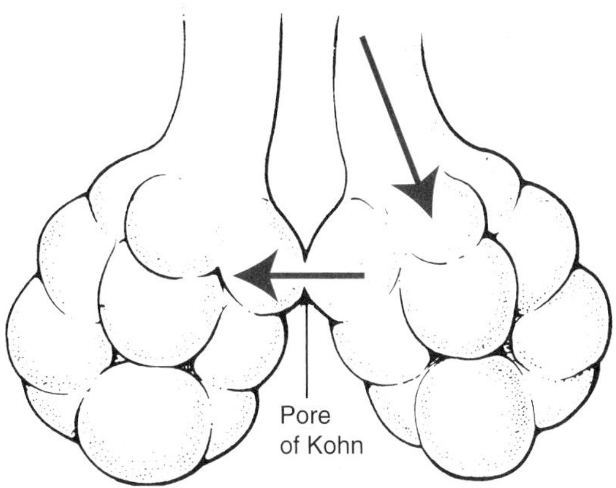

FIGURE 19-5. Interconnecting alveoli through the pore of Kohn.

branes. These substances, **surfactant** and **alpha 1-antitrypsin**, must be present in sufficient quantities to promote alveolar health.

SURFACTANT. When water and air come in contact with each other, the water molecules on the surface have a strong attraction to one another and continually try to contract in size. This characteristic is termed **surface tension**. In the lungs, there are millions of air spaces (alveoli), each with a similar air–liquid interface that, without surfactant and other pulmonary dynamics, would continuously try to contract. Surfactant is a liquid mixture of phospholipids composed primarily of dipalmitoyl phosphatidylcholine (lecithin) and phosphatidylglycol. It is synthesized in the alveolar type II epithelial cells and is secreted to form a film across the alveolar surface. The presence of surfactant within the alveoli acts to lower surface tension and thus prevents collapse of the alveoli.[4]

The volume of surfactant varies according to the diameter of the alveoli itself. As the alveoli inflate, the surfactant spreads out over the surface of the alveolar membrane. As the alveoli empty, the surfactant layer becomes thicker in relation to the decreased space. Smaller alveoli have a thicker layer, whereas larger alveoli have a thinner layer. This promotes expansion and stability of the alveoli.[3]

The surfactant layer must be replenished continually. The half-life of pulmonary lecithin is 14 hours, which suggests that active synthesis must be continuous. Oxygen is also needed for its production. In the event of hypoventilation, there may be alveolar collapse due to a deficiency of surfactant.

Surfactant also functions as a protective, waterproof material that may prevent the movement of fluid across the alveolar-capillary membrane during the respiratory cycle. The absence of surfactant leads to a tendency to pull fluid into the alveoli, which interferes with gas exchange significantly.

ALPHA 1-ANTITRYPSIN. Alpha 1-antitrypsin is a glycoprotein produced by the liver that plays a significant role in the maintenance of the pulmonary tissue. The primary function of alpha 1-antitrypsin is to inhibit natural proteolytic enzymes, such as elastase, collagenase, trypsin, and chymotrypsin, that normally reside in the lung. Deficiency of this enzyme tips the balance in favor of the proteolytic enzymes and leads to excessive tissue destruction.[11]

The Pleura and Pleural Space

A double-layer membrane called the *pleurae* surrounds the lungs. The pleurae provide a cover for the lungs and line the thoracic wall. They are composed of two distinct layers: (1) the *visceral pleurae,* which cover the lung parenchyma, and (2) the *parietal pleurae,* which cover the outside of the lungs and are in contact with the thoracic cage. Between these layers is a small space, called the *pleural space,* which contains serous fluid that allows the layers to move easily and without friction during normal ventilation. The pressure within this space is sub-atmospheric (−5 cm H_20) at rest, and it becomes even more sub-atmospheric (−8 cm H_20) during inspiration. This essential negative pressure is a major factor in maintaining lung expansion (see p. 537).

The Thoracic Cage

The lungs are surrounded and protected by the ribs and connective tissues, which constitute the bony thorax or thoracic cage. Twelve pairs of ribs encircle the lungs and play an integral role in maintaining pressures and tensions that are necessary for normal ventilation. The anterior structures of the thorax are composed of the *manubrium, sternum,* and *xyphoid process* (Fig. 19-6A). The first seven ribs attach to the sternum anteriorly by means of costal cartilage. The eighth, ninth, and ten ribs do not attach to the sternum but, rather, are attached to the costal cartilage of the rib immediately above. The eleventh and twelfth ribs, also called the "floating ribs," do not attach to any anterior structures. Posteriorly, the ribs are connected to the thoracic vertebrae (Fig. 19-6B). The thoracic cage contains the thoracic cavity, which houses the lungs, pleura, and pleural space and mediastinum.

Mediastinum

The mediastinum is an anatomic region or body cavity that is located between the lungs. It is bordered by the sternum anteriorly, by the pleural surfaces of the lung laterally, by the diaphragm inferiorly, and by the thoracic vasculature superiorly. The mediastinum houses

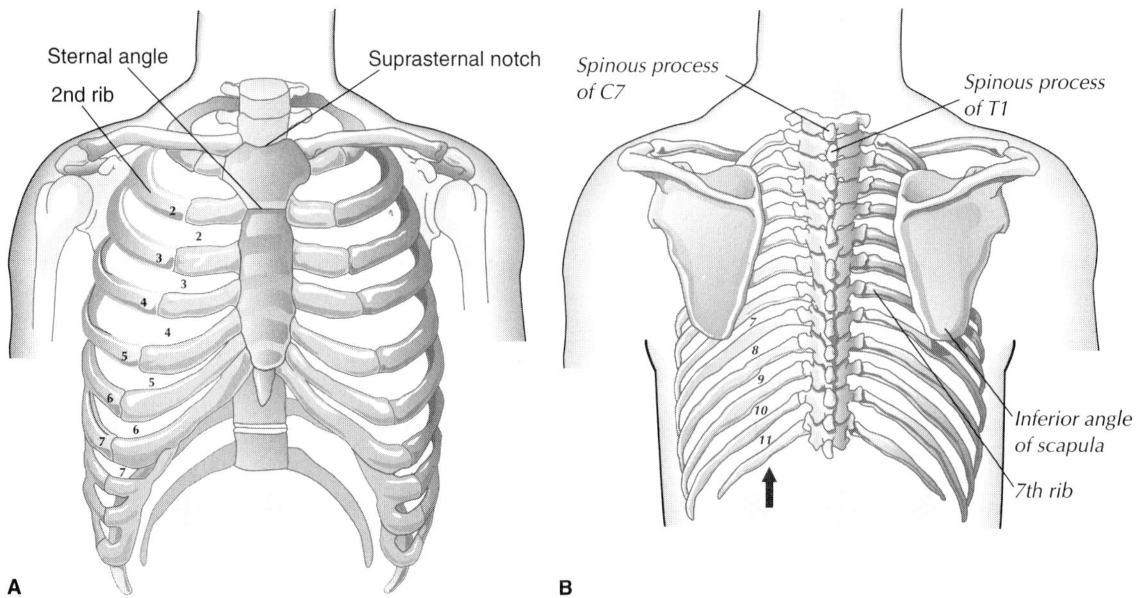

FIGURE 19-6. The bony structures of the chest form a protective expandable cage around the lungs and heart. **A.** Anterior view. **B.** Posterior view.

the trachea, esophagus, heart, pulmonary lymphatics, great blood vessels, and thymus gland.

Respiratory Muscles

The muscles of ventilation can be classified as either inspiratory or expiratory. The diaphragm, external intercostals, and accessory muscles are inspiratory muscles. The abdominal and internal intercostal muscles are expiratory muscles (Fig. 19-7). The act of inspiration is an active process that requires coordinated contraction of the inspiratory muscles. Expiration is normally a passive process, but if expiration is forced, then the expiratory muscles will contract (see below).

INSPIRATORY MUSCLES

The major muscle in the act of breathing is the *diaphragm.* It is divided into halves or hemidiaphragms, which are flat, dome-shaped muscles interconnected by a tendon. These muscles are able to facilitate lung expansion by moving downward during inspiration. Diaphragmatic innervation is via the *phrenic nerve,* which originates mainly from the fourth cervical nerve of the respective thoracic side. During quiet breathing the diaphragm descends approximately 1 cm, but during forced inspiration it can descend by as much as 10 cm. Normal diaphragmatic contraction temporarily compresses the abdominal contents. Consequently, the movement of the diaphragm can be impeded by abnormalities in the abdominal cavity (such as abdominal distension).

The *external intercostal muscles,* located between the ribs, are able to further enlarge the thorax during inspiration by creating an upward and outward motion of the lower ribs. The upper ribs can also move outward. The ribs are attached to the vertebrae in such a way that they rotate on an axis as they are moved by these muscles.

The *scalene* and *sternocleidomastoid muscles,* located in the neck, are called accessory respiratory muscles. They can be used during labored breathing to raise the first two ribs and sternum in an effort to increase the size of the thoracic cavity.

EXPIRATORY MUSCLES

During expiration inspiratory muscles relax, allowing the lungs and chest walls to passively return to their resting size. The pressure in the thorax increases and allows air to move out of the lungs. Forced expiration, however, requires the contraction of the *internal intercostal muscles,* which are located between the ribs, running at opposite angles to the external intercostals.

The muscles of the abdominal wall can be powerful aids to forced expiration. Normally, they are only used to generate the explosive pressure that is necessary for coughing. They can also be used to control the expiratory process during such activities as singing.

Blood Supply of the Pulmonary System

The pulmonary system has two blood supplies: bronchial circulation and pulmonary circulation.

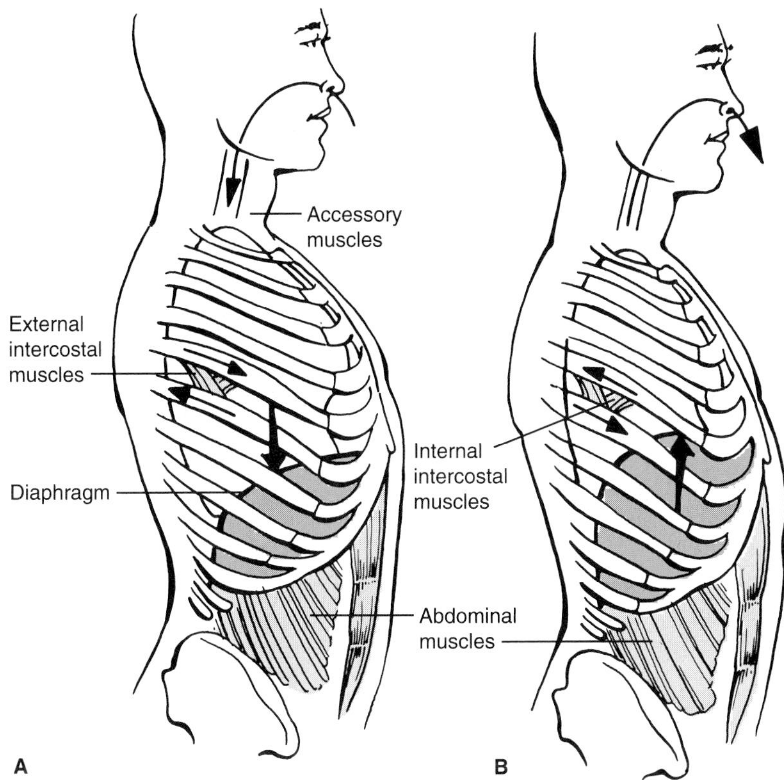

FIGURE 19-7. **Muscles of ventilation. A. Inspiratory muscles. B. Expiratory muscles.**

BRONCHIAL CIRCULATION

Bronchial circulation arises from the thoracic aorta and upper intercostal arteries and consists of a bronchial artery network. Serving as part of the systemic blood supply, these arteries nourish the trachea and bronchi to the level of the respiratory bronchioles. After forming capillary plexuses, this bronchial circulation returns through a pulmonary vein to the left atrium. Bronchial blood flow amounts to about 1% to 2% of the total cardiac output.[4]

The bronchial circulation supplies the lung's supporting tissues, its nerves, and the outer layers of the pulmonary arteries and veins. Normally, it does not supply the respiratory bronchioles, alveolar ducts, or alveolar walls. In the event of interruption of the pulmonary circulation, the bronchial circulation can support the metabolic needs of these tissues, but the affected tissues lose their ability to participate in gas exchange.

PULMONARY CIRCULATION

The pulmonary circulation provides blood flow, which is called **perfusion**, to the **alveolar-capillary membrane**. Normally the pulmonary artery delivers the entire output of the right ventricle to the lungs. This stroke volume is approximately 70 mL of blood with each heartbeat. This volume is spread over the surface area of the lung (70 m^2), which allows for rapid diffusion of gases. Blood circulates through the small pulmonary capillaries that make up the pulmonary capillary bed (PCB). After it circulates through the PCB, oxygenated blood is returned to the left heart by way of the pulmonary veins (Fig. 19-8). In addition to delivering blood to the alveolar-capillary membrane for gas exchange, the pulmonary circulation also provides a reservoir for blood, filters small thrombi, and traps white blood cells.

The pulmonary circulation is a low-pressure system with pressures much lower than those in the systemic circulation. The normal mean pulmonary artery pressure is 14 mm Hg. Because the mean left atrial pressure of the heart is about 5 mm Hg, the driving pressure across the pulmonary bed is only about 9 mm Hg.

RECRUITMENT. Approximately 10% to 20% of the total blood volume stays in the pulmonary vascular bed at any given time. The pulmonary circulation is capable of accepting several times this amount, which allows it to accommodate variations in cardiac output or blood volume. The distensibility of the bed is accomplished both by dilating pulmonary vessels and by opening closed or unused vessels. This is called *recruitment*. Dis-

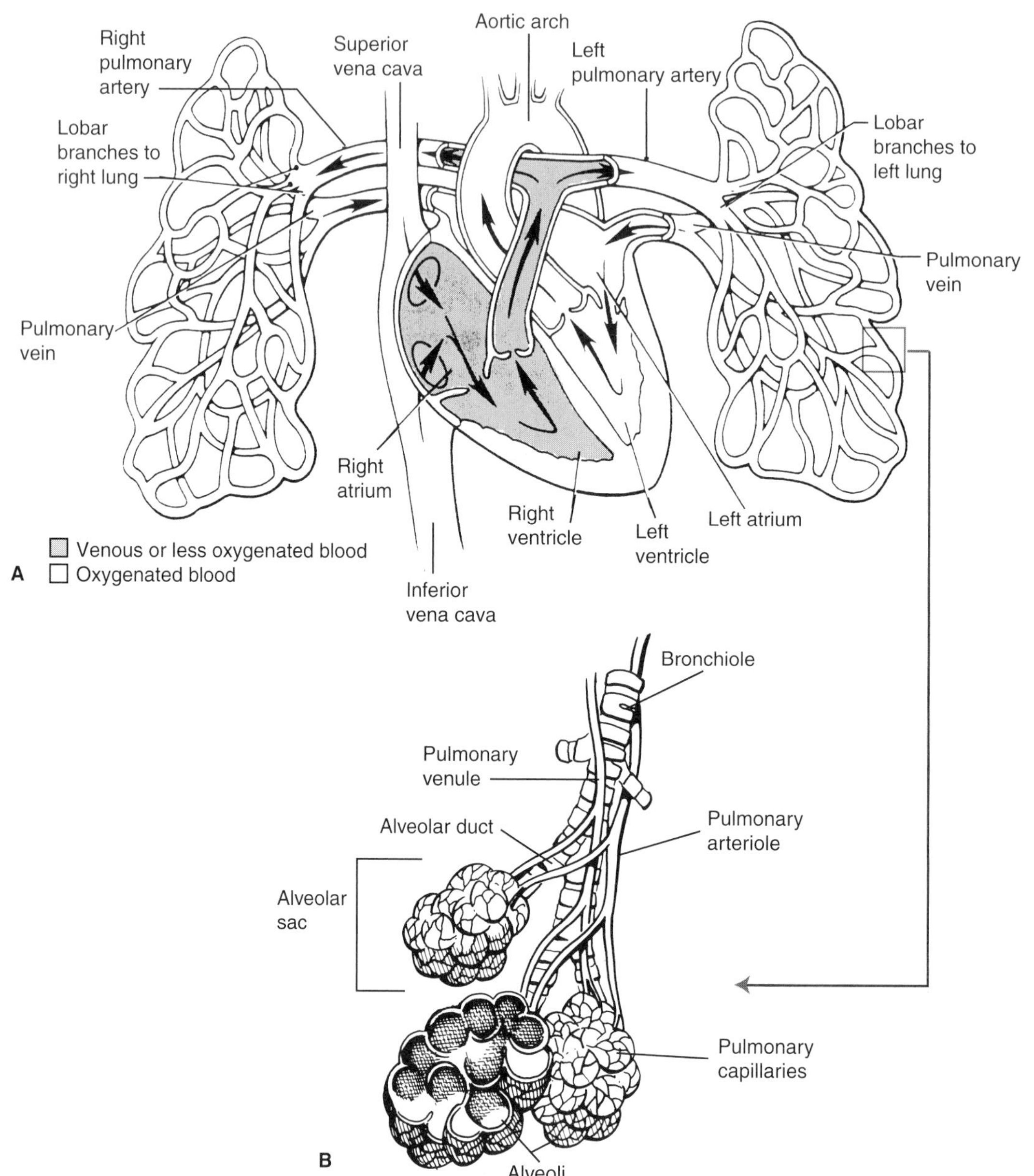

FIGURE 19-8. **A.** Circulation from the right heart to the lungs to the left heart. **B.** Pulmonary arterioles, capillaries, and venules at the bronchioles and alveolar sacs.

tension of the pulmonary vascular bed reduces pulmonary vascular resistance until its capacity is reached. This ability to accommodate large amounts of blood flow during exercise, for example, helps to prevent a significant rise in pulmonary capillary pressure.[4]

Lymphatic Drainage

Lymphatic drainage in the lungs is extensive, extending from all of the supportive tissues of the lungs and terminating mainly in the right lymphatic duct. Drainage is through superficial and deep plexuses. Larger lymphatic vessels lead to lymph nodes, which filter potentially harmful particles from lymph before it is returned to the blood stream through the collecting ducts. In the thoracic cavity, the lymph nodes are found within the mediastinum and along the trachea and bronchi.[9]

Nervous Control of the Pulmonary System

The major nerve supply to the diaphragm is through the two *phrenic nerves*, which supply each half of the diaphragm separately. The 11th cranial nerve, also known as the *accessory*, innervates most of the larynx and pharynx. The trachea is supplied by branches of the vagus nerve, as well as the recurrent laryngeal nerves and the sympathetic trunks. Several cranial nerves are involved with nervous control to the nose and oral cavity. These include the first pair (the *olfactory*), the fifth pair (the *trigeminal*), the seventh pair (the *facial*), the ninth pair (the *glossopharyngeal*), and the tenth pair (the *vagi*) (see p. 908). Sensory pain fibers are also diffuse in these areas.

Autonomic nerve fibers transmit to and from the lungs through pulmonary plexuses at the root of each lung. The plexuses contain branches of sympathetic trunks as well as parasympathetic fibers from the vagus nerve. Bronchial smooth muscle wraps around the bronchi and is innervated by both the sympathetic and parasympathetic nervous systems. Increased parasympathetic (vagal) activity promotes bronchoconstriction, whereas increased sympathetic stimulation results in bronchodilation.

Intercostal nerves from the thoracic cord region innervate the intercostal muscles of respiration. The parietal pleura is supplied by the intercostal nerves and phrenic nerves. The visceral pleura is supplied through the pulmonary plexus.

RESPIRATORY CENTERS

The respiratory centers, located in the medulla, the pons, and the peripheral arteries, adjust **alveolar ventilation** according to the demands of the body. Their location is illustrated in Figure 19-9, and their function is described below.

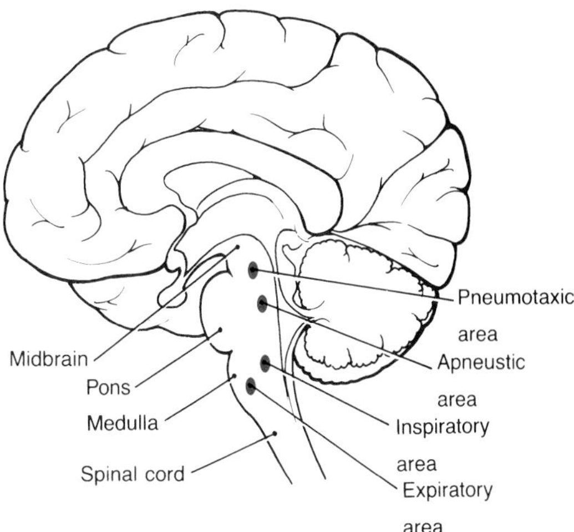

FIGURE 19-9. **Location of respiratory centers.**

NORMAL FUNCTION OF THE PULMONARY SYSTEM

The pulmonary system is responsible for gas ex-change, which is accomplished through ventilation and gas transport. In harmony with the circulatory system, it provides for exchange of oxygen and car-bon dioxide in the systemic tissues. The system has critical importance in acid-base balance and in immune defense.

Ventilation

Gas exchange requires the movement of gases into and out of the lungs. Various control mechanisms and forces interplay in the two phases of ventilation: inspiration and expiration. Inspiration is the process of moving air into the lungs; expiration moves it out.

VENTILATORY CONTROL MECHANISMS

Control of ventilation is through central and peripheral receptors that relay messages to the nervous system. The central receptors are found mainly in the medulla oblongata and pons, whereas the peripheral receptors are found in the aortic arch and internal carotid arteries. Conscious control of ventilation is exerted through cerebral cortex overriding of the normal breathing pattern, which accounts for breath holding and reactions to various external stimuli.

Central Respiratory Centers Affecting Ventilation

The nervous system makes adjustments in alveolar ventilation according to physiologic demands. This is coordinated and controlled through the respiratory centers located in the medulla oblongata and the pons (see Fig. 19-9). On the basis of information received from various receptors, these centers send messages to the respiratory muscles, stimulating them to contract or relax. Within the respiratory centers, there are four distinct groups of neurons:[2]

- *Dorsal respiratory group* (DRG): Found in medulla; sets basic automatic rhythm of respiration; sends signals to diaphragm and inspiratory intercostal muscles; receives message from peripheral chemoreceptors, baroreceptors (pressure receptors), and various lung receptors

- *Ventral respiratory group* (VRG): Located in medulla; inactive during quiet breathing; becomes active when ventilatory demands are increased; can affect inspiration and expiration
- *Pneumotaxic center*: Located in upper pons; limits respiration by modifying inspiratory rate and depth
- *Apneustic center*: Located in lower pons; function thought to be associated with the pneumotaxic center to control the depth of inspiration

Central Chemoreceptors

Respiratory neurons located in the medulla oblongata are chemosensitive structures and thus are called **chemoreceptors**. These receptors, through their sensitivity to carbon dioxide, provide the majority of control over ventilation. Carbon dioxide diffuses across the blood–brain barrier, combining with water to form carbonic acid (H_2CO_3) which then quickly dissociates into bicarbonate (HCO_3^-) and a hydrogen ion (H^+). These receptors detect changes in hydrogen ion concentrations in the cerebrospinal fluid.[4] Even a very small derivation from normal results in stimulation of the respiratory center to increase rate and depth of ventilation when hydrogen ion concentrations are high, or to depress ventilation if hydrogen ions concentrations are low.[5]

Peripheral Chemoreceptors and Baroreceptors Affecting Ventilation

Peripheral chemoreceptors, located in the carotid bodies at the bifurcations of the common carotid arteries and aortic bodies at the arch of the aorta, monitor arterial oxygen, carbon dioxide and pH levels (Fig. 19-10). They are sensitive to decreased oxygen tension levels, which when detected cause a message to be sent to the respiratory center. This center then stimulates an increase in ventilation.[4] If the carbon dioxide level is also increased, this will serve as an even stronger stimulus.

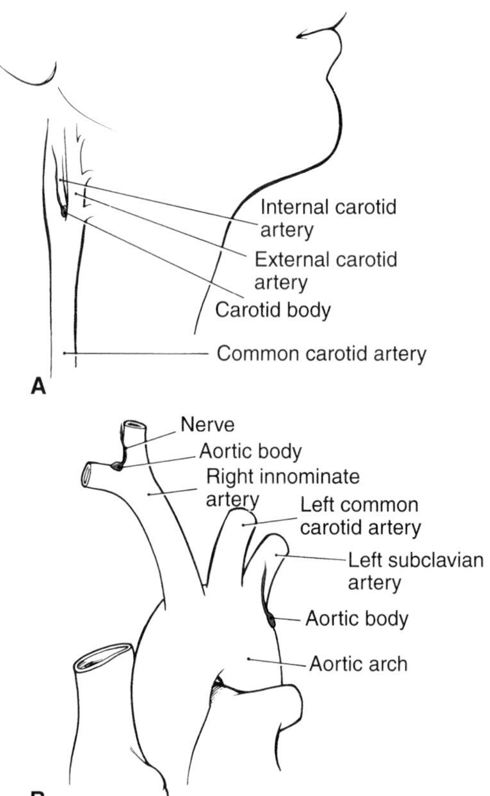

FIGURE 19-10. **Location of peripheral chemoreceptors in (A) carotid sinus area and (B) aortic arch area.**

Inflation Reflex

If the lung becomes over-stretched, the **Hering-Breuer reflex** is activated and a feedback signal inhibits further inspiration. This very important reflex serves to regulate the depth of breathing by limiting lung inflation. The stretch receptors in the pleura, bronchioles, and alveoli travel through the vagus nerves to the pneumotaxic area, which shortens the duration of inspiration.[9]

LUNG MECHANICS ASSOCIATED WITH VENTILATION

Normal gas exchange is dependent on how effectively gases move into and out of the body. The lung mechanics that accomplish this are dependent upon several factors: **compliance**, **elastance**, inspiratory and expiratory lung pressures, **airway** and **tissue resistance**, and the work of breathing. Pulmonary function testing is used to measure lung volume, flow rates, and resistance, which are important factors in evaluating pulmonary and cardiac diseases (see Appendix Table A).

Compliance and Elastance

Compliance is a measurement of distensibility or the ease by which a tissue can be stretched. The fewer elastic forces to be overcome to achieve stretch, the more compliant the tissue. Compliance measurements are derived by calculating the amount of pressure needed to effect a change in volume. The ease of inflating a previously inflated balloon compared with the effort needed to inflate a new balloon illustrates this concept nicely. In the old balloon, less pressure is needed to make a large volume change. Conversely, more pressure is required to make a smaller volume change in a new balloon. More compliant tissue, such as the old balloon, requires less pressure to achieve stretch/inflation. This is true because the compliant tissues have fewer elastic forces to overcome. Box 19-1 illustrates this concept, using the balloon analogy and assigning arbitrary numbers.

Compliance of the lungs is determined by the flexibility of the chest wall and the lung tissue itself. If there has been scarring of the lungs, such as in pulmonary fibrosis, the lungs become less compliant; consequently, respiratory effort, or work of breathing, increases.[11] In-

BOX 19-1 CALCULATING COMPLIANCE

Using delta (Δ) as a symbol for change, compliance (C) is expressed as follows:

C = (Δ) Volume (V)/(Δ) Pressure (P)

Balloon analogy—assigning arbitrary numbers.

Old Balloon

Small pressure needed: 1
Large volume change: 10
C = 10/1
C = 10

New Balloon

Large pressure needed: 10
Small volume change: 3
C = 3/10
C = 0.30
The old balloon is much more compliant than the new one.

BOX 19-2 CALCULATING ELASTANCE

Using delta (Δ) as a symbol for change, elastance (E) is expressed as follows:

E = (Δ) Pressure/(Δ) Volume

Rubber Band

- A thick rubber band requires more work to stretch it, so is less compliant and more elastant.
- A thin rubber band requires less work to stretch, so is more compliant and less elastant.

creased compliance, such as in emphysema, can be equally problematic since the lungs can be readily inflated but when exhalation occurs, the airways tend to collapse and close prematurely, resulting in air trapping (see p. 558).

Elastance is the opposite of compliance. Whereas compliance refers to the forces that effect expansion of the lung, elastance reflects the forces that seek to return the tissue to the resting or relaxed position. Compliance and elastance are closely related in pulmonary dynamics. The lungs inherently tend to return to their natural state, so without forces and action to effect expansion, they will tend to collapse. Rubber bands serve as a good example of this concept. A thick rubber band requires much more work to stretch, and it returns to its original shape rather easily. A thin rubber band is much easier to stretch but assumes its resting shape more slowly. Therefore, the thick rubber band is less compliant and more elastant, compared with the thin one. Box 19-2 gives the formula used to calculate elastance.

The chest wall also has the properties of elastance and compliance, but they differ from those associated with the lungs. To illustrate this difference, one can imagine that the lungs and chest wall could be separated but remain as living and moving structures retaining all of their properties. Each of the two structures could be separated from the pull of the other and could seek its own resting size, which would represent an equilibrium between elastance and compliance. In the case of the chest wall freed from the lungs, it would seek a much larger resting size than when it was attached to the lungs. Without the inward pull of the lungs, the chest wall would be abnormally large. Conversely, the lungs separated from the chest wall would tend to relax to a much smaller size compared with when they rested against the chest wall.

Considering the dynamic properties of the lungs and chest wall collectively, it can be seen that elastance of the lungs prevents over-distension of the thorax, whereas chest wall compliance prevents collapse of the lungs.

Inspiratory Lung Pressures

The flow of air into and out of the lung involves an interrelationship among intrapulmonic, intrapleural, and atmospheric pressures. **Intrapulmonic pressure** refers to pressure within the lungs themselves. **Intrapleural pressures** are those of the pleural space, which remain negative to atmospheric pressures. Atmospheric pressures are those of the outside air or atmosphere; at sea level this is 760 mm Hg.

Inspiration is initiated through contraction of the diaphragm. Diaphragmatic and inspiratory muscle contraction results in a downward movement of the lungs and increases the size of the thoracic cage. As a result, the intrapleural space becomes larger and the pressure becomes more negative. The intrapulmonic pressure becomes negative because the thoracic cage increases in size, the alveoli also increase in size, and the pressure within them becomes slightly sub-atmospheric. A pressure gradient between the mouth and the alveoli develops. Gas flows from the higher to lower pressure into the lungs and the lungs inflate (Fig. 19-11).

Expiratory Lung Pressures

During expiration, the opposite occurs from inspiration. At the end of active effort, the diaphragm relaxes and moves upward, which increases intrapulmonic pressures to exceed atmospheric level, resulting in passive movement of air out of the lungs. During expiration the intrapleural pressures becomes less negative but still remains negative (see Fig. 19-11). As lung volumes decrease, the size of the airways and alveolar ducts is reduced. During quiet ventilation, some of the

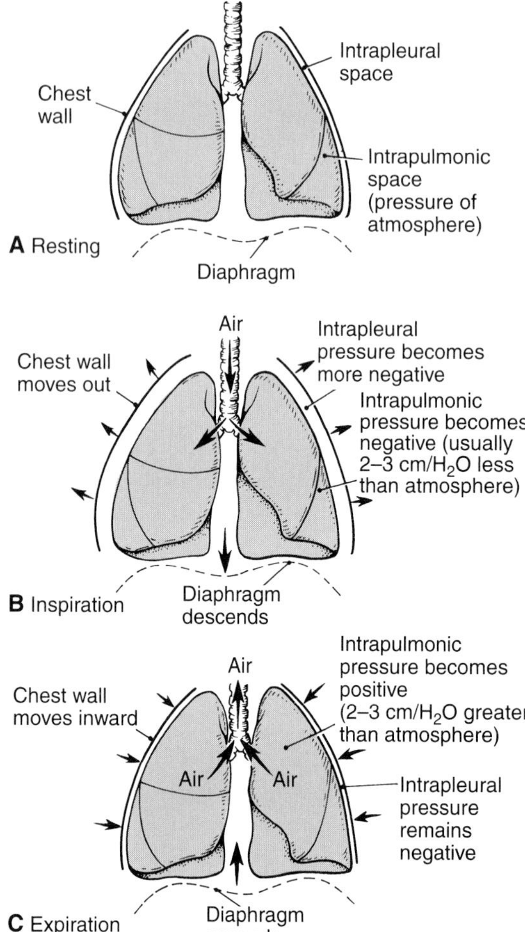

FIGURE 19-11. **Phases of ventilation. A. No air movement (resting). B. Air moves from the environment to the intrapulmonic space (inspiration). C. Air moves from the intrapulmonic space to the environment (expiration).**

smaller airways close during expiration. Because of the effects of gravity, airway closure is more pronounced in the supine position.

AIRWAY RESISTANCE

Airways provide an important conduit for air to travel to the alveoli, but also offer some resistance to ventilation. A significant increase in resistance results in increased work of breathing overall. Because the respiratory tree is a series of branching tubes of varying sizes, the resistances vary.

Airway resistance is influenced by many factors. A sigh or deep inspiration usually reduces resistance, whereas forced expiration, even in the healthy person, increases it. This is usually due to airway compression but may be due to mucus or inflammation of the airway.

The pattern of airflow also affects airway resistance. Figure 19-12 shows two major airflow patterns within tubes, the **laminar** and **turbulent** patterns. In laminar (or streamline) flow, the gas flow through the airways is like very thin cylinders moving inside each other. The cylinder on the outside moves slowly as it has to contend with the frictional forces imposed by the wall of the tube. More central cylinders of air are able to move comparatively faster. Gas density has no influence on the velocity of this type of flow. Gas that flows along a straight line encounters relatively little friction. When airway caliber changes, however, the laminar pattern is altered. Additional pressure may be required to reaccelerate the gas and to reestablish a laminar flow pattern.

When flow rates are high or when airways are partially obstructed or collapsed, airflow becomes turbulent. In normal lungs, turbulent flow occurs in the large central airways because of molecular collision and resistance imposed by the airway walls.

Much of the airflow in the lungs is probably transitional between turbulent and laminar. The work required for maintaining turbulent airflow is greater than that required to maintain laminar flow.

Tissue Resistance

In addition to airway resistance, some resistance is imposed by the lung and chest wall tissues; this is referred to as tissue resistance. Although the frictional resistance of tissue movement cannot be measured directly, it can be calculated and normally accounts for about 20% of total pulmonary resistance. Tissue resistance is rarely increased to the point of being limiting by itself. Diseases that cause lung tissue damage, such as pulmonary fibrosis, cause increased tissue resistance.

Work of Breathing

The act of breathing (or ventilation) requires muscular work to overcome airway resistance, tissue resistance, and the elastic forces of the lungs and chest wall. The work of breathing is defined as the energy required for the process of inspiration, since the act of expiration is normally a passive process.

The work of breathing is proportional to the pressure changes times the volume change. Volume change is the amount of air moved in or out with each normal breath, called **tidal volume**. The pressure change is that pressure needed to overcome the elastic and resistive forces. The elastic forces are mainly the elastic recoil of the chest wall and lungs themselves. Resistive forces are mainly those

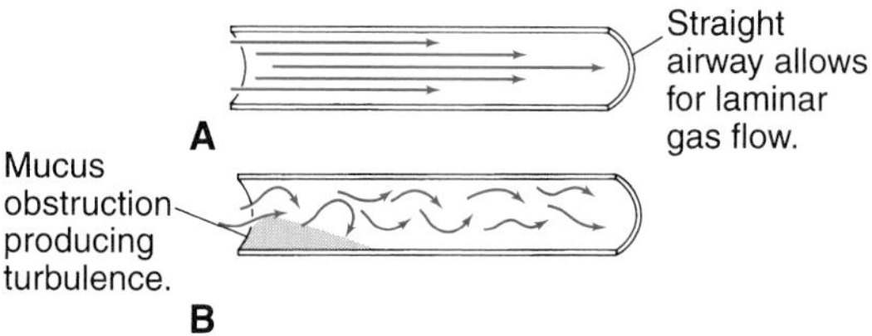

FIGURE 19-12. **A. Schematic representation of laminar gas flow. B. Representation of turbulent gas flow.**

of airway and tissue resistance, which are greatly altered by airway width. When airways widen, resistance is greatly diminished and air flows through easily. When airways narrow, such as with bronchospasm, resistance is increased and air movement is much more difficult, since it takes more pressure to move air through a narrow airway than a wide one. In areas of laminar flow, if airway radius is reduced by one half, resistance is increased by 16 times.[12] Because airways normally widen on inspiration and narrow on expiration, resistance is greater during expiration than during inspiration. This normal change in resistance helps to explain why air tends to become trapped on expiration in asthma or other chronic obstructive lung diseases. During quiet breathing, 65% of the work done overcomes elastic forces and 35% overcomes frictional resistance.[7] Work of breathing is minimal at normal breathing frequency but increases significantly at higher rates.

The work of breathing consumes oxygen. At rest, respiration accounts for only 1% of the body's energy expenditures. With moderate exercise, it only accounts for 3% of energy use.[9] This increases moderately with normal ventilatory changes, but with significant respiratory pathology the work of breathing may increases many times. In advanced disease states, the oxygen cost of ventilation can be 25% to 30% of the total metabolic rate.[11,13] In this situation, the ventilatory effort may cost the person more oxygen than it delivers and may produce more carbon dioxide than can be eliminated. It becomes a problem of supply and demand, and the natural balance of delivery and consumption is disrupted. If this process continues unabated, respiratory failure ensues.

VENTILATION-PERFUSION RELATIONSHIPS

Arterial oxygenation is affected by ventilation and perfusion (see p. 541). Abnormalities in pulmonary blood flow or in relationships between ventilation ($\dot{V}$) and perfusion ($\dot{Q}$) alter arterial oxygen tension and, subsequently, oxygenation of body tissues. A perfect ventilation-perfusion relationship, or ratio, is represented by the numeral 1. Ventilation and perfusion within the normal lungs are not evenly matched. This is referred to as **ventilation-perfusion mismatching** and is largely influenced by the effect of gravity and body position.[12]

VENTILATION-PERFUSION ZONES

The ventilation-perfusion ratios within the lung can be divided into three zones. These zones, in an upright individual, are represented in Figure 19-13. The upper lung zones receive more ventilation and less perfusion in comparison to the other zones. The middle zones are matched in terms of ventilation and perfusion. At the lung bases, there is better perfusion than ventilation. If the individual is in the upright position, pulmonary blood flow increases linearly from top to bottom due to gravitational forces. At the apex, the pulmonary arterial pressure is just sufficient to raise minimal amounts of blood to the top of the lungs and perfuse the apices.[4,12] Because capillary pressure is very low, if blood volume is reduced for some reason, such as systemic loss or pulmonary capillary destruction, apical perfusion may decrease or cease altogether.[13]

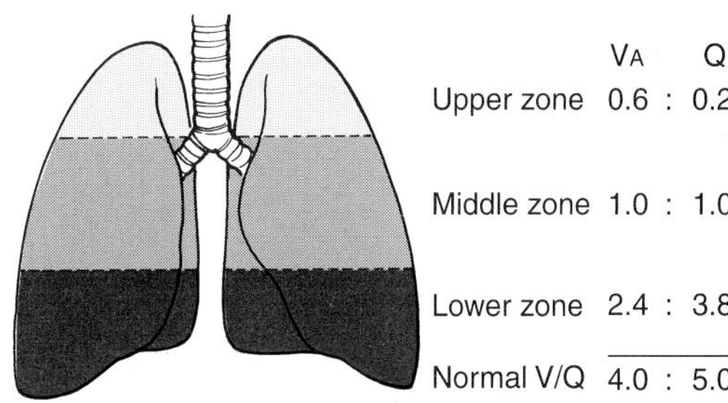

FIGURE 19-13. **The lungs can be divided into three zones. Ventilation-perfusion ($\dot{V}/\dot{Q}$) differs according to the position assumed. In the upright position the upper segments are hypoperfused, and in the lower segments they are hypoventilated. The relationship between ventilation and perfusion varies in the zones.**

Blood flow to the lungs changes with exercise and position. During exercise, all areas of the lung receive increased blood flow. When an individual lies down, flow from apices to bases becomes more uniform. In the case of pathology involving one lung, if an individual is positioned with the affected side dependent, oxygenation may be adversely affected as this increases perfusion to an already compromised lung.

DEAD SPACE

Ventilation and perfusion are also influenced by **anatomic dead space.** During normal ventilation, a portion of the air inspired does not come in contact with the alveoli and does not participate in gas exchange. Examples of anatomic dead space include the trachea and bronchi.

Alveolar dead space refers to areas of alveoli that are not participating in blood–gas exchange (Fig. 19-14). In the healthy lung, some of the alveoli are not actively functioning. Added together, anatomic and alveolar dead space are called *physiologic dead space.* Inspired air that does not participate in gas exchange, whether due to anatomic or alveolar dead space, is called *wasted ventilation.* During a pulmonary illness, the amount of alveolar dead space is usually increased. This results in an increase in $\dot{V}/\dot{Q}$ mismatching above normal physiologic baseline.

SHUNTING

The physiologic opposite of dead space ventilation is **shunting**. Shunting occurs when blood in the pulmonary capillary bypasses normal gas-exchange mecha-

FOCUS ON CELLULAR PHYSIOLOGY

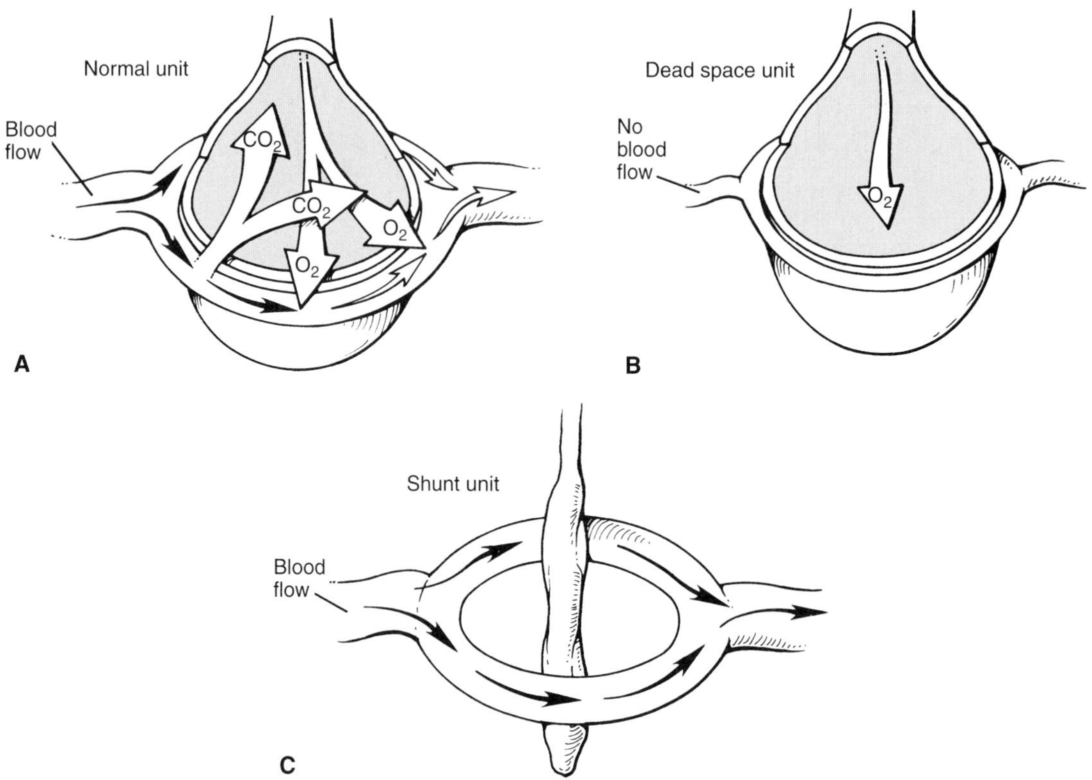

FIGURE 19-14. **A.** Schematic representation of normal alveolar-capillary unit. **B.** Representation of ventilation without perfusion. **C.** Representation of perfusion without ventilation.

nisms; thus, blood returns to the heart without picking up oxygen or releasing carbon dioxide. This occurs when a portion of the lung is perfused but not ventilated. This phenomenon is demonstrated by Figure 19-14C. A small amount of shunting, usually less than 2.5% of cardiac output, is normal. This accounts for the fact that normal oxygen saturation of hemoglobin in arterial blood gases is 96% to 98%. Abnormal amounts of shunting may be caused by problems associated with reduced or non-ventilation, such as occurs with atelectasis or pneumonia (see Chapter 20).

Blood returning to the heart from shunted areas is mixed with blood returning from the normal areas, thus creating an admixture of oxygenated and poorly oxygenated blood. This reduces oxygen content of the arterial blood that is pumped throughout the body. If shunting is not severe, the body can compensate for the amount of carbon dioxide that has not been exchanged within the shunted areas. Usually, hyperventilation of the unaffected areas can effectively blow off enough carbon dioxide to compensate. However, oxygen exchange cannot be compensated for so readily. As compensation continues, it eventually results in an arterial blood gas pattern of normal carbon dioxide levels but reduced oxygenation. If the body is unable to compensate adequately for the carbon dioxide exchange, blood gases show acidemia, hypoxemia, and hypercapnia.[1,13]

LUNG FLUID BALANCE

In the normal lung, the movement of fluid is determined by both capillary hydrostatic and protein osmotic pressures within the vessels. These forces, referred to as **Starling forces**, are responsible for preventing undesired leakage of fluids out of the pulmonary capillary. When there is abnormal permeability of the capillary membrane, either due to changes in hydrostatic pressure secondary to volume overload or due to osmotic derangements, fluid can leak into the alveoli and tissue interstitium. This impairs ventilation and gas exchange as the alveoli become flooded with fluid and decreases normal diffusion of gases.

Gas Exchange

Exchange of oxygen and carbon dioxide occurs both at the alveolar and tissue levels (Fig. 19-15). Gases are exchanged by the process of diffusion, the movement of

FOCUS ON CELLULAR PHYSIOLOGY

O_2 (100 mm Hg)
O_2 (100 mm Hg)
CO_2 (40 mm Hg)
Lung capillary
CO_2 (40 mm Hg)
Alveolus
O_2 (37 mm Hg)
CO_2 (46 mm Hg)
Direction of blood flow
A

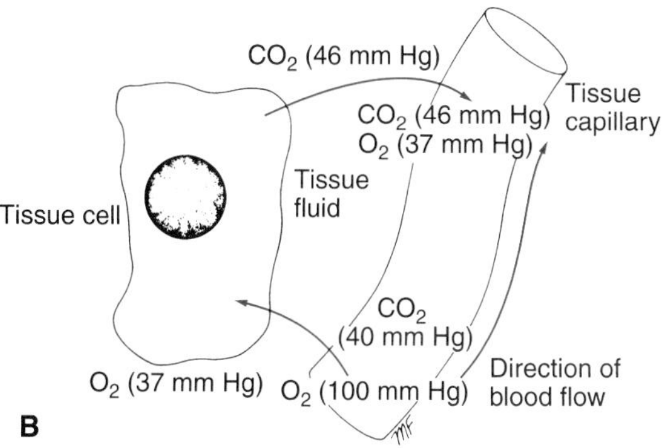

FIGURE 19-15. **A.** **Schematic representation of gas exchange at alveolus. B. Representation of gas exchange at tissue level.**

gases from an area of higher concentration to an area of lower concentration.

GAS EXCHANGE AT THE ALVEOLAR-CAPILLARY LEVEL

Effective ventilation requires that the gas be exchanged in the pulmonary capillary bed. Figure 19-15A shows the movement and partial pressures of gases as they diffuse between the pulmonary capillary and the alveoli. Although the pulmonary capillaries are very small here, they are large enough to accommodate red blood cells (RBCs). The capillary and alveolar walls are each only one cell thick, rendering a very thin diffusion membrane; therefore, gases diffuse across the membrane with little difficulty. Each RBC stays in the pulmonary capillary bed for about 1 second and exchanges gases with two or three alveoli during this time. Approximately 70 mL of blood is normally exchanging gases at a given moment in the pulmonary capillary bed of an adult. The principal exchange of gases here involves the movement of oxygen from the alveoli into the pulmonary capillary and, at the same time, the movement of carbon dioxide out of the pulmonary capillary and into the alveoli.

GAS EXCHANGE AT THE TISSUE LEVEL

Oxygen is carried to the tissues through the arterial circuit; Figure 19-15B demonstrates the partial pressures and exchange of gases at the tissue level. Here, oxygen diffuses out of the blood vessel and into the tissues, while carbon dioxide from the tissues moves into the blood vessel to be carried to the lungs for removal.

Gas Transport

Gases may be dissolved in plasma, bound to substances such as hemoglobin, or be transported in other forms such as carbonic acid or bicarbonate. A key to understanding normal gas exchange is the concept of fractional gas concentrations. The oxygen content of dry air at sea level is approximately 21%. Nitrogen accounts for 78% of ambient air, and the remainder is composed of carbon dioxide (approximately 0.02%) and other minute amounts of other trace gases, such as argon, neon, and helium.[4,7] The pressure each gas exerts is referred to as the *partial pressure.*

OXYGEN TRANSPORT AND DIFFUSION

Oxygen tension, or partial pressure of oxygen at sea level, is equal to the barometric pressure of 760 mm Hg multiplied by the fraction of oxygen in dry air (20.93%), which equals 160 mm Hg.[5] As the inspired air is warmed and humidified in the upper airways, it becomes diluted by water vapor; this causes the oxygen tension to fall to 149.3 mm Hg. Inspired air is then further diluted when it mixes with other gases in the lower airways and alveoli. Factors that lower inspired oxygen concentration or that raise alveolar carbon dioxide levels also lower alveolar oxygen levels and, hence, lower arterial blood oxygen tension. The end result is a reduction of oxygen available for delivery to tissues. Normal arterial blood gas values are found in Appendix Table B.

In the lungs, oxygen diffuses from areas of higher concentration to areas of lower concentration. The speed of diffusion is dependent on the concentrations of gas involved and the characteristics of the *diffusion barrier,* which is the alveolar-capillary membrane and associated interspace. This membrane is very thin (0.1 to 0.5 microns), thus making diffusion of O_2 very easy.[2]

Inhaled air has a higher partial pressure of oxygen than that in pulmonary capillary blood, so oxygen molecules diffuse from the alveolus, into the alveolar-capillary interspace, and then into the pulmonary capillary blood. Once in the pulmonary capillary blood, the majority of diffused oxygen binds with **hemoglobin,** a complex spherical molecule on the red blood cell, and thus becomes available for transportation to body tissue. The hemoglobin molecule is composed of four heme groups, which are the substances that actually combine with the oxygen molecule. Each hemoglobin molecule has the capacity to carry four oxygen molecules. Hemoglobin combined with oxygen is called **oxyhemoglobin**. This combining action occurs readily and is reversible.

In the adult, the average hemoglobin level is 15 g/dL of blood. Each gram of fully saturated hemoglobin can carry 1.34 mL of oxygen.[4] Each milliliter of blood with an oxygen tension of 100 mm Hg can carry about 0.03 mL of dissolved oxygen. This means that 100 mL of blood with a hemoglobin of 15 g and 100% saturation has an oxygen content of about 20 mL of oxygen, which is expressed as "volumes percent" (vol. %). A very small percentage of oxygen is carried dissolved in the plasma (.29%), so hemoglobin is by far the most important method of oxygen transport in the blood.

Oxygen is essential for cellular metabolism, but the cells have no capability to store it. Without constant delivery of oxygen, **tissue hypoxia** and anaerobic metabolism result. Tissue hypoxia is defined as inadequate critical oxygen tension to meet the needs of the cell. **Critical oxygen tension** is the level of cellular oxygen tension that results in mitochondrial dysfunction.[13]

Oxyhemoglobin Dissociation Curve

The relationship between oxygen and hemoglobin is nonlinear. The affinity of hemoglobin for oxygen is plotted on the **oxyhemoglobin dissociation curve** shown in Figure 19-16. This S-shaped curve is derived by plotting oxyhemoglobin saturation (the percentage of hemoglobin that has combined with oxygen) against the oxygen tension (mm Hg) to which it is exposed. Since oxyhemoglobin dissociation is readily reversible, the curve reflects the ease with which hemoglobin gives up oxygen as well as the ease with which it takes up oxygen. This is important because, to a large extent, oxygen delivery to the tissues depends on the ease with which hemoglobin gives up its oxygen once it reaches the tissues.

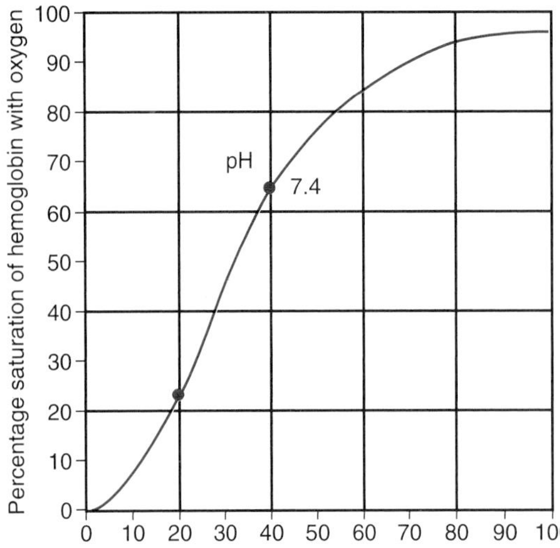

FIGURE 19-16. The oxyhemoglobin dissociation curve at an arterial pH of 7.4.

The upper portion of the oxyhemoglobin dissociation curve is flat, showing that when the oxygen tension is 70 mm Hg or above, hemoglobin becomes nearly fully saturated. However, when oxygen tension begins to fall below 60 mm Hg, the degree of saturation also falls rapidly (see Fig. 19-16). When oxygen tension falls to 40 mm Hg, the saturation of hemoglobin is about 70% or approximately the level of venous blood. At oxygen tension of 20 mm Hg, the saturation is less than 30%, which is insufficient to sustain life.

Many factors alter the affinity of hemoglobin for oxygen. An increase in hemoglobin affinity for oxygen makes the curve shift to the left, and oxygen is given up less readily to the tissues. Alkalemia, hypothermia, and hypocarbia are among factors that can cause a leftward shift. Conversely, acidemia, hypercarbia, and hyperthermia reduce the affinity of hemoglobin for oxygen and result in increased oxygen availability to the tissues. This causes the curve to shift to the right. Figure 19-17 shows the effects of pH, pCO_2, and body temperature on the affinity of hemoglobin for oxygen.

Tissue Oxygenation

The factors that affect tissue oxygenation are summarized in Box 19-3. Oxygen content of arterial blood is determined by a combination of alveolar oxygenation, hemoglobin content, saturation, and affinity for oxygen. Oxygen delivery to the tissues depends on adequacy of blood flow to the tissue, the diffusion of oxygen into the tissues, and movement of carbon dioxide out of the tissue. Also, oxygen delivery to the tissues is markedly influenced by arterial blood pH and body temperature.

CARBON DIOXIDE DIFFUSION AND TRANSPORT

Carbon dioxide is the by-product of metabolic activity and travels a pathway opposite to oxygen. Tissue carbon dioxide diffuses rapidly into the venous end of the capillaries with a gradient of less than 1 mm Hg. It diffuses about 20 times more readily than oxygen. The systemic venous blood eventually returns carbon dioxide to the pulmonary capillary bed via the pulmonary artery and pulmonary arterioles. Following pressure gradients, carbon dioxide in pulmonary capillary blood diffuses across the alveolar-capillary interspace and into the alveolus. The carbon dioxide is then removed from the alveolus during expiration. The movement of

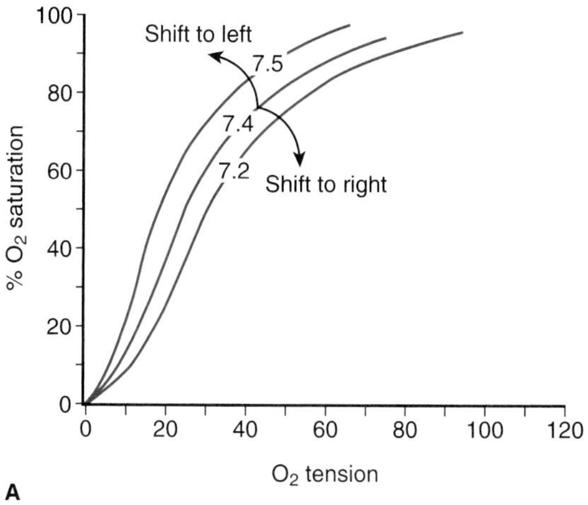

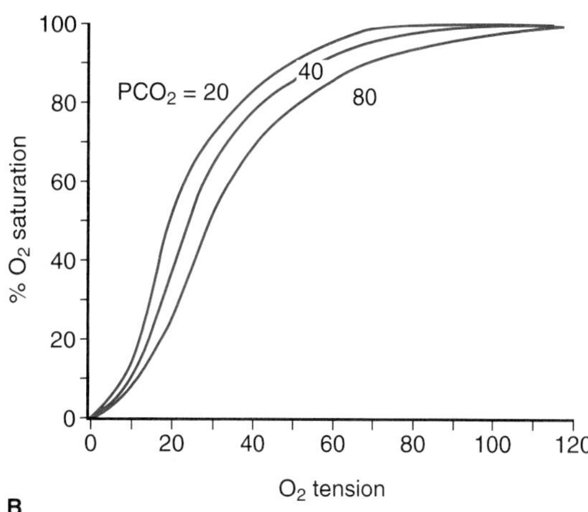

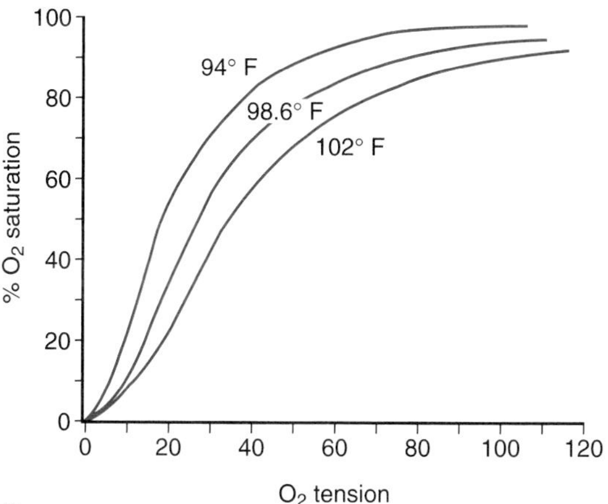

FIGURE 19-17. Effects of **(A)** pH, **(B)** PCO_2, and **(C)** temperature on the oxyhemoglobin dissociation curve.

> **BOX 19-3 FACTORS THAT AFFECT TISSUE OXYGENATION**
>
> Oxygen tension arterial blood
> Hemoglobin content
> Hemoglobin saturation
> Blood flow to tissues
> Diffusion of oxygen to tissues
> Diffusion of carbon dioxide
> Arterial pH
> Body temperature

oxygen and carbon dioxide across the alveolar-capillary membrane due to ventilation, diffusion, and perfusion is depicted in Figure 19-15A.

Carbon dioxide transport occurs in two forms: in RBCs (89%) and in the plasma (approximately 11%). In the RBC the majority of the carbon dioxide is carried as bicarbonate (63%). It may also be carried as **carbaminohemoglobin** (carbon dioxide combined with hemoglobin, 21%) or dissolved (5%). In the plasma, it is carried as bicarbonate (5%) as a *carbamino compound* (1%) or dissolved (5%).[2]

Figure 19-18 illustrates the reaction of carbon dioxide as it is carried dissolved in the RBCs. It is important to note that this is a reversible reaction that occurs rapidly at the tissue level, where carbon dioxide is picked up, and in the lungs, where it is released. Most carbon dioxide diffuses into RBCs, is combined with

FOCUS ON CELLULAR PHYSIOLOGY

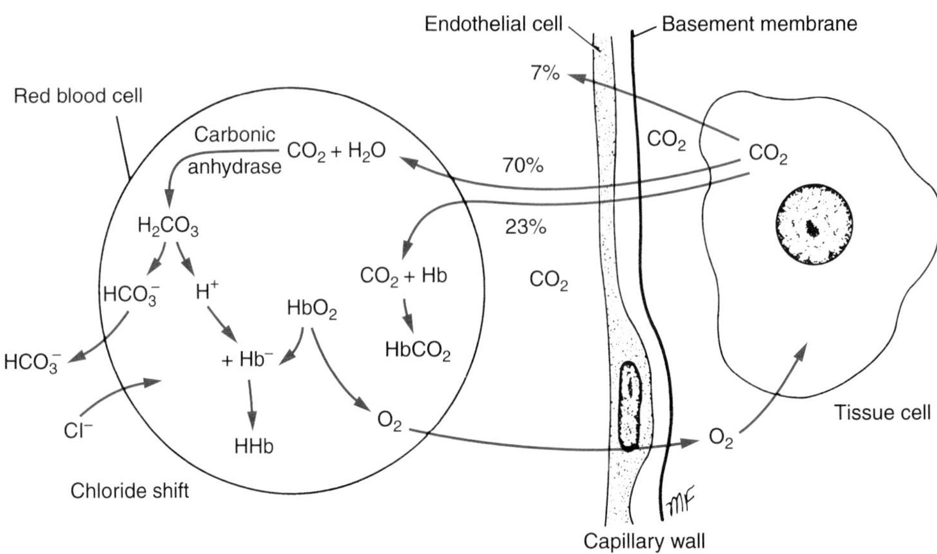

FIGURE 19-18. **Methods of carbon dioxide transport in the red blood cell (RBC). Seventy percent of CO_2 is combined with H_2O to form carbonic acid and bicarbonate, 23% is carried in combination with Hb, and 7% is carried in the plasma.**

water, and, through the action of a catalyst called *carbonic anhydrase*, forms *carbonic acid* (H_2CO_3). Carbonic acid immediately dissociates into hydrogen ions (H^+) and bicarbonate ions (HCO_3^-) that can diffuse back into the plasma or stay in combination with a positive ion in the RBCs. The excess hydrogen ion formed in this reaction usually binds with the hemoglobin molecule to form **hydrogen hemoglobin.** If significant amounts of bicarbonate ions diffuse into the plasma, a negative ion is drawn into the RBCs to equalize the electrochemical gradient. This ion is usually chloride, and the mechanism of its movement is called the *chloride shift*.[4,10] This process can provide bicarbonate to the plasma when the pH is decreased. Normally, in the lungs a reverse process occurs very rapidly. Hydrogen is released from hemoglobin and recombines with bicarbonate to form carbonic acid, which dissociates into carbon dioxide and water. Carbon dioxide diffuses out of the RBCs into the alveolar-capillary interspace and is blown off in the exhaled air.

Under normal alveolar ventilation conditions, alveolar carbon dioxide (P_ACO_2) of 40 mm Hg is in equilibrium with the resulting arterial carbon dioxide (PaO_2) of 40 mm Hg. The levels of both alveolar and arterial carbon dioxide are directly and inversely proportional to the volume of alveolar ventilation. Thus, in alveolar hypoventilation, halving the alveolar ventilation from 4 to 2 L/minute doubles the $PaCO_2$ from 40 to 80 mm Hg. In hyperventilation, doubling the alveolar ventilation from 4 to 8 L/minute halves the $PaCO_2$ to 20 mm Hg.[2,5]

Respiratory Regulation of Acid-Base Equilibrium

As is described in Chapter 6, the major blood buffers are hemoglobin, the plasma proteins, and the carbonic acid–bicarbonate system. The amounts of carbon dioxide and hydrogen ion present affect the blood pH significantly. Any increase in blood carbon dioxide concentration causes a shift in pH to the acidic side (pH <7.35). Any decrease in carbon dioxide content causes a shift to the alkaline side (pH >7.45). Carbon dioxide, usually in the form of carbonic acid (H_2CO_3), is closely regulated by the physiologic buffer system of the lungs.

If the metabolic rate increases, such as during exercise or with fever, the rate of carbon dioxide formation increases. Conversely, if the rate of metabolism decreases, the formation of carbon dioxide also decreases. Alveolar ventilation changes according to nervous control of respiration through the chemoreceptors in the medulla. As described on page 536, these chemoreceptors are extremely sensitive to minute changes in the carbon dioxide (and hydrogen) level and stimulate an increase or decrease in the respiratory rate. Thus, the respiratory rate and depth of respiration seek to either retain or blow off excess carbon dioxide according to the pH of blood.

The two major alterations in acid-base balance related to pulmonary function are **respiratory acidosis** and **respiratory alkalosis**. These alterations are discussed in Chapter 6.

DEFENSES OF THE AIRWAYS AND LUNGS

Defenses of the lungs include mechanisms designed to remove debris and anti-microbial agents. All of the mechanisms have as their purpose the protection of the lower airways.

Defenses Against Particulates in the Airways

Under normal conditions, an individual inspires 10,000 to 12,000 L of air daily. Each liter of urban air may have several million particles suspended in it, most of which are deposited along the respiratory tract and are cleansed by the defenses of the airways. Particles smaller than 0.5 mm in diameter usually remain suspended in inhaled air and are expelled from the lungs during expiration.

The first site of deposition of particulates in the airway is the nose (Fig. 19-19). Particulates larger than 10 mm in diameter are filtered out in the nose or trapped in the nasal mucosa. The inertia of large particles determines deposition at these sites. Their large mass and high linear velocity force them to rain out or be deposited in the nasal mucosa.

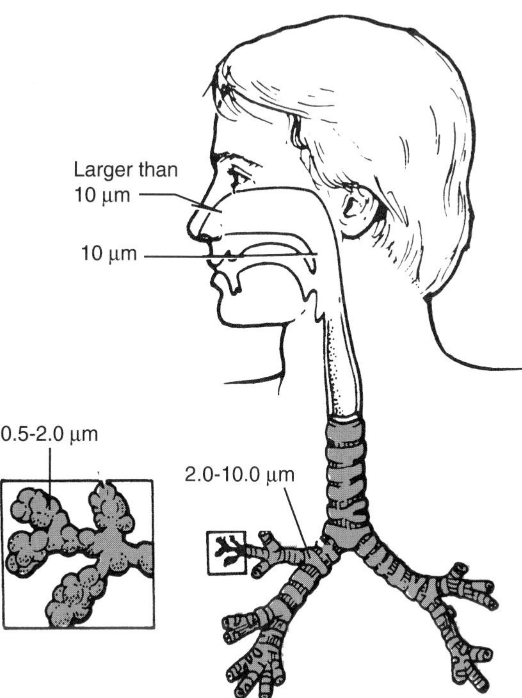

FIGURE 19-19. Deposition of particulates in the airways depends on their size.

As the inhaled air flows over the tonsils and adenoids, particulates are deposited by impaction. These structures are ideally located in the airway to entrap debris that passes over them. In addition to mechanical defense, the tonsils and adenoids may function in immunologic responses. Farther along the respiratory tract, linear velocity of air decreases as the surface area increases, which allows particulates in the range of 2 to 10 mm to be deposited on the *mucociliary blanket* by means of sedimentation (settling out). Particulates smaller than 2 mm reach the alveoli either by gravitational forces or, to a lesser extent, by random movement of molecules due to thermal energy, called **Brownian movement**. These particulates are removed primarily by mucociliary transport and phagocytosis. Smaller particles may present more of a threat to the lungs than larger ones, because they are able to penetrate more deeply and remain in the tissue longer.

Mucociliary Transport

The **mucociliary escalator system**, or mucous blanket, is the major non-specific defense mechanism for the respiratory tract. The key components of this system are the *mucus-secreting goblet cells* found in the bronchi, the *ciliated epithelial cells*, and the mucus itself (Fig. 19-20A).

The ciliated epithelial cells of the respiratory tract help keep the airways clear by continuously propelling a *mucous blanket* toward the mouth. These cells line the entire respiratory tract with the exception of the anterior onethird of the nose, part of the pharynx, and the alveoli. The surface of each ciliated cell contains about 200 cilia.[2] The cilia move in a synchronous, continuous, wavelike motion in an effort to carry mucus and debris up the airway, through the larynx, and to the mouth (Fig. 19-20B).

From an upright position, the cilia sweep forward about 30 to 35 degrees and then bend to make their recovery. The movement has been likened to the strokes of a boat's oars. Each cilium makes a forceful, fast effector stroke forward, followed by a less forceful, slower stroke backward. Beating in sequential waves as high as 1,000 cycles per minute, cilia move mucus up the airway. The beat is rapid, thus preventing recoil of the mucus layer between beats.

Mucus is produced primarily by the goblet or mucus-secreting cells that line the tracheobronchial tree. Mucus is normally composed of water, electrolytes, and several types of mucopolysaccharides, which account for its viscosity. The respiratory tract produces about 100 mL/day of mucus.[2]

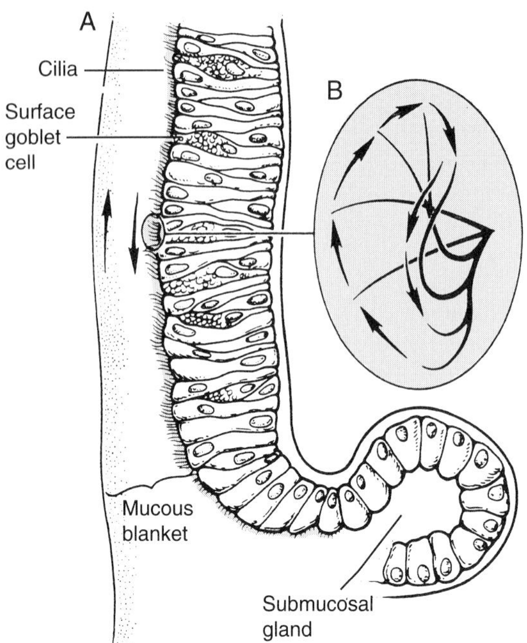

FIGURE 19-20. **A.** The mucociliary escalator. **B.** Conceptual scheme of ciliary movement, which allows forward motion to move the viscous gel layer and backward motion to occur entirely within the more fluid sol layer.

The mucous blanket consists of two layers: the *sol layer*, which surrounds the cilia, and the *gel* or *surface layer*. The less viscous sol layer provides a medium in which the cilia can move. With power strokes, the tips of the cilia strike the bottom of the gel layer and propel it toward the mouth to either be swallowed or expectorated.[8] Cells in the alveoli may also contribute secretions to the mucous blanket.

The mucous layers retain a constant depth, and the rate of transport of mucus increases rapidly as the mucus moves toward the trachea. Some mucus is reabsorbed in the large airways to maintain a constant depth. The efficiency of the mucociliary transport system can be altered by depressed ciliary activity, changes in the property of mucus, and injury to the respiratory epithelium cells. Cigarette smoke is known to paralyze cilia and injure airway epithelium.

Alveolar Clearance

Mucociliary transport, lymphatic drainage, blood flow, and phagocytosis all play a role in creating a sterile environment within the alveoli. *Pulmonary alveolar macrophage* (PAM) activity is the principal alveolar defense against particulates. As shown in Figure 19-21, PAMs regularly scavenge the surface of the epithelium, engulfing and digesting foreign material. PAMs originate from bone marrow and, in addition to phagocytosis, have several additional functions. They can help process and prepare inhaled antigens for immunologic attack and secrete granulocyte-attracting substances.[3]

FOCUS ON CELLULAR PHYSIOLOGY

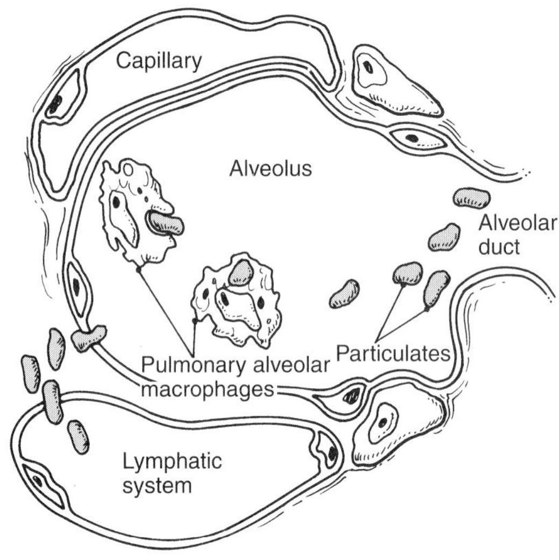

FIGURE 19-21. Alveolar clearance effected by macrophage ingestion of particulate matter, particles traveling in the alveolar duct, lymphatic clearance of particulate matter, blood flow clearance, and carriage of particulates within the macrophages.

Some particulates are removed by the perivascular, peribronchial, and hilar lymph systems. The lymphatics probably transport the particulates that have been successfully engulfed in macrophages. It is unclear to what extent blood flow is responsible for alveolar clearance.

Some particulates remain in the lungs for protracted periods, whereas others stay for only an intermediate period and are then cleared. The period of time particulates remain in the lung depends upon a number of factors, including deposition site, the nature of the particulate, and host resistance. Some particulates can remain in the lungs indefinitely (e.g., asbestos, silica, and carbon) and may, over time, stimulate undesirable fibroblast proliferation.

Reflexes of the Airways

In addition to mechanical defenses, the respiratory tract is equipped with several protective reflex mechanisms.

Sneeze Reflex

The sneeze reflex is one of the defenses against irritant materials. Particulates or irritants stimulate the trigeminal nerve, which results in the sneeze response. The sneeze is characterized by a deep inspiration, followed by a violent expiratory blast through the nose.

Cough Reflex

The cough reflex is important in clearing the trachea and large bronchi of foreign matter. Irritants trigger stimulatory impulses to be sent from the vagus nerve to the medulla. The cough reflex starts by initiating a deep inspiration. Next, the glottis closes, the diaphragm relaxes, and the expiratory and abdominal muscles contract against the closed glottis. Maximal intrathoracic and intra-airway pressures are produced that cause the trachea to narrow. When the glottis opens, the large pressure differential between the airways and the atmosphere, coupled with tracheal narrowing, creates airflow through the trachea at velocities as high as 100 miles an hour.[4] This is very effective in propelling secretions toward the mouth. Although the cough is more effective in clearing the major airways, it also may help clear the peripheral airways through a milking action created by the high intrathoracic pressures generated. This may also aid in the delivery of secretions from the peripheral airways to the main bronchi for expulsion by coughing. An individual may also consciously initiate a cough at any time.

Reflex Bronchoconstriction

Reflex **bronchoconstriction** protects the upper and lower airways from mechanical and chemical irritants. Both cough and reflex bronchoconstriction stimuli are initiated by subepithelial airway receptors in response to irritants. For example, when the receptors are exposed to dust, a reflex narrowing of the airway, along with a cough, increases the linear velocity of airflow and assists in the removal of dust from the airways. Reflex bronchoconstriction also protects the alveoli from harmful fumes and prevents gases from entering the lower airways.

Removal of gases from the inspired air depends on their solubility in water. Highly soluble gases, such as sulfur dioxide and acetone, are removed in the upper respiratory tract. Less soluble gases, such as nitrous oxide and ozone, are able to reach the peripheral lung tissue. The protection offered by reflex bronchoconstriction is dose related and time related, which means that if exposure to the toxic fumes is brief or of low concentration, reflex bronchoconstriction may protect the lungs adequately. However, if the concentration of gas is high or the period of exposure is prolonged, the protective mechanisms may not be effective.

Hering-Breuer Reflex

If the lung becomes overstretched, the Hering-Breurer reflex is activated. This important reflex serves as a protective mechanism to limit lung inflation.

Defense Against Microbial Agents

Invasion of the lungs by microbial agents is an ever-present danger. Microorganisms have the ability to replicate themselves, and, conceivably, one organism could multiply and extensively infiltrate lung tissue. The defenders against infectious agents must act quickly to kill the organisms before they have sufficient opportunity to proliferate.

Under normal circumstances, the pulmonary alveolar macrophage system is the primary bactericidal mechanism for clearing infectious agents from the lungs.[6] Pulmonary alveolar macrophages ingest bacteria at such a rapid rate that most are destroyed in situ. The rate of bacterial killing in the lungs usually exceeds the rate at which the bacteria are transported out of the lungs. This is known as **net bacterial lung clearance**. Three factors contribute to this process: (1) physical transport of bacteria out of the lung, (2) in situ bacterial killing, and (3) bacterial multiplication.[13]

The rate of macrophage bactericidal activity is influenced by the type of offending bacteria involved. Some organisms are readily inactivated by phagocytosis, whereas others appear resistant to this process. *Klebsiella pneumonia* and *Pseudomonas aeruginosa*, for example, are slowly killed in the lungs, resulting in a net increase, rather than a net clearance, of organisms.[13] Adverse metabolic conditions, such as hypoxia, acidosis, and high levels of cortisol, slow net bacterial lung clearance.

The dynamics of different responses to bacteria, fluctuations in host resistance, and environmental changes may permit an organism to multiply at any given time. All of these factors influence the fate of the microorganism.

Immunologic Defense

Closely associated with the macrophage system is the *immunologic defense system of the lungs*. The cells involved in the specific immune response are described in Chapter 10. These include the T lymphocytes (thymic-dependent) and B lymphocytes (bone marrow–derived), which, in a complex, interacting pattern provide immunity and defend the body against foreign invasion.

Specialized B lymphocytes become immunoglobulin-secreting plasma cells and can assist pulmonary alveolar macrophages in inactivating infectious material. This humoral response involves five classes of immunoglobulins: IgG, IgM, IgA, IgD, and IgE. The first three classes are important in the control of infectious diseases. Both IgM and IgG provide the primary and secondary antibody responses against pathogens by facilitating opsonization and phagocytosis of bacteria. IgA is a secretory immunoglobulin and can be found in bronchial secretions.[3] IgA protects the lungs against viral and bacterial invasion. It may also inhibit the ability of the organisms to adhere to the mucosal surfaces.

The T lymphocytes provide for cell-mediated immunity. They play a major role in attracting macrophages to the site of an infection. Tuberculosis is an excellent prototype for understanding this response. Inhaled tuberculosis bacilli travel from the lungs to the lymph nodes, where the macrophages engulf, process, and concentrate the antigens of the bacilli. A few T lymphocytes bearing receptors for tuberculin antigens react with the bacillus and undergo multiplication. These T cells circulate back to the lungs and release chemical mediators that induce macrophages and other leukocytes to kill the bacteria (see p. 558).

REFERENCES

1. Des Jardines, T. (1998). *Cardiopulmonary anatomy and physiology: Essentials for respiratory care* (3rd ed.). Albany, NY: Delmar Publishers.
2. Ganong, W. F. (1997). *Review of medical physiology* (18th ed.). Los Altos, CA.: Appleton & Lange.
3. Grippi, M. A. (1995). *Pulmonary pathophysiology.* Philadelphia: J. B. Lippincott.
4. Guyton, A. C. (1996). *Textbook of medical physiology* (9th ed.). Philadelphia: W. B. Saunders.
5. Guyton, A. C. & Hall, J. E. (1997). *Human physiology and mechanisms of disease* (6th ed.). Philadelphia: W.B. Saunders.
6. Martin, D., & Youtesy, J. (1998). *Respiratory anatomy and physiology.* St. Louis: C. V. Mosby.
7. Nunn, J. F. (1993). *Applied respiratory physiology* (4th ed.). London: Butterworths.
8. Seaton, A., Seaton, D., & Leitch, A. (1989). *Crofton and Douglas's respiratory diseases* (4th ed.). Oxford: Blackwell Scientific.
9. Shier, D., Butler, J., & Lewis, R. (1996). *Hole's human anatomy and physiology* (7th ed.). Dubuque, IA: Wm. C. Brown.
10. Staub, N. C. (1998). The respiratory system. In R. M. Berne and M. N. Levy, *Physiology* (4th ed.). St. Louis: Mosby.
11. Travis, W. D., Farber, J. L., & Rubin, E. (1999). The respiratory system. In E. Rubin & J. L. Farber, *Pathology* (3rd ed.). Philadelphia: Lippincott Williams & Wilkins.
12. West, J. B. (1990). *Respiratory physiology: The essentials* (4th ed.). Baltimore: Williams & Wilkins.
13. West, J. B. (1998). *Pulmonary pathophysiology* (5th ed.). Baltimore: Williams & Wilkins.

Chapter

20

Altered Pulmonary Function

Lynda A. Mackin / Barbara L. Bullock

KEY TERMS

air trapping
alveolitis
atelectasis
atopy
barotrauma
bronchogenic
cardiogenic pulmonary edema
cor pulmonale
embolus
empyema
flail chest
granuloma
Ghon complex
hematogenous spread
hypercapnic
hypoxemic
interstitial edema
kyphoscoliosis
non-cardiogenic pulmonary edema
paradoxical movement
paraneoplastic syndrome
parapneumonic effusion
pectus carinatum
pectus excavatum
Pickwickian syndrome
pneumothorax
primary tuberculosis
pleural effusion
pleuritis
pyothorax
shunting
splinting
thrombus
tubercle
tuberculous bacillemia
vascular redistribution
Virchow's triad

Pathologies that affect the respiratory system include common respiratory tract infections, obstructive diseases, restrictive disorders, and pleural, vascular, and malignant disruptions. These conditions can interfere with oxygen intake or transport, and the clinical manifestations may exhibit common features.

RESPIRATORY INFECTIONS

Infectious processes can involve either the upper or lower respiratory tract or both. These processes may be caused by viruses, bacteria, fungi, or protozoa and can range from mild and self limiting to debilitating or fatal.

Upper Respiratory Tract Infections

The majority of upper respiratory tract infections are viral in etiology. Most cases are due to rhinovirus, respiratory syncytial virus, adenovirus, and parainfluenza.[47] These viruses can be quite contagious and are spread by hand-to-hand contact or by inhalation of the pathogen into the upper respiratory tract. Bacterial infections also can occur and may be caused by *Streptococcus pneumoniae*, other streptococci, or *Hemophillus influenzae*.[21] Approximately 60% of infections involving the pharynx are viral in etiology, but about 30% of cases are due to the bacteria *Chlamydia*, and 5% to 10% are due to mycoplasma or Group A streptococcus.[47] Upper respiratory infections occur more frequently during the fall and winter season, since this is when people tend to spend more time in enclosed spaces.

PATHOPHYSIOLOGY AND CLINICAL MANIFESTATIONS

Infection occurs when the pathogen gains entry into the upper respiratory tract, proliferates, and initiates an inflammatory reaction. The pathophysiologic changes seen in upper respiratory infections in general are characterized by an acute inflammation of the upper airway structures, including the sinuses, nasopharynx, pharynx, larynx, and trachea. The presence of the pathogen triggers infiltration of the mucous membranes by inflammatory and infection-fighting cells. The cellular infiltration leads to mucosal swelling and secretion of a serous or mucopurulent exudate, which may be clear or discolored. Secondary bacterial infection can occur when the normal drainage pathways and mechanisms of the upper airway become obstructed.

VIRAL RHINITIS (COMMON COLD)

Viral rhinitis, often referred to as the common cold, is an acute viral infection of the upper airway, including the sinuses and pharynx. Symptoms typically include headache, watery *rhinorrhea* (runny nose), general malaise, sneezing, and a scratchy, irritated throat. Discolored nasal discharge may indicate a secondary bacterial infection. Examination of the nasal mucosa or oropharynx may reveal some generalized redness.

SINUSITIS

Sinusitis is usually a bacterial infection of the sinuses/paranasal sinuses that occurs following viral rhinitis. The virus-induced inflammation of the sinus mucosa causes obstruction of the normal drainage pathways, thus creating an ideal site for bacterial proliferation. The most common organisms causing this condition are group A *Streptococcus pyogenes, Staphylococcus aureus,* and *Haemophilus influenzae.* Constitutional symptoms include purulent nasal discharge, sinus congestion, tenderness over the sinus cavity, headache, post-nasal drip, cough, sore throat, and possible fever. Sinus infections that become longstanding are termed *chronic sinusitis.*

PHARYNGITIS

Pharyngitis is an acute inflammatory infection of the upper airway/pharynx that is commonly referred to as a "sore throat." It is usually caused by viral or bacterial invasion of the pharynx. Common symptoms include sore throat, discomfort with swallowing, hoarse voice (if infection includes larynx), tonsillitis, and sometimes lymph node swelling in the neck. The majority of cases are self limiting and do not require any specific treatment beyond comfort measures.

Lower Respiratory Tract Infection

In order for an infection of the lower respiratory tract to occur, at least one of the following three conditions must be present:[4]

- Host defenses are weakened or impaired.
- An inoculum (large number) of pathogenic organisms must gain entry and overwhelm the natural defenses of the lower respiratory tract.
- The organism must be sufficiently virulent (strong enough to cause infection).

Different types of lower respiratory tract infections cause various effects. Examples of lower respiratory tract infections include acute bronchitis, pneumonia, and tuberculosis.

ACUTE BRONCHITIS

Acute bronchitis is a common, usually self-limiting, viral, or bacterial infection of the tracheobronchial tree. In otherwise healthy individuals, the etiologic agent is usually viral such as rhinovirus, respiratory syncytial virus (RSV), parainfluenza virus, coronavirus, adenovirus, and influenzae A and B viruses. Bacterial agents include *Mycoplasma pneumoniae, Chlamydia pneumoniae,* and *Bordetella pertussis.* Occasionally, fungal etiologies can be found in individuals with co-morbid conditions, such as immune deficiency.[39]

Pathophysiology and Clinical Manifestations

Etiologic agents gain entry into the respiratory tract through either inhalation or aspiration of secretions. The pathogen creates a localized inflammatory reaction on the airway mucosa that results in swelling and increased mucus production. Significant inflammation and obstruction may result in wheezing.

Presenting symptoms at onset can be similar to those experienced with an upper respiratory tract infection. These may include sore throat, general malaise, chest congestion, cough (productive or nonproductive), chest tightness, retrosternal discomfort, and, in some cases, wheezing. Fever may or may not be present, but the individual usually does not appear acutely ill.[39] Time periods for symptoms vary but generally last 3 to 10 days. A residual cough may persist for several weeks following infection.

PNEUMONIA

Pneumonia is an inflammation of the lung in which some or all of the alveoli, interstitial tissue, and bronchioles become edematous and filled with fluid or blood cells as a result of infection or irritation by chemical agents.[17] Proliferation of infecting pathogens can lead to a variety of pathologic and clinical features, depending on host resistance and virulence of the organism. The immunocompromised, hospitalized, very young, and very old are at greatest risk for serious lower respiratory tract infections.

Classification

Pneumonia can be classified as to the infectious causative agent, according to the location of causation, or as due to aspiration (Table 20-1). The infectious causative agents may be bacterial, viral, or other types of organisms and may involve virulent or "opportunistic" organisms. These organisms may also be classified as "typical" or "atypical" infections according to

TABLE 20-1

VARIOUS CLASSIFICATIONS OF PNEUMONIA

CLASSIFICATION	EXAMPLES	SIGNIFICANCE
INFECTIOUS		
Bacterial	*Streptococcus pneumoniae* (pneumococcus)	*S. pneumoniae* most common cause of community-acquired pneumonia; prototype of "typical" pneumonias
Viruses	Rhinoviruses Respiratory syncytial virus Influenza viruses	Cause common cold, bronchiolitis in children, croup, pneumonia and Reye syndrome
Fungal	*Pneumocystis carinii* (PCP) coccidioidomycosis, histoplasmosis, cryptococcus	PCP causes pneumonia in individuals with a weakened immune system; other fungi cause pneumonia by inhalation of infected material
Rickettsia	*Coxiella burnetti*	Causes pneumonia through inhalation of dust particles; grows in macrophages
Nontubercular mycobacteria (NTMB)	*M. Kansasii* *M. avium intracellulare*	Cause pneumonia in immune-suppressed persons
Chlamydia	*Chlamydia pneumoniae* *Chlamydia psittaci*	Organisms grow within host cells
ATYPICAL BACTERIA		
Organisms that multiply within a host cell and can infect the respiratory system	*Mycoplasma pneumoniae* *Chlamydia pneumoniae* *Chlamydia psittaci* *Legionella pneumophilia*	Most pneumonia caused by *M. pneumoniae;* which is transmitted by respiratory secretions of infected persons and colonizes on mucosa that lines the airways, causing bronchopneumonia Legionella organisms are inhaled and ingested by resident macrophages, grows and cause flu-like syndromes and pneumonia
HOSPITAL ACQUIRED (HAP)	Gram-negative organisms such as *Escherichia coli, Klebsiella pneumoniae*	Diagnosed after hospital admission; usually results following surgical procedures, intravenous catheters, endotracheal tubes
COMMUNITY ACQUIRED (CAP)	Virulent bacteria, especially *Streptococcus pneumoniae*	Contracted in the community with person-to-person contact
ASPIRATION PNEUMONIA	Chemical pneumonitis Bacterial pathogens Inert substances	Occurs when secretions of foreign substances are inhaled into the tracheobronchial tree Toxic substances such as stomach acids, bile, and mineral oil cause chemical pneumonitis and acute lung injury Aspiration of bacterial pathogens a common method of developing bacterial pneumonia Inert substances such as teeth, food, and water may cause bronchial obstruction or pneumonitis of lungs

the method of disease causation. *Community-acquired pneumonia* (CAP) and *hospital-acquired pneumonia* (HAP) are terms used to describe pneumonia according to the location where it was contracted. These pneumonias are usually caused by bacteria and are discussed with bacterial pneumonias.[4] Aspiration pneumonia can also occur following aspiration of fluids or inert substances.

Bacterial Pneumonia

Bacterial pneumonia is the most common type of lung infection and may be manifested by consolidation of an entire lobe or scattered areas in the same or several lobes. It is often contracted in the community, and etiologic agents vary according to the age and overall health status of the host (Box 20-1). *Streptococcus pneumoniae* is the most common pathogen, accounting for 30% to 50% of all CAP cases.[3,46] The responsible pathogen, however, is determined only in about 50% of cases of CAP. It is estimated that there are 4 million cases of CAP in the United States annually. Outpatient mortality for CAP is 1% to 5%.[4]

Hospital-acquired pneumonia (HAP) is a leading cause of death from nosocomial infections. There are many pathogenic etiologies for HAP, especially several gram-negative species (Box 20-2). HAP has an estimated occurrence rate of 5 to 10 cases per 1000 hospital admissions, and mortality rates can be as high as 70%.[4]

There is an increased risk for morbidity and mortality with any type of pneumonia when there is associated cardiac disease, chronic obstructive pulmonary disease, cirrhosis of the liver, malignancies, and asplenia (absence of the spleen).[51] Specific risk factors have been identified in the pathogenesis of HAP (Box 20-3). The severity of underlying illness at time of presentation and the role of aspiration of gram-negative bacteria from oropharyngeal secretions continue to be investigated.[14,38]

PATHOPHYSIOLOGY. Most bacteria that cause pneumonia are normally found in the oropharynx and nasopharynx and gain entry into the respiratory tract though aspiration of oropharyngeal secretions.[23] Normally, foreign particulates or substances are cleared by means of the mucociliary escalator mechanisms. If the cilia are injured in some way, such as in chronic bronchitis, the escalator is less effective. Pneumonia can also occur due to **hematogenous spread** of bacteria from an extra-pulmonary infection site—that is, bacteria from another infected site can be carried in the blood to the lungs and cause pneumonia.

BOX 20-1 MOST COMMON COMMUNITY-ACQUIRED PNEUMONIA PATHOGENS

Outpatients, Age < 60, No Co-morbidities

Streptococcus pneumoniae
Mycoplasma pneumonia
Respiratory viruses
Chlamydia pneumoniae
Hemophillus pneumoniae

Miscellaneous

Legionella species
S. aureus
M. tuberculosis
Endemic fungi
Aerobic gram-negative bacilli

Outpatients, Age < 60, With Co-morbidities

S. pneumoniae
Respiratory viruses
H. influenzae
Aerobic gram-negative bacilli
S. aureus

Miscellaneous

Moraxella catarrhalis
Legionella species
M. tuberculosis
Endemic fungi

(American Thoracic Society Statement [1993]. Guidelines for the initial management of adults with community-acquired pneumonia: Diagnosis, assessment of severity, and initial antimicrobial therapy. *American Review of Respiratory Disease, 148*, 1418–1426.)

BOX 20-2

MOST COMMON HOSPITAL-ACQUIRED PNEUMONIA PATHOGENS

Acinetobacter species
Enterobacteriae
Enterobacter species
Escherichia coli
Klebsiella pneumoniae
Serratia marcescens
Pseudomonas aeruginosa
Pseudomonas (Burkholderia) cepacia
Stenotrophomonas (Xanthomona) maltophilia

Gram-positive cocci:

Streptococci
Group D *streptococci*
Staphylococcus aureus
Methacillin-resistant *S. aureus* (MRSA)
Coagulase-negative *Staphylococci* (*S. epidermis*)

(Lynch, J. P. [1997]. Bacterial pneumonia. In M. G. Khan, & J. P. Lynch [Eds.], *Pulmonary disease diagnosis and treatment.* Baltimore: Williams & Wilkins.)

BOX 20-3

RISK FACTORS FOR HOSPITAL-ACQUIRED PNEUMONIA

Intensive care unit admission
Intracranial pressure monitoring
Stress ulcer prophylaxis with acid-inhibiting medications
Mechanical ventilator circuit changes every 24 hours
Fall-winter season
Underlying chronic lung disease
Altered level of consciousness
Endotracheal intubation
Nasogastric tubes
Gastric content aspiration
Thoracoabdominal surgery
Inappropriate antibiotic use

(American Thoracic Society Statement. [1995]. Hospital-acquired pneumonia in adults: Diagnosis, assessment of severity, initial antimicrobial therapy, and preventative strategies. *American Journal of Respiratory and Critical Care Medicine, 153,* 1711–1725.)

Once the pathogen has gained entry into the lung, the resulting inflammatory process and subsequent infection begins with a change in airway epithelial cells that allows for enhanced bacterial adherence. Different bacteria affect the lung tissue in different ways. For example, pneumonia due to *S. pneumoniae* (pneumococcus) causes an acute inflammatory response with polymorphonuclear leukocytes (PMNs) and congestion, whereas pneumonia due to *S. aureus* is characterized by the development of multiple small or large abscesses. The pathogen must reach the alveoli and destroy the defense mechanisms of the alveolar macrophages to cause disease. The pathogen can also move into the interstitium via the terminal bronchioles and be carried away by lymphatic drainage to lodge on the pleural surface or in regional lymph nodes.

The initial inflammatory response varies with the infecting bacteria. It often results from protein-rich, bacteria-laden edematous fluid, which attracts PMNs, circulating monocytes, and plasma proteins to the alveoli. PMN neutrophils accumulate within the alveolar air spaces within hours from initiation of the inflammatory process and remain for approximately 3 days. Circulating peripheral blood monocytes arrive at the site of infection 1 to 2 days after infection. These monocytes then mature into functional macrophages. Lymphocytes can be found in the alveolar air spaces from 5 to 7 days after infection.

On a macroscopic level, there are several stages of consolidation that may be seen with pneumococcal and streptococcal pneumonias.[55] Within a few hours after insult, the alveolar epithelium becomes blood tinged due to swollen capillaries. The alveolar air spaces become engorged with edematous fluid, red blood cells, and desquamated epithelial cells. Fibrin mesh deposits, erythrocytes, PMNs, and mononuclear leukocytes in the alveolar air spaces cause the lung tissue to take on a dry, granular, dark reddish-brown appearance. This is referred to as "red hepatization" and normally lasts for about 2 to 3 days. This phase is followed by "gray hepatization," which is characterized by dense, friable lung tissue, which includes alveolar exudates, fibrin, and macrophages. This stage persists for 2 or more days.[50] The pathology of pneumonia due to pneumococcal pneumonia is summarized in Figure 20-1.

The end result of this complex inflammatory process is poor lung ventilation of the affected areas due to cellular infiltration and congestion. The filling of alveoli with exudate, or consolidation, causes them to become airless. Sustained perfusion with poor ventilation occurs in the consolidated area. Focal pneumonia (also referred to as *lobar, bronchopneumonia, bronchial* or *bronchiolar pneumonia*) indicates that the respiratory bronchioles, alveolar ducts, and alveoli are involved. The infection is spread from the bronchial tree from one lobule to another and from segment to segment and lobe to lobe. Extension of the infection into the alveoli may occur through the pores of Kohn. In lobar pneumonias, the infection spreads between alveoli until it is contained by the segments of the lungs. In bronchopneumonias, the pathologic process is not confined by

FOCUS ON CELLULAR PATHOPHYSIOLOGY

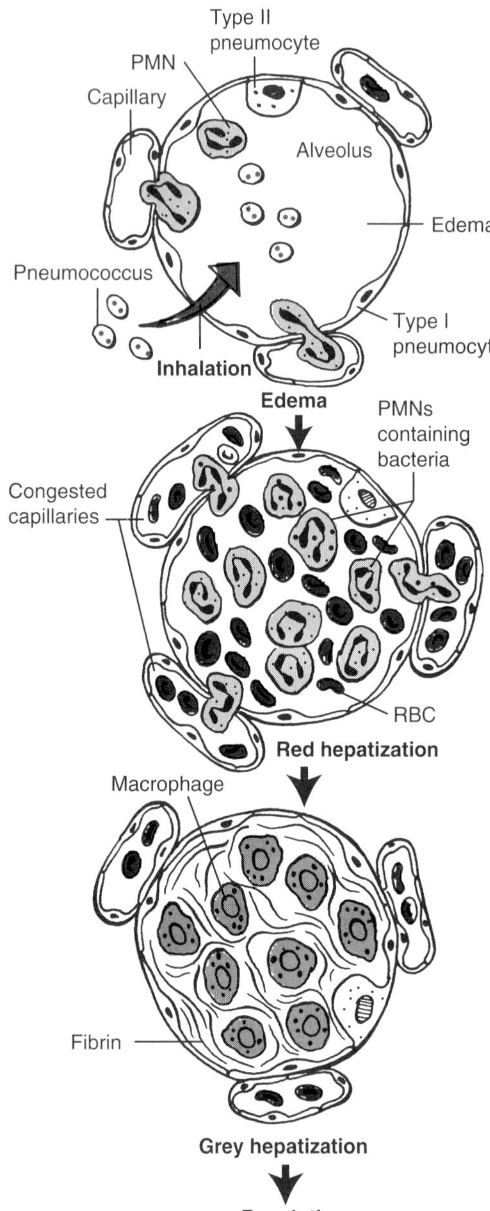

FIGURE 20-1. Pathogenesis of lobar pneumococcal pneumonia. Pneumococci, characteristically in pairs (diplococci), multiply rapidly in the alveolar spaces and produce extensive edema. They incite an acute inflammatory response, in which polymorphonuclear leukocytes and congestion are prominent (red hepatization). As the inflammatory process progresses, macrophages replace the polymorphonuclear leukocytes and ingest debris (gray hepatization). The process usually resolves, but complications may ensue. (Rubin, E. & Farber, J. [1999]. *Pathology* [3rd ed.] Philadelphia: Lippincott Williams & Wilkins.)

anatomic barriers and extends to nearby areas of the lungs, creating a patchy appearance in more than one area of the lung.[43] Necrotizing pneumonias or lung abscesses can occur when proteolytic or elastolytic enzymes are released by bacteria or inflammatory cells. *S. aureus*, *Streptococcus pyrogens*, enteric gram-negative bacteria, and *Pseudomonas aeruginosa* all have this potential.

A number of complications may be associated with acute bacterial pneumonia, including **pleuritis** (inflammation of the pleura), **pleural effusion**, **pyothorax** (pus in the pleural cavity), **empyema** (the pyothorax organizes and has fibrous walls), and bacteremia (circulating bacteria may lead to endocarditis or meningitis).[50]

CLINICAL MANIFESTATIONS. The clinical time course of pneumonia varies widely. In acute bacterial pneumonia, the inflammatory process occurs over a period of 5 to 10 days. In 70% of cases this coincides with symptoms, but the inflammation and symptoms can extend for as long as 2 to 3 weeks or the complications can cause a degenerating picture.[35]

The "typical" clinical presentation of CAP includes fever of abrupt onset, chills, sweats, cough, purulent (often rust-colored) sputum, pleuritic pain, and fatigue. It should be noted, however, that clinical presentations can vary widely. In the elderly, presenting symptoms may be very subtle and may only be heralded through a change in mental status, poor appetite, or an apparent deterioration of an underlying disorder such as chronic obstructive lung disease.

To be labeled HAP, the following criteria must be met:[29,48]

- Onset of symptoms at least 48 hours after hospital admission
- Infectious process not present on admission to hospital
- Temperature >38°C
- Blood leukocytosis
- Chest radiograph demonstrating new pulmonary infiltrates consistent with an infectious process
- Purulent endotracheal secretions

Pneumocystis carinii Pneumonia

Pneumocystis carinii is an organism that was thought to be a protozoa but is probably a fungus.[43,56] *Pneumocystis carinii* pneumonia (PCP) is an "opportunistic" lower respiratory tract infection that causes disease in individuals who have a weakened immune system, such as those with acquired immunodeficiency syndrome (AIDS) or receiving immunosuppressive therapy (e.g., chemotherapy or steroids). The epidemiology of PCP is not completely understood. It is believed that during early childhood, exposure causes a clinically inapparent illness that results in low-level antibodies. *P. carinii* is of low virulence and, in the presence of normal immune function, does not cause disease. When there is an alteration in immune function affecting T-cell immunity, reactivation of infection or increased susceptibility to infection can occur. Whether the infection can be spread from one susceptible person to another remains controversial but has been described in cohorts of immunosuppressed patients, the elderly, and severely malnourished infants.[30]

CLINICAL MANIFESTATIONS. Clinical presentation is dependent upon the underlying etiology of the immune dysfunction.[30] When infection occurs in a non-human immunodeficiency virus (HIV)–infected host, the clinical course is quite different from that seen in an HIV-infected host. The non-HIV-infected individual presents with fever, nonproductive cough, dyspnea, tachypnea, and pulmonary congestion. Infection in this population is rapid and progressive, resulting in diffuse alveolar and interstitial infiltrates on chest radiograph. Within 4 to 15 days, symptoms progress to hypoxemia and respiratory failure. In the HIV-infected host, the presenting symptoms are similar but the progression is much more insidious.[30] There may be a low-grade fever, mild cough, and weight loss. The chest radiograph may show only subtle interstitial infiltrates, if any at all. As the infection progresses in this population, tachypnea increases and eventually hypoxemia becomes evident. During the acute phase of illness, arterial blood gases demonstrate respiratory alkalosis. In the terminal stages, there is severe respiratory acidosis.

Pneumonias Caused by Other Pathogens

Pneumonia may be caused by other pathogens, including viruses, fungi, rickettsia, and non-tubercular mycobacteria. "Atypical" pneumonia is usually caused by *Mycoplasma pneumoniae*, but *Chlamydia pneumoniae, Chlamydia psittaci,* and *Legionella pneumophila* are special types of bacteria that can cause the disease.[3]

VIRUSES. Viruses are the suspected etiology in approximately 8% of adult pneumonia cases and account for up to 16% of cases in children, including bronchiolitis and pneumonia.[19] Epidemics of this viral infection occur in winter and often affect young children and infants. The common types of viruses associated with viral pneumonia are influenza, adenovirus, chickenpox virus, and respiratory syncytial virus. In adults, viral pneumonia may affect the alveolar epithelial cells, causing interstitial inflammation and intra-alveolar edema. The presence of mononuclear cells is characteristic.[50] The course may be very rapid, causing an acute clinical picture of respiratory distress with or without fever. The terminal and respiratory bronchioles may become damaged and thus susceptible to secondary bacterial invasion that spreads to the surrounding alveoli.

FUNGI. Various potentially pathogenic fungi exist in soils and some natural substances throughout the United States. Fungal pneumonia can occur if coccidioidomycosis, histoplasmosis, cryptococcus, and a variety of other fungi are introduced through inhalation of infected dust particles into the respiratory tract. The clinical picture may be one of chronic infection or lesions similar to the Ghon complex of tuberculosis (see p. 557).

RICKETTSIA. "Q fever," caused by *Coxiella burnetii*, is an example of a rickettsial pneumonia that can be spread from animals or through inhalation of infected dust particles. It grows in the macrophages of the lung, liver, bone marrow, and spleen and stimulates the formation of granulomas.[43]

NON-TUBERCULAR MYCOBACTERIA. Non-tubercular mycobacteria (NTMB) such as *Mycobacteria kansasii* or *Mycobacteria avium intracellulare* (MAC) are also capable of causing significant infections, which often resemble tuberculosis. These organisms cause pneumonia with greater frequency in individuals who are immunosuppressed or immunocompromised.

ATYPICAL PNEUMONIAS. *Myoplasma pneumoniae* is the main organism that causes "atypical pneumonia." The pneumonia develops gradually, with respiratory symptoms progressing to the development of patchy intra-alveolar pneumonia. The clinical course is often prolonged but rarely fatal.[50]

Chlamydia pneumoniae commonly causes pneumonia and upper respiratory tract disease. Because chlamydia must grow within host cells, the eradication of the organism requires long-term treatment with a broad-spectrum antibiotic.

Psittacosis, caused by *Chlamydia psittaci,* a small bacteria that can only grow inside host cells, is transmitted from birds and sheep. It causes a flulike disease that may progress to irregular consolidation and interstitial pneumonia.[50]

Legionella pneumophila was first described at an American Legion convention in Philadelphia in 1976, and the organism was identified as a fastidious bacterium that lives in aquatic environments. Outbreaks of the disease have been traced to air-conditioning cooling towers and evaporative condensers. The organism rapidly grows in the lungs and causes fibrin and inflammatory cells in the alveoli; often, the picture is complicated by empyema. The symptoms of the disease include fever, cough, and chest pain, with a mortality rate of 10% to 20%.[50]

Aspiration Pneumonia

Aspiration pneumonia occurs when secretions or inert substances are inhaled into the tracheobronchial tree. Aspiration of oropharyngeal secretions occurs relatively frequently in healthy humans during sleep, and aspiration episodes occur with much greater frequency in individuals with oropharyngeal or neurologic dysfunction. Medications, alcohol, or altered levels of consciousness are among factors that can increase the incidence of aspiration (Box 20-4). Three aspiration syndromes include chemical pneumonitis, aspiration of bacterial pathogens, and aspiration of inert substances.[27] These are classified according to their cause.

Chemical pneumonitis occurs when toxic substances (such as gastric acid, bile, hydrocarbon fats, or mineral oil) are introduced into the lung. Acute lung injury and inflammation may lead to necrosis and fibrosis of the airways. Secondary bacterial pneumonia occurs in only about 50% of chemical pneumonitis cases.[27] Symptom onset is rapid (2–5 hours) and includes cyanosis, tachypnea, dyspnea, tachycardia, hypotension, bronchospasm, congestion, and frothy sputum.

Aspiration of bacterial pathogens results in bacterial pneumonia, as discussed above. The most common source of bacterial pathogens is from the oropharynx.

Aspiration of inert substances such as foreign bodies (teeth, food) or large amounts of water (near drowning) may cause bronchial obstruction and/or pneumonitis of the lung. Coughing and cyanosis may be present, and localized wheezing on chest auscultation may indicate a partial airway obstruction.[27] Water will cause a dilution of surfactant and may promote atelectasis and adult respiratory distress syndrome.

Pulmonary Tuberculosis

Pulmonary tuberculosis (TB) is a major cause of death from infectious disease worldwide. In the United States, from 1950 until 1985 TB cases declined at an annual rate of 5% per year.[11] However, beginning in 1985, the number of reported cases increased by 18% annually. This case increase was thought to be due to the emergence of HIV, decreased federal funding for TB-control programs, and an increase in the number of immigrants from countries where TB is endemic. Fortunately, more recent data analysis indicates a decline in cases reported. The Centers for Disease Control (CDC) reported that 1997 data indicated a 7% decrease from 1996 and a 26% decrease since 1992.[12] In 1997, six states (California, Florida, Illinois, New Jersey, New York, and Texas) accounted for 57% of all TB cases reported.[12]

Specific populations are at increased risk for TB infection (Box 20-5). Underlying or concurrent medical conditions can also increase the risk for TB (Box 20-6).

ETIOLOGY

Pulmonary TB is caused by *Mycobacterium tuberculosis* (*M. TB*). *M. TB* is an aerobic, rod-shaped, acid-fast bacilli that can be spread by aerosolized droplet nuclei produced by an infected individual. These droplets are expelled into the environment by the infected host through activities such as coughing, laughing, sneezing, and singing. If these droplets successfully gain entry into the airways and begin to proliferate within a new host, tuberculous infection ensues. In most normal hosts, immune system activity is sufficient to effectively contain and suppress the infection, rendering it inactive or dormant. However, if the immune system is unable to effectively contain the initial infection, progression to clinical disease occurs. This is referred to as

BOX 20-4 RISK FACTORS FOR ASPIRATION PNEUMONIA

Advanced age
Decreased level of consciousness
Seizures
Cerebral vascular accidents
Dysphagia
Impaired gastroesophageal motility
Gastroesophageal reflux
Endotracheal intubation
Anesthesia
Naso- or orogastric tubes
Enteral feedings
Tracheostomy
Gastrostomy tubes
Jejunostomy
Alcohol use/abuse

(Adapted from Lomaton, J. R., George, S. S. & Brandstetter, R. D. [1997]. Aspiration pneumonia. *Postgraduate Medicine, 102*[2], 225–231.)

BOX 20-5 POPULATIONS AT RISK FOR TUBERCULOUS INFECTION

Close contacts of infectious TB cases
HIV infected
Homeless
Medically underserved or low-income groups
Substance abusers (alcohol or street drugs)
Residents and employees of medical institutions, shelters, or correctional facilities
Recent immigrants from countries where TB is prevalent
High-risk ethnic groups
Infants, children, and adolescents in contact with high-risk adults

(Centers for Disease Control [1995]. Screening for tuberculosis and tuberculosis infection in high-risk populations: Recommendations of the Advisory Council for the Elimination of Tuberculosis. *Morbidity and Mortality Weekly Report, 44* [No. RR-11], 19–33.)

BOX 20-6

MEDICAL RISK FACTORS FOR TUBERCULOUS INFECTION

Diabetes mellitus
Chronic renal failure
Silicosis
Hematologic disorders (lymphoma, leukemia)
Body weight 10% below ideal
Immunosuppressed (post-bone marrow or organ transplant)
Individuals on long-term high-dose corticosteroid treatment
Some head and neck malignancies
History of gastrectomy or jejunoileal bypass surgery

(Centers for Disease Control [1995]. Screening for tuberculosis and tuberculosis infection in high-risk populations: Recommendations of the Advisory Council for the Elimination of Tuberculosis. *Morbidity and Mortality Weekly Report, 44* [No. RR-11], 19–33.)

primary TB. Once the bacilli have been introduced into the host, and even if immune system containment is successful, there is a 5% to 10% risk over an individual's lifetime of reactivation of infection leading to active TB infection.[23,43]

PATHOPHYSIOLOGY

The ability of *M. TB* to cause disease is related to its ability to escape killing by macrophages and to induce a Type IV hypersensitivity response (see p. 318). The organisms can elude destruction from the defensive phagocytes by not allowing the lysosomes to destroy them.[42] The stages of the disease are usually described in terms of primary infection and secondary/disseminated infection.

Primary Infection

The small size of the droplet nuclei allows the organism to evade most of the protective mechanisms of the lung as it is inhaled into the alveoli. The organisms lodge in the periphery of the lung and are phagocytosed by alveolar macrophages, which transport them to hilar lymph nodes.[42] The successful establishment of infection depends both on the number of organisms introduced and on the microbicidal activity of the alveolar macrophages. The macrophages are often unsuccessful in killing the mycobacteria but can form giant cells to contain them. T lymphocytes interact with macrophages to form granulomas, which can sometimes kill the mycobacteria. The residual effect of the primary infection usually is a healed calcified lesion known as a **Ghon complex.** Within and around the lesion, tissue necrosis and scarring usually occurs.

The T cell–mediated immune response takes 4 to 6 weeks and results in demonstrable immunity through a positive purified protein derivative (PPD) test reaction. In the minority of cases, especially in infants or immunodeficient adults, there is progressive spread with cavitation, tuberculous pneumonia, or miliary TB that follows primary infection.[23]

Secondary or Reactivation Tuberculosis

Most cases of secondary pulmonary TB develop due to reactivation of a primary infection, which may have produced disseminated organisms that did not produce a clinical infection.[23]

The cellular response to the organisms leads to the formation of many **granulomas** and extensive tissue necrosis. Poorly defined lesions, called **tubercles,** develop, which usually have central areas of caseous necrosis. These areas may heal, or they may erode into a bronchus and then drain out infected material. These cavities may be very large and tend to be situated in the apices of the lung (Fig. 20-2).[50]

The organism can also be transported across alveolar walls, into the lymphatic system, and thus into the blood stream, causing a **tuberculous bacillemia.** As a result of the bacillemia, extra-pulmonary infection, such as in the bone, gut, or urinary tract occurs. This complication is called *miliary TB.*

CLINICAL MANIFESTATIONS

Typical symptoms of active TB include constitutional symptoms such as fever, fatigue, weight loss, night sweats, malaise, cough, sputum production, and, occasionally, vague chest pain and hemoptysis. Often the physical examination will be normal unless there is an

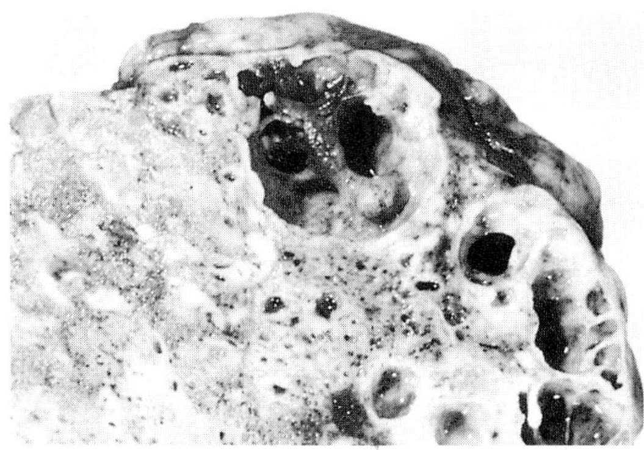

FIGURE 20-2. Tuberculous cavities. The apex of the left upper lobe shows tuberculous cavities surrounded by consolidated and fibrotic pulmonary parenchyema. (Rubin, E. & Farber, J. [1999]. *Pathology* [3rd ed.]. Philadelphia: Lippincott Williams & Wilkins.)

active lung infiltrate, pleural effusion, or general evidence of chronic infection, such as wasting.

An indurated (raised) skin reaction to the purified protein derivative (PPD) skin test at least 48 hours after intradermal placement suggests the presence of memory T cells for *M. Tb.* An erythematous reaction of 10 mm or larger is necessary to be considered positive, but this depends upon multiple factors such as age, immune competence, geographic location, and medications.[44] The test is not 100% sensitive or reliable and does not distinguish between recent and past infection.

Many acid-fast bacilli (AFB) organisms may be seen on an initial sputum smear. The specimen is then termed "smear positive." Although the smear status does not confirm that the bacterium is tuberculous, it does indicate a heavy bacterial load and a strong potential for contagion.

Radiographic manifestations of pulmonary tuberculous infections include infiltrates, particularly in the upper lobes or superior segments of the middle or lower lobes, and cavities or calcified nodular lesions in cases of past infection. In the immunocompromised host, the chest radiograph may appear completely normal even in the presence of active infection.

OBSTRUCTIVE DISORDERS

Obstructive lung disorders are diseases that interfere with the normal flow of air out of the lungs during expiration. Obstructive disorders have the potential to be life threatening.

Asthma

Regardless of severity, asthma is defined as "a chronic inflammatory disorder of the airways."[36] This chronic disease is characterized by reversible airway bronchospasm, mucus hypersecretion, and airway edema. The reversibility of the disorder is what separates it from disorders classified as "chronic obstructive pulmonary diseases," since the asthmatic individual can potentially enjoy symptom-free intervals.

ETIOLOGY

The etiology of asthma is multifactorial and is somewhat dependent upon age of presentation. Child-onset asthma is frequently associated with **atopy** (see p. 312). Atopy is defined as a genetic propensity to produce IgE proteins that are directed towards common environmental allergens such as house-dust mites, fungi, and animal proteins.[36] The likelihood of developing adult asthma is increased in infants or young children with a history of allergy or wheezing associated with viral infection, or a family history of allergies.[31]

In adults, allergies may also play a significant role; however, IgE antibodies and a family history are not as common compared with child-onset disease. The coexistence of respiratory tract infections, nasal polyps, and sinusitis with adult asthma is also frequently reported.

Occupational asthma is a disorder that occurs when an individual develops asthma symptoms due to exposures in the work environment. Pollution in the environment may also provide a trigger for an asthma attack. Occupational asthma triggers include dusts, fumes, animal danders, and molds.

Drug-induced asthma is a term used to describe asthma-like symptoms due to hypersensitivity to various drugs. Aspirin commonly causes this reaction, but other drugs such as propranolol and nonsteroidal anti-inflammatory agents may also elicit this response.

Exercise-induced asthma may occur in individuals who have no other trigger for the asthma, or exercise may provoke a response in a known asthmatic. It is apparently due to heat or water loss from the epithelium of the airways.[50] Emotional factors can aggravate or precipitate an asthmatic attack and are seen in approximately half of all asthmatics.[50]

PATHOPHYSIOLOGY

Airway inflammation is considered to be the most important pathophysiologic factor in asthma.[36] Frequently, the inflammation occurs in response to exposure to an allergen or infection. Other important pathophysiologic changes thought to be associated with this inflammation include:

- Airway hyperresponsiveness (or "twitchiness") that results in airflow limitations, symptoms, and chronic disease
- Bronchospasm (an involuntary tightening of the airway smooth muscles), which also contributes to airflow limitations
- Airway edema, airway wall remodeling, and mucus plug formation, which all contribute to bronchial obstruction
- Immunologic responses, such as mast cell activation and infiltration of inflammatory cells such as neutrophils, eosinophils, and lymphocytes that account for the inflammatory feature of the disease
- Denudation (or stripping) of airway epithelium and collagen deposition below the basement membrane, which contribute to chronic airway changes seen in long-standing asthma

CLASSIFICATION

Asthma is classified by its severity. The severity ratings are as follows: mild intermittent, mild persistent, moderate persistent, and severe persistent.[36] Assessment of symptom severity is based on frequency of symptoms, frequency and character of attacks, use of medications, presence or absence of night-time symptoms, and pulmonary function values (see Appendix Table A). Table 20-2 summarizes the classification of asthma severity.

TABLE 20-2
CLASSIFICATION OF ASTHMA SEVERITY

	SYMPTOMS	NIGHT-TIME SYMPTOMS	LUNG FUNCTION
Mild intermittent	Symptoms 2× or less/wk Asymptomatic between attacks; exacerbations brief, may intensify	≤2/month	FEV_1 or PEF ≥ 80% predicted PEF variability <20%
Mild persistent	Symptoms greater than 2×/wk Attacks may affect activity	>2/month	FEV_1 or PEF ≥ 80% predicted PEF variability 20–30%
Moderate persistent	Daily Symptoms Daily use of short-acting medications Attacks affect activity Attacks greater than 2×/week, may last days	> 1/week	FEV_1 or PEF > 60–<80% pred. PEF variability >30%
Severe persistent	Continual symptoms Limited physical activity Frequent attacks	Frequent	FEV_1 or PEF ≤ 60% predicted PEF variability > 30%

(Adapted from National Institutes of Health: National Heart, Lung and Blood Institute. [1997]. *Expert Panel Report II: Guidelines for the diagnosis and management of asthma.* NIH Publication No. 97-4051, p. 8. Washington; DC: NIH.)

CLINICAL MANIFESTATIONS

Acute, sometimes abrupt, onset of cough, wheezing, chest tightness, tachypnea, tachycardia, and increased work of breathing are the characteristic initial symptoms of an asthma attack. In asthma that is triggered by exposure to an antigen, a "late-phase reaction" can occur 4 to 8 hours following initial symptom onset and coincides with the inflammatory response. When an asthmatic attack is associated with atopic disease, individuals may also demonstrate concurrent allergic symptoms such as rhinitis, nasal polyps, sinusitis, and eczema.

The use of accessory muscles for breathing may be noted during an acute attack. In severe cases, hypoxemia and respiratory fatigue can ensue. If it is accompanied by hypercarbia, acute respiratory failure is imminent.

During an acute attack, pulmonary function testing demonstrates decreased forced expiratory flows due to the obstruction of the airways imposed by inflammation, swelling, excess mucus, and bronchospasm. FEV_1 and PEF (peak expiratory flow) are two measures that are helpful in assessing asthma activity and severity (see Appendix Table A).

Chronic Obstructive Pulmonary Disease

Chronic obstructive pulmonary disease (COPD) is defined as a disease state characterized by the presence of airflow obstruction that is generally progressive, may be accompanied by airway hyperreactivity, and may be partially reversible.[5] COPD is a global term used to identify a group of overlapping heterogeneous disorders. The individual disorders include emphysema, chronic bronchitis, and bronchiectasis. These are distinguished by their anatomic and clinical characteristics (Table 20-3).

It is estimated that 14 million American suffer from some form of COPD. The death rate is estimated to be approximately 18.6 per 100,000 people.[5] Exposure to tobacco smoke is the primary cause for COPD. Typically, the individual with COPD has at least a 20 pack-year (average number of packs per day multiplied by number of years of smoking) history of smoking and presents for medical advice during the fifth decade of life, usually in the context of an acute or recurrent chest illness or productive cough.[5] In the sixth to seventh decades, dyspnea becomes a constant feature. The risk factors for COPD are presented in Box 20-7.

The etiologic, pathophysiologic, and clinical features of different types of COPD overlap but also can cause distinct pictures. With this concept established, each entity is described below.

EMPHYSEMA

Emphysema is characterized by abnormal and permanent enlargement of the airspaces distal to the terminal bronchioles, which results in destruction of the walls of the alveoli.[23] It is defined according to the anatomic change brought about by the destruction. Box 20-8 describes the types of emphysema. The most severe type of emphysemas occur in men who smoke heavily.[23]

Pathophysiology

The pathophysiologic changes associated with emphysema are characterized by permanent destruction

TABLE 20-3

CHRONIC OBSTRUCTIVE PULMONARY DISEASE

CONDITION	ANATOMIC SITE	MAJOR PATHOLOGIC CHANGES	ETIOLOGY	SIGNS/SYMPTOMS
Chronic bronchitis	Bronchus	Mucous gland hyperplasia, hypersecretion	Tobacco smoke, air pollutants	Cough, sputum production
Bronchiectasis	Bronchus	Airway dilation and scarring	Persistent or severe infections	Cough; purulent sputum; fever
Emphysema	Acinus	Airspace enlargement; wall destruction	Tobacco smoke	Dyspnea

(Adapted from Cotran, R. S., Kumar, V. & Collins, T. [1999]. *Robbins' pathologic basis of disease* [6th ed.]. Philadelphia: W. B. Saunders.)

of air spaces. The alveolar walls are destroyed without any obvious evidence of fibrosis.[15] The loss of alveolar walls also leads to a significant hyperinflation accompanied by a decrease in functional alveolar capillary bed surface area. This change directly affects efficiency of gas exchange.

As a direct consequence of the pathologic destruction, the small airways are no longer supported and eventually become distorted and deformed. The airway changes result in **air trapping** due to premature small airway closure during exhalation.

Clinical Manifestations

Clinical manifestations do not usually appear until at least one third of the functioning pulmonary parenchyma is destroyed.[23] The first symptom is dyspnea that becomes steadily more pronounced. Cough and wheezing may be present, especially if there is associated bronchitis.

The individual with emphysema often displays a cachectic body habitus, increased anterior-posterior chest diameter (barrel chest appearance), obvious prolongation of the expiratory cycle, and use of accessory muscles in forced expiration. The skin color is often florid, even in the face of severe pulmonary damage, with arterial blood gases demonstrating only moderate hypoxemia until late stages of the disease. This has been termed the "pink puffer" appearance. When hypoxemia does occur it may lead to erythrocytosis (described below). The individual with emphysema will complain of shortness of breath, especially with activity, but may have very little sputum production. On chest auscultation, the breath sounds are somewhat quiet and distant. The long-term energy cost of this pulmonary disease is a common cause of respiratory failure (see p. 579). Table 20-4 differentiates the predominant emphysema from the predominant bronchitis clinical picture.

CHRONIC BRONCHITIS

Chronic bronchitis is defined as the presence of a continual productive cough for more than half the time over a period of 2 years.[50] In 90% of cases, chronic bronchitis is caused by cigarette smoking, but it may be associated with other risk factors (see Box 20-7). The cellular alterations are variable but mainly result from an increase in mucus secretion by the goblet cells of the bronchial mucous glands.

BOX 20-7

RISK FACTORS FOR COPD

- Cigarette smoking
- Passive smoke exposure
- Male sex
- Nonwhite race
- Low socioeconomic status
- Alpha 1-antitrypsin deficiency
- Air pollution
- Occupational exposure
- Hyper-responsive airways

BOX 20-8

TYPES OF EMPHYSEMA

Centrilobular Emphysema

Dilatation and destruction involve central part of acinus.

Panacinar Emphysema

Dilatation and destruction involve entire acinus.

Results from some genetic conditions in which there is deficiency of alpha 1-antiprotease (alpha 1-antitrypsin); causes early onset of emphysema.

TABLE 20-4

CLINICAL COMPARISON OF PREDOMINANT BRONCHITIS AND EMPHYSEMA

	PREDOMINANT BRONCHITIS	PREDOMINANT EMPHYSEMA
Age (yr)	40–45	50–75
Dyspnea	Mild; late	Severe; early
Cough	Early; copious sputum	Late; scanty sputum
Infections	Common	Occasional
Respiratory insufficiency	Repeated	Terminal
Cor pulmonale	Common	Rare; terminal
Airway resistance	Increased	Normal or slightly increased
Elastic recoil	Normal	Low
Chest radiograph	Prominent vessels; large heart	Hyperinflation; small heart
Appearance	*Blue bloater*	*Pink puffer*

(Cotran, R. S., Kumar, V. & Collins, T. [1999]. *Robbins' pathologic basis of disease* [6th ed.]. Philadelphia: W. B. Saunders.)

Pathophysiology

Pathophysiologic changes seen in chronic bronchitis generally involve the airways rather than the alveoli. Goblet cells in the airways multiply and secrete excessive amounts of mucus. Areas of squamous metaplasia of bronchial epithelium and hypertrophy of airway smooth muscle can also be seen. The basal cells of the epithelium become hyperplastic and the basement membrane thickens. Lymphocytes and macrophages are attracted due to chronic inflammation and infection. The small airways become distorted and can become plugged with secretions. The airways eventually lose their structural integrity due to damage of the supporting structures (cartilage) and thus close prematurely during exhalation. This promotes air trapping.[5] Morphologic changes associated with chronic bronchitis are shown in Figure 20-3.

In severe cases there is sustained hypoxia, which stimulates the kidneys to increase production of erythropoietin. Erythropoietin release stimulates RBC production, which eventually leads to an increase in the number of circulating RBCs. The increased number of RBCs, termed *erythrocytosis*, attempts to increase oxygen delivery to the tissues in order to offset hypoxemia imposed by the underlying pulmonary disease. This excessive number of circulating RBCs increases blood viscosity and can interfere with circulation.

Clinical Manifestations

Initially sputum production is primarily mucoid and may increase in quantity and become purulent during respiratory infections. Most of the expectoration occurs in the morning hours. Superimposed acute chest illnesses occur intermittently and increase in frequency in the later stages of the disease process.[10]

As the condition becomes chronic, productive cough, chest congestion, and shortness of breath at rest and with activity are experienced. Later signs in chronic bronchitis include fluid retention in the periphery, manifesting as edema (see Table 20-4). Symptoms of right heart failure, called **cor pulmonale**, and a cyanotic appearance of the skin have been described as the "blue bloater" appearance. The chronic bronchitic often retains carbon dioxide and thus exhibits hypercarbia as well as hypoxemia on arterial blood gas analysis. On chest auscultation, the breath sounds may reveal crackles, wheezes, and rhonchi.

BRONCHIECTASIS

Bronchiectasis is a disorder that is characterized by permanent dilation and destruction of cartilage-containing airways. The term identifies an anatomic finding that is the result of multiple pulmonary insults rather than a specific disease entity.[8]

Etiology

Over time, inflammation from repeated infection, toxic exposure, or a foreign body impairs mucociliary clearance mechanisms within the airways, resulting in the airway abnormalities. Bronchiectatic airway changes can also occur as a residual of pulmonary tuberculous infections, fungal infections, or genetic disorders such as cystic fibrosis. Prior to the discovery of effective antibiotic treatments for respiratory tract infections, bronchiectasis was a common disease.

FOCUS ON CELLULAR PATHOPHYSIOLOGY

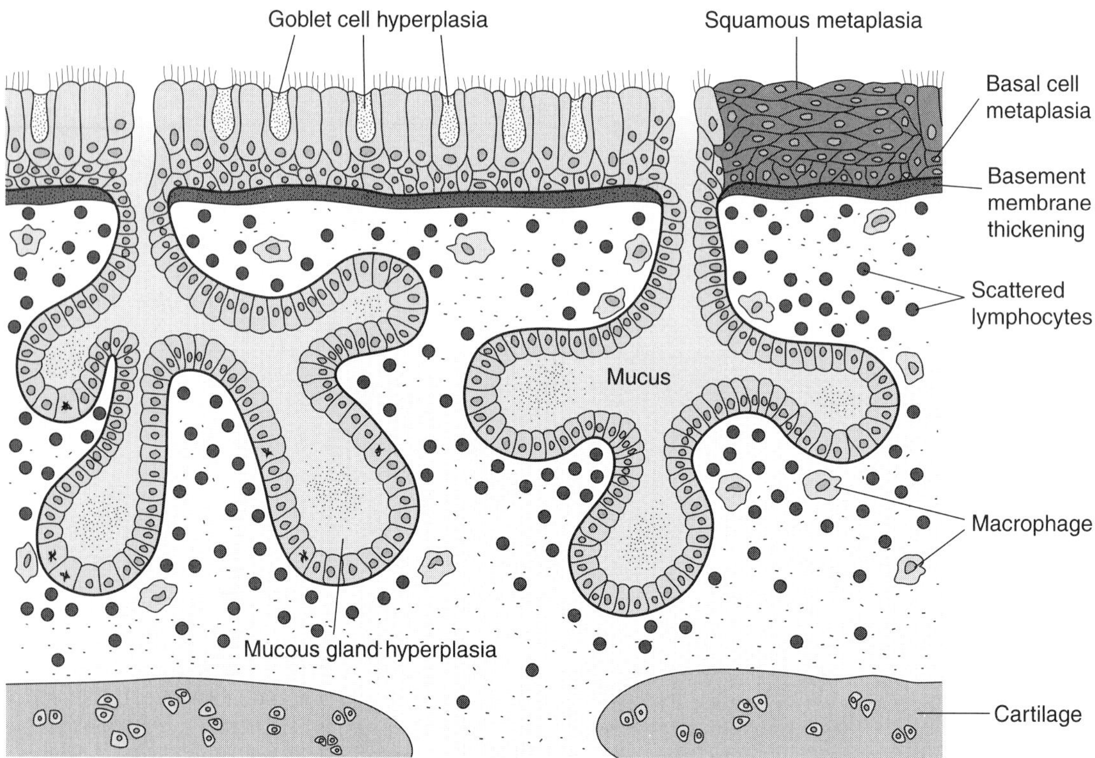

FIGURE 20-3. Morphologic changes in chronic bronchitis. (Rubin, E. & Farber, J. *Pathology* [3rd ed.]. Philadelphia: Lippincott Williams & Wilkins).

Pathophysiology

As a result of the insults described above, the distal airways become permanently deformed and dilated. Most individuals have bronchiectatic changes confined to one or two neighboring lobes. The left lower lobe is the most common site of involvement.[8] Inflammation and denuding of the airway epithelium are common histologic findings. As a direct result of this process, the cartilage and elastic tissue that support the airways are damaged. Areas of peribronchial pneumonia or atelectasis can be found around bronchiectatic segments. Inflammatory infiltration of small airways can result in obstruction. Fibrosis occurs in severe cases.[8] The bronchiectatic deformations provide ideal sites for proliferation of bacteria and recurrent infection, thus potentially perpetuating the problem.[54]

Clinical Manifestations

Chronic, persistent cough with copious amounts of purulent sputum (which can amount to more than 100 cc/day[8]) is the most common presenting symptom. In cases of congenital disorders, symptoms may start as early as age 2 to 7 years. If bronchiectasis is of a post-infectious type, the onset of symptoms may be more insidious, but often the individual can relate a history of childhood infections. If associated with systemic or genetic disorders (such as cystic fibrosis), other symptoms such as sinus disease or malabsorption may also be apparent. Hyperresponsive airways and associated wheezing are not uncommon. On auscultation, coarse inspiratory and expiratory crackles are heard but may clear with coughing. A chest radiograph can demonstrate abnormally enlarged airways.[18] Pulmonary function tests and arterial blood gases are similar to those associated with chronic bronchitis.

Cystic Fibrosis

Cystic fibrosis (CF) is an inherited autosomal recessive exocrine disorder that affects 1 in 1500 to 1 in 4000 live births.[45,48] The pulmonary manifestations of the disease are due to viscous mucus secretions and obstruction and infection of the airways. The disease affects respiratory, gastrointestinal, and reproductive function and is also discussed on page 772.

This disorder occurs when the CF gene appears on the long arm of chromosome 7.[40] Different combinations of gene abnormalities will result in varying disease characteristics of organ involvement in a given individual. Not all individuals diagnosed with CF manifest significant pulmonary involvement.

PATHOPHYSIOLOGY

The pathophysiologic features of CF are due to dysfunction of epithelial chloride ion channels.[1] The chloride channels either do not open up or are completely absent. In the lung, this causes excessive sodium reabsorption and decreased chloride excretion, leading to dehydration of the mucous layer, defective mucociliary action, and mucus plugging of airways.[40] The airways of many CF sufferers are colonized with *Pseudomonas aeruginosa* species, particularly a mucoid form that resists antibiotics. Bronchiectasis results secondarily in response to chronic and recurrent infections.

CLINICAL MANIFESTATIONS

Pulmonary manifestations of CF include cough, chest congestion, copious sputum, and shortness of breath. Symptoms often begin in infancy. Progressive obstruction, deterioration of pulmonary function, dyspnea, hemoptysis, hypoxemia, and complex bacterial infections are all part of the usual progression of this disorder. Respiratory failure is the cause of death in 95% of cases.[1]

RESTRICTIVE DISORDERS

Restrictive pulmonary disorders are diseases or conditions such as atelectasis or pneumothorax that result in inhibition of normal expansion of the lung. As opposed to obstructive disorders, difficulties are experienced during the inspiratory phase of respiration. Table 20-5 classifies the conditions and their pathogenesis.

Atelectasis

Atelectasis is a common, acute, restrictive disorder that occurs when previously expanded lung tissue collapses. The end result is a shrunken, airless state of the alveoli that does not participate in gas exchange. It may be classified as obstruction (reabsorption), compression, or contraction atelectasis.[23]

CLASSIFICATION

Reabsorption atelectasis is the result of bronchial or bronchiolar obstruction by mucosal edema, an airway tumor, or retained secretions. Gases trapped distal to the obstruction become reabsorbed, leading to collapse of the lung units. Any condition that promotes supine positioning, immobility, decreased depth of respiratory excursions, and decreased cough can cause reabsorption atelectasis. Prolonged inhalation of 100% oxygen can also promote atelectasis, as the high concentration of inspired air dilutes the concentration of other alveolar gases that normally help to keep air spaces open.

Compression atelectasis occurs secondary to a space-occupying process such as a pneumothorax, pleural effusion, or large mass. The lesion causes crowding of the lung tissue and prevents normal expansion.

Contraction atelectasis results from localized or generalized fibrotic changes in the lung or pleura that prevent the lung from expanding fully.[23] This may be seen in various forms of pulmonary fibrosis.

PATHOPHYSIOLOGY

The natural tendency of the lungs and alveoli is to collapse as elastic forces are constantly trying to force the lung tissue inward. These forces are opposed by the negative intrapleural forces and chest wall expansion (see p. 536). When airflow into the alveoli is disrupted, alveolar sacs collapse. In the collapsed state, little or no surfactant is produced since it has a short half-life and requires oxygen to replenish itself. The collateral communication through the pores of Kohn becomes ineffective in preventing collapse when airways to adjacent alveoli also become obstructed.

Perfusion to the collapsed airways is not affected, so blood continues to flow by airless alveoli. No gases are exchanged and blood does not become oxygenated. This perfusion without ventilation is referred to as a *shunt* or **shunting**. Because the flow of deoxygenated blood passes through the pulmonary capillary bed without being oxygenated, it is termed a *right-to-left shunt* within the lung (Fig. 20-4). If atelectasis involves a significant part of the lung, the normal ventilation-perfusion ratio is disturbed, and hypoxemia will result (see p. 539).

CLINICAL MANIFESTATIONS

Clinical symptoms depend on the amount of lung tissues affected. If only a small portion of the lung is involved, clinical manifestations may not be evident. Significant portions of affected lung tissue may cause tachypnea, cough, fever, and a complaint of dyspnea. Decreased chest wall expansion may be seen, and chest auscultation may reveal focal decreased breath sounds or increased crackles at the lung bases. Arterial blood gas analysis may reveal hypoxemia, and a chest radiograph will demonstrate decreased lung volume or an area of collapse in the atelectatic area.

Retained secretions and decreased depth of respiratory excursions are commonly seen following surgical procedures. Sedating medications and postoperative pain often depress the individual's protective cough reflex and decrease the sigh mechanism. Inadequate

(text continues on page 566)

TABLE 20-5

RESTRICTIVE LUNG DISEASES

CATEGORY	EXAMPLES	PATHOGENESIS	CLINICAL MANIFESTATIONS
Respiratory center depression	Narcotic and barbiturate dependence	Direct depression of respiratory center	Respiratory rate: < 12/min; associated signs of hypoventilation
	Central nervous systems lesions, head trauma	Injury to or impingement on respiratory centers	Hyper- or hypoventilation; cerebral edema and its signs
Neuromuscular	Guillain-Barré syndrome	Acute toxic polyneuritis; intercostal paralysis leads to diaphragmatic breathing; vagal and SNS paralysis lead to reduced ability of bronchioles to constrict, dilate, react to irritants	Reduced negative inspiratory pressure, V_T, V_C, compliance, breath sounds; hypoxemia, hypercapnia
	Duchenne muscular dystrophy	Genetic; thoracoscoliosis; paralysis of intercostals, abdominal muscles, diaphragm, accessory muscles	Pulmonary symptoms appear late; reduced IC, ERV, V_C, V_T, FRC, compliance PO_2; elevated PCO_2; abnormal respiratory patterns
Restriction of thoracic excursion			
Thoracic deformity	Kyphoscoliosis, pectus excavatum	Deformity of chest compresses lung tissue and limits thoracic excursion	Reduced breath sounds in affected areas, probably with rales; reduced compliance, TLC, V_C, ERV; signs of hypoventilation, hypoxemia, increased work of breathing
Traumatic chest wall instability	Flail chest	Fracture of a group of ribs leads to unstable chest wall; reduced intrathoracic pressure on inspiration pulls area in and causes pressure on parenchyma; this increases work of breathing and hypoventilation	Obvious flail, unequal chest excursion, bruising, skin injuries, localized pain on inspiration, dyspnea, reduced breath sounds with rales and rhonchi; reduced compliance, ERV, TLC, V_C, PO_2
Obesity	Obesity hypoventilation syndrome (Pickwickian syndrome)	Excess abdominal adipose tissue impinges on thoracic space and diaphragmatic excursion; reduced respiratory drive; increased weight of chest restricts thoracic excursion	Somnolence, twitching, periodic respirations, polycythemia, right ventricular hypertrophy/failure; reduced compliance, ERV, TLC, V_C, PO_2; elevated PCO_2; distant breath sounds
Pleural disorders	Pleural effusion	Accumulation of fluid in pleural space secondary to altered hydrostatic or oncotic forces	Unequal chest expansion; dullness and reduced breath sounds in affected area; may be constant chest discomfort; dyspnea if amount of fluid large; if over 250 mL, shows on radiographs; if large, bulging of intercostal space
	Pneumothorax	Accumulation of air in pleural space with proportional lung collapse	Hyperresonance; reduced breath sounds; tracheal deviation away from pneumothorax side;

TABLE 20-5

RESTRICTIVE LUNG DISEASES (Continued)

CATEGORY	EXAMPLES	PATHOGENESIS	CLINICAL MANIFESTATIONS
			tachycardia; unequal chest expansion; breath sounds reduced or absent; shows on radiographs
Disorders of lung parenchyma	Pulmonary fibrosis	Many possible causes: occupational, sarcoidosis, medications	Reduced compliance, hypoxemia, hypercapnia, and their consequences
	Tuberculosis	Bacterial invasion leads to scarring, reduced compliance, and reduced lung function	Visible on films; positive skin test, sputum; malaise, weight loss, fatigue, evening fever with night sweats, cough, hemoptysis
	Atelectasis	Obstruction of bronchioles, shrunken airless alveoli; reduced compliance; right-to-left shunting	Dyspnea, tachycardia, cough, fever, decreased chest wall expansion, hypoxemia, radiologic evidence
	Adult respiratory distress syndrome (ARDS)	Widespread atelectasis; loss of surfactant; interstitial edema, formation of hyaline membrane.	Dyspnea, tachypnea, grunting, labored respirations, hypoxemia, occasional hypercapnia, cyanosis; radiographs show bilateral patchy infiltrates
	Pulmonary edema	Increased pulmonary capillary pressure leads to interstitial and alveolar edema	Hypoxemia, tachypnea; signs of congestive heart failure, radiologic butterfly infiltrates, rales
	Aspiration pneumonia	Chemical irritant from aspirant leads to bronchoconstriction, necrosis, and fibrosis of airways	Hypoxemia, signs of ARDS, wheezing, tachypnea, tachycardia
	Pneumoconiosis	Inhalation of pollutants, results in scarring, fibrosis, and secondary emphysema	Slow developing pulmonary signs of dyspnea, hypoxemia, hypercapnia, cor pulmonale
	Bacterial pneumonia	Virulent bacteria, especially pneumococcal; inflammatory exudate with congestion and edema; poor ventilation in consolidated areas	Rapidly developing fever, chest pain, cough, blood-streaked or rust-colored sputum; responds well to antibiotic treatment
	Viral pneumonia	Rapid onset of inflammation in alveoli and terminal and respiratory bronchioles; secondary bacterial infection common	Respiratory distress with or without fever; much more severe in children with fever, dehydration, and respiratory failure, especially under 2 y of age
Interstitial lung diseases	Pulmonary fibrosis	Scarring and fibrosis of lung parenchyema	Gradual onset of dyspnea, dry cough, tachypnea, fine inspiratory crackles, lung base reduced TLC, V_C, compliance

FOCUS ON CELLULAR PATHOPHYSIOLOGY

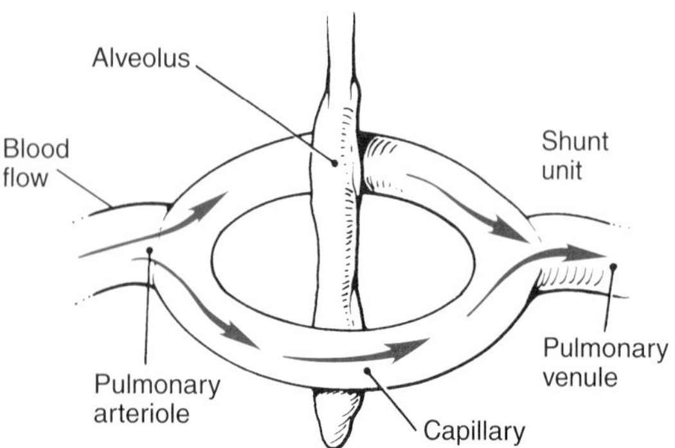

FIGURE 20-4. Schematic demonstration of a right-to-left shunt across the pulmonary bed.

alveolar expansion and retained secretions in dependent areas of the lung promote atelectasis.

Chest Wall Abnormalities

As an individual ages, the anterior-posterior diameter of the thorax tends to increase, but this does not significantly influence pulmonary function. Examples of chest wall abnormalities that can interfere with lung function include rib fractures and abnormal spine, sternal, or rib curvatures, such as **kyphoscoliosis** or **pectus excavatum**. Some congenital chest wall abnormalities are evident early in life; others become more apparent as a child grows. Although most mild deformities do not interfere with gas exchange, severe deformities are capable of doing so. Kyphoscoliosis is present when there is an abnormal curvature of the upper spine, thus deforming the thoracic cage. Pectus excavatum, or funnel chest, is a deformity of the lower end of the sternum. The sternum is caved in because of attachment to the spine by thick fibrous bands. **Pectus carinatum** (pigeon breast) is an abnormal prominence of the sternum (Fig. 20-5).

ETIOLOGY

The majority of significant chest wall abnormalities are due to congenital deformities. Osteoporotic changes in the spine can also contribute to worsening of kyphosis in elderly individuals.

PATHOPHYSIOLOGY

The degree of respiratory impairment, whether it is due to a deformity or rib fracture, varies widely and depends upon the extent of the deformity or injury. The abnormal curvature of the spine results in restrictive ventilation and lung tissue compression/crowding on the affected side. Function of the pulmonary vascular bed in the affected areas is also impaired, which over time results in increased work of breathing, alveolar hypoventilation, and hypoxemia.

CLINICAL MANIFESTATIONS

Significant chest wall abnormalities are usually evident on inspection. Lung compliance, total lung capacity, vital capacity, and other volume measurements are reduced (see Appendix Table A). Breath sounds over the compressed lung tissue may be decreased or demonstrate crackles. Musculoskeletal pain may occur as a consequence of the imposed postural changes associated with severe deformities. If the abnormality is sufficient to result in chronic hypoventilation, carbon dioxide retention and chronic respiratory failure can ensue. Often, a significant deformity will promote sputum retention, decreased airway clearance, atelectasis, and pneumonia.

Chest Wall Injuries

Examples of chest wall injuries include rib fracture and flail chest. Acute injuries of the chest wall can occur as a consequence of blunt or penetrating trauma or, in the case of a bony malignancy, a pathologic fracture. The injuries may be simple, such as a rib fracture, or as serious as flail chest abnormality.

PATHOPHYSIOLOGY

The most common chest wall injury is a simple rib fracture. Because it causes profound inspiratory pain, there is voluntary splinting, which results in restricted tidal volume and an increased respiratory rate. The victim also voluntarily inhibits the urge to cough in an effort to avoid pain. A young, otherwise healthy individual usually tolerates a fractured rib well, but if the patient is elderly or if the injury is superimposed on pre-existing pulmonary disease, impaired clearance of secretions, atelectasis, pneumonia, and even respiratory failure can occur. The respiratory drive and the cough reflex may be depressed by administration of narcotic analgesics. Potential complications include lung contusion or lung puncture resulting in pneumothorax (see p. 573).

If several adjacent ribs are fractured, the rib fracture becomes uncoupled from the chest wall and the stability of the chest wall is lost. This is termed a **flail chest** and is common in steering wheel injuries (Fig. 20-6).[32] During inspiration, as pleural pressure becomes increasingly negative, the injured area of the chest wall is sucked inward. Consequently, the underlying lung tissue does not expand, lung compliance is reduced, work of breathing is increased, and gas exchange is impaired due to hypoventilation. During expiration, the affected area of the chest moves outward due to the increased pleural pressure. This phenomenon is referred to as **paradoxical movement** and is a reflection of the changes in pleural pressure. The end result is ineffective ventilation and in-

A. FUNNEL CHEST *(Pectus Excavatum)*

Cross Section of Thorax

B. THORACIC KYPHOSCOLIOSIS

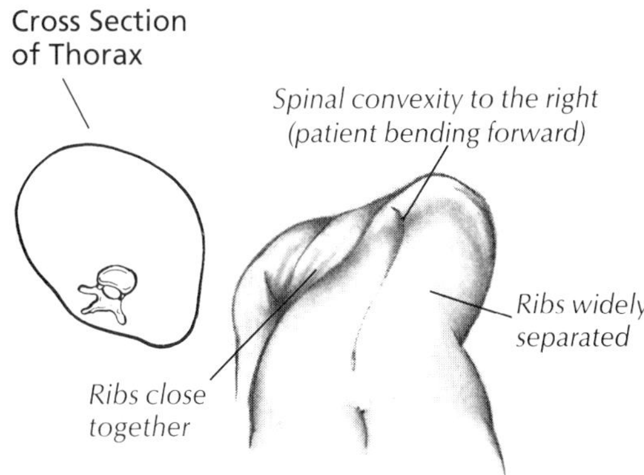

C. PIGEON CHEST *(Pectus Carinatum)*

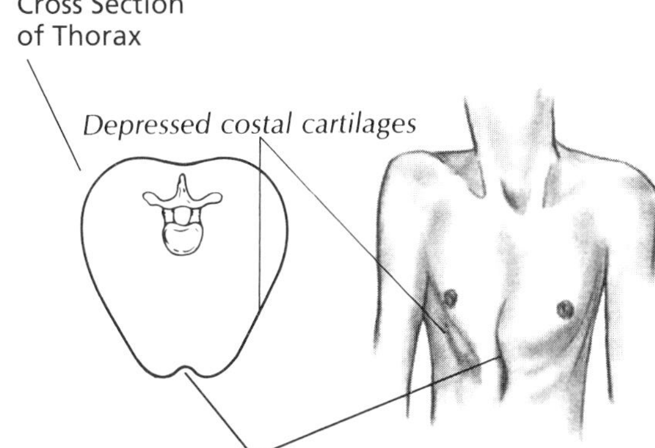

FIGURE 20-5. Thoracic deformities. **A.** A funnel chest is characterized by a depression in the lower portion of the sternum. Compression of the heart and great vessels may cause murmurs. **B.** In thoracic kyphoscoliosis, abnormal spinal curvatures and vertebral rotation deform the chest. Distortion of the underlying lungs may make interpretation of lung findings very difficult. **C.** In a pigeon chest, the sternum is displaced anteriorly, increasing the anteroposterior diameter. The costal cartilages adjacent to the protruding sternum are depressed. (Bates, B. [1999]. *A guide to physical examination and history taking* [7th ed.] Philadelphia: Lippincott Williams & Wilkins.)

creased energy demands from respiratory muscles due to the flail segment.

The more the injured individual works to maintain adequate ventilation, the more paradoxical the respiratory efforts become. In severe cases, a pendulum movement of the mediastinum may occur with each breath, putting pressure on the otherwise unaffected lung. The paradoxical motion may impair venous return to the heart, resulting in decreased cardiac output, systemic blood pressure, and shock.

CLINICAL MANIFESTATIONS

Clinical manifestations of rib fracture include point tenderness of the chest wall, shortness of breath, and pain on inspiration. Bruising over the injured area may be evident. **Splinting** (the intentional restriction of inspiratory depth to prevent pain) may be observed. Breath sounds over the injured area are decreased or may demonstrate crackles and/or rhonchi. Pulmonary function testing is rarely performed under these circumstances but would reveal decreased compliance and decreased lung volumes, depending on the location and extent of the injury.

Clinical manifestations of flail chest include the obvious signs of chest wall trauma, flail (paradoxical) chest wall movement, a complaint of severe dyspnea, pain (especially on inspiration), and crackles or diminished breath sounds on auscultation. Chest radiographs show evidence of fractured ribs, and blood gases may indicate hypoxemia and impending respiratory failure.[32]

Acute Respiratory Distress Syndrome

Acute respiratory distress syndrome (ARDS) is a secondary pathologic process that is characterized by progressive deterioration of oxygenation, resulting in respiratory difficulty and eventually, respiratory failure (see p. 579). It is considered to be the respiratory part of multisystem organ dysfunction syndrome (MODS)

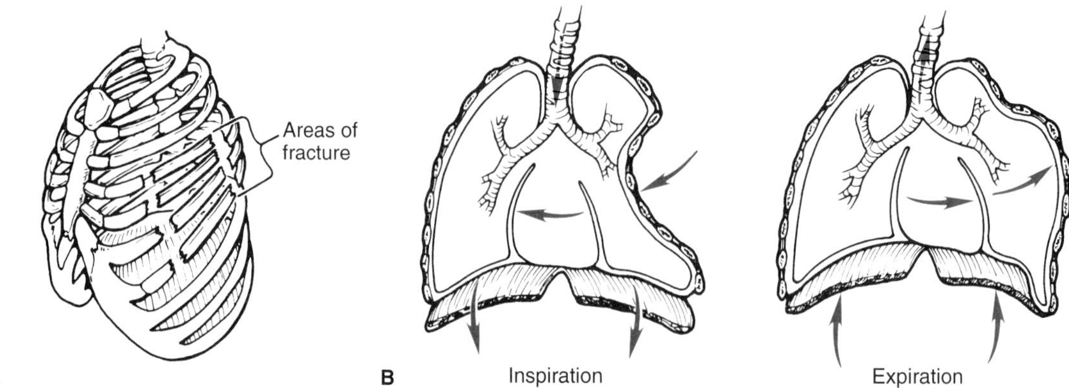

FIGURE 20-6. **A.** Chest wall injury that can produce flail chest abnormality. **B.** Physiology of flail chest abnormality resulting in paradoxical breathing.

(see p. 517). ARDS is considered to be the most severe manifestation of acute lung injury (ALI) in adults.[9] The term acute lung injury is used to delineate injury to the alveolar-capillary barrier from a variety of insults such as aspiration, hypoxemia, and septicemia. It represents a continuum of early injury, which may progress to the damaging response seen with ARDS.

Risk factors for ALI and ARDS are divided into two groups: (1) direct lung injury such as diffuse pulmonary infection, gastric aspiration, or near drowning and (2) indirect injuries such as sepsis syndrome, multiple transfusions, or thoracic trauma (Table 20-6).[33]

PATHOPHYSIOLOGY

ARDS is characterized by increased alveolar-capillary barrier permeability, decreased lung compliance, intrapulmonary shunting, ventilation/perfusion mismatch, and eventually increased pulmonary vascular resistance.[33] Three overlapping phases of injury have been described: (1) acute phase, (2) subacute or proliferative phase, and (3) chronic phase.

The acute phase lasts for approximately 1 week and is characterized by increased permeability of the alveolar-capillary membrane. Protein-rich fluid from the alveolar capillaries leaks into the interstitial space. Interstitial and alveolar edema occurs when leukocytes, RBCs, and cellular debris collect in the alveolar spaces. The alveolar type I cells become damaged and die and fluid moves into the alveolar spaces, causing the deposition of plasma proteins and formation of fibrin-containing precipitates (hyaline membranes).[50] Proliferation of type II cells replaces the normal epithelial lining of the alveoli. Severe hypoxemia is the hallmark of the disorder and is due to intra-alveolar accumulation of proteinaceous fluid, alveolar-capillary membrane damage, and areas of atelectasis that create a large intrapulmonary shunt.

The small pulmonary vasculature becomes engorged and microvascular thromboemboli form. The subacute or proliferative phase is from days 4 to 10. Fibroblasts also begin to appear in the alveolar fluid and deposit collagen in the alveolar walls. When fibroblasitc proliferation ceases, the alveolar exudate and hyaline membranes are reabsorbed, with normal alveolar function slowly returning.

During the late phase, which lasts beyond day 8, if resolution does not occur, fibroproliferation continues and the lung parenchyma becomes remodeled. As a direct result of this proliferation, diffuse fibrosis begins to develop and subsequent capillary obliteration occurs. The resulting ventilatory pattern is that of decreased compliance and restriction. In addition, persistent hypoxemia promotes pulmonary vascular hypertension, which increases right-sided cardiac workload (Fig. 20-7).[28,33]

Throughout this entire process there is a complex cascade of immune responses and inflammatory cell activity that directly influences the pathophysiologic manifestations of the syndrome. Key components of the cascade and physiologic response/changes are illustrated in Flowchart 20-1.

CLINICAL MANIFESTATIONS

Clinical manifestations include dyspnea, increased respiratory effort, tachypnea, hypoxemia unresponsive to increasing fractions of inspired oxygen (FiO_2), and eventually exhaustion and acute respiratory failure. Initial arterial blood gases may show moderate hypoxemia and respiratory alkalosis due to the compensatory tachypnea, but as the syndrome progresses the above-described blood gas alterations are seen. Intubation and mechanical ventilation are necessary in nearly all cases. A chest radiograph demonstrates bilateral patchy infiltrates. Mortality is reportedly between 30% and 60%, with the greatest risk being when three or more organ

TABLE 20-6

CONDITIONS LEADING TO ALI AND ARDS

PREDISPOSING FACTORS	INCIDENCE OF ARDS (%)
Direct lung insults	
Aspiration of gastric contents	30–36
Pneumonia	12
Inhalation lung injury (smoke, crack cocaine)	
Near drowning	
High-altitude pulmonary edema	
Pulmonary contusion	
Reexpansion lung injury	
Radiation	
Systemic insults	
Sepsis syndrome	25–43 (ALI in 60%)
Shock	
Nonthoracic trauma	17–40
Burns	
Pancreatitis	2
Uremia	
Diabetic ketoacidosis	
Acute neurologic insult (e.g., SAH, head trauma)	
Disseminated intravascular coagulation	22
Multiple transfusions	5–40
Cardiopulmonary bypass	
Systemic drug toxicity	
Oxygen toxicity	
Thromboembolism	
Fat embolism	
Air embolism	
Complications of pregnancy	
Carcinomatosis	

(Mehrad: B., & Weg, J. G. [1997]. Acute lung injury and acute respiratory distress syndrome. In M. G. Khan & J. P. Lynch [Eds.], *Pulmonary disease diagnosis and therapy.* Baltimore: Williams & Wilkins.)

system disorders are present concurrently.[33] Survivors may demonstrate a restrictive pattern and decreased diffusing capacity on subsequent pulmonary function testing for several months after hospitalization.

Respiratory Distress Syndrome of the Newborn

Respiratory distress syndrome of the newborn (also known as hyaline membrane disease) is a disorder characterized by poor gas exchange and ventilatory failure due to insufficient surfactant.

The pathophysiologic mechanisms of respiratory distress syndrome (RDS) in the newborn are quite different from those seen in the adult. RDS is associated with premature birth, but lung maturity at time of birth rather than gestational age is thought to be the most important factor.[20] In the preterm neonate the lungs may not be fully developed, and therefore there is insufficient surfactant available to promote optimal gas exchange and ventilatory function.

PATHOPHYSIOLOGY

The lack of surfactant results in atelectasis, increased work of breathing, hypoxemia, and respiratory acidosis.[20] Pulmonary vasoconstriction and pulmonary vascular resistance increase, resulting in hypoperfusion that leads to capillary damage and necrosis of the alveoli. The ischemic injury allows fluid to leak into interstitial and alveolar spaces and hyaline membrane formation. The intrapulmonary shunting seen is a direct result of lung collapse and altered pulmonary circulation (Flowchart 20-2). In addition, elevated pulmonary circulatory pressures create high pressures on the right side of the heart. This high pressure perpetuates fetal circulation by keeping the foramen ovale and the ductus arteriosus patent, further exacerbating hypoxemia through a right-left shunting mechanism (see p. 563).

CLINICAL MANIFESTATIONS

Clinical manifestations are evident immediately at time of birth. Rapid, shallow respirations, rib retrac-

FOCUS ON CELLULAR PATHOPHYSIOLOGY

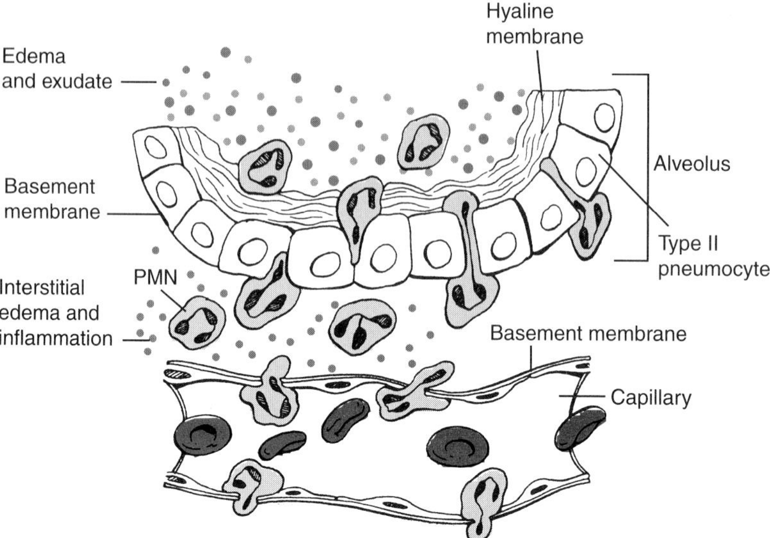

FIGURE 20-7. Diffuse alveolar damage in ARDS. In ARDS, type I cells die as a result of diffuse alveolar damage. Intra-alveolar edema follows, after which there is formation of hyaline membranes composed of proteinaceous exudate and cell debris. In the acute phase, the lungs are markedly congested and heavy. Type II cells multiply to line the alveolar surface. Interstitial inflammation is characteristic. The lesion may heal completely or progress to interstitial fibrosis. (Rubin, E. & Farber J. [1999]. *Pathology* [3rd ed.]. Philadelphia: Lippincott Williams & Wilkins.)

tion, nasal flaring, and inspiratory grunting can be seen. Despite advances in pre- and post-delivery therapeutic options and care, mortality remains high. Up to 70% of all preterm deaths are attributable to RDS.[20]

HYPOVENTILATION DISORDERS

Alveolar hypoventilation is defined as a state in which alveolar ventilation decreases and, consequently, alveolar CO_2 increases.[24] A variety of physiologic alterations can lead to hypoventilation, including central nervous system depression, restrictive ventilatory disorders secondary to chest wall abnormalities, obesity, obstructive sleep apnea, and neuromuscular disorders. Neuromuscular hypoventilation disorders are discussed on page 945.

Central Nervous System Depression

Central control of breathing is located in the medulla oblongata. Higher centers, such as the pons (which is responsible for smooth respiratory patterns) and the cortex (which is the behavioral control center), provide input to the central controllers. Central and peripheral chemoreceptors provide sensory feedback to the central controllers regarding PCO_2 and PO_2 concentrations, respectively. Any insult to the central nervous system, such as head trauma, general anesthesia, or narcotic overdose, can cause alterations in the feedback mechanism and result in respiratory depression.

Clinical manifestations include abnormal breathing patterns (shallow or discordant efforts) and decreased PaO_2 with increased $PaCO_2$. Pulmonary function studies will show reduced inspiratory capacity, vital capacity, tidal volume, functional residual capacity, and expiratory reserve volumes (see Appendix Table A).

Obesity Hypoventilation Syndrome

Excess adipose tissue imposes increased work of breathing and pressures needed to effect ventilation substantially. The etiology of obesity hypoventilation syndrome (OHS), also referred to as **Pickwickian syndrome**, is not completely understood but is thought to be due to two physiologic alterations. Pulmonary function testing has revealed that in individuals with OHS there is a decrease in inspiratory muscle strength, decreased total lung capacity, and decreased maximum voluntary ven-

FLOWCHART 20-1 **Pathophysiology of Acute Respiratory Distress Syndrome**

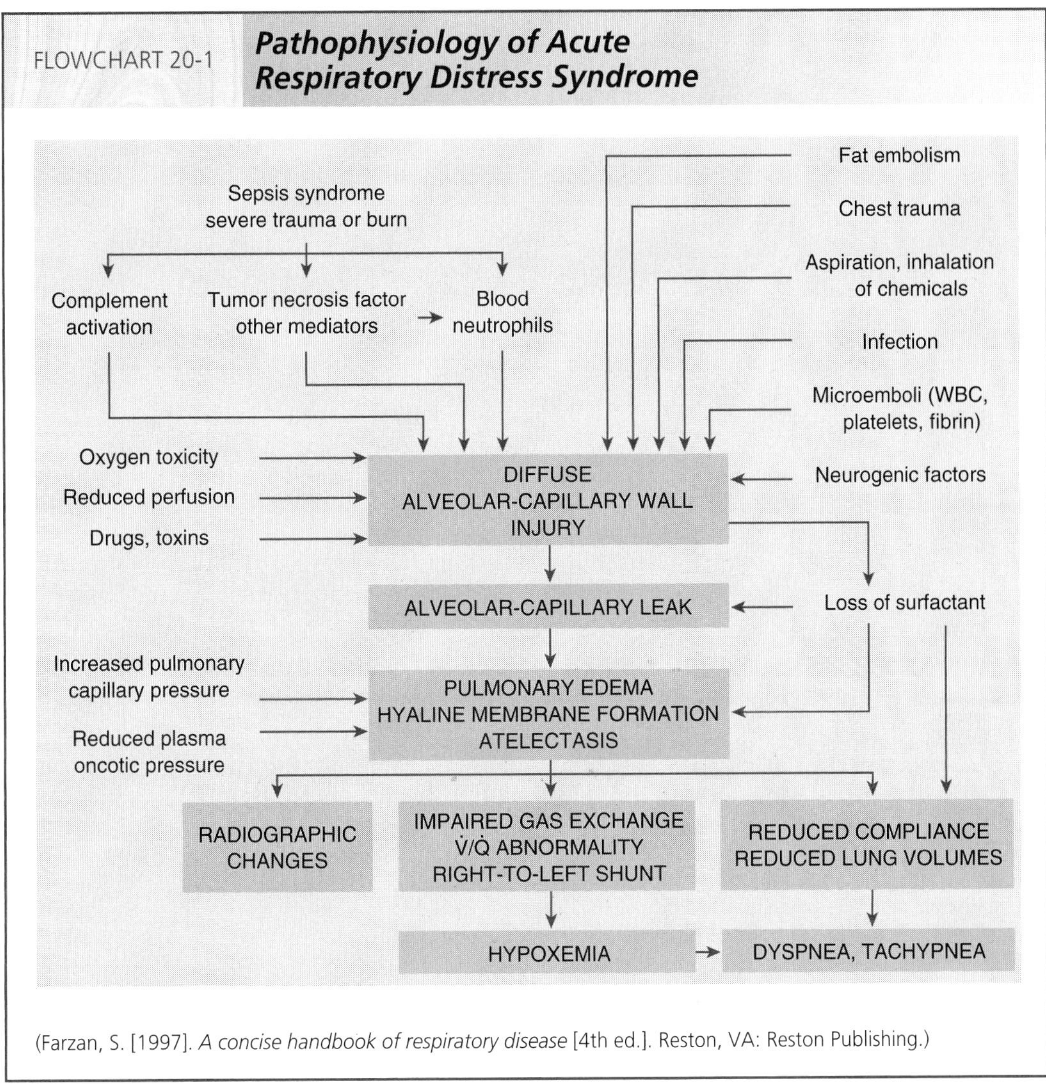

(Farzan, S. [1997]. *A concise handbook of respiratory disease* [4th ed.]. Reston, VA: Reston Publishing.)

tilation rates. In addition, a decreased ventilatory response to high CO_2 or hypoxia has been observed.

During sleep, individuals with OHS also exhibit obstructive sleep patterns, which worsen baseline hypoxemia. Somnolence, twitching, abnormal respiratory patterns, and polycythemia may be present. Right ventricular hypertrophy and eventual failure may ensue. Pulmonary function testing reveals decreased compliance, expiratory reserve volume, total lung capacity, and vital capacity. Arterial blood gas analysis reveals hypercapnia and mild to moderate hypoxemia.

INTERSTITIAL LUNG DISEASES

Interstitial lung diseases are a heterogeneous group of restrictive disorders that collectively result in scarring and fibrosis of the lung. Examples include sarcoidosis and idiopathic pulmonary fibrosis.

Etiology

The etiology can be identified in only a minority of the cases found. Some cases are associated with other systemic disorders such as connective tissue diseases (e.g., rheumatoid arthritis and systemic lupus erythematosus). In other cases it may be due to inhalation of particles, such as with pulmonary fibrosis associated with asbestosis.

The interstitial lung diseases are divided into two distinct groups: those of known cause and those of unknown cause. Table 20-7 summarizes the major categories using this classification system.

FLOWCHART 20-2 **Pathophysiology of Respiratory Distress of the Newborn**

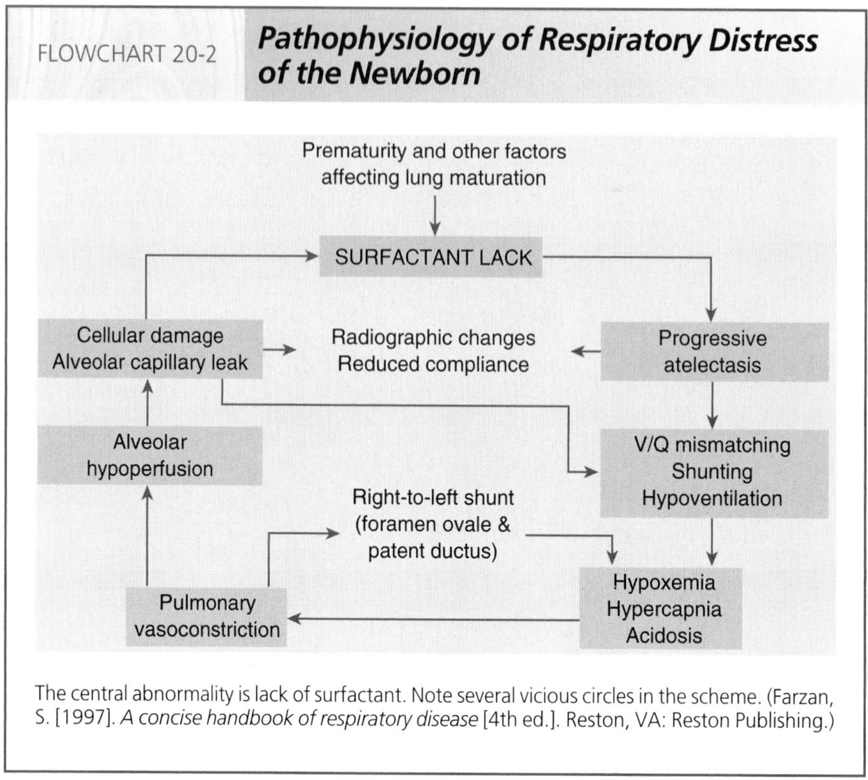

The central abnormality is lack of surfactant. Note several vicious circles in the scheme. (Farzan, S. [1997]. *A concise handbook of respiratory disease* [4th ed.]. Reston, VA: Reston Publishing.)

Pathophysiology

The exact pathophysiologic mechanism of interstitial lung diseases is largely unknown. It is believed that the lung sustains an injury that leads to inflammation of the inter-alveolar septum. This is referred to as **alveolitis**. The persistence of this inflammation ultimately leads to the development of irreversible interstitial scarring and fibrosis.[23]

Clinical Manifestations

Despite the heterogenicity of this group of diseases, the clinical presentations are similar. Typically, individuals complain of a gradual onset of dyspnea and dry cough. Clubbing of the digits, due to chronic hypoxia, may also be observed. Tachypnea and reduced tidal volume are common. On auscultory examination, fine inspiratory crackles may be heard at the lung bases. Resting oxygenation may be preserved initially, but exercise-induced hypoxemia is evident and eventually is present at rest as well. Depending on the etiology, the condition may be characterized by progressive respiratory insufficiency and failure. Pulmonary function tests reveal a restrictive pattern characterized by decreased compliance, reduced lung volumes, and decreased vital capacity.

DISEASES AND DISORDERS OF THE PLEURAL SPACE

Conditions that alter the pleural space are often secondary to other systemic problems. These may result in pleuritis, pleural effusion, and pneumothorax. The pleura may also develop benign or malignant tumors, but these occur rarely or may be due to metastatic spread from another site (see p. 579).

Pleural Effusion

An excessive accumulation of pleural fluid is called a pleural effusion. It may accompany various disease conditions.

ETIOLOGY AND PATHOPHYSIOLOGY

Pleural effusions mainly fall into one of two categories: (1) *transudative* or (2) *exudative*.[7] Other mechanisms that can cause accumulation of fluid in the pleural area include bleeding or infection. Pleural fluid laboratory analysis is used to determine the underlying mechanism.

Transudative pleural effusions occur when excess pleural fluid accumulates secondary to increased hydrostatic pressure in the pleural capillaries, decreased colloid osmotic pressure in the systemic circulation, or

TABLE 20-7

CLASSIFICATIONS OF INTERSTITIAL LUNG DISEASES

KNOWN CAUSES	UNKNOWN CAUSES
Inorganic dusts	Crytogenic fibrosis alveolitis (idiopathic pulmonary fibrosis)
Organic dusts	Sarcoidosis
Gases, fumes, vapors	Langerhans cell granulomatosis
Drugs	Rheumatic disease–associated
Poisons	Goodpasture's syndrome
Radiation	Idiopathic pulmonary hemosiderosis
Infections	Wegener's granulomatosis
Residue of any active infection	Lymphoid granulomatosis
Pulmonary edema	Churg-Strauss syndrome
Lymphangitic carcinoma	Angioimmunoblastic lymphadenopathy
	Inherited diseases (tuberous sclerosis, neurofibromatosis)
	Pulmonary veno-occlusive disease
	Ankylosing spondylitis
	Amyloidosis
	Chronic eosinophilic pneumonia
	Pulmonary lympangiomyomatosis
	Whipple's disease
	Alveolar proteinosis
	Inflammatory bowel disease–associated

(Adapted from Stauffer, J. L. [1998]. Lung: interstitial lung diseases. In L. M. Tierney, S. J. McPhee, & M. A. Papadakis [Eds.], *Current medical diagnosis and treatment* [37th ed.]. Stamford, CT: Appleton & Lange.)

both. Transudative effusions are the result of disorders other than in the lung itself. Examples include pleural effusions associated with congestive heart failure or low serum protein states such as those seen in liver disease or nephrotic syndrome. Laboratory analysis of transudative fluid typically reveals a low protein content.

Exudative pleural effusions occur due to increased permeability of the pleural capillary membrane, lung parenchymal diseases, inflammation, infection, or malignancy. Exudative effusions can occur secondary to neoplasms, collagen vascular disorders, pulmonary emboli, gastrointestinal diseases such as pancreatitis, esophageal perforation or abdominal surgery, or as a reaction to medications.[7] Exudative fluid typically has a high protein or lactic dehydrogenase (LDH) content and a high cell count.[7]

Accumulation of fluid can also occur due to bleeding into the pleura space from surgical intervention or trauma to the chest wall, diaphragm, lung, blood vessels, or mediastinum (referred to as a *hemothorax*). When an infection or injury results in the formation of fibrinous tissue around the visceral pleura, this is identified as a *fibrothorax*. If pneumonia has extended into the pleural space and triggers an accumulation of pleural fluid, a **parapneumonic effusion** occurs. If the infection becomes organized and fibrotic sheets create partitions around the lesion, the infection has become an empyema. The impact on pulmonary function is one of restriction. The presence of excessive amount of pleural fluid compresses the lung tissue it surrounds and, therefore, compromises gas-exchange capacity and efficiency. Intrapleural fluid occupies space and displaces lung tissue, resulting in compression atelectasis, altered gas exchange, decreased lung compliance, and ventilatory restriction (Fig. 20-8).

CLINICAL MANIFESTATIONS

Clinical manifestations of pleural effusions include dyspnea, cough, chest pain, tachypnea, and complaints of difficulty in taking a deep breath.[7] Asymmetric chest expansion can be observed as well as decreased breath sounds in the affected area. Ventilation-perfusion mismatching occurs due to compression of surrounding lung tissue, resulting in arterial hypoxemia. In some cases, the individual may be completely asymptomatic.

Pneumothorax

Pneumothorax is defined as the presence of atmospheric air in the pleural space. Some pneumothoraces are small and may be asymptomatic; others can be life threatening and require rapid identification and intervention. Some occur following a chest wall injury, whereas others occur spontaneously.

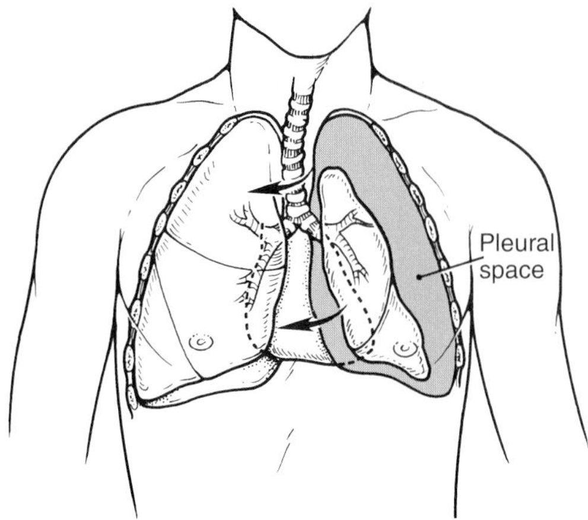

FIGURE 20-8. Pleural effusion. *Shaded area* shows fluid collection in the pleural space. Lung tissue is displaced and mediastinal structures are compressed.

ETIOLOGY

As illustrated in Figure 20-9A, atmospheric air enters the pleural space when an opening is created either between the pleura and the environment or from an abnormal communication within the thoracic cavity itself. Traumatic chest injuries, whether penetrating or non-penetrating, are common etiologies.[25] Gunshot or stab wounds are examples of penetrating injuries. Non-penetrating injuries can occur by laceration of the parietal pleura from a rib fracture or dislocation or by sudden compression of the chest wall and alveolar rupture. *Iatrogenic pneumothoraces* may result as a complication of central venous catheter placement or transthoracic needle biopsy procedures. Pneumothoraces can also occur due to **barotrauma** induced by excessively high mechanical ventilator pressures. A *primary spontaneous pneumothorax* can occur in an otherwise healthy individual and is probably due to the sudden rupture of a previously unrecognized bleb.[50] *Secondary pneumothoraces* occur secondary to underlying lung disease, such as rupture of a subpleural emphysematous bleb or a tear in the tracheobronchial tree, or due to anatomic alterations associated with COPD, cystic fibrosis, asthma, *P. carinii* pneumonia, and TB. Thoracic surgery procedures always result in surgical pneumothoraces.

PATHOPHYSIOLOGY

During normal ventilation, pleural pressure is more sub-atmospheric than intra-alveolar pressure. Therefore, if there is a break in either the integrity of the lung through the visceral pleura or the chest wall through the parietal pleura, air rushes into the area of lowest pressure, which is the pleural space. In the case of a penetrating chest wound, the movement of air into the thorax continues as long as the opening is maintained. The underlying lung becomes compressed and can no longer participate in gas exchange.

Sometimes air is sucked into the pleural space on inspiration, but the opening self-seals on expiration. With each subsequent breath, this one-way valve allows intrapleural pressures to continue to increase. This is termed a *tension pneumothorax* and is a life-threatening condition (Fig. 20-9B). The increasing thoracic pressure compresses the heart, lungs, and vascular structures, severely impairing function.

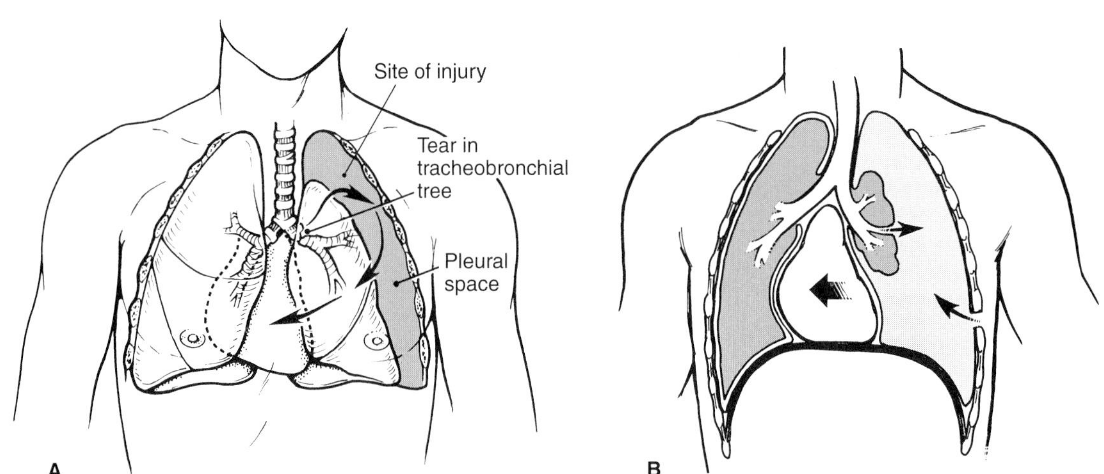

FIGURE 20-9. Pneumothorax. **A.** Atmospheric air entering the pleural space through a tracheobronchial tear. Compression of lung tissue occurs. **B.** Tension pneumothorax occurs with compression and shifting of mediastinal structures. Entry site is an opening in the chest wall.

CLINICAL MANIFESTATIONS

The size and severity of a pneumothorax will dictate the severity of signs and symptoms. A significant pneumothorax may present with sudden onset of dyspnea, chest pain, asymmetric chest expansion, and reduced or absent breath sounds on the affected side.[25] Tracheal deviation toward the unaffected side may also be observed, and breath sounds are reduced. Arterial blood gases may reveal acute hypoxemia at the outset. Symptoms of a tension pneumothorax are dramatic and include rapidly increasing respiratory distress, cyanosis, bulging sternum, distended neck veins, elevated central venous pressure, and systemic hypotension.

BOX 20-9 RISK FACTORS FOR DEEP VEIN THROMBOSIS

- Prolonged bed rest
- Surgery (especially hip/orthopedic, lower abdominal)
- Childbirth
- Stroke
- Cardiac disorders
- Obesity
- Multiple trauma
- Malignancy
- Varicose veins
- Advanced age
- Fractures of hip or femur

DISORDERS OF VASCULAR ORIGIN

Some pulmonary disorders arise from vascular and cardiac pathology outside the lungs, and some arise from vascular pathology within the lung beds themselves. The more common conditions are pulmonary embolism, pulmonary hypertension, and pulmonary edema. Pulmonary edema was discussed on page 478 and will be briefly discussed in this section.

Pulmonary Embolism

Pulmonary embolism is the occlusion of a part of the pulmonary vasculature due to blockage by a foreign substance from a distant source. Pulmonary embolisms are associated with as many as 100,000 deaths in the United States each year. Mortality in untreated cases is as high as 30%.[13]

ETIOLOGY

Pulmonary emboli usually arise from one of three sources: (1) a thromboembolism from the systemic venous system or right side of the heart; (2) a tumor embolism from a tumor that has invaded the circulatory system; or (3) other types of foreign substances such as amniotic fluid, air, materials injected intravenously, or fat or bone marrow (both from a long bone fracture).[48] The majority of pulmonary emboli arise from deep vein thromboses (DVTs) in the lower extremities.

Several factors relating to conditions within the venous system have been identified as risk factors. Intimal injury to the venous epithelium, venous stasis (such as occurs during periods of immobility), and hypercoagulable states (such as those associated with some malignancies and blood disorders or secondary to oral contraceptive use) are the factors referred to as **Virchow's triad.**[6] Clinical risk factors for developing DVT are presented in Box 20-9.[6,48] Venous thromboembolism is relatively rare in the non-hospitalized population; the majority of cases occur in hospitalized or recently hospitalized patients.[6]

PATHOPHYSIOLOGY

The majority of emboli originate from deep veins in the lower extremities. Initially a blood clot, or **thrombus**, forms in a portion in the deep venous system. The clot becomes an **embolus** when it becomes dislodged from its site of origin and travels through the systemic venous system, through the right chambers of the heart, and into the pulmonary circulation. Within the pulmonary circulation system, the clot eventually lodges in a branch of the circulatory system and blocks flow of blood distal to the obstruction. A large blockage can result in occlusion of a large portion of the pulmonary circulation and sudden death. Infarction of the lung tissue can result when the embolus is large enough to occlude a blood vessel, causing tissue death to lung tissue distal to the obstruction. The clot can occlude a small vessel, causing temporary symptoms until the fibrinolytic system destroys it. It can also manifest as a showering of multiple small pulmonary emboli that may be recurrent or chronic.

Pathophysiologic consequences, depending upon severity, can include hypoxic vasoconstriction, pulmonary edema, atelectasis due to decreased surfactant, and release of various neurohumoral substances, including histamine. Dead space ventilation increases as the corresponding affected lung units continue to be ventilated but are not perfused (see p. 539). Longstanding, large emboli eventually lead to elevated pulmonary circulation pressures.

CLINICAL MANIFESTATIONS

If the clot source is in the lower extremity, signs and symptoms consistent with venous occlusion, such as calf asymmetry, duskiness, swelling, localized tenderness, or calf pain with dorsiflexion of the foot, may be present. Pulmonary clinical presentation can be somewhat nonspecific. Pulmonary symptoms may include any or all of the following: tachypnea, tachycardia, chest pain, wheezing, apprehension, coughing, hemoptysis, hypoxemia associated with respiratory alkalosis, systemic hypotension/shock, pulmonary hypertension, and eventual right heart failure. Chest auscultation may be normal or reveal localized decreased breath sounds or a pleural friction rub. Small emboli may be asymptomatic and have little physiologic consequence. However, when pulmonary symptoms are severe, cardiopulmonary arrest and death may be imminent. The extent of physiologic insult is largely dependent upon the extent of the lung involved and the presence or absence of coexisting cardiopulmonary disease.[49]

Pulmonary Hypertension

Pulmonary hypertension is an abnormal increase in pulmonary artery pressures. The term is usually reserved for long-term problems resulting from the elevated pressures.

ETIOLOGY AND CLASSIFICATION

Because the majority of resistance within the pulmonary circulation comes from the pulmonary capillary network, an abnormality in any part of the vascular network (such as capillaries, venules, veins, or arteries) can adversely affect pulmonary artery pressures.[35]

Pulmonary hypertension is classified as either primary or secondary. Pulmonary hypertension caused by an underlying cardiac or pulmonary disease is referred to as secondary pulmonary hypertension. Several physiologic conditions or disorders can predispose pulmonary hypertension (Box 20-10).

Primary pulmonary hypertension (PPH) is a relatively rare but serious disorder that primarily affects women between the ages of 20 and 30 years. Its etiology is largely unknown. Appetite-suppressant drugs have been suspected of causing PPH in some individuals. Familial PPH accounts for approximately 6% of the cases reported to the Primary Pulmonary Hypertension National Registry.[41] Portal hypertension, HIV infection, and cocaine inhalation have also been implicated in some cases.[41] Diagnostic criteria for PPH require a resting mean pulmonary artery pressure (PAP) of greater than 20 mm Hg and that other potential causes (such as heart or lung disease) have been ruled out.[41]

BOX 20-10 CAUSES OF PULMONARY HYPERTENSION

- Secondary to pulmonary venous hypertension
- Secondary to hypoxia
- Secondary to systemic disease
- Secondary to congenital cardiac disease
- Secondary to emboli
- Primary pulmonary hypertension

(Adapted from Albert, R. K. [1996]. Pulmonary hypertension and chronic cor pulmonale as viewed by the pulmonologist. In J. W. Hurst [Ed.], *Medicine for the practicing physician* [4th ed.]. Stamford, CT: Appleton & Lange.)

PATHOPHYSIOLOGY

The pathophysiologic basis for secondary pulmonary hypertension has been related to several factors, which may occur singly or in combination. These include chronic left heart failure, especially that resulting from mitral valve disease or cardiomyopathy; congenital heart conditions that result in overloading of the pulmonary vascular circuit, such as atrial septal defect, patent ductus arteriosus, or ventricular septal defect; chronic hypoxemia that causes vasoconstriction of the pulmonary vascular bed; and damage to or obstruction of the pulmonary capillary bed.

If the elevated pulmonary pressures are not lowered through treatment of the underlying cause, the blood vessels become rigid and more force is needed to propel blood though the vasculature. As a consequence, the right ventricle hypertrophies. Cor pulmonale or pulmonary heart disease then develops.

The pathophysiologic basis for PPH has been described in terms of three elements: vasoconstriction, vascular-wall remodeling, and thrombosis in situ.[41] The earliest pathologic finding is that of medial hypertrophy of the vessels, termed *hypertrophic muscularis.* Alterations in the pulmonary vascular endothelium are also suspected. Thrombosis is believed to occur secondarily to intimal injury of the pulmonary vasculature, abnormal fibrinolysis, excessive procoagulant activity, or platelet abnormalities. Late in the disease process, there is extensive intimal fibrosis and muscle thickening.[41] The pathophysiologic changes associated with PPH are illustrated in Figure 20-10. These changes are irreversible.

CLINICAL MANIFESTATIONS

In many cases, primary or secondary pulmonary hypertension may not be detected until the pulmonary artery pressure has increased to levels similar to that of systemic blood pressure. An enlargement of the right heart seen on a chest radiograph may be the first indication of disease. Physical complaints such as fatigue, chest pain, and dyspnea (especially on exertion), syncope, near-syncope, or lightheadedness may be reported, particularly in later stages.[2] In secondary pulmonary hypertension, there may be symptoms of the underlying condition.

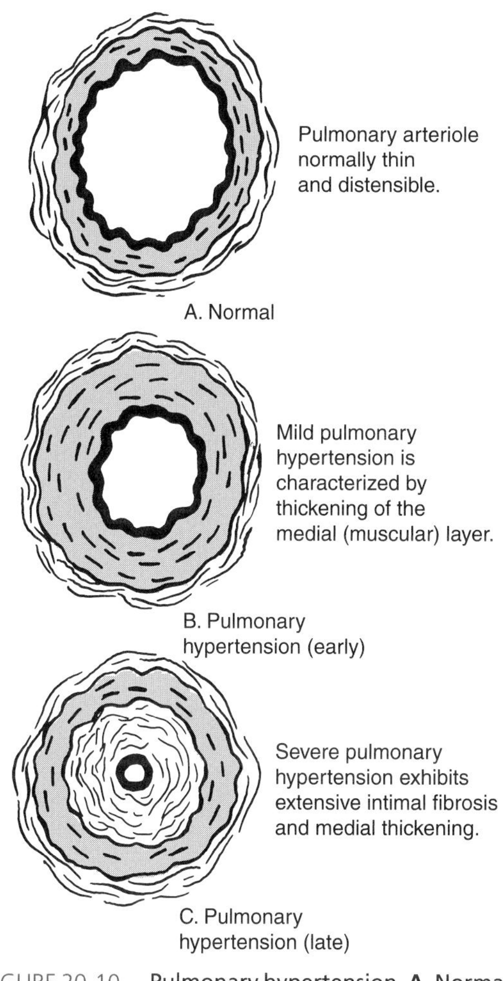
Pulmonary arteriole
normally thin
and distensible.
A. Normal
Mild pulmonary
hypertension is
characterized by
thickening of the
medial (muscular) layer.
B. Pulmonary
hypertension (early)
Severe pulmonary
hypertension exhibits
extensive intimal fibrosis
and medial thickening.
C. Pulmonary
hypertension (late)

FIGURE 20-10. **Pulmonary hypertension. A. Normal pulmonary arteriole. B. Early pulmonary hypertension. C. Late, obliterative pulmonary hypertension. (Modified from Rubin, E. & Farber, J. [1999] *Pathology* [3rd ed.]. Philadelphia: Lippincott Williams & Wilkins.)**

In cor pulmonale, the symptoms may be masked by those associated with the lung disorder itself. Initially, elevated pulmonary pressures become severe only during exercise; later they persist at rest as well. The individual may complain of chest pain or increased dyspnea. Signs and symptoms of right heart failure such as peripheral edema, hepatic congestion, and jugular venous distention occur in later stages of the disorder.[2]

Pulmonary Edema

The pulmonary vascular system has the capacity to accommodate volumes of blood up to three times normal. However, once a critical volume is achieved or if there is abnormally increased permeability at the level of the alveolar-capillary membrane, flooding of the alveoli and lung tissue (interstitium) can occur. This is referred to as *pulmonary edema.*

ETIOLOGY

Pulmonary edema can be a complication of an abnormality or a consequence of lung disease or extrapulmonary dysfunction. The underlying etiology of pulmonary edema is multifold. If there is significant cardiac dysfunction due to decreased contractility or valvular disease, left ventricular volume exceeds pumping ability and blood begins to dam back into the pulmonary vascular system. This is an example of **cardiogenic pulmonary edema** (discussed on p. 478).

If toxic exposure, aspiration, or infection has triggered abnormally increased permeability, **non-cardiogenic pulmonary edema** may ensue. In cases of central nervous system insult, the exact etiology of pulmonary edema is unclear but is thought to be related to increased sympathetic nervous system activity. Common causes of non-cardiogenic pulmonary edema are presented in Table 20-8.

TABLE 20-8

CAUSES OF NON-CARDIOGENIC EDEMA

CAUSE	RESULTS
Alveolar damage and increased capillary permeability	Acute inflammation; septicemia; inhalation of poisonous gases, smoke fumes, and particulates; aspiration of toxic fluids
Drug-induced injury	Chemotherapeutic agents produce toxic oxygen radicals; alveolar-capillary cytotoxicity may result from heroin, oxygen toxicity; alveolar-capillary permeability is increased by antibiotics, inhalants, radio-opaque media
High attitude	Mechanism unknown; causes diffuse pulmonary edema
Post head injury	Autonomic nervous system stimulation
Lymphatic obstruction/ insufficiency	Diffuse infiltration of lymphatic channels with malignant processes; silicosis
Decreased colloid osmotic pressure	Severe hypoalbuminemia from severe liver, kidney, or protein-wasting diseases

PATHOPHYSIOLOGY

Under normal physiologic conditions, fluid movement across the alveolar-capillary membrane is prevented due to Starling forces (see p. 540). Pulmonary edema occurs when there is a net increase in Starling's forces or because of increased permeability at the alveolar-capillary membrane.[35]

Lymphatic vessels can initially remove some of the excess fluid; however, when this capacity is exceeded, excess water leaks into the pericapillary interstitial spaces.[35] Only a small amount of fluid can be accommodated within these spaces. Larger amounts of fluid can collect in the peri-bronchovascular interstitial spaces. When the capacity of these spaces is exceeded and the rate of filtration continues to exceed removal, alveolar filling occurs. Despite increased filtration rates, the peribronchial spaces continue to fill and a small amount of fluid accumulates in the interalveolar walls. Once the lymphatic system becomes completely overwhelmed, it bypasses its own system and continues to fill peribronchial spaces, following an interstitial pressure gradient. This is termed transudation or **interstitial edema**. Fluid can also spill into the pleural spaces.

CLINICAL MANIFESTATIONS

The clinical presentation of pulmonary edema is striking. The symptoms of cough (initially dry and later productive of frothy or bloody fluid), dyspnea, and tachypnea often occur relatively abruptly. The individual will complain of inability to breathe comfortably or "get enough air." A redistribution of blood flow to the upper lung zone vessels also occurs. This is referred to as **vascular redistribution** and can be appreciated on the chest radiograph. Sometimes enlargement of the heart can also be observed on chest radiograph. Chest auscultation reveals coarse and fine crackles, initially at the bases of the lung. This fluid, left untreated, will progressively extend upward.

RESPIRATORY TRACT MALIGNANCIES

Although some tumors of the respiratory tract are benign, malignant tumors are more common and cause significant morbidity and mortality. The locations of respiratory tract malignancies can be in any portion of the system, with laryngeal and parenchymal lung tumors being the most common. Pleural malignancies are rare but closely associated with asbestos exposure.

Most respiratory tract malignancies are related to cigarette smoking. Cigarette smoke is known to have multiple organ-specific carcinogens and has been causally linked to cancers in the mouth, larynx, esophageal, lung, and bladder.

Laryngeal Cancer

Laryngeal cancer accounts for 1% to 2% of all cancers reported in the United States, with the majority of cases in men between the ages of 50 and 75 years.[52] Tobacco smoking increases the risk of developing laryngeal cancer, and concomitant use of alcohol is thought to further heighten risk. Human papilloma virus types 6, 8, and 16 have also been suspected as etiologic agents.[16]

Malignancies of the true vocal cords are more common compared with those involving supraglottic structures. Tumors in the subglottic area are rare. Squamous cell type carcinomas are more common than small cell carcinomas. Metastasis to the regional lymph nodes usually occurs first, but it may also involve the lung.[23] Classifications are based on anatomic location, being either supraglottic or subglottic, as well as on cell type.

CLINICAL MANIFESTATIONS

The typical presenting symptoms include persistent, progressive hoarseness, dyspnea, and cough. In some cases the voice is lost. Dyspnea occurs more frequently when subglottic lesions are present. Sore throat and pain is more likely with supraglottic lesions. Cough may occur after swallowing. Occasionally individuals may complain of general neck problems. Hemoptysis is rare.[16]

Lung Cancer

Lung cancer accounts for 32% of all cancer deaths in men and 25% in women.[34] Most cases are diagnosed between the ages of 50 and 70 years of age; rarely are cases found in individuals younger than 40.[34]

ETIOLOGY

Cigarette smoking is thought to be the most important cause of lung cancer in men and women. The risk of developing lung cancer increases by 13-fold in the smoker and by 1.5-fold for the person exposed to second-hand smoke.[34] In addition, the frequency of lung cancer is increasing in women, who may be more susceptible than men to the carcinogens found in cigarette smoke. There is clearly a *dose–response relationship*, meaning that the more cigarettes smoked over time, the greater the risk of developing the malignancy. Other possible etiologic agents include ionizing radiation, industrial carcinogens and gases, heavy metals, and asbestos. Smoking and such environmental exposures probably act as co-carcinogens.[34] Genetic factors, air pollution, and lung scars are also suspected factors, but the correlation has not been as well established.

CLASSIFICATIONS

The four major histologic classifications of lung carcinomas are as follows: squamous cell carcinoma, small cell carcinoma, large cell carcinoma, and adenocarcinoma (including bronchoalveolar cell carcinoma). For clinical purposes, however, the carcinomas are classified as small cell lung cancer (SCLC) or non-small cell lung cancer (NSCLC) (Box 20-11). Small cell carcinomas have a strong correlation to cigarette smoking and carry a poor prognosis. Survival time after SCLC diagnosis, if left untreated, is approximately 9 to 10 months, with only 5% of individuals alive after 5 years.[34] Squamous cell carcinomas usually arise in the central portion of the lung from the bronchial tissue. These well-differentiated tumors are readily shed in the sputum.[50] Box 20-11 presents these classifications and the relative frequency of each tumor type.

PATHOPHYSIOLOGY

A lung cancer lesion begins with the transformation of one airway epithelial cell.[22] Some of the lung cancers originate in the bronchi and are thus termed **bronchogenic**. Specific portions of the bronchi, such as the segmental bifurcations and sites of mucus production, are thought to be more vulnerable to injury secondary to carcinogens.[50]

As the tumor grows it can partially obstruct the airway lumen or grow to an extent that it completely blocks the airway, resulting in post-obstructive lobar collapse distal to the lesion. The tumor can also hemorrhage, resulting in hemoptysis. Metastasis, in most tumors, occurs early to other thoracic structures such as hilar lymph nodes or the mediastinum. Distant metastasis to other organs such as the brain, liver, bone, and adrenals frequently occurs. Small cell carcinomas can also trigger the release of an excessive amount of hormones, particularly adrenal hormones, that result in significant endocrine derangements. This phenomenon represents a classic **paraneoplastic syndrome** (see p. 84).

BOX 20-11 CLASSIFICATION OF LUNG CARCINOMAS

Non-small Cell Carcinomas	
Squamous cell carcinomas	25–35% of total
Large Cell Carcinomas (undifferentiated)	5–20%
Adenocarcinoma	25–35%
Small Cell (Oat Cell) Carcinoma (Undifferentiated)	10–25%

(Summarized from Chandrasoma, P. & Taylor, C. R. [1998]. *Concise pathology* [3rd ed.]. Stamford, CT: Appleton & Lange.)

CLINICAL MANIFESTATIONS

Most tumors grow asymptomatically. Once the tumor is large enough to interfere with airway function, symptoms such as cough, sputum production, hemoptysis, pneumonia, airway obstruction, and pleural effusions can become apparent. Many lung cancers are diagnosed without any presenting symptoms, being detected when a chest x-ray is performed for some other reason. If the individual is symptomatic when medical advice is sought, the tumor is usually in an advanced stage. Weight loss, fatigue, and dyspnea ensue as the malignancy progresses.

Pleural Malignancies

The majority of primary pleural malignancies are related to asbestos exposure. This type of pleural malignancy is called *malignant mesothelioma*. Some mesotheliomas are not malignant, but the vast majority are. Malignant mesotheliomas are relatively rare, accounting for only 2000 cases per year in the United States.[26] Pleural malignancies can also be metastatic from other thoracic malignancies.

PATHOPHYSIOLOGY

Malignant mesotheliomas arise directly from the mesothelial cells in the pleural lining and grow slowly. The malignant cells spread throughout the pleural lining, eventually encasing the pleura as a whole, and lead to contraction of the affected lung. Pleural effusions are present in 50% of cases at time of presentation. Distant metastasis, including to the bone, can occur.[26]

CLINICAL MANIFESTATIONS

The most common presenting symptoms are chest pain and cough. The presence of pleural effusion is common. Fatigue, weight loss, and progressive dyspnea are also experienced. The prognosis in malignant mesothelioma is very poor.[26]

RESPIRATORY FAILURE

Respiratory failure is the inability of the lungs to meet the basic demands for tissue oxygenation at rest. It may result from a wide variety of intrapulmonary or nonpulmonary disorders. It often occurs with gradual onset

FOCUS ON THE PERSON WITH ASTHMA

D. D., a 14 year-old African-American female with a history of seasonal hay-fever symptoms and eczema, has been troubled recently by chest tightness, wheezing, and cough. The cough is only minimally productive of white sputum. There is a strong family history of allergies, and D. D. received "allergy shots" when she was younger. She tells her mother that when she visits a friend's home where a cat resides, the symptoms seem to be much worse. Concerned about her daughter's complaints, D. D.'s mother takes her to the family clinic, where a diagnosis of asthma is eventually established.

Questions

1. What historical factors would raise concern that D. D. may have asthma?
2. What environmental factors could potentially exacerbate her condition?
3. What is the main pathophysiologic process in the airways that is responsible for the clinical manifestations of asthma?

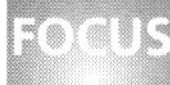

FOCUS ON THE PERSON WITH CHRONIC OBSTRUCTIVE LUNG DISEASE

Mr. S. is an 82-year-old male with a history of chronic obstructive pulmonary disease and stable angina associated with coronary artery disease. He was hospitalized 6 months ago for an episode of congestive heart failure but has done well since discharge. Mr. S. lives in a cottage behind his daughter's home, joins her family for dinner each night and, despite his chronic illnesses, remains independent. Over the past few days, the daughter has noticed that Mr. S. has been eating poorly and seems a little confused about recent events. Concerned that there may be something wrong with his heart, she asks about chest pain or cough, both of which he denies. The next day she notices that he misses his Tuesday morning bridge club meeting and his breathing appears to require more effort when compared with his baseline. Despite his insistence that nothing is wrong other than being "a little tired," he eventually agrees to see his primary care provider. Physical examination reveals normal vital signs and cardiac exam, but crackles are noted at the left lower lung field. A chest radiograph confirms left lower lobe pneumonia.

Questions

1. What subtle changes may have signaled a problem in this individual?
2. What pathophysiologic processes account for the findings on physical examination?

of symptoms of hypoxemia and hypercapnia. As respiratory failure ensues, the pCO_2 begins to rise, which leads to significant respiratory acidosis. If the process is gradual, the kidneys will compensate for the increased acid load (see p. 180).

Acute Respiratory Failure

This disorder is a sudden and life-threatening deterioration of gas exchange that occurs when there is inadequate oxygen production and carbon dioxide removal. It may be associated with a variety of pulmonary and non-pulmonary diseases (infections, neurologic disorders/injuries, and cardiac failure). Acute respiratory failure is defined broadly as a PaO_2 less than 50 mm Hg or a $PaCO_2$ greater than 50 with an arterial pH less than 7.35.[37] It is further defined as either **hypoxemic** or **hypercapnic** despite treatment with supplemental oxygen. Generally this is characterized by a PaO_2 less than 50 mm Hg while receiving an FiO_2 0.6 or more. Hypercapnic respiratory failure is associated with a $PaCO_2$ greater than 50 mm Hg. Both hypoxemic and hypercapnic respiratory failure may occur in acute and chronic forms. Acute forms develop quickly, and chronic forms over several days or weeks.

Chronic Respiratory Failure

This disorder is a late manifestation of chronic bronchitis and emphysema. It is defined as a deterioration of gas exchange that has been gradual or persistent following an episode of acute respiratory failure.[37] In cases of COPD this occurs due to the weakened nature of the inspiratory muscles, increased airway resistance, and hypoxemia. Arterial blood gases typically reveal a $Pa0_2$ less than 55 mm Hg, a $PaCO_2$ greater than 50 mm Hg, and a pH less than 7.35.[37]

REFERENCES

1. Aitken, M. (1997). Cystic fibrosis. In W. N. Kelley (Ed.), *Textbook of internal medicine* (3rd ed.). Philadelphia: Lippincott-Raven.
2. Albert, R. K. (1996). Pulmonary hypertension and chronic cor pulmonale as viewed by the pulmonologist. In J. W. Hurst (Ed.), *Medicine for the practicing physician* (4th ed). Stamford, CT: Appleton & Lange.
3. American Thoracic Society Statement (1993). Guidelines for the initial management of adults with community-acquired pneumonia: Diagnosis, assessment of severity, and initial antimicrobial therapy. *American Review of Respiratory Disease, 148*, 1418–1426.
4. American Thoracic Society Statement. (1995). Hospital-acquired pneumonia in adults: Diagnosis, assessment of severity, initial antimicrobial therapy, and preventative strategies. *American Journal of Respiratory and Critical Care Medicine, 153*, 1711–1725.
5. American Thoracic Society. (1995). Standards for the diagnosis and care of patients with chronic obstructive pulmonary disease. *American Journal of Respiratory and Critical Care Medicine, 152*, S77–S120.

6. Anderson, F. A. & Wheeler, H. B. (1995). Venous thromboembolism. *Clinics in Chest Medicine, 16*(2), 236–251.
7. Andrews, C. O. & Gora, M. L. (1994). Pleural effusions: Pathophysiology and management. *Annals of Pharmacotherapy, 28,* 894–902.
8. Beaty, C. D. (1997). Bronchiectasis. In W. N. Kelley (Ed.), *Textbook of internal medicine* (3rd ed.). Philadelphia: Lippincott-Raven.
9. Bernard, G. R., Artigas, A., Brigham, K. L., Carlet, J., Falke, K., Hudson, L., Lamy, M., Legall, J. R., Morris, A., Spragg, R. and the Consensus Committee. (1994). The American-European Consensus Conference on ARDS: Definitions, mechanisms, relevant outcomes, and clinical trial coordination. *American Journal of Respiratory and Critical Care Medicine, 149,* 818–824.
10. Celli, B. R. (1997). Chronic obstructive pulmonary disease. In M. G. Khan & J. P. Lynch (Eds.), *Pulmonary disease diagnosis and treatment.* Baltimore: Williams & Wilkins.
11. Centers for Disease Control. (1997). Tuberculosis morbidity—United States 1996. *Morbidity and Mortality Weekly Report, 46*(3), 695–700.
12. Centers for Disease Control. (1998) Tuberculosis morbidity—United States, 1997. *Morbidity and Mortality Weekly Report, 47*(13).
13. Chan, C. K. & Matthay, R. A. (1998). Pulmonary thromboembolism. In J. H. Stein, *Internal medicine* (5th ed.). St. Louis: Mosby.
14. Garrouste-Orgeas, M., Chevret, S., Arlet, G., Marie, O., Rouveau, M., Popoff, N. & Schlemmer, B. (1997). Oropharyngeal gastric colonization and nosocomial pneumonia in adult intensive care unit patients. *American Journal of Respiratory and Critical Care Medicine, 156,* 1647–1655.
15. Gurney, J. W. (1998). Pathophysiology of obstructive airway disease. *Radiologic Clinics of North America, 36*(1), 15–27.
16. Gussack, G. S. (1996). Carcinoma of larynx. In J. W. Hurst (Ed.), *Medicine for the practicing physician* (4th ed). Stamford, CT: Appleton & Lange.
17. Guyton A. C. & Hall, J. E. (1997). Regulation of respiration and respiratory insufficiency. In A. C. Guyton & J. E. Hall (Eds.), *Human physiology and mechanism of disease* (6th ed.). Philadelphia: W. B. Saunders.
18. Hammond, D. I., Don, C. & Khan, M. G. (1997). Interpretation of the chest radiograph. In M. G. & J. P. Lynch (Eds.), *Pulmonary disease diagnosis and treatment.* Baltimore: Williams & Wilkins.
19. Hayden, F. G. & Gwaltney, J. M. (1994). Viral infections. In J. F. Murray & J. A. Nadel (Eds.), *Textbook of respiratory medicine* (2nd ed.). Philadelphia: W. B. Saunders.
20. Hicks, M. A. (1995). A systematic approach to neonatal pathophysiology: Understanding respiratory distress syndrome. *Neonatal Network, 14*(1), 29–35.
21. Jackler, R. K. & Kaplan, M. J. (1998). Ear, nose and throat. In L. M. Tierney, S. J. McPhee & M. A. Papadakis (Eds.), *Current medical diagnosis and treatment* (37th ed.). Stamford, CT: Appleton & Lange.
22. Kern, J. A. & Clamon, G. (1997). Lung cancer. In W. N. Kelley (Ed.), *Textbook of internal medicine* (3rd ed.). Philadelphia: Lippincott-Raven.
23. Kobitz, L. (1999). The lung. In R. S. Cotran, V. Kumar, and T. Collins, *Robbins' pathologic basis of disease* (6th ed.). Philadelphia: W. B. Saunders.
24. Krachman, S., & Criner, G. J. (1998). Hypoventilation syndromes. *Clinics in Chest Medicine, 19*(1), 139–155.
25. Light, R. W. (1994). Pneumothorax. In J. F. Murray & J. A. Nadel (Eds.), *Textbook of respiratory medicine* (2nd ed.). Philadelphia: W. B. Saunders.
26. Light, R. W. (1994). Tumors of the pleura. In J. F. Murray & J. A. Nadel (Eds.), *Textbook of respiratory medicine* (2nd ed.). Philadelphia: W. B. Saunders.
27. Lomaton, J. R., George, S. S. & Brandstetter, R. D. (1997). Aspiration pneumonia. *Postgraduate Medicine, 102*(2), 225–231.
28. Luce, J. M. (1998). Acute lung injury and the acute respiratory distress syndrome. *Critical Care Medicine, 26*(2), 369–376.
29. Lynch, J. P. (1997). Bacterial pneumonia. In M. G. Khan & J. P. Lynch (Eds.), *Pulmonary disease diagnosis and treatment.* Baltimore: Williams & Wilkins.
30. Lynch, J. P., & Toews, G. B. (1997). Fungal, mycobacterial and viral pulmonary infections. In M. G. Khan & J. P. Lynch (Eds.), *Pulmonary disease diagnosis and treatment.* Baltimore: Williams & Wilkins.
31. Martinez, F. D., Wright, A. L., Taussing, L. M., Holberg, C. J., Halonen, M., & Morgan, W. J. (1995). Group Health Medical Associates. Asthma and wheezing in the first six years of life. *New England Journal of Medicine, 332,* 133–138.
32. McCool, F. D. & Rochester, D. F. (1994). The lungs and chest wall diseases. In J. F. Murray & J. A. Nadel (Eds.), *Textbook of respiratory medicine* (2nd ed.). Philadelphia: W. B. Saunders.
33. Mehrad, B. & Weg, J. G. (1997). Acute lung injury and acute respiratory distress syndrome. In M. G. Khan & J. P. Lynch (Eds.), *Pulmonary disease diagnosis and treatment.* Baltimore: Williams & Wilkins.
34. Minna, J. D. (1998). Neoplasms of the lung. In A. S. Fauci, E. Braunwald, K. J. Isselbacher, J. D. Wilson, J. B. Martin, D. L. Kasper, S. L. Hauser, & D. L. Longo (Eds.), *Harrison's principles of internal medicine* (14th ed.). New York: McGraw-Hill.
35. Murray, J. F. (1994). General principles and diagnostic approach. In J. F. Murray & J. A. Nadel (Eds.), *Textbook of respiratory medicine* (2nd ed.). Philadelphia: W. B. Saunders.
36. National Institutes of Health: National Heart, Lung and Blood Institute. (1997). *Expert Panel Report II: Guidelines for the diagnosis and management of asthma.* NIH Publication No. 97-4051. Washington, DC: NIH.
37. Powell, C. A. & Joyce-Brady, M. F. (1997). Acute and chronic respiratory failure. In R.H. Goldstein, J. J. O'Connell, & J. B. Karlinsky (Eds.), *A practical approach to pulmonary medicine.* Philadelphia: Lippincott-Raven.
38. Rello, J., Rue, M., Jubert, P., Muses, G., Sonora, R., Valles, J., & Niederman, M. S. (1997). Survival in patients with nosocomial pneumonia: Impact of the severity of illness and etiological agent. *Critical Care Medicine, 25*(11), 1862–1867.
39. Robles, A. M. (1996). Acute infectious bronchitis. In J. W. Hurst (Ed.), *Medicine for the practicing physician* (4th ed.). Stamford, CT: Appleton & Lange.
40. Rubin, E. & Farber, J. L. (1999). Developmental and genetic disease. In E. Rubin and J. L. Farber, *Pathology* (3rd ed.). Philadelphia: Lippincott-Raven.
41. Rubin, L. J. (1997). Primary pulmonary hypertension. *The New England Journal of Medicine, 336*(2), 111–117.
42. Samuelson, J. (1999). Infectious diseases. In R. S. Cotran, V. Kumar, & T. Collins, *Robbins' pathologic basis of disease* (6th ed.). Philadelphia: W. B. Saunders.
43. Schaecter, M., Medoff, G. & Eisenstein, B. I. (1998). *Mechanisms of microbial disease* (3rd ed.). Baltimore: Williams & Wilkins.
44. Sheehan, C. (1997). *Clinical immunology* (2nd ed.). Philadelphia: Lippincott.
45. Schofield, D. (1999). Diseases of infancy and childhood. In R. S. Cotran, V. Kumar, & T. Collins, *Robbins' pathologic basis of disease* (6th ed.). Philadelphia: W. B. Saunders.
46. Simon, H. B. (1995). Approach to the patient with acute bronchitis or pneumonia in the ambulatory setting. In A. H. Goroll, L. A. May, & A. G. Mulley (Eds.), *Primary care medicine* (3rd ed.). Philadelphia: J.B. Lippincott.
47. Simon, H. B. (1995). Management of the common cold. In A. H. Goroll, L. A. May, & A. G. Mulley (Eds.), *Primary care medicine* (3rd ed.). Philadelphia: J. B. Lippincott.

48. Stauffer, J. L. (1998). Lung. In L. M. Tierney, S. J. McPhee, & M. A. Papadakis (Eds.), *Current medical diagnosis and treatment* (37th ed.). Stamford, CT: Appleton & Lange.
49. Tino, G. & Kelley, M. A. (1997). Pulmonary thromboembolism. In W. N. Kelley (Ed.), *Textbook of internal medicine* (3rd ed.). Philadelphia: Lippincott-Raven.
50. Travis, W. D., Farber, J. L. & Rubin, E. (1999). The respiratory system. In E. Rubin & J. L. Farber, *Pathology* (3rd ed.). Philadelphia: Lippincott-Raven.
51. Vallen-Mashikian, M. A. & Menenghetti, A. (1997). Community-acquired pneumonia. In R. H. Goldstein, J. J. O'Connell, & J. B. Karlinsky (Eds.), *A practical approach to pulmonary medicine.* Philadelphia: Lippincott-Raven.
52. Vokes, E. E. (1998). Head and neck cancer. In A. S. Fauci, E. Braunwald, K. J. Isselbacher, J. D. Wilson, J. B. Martin, D. L. Kasper, S. L. Hauser, & D. L. Longo (Eds.), *Harrison's principles of internal medicine* (14th ed.). New York: McGraw-Hill.
53. Wagenvoort, C. A. (1995). Pathology of pulmonary thromboembolism. *Chest, 107,* 10S–17S.
54. Weg, J. G. (1996). Bronchiectasis. In J. W. Hurst (Ed.), *Medicine for the practicing physician* (4th ed.). Stamford, CT: Appleton & Lange.
55. Winn, W. C. & Chandler, F. W. (1994). Bacterial infections. In D. H. Dail & S. P. Hammar (Eds.), *Pulmonary pathology* (2nd ed.). New York: Springer-Verlag.
56. Young, L. S. (1994). *Pneumocystis carinii.* In J. E. Pennington (Ed.), *Respiratory infections, diagnosis and management* (3rd ed.). New York: Raven Press.

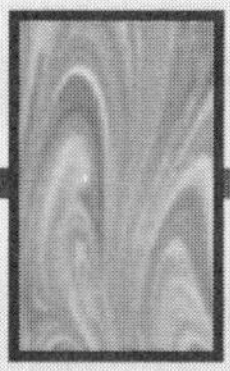

UNIT 5: CASE STUDY

Pulmonary Tuberculosis

Introduction to the Patient

Mr. A. is a 55-year-old male, recent immigrant from the Philippines who presents to the Emergency Department with a complaint of hemoptysis for 2 days. He reports that he had a "little cough" for about 3 months, but it was rarely productive of any sputum until the onset of hemoptysis yesterday. He also admits to a 10-lb. weight loss and a general sense of fatigue over the past 2 months. He attributed the fatigue to working the night shift. He has also been awakened from sleep with fever and sweating profusely.

Social History

Mr. A. works nights at the local airport. He smokes filtered cigarettes, about one pack per day for more than 30 years (30 pack years). He has been considering quitting smoking because of the chronic cough. He does not take any medications. Mr. A. is married and supports his family, a wife and three preteen boys, in the Philippines.

Past Medical and Family History

There is no significant history of heart disease, cancer, or diabetes, but Mr. A.'s father and older brother reportedly were diagnosed and treated for tuberculosis. He also reports that the father was diagnosed with pulmonary emphysema, which caused his death at age 75. Mr. A.'s mother is living and has no particular complaints except "stiffness" of the joints.

Physical Examination

Mr. A. appeared pale and thin. He was 5 ft. 4 in. tall and weighed 130 lb. He was alert and oriented but very anxious. Blood pressure on admission was 142/76 and pulse 102. Breath sounds were very quiet, and the chest wall had a barrel-shaped appearance. No pulmonary rales were appreciated. The exam was otherwise unremarkable.

Diagnostic Tests

Blood work ordered included complete blood count, chem 13, and arterial blood gases. The CBC included the following: Hct 51, Hgb 16.5, WBC 10,200. The Chem 13 included a sodium of 132, a potassium of 4.8, and other values were normal. The arterial blood gases were as follows: pH 7.34, $PaCO_2$ 48, PaO_2 68, O_2 Sat 88%, HCO_3 28.

Chest x-ray PA and lateral showed a round lesion in the apex of the right lung. Evidence of a right-sided pleural effusion was also noted. Radiographic evidence indicated possible chronic obstructive lung disease.

Clinical Course

Mr. A. was admitted to a private, negative-pressure room with respiratory precautions. His admitted diagnosis was "Possible active pulmonary tuberculosis" and "Rule-Out COPD." A tuberculin skin test was placed on his right forearm.

CRITICAL THINKING QUESTIONS

1. What clues in this patient's history suggest tuberculosis as a possible etiology for his illness?
2. Considering the results of his blood work and radiographic test, what are some of the possible other conditions that could be considered?
3. Describe, in detail, the pathophysiology of *Mycobacterium tuberculosis.* Discuss the implications of his smoking habit in the etiology of this disease.
4. Discuss the pathophysiology and clinical course of chronic obstructive pulmonary disease. What would be the evidence for this condition on the x-ray examination?
5. Outline the plan of care for this patient, including diagnosis of *M. tb* and possible COPD. Consider the medical, pharmacologic, nutritional, and nursing aspects of this plan of care.
6. What are the important long-term teaching aspects necessary in the management of this patient's plan of care?

Besides your pathophysiology text, you will need a good pharmacology textbook, a medical infectious disease textbook, a medical pulmonary textbook, a pathology text, and nursing or other research articles to guide your completion of this case study.

Suggested references include:

Karch, A. M. (2000). *Focus on nursing pharmacology.* Philadelphia: Lippincott Williams & Wilkins.

Gantz, N. M., Brown, R. B., Berk, S. L., Esposito, A. L. & Gleckman, R. A. (1999). *Manual of clinical problems in infectious disease* (4th ed.). Philadelphia: Lippincott Williams & Wilkins.

Burton, G. G., Hodgkin, J. E., Ward, J. J., et al. (1997). *Respiratory care: A guide to clinical practice* (4th ed.). Philadelphia: Lippincott-Raven.

Rubin, E. & Farber, J. (1999). *Pathology* (3rd ed.). Philadelphia: Lippincott Williams & Wilkins.

UNIT 5 APPENDIX A

PULMONARY FUNCTION TESTS

TEST	NORMAL ADULT VALUES	SIGNIFICANCE
LUNG VOLUMES		
1. Tidal volume (V_t)	Approximately 500 mL	The volume of gas moved in and out of the lungs with each breath. The V_t represents only a small percentage of the amount of air that the lungs are capable of moving.
2. Expiratory reserve volume (ERV)	(± 1,200 mL)	The additional amount of gas or air that can be forcefully exhaled after a normal expiration is complete.
3. Residual volume (RV)	(± 1,200 mL)	The amount of air remaining in the lungs after a forced expiration. Since it is physiologically impossible to completely empty one's lungs, this measurement is taken indirectly.
4. Inspiratory reserve volume (IRV)	(± 3,100 mL)	The maximum volume of air that can be inhaled after a normal resting inspiration.
LUNG CAPACITIES		
1. Total lung capacity (TLC)	Adult TLC equals approximately 6,000 mL	The maximum volume of gas that the lungs can hold. Not all of this inspired gas is available for exchange, because this measurement includes dead space gas. The TLC equals the IRV plus the V_t plus the ERV plus the RV (TLC = IRV + V_t + ERV + RV).
2. Functional residual capacity (FRC)	Approximately 2,400 mL.	Refers to the volume of gas remaining in the lungs at the end of a spontaneous expiration and includes the ERV and the RV (FRC = ERV + RV).
3. Vital capacity (VC) measured either as expiratory or inspiratory	About 5,000 mL in adult males.	Expiratory vital capacity is the maximum volume of gas that can be exhaled after the deepest possible inspiration. Inspiratory vital capacity is the maximum amount of gas that can be inhaled after the fullest possible exhalation. Usually, expiratory vital capacity equals inspiratory vital capacity. Total vital capacity, therefore, equals IRV plus V_t plus ERV (VC = IRV + V_t + ERV). The vital capacity increases with height, usually is greater in men, and is roughly proportional to lean body weight in young adults. It decreases slightly in the supine position due to the splinting of posterior rib movement and reduced diaphragmatic action. On quiet breathing, the lungs are roughly one-third inflated in the supine position and one-half inflated in the upright position. This test is a common part of spirometric testing and is called the forced vital capacity (FVC).
4. Inspiratory capacity (IC)	Approximately 3,600 mL of air	The maximum volume of air that can be inhaled from a resting position. It equals the V_t plus the IRV (IC = V_t + IRV). The RV, TLC, VC, and FRC are not anatomically fixed but depend on elastic characteristics and muscle forces. All lung volumes and capacities change with aging due in part to a decrease in elastic recoil in the elderly. Therefore, with age, the RV and FRC increase slightly and the VC decreases. This decrease is partially due to stiffening of the thoracic cage and decreased chest mobility.

(continued)

UNIT 5 APPENDIX A

PULMONARY FUNCTION TESTS (Continued)

TEST	NORMAL ADULT VALUES	SIGNIFICANCE
MEASUREMENTS THAT SHOW RELATIONSHIP BETWEEN FLOW AND VOLUME		
1. Forced expiratory flow in 1 second (FEV_1)	The normal individual should be able to exhale 80% of his or her FVC in 1 second	The amount of air that can be forced out of the lungs on expiration in 1 second. The flow rates can be plotted by comparing expired air volume over time. Occasionally this measurement is made at 3 seconds as well.
2. Peak expiratory flow (PEF)	≥ 80% of predicted normal Highest rate of flow sustained for 10 msec or more during which air can be expelled from the lungs	Decreased PEF results from obstruction of small airways; related to age, sex, and smoking behaviors The amount of gas actually reaching the exchange area, the tidal volume (V_t) minus the dead space.
3. Alveolar ventilation	Estimated from standard tables, usually equals adult's ideal weight in pounds	Dead space (V_D) is usually estimated from standard tables, but it can be approximated to equal an adult's ideal weight in pounds.
4. Minute ventilation		The total amount of air entering or leaving the body per minute, calculated by multiplying the tidal volume by the respiratory rate. It includes the anatomic dead space.

UNIT 5 APPENDIX B

DIAGNOSTIC TESTS

TEST	NORMAL VALUES	SIGNIFICANCE
ARTERIAL BLOOD GAS ANALYSIS (BAGS)		
PO_2	80–100 mmHg	Oxygen available for saturation
PCO_2	35–45 mmHg	Pressure of carbon dioxide in arterial blood
O_2 saturation	95–98%	Percent of hemoglobin saturated with oxygen
HCO_3^-	22–26 mEq/L	Amount of bicarbonate in arterial blood
Base excess (BE)/base deficit (BD)	+2/–2	The deviation of HCO_3^- from 24 mEq/L
CHEST RADIOGRAPHS (CHEST X-RAYS)	Clear, with normal thoracic structures identified	Evaluate thoracic bony structures, lung tissue, mediastinal structures, heart size, pleura, large airways and major thoracic blood vessels; usually taken in two views: posterior-anterior (PA) and lateral
PULSE OXIMETRY	94–100%	Noninvasive technique using light reflection technology that determines degree (%) of oxygen saturation of RBCs in arterial blood
FINE-NEEDLE BIOPSY	Negative	Small needle passes into the chest to sample tissue or fluid from an unknown mass
SPUTUM CULTURE	Negative for pathogenic species	Microbial culture of respiratory secretions to determine etiology and antibiotic sensitivity; may be helpful in diagnosing pneumonia or tuberculosis

UNIT BIBLIOGRAPHY

Bernard, S. I. (1998). COPD: Overview of definitions, epidemiology, and factors influencing its development. *Chest, 113*(4 supp), 235S–241S.

Binkin, N. J., Zuber, P. L., Wells, C. D., Tipple, M. A. & Castro, K. G. (1996). Overseas screening for tuberculosis in immigrants and refugees to the United States: Current status. *Clinical Infectious Diseases, 23,* 1226–1232.

Chastre, J., Trouillet, J. L., Vuagnat, A., Joly-Guillou, M. L., Clavier, H., Dombret, M. C. & Gibert, C. (1998). Nosocomial pneumonia in patients with acute respiratory distress syndrome. *American Journal of Respiratory and Critical Care Medicine, 157,* 1165–1172.

Correa, A. G. (1997). Unique aspects of tuberculosis in the pediatric population. *Clinics in Chest Medicine, 18*(1), 89–98.

Daley, C. J., Hahn, J. A., Moss, A. R., Hopewell, P. C. & Schecter, G. F. (1998). Incidence of tuberculosis in injection drug users in San Francisco. *American Journal of Respiratory and Critical Care Medicine, 157,* 19–22.

DeBock, G. H., Dekker, F. W., Stolk, M. P., Springer, J. K. & van Houwelingen, J. C. (1997). Anti-microbial treatment in acute maxillary sinusitis: A meta-analysis. *Journal of Clinical Epidemiology, 50*(8), 881–890.

Fagon, J., Chastre, J., Vuagnat, A. Trouillet, J., Novara, A. & Gilbert, C. (1996). Nosocomial pneumonia and mortality among patients in Intensive Care Units. *Journal of the American Medical Association, 275*(11), 866–869.

Fine, M. J., Auble, T. E., Yealy, D. M., Hanusa, B. H., Weissfeld, L. A., Singer, D. E., Coley, C. M., Marrie, T. J. & Kapoor, W. N. (1997). A prediction rule to identify low-risk patients with community-acquired pneumonia. *New England Journal of Medicine, 336*(4), 243–250.

Giuntini, C., Di Rocco, G., Marini, C., Melillo, E, & Palla, A. (1995). Epidemiology (of thromboembolism). *Chest, 107* (1 supp), 3S–9S.

Kankam, C. G. & Sallis, R. (1997). Acute sinusitis in adults. *Postgraduate Medicine, 102*(2), 253–258.

Kennedy, D. W., Gwaltney, J. M. & Jones, J. G. (1995). Medical management of sinusitis: Educational goals and management guidelines. *Annals of Otolaryngology, Rhinology & Laryngology,* (Supplement), *167,* 22–30.

Leiberman, D., Porath, A., Schlaeffer, F., Liberman, D. & Boldur, I. (1996). *Legionella* species community-acquired pneumonia: A review of 56 hospitalized adult patients. *Chest, 109*(5), 1243–1249.

Leiner, S. & Mays, M. (1996). Diagnosing latent and active pulmonary tuberculosis: A review for clinicians. *Nurse Practitioner, 21*(2), 86–111.

Mendel, L. A., & Campbell, D. (1998). Nosocomial pneumonia guidelines: An international perspective. *Chest, 113* (supp. 3), 188S–193S.

Marfan, A. A., Sporrer, J., Moore, P. S. & Stefkin, A. D. (1995). Risk factors for adverse outcome in persons with pneumococcal pneumonia. *Chest, 107*(2), 457–462.

Marrie, T. J., Fine, M. J. & Coley, C. M. (1996). Ambulatory patients with community-acquired pneumonia: The frequency of atypical agents and clinical course. *American Journal of Medicine, 101,* 508–515.

Miller, K. S. & Miller, J. M. (1996). Tuberculosis in pregnancy: Interactions, diagnosis, and management. *Clinical Obstetrics and Gynecology, 39*(1), 120–142.

Moffitt, M. P. & Wisinger, D. B. (1996). Tuberculosis: Recommendations for screening, prevention, and treatment. *Postgraduate Medicine, 100*(4), 201–218.

National Lung Health Education Program Executive Committee. (1998). Strategies in preserving lung health and preventing COPD and associated diseases. *Chest, 113*(2), 123S–135S.

Newman, L. S., Rose, C. S. & Maier, L. A. (1997). Sarcoidosis. *New England Journal of Medicine, 17,* 1124–1234.

Niederman, M. S. (1998). Community-acquired pneumonia: A North American perspective. *Chest, 113*(supp. 3), 179S–182S.

Stulbarg, M. S. & Frank, J. A. (1998). Obstructive pulmonary disease: The clinician's perspective. *Radiologic Clinics of North America, 36*(1), 1–13.

Thomason, M. H., Payseur, E. S., Hakenewerth, A. H., Norton, J., Mehta, B., Reeves, R., Moore-Swartz, M. W., & Robbins, P. I. (1996). Nosocomial pneumonia in ventilated trauma patients during stress ulcer prophylaxis with sucralfate, antacid, and ranitidine. *Journal of Trauma: Injury, Infection and Critical Care, 41*(3), 503–508.

Woodhead, M. (1998). Community-acquired pneumonia guidelines: An international comparison; a view from Europe. *Chest, 113*(supp. 3), 183S–187S.

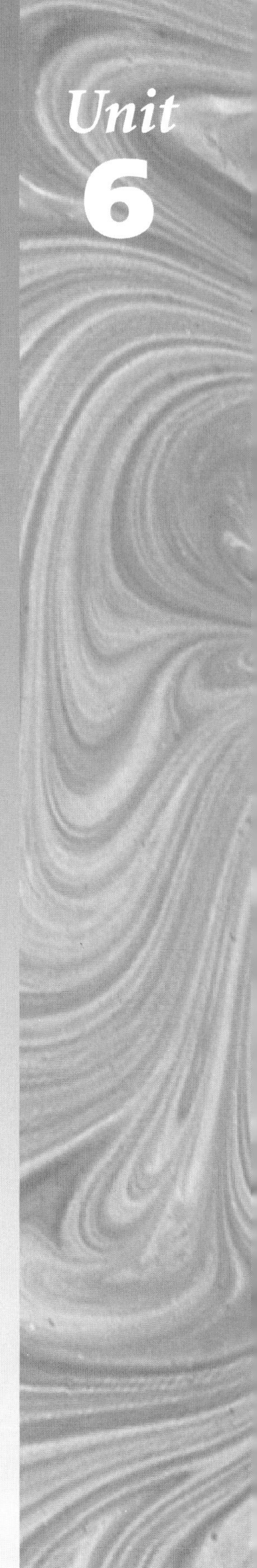

Urinary Excretion

FOCUS ON
Urinary Tract Changes Through the Life Span

INFANT (1–12 MONTHS):

Kidney and urinary tract structure is present at birth. By age 5 months, the tubules have adult-like proportions in size and shape. Renal function is not mature until about age 12 months, with renal excretion of excessive proteins not developed until that time. Urine has low specific gravity of 1.000 to 1.010.

TODDLER AND PRESCHOOL AGE (1–5 YEARS):

Renal function relatively mature by latter half of second year. Urine is concentrated on an adult level. Bladder capacity increases and voluntary bladder control usually occurs due to maturation of the nervous system, with the ability to retain urine for up to 2 hours. Occasional accidents and bedwetting are possible.

SCHOOL AGE (6–12 YEARS):

Bladder capacity increases and control is complete. Normal adult renal function is seen.

ADOLESCENCE (13–19 YEARS):

Bladder capacity increases with voiding amounts of approximately 1500 mL per day. Renal function is like that of an adult. Females who are sexually active have an increased risk for urinary tract infections.

YOUNG ADULT AND ADULT (20–45 YEARS):

Renal function is normal unless congenital or infectious problems occur. Increased sexual activity or pregnancies may lead to increased risk of urinary tract infections. Polycystic disease may lead to early onset of renal failure.

MIDDLE-AGED ADULT (46–64 YEARS):

Glomerular filtration rate and tubular function begin to gradually decline. Renal reserve also begins to decline, so the kidney does not compensate as well for acute metabolic changes. Stress incontinence and bladder prolapse are common in women.

LATE ADULTHOOD (65–100+ YEARS):

Filtration and excretion slow. Drugs are excreted more slowly. Decreased blood flow due to arteriosclerosis and hypertension may alter renal function. Bladder muscles weaken and bladder capacity decreases to less than 50% of that of young adults. Micturition reflex is delayed. Ability to store urine decreases. Frequent urination and urgency are common problems. Prostatic hypertrophy in males and bladder prolapse in females are common dysfunctions. Tubules decrease in length and volume. Nephrons decrease in size and number. Sixty-four percent of the nephrons are nonfunctional in the very elderly. Stress of illness often leads to renal dysfunction.

Chapter 21

Normal Renal Function and Urinary Excretion

Anita Tesh

KEY TERMS

afferent arteriole
Bowman's capsule
capsular hydrostatic pressure (CHP)
collecting duct
countercurrent exchanger
countercurrent mechanism
countercurrent multiplier
distal convoluted tubule (DCT)
efferent arteriole
erythropoietin
glomerular blood hydrostatic pressure (GBHP)
glomerular filtrate
glomerular filtration rate (GFR)
glomerulus
juxtaglomerular apparatus
loop of Henle
nephron
net filtration pressure (NFP)
proximal convoluted tubule (PCT)
renal artery
renal corpuscle
renin–angiotensin–aldosterone system
specific gravity
threshold, renal
transport maximum
tubular reabsorption
tubular secretion
vasa recta

The urinary system is composed of two kidneys, two ureters, the urinary bladder, and the urethra. This system removes waste products from the blood, maintains the body's levels of water and electrolytes, and plays critical roles in the body's homeostatic balance. This chapter will discuss structure and function related to the production and flow of urine, as well as selected other functions of the kidneys.

STRUCTURE OF THE KIDNEYS

The kidneys are located in the abdomen on either side of the vertebral column, behind the peritoneum (retroperitoneal space), as illustrated in Figure 21-1. Each bean-shaped kidney weighs about 150 g and is about the size of a closed fist.[5] The right kidney is slightly lower than the left because the liver is located above it. The kidneys are surrounded by a layer of perirenal fat that helps protect and support them. A layer of connective tissue called the *renal fascia* encapsulates and anchors the kidneys in place. A notch called the hilum is located at the concave portion of each kidney facing the vertebral column. The renal artery and vein, lymphatics, nerves, and a funnel-shaped extension of the upper ureter called the renal pelvis constitute the hilum.

The kidneys are divided into three regions: (1) the *cortex*, or outer portion; the (2) *medulla*, or inner portion; and (3) the *renal pelvis*. The medulla contains 8 to 18 triangular *renal pyramids*, which appear striated due to the collecting ducts, nephrons, and blood vessels that compose them. The renal pyramids are separated by the *columns of Bertin*, portions of cortical tissue that extent into the medulla.[6,10] The renal pyramids and associated cortical tissue form the *lobes* of the kidney. The apex of each pyramid is called the *papilla*.

The renal pelvis collects urine and provides a passageway for urine to the bladder (Fig. 21-2). Cuplike extensions called the minor *calices* surround the **collecting ducts** of the papilla. Shown in Figure 21-2, the *minor calices* empty urine into the *major calices*, from which it flows into the renal pelvis, then leaves the kidney to flow into the ureters.

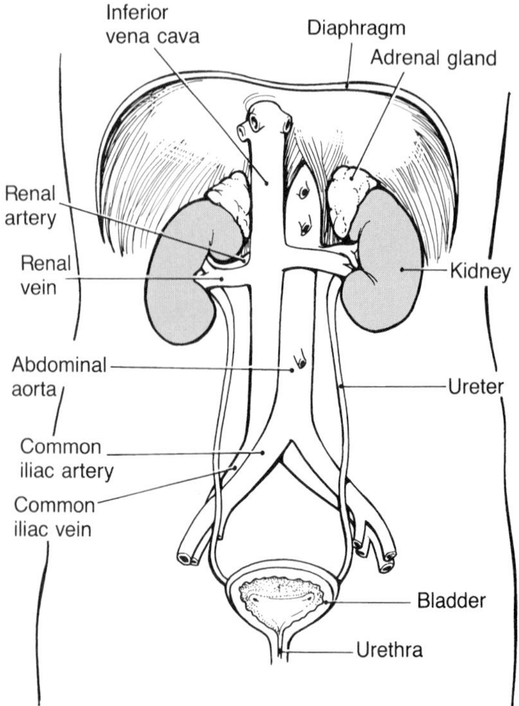

FIGURE 21-1. Urinary system, with blood vessels.

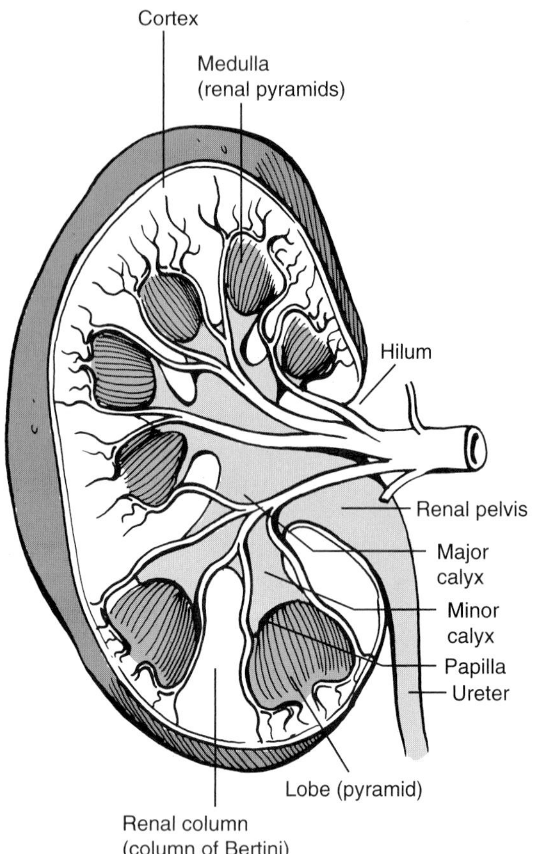

FIGURE 21-2. Macroscopic organization of the kidney.

Microscopic Anatomy

Understanding renal function requires an awareness of the interrelationship of certain microscopic elements of the kidney: (1) the nephron, (2) the glomerulus, and (3) the juxtamedullary apparatus. These will be discussed in the following sections.

THE NEPHRON

The **nephron** is the basic functional unit of the kidney. Each kidney contains about 1.2 million nephrons.[2] Kidneys cannot regenerate nephrons; therefore this number decreases with illness, injury, and normal aging.[5] Each nephron is composed of four parts: (1) Bowman's capsule, (2) the proximal convoluted tubule (PCT), (3) the loop of Henle, and (4) the distal convoluted tubule (DCT). Figure 21-3 shows these structures as well as the glomerulus.

Bowman's capsule is a cuplike structure that surrounds a capillary network called the **glomerulus,** which is further discussed below. Together the two are called the **renal corpuscle**. Water and solutes from blood in the glomerulus pass into Bowman's capsule to form the **glomerular filtrate**, a fluid similar to plasma but without plasma proteins.

The proximal convoluted tubule (PCT), loop of Henle, and distal convoluted tubule (DCT) constitute the tubular portion of the nephron, which transports, reabsorbs, and secretes the glomerular filtrate. The **proximal convoluted tubule** is the coiled portion of the tubule, which is proximal to the Bowman's capsule. The microvilli on the inner surface of the PCT increase the surface area available for secretion and absorption of fluids and solutes. Mitochondria also are located in the PCT. From 65% to 80% of the glomerular filtrate is reabsorbed from the PCT back into the bloodstream. The remaining 20% to 35% proceeds to the loop of Henle.[5]

The **loop of Henle**, shown in Figure 21-3, is the uncoiled portion of the tubule connected to the PCT. The loop of Henle comprises descending and ascending limbs. The upper portion of each limb is thick, and the lower portion is thinner. The descending limb makes a tight hairpin turn upward, where it becomes the thin portion of the ascending limb.

The **distal convoluted tubule** is the coiled distal portion of the tubule connected to the loop of Henle, as illustrated in Figure 21-3. The DCT also contains mitochondria and microvilli. Two or more DCTs join together to form the collecting duct.

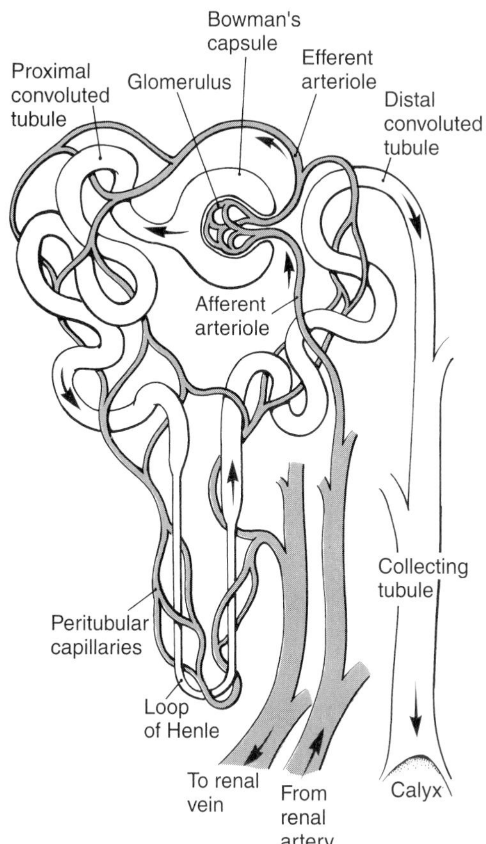

FIGURE 21-3. **Structure of the nephron and glomerulus.**

There are two types of nephrons: (1) cortical (also called superficial) and (2) juxtamedullary. These are illustrated in Figure 21-4. Bowman's capsule lies in the cortex in both types of nephrons. The tubules of the cortical nephrons (85% of all nephrons) penetrate the cortex and only into the outer region of the medulla, whereas the juxtamedullary nephrons contain longer loops of Henle that extend deep into the medulla, making these nephrons more effective in altering urine concentration.[2,8]

THE GLOMERULUS AND THE BLOOD SUPPLY TO THE KIDNEYS

The kidneys are highly vascular; although they make up only about 5% of body weight, they receive about 25% of the cardiac output.[1] The cortex is more richly supplied with blood than the medulla. The anatomical arrangement of renal blood vessels makes the kidney, especially the medullary area, very susceptible to ischemic damage.[1] From the aorta, blood enters the hilum of the kidney by way of the **renal artery**, which branches into segmental arteries. These arteries successively subdivide into interlobar, arcuate, and interlobular arteries, which give rise to the afferent arterioles. **Afferent arterioles** subdivide into tufts of capillaries called glomeruli.

The glomerulus loops into Bowman's capsule. In order to permit the free flow of water and soluble material to Bowman's capsule, the glomerular capillary membrane is composed of three main layers illustrated in Figure 21-5: (1) the endothelial layer, (2) the glomerular basement membrane, and (3) the epithelial layer. The thin inner endothelial layer has thousands of pores (fenestrations) that provide for membrane permeability. The middle layer, the glomerular basement membrane, is a continuous meshwork of collagen, glycoproteins, and mucopolysaccharides that prevents large proteins and molecules from passing into Bowman's capsule. The epithelial layer is composed of cells called podocytes, which have projections called pedicles (foot processes) that cover the glomerular basement membrane. Figure 21-5 illustrates narrow slit pores (filtration slits) between the pedicles, through which small proteins can pass. Plasma proteins are too large to pass through the silt pores.[1]

Efferent arterioles carry blood away from the glomeruli and form a second network of capillaries, the *peritubular capillary network*, that encircles the nephron. The peritubular network of the deeper-lying juxtamedullary glomeruli also forms sets of capillaries called the **vasa recta**. The vasa recta, illustrated in Figure 21-4, extend into the medulla near the ascending and descending loops of Henle.[1,2] Interlobular veins are formed from the peritubular capillary network. These veins converge into the arcuate veins, then the interlobar veins, and then the renal vein. Blood from the renal vein leaves the kidneys to drain into the inferior vena cava.

JUXTAGLOMERULAR APPARATUS

The **juxtaglomerular apparatus**, which is shown in Figure 21-6, is a small endocrine gland located where the DCT is adjacent to the glomerulus. It is composed of: (1) the macula densa, a set of specialized cells in the DCT, and (2) the juxtaglomerular cells in the afferent arteriole. The juxtaglomerular apparatus produces *renin*, which transforms angiotensinogen to angiotensin I. The macula densa cells contribute to the control of the glomerular filtration rate.[1]

Innervation of the Kidneys

Nerve fibers reach the kidney through the renal plexus, which extends along the renal artery and enters the kidney at the hilum. The kidney's nerve supply generally follows the distribution of the arterial vessels. The kidneys are innervated primarily by the sympathetic

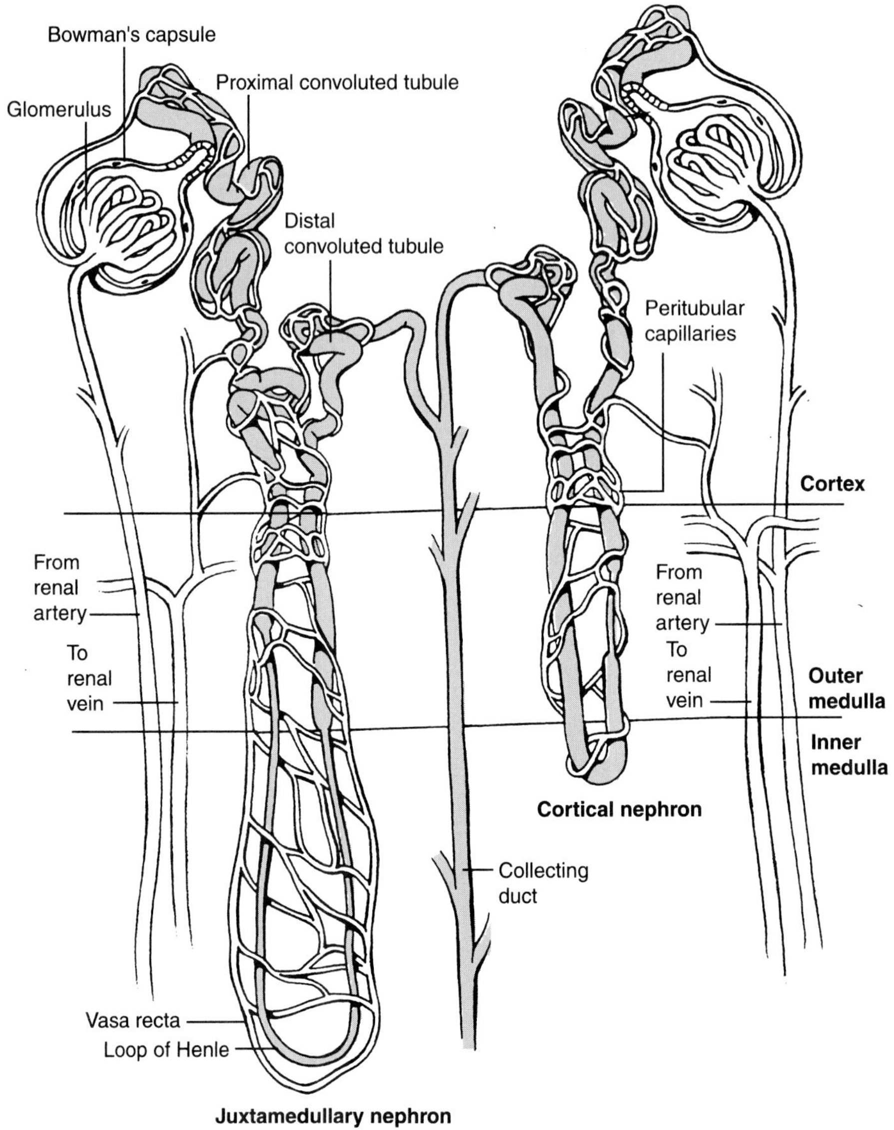

FIGURE 21-4. **Structure of cortical and juxtamedullary nephrons.**

division of the autonomic nervous system. Stimulation of the sympathetic nerves constricts the afferent arterioles and causes release of renin.[10] The parasympathetic system has important effects on the ureters and urinary bladder but no noted effects on the kidneys.[7,8]

FUNCTION OF THE KIDNEYS

The kidneys maintain plasma composition within narrow limits by removing some substances from the blood and adding others back to it, thus altering the composition of the urine. The large number of nephrons in a healthy kidney provides a large reserve in renal function. The kidneys use three major mechanisms to maintain this balance of plasma composition that results in urine formation: (1) glomerular filtration, (2) tubular reabsorption, and (2) tubular secretion. These are illustrated in Figure 21-7 in the pertinent portions of the nephron. In addition to maintaining plasma composition, the kidneys also have hormonal functions in regulation of blood pressure, erythropoiesis, and vitamin D activation. Finally, the kidneys are also capable of gluconeogenesis in prolonged fasting. The functions of the kidney are highlighted in Box 21-1.

FOCUS ON CELLULAR PHYSIOLOGY

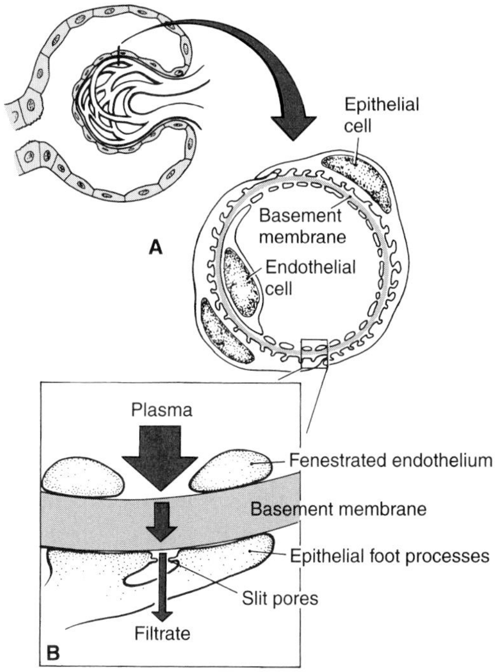

FIGURE 21-5. **A.** Schematic illustration of the three layers of the glomerular capillary. **B.** The dense layer of the glomerular basement membrane (GBM) prevents passage of large molecules into the ultrafiltrate.

Glomerular Filtration

Glomerular filtration, the first step in urine formation, is the movement of fluids and solutes from the blood in the glomerular capillary into Bowman's capsule (Fig. 21-8). As blood passes through the glomerulus, water and small solutes are able to permeate the glomerular capillary walls. Larger molecules, such as plasma proteins and blood cells, are unable to permeate the glomerular membrane. The resulting fluid is glomerular filtrate, a relatively protein-free fluid. The quantity of glomerular filtrate produced each minute, the **glomerular filtration rate** (GFR), is typically about 125 mL per minute.

The unique arrangement of capillaries between arterioles allows a higher pressure to be maintained in the glomerulus. The efferent arterioles are smaller in diameter than the afferent arterioles, which contributes to higher glomerular pressure because of increased vascular resistance in the efferent arteriole. Figure 21-9 summarizes the filtration process, which depends on the interaction of forces that contribute to the outward flow of filtrate into Bowman's capsule and the retention of fluid within the glomerulus.

FOCUS ON CELLULAR PHYSIOLOGY

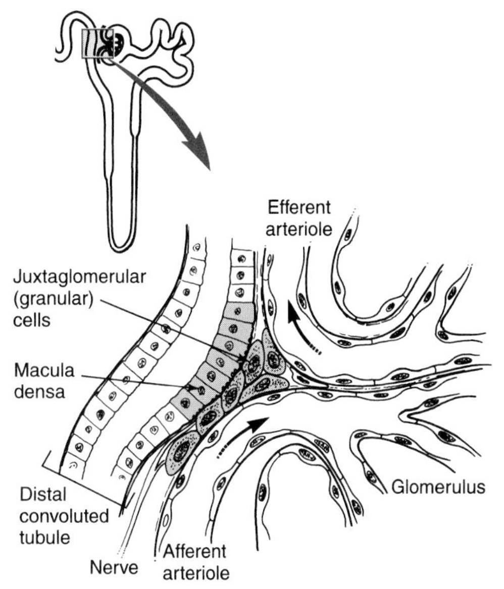

FIGURE 21-6. The relation of the juxtaglomerular apparatus, the distal convoluted tubule, and the glomerulus.

The pressure chiefly responsible for filtration is the **glomerular blood hydrostatic pressure (GBHP)**. This pressure, created by the systemic blood pressure, forces filtrate out of the glomerulus into Bowman's capsule. GBHP normally is equal to the mean arterial pressure (MAP), approximately 60 to 80 mm Hg. If it falls to 42 mm Hg, filtration usually does not take place.

Working in opposition to the GBHP is the hydrostatic pressure in Bowman's capsule, called the **capsular hydrostatic pressure (CHP)**. This pressure, normally about 18 mm Hg, is exerted by the walls of Bowman's capsule and the fluid in the renal tubule. CHP resists filtration, and increased CHP will cause the GFR to decrease.[5] Another pressure that works in opposition to GBHP and resists filtration is the *blood colloidal osmotic pressure* (BCOP), normally about 30 mm Hg. This pressure, also called the *oncotic pressure,* is the inward force exerted by plasma proteins. Since blood contains more protein than filtrate does, the colloidal pressure works to retain fluid in the glomerulus.

The net result of all these pressures—glomerular, capsular, and colloidal osmotic—is the **net filtration pressure (NFP)**. The NFP is equal to the forces inducing filtration (the GBHP) minus the forces opposing filtration (the CHP and BCOP):

$$\text{NFP} = \text{GBHP} - (\text{CHP} + \text{BCOP})$$

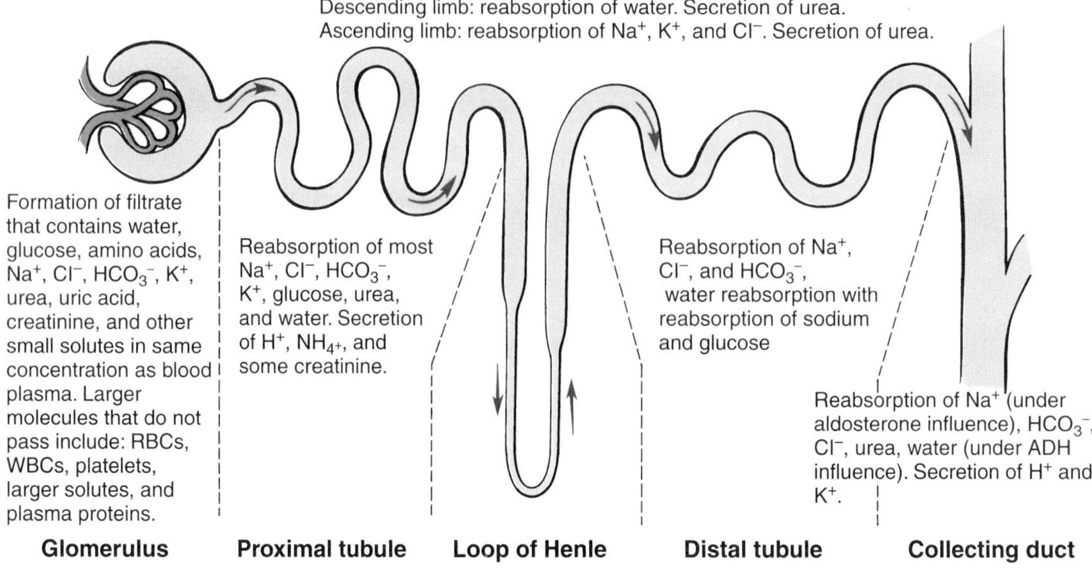
Descending limb: reabsorption of water. Secretion of urea.
Ascending limb: reabsorption of Na+, K+, and Cl−. Secretion of urea.
Formation of filtrate that contains water, glucose, amino acids, Na+, Cl−, HCO3−, K+, urea, uric acid, creatinine, and other small solutes in same concentration as blood plasma. Larger molecules that do not pass include: RBCs, WBCs, platelets, larger solutes, and plasma proteins.
Reabsorption of most Na+, Cl−, HCO3−, K+, glucose, urea, and water. Secretion of H+, NH4+, and some creatinine.
Reabsorption of Na+, Cl−, and HCO3−, water reabsorption with reabsorption of sodium and glucose
Reabsorption of Na+ (under aldosterone influence), HCO3−, Cl−, urea, water (under ADH influence). Secretion of H+ and K+.
Glomerulus
Proximal tubule
Loop of Henle
Distal tubule
Collecting duct

FIGURE 21-7. Functions in each portion of the nephron.

where NFP is the net filtration pressure, GBHP is the glomerular capillary hydrostatic pressure, CHP is the hydrostatic pressure in Bowman's capsule, and BCOP is the oncotic or colloid osmotic pressure in glomerular-capillary plasma.[2,5] For example, if the GBHP is 60 mm Hg, the CHP is 15, and the BCOP is 27, the NFP will be 60 − (15 + 27), or 18 mm Hg. Many factors can alter the GFR, such as changes in blood pressure, plasma proteins, and sympathetic nervous system stimulation.

GLOMERULAR FILTRATION RATE

Glomerular filtration rate is used to evaluate renal function. It can be calculated from the rate at which the kidneys can clear the plasma of a substance which is freely filtered from the blood and not reabsorbed by the tubules. The plant-derived polysaccharide *inulin* is most often used for this determination.[2] Based on a 24-hour urine specimen and blood sample, the GFR is calculated as:

$$\text{GFR} = \frac{[U_s V]}{P_s}$$

where U_s is the amount of substance (mg/dL) excreted in the urine in 24 hours, V is the volume of urine produced in mL/min (total volume excreted during the 24-hour period divided by 1440 minutes), and P_s is the serum level of the substance in mg/dL.[2,5]

The use of inulin and similar substances is inconvenient clinically because they must be given over several hours, so another substance, creatinine, is used to estimate it. Creatinine is produced by the body and almost totally excreted in the urine. However, since some creatinine is excreted by the tubules, using it to estimate the GFR usually gives a value slightly higher than, but very close to, the true GFR[3]. For example, if 1,800 mL of urine is excreted in 24 hours, V = 1,800 mL/ 1440 minutes = 1.25 mL/min. If the concentration of creatinine is 104 mg/dL in the urine and 1.0 mg/dL in the blood, the above formula could be used to estimate GFR as follows:

$$\text{Estimated GFR} = \frac{(104 \times 1.25)}{1.0} = 130 \text{ mL/min}$$

BOX 21-1 MAJOR FUNCTIONS OF THE KIDNEYS

- Regulation of water balance
- Regulation of electrolyte balance
- Regulation of acid-base balance
- Excretion of foreign chemicals and metabolic waste materials
- Synthesis and activation of renin, erythropoietin, vitamin D, and prostaglandins
- Gluconeogenesis
- Degradation of polypeptide hormones

Tubular Reabsorption

The kidneys change the composition of filtrate and thereby control the composition of plasma by excreting different concentrations of substances.[5] This is achieved by tubular reabsorption and secretion. For example, if a person drinks a large volume of water, the urine becomes very dilute. In a dehydrated state, urine output is

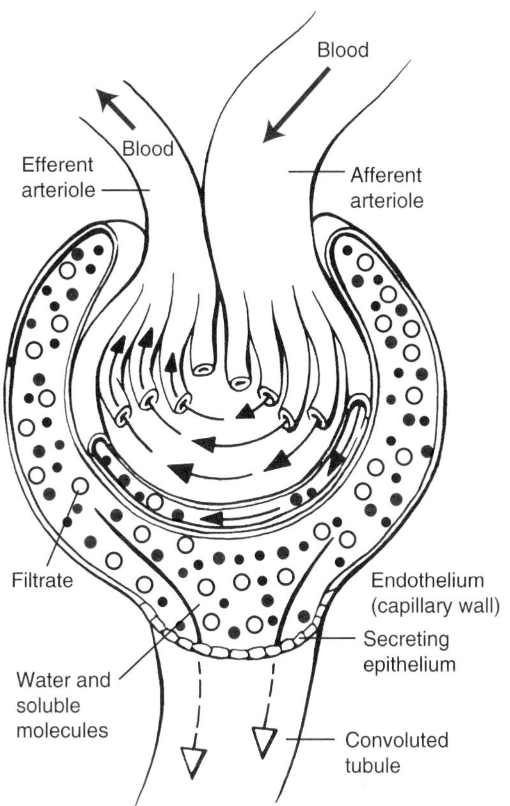

FIGURE 21-8. The process of filtration in the formation of urine. The high pressure inside the capillaries of the glomerulus forces dissolved substances (but not plasma proteins) and much water into the space inside Bowman's capsule. The smaller caliber of the efferent vessel as compared with that of the larger afferent vessel causes this pressure.

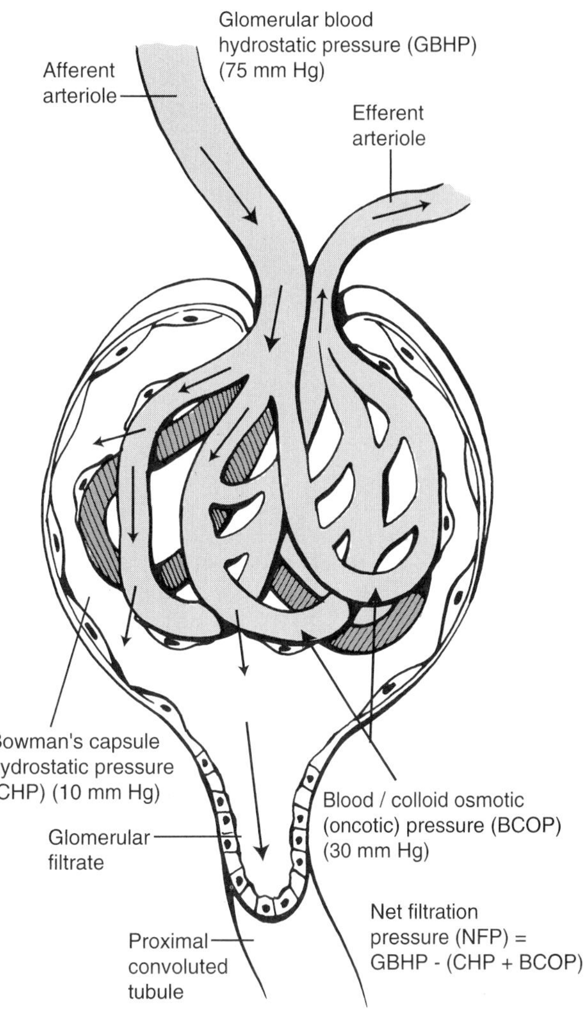

FIGURE 21-9. Schematic representation of the relation between hydrostatic pressure and colloid osmotic pressure. The end result is the net filtration pressure, which forms the glomerular filtrate.

markedly decreased and the urine is very concentrated. **Tubular reabsorption**, the second step of urine formation, requires movement of solutes from the filtrate back into the blood in the vasa recta and peritubular capillaries. As noted previously, about 125 mL of glomerular filtrate are formed each minute; this adds up to 180 L per day. Since urine output is normally about 1 to 2 L per day, the tubules and peritubular capillaries must reabsorb approximately 179 of the 180 L of filtrate produced each day. Many filtered substances identified in Table 21-1 are later reabsorbed.[5]

REABSORPTION IN THE PROXIMAL CONVOLUTED TUBULES

Approximately 70% of glomerular filtrate is reabsorbed in the proximal convoluted tubules. This reabsorption is accomplished by active and passive transport. Some ions passively follow the active transport of other ions.[6,10]

Active Transport

Active transport, the movement of molecules against a concentration gradient, requires expenditure of energy. The PCTs are able to carry on active transport because their epithelial cells contain mitochondria. The microvilli on these cells also increase the surface area for reabsorption and secretion. Some of the substances that depend on active transport include glucose, many electrolytes, amino acids, proteins, and vitamins.[4–6]

Glucose is actively transported from the PCT into the plasma, and normally none appears in the urine. Glucose binds with the same carrier that transports

TABLE 21-1

FILTRATION, REABSORPTION, AND EXCRETION RATES OF SELECTED SUBSTANCES BY THE KIDNEYS

	AMOUNT FILTERED	AMOUNT REABSORBED	AMOUNT EXCRETED	% OF FILTERED LOAD REABSORBED
Glucose (gm/day)	180	180	0	100
Bicarbonate (mEq/day)	4,320	4,318	2	> 99.9
Sodium (mEq/day)	25,560	25,410	150	99.4
Chloride (mEq/day)	19,440	19,260	180	99.1
Urea (gm/day)	46.8	23.4	23.4	50
Creatinine (gm/day)	1.8	0	1.8	0

(Guyton, A., & Hall, J. [1997]. *Human physiology and mechanisms of disease* [6th ed.]. Philadelphia: W. B. Saunders.)

sodium ions.[4] This movement is limited by the **transport maximum**, the maximum amount of a substance that can be reabsorbed at any time.[5,6] If the plasma glucose level exceeds the **threshold** of approximately 175 mg/dL or 220 mg/min, the transport mechanism becomes saturated with glucose.[5] Glucose is then left in the tubules and appears in the urine (glycosuria). The transport maximum varies between individuals, especially if there is a chronic increase in glucose load (as often happens in diabetes mellitus).

Sodium and potassium are actively transported from the PCT into the plasma of the peritubular capillaries through the channels in the epithelial cells. Sodium ions (Na^+) and potassium ions (K^+) are positive, and their movement allows negative ions, such as chloride (Cl^-) and phosphate (HPO_4^{2-}), to follow passively.[5]

Proteins are reabsorbed in the PCT through the active process of *endocytosis*.[4] The proteins attach to microvilli of the PCT, are ingested by the tubular cells, and are broken down into amino acids, which are transported into the plasma.

Passive Transport

Passive transport (osmosis and diffusion) is movement of substances across a membrane without the expenditure of energy. In the PCT the electrical gradient caused by active transport of positive ions, mainly sodium, allows negative ions such as Cl^- and bicarbonate (HCO_3^-) to diffuse across the tubular membrane. This maintains equal osmotic pressures of fluid inside the tubules and in the plasma. When solutes are actively reabsorbed into the plasma, fluid in the tubules becomes less concentrated and fluid in the peritubular capillaries becomes more concentrated. This causes water to move into the peritubular capillaries. Excretion of excess water or conservation of water by the kidneys maintains the plasma osmolarity at a fixed specific gravity of 1.010. This regulation is strongly influenced by the action of antidiuretic hormone on the DCT and collecting tubules (see p. 598).

CONCENTRATION OF URINE IN THE LOOP OF HENLE

The main function of the loop of Henle is to concentrate the filtrate. The juxtamedullary nephrons, whose loops of Henle extend into the medulla of the kidney, are most active in urine concentration. The loops of Henle and the vasa recta that surround them work together to concentrate urine in a system called the **countercurrent mechanism**. The two components of this mechanism are the countercurrent multiplier and the countercurrent exchanger.

Function of the countercurrent mechanism depends on the anatomic relations of the loop of Henle, the vasa recta, and the collecting tubules and ducts. It also depends on the presence of an osmolar gradient in the interstitial fluid of the medulla, in which osmolarity increases with depth. The loops of Henle, collecting tubules and ducts, and vasa recta are surrounded by this osmolar gradient as shown in Figure 21-10.

Glomerular filtrate normally is iso-osmotic, about 300 mOsm/L, as it passes from the PCT into the loop of Henle. As it moves down the descending limb of the loop, it is exposed to the increasingly high osmolarity of the interstitial fluid of the medulla. The descending limb is freely permeable to water, Na^+, and Cl^-. The high osmolarity of the medulla causes water to move out of the filtrate by osmosis and Na^+ and Cl^- to diffuse in until the filtrate reaches equilibrium with the surrounding interstitial fluid. The filtrate becomes hyperosmolar and reaches a concentration of about 1200 mOsm/L as it rounds the hairpin turn at the bottom of the loop of Henle.

This hyperosmolar filtrate next moves into the ascending limb of the loop of Henle, where Na^+, Cl^-, and K^+ are avidly reabsorbed. Since the ascending limb is impermeable to water, it remains in the filtrate. This causes osmolarity of the filtrate to fall as it moves up the ascending limb.

The filtrate is hypo-osmolar when it enters the DCT. More Na^+ and Cl^- are reabsorbed in the DCT and collecting tubules. Final urine concentration is regulated by the action of ADH on the DCT, collecting tubules, and ducts. In the absence of ADH, these structures are impermeable to water and a large volume of dilute urine is formed. The presence of ADH makes the DCT, collecting tubules, and ducts permeable to water. This allows water to diffuse out of these structures into the interstitium, resulting in formation of a small volume of concentrated urine.[3,5] The kidneys have a tremendous capacity to alter the proportions of water and solutes in the urine in response to the body's needs. Urine osmolarity can vary from as low as 50 mOsm/L when there is excess water in the body to as high as 1400 mOsm/L when body water is low.[5]

Countercurrent Multiplier

The osmolar gradient in the renal medulla is essential for formation of concentrated urine. The gradient is caused by the accumulation of solutes in the medullary interstitial fluid. This solute buildup is accomplished by transport of Na^+ and other ions into the interstitium from the thick portion of the ascending loop of Henle and the collecting ducts, and by passive diffusion of large amounts of urea from the collecting ducts into the interstitium. The hairpin turn that the loop of Henle makes as it passes through the medulla allows these processes to gradually trap solutes in the interstitium of the medulla. Since this multiplies the concentration gradient established by transport of ions, it is called the **countercurrent multiplier**.[5]

Countercurrent Exchanger

Without a special pattern of blood flow, the solutes accumulated in the medulla would be quickly dispersed. The vasa recta serve an important role in protecting the osmotic gradient in the renal medulla, through a mechanism called the **countercurrent exchanger**. The unusual U shape of the vasa recta capillary as it follows the loop of Henle means that it also is subjected to the osmotic gradient in the medulla. In response to the gradient, blood flowing through the vasa recta becomes progressively more concentrated as it descends the U, then more dilute as it moves back up. Although water and solutes move in and out of the vasa recta, there is little net effect on the osmotic gradient of the medulla because of the U shape of these capillaries. The osmotic gradient is further protected by the fact that blood flow to the medulla is sluggish compared with that of the cortex. Also, most

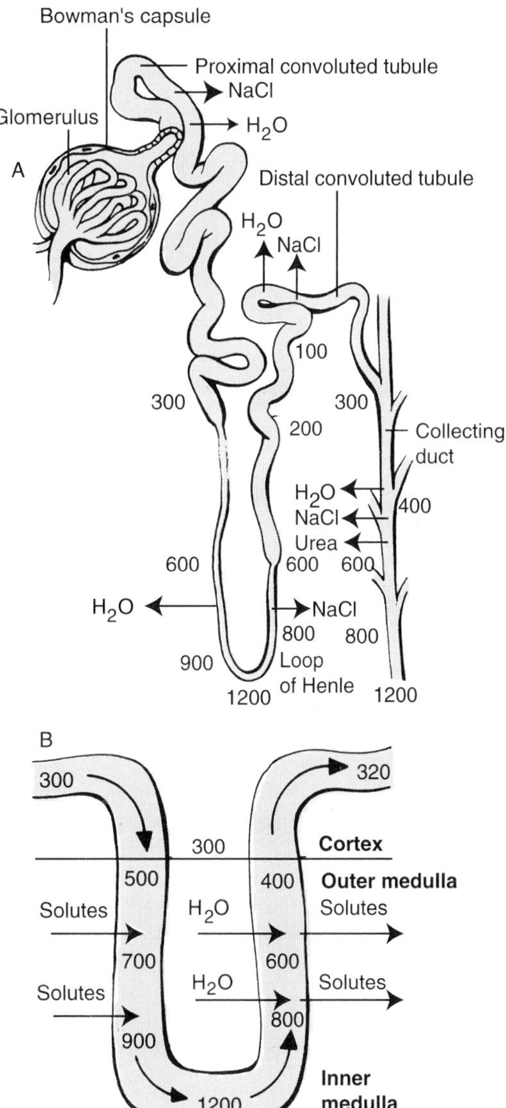

FIGURE 21-10. Mechanism of urine concentration. **A.** Countercurrent multiplier. **B.** Recycling of salts and urea in the vasa recta: countercurrent exchanger. Concentrations are in milliosmoles per liter (mOsm/L).

water reabsorbed in response to ADH exits from portions of tubules in the cortex rather than the medulla. The vasa recta carries away water reabsorbed in the medulla, further protecting the gradient.[5] The osmotic gradient can be damaged by changes in renal blood flow, osmotic diuresis, and other conditions that alter the amounts of water and solute present in the medulla. Such changes hinder function of the countercurrent mechanism and impair the ability to concentrate urine.

REABSORPTION IN THE DISTAL CONVOLUTED TUBULES

Sodium, Chloride, and Potassium Reabsorption

The DCT and collecting tubules reabsorb smaller amounts of Na^+ than do the loops of Henle. The hormone *aldosterone* affects Na^+ reabsorption at the DCT. Release of aldosterone is triggered by the renin–angiotensin–aldosterone system or by an increase in serum K^+ levels. Aldosterone causes retention of Na^+ and excretion of K^+.

Chloride is reabsorbed both passively (following sodium) and actively. Active Cl^- transport is usually linked with bicarbonate ion movement, and may involve reabsorption of Cl^- with loss of bicarbonate, or reabsorption of bicarbonate with loss of Cl^-.[3,9] Almost all the initially filtered sodium and chloride is eventually reabsorbed.[3]

Water Reabsorption

Water reabsorption in the DCT and collecting tubules is regulated by *antidiuretic hormone (ADH; vasopressin)*, which controls permeability of the tubules to water. Antidiuretic hormone is produced by the hypothalamus and stored in the posterior pituitary gland. It is released when osmoreceptors in the anterior hypothalamus detect increased osmolarity of the plasma. Increased ADH levels in the blood allow water to move osmotically from the tubules into the capillaries. This results in more concentrated urine and returns water to the plasma. Absence of ADH results in decreased tubular permeability, causing water to stay in the tubules and urine to be very dilute.

Tubular Secretion

Tubular secretion, the final step in urine formation, is the movement of fluid and solute from the blood back into the glomerular filtrate. Active and a few passive secretory mechanisms are present at various points in the PCT, DCT, and collecting tubules.

HYDROGEN IONS

Hydrogen ions (H^+) are actively secreted in the PCT, DCT, and collecting tubules. The number of H^+ ions secreted depends on (1) the pH of the extracellular fluid and (2) the amount of buffer in the glomerular filtrate. This is an important component of the body's acid-base regulation. If the plasma hydrogen ion concentration is high (low pH), large quantities of H^+ are secreted. Low plasma concentrations (high pH) cause decreased H^+ secretion. If the urine becomes highly acidic (low pH), H^+ secretion is inhibited.

The mechanisms whereby excess H^+ ions are removed include (1) formation of CO_2 and H_2O from HCO_3 and H^+ reactions in the tubule lumen, (2) the formation of $H_2PO_4^-$ from H^+ and HPO_4^{--}, and (3) formation of NH_4 (ammonium) from NH_3 (ammonia) reactions. These mechanisms are illustrated and further described in Figure 21-11.

POTASSIUM

Less than 10% of potassium in the initial glomerular filtrate arrives at the distal tubules. Potassium ions are reabsorbed primarily from the PCT and loop of Henle, with some additional reabsorption at the DCT.[5] Excretion of excess K^+ requires active secretion of K^+ from the capillaries into the cortical and collecting ducts. This is partly controlled by aldosterone. Reabsorption of Na^+ leaves a negative electrochemical gradient in the tubules. To maintain electrochemical neutrality, positive K^+ moves into the filtrate to take the place of Na^+. Since excess potassium is often ingested in the normal diet, the secretion method for potassium excretion is essential to maintain normal serum levels of 3.5 to 5.0 mEq/L.

If serum potassium is low, the cortical collecting ducts do not secrete potassium and the medullary collecting ducts reabsorb some potassium. This is the only mechanism for conservation of potassium, causing its value to be depleted rather easily in dietary deficiency or when osmotic diuretics are administered.

Physical Characteristics of Urine

Urine is composed of 95% water and 5% dissolved solids and gases. Table 21-2 summarizes some specific characteristics of urine. Variations relate to diet and fluid intake. Abnormal constituents or high concentrations of normal constituents may affect the appearance and odor of urine. Urine concentration may be increased by the presence of increased amounts of urea, creatinine, uric acid, potassium, or other substances. Urine concentration is usually assessed by measurement of specific gravity. **Specific gravity** is a measure of solute concentration of the urine. However, usual methods of determining specific gravity actually measure urine density, not urine concentration, and hence may be misleading. For example, protein in the urine can cause an increased urine density without a significant change in osmolarity. The color of urine normally ranges from pale yellow to amber, which is the result of the pigment urochrome. Urine often is more deeply colored when the specific gravity is increased. The urine may become discolored from certain disease conditions or from foods or medicines. Dark or bright red urine typically comes from bleeding along the upper or lower urinary tract. Dark yellow

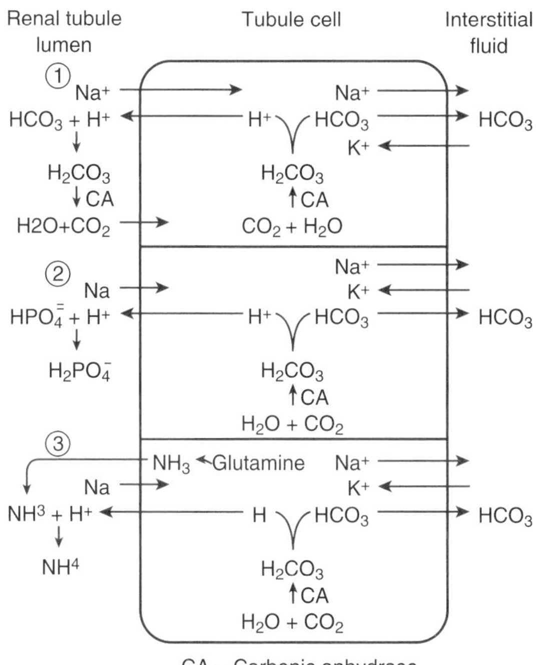

FIGURE 21-11. Mechanisms of H^+ secretion. Note that Na^+ is reabsorbed for each H^+ secreted. (1) Reabsorption of filtered HCO_3^- and secretion of H^+. Secreted H^+ combines with HCO_3^- in the renal tubule, forming H_2CO_3. Carbonic anhydrase (CA), a catalytic enzyme, facilitates the formation of H_20 and CO_2 from H_2CO_3 in the renal tubule. CO_2 diffuses across the cell membrane and reacts with H_20 to form H_2CO_3. In the renal tubule cell; CA facilitates the formation of H_2CO_3, which dissociates into H^+ and HCO_3^- and begins the cycle over again. Most of the HCO_3^- is absorbed in the proximal tubule. (2) Titratable acid formation: The H^+ secreted into the tubule lumen reacts with a dibasic phosphate (HPO_4^{--}) to form a monobasic phosphate ($H_2PO_4^-$). (3) Ammonium formation. Diffused ammonia (NH_3), which has been formed from glutamine in the cell, reacts in the tubule lumen with H^+ to form ammonium (NH^+_4), which is excreted. New HCO_3^- is formed and reabsorbed with each NH^+_4 excreted.

urine may be associated with increased concentration of conjugated bilirubin in the blood. Drugs such as phenazopyridine and phenytoin can produce a pink, red, or red-brown urine. Severe Pseudomonas infection, especially of the entire urinary tract, may produce a blue-green or green, often cloudy, urine.

Endocrine Function of the Kidney

In addition to producing urine, the kidneys serve as endocrine organs, producing **renin**, **erythropoietin**, activated *Vitamin D*, prostaglandins, kinins, and several other hormones and locally acting substances.[2,8] The first three of these will be summarized below.

TABLE 21-2

PHYSICAL CHARACTERISTICS OF URINE

Appearance	Clear, amber yellow
pH	4.6–8.0
Odor	Aromatic to ammonia-like
Specific gravity	1.005–1.030
Ketones	Negative
Protein	50–80 mg/24 hours at rest <250 mg/24 hours after strenuous exercise
Glucose	Negative <0.5 g/day or <2.78 mmol/day
Red blood cells	<2 per microscopic slide 0 red blood cell casts
Bacteria	Negative culture and sensitivity
Urobilinogen	0–4 mg/24 hours

RENIN: BLOOD PRESSURE REGULATION BY THE KIDNEYS

Kidney functions are vital to blood pressure regulation. This regulation involves control of plasma sodium and water levels, discussed earlier, as well as the **renin–angiotensin–aldosterone system,** which is summarized in Flowchart 21-1.

The enzyme renin is produced and secreted by juxtaglomerular cells (shown in Fig. 21-6) within the juxtaglomerular apparatus. Renin causes the plasma protein angiotensinogen to convert to angiotensin I, which is transformed into angiotensin II in the lungs. Angiotensin II causes vasoconstriction throughout the body, raising blood pressure. It also stimulates the adrenal cortex to release aldosterone, which causes sodium to be reabsorbed from the tubules into the blood. Water passively follows the reabsorbed sodium. Angiotensin II also increases thirst through the hypothalamus and stimulates the release of antidiuretic hormone from the posterior pituitary.[5] Thus, the renin–angiotensin–aldosterone system results in an increase of both blood pressure and blood volume.

The rate of renin secretion by the juxtaglomerular cells is controlled by baroreceptors in the kidney's arterioles, osmoreceptors in the macula densa, and the sympathetic nervous system. The baroreceptors vary renin secretion in response to perfusion pressure, secreting more renin when the pressure is low and less when the pressure is higher. The macula densa responds to increased concentrations of sodium or chloride by inhibiting renin release, and to decreased concentrations by stimulating renin release. Stimulation of renal sym-

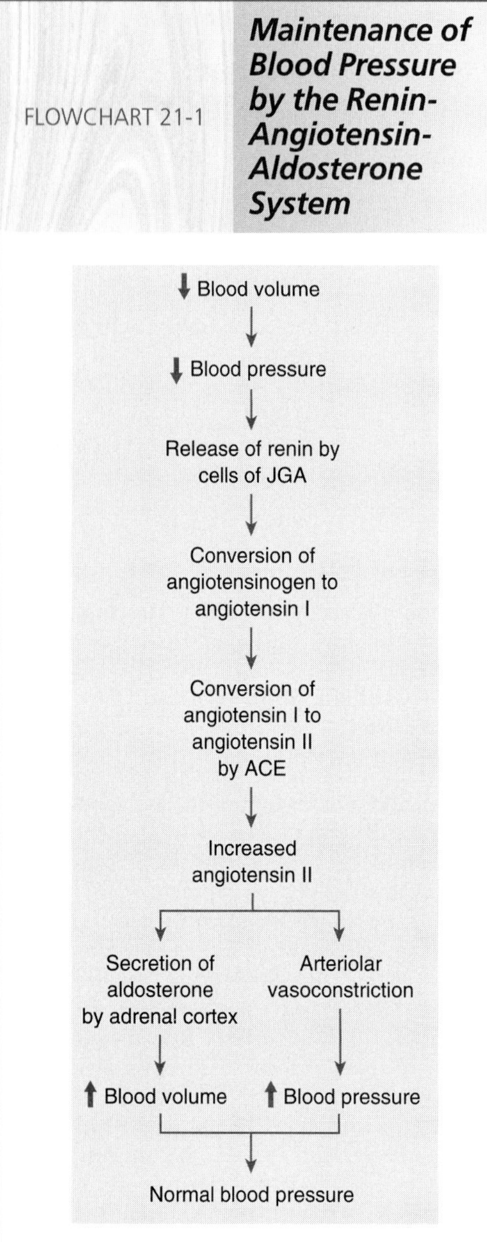

Mechanism by which renin, angiotensin, and aldosterone function to restore blood pressure. ACE, angiotensin converting enzyme in lungs; JGA, juxtaglomerular apparatus.

pathetic nerves causes renin release, causing renal vasoconstriction, which also triggers the baroreceptor response. Since the baroreceptors and osmoreceptors are located within the kidney, the same mechanisms by which the kidney controls blood pressure also help keep renal perfusion pressure within optimal limits.[2]

ERYTHROPOIETIN SECRETION

The hormone erythropoietin is a major factor in the control of erythrocyte (red blood cell) production. In adults most erythropoietin is produced by the kidneys in response to hypoxia of renal cells. The exact kidney cells that produce the hormone have not been identified.[2] Small amounts of erythropoietin also are produced by the liver. Erythropoietin stimulates the bone marrow to increase *erythropoiesis* (production of red blood cells). Absence of this hormone, such as seen in end-stage renal failure, results in severe anemia.[2] Chronic hypoxia, such as seen with COPD, smoking, or living at high altitudes, causes increased erythrocyte production.

SECRETION OF ACTIVATED VITAMIN D

Vitamin D is either produced by the effects of ultraviolet light on the skin or ingested in foods. It must undergo several changes before it can stimulate absorption of calcium by the intestine. It is hydroxylated first in the liver, then in the kidney, to form activated vitamin D (1,25-dihydroxycholecalciferol). This process is controlled by parathyroid hormone (PTH) and is discussed further in Chapter 23. Effects of vitamin D on calcium balance are discussed on page 799.

ACCESSORY URINARY STRUCTURES

Accessory structures include the ureters, bladder, and urethra. These organs store and transport urine and do not have an effect on the characteristics of urine. When urine is excreted from the kidneys, it is transported through the ureters into the bladder and exits the body through the urethra.

Ureters

The ureters are composed of three layers of smooth muscle and are lined with a layer of mucous membrane. The mucous secretions of this layer protect the ureters from the constituents of urine. The ureters are innervated by both sympathetic and parasympathetic nerves. Each has an intramural plexus of nerve fibers that extend along its entire length.[5] The pressure of urine flowing from the collecting ducts initiates peristaltic movement, which forces the urine down the ureter toward the bladder. As with other visceral smooth muscles, parasympathetic stimulation enhances this peristalsis and sympathetic stimulation inhibits it.[5]

The ureters enter the bladder in an area at the base of the bladder called the *trigone*, shown in Figure 21-12.

The muscular tone of this area normally prevents backflow of urine into the ureters.

Bladder

The bladder is a hollow, muscular organ located behind the symphysis pubis. When empty, the inner wall of the bladder has numerous folds, called *rugae*. When filled with urine, it smooths, thins, and rises into the abdomen. It is composed of several layers: (1) the mucosa, (2) the detrusor muscle, and (3) the serous layer. The mucosal layer contains transitional epithelium, which, along with the rugae, allows the bladder to stretch during filling.[6] The serous layer coats the superior portion of the bladder and is formed by the peritoneum. The detrusor muscle is composed of longitudinal and circular muscles. Contractions of this muscle causes bladder emptying.[7]

As shown in Figure 21-12, *internal* and *external urethral sphincters* are located between the bladder and the urethra. These sphincters are formed by circular muscles and, when stimulated, allow urine to pass from the bladder into the urethra. The principal nerve supply to the bladder is through the sacral plexus, which connects mainly with spinal cord segments S2 to S4.[7] Sensory fibers respond to stretching of the bladder walls. The motor nerve fibers are mainly parasympathetic. Sympathetic fibers connect with the lumbar spinal cord segments and mainly innervate bladder blood vessels. The pudendal nerves supply the external urethral sphincter.[5]

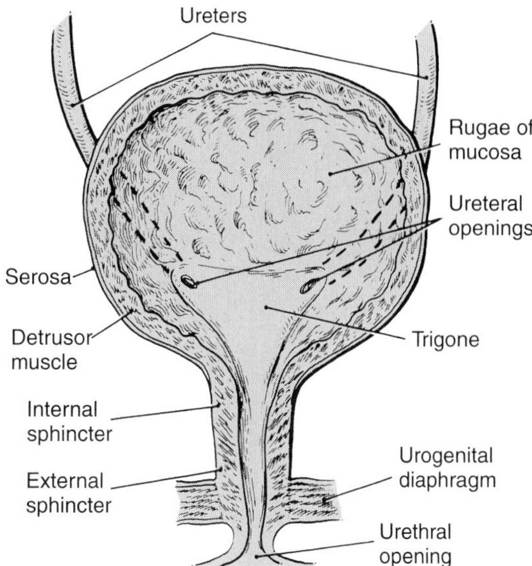

FIGURE 21-12. **Structure of the bladder and its internal and external urethral sphincters.**

Urethra

The urethra also exits the bladder at the trigone and opens to the exterior at the *urinary meatus.* The female urethra, pictured in Figure 21-13, is located posteriorly to the symphysis pubis and anteriorly to the vagina. The urethra is approximately 3.75 cm long and is composed of smooth muscle.

As Figure 21-14 shows, when the male urethra leaves the bladder, it passes through the prostate gland, then between a membranous portion that extends from the prostate to the corpus spongiosum of the penis. Finally, the urethra passes through the corpus spongiosum and

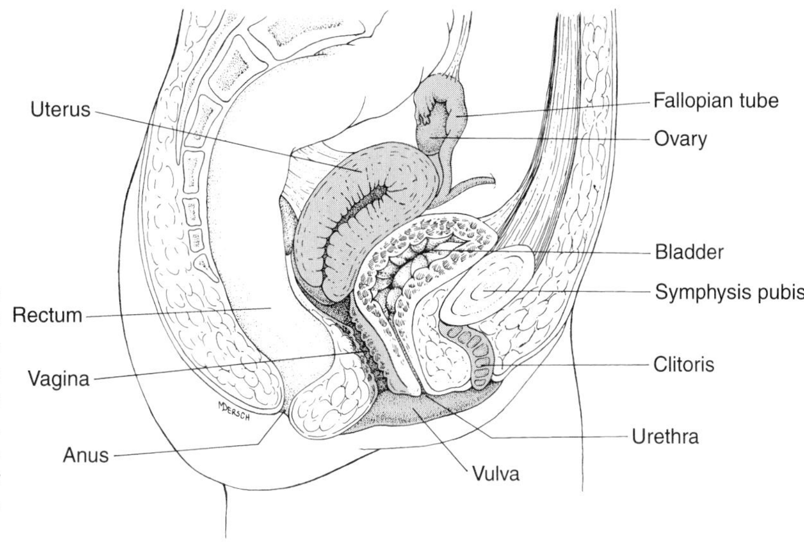

FIGURE 21-13. **Female genitourinary structure as seen in sagittal section. Notice the proximity of the urethral opening to the vaginal and anal openings. (Reeder, S. J., Martin, L. L., & Koniak, D. [1997]. *Maternity nursing* [18th ed.]. Philadelphia: Lippincott.)**

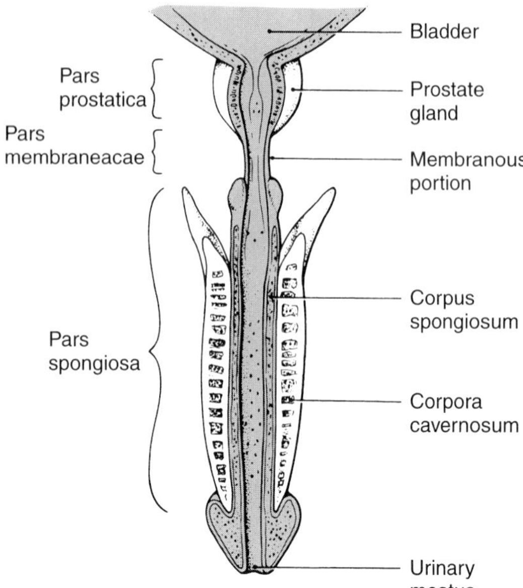

FIGURE 21-14. **Structure of the male genitourinary anatomy.**

terminates at the urinary meatus. The male urethra is approximately 20 cm long and transports both urine and semen.

MICTURITION REFLEX

The micturition reflex is composed of spinal cord, bladder, and urethral nerve structures and allows for micturition (voiding). Sensory receptors in the bladder and urethra transmit signals via pelvic nerves to the sacral spinal cord when these structures are stretched by urine. The parasympathetic nervous system reflexively transmits back to the bladder via the same nerves, resulting in micturition. The micturition reflex results in contraction of the detrusor muscle and relaxation of the internal sphincter. Urination proceeds unless it is stopped by voluntary contraction of the external sphincter, which is under cerebral control. The cerebral centers keep the micturition reflex partly inhibited until micturition is desired. The higher centers also can facilitate the micturition reflex by relaxing the external sphincter.[5]

REFERENCES

1. Cotran, R. S., Kumar, V., & Collins, J. (1999). *Robbins' pathologic basis of disease* (6th ed.). Philadelphia: W. B. Saunders.
2. Greger, R. (1996). Introduction to renal function, renal blood flow and the formation of urine. In R. Greger & U. Windhorst, *Comprehensive human physiology: From cellular mechanisms to integration*. New York: Springer.
3. Greger, R. (1996). Principles of renal transport: Concentration and dilution of urine. In R. Greger & U. Windhorst, *Comprehensive human physiology: From cellular mechanisms to integration*. New York: Springer.
4. Greger, R. (1996). Renal handling of the individual solutes of glomerular filtrate. In R. Greger & U. Windhorst, *Comprehensive human physiology: From cellular mechanisms to integration*. New York: Springer.
5. Guyton, A. C. & Hall, J. E. (1997). *Human physiology and mechanisms of disease* (6th ed.). Philadelphia: W.B. Saunders.
6. Hole, J. W. (1995). *Essentials of human anatomy and physiology* (5th ed.). Boston: William Brown Publishers.
7. Janig, W. (1996). Regulation of the lower urinary tract. In R. Greger & U. Windhorst, *Comprehensive human physiology: From cellular mechanisms to integration*. New York: Springer.
8. Koeppen, B. M. & Stanton, B. A. (1997). *Renal physiology* (2nd ed.). St. Louis: Mosby.
9. Lang, F. (1996). Acid-base balance. In R. Greger & U. Windhorst, *Comprehensive human physiology: From cellular mechanisms to integration*. New York: Springer.
10. Stanton, B. A. & Koeppen, B. M. (1998). Elements of renal function. In R.M. Berne & M. N. Levy, *Physiology*. St. Louis: Mosby.

Chapter

22

Altered Renal Function and Urinary Excretion

Anita Tesh

KEY TERMS

acute tubular necrosis
azotemia
chronic analgesia nephritis
cystitis
diabetic nephropathy
glomerulonephritis
HIV nephropathy
hypercalcemia
hypercalciuria
hyperoxaluria
hyperuricemia
hyperuricosuria
hypocitraturia
interstitial nephritis
nephritic disease
nephritis
nephrolithiasis
nephrosis
nephrotic syndrome
pyelonephritis
renal failure
renal osteodystrophy
renal tubular acidosis
uremia
uremic syndrome
urolithiasis
vesicoureteral reflux
Wilms' tumor

Many factors affect the genitourinary system. These include functional and structural abnormalities, infections, obstructions, ischemia, and immune reactions. The resulting genitourinary problems range from relatively minor dysfunctions to severe or progressive conditions that can lead to renal failure. These concepts are presented in this chapter.

DISORDERS OF MICTURITION

Voiding difficulties are among the most common problems brought to medical attention. Many voiding problems probably remain unreported because of the embarrassing nature of the problem. Voiding requires an intact central nervous system, functional sphincter and bladder muscles, and an unobstructed pathway exiting the body. Control of voiding and continence can be severely impaired by disorders of any of these components.[20]

Interference With Emptying the Bladder

Interference with emptying the bladder includes difficulty starting and maintaining a urinary stream and urinary retention (incomplete emptying of the bladder). Many of the conditions linked with interference with bladder emptying are associated with those that narrow or obstruct the urine outflow channels, such as inflammatory conditions or tissue hyperplasia, or with those that result from or cause dysfunction in neural innervation or bladder muscle tone. Difficulty starting and maintaining a urinary stream is a common symptom of benign prostatic hyperplasia (BPH) (discussed later in this chapter). Individuals who have had prostatic surgery, prostatitis, or denervation injury also may have this problem, as may persons with congenital or acquired urethral stenosis.

Urinary retention may occur as a result of numerous conditions enumerated in Box 22-1.[1] It is important to distinguish frank urinary retention (absolute inability to void) from increased residual urine (a postvoid residual volume of approximately 50 mL in adults). Frank urinary retention, which may manifest as "overflow incontinence," requires immediate attention. Increased postvoid volume may be clinically insignificant.[1]

Interference With Urine Storage in the Bladder

Frequency and incontinence are common problems that affect both men and women, especially after the age of 50. The problems can be transient or persistent

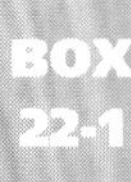

BOX 22-1

CAUSES OF URINARY RETENTION

Obstructive
- Benign prostatic hypertrophy
- Urethral edema
- Urethral scarring
- Urethral stenosis
- Fecal impaction

Cystocele

Bedridden state/immobility

Drugs
- Anticholinergics
- Antihistamines
- Tricyclic antidepressants
- Surgical anesthetics
- Opioid analgesics

Detrusor muscle dysfunction
- Overstretching of detrusor muscle
- Diabetic cystopathy (detrusor areflexia)
- Age-related detrusor hyporeflexia

Nervous system dysfunction
- Spinal cord injury or lesions
- Brain injury or lesions

and may be related to conditions such as urinary tract infections or prostatic problems.

Dysuria refers to difficulty or discomfort on voiding. Persons affected often also complain of frequency (voiding more often than every 2 hours), urgency (intense need to void), or incontinence (involuntary voiding). Most conditions producing these symptoms arise from irritation of the bladder or urethra.[13] *Urinary incontinence* is a very common health problem, especially among the elderly. Incidence increases with age and disability.[1] Incontinence is associated with numerous disorders and dysfunctions. It can be divided into overlapping types of stress, urge, overflow, and functional incontinence. Manifestations of each of these types of incontinence are discussed in Table 22-1.[1,29] Course and prognosis depend on the underlying condition.

STRUCTURAL ABNORMALITIES OF THE URINARY SYSTEM

Congenital Disorders of the Urinary System

Malformations of the urinary system are very common at birth. Some are severe, some do not cause clinical problems until adult life, and others are asymptomatic. Most congenital urinary system abnormalities are due to developmental defects arising during gesta-

TABLE 22-1

CAUSES OF URINARY INCONTINENCE

TYPE	CLINICAL PRESENTATION	PATHOPHYSIOLOGIC MECHANISM	COMMON CAUSES
Stress urinary incontinence	Involuntary loss of urine (usually small amounts) on physical effort, that increases intra-abdominal pressure: sneezing, coughing, walking	Pressure in bladder (without detrusor contraction) exceeds pressure generated by urinary sphincter	Decreased muscular support of bladder and urethral distention caused by age-related changes, postmenopausal changes, multiple childbirth, surgery, and recurrent bladder infections
Urge incontinence	Inability to delay voiding after fullness perceived	Pressure generated in bladder by detrusor contraction exceeds pressure generated by external urinary sphincter (under voluntary control)	Detrusor hyperreflexia Bladder infections, stones, or tumors CNS disorders (stroke, dementia, Parkinson's disease) Spinal cord lesions Pelvic plexus trauma
Overflow incontinence	Loss of small amounts of urine when bladder is full	Urinary retention causes pressure in overdistended bladder to exceed sphincter pressure without full detrusor contraction	Neurogenic bladder from cord injury or diabetes mellitus Multiple sclerosis
Functional incontinence	Voiding not consciously controlled	Urine loss occurs reflexively when bladder distention initiates detrusor muscle contraction	Severe CNS disorders Severe dementia or psychological dysfunction

tion rather than hereditary defects. The hereditary polycystic kidney diseases, discussed below, are exceptions to this.[11]

Common congenital abnormalities, and the problems associated with them, are listed in Table 22-2. As noted in the table, the congenital bladder conditions all predispose to infection, and several predispose to cancer. Congenital abnormalities of the ureters are found in about 2% to 3% of all autopsies.[11] Many have little clinical significance; an exception is abnormality of the vesicoureteral junction, which impairs the one-way valve that normally prevents backflow of urine from the bladder toward the kidneys. This defect results in **vesicoureteral reflux,** a major contributor to kidney infections.[11] Most congenital abnormalities of the kidney involve structural malformations, although congenital metabolic defects also occur, such as those associated with *polycystic disease.*

Cystic Diseases of the Kidney

Several conditions exist that involve the presence of cysts in the kidney. These include hereditary polycystic disease, simple cortical cysts, medullary sponge kidney, and nephronophthisis-uremic medullary cystic disease (UMCD). Some of these are benign, but others are associated with significant pathology.

HEREDITARY POLYCYSTIC DISEASE

Hereditary polycystic diseases involve significant pathology. Two forms of inherited polycystic kidney disease exist: (1) autosomal dominant (adult) polycystic disease and (2) autosomal recessive (childhood) polycystic disease. In both types, the kidneys are enlarged, infiltrated with cysts, and have decreased numbers of functioning nephrons bilaterally. The formation and distribution of the cysts differ between the two types. Both types are associated with the presence of cysts in the liver. The adult form is also associated with intracranial aneurysms and accounts for 6% to 12% of renal transplantations or chronic dialysis. The age at onset of symptoms for the adult form is quite variable, but is usually in the fourth or fifth decade of life. The childhood form is much less common than the adult form. Infants with this condition are usually symptomatic at birth and rapidly develop renal failure.[11]

OTHER CYSTIC KIDNEY DISEASES

Simple cysts, usually in the cortex, are common postmortem findings and are usually without clinical significance. For unknown reasons, cysts also sometimes develop in the cortex and medulla of persons receiving prolonged hemodialysis. These cysts may bleed and are associated with renal carcinomas. *Medullary sponge kidney,* in which there are multiple cysts in the medulla, is typically a benign condition of adults of unknown cause. However, another group of diseases involving medullary cysts, the *nephronophthisis-uremic medullary cystic disease* (UMCD) complex, is severe and typically progresses to renal failure. There are four recognized variants of UMCD diseases, three of which are hereditary. In all four types, the medullary cysts are accompanied by tubular atrophy and interstitial fibrosis, and the onset of symptoms is typically in childhood.[11]

TABLE 22-2

COMMON CONGENITAL MALFORMATIONS OF THE URINARY SYSTEM

ABNORMALITY	ASSOCIATED PROBLEMS
Diverticula of bladder	Infections, calculi formation, vesicoureteral reflux, carcinoma (rare)
Exstrophy of bladder (exposure on surface of body)	Infections, carcinoma
Fistulas between bladder and vagina, rectum, uterus, or umbilicus	Infection
Abnormality of vesicoureteral junction	Vesicoureteral reflux, infections
Agenesis of kidneys (failure to develop)	Bilateral: incompatible with life; unilateral: glomerulosclerosis and renal failure
Hypoplasia of kidneys (abnormally small size, usually unilateral)	Renal insufficiency, infection
Ectopic kidneys (displaced to pelvis or abdomen)	Infections, obstruction due to kinking of ureters
Horseshoe kidney (kidneys joined at lower pole)	Obstruction of ureters
Fused pelvic kidney (pancake kidney)	Obstruction
Autosomal dominant (adult) polycystic disease	Hematuria, proteinuria, hypertension, renal failure, cysts of liver, cerebral aneurysms
Autosomal recessive (childhood) polycystic disease	Renal failure, cysts of liver

INFECTIONS OF THE GENITOURINARY TRACT

Although the urinary tract is normally sterile, urinary tract infections (UTIs) are very common. UTIs may involve infection of the urinary bladder (cystitis) or of the kidney (pyelonephritis) and may be symptomatic or asymptomatic.[11] UTIs are diagnosed by culture of the causative microorganism. Active infection is usually considered to be present when more than 100,000 bacteria/mL of urine appear in a clean-voided specimen. The most common cause of urinary tract infection is *Escherichia coli*, a gram-negative aerobic organism present in the lower intestinal tract. Infections also may be caused by other organisms, such as *Klebsiella*, *Proteus*, and *Staphylococcus* species, especially in the presence of an indwelling catheter. Recurrent infections are more often caused by these organisms.

Cystitis

The most common genitourinary disease is **cystitis**, or inflammation of the bladder mucosa. Risk factors for cystitis are shown in Box 22-2. Numerous subtypes of cystitis exist, based on cause or pathology exhibited.[21] The term *hemorrhagic cystitis* is used when bloody urine is present; this is often seen following chemotherapy or radiation therapy over the bladder area. *Suppurative cystitis* occurs when suppurative exudate accumulates on the endothelial lining of the bladder; ulcerations of the mucosa may be also develop. *Chronic interstitial cystitis* is associated with chronic, nonbacterial inflammation and suprapubic pain. In some cases ulcer formation (Hunner ulcers) occurs; these are susceptible to bleeding. It involves all layers of the bladder, occurs more often in women, and is of unknown etiology.

BOX 22-2 RISK FACTORS FOR CYSTITIS

Female gender
Sexual intercourse
Urethral trauma
Pregnancy
Poor hygiene
Indwelling catheter
Neurogenic bladder
Kidney disease
Obstructive conditions
Chemotherapy
Radiation therapy
Diabetes mellitus

ETIOLOGY

Normally, any organisms that gain access to the bladder are rapidly expelled by voiding and inhibited by the acidity of urine. Decreased urinary stream, increased bacterial colonization, and a susceptible host contribute to inadequate bacterial expulsion. Urinary pH varies with systemic metabolic conditions. A less acid urine may support bacterial colonization.

Cystitis is much more common in women than in men because of the shortness of the urethra and the proximity of the urethral opening and vagina to the anal area. In women, sexual intercourse may traumatize the urethra and allow bacteria to migrate to the bladder. Cystitis often develops in persons with indwelling urethral catheters, even when they are receiving antimicrobial therapy. Any individual who has an indwelling catheter for more than 96 hours is at high risk for developing cystitis with organisms that may become resistant to antimicrobial therapy.[21] Nearly 100% of chronically catheterized persons develop UTIs.[1]

CLINICAL MANIFESTATIONS

Cystitis is usually caused by organisms that gain access to the bladder from the urethra. Significant bacteriuria is present in 60% to 70% of cases of cystitis. However, some persons may have symptomatic cystitis without demonstration of a causative organism by culture.[11] Cystitis may be (1) acute or (2) chronic. *Acute cystitis* is typically accompanied by frequent, painful urination, urinary urgency, and suprapubic pain. *Chronic cystitis* may have no symptoms besides *pyuria* (white blood cells in the urine).

Pyelonephritis

Inflammation of the renal pelvis, called **pyelonephritis**, is mainly caused by bacterial infection.[32] Ascending infection from the bladder is the most common cause of pyelonephritis.[11] As with cystitis, the infection usually is caused by gram-negative bacteria. Urinary tract obstructions and vesicoureteral reflux also contribute to development of kidney infections. Vesicoureteral reflux involves retrograde flow of urine from the bladder into the ureters. It may result from a structural abnormality of the urinary tract or develop following a UTI.

Pyelonephritis may be either (1) acute or (2) chronic.

ACUTE PYELONEPHRITIS

Clinical manifestations of *acute pyelonephritis* usually include the sudden onset of fever, chills, nausea, vomiting, diarrhea, and pain at the costovertebral angle. Leukocytosis and pyuria are common. Some hematuria may be present initially. The urine may show organisms or may actually be sterile.[35] Acute pyelonephritis may follow symptomatic or asymptomatic cystitis or, less commonly, a blood-borne infection (septicemia).[12]

The symptoms of acute pyelonephritis subside with or without treatment, but urine colonization by organisms may persist for weeks or months. Acute pyelonephritis causes abscesses on the cortical surface of the kidney. Although damage to the glomeruli is rare, tubules may rupture. Healing usually involves replacement of affected areas of the cortical surface by scar tissue.

CHRONIC PYELONEPHRITIS

Chronic pyelonephritis involves chronic tubular and interstitial inflammation and scarring. It can result from various diseases and conditions that are associated with infections, obstructions, and reflux nephropathy. Chronic pyelonephritis may follow symptomatic or asymptomatic UTIs or vascular and hypertensive conditions that affect the glomeruli. It is a common cause of chronic renal failure. As noted in Figure 22-1, severe vesicouteral reflux or obstruction may result in renal damage in the absence of infection.[11] Pathologically, the kidneys become scarred and irregular, and the calices and renal pelvis become deformed (see Fig. 22-1). Gradual atrophy and destruction of the tubules lead to chronic renal failure.[11,32]

Clinical manifestations include either recurrent episodes of acute pyelonephritis or a gradual onset of renal insufficiency. Recurrent pyuria, bacteriuria, back pain, fever, and mild proteinuria with lymphocytes and plasma cells may be observed. Chronic pyelonephritis associated with vesicoureteral reflux may lack clinical manifestations until late in the course of the disease.

DAMAGE TO RENAL STRUCTURES

Conditions of kidney dysfunction are often divided into those that affect (1) the glomeruli and (2) the renal tubules and interstitium. Some conditions affect more than one structure, and damage to one structure almost always eventually affects the others.

Glomerular Disease

Glomerular injury is the most common cause of chronic renal failure. Numerous forms of glomerular disease exist; some are primary conditions, whereas others are secondary to systemic or hereditary diseases. Glomerular injury may also result from chemicals, drugs, irradiation, hypoxemia, and other agents.

PATHOPHYSIOLOGY AND ETIOLOGY

Glomerular disease may be (1) nephritic or (2) nephrotic, or both. In **nephritic disease**, also called **nephritis**, there is active proliferation of glomerular cells and an extensive inflammatory process. The inflammation leads to a decrease in glomerular filtration rate (GFR), which may be transient or progress to renal failure.[9] Decreased GFR, with retention of sodium and water, may lead to hypertension. When damage to the glomerulus causes increased permeability of the glomerular basement membrane (GBM),

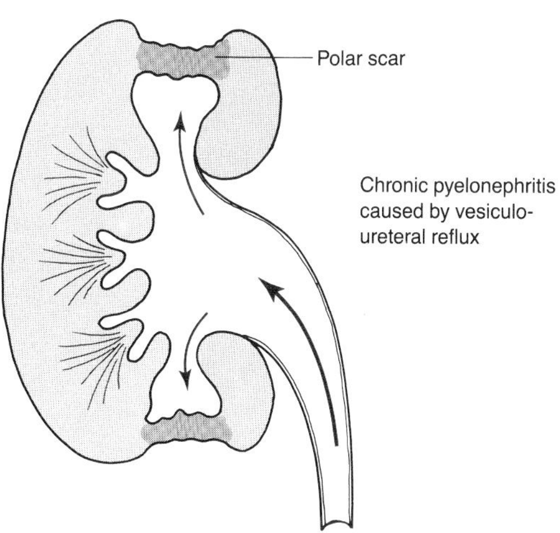

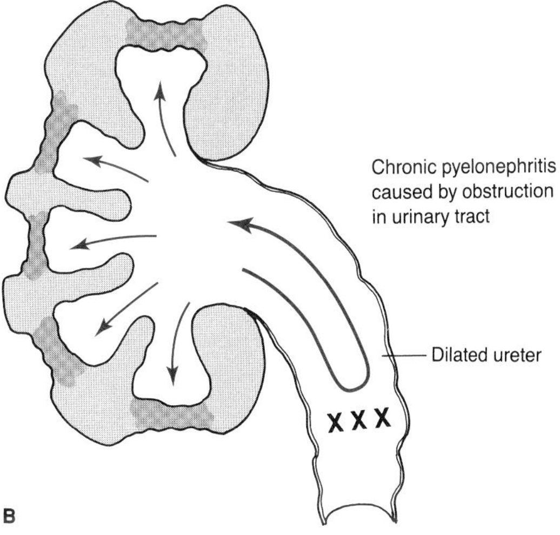

FIGURE 22-1. The two major types of chronic pyelonephritis. **A.** Vesiculoureteral reflux causes infection of the peripheral compound papillae and scars in the poles of the kidney. **B.** Obstruction of the urinary tract leads to high-pressure backflow of urine, which causes infection of all papillae, diffuse scarring of the kidney, and thinning of the cortex. (Rubin, E., & Farber, J. L. [1999]. *Pathology* [3rd ed.]. Philadelphia: Lippincott.)

proteinuria and hematuria result.[11] **Nephrosis,** also called **nephrotic syndrome**, occurs when damage to the GBM results in severe protein loss in the urine, leading to hypoalbuminemia. A serum albumin level of less than 3 g/dL results in generalized body edema (anasarca), as described in Flowchart 22-1. In many cases, the decreased serum protein levels stimulate lipoprotein synthesis by the liver, leading to hyperlipidemia and lipiduria (lipids in the urine).[11]

Immune mechanism are responsible for the glomerular damage in most forms of primary glomerular disease and many forms of secondary disease.[11] Injuries related to antigen-antibody reactions are the most common cause of damage, although cell-mediated and other immune mechanisms also play roles. The antigens in these reactions may be exogenous (such as infectious agents) or endogenous (as seen in certain autoimmune diseases and malignancies). Antigen-antibody–associated injury may occur in either of two ways: first, antigen-antibody complexes circulating in the blood become trapped in the glomeruli. These trapped complexes block the glomeruli and lead to inflammation and structural damage. Second, antibodies react to antigens within the glomerular membranes. These antigens may be parts of the glomerulus itself or parts of molecules that have previously bound to the glomerulus, such as drugs or parts of infectious agents. These reactions may trigger other immune mechanisms (such as activation of complement) and lead to glomerular damage.[11]

Glomerulonephritis, an inflammatory disease of the glomerulus, is a form of nephritis and presents in different forms. Table 22-3 summarizes the etiology, pathology, and clinical manifestations of common types of glomerulonephritis.

FLOWCHART 22-1 **Development of Edema In Nephrosis**

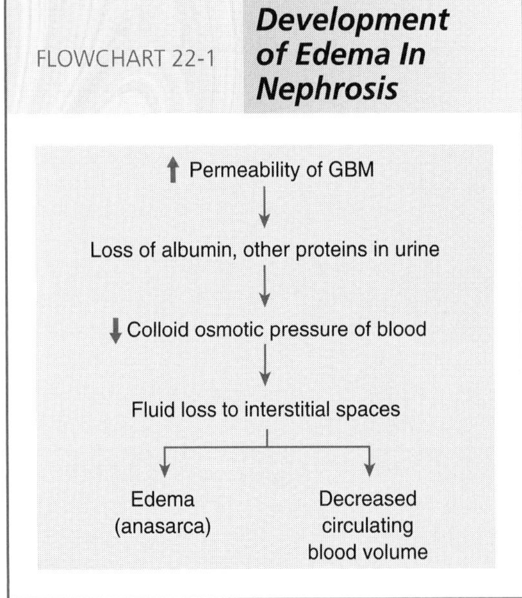

ACUTE GLOMERULONEPHRITIS

Acute glomerulonephritis usually has an abrupt onset. It includes acute poststreptococcal glomerulonephritis and nonstreptococcal acute glomerulonephritis.

Acute Poststreptococcal Glomerulonephritis

Acute glomerulonephritis occurs most often in children and is associated with group A, β-hemolytic streptococcal infection of the nasopharynx or, occasionally, the skin. Development of poststreptococcal glomerulonephritis (PSGN) typically occurs 1 to 2 weeks after infection and requires individual sensitivity to β-hemolytic streptococci. PSGN is caused by trapping of complexes of antibodies and streptococci-associated antigens in the glomeruli, not by active infection of the glomeruli by the bacteria.

The pathophysiology associated with PSGN reveals that the glomeruli become enlarged and hypercellular, with proliferation of cells on the epithelial side of the GBM. Infiltration of the area with leukocytes is followed by interstitial edema and inflammation. "Humps," which probably represent precipitated antigen-antibody complexes, form on the GBM.[35] Increased permeability of the GBM results in loss of red blood cells and protein in the urine. A decrease in GFR leads to retention of sodium and water. The precipitated complexes may contain large amounts of complement, resulting in *hypocomplementemia.*

Clinical manifestations of PSGN include the acute onset of edema, oliguria, proteinuria (which occasionally reaches nephrotic levels), anemia, and a characteristic cocoa-colored urine with red blood cell casts. Hypertension is usual and probably results from fluid retention. Elevated titers to streptococcal coenzymes indicate the presence of antibodies due to recent streptococcal infection. The erythrocyte sedimentation rate is usually increased.

Acute PSGN in children generally resolves within a week, then exhibits immunity to further infection. Adults with PSGN are more likely to show persistent proteinuria, hematuria, and hypertension.[11] Occasionally, PSGN converts to a progressive form of glomerulonephritis, resulting in renal failure.

Nonstreptococcal Acute Glomerulonephritis

Acute glomerulonephritis is occasionally seen following infection with viruses, parasites, or bacteria other than *Streptococcus.* This glomerulonephritis is similar in clinical presentation and course to PSGN. It is also presumably caused by the trapping of immune complexes that lead to similar glomerular lesions.[12]

RAPIDLY PROGRESSIVE GLOMERULONEPHRITIS

Rapidly progressive glomerulonephritis (RPGN) leads to renal failure over weeks to months. It may occur as an idiopathic (primary) condition or as a complication

TABLE 22-3

COMMON TYPES OF GLOMERULONEPHRITIS

DISORDER	COMMON CLINICAL MANIFESTATIONS	LIKELY PATHOLOGIC MECHANISM	ETIOLOGIC OR ASSOCIATED FACTORS
Acute poststreptococcal glomerulonephritis	Acute nephritis, sometimes with nephrosis and hypocomplementemia	Trapped immune complexes IgG and C3 in GBM	Streptococci
Nonstreptococcal acute glomerulonephritis	Acute nephritis, sometimes with nephrosis and hypocomplementemia	Trapped immune complexes	Other bacteria, parasites, viruses
Rapidly progressive glomerulonephritis	Nephritis, crescent formation	Trapped immune complexes and other immune mechanisms	Idiopathic, streptococci, systemic lupus erythematosus
		Anti-GBM antibodies	Goodpasture's syndrome
IgA nephropathy (Berger's disease)	Nephrosis, hematuria	Trapped immune complexes (IgA, sometimes with C3, IgG and IgM))	?Infections, exercise
Minimal change disease (lipoid nephrosis)	Nephrosis	Undetermined immune mechanism	?Infections, immunizations, atopic disorders
Focal segmental glomerulosclerosis	Nephrosis, or proteinuria without nephrotic syndrome	? Trapped immune complexes (IgM and C3)	HIV infection, heroin addiction
Membranous glomerulonephritis (membranous nephropathy)	Nephrosis	Formation of immune complexes in situ (IgG and C3)	Systemic lupus erythematosus; certain tumors and infections; exposure to certain drugs, gold, or mercury
Membranoproliferative glomerulonephritis (mesangiocapillary glomerulonephritis)	Slowly progressive nephritis, or sometimes nephrosis	Variable: alternative complement pathway activation, or immune complex	Hepatitis B and C, systemic lupus erythematosus, liver disease, certain cancers
Chronic Glomerulonephritis	Progressive renal insufficiency	Variable	Other types of glomerulonephritis; hereditary or multisystem disease

of infection or multisystem diseases, such as systemic lupus erythematosus (SLE) or Goodpasture's syndrome.[5] RPGN is characterized by the presence of *crescents*, which are formed by proliferation of glomerular cells and the migration of monocytes and macrophages into the Bowman's space.[12] Fibrin is deposited between the crescents. The crescents, which may be associated with necrosis, compress the glomerulus and eventually obliterate the Bowman's space.[11] The GBM is ruptured, and interstitial edema with infiltration of leukocytes leads to degenerative changes of the tubules.

Idiopathic RPGN accounts for almost half of all cases of RPGN. Since some cases show evidence of various immune deposits and others show evidence of cytotoxic changes, it is thought that several different pathogenic mechanisms may be associated with idiopathic RPGN.[11] Clinical manifestations include a rapid, progressive decline in renal function with severe oliguria or anuria. Hypertension, proteinuria, and hematuria are common. Irreversible renal failure often occurs in weeks or months.[5]

Goodpasture's syndrome is RPGN caused by anti-GBM antibodies. This rare autoimmune disorder usually affects young men, who may have genetic predisposition to the disease. It is often preceded by exposure to hydrocarbon solvents or viruses, although various drugs and cancers have also been implicated. Antibodies (usually IgG) against the GBM are seen in more than 95% of cases.[11,12] The glomeruli may show crescent formation or be nearly normal. The anti-GBM antibodies also may bind to the alveolar basement membrane, causing alveolar damage and pulmonary hemorrhage. Smokers develop pulmonary complications more often than nonsmokers.[11] Clinical manifestations include hematuria, proteinuria, and nephrosis. Pulmonary bleeding may be fatal even without evidence of renal disease.[12] The disease may progress rapidly, or it may exhibit long remissions. Pulmonary hemorrhage usually decreases after bilateral nephrectomy.

IgA NEPHROPATHY (BERGER'S DISEASE)

IgA nephropathy (Berger's disease) is thought to be the most common form of glomerulonephritis worldwide.[5,11] The disease is thought to result from an abnormality of immune regulation. It is characterized by IgA deposits in the mesangial cells, which are glomerular cells thought to help regulate filtration.[15,16] IgG or IgM may also be deposited in the mesangial cells. The trapped IgA activates complement, leading to damage to the glomeruli.[11] This disease presents with either asymptomatic microscopic hematuria and/or proteinuria (usually in adults) or gross hematuria following infections or exercise (usually in children).[5] It is typically slowly progressive and may be associated with minimal change disease (discussed below).

MINIMAL CHANGE DISEASE (LIPOID NEPHROSIS)

Minimal change disease (MCD) is the most frequent cause of nephrotic syndrome in children and a common cause in adults.[5,11] It results in decreased glomerular filtration rate and loss of binding together of glomerular foot processes.

Etiology and Pathophysiology

MCD is thought to be a hypersensitivity reaction because it often follows respiratory infections or routine immunization, responds to corticosteroids and immunosuppressive drugs, and is associated with other atopic disorders.[11] It is characterized by diffuse flattening and swelling of the foot processes (pedicles) of the GBM; otherwise, the glomeruli appear normal.[11] The injury to the pedicles allows albumin and lipids to leak into the urine. The cells of the proximal tubules may fill with lipids, thus the name *lipoid nephrosis.*

Clinical Manifestations

The clinical course is variable, characterized by periods of remission and exacerbation. Generally, the prognosis is good. Although MCD involves massive proteinuria, renal function usually remains good. Hypertension and hematuria are rare. A few persons with MCD become corticosteroid-dependent. MCD occasionally progresses to focal glomerulosclerosis and renal failure.

FOCAL SEGMENTAL GLOMERULOSCLEROSIS

Focal segmental glomerulosclerosis (FSG) involves sclerosis (thickening and hardening) of some, but not all, of the glomeruli. In the affected glomeruli, only portions (segments) of the capillaries are involved. The disease typically starts with the juxtamedullary glomeruli but then becomes generalized. Pathologically, the sclerotic segments show collapse of the GBM, with deposits of IgM and complement fragments in the sclerosing lesions. Changes in the foot-processes similar to those in MCD may occur. FSG may be primary or secondary to other conditions or diseases, such as heroin abuse or human immunodeficiency virus (HIV) infection. FSG is sometimes considered a severe form of MCD rather than a separate disease. FSG progresses at variable rates, with about 20% of affected persons developing renal failure within 2 years.[11]

Clinical manifestations are associated with nephrotic syndrome, with large loss of protein in the urine. Generally the prognosis is poor, with renal failure occurring in 2 to 3 years. Response to corticosteroids in FSG is poor.

MEMBRANOUS GLOMERULONEPHRITIS

Membranous glomerulonephritis (MGN; *membranous nephropathy*) is a common cause of nephrotic syndrome in adults.[5,11] In MGN the glomerular capillary wall becomes diffusely thickened and develops deposits, which usually contain IgG and complement. Immune damage to the GBM allows loss of protein in the urine.[11] Edema, hypoalbuminemia, hematuria, and mild hypertension may result. MGN is usually idiopathic but may be associated with SLE, exposure to inorganic (gold or mercury) or organic (penicillamine, captopril) drugs, tumors, and some infections. The clinical course is extremely variable. It may progress to renal failure, show repeated exacerbations and remissions, or show a spontaneous, complete remission.

MEMBRANOPROLIFERATIVE GLOMERULONEPHRITIS (SLOWLY PROGRESSIVE GLOMERULONEPHRITIS, MESANGIOCAPILLARY GLOMERULONEPHRITIS)

In membranoproliferative glomerulonephritis (MPGN), the GBM thickens and mesangial cells grow out along the capillary wall, sometimes extending processes into the GBM.[5,11] Deposits containing IgG and complement may be present in the glomerular cells. MPGN may be primary or associated with various conditions such as hepatitis B and C, SLE, chronic liver disease, and certain malignancies. It accounts for 5% to 10% of all cases of idiopathic nephrotic syndrome.[11]

MPGN may present with any of the manifestations of nephrotic syndrome and may include hypocomplementemia.[12] MPGN assumes several forms, all of which are slowly progressive and unremitting. About half of affected persons develop chronic renal failure within 10 years.[11]

GLOMERULONEPHRITIS CAUSED BY HEREDITARY OR MULTISYSTEM DISEASE

Many systemic conditions are associated with glomerular injury. This causes major clinical complications in some diseases. Many of these conditions are discussed in other chapters of this text, but some of the renal pathology is discussed here.

DIABETIC GLOMERULOSCLEROSIS. This condition is a major cause of end-stage renal disease. The most common lesions involve the glomeruli and cause proteinuria, nephrotic syndrome, and chronic renal failure. Diabetes also causes sclerosis of the renal arterioles, increased susceptibility to infection, and tubular lesions. The conglomerate of renal lesions associated with diabetes is called **diabetic nephrophathy.**[11]

LUPUS NEPHRITIS. This condition is a very common complication of SLE and presents in several patterns. It is probably caused by trapped immune complexes in the GBM that produce destruction and nephrosis, with different patterns of presentation reflecting different sites and amounts of GBM damage.[6] SLE is associated with RPGN, MPGN, chronic glomerulonephritis, and chronic renal failure. Pathology in the kidneys can vary from minimal changes to extensive damage with crescent formation.[6,11]

HIV NEPHROPATHY. **HIV nephropathy** is associated with HIV infection. It involves diffuse sclerosis and collapse of glomeruli, accompanied by extensive inflammation and damage to renal tubules and the interstitium. It progresses rapidly to renal failure. Infection with HIV is also associated with other forms of renal disease, including MCD, mesangial hyperplasia, and IgA deposition.[5] The mechanism behind these renal changes is unclear.[6]

HENOCH-SCHÖNLEIN PURPURA. This syndrome is characterized by IgA deposits in various body tissues. These deposits lead to purpuric skin lesions, abdominal pain, vomiting, intestinal bleeding, joint pain, and renal damage.[6,11] The renal pathology is similar to that of IgA nephropathy. The syndrome often follows upper respiratory tract infection. It is more common in children, but renal complications are often more severe in adults. The extent of renal damage and the clinical course of the disease are quite variable.[11]

AMYLOIDOSIS. This condition may produce glomerulonephritis by precipitation of amyloid within the glomeruli. Amyloidosis often results in proteinuria, nephrotic syndrome, and chronic renal failure.[11]

HEREDITARY NEPHRITIS. This refers to a group of hereditary diseases that result in defective synthesis of the GBM. The best known of these conditions is *Alport's syndrome*, which also includes hearing loss and eye abnormalities. Inheritance is typically X-linked, but autosomal recessive and dominant patterns are also seen.[26]

CHRONIC GLOMERULONEPHRITIS

Chronic glomerulonephritis (CGN) is an insidious progressive disorder. It may result from any type of glomerular disease, as shown in Figure 22-2, and may exhibit both nephrotic and nephritic characteristics. The glomeruli become scarred and may be totally obliterated. The tubules atrophy. The glomeruli and renal capsules become infiltrated with lymphocytes and plasma cells. Sclerosis of the arteries and arterioles probably contributes to the hypertension almost always seen in this disease. The course of CGN is related to the underlying disorder, but it almost always progresses to renal failure after years of declining renal function. Proteinuria, hypertension, and azotemia are common late manifestations.

Tubular and Interstitial Diseases

Disorders of the renal tubules and interstitium, called **interstitial nephritis (IN)**, can be either acute or chronic, and are caused by many factors.[27] If the cause

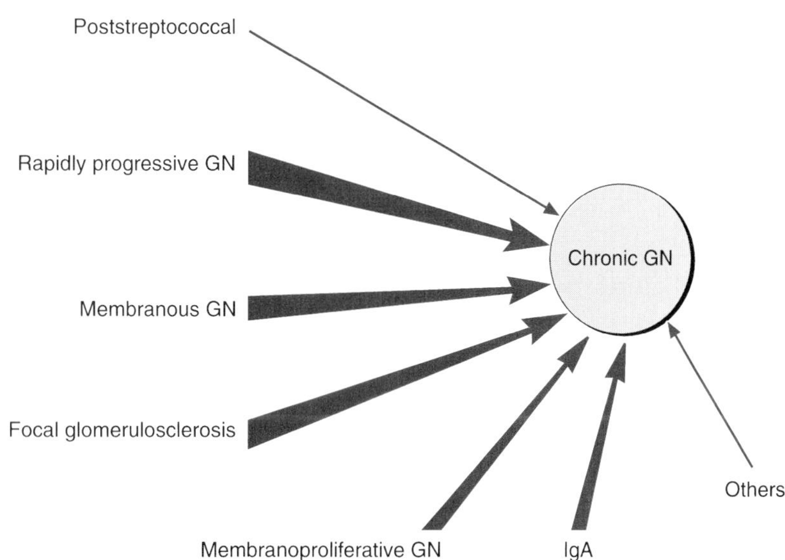

FIGURE 22-2. Primary glomerular diseases leading to chronic glomerulonephritis (GN). The thickness of the arrows reflects the approximate proportion of patients in each group who progress to chronic GN. Poststreptococcal, 1%–2%); rapidly progressive (crescentic), 90%; membranous, 50%; focal glomerulosclerosis, 50%–80%; membranoproliferative, 50%; IgA nephropathy, 30%–50%. (Cotran, R., Kumar, V. and Collins, J. [1999]. *Robbins' pathologic basis of disease* [6th ed.]. Philadelphia: W. B. Saunders.)

BOX 22-3 CAUSES OF ACUTE INTERSTITIAL NEPHRITIS

- Nephrotoxins
  - Antibiotics
    - Penicillins
    - Rifampin
    - Aminoglycosides
    - Sulfonamides
    - Cephalosporins
    - Cyclosporin A
    - Others
  - Nonsteroidal anti-inflammatory drugs
  - Miscellaneous drugs
    - Amphotericin-B
    - Allopurinal
    - Sulfonamide diuretics
    - Furosemide
    - Thiazide diuretics
    - Radiographic contrast agents
    - Many others
  - Organic solvents
- Systemic infections
  - *Streptococcus* infections
  - Rocky Mountain spotted fever
  - Legionnaires' disease
  - Others
- Primary renal infections
  - Primary pyelonephritis
  - Renal tuberculosis
  - Fungal nephritis
- Immune disorders
  - Systemic lupus erythematosus
  - Rejection of renal transplant
  - Sarcoidosis
  - Others

BOX 22-4 CAUSES OF CHRONIC INTERSTITIAL NEPHRITIS

- Persistent or progressive acute interstitial nephritis
- Chronic urinary tract obstruction
- Urinary reflux
- Chronic bacterial pyelonephritis or renal tuberculosis
- Arteriolar nephrosclerosis
- Nephrotoxins
  - Drugs
    - Analgesics
    - Cisplatin
    - Others
  - Metals
    - Copper
    - Lead
    - Lithium
    - Mercury
- Metabolic imbalances
  - Hypercalcemia
  - Hypokalemia
  - Hyperoxaluria
  - Hyperuricemia
- Radiation
- Systemic disorders
  - Immune diseases
    - Systemic lupus erythematosus
    - Chronic transplant rejection
  - Neoplasia
    - Leukemia
    - Lymphoma
    - Multiple myeloma
  - Others
    - Amyloidosis
    - Diabetes mellitus
    - Sickle cell anemia
    - Others

is infectious, the term pyelonephritis is usually used to describe the process. Some causes of acute IN are shown in Box 22-3; causes of chronic IN are identified in Box 22-4. Four mechanisms of tubular and interstitial disease are discussed here: (1) toxic mechanisms, (2) metabolic imbalances, (3) tubular acidosis, and (4) acute tubular necrosis.

TOXIC MECHANISMS

The profuse renal blood supply and the concentration of nephrotoxic substances in the tubules facilitate damage to the tubules and parenchyma. Toxins can cause either acute or chronic damage. The number of substances, particularly drugs, found to be nephrotoxic continues to grow.[11,27] Toxins can cause renal damage either through immune mechanisms or by other direct damage to the tubules.[11]

Immune mechanisms appear to underlie the toxic effects of many drugs. *Acute drug-induced interstitial nephritis* typically begins about 15 days after drug exposure and may be accompanied by fever, eosinophilia, skin rash, hematuria, proteinuria, and sterile pyuria.[3,11] Pathologically, this appears to be a delayed-hypersensitivity (allergic) reaction and is not dose-dependent. The interstitium develops pronounced edema and inflammation and becomes infiltrated with leukocytes. IgE- and cell-mediated immunity reactions also damage tubular cells. Recovery usually is complete after the drug is discontinued.[11,35]

Chronic analgesia nephritis occurs most often in persons who ingest large quantities of analgesic mixtures. These mixtures usually contain phenacetin, often in combination with aspirin, caffeine, acetaminophen, or codeine. Disease prevalence reflects patterns of analgesic use. In the United States, it is more common in the Southeast.[11] The mechanism of injury may include renal ischemia caused by aspirin inhibiting the vasodilatory effects of prostaglandins. Phenacetin may have a direct toxic effect on the vasa recta, or it may cause papillary necrosis. The result is fibrosis, necrosis, calcification, fragmentation, and sloughing of the papillae. The kidneys lose the ability to concentrate urine. Headache, anemia, gastrointestinal symptoms, hypertension, and urinary tract infections also can occur. The disease can progress to chronic renal failure; however, withdrawal of the drugs can lead to stabilized or improved renal function. The disease also is associated with development of a carcinoma of the renal pelvis.[11]

METABOLIC IMBALANCES

Abnormal body metabolism can lead to states that are toxic to the renal tubules. The imbalances that most frequently cause renal dysfunction are (1) **hyperuricemia**, (2) **hypercalcemia**, (3) hypokalemia, and (4) **hyperoxaluria**.

HYPERURICEMIA. Elevated uric acid levels may cause either acute or chronic IN and are also associated with formation of kidney stones. Acute IN is usually caused by the precipitation of uric acid crystals in the tubules, causing intrarenal obstruction, inflammation, fibrosis, and possibly acute renal failure. Acute uric acid damage is most often seen in persons undergoing chemotherapy for leukemia or lymphoma. Dehydration, as after severe vomiting, can contribute to the process.[3]

Chronic urate nephropathy results from prolonged elevations of serum uric acid, usually due to gout. In gouty nephropathy, urate crystals deposit in the distal tubules, collecting ducts, and interstitium. Tophi, large aggregates of urate crystals surrounded by leukocytes and areas of intense inflammation, may form. This may result in tubular obstruction, with cortical atrophy and scarring, and may lead to chronic renal failure. Lead exposure (as through drinking "moonshine" whiskey) increases the risk of development of gouty nephropathy.[11]

HYPERCALCEMIA. Hypercalcemia can lead to formation of calcium deposits in the tubules and interstitium, as well as formation of kidney stones. Intracellular accumulation of calcium can disrupt cellular processes, causing cell death and consequent obstruction of nephrons by cellular debris. Hypercalcemia also causes renal vasoconstriction and lowers permeability of the glomerular capillary wall, impairing GFR.[6]

HYPOKALEMIA. Moderate to severe hypokalemia that persists for several weeks can lead to damage to renal tubules. Tubular cells develop numerous vacuoles, and glomeruli may shrink and become sclerotic. This results in a decreased ability to concentrate urine, which usually returns to normal after potassium levels are restored.[18,22]

HYPEROXALURIA. Oxalate nephropathy can occur from inherited enzyme deficiencies, from defective glyoxylic acid metabolism, and from ethylene glycol (antifreeze), methoxyflurane, and massive ascorbic acid overdose.[3] It produces progressive interstitial fibrosis and recurrent renal stones. Systemic poisoning with ethylene glycol resembles acute alcohol intoxication but can cause chronic tubulointerstitial nephritis.[3]

ACUTE TUBULAR NECROSIS

Acute tubular necrosis (ATN) is a syndrome of destruction of tubular epithelial cells leading to acute impairment of renal function. It is the most common cause of acute renal failure.[11,35] ATN is typically due to either (1) ischemia or (2) exposure to nephrotoxic agents. Ischemic and nephrotoxic causes are identified in Box 22-5. Ischemia is the more frequent cause, with its severity and duration affecting the extent of damage and the prognosis.[17,30] However, the likelihood that ATN will develop in a given situation is difficult to predict, in part because multiple predisposing factors may occur together (such as ischemia plus hemoglobinuria).[6]

Ischemic ATN most often appears after an episode of shock, usually subsequent to conditions such as sep-

BOX 22-5 ISCHEMIA AND NEPHROTOXINS IMPLICATED IN ACUTE TUBULAR NECROSIS

Ischemia

Severe congestive heart failure: cardiogenic shock
Hemorrhagic, septic, neurogenic shock
Burns
Dehydration
Hepatic failure with ascites
Complications of pregnancy: toxemia

Nephrotoxins

Antibiotics such as gentamicin
Antibacterials such as sulfonamides
Diuretics such as furosemide
Antineoplastic drugs such as methotrexate
Contrast media, especially those containing iodine
Organic solvents such as carbon tetrachloride
Hemoglobin/myoglobin products
Fungicides such as amphotericin B
Heavy metals such as gold therapy
Anesthetic agents such as methoxyflurane
Antitubercular drugs such as isoniazid
Narcotic analgesics such as heroin
Antigout drugs such as colchicine
Anti–heavy metal poisoning agents such as calcium edetate disodium

sis, burns, crushing injuries, peripheral circulatory collapse, and postoperative hypotension.[6,35] Pathologically, ischemia causes numerous structural and functional changes in the tubular epithelial cells, including cellular energy depletion, intracellular calcium accumulation, and free radical damage to cell membranes.[6] In ischemic ATN, patchy necrosis occurs at multiple points in the tubules, particularly the straight portion of the proximal tubules, as shown in Figure 22-3A. The basement membrane may be ruptured and the tubular lumen occluded by casts and debris. Damage to the brush border of the proximal tubule cells also results. Other abnormalities include leukocytes in the vasa recta and interstitial edema. Often there is also simultaneous evidence of cellular regeneration. If the episode of ATN is not fatal, this regeneration eventually completely reverses the damage.[6,11]

Nephrotoxic ATN may occur after exposure to numerous agents (see Box 22-5) or following hemolysis or skeletal muscle breakdown, which results in hemoglobin or myoglobin precipitating in urine.[6] Nephrotoxic agents destroy tubular cells through a number of mechanisms, including direct cellular toxic effects, lysis of red blood cells, intravascular coagulation, precipitation of oxalate and uric acid crystals, disruption of cellular ion balances, occlusion of tubules, and tissue hypoxia.[6,35] Susceptibility to nephrotoxicity of agents is increased by dehydration and preexisting renal disease. The decline in the number of functioning nephrons seen with aging makes older persons particularly susceptible to nephrotoxic damage.

In nephrotoxic ATN, most necrosis is concentrated in the proximal tubules, although lesions may also occur in distal tubules (see Fig. 22-3B). Some toxins cause specific patterns of damage.[11] Pathologically, less basement membrane disruption typically occurs than in ischemic ATN.[17] Casts and cellular debris obstruct the distal tubules, and necrosis is present in all nephrons. Interstitial edema, leukocytes in the vasa recta, and inflammatory cells in the interstitium are characteristic.

Clinical Manifestations

The clinical course of ATN is divided into (1) initiating, (2) maintenance, and (3) recovery phases. In the *initiating phase* (usually about the first 36 hours), tubular damage is occurring but the only clinical signs may be a slight decline in urine output and rise in BUN. The *maintenance phase* is characterized by rising BUN, hyperkalemia, metabolic acidosis, and, in many cases, oliguria with salt and water retention. Persons who survive this phase enter the *recovery phase*, during which urine volume steadily increases. The tubules are still damaged, so the kidneys lose large amounts of water and electrolytes. Hypokalemia becomes a problem. Eventually, BUN and creatinine levels return to normal and the kidneys recover the ability to concentrate urine. Impairment of tubular function may last for months, but most persons who reach the recovery phase even-

FOCUS ON CELLULAR PATHOPHYSIOLOGY

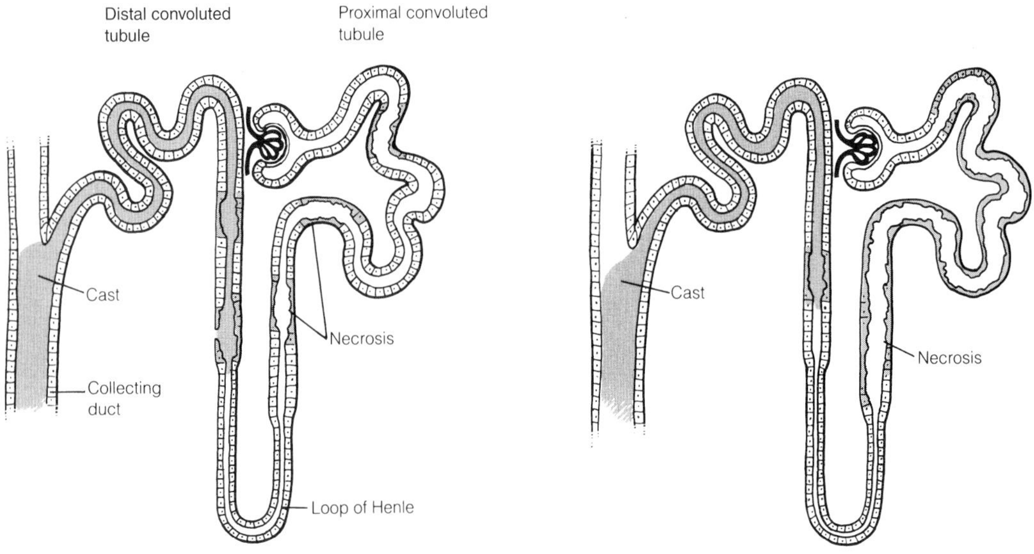

FIGURE 22-3. **A.** Patchy ischemic necrosis of the proximal tubules. **B.** Characteristic nephrotoxic injury of large segments of proximal tubule.

tually fully recover. In ischemic ATN, survival also depends on other damage done by the cause of ischemia. In nephrotoxic ATN, survival also depends on whether the toxin has damaged other organs in the body.[6,11]

RENAL TUBULAR ACIDOSIS

The term **renal tubular acidosis** (RTA) refers to a group of disorders characterized by normal glomerular filtration accompanied by impairment of renal acidification. RTA is divided into two types: Type I (distal RTA) and Type II (proximal RTA). Numerous conditions, which are listed in Table 22-4, can produce RTA.[6] In *Type I RTA* the collecting tubules are unable to secrete hydrogen ions. This causes hyperchloremic metabolic acidosis and increased pH of the urine (usually above 5.3). Hypokalemia and formation of kidney stones are common complications of Type I RTA.

Type II RTA is caused by a decreased ability of the proximal tubules to reabsorb bicarbonate ions. Metabolic acidosis, potassium wasting, and alkaline urine initially result. Eventually, however, the serum bicarbonate level falls to the point where the remaining bicarbonate can be reabsorbed. Bicarbonate and potassium wasting then stop, and a new acid-base balance is developed.[6]

TABLE 22-4

ETIOLOGY OF RENAL TUBULAR ACIDOSIS

TYPE I (DISTAL)	TYPE II (PROXIMAL)
Primary idiopathic hereditary disorders	Primary idiopathic hereditary disorders
Familial	Cystinosis
Marfan's syndrome	Galactosemia
Sickle cell anemia	Tyrosinemia
Wilson's disease	Wilson's disease
Others	Pyruvate carboxylase deficiency
Drugs and toxins	Drugs and toxins
Amphotericin B	Lead
Lithium	Cadmium
Toluene	Mercury
Calcium disorders	Copper
Hypercalcemia	Acetazolamide
Hypercalciuria	Ifosfamide
Hypervitaminosis D	Outdated tetracycline
Chronic hyper-parathyroidism	Others
Systemic and auto-immune diseases	Systemic disorders
Thyroiditis	Multiple myeloma
Cirrhosis	Vitamin D deficiency
Amyloidosis	Nephrotic syndrome
Multiple myeloma	Amyloidosis
Medullary sponge kidney	Renal transplant rejection
Others	Others
Associated with hyperkalemia	
Sickle cell anemia	
Systemic lupus erythematosus	
Urinary tract obstruction	
Renal transplant rejection	
Hyperaldosteronism	

OBSTRUCTION OF THE GENITOURINARY TRACT

Untreated obstructive disorders can cause considerable renal dysfunction, including hemorrhage and renal failure. The principal obstructive conditions are prostatic hyperplasia, renal calculi, and renal tumors.

Conditions of the Prostate

The prostate consists of four lobes that surround the urethra. Common conditions that affect the prostate include benign prostatic hyperplasia, inflammation of the prostate, and cancer of the prostate. Prostatic hyperplasia and cancer of the prostate are briefly discussed below and in Chapter 36. Prostatitis is discussed in Chapter 36.

BENIGN PROSTATIC HYPERPLASIA (NODULAR HYPERPLASIA)

Benign prostatic hyperplasia (BPH) is hyperplasia of glandular and cellular tissue resulting in enlargement of the prostate. BPH affects most men over 50 years of age. The prostate normally weighs about 20 g; in BPH, it typically weighs 60 to 100 g but may weigh over 200 g.[11]

Etiology and Pathophysiology

The cause of BPH is unknown, but it is believed to result from changes in the sex hormones, as discussed in Chapter 36. As shown in Figure 22-4, the periurethral lobes enlarge and normal tissues and the urethra are compressed, obstructing urine outflow.[11]

Clinical Manifestations

Obstruction by BPH can cause urinary frequency, decrease in force and size of the stream, straining to urinate, difficulty in starting and stopping the stream, and incomplete bladder emptying. Complications of BPH include hydroureter, acute renal failure, hematuria, calculi, reflux, UTI, thickening of the bladder muscles, and sudden onset of acute urinary retention. BPH does not predispose to development of prostate cancer.[33]

CANCER OF THE PROSTATE

Carcinoma of the prostate is the most common form of cancer in men. It is typically a disease of men over age 50, and its incidence increases with age. The etiology

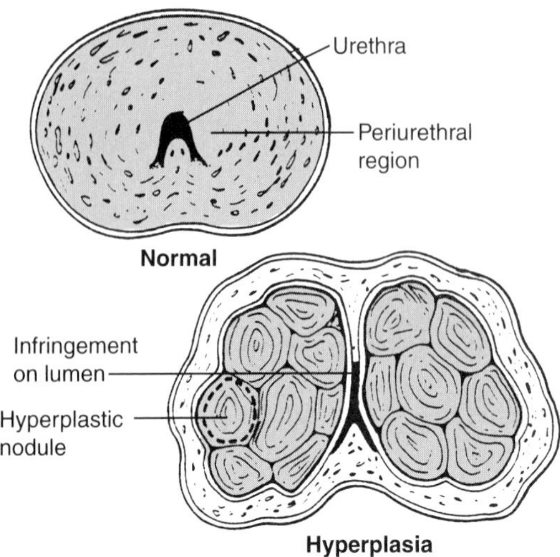

FIGURE 22-4. Relation to the urethra of normal and of hyperplastic prostate. Notice infringement on the lumen in the latter.

of prostatic cancer is unclear, although age, race, family history, hormone levels, and environmental factors appear to play roles.[11] Prostatic cancer often initially presents with symptoms of urethral obstruction. Usually, metastasis has already occurred when these symptoms arise. Prostatic cancer typically arises in the posterior lobe but then invades the medial and lateral areas where BPH originates. Thus, it may produce urethral obstruction identical to that seen in BPH. It also can obstruct the ureters by extending directly into the bladder or by invading the seminal vesicles behind the bladder. Obstruction of the ureters leads to development of uremia.[36] For more information on prostatic cancer see Chapter 36.

Calculi

Urinary stones or calculi are common in the United States. Calculi can form anywhere in the urinary system, but most form in the kidney.[11] Calculi formation in the renal pelvis or calices is called **nephrolithiasis. Urolithiasis** refers to stones anywhere in the urinary tract, including those in the kidney. Symptoms of urolithiasis vary from hematuria or oliguria to renal colic. However, the hallmark of urolithiasis is pain, which is usually associated with small stones in the ureters. The ureters contract in an attempt to pass the stone; this results in the colic-type pain in the flank or costovertebral angle, which often radiates to the abdomen and groin. Large stones in the kidney cannot be passed through the small ureter and usually do not cause pain. Hematuria results from the damage done by the stone in the urinary tract. Oliguria may result when the stone obstructs the flow of urine.

STRUCTURE AND COMPOSITION

Calculi vary in shape and size. Some are as small as grains of sand; others entirely fill the renal pelvis, such as the staghorn calculi shown in Figure 22-5. Calculi also vary in color, texture, and composition. Stones may be either unilateral or bilateral and may be single or multiple. Stones contain an organic matrix, or framework, and crystalloids such as calcium, oxalate, phosphate, urate, uric acid, struvite, and cystine.[11]

FACTORS THAT PROMOTE STONE FORMATION

The incidence of urolithiasis is higher in men, in persons leading a sedentary lifestyle, and in families with a history of stones. In the United States, the incidence is

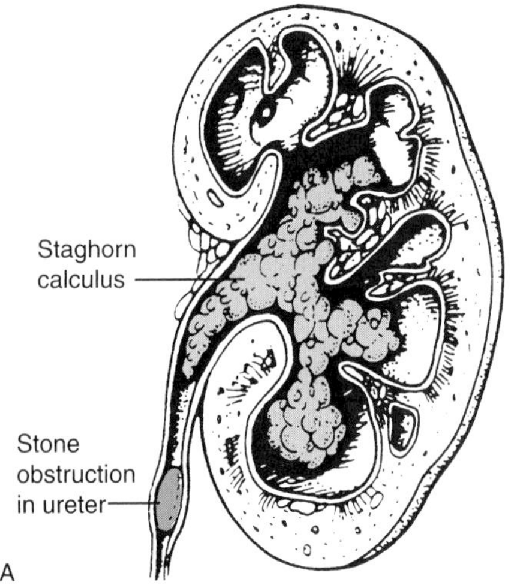

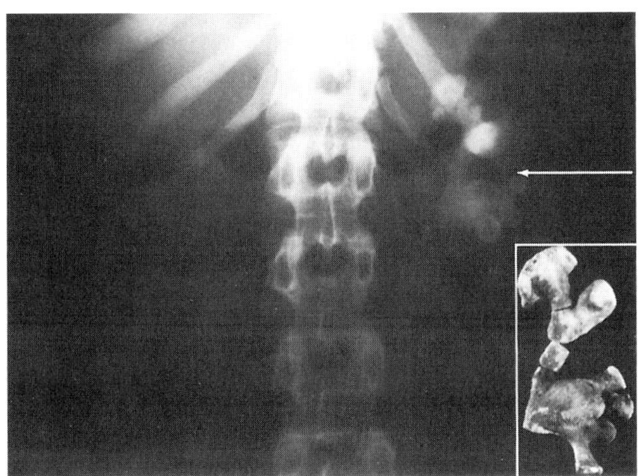

FIGURE 22-5. **A.** Staghorn calculus obstructing the entire renal pelvis. **B.** Radiologic appearance of a large staghorn calculus. *Arrow* shows location of stone. Inset shows actual appearance on removal.

highest in the Southeast.[19] Some stones are associated with certain types of urinary tract infection. The average age for the occurrence of renal stones is between 20 and 30 years, but they can occur at any age.[11] Stone formation may result from alteration in urine pH, decrease in inhibitors, or supersaturation of urine. The urine almost always shows an increased concentration of the stones' constituents. However, some individuals have hypercalciuria, hyperoxaluria, or hyperuricosuria without developing clinically apparent stones.[11]

SUPERSATURATION OF URINE. The concentration of stone constituents in the urine is the most important factor in urolithiasis.[11] Stone formation typically begins when the urine concentration passes a critical point at which urine can no longer keep the substance in solution (supersaturation). Hypovolemia and low urine production promote concentration of substances in the urine. Urine saturation also is affected by serum levels of the substance and by renal excretion and reabsorption.

ALTERATIONS IN PH. The solubility of crystalloids is affected by pH. Alterations in pH may cause substances to leave the urine, attach to the matrix, and crystallize. Stones that form in an acid urine contain uric acid, cystine, oxalate, or xanthine. Most stones formed in alkaline urine contain calcium phosphate or struvite. Urinary pH, and the risk of stone formation, may be affected by diet or persistent use of some medications, such as those containing aluminum hydroxide, calcium carbonate, ascorbic acid, and sodium bicarbonate.

DECREASE IN INHIBITORS. A decrease in factors that inhibit the formation of crystals in the urine may cause stone formation, even in persons who do not have elevated urine levels of the stone's constituents.[11] The list of inhibitors is long and includes magnesium, sodium, pyrophosphate, urea, citrate, amino acids, and trace metals. Urine contains inhibitors for calcium oxalate and calcium phosphate but not for uric acid, cystine, or struvite.[10]

TYPES OF STONES

Many stones are composed of mixtures of substances. Most fall into one of four types. Table 22-5 lists these, their characteristics, and factors associated with their formation.[6,11,19,24]

TABLE 22-5

COMMON TYPES OF URINARY STONES

CONSTITUENT	% OF ALL STONES	APPEARANCE	URINE pH FAVORING FORMATION	FACTORS FACILITATING FORMATION	ASSOCIATED CONDITIONS
Calcium stones (calcium oxalate, calcium phosphate)	75–80	White to gray, small, soft, radiopaque	Alkaline	Hypercalcemia Hypercalciuria Hyperuricosuria Hyperoxaluria Hypocitraturia	(See Box 22-6) Dehydration, gout, high-oxalate diet; hereditary disease; small-bowel disease/surgery, chronic diarrhea
Struvite (Mg^{++}, NH_3, Ca^{++}, PO_4)	10–15	Large to staghorn, rapidly growing, usually radiopaque	Alkaline	UTI by urea-splitting bacteria	Catheterization, cystoscopy, long-term antibiotic use
Uric acid	5–10	Yellow to brown, small to staghorn, soft, radiolucent	Acidic	Hyperuricemia Hyperuricosuria	Gout, dehydration, chemotherapy, leukemia, polycythemia vera, chronic diarrhea, aspirin or probenecid use, hereditary disease
Cystine	1–2	White or yellow, soft, hexagonal crystals, variable size, poorly radiopaque	Acidic	Hypercystinuria	Hereditary disease

Calcium Stones

Calcium stones are often formed in the presence of hypercalcemia or hypercalciuria. Hypercalcemia is caused by numerous factors (Box 22-6). **Hypercalciuria** occurs with increased excretion of urinary calcium due to hypercalcemia, increased calcium absorption from the gut (as seen in hyperparathyroidism), excess bone reabsorption (as seen in immobility), or a renal defect. A renal defect that causes hypercalciuria is usually a tubular defect resulting in a calcium leak. For example, in renal tubular acidosis the distal convoluted tubule and collecting duct are not able to maintain acid urine. Since calcium is not as soluble in alkaline urine, it may precipitate to form stones.

The vast majority of calcium-containing stones are composed of calcium oxalate.[6,19] **Hyperuricosuria** is also associated with formation of calcium oxalate stones; uric acid crystals may serve as the nucleus around which calcium stones form.[11,19] Even mild hyperoxaluria also increases the risk of calcium oxalate stone formation.[6] Oxalates are present in certain green leafy vegetables, and stones may be related to excess consumption of these foods.[11,19] Hyperoxaluria also may occur after bowel surgery and with small bowel disease.

Urinary citrate appears to inhibit formation of calcium stones; conversely, the lack of urinary citrate seems to foster the formation of calcium stones. This is evidenced by common findings of **hypocitraturia** in persons who form calcium stones.[19] Excess consumption of certain soft drinks may contribute to hypocitraturia.[6] Some persons with normal urinary pH, serum electrolyte, and urine values develop calcium stones of unknown cause.[11] Many times these persons have recurrent stone disease.

BOX 22-6 CAUSES OF HYPERCALCEMIA

- Primary hyperparathyroidism
- Cancer
  - Parathyroid hormone-related protein
  - Ectopic production of 1,25-dihydroxy vitamin D_3
  - Other factors produced ectopically
  - Lytic bone metastases
- Nonparathyroid endocrine disorders
  - Thyrotoxicosis
  - Pheochromocytoma
  - Adrenal insufficiency
  - Vasoactive intestinal polypeptide hormone–producing tumor
- Granulomatous diseases (1,25-dihydroxy vitamin D_3 excess)
  - Sarcoidosis
  - Tuberculosis
  - Histoplasmosis
  - Coccidioidomycosis
  - Leprosy
- Medications
  - Thiazide diuretics
  - Lithium
  - Estrogens and antiestrogens
- Milk-alkali syndrome
- Vitamin A intoxication
- Vitamin D intoxication
- Familial hypocalciuric hypercalcemia
- Immobilization
- Parenteral nutrition
- Acute and chronic renal insufficiency

(Stein, J. [Ed]. [1998]. *Internal medicine* [5th ed.]. St. Louis: Mosby.)

Struvite Stones (Magnesium Ammonium Phosphate Stones)

Struvite stones are caused by urinary tract infection with urea-splitting bacteria. This process is depicted in Flowchart 22-2. The bacteria use the enzyme urease to split urea into ammonia. This causes an elevated urinary pH, allowing large struvite stones, which may fill the renal pelvis (staghorn calculi), to form.[11] The UTI may follow catheterization, cystoscopy, or long-term antibiotic use. It is most often caused by *Proteus* species but may also be due to *Klebsiella, Pseudomonas, Serratia, Enterobacter*, or *Staphylococcus*.[6,24] Struvite stones are more frequent in women and tend to be recurrent.

Uric Acid Stones

Both hyperuricemia and urine pH play important roles in the formation of uric acid stones. Hyperuricemia and hyperuricosuria greatly increase the risk of uric acid stone formation. Hyperuricosuria is common in gout and conditions of rapid cell turnover, such as leukemia and some chemotherapy. These conditions cause cell necrosis, which results in hyperuricosuria because purines convert mostly to uric acids.

FLOWCHART 22-2 **Formation of Struvite Stones**

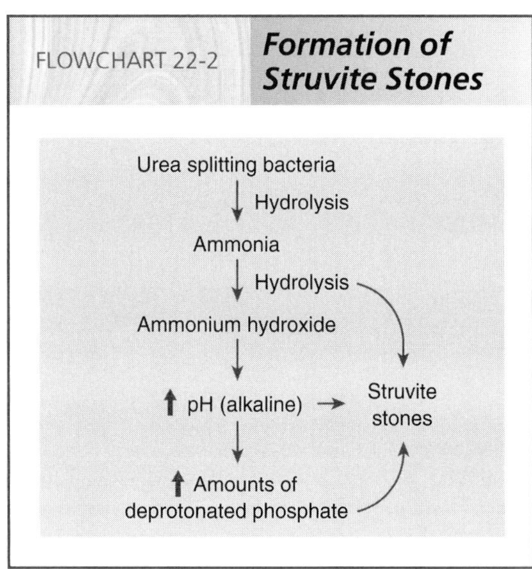

More than half of persons who form uric acid stones have neither hyperuricemia nor hyperuricosuria.[11] Urine pH may account for formation of some of these stones. Urine acidity decreases the solubility of uric acid.[6,19] Persons with uric acid stones often excrete less urinary ammonia than normal, which results in acidic urine.[6] Decreased ammonia production and urine acidity may contribute more than hyperuricemia to the high number of stones seen in persons with gout.[6]

Cystine Stones

Cystine stones are typically due to cystinuria caused by an autosomal recessive disorder. This disorder causes impaired transport of cystine and other amino acids in the renal tubules. Since cystine is less soluble than the other amino acids, small hexagonal crystals of cystine may form. These may eventually form large or even staghorn calculi.[6]

Tumors

TUMORS OF THE BLADDER

Most tumors of the bladder are malignant, and the benign tumors that occur are difficult to distinguish from malignant lesions.[11,34] Carcinoma of the bladder usually affects the transitional epithelium, and 90% of bladder cancers are classified as transitional cell carcinomas. Other forms seen include transitional cell papilloma, squamous cell, and adenocarcinoma. About half of bladder cancers are aggressive, highly anaplastic lesions. They may be invasive or noninvasive.[11] Appearance of the neoplasm typically is preceded by a long period of progressively atypical cells.

Etiology

Bladder cancer has long been associated with industrial exposure to aromatic amines and certain dyes and pigments, with cancers appearing 15 to 40 years after exposure.[11] In the United States today, workplace exposures are minimized and tobacco is the most important risk factor.[34] In men, 80% of cases may be due to cigarette smoking.[11] Worldwide, the parasite *Schistosoma haematobium* accounts for many cases, particularly in areas such as Egypt where the condition is endemic.[34] Box 22-7 lists other risk factors.[11,14,34] The exact mechanism by which these factors induce neoplasia is not known.[11]

Clinical Manifestations

The clinical manifestation of bladder cancer usually is painless gross or microscopic hematuria. Less often, dysuria, urinary frequency, or urgency is seen. If the ureteral orifice is involved, pyelonephritis or hydronephrosis (distention of renal pelvis with urine) may follow. Other manifestations are rare until late in the course of the disease. About 70% of neoplasms are localized to the bladder when first discovered. Bladder cancers have a pronounced tendency to recur after excision.[11]

BOX 22-7 RISK FACTORS FOR BLADDER CANCER

Established Factors

Male gender
Age over 50 years
Urban dwelling
Industrialized country
Workplace exposure to aromatic amines or dyes and pigments used in textile, printing, paint, plastic, rubber, and cable industries
Tobacco use
Long-term use of phenacetin
Long-term use of cyclophosphamide
Chronic, recurrent nephrolithiasis
Recurrent upper respiratory tract infection
Bladder infection, with *Schistosoma haematobium*

Suggested Influences

Excessive coffee or caffeine use
Long-term use of saccharin or cyclamates
Chronic alcohol use
Hereditary predisposition

RENAL TUMORS

Many renal tumors are clinically silent and incidentally found at autopsy. They have been associated with genetic transmission, cigarette smoking, obesity, analgesic nephropathy, and cystic disease of the kidney. Renal tumors can cause damage to the renal parenchyma. Clinical manifestations are usually late in developing and may include hematuria or complaints of dull pain in the flank area. Palpable tumors are usually larger than those discovered on routine radiologic examination. Renal tumors are classified as (1) benign or malignant and (2) by area of involvement.

Benign Tumors

Cortical adenomas are the most common benign tumors of the kidneys. They are usually small (<2 cm in diameter) and asymptomatic. Many are found during postmortem examination of elderly people, although some are detected during surgery or radiologic examination. These adenomas are believed to originate from the tubular epithelium and may be difficult to distinguish histologically from renal cell carcinomas.[11] *Oncocytomas* are well-encapsulated benign tumors composed of large eosinophilic cells. They are derived from proximal tubular epithelial cells. They may grow to a large size, and biopsy is essential to differentiate them from renal cell carcinomas.[11] Clinical manifestations of large tumors are similar to other forms of renal tumors and include flank pain and hematuria.

Hamartomas or *angiomyolipomas* are rare benign tumors composed of vascular, smooth muscle, and adipose tissues. They are often seen in persons with tuberous sclerosis, a syndrome of cerebral cortex lesions, epilepsy, mental retardation, and skin abnormalities.[11]

Malignant Tumors

Renal cell carcinomas, Wilms' tumor, and tumors of the renal pelvis are malignant tumors of the renal system. Generally renal cell carcinomas and tumors of the renal pelvis are considered adult cancers, whereas Wilms' tumor is considered an embryonic kidney tumor.

RENAL CELL CARCINOMAS. Renal cell carcinomas account for 85% to 90% of tumors of the kidney. Renal carcinomas develop in nearly two-thirds of persons with *von Hippel-Lindau disease*, a hereditary disorder involving angiomas of the retina and cerebellum. Box 22-8 lists other risk factors for renal cell carcinomas.[11,14,34]

Renal carcinomas arise from tubular epithelium and can occur anywhere in the kidney. They vary in size from a few to several centimeters. The tumor margins are usually clearly defined, and the tumors include areas of ischemia, necrosis, and focal hemorrhage. Tumor cells vary from well differentiated to very anaplastic. They may proliferate throughout the kidneys, hilum, and ureters. These tumors tend to invade the renal vein, and a continuous cord of tumor cells may even extend through the vena cava to the right side of the heart. Renal cell carcinomas may grow to a large size without producing symptoms.[11] A third have metastasized by the time they are first detected.[34] They typically spread by vascular routes to the lungs, bone, lymph nodes, liver, and brain.

Renal cell carcinomas often produce hormones or hormone-like substances such as erythropoietin, parathyroid-like hormone, renin, gonadotropins, and glucocorticosteroids.[11] These secretions produce *paraneoplastic syndromes,* which may be the first indications of disease. The behavior of the tumors is unpredictable; rapid growth and metastases may be followed by years of slow growth. Clinical manifestations are variable; microscopic or macroscopic hematuria is the most consistent.[34] Other manifestations include flank pain, fever, weight loss, and a palpable mass. The combination of hematuria, flank pain, and palpable mass is labeled "the classic triad" but appears in fewer than 10% of cases.[11,34] As noted in Table 22-6, prognosis is based on several factors, including staging, the number of metastases, cell type, and size of the tumor.[34]

WILMS' TUMOR. **Wilms' tumor** is a malignant tumor that occurs primarily in children between 2 and 5 years of age.[11,34] The risk for developing the tumor is associated with at least three syndromes of congenital

BOX 22-8

RISK FACTORS FOR RENAL CELL CARCINOMA

Von Hippel-Lindau disease
Family history of renal cell carcinoma
Male gender
Age over 50 years
Tobacco use
Obesity
Excessive use of phenacetin
Dialysis-associated cystic disease
Adult polycystic kidney disease
Exposure to Thorotrast contrast medium
Occupational exposure to:
- Asbestos
- Cadmium
- Leather tanning
- Gasoline or other petroleum products

TABLE 22-6

PROGNOSIS FOR RENAL CELL CARCINOMA

DESCRIPTION OF TUMOR	TNM STAGE	T	N	M	5-YEAR SURVIVAL (%)
Confined to renal parenchyma	I	1	0	0	66–88
Confined to renal parenchyma	II	2	0	0	66–88
Invades perinephric fat	III	3a	1	0	47–68
Invades renal vein or vena cava	III	3b	1	0	35–60
In regional lymph nodes	III	1–3	1–3	0	15–30
In adjacent or distant organs	IV	4 Any T	1–3 Any N	1	2–13

T, tumor; N, node; M, metastasis
(Adapted from DeVita, V. T., Hellman, S., & Rosenberg, S. A. [1993]. *Cancer: Principles and practice of oncology* [4th ed.]. Philadelphia: Lippincott.)

malformation. Risk has also been tied to defects in at least two different chromosomal loci, with evidence of involvement of a third locus.[11]

By the time the tumor is discovered, a very large abdominal mass is often palpable. Symptoms may include microscopic hematuria, pain, fever, vomiting, and hypertension resulting from renal ischemia. Pulmonary metastasis is often present at the time of diagnosis.[11,34]

Wilms' tumors usually are well circumscribed and frequently have necrotic, cystic, and hemorrhagic areas. Tumors may be bilateral. Histologically, they contain proliferating embryonic connective tissue. The glomeruli and tubules are primitive.[11] Numerous factors determine the prognosis for this tumor, but long-term survival rates are up to 90% with treatment by chemotherapy, radiotherapy, and surgery.[11,34]

TUMORS OF THE RENAL PELVIS. Tumors of the renal pelvis account for 5% to 10% of primary renal tumors.[11] Almost 90% are transitional cell carcinomas, but as with bladder cancer, it is often difficult to distinguish benign from malignant tumors.[11,14] Risk factors for carcinoma of the renal pelvis include analgesia-induced nephropathy, in addition to those for bladder cancer.[14] These tumors produce hematuria early and so are usually small when discovered. However, infiltration of the pelvic wall and renal calices is common, as is renal vein involvement. Hence, the prognosis is often poor despite the small size of the tumor.[11,14]

RENAL FAILURE AND UREMIA

Renal failure occurs when the kidneys are unable to remove the waste products of metabolism from the blood. It can occur abruptly, as in *acute renal failure* (ARF), or over a long period, as in *chronic renal failure* (CRF).[9] Renal failure causes alterations in electrolyte, acid-base, and water balance and the accumulation of substances normally excreted by the body. These alterations can result in **uremia**, a toxic condition that affects all body systems.

Acute Renal Failure

Acute renal failure (ARF) is a fairly common, and often reversible, complication of acute illness. ARF is characterized by **azotemia**, the accumulation of nitrogenous waste products in the blood. *Oliguria* (urine output of less than 400 mL per 24 hours) or *anuria* (no urine production) occurs in about half of patients.[7,30]

ARF occurs when there is sudden suppression of kidney function. It can result from many different causes, which are categorized as (1) prerenal, (2) intrarenal/intrinsic, and (3) postrenal obstructive diseases. The etiologic basis of each of these is listed in Box 22-9.[7,28]

BOX 22-9

ETIOLOGY OF ACUTE RENAL FAILURE

Prerenal

- Hypovolemia
  - Hemorrhage
  - Skin/wound losses
  - GI losses
  - Renal losses
  - Extravascular pooling
  - Inadequate intake
- Low cardiac output/hypotension
  - Dysrhythmias
  - CHF
  - Myocardial disease
  - Valvular disease
  - Cardiac tamponade
  - Pulmonary embolism
  - Positive-pressure mechanical ventilation
  - Sepsis
  - Anaphylaxis
  - Shock
  - Liver failure
  - Anesthesia
- Renal hypoperfusion/vasoconstriction
  - Arterial embolism
  - Aortic or renal artery aneurysm
  - Norepinephrine, epinephrine
  - Hypercalcemia

Intrarenal/Intrinsic

- Glomerular/microvascular injury
  - Glomerulonephritis
  - DIC
  - Vasculitis
  - Hypertension
  - Toxemia of pregnancy
- Interstitial nephritis
  - Toxic
  - Metabolic imbalances
  - Infective
- Acute tubular necrosis
  - Ischemic
  - Nephrotoxic
- Renal transplant rejection

Postrenal Obstructive

- Ureteral obstruction
  - Calculi
  - Clots
  - Neoplasms
  - External compression
- Urethral obstruction
  - Prostatitis
  - Prostatic hyperplasia
  - Clots
  - Calculi
  - Neoplasms
  - Phimosis
  - Stricture
  - Foreign objects
- Venous occlusion
  - Thrombosis
  - Neoplasm

Prerenal disease ARF refers to conditions that diminish renal perfusion pressure. *Intrarenal ARF* results from acute parenchymal changes that damage the nephrons. *Postrenal obstructive ARF* includes conditions that obstruct excretion of normally formed urine. Either prerenal or postrenal ARF can evolve into intrarenal ARF. For example, renal ischemia (prerenal) that lasts more than a few hours can damage tubular epithelial cells, leading to intrarenal ARF. Ischemia is the most common cause of ARF. Acute tubular necrosis (discussed earlier in this chapter), which may result from either ischemia or nephrotoxicity, is the most common form of ARF.

PATHOPHYSIOLOGY

Depending on the cause, several different pathophysiologic mechanisms may operate in ARF. These include (1) tubular obstruction, (2) back-leak of filtrate through damaged tubules, and (3) hemodynamic (vascular) alterations.[23] Oliguria due to tubular abnormality is believed to result from either back-leakage or intratubular obstruction. The underlying process results in the renal injury, leading to acute suppression of renal function.

Tubular Obstruction

Tubular factors are primary elements in renal insufficiency, as shown in Flowchart 22-3.[30] *Tubular obstruction* may be caused by casts, debris, or interstitial edema. It can occur as a result of tubular ischemia, which causes swelling and necrosis of the tubular cells. The necrotic cells are sloughed off, causing obstruction of the tubules and increased pressure in Bowman's capsule. This pressure opposes the glomerular hydrostatic pressure and results in a decreased GFR. Oliguria results and may progress to anuria. There is also impairment of the ability to excrete urea, creatinine, potassium, sodium, and water.

Back Leak Theory of Increased Permeability

The *back-leak theory of increased permeability* proposes that oliguria sometimes is caused by disruption of tubular epithelium, rather than a decrease in GFR. This abnormality allows substances to be reabsorbed from the tubular lumen and interstitium into the peritubular circulation.

Hemodynamic Alterations

Oliguria also may result from vascular changes, especially renal artery vasoconstriction. In early stages of ARF, vasoconstriction occurs in the renal cortex, causing a reduction in GFR and leading to oliguria. The renin–angiotensin–aldosterone system also may contribute to the vasoconstriction and oliguria. Renin is released when renal perfusion pressure is low, causing conversion of angiotensinogen to angiotensin and ultimately leading to vasoconstriction (see Flowchart 22-3).

FLOWCHART 22-3 **Results of Damage to Renal Tubules**

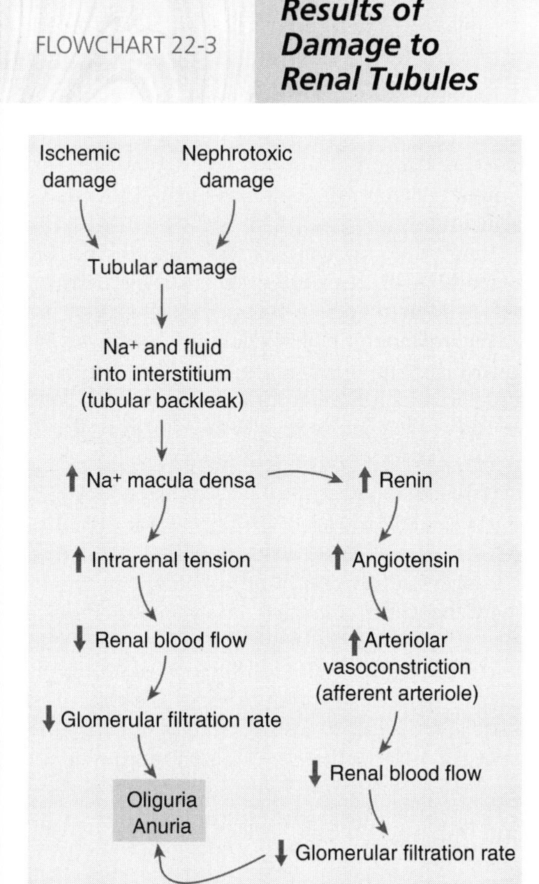

Damage to the renal tubules may be produced by ischemic or nephrotoxic damage. Tubular damage can lead to decreased glomerulofiltration through increased intrarenal tension and decreased blood flow.

The arterial vasoconstriction also may be enhanced by the loss of the vasodilatory effects of some prostaglandins.[11] Autoregulation normally retains blood flow through the kidneys and prevents tubular necrosis, partly through the effects of prostaglandins. With persistent vasoconstriction, this mechanism may be lost. The GFR is sometimes decreased out of proportion to renal blood flow in ARF. This may be due to loss of renal autoregulation and disruption of the renin–angiotensin–aldosterone system.

STAGES OF ACUTE RENAL FAILURE

The course of ARF can vary tremendously. The three stages of ARF are the same as discussed earlier with ATN: initiation, maintenance, and recovery.

Initiation Stage

The *initiation stage* begins with the event that initiates suppression of renal function. The course of ARF is related to the magnitude of the initiating insult and the length of time that renal hemodynamics and cellular dynamics are altered. Survival also depends on the extent of damage to other body systems by the initiating insult.[11]

Maintenance Stage

The *maintenance stage* is characterized by electrolyte imbalances and, typically, oliguria. Urine specific gravity often remains at about 1.010, which is the same as plasma. Water excess may result from administration of fluids during the initiation stage or from water produced during fat catabolism. Hyponatremia is caused by dilution of extracellular fluid with excess water. Elevations of potassium, creatinine, phosphate, and urea result from breakdown of muscle protein and renal inability to excrete metabolites. Metabolic acidosis results from impaired excretion of hydrogen by the kidneys. After 2 to 3 days of ARF, most persons develop moderate to severe anemia because of suppressed erythropoiesis (probably caused by lack of erythropoietin and uremic toxins).

Recovery Stage

The *recovery stage* is characterized by gradually increasing urine output and normalizing laboratory values. Diuresis may begin as early as 24 hours after the onset of ARF, or much later. Despite the increased output (as much as 6 L/day), tubular function remains impaired. Serum urea, creatinine, and other accumulated substances continue to rise during the first days of diuresis and act as osmotic diuretics. Large amounts of sodium and potassium are lost in urine. Dehydration may occur as a result of the inability to conserve water. Wide fluctuations in fluid and electrolyte balance are common during this stage. Recovery is gradual, with GFR, renal blood flow, and tubular function improvement occurring over a 6- to 12-month period.

Chronic Renal Failure

Chronic renal failure (CRF) is a slowly progressive condition characterized by irreversible reduction in the GFR and renal impairment. The conditions that cause CRF (Box 22-10) primarily affect the renal parenchyma, resulting in progressive damage to the nephrons and glomeruli.[6,8,37] This damage may be focal or diffused throughout the kidneys. CRF passes through four stages, which are identified in Table 22-7. In these stages there is progressive loss of nephrons, which leads to greater dysfunction and more difficulty in maintaining fluid and electrolyte balance. Systemic effects ultimately occur in all of the organs of the body. The progression toward **uremia** (symptomatic end-stage renal failure) usually is gradual because it can be controlled by diet and fluid restrictions for long periods. When the kidneys can no longer maintain fluid and electrolyte balance, either dialysis therapy or transplantation is necessary for survival.

BOX 22-10 COMMON CAUSES OF CHRONIC RENAL FAILURE

Diabetic nephropathy
Hypertension
Vascular disease
Cystic renal disease
Chronic pyelonephritis
Tubulointerstitial disease
Chronic vesicoureteral reflux
Chronic obstruction
Chronic glomerulonephritis (from many causes; see Fig. 22-2)

PATHOPHYSIOLOGY

The renal impairment in CRF is due to a decrease in the number of correctly functioning nephrons, rather than the number of diseased nephrons.[25] A crucial feature of this intact nephron theory is that the balance between glomeruli and tubules must be maintained. As the nephrons receive more filtrate, they also must be able to reabsorb more to maintain the steady state.

The progressive nature of nephron loss accounts for the body's ability to maintain homeostasis in the early stages of CRF: renal reserve allows for compensatory increases in reabsorption and excretion. The number of functioning nephrons eventually declines to a level inadequate to sustain the homeostatic balance, and physiologic disruptions occur. Renal failure eventually results in uremia, a condition that affects all body systems. The pathophysiology of chronic renal failure is summarized in Flowchart 22-4 and discussed below.

FLUID IMBALANCE. Early in CRF, the kidneys lose the ability to concentrate urine appropriately, resulting in excess water loss. The solute load per nephron is increased, and normal solute concentration in the blood is maintained until the GRF is reduced to about 25% of normal or less.[25] Osmotic diuresis and dehydration may result. Loss of greater numbers of nephrons leads to inability to dilute urine. This results in *isosthenuria*, a condition in which urine and plasma have the same osmolality (about 1.010), called a *fixed specific gravity.* This indicates severe renal damage. Anuria and fluid overload may result when the GFR decreases to less than 5 mL/min.

SODIUM IMBALANCE. Sodium balance is a serious problem in CRF. Since damaged nephrons are unable to exchange sodium, the intact nephrons receive an excess, causing an excess amount to be excreted in the

TABLE 22-7

STAGES OF CHRONIC RENAL FAILURE

STAGE	DESCRIPTION
1. Decreased renal reserve	Homeostasis maintained; no symptoms; residual renal reserve 40% of normal
2. Renal insufficiency	Decreased ability to maintain homeostasis; mild azotemia and anemia; may be unable to concentrate urine and conserve H_2O; residual renal function 15%–40% of normal; GFR decreases to 20 mL/min (normal 100–120 mL/min)
3. Renal failure	Azotemia and anemia severe; nocturia, electrolyte and fluid disorders; residual renal function 5%–15% of normal
4. Uremia (end-stage renal disease)	No homeostasis; becomes symptomatic in many systems, residual renal function less than 5% of normal

GFR, glomerular filtration rate.

urine. This increased elimination is accompanied by osmotic diuresis, which may cause dehydration. Hyponatremia and dehydration may be exacerbated by vomiting and diarrhea. Careful sodium and water restriction may allow maintenance of sodium balance, however. If water intake is excessive, dilutional hyponatremia, edema, and weight gain may occur.[8] Since the damaged kidney is unable to respond quickly to changes in serum sodium, increased intake may cause hypernatremia, volume overload, and hypertension.[37]

POTASSIUM IMBALANCE. If water balance is maintained and metabolic acidosis is controlled, hyperkalemia seldom becomes a problem until end-stage renal failure. Potassium balance is believed to result from adaptations made to the increased potassium presented to each functioning nephron. The mechanism for maintaining potassium balance is not understood, but it may be related to enhanced aldosterone secretion. However, hyperkalemia may result from excessive intake of potassium, certain medications, hypercatabolic illness (infection), hyponatremia, or acute acidosis. El-

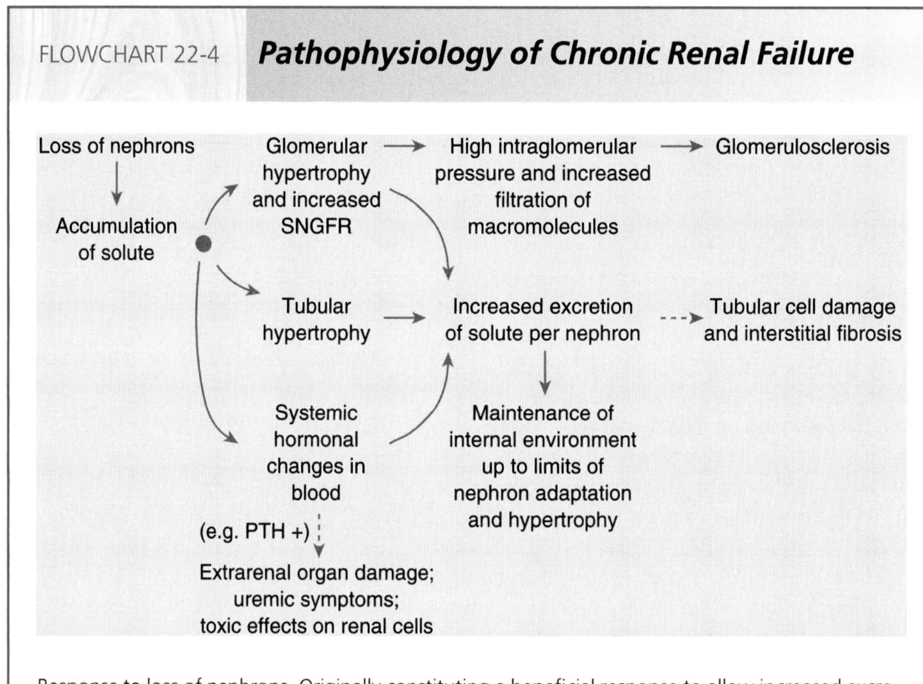

Response to loss of nephrons. Originally constituting a beneficial response to allow increased excretion through remaining intact nephrons, these changes ultimately lead to continuing nephron loss independent of the initial injury or disease (nephron trade-off). PTH, parathyroid hormone, SNGFR, single nephron glomerular filtration rate. (Stein, J. [Ed.] [1998]. *Internal medicine* [5th ed.]. St. Louis: C. V. Mosby.)

evated serum potassium also is characteristic of uremia or end-stage renal disease.

Hypokalemia is uncommon in CRF but can occur in association with inadequate intake, diuretic therapy, hyperaldosteronism, vomiting, excessive diarrhea, and renal tubular acidosis.[8] Hypokalemia further impairs the ability of the nephrons to concentrate urine.

ACID-BASE IMBALANCE. Metabolic acidosis develops in CRF because of loss of ability of the renal tubules to excrete hydrogen ions. Acids, which are continually being formed by metabolism, are not filtered as effectively through the GBM; the production of ammonia decreases, and the tubular cells become dysfunctional. Failure to form bicarbonate also may contribute to this imbalance. Part of the excess serum hydrogen is buffered by the bone salts. As a result, chronic metabolic acidosis increases the possibility of osteodystrophy.[8,11,37]

MAGNESIUM IMBALANCE. The magnesium level is normal in early CRF, but progressive reduction in urinary excretion may cause accumulation. A combination of decreased excretion and high intake (as from antacids) may cause neuromuscular depression and cardiac or respiratory arrest.[31,37]

PHOSPHORUS AND CALCIUM IMBALANCE. Normally, calcium and phosphorus levels are maintained by parathyroid hormone, which causes renal reabsorption of calcium by the kidneys, mobilization of calcium from bone, and depression of tubular reabsorption of phosphorus. Activated vitamin D enhances calcium absorption from the gastrointestinal tract. When renal function deteriorates to 20% to 25% of normal, less activated vitamin D is formed, leading to hypocalcemia. Hyperphosphatemia occurs due to decreased renal excretion. Hyperphosphatemia and hypocalcemia lead to secondary hyperparathyroidism. If prolonged, this results in a pattern of bone pathology called renal osteodystrophy, which is detailed in Flowchart 22-5.

ANEMIA. Anemia in CRF results from several factors, the most important of which is decreased erythropoeitin formation.[6,37] Uremic plasma shortens the lifespan of RBCs by impairing the ability of the cell membrane to pump sodium out, leading to swelling and hemolysis. Other factors that contribute to anemia include: (1) loss of RBCs through gastrointestinal ulceration, dialysis, and blood taken for laboratory analysis; (2) dialysis-induced folate deficiency; (3) iron deficiency; and (4) elevated levels of parathyroid hormone, which stimulates osteitis fibrosis (fibrous tissue replacing bone marrow).[4] This results in a normocytic, normochromic anemia, with hematocrits in the range of 15% to 30%.[6,8,37]

BLEEDING DISORDERS. Bleeding disorders are common in CRF and are mainly caused by thrombocytopenia or platelet dysfunction. As the nitrogenous wastes accumulate, there is increased risk of hemorrhage.

UREA AND CREATININE ALTERATIONS. Urea, a byproduct of protein metabolism, accumulates as renal function declines. The blood urea nitrogen (BUN) level is not an adequate indicator of renal disease because it may be elevated by other factors such as increased protein intake, shock, and dehydration. Serum creatinine level is a better indicator of renal function because urinary excretion of creatinine normally equals the amount produced in the body. With normal renal function, an increase of serum creatinine from 1 to 2 mg/dL represents a fall of GFR from 120 to 60 mL/min. With severe renal failure, plasma creatinine stabilizes at about 10 mg/dL.

The serum creatinine and BUN levels are referred to as *renal function studies*. If the BUN is elevated and the creatinine is normal, the source is not renal. Elevation of both values indicates renal dysfunction. Because BUN is formed by the liver as an end product of protein metabolism, it may be low in liver disease and it does not elevate in hepatorenal syndrome, but the creatinine does increase. These and other renal diagnostic studies are summarized in Unit 6 Appendix A.

CARBOHYDRATE INTOLERANCE. Carbohydrate intolerance can occur in persons with CRF. It may be caused by impaired renal clearance of insulin and peripheral resistance to insulin. Uremia toxins may interfere with the actions of insulin, and insulin binding is decreased in uremia. Insulin levels typically are normal or increased.[37]

UREMIC SYNDROME

Uremic syndrome represents the fourth stage of CRF, or end-stage renal disease (see Table 22-7). Uremia is associated with metabolic events and complications in all body systems. Urea is not the only toxin responsible for uremic syndrome; other accumulated metabolites and parathyroid hormone also contribute.[15] As noted in Figure 22-6, uremia affects all body systems.

Clinical Manifestations

The clinical manifestations of chronic renal failure involve all body systems. Unchecked, these culminate in uremic syndrome.

NEUROLOGIC ALTERATIONS. Some form of neuropathy occurs in at least 50% of all persons who have end-stage renal disease or are on long-term hemodialysis.[25] Peripheral neuropathy is common in CRF. It typically begins in the lower extremities and includes delayed sensory and motor responses, burning sensations, and numbness in the feet and legs. It may be generalized or occur in isolated areas. Complaints of a crawling sensation, prickling, or pruritus are common, as is discomfort and frequent movement of the legs (restless leg syndrome).[6] Autonomic dysfunction (e.g., hypotension or impotence) may be present with or without peripheral neuropathy. No specific uremic neurotoxin has been identified.[2]

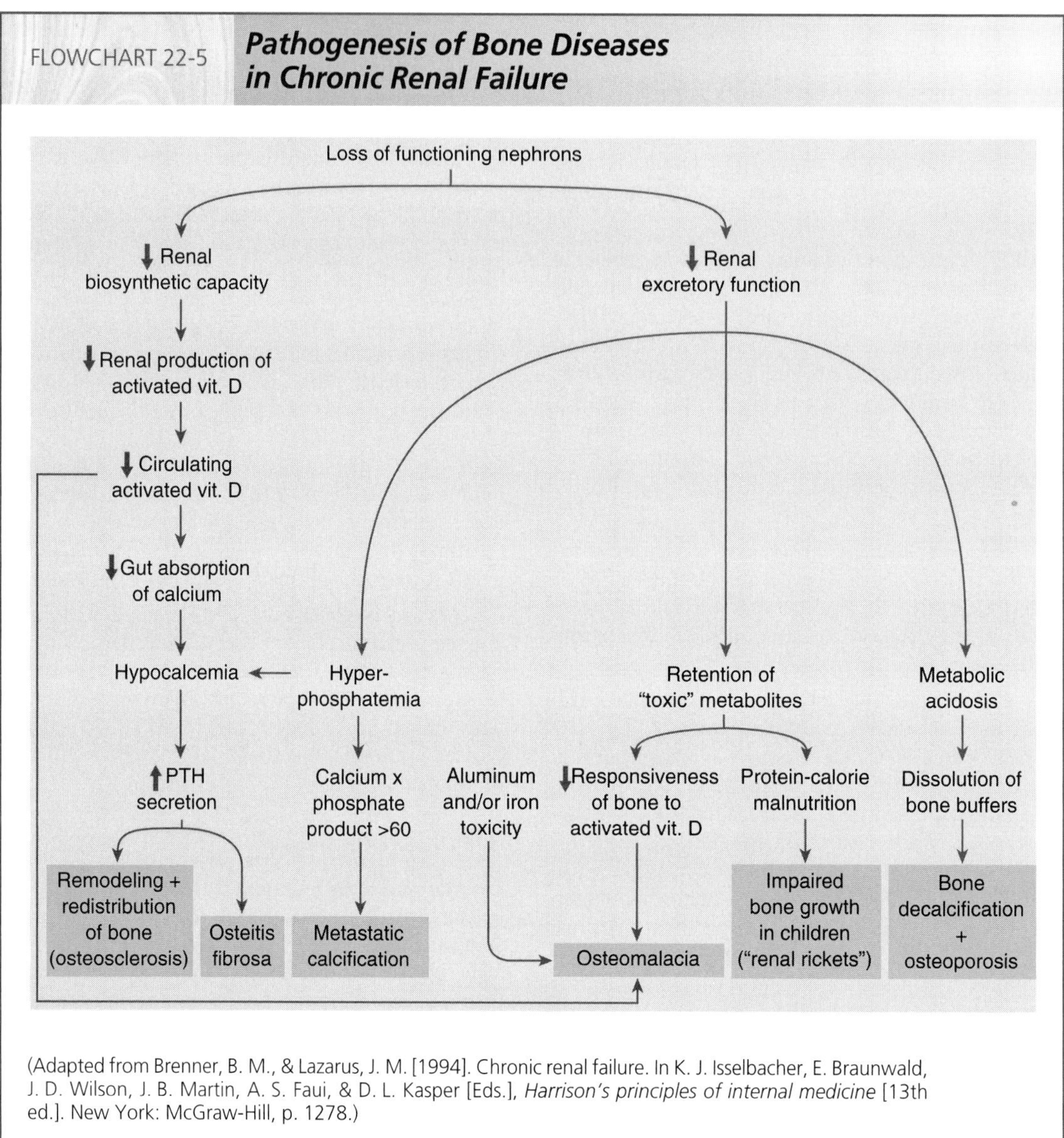

FLOWCHART 22-5 ***Pathogenesis of Bone Diseases in Chronic Renal Failure***

(Adapted from Brenner, B. M., & Lazarus, J. M. [1994]. Chronic renal failure. In K. J. Isselbacher, E. Braunwald, J. D. Wilson, J. B. Martin, A. S. Faui, & D. L. Kasper [Eds.], *Harrison's principles of internal medicine* [13th ed.]. New York: McGraw-Hill, p. 1278.)

As renal failure progresses, central nervous system effects develop, including drowsiness, sleep pattern disturbances, inability to concentrate, poor memory, hallucinations, seizures, and coma. This is sometimes called *uremic encephalopathy*. The alterations are believed to be related to a number of factors, including the accumulation of uremic toxins and parathyroid hormone, deficiency of ionized calcium in spinal fluid with retention of potassium and phosphates, hypertensive crises, and altered fluid loads.[6] Dialysis dementia is a progressive condition that affects some persons on long-term hemodialysis. The cause of the condition is unclear, but it has been linked with aluminum intoxication and, in the growing child, exposure of developing brain tissue to uremia. Personality changes, dementia, seizures, and death may result.[2,8]

CARDIOVASCULAR ALTERATIONS. Hypertension is present in most persons with uremia; it may result from vascular changes (nephrosclerosis), increased renin secretion, or fluid overload. Congestive heart failure and pulmonary edema may also result from fluid overload. Other cardiovascular diseases associated with uremia include stroke, accelerated atherosclerosis, myocardial infarction, cardiomyopathy, pericarditis, and cardiac tamponade. Pericarditis may be caused by the uremia, or it may result after dialysis.[6,37]

RESPIRATORY ALTERATIONS. In uremia, pulmonary congestion may occur even in the absence of fluid overload. This congestion shows a characteristic "bat wing" or "butterfly wing" pattern on radiologic examination. It is sometimes called *uremic lung* or *uremic pneumonitis*.[8,25] Pneumonia also is a major threat in

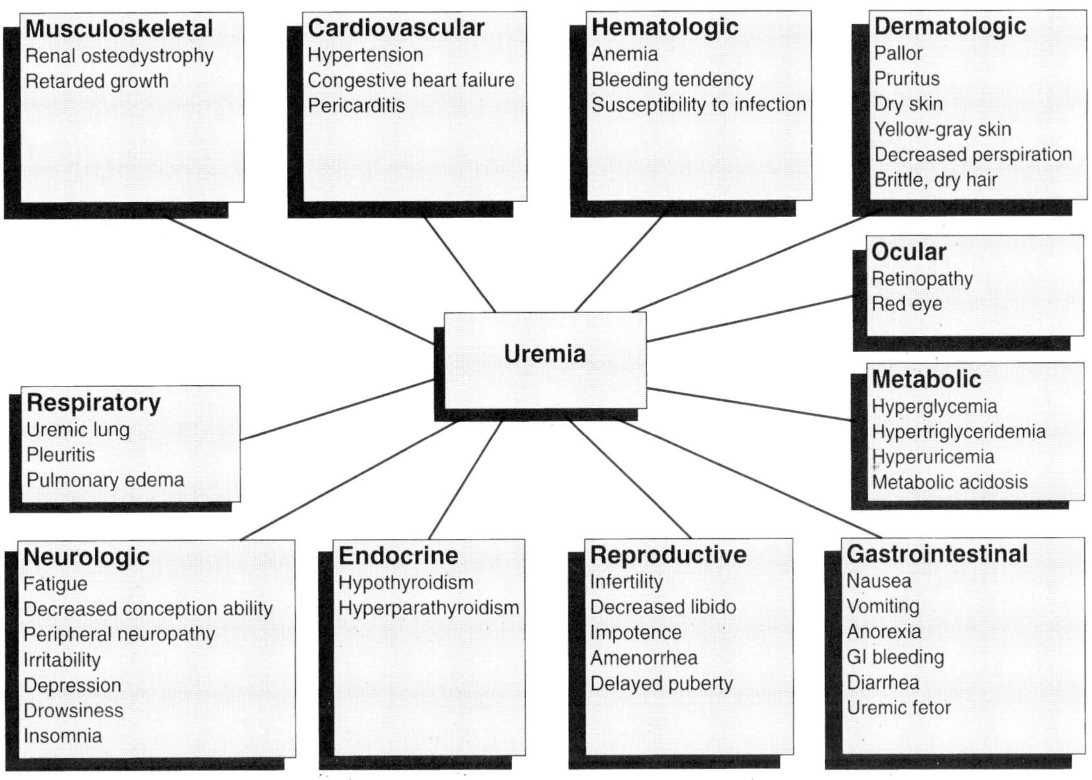

FIGURE 22-6. Uremia affects all body systems.

CRF because the uremic environment depresses the immune response.

GASTROINTESTINAL ALTERATIONS. Nausea, vomiting, hiccups, and anorexia are common in CRF. Their cause is not well understood, but they are related to the degree of uremia and may improve if hydration is maintained and protein restrictions are followed.[8] *Uremic fetor*, or urine breath, occurs when the salivary urea is broken down to ammonia, causing an unpleasant metallic taste. The oral mucosa often is dry, and the tongue is yellow-brown. Gastritis, peptic ulcer disease, esophagitis, colitis, and ulcers of the oral mucosa (uremic stomatitis) are common.[11] Gastrointestinal bleeding may result from ulcerations and capillary fragility.

MUSCULOSKELETAL ALTERATIONS. In uremia, faulty bone metabolism called **renal osteodystrophy** is caused by a combination of hyperparathyroidism, calcium and phosphorus alterations, decreased synthesis of the active form of vitamin D, and metabolic acidosis (see Flowchart 22-5). As noted earlier, these imbalances are common in CRF. Renal osteodystrophy develops in almost all persons with uremia and causes an increased tendency to spontaneous fractures.

Several bone lesions may result from renal osteodystrophy, including (1) osteomalacia, (2) osteitis fibrosa, (3) metastatic soft-tissue calcification, and (4) osteosclerosis. *Osteomalacia* is the accumulation of osteoid material after calcification has ceased, leading to soft, brittle bones. It may result from poor tissue use of vitamin D or from excess aluminum intake (e.g., from antacids).[6] *Osteitis fibrosa,* which occurs when fibrous tissue replaces bone tissue, may result from secondary hyperparathyroidism. Soft-tissue *metastatic calcification* refers to the deposition of calcium and phosphate crystals in the synovial tissues and soft tissues of the eyes, joints, muscles, and lungs. *Osteosclerosis* is caused by bone redistribution and remodeling and leads to increased bone density, mainly affecting the face, skull, and spine.

HEMATOLOGIC ALTERATIONS. In uremia, the normochromic, normocytic anemia typically seen in CRF becomes quite severe.[6,25] Coagulation disorders, caused by platelet defects, occur in most persons with uremia. This may cause a wide range of problems, including epistaxis, purpura, and hemorrhage with trauma or surgery.[6] Depressed immune response, particularly of phagocytosis, leads to a high incidence of serious infections in uremia.[25,37]

DERMATOLOGIC ALTERATIONS. The most common dermatologic disorders associated with uremia include pruritus, dry skin, and skin discoloration or pigmenta-

FOCUS ON THE PERSON WITH ABNORMAL KIDNEY FUNCTION

Ms. M. L., a 49-year-old secretary, was seen by her physician for complaints of fatigue, weight gain, and anorexia. She related a history of glomerulonephritis as a child with no apparent residual problems. Urinalysis showed marked proteinuria. Her blood pressure was 150/105 and serum creatinine was 4.1 mg/dL, with a blood urea nitrogen of 56 mg/dL.

Questions

1. If this condition is related to the glomerulonephritis seen in childhood, why did it manifest so many years later?
2. Describe the different types of glomerular diseases that may lead to this condition.
3. Describe the pathophysiology of the condition.
4. What measures can be utilized to delay the ultimate outcome of this condition?
5. What are appropriate treatments that may be used during the various stages?

See Appendix A for discussion.

FOCUS ON THE PERSON WITH DECREASED URINE OUTPUT

Ms. S. J. is a 20-year-old female who was brought to the emergency room in a comatose state following the ingestion of a large amount of barbiturate drugs and alcohol in an apparent suicide attempt. At the time of admission her blood pressure was 50/32, pulse weak and thready at 118, apneic and supported by ventilatory assistance. Despite routine therapeutic measures her blood pressure remained low during the first 36 hours after admission. Her renal output decreased from 20 mL/hour to 1–2 mL/hour. Serum creatinine became elevated to 5.2 mg/dL and blood urea nitrogen 76 mg/dL. Serum potassium climbed from 4.8 to 6.5 in this period of time.

Questions

1. As far as renal status is concerned, what is the apparent diagnosis of the problem described?
2. Describe, in detail, the pathophysiology of the diagnosis selected.
3. Considering the laboratory results, is there any emergent problem seen? If so, what is the danger and what should be done to prevent complications?
4. What are the possible ultimate outcomes of the condition described above?
5. Select some appropriate treatment options and indicate a rationale for their institution.

See Appendix A for discussion.

tion. Uremia is characterized by a sallow, yellow pigmentation of the skin due to the pallor of anemia combined with deposition of pigmented urochromes in the subcutaneous fat. Dryness of the skin, or xerosis, is caused by atrophy of the sweat glands and dehydration. *Uremic pruritus* (itching) is unexplained but possibly is related to excess parathyroid hormone, skin deposits, or peripheral neuropathy.[6] *Uremic frost* may occur in advanced uremia when the urea deposits are excreted in sweat and crystallize.

OTHER SYSTEM ALTERATIONS. Other organ and system alterations also occur. Uremia does not spare any system, so endocrine, reproductive, ocular, and other effects may be manifested; they are listed in Figure 22-6.

REFERENCES

1. Ahronheim, J. C. (1996). Special problems in the geriatric patient. In J. C. Bennett & F. Plum (Eds.), *Cecil textbook of medicine*. Philadelphia: W. B. Saunders.
2. Arieff, A. I. (1994). Neurologic manifestations of uremia. In B. M. Brenner & F. C. Rector (Eds.), *The kidney* (5th ed.). Philadelphia: Ardmore.
3. Albert, S., & Neilson, E. G. (1994). Tubulointerstitial diseases. In J. Stein (Ed.), *Internal medicine* (4th ed.). St. Louis: Mosby.
4. Anagnostou, A., & Kurtzman, M. A. (1994). Hematologic consequences of renal failure. In B. M. Brenner & F. C. Rector (Eds.), *The kidney* (5th ed.). Philadelphia: Ardmore.
5. Appel, G. B. (1996). Glomerular disorders. In J. C. Bennett & F. Plum (Eds.), *Cecil textbook of medicine*. Philadelphia: W. B. Saunders.
6. Black, R. M. (1996). *Rose & Black's clinical problems in nephrology*. Boston: Little, Brown.
7. Brady, H. R., & Brenner, B. M. (1994). Acute renal failure. In K. J. Isselbacher, E. Braunwald, J. D. Wilson, J. B. Martin, A. S. Faui, & D. L. Kasper (Eds.), *Harrison's principles of internal medicine* (13th ed.). New York: McGraw-Hill.
8. Brenner, B. M., & Lazarus, J. M. (1994). Chronic renal failure. In K. J. Isselbacher, E. Braunwald, J. D. Wilson, J. B. Martin, A. S. Faui, & D. L. Kasper (Eds.), *Harrison's principles of internal medicine* (13th ed.). New York: McGraw-Hill.
9. Coe, F. L. & Brenner, B. M. (1994). Approach to the patient with diseases of the kidneys and urinary tract. In K. J. Isselbacher, E. Braunwald, J. D. Wilson, J. B. Martin, A. S. Faui, & D. L. Kasper (Eds.), *Harrison's principles of internal medicine* (13th ed.). New York: McGraw-Hill.
10. Coe, F. L., & Favus, M. J. (1994). Disorders of stone formation. In B. M. Brenner & F. C. Rector (Eds.), *The kidney* (5th ed.). Philadelphia: Ardmore.
11. Cotran, R. S., Kumar, V., & Collins, J.(1999). *Robbins' pathologic basis of disease* (6th ed.). Philadelphia: W. B. Saunders.
12. Couser, W. C. (1994). Glomerular diseases. In J. Stein (Ed.), *Internal medicine* (4th ed.). St. Louis: Mosby.
13. Forland, M. Dysuria and frequency. In S. G. Massry & R. J. Glassock (Eds.), *Textbook of nephrology* (3rd ed.). Baltimore: Williams & Wilkins.
14. Garnick, M. B., & Brenner, B. M. (1994). Tumors of the urinary tract. In K. J. Isselbacher, E. Braunwald, J. D. Wilson, J. B. Martin, A. S. Faui, & D. L. Kasper (Eds.), *Harrison's principles of internal medicine* (13th ed.). New York: McGraw-Hill.

15. Greger, R. (1996). Introduction of renal function, renal blood flow and the formation of urine. In R. Greger & U. Windhorst (Eds.), *Comprehensive human physiology: From cellular mechanisms to integration.* New York: Springer.
16. Greger, R. (1996). Renal handling of the individual solutes of glomerular filtration. In R. Greger & U. Windhorst (Eds.), *Comprehensive human physiology: From cellular mechanisms to integration.* New York: Springer.
17. Harris, R. C., Meyer, T. W., & Brenner, B. M. (1994). Nephron adaptation to renal injury. In B. M. Brenner & F. C. Rector (Eds.), *The kidney* (5th ed.). Philadelphia: Ardmore.
18. Hostetter, T. H. & Brenner, B. M. (1994). Tubulointerstitial diseases of the kidney. In K. J. Isselbacher, E. Braunwald, J. D. Wilson, J. B. Martin, A. S. Faui, & D. L. Kasper (Eds.), *Harrison's principles of internal medicine* (13th ed.). New York: McGraw-Hill.
19. Hruska, K. (1996). Renal calculi (nephrolithiasis). In J. C. Bennett & F. Plum (Eds.), *Cecil textbook of medicine.* Philadelphia: W. B. Saunders.
20. Janig, W. (1996). Regulation of the lower urinary tract. In R. Greger & U. Windhorst (Eds.), *Comprehensive human physiology: From cellular mechanisms to integration.* New York: Springer.
21. Kaye, D., Tunkel, A. R., & Fournier, G. R. (1994). Urinary tract infections. In J. Stein (Ed.), *Internal medicine* (4th ed.). St. Louis: Mosby.
22. Kokko, J. P. (1996). Disorders of fluid, electrolyte, and acid-base balance. In J. C. Bennett & F. Plum (Eds.), *Cecil textbook of medicine.* Philadelphia: W. B. Saunders.
23. Kumar, S. & Stein, J. H. (1994). Acute renal failure. In J. Stein (Ed.), *Internal medicine* (4th ed.) St. Louis: Mosby.
24. Lemann, J. (1994). Nephrolithiasis. In J. Stein (Ed.), *Internal medicine* (4th ed.). St. Louis: Mosby.
25. Luke, R. G., & Strom, T. B. (1994). Chronic renal failure. In J. Stein (Ed.), *Internal medicine* (4th ed.). St. Louis: Mosby.
26. Martinez-Maldonado, M. (1996). Hereditary chronic nephropathies. In J. C. Bennett & F. Plum (Eds.), *Cecil textbook of medicine.* Philadelphia: W. B. Saunders.
27. McKinney, T. D. (1996). Tubulointerstitial diseases and toxic nephropathies. In J. C. Bennett & F. Plum (Eds.), *Cecil textbook of medicine.* Philadelphia: W. B. Saunders.
28. Mitch, W. E. (1996). Acute renal failure. In J. C. Bennett & F. Plum (Eds.), *Cecil textbook of medicine.* Philadelphia: W. B. Saunders.
29. O'Donnell, P. D. (1997). *Urinary incontinence.* St. Louis: Mosby.
30. Olsen, S. & Solez, K. (1994). Acute tubular necrosis and toxic renal injury. In C. G. Tisher & B. M. Brenner (Eds.), *Renal pathology with clinical and functional correlates* (2nd ed.). Philadelphia: J.B. Lippincott.
31. Quamme, G. A., & Dirks, J. H. (1994). Magnesium metabolism. In R. G. Narins, *Maxwell and Kleeman's clinical disorders of fluid and electrolyte metabolism* (5th ed.). New York: McGraw-Hill.
32. Rubin, R. H., Tolkoff-Rubin, N. E., & Cotran, R. S. (1994). Urinary tract infection, pyelonephritis, and reflux nephropathy. In B. M. Brenner & F. C. Rector (Eds.), *The kidney* (5th ed.). Philadelphia: Ardmore.
33. Sagalowsky, A. I., & Wilson, J. D. (1994). Hyperplasia and carcinoma of the prostate. In K. J. Isselbacher, E. Braunwald, J. D. Wilson, J. B. Martin, A. S. Faui, & D. L. Kasper (Eds.), *Harrison's principles of internal medicine* (13th ed.). New York: McGraw-Hill.
34. Shapiro, C. L., Garnick, M. B., & Kantoff, P. W. (1996). Tumors of the kidney, ureter, and bladder. In J. C. Bennett & F. Plum (Eds.), *Cecil textbook of medicine.* Philadelphia: W. B. Saunders.
35. Spargo, B. H., & Haas, M. (1994). The kidney. In E. Rubin & J. L. Farber, *Pathology* (2nd ed.). Philadelphia: J. B. Lippincott.
36. Steinberg, G. D., & Brendler, C. B. (1996). Diseases of the prostate. In J. C. Bennett & F. Plum (Eds.), *Cecil textbook of medicine.* Philadelphia: W. B. Saunders.
37. Warnock, D. G. (1996). Chronic renal failure. In J. C. Bennett & F. Plum (Eds.), *Cecil textbook of medicine.* Philadelphia: W. B. Saunders.

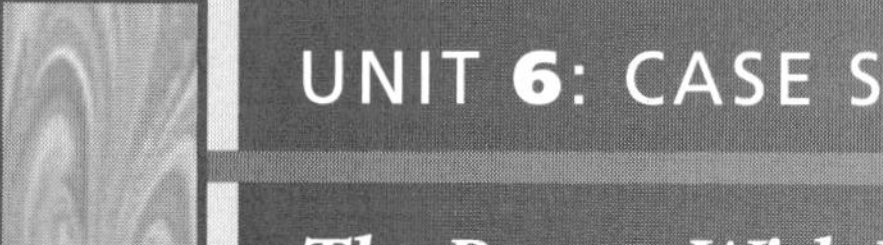

UNIT 6: CASE STUDY

The Person With Back Pain and Hematuria

Introduction to the Patient

J. K. is a 42-year-old male who arrives in the emergency department complaining of severe back pain off and on for the past 6 hours. He also reports difficulty urinating, stating that "It feels like I have to urinate, but then when I try, I only pass a small amount of urine and it has some blood in it."

Present Illness

Approximately 6 hours ago, Mr. K. noticed a sharp, stabbing pain in his lower left back that radiated to the left flank, abdomen, groin, and thigh. After approximately 20 minutes, the pain subsided but then reappeared about 2 hours later, just as severe. He complains of frequency and urgency, voiding only small amounts of reddish urine, with difficulty. He also reports some nausea and vomiting associated with the pain episodes and taking two doses of ibuprofen 400 mg with minimal relief.

Social History

Mr. K., a single male who lives alone, works full time for a construction company. He denies any history of tobacco or recreational drug use. He does report occasional social drinking, having "one or two beers after work, maybe two to three times a month with his buddies." J. K. states that he usually eats three meals a day and exercises regularly. His favorite foods are milk, ice cream, and cheese. "I love to have a dish of ice cream every night while watching television before I go to bed."

Past Medical History

J. K. states that he is in fairly good health, except for occasional sinus headaches relieved with over-the-counter pseudoephedrine and ibuprofen. He reports a previous episode of kidney stones approximately 5 years ago, which he was "able to pass." He denies any other previous history of medical problems. Prior to this episode, he had no complaints of difficulty voiding and his urine was clear yellow.

Family History

J. K. is the second of four children. He has an older brother, age 45, and two younger sisters, ages 38 and 35. All are alive and "relatively healthy." His brother and father have a history of kidney stones. His father required surgery (approximately 20 years ago) to remove two large stones from his kidney.

Physical Examination

J. K. is a well-developed, athletic male who appears pale and diaphoretic. He is oriented to person, place, and time. His vital signs are: temperature—99.2°F; pulse—96 and regular; respirations—22; blood pressure—128/78. Lungs are clear to auscultation. Abdomen is soft, slightly distended. Bowels sounds active in all four quadrants. No bruits heard on auscultation. Abdominal tenderness is noted in the left lower quadrant groin area. Slight left CVA tenderness is noted on palpation. Some dullness is present over the suprapubic area on percussion. Prostate examination unremarkable.

Diagnostic Tests

Urinalysis: reddish-brown urine; pH 8; positive for red blood cells, white blood cells, and crystals
Urine C&S: negative
Urine calcium level: elevated
Polarizing microscopy: positive for calcium oxalate crystals
Serum uric acid: 6.7 mg/dL
Serum BUN and creatinine: within normal limits
KUB: two 5-mm-sized opacities in left ureter
IVP: confirmation of findings of KUB; slight distention of left ureter proximal to opacities

CRITICAL THINKING QUESTIONS

1. Explain the underlying pathophysiologic mechanisms involved with J. K.'s complaints of pain and hematuria.
2. Describe the possible factors that may contribute to J. K.'s risk for renal calculi.
3. Propose possible strategies that might be used to relieve J. K.'s pain.
4. J. K. was discharged with a prescription for chlorthalidone (thiazide diuretic) to decrease intestinal calcium absorption and reduce renal excretion. Construct a list of instructions to include when teaching J. K. how to prevent a recurrence.

Besides your pathophysiology text, you'll need a good pharmacology text, a nephrology/urology text, a medical-surgical nursing text, and current research to complete this case study. Suggested references follow:

Goldfarb, S. (1999). Beverages, diet, and prevention of kidney stones. *American Journal of Kidney Diseases, 33*(2), 398–403.

Greenberg, A. (1998). *Primer on kidney diseases.* New York: Academic Press.

Herwig, K. (1996). Urinary stones: Hypercalciuria. In R. Rakel, *Saunders' manual of medical practice.* Philadelphia: W. B. Saunders.

Karch, A. M. (1999). *1999 Lippincott's nursing drug guide.* Philadelphia: Lippincott-Raven.

Marangella, M., Vitale, C., Bagnes, C., Bruno, M., & Ramillo, A. (1999). Idiopathic calcium nephrolithiasis. *Nephron, 81*(1), 38–44.

Smeltzer, S. & Bare, B. (2000). *Brunner and Suddarth's textbook of medical-surgical* nursing (9th ed.). Philadelphia: Lippincott Williams & Wilkins.

Website Resources:

Kidney Stones—Rocks that Don't Always Roll http://www.mayohealth.org/mayo/9706/htm/k_stones.htm

National Kidney Foundation http://www.kidney.org

Nephrolithiasis http://uhs.bsd.uchicago.edu/uhs/topics/nephro.html

UNIT 6 APPENDIX A

DIAGNOSTIC TESTS

TEST	PURPOSE/NORMAL FINDINGS	SIGNIFICANCE
Urinalysis	Routine method for evaluating kidney function and detecting conditions that might affect the kidney or urinary tract	Urinalysis is routinely done on admission and prior to elective surgery
	Normal findings:	
	Pale yellow to amber color	Nearly colorless urine may indicate a large fluid intake or chronic interstitial nephritis. Orange-colored urine may indicate concentrated urine. Some urinary tract medications may turn the urine orange. Red to reddish brown color may suggest hemoglobinuria. Brown to black urine may be a result of large amounts of hemoglobin in the urine. A smoky color may be indicative of red blood cells (RBCs) in the urine.
	Clear to slightly hazy appearance	Turbid urine is common with urinary tract infections (UTIs). However, hazy or turbid appearance may occur if the specimen has been refrigerated or left standing at room temperature. Semen or vaginal drainage, when mixed with urine, may cause it to appear turbid. Cloudy urine may result from a change in the urine pH, but this is not abnormal. Cloudy urine typically indicates RBCs, white blood cells (WBCs), or bacteria.
	pH ranging from 4.6 to 8 (average of 6)	pH less than 7 occurs with acidosis. pH greater than 7 may indicate UTI, renal tubular acidosis, or chronic renal failure. pH value must be evaluated in light of other diagnostic tests. pH increases if the specimen is left standing for a prolonged period of time.
	Negative for protein, glucose, ketones, and bacteria	Proteinuria usually results from an increased glomerular filtration rate secondary to glomerulonephritis. If persistent, it usually indicates some degree of renal disease such as glomerulonephritis, nephrosis, polycystic kidney disease, or chronic urinary tract obstruction. Increased glucose levels may indicate diabetes mellitus or inflammatory renal disease. Stress or excitement may result in false-positive glucosuria. Ketonuria may indicate metabolic disorders, such as diabetes or renal glycosuria; dietary problems, such as starvation or prolonged vomiting; or increased metabolic states such as fever or pregnancy. Twenty or more bacteria/high-power field (HPF) suggests UTI.
	Urine sediment: RBCs 0 to 2 /HPF without RBC casts	Increased RBCs may indicate pyelonephritis, cystitis, genitourinary tract conditions. RBC casts indicate hemorrhage secondary to acute inflammatory or vascular disorders of the glomerulus.

(continued)

UNIT 6 APPENDIX A **(Continued)**

DIAGNOSTIC TESTS

TEST	PURPOSE/NORMAL FINDINGS	SIGNIFICANCE
	WBC 0 to 4 /HPF without WBC casts	Increased WBCs indicate infection. WBC greater than 50/HPF suggest an acute bacterial infection. WBC casts suggest infection of the renal parenchyma with pyelonephritis as the most common cause.
	Epithelial cells 0 to 2	Squamous epithelial cells are found normally in urine. Large numbers of epithelial cells may suggest acute tubular damage, acute glomerulonephritis. If epithelial casts are found, they suggest damage to the tubular epithelium from nephrosis, glomerulonephritis, or acute tubular necrosis.
	Hyaline and granular casts 0 to 2 /low-power field (LPF); negative for waxy casts	Hyaline casts suggest damage to the capillary membrane of the glomerulus. Granular casts may indicate acute tubular necrosis, advanced glomerulonephritis, pyelonephritis, or malignant nephrosclerosis. Waxy casts indicate severe renal disease.
	Crystals variable with urine pH and temperature	Large amounts of calcium oxalate crystals may suggest chronic renal disease. Large amounts of calcium phosphate crystals may be seen with chronic cystitis, prostatic hypertrophy, or hyperparathyroidism. Large amounts of urate crystals occur with high serum uric acid levels (gout).
Urine specific gravity	Evaluation of concentration function of the kidneys measuring the number and size of the particles in the urine Normal findings: 1.001 to 1.035 (usual range of 1.010 to 1.025)	High values indicate concentrated urine such as with dehydration, SIADH, decreased renal blood flow, x-ray contrast media, and glycosuria. Low values support more dilute urine, such as with volume overload, diabetes insipidus, and acute tubular necrosis (ATN). In ATN, specific gravity becomes fixed near 1.010.
Urine culture and sensitivity (C&S)	Urine specimen collection into a sterile container for detecting specific organisms and identifying the organism's response to different antibiotics Normal findings: fewer than 10,000 bacteria/mL	Specimen contamination may be responsible for bacterial count. Counts of 100,000 bacteria/mL or more are strongly suggestive of a UTI. Specimens left standing at room temperature for prolonged periods may reveal an increased number of many different organisms.
Urine osmolality	Precise measurement of the exact urine concentration to evaluate the kidney's ability to concentrate and dilute urine; influenced by the number of particles present Normal finding: 300 to 900 mOsm/kg in 24 hours (or 50 to 1200 mOsm/kg in a random specimen)	Increased osmolality may suggest SIADH or hypernatremia. Decreased osmolality may indicate diabetes insipidus, hypokalemia, hypercalcemia, or ATN. Typically a serum osmolality is obtained at the same time to compare the ratio of urine to serum and provide more definitive information about renal function.
Urine electrolytes	Indication of the kidney's ability to regulate fluid and electrolyte balance; values vary greatly with dietary intake; large ranges may be seen	

(continued)

UNIT 6 APPENDIX A **(Continued)**

DIAGNOSTIC TESTS

TEST	PURPOSE/NORMAL FINDINGS	SIGNIFICANCE
	Normal findings:	
	Sodium: 40 to 220 mEq/L/24 hours	Increased urine sodium levels may suggest renal tubular acidosis or ATN. Decreased urine sodium levels may suggest nephrotic syndrome, pre-renal azotemia, or acute hypovolemia. Diuretics and caffeine may increase urine sodium levels.
	Potassium: 25 to 125 mEq/L/24 hours	Increased urine potassium levels may suggest primary renal disease. Decreased urine potassium levels may be seen with pyelonephritis and glomerulonephritis.
	Calcium: 100 to 300 mg/24 hours	Increased urine calcium levels may be seen with bladder cancer and renal tubular acidosis. With increased urine calcium levels, the patient's risk for nephrolithiasis increases.
	Magnesium: 6.0 to 10.0 mEq/24 hours	Decreased urine magnesium levels may suggest chronic renal disease. Thiazide diuretics may result in increased urine magnesium levels.
Serum creatinine	Evaluation of kidneys' ability to excrete creatinine, a breakdown product of muscle metabolism Normal findings: 0.6 to 1.3 mg/dL	Creatinine is a more specific and sensitive indicator of renal function. Increased creatinine levels may suggest impaired renal function, suggesting chronic nephritis or obstruction of the urinary tract. It also may be elevated in shock and severe dehydration.
Serum blood urea nitrogen (BUN)	Method to evaluate gross renal function by measuring urea (end-product of protein metabolism) levels excreted by the kidneys Normal findings: 7 to 18 mg/dL; 8 to 20 mg/dL (in adults over age 60)	Elevated BUN levels may suggest impaired renal function. Amount of BUN excreted varies with protein intake. Excessive protein intake or catabolism may increase BUN.
Creatinine clearance	Urine and serum specimens obtained to evaluate glomerular filtration Normal findings (mL/min/1.73m^2): dependent on sex and age: 20 to 30 yrs: 88–146 (male)/81–134 (female) 30 to 40 yrs: 82–140 (male)/75–128 (female) 40 to 50 yrs: 75–133 (male)/69–122 (female) 50 to 60 yrs: 68–126 (male)/64–116 (female) 70 to 80 yrs: 55–113 (male)/52–105 (female)	Decreased creatinine clearance suggests impaired renal function, intrinsic renal disease, glomerulonephritis, nephrotic syndrome, or acute tubular necrosis. Exercise and pregnancy may increase creatinine clearance levels. Numerous drugs such as barbiturates and thiazide diuretics may decrease creatinine clearance; others, such as aminoglycosides and cephalosporins, may increase creatinine clearance values.
Serum uric acid	Method to evaluate breakdown product of purine metabolism and the kidneys' ability to excrete it Normal finding: 3.5–7.2 mg/dL (male)/2.6–6.0 mg/dL (female)	Increased levels may be seen in renal disease, renal failure, gout, pre-renal azotemia, and leukemia. Most commonly, renal failure is associated with increased levels in patients who are hospitalized.
Prostate-specific antigen (PSA)	Measurement of a marker for evaluating prostatic cancer and effectiveness of treatment Normal findings: 04.0 ng/mL	In most patients with prostatic cancer, PSA is increased. PSA is found in both normal epithelial and cancerous cells of the prostate. Levels of 4–8 ng/dL suggest benign prostatic hypertrophy. Values greater than 8 ng/dL are highly suggestive of prostatic cancer.

(continued)

UNIT 6 APPENDIX A **(Continued)**

DIAGNOSTIC TESTS

TEST	PURPOSE/NORMAL FINDINGS	SIGNIFICANCE
Kidneys, ureters and bladder (KUB)	Radiographic depiction of the size, shape, and position of the structures to detect any abnormalities or displacement Normal findings: structures of normal size, shape and position; no displacement seen	Calculi may be visible even if ureters are not clearly seen. Urinary bladder typically casts a shadow on the film.
Intravenous urography (IVU; excretory urography or intravenous pyelography [IVP])	Set of x-rays under fluoroscopy taken at predetermined intervals following intravenous injection of contrast medium Normal findings: • Urinary structures normal in shape, size, and position • Kidney outline appearing within 2 to 5 minutes after injection of contrast medium • Renal pelvis visualized 5 to 7 minutes after injection • Ureter and bladder seen as contrast medium enters lower urinary tract • No residual urine noted in post-voiding x-ray	Length of time for contrast medium to first appear and then be excreted determines renal function. A delay in noting contrast medium suggests renal dysfunction. Contrast medium not appearing suggests poor or absent renal function. Stones, abnormalities in size, shape, or position, or tumors may be revealed. Enlargement may suggest obstruction or polycystic disease. Normal-sized kidney in the presence of renal failure suggests an acute process. Irregular scarring may indicate chronic pyelonephritis.
Renal ultrasound	Use of high-frequency sound waves to visualize kidney parenchyma and other structures, including renal blood vessels Normal finding: normal image pattern reflecting normal size and position of the kidneys	Ultrasound provides differentiation between bilateral hydronephrosis, polycystic kidney disease, and small end-stage changes from glomerulonephritis or pyelonephritis. Fluid collections such as abscesses or hematomas may be seen. Solid masses can be differentiated from cystic masses.
Computed tomography (CT) and magnetic resonance imaging (MRI)	Visualization of abnormalities not readily seen on routine x-rays; provide a three-dimensional view of the structures Normal findings: air appearing black; bone appearing white; soft tissue appearing gray with shading correlating to tissue density	Special contrast medium is usually administered prior to test to allow visualization of the bowel and help differentiate it from other structures. Clearly defined area of consistent density suggests an encapsulated tumor.
Renal scan	Use of intravenously injected radioisotopes and imaging to evaluate blood flow, structure, and/or function Normal findings: • Normal blood flow bilaterally with blood flow equal in both kidneys • Normal shape, size, position, and function • 50% of radioisotope excreted in 10 minutes	Increased blood flow to a vascular tumor or decreased blood flow secondary to transplant rejection may be seen. Cold areas may indicate tumor, cyst, or abscess.
Renal angiography	Visualization of renal arteries via x-ray after injection of contrast medium via catheter inserted into a major artery Normal finding: blood flow dynamic with intact vasculature; negative for narrowing, obstruction, or occlusion	Renal cysts can be differentiated from renal tumors. Abnormalities in vessel structure such as narrowing or occlusion may be revealed. The study can be used to screen for renovascular hypertension.
Cystoscopy	Endoscopic exam of the lower urinary tract providing views of the interior bladder, urethra, prostatic urethra, and ureteral orifices Normal findings: normal structure and function of the bladder, urethra, and orifices	This test may be used to crush or retrieve small stones or other material from the urethra, ureters, and bladder or to open strictures and fulgurate bladder tumors. Retrograde pyelography (contrast medium introduced via ureteral catheter inserted into the renal pelvis through the ureters) is

(continued)

UNIT 6 APPENDIX A **(Continued)**

DIAGNOSTIC TESTS

TEST	PURPOSE/NORMAL FINDINGS	SIGNIFICANCE
		often performed in conjunction to evaluate the collecting system and detect possible ureteral obstruction. A brash biopsy also may be done to collect cells for histologic examination.
Urodynamic studies	Series of procedures to evaluate the motor and sensory function of the bladder (the neuroanatomic connections between the brain, spinal cord, and bladder), specifically the detrusor muscle and external sphincter reflex: • Uroflowmetry (determination of the volume of urine passing through the urethra per minute) • Cystometrogram (graphic recording of pressures in the bladder at various phases of filling and emptying in conjunction with the patient's sensations of fullness and need to void) • Urethral pressure profile (measurement of urethral pressure along the length of the urethra) • Cystourethrogram (visualization of the urethra and bladder for evaluation of stress incontinence and bladder wall or urethral abnormalities) • Rectal electromyogram (EMG) (evaluation of neuromuscular function using electrodes placed near the anus or pelvic floor musculature) Normal findings: • Reports of sensation of fullness, heat, and cold • Bladder capacity of 400 to 500 mL; residual urine less than 30 mL • First desire to void at 175–250 mL, with fullness sensed at 350–450 mL • Strong, uninterrupted urine stream on voiding • Low voiding pressures • Ability to suppress detrusor reflex on command • Normal urethral closing mechanism with normal rectal EMG readings	Vesical sphincter incoordination is the most common cause of incontinence. Benign prostatic hypertrophy may be indicated by urethrovesical hyperreflexia. Absence of residual urine after voiding and difficulty initiating voiding may indicate detrusor areflexia. In post-menopausal women, urethral pressure profile may be abnormal secondary to lack of estrogen to mucosal sphincter.
Renal biopsy	Tissue specimen obtained via open (nephrostomy) or closed technique to evaluate for malignant cells Normal findings: no evidence of malignant cells	Tissue type and definitive data about the lesion are provided to guide treatment.

UNIT BIBLIOGRAPHY

Agency for Health Care Policy and Research (1996). *Clinical practice guideline number 2: Urinary incontinence in adults: Acute and chronic management.* Rockville, MD: U.S. Department of Health and Human Services.

Agency for Health Care Policy and Research (1994). *Clinical practice guideline: Benign prostatic hyperplasia: Diagnosis and treatment.* Rockville, MD: U.S. Department of Health and Human Services.

Brenner, B. M. & Rector, F. C. (Ed.) (1996). *Brenner and Rector's the kidney* (5th ed.). Philadelphia: W. B. Saunders.

Cantanzaro, J. (1996) Managing incontinence. An update. *RN, 59*(10), 38–44.

Churg, J., Bernstein, J. & Glassock, R. J. (1995). *Glomerular diseases* (2nd ed.). New York: Igaku-Shoin.

Crowley, L. V. (1997) *Introduction to human disease* (4th ed.). Boston: Jones and Bartlett.

Ferris, T. F. (1994) Renal diseases and hypertension. In J. A. Barondess & C. C. Carpenter (Eds.), *Differential diagnosis.* Philadelphia: Lea & Febinger.

Gillenwater, J. Y., Grayhack, J. T., Howards, S. S., & Duckett, J. W. (Eds.) (1996). *Adult and pediatric urology* (3rd ed.). Baltimore: Mosby.

Greenberg, A. (Ed.) (1998). *Primer on kidney diseases* (2nd ed.). San Diego: Academic Press.

King, B. (1997). Preserving renal function. *RN, 60*(8), 34–39.

Kobrin, S. & Aradhey, S. (1997). Preventing progression and complications of renal disease. *Hospital Medicine, 33*(11), 11–12, 17–18, 20, 29–31, 35–36, 39–40.

Koeppen, B. M. & Stanton, B. A. (1997). *Renal pathophysiology* (2nd ed.). St. Louis: Mosby–Year Books.

Kopple, J. D. & Massry, S. G. (Eds.) (1997). *Nutritional management of renal diseases.* Baltimore: Williams & Wilkins.

Krane, R. J., Fitzpatrick, M., & Siroky, J. M. (1994). *Clinical urology.* Philadelphia: J.B. Lippincott.

Massry, S. G. & Glassock, R. J. (Eds.) (1995). *Textbook of nephrology* (3rd ed.). Baltimore: Williams & Wilkins.

Murphy, W. M. (1997). *Urological pathology* (2nd ed.). Philadelphia: W. B. Saunders.

Narins, R. G. (1994). *Maxwell and Kleeman's clinical disorders of fluid and electrolyte metabolism* (5th ed.). New York: McGraw-Hill.

Neilson, E. G. & William, G. C. (Eds.) (1997). *Immunologic renal diseases,* Philadelphia: Lippincott-Raven.

O'Donnell, P. D. (Ed.) (1994). *Geriatric urology.* Boston: Little, Brown.

Raz, S. (Ed.) (1996). *Female urology* (2nd ed.). Philadelphia: W. B. Saunders.

Rose, B. D. & Rennke, H. G. (1994). *Renal pathophysiology: The essentials.* Baltimore: Williams & Wilkins.

Ross, L. M. (Ed.) (1997). *Kidney and urinary tract diseases and disorders sourcebook.* Detroit, MI: Omnigraphics.

Rubin, E., & Farber, J. L. (1999) *Pathology* (3rd ed.). Philadelphia: Lippincott Williams & Wilkins.

Sant, G. R. (1994). *Pathophysiologic principles of urology.* Boston: Blackwell Scientific Publications.

Schrier, R. W. (Ed.) (1997). *Renal and electrolyte disorders* (4th ed.). Philadelphia: Lippincott.

Schrier, R. W. & Gottschalk, C. W. (Eds.) (1997). *Diseases of the kidney* (6th ed.). Boston: Little, Brown.

Stein, J. (Ed.) (1994). *Internal medicine* (4th ed.). St. Louis: Mosby.

Stockert, P. (1999). Getting UTI patients back on track. *RN, 62*(3), 49–54.

Suki, W. N. & Massry, S. G. (Eds.) (1997). *Suki and Massry's therapy of renal diseases and related disorders* (3rd ed.). Boston: Kluwar Academic Press.

Tamparo, C. D. & Lewis, M. A. (1995). *Diseases of the human body.* Philadelphia: F. A. Davis.

Tischer, C., & Brenner, B. M. (1999). *Renal pathology with clinical and functional correlations* (2nd ed.). Philadelphia: J. B. Lippincott.

Toto, K. H. (1996). The kidney in multiple organ dysfunction syndroms. In V. H. Secor (Ed.), *Multiple organ dysfunction & failure: Pathophysiology and clinical implications.* St. Louis: Mosby.

Watson, M. L. & Torres, V. E. (Eds.) (1996). *Polycystic kidney diseases.* New York: Oxford University Press.

CANCER

Ernstoff, M. S., Heaney, J. A. & Peschel, R. E. (Eds.) (1997). *Urologic cancer.* Cambridge, MA: Blackwell Scientific.

McKinney, B. (1996). When this rare cancer strikes. *RN, 59*(12), 36–40.

Oesterling, J. E. & Richie, J. P. (Eds.) (1997). *Urologic oncology.* Philadelphia: W.B. Saunders.

Vogelzany, W. J., Shipley, W. U., Scardino, P. T. & Coffes, D. S. (Eds.) (1996). *Comprehensive textbook of genitourinary oncology.* Baltimore: Williams & Wilkins.

KIDNEY STONES

Coe, F. L., Favus, M. J., Pak, C. Y, Parks, J. H., & Preminger, G. M. (Eds.) (1996). *Kidney stones: Medical and surgical managements.* Philadelphia: Lippincott-Raven.

Singer, A. J. (1995). Pitfalls in the diagnosis of urolithiasis. *Infections in Urology.* 8(4), 102, 125.

Sosa, R. E. & Martin, T. V. (1996). Critical challenges of renal calculi in women. *Medscape Women's Health, 1*(8).

Wehle, M. J. & Segura, J. W. (1998). Acute ureteral stones: Clues to the diagnosis and initial treatment. *Hospital Medicine, 34* (5), 47–48, 51–55.

RENAL FAILURE

Cameron, J. S. (1996). *Kidney failure.* New York: Oxford University Press.

Jacobs, C., Kjellstrand, C. M., Koch, K. M., & Winchester, J. F. (Eds.) (1996). *Replacement of renal function by dialysis* (4th ed.). Boston: Kluwer Academic Press.

Kelly, M. (1997). Clinical snapshot: Acute renal failure. *American Journal of Nursing, 97*(3), 32–33.

McGee, H. M. & Bradly, C. (Eds.) (1994). *Quality of life following renal failure: Psychosocial challenges accompanying high technology Medicine,* Langhorne, PA: Harwood Academic Publishers.

Sosa-Guerrero, S., & Gomez, N. J. (1997). Dealing with end-stage renal disease. *American Journal of Nursing, 97*(10), 44–51.

Stark, J. (1997). Dialysis choices: Turning the tide in acute renal failure. *Nursing, 27*(2), 41–46.

RENAL TRANSPLANTATION

Forbes, A. J. (Ed.) (1998). Is corticosteroid withdrawal after kidney transplantation a good idea? *Drugs and Therapy Perspectives, 11*(6), 13–16.

Forbes, A. J. (Ed.) (1998). Renal transplant patients have a good quality of life. *Drugs and Therapy Perspectives, 11*(8), 13–16.

Rao, V. K. (1998). *Renal transplantation. Surgical Clinics of North America, 78*(1).

Shapiro, R. Simmons, R. L. & Starzl, T. (Eds.) (1997). *Renal transplantation.* Stanford, CT: Appleton & Lange.

ON-LINE RESOURCES

American Association of Kidney Patients *http://www.aakp.org*

American Foundation for Urologic Diseases *http://www.afud.org*

Health Oasis Mayo Clinic *http://www.mayohealth.org*

The Kidney Transplant/Dialysis Association, Inc. *http://www.ultranet.com/~kdta/index.shtml*

National Association for Continence (NAFC) *http://www.nafc.org*

National Institute of Diabetes and Digestive and Kidney Diseases *http://www.aiddk.nih.gov*

National Kidney Foundation *http://www.kidney.org*

The Urology Center *http://www.urostar.com*

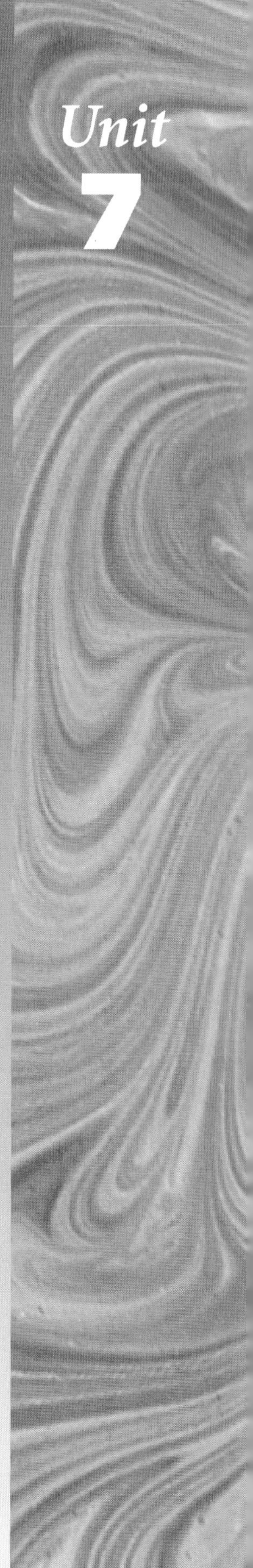

Endocrine Regulation

FOCUS ON Endocrine Changes Through the Life Span

INFANT (1–12 MONTHS):

The pituitary gland and adrenal cortex are somewhat immature, possibly affecting fluid and electrolyte balance and ability to respond to stress effectively. Growth and metabolism are dependent on growth hormone secretion and thyroid function. Production of glucagon and insulin is limited, causing variations in blood sugar levels.

TODDLER AND PRESCHOOL AGE (1–5 YEARS):

Endocrine function begins to stabilize. Growth is dependent on growth hormone, thyroxin, and insulin secretion. Adrenocortical secretions increase and stabilize.

SCHOOL AGE (6–12 YEARS):

Growth hormone and other hormones are necessary for growth spurts that occur during this phase. Endocrine functions reach adult capacity. Anterior pituitary gland begins to produce gonadotropic hormones. As puberty begins, sex hormones are secreted, which account for the beginning secondary sex characteristics.

ADOLESCENCE (13–19 YEARS):

Growth spurts occur, usually between ages 9 to 14 years in females and ages 10 to 17 years in males. Growth hormone, thyroxin, and insulin play important roles in the growth process. Sex hormones, secreted in increased amounts, are essential in influencing the structure and function of the sex organs and in the onset of secondary sex characteristics.

YOUNG ADULT AND ADULT (20–45 YEARS):

Physical maturation is complete during the early adult period under the influence of hormones. The normal feedback for hormone secretion is maintained, and hormonal balance is attained for physiologic functioning. Sex hormone function peaks. Basal metabolic rate reaches its maximum at age 30 years and then gradually declines.

MIDDLE-AGED ADULT (46–64 YEARS):

Basal metabolism declines at a rate of 2% per decade. A decrease in the production of neurotransmitters that stimulate pituitary release of sex hormones leads to decreased estrogen and testosterone production. The thyroid gland begins to fibrose, resulting in decreased thyroid gland activity and thyrotropin secretion and release. Excretion of 17-ketosteroids begins to decline. ACTH secretion also begins to decline, accompanied by a decrease in adrenal secretory activity.

LATE ADULTHOOD (65–100+ YEARS):

Gradual decline in hormonal levels may result in more problems with stress and illness adaptation, particularly due to decreased adrenal hormones. Pituitary gland volume decreases by 20%. Growth hormone secretion is maintained. However, blood levels may be lower. Thyroid function is often decreased. Parathyroid function is maintained unless there is a change in plasma calcium levels from other conditions or disorders of other glands. Release of insulin by the beta cells is delayed and insufficient. A decreased sensitivity to insulin also occurs. The ability to metabolize glucose diminishes, leading to higher blood glucose concentrations. Circadian patterns of hormonal secretions are altered. Continued effects of decreased sex hormones are seen.

Chapter 23

Normal Endocrine Function

Joan Parker Frizzell

KEY TERMS

anabolic
counter-regulatory
gluconeogenesis
glycogenolysis
glycolysis
homeostasis
hormone
limbic system
lipogenesis
lipolysis
negative feedback
neocortex
non-vesicular hormone secretion
positive feedback
reticular activating system
thermogenesis
tropic hormone
vesicular hormone secretion
vitiligo

This chapter will introduce the concepts basic to endocrinology and provide an overview of the normal functions of the endocrine system. The endocrine system is a complex system that maintains a stable internal milieu despite potential alterations from both internal and external stimuli. Through secretions of substances called **hormones**, which are capable of signaling target cells to respond in a desired manner, the endocrine system maintains **homeostasis** and regulates physiologic activity. Additionally it is responsible for the physiologic functions of growth, development, maturation, and reproduction.

HORMONES

Figure 23-1 presents an overview of the hormones of the endocrine system and shows their relationship to the nervous system. Additionally, the targets of each of the hormones are identified. Hormones travel to their target glands, organs, or cells in response to specific signals.

Hormone Synthesis

Hormones exert physiologic effects on other cells. As biochemical structures, hormones are similar to other physiologic molecules. Thus they can be categorized according to their basic structure as (1) peptide and protein hormones, (2) amine and amino acid hormones, or (3) steroid hormones. Their synthesis is also comparable to that of similar biologic molecules. The following is an overview of hormonal synthesis. Figure 23-2 identifies precursors of some common hormones.

PEPTIDE AND PROTEIN HORMONES

The process of protein synthesis describes the production of both peptide and protein hormones. Hormones in this category include thyrotropic stimulating hormone (TSH), insulin, and adrenocorticotropic hormone (ACTH). Through the actions of deoxyribonucleic acid and ribonucleic acid, the protein is produced at ribosomes. The initial protein is often larger than the final hormone and is referred to as a *preprohormone*. The preprohormone contains a signal peptide that directs its transfer to the endoplasmic reticulum.[3] As the preprohormone is transferred from the ribosome to the endoplasmic reticulum, the signal peptide is removed. At this point it is referred to as a *prohormone*. The prohormone is transferred to the Golgi apparatus. Further processing converts the prohormone into the actual hormone that will be secreted by the cells of the endocrine gland. This processing may include cleavage of the prohormone into smaller units or the addition

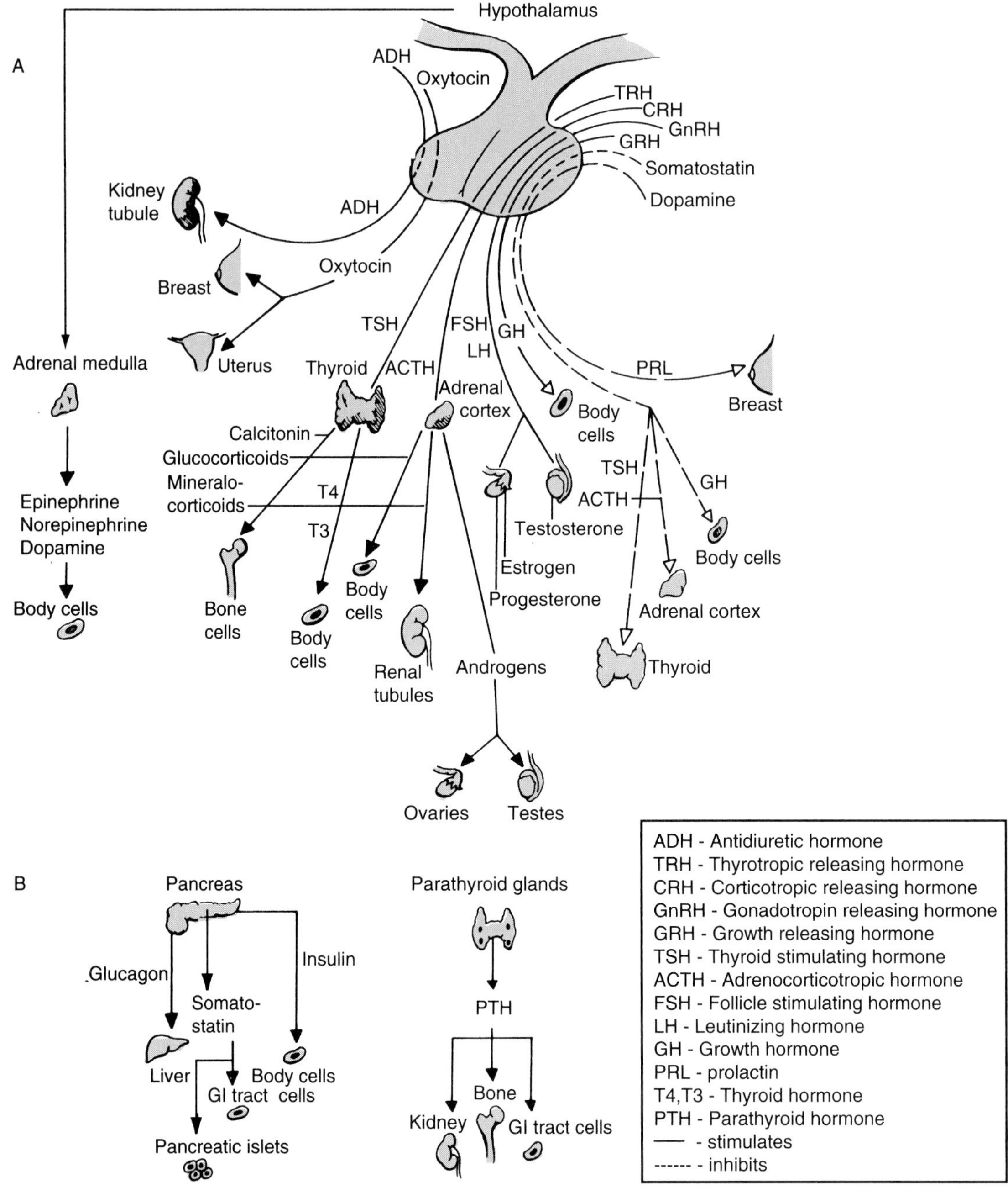

FIGURE 23-1. **Overview of the endocrine system hormones and their target organs. A. Endocrine system under neural influence. B. Endocrine system not under neural influence.**

of carbohydrate units. The completed hormone is stored in a secretory granule together with its coproducts. An example of this processing is seen in the production of insulin. The connecting peptide, or C peptide, is removed from the proinsulin during processing by the Golgi apparatus. However, both insulin and the C peptide are released together from the secretory granule. The C peptide produced during insulin synthesis has no known biologic function.[21] In contrast to this, the prohormone pro-opiomelanocortin has several biologically active segments, including melanocyte stimulating hormone (MSH), ACTH, and β endorphin.

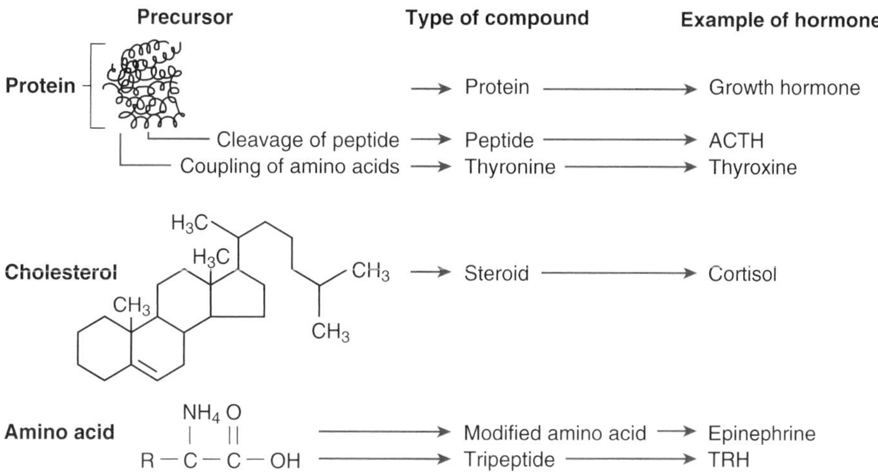

FIGURE 23-2. Precursors of hormones. Shown are representations of the source of the major hormones, with examples of the molecular types of derivatives and hormones that reflect each chemical type. (Adapted from Baxter, J. D. [1997]. Introduction to endocrinology. In F. S. Greenspan & G. S. Strewler. *Basic and clinical endocrinology* [5th ed.]. Stamford, CT: Appleton-Lange.)

AMINES AND AMINO ACIDS

Catecholamines and thyroid hormones are examples of amines/amino acids. Their synthesis will be discussed below.

Catecholamines are synthesized by a series of enzymatic reactions from the amino acid tyrosine. This synthesis can occur both in the adrenal medulla and in neuronal tissues. However, epinephrine, in contrast to norepinephrine and dopamine, is synthesized only in the adrenal medulla and accounts for 80% of the catecholamines secreted by the medulla.[13] Catecholamines are stored in secretory granules prior to their release.

Thyroid hormone synthesis involves the iodination of the amino acid tyrosine. The monoiodotyrosine (MIT) molecules are combined to form diiodotyrosine (DIT). Additional coupling results in the formation of triiodothyronine (T_3) and tetraiodothyronine (T_4). Further processing of the hormone occurs in the thyroid gland or, after being secreted, by the peripheral tissues. Deiodination of T_4 occurs, converting it to T_3, the more active form.[2] Tyrosine is linked by peptide bonding to a larger protein, thyroglobulin. Thus, T_3 and T_4 are highly protein bound.

STEROID HORMONES

A series of enzymatic reactions results in the synthesis of steroid hormones from cholesterol. Examples of lipid-derived steroid hormones are glucocorticoids and estrogen. Since intracellular storage of these hormones is limited, the entire synthesis sequence must be initiated for steroid secretion to occur. Thus cholesterol is the intracellular storage form of steroid hormones.[3] Additionally, all steroid hormones are bound to plasma proteins. For example, more than 90% of total cortisol is protein bound.[2]

Secretion

In order to exert the desired effects on the target cells, the hormones must be secreted from cells that synthesized them. There are two basic types of hormonal secretion: (1) **vesicular** and (2) **non-vesicular**. These are illustrated in Figure 23-3. Hormones such as the steroid hormones are secreted as they are synthesized. There is no storage or hormonal reserve within the endocrine glands. In contrast to this, the protein and peptide hormones are sequestered in storage vesicles similar to those seen with neurotransmitters. Like neurotransmitters, they are released when a stimulus causes an increase in intracellular calcium levels. The hormonal vesicles move along microtubules to the plasma membrane, where they are released by the process of exocytosis.

Protein Binding

Movement of the hormone from the synthesizing cell to the target cell enables the hormone to exert its effects. The ability of the hormone to both move into and out of the general circulation is also important. Hormones that are highly protein bound remain within the blood stream. Only the unbound portion can move freely into the interstitial spaces and thus reach the target cells. The unbound portion is considered the free hormone and therefore bioactive. The bound portion is unable to exert its desired effects. For example, only 0.04% of T4 and 0.4% of T3 are not protein bound. It is those frac-

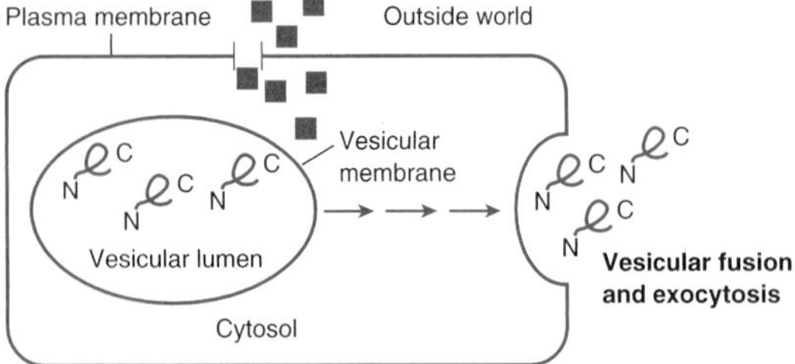

FIGURE 23-3. Vesicular and nonvesicular modes of hormone secretion. Schematic diagram of a cell, indicating that some hormones are transported in vesicles to the cell surface and released in quanta upon fusion of the vesicle with the plasma membrane, while other hormones are transported directly across the plasma membrane either by specific transporters or by diffusion. Vesicular secretion can be regulated separately at the level of synthesis and of release, while control over synthesis is the only known way to regulate hormones released in a nonvesicular manner. Examples of hormones secreted in a vesicle-mediated fashion are most polypeptide hormones and catecholamines. Examples of the hormones released in a nonvesicular manner are the eicosanoids, steroids, and thyroid hormones. (Lingappa, V. R. & Mellon, S. H. [1997]. Hormone synthesis and release. In F. S. Greenspan & G. S. Strewler. *Basic and clinical endocrinology* [5th ed.]. Stamford, CT: Appleton-Lange.)

tions that are responsible for thyroid hormonal activity. Additionally, the bound and unbound portions are in equilibrium, so that as the free portion is reduced, some of the bound portion is released from the protein.

Signaling

The action of the hormones on the target cells may occur in one of four modes: (1) autocrine, (2) paracrine, (3) endocrine, and (4) neurocrine (Fig. 23-4). *Autocrine* influence occurs when the hormones are able to modify the secretory activity of the cells that produces them. *Paracrine* influence is the result of the hormones acting locally by diffusion on neighboring cells within the same gland. *Endocrine* influence is carried out by hormones that are secreted into and carried by circulating body fluids to the target cells. *Neurocrine* action refers to the production of hormones by neuronal tissue. However, the hormones are transported from the tissue of origin and stored in an endocrine gland for subsequent release. An example of this would be the synthesis of antidiuretic hormone by hypothalamic nuclei with subsequent storage in the posterior pituitary gland.

Mechanisms of Hormonal Action

The effects seen from hormonal activity, shown in Figure 23-5, occur through two basic mechanisms of action: (1) specific cell surface receptors and (2) through forming intracellular receptor complexes. When hormones such as catecholamines and TSH are released, they bind to specific cell surface receptors, initiating a relatively faster "second messenger" response.[3] These receptors are coupled to a G protein complex that activates adenylyl cyclase. This then causes an increase in formation of cyclic adenosine monophosphate (cAMP), the second messenger. As a second messenger, cAMP initiates many other intracellular activities. These intracellular activities cause the end-organ responses associated with the particular hormonal activity.[10] There are several second messengers, including diacylglycerol and inositol triphosphate. The duration of action for these effects is relatively short, since many of the hormones that utilize this mechanism of action have very short half-lives.

Steroid hormones are lipid soluble. Thus, they are able to move through the cell membranes of target tissues and exert their action intracellularly. This is a relatively slower mechanism of action than the previously described second messenger systems. This process, which is shown in Figure 23-6, is initiated when the hormone binds with a specific receptor protein.[19] The hormone-receptor protein complex becomes activated, traveling to the nucleus to exert its effects on the cell. Activation exposes a site on the complex with affinity for DNA. This initiates a transcription process that produces new messenger RNA (mRNA).[28] The mRNA directs the formation of new proteins by the ribosomes. It is these newly formed proteins that are responsible for the "hormonal effects" of the steroid hormones. The effects take longer to occur. However, the half-life of steroid hormones is fairly long.

Receptor responses vary in terms of the amount of stimulation to the receptor. Prolonged stimulation of receptors results in a decrease in the number of receptors, or *down regulation*. Conversely, decreased receptor stimulation can cause an increase in the number of the receptors, or *up regulation*. An example of this physiologic effect is observed when hormone levels fluctuate from pathologic processes or when hormones are administered exogenously. Many hormones are secreted in a pulsatile manner. It has been observed that when there is a constant blood level of those hormones, the actual response is reduced. This is due to down regulation of the hormone receptors.

Feedback Mechanisms

Hormones are secreted as needed to maintain biologic function and physiologic homeostasis. Normally the

FOCUS ON CELLULAR PHYSIOLOGY

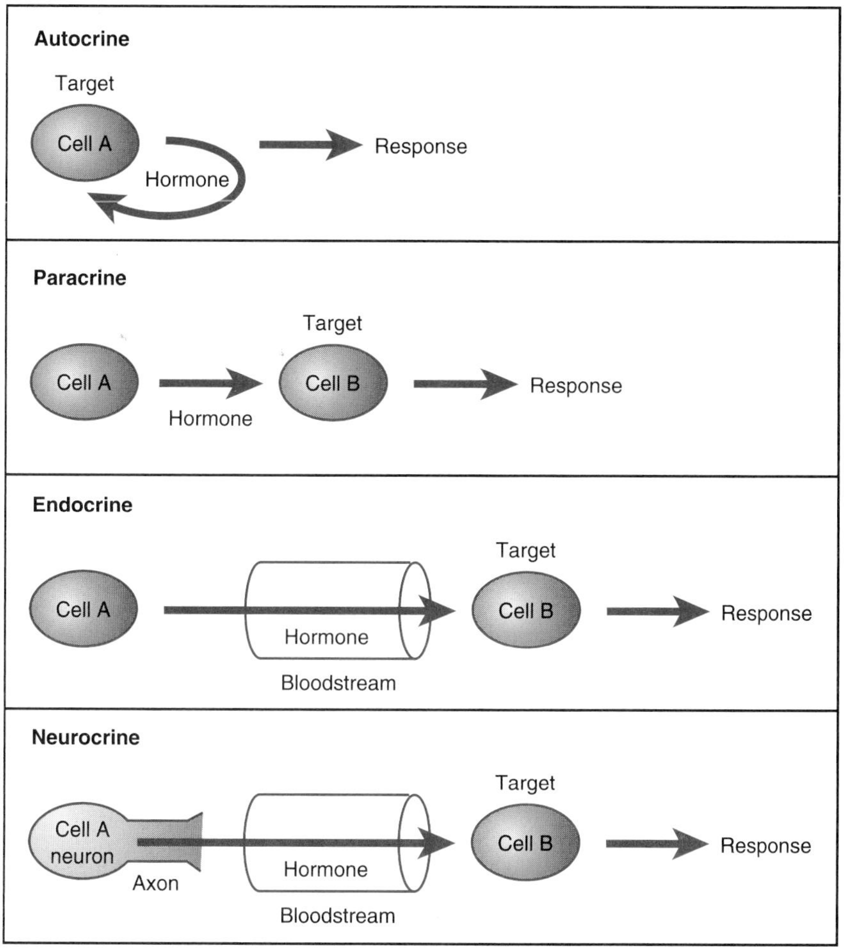

Autocrine

Target

Cell A

Hormone

Response

Paracrine

Target

Cell A

Cell B

Hormone

Response

Endocrine

Target

Cell A

Hormone

Cell B

Response

Bloodstream

Neurocrine

Target

Cell A neuron

Axon

Hormone

Cell B

Response

Bloodstream

FIGURE 23-4. Examples of cell-to-cell signaling through hormone molecules. In autocrine function the hormone signal acts back on the cell of origin or adjacent identical cells. In paracrine function the hormone signal is carried to an adjacent target cell over short distances via the interstitial fluid. In endocrine function the signal is carried to a distant target via the bloodstream. In neurocrine function the hormone signal originates in a neuron and after axonal transport to the bloodstream is carried to a distant target cell (Berne, R. M. & Levy, M. N. [1996]. *Principles of physiology* [2nd ed.]. St. Louis: C. V. Mosby.)

secretion is controlled by feedback mechanisms that maintain appropriate hormonal levels. The feedback mechanism may be a negative or positive feedback response. In addition to the feedback mechanism, hormonal secretion patterns may follow specific rhythms.

NEGATIVE FEEDBACK RESPONSE

Most often, hormonal secretion is controlled through a **negative feedback** response as shown in Flowchart 23-1. Thus, elevated levels of a particular hormone prevent further release of the hormone. In the neuroendocrine axis, elevated levels of target organ hormones decrease the secretion of releasing hormones from the hypothalamus and **tropic hormones** from the anterior pituitary. This maintains normal levels of endocrine activity.

One exception in the tropic hormones to the negative feedback response is the secretion of prolactin. Its secretion is inhibited by dopamine secretion from the

FOCUS ON CELLULAR PHYSIOLOGY

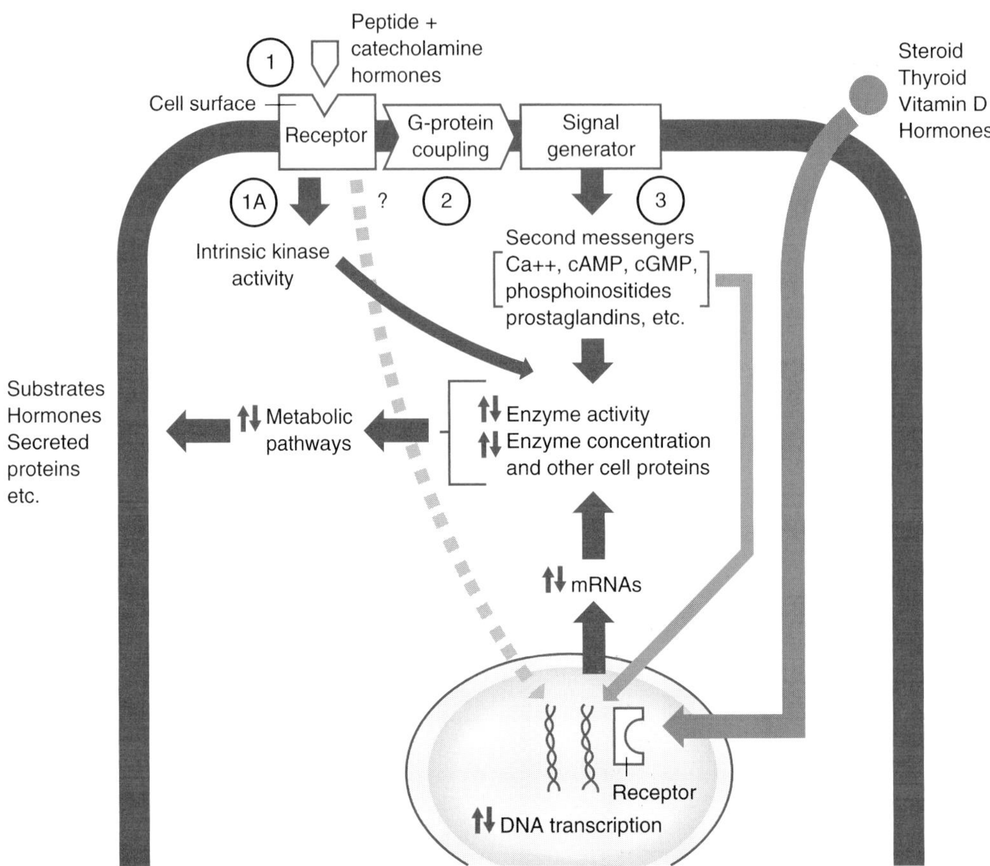

FIGURE 23-5. Overview of hormonal action on target tissues. Hormones may interact with either plasma membrane of intracellular receptors or they may generate second messengers within the cytoplasm or the nucleus. Metabolic pathways may be regulated by altering the activities or the concentrations of enzymes. Cell growth and architecture may also be modulated. (Berne, R. M. & Levy, M. N. [1996]. *Principles of physiology* [2nd ed.]. St. Louis: C. V. Mosby.)

hypothalamus. Dopamine acts as a prolactin-inhibiting hormone to block the secretion of prolactin from the anterior pituitary. Thus, anything that blocks dopaminergic activity, including medications such as haloperidol, can promote prolactin secretion. Additionally, elevated levels of prolactin and breastfeeding an infant will increase prolactin secretion.

POSITIVE FEEDBACK RESPONSE

The process of **positive feedback** is much less common and is seen in the regulation of ovarian hormones. Positive feedback refers to the presence of a hormone stimulating increased secretion of that same hormone or other related hormones. In the normal menstrual cycle, the presence of estrogen promotes the release of gonadotropin releasing hormone (GnRH). The increased levels of GnRH effect the secretion of luteinizing hormone (LH) and follicle stimulating hormone (FSH). These hormones then stimulate the ovaries to secrete estrogen. This process suggests that estrogen exerts a positive feedback effect on this portion of the menstrual cycle.[1]

Hormone Cycles

Hormone secretion varies over a period of time and may follow a specific rhythm. Hormones such as cortisol have a diurnal variation, and ovarian hormonal levels have a monthly pattern of secretion. Other factors

FOCUS ON CELLULAR PHYSIOLOGY

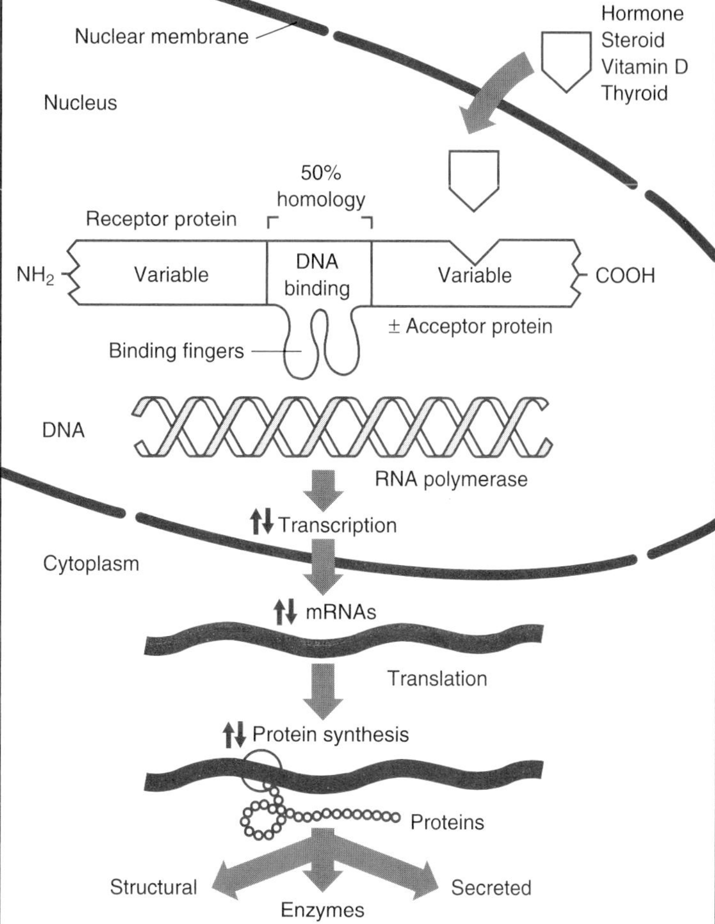

FIGURE 23-6. Overview of steroid and thyroid hormonal action. The hormone combines with a nuclear protein receptor. The carboxy-terminal portion of the receptor varies for each hormone. The midportion of the receptor molecule has considerable similarity among hormones. The midportion contains DNA-binding fingers. Binding of the hormone receptor complex to hormone regulatory elements in DNA molecules either stimulates or suppresses transcription of target genes. The result is increased or decreased synthesis of cell proteins. (Berne, R. M. & Levy, M. N. [1996]. *Principles of physiology* [2nd ed.]. St. Louis: C. V. Mosby.)

that can influence hormonal release include seasonal variations[3] and stages of development such as puberty and senescence. Pain and emotional responses such as stress and fright also alter hormonal levels through complex neuronal interactions.

ENDOCRINE INTERACTIONS WITH OTHER SYSTEMS

Recently, research has demonstrated interactions between the endocrine system, the immune system, and the nervous system. Examples of these interactions include the physiologic responses to hypoglycemia and stress. The physiologic stress response is reviewed in Chapter 5. The response to hypoglycemia is presented in conjunction with the function of the endocrine pancreas in this chapter.

Interaction With the Immune System

The interaction between the endocrine system and the immune system is a topic that is the focus of much health-related research and is important to the understanding of endocrine pathophysiology. This is evidenced by examples of endocrine diseases such as Graves' disease and type 1 diabetes mellitus, which are the result of an autoimmune response. Additionally, hormones such as glucocorticoid cortisol have been shown to decrease inflammatory and immunologic responses. It also appears that humoral factors from lymphocytes influence ACTH levels.[36] Activated lymphocytes and certain macrophages are capable of producing pro-opiomelanocortin and its end products ACTH and β-endorphin. This synthesis is apparently stimulated by corticotropin releasing hormone (CRH) from the hypothalamus and inhibited by glucocorti-

FLOWCHART 23-1 **Negative Feedback for Hormonal Regulation**

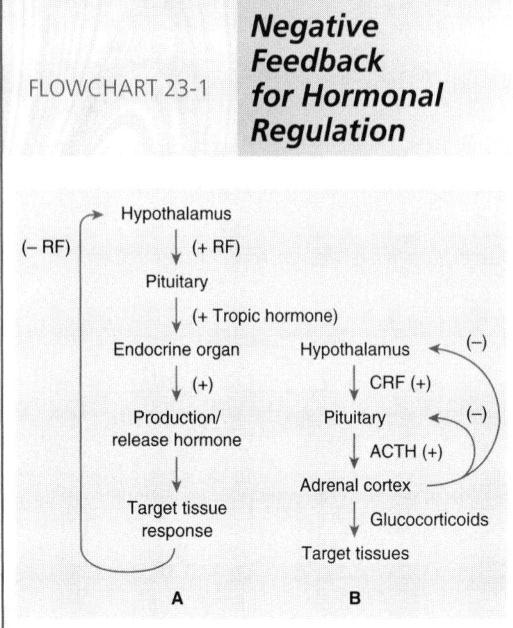

A. Possible mechanism of a negative feedback system for maintenance of hormone balance. **B.** Negative feedback mechanism regulating secretion of adrenocorticotropin (ACTH). The hypothalamus secretes corticotropin releasing factor (CRF), which stimulates release of ACTH by the pituitary. ACTH stimulates glucocorticoid secretion by the adrenal cortex. Glucocorticoids have a negative feedback on the pituitary and on the hypothalamus.

coids.[28] Additionally, Interleukin 1 produced by macrophages has been shown to stimulate hypothalamic activity promoting CRH secretion, ultimately increasing levels of glucocorticoids.[11]

Neuroendocrine Interactions

The relationship between the endocrine system and the nervous system is unique. The responses seen in both systems involve the similar mechanism of receptor activation. Many of the same stimuli that trigger an endocrine response also trigger a response in the nervous system, as shown in Figure 23-7. Some biological molecules have both neurotransmitter and endocrine activity. This action is seen in the physiologic responses to stress and hypoglycemia. For example, epinephrine functions as a neurotransmitter, stimulating beta-adrenergic effects. It also promotes gluconeogenesis by the liver to elevate blood glucose levels. Additionally, catecholamines and thyroid hormones have a synergistic effect on the cardiovascular system. Glucocorticoids enhance the vascular response to catecholamines.[10] Thus, the interaction between the endocrine system and the nervous system is important in maintaining physiologic homeostasis.

HYPOTHALAMUS

The hypothalamus is an area of the brain that consists of the floor and the lateral walls of the third ventricle. It is composed of nuclei, which are actually the cell bodies of clusters of neurons (Fig. 23-8). The hypothalamus is connected to the pituitary gland by the pituitary stalk or infundibulum.

The *neuroendocrine axis* describes the relationship between the hypothalamus, the anterior pituitary gland, and the target organ's endocrine effects. This is the link between the central nervous system and the endocrine-mediated activities of the body. There is a direct anatomic, vascular link between the hypothalamus and the anterior pituitary gland (adenohypophysis). Figure 23-8 diagrams this relationship. The hypothalamic–hypophyseal portal system enables the hypothalamus to modulate the secretion of the hormones produced in the anterior pituitary gland.

Unique to the hypothalamus, as compared with the rest of the brain, are fenestrations or openings in its capillaries. Thus the blood–brain barrier is not intact, resulting in greater access to circulating blood. This accounts for the increased sensitivity of the hypothalamus to chemical stimuli in the blood stream.

Hypothalamus Function

The hypothalamus is responsible for many homeostatic integrative functions. Interactions between the autonomic nervous system (ANS) and the endocrine system are coordinated with information from other areas in the brain.

The hypothalamus receives input from the **neocortex** and **limbic systems** as well from the **reticular activating system** (see Chaps. 29 and 30 for a description of these areas of the brain). As a result of this input, the hypothalamus coordinates and integrates emotional, behavioral, and physiologic activity. The functions of the hypothalamus include the following:

- Temperature regulation
- Neuroendocrine control of catecholamine secretion
- Fluid volume regulation
- Stimulation of hunger and thirst
- Regulation of sexual behavior
- Regulation of growth and development
- Defensive reactions such as fear and rage
- Control of various endocrine activity rhythms

Hormones of the Hypothalamus

The hormones of the hypothalamus are divided into two categories: (1) posterior pituitary and (2) hypophyseal tropic. Table 23-1 provides a list of these hormones, including a description of their role in endocrine function.

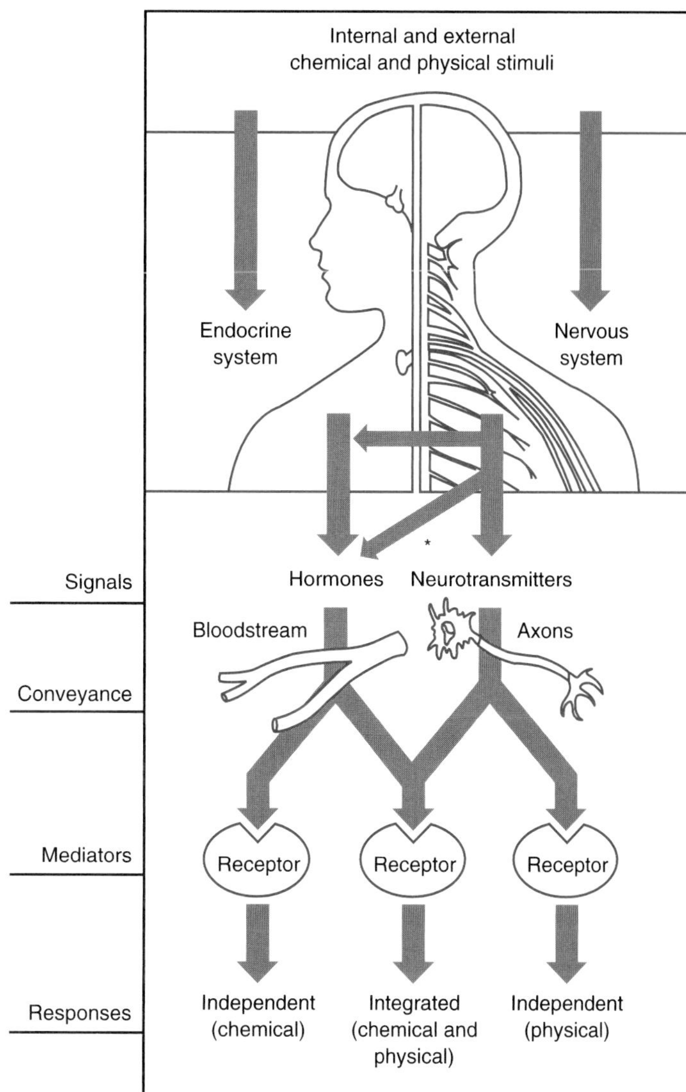

FIGURE 23-7. Overview of the relationship between the nervous system and the endocrine system. Similar activity may elicit activity of both systems. Hormones secreted by endocrine cells and conveyed via the bloodstream are analogous to neurotransmitters released by neurons after being conveyed by axons. Neurotransmitters may stimulate hormone release and themselves act as hormones. Responses are mediated by receptors in each system and may consist of either chemical or physical changes. (Berne, R. M. & Levy, M. N. [1996]. *Principles of physiology* [2nd ed.]. St. Louis: C. V. Mosby.)

The posterior pituitary hormones are produced by the hypothalamus, travel to the posterior pituitary via the hypothalamic hypophyseal tract,[10] and are stored and secreted by the posterior pituitary gland. The hypophyseal tropic hormones enter the hypothalamic–hypophyseal portal system, exerting their effects on the anterior pituitary gland. The hypophyseal tropic hormones are considered to be either releasing or inhibiting hormones. In terms of prolactin release from the anterior pituitary, there is no specific releasing hormone from the hypothalamus. However, TRH and another hypothalamic peptide, vasoactive intestinal polypeptide (VIP), appear to stimulate prolactin secretion. It is also possible that serotonergic stimulation may contribute to this as well.

The hypophyseal tropic hormones are released in a pulsatile manner to generate a response from the anterior pituitary gland. Clinical experience has demonstrated that continuous release of these hormones results in a decreased anterior pituitary response due to down regulation of receptors. The mechanism of action of the hypophyseal tropic hormones is through activation of second messenger systems. These second messengers regulate gene expression and hormonal secretion from the anterior pituitary gland.[3]

PITUITARY GLAND

The pituitary gland, often referred to as the master gland, is controlled by the hypothalamus. It is located in a small depression of the sphenoid bone called the sella turcica, or Turkish saddle. It is surrounded by the dura

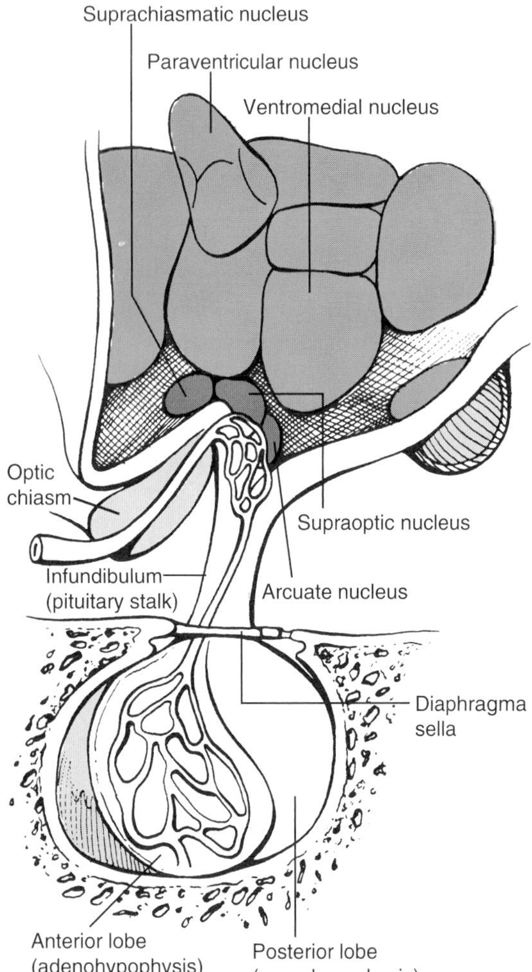

FIGURE 23-8. **Diagram of the hypothalamic nuclei and the portal-hypophyseal vessels. (Modified from Ganong, W. F. [1997]. *Review of medical physiology* [18th ed.]. Norwalk, CT: Appleton and Lange.)**

mater. As illustrated in Figure 23-8, the top of the gland is separated from the brain by a portion of the dura referred to as the diaphragma sellae. Because of the diaphragma sellae, the arachnoid membrane and thus cerebrospinal fluid is prevented from entering the sella turcica.[1] There is an opening in the diaphragma sellae for the pituitary stalk. The optic chiasm is in front of the pituitary stalk, about 5 mm above the diaphragma sellae.

The pituitary gland is divided into two parts: the anterior pituitary and the posterior pituitary, as shown in Figure 23-9. The posterior pituitary gland, or *neurohypophysis*, is composed of axons whose cell bodies are located in the supraoptic and paraventricular nuclei of the hypothalamus. The anterior pituitary, or *adenohypophysis*, is composed of secretory cells that respond to the releasing and inhibiting hormones of the hypothalamus.

There is a small portion between the anterior and posterior pituitary referred to as the intermediate lobe or pars intermedia. This section is rudimentary in humans. Some of its cells appear to be similar to those of the anterior pituitary. However, it is considered to be the site of MSH secretion.[10] MSH stimulates melanin synthesis. Both MSH and ACTH are produced from the same prohormone; therefore, MSH activity is linked to circulating levels of ACTH. Abnormalities in pigmentation such as **vitiligo** are often due to alterations in pituitary function. Skin pallor is associated with hypopituitarism.

Pituitary Function

The pituitary gland functions to secrete hormones that are important in the control of metabolic activities throughout the body. Its control comes through complex vascular and neural connections with the nervous system as well as through feedback loops from target glands and organs.

Hormones of the Anterior Pituitary

Traditionally, the cells of the anterior pituitary gland were classified on the basis of their staining properties. However, recent advances in immunochemistry and electron microscopy have identified five cell types:[10]

1. Somatotropes
2. Lactotropes
3. Thryotropes
4. Gonadotropes
5. Corticotropes

The anterior pituitary gland secretes six hormones from these cells: TSH, ACTH, GH, FSH, LH, and PRL. The first five are considered tropic hormones, that is, they stimulate other glands or organs to secrete hormonally active substances. The sixth hormone, prolactin, acts directly on breast tissue to stimulate milk production. The function of an additional anterior pituitary hormone, lipotropin, is unknown at this time. Table 23-2 lists the hormones of the anterior pituitary gland. Their secretion is regulated by the releasing and inhibiting hormones of the hypothalamus. The tropic hormones are also controlled through feedback mechanisms. Both TSH and ACTH will be discussed later in this chapter in the context of their respective tropic glands. The roles of FSH and LH in male and female development are reviewed in Chapters 36 and 37. Prolactin is also reviewed in Chapter 37.

GROWTH HORMONE

Growth hormone (GH), also referred to as somatotropin, is produced by the somatotrophs, the most numerous cells of the anterior pituitary gland. Although its synthesis and secretion are stimulated by GRH, its synthesis is also stimulated by thyroid hormones and cortisol.[3] Like its releasing hormone, GRH, GH is secreted in a pulsatile manner. Somatostatin, as an inhibitor of GH secretion, decreases the frequency and amount of GH

TABLE 23-1

HYPOTHALAMIC HORMONES

HORMONE	CATEGORY	FUNCTION
Antidiuretic hormone (ADH)	Posterior pituitary	Regulation of water balance; potent vasoconstrictor
Oxytocin	Posterior pituitary	Stimulation of lactation; contraction of uterus during childbirth
Thyrotropin-releasing hormone (TRH)	Hypophyseal tropic	Stimulates secretion of thyroid-stimulating hormone (TSH)
Somatostatin	Hypophyseal tropic	Inhibits the secretion of growth hormone (GH) and TSH
Growth hormone releasing hormone (GRH)	Hypophyseal tropic	Stimulates secretion of GH
Dopamine	Hypophyseal tropic	Prolactin (PRL)-inhibiting hormone
Corticotropin-releasing hormone (CRH)	Hypophyseal tropic	Stimulates secretion of ACTH and other products of its prohormone
Gonadotropin-releasing hormone (GnRH)	Hypophyseal tropic	Secretion of LH and FSH

secretion. Table 23-3 summarizes the physiologic factors that influence GH secretion. These can be considered in terms of neurogenic, metabolic, and hormonal. The metabolic stimuli include reduced levels of glucose and free fatty acids.[3] Short-term fasting increases GH secretion, whereas obesity decreases it. Its secretion is also controlled by a negative feedback mechanism, since elevated GH levels stimulate somatotropin release. However, the final determination of secretion is an increase of GRH and a decrease in somatostatin.

There is a diurnal rhythm in the pulsatile secretions of GH. Growth hormone levels are greatly increased after about 1 to 2 hours of deep sleep. Light sleep and rapid eye movement (REM) sleep inhibit GH release. Loss of this diurnal rhythm can be indicative of either hypothalamic or pituitary dysfunction. Stress, trauma, surgery, and exercise influence GRH and thus increase the release of GH. As expected, there is also a variation in GH levels based on age. Children have higher levels than the elderly.

Functions of GH

The actions of GH are **anabolic**. Protein synthesis is increased through stimulation of the actions of DNA and RNA. As a result of this action, the total body nitrogen balance becomes positive. The amount of body fat decreases while lean muscle mass increases. Linear bone growth occurs from stimulation of the chondrocytes, the cartilage-forming cells. Most body tissues have an anabolic response to GH. Thus, there is improved functioning of major body organs.

In terms of overall metabolic activity, GH could be considered a diabetogenic hormone. It promotes insulin resistance in muscle and adipose tissue. Therefore, plasma glucose levels increase with a concomitant increase in insulin levels. Usually insulin promotes **lipogenesis**. However, GH antagonizes this and causes **lipolysis** to occur. This causes an increase in free fatty acids with the formation of ketoacids. However, in healthy individuals, there is coordinated activity between insulin and GH. Therefore, the diabetogenic activity of GH is balanced by the effects of insulin. The following is a description of the coordinated metabolic activity of GH and insulin:

- With protein intake, both GH and insulin are secreted. The antagonistic effects of GH prevent hypoglycemia, which could occur since carbohydrates were not ingested.
- When only carbohydrates are ingested, only insulin is secreted. Since insulin is needed for carbohydrate metabolism, GH is not needed.
- With fasting, GH secretion is increased. However, levels of both insulin and somatomedins are reduced. This enables lipolysis to occur since free fatty acids will be used as an energy source.

When both GH and insulin are secreted as needed, plasma glucose levels remain within normal limits. As indicated previously, GH is essential not only for the regulation of metabolic activity but also for somatic growth. Thus its synthesis and release are essential to maintain bodily functions throughout life.

Hormones of the Posterior Pituitary

The synthesis and secretion of posterior pituitary hormones is under direct neural control of the hypothalamus. First, a prohormone is synthesized in the supraoptic and paraventricular nuclei of the hypothalamus. The prohormone is transported by way of neurosecretory granules down the neuronal fibers of the hypothalamic–hypophyseal tract to the posterior pituitary gland. As the prohormone travels to the posterior

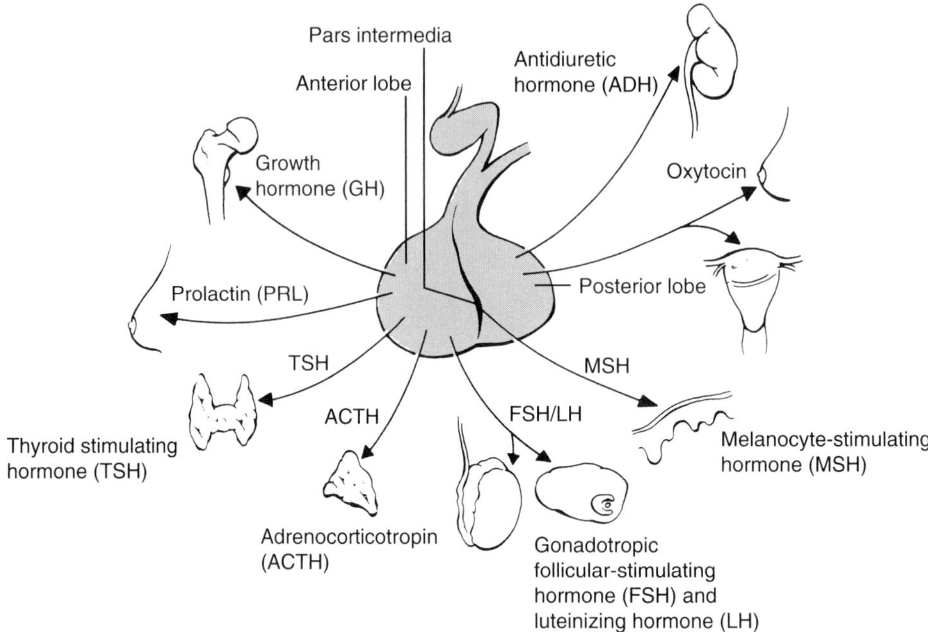

FIGURE 23-9. Diagram of anatomic and functional relationship between the hypothalamus and the pituitary gland. Note that the posterior pituitary gland is an extension of neural tissue that stores neurohormones and has its own arterial blood supply. In contrast, the anterior pituitary gland is endocrine tissue with a blood supply largely derived from veins that first drain neural tissue in the median eminence. By this arrangement the endocrine cells are exposed to high concentrations of neurohormones originating in the hypothalamus and stored in the median eminence. The hormones secreted by the anterior and posterior pituitary gland reach and act on peripheral target cells. (Berne, R. M. & Levy, M. N. [1996]. *Principles of physiology* [2nd ed.]. St. Louis: C. V. Mosby.)

pituitary gland, it is metabolized to the hormone. The hormone is stored in the posterior pituitary until it is secreted. The secretion of the hormone occurs when an action potential is initiated by the hypothalamic cell bodies. The two hormones secreted by the posterior pituitary are antidiuretic hormone (ADH) and oxytocin. Oxytocin, which causes uterine contraction and milk expression, will be discussed in Chapter 37 in relation to the female reproductive system. The action of ADH will be reviewed below.

ANTIDIURETIC HORMONE (ADH)

Changes in plasma osmolarity are the major stimuli for ADH (vasopression) secretion. An osmolarity of 280 mOsm/kg is the threshold for this response. There are osmoreceptors in the hypothalamus that are located outside of the blood–brain barrier.[4] Thus they are exquisitely sensitive to changes as minute as 1% or 2% in plasma osmolarity and are able to regulate the synthesis and release of ADH. Increased osmolarity of the surrounding plasma causes shrinkage of the osmoreceptors since water moves out of them. This response stimulates the hypothalamus, initiating the electrical impulse that results in the secretion of ADH. Thirst and water intake are regulated by comparable mechanisms.[10]

In addition to increased osmolarity, a variety of other factors regulate the release of ADH, which are enumerated in Table 23-4. Volume receptors in the thoracic cavity sense changes in circulating vascular volume. Decreases in circulating volume are accompanied by ADH release. Arterial baroreceptors and atrial stretch receptors sense changes in circulating blood volume and blood pressure. They then transmit this information through the vagus and glossopharyngeal nerves to the medulla. Fibers in the medulla transmit the signal to the hypothalamus, stimulating ADH secretion.[4] Additionally, positive pressure ventilation decreases blood volume in the great vessels in the thorax, also promoting ADH release. Trauma, pain, anxiety, and drugs such as nicotine and opioid analgesics stimulate ADH secretion. In contrast to this, alcohol inhibits ADH, which partially accounts for the diuresis associated with excess intake of alcohol.

Function of ADH

Antidiuretic hormone's principal physiologic effect is the retention of water by the kidney. This action

TABLE 23-2

HORMONES OF THE ANTERIOR PITUITARY GLAND

NAME AND SOURCE	PRINCIPAL ACTIONS
Thyroid-stimulating hormone (TSH, thyrotrope)	Stimulates growth of thyroid gland and secretion of T_3 and T_4
Adrenocorticotropic hormone (ACTH, corticotrope)	Stimulates the growth of the adrenal cortex and the secretion of adrenal steroids, primarily glucocorticoids.
Follicle-stimulating hormone (FSH, gonadotrope)	Female: Ovarian follicle growth; stimulates estrogen secretion Male: Spermatogenesis
Luteinizing hormone (LH, gonadotrope)	Female: Ovulation and luteinization of ovarian follicles; stimulates progesterone secretion Male: Testosterone secretion
Growth hormone (GH, somatotrope)	Stimulates body growth and secretion of insulin-like growth factors (IGF) Increases hepatic glucose output Anti-insulin effect in muscle
Prolactin (PRL, lactotrope)	Stimulates milk secretion and maternal behavior
Lipotropin (LPH, corticotrope)	Action unknown

(Modified from Ganong, W. F. [1997]. *Review of medical physiology* [18th ed.]. Stamford, CT: Appleton & Lange.)

occurs through stimulation of V_2 receptors. The V_2 receptors are located on the luminal membrane of the nephron's collecting tubules. Stimulation of the V_2 receptors triggers the insertion of water channels called aquaporins, which promote water retention. Thus ADH increases the permeability of the tubules to water, enabling water conservation and concentration of urine.

The other major physiologic action of ADH is to act as a powerful vasoconstrictor through the activation of the V_{1A} receptors.[16] Stimulation of these receptors in the peripheral arterioles mediates vasoconstriction and

TABLE 23-3

SUMMARY OF FACTORS THAT AFFECT GROWTH HORMONE SECRETION

FACTOR	ENHANCED SECRETION	INHIBITED SECRETION
Neurogenic	Stage III and Stage IV sleep Trauma, surgery, inflammation Alpha-adrenergic, dopamine, and acetylcholine agonists Beta-adrenergic antagonists	REM sleep Beta-adrenergic agonists Alpha-adrenergic and acetylcholine antagonists
Metabolic	Hypoglycemia and fasting Uncontrolled DM Uremia Hepatic cirrhosis	Hyperglycemia Elevated fatty acids Obesity
Endocrine	GRH Estrogen Glucagon ADH	Somatostatin Hypothyroidism Elevated glucocorticoid levels

(Modified from Thorner, M. O. et al. [1992]. The anterior pituitary. In J. D. Wilson & D. W. Foster Jr. [Eds.], *William's textbook of endocrinology* [8th ed.]. Philadelphia: W. B. Saunders.)

TABLE 23-4

SUMMARY OF FACTORS THAT AFFECT ADH SECRETION

SECRETION INCREASED	SECRETION DECREASED
Increased plasma osmolarity due to either loss of free water or infusion of hypertonic fluids	Decreased plasma osmolarity
Pain, emotion, and stress	Increased extracellular fluid volume
Nausea and vomiting	Alcohol
Standing and changes in blood pressure	Trauma
Angiotensin II	Neoplasms
Drugs, including carbamazepine, epinephrine, opioids, chlorpropamide, cyclophosphamide	Infections

increases peripheral vascular resistance. The V_{1A} receptors are also found in the liver and brain. In the liver, they promote **glycogenolysis.**[10] Vasopressin (ADH) is a neurotransmitter in the brain and spinal chord.[3]

The physiologic effects of hormone occur fairly rapidly. However, it has a half-life of approximately 18 minutes. Thus these effects are of a relatively short duration.

THYROID GLAND

The thyroid gland, which regulates many physiologic functions, is located in the anterior neck, between the larynx and the trachea (Fig. 23-10). It is composed of two lobes located on either side of the trachea. The lobes are connected by a bridge or isthmus, which lies just below the cricoid cartilage of the trachea. Characteristically, the superior portion of each lobe is somewhat pointed, whereas the inferior portion is rounded and blunt.

Microscopic examination of the thyroid gland reveals that it is composed of a series of follicles. The follicles contain a pink-staining material called colloid. The follicular cells are the targets of TSH. When stimulated by TSH, they have a columnar appearance as shown in Figure 23-11. Conversely, they appear flattened and cuboidal when resting.[3,17] The follicular cells produce thyroglobulin that is secreted into the lumen of the follicle. The thyroid hormones, T_3 and T_4, are synthesized at the cell–colloid interface. The thyroglobulin is brought into the follicular cell by endocytosis. It is then hydrolyzed to release the thyroid hormones. The effects of thyroid hormones are summarized in Table 23-5 and discussed below.

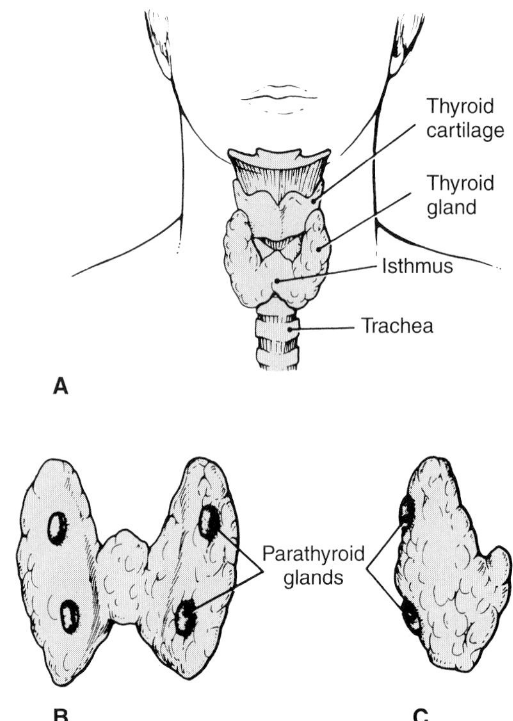

FIGURE 23-10. Structure of the thyroid gland. **A.** Anterior view. **B.** Posterior view showing parathyroid glands. **C.** Lateral view.

FOCUS ON CELLULAR PHYSIOLOGY

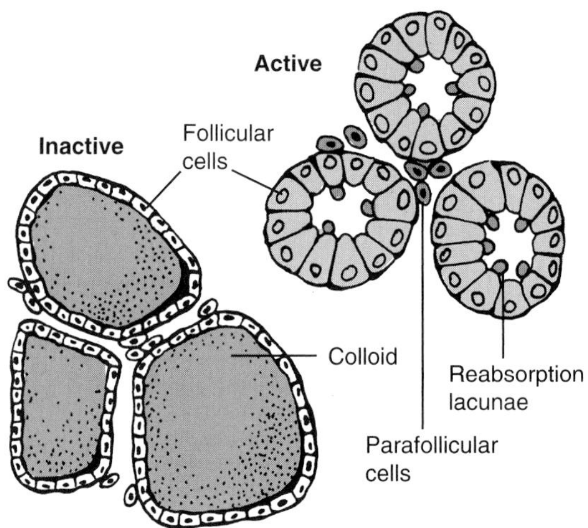

FIGURE 23-11. Histology of the thyroid gland. (Ganong, W. F. [1997]. *Review of medical physiology* [18th ed.]. Norwalk, CT: Appleton and Lange.)

TABLE 23-5

PHYSIOLOGIC EFFECTS OF THYROID HORMONE

TARGET TISSUE	EFFECT	MECHANISM
Heart	Chronotropic	Increase number and affinity of beta-adrenergic receptors
	Inotropic	Enhance response to catecholamines
Adipose tissue	Catabolic	Stimulate lipolysis
Muscle	Catabolic	Increase protein breakdown
Bone	Developmental and metabolic	Promote normal growth Accelerate bone turnover
Nervous system	Developmental	Promote normal development
Gut	Metabolic	Increase rate of carbohydrate absorption
Lipoprotein	Metabolic	Stimulate formation of LDL receptors
Other	Calorigenic	Stimulate and increase metabolic rate

(Modified from McPhee, S. J., & Bauer, D. C. [1997]. Thyroid disease. In S. J. McPhee, V. R. Lingappa, W. F. Ganong, & J. D. Lange [Eds.], *Pathology of disease* [2nd ed.]. Stamford, CT: Appleton & Lange.)

Hormones of the Thyroid

The thyroid gland produces three hormones: triiodothyronine (T3), thyroxine (T4), and calcitonin. Most of the hormone produced is T4, which is converted into T3 in the peripheral tissues such as the liver and kidney. T3 exerts a significantly more powerful effect than T4. T3 and T4 together are referred to as thyroid hormone. Thyroid hormone controls cellular metabolism, thereby promoting normal growth and development and regulating heat and energy production. Calcitonin functions in calcium and phosphorus regulation.

THYROID HORMONE: T3 AND T4

Thyroid hormonal secretions are regulated primarily by TRH, TSH, and a negative feedback system with the neuroendocrine axis, which is depicted in Figure 23-12. This axis results in pulsatile secretion of TSH with relatively steady levels of T_3 and T_4. However, there is also autoregulation by the thyroid gland in relation to available iodine. Additionally, thyroid function can be stimulated or inhibited by TSH receptor antibodies. TSH produces a variety of effects on the thyroid cells. Stimulation of TSH generates the formation of cAMP as a second messenger. This stimulates iodine metabolism and synthesis and release of the thyroid hormones, T_3 and T_4. In contrast to TSH, T_3 and T_4 work via an intracellular mechanism binding to intranuclear receptors. The hormonal activity is dependent upon DNA and mRNA transcription. Thus it may take 12 to 48 hours to achieve full effects.[3,17]

Most of the time the thyroid hormone circulates in plasma bound to plasma proteins, primarily thyroid-binding globulin. However, the free hormone is the fraction that is bioactive; the larger protein-bound portion is not readily accessible. The free hormone enters the cell by either passive diffusion or a specific carrier mechanism. Once inside the cell T_4 is converted to T_3, suggesting that T_3 is the active form of the hormone.[17] Thyroid hormone effects on various structures are summarized in Table 23-5.

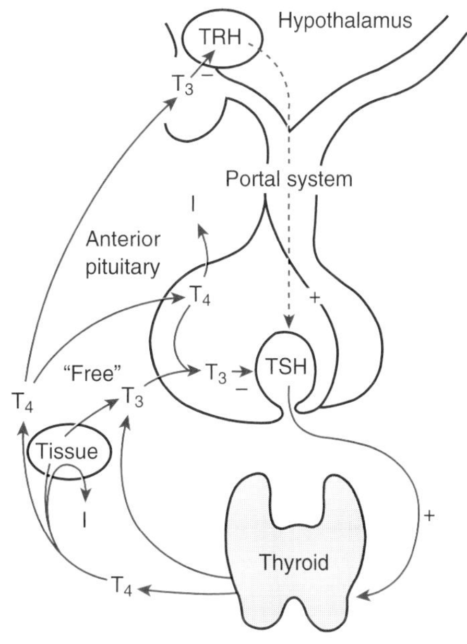

FIGURE 23-12. Hypothalamic-pituitary-thyroid axis. (Redrawn from Martin, J. B., Reichlin, S., & Brown, G. M. [1987]. *Clinical neuroendocrinology*. New York: Oxford University Press. Used by permission of Oxford University Press, Inc.)

Role in Fetal Development

Fetal thyroid function begins at about 11 weeks gestation.[17] Until that time, the developing fetus is entirely dependent upon the small amount of hormone that crosses the placenta. Adequate hormonal levels are essential for brain development and skeletal maturation.

Metabolic Activity

Thyroid hormones mediate various metabolic activities. Oxygen consumption and heat production are increased, possibly due to stimulation of Na^+/K^+ ATPase. This contributes to an increase in the total basal metabolic rate.[17]

Cholesterol synthesis and degradation are enhanced. This is due in part to an increase in hepatic low density lipoprotein (LDL) receptors. There is an increase in both lipogenesis and lipolysis.[5] Gluconeogenesis, glucogenolysis, and intestinal glucose absorption are also increased.

Cardiovascular and Pulmonary Effects

Thyroid hormones enhance myocardial contractility and increase the heart rate. These factors ultimately influence cardiac output.[5,30] Normal hypoxic and hypercapnic drive are dependent upon the action of thyroid hormones.

Neuromuscular Effects

Thyroid hormones are necessary for normal development and function of the central nervous system.[17] There is a direct relationship between the speed of muscle contraction and relaxation and the level of thyroid hormones. Hyperreflexia is seen in hyperthyroidism. Additionally, TRH may also function as a neurotransmitter. It has been shown to stimulate sympathetic outflow within the central nervous system.[30]

Endocrine Effects

The rate of metabolism of many hormones and pharmacologic agents is dependent upon thyroid hormonal activity. For example, the half-life of cortisol is markedly reduced in a hyperthyroid individual. The converse is true for hypothyroidism. Additionally, both hypo- and hyperthyroidism result in female infertility since ovulation is altered.

IODIDE METABOLISM

Iodide is essential to the normal function of the thyroid gland. When iodine is ingested, it is converted to iodide and absorbed into the bloodstream. Iodide is taken up by the thyroid gland and the excess is excreted by the kidney. Thyroid removal of iodide from the circulation is accomplished by means of an iodide pump or iodide trapping. The process is influenced by TSH. Iodide is taken into the follicular cells against both an electrical and a concentration gradient as part of a sodium iodide (Na^+/I^-) cotransport system.[17,31] The energy for this cotransporter is generated by Na^+/K^+ ATPase, which drives the Na^+/K^+ pump.[17] This active transport process provides an iodide concentration 30 to 40 times greater than that of the blood stream. The biosynthesis of thyroid hormones is shown in Figure 23-13. The formation of the thyroid hormones occurs at the cell–colloid interface. Iodide is oxidized and incorporated into tyrosine in thyroglobulin, forming monoiodothyronine.[17] Coupling of monoiodothyronine (MIT) produces diiodothyronine (DIT). Combinations of DIT and MIT unite within the thyroglobulin molecule to form triiodothyronine (T_3) and tetraiodothyronine (T_4).

CALCITONIN

Calcitonin is produced by the parafollicular cells of the thyroid gland. It is also found in nervous tissue. There it appears to function as a neuromodulator and an analgesic. However, its major physiologic action is to decrease plasma calcium levels. The major stimulus for calcitonin secretion is a rise in plasma calcium levels. It accomplishes this through antagonizing the action of parathyroid hormone on bone, inhibiting osteoclast-mediated resorption.[35] Thus the rate of bone turnover or remodeling is decreased.[3] It also antagonizes the effects of parathyroid hormone on the kidneys, allowing calcium to be excreted in the urine. Furthermore, it inhibits the renal reabsorption of phosphate and induces excretion of sodium and water.[35]

Although the actions of calcitonin include an interaction with other hormones in the regulation of plasma calcium levels, it is not an essential hormone. Plasma calcium levels do not change with either an excess or a deficit in calcitonin levels. However, it may be a factor in skeletal development. More of the hormone is secreted in younger patients. It may also protect the bones of pregnant women and nursing mothers from excessive calcium loss. Both lactation and fetal bone development require large amounts of calcium.[10] Calcitonin is also useful clinically as an inhibitor of osteoclastic bone resorption; thus it is being used to treat osteoporosis and Paget's disease.

PARATHYROID GLANDS

The parathyroid glands consist of four small glands embedded in the posterior aspect of the thyroid gland (see Fig 23-10). There is one parathyroid gland in each superior and inferior lateral area of the thyroid. Each gland is small, about the size of a pea, and weighs approximately 40 mg. The two cell types in the parathyroid gland are the oxyphil cell and the chief, or principal, cell. These are illustrated in Figure 23-14. Chief cells are responsible for the synthesis and secretion of parathyroid hormone. The oxyphil cells appear after puberty. Since the number

FOCUS ON CELLULAR PHYSIOLOGY

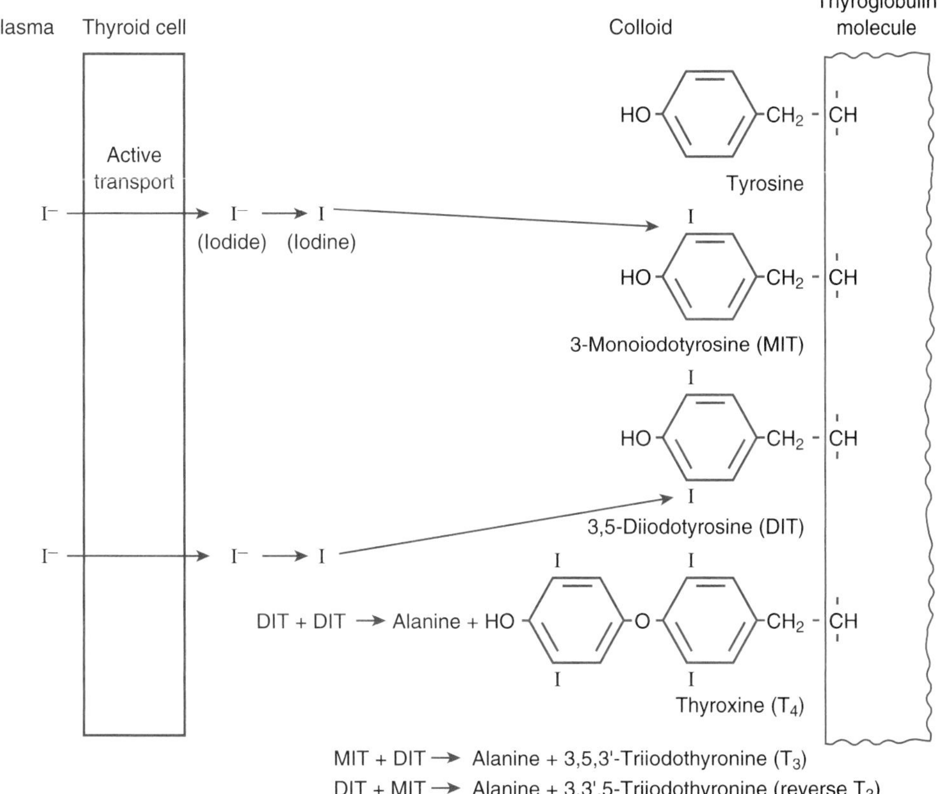

FIGURE 23-13. **Outline of thyroid hormone synthesis. Iodination of tyrosine takes place at the apical border of the thyroid cells while the molecules are bound in peptide linkage in thyroglobulin. (Ganong, W. F. [1997].** ***Review of medical physiology*** **[18th ed.]. Norwalk, CT: Appleton and Lange.)**

of oxyphil cells increases with age, they may actually be degenerated chief cells.[10]

Parathyroid Hormone

The parathyroid glands secrete parathyroid hormone (PTH), which helps to regulate calcium metabolism. The unbound portion, or ionized calcium, is the major stimulus for parathyroid hormone (PTH) synthesis and secretion.[10] A decrease in the level of circulating ionized calcium stimulates PTH secretion. Conversely, an increase in ionized calcium inhibits its secretion. The parathyroid gland is extremely sensitive to changes in calcium levels. The rate of PTH secretion can change within seconds of alteration in calcium levels.[33] Other factors that influence the rate of secretion of PTH include catecholamines and serum magnesium levels. Hypermagnesia inhibits its secretion, whereas catecholamines stimulate its secretion.[35] In contrast to other endocrine glands such as the pancreas and thyroid gland, the parathyroid glands contain a limited amount of hormone. Thus PTH must continually be synthesized and secreted.[15] Additionally, PTH has a very short half-life—about 2 to 4 minutes.[35] The parathyroid gland also differs in terms of the cation required for exocytosis of secretory vesicles. Usually this is a calcium-dependent process. However, PTH must be secreted when calcium levels are low and magnesium replaces calcium in promoting the exocytosis of PTH secretory vesicles.[35]

PARATHYROID HORMONE FUNCTION

As illustrated in Figure 23-15, parathyroid hormone maintains calcium levels by acting directly on the kidneys and bone and indirectly on the gastrointestinal tract. In the kidneys, PTH increases the reabsorption of calcium in the ascending loop of Henle and the distal tubule. However, the reabsorption of phosphate is blocked in the proximal and distal tubules. Thus the balance between calcium and phosphate levels is main-

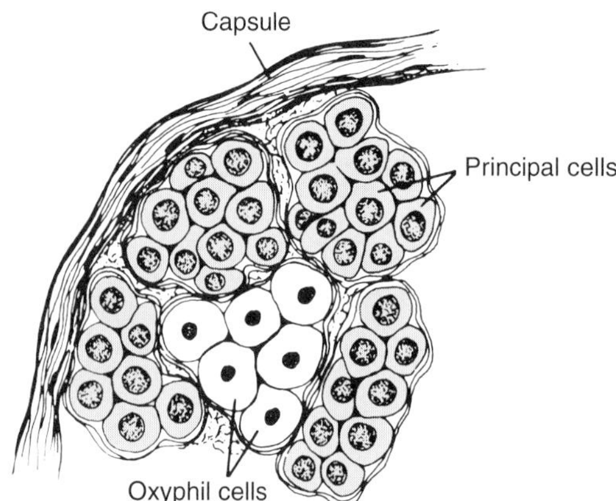

FIGURE 23-14. **Histology of parathyroid gland. The cells are arranged in cords by loose connective tissue. The principal cells are predominant in number. Oxyphil cells are recognized by their smaller, more condensed nuclei and larger relative cytoplasmic volume. (Borysenko, M. et al. [1984]. *Functional histology* [2nd ed.]. Boston: Little, Brown.)**

tained through renal excretion.[3] Additionally, renal synthesis of vitamin D is stimulated by PTH. Vitamin D is necessary for calcium absorption from the gastrointestinal tract. Thus, this provides an indirect action of PTH on the gastrointestinal tract.

The net effect of PTH on bone is to promote the removal of calcium. When osteocytes are stimulated by PTH, they remove calcium from the bone canalicular fluid, transferring it into the interstitial fluids.[3] However, its effects on osteoclasts are much more dramatic. Parathyroid hormone increases the number and size of osteoclasts by stimulating their production from precursor cells. The osteoclasts are then actively involved in bone resorption. Usually, osteoblasts work in concert with osteoclasts, forming new bone as part of the remodeling process. However, PTH inhibits this action by the osteoblasts. It is through these actions that PTH is able to rapidly restore normal calcium levels.

Calcium Metabolism

Calcium is ingested in food. Three major organs are responsible for maintaining adequate blood levels: kidneys, bone, and intestines. Only about one third of the daily intake of calcium is absorbed from the intestines. The remainder is excreted in the feces by the kidneys. However, most calcium in the kidneys is reabsorbed by active transport in the renal tubules. Homeostatic mechanisms, from bone remodeling, cause a turnover of about 500 mg of calcium per day.

Calcium is absorbed from the gastrointestinal tract by both active transport and passive diffusion. When intake is low, active transport is the predominant mechanism of absorption since passive diffusion is insufficient for physiologic needs. Vitamin D enhances the production of calcium-binding proteins by intestinal mucosal cells, increasing their capacity for calcium transport. The inactive form is activated by the kidney, with PTH being the major stimulus for this activation. Thus a decrease in calcium levels, promoting secretion of PTH, ultimately results in an increased activation of vitamin D. Additionally, a decrease in inorganic phosphorus also increases vitamin D activation.[3]

Bone Remodeling

Throughout the life span, bone is constantly being remodeled; older bone is being resorbed and new bone is formed. As part of that process, calcium is turned over at a rate of 18% per year in adults and 100% in infants.[10] Parathyroid hormone secreted by the parathyroid gland assists in the regulation of this process, in conjunction with vitamin D. As part of the remodeling process, bone reabsorption and formation are closely integrated, involving the activity of the bone cells, which are discussed on page 799.

ADRENAL GLAND

The adrenal, or suprarenal, glands are located on the superior pole of each kidney in the retroperitoneal space, as shown in Figure 23-16. A thick fibrous capsule surrounds the glands. The outermost portion and largest portion of each gland is the cortex. The cortex surrounds the smaller medulla, which is more medially located.

The adrenal glands are responsible for a wide variety of physiologic functions. Their actions include blood glucose regulation, maintenance of fluid and electrolyte homeostasis, and production and secretion of catecholamines.

Effects of ACTH on Adrenal Cortex

ACTH is produced by the anterior pituitary gland, and its release is controlled primarily by CRH. Other factors influence the release of ACTH. Some of them, such as vasoactive intestinal peptide (VIP), work synergistically with CRH to increase ACTH levels. Others, such as vasopressin, not only work with CRH but also have some independent action in stimulating ACTH release. Table 23-6 provides a list of factors that influence the secretion of ACTH.

ACTH regulates the growth and function of the adrenal cortex and the release of its hormones: glucocorticoids, mineralocorticoids, and androgens. ACTH also has an effect on immune function. It is able to influence the immune response by binding to leukocytes and modulating B-cell and T-cell activity. Additionally, β-endorphin, which is derived from the same prohormone as ACTH, appears to suppress anti-

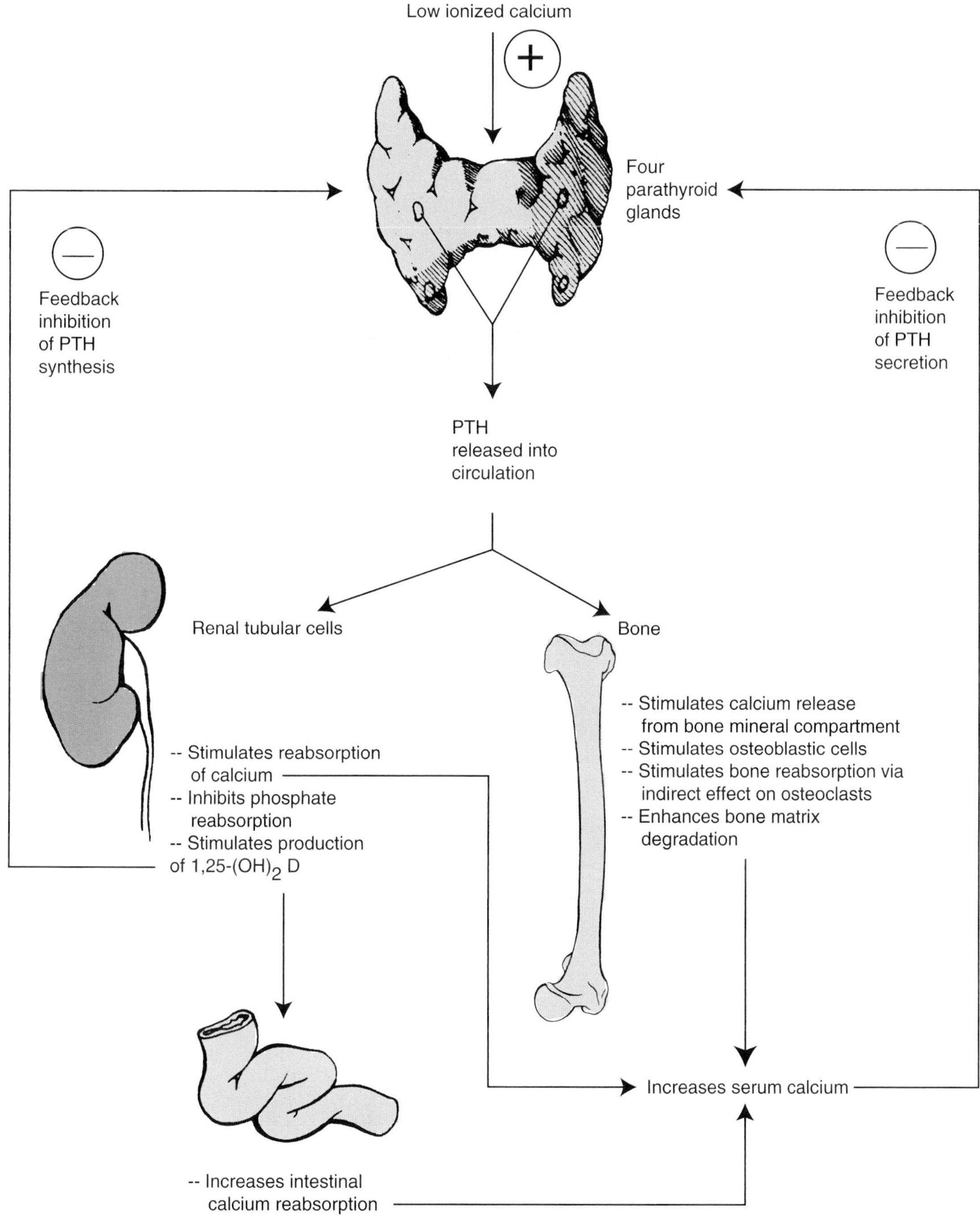

FIGURE 23-15. **Main functions of parathyroid hormone. (Modified from Chandrasoma, P., & Taylor, C. E. [1998].** ***Concise pathology*** **[3rd ed.]. Stamford, CT: Appleton and Lange).**

body formation.[28] However, it has also been shown to enhance natural killer cell activity.[20,29]

Hormones of the Adrenal Cortex

The adrenal cortex comprises three distinct layers: (1) the zona glomerulosa, (2) the zona fasiculata, and (3) the zona reticularis. The adrenal cortex secretes three types of steroid hormones: (1) glucocorticoids, (2) mineralocorticoids, and (3) androgens, or sex steroid precursors. The zona fasiculata and the zona reticularis are stimulated by ACTH to produce glucocorticoids and androgens. Mineralocorticoid production is associated with the zona glomerulosa. The following is a description

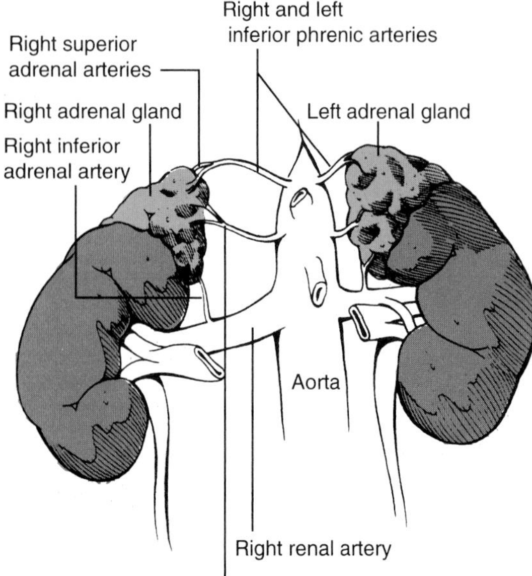

FIGURE 23-16. **Anatomy of the adrenal glands.**

of the physiologic functions of the major hormones of the adrenal cortex:

- Glucocorticoids: Regulation of carbohydrate and protein metabolism; regulation of the inflammatory response; promotion of adaptation as part of the physiologic stress response. The primary glucocorticoid is cortisol (see Chap. 5).
- Mineralocorticoids: Regulation of sodium and water reabsorption by the renal tubules. The primary mineralocorticoid is aldosterone.
- Androgens: Promotion of secondary sexual characteristics. Androgens are precursors to testosterone and estrogen.

TABLE 23-6

FACTORS THAT STIMULATE ACTH SECRETION

FACTOR	SOURCE
Corticotropin-releasing hormone	Hypothalamus
Vasoactive intestinal peptide	Hypothalamus
Vasopressin	Posterior pituitary
Humoral factors	Macrophages Lymphocytes
Catecholamines	Sympathetic nervous system Adrenal medulla

(Compiled from Reisine,T. [1988]. Neurohumoral aspects of ACTH. *Hospital Practice, 23*(3),77–96.)

GLUCOCORTICOIDS

Cortisol, cortisone, and corticosterone are glucocorticoids produced by the adrenal cortex. Cortisol is the primary glucocorticoid with the most potent effect and will be discussed below. Its secretion is controlled by the neuroendocrine axis through a negative feedback mechanism. The releasing hormone, corticotropin releasing hormone (CRH), stimulates the anterior pituitary gland to secrete ACTH, which in turn promotes the synthesis and secretion of glucocorticoids.

Cortisol exerts its physiologic effects by a relatively slower, intracellular mechanism. This process is initiated when the hormone binds with a specific receptor protein, enabling it to enter the cell. The hormone–receptor protein complex must become activated and reach the nucleus to actually exert its effects on the cell. Activation exposes a site on the complex with affinity for DNA. This activates a transcription process that produces new messenger RNA (mRNA).[28] The mRNA directs the formation of new proteins by the ribosomes. It is these newly formed proteins that are responsible for the "hormonal effects" of the steroid hormones.

Cortisol is secreted in pulsatile bursts in a diurnal rhythm. It peaks at around 6 AM with levels of 9 to 25 μg/dL[18] and decreases to 5 μg/dL in the evening.[3] This pattern of secretion is associated with sleep/wake cycles and can be shifted when sleep/wake cycles are altered. A shift can also occur with changes in light-dark exposure and meal times. Other factors that can affect this diurnal rhythm include physical stressors such as surgery or trauma and psychologic stressors such as severe anxiety and depression.[8]

Function of Glucocorticoids

Glucocorticoids are necessary for survival, as illustrated in Figure 23-17. Their secretion is increased during stress, pain, and prolonged exercise. Their major effects include regulating the metabolic function of the body and controlling the inflammatory response. However, many tissues also are affected by glucocorticoid activity; they are identified in Table 23-7.

In most tissues, protein synthesis is inhibited and protein catabolism is enhanced by glucocorticoids. The net effect is to provide substrates for gluconeogenesis. Anabolic activity in the liver is increased. Gluconeogenesis and glycogen synthesis and storage also increase. Since glucose uptake is inhibited in muscle cells, circulating blood glucose levels increase. This enables glucocorticoids to function as a **counter-regulatory** hormone in maintaining glucose homeostasis. Additionally, glucocorticoids increase lipolysis with the release of glycerol and free fatty acids.

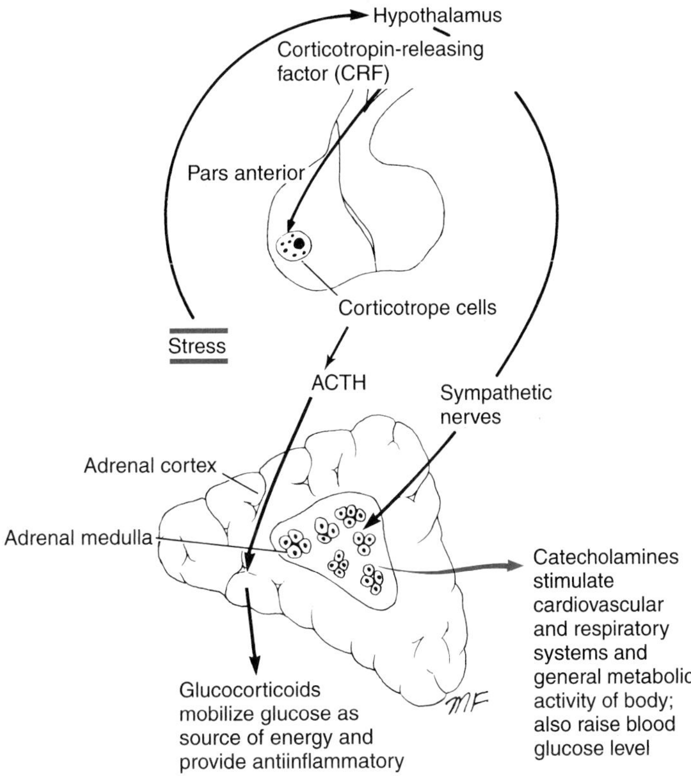

FIGURE 23-17. **Hypothalamic–pituitary–adrenal axis, showing the effects of stress on the activities of the adrenal gland.**

TABLE 23-7

EFFECTS OF GLUCOCORTICOIDS

TISSUE	EFFECT	MECHANISM
Muscle	Catabolic	Inhibit glucose uptake and metabolism Decrease protein synthesis Increase release of amino acids and lactate
Adipose	Lipolytic	Stimulate lipolysis Increase release of free fatty acids
Liver	Synthetic	Increase gluconeogenesis Increase glycogen synthesis and storage
Immune system	Suppression	Reduce number of circulating lymphocytes, monocytes, eosinophils, and basophils Interfere with antigen processing Interfere with antibody production
	Anti-inflammatory	Decrease migration of neutrophils, monocytes, and lymphocytes
Cardiovascular	Increase peripheral vascular tone	
Renal	Increase glomerular filtration rate Regulation of water and electrolyte balance	

(Modified from McPhee, S. J. [1997]. Disorders of the adrenal cortex. In S. J. McPhee, V. R. Lingappa, W. F. Ganong, & J. D. Lange [Eds.], *Pathophysiology of disease* [2nd ed.]. Stamford, CT: Appleton & Lange.)

In connective tissue, glucocorticoids inhibit fibroblasts, leading to loss of collagen and connective tissue. Glucocorticoids directly inhibit bone formation by decreasing cellular proliferation and synthesis of RNA. Additionally, they reduce intestinal reabsorption of calcium, in part due to impaired vitamin D synthesis.[3] In fluid and electrolyte balance, glucocorticoids promote sodium and water reabsorption. This effect is the result of interaction with mineralocorticoid receptors. In the eyes, intraocular pressure increases and decreases according to the diurnal variations in glucocorticoid levels.[8]

MINERALOCORTICOIDS

Aldosterone is a mineralocorticoid that regulates fluid and electrolyte levels. Its secretion is regulated by the renin–angiotensin system (RAS) and to a much lesser extent by ACTH (see Chap. 29 for a more complete discussion of the RAS). Essentially, decreased sodium levels and a decrease in plasma volume trigger the secretion of renin by the renal juxtaglomerular cells. Renin promotes the conversion of angiotensinogen to angiotensin I. Specific angiotensin-converting enzymes (ACE) convert angiotensin I to angiotensin II, a powerful vasoconstrictor. Angiotensin II binds to receptors in the adrenal cortex, stimulating the synthesis and secretion of aldosterone. When sodium and plasma volume return to normal levels, aldosterone secretion is reduced.

Function of Mineralocorticoids

Aldosterone, the primary mineralocorticoid, acts in the distal convoluted tubule and the collecting duct of the nephron. Sodium reabsorption is promoted by two different mechanisms: (1) an increase in the number of sodium channels on the luminal membrane of the tubular cells for reabsorption, and (2) an increase in the action of Na^+/K^+ ATPase to move sodium out of the cell into the interstitial fluid.[3] It is also theorized that aldosterone enhances mitochondrial activity to supply additional ATP for the Na^+/K^+ pump.[12] Since water is passively absorbed with the sodium, the plasma sodium level is only slightly increased. Additionally, as sodium is reabsorbed, potassium is excreted. Thus, the net effect is an isotonic volume expansion.[3]

ANDROGENS

Several steroids with sex hormone activity are secreted by the adrenal cortex. However, only the androgen *dehydroepiandrosterone* (DHEA) is produced in significant amounts. Like other androgens, it exerts masculinizing effects and promotes protein anabolism and growth. Another adrenal androgen, *androstenedione*, is converted to estrogen in the circulation. This becomes a source of estrogen for menopausal women. The secretion of adrenal androgens is controlled by ACTH, not the gonadotropins.

Adrenal Medulla

Located in the interior portion of the gland, the adrenal medulla secretes catecholamines, which include epinephrine, norepinephrine, and dopamine. Of these, epinephrine is the primary catecholamine. Norepinephrine and dopamine are produced mostly in the peripheral tissues of the sympathetic nervous tissue. The adrenal medulla can be considered an extension of the sympathetic nervous system since it is essentially a specialized sympathetic ganglia.[3] However, the cells of the medulla do not have axons or synaptic bulbs. They consist of chromaffin cells innervated by preganglionic fibers from the splanchnic nerve. These cells discharge the catecholamines that they produce directly into the blood stream in a manner similar to that of endocrine tissues. The adrenal medulla is an example of the interelationship between the nervous system and the endocrine system.[13]

Functions of Catecholamines

Adrenal medullary secretions play an important role in the "fight or flight" portion of the physiologic stress response. Flowchart 23-2 shows the sympathetic adrenal medullary response in stress. Epinephrine secretion as

FLOWCHART 23-2 **Sympathetic Adrenal-Medullary Response**

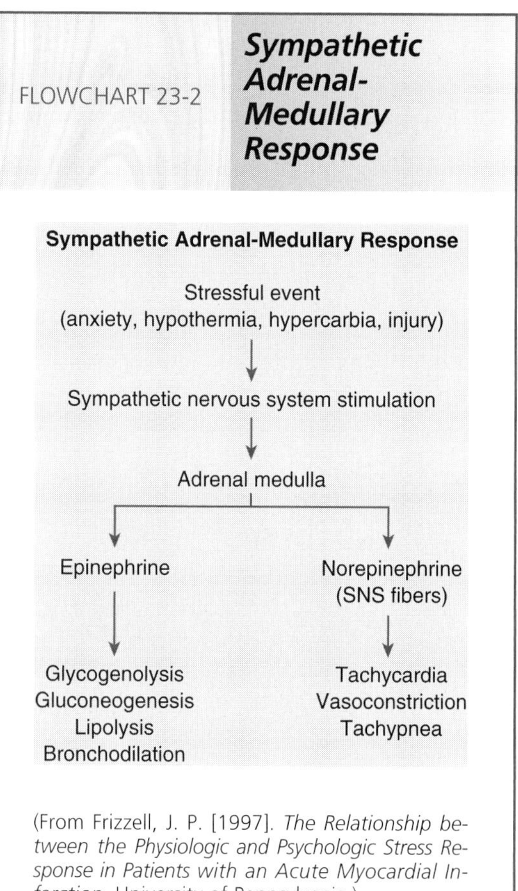

(From Frizzell, J. P. [1997]. *The Relationship between the Physiologic and Psychologic Stress Response in Patients with an Acute Myocardial Infarction.* University of Pennsylvania.)

part of this response is capable of producing adrenergic effects in all tissues with adrenergic receptors.

The metabolic effects of catecholamines are profound. Mobilization of glucose stores occurs through increased glycogenolysis. Additionally, there is increased gluconeogenesis. Epinephrine inhibits the secretion of insulin so that blood glucose levels are increased. In this manner, epinephrine functions as a counter regulatory hormone to maintain glucose homeostasis. Catecholamines also increase the basal metabolic rate. This produces a nonshivering **thermogenesis**, which is an important response to cold exposure.[3]

Catecholamines also indirectly regulate fluid and electrolyte levels through stimulating renin secretion by the juxtaglomerular cells of the nephron. Beta-adrenergic effects also increase the movement of potassium into muscle cells. Thus sodium and potassium balance is maintained.[3] Other effects of catecholamines are those associated with the sympathetic nervous system and listed in Table 29-11.

ENDOCRINE PANCREAS

The pancreas is a fish-shaped organ located in the upper portion of the posterior abdominal wall, behind the stomach (Fig. 23-18). It has a characteristic lobular appearance. The endocrine cells of the pancreas, islets of Langerhans, are embedded like small islands between the exocrine acinar cells (Fig. 23-19). The islets of Langerhans have specific cell types that synthesize and secrete hormones that promote and maintain glucose utilization and cellular metabolism.

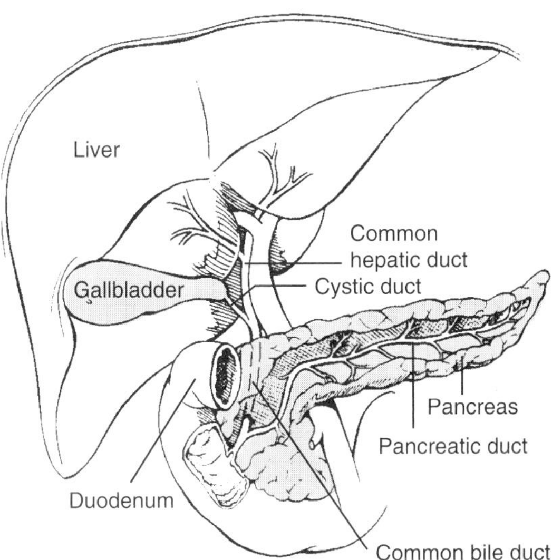

FIGURE 23-18. Anatomy of pancreas. (Memmler, R. L., Cohn, B. J., & Wood, D. L. [1996]. *The human body in health and disease* [8th ed.]. Philadelphia: J. B. Lippincott.)

The pancreas has both exocrine and endocrine functions. The endocrine activity of the pancreas will be presented in this chapter. The exocrine functions of the pancreas are reviewed in Chapter 26.

Function of the Endocrine Pancreas

The major function of the endocrine pancreas is glucose homeostasis. In the healthy individual, blood glucose levels range from 80 to 100 mg/dL. This concentration changes to 120 to 140 mg/dL after a meal. The feedback system to the endocrine pancrease returns the concentration to normal within about 2 hours after the last absorption of carbohydrates.

The blood glucose level is vital in maintaining normal functioning in the brain and major organs. The brain is almost exclusively dependent upon glucose as its energy source. It can store only a small amount of glycogen and cannot synthesize glucose.[6] Interestingly enough, it is one of the few areas of the body with glucose transporters that function independently of insulin. However, when blood glucose levels are reduced, the brain still needs to have adequate amounts of glucose to function. Although insulin is the only hormone whose action results in lowered blood sugar levels, there are several counter-regulatory hormones that are capable of elevating blood glucose. This response is accomplished by mobilizing glucose stores through glycogenolysis or by producing new glucose by **gluconeogenesis** (the production of glucose from noncarbohydrate sources). Thus, normal levels of blood glucose are maintained. Once glucose is absorbed, 50% of it undergoes **glycolysis** (the metabolism of glucose) to become an immediate source of energy. The remainder is stored for future energy needs (30% to 40% is converted to fat, with 10% stored as glycogen).[14]

As discussed in Chapter 24, the physiologic response to reduced glucose levels utilizes several hormones to correct hypoglycemia and prevent cellular injury. These hormones also work synergistically with the ANS to restore glucose homeostasis.

Hypoglycemia is sensed in the brain and stimulates a series of responses. These responses include the secretion of the counter-regulatory hormones, reduction of insulin secretion, and activation of the ANS. ANS effects include the hemodynamic changes and neurogenic symptoms characteristic of hypoglycemia (see Chap. 24). These include tachycardia, tremors, pallor, and diaphoresis. Additionally, epinephrine is released by the ANS to mobilize glucose stores. The counter-regulatory hormones secreted during hypoglycemia include glucagon, growth hormone, and cortisol.[6,7,10] Their roles in glucose homeostasis include the following:

- Glucagon: Actions oppose insulin. Primary hormone to restore glucose homeostasis by stimulating glycogenolysis, lipolysis, and gluconeogenesis.

FOCUS ON CELLULAR PHYSIOLOGY

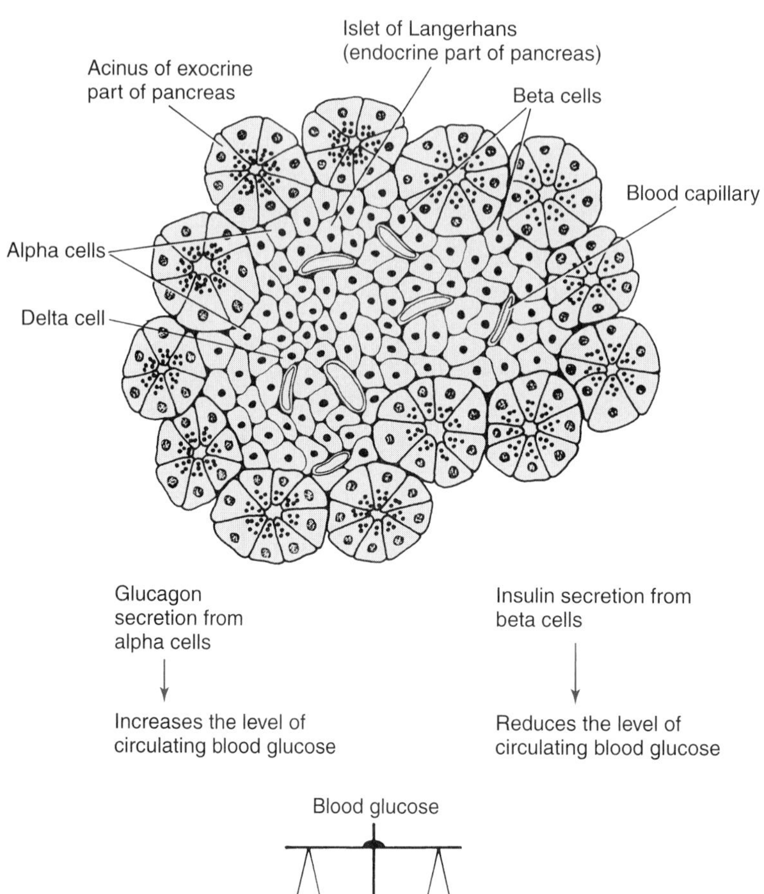

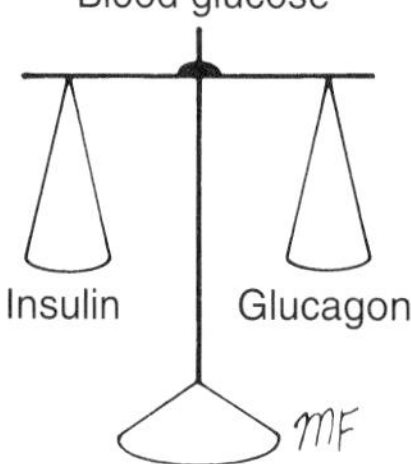

FIGURE 23-19. **Histology of the pancreas.**

- Epinephrine: Secreted as part of ANS activation. Mobilizes glucose stores through glycogenolysis. Increases circulating free fatty acids.
- Growth hormone: Decreases glucose uptake by tissues, possibly through decreasing the number of insulin receptors. Mobilizes free fatty acids.
- Glucocorticoids: Primarily cortisol. Support actions of glucagon. Decrease peripheral glucose utilization. Promote glycogenolysis and gluconeogenesis.

These counter-regulatory actions are essential in maintaining glucose homeostasis and preventing complications from hypoglycemia.

Pancreatic Hormones

The cell types of the pancreas have previously been identified using the Greek alphabet. Recently, however, many endocrinologists have replaced these designations with letters from the English alphabet.[10,21] The cell types and their respective hormones are described below.

- B cells (beta cells) are most abundant and secrete insulin. This is the major hormone secreted by the endocrine pancreas. Its physiologic action is to promote cellular uptake and utilization of glucose. It is an anabolic hormone that integrates the utilization of the major metabolic sources of energy, glucose, fats, and proteins. Its effects on various tissues are listed in Table 23-8.
- A cells (alpha cells) secrete glucagon. This is the major counter-regulatory hormone. Since it increases blood sugar levels through glycogenolysis, it has a physiologic effect that is opposite to that of insulin.
- D cells (delta cells) secrete somatostatin. This hormone inhibits the secretion of insulin, glucagon, and

TABLE 23-8

EFFECTS OF INSULIN ON VARIOUS TISSUES

TISSUE	INSULIN EFFECTS
Adipose tissue	Increased glucose entry Increased fatty acid synthesis Increased triglyceride deposition Increased potassium uptake
Muscle tissue	Increased glucose entry Increased glycogen synthesis Increased amino acid uptake Increased protein synthesis Decreased protein catabolism Increased potassium uptake
Liver	Decreased ketogenesis Increased protein synthesis Increased lipid synthesis Increased glycogen synthesis
General	Increased cell growth

(Modified from Ganong, W. F. [1997]. *Review of medical physiology* [18th ed.]. Stamford, CT: Appleton & Lange.)

pancreatic polypeptide. Additionally, it reduces the secretion of many digestive enzymes such as pepsin and gastrin.

- F cells secrete pancreatic polypeptide. The exact physiologic activity of this polypeptide is not known; however, it is secreted in response to a high-protein meal, fasting, exercise, and acute hypoglycemia. It is speculated that it exerts effects on gastrointestinal secretion.

INSULIN

Insulin is formed from a preproinsulin that is further synthesized to a proinsulin composed of two complex chains of polypeptides, referred to as A and B chains. The two chains are linked together by two disulfate bonds and a C peptide. Before secretion, the C peptide is removed and released from the B cells along with insulin. The C peptide has no known biological activity. Both insulin and the C peptide are secreted from secretory granules in approximately equal amounts, along with a small amount of proinsulin.

The average daily secretion of insulin is about 40 to 50 units per day. Insulin secretion occurs in two modes: (1) basal insulin secretion and (2) stimulated insulin secretion. *Basilar insulin* secretion is the amount needed to maintain homeostasis and occurs without stimulation. *Stimulated insulin* secretion occurs in response to food intake. However, glucose is the strongest stimulus for insulin secretion. The threshold for insulin secretion is a glucose level of 80 to 100 mg/dL. Insulin secretion occurs approximately 8 to 10 minutes after food intake, reaching a peak concentration at about 30 to 45 minutes. It returns to baseline values at about 90 to 120 minutes after food intake. Insulin has a half-life of 3 to 5 minutes and is metabolized by the liver, kidney, and placenta.[14,21]

The pancreatic B cells are able to absorb glucose through the action of a specific glucose transporter (GLUT-2). Once inside the cell, glucose is phosphorylated in preparation for glucose metabolism. Figure 23-20 depicts glucose metabolism–mediating changes in the B cells' second messenger systems. This ultimately changes the cell membrane action potential, causing depolarization. As calcium enters the cell through voltage gated channels, insulin is secreted.[3,7,22]

Other factors, such as vagal stimulation, can also promote insulin secretion. However, glucose is the major stimulus for insulin secretion. Once insulin secretion has been initiated, the amount of insulin secreted can be increased. This occurs through beta-adrenergic activation or through the action of hormones such as cholecystokinin and gastrin.[21] As mentioned previously, somatostatin inhibits insulin secretion. In addition, alpha-2 adrenergic activity and prostaglandin E_2 inhibit insulin secretion.[22] Hypokalemia is also associated with reduced insulin secretion.[10]

Function of Insulin

Insulin facilitates the transport of glucose into cells through the action of glucose transporters (Fig. 23-21). There are several different types of glucose transporters. The glucose transporters for the brain (GLUT-1 and GLUT-3) and pancreatic B cells (GLUT-2) are able to independently absorb glucose from the blood stream. The glucose transporter (GLUT-4) for adipose tissue, skeletal and cardiac muscle is an insulin-dependent transporter. Insulin, through interaction with its receptor, promotes the mobilization of glucose transporters to the cell surface. This action ultimately increases the amount of glucose absorbed by the cell through facilitated diffusion.[10,21]

The major actions of insulin are metabolic, promoting the storage of energy substrates. As a result, plasma concentrations of glucose, free fatty acids, and certain amino acids decrease. This occurs through coordinated regulation of metabolism. Insulin stimulates the transport of glucose into the cells, enabling it to become the primary energy source. It also stimulates the conversion of glucose to glycogen.

Insulin promotes the storage of fat in adipose tissue. Since glucose is the primary energy source, there is less movement of free fatty acids from adipose tissue. Lipolysis is decreased. Triglyceride synthesis and storage is increased, promoting weight gain. Insulin also stimulates the formation of free fatty acids from glucose.

Insulin stimulates the cellular uptake of amino acids. Overall anabolic activity is increased. Protein and other

FOCUS ON CELLULAR PHYSIOLOGY

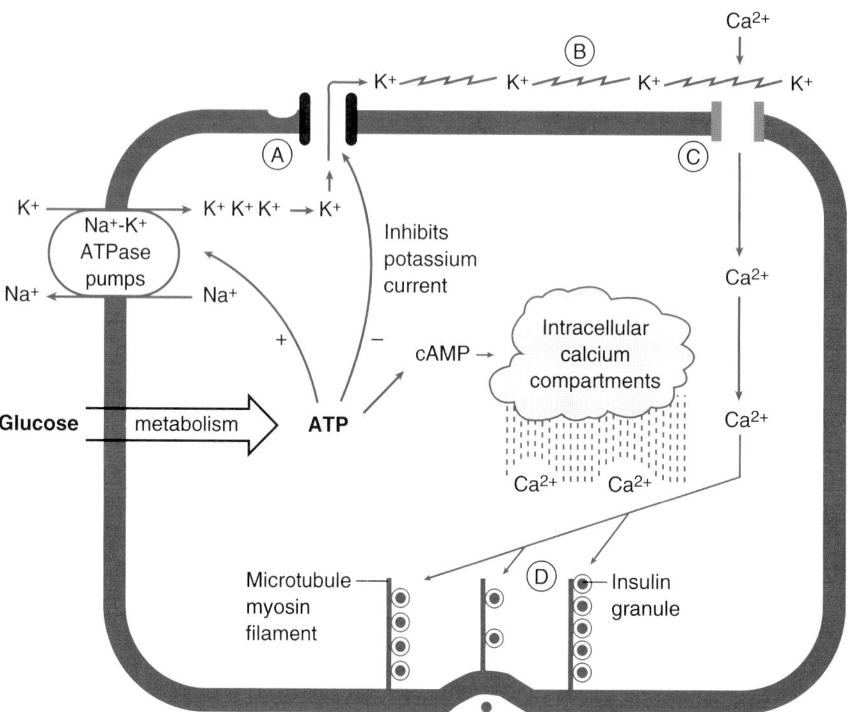

FIGURE 23-20. **Regulation of insulin by glucose. A.** "Resting" beta cell (blood glucose, <100 mg/dl). The ADP/ATP ratio is high enough so that ATP-sensitive potassium channels (*ASKC*) are open, and the membrane potential is about −70 mV. The voltage-sensitive calcium channels (*VSCC*) and calcium-sensitive potassium channels (*CSKC*) are closed. **B.** The beta cell response to increased blood glucose. In response to the increased glucose entry and metabolism, the ratio of ADP/ATP decreases, and the ATP-sensitive potassium channels close. The VSCC are activated; calcium enters and stimulates insulin secretion. Increased cytosolic calcium inhibits the VSCC and activates the CSKC, thereby allowing the cell membrane to repolarize and the calcium channels to close. The persistence of high glucose levels results in repeated spiking of electrical discharges and oscillation of intracellular calcium concentrations. (Goodman, H.M. [1994]. *Basic medical endocrinology* [2nd ed.]. New York: Raven.)

macromolecule synthesis is increased. Thus there is enhanced cellular growth, tissue regeneration, and bone remodeling.[3]

Insulin has other actions in addition to its metabolic activity. This effect occurs through the enhancement of growth factor activity. For example, platelet-derived growth factor (PDGF) action is increased in the presence of insulin. Insulin may also regulate gene expression. Decreases in the level of enzymes necessary for gluconeogenesis have been observed after insulin administration.[14] Additionally, insulin is able to promote potassium entry into cells, possibly by increasing the activity of Na^+/K^+ ATPase. Cellular uptake of phosphorus and magnesium also increase.[3] Increased renal reabsorption of potassium, phosphate, and sodium is the result of insulin activity on the renal tubules. Insulin also has paracrine effects, inhibiting the secretion of glucagon by the A cells.[14]

GLUCAGON

Glucagon is an important counter-regulatory hormone. Its action is opposite to that of insulin, and its secretion results in an increase in blood glucose concentration. Glucagon stimulates glycogenolysis and gluconeogenesis in the liver.

The secretion of glucagon is regulated by blood glucose levels, ingested proteins, amino acids, and insulin. These exert a feedback effect on glucagon activity. Glucagon is secreted when blood glucose levels fall or

FOCUS ON CELLULAR PHYSIOLOGY

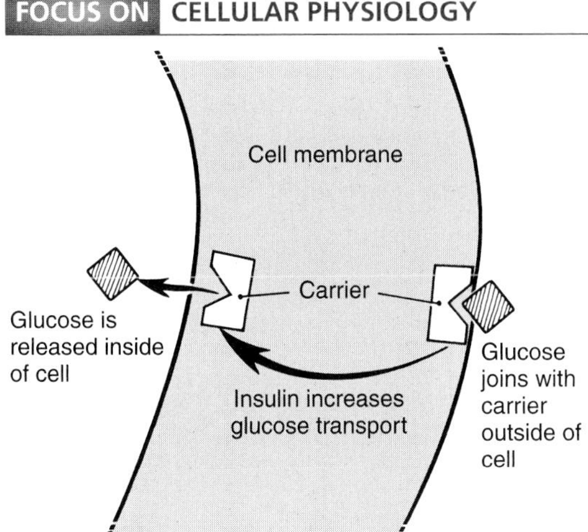

FIGURE 23-21. Diagram of glucose transporter.

a protein meal is ingested, supplying amino acids for gluconeogenesis. In contrast to this, fatty acids, another source of energy, suppress glucagon secretion.[10] As previously mentioned, both insulin and somatostatin suppress glucagon secretion.[3]

SOMATOSTATIN

Somatostatin is a neuropeptide that is produced in both the hypothalamus and the pancreatic D cells. It inhibits the secretion of insulin, glucagon, and pancreatic polypeptide. Metabolically, it decreases the rate of digestion and the absorption of nutrients from the gastrointestinal tract. Additionally, it reduces the secretion of gastrointestinal enzymes that are essential for digestion. Somatostatin secretion is stimulated by some of the same substances that stimulate insulin secretion—glucose and amino acids. Its secretion is stimulated by cholecystokinin and inhibited by insulin.[3,10]

REFERENCES

1. Aron, D. C., Findling, J. W., & Tyrrell, J. B. (1997). Hypothalamus and pituitary. In F. S. Greenspan and G. J. Strewler (Eds.), *Basic and clinical endocrinology* (5th ed.). Stamford, CT: Appleton & Lange.
2. Baxter, J. D. (1997). Introduction to endocrinology. In F. S. Greenspan & G. J. Strewler (Eds.), *Basic and clinical endocrinology* (5th ed.). Stamford, CT: Appleton & Lange.
3. Berne, R. M. & Levy, M. N. (1996). *Principles of physiology* (2nd ed.). St. Louis: C. V. Mosby.
4. Blevins, L. S., & Wand, G. S. (1992). Diabetes insipidus. *Critical Care Medicine, 20*(1), 69–79.
5. Brent, G. A. (1994). The molecular basis of thyroid hormone action. *New England Journal of Medicine, 331*(13), 847–853.
6. Cryer, P. E., Fisher, J. N., & Shamoon, H. (1994). Hypoglycemia. *Diabetes Care, 17*(7), 734–755.
7. Feingold, K. R. & Funk, J. L. (1997). Disorders of the endocrine pancreas. In S. J. McPhee, V. R. Lingappa, W. F. Ganong, & J. D. Lange (Eds.), *Pathology of disease* (2nd ed.). Stamford, CT: Appleton & Lange.
8. Findling, J. W., Aron, D. C., & Tyrell, J. B. (1997). Glucocorticoids and adrenal androgens. In F. S. Greenspan & G. J. Strewler (Eds.), *Basic and clinical endocrinology* (5th ed.). Stamford, CT: Appleton & Lange.
9. Frizzell, J. P. (1997). *The relationship between the physiologic and psychologic response to stress in patients with an acute myocardial infarction* [dissertation]. Philadelphia: University of Pennsylvania.
10. Ganong, W. F. (1997). *Review of medical physiology* (18th ed.). Stamford, CT: Appleton & Lange.
11. Glaser, R., Kennedy, S., Lafuse, W., Bonneau, R., Speicher, C., Hillhouse, J., & Kiecolt-Glaser, J. (1990). Psychologic stress-induced modulation of interleukin 2 receptor gene expression and interleukin 2 production in peripheral blood leukocytes. *Archives of General Psychiatry, 47*, 707–712.
12. Granner, D. K. (1996). Hormones of the adrenal cortex. In R. K. Murray, K. Granner, P. A. Mayes, & V. W. Rodwell (Eds.), *Harper's biochemistry* (24th ed.). Stamford, CT: Appleton & Lange.
13. Granner, D. K. (1996). Hormones of the adrenal medulla. In R. K. Murray, K. Granner, P. A. Mayes, & V. W. Rodwell (Eds.), *Harper's biochemistry* (24th ed.). Stamford, CT: Appleton & Lange.
14. Granner, D. K. (1996). Hormones of the pancreas and the gastrointestinal tract. In R. K. Murray, K. Granner, P. A. Mayes, & V. W. Rodwell (Eds.), *Harper's biochemistry* (24th ed.). Stamford, CT: Appleton & Lange.
15. Granner, D. K. (1996). Hormones that regulate calcium metabolism. In R. K. Murray, K. Granner, P. A. Mayes, & V. W. Rodwell (Eds.), *Harper's biochemistry* (24th ed.). Stamford, CT: Appleton & Lange.
16. Granner, D. K. (1996). Pituitary and hypothalamic hormones. In R. K. Murray, K. Granner, P. A. Mayes, & V. W. Rodwell (Eds.), *Harper's biochemistry* (24th ed.). Stamford, CT: Appleton & Lange.
17. Greenspan, F. S. (1997). The thyroid gland. In F. S. Greenspan & G. J. Strewler (Eds.), *Basic and clinical endocrinology* (5th ed.). Stamford, CT: Appleton and Lange.
18. Grinspoon, S. K. & Biller, B. M. K. (1994). Laboratory assessment of adrenal insufficiency. *Journal of Clinical Endocrinology and Metabolism, 79*(4), 931–932.
19. Guyton, A. C. (1991). *Textbook of medical physiology* (8th ed.). Philadelphia: W. B. Saunders.
20. Houldin, A. D., Lev, E., Prystowsky, M. B., Redei, E., & Lowery, B. J. (1991). Psychoneuroimmunology: A review of literature. *Holistic Nursing Practice, 5*(4), 10–20.
21. Karam, J. H. (1997). Pancreatic hormones and diabetes mellitus. In F. S. Greenspan & G. J. Strewler (Eds.), *Basic and clinical endocrinology* (5th ed.). Stamford, CT: Appleton and Lange.
22. Laychock, S. G. (1990). Glucose metabolism, second messengers and insulin secretion. *Life Sciences, 47*(25), 2307–2316.
23. Leibowitz, S. F. (1994). Specificity of hypothalamic peptides in the control of behavior and physiologic processes. *Annals of the New York Academy of Sciences, 739*, 12–35.
24. Lingappa, V. R. (1997). Disorders of the hypothalamus and pituitary gland. In S. J. McPhee, V. R. Lingappa, W. F. Ganong, & J. D. Lange (Eds.), *Pathology of disease* (2nd ed.). Stamford, CT: Appleton & Lange.

25. Marcinek, M. B. (1977). Stress in the surgical patient. *American Journal of Nursing, 77*(11), 1809–1811.
26. McPhee, S. J. (1997). Disorders of the adrenal cortex. In S. J. McPhee, V. R. Lingappa, W. F. Ganong, & J. D. Lange (Eds.), *Pathology of disease* (2nd ed.). Stamford, CT: Appleton & Lange.
27. McPhee, S. J. & Bauer, D. C. (1997). Thyroid disease. In S. J. McPhee, V. R. Lingappa, W. F. Ganong, & J. D. Lange (Eds.), *Pathology of disease* (2nd ed.). Stamford, CT: Appleton & Lange.
28. Munck, A. & Guyre, P. M. (1991). Glucocorticoids and immune function. In R. Ader, D. Felton, & N. Cohen (Eds.), *Psychoneuroimmunology.* New York: Academic Press.
29. O'Leary, A. (1990). Stress, emotion, and human immune function. *Psychological Bulletin, 108*(3), 363–382.
30. Polikar, R., Burger, A., G., Scherrer, U., & Nicod, P. (1993). The thyroid and the heart. *Circulation, 87*(5), 1435–1441.
31. Reasner, C. A., & Talbert, R. I. (1997). Thyroid disorders. In J. R. Dipiro, R. L. Talbert, G. C. Yee, G. R. Matzke, B. G. Wells, & L. M. Posey, *Pharmacotherapy: A pathophysiologic approach* (3rd ed.). Stamford, CT: Appleton & Lange.
32. Reisine, T. (1988). Neurohumoral aspects of ACTH. *Hospital Practice, 23*(3), 77–96.
33. Shoback, D. M. & Strewler, G. J. (1997). Disorders of the parathyroids and calcium metabolism. In S. J. McPhee, V. R. Lingappa, W. F. Ganong, & J. D. Lange (Eds.), *Pathology of disease* (2nd ed.). Stamford, CT: Appleton & Lange.
34. Stephenson, C. A. (1977). Stress in critically ill patients. *American Journal of Nursing, 77*(11), 1806–1809.
35. Strewler, G. J. (1997). Mineral metabolism and metabolic bone disease. In F. S. Greenspan & G. J. Strewler (Eds.), *Basic and clinical endocrinology* (5th ed.). Stamford, CT: Appleton and Lange.
36. Thorner, M. O. et al. (1992). The anterior pituitary. In J. D. Wilson and D. W. Foster Jr. (Eds.), *William's textbook of endocrinology* (8th ed.). Philadelphia: W. B. Saunders.
37. Weissman, C. (1990). The metabolic response to stress: An overview and update. *Anesthesiology, 73*(2), 308–327.

Chapter 24

Altered Endocrine Function

Joan Parker Frizzell

KEY TERMS

acromegaly
acquired hypothyroidism
Addison's disease
Chvostek's sign
congenital hypothyroidism
craniopharyngioma
cretinism
Cushing's disease
Cushing's syndrome
diabetes insipidus
diabetic nephropathy
empty sella syndrome
gastrinoma
gigantism
goiter
goitrogen
glucagonoma
glucocorticoid
hyperparathyroidism
hyperprolactinemia
insulinitis
insulinoma
mineralocorticoid
molecular mimicry
myxedema
onycholysis
polyuria
prolactinemia
pseudohypoaldosteronism
psychogenic polydipsia
retinopathy
somatostatinoma
thyroid dermopathy
thyroid osteopathy
thyrotoxicosis
Trousseau's sign

Endocrine disorders are very complex because many endocrine hormones have a variety of physiologic effects. Additionally, as in the case of the *neuroendocrine axis,* the function of one endocrine gland influences the function of other glands. However, most endocrine disorders can be considered in terms of an excess or a deficiency of hormonal levels. This is most often the result of hyperfunction or hypofunction of the endocrine gland. In some circumstances the disease process may be due to a problem outside the gland that affects glandular activity. Alterations in target tissue receptor responsiveness to the hormone may also present as endocrine hypofunction or hyperfunction. Figure 24-1 provides an overview of endocrine dysfunction, and Table 24-1 presents common manifestations associated with endocrine disorders.

This chapter presents an overview of the basic pathophysiology common to most endocrine disorders and discusses dysfunction of each endocrine gland.

HYPOFUNCTION

Endocrine hypofunction is an alteration in endocrine activity that presents with manifestations of hormonal deficit. This can be due to (1) glandular disorders that result in a decrease in hormonal secretion, (2) extraglandular disorders that modify glandular activity, or (3) defects in hormonal synthesis.

Glandular Disorders

The most common reason for endocrine hypofunction is destruction of the endocrine gland. There are four basic mechanisms responsible for this: (1) autoimmune destruction, (2) damage from neoplasms, (3) damage from infection, and (4) damage from ischemia/hemorrhage.[10]

AUTOIMMUNE DESTRUCTION

Many factors lead to susceptibility to autoimmune endocrine dysfunction. However, there appears to be a genetic predisposition to a particular autoimmune disorder. For example, Type 1 diabetes mellitus (DM) has a strong genetic component, as has been shown by studying families with the disease. Specific human

(text continues on page 671)

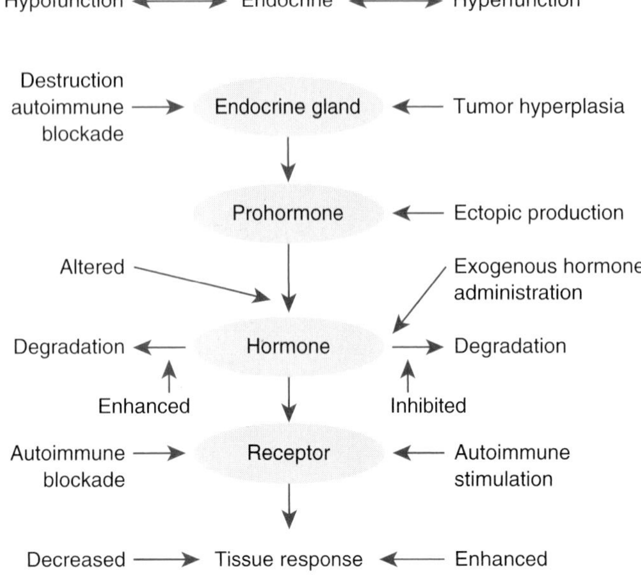

FIGURE 24-1. Etiology of endocrine hypofunction and hyperfunction. (Summarized from Baxter, J. D. [1985]. In J. B. Wyngaarden & L. H. Smith [Eds.], *Cecil's textbook of medicine*. Philadelphia: Saunders; and Baxter, J. D. [1997]. Introduction to endocrinology. In F. S. Greenspan & G. J. Strewler [Eds.], *Basic and clinical endocrinology* [5th ed.]. Stamford, CT: Appleton & Lange.)

TABLE 24-1

MANIFESTATIONS OF ENDOCRINE DISORDERS

SYMPTOM	ASSOCIATED ENDOCRINE DISORDERS
Abdominal pain	Addisonian crisis, diabetic ketoacidosis, hyperparathyroidism
Decreased menstruation	Adrenal insufficiency, Cushing's syndrome, hyperprolactinemia, hypopituitarism, hypothyroidism
Anemia	Adrenal insufficiency, hypothyroidism, hyperparathyroidism, panhypopituitarism
Constipation	Diabetic neuropathy, hypothyroidism, pheochromocytoma
Depression	Adrenal insufficiency, Cushing's syndrome, hypoglycemia, hypothyroidism
Diarrhea	Hyperthyroidism
Fever	Adrenal insufficiency, hyperthyroidism, hypothalamic disease
Hair changes	Decreased body hair: hypothyroidism, hypopituitarism Hirsutism: androgen excess states, acromegaly
Polyuria	Diabetes insipidus, diabetes mellitus
Skin changes	Dry: hypothyroidism Hyperpigmentation: adrenal insufficiency Hypopigmentation: panhypopituitarism
Fatigue	Addison's disease, Cushing's syndrome, hypothyroidism, panhypopituitarism
Weight changes	Gain: Cushing's syndrome, hypothyroidism, pituitary tumors Loss: adrenal insufficiency, hyperthyroidism, diabetes mellitus

(Modified from Baxter, J. D. [1997]. Introduction to endocrinology. In F. S. Greenspan & G. J. Strewler (Eds.), *Basic and clinical endocrinology* [5th ed.]. Stamford, CT: Appleton & Lange.)

leukocyte antigens (HLA) have been linked to the development of DM.[69]

It has also been demonstrated that viral infections may precede the development of an autoimmune endocrine disorder such as DM. This relationship may be explained by one of the three following mechanisms:

1. The activation of the immune system that occurs in combating an infectious agent may result in the activation of an autoreactive immune cell. This activation ultimately leads to autoimmune destruction of the endocrine cells.
2. The polypeptide sequences of the foreign antigen may be similar to self proteins. As the immune response is triggered against the foreign antigen, destruction of self antigens also occurs. Indeed, a similarity has been noted between the peptides of pancreatic enzymes and coxsackie virus B. This response is also referred to as molecular mimicry.[69,79]
3. Finally, it is theorized that the tissue itself is altered, either from injury or medications. The resultant inflammatory response may release large amounts of self antigen at a level high enough to trigger an autoimmune response.[69]

Other Causes of Endocrine Hypofunction

Neoplasms can destroy the gland by replacing glandular tissue with neoplastic cells, by inhibiting blood supply to the gland, or by compressing the gland and preventing normal secretory function, such as in pituitary hypofunction.[3] *Infections* and the associated *inflammatory response* can damage endocrine glands and impair their function. For example, many opportunistic infections seen in individuals with acquired immunodeficiency syndrome (AIDS), such as cytomegalovirus, result in adrenal insufficiency.[21] *Ischemic damage* such as that associated with profound hypotension can lead to necrosis with loss of endocrine function.

Extraglandular disorders may influence action of the endocrine gland. For example, damage to the renal juxtaglomerular cells decreases renin release and ultimately reduces the amount of aldosterone secreted by the adrenal cortex.[10] *Alterations in hormonal synthesis* can produce symptoms comparable to endocrine hypofunction. For example, hypothyroidism can occur from inherited synthesis defects or from decreased dietary iodine, resulting in clinical manifestations of goiter and symptoms of hypothyroidism.[32]

HYPERFUNCTION

Endocrine hyperfunction occurs when there is an excess of hormonal activity. The associated clinical manifestations are those of hormonal excess. Although secretory tumors are the most common cause of endocrine hyperfunction, it can also occur due to autoimmune stimulation and/or administration of exogenous hormones.

Neoplasia and Hyperplasia

Secretory tumors can occur in any of the endocrine glands. In addition to excessive production of hormones by the gland, tumors may also secrete hormones not usually associated with their tissue type. For example, antidiuretic hormone secretion occurs with small cell carcinoma of the lung.[7,68]

Hyperplasia, an increase in the size of the gland from idiopathic or extraglandular processes, results in an increase in the number of hormone-synthesizing and -secreting cells. This results in glandular hyperfunction.

Autoimmune Stimulation

The pathophysiologic mechanisms resulting in autoimmune endocrine hyperfunction are similar to those of autoimmune endocrine hypofunction. However, the antibodies produced are stimulatory rather than inhibitory.

The most common form of hyperthyroidism, Graves' disease, is the classic example of autoimmune stimulation producing glandular hyperfunction. In this disease, antibodies have the ability to stimulate the TSH receptor, promoting increased thyroid cell growth and increased thyroid hormone secretion.[61]

Exogenous Hormone Administration

Traditionally, hormonal therapy is given at physiologic doses as replacement therapy for hormone deficiency.[24] When pharmacologic doses are administered, the patient may exhibit symptoms of hormonal excess consistent with endocrine hyperfunction. For example, symptoms of glucocorticoid excess, Cushing's syndrome, accompany the use of these hormones when they are administered for anti-inflammatory and immunosuppressant effects.

Alterations in Target Tissue Responsiveness

A number of endocrine disorders are associated with alterations in target tissue responsiveness or tissue receptor sensitivity. It is theorized that these alterations may be due to genetic mutations. An example is the "syndrome X" phenomenon, which is associated with insulin resistance, hyperlipidemia, and hypertension.[10] Another example is Type 2 DM, which is associated with insulin resistance and possibly with down regulation of insulin receptors (see Chapter 23).[7,37]

ALTERATIONS IN HYPOTHALAMIC PITUITARY FUNCTION

The hypothalamic pituitary axis regulates many physiologic functions and therefore affects the functioning of the other endocrine organs. Because of this, dysfunction of the hypothalamic pituitary axis is difficult to distinguish from other disorders since the symptoms can be varied. The symptoms can be both endocrine and non-endocrine in nature. Endocrine symptoms are those of either decreased or increased secretion of the pituitary hormones. Non-endocrine symptoms are frequently neurologic in nature and are described in Chapter 32. They are associated with either an intracranial lesion or trauma, since head trauma can also precipitate neuroendocrine dysfunction.

Hypothalamic Dysfunction

Due to the unique interaction between the hypothalamus and the pituitary gland, hypothalamic dysfunction is often associated with alterations in pituitary function. However, as mentioned in Chapter 23, the hypothalamus is responsible for many homeostatic regulatory functions. Therefore, alterations can also occur in behavior, appetite, and temperature regulation.

ETIOLOGY

Tumors are the most common cause of hypothalamic dysfunction. In young adults, adolescents, and children the most common tumor is **craniopharyngioma**, a tumor of congenital origin that arises from the remnants of the Rathke pouch or the hypophyseal stalk.

CLINICAL MANIFESTATIONS

Although the symptoms of craniopharyngioma are initially endocrine in nature, they are often not identified until neurologic manifestations, such as visual disturbances and increased intracranial pressure, become evident. At diagnosis, more than 80% of individuals have symptoms of neuroendocrine dysfunction, such as growth hormone deficiency and growth retardation in children and hypogonadism, diabetes insipidus, and hyperprolactinemia in adults.[3]

Pituitary Dysfunction

Like hypothalamic dysfunction, pituitary disorders are associated with both endocrine and non-endocrine, or neurologic, alterations. The neurologic alterations are the result of the space-occupying aspect of a tumor. Disorders of the anterior pituitary gland include syndromes associated with either endocrine hypofunction or hyperfunction. In contrast, posterior pituitary dysfunction involves alterations in antidiuretic hormone activity. Table 24-2 describes disorders associated with pituitary dysfunction.

Empty Sella Syndrome

The **empty sella syndrome** refers to the extension of the subarachnoid space into the sella turcica, partially filling it with cerebrospinal fluid (CSF). As a result, there is flattening of the pituitary gland with enlargement of the sella turcica. Figure 24-2 demonstrates the anatomic changes seen in empty sella syndrome.

ETIOLOGY

Empty sella syndrome is classified as either (1) primary or (2) secondary, according to the underlying cause. *Primary*, or *idiopathic*, empty sella syndrome is the most

TABLE 24-2

DISORDERS ASSOCIATED WITH PITUITARY DYSFUNCTION

HORMONE	REDUCED SECRETION	INCREASED SECRETION
Growth hormone (GH)	Prepubertal dwarfism, hypoglycemia, postpubertal hypoproteinemia	Prepubertal gigantism, postpubertal acromegaly
Thyroid-stimulating hormone (TSH)	Hypothyroidism, cretinism	Hyperthyroidism, thyrotoxicosis
Adrenocorticotropic hormone (ACTH)	Addison's disease, hypoglycemia	Cushing's disease
Prolactin	Inability to produce milk postpartum, amenorrhea, parturition	Galactorrhea, functional hypogonadism
Follicle-stimulating hormone (FSH)	Hypogonadism, sterility, impotence, loss of secondary sexual characteristics, amenorrhea	Precocious puberty, primary gonadal failure, castration, climacteric, hirsutism, polycystic ovarian disease
Luteinizing hormone (LH)	Hypogonadism, sterility, impotence, loss of secondary sexual characteristics, ovarian failure	Precocious puberty, primary gonadal failure, castration, climacteric, hirsutism, polycystic ovarian disease
Melanocyte-stimulating hormone (MSH)	Paleness, panhypopituitarism	Vitiligo, darkening of the skin
Antidiuretic hormone (ADH)	Diabetes insipidus	Syndrome of inappropriate ADH secretion, water intoxication, dilutional hyponatremia
Oxytocin	Infertility, inability to breastfeed newborn infant	Galactorrhea, amenorrhea

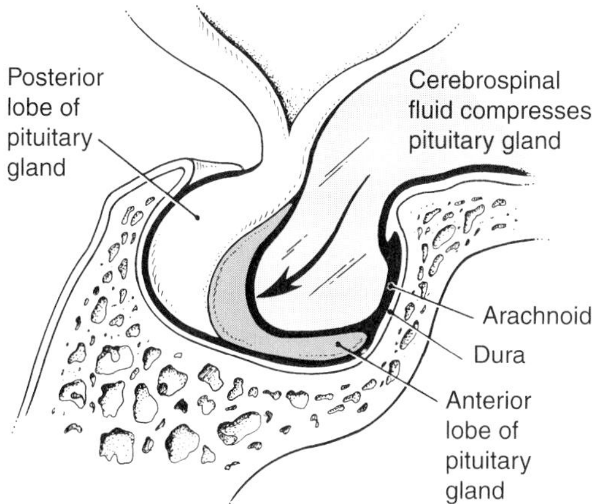

FIGURE 24-2. Empty sella syndrome.

common cause of an enlarged sella turcica and results from an abnormally large opening through which the hypophyseal stalk passes, the diaphragma sella. This is often a developmental defect.[3]

Secondary empty sella syndrome can develop as a result of spontaneous infarctions or regression of a pituitary tumor. Prolactin and GH-secreting pituitary adenomas may develop hemorrhagic infarction. This permits downward movement of the overlying structures into the sella turcica. Empty sella syndrome can also occur following ablation of the pituitary gland by irradiation or surgery. It can also be seen in multiparous women; the tendency of the pituitary to enlarge during pregnancy and regress afterward may be the basis of pathogenesis.

CLINICAL MANIFESTATIONS

Although headache is a common symptom, empty sella syndrome is most often asymptomatic. Serious symptoms occur rarely but may include CSF rhinorrhea, visual field deficits, and intracranial hypertension.[3] It is diagnosed most often in obese, hypertensive, middle-aged women who have borne many children.

Pituitary Adenoma

The most common cause of pituitary dysfunction is a pituitary adenoma, or primary pituitary tumor. Pituitary adenomas may be classified according to (1) the predominant cell type or (2) their secretory qualities. They may interfere with pituitary functions by virtue of their space-occupying properties or by the secretory variations of their hormones. Pituitary adenomas are discussed further in Chapter 33.

CLINICAL MANIFESTATIONS

Typically the endocrine symptoms are those associated with excessive secretion of the specific pituitary hormones. However, expansion of the adenoma, infarction, or hemorrhage into the gland can impair normal secretion. Thus the patient may not synthesize or secrete one or more of the pituitary hormones. The typical endocrine dysfunction seen in pituitary adenoma includes hypersecretion of adrenocorticotropic hormone, growth hormone, and prolactin. Although prolactin-secreting adenomas, **prolactinomas**, account for 60% of all primary pituitary tumors, they are also found incidentally in approximately one fourth of all individuals who have autopsies.[17,40]

In general, problems stemming from the space-occupying factor are the result of destruction or suppression of surrounding tissue. Thus, depending on the size and location of the adenoma, neurologic symptoms and visual disturbances may also occur. Adenomas that are larger than 10 mm can exert pressure on the segment of the optic tract that crosses anteriorly to the pituitary gland (the optic chiasm). They can also exert pressure on the sinuses laterally.[40] Adenomas that are smaller often produce symptoms of hormonal excess without concomitant neurologic symptoms.

The occurrence of a nonsymptomatic adenoma is referred to as an incidentaloma. These are often discovered during an MRI or CT scan or at the time of death on autopsy.[17]

The neurologic symptoms that are seen with pituitary adenoma include the following:

- Headache
- Visual field deficits
- Cranial nerve palsy
- Temporal lobe epilepsy
- CSF rhinorrhea

Hypopituitarism

Hypopituitarism, or pituitary insufficiency, includes hyposecretion of one or more of the pituitary hormones. Panhypopituitarism refers to the failure of all cell types in the pituitary gland to synthesize and secrete their hormones. This hyposecretion persists despite hypofunction of one or more of its target organs in the neuroendocrine axis.

ETIOLOGY

The most common cause of hypopituitarism is a space-occupying lesion such as a pituitary adenoma or brain tumors. A pituitary tumor may also be part of a syndrome referred to as *multiple endocrine neoplasia,* in which there are concomitant tumors of the parathyroid glands and pancreas.[23] Additionally, anorexia nervosa may result in hypopituitarism. However, in this instance the thyroid and adrenal hormones are not usually affected.[23] Other causes of hypopituitarism are listed in Box 24-1.

To determine the etiology of hypopituitarism, pituitary hormonal hyposecretion must be differenti-

PITUITARY LESIONS CAUSING HYPOPITUITARISM

Tumors
Pituitary adenoma
Craniopharyngioma
Metastatic carcinoma
Primary pituitary carcinoma
Meningioma

Pituitary Infarction
Pituitary apoplexy (pituitary tumor)
Postpartum pituitary necrosis (Sheehan's syndrome)
Diabetes mellitus
Shock
Sickle cell anemia (crisis)
Infections (malaria, epidemic hemorrhagic fever)
Cavernous sinus thrombosis
Vasculitis (temporal arteritis, Takayasu's arteritis)
Trauma (stalk section or sella fracture)

Infiltrative Diseases
Sarcoidosis
Tuberculosis
Leukemia
Lymphoma
Hemochromatosis
Autoimmune hypophysitis

Miscellaneous
Hypophysectomy
Radiation necrosis
Carotid artery aneurysm
Pituitary abscess
Congenital anomalies (hypoplasia, aplasia)

(Kelley, W. N. [1996]. *Textbook of internal medicine* [3rd ed.]. Philadelphia: Lippincott.)

ated from primary or target organ hypofunction. Thus, anterior pituitary hormonal levels need to be compared with target hormonal levels. Table 24-3 lists the relationship between primary and secondary endocrine dysfunction for the thyroid and adrenal glands. Provocative hormonal testing may also be necessary to fully evaluate the extent of endocrine hypofunction.[3]

CLINICAL MANIFESTATIONS

The clinical manifestations are those of the target organ deficiency syndromes. The patient will have symptoms comparable to adrenal insufficiency, hypothyroidism, and diabetes insipidus. The consequences of decreased ACTH and antidiuretic hormone (ADH) may become life threatening. An impaired physiologic stress response can result so that even a mild stress could become lethal. Additionally, with loss of ADH, adequate fluid balance will not be maintained and complications of dehydration and hypernatremia will develop (see Chapter 6).

Signs and symptoms of hypopituitarism may depend on the age of the patient, the underlying destructive process, and the extent and rapidity of hormone loss. Typical clinical manifestations include the following:[23]

- Sexual dysfunction; weakness; cold intolerance; loss of axillary and pubic hair; genital atrophy; skin pallor
- Hypotension; bradycardia
- Low level of thyroid hormones; decreased response to ACTH stimulation
- Male low testosterone; female amenorrhea; elevated prolactin level; decreased FSH and LH levels
- Prepubertal shortness of stature

Altered Growth Hormone Secretion

Alterations in growth hormone secretion can affect the stature of a child, alter the appearance of an adult, and alter carbohydrate metabolism. The clinical manifestations of these affects depend on whether the individual has completed linear bone growth.

GROWTH HORMONE EXCESS

The physiologic response to growth hormone (GH) excess is different in children than in adults. In children and adolescents, if the GH hypersecretion occurs prior to the closure of the epiphyseal plates (growth plates), the result is **gigantism**. In adults, and after closure of the epiphyseal plates, the result is **acromegaly**. Table 24-4 describes the effects of growth hormone excess.

Etiology

The most common cause of GH excess is a secretory pituitary adenoma. Hypersecretion of GH can also occur in acute illness, chronic renal failure, and cirrhosis. Occasionally, GH excess is the result of ectopic secretion of growth hormone–releasing hormone from carcinoid or islet cell tumors.[3]

Gigantism

In gigantism, there is symmetric excessive linear growth, exceeding three standard deviations above the mean height for age. Hypogonadism is often associated with gigantism and leads to delayed epiphyseal closure. If GH excess continues through adolescence and into adulthood, there will also be symptoms of acromegaly.

Acromegaly

In acromegaly, linear growth of bones is no longer possible due to epiphyseal closure. Thus, the tissues thicken and growth takes place in the acral areas (hands, feet, nose, and mandible). The clinical signs and symptoms associated with acromegaly, illustrated in Figure

TABLE 24-3

HORMONAL LEVELS IN PRIMARY AND SECONDARY ENDOCRINE DYSFUNCTION

	ENDOCRINE HORMONE	PITUITARY HORMONE
PRIMARY HYPOFUNCTION		
Adrenal gland	Decreased cortisol level	Elevated ACTH
Thyroid gland	Decreased T_3 and T_4	Elevated TSH
SECONDARY HYPOFUNCTION		
Adrenal gland	Decreased cortisol level	Decreased ACTH
Thyroid gland	Decreased T_3 and T_4	Decreased TSH
PRIMARY HYPERFUNCTION		
Adrenal gland	Increased cortisol level	Decreased ACTH
Thyroid gland	Increased T_3 and T_4	Decreased TSH
SECONDARY HYPERFUNCTION		
Adrenal gland	Increased cortisol level	Elevated ACTH
Thyroid gland	Increased T_3 and T_4	Elevated TSH

24-3, result from local effects of tumor growth and the effects of hypersecretion of GH. There is also concomitant hypersecretion of prolactin in 20% to 40% of individuals with acromegaly.[32]

The physiologic changes associated with acromegaly progress slowly and insidiously. It often goes undetected for years. Affected persons may first notice a progressive increase in ring, shoe, and glove sizes. Acromegalic arthritis develops from proliferation of joint cartilage. This affects the joints of the long bones and the spine. Osteoporosis develops from increased bone absorption.

Although excessive growth is the classic feature of this disorder, GH excess causes a generalized systemic disorder. The lungs, liver, spleen, kidneys, and intestines enlarge. Hypertension, coronary artery atherosclerosis, and marked cardiomegaly occur. Congestive heart failure often develops. The adrenal, thyroid, and parathyroid glands become enlarged. There is insulin resistance and carbohydrate intolerance.[6]

Typical clinical manifestations include the following:[23]

- Excessive growth of the hands, feet, jaw, and internal organs; increased glove and ring size; increased shoe size; protrusion of lower jaw (prognathism)
- Coarse facial features
- Amenorrhea; headaches; visual field deficits; sweating; weakness
- Serum GH remains elevated following oral glucose administration
- Elevated levels of insulin-like growth factor 1 (IGF-1)

GROWTH HORMONE DEFICIT

A deficiency in GH levels can be either (1) congenital or (2) acquired. The clinical manifestations depend on the age at which the GH deficit occurs.

Congenital

In congenital growth hormone deficiency, the infant has a normal birth length. The growth disorder becomes apparent during the first or second year of life. Typically these children have the following characteristics:[70]

- Short stature (below the third percentile)
- Obesity; immature appearance
- Immature voice pitch
- Delay in skeletal maturation
- Hyperlipidemia; elevated cholesterol levels

In contrast to children whose growth failure is due to congenital primary hypothyroidism, these children are of normal intelligence.

If GH is the only pituitary hormone that is reduced, the problem may be due to hyposecretion of growth hormone–releasing hormone by the hypothalamus. In this instance, the response to growth hormone may be normal.

Acquired

Acquired GH deficiency is associated with abnormalities of the hypothalamus and the pituitary gland. Conditions associated with GH deficiency include:[70]

- Craniopharyngioma
- Germinoma
- Glioma

TABLE 24-4

EFFECTS OF GROWTH HORMONE EXCESS

LOCATION	SYMPTOMS	SIGNS
General	Fatigue Increased sweating Heat intolerance Weight gain Possible increased malignancy risk	Glucose intolerance Hypertriglyceridemia
Skin and subcutaneous tissue	Enlarging hands, feet Coarsening facial features Oily skin Hypertrichosis	Moist, warm, fleshy, doughy handshake Skin tags Acanthosis nigricans Increased heel pad
Head	Headaches	Parotid enlargement Frontal bossing
Eyes	Decreased vision	Visual field defects
Ears		Otoscope speculum cannot be inserted
Nose, throat, paranasal sinuses	Sinus congestion Increased tongue size Malocclusion Voice change	Enlarged furrowed tongue Tooth marks on tongue Widely spaced teeth Prognathism
Neck		Goiter Obstructive sleep apnea due to visceromegaly
Cardiorespiratory system	Congestive heart failure	Hypertension Cardiomegaly, cardiomyopathy Left ventricular hypertrophy
Genitourinary system	Decreased libido Impotence Oligomenorrhea Infertility Renal colic	Urolithiasis
Neurologic system	Paresthesias Hypersomnolence	Carpal tunnel syndrome Nerve root compression due to bone and cartilage growth
Muscles	Weakness	Proximal myopathy
Skeletal system	Joint pains (shoulders, back, knees)	Osteoarthritis Increased 1,25-$(OH)_2D_3$ due to increased 1α-hydroxylase, resulting in increased Ca^{2+} absorption from gut and excretion in urine, increased bone density and turnover

(Modified and reproduced, with permission from Daniels, G. H., Norton, I. B. [1991]. Neuroendocrine regulation and diseases of the anterior pituitary and hypothalamus. In J. Wilson et al. [Eds.], *Harrison's principles of internal medicine* [12th ed.]. New York: McGraw-Hill).

- Empty sella syndrome
- Delay in skeletal maturation

In adulthood the typical clinical manifestations include obesity, asthenia, and reduced cardiac output.

Hyperprolactinemia

Hyperprolactinemia is excess secretion of prolactin by the anterior pituitary gland. It is the most common anterior pituitary disorder.

ETIOLOGY

Etiologies of hyperprolactinemia includes a prolactin-secreting adenoma, excess administration of dopamine receptor antagonists, primary hypothyroidism, and other factors. Prolactin-secreting pituitary adenomas account for as many as 65% of all pituitary tumors.

Several systemic disorders can promote hyperprolactinemia. Renal disease and liver disease should be eliminated as potential causes of the disorder. Endocrine

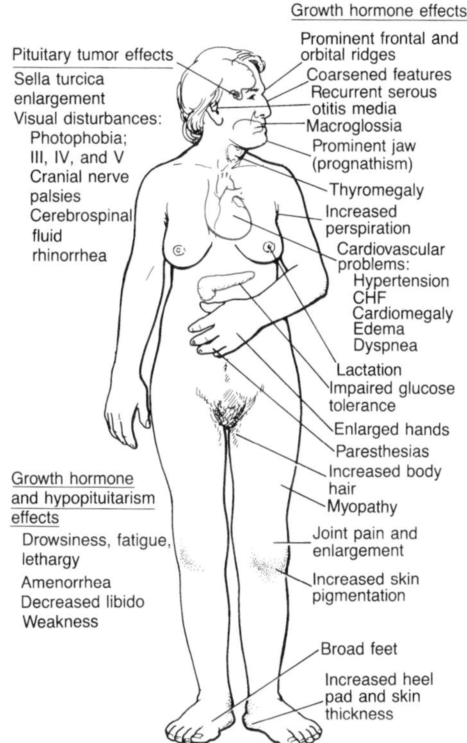

FIGURE 24-3. **Appearance of acromegaly. Clinical manifestations relate to growth hormone secretion and effects from tumor encroachment on small pituitary space.**

evaluation should also examine thyroid function. Primary hypothyroidism is a common endocrine disorder associated with hyperprolactinemia. As noted in Chapter 23, excessive thyrotropin releasing–hormone (TRH) secretion can stimulate both thyrotropes and lactotropes. Additionally, the prolactin response to TRH is exaggerated in individuals with primary hypothyroidism. The resultant effect is hyperplasia of both thyrotropes and lactotropes with significant pituitary enlargement. This can be mistaken for a prolactin-secreting pituitary adenoma.[3]

CLINICAL MANIFESTATIONS

The clinical manifestations of hyperprolactinemia are different in women than in men. The primary symptoms for women are galactorrhea and amenorrhea. Apparently, prolactin induces amenorrhea by blocking the action of gonadotropins, FSH and LH. Infertility occurs since elevated prolactin levels inhibit the normal pulsatile secretion of FSH and LH, preventing ovulation. Thus, in women there is hypogonadism with associated osteoporosis due to estrogen deficiency. Other concomitant symptoms, such as vaginal dryness, are associated with decreased estrogen levels. However, women with hyperprolactinemia also develop hirsutism, anxiety, and depression.[3]

In men, the usual clinical manifestations are hypogonadism, impotence, and infertility. Many also have decreased libido. Serum testosterone levels are low while gonadotropin (FSH and LH) levels are either normal or elevated.[3,23]

Diabetes Insipidus

Diabetes insipidus (DI) is the result of either decreased synthesis and secretion of antidiuretic hormone (ADH; vasopressin) or the inability of the kidney to respond to ADH. The former is referred to as *central or neurogenic diabetes insipidus*; the latter is referred to as *nephrogenic diabetes insipidus*. The diagnosis and treatment of these must also be differentiated from other causes of polyuria, such as osmotic diuresis and **psychogenic polydipsia**. Psychogenic polydipsia, also referred to as primary polydipsia or compulsive water drinking, is a psychogenic alteration in the thirst stimulus characterized by water intake as great as 5 L/day, which contributes to fluid volume overload, inhibition of ADH secretion, and water diuresis.[3]

Diabetes insipidus is characterized by the passage of large quantities of urine of low specific gravity. This **polyuria** is accompanied by polydipsia in an effort to maintain water balance. Increased water loss produces an elevation in plasma osmolality. Elevated plasma osmolarity, in the normal individual, stimulates thirst and ADH synthesis and secretion.

NEUROGENIC DIABETES INSIPIDUS

The most common cause of neurogenic DI is damage to the hypothalamic neurohypophyseal system from head trauma or malignancy or following intracranial surgery. Box 24-2 provides a more complete etiology of DI. Regardless of the etiology, ADH synthesis and secretion is reduced. Often the stimulus for thirst is intact. However, if it is not or if the patient is unable to maintain adequate intake, dehydration may develop.

The clinical manifestations of DI include the symptoms associated with its etiology, in addition to polydipsia, polyuria, and hypotonic urine with a specific gravity of less than 1.006. Urine osmolality will be less than 200 mOsm/kg. If adequate fluid intake is not maintained, the patient will develop hypernatremia with the concomitant central nervous system symptoms seen in hypernatremia and severe dehydration.[3,9]

NEPHROGENIC DIABETES INSIPIDUS

The loss of renal responsiveness to ADH may be induced by medication or due to alterations in the ADH receptors. The alteration can be to either the V_2 receptor

CAUSES OF DIABETES INSIPIDUS

- I. Vasopressin deficiency (neurogenic or central diabetes insipidus)
  - A. Decreased secretion
    - 1. Idiopathic
      - a. Sporadic (? autoimmune)
      - b. Familial (autosomal dominant inheritance)
    - 2. Traumatic (accidental or surgical)
    - 3. Malignancy
      - a. Primary (craniopharyngloma, germinoma, meningioma, pituitary adenoma with suprasellar extension)
      - b. Metastatic (lung, breast, leukemia)
    - 4. Granuloma (sarcoid, histiocytosis, xanthoma dissemination)
    - 5. Infectious (meningitis, encephalitis, syphilis)
    - 6. Vascular (aneurysm, Sheehan's syndrome, cardiac arrest, vasculitis)
    - 7. Psychobiologic (anorexia nervosa)
    - 8. Toxic (carbon monoxide)
    - 9. Congenital malformations
  - B. Increased metabolism
    - 1. Pregnancy
- II. Vasopressin resistance (nephrogenic diabetes insipidus)
  - A. Idiopathic
    - 1. Sporadic
    - 2. Familial (X-linked recessive inheritance)
  - B. Post obstructive
  - C. Malignancy (retroperitoneal fibrosarcoma)
  - D. Granuloma (sarcoid)
  - E. Infectious (pyelonephritis)
  - F. Vascular (sickle cell disease or trait)
  - G. Metabolic (hypokalemia, hypercalciuria)
  - H. Toxic (lithium, demeclocycline, methoxyflurane, methicillin)
  - I. Malformations (polycystic disease)
  - J. Pregnancy
- III. Excessive water intake (primary polydipsia)
  - A. Psychogenic (schizophrenia, affective disorders)
  - B. Dipsogenic
    - 1. Idiopathic
    - 2. Traumatic
    - 3. Granuloma (neurosarcoidosis)
    - 4. Infectious (meningitis)
    - 5. Other (multiple sclerosis)

(Stein, J. [Ed.] [1994]. *Internal medicine* [4th ed.]. St. Louis: C.V. Mosby.)

located in the renal-collecting tubules, impairing its function, or in the aquaporin water channels.[27,40] Thus, the ability to concentrate urine and to conserve water is lost. In addition to polyuria, individuals with nephrogenic DI often have hypercalcemia and hypokalemia.[9]

CLINICAL MANIFESTATIONS

The typical clinical manifestations include symptoms associated with both dehydration and hypernatremia. These include tachycardia, hypotension, muscle cramps, and lethargy.[23]

Individuals with DI lack the ability to conserve water and concentrate urine. In the normal individual, water deprivation increases plasma osmolality, promoting thirst and ADH secretion. In contrast, individuals with DI will demonstrate weight loss as well as no change in urine osmolality.[9]

Although both DI and psychogenic polydipsia present with excessive urinary excretion, there are differences in both urinary and plasma osmolality and sodium levels. Simultaneous samples of both urine and plasma demonstrate that the urine is more dilute than the plasma in DI. However, in psychogenic polydipsia both the urine and the plasma are dilute. Table 24-5 provides differential diagnostic information for DI.

Syndrome of Inappropriate Antidiuretic Hormone

The syndrome of inappropriate ADH secretion (SIADH) refers to disorders associated with the secretion of ADH unrelated to plasma osmolality or volume deficit.

ETIOLOGY

Syndrome of inappropriate ADH secretion results from a hypoactive or inactive feedback inhibition of the posterior pituitary, which causes continued release of ADH. The syndrome may occur from an alteration to the hypothalamic neurohypophyseal system or from other alterations. Box 24-3 provides information on the etiology of SIADH. It may occur as a result of a paraneoplastic syndrome in which nonendocrine tumors demonstrate inappropriate secretion of ADH. For example carcinomas, such as small cell carcinoma of the lung synthesize ADH. Additionally, several medications promote ADH secretion. Fluoxetine (Prozac) is a common cause of SIADH in the elderly.[55] Box 24-4 lists other medications associated with SIADH. Endocrine disorders such as adrenal insufficiency, severe hypothyroidism, and anterior pituitary insufficiency may be associated with increased ADH levels.[3]

TABLE 24-5

DIFFERENTIAL DIAGNOSTIC STUDIES FOR POLYURIA

DIAGNOSTIC TEST	NEUROGENIC DI	NEPHROGENIC DI	PSYCHOGENIC POLYDIPSIA
Plasma osmolality	Increased	Increased	Decreased
Urine osmolality	Decreased	Decreased	Decreased
Urine osmolality during water deprivation	No change	No change	Increased

(Modified from Aron, D. C. Findling, J. W. & Tyrell, J. B. [1997]. Hypothalamus and pituitary. In F. S. Greenspan & G. J. Strewler (Eds.), *Basic and clinical endocrinology* [5th ed.]. Stamford, CT: Appleton & Lange.)

PATHOPHYSIOLOGY

There are four types of osmoregulatory defects associated with SIADH:

1. Type A, occurring in 20% of individuals with SIADH, is characterized by erratic and irregular secretion of ADH unrelated to plasma osmolality.
2. Type B, occurring in about 35% of individuals, is associated with excessive secretion of ADH but in a pattern proportional to plasma osmolality.
3. Type C, occurring in another 35% of the individuals, is associated with a high baseline level of ADH that increases with plasma osmolality.
4. Type D appears to be associated with a change in renal sensitivity to ADH. This type accounts for less than 10% of the population with SIADH.

CLINICAL MANIFESTATIONS

Continuous release of ADH results in excessive reabsorption of water in the renal system and excessive retention of water with expansion of fluid volume. The resulting clinical manifestations in SIADH include the following:[3,40,55]

- Fluid volume overload
- Hyponatremia or hypertonic urine

ETIOLOGY OF SIADH

Neoplasms
 Lung (small cell in 80%), pancreas, duodenum, lymphoma, ureter, prostate, Ewing's sarcoma
Pulmonary
 Infection (viral, bacterial, fungal), abscess, asthma, respirator therapy
Central nervous system
 Trauma, neoplasms, infections, vascular degenerative diseases (including aging), psychoses
Cardiac
 Atrial tachycardias, post-mitral-commissurotomy syndrome
Metabolic
 Myxedema, adrenal insufficiency, acute porphyria, anterior pituitary insufficiency, angiotensin II
Stress
Drugs
 Hypoglycemic agents (chlorpropamide, tolbutamid), and neoplastic drugs (cyclophosphamide, vincristine) narcotics (morphine, barbiturates), psychotropics (phenothiazine derivatives)

(Stein J. [ed.] [1998]. *Internal medicine* [5th ed.]. St. Louis: C.V. Mosby.)

CAUSES OF DRUG-INDUCED SIADH

Increased ADH Production

Antidepressants

Amitriptyline, clomipramine, desipramine, imipramine, fluoxitine
Monoamine oxidase inhibitors

Antineoplastics

Cyclophosphamide, vincristine, vinblastine

Neuroleptic agents

Thiothixene, thioridazine, fluphenazine, haloperidol, trifluoperazine

Other

Carbamazipine, clofibrate

Potentiated ADH Action

Carbamazepine, chlorpropamine, tolbutamide, cyclophosphamide, NSAIDs, somatostatin, and analogues

(Modified from Okuda, T., Kurokawa, K. & Papdakis, M. A. [1998]. Fluid and electrolyte disorders. In L. M. Tierney, Jr., S. J. McPhee, & M. A. Papadakis, *Current medical diagnosis and treatment* [35th ed.]. Stamford, CT: Appleton & Lange.)

- Hemodilution
- Decreased plasma osmolality (<280 mOsm/kg) with increased urinary osmolality (>150 mOsm/kg)
- Sodium loss or salt wasting, due to increased fluid volume and subsequent decreased aldosterone secretion[27]
- Increased urinary sodium (>20 mEq/L)
- Neurologic symptoms associated with hyponatremia and fluid volume overload

ALTERATIONS IN THYROID FUNCTION

The physiologic effects of the thyroid gland are widespread and influence all major body systems; thus, alterations in thyroid function can have profound effects. Changes are seen in mentation, cardiac function, and energy utilization. Symptoms are often insidious and nonspecific, making diagnosis difficult.

Goiter

Various types of disorders can alter the size and state of the thyroid. An enlarged thyroid is referred to as a **goiter**. Figure 24-4 provides an example of the physical appearance of a goiter. The presence of a goiter is not necessarily indicative of thyroid dysfunction. Without the presence of identifiable clinical manifestations, an enlarged thyroid gland is referred to as a *nontoxic goiter. Endemic goiter* refers to an enlargement of the thyroid gland in at least 10% of the area population. This often occurs in a region with dietary iodine deficiency.

ETIOLOGY

Diffuse enlargement of the thyroid is most commonly caused by prolonged stimulation by TSH. As previously mentioned, insufficient iodine intake is the most common reason for increased TSH secretion. Thus, the gland enlarges in an attempt to produce sufficient amounts of thyroid hormones.[49]

Additionally, goiter may be due to foods or medications that can promote thyroid gland enlargement. These are referred to as **goitrogens**. However, dietary goitrogens such as cassava and cabbage are a rare cause of goiter. Medications such as amiodarone and kelp tablets, which contain large amount of iodine, may also produce goiter. Lithium carbonate is a well-known goitrogen.[32]

Nodular goiters may result from malignancy or benign processes such as dietary iron deficiency or Graves' disease. Although nodular goiters may also be the result of dietary iodine deficiency, further evaluation is necessary to eliminate other pathologies. A solitary thyroid nodule may be indicative of a malignancy. The presence of multiple nodules is likely to represent a benign process.

CLINICAL MANIFESTATIONS

Symptoms of thyroid goiter, with or without nodules, include hypothyroidism and hyperthyroidism as well as dysphagia and dyspnea from an extremely large goiter. Figure 24-5 demonstrates the cellular changes that are seen in thyroid disease.

Hypothyroidism

Hypothyroidism is the result of a deficiency of thyroid hormone, leading to a decreased rate of body metabolism and a general slowing of physiologic processes.

ETIOLOGY

Hypothyroidism may be **congenital** or **acquired** or result from certain medications (Box 24-5). Ninety-five percent of individuals with hypothyroidism have the

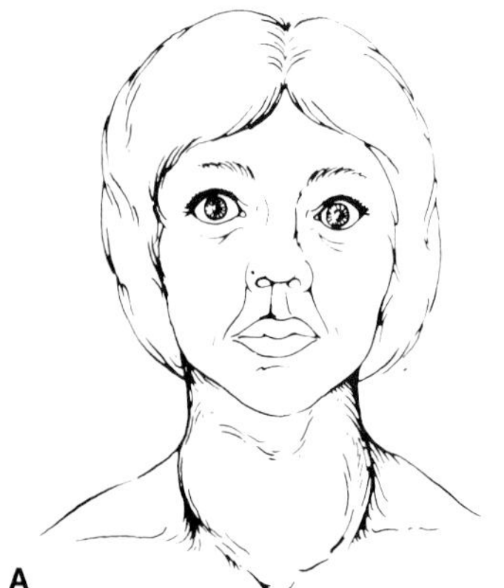

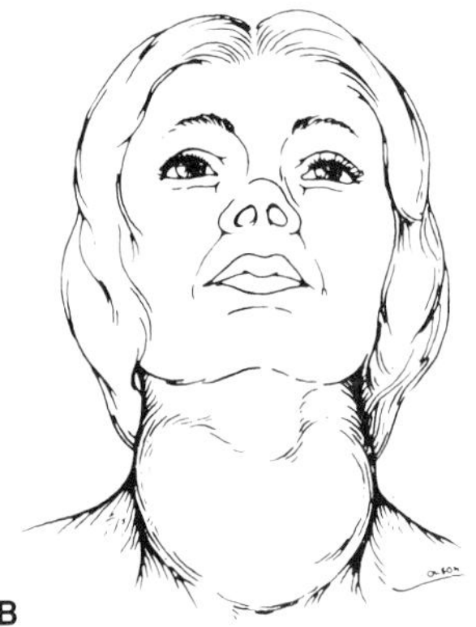

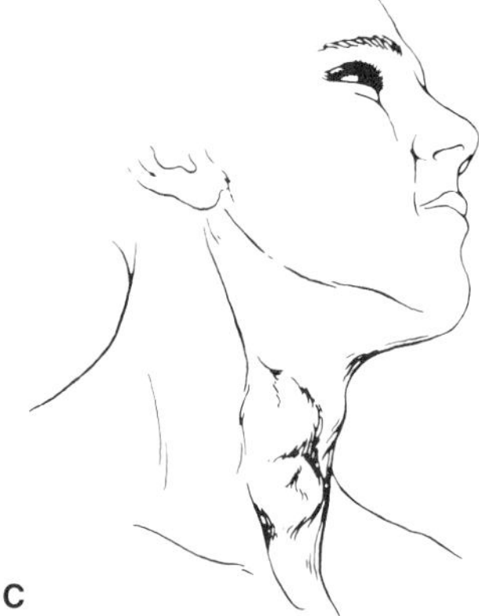

FIGURE 24-4. Thyroid abnormalities. **A.** Diffuse toxic goiter (Graves' disease) with exophthalmos. **B.** Diffuse non-toxic goiter. **C.** Nodular goiter. (Judge, R. D. Zelenock, G. B., & Zuidema, G. D. [Eds.] [1997]. *Clinical diagnosis* [5th ed.]. Philadelphia: Lippincott-Raven.)

FOCUS ON CELLULAR PATHOPHYSIOLOGY

Normal

Active

Inactive

Colloid

Parafollicular cells

Follicular epithelial cells

Graves' disease

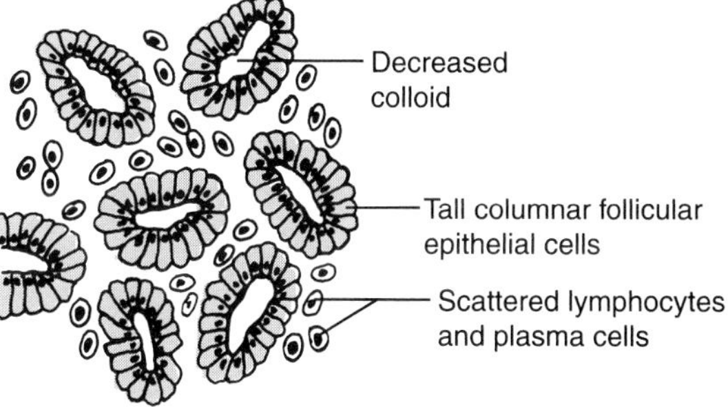

Hashimoto's thyroiditis

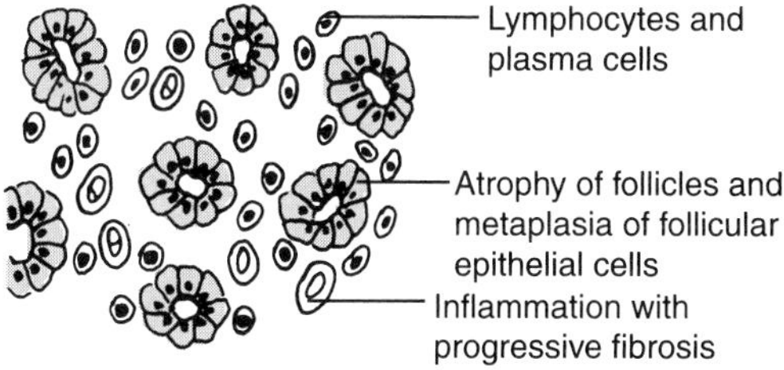

FIGURE 24-5. Normal and abnormal thyroid histology.

BOX 24-5

ETIOLOGY OF HYPOTHYROIDISM

Congenital
Aplasia or hypoplasia of thyroid gland
Defects in hormone biosynthesis or action

Acquired
Hashimoto's thyroiditis
Severe iodine deficiency
Lymphocytic ablation
Thyroid ablation from surgery or radiation

Medications
Iodine
Propylthiouracil, methimazole
Potassium percholarate
Thiocyanate
Lithium

(Modified from McPhee, S. J. & Bauer, D. C. [1997]. Thyroid disease. In S. J. McPhee, V. R. Lingappa, W. F. Ganong, & J. D. Lange [Eds.], *Pathology of disease* [2nd ed.]. Stamford, CT: Appleton & Lange.)

primary form (disorder of the gland itself).[35] Hypothyroidism can also be secondary due to alterations in pituitary and hypothalamic function. The most common cause of hypothyroidism is Hashimoto's thyroiditis, an autoimmune destruction of the thyroid gland.

CLINICAL MANIFESTATIONS

The clinical manifestations in hypothyroidism may vary from mild symptoms to **myxedema**, a potentially life-threatening complication of hypothyroidism. When hypothyroidism occurs during developmental stages of infancy and childhood, it can result in reduced growth and mental retardation. In the adult, the symptoms represent a generalized physiologic slowing and a decrease in the basal metabolic rate.[32] Typical clinical manifestations include the following:[23]

- Weakness, fatigue, cold intolerance, constipation
- Dry skin, bradycardia, delayed deep tendon reflexes
- Anemia, hyponatremia
- Depression

Clinical manifestations of hypothyroidism are further summarized in Table 24-6.

Altered facies are often seen in hypothyroidism due to a combination of several factors. The skin appears yellowish since the conversion of carotene to vitamin A is reduced. There is an increase in the deposition of protein polysaccharide complexes. As these accumulate, sodium and water retention is increased. This promotes the development of the characteristic puffiness seen in hypothyroidism. The accumulation of mucopolysaccharides in the larynx is associated with hoarseness.[49]

Physiologic alterations include decreased secretion of growth hormone with a concomitant reduction in IGF I concentrations.[10] Plasma cholesterol and triglyceride levels are elevated, with decreased formation of LDL receptors. Thyroid-stimulating hormone levels are elevated in primary hypothyroidism. However, TSH and T_3 and T_4 levels are decreased in secondary hypothyroidism. Measurement of free thyroxine levels

TABLE 24-6

CLINICAL MANIFESTATION OF HYPOTHYROIDISM

	SYMPTOMS	SIGNS
General	Cold intolerance Fatigue Mild weight gain	Hypothermia
Nervous system	Lethargy Memory defects Poor attention span Personality change	Somnolence Slow speech Myxedema with psychopathology: myxedema madness Diminished hearing and taste Cerebellar ataxia
Neuromuscular	Weakness Muscle cramps Joint pain	Delayed relaxation of deep tendon reflexes Carpal tunnel syndrome
Gastrointestinal	Nausea Constipation	Large tongue Ascites
Cardiorespiratory	Decreased exercise tolerance	Hoarse voice Bradycardia Mild hypertension Pericardial effusion Pleural effusion
Reproductive	Decreased libido Decreased fertility Menstrual disorders	
Skin and appendages	Dry, rough skin Puffy facies Hair loss Brittle nails	Nonpitting edema of hands, face, and ankles Periorbital swelling Pallor Yellowish skin carotenemia) Coarse hair Dry axillae

(Becker, K. L. et al. [1995]. *Principles and practice of endocrinology and metabolism* [2nd ed.]. Philadelphia: Lippincott.)

(FT_4) levels is preferred since they directly measure the free or unbound portion of thyroxine (tetraiodothyronine). Since thyroxine is highly protein bound, FT_4 represents only about 0.025% of the total T_4. However, it is the unbound portion that is biologically active.[23]

Hypothyroid individuals are often anemic due to decreased erythropoiesis.[49] Medication distribution and metabolism is also reduced; thus, the therapeutic effects of many medications can be achieved with lower doses. There is an increased sensitivity to barbiturates, phenothiazines, and opioid analgesics.[57]

Complications usually consist of cardiopulmonary symptoms. Slow, shallow respirations are seen with altered ventilatory responses to hypercapnia or hypoxia. There is also an increased incidence of sleep apnea in hypothyroid individuals.[49] Cardiomegaly may be present with an increased risk of pericardial effusion. The risk of coronary artery disease is also increased.[32]

HASHIMOTO'S THYROIDITIS

The most common cause of hypothyroidism is Hashimoto's thyroiditis, an autoimmune destruction of the thyroid gland. It is theorized that an alteration in T cell suppressor function permits helper T cells to produce autoantibodies. The resultant immune response destroys the thyroid gland.[54] The clinical manifestations of this disorder vary as the disease progresses. Initially, there is the development of a nodular goiter. In later stages, the gland atrophies and becomes fibrotic. Eventually hypothyroidism becomes evident.

There appears to be a familial tendency to develop Hashimoto's thyroiditis. It occurs more frequently in families that have at least one other person with an autoimmune thyroid disease. It is associated with other autoimmune disorders as well, and is also associated with class II human leukocyte antigens (HLA) DR4 and DR5.[5]

The clinical manifestations are those of hypothyroidism. However, differences are noted both on biopsy of the gland and during serologic evaluations. Microscopic examination demonstrates lymphocytic penetration into glandular tissue (see Fig. 24-5). Additionally, the ratio of T cells to B cells is altered: there is a decrease in T cells with an associated increase in B cells.[41] Serologically, the following auto antibodies are identified: thyroglobulin antibody, thyroidal peroxidase antibody, and the TSH receptor–blocking or antagonist antibody (TSH R[block] Ab).

CRETINISM

Thyroid hormone deficiency during embryonic and neonatal life results in a state known as **cretinism** in infants. The incidence of neonatal hypothyroidism in the white population is 1:5000, whereas the incidence is only 1:32,000 in the African-American population.[32] This disorder can occur due to congenital abnormalities of the neuroendocrine axis. However, thyroid hormones can cross the placenta, so if the mother is euthyroid, the infant will be normal at birth. The placental transfer of TSH R[block] Ab may result in lack of thyroid gland development. This is referred to as *athyreotic cretinism.*[32]

Clinical Manifestations

The deficiency may not be readily apparent at birth because sufficient hormones have been provided by the mother. In the newborn, there is the characteristic puffy appearance often accompanied by deaf mutism and extrapyramidal symptoms. The newborns often have respiratory difficulties, cyanosis, jaundice, an umbilical hernia, and lack of bone maturation. Lack of tibial and femoral epiphysis in a newborn is indicative of cretinism.[49]

The infant is sluggish and falls behind the normal rate of growth and development. Mental retardation and delayed growth patterns are characteristic throughout childhood. The arms and legs of children are short in relation to the trunk; the face and hands are broad and puffy; and the abdomen is protuberant, often with an umbilical hernia (Fig. 24-6). Precocious puberty may occur in the adolescent. In addition, radiographic examination demonstrates an enlargement of the sella turcica. This may be indicative of pituitary hypertrophy in an effort to increase TSH secretion.[32]

MYXEDEMA COMA

Untreated hypothyroidism can progress to myxedema coma. This disorder can be triggered by an external factor. Successful treatment involves not only providing appropriate hormonal replacement therapy, but also identifying and treating the precipitating factor. This can include the following: infections, surgery, acute medical illnesses, neurologic disorders, medications such as sedatives and hypnotics, trauma, and hypothermia.[66]

The mortality rate for myxedema coma is high; thus, it is a true medical emergency. Additionally, a low T_4 in any critically ill individual is potentially fatal.[66]

Although the clinical manifestations of myxedema coma are similar to those of hypothyroidism, the symptoms are much more pronounced (Table 24-7). Some individuals may also have SIADH. The typical clinical manifestations are as follows:[32,49]

- Puffy facies with yellowish skin; alveolar hypoventilation
- Progressive weakness, hypoglycemia, hyponatremia
- Elevated CSF protein
- Confusion, paranoia, and mania (myxedema madness)

Hyperthyroidism

Hyperthyroidism, also known as **thyrotoxicosis**, is a disorder related to excessive secretion of the thyroid glands. Hyperthyroidism is characterized by increased synthesis and secretion of T_3 and T_4, leading to an increased metabolic rate.

ETIOLOGY

Hyperthyroidism may be primary, originating in the thyroid gland, or secondary, due to increased stimulation from TSH. However, the most common etiology of hyperthyroidism is Graves' disease. Box 24-6 provides a more complete list of the etiologies of hyperthyroidism.

CLINICAL MANIFESTATIONS

The severity of the disease may be affected by the person's age, duration of hyperthyroid function, and the presence of other disease processes in any other organ system. Because of the increased amount of thyroid hormones reaching the cells, all metabolic activities are accelerated. The basal metabolism rate rises, energy expenditure is increased, and heat production rises.

The clinical manifestations of hyperthyroidism can be considered an exaggerated expression of the physiologic activity of the thyroid hormones. Table 24-8 describes the manifestations of hyperthyroidism. The increase in physiologic activity places a considerable burden on the cardiovascular system. There is an increased occurrence of cardiac arrhythmias with decreased peripheral vascular resistance. The individual is then at risk for the development of high-output cardiac failure.[27]

Hyperthyroidism is characterized by increased cardiovascular and metabolic sensitivity to catecholamines. This is most probably due to an increase in the number

(text continues on page 685)

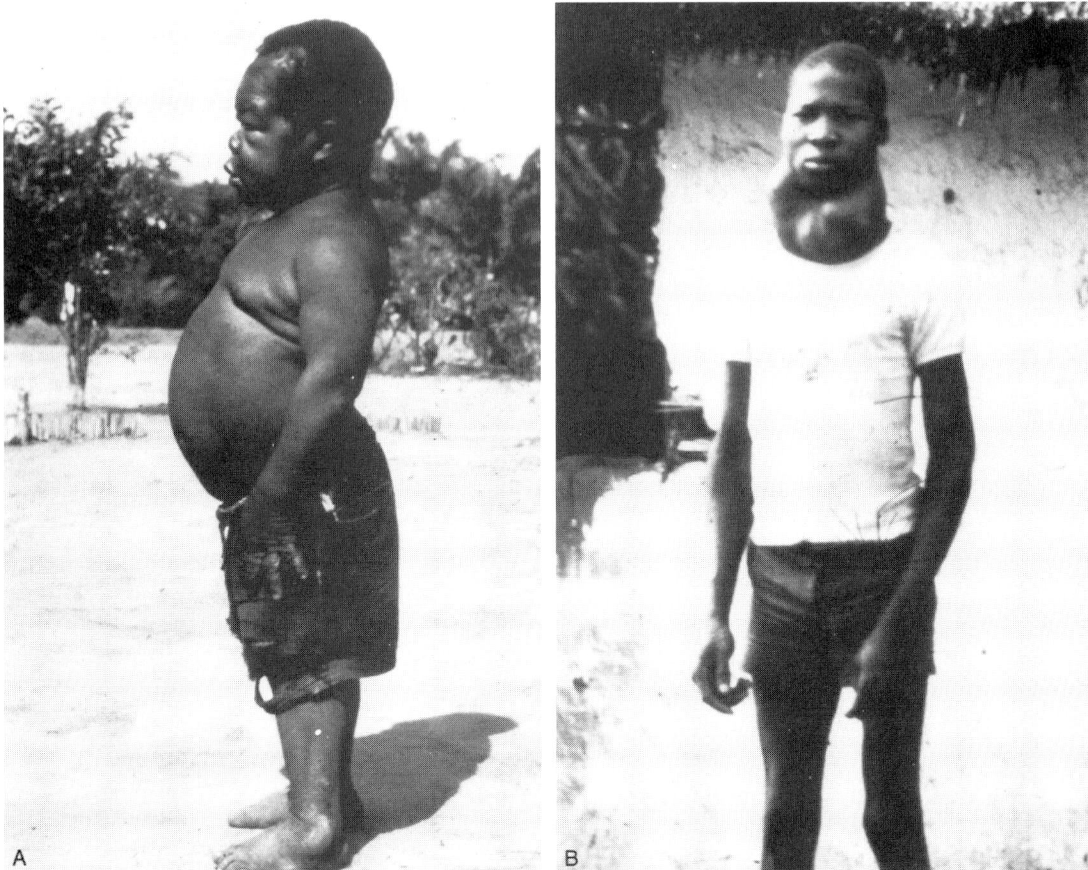

FIGURE 24-6. Cretin and euthyroid with goiter. **A.** Endemic cretin of Zaire. These children, born in areas of severe iodine deficiency, have marked mental retardation, short stature, muscle weakness, and motor incoordination. Note the obesity and protuberant abdomen. **B.** Other members of the community are clinically euthyroid, but, as in this youth, some of them have very large, multinodular goiters. (Becker, K. D. et al. [1995]. *Principles and practice of endocrinology and metabolism* [2nd ed.]. Philadelphia: Lippincott.)

TABLE 24-7

CLINICAL FEATURES OF HYPOTHYROIDISM AND MYXEDEMA COMA

SYSTEM	HYPOTHYROIDISM	MYXEDEMA COMA
Central nervous system	Fatigue, slowed mentation; Delayed deep tendon reflexes	Psychosis, obtundation, coma
Cardiovascular	Bradycardia, hypertension	Bradycardia
Gastrointestinal	Constipation	Ileus
Thermoregulation	Cold intolerance, cool, dry skin	Hypothermia

(Smallridge, R. C. [1992]. Metabolic and anatomic thyroid emergencies. *Critical Care Medicine, 20*(2), 276–291.)

ETIOLOGY OF HYPERTHYROIDISM

Graves' disease
Thyroid adenoma
Overproduction of TSH
Thyroiditis
Excessive thyroid hormone replacement
Toxic multinodular goiter

(Modified from Ganong, W. F. [1997]. *Review of medical physiology* [18th ed.]. Stamford, CT: Appleton & Lange.)

and reactivity of beta and alpha adrenergic receptors, since catecholamine levels are not elevated. Additionally, beta adrenergic antagonists effectively treat the tachycardia, arrhythmias, and tremors associated with hyperthyroidism.[39,56] The wide-eyed stare (exophthalmos) often seen in hyperthyroidism (Fig. 24-7) may also be associated with increased sympathetic tone.

As in hypothyroidism, there are psychological alterations associated with hyperthyroidism. Many individuals demonstrate nervousness and emotional lability. This can progress to mania and psychosis.

Serologically, a decrease in TSH levels is observed as part of the normal negative feedback response due to excessive secretion of T3 and T4 in primary hyper-

TABLE 24-8

CLINICAL MANIFESTATIONS OF HYPERTHYROIDISM

SYSTEM	CLINICAL MANIFESTATION
General	Nervousness, insomnia, fatigue, tremulousness, heat intolerance, weight loss
Skin	Warm and moist, hyperhidrosis, alopecia, hyperpigmentation, onycholysis, acropachy, pretibial myxedema, preradial myxedema, urticaria, pruritis, vitiligo
Eyes	Exophthalmos, conjunctivitis, chemosis, ophthalmoplegia, optic nerve involvement
Cardiovascular	Tachycardia, shortness of breath, palpitations, atrial fibrillation, heart block, high output congestive heart failure, angina pectoris, increased pulse pressure, Means-Lerman "scratch" murmur
Gastrointestinal	Tremor of tongue, hyperphagia increased thirst, diarrhea or hyperdefecation, elevated liver function tests, hepatomegaly
Metabolic	Elevated serum calcium, decreased serum magnesium, increased osseous alkaline phosphatase, hypercalciuria
Neuromuscular	Fine tremor of hands, weakness of proximal muscles, myopathy, muscle atrophy, creatinuria, periodic paralysis
Osseous	Osteoporosis
Neurologic	Fever, delirium, stupor, coma, syncope, choreoathetosis
Reproductive/sexual	Irregular menses, gynecomastia, decreased fertility
Hematopoietic	Anemia (usually normochromic, normocytic), lymphocytosis, lymphadenopathy, enlarged thymus, splenomegaly
Mental	Restlessness, irritability, anxiety, inability to concentrate, lability, depression, psychiatric reactions
Influence on vitamins	Decreased serum vitamin A, prealbumin, and retinol-binding protein; increased requirement for pyridoxine and thiamine; decreased serum 1,25-vitamin D_2

(Becker, K. L. et al. [1995]. *Principles and practice of endocrinology and metabolism* [2nd ed.]. Philadelphia: Lippincott.)

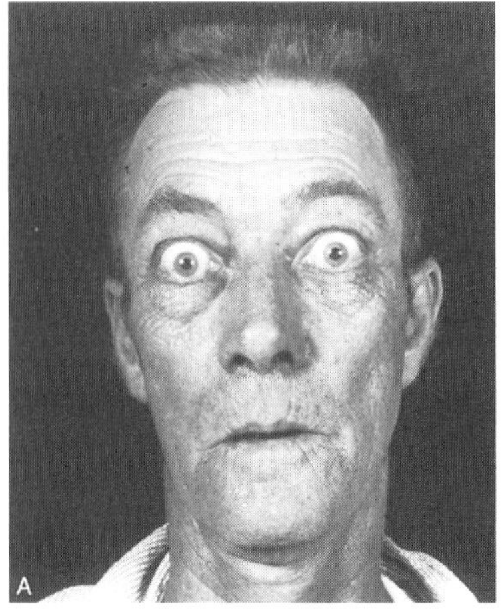

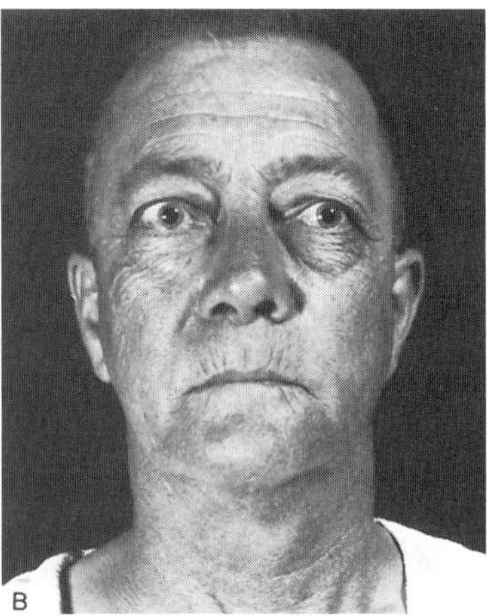

FIGURE 24-7. Patient with Graves' disease. **A.** Appearance before therapy with an antithyroid drug. **B.** Four months after the commencement of therapy. Note the markedly decreased stare. (Braverman, L. E. & Utiger, R. D. [1996]. *Werner and Ingbar's the thyroid: A fundamental and clinical text* [7th ed.]. Philadelphia: Lippincott.)

thyroidism. However, inappropriate pituitary secretion of TSH is seen in secondary hyperthyroidism. Additionally, excessive thyrotropic-releasing hormone (TRH) secretion occurs in tertiary hyperthyroidism.

GRAVES' DISEASE

Graves' disease, an autoimmune disorder, is the most common cause of hyperthyroidism. About 15% of individuals with Graves' disease have a relative with the same disorder. Women have a higher incidence of the disease than men. The peak age for its occurrence is from 20 to 40 years.

Etiology

It is theorized that stress or a viral infections may trigger the development of this disorder. The T cell lymphocytes become sensitized to thyroid antigens and stimulate the B cell lymphocytes to secrete autoantibodies. It is also theorized that an alteration in T cell lymphocyte suppressor function enables the secretion of autoantibodies. A TSH receptor antibody (TSH R [Stim] Ab) stimulates the TSH receptor, increasing cell growth and hormonal synthesis in a manner analogous to TSH activity. The presence of TSH R (Stim) Ab is useful in terms of both diagnosis and treatment.[32,49]

Clinical Manifestations

In addition to the symptoms seen in hyperthyroidism, the clinical manifestations of Graves' disease includes exophthalmos, pretibial myxedema, and goiter with or without bruit.[23,32] **Onycholysis**, or separation of the nail from the nailbed, is also found with Graves' disease.[32,49]

The signs associated with exophthalmos have been classified by the American Thyroid Association. The mnemonic "NO SPECS" is formed by the first letters of each class, as shown in Box 24-7.[35] Typically, the white sclera is visible both above and below the iris. Periorbital edema is also present, with swelling of the extraocular muscles and of the connective tissue within the orbits due to infiltration of lymphocytes, mucopolysaccharides, and edema. This pushes the eye forward. Sight loss occurs from either pressure on the optic nerve or keratitis from corneal exposure.[27,49] Figure 24-7 shows exophthalmos in an individual with Graves' disease.

Pretibial myxedema, also called **thyroid dermopathy**, is due to the accumulation of glycosaminoglycans. The skin becomes thickened and develops a nonpitting edema. Bony involvement, or thyroid **osteopathy**, also occurs. This consists of periosteal swelling, usually in the proximal phalanges of the hands.

Microscopic examination of the thyroid gland demonstrates scattered lymphocytes throughout the

BOX 24-7

CLASSIFICATION OF EYE CHANGES IN GRAVES' DISEASE

Class	Definition
0	**N**o signs or symptoms
1	**O**nly signs, no symptoms. (Signs limited to upper lid retraction, stare, lid lag)
2	**S**oft tissue involvement
3	**P**roptosis
4	**E**xtraocular muscle involvement
5	**C**orneal involvement
6	**S**ight loss (optic nerve involvement)

(Werner, S. C. [1977]. Classification of the eye changes of Graves' disease. *Journal of Clinical Endocrinology and Metabolism, 44,* 302.)

interstitial spaces. The amount of colloid is reduced. The surrounding follicles have a tall columnar epithelium (see Fig. 24-5).[49]

THYROTOXIC CRISES

Prolonged, untreated hyperthyroidism may decompensate to thyrotoxic crisis, or thyroid storm. This disorder may be triggered by a concomitant illness or surgery. Box 24-8 provides a more complete list of the triggers of thyroid storm. The typical clinical manifestations in thyrotoxic crisis are contrasted with hyperthyroidism in Table 24-9.

It is theorized that there is an increased availability of bioactive hormone for the target cells. There is an increase in FT_4 in individuals with thyroid storm as compared with other individuals, despite comparable total T_3 and T_4 levels. Thus, the clinical appearance is of an exaggerated hyperthyroid state. There is also an enhanced catecholamine response, possibly due to an increase in target cell beta adrenergic receptor density.[11]

ALTERATIONS IN PARATHYROID FUNCTION

The major physiologic effects of the parathyroid hormones are directed toward maintaining calcium homeostasis. Parathyroid hormone promote renal calcium reabsorption and stimulates the synthesis of vitamin D, which increases the absorption of calcium and phosphate from the gastrointestinal tract. Thus, the signs and symptoms of altered parathyroid function are related to alterations in calcium levels.

BOX 24-8

KNOWN PRECIPITANTS OF THYROID STORM

Conditions Associated with a Rapid Rise in Thyroid Hormone Levels

- Thyroid surgery
- Withdrawal of antithyroid drug therapy
- Radioiodine therapy
- Vigorous thyroid palpation
- Iodinated contrast dyes

Conditions Associated with an Acute or Subacute Nonthyroid Illness

- Nonthyroid surgery
- Infection
- Cerebrovascular accident
- Pulmonary thromboembolis
- Parturition
- Diabetic ketoacidosis
- Emotional stress
- Trauma

(Burch, H. B. & Wartofsky, L. [1993]. Life-threatening thyrotoxicosis: Thyroid storm. *Endocrinology and Metabolism Clinics of North America, 22*(2), 263–277.)

Hyperparathyroidism

Hyperparathyroidism is characterized by enhanced activity of the parathyroid glands.

ETIOLOGY

Primary hyperparathyroidism is seen in about 0.1% of adults.[28] It is usually the result of a parathyroid chief cell adenoma but may also be due to hyperplasia or carcinoma. Parathyroid hyperplasia is also seen as part of an autosomal dominant multiple endocrine neoplasia syndrome (MEN) (Box 24-9). *Secondary hyperparathyroidism* refers to altered parathyroid function as the result of impaired physiologic processes that affect the gland, such as those in individuals with chronic renal failure. Decreased synthesis of vitamin D and renal phosphate retention promote hyperplasia of the parathyroid gland, with increased synthesis and secretion of PTH. Secondary hyperparathyroidism is also seen in disorders such as rickets in which the ionized calcium level is chronically reduced.[27,62]

CLINICAL MANIFESTATIONS

Hyperparathyroidism results in hypersecretion of parathyroid hormone (PTH). The physiologic result of increased PTH is (1) an elevation in serum calcium levels and (2) excessive secretion of phosphorus by the kidneys. This can result in renal stone formation, which is often the only major presenting symptom. Most individuals are asymptomatic, with hypercalcemia being discovered during a routine physical examination. However, the clinical manifestations of hyperparathyroidism may include the following:[23,69]

- Fatigue and changes in mentation
- Hypertension
- Constipation
- Renal stones and polyuria with gradual loss of renal function
- Bone pain and pathologic fractures

Osteitis fibrosa cystica is the classic form of bone disease seen with hyperparathyroidism. Bone remodeling is increased due to an increase in bone-resorbing osteoclasts. Bone resorption is greater than the bone formation. The bone marrow becomes fibrotic. Osteoporosis occurs with increased loss of cortical bone as opposed to trabecular bone. This produces a "salt and pepper" appearance on x-rays. The result is bone pain with the occurrence of pathologic fractures.[62]

TABLE 24-9

CLINICAL MANIFESTATIONS OF HYPERTHYROIDISM AND THYROTOXIC CRISIS

SYSTEM/FUNCTION	HYPERTHYROIDISM	THYROTOXIC CRISIS
Central nervous system	Emotional lability, short attention span, tremor, weakness	Apathy, agitation, emotional lability, delirium, coma
Cardiovascular	Tachycardia, systolic hypertension	Congestive heart failure, arrhythmias
Gastrointestinal	Hyperdefecation	Vomiting, diarrhea, jaundice
Thermoregulation	Warm, moist skin, heat intolerance	Fever
Nutrition	Increased appetite, weight loss	Severe weight loss, vitamin deficiencies

(Modified from Smallridge, R. C. [1992]. Metabolic and anatomic thyroid emergencies. *Critical Care Medicine, 20*(2), 276–291.)

In addition to elevated parathyroid hormone levels, both serum and urine calcium levels are also increased. Since calcium is highly protein bound, ionized calcium levels should be used in evaluation of serum calcium levels. Serum phosphate levels are decreased. If osteitis fibrosa cystica is present, the alkaline phosphatase will be elevated. Biochemical alterations also may include hyperchloremia with hyperchloremic metabolic acidosis.[23,69]

BOX 24-9

CLINICAL FEATURES OF MULTIPLE ENDOCRINE NEOPLASIA (MEN) SYNDROMES

Men 1

- Benign parathyroid tumors
- Pancreatic tumors
  - Gastrinoma
  - Insulinoma
- Pituitary tumors
  - Growth hormone secreting
  - Prolactin secreting
  - ACTH secreting

Men 2a

- Medullary carcinoma of the thyroid
- Pheochromocytoma
- Hyperparathyroidism

Men 2b

- Medullary carcinoma of the thyroid
- Pheochromocytoma
- Mucosal neuromas

(Modified from Shoback, D. M. & Strewler, G. J. [1997]. Disorders of the parathyroids and calcium metabolism. In S. J. McPhee, V. R. Lingappa, W. F. Ganong, & J. D. Lange [eds.], *Pathology of disease* [2nd ed.]. Stamford, CT: Appleton & Lange.)

Hypoparathyroidism

Hypoparathyroidism is the result of decreased secretion of PTH or decreased hormonal response at the level of the tissues.

ETIOLOGY

Hypoparathyroidism is usually due to removal or destruction of the parathyroid gland during neck surgery. However, it can also occur as a result of autoimmune destruction of the gland. Acquired hypoparathyroidism is also seen in association with other endocrine disorders such as adrenal insufficiency. Additionally, hypomagnesemia may impair parathyroid function.

CLINICAL MANIFESTATIONS

Due to lack of circulating PTH, calcium is not resorbed from bone, kidneys, or intestines. The result is a decrease in serum calcium levels. This in turn causes increased neuromuscular activity and the symptoms of tetany. Therefore, all of the clinical manifestations, such as **Chvostek's sign** (Fig. 24-8) and **Trousseau's sign** (Fig. 24-9), result from decreased levels of serum calcium. Serum phosphate levels are often elevated in hypoparathyroidism. Typical clinical manifestations include the following:[23]

- Personality changes, lethargy, and anxiety
- Tetany
- Tingling of the lips and hands
- Muscle and abdominal cramps
- Defective nails and teeth
- Cataracts

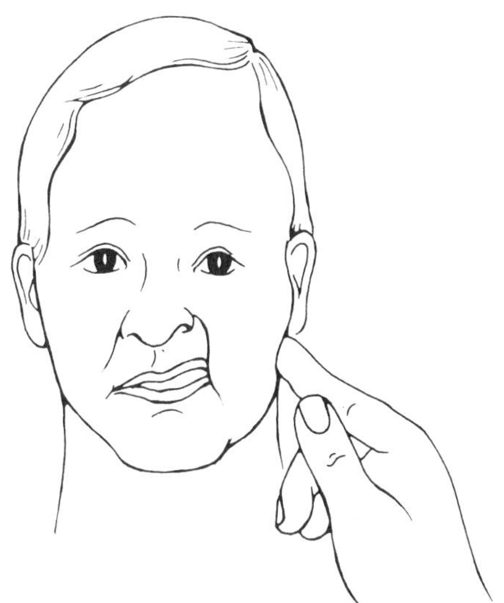

FIGURE 24-8. Chvostek's sign. Tapping the facial nerve approximately 2 cm anterior to the earlobe will elicit Chvostek's sign (unilateral twitching of the facial muscles) in some individuals with hypocalcemia. (Metheny, N. M. [1996]. *Fluid and electrolyte balance* [3rd ed.]. Philadelphia: Lippincott-Raven.)

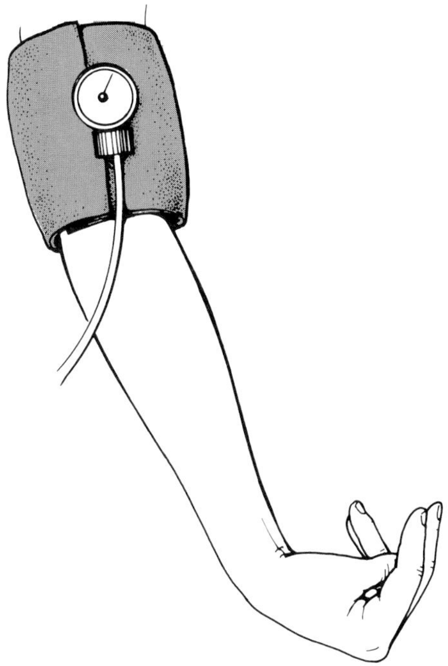

FIGURE 24-9. Trousseau's sign. Carpopedal spasm in hypocalcemia is elicited when blood supply is occluded to the arm for 3 minutes. It is a characteristic sign of hypocalcemia.

The complications occurring from hypoparathyroidism may be life threatening. Acute tetany accompanied by vocal chord palsy and stridor as well as seizures may occur in cases of severe hypocalcemia. Parkinsonian symptoms may appear.

Pseudohypoparathyroidism

Pseudohypoparathyroidism is an inheritable disorder of tissue resistance to PTH. Despite elevated PTH levels, the biochemical presentation is comparable to that of hypoparathyroidism. There is hypocalcemia with hyperphosphatemia. The clinical manifestations include short stature, round face, obesity, and mental retardation. The fourth fingers are shortened due to shortening of the metacarpal bones. The affected hands have a dimple in place of a knuckle.[23,69]

ALTERATIONS IN ADRENOCORTICAL FUNCTION

The hormones of the adrenal cortex regulate physiologic functions that are essential for life. The **glucocorticoids** protect against hypoglycemia by promoting gluconeogenesis and glycogenolysis. They also have inherent anti-inflammatory actions and are an important part of the physiologic stress response. The **mineralocorticoids** stimulate sodium and water retention to maintain normal fluid and electrolyte balance. Changes in adrenocortical function are manifested by altered fluid balance, altered glucose levels, and an impaired stress response.

Hypofunction

Hypofunction of the adrenocortical glands may lead to adrenal insufficiency, adrenal crisis, or hypoaldosteronism.

ADRENAL INSUFFICIENCY

Adrenal insufficiency refers to a reduction in one or more of the hormones secreted by the adrenal cortex as the result of dysfunction of the hypothalamic-pituitary-adrenal axis. It may be *primary*, due to the destruction or dysfunction of the adrenal cortex, or *secondary*, from the lack of ACTH secretion from the anterior pituitary gland. There is also a congenital defect of hormonal synthesis that can result in reduced cortisol secretion. The etiologies of adrenal insufficiency are listed in Box 24-10. The symptoms are essentially those of hormonal deficit, ranging from hemodynamic compromise to subtle dysfunction appearing only with stress. However, since mineralocorticoid deficit is not always seen

ETIOLOGY OF ADRENOCORTICAL INSUFFICIENCY

Primary Adrenocortical Insufficiency

Major Causes

Autoimmune (80%)
Tuberculosis (20%)

Minor Causes

Adrenal hemorrhage and infarction
Histoplasmosis
Metastatic carcinoma
AIDS
Radiation therapy
Adrenalectomy
Medications: metyrapone, ketoconazole, mitotane

Secondary Adrenocortical Insufficiency

Exogenous glucocorticoid therapy
Pituitary tumor
Hypothalamic tumor

(Modified from McPhee, S. J. [1997]. Disorders of the adrenal cortex. In S. J. McPhee, V. R. Lingappa, W. F. Ganong, & J. D. Lange [eds.], *Pathology of disease* [2nd ed.]. Stamford, CT: Appleton & Lange.)

in secondary adrenal insufficiency, there may be some variation in clinical manifestations.[34,47]

Primary Insufficiency

Primary adrenal insufficiency is due to decreased adrenocortical activity. The hypothalamic and anterior pituitary functions are basically intact.

ETIOLOGY. Primary insufficiency, also referred to as **Addison's disease**, is the result of adrenocortical dysfunction. It is more common in women than in men and is usually diagnosed in the third to fifth decades of life. The most common cause of primary adrenal insufficiency is adrenal atrophy due to autoimmune adrenalitis. The loss of 90% of both adrenal cortices results in adrenal insufficiency. Altered adrenal function develops gradually with the clinical manifestations of a decreased adrenal reserve. The individual appears stable until an illness or other stressor precipitates adrenal crisis.[21,27]

CLINICAL MANIFESTATIONS. As adrenal secretion of cortisol decreases, pituitary section of ACTH increases due to the lack of negative feedback inhibition of the neuroendocrine axis. Physically the individual develops marked (1) hyperpigmentation, (2) hypoglycemia, (3) hypotension, and a (4) decrease in cardiac size. Hyperpigmentation is due to increased melanocyte-stimulating hormone activity from increased synthesis and secretion of ACTH. Decreased gluconeogenesis can lead to hypoglycemia. Chronic hypotension with reduced cardiac workload results in a decrease in cardiac size. Decreased secretion of adrenal androgens causes amenorrhea in women.[21,27,47]

Other clinical manifestations include the following:[21,23]

- Weakness, fatigue, anemia
- Anorexia, weight loss
- Abdominal pain, nausea, vomiting, and diarrhea
- Sparse axillary and pubic hair, amenorrhea
- Muscle and joint pains

Decreased mineralocorticoid activity occurs concomitantly to decreased glucocorticoid activity in primary adrenal insufficiency, resulting in the following fluid and electrolyte abnormalities and changes in white blood cell ratios:[23]

- Hyponatremia and hyperkalemia
- Elevated calcium and urea nitrogen
- Neutropenia, eosinophilia
- Relative lymphocytosis

Secondary Insufficiency

ETIOLOGY. The most common cause of secondary adrenal insufficiency is depression of the neuroendocrine axis due to administration of exogenous glucocorticoids at pharmacologic doses. If treatment with exogenous glucocorticoids continues for more than 4 or 5 weeks, there is prolonged suppression of CRH, ACTH, and endogenous glucocorticoid secretion. Adrenal atrophy may occur. The neuroendocrine axis becomes nonresponsive. Pharmacologic doses of glucocorticoids must be slowly tapered down to avoid the development of symptoms of adrenal insufficiency. Once pharmacologic doses of glucocorticoids have been discontinued, there is a prolonged alteration in the neuroendocrine axis. It may take 23 months for the anterior pituitary to respond to changes in glucocorticoid levels. However, it may be another 69 months for glucocorticoid levels to return to normal.[29] If during this time the individual becomes seriously ill or suffers a major trauma or stressor, adrenal crisis can occur since the adrenal function is altered.[47]

Secondary adrenal insufficiency also occurs from deficient ACTH secretion. This is often due to either a pituitary or a hypothalamic tumor. The lack of ACTH leads to decreased cortisol and adrenal androgen secretion.

CLINICAL MANIFESTATIONS. The signs and symptoms of secondary adrenal insufficiency are comparable to that of primary adrenal insufficiency. However, aldosterone secretion is usually normal. Additionally, since ACTH is reduced, hyperpigmentation does not occur.[21,47]

The presence of cushingoid features in conjunction with the manifestations of adrenal insufficiency is suggestive of secondary adrenal insufficiency due to administration of exogenous glucocorticoids.[21,29,47]

Hypothalamic or pituitary tumors may have concomitant loss of other pituitary hormones. Thus, there may also be evidence of hypogonadism and hypothyroidism. However, a pituitary adenoma may also have associated hypersecretion of GH or prolactin.[21]

There are differences in hormonal levels between primary and secondary adrenal insufficiency. An elevated ACTH level with a depressed cortisol level is suggestive of a primary disorder. If both hormonal levels are depressed, the results are suggestive of a secondary or tertiary (hypothalamic) etiology. Additionally, ACTH stimulation produces an increase in cortisol in secondary adrenal hypofunction. In contrast, there is no concomitant increase in cortisol levels with ACTH stimulation in primary hypofunction. Table 24-10 summarizes the hormonal changes seen in primary and secondary adrenal insufficiency. Aldosterone secretion is usually maintained at normal levels in secondary adrenal insufficiency.[21,34,47]

ADRENAL CRISIS

Acute adrenal crisis occurs as the result of insufficient glucocorticoids and is precipitated by severe infection, trauma, surgery, dehydration, and other factors. It often presents as unexplained hypotensive shock in conjunction with a relative resistance to resuscitative efforts with beta adrenergic stimulants (vasopressors and isotopes). There is a synergistic relationship between glucocorticoids and vascular responsiveness to catecholamines. Therefore, the loss of glucocorticoid activity in adrenal crisis can lead to cardiovascular collapse.[12,21,23] Flowchart 24-1 demonstrates the pathogenesis and additional clinical manifestations of adrenal crisis.

Typical clinical manifestations in adrenal crisis include the following:[21,23]

- Confusion, depressed mentation, coma
- Headache, lassitude, weakness
- Abdominal pain, nausea, vomiting, diarrhea, anorexia
- Hypotension, shock, fever
- Hypoglycemia, hyperkalemia, hyponatremia
- Dehydration, volume depletion

HYPOALDOSTERONISM

An isolated reduction in aldosterone secretion is seen in renal disease when renin levels are decreased. Additionally, it can also occur with enzyme deficiencies seen in adrenogenital syndrome. Reduced aldosterone synthesis and secretion is also observed with long-term use of heparin. **Pseudohypoaldosteronism** refers to a syndrome in which there is resistance to hormonal activity.[12,27] Hypoaldosteronism associated with renal disease is most often diagnosed in men in the fifth to seventh decades of life. Frequently there is evidence of pyelonephritis, diabetes mellitus, or gout.[47]

Clinical manifestations include the following:[27]

- Hyperkalemia, hyponatremia
- Excess loss of urinary sodium
- Hypotension
- Hyperchloremic metabolic acidosis

Hyperfunction

Hyperfunction occurs as the result of excessive secretion of the hormones of the adrenal cortex. Although this typically refers to excessive glucocorticoid activity, excessive secretion of aldosterone can also occur.

HYPERCORTICALISM

Hypercorticalism occurs from excessive levels of glucocorticoids. This leads to a typical appearance, referred to as cushingoid manifestations. **Cushing's disease** occurs from elevated levels of endogenous glucocorticoids as a result of excessive pituitary ACTH secretion. **Cushing's syndrome** refers to the physical and physiologic manifestations of excessive glucocorticoid levels as a result of several mechanisms. Unfortunately, these terms are often used interchangeably.

Cushing's Disease

About 70% of individuals with cushingoid manifestations have Cushing's disease due to hypersecretion of ACTH from a pituitary adenoma. These adenomas are eight times more common in women.[40,47] Less commonly, the pituitary hypersecretion of ACTH is due to

TABLE 24-10

HORMONAL LEVELS IN PRIMARY AND SECONDARY ADRENAL INSUFFICIENCY

	CORTISOL LEVEL	ACTH LEVEL
Primary hypofunction	Decreased	Elevated
Secondary hypofunction	Decreased	Decreased
ACTH stimulation in primary hypofunction	Decreased	Not applicable
ACTH stimulation in secondary hypofunction	Elevated	Not applicable

FLOWCHART 24-1 **Pathogenesis of Adrenal Crises**

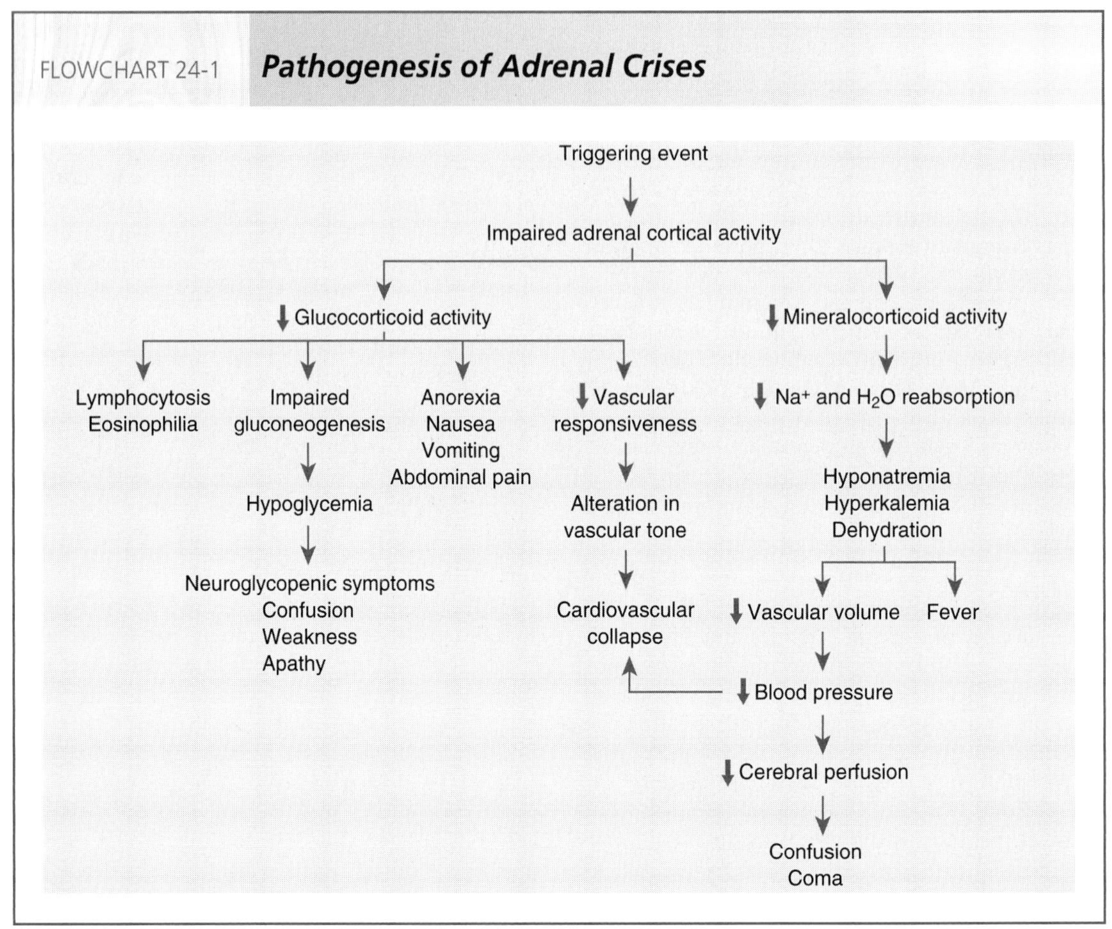

excessive CRH from the hypothalamus. In this case, the pituitary gland demonstrates diffuse hyperplasia rather than evidence of an adenoma. In either circumstance, the excessive ACTH hypersecretion promotes adrenal hyperplasia. This hyperplasia is either non-nodular or micronodular.[21]

Ectopic CRH secretion promotes increased ACTH synthesis and secretion by the anterior pituitary gland. Thus, the increased ACTH stimulates adrenocortical hypersecretion of glucocorticoids. Although rare, ectopic CRH secretion has been observed in bronchial carcinoid tumors.[47]

Cushing's Syndrome

The excessive levels of glucocorticoids seen in Cushing's syndrome are the result of (1) pharmacologic doses of exogenous glucocorticoids; (2) secretory adrenocortical tumors, which stimulate the adrenal cortex to increase its production of hormones despite adequate production; or (3) ectopic ACTH secretion by non-pituitary tumors, which leads to spontaneous Cushing's syndrome.[21,23,47]

Ectopic ACTH hypersecretion is most frequently seen in conjunction with small cell carcinoma of the lung. However, other tumors, such as thymomas and pancreatic islet cell tumors, may also secrete ACTH.

As in Cushing's disease, the elevated ACTH levels promote adrenal hyperplasia. Additionally, chronic ectopic ACTH secretion results in suppression of pituitary ACTH and reduced hypothalamic secretion of CRH. The clinical manifestations often include hyperpigmentation.[21,47]

Hypersecretion of glucocorticoids occurs from both adrenocortical adenomas and carcinomas. Additionally, hypersecretion of adrenal androgens may be seen. This hypersecretion is not dependent upon ACTH secretion. If adrenal androgens are elevated, the clinical manifestations will also include hirsutism and virilization.[21] Gonadal dysfunction also occurs with elevated adrenal androgens. This is demonstrated by amenorrhea and infertility in women and by decreased libido in men.[47]

Clinical Manifestations

Elevated glucocorticoid levels are associated with certain characteristic physical changes, such as the moon facies due to accumulation of facial fat. Figure 24-10 shows physical changes over time in an individual with

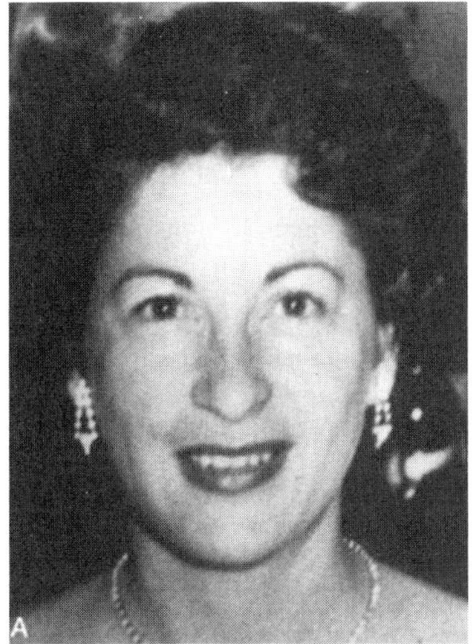

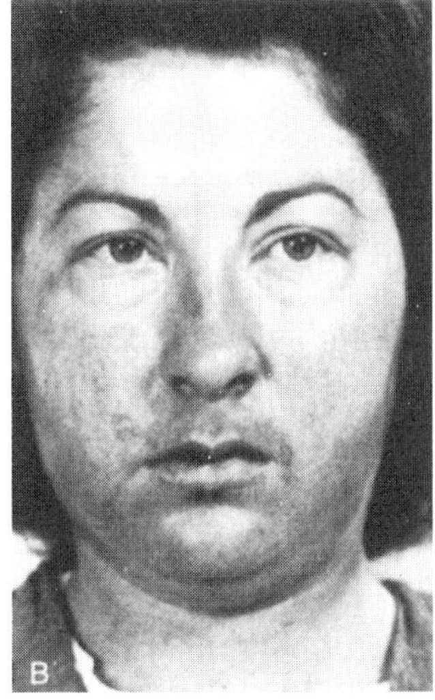

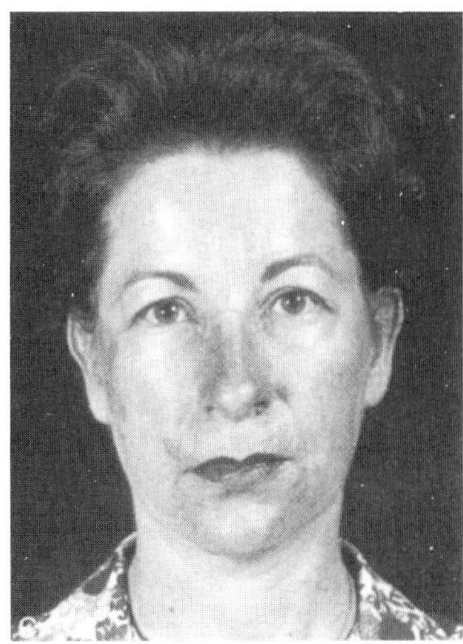

FIGURE 24-10. **Progressive facial changes in a woman with Cushing's disease. A. Prior to onset of the illness. B. Preoperative. C. One year after surgery. (Becker, K. D. et al. [1995]. *Principles and practice of endocrinology and metabolism* [2nd ed.]. Philadelphia: Lippincott.)**

Cushing's syndrome. In addition to the clinical manifestations of Cushing's syndrome, noted in Figure 24-11, elevated glucocorticoids levels result in the following:[21,47]

- Euphoria, emotional lability, anxiety, depression, sleep disorders
- Osteoporosis
- Increased risk of infection
- Hyperglycemia, glycosuria, leukocytosis, lymphocytopenia, hypokalemia
- Hypertension

There is loss of the normal diurnal rhythm of glucocorticoid secretion. Additionally, glucocorticoid excess promotes increased gluconeogenesis and antagonism of the action of insulin. This leads to elevated glucose levels with the symptoms of DM. Indeed, DM occurs in about 10% to 15% of individuals with glucocorticoid excess.

The action of fibroblasts is also inhibited by glucocorticoid excess. This contributes to loss of collagen and connective tissue. There is thinning of skin and poor wound healing. This promotes an increased risk of wound dehiscence following surgery.

The normal inflammatory response is also impaired due to inhibition of phospholipase A in releasing arachidonic acid from tissue phospholipids. This results in a decrease in the metabolites of arachidonic acid that mediate inflammation and clotting (see Chapters 10 and 15). Antibody formation is also impaired, increasing the risk of infection.

Hypertension, also seen, appears to have a variety of contributory factors. Mineralocorticoid effects are seen when glucocorticoid levels are elevated; thus, sodium and water retention is increased. Angiotensin II, a powerful vasoconstrictor, is also elevated, possibly as a result of increased hepatic synthesis. Additionally, glucocorticoids increase vascular responsiveness to catecholamines.[21]

Cushing's syndrome is classified as either (1) ACTH dependent or (2) ACTH independent. Elevated ACTH levels are seen in pituitary, hypothalamic, and ectopic etiologies of glucocorticoid excess. In contrast, ACTH levels are decreased in instances of adrenal Cushing's syndrome. Table 24-11 shows hormonal levels typically seen in hypercorticolism. ACTH levels are decreased in ACTH-independent adrenal hypersecretion following administration of Dexamethasone. Both ACTH and cortisol levels are elevated in Cushing's disease after administration of CRH.

HYPERALDOSTERONISM

Hyperaldosteronism is the result of excessive secretion of aldosterone. Primary hyperaldosteronism occurs from an abnormality in the adrenal cortex. Secondary hyperaldosteronism is the result of pathologic activity that stimulates increased aldosterone synthesis and secretions.

Etiology

Although primary hyperaldosteronism can occur from hyperplasia of the zona glomerulosa tissue of the adrenal cortex, the most common cause is excessive secretion from an adenoma. Aldosterone-secreting adenomas are more common than cortisol-secreting adenomas. However, they are often discovered only incidentally, since they usually are small and may be missed on CT scans.

(text continues on page 695)

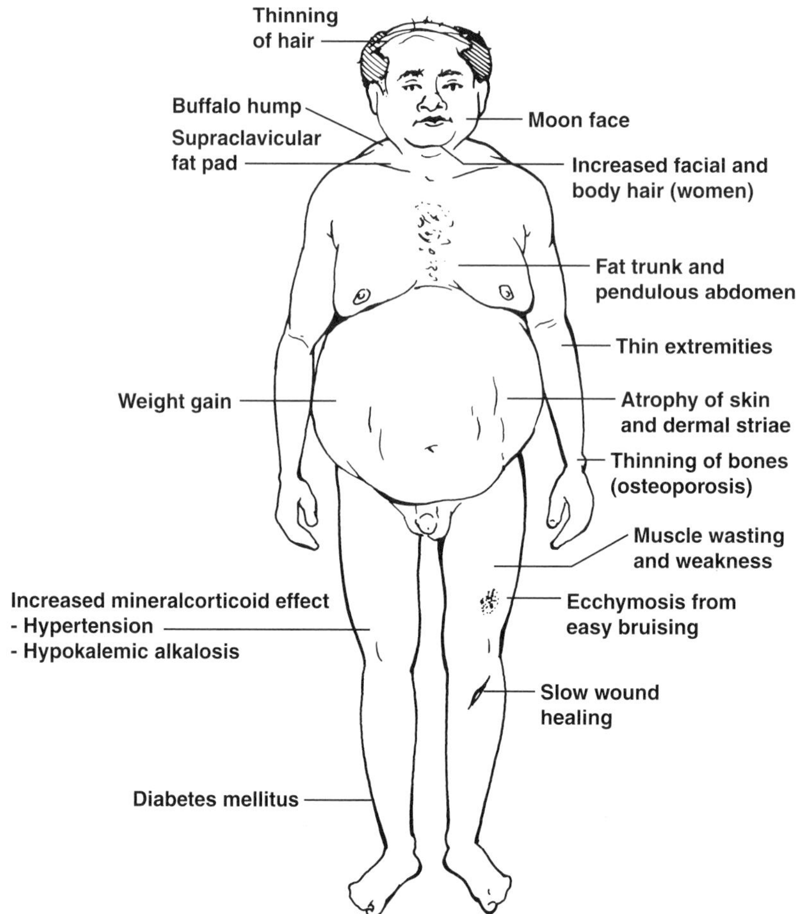

FIGURE 24-11. Major clinical manifestations of Cushing's syndrome.

TABLE 24-11

HORMONAL LEVELS FOR EVALUATION OF HYPERCORTISOLISM

	CORTISOL LEVEL	ACTH LEVEL
BASELINE LEVELS		
Non–ACTH-dependent adrenal hypersecretion	Elevated	Decreased
ACTH-dependent adrenal hypersecretion	Elevated	Elevated
DEXAMETHASONE TEST		
Non–ACTH-dependent adrenal hypersecretion	Elevated	Decreased
ACTH-dependent adrenal hypersecretion	Elevated	Elevated
CRH TEST		
Non–ACTH-adrenal hypersecretion	No change from baseline	No change from baseline
Pituitary ACTH hypersecretion	Markedly elevated	Markedly elevated
Ectopic ACTH hypersecretion	No change from baseline	No change from baseline

Secondary hyperaldosteronism is seen in many individuals with congestive heart failure, nephrosis, or cirrhosis of the liver. It is due to excessive secretion of renin by the juxtaglomerular apparatus of the kidney. These conditions are associated with either sodium wasting or decreased renal perfusion, situations that increase renin secretion. Secondary hyperaldosteronism is rarely due to a renin-secreting tumor.[8,21,27,47]

Clinical Manifestations

Since there is potassium depletion, many of the symptoms are those of profound hypokalemia. Excess mineralocorticoid secretion results in the following:[27,47]

- Hypokalemia, hypernatremia
- Hypertension
- Tetany
- Polyuria, thirst
- Metabolic alkalosis

A hallmark of hyperaldosteronism is an increase in the ratio of aldosterone to renin activity to greater than 25.[21]

Adrenal Androgen Syndromes

Adrenal androgen syndromes are the result of abnormalities in the secretion of androgens such as androstenedione. Since these hormones are precursors to testosterone and dihydrotestosterone, the effects are different in males and females. As part of these syndromes, female pseudohermaphroditism and feminizing estrogen-secreting tumors are also seen.[21,27]

ETIOLOGY

Elevated androgens can occur from excessive adrenal or ovarian secretion or due to enhanced peripheral conversion. Adrenal hypersecretion can be caused by Cushing's syndrome, adrenal carcinoma, or congenital adrenal hyperplasia due to hereditary defects in cortisol synthesis.[21,23]

CLINICAL MANIFESTATIONS

Excess androgen secretion is associated with masculinization, hirsutism, and precocious pseudo-puberty.[21,27,47] Prenatal exposure to excessive androgens presents differently in males than in females: Males appear normal whereas females have virilization. Postnatally, symptoms of androgen excess are seen. Thus, lifelong hormonal replacement therapy is needed to ensure normal puberty and fertility.[47]

ALTERATIONS IN ADRENAL-MEDULLARY FUNCTION

The adrenal medulla synthesizes and secretes the catecholamines epinephrine and norepinephrine. Therefore, alterations in adrenal-medullary function are related to epinephrine excess or deficit.

Hypofunction

Hypofunction of the adrenal medulla, with loss of adrenal catecholamine secretion, is seen following bilateral adrenalectomy. If the sympathetic nervous system is intact, individuals usually are asymptomatic. However, in autonomic insufficiency, lack of adrenal epinephrine is associated with decreased recovery from hypoglycemia. This is due to the loss of the counterregulatory effect of epinephrine in glucose homeostasis. These individuals often have a reduction in the warning signs of hypoglycemia. Many of these signs are neurogenic in nature, being related to epinephrine secretion.

Symptomatic orthostatic hypotension is also associated with autonomic insufficiency. This is due to the interruption of the reflex mechanisms that control blood pressure during position changes.

Hyperfunction: Pheochromocytoma

Adrenal medullary hyperfunction is excessive secretion of epinephrine or norepinephrine, or both, and in some cases dopamine.

ETIOLOGY

Pheochromocytoma, which is the primary cause of adrenal-medullary hyperfunction, is a potentially life-threatening secretory adrenal tumor arising from the chromaffin cells. The tumors have been found in both sexes of all ages. They can be either benign or malignant and may be seen as part of multiple endocrine neoplasia syndromes. Adrenal hyperfunction rarely occurs from adrenal-medullary hyperplasia. However, when it does, it is often associated with multiple endocrine neoplasia.[28]

CLINICAL MANIFESTATIONS

Pheochromocytoma leads to an excessive secretion of epinephrine, norepinephrine, and sometimes dopamine. Thus, the symptoms are those of catecholamine excess.

Although symptoms can be prevalent all of the time, many individuals have episodic or sporadic periods of varying intensity, including periods when they are relatively asymptomatic. The episodes are related to a sudden increase in catecholamine secretion from the tumor. Thus, the symptoms of the episodes resemble those that would occur following an injection of epinephrine or norepinephrine. Typical clinical manifestations seen during an episode include the following:[21,28]

- Hypertension
- Headache, nervousness, anxiety
- Visual disturbances
- Diaphoresis
- Palpitations, chest pain
- Abdominal pain, nausea, and vomiting

The complications of untreated pheochromocytoma are extensive. These include hypertensive retinopathy, nephropathy, myocardial infarction, and intracranial hemorrhage. Thus, it is important to identify and treat this disorder.

Elevated levels of metanephrines and vanillylmandelic acid are seen in 24-hour urinary collections.[31] Plasma catecholamine levels are also elevated during symptomatic episodes. Individuals with pheochromocytoma also have a different response to clonidine, a centrally acting alpha-2 agonist often used to treat hypertension. In pheochromocytoma, there is no change in either blood pressure or plasma catecholamine levels. However, in essential hypertension, clonidine decreases plasma norepinephrine levels.[48]

ALTERATIONS IN THE FUNCTION OF THE ENDOCRINE PANCREAS

Although DM is the major disorder associated with dysfunction of the endocrine pancreas, there are disorders associated with the other secretory pancreatic cells.

Secretory Islet Cell Tumors

The various cell types of the pancreatic islets may develop secretory neoplasms, which may be benign or malignant. However, the clinical manifestations are related to hypersecretion of the particular hormone. Islet cell tumors secrete excessive amounts of gastrin, somatostatin, insulin, and glucagon.

Insulinomas secrete excessive amounts of insulin, C peptide, and proinsulin. The tumors may be multiple and may be part of MEN. The major presenting symptom of insulinomas is hypoglycemia.

Gastrinomas stimulate hypersecretion of gastric acid, promoting peptic ulceration. This syndrome is referred to Zollinger-Ellison syndrome. Gastrinomas are usually benign. They are also found as part of MEN.

Glucagonomas secrete excessive glucagon. Typical clinical manifestations include glucose intolerance, rash, anemia, and weight loss.

Somatostatinomas are very rare secretory neoplasms. They are associated with weight loss, DM, malabsorption of fats, gall bladder disease, and hypochlorhydria.

Diabetes Mellitus

Diabetes mellitus refers to a group of metabolic diseases characterized by an elevation in blood glucose levels (hyperglycemia). The American Diabetes Association estimates that 16 million people living in the United States have DM. However, more than one third are not yet diagnosed. Diabetes mellitus is the silent killer, since many people are not aware that they have DM until they develop one of the life-threatening complications. It has become the seventh leading cause of death in the U.S. In 1992, the direct and indirect cost of DM was estimated to be $92 billion.[1,2,59]

The prevalence of DM increases with age.[7] Over 10% of individuals over the age of 65 have DM as compared with 0.8% of individuals younger than 38. The incidence is also greater in women (55%) than men (45%). Within the population of people in the U.S., the incidence varies by ethnic group: Mexican American and Puerto Rican descent, 14.3%; non-Hispanic African Americans, 10.1%; and Cuban Americans and non-Hispanic whites 5.9%. The highest rate of DM in the United States is found in the Pima Indians of Arizona. The incidence in that population for the age group 30 to 64 years of age is 50%. Finland has the highest rate of DM in the world, more than 35 per 100,000 people.[2]

The risk factors for DM include the following:[1,18]

- Overweight (>120% of desirable body weight)
- Hypertension
- HDL cholesterol level <35 mg/dL, triglyceride level >250 mg/dL)
- Lack of exercise
- Family history of DM
- Age 45 or older
- Women who have given birth to an infant weighing more than 9 pounds at birth
- Member of high-risk ethnic group: African American, Hispanic, American Indian

CLASSIFICATION AND ETIOLOGY

As mentioned previously, the term diabetes mellitus refers to a group of disorders. The etiology, clinical manifestations, and treatment of these disorders can vary considerably. For this reason, the 1997 Expert Committee on the Diagnosis and Classification of Diabetes Mellitus published a revised classification system based on the etiology of the hyperglycemia. The general categories of this revised list are shown in Box 24-11. This is a dramatic change from the prior classification system, that was more or less treatment focused.[18]

The new classification system takes into consideration hyperglycemia induced by a variety of mechanisms. Typically the largest percentage of the population with hyperglycemia will be classified as either Type 1 or Type 2. Type 1 refers to hyperglycemia as the result of autoimmune destruction of the pancreatic B cells. Hyperglycemia due to a range of insulin-related alterations, such as insulin deficiency and insulin resistance, characterizes Type 2. The other specific types include hyperglycemia as a result of dysfunction of the exocrine pancreas, endocrine dysfunction, and medications. Gestational DM is listed as Type IV.[18] Type 1 and Type 2 will be discussed in detail in this chapter.

BOX 24-11

ETIOLOGIC CLASSIFICATION OF DIABETES MELLITUS

I. Type 1 Diabetes (B-cell destruction usually associated with absolute insulin deficiency)
   Immune mediated
   Idiopathic
II. Type 2 diabetes (may range from mostly insulin resistance with relative insulin deficiency to predominantly secretory defect with insulin resistance)
III. Other specific types
   Genetic defects of B-cell function
   Genetic defects in insulin action
   Diseases of the exocrine pancreas
   Endocrinopathies
   Drug or chemical induced
   Infection
   Uncommon forms of immune-mediated diabetes
   Other genetic syndromes sometimes associated with diabetes
IV. Gestational diabetes

(Modified from The Expert Committee on the Diagnosis and Classification of Diabetes Mellitus. [1997]. The report of the Expert Committee on the Diagnosis and Classification of Diabetes Mellitus. *Diabetes Care, 20*(7), 1185.)

BOX 24-12

CRITERIA FOR THE DIAGNOSIS OF DIABETES MELLITUS

1. Symptoms of diabetes plus casual plasma glucose concentration ≥ 200 mg/dL (11.1 mmol/L). Casual is defined as any time of day without regard to time since last meal. The classic symptoms of diabetes include polyuria, polydipsia, and unexplained weight loss, or
2. Fasting plasma glucose ≥ 126 mg/dL (7.0 mmol/L). Fasting is defined as no caloric intake for at least 8 hours, or
3. 2-hour postprandial glucose ≥ 200 mg/dL during an oral glucose tolerance test (OGTT). The test should be performed as described by the World Health Organization using a glucose load containing the equivalent of 75 g anhydrous glucose dissolved in water.

In the absence of unequivocal hyperglycemia with acute metabolic decompensation, these criteria should be confirmed by repeat testing on a different day. The third measure, OGTT, is not recommended for routine clinical use.

(The Expert Commitee on the Diagnosis and Classification of Diabetes Mellitus. [1997]. The report of the Expert Commitee on the Diagnosis and Classification of Diabetes Mellitus. *Diabetes Care, 20*(7), 1190.)

Gestational diabetes is a complication of pregnancy, occurring in 2% to 6% of pregnancies. Uncontrolled gestational diabetes is associated with increased infant morbidity and mortality, macrosomia, and cesarean deliveries and is a strong marker for the future development of maternal DM. Glucose utilization is altered, despite the fact that hyperinsulinism is common in normal pregnancy. It appears to be related to anti-insulin effects of progesterone, cortisol, and human placenta lactogen. This increases the amount of insulin needed to maintain glycemic control. As a result of these factors, there in an increased risk of hypoglycemia and ketoacidosis in these women (see Chapter 4).[42]

In addition to revising the classification system, the expert committee also established new criteria for the diagnosis of DM (Box 24-12). These criteria are based on threshold blood glucose levels related to the development of complications from hyperglycemia. For example, the incidence of complications was markedly increased in individuals with fasting blood glucose levels of greater than or equal to 126 mg/dL in many research studies. Additionally, a 2-hour postprandial plasma glucose level greater than or equal to 200 mg/dL is associated with a marked increase in microvascular complications.[18]

Type 1 Diabetes Mellitus

Type 1 DM is an autoimmune disorder characterized by destruction of pancreatic B cells. If untreated, it ultimately leads to ketosis. The pathophysiologic process that leads to its development begins prior to the onset of hyperglycemia. Indeed, 80% to 90% of islet B cell function must be destroyed. **Insulinitis**, a chronic inflammatory process, occurs as part of autoimmune destruction of the B cells. With insulinitis, the islets contain variable numbers of degranulated B cells and an inflammatory infiltrate consisting of CD8 and CD4 cells, macrophages, and natural killer cells (see Chapter 11). The distribution of the affected islets within the pancreas is unusual in that one pancreatic lobule will be affected while another may appear to be normal.[4,60]

Although cell-mediated immune mechanisms are implicated as part of the insulinitis phase, humoral responses also are associated with the development DM. Specific autoantibodies have been identified, including islet cell and insulin autoantibodies. The combination of these two autoantibodies is highly predictive for the development of Type 1 DM. These antibodies have been detected as early as 10 years before the onset of the disease.[19,60,65]

Genetic factors play a role in the development of Type 1 DM. The occurrence of DM in the twin sibling is much greater for monozygotic twins than for dizygotic twins. Additionally, specific human leukocyte antigens (HLA) on the sixth chromosome are associated with the development of Type 1 DM. These HLA antigens are apparently linked to immune response genes that promote a genetic susceptibility for DM.[19,60,65]

Environmental factors and exposure to viruses are also related to the occurrence of Type 1 DM in genetically susceptible individuals. As previously mentioned, the islet cell antigen glutamic acid decarboxylase (GAD) has some similarity with coxsackie B virus. This is referred to as **molecular mimicry**. Thus, it is hypothesized that the immune response to this foreign protein may also trigger islet B cell destruction. Comparable molecular mimicry is also seen between bovine serum albumin from cow's milk and a pancreatic islet B cell surface antigen.[19,37,60,65]

Type 2 Diabetes Mellitus

Type 2 DM is characterized by insulin resistance alone or in conjunction with a reduction in insulin synthesis and secretion. In contrast to Type 1 DM, it is essentially a nonketotic form of DM. Although there is a strong genetic predisposition, it is not linked to HLA markers on the sixth chromosome. Additionally, there is no autoimmune destruction of the pancreatic islet B cells. Because the hyperglycemia develops gradually, Type 2 DM frequently is not diagnosed in the early stages of the disease.[18,37]

It appears that a combination of genetic and environmental factors contributes to the development of Type 2 DM. Although the exact mechanisms are unknown, there is a link between diet and exercise. In obese individuals, there is increased insulin resistance, often with a compensatory hyperinsulinemia.[18,59]

In terms of genetic susceptibility, there is a stronger genetic link in Type 2 DM than in Type 1 DM. The occurrence of Type 2 DM in a child whose parent also has the disease is about 33%. The incidence with monozygotic twins is between 34% and 72%.[19] However, the hereditary pattern appears to be complex, involving multiple genetic factors rather than one specific type of heredity pattern. Additionally, environmental factors such as obesity and exercise affect the development of DM in susceptible individuals.[59]

It is theorized that insulin resistance is the initial dysfunction in Type 2 DM. Thus, insulin resistance rather than hyperglycemia promotes hyperinsulinemia. The increased demand for insulin leads to progressive loss of pancreatic islet B cell function. Additionally, there appears to be decreased secretion of insulin from the B cell due to glucose nonresponsiveness. It also appears that hyperglycemia itself promotes the unresponsiveness of the pancreatic B cell.[19,59,60]

CLINICAL MANIFESTATIONS AND PATHOPHYSIOLOGY

Despite differences in etiology, the presenting symptoms are related to hyperglycemia due to some type of alteration in insulin secretion and/or function. The physiologic and metabolic alterations depend upon the percentage of loss of insulin action. Thus, there are both similarities and differences seen in the clinical manifestations of individuals with Type 1 DM as compared with Type 2 DM (Table 24-12).

Weight loss despite increased appetite is a common feature in Type 1 DM. This is due both to loss of fluids from osmotic diuresis and to loss of muscle and fat stores from gluconeogenesis and fatty acid metabolism. The use of fats as an alterative energy source also leads to the development of ketosis. Loss of fluids predisposes individuals to orthostatic hypotension. Protein catabolism leads to a negative nitrogen balance (see Chapter 7).[45]

In contrast to Type 1 DM, individuals with Type 2 DM do not have a marked reduction in body weight. Since adipose tissue is very sensitive to insulin effects, there may be enough insulin to prevent lipolysis and promote fat storage. Fat distribution is often more central in the upper part of the body; thus, there is an increased waist-to-hip ratio. Hypertension is also often seen.[19,37]

TABLE 24-12

MANIFESTATIONS OF TYPE 1 AND TYPE 2 DIABETES MELLITUS

CHARACTERISTIC	TYPE 1 DM	TYPE 2 DM
Body weight	Markedly reduced	No major change
Fat distribution	No particular pattern	Central or upper body
Ketosis	Common	Rare
Lipolysis	Present	Absent
Blood pressure	Orthostatic hypotension	Hypertension

Typical clinical features that are common to both Type 1 and Type 2 DM include the following:[37]

- Polyuria and thirst
- Recurrent blurred vision
- Paresthesias
- Fatigue
- Vulvovaginitis in women

In both Type 1 and Type 2 DM there is an alteration in the glucagon–insulin ratio. It is higher than normal and is similar to that seen in fasting. Thus, there is insufficient insulin to counterbalance the effects of glucagon. Glucagon stimulates hepatic glucose production (gluconeogenesis). Normally, insulin promotes glucose utilization through stimulation of insulin-dependent glucose transporters. However, in DM there is either a lack or deficiency of insulin, resulting in decreased glucose utilization. When the glucagon–insulin ratio is elevated, the result is an elevation in blood glucose.[19]

The metabolic alterations depend on the amount of insulin available. Individuals with residual insulin secretion in conjunction with insulin resistance may present with a normal fasting blood glucose but an elevated postprandial hyperglycemia. With additional loss of insulin, glucagon's effects are not counterbalanced and both fasting and postprandial hyperglycemia occur.[19]

Lipolysis occurs from insulin deficiency, since gluconeogenesis depends on fatty acid metabolism. Fatty acid metabolism produces ketone bodies, acetoacetic acid, and 3-hydroxybuteric acid.[45] These then become part of the very-low-density lipoproteins (VLDL). The insulin deficiency also reduces the amount of available lipoprotein lipase, the enzyme that hydrolyses VLDL. The end result is an increase in VLDLs due to increased synthesis and decreased clearance.[19]

Any concomitant illness or stressful condition can increase the amount of counter-regulatory hormones such as glucocorticoids and epinephrine (see Chapter 23). These also elevate blood glucose levels. Since insulin levels are insufficient in a non-stressed state, the physiologic stress response can have dramatic consequences for individuals with DM. The metabolic alterations become exaggerated and can induce ketoacidosis.[19]

ACUTE COMPLICATIONS

Diabetes mellitus causes a variety of complications, which are responsible for the morbidity and mortality associated with the disease. In terms of acute or chronic complications, the acute complications can be life threatening and require immediate treatment. In contrast, the chronic complications appear to be due to prolonged hyperglycemia.

Hyperglycemia

ETIOLOGY. Hyperglycemia, the hallmark of DM, may result from (1) an alteration in insulin secretion, (2) impaired insulin action, or (3) a combination of both of these changes.

CLINICAL MANIFESTATIONS. As a result of hyperglycemia, there are several physiologic manifestations. The glucose level can be greater than the reabsorptive capacity of the renal tubules, resulting in glucosuria. This promotes an *osmotic diuresis* with loss of both fluid and electrolytes. This is demonstrated clinically with both polyuria and *nocturia*. Excessive loss of fluids stimulates thirst and polydipsia. Glucosuria can result in a significant loss of calories since glucose loss can exceed 75 gm/day. Decreased responsiveness in the satiety center of the hypothalamus promotes *polyphagia*. Thus, the symptoms of both Type 1 and Type 2 DM (polyuria, polydipsia, and polyphagia) are the result of hyperglycemia.[19]

Plasma osmolality is increased as a result of hyperglycemia. This can promote changes in the water content of the lens of the eye, leading to blurred vision. Glucosuria increases the incidence of candidal infections. Candidal vulvovaginitis is often a presenting symptom in women with DM. Likewise, candidal balanitis (an infection of the glans penis) is seen in uncircumcised men.[19]

Two patterns of hyperglycemia are seen as a result of treatment of DM: the *Somogyi effect* and the *dawn phenomenon*. Table 24-13 lists the associated blood glucose patterns seen in these circumstances. The Somogyi effect is an episode of nighttime hypoglycemia that induces a surge of counter-regulatory hormones. Thus, despite a very low nocturnal blood glucose level, pre-breakfast or fasting blood glucose levels can be elevated. The dawn phenomenon is characterized by a reduced sensitivity to insulin in the early morning or dawn (between 5 and 8 AM). It may also be related to an early-morning pulsatile secretion of growth hormone. However, a more common etiology for early-morning hyperglycemia is a decrease in available insulin.[37]

Diabetic Ketoacidosis

ETIOLOGY. Diabetic ketoacidosis (DKA) is a serious complication of uncontrolled Type 1 DM. However, it can occur in both Type 1 and Type 2 DM in any circumstance, such as illness or trauma that leads to increased secretion of counter-regulatory hormones. It is the result of a profound insulin deficiency, and glucose levels can be as high as 500 mg/dL (27.8 mmol/L).[19,37]

CLINICAL MANIFESTATIONS. The typical clinical manifestations include the following:[37,71]

- Fatigue, visual disturbances, altered level of consciousness
- Rapid, deep respirations (Kussmaul respirations)
- Fruity or "acetone" breath
- Flushed dry skin, dry mucous membranes
- Abdominal cramps, nausea, vomiting

TABLE 24-13

PATTERNS OF OVERNIGHT BLOOD GLUCOSE LEVELS

	BLOOD GLUCOSE LEVELS (mg/dL)		
	10 PM	3 AM	7 AM
Somogyi effect	90	40	200
"Dawn phenomenon"	110	110	150
Waning of circulating insulin levels plus "dawn phenomenon"	110	190	220
Waning of circulating insulin levels plus "dawn phenomenon" plus Somogyi effect	110	40	380

(Modified from Karam, J. H. [1997]. Pancreatic hormones and diabetes mellitus. In F. S. Greenspan & G. J. Strewler [Eds.], *Basic and clinical endocrinology* [5th ed.]. Stamford, CT: Appleton & Lange.)

- Tachycardia, hypotension
- Glucosuria, ketonuria
- Decreased plasma pH (<7.3) and bicarbonate levels (<15 mEq/L)
- Increased anion gap

The physiologic and metabolic alterations that occur are the result of both increased fatty acid metabolism and increased plasma osmolality due to hyperglycemia. The increased osmolality promotes water movement from the intracellular space into the extracellular space, resulting in fluid and electrolytes loss through *osmotic diuresis.* Profound dehydration occurs.[71] Flowchart 24-2 summarizes the pathogenesis of DKA.

The high glucagon–insulin ratio stimulates fatty acid metabolism, producing higher levels of ketoacids. These are moderately strong acids and are buffered in the blood. Urinary excretion of ketoacids includes the loss of buffering cations, depleting the alkali reserve and causing acidosis.[45]

Both sodium and potassium are lost through osmotic diuresis. Sodium decreases by approximately 1.6 mEq/L for every 100 mg/dL increase in blood glucose levels. Additionally, acidosis promotes a shift of potassium from the intracellular space to the extracellular space (see Chapter 6). This increases the amount of potassium depletion occurring through osmotic diuresis. Potassium shift may result in elevated serum potassium levels even though the overall body levels of potassium are depleted. Phosphate depletion also occurs in DKA.[19,37,71]

The alteration in the level of consciousness is related to increased plasma osmolality. Coma is most probably a sign of brain dehydration. This can be seen when plasma osmolality approaches 340 mOsm/kg.[19,71]

Hyperglycemic Hyperosmolar Nonketosis

ETIOLOGY. Hyperglycemic hyperosmolar nonketosis (HHNK) is a hyperglycemic emergency that occurs in Type 2 DM. It can occur in conjunction with renal insufficiency or heart failure. There is often a precipitating event, such as pneumonia, cerebral vascular accident, or trauma. Additionally, the development of HHNK has been linked to certain medications such as glucocorticoids, thiazide diuretics, and phenytoin. Certain procedures such as peritoneal dialysis have been associated with HHNK. Hypertonic solutions for parenteral hyperalimentation and enteral feedings increases the risk of developing HHNK.[19,37,64,71]

CLINICAL MANIFESTATIONS. Typical clinical manifestations of HHNK include the following:[36,37,71]

- Weakness, lethargy, changing level of consciousness
- Polyuria, polydipsia
- Dehydration, dry mucous membranes, decreased skin turgor
- Orthostatic hypotension
- Plasma glucose levels greater than 800 mg/dL (44.4 mmol/L)
- Plasma osmolality greater than 300 mOsm/kg
- No acidosis, pH greater than 7.3
- Bicarbonate levels greater than 15 mEq/L
- Normal anion gap

Although the amount of insulin is insufficient to promote glucose homeostasis, there is enough to prevent the development of ketosis. Only minimal levels of insulin are needed to prevent lipolysis. Thus, fatty acids are not utilized as an alternative energy source. Increased glucagon levels stimulate gluconeogenesis and the mobilization of glucose stores. As a result there is a profound hyperglycemia. As in DKA, the hyperglycemia promotes osmotic diuresis, leading to dehydration and an increase in plasma osmolality. As osmolality exceeds

FLOWCHART 24-2 **Pathogenesis of Diabetic Ketoacidosis**

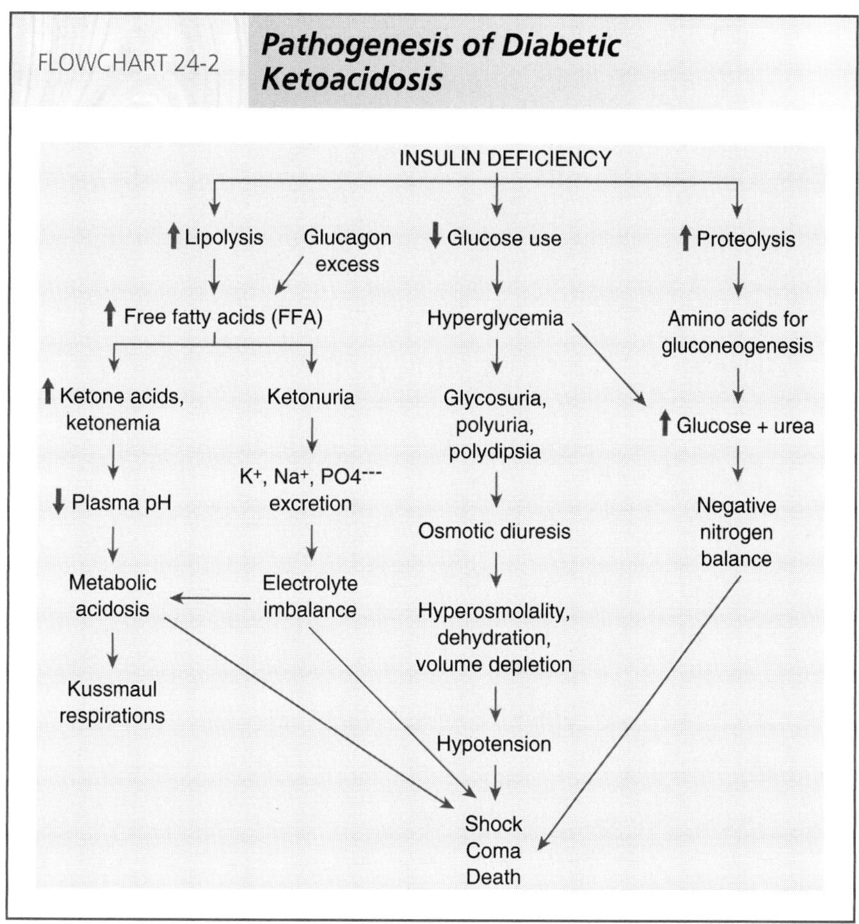

300 mOsm/kg, there are changes in the level of consciousness. Coma can occur with a plasma osmolality of greater than 330 mOsm/kg.[19,37,71] Flowchart 24-3 illustrates the pathogenesis of HHNK.

Hypoglycemia

ETIOLOGY. Hypoglycemia is a complication of treatment for DM. Although it also can occur from an insulinoma, a secretory islet cell tumor, it is most frequently the result of administration of insulin in an amount greater than the glucose load requires. Occasionally, hypoglycemia also occurs from an increased dose of an oral hypoglycemic agent, such as a sulfonylurea. Individuals who are at greatest risk for hypoglycemia have one or more of the following features:[14,19,37]

- Excessive insulin administration
- Reduced glucose intake
- Increased glucose need
- Consumption of alcoholic beverages
- Decreased clearance of medication

CLINICAL MANIFESTATIONS. Symptoms can be divided into two categories: those that are the result of neuroglycopenia and those that are the result of stimulation of the autonomic nervous system. The secretion of epinephrine, a counter-regulatory hormone, is increased in hypoglycemia (see Chapter 23). Additionally, hypoglycemia that occurs during sleep presents with early morning symptoms. Box 24-13 describes the signs and symptoms of hypoglycemia.

Individuals who are taking beta-adrenergic antagonists are at particular risk. These medications block the catecholamine-mediated warning symptoms. Thus, these individuals may not experience the symptoms associated with hypoglycemia and not respond rapidly enough to treat their hypoglycemia. It appears that individuals with Type 1 DM have an impaired counter-regulatory response in maintaining glucose homeostasis. Within the first few years of DM, the glucagon response becomes altered. The reduced secretion of glucagon is not related to any currently detectable pathology of the pancreatic A cells. Since glucagon is the primary counter-regulatory hormone, physiologic recovery from hypoglycemia is impaired. Additionally, with advanced age, the catecholamine response is also reduced. Thus, as many as 50% of individuals with long-standing Type 1 DM may have an impaired counter-regulatory response to hypoglycemia.[14,37]

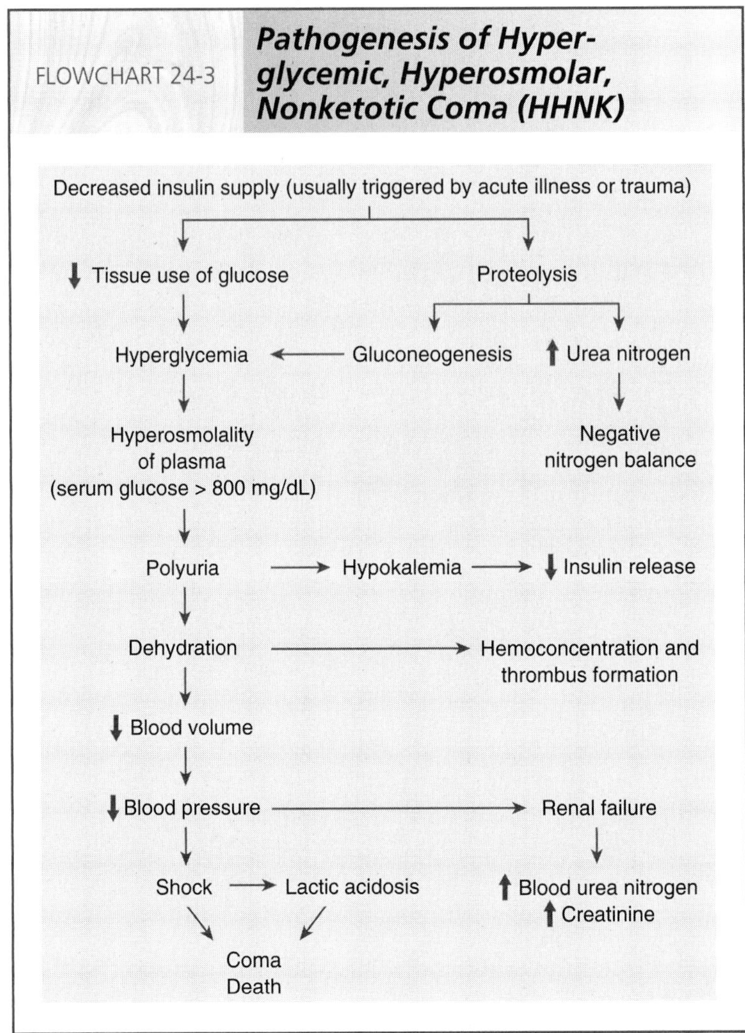

The detrimental effect of hypoglycemia on the central nervous system are profound. The brain depends exclusively on glucose for energy production; it cannot store or synthesize glucose. Thus, hypoglycemia causes cognitive alterations. Frequent episodes of hypoglycemia have been associated with lower IQ. If hypoglycemia is untreated, stupor, coma, and even death may occur.[14,37]

CHRONIC COMPLICATIONS

Chronic complications of DM contribute to the high morbidity and mortality associated with this disease. The complications include (1) microvascular disease, (2) macrovascular disease, and (3) neuropathy. The development of these chronic complications increases with the duration of the disease, potentially impairing the function of various organs and altering circulation and sensation. Thus, over time almost every system of the body is affected. It is theorized that prolonged hyperglycemia leads to the development of these complications.[13,19,53] Table 24-14 describes the chronic complications associated with DM.

Recent research with the Diabetes Control and Complications Trial has demonstrated a 60% reduction in the development of chronic complications in individuals who maintained mean glucose levels of 155 mg/dL and mean levels of glycosylated hemoglobin (HbA_{1C}) of 7.2%. However, these individuals also had a greater risk for the occurrence of hypoglycemic episodes.[13,15,36]

Microvascular Disease

Microvascular disease affects the smallest blood vessels, the capillary and the precapillary arterioles. It includes retinopathy and nephropathy. It is characterized by thickening and increased amounts of collagen in the basement membranes of small vessels.[36]

ETIOLOGY. The pathogenesis of microvascular disease is theorized to occur through two major mechanisms: (1) the formation of advanced glycosylation end

BOX 24-13

SIGNS AND SYMPTOMS OF HYPOGLYCEMIA

Symptoms Associated With Catecholamine Secretion

Sweating	Tremor
Weakness	Shakiness
Hunger	Anxiety
Faintness	Palpitations
Tachycardia	

Symptoms Associated With Neuroglycopenia

Confusion	Inappropriate affect
Abnormal behavior	Irritability
Coma	Headaches
Weakness	

Symptoms Associated With Nocturnal Hypoglycemia

Morning headache	Difficulty awakening
Lassitude	Nightmares
Night sweats	Loud respirations

TABLE 24-14

CHRONIC COMPLICATIONS OF DIABETES MELLITUS

SYSTEM	COMPLICATIONS
Eyes	Diabetic retinopathy Cataracts
Unusual Infections	Necrotizing fasciitis Necrotizing myositis Mucor meningitis Emphysematous cholecystitis
Cardiovascular	Myocardial infarction Cardiomyopathy
Kidneys	Intracapillary glomerulosclerosis Infection Renal tubular necrosis
Skin	Candidiasis Foot and leg ulcers
Nervous System	Peripheral neuropathy Cranial neuropathy (CN III, IV, VI, VII) Autonomic neuropathy Loss of sweating Gastroparesis Urinary bladder atony

(Modified from Karam, J. H. [1997]. Pancreatic hormones and diabetes mellitus. In F. S. Greenspan & G. J. Strewler [Eds.], *Basic and clinical endocrinology* [5th ed.]. Stamford, CT: Appleton & Lange.)

products and (2) the accumulation of fructose and sorbitol through the sorbitol pathway. It is also theorized that vasodilation and impaired vascular responsiveness may contribute to microvascular disease.[13,19,44,53]

Advanced glycosylation end products (AGE) occur as a result of hyperglycemia. These are irreversibly glycated proteins that are formed when glucose reacts with the amino acid groups in proteins. This is the process involved in the formation of HbA_{1C}, which is used to evaluate glycemic control. Since red blood cells circulate for approximately 120 days, HbA_{1C} is reflective of glucose levels for the preceding 8 to 12 weeks.[22,37] The AGE can also bind to basement membranes, vessel walls, and specific receptors or macrophages. This action may account for the alterations seen in small vessels.[19,53]

Increased activation of the *sorbitol pathway* occurs in hyperglycemia with accumulation of both sorbitol and fructose. However, there is a greater concentration of sorbitol. This action is seen in tissues that are not insulin dependent, such as the lens, peripheral nerves, and renal glomeruli. The accumulation of sorbitol leads to increased cellular osmolality, decreased Na^+/K^+ ATPase activity, and decreased nerve conduction. This may be a major component in the development of neuropathies, renal and eye disease.[19,44,53]

RETINOPATHY. **Retinopathy,** or eye disease, associated with DM is the major cause of blindness in the U.S. It is the result of microvascular changes associated with hyperglycemia. Two distinct patterns develop in DM retinopathy: (1) non-proliferative or background retinopathy and (2) proliferative retinopathy. Nonproliferative retinopathy represents the earliest type of eye involvement. The changes associated with nonproliferative retinopathy include microaneurysms, exudates, and retinal edema. The microaneurysms appear as red dots on the retina. Increased vascular permeability leads to leakage of fats and fluids. The fats appear as shiny yellow spots with distinct borders or hard exudates. Retinal ischemia is visible as hazy yellow areas with indistinct borders or cotton wool spots. Proliferative retinopathy includes neovascularization with the growth of new capillaries. Since these capillaries can exert an abnormal traction on the retina, there is an increased risk of retinal detachment. Figure 24-12 depicts the alterations seen in diabetic retinopathy.[19,37]

NEPHROPATHY. Diabetes is the leading cause of end-stage renal disease in the U.S. **Diabetic nephropathy** is the result of an alteration in glomerular function. It is characterized by proteinuria, hypertension, and progressive renal insufficiency. There is thickening of the basement membranes of the glomerular capillaries, leading to the development of glomerular sclerosis. These changes in the glomeruli are accompanied by a small urinary loss of albumin. However, over time this can progress to proteinuria. Hypertension develops as

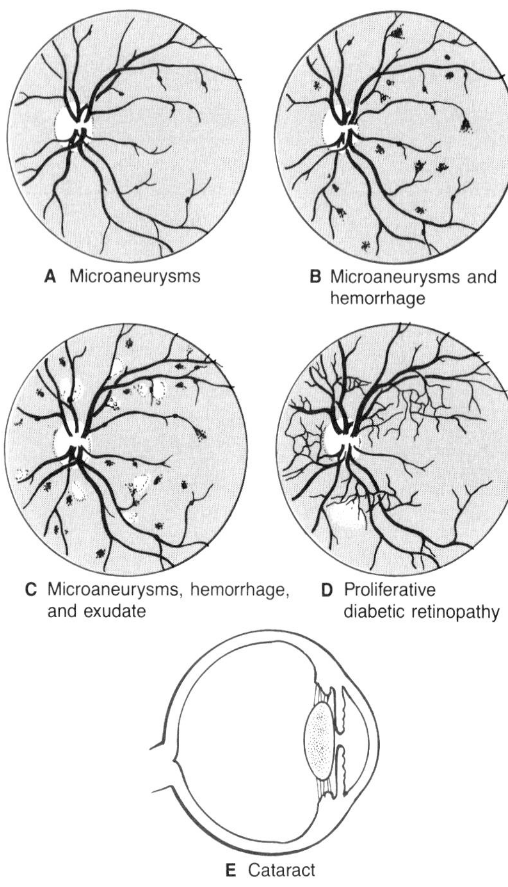

FIGURE 24-12. **Eye changes of diabetes: A. Microaneurysms; B. microaneurysms and hemorrhage; C. microaneurysms, hemorrhage, and exudate; D. proliferative diabetic retinopathy; E. cataract.**

the renal disease progresses. However, hypertension can also increase the progression of diabetic nephropathy; thus, the control of hypertension becomes an important part of treatment for diabetic nephropathy.[6,19,37]

Macrovascular Disease

Macrovascular, or large vessel, disease is a cardiovascular complication that increases the risk of myocardial infarction, cerebrovascular accident, claudication, and gangrene of the lower extremities. Essentially there is an acceleration in the development of atherosclerosis in individuals with DM. This is due to many different factors. As mentioned previously, the physiologic and metabolic alterations in DM lead to an increase in VLDL. Additionally, there is an alteration in the balance between thrombotic and fibrinolytic factors. Thus, the thrombotic activity is enhanced while the fibrinolytic activity is decreased. Increased foam cell activity also promotes the development of atherosclerosis. The combination of all of these factors promotes the cardiovascular disease that is seen in DM.[19,26,37]

Neuropathy

The proposed mechanism for the alteration in neuropathy appears to be a combination of altered metabolism and vascular insufficiency. As mentioned previously, hyperglycemia enhances the activity of the sorbitol pathway, promoting sorbitol excess. This changes the cellular osmolality, ultimately impairing cellular physiologic activity. The activity of Na^+/K^+ ATPase is decreased, compromising neuronal function. The injured cells are unable to remove free radicals, so that additional tissue damage occurs. Impaired blood flow reduces oxygen delivery to the nerves, further compromising them. There is also atrophy of the nerve axon with loss of myelin. Thus, the neuronal damage

FOCUS ON ADRENAL CRISIS: A WOMAN WITH HYPOTENSION

D. W. is a 55-year-old female who is admitted after a fall with a fracture of the neck of the right femur. Following surgery, she is nauseous and vomiting, complaining of abdominal pain. She is also profoundly hypotensive.

She has had ulcerative colitis for more than 15 years. She has previously been treated with systemic steroids for several years. However, she was able to discontinue the steroid therapy and has been taking olsalazine for the past 3 or 4 months. She is menopausal.

She has a younger sister with Crohn's disease. Her mother has Type 1 DM and coronary artery disease. Her father is apparently healthy with no known medical problems.

Her parents divorced when she was young. She has had minimal contact with her father. She is employed as a secretary for a major real estate management company. Her life style is fairly sedentary. She does not really socialize with friends—only work-related activities.

Temperature: 101 Pulse: 100 Respirations: 22 Blood pressure: 80/palpable Height: 5 ft 3 in. Weight 160 lb.

Weak and lethargic. Lungs are clear. Heart rate is rapid with occasional irregular beats. Lungs are clear, but her breath sounds are decreased. Abdomen is firm and diffusely tender. Appears to be dehydrated despite intravenous hydration during surgery. Diagnostic studies: Hematocrit and BUN are elevated. Glucose 80 mg/dL. Hyperkalemia, hyponatremia.

Questions

1. What are the potential risk factors for the development of adrenal crisis?
2. What are the major pathologic changes associated with her clinical manifestations?
3. How can primary adrenal insufficiency be differentiated from secondary adrenal insufficiency?

seen in diabetic neuropathy is most probably due to a combination of factors.[19,20,75]

The alterations associated with diabetic neuropathy, either alone or in combination with the other previously mentioned complications, lead to the development of a variety of problems. The accompanying sensory loss seen in both hands and feet (glove and stocking syndromes) not only alter the life style of individuals with DM but also contribute to chronic problems such as foot ulcers. Autonomic neuropathy is associated with tachycardia, orthostatic hypotension, impotence, and incontinence. Impairment of specific cranial nerves causes headaches, ptosis, and impaired eye movement (see Chapters 29 and 30).[19,37,75]

REFERENCES

1. American Diabetes Association (1997). *Diabetes fact sheet.* :Author.
2. American Diabetes Association (1997). *Diabetes 1996: Vital statistics.* Alexandria, VA: Author.
3. Aron, D. C., Findling, J. W., & Tyrrell, J. B. (1997). Hypothalamus and pituitary. In F. S. Greenspan & G. J. Strewler (Eds.), *Basic and clinical endocrinology* (5th ed.). Stamford, CT: Appleton & Lange.
4. Atkinson, M. A. & Maclaren, N. K. (1994). The pathogenesis of insulin dependent diabetes mellitus. *New England Journal of Medicine, 331*(21), 1428–1436.
5. Baker, J. R. (1991). Endocrine diseases. In D. P. Stites and A. I. Terr, *Basic and clinical immunology.* Stamford, CT: Appleton & Lange.
6. Bauer, J. H. (1994). Diabetic nephropathy: Can it be prevented? Are there renal protective antihypertensive drugs of choice? *Southern Medical Journal, 87*(10), 1043–1053.
7. Baxter, J. D. (1997). Introduction to endocrinology. In F. S. Greenspan & G. J. Strewler (Eds.), *Basic and clinical endocrinology* (5th ed.). Stamford, CT: Appleton & Lange.
8. Biglieri, E. G., Kater, C. E. & Ramsay, D. J. (1994). Endocrine hypertension. In F. S. Greenspan & J. D. Baxter, *Basic and clinical endocrinology.* Stamford, CT: Appleton & Lange.
9. Blevins, L. S. & Wand, G. S. (1992). Diabetes insipidus. *Critical Care Medicine, 20*(1), 69–79.
10. Brent, G. A. (1994). The molecular basis of thyroid hormone action. *New England Journal of Medicine, 331*(13), 847–852.
11. Burch, H. B. & Wartofsky, L. (1993). Life-threatening thyrotoxicosis: Thyroid storm. *Endocrinology and Metabolism Clinics of North America, 22*(2), 263–277.
12. Chin, R. (1991). Adrenal crisis. *Critical Care Clinics, 7*(1), 23–42.
13. Clark, C. M. & Lee, D. A. (1995). Prevention and treatment of the compications of diabetes mellitus. *New England Journal of Medicine, 332*(18), 1210–1217.
14. Cryer, P. E., Fisher, J. N., & Shamoon, H. (1994). Hypoglycemia. *Diabetes Care, 17*(7), 734–755.
15. The Diabetes Control and Complications Trial Research Group (1993). The effect of intensive treatment of diabetes on the development and progression of long-term complications in insulin-dependent diabetes mellitus. *New England Journal of Medicine, 329*(14), 786.
16. Daitch, J. A., Goldfarb, D. A., & Novick, A. C. (1997). Cleveland Clinic experience with adrenal Cushing's syndrome. *Journal of Urology, 158,* 2051–2055.
17. Donovan, L. E. & Corenblum, B. (1995). The natural history of the pituitary incidentaloma. *Archives of Internal Medicine, 155,* 181–183.
18. The Expert Commitee on the Diagnosis and Classification of Diabetes Mellitus (1997). The report of the Expert Commitee on the Diagnosis and Classification of Diabetes Mellitus. *Diabetes Care, 20*(7), 1183–1197.
19. Feingold, K. R., & Funk, J. (1997). Disorders of the endocrine pancreas. In S. J. McPhee, V. R. Lingappa, W. F. Ganong, & J. D. Lange (Eds.), *Pathology of disease* (2nd ed.). Stamford, CT: Appleton & Lange.
20. Feldman, E. L., Stevens, M. J. & Greene, D. A. (1997). Pathogenesis of diabetic neuropathy. *Clinical Neuroscience, 4,* 365–370.
21. Findling, J. W., Aron, D. C., & Tyrrell, J. B. (1997). Glucocorticoids and adrenal androgens. In F. S. Greenspan & G. J. Strewler (Eds.), *Basic and clinical endocrinology* (5th ed.). Stamford, CT: Appleton & Lange.
22. Fischbach, F. (1992). *A manual of laboratory and diagnostic tests* (4th ed.). Philadelphia: J. B. Lippincott.
23. Fitzgerald, P. A. (1998). Endocrinology. In L. M. Tierney, Jr., S. J. McPhee, & M. A. Papadakis, *Current medical diagnosis and treatment* (35th ed.). Stamford, CT: Appleton & Lange.
24. Fitzgerald, P. A. & Klonoff, D. C. (1998). Hypothalamic and pituitary hormones. In B. G. Katzung, *Basic and clinical pharmacology* (7th ed.). Stamford, CT: Appleton & Lange.
25. Frizzell, J. P. (1998). Avoiding lab test pitfalls. *American Journal of Nursing, 98*(2), 34–37.
26. Fujii, S. (1997). Advances in the understanding of diabetic vascular disease. *Journal of Cardiovascular Risk, 4*(2), 67–69.
27. Ganong, W. F. (1997). *Review of medical physiology* (18th ed.). Stamford, CT: Appleton & Lange.
28. Goldfien, A. (1997). Adrenal medulla. In F. S. Greenspan & G. J. Strewler (Eds.), *Basic and clinical endocrinology* (5th ed.). Stamford, CT: Appleton & Lange.
29. Goldfien, A. (1998). Adrenocorticosteroids and adrenocortical antagonists. In B. G. Katzung, *Basic and clinical pharmacology* (7th ed.). Stamford, CT: Appleton & Lange.
30. Grady, H. J., Jacobs, D. S. & Olsowka, E. S. (1996). Chemistry. In D. S. Jacobs, W. R. DeMott, H. J. Grady, R. T. Horvat, D. W. Huestis, & G. L. Kasten, *Laboratory test handbook* (4th ed.). Cleveland: LexiComp.
31. Granner, D. K. (1996). Hormones of the adrenal medulla. In R. K. Murray, D. K. Granner, P. A. Mayes, & V. W. Rodwell, *Harper's biochemistry* (24th ed.). Stamford, CT: Appleton & Lange.
32. Greenspan, F. S. (1997). The thyroid gland. In F. S. Greenspan & G. J. Strewler (Eds.), *Basic and clinical endocrinology* (5th ed.). Stamford, CT: Appleton & Lange.
33. Greenspan, F. S. & Dong, B. J. (1998). Thyroid and antithyroid drugs. In B. G. Katzung, *Basic and clinical pharmacology* (7th ed.). Stamford, CT: Appleton & Lange.
34. Grinspoon, S. K. & Biller, B. M. K. (1994). Laboratory assessment of adrenal insufficiency. *Journal of Clinical Endocrinology and Metabolism, 79*(4), 923–931.
35. Heitman, B., & Irizarry, A. (1995). Hypothyroidism: Common complaints, perplexing diagnosis. *Nurse Practitioner, 20*(3), 540–560.
36. Karam, J. H. (1998). Diabetes mellitus and hypoglycemia. In L. M. Tierney, Jr., S. J. McPhee, & M. A. Papadakis, *Current medical diagnosis and treatment* (35th ed.). Stamford, CT: Appleton & Lange.
37. Karam, J. H. (1997). Pancreatic hormones and diabetes mellitus. In F. S. Greenspan & G. J. Strewler (Eds.), *Basic and clinical endocrinology* (5th ed.). Stamford, CT: Appleton & Lange.
38. Kaye, T. B. & Crapo, L. The Cushing syndrome: An update on diagnostic tests. *Annals of Internal Medicine, 112,* 434–444.
39. Levy, G. S. (1990). Catecholamine–thyroid hormone interactions and the cardiovascular manifestations of hyperthyroidism. *American Journal of Medicine, 88,* 642–645.

40. Lingappa, V. R. (1997). Disorders of the hypothalamus and pituitary gland. In S. J. McPhee, V. R. Lingappa, W. F. Ganong, & J. D. Lange (Eds.), *Pathology of disease* (2nd ed.). Stamford, CT: Appleton & Lange.
41. Livolsi, V. A. (1994). The pathology of autoimmune thyroid disease: A review. *Thyroid: Official Journal of the American Thyroid Association, 4*, 333–339.
42. Martin, M. C., Taylor, R. N., & Kitzmiller, J. L. (1991). The endocrinology of pregnancy. In F. S. Greenspan & J. D. Baxter, *Basic and clinical endocrinology*. Stamford, CT: Appleton & Lange.
43. Mason, J. W. (1968). Organization of psychoendocrine mechanisms: The scope of psychoendocrine research. *Psychosomatic Medicine, 30*, 565–575.
44. Mayes, P. A. (1996). The pentose phosphate pathway and other pathways of hexose metabolism. In R. K. Murray, D. K. Granner, P. A. Mayes, & V. W. Rodwell, *Harper's biochemistry* (24th ed.). Stamford, CT: Appleton & Lange.
45. Mayes, P. A. (1996). Oxidation of fatty acids: Ketogenesis. In R. K. Murray, D. K. Granner, P. A. Mayes, & V. W. Rodwell, *Harper's biochemistry* (24th ed.). Stamford, CT: Appleton & Lange.
46. McFarland, K. F. (1997). Type 2 diabetes: Stepped-care approach to patient management. *Geriatrics, 52*(10), 22–39.
47. McPhee, S. J. (1997). Disorders of the adrenal cortex. In S. J. McPhee, V. R. Lingappa, W. F. Ganong, & J. D. Lange (Eds.), *Pathology of disease* (2nd ed.). Stamford, CT: Appleton & Lange.
48. McPhee, S. J. (1997). Disorders of the adrenal medulla. In S. J. McPhee, V. R. Lingappa, W. F. Ganong, & J. D. Lange (Eds.), *Pathology of disease* (2nd ed.). Stamford, CT: Appleton & Lange.
49. McPhee, S. J. & Bauer, D. C. (1997). Thyroid disease. In S. J. McPhee, V. R. Lingappa, W. F. Ganong, & J. D. Lange (Eds.), *Pathology of disease* (2nd ed.). Stamford, CT: Appleton & Lange.
50. Mills, P. J. & Dimsdale, J. E. (1988). The promise of receptor studies in psychosomatic research. *Psychosomatic Medicine, 50*, 555–566.
51. Mills, P. J. & Dimsdale, J. E. (1993). The promise of receptor studies in psychosomatic research II: Applications, limitations, and progress. *Psychosomatic Medicine, 55*, 448–457.
52. Moore, R. E. (1994). Immunochemical methods. In K. D. McClatchey (Ed.), *Clinical laboratory medicine*. Philadelphia: Williams & Wilkins.
53. Nathan, D. M. (1996). The pathophysiology of diabetic complications: How much does the glucose hypothesis explain? *Annals of Internal Medicine, 124*(1 pt. 2), 86–89.
54. O'Connor, A. L. (1993). A joint venture between laboratory and nursing towards quality assurance in bedside blood glucose monitoring. *Canadian Journal of Medical Technology, 55*, 86–96.
55. Okuda, T. Kurokawa, K. & Papadakis, M. A. (1998). Fluid and electrolyte disorders. In L. M. Tierney, Jr., S. J. McPhee, & M. A. Papadakis, *Current medical diagnosis and treatment* (35th ed.). Stamford, CT: Appleton & Lange.
56. Polikar, R., Burger, A. G., Scherrer, U., & Nicod, P. (1993). The thyroid and the heart. *Circulation, 87*(5), 1435–1441.
57. Reasner, C. A. & Talbert, R. L. (1997). Thyroid disorders. In J. T. Dipiro, R. L. Talbert, G. C. Yee, G. R. Matzke, B. G. Wells, & L. M. Posey, *Pharmacotherapy: A pathophysiologic approach* (3rd ed.). Stamford, CT: Appleton & Lange.
58. Sacher, R. A. & McPherson, R. A. (1991). *Widmann's clinical interpretation of laboratory tests* (10th ed.). Philadelphia: F. A. Davis.
59. Sacks, D. B., & McDonald, J. M. (1996). The pathogenesis of type II diabetes mellitus. *American Journal of Clinical Pathology, 105*, 149–156.
60. Shamoon, H. (1992). Pathophysiology of diabetes. *Drugs, 44* (Suppl. 3), 112.
61. Shizuru, J. A. (1997). Autoimmunity and endocrine disease. In F. S. Greenspan & G. J. Strewler (Eds.), *Basic and clinical endocrinology* (5th ed.). Stamford, CT: Appleton & Lange.
62. Shoback, D. M. & Strewler, G. J. (1997). Disorders of the parathyroids and calcium metabolism. In S. J. McPhee, V. R. Lingappa, W. F. Ganong, & J. D. Lange (Eds.), *Pathology of disease* (2nd ed.). Stamford, CT: Appleton & Lange.
63. Singer, I., Oster, J. R., & Fishman, L. M. (1997). The management of diabetes insipidus in adults. *Archives of Internal Medicine, 157*, 1293–1301.
64. Siperstein, M. D. (1992). Diabetic ketoacidosis and hyperosmolar coma. *Endocrinology and Metabolism Clinics of North America, 21*(2), 415–432.
65. Skyler, J. S. & Marks, J. B. (1993). Immune intervention in type I diabetes mellitus. *Diabetes Reviews, 1*(1), 15–42.
66. Smallridge, R. C. (1992). Metabolic and anatomic thyroid emergencies. *Critical Care Medicine, 20*(2), 276–291.
67. Steil, C. F. (1997). Diabetes mellitus. In J. T. Dipiro, R. L. Talbert, G. C. Yee, G. R. Matzke, B. G. Wells, & L. M. Posey, *Pharmacotherapy: A pathophysiologic approach* (3rd ed.). Stamford, CT: Appleton & Lange.
68. Strewler, G. J. (1997). Humoral manifestations of malignancy. In F. S. Greenspan & G. J. Strewler (Eds.), *Basic and clinical endocrinology* (5th ed.). Stamford, CT: Appleton & Lange.
69. Strewler, G. J. (1997). Mineral metabolism and metabolic bone disease. In F. S. Greenspan & G. J. Strewler (Eds.), *Basic and clinical endocrinology* (5th ed.). Stamford, CT: Appleton & Lange.
70. Styne, D. (1997). Growth. In F. S. Greenspan & G. J. Strewler (Eds.), *Basic and clinical endocrinology* (5th ed.). Stamford, CT: Appleton & Lange.
71. Suave, D. O. & Kessler, C. A. (1992). Hyperglycemic emergencies. *AACN Clinical Issues in Critical Care Nursing, 3*(2), 350–360.
72. Swift, R. M., Griffiths, W., & Camara, P. (1991). Special technical considerations in laboratory testing for illicit drugs. In A. Stoudemire & B. S. Fogel (Eds.), *Medical psychiatric practice*. Washington, D. C.: American Psychiatric Press.
73. Tremblay, M. S., Chu, S. Y., & Mureika, R. (1995). Methodological and statistical considerations for exercise-related hormone evaluations. *Sports Medicine, 20*(2), 90–108.
74. Van Noort, J. V., & Amor, S. (1998). Cell biology of autoimmune diseases. *International Review of Cytology, 178*, 127–206.
75. Vinik, A., Holand, M. T., LeBeau, J. M., Liuzzi, F. J., Stansberry, K. B., & Colen, L. B. (1992). Diabetic neuropathies. *Diabetes Care, 15*(12), 1926–1975.

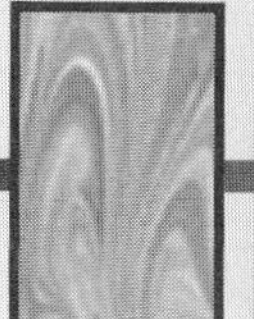

UNIT 7: CASE STUDY

The Person With Fruity Breath Odor

Introduction to the Patient

A. M. is a 66-year-old African American female who is recovering slowly from viral pneumonia. When her daughter came to check on her, she found A. M. in bed complaining of weakness, constant fatigue, and abdominal cramps.

Present Illness

For the past few weeks, A. M. has been complaining of thirst and frequent urination. She also reports that she cannot see very well. Additionally, A.M. has recently lost approximately 4 pounds over the last 3 weeks.

Social History

A. M. lives alone since the death of her husband 8 months ago. They had been married for 44 years. She is a homemaker who has never worked outside of the home. She states that she "doesn't get out much, except to the grocery store and church." Her day is spent doing some light housework and "watching her soaps" on the television. Her children are all grown and live near her. She does not smoke but admits to being a social drinker.

Past Medical History

A. M. reports a history of "arthritis" and occasionally takes an over-the-counter arthritis medication with relief. She complains of some early morning joint pain on arising, which improves throughout the day. "It takes me a little while to get going in the morning." She was diagnosed with diabetes mellitus (DM) Type 2 approximately 2 years ago. Currently, she takes glipizide 5 mg every morning before breakfast and is on a 1800-cal ADA diet.

Family History

A. M.'s father had Type 2 diabetes and peripheral vascular disease. He died at the age of 59 from a myocardial infarction.

Physical Examination

A. M. is 5 ft, 4 in. and weighs 170 pounds. Her vital signs are as follows: temperature—99.4° F; pulse—112; respirations—28; blood pressure—118/58 (lying), 96/50 (sitting).

Skin is dry and warm, with poor turgor. Mucous membranes dry. Sweet fruity odor of breath (acetone) is noted. A. M. is oriented × 3 but slightly lethargic and sleepy. Respirations are deep and rapid with rhonchi auscultated bilaterally. Abdomen is soft, non-tender, with bowel sounds present in all four quadrants. Claudication and numbness present in lower extremities. Small, dime-sized, reddened area is present on lateral aspect of the right great toe. Pedal pulses faint but present bilaterally. Ophthalmologic examination reveals several small microaneurysms.

Diagnostic Tests

Arterial blood gases: pH—7.25; $PaCO_2$—30 mm Hg; HCO_3^-—14 mEq/L
Hematocrit and BUN: elevated
Serum potassium (K+): 6.2 mEq/L
Serum sodium (Na): 150 mEq/L
Serum osmolality: 305 mOsm/kg
Serum glucose: 540 mg/dL
Glycosylated hemoglobin ($HgbA_{1c}$): 13%

CRITICAL THINKING QUESTIONS

1. Describe the risk factors evidenced in A. M.
2. Summarize the major pathophysiologic changes responsible for A. M.'s clinical manifestations.
3. Contrast the pathophysiology of Type 1 and Type 2 diabetes.
4. Analyze the benefit of following A. M. with glycosylated hemoglobin levels.
5. Develop a checklist of teaching topics for A. M. to minimize her risk for a recurrence of this situation.

Besides your pathophysiology text, you'll need a good pharmacology text, an endocrinology/diabetes text, a diagnostic/laboratory test text, a medical-surgical nursing text, and current research to complete this case study. Suggested references follow:

Davidson, M., Davidson, A., & Zorab, R. (Eds.) (1998). *Diabetes mellitus: diagnosis and treatment.* Philadelphia: W.B. Saunders.

Fischbach, F. (1996). *A manual of laboratory and diagnostic tests* (5th ed.). Philadelphia: Lippincott-Raven.

Joslin, E., Ronald, C., Kakn, M., & Weir, G. (1994). *Joslin's diabetes mellitus.* Philadelphia: Lea and Febiger.

Karch, A. M. (1999). *1999 Lippincott's nursing drug guide.* Philadelphia: Lippincott-Raven.

Mayfield, J. A., Reiber, G. E., Sanders, L. J., Janesse, D., & Pogach, L. M. (1998). Preventive foot care in people with diabetes. *Diabetes Care, 21,* 2161–2177.

Smeltzer, S. & Bare, B. (2000). *Brunner and Suddarth's textbook of medical-surgical nursing* (9th ed). Philadelphia: Lippincott, Williams & Wilkins.

Website Resources:

American Diabetes Association *http://www.diabetes.org*

American Diabetes Association Clinical Practice Recommendations *http://www.diabetes.org/Diabetescare/supplement198/*

Diabetes Center *http://www.endocrineweb.com/diabetes*

National Institute of Diabetes and Digestive and Kidney Disease (NIDDK) *http://www.niddk.nih.gov*

UNIT 7 APPENDIX A

DIAGNOSTIC TESTS

TEST	PURPOSE/ NORMAL FINDINGS	SIGNIFICANCE
THYROID		
Free T3 (FT3)	Evaluation of thyroid function by measuring the fraction of circulating T3 that exists in a free state, unbound to protein Normal findings: 260 to 480 pg/dL	FT3 levels may be elevated in hyperthyroidism or T3 thyrotoxicosis. FT3 levels may be decreased in hypothyroidism or the third trimester of pregnancy.
Free T4 (FT4)	Evaluation of T4, the metabolically active form available to the tissues to determine thyroid status Normal findings: 0.8 ng/dL	Increased FT4 levels may be seen in Graves' disease and thyrotoxicosis. Decreased FT4 levels may be associated with primary or secondary hypothyroidism and T3 thyrotoxicosis. FT4 levels are lower in adolescents as compared with adults.
Total T3	Quantitative measurement of the total T3 concentration, usually performed by radioimmunoassay (RIA) Normal findings: 80 to 200 ng/dL (over age 24 years)	T3 levels are the diagnostic test of choice for determining T3 thyrotoxicosis. Increased T3 levels may be associated with hyperthyroidism, T3 thyrotoxicosis, and acute thyroiditis. Decreased T3 levels may be associated with hypothyroidism (although the level may be normal) and starvation. Drugs such as anabolic steroids, salicylates (large doses), and phenytoin may decrease T3 levels. Drugs such as estrogen, methadone, and heroin may increase T3 levels.
Total T4	Direct evaluation of the concentration of T4 in the blood, usually performed by RIA Normal findings: 5.4 to 11.5 ug/dL	T4 levels increase during the last half of pregnancy. Increased T4 levels may suggest hyperthyroidism, acute thyroiditis, or hepatitis. Decreased levels may suggest hypothyroidism or hypoproteinemia. Drugs such as estrogens, methadone, and heroin may increase T4 levels. Drugs such as salicylates and anticoagulants may decrease T4 levels.
T3 uptake	Indirect measurement of the amount of unsaturated thyroxine-binding globulin in the blood (inversely proportional to thyroxine-binding globulin level) expressed as a ratio of the specimen to the standard control Normal findings: 0.8 to 1.3 with 25% to 35% uptake	This test is useful only when viewed with the results of T4 levels. Decreased T3 uptake occurs normally in pregnancy and with drugs such as estrogens, methadone, and heparin. Increased T3 uptake occurs with drugs such as anabolic steroids, phenytoin, and salicylates (large doses).
Thyroglobulin (Tg)	Measurement of the glycoprotein and iodinated secretions of the thyroid gland containing the precursors of T3 and T4 and also these hormones Normal findings: 3 to 42 ng/mL	Increased levels may indicate thyroid cancer, hyperthyroidism, or subacute thyroiditis. Decreased levels may indicate thyrotoxicosis factitia.
Thyroid-stimulating hormone ([TSH] Thyrotropin)	Measurement of the anterior pituitary gland's production of TSH based on the feedback system Normal findings: 0.2 to 5.4 ug/mL	TSH is the most sensitive test to detect primary hypothyroidism; usually performed with T3 and T4 RIA. A rise in TSH represents the pituitary's response to a drop in circulating thyroid hormone, usually the first indication of thyroid gland failure.

(continued)

UNIT 7 APPENDIX A

DIAGNOSTIC TESTS (Continued)

TEST	PURPOSE/ NORMAL FINDINGS	SIGNIFICANCE
		Increased levels of TSH may indicate primary hypothyroidism, thyrotoxicosis, or a thyrotropin-producing tumor. Decreased levels may suggest secondary or tertiary hypothyroidism or hyperthyroidism.
Thyrotropin-releasing hormone (TRH) stimulation test	Intravenous injection of TRH to increase pituitary secretion of TSH Normal findings: After injection, at least twice the baseline value (baseline—0.2 to 5.4 uIU/L)	This test helps to differentiate the type of hypothyroidism. A slight increase or no response suggests hyperthyroidism. An elevated baseline, followed by an increase of two or more times the value, suggests primary hypothyroidism. No response may suggest secondary hypothyroidism; a delayed response may suggest tertiary hypothyroidism.
Thyroxine-binding globulin (TBG)	Measurement of the protein-bound thyroxine, which has a significant effect on the amount of bound and metabolically active forms of T3 and T4 Normal findings: 15 to 30 ug/dL (males) 1.5 to 32.2 ug/dL (females [nonpregnant])	Increased levels may suggest hypothyroidism, hepatic disease, or estrogen-producing tumor. Decreased levels may suggest nephrotic syndrome, acromegaly, severe acidosis, malnutrition, or hepatic disease.
Radioactive iodine uptake test	Measurement of the thyroid gland's ability to concentrate and metabolize iodine at 2, 6, and 24 hours after oral administration of radioactive iodine Normal findings: 1% to 3% absorbed after 2 hrs 5% to 20% absorbed after 6 hrs 15% to 40% absorbed after 24 hrs	This test is usually performed in conjunction with a thyroid scan. Increased uptake may suggest hyperthyroidism. Decreased uptake may suggest hypothyroidism. Uptake may be low in severe diarrhea or with rapid diuresis even though the gland function is normal. Uptake may be enhanced by pregnancy, cirrhosis, renal failure, and certain drugs such as barbiturates and lithium. Uptake may be lowered with the intake of iodine-containing foods and drugs, antithyroid agents, thyroid agents (used within 1 to 2 weeks of the test), and other drugs such as nitrates, corticosteroids, antihistamines, coumarin derivatives, and sulfonamides.
Thyroid scan	Measurement of thyroid gland's ability to concentrate radioactive isotope to determine size, position, and function Normal findings: even distribution of radioactive isotope with normal size, position, shape, and absence of nodules	Cold nodules (areas of decreased uptake) may suggest thyroid cancer or hypothyroidism. Hot nodules (areas of increased uptake) may indicate hyperthyroidism or Graves' disease.
PARATHYROID		
Urine calcium (quantitative Sulkowitch)	24-hour urine specimen to evaluate parathyroid function Normal finding: 100 to 300 mg/day (normal diet)	The amount of calcium excreted varies with the amount of calcium ingested in the diet. Increased levels may suggest hyperparathyroidism, Paget's disease, renal

UNIT 7 APPENDIX A

DIAGNOSTIC TESTS (Continued)

TEST	PURPOSE/ NORMAL FINDINGS	SIGNIFICANCE
	50 to 150 mg/day (low-calcium diet)	tubular acidosis, vitamin D intoxication, diabetes, or thyrotoxicosis. Increased urine calcium levels almost always are associated with increased serum calcium levels. Decreased levels may suggest hypoparathyroidism, vitamin D deficiency, pre-eclampsia, acute nephrosis, or metastatic prostate cancer. Corticosteroids, immobilization, or excessive milk intake may falsely elevate urine calcium levels. Thiazide diuretics or antacids may falsely depress urine calcium levels.
Parathyroid hormone (PTH) assay	Measurement of the three molecular forms of PTH (NH2-terminal, COOH-terminal, and intact molecule) to evaluate calcium metabolism and establish hyperparathyroidism and differentiate the cause of hypercalcemia Normal findings: NH2-terminal—8 to 24 pg/mL COOH-terminal—50 to 330 pg/mL Intact molecule—10 to 65 pg/mL	Increased PTH levels may suggest primary or secondary hyperparathyroidism. Decreased PTH levels may indicate Graves' disease, secondary hypoparathyroidism, magnesium deficiency, or hyperthyroidism. Elevated blood lipid levels may interfere with the results.
Parathyroid scan	Injection of radioisotope to visualize parathyroid gland Normal findings: absences of increased perfusion or uptake in the gland	Abnormal concentrations of isotope may suggest benign or malignant parathyroid tumors.
ADRENALS		
Serum cortisol	Measurement of adrenal hormone function based on diurnal variations Normal findings: 8 AM—5 to 23 ug/dL 4 PM—3 to 16 ug/dL	Decreased cortisol levels may suggest adrenal hyperplasia, Addison's disease, or hepatitis. Increased cortisol levels may indicate hyperthyroidism, stress, or adrenal adenomas. Increased levels on arising without variation later in the day may indicate Cushing's syndrome.
Cortisol suppression test	Measurement of adrenal function after administration of dexamethasone Normal findings: 8 AM—5 to 23 ug/dL 4 PM—3 to 16 ug/dL	Patients with Cushing's syndrome typically reveal no suppression or diurnal variation. Falsely positive results may occur with pregnancy, dehydration, trauma, fever, or uncontrolled diabetes.
Cortisol stimulation test	Measurement of adrenal function after intramuscular injection of cosyntropin (a synthetic form of ACTH) Normal findings: an increase of at least 10 ug/dL above baseline (or at least 5 ug/dL)	Prolonged administration of steroids may interfere with the results. Failure of the level to rise may suggest adrenal insufficiency.
Total plasma catecholamines	Measurement of norepinephrine and epinephrine concentrations with the patient in the supine position and resting for at least 30 minutes prior to specimen collection	Caffeine, tobacco, drugs such as amphetamines, and over-the-counter nasal sprays and decongestants may result in increased catecholamine levels.

(continued)

UNIT 7 APPENDIX A

DIAGNOSTIC TESTS (Continued)

TEST	PURPOSE/ NORMAL FINDINGS	SIGNIFICANCE
	Normal findings: Epinephrine—100 pg/mL Norepinephrine—less than 100 to 550 pg/mL	Epinephrine values above 400 pg/mL or norepinephrine values above 2000 pg/mL may suggest pheochromocytoma.
Urine catecholamines	Measurement of adrenal function by determining the amount of metabolites (vanillylmandelic acid [VMA], epinephrine, norepinephrine, and metanephrine) excreted in the urine over 24 hours Normal findings (per 24 hours): Total catecholamines—14 to 110 ug VMA—up to 2 to 7 mg Epinephrine—0 to 20 ug Norepinephrine—15 to 80 ug Dopamine—64–400 ug	VMA is the primary urine metabolite excreted and the easiest to detect. This test is performed primarily for detecting pheochromocytoma as a cause of hypertension. High VMA levels may indicate pheochromocytoma. Slight to moderate elevations of VMA may suggest neuroblastomas or ganglioneuromas. Elevated urinary catecholamines may indicate pheochromocytoma, myocardial infarction, hypothyroidism, or DKA. Hypoglycemia and foods such as tea, caffeine, chocolate, bananas, chewing gum, licorice, and salad dressing may increase the levels of VMA.
Urine steroids	Measurement of adrenal function by measuring the three groups of steroids excreted in the urine over 24 hours Normal findings (over 24 hours): 17-ketosteroids (KS)—8 to 20 mg (males)/6 to 15 mg (females) 17-hydroxycorticosteroids (OHCS)—3 to 10 mg (males)/2 to 6 mg (females) 17-ketogenic steroids (KGS)—5 to 24 mg (males)/5 to 15 mg (females)	Increased levels of 17-KS may suggest Cushing's syndrome, adrenal cancer, or congenital renal hyperplasia. Decreased levels of 17-KS may indicate Addison's disease, myxedema, nephrosis, or hypogonadism. Increased levels of 17-OHCS may indicate acute illness, Cushing's syndrome, severe hypertension, thyrotoxicosis, or obesity. Decreased levels of 17-OHCS may suggest Addison's disease or hypothyroidism. Increased levels of 17-KGS may indicate adrenal hyperplasia or Cushing's syndrome. Decreased levels of 17-KGS may be seen with Addison's disease, cretinism, or cessation of corticosteroid therapy.
Adrenal scan	Nuclear imaging evaluation of the adrenal medulla for tumors or sites of hormone over-secretion after injection of radioisotope with follow-up scans on the second, third, and fourth days or more if necessary Normal findings: absence of tumor or sites of hormonal over-secretion	The majority of pheochromocytomas occur in the abdomen and are visualized with this scan.
PITUITARY		
Serum antidiuretic hormone (ADH)	Measurement of the hormone produced by the posterior pituitary gland to evaluate for disorders involving urine concentration Normal findings: 0 to 4.7 pg/mL	Increased levels may suggest SIADH, Guillain-Barré syndrome, nephrogenic diabetes insipidus (DI), or brain injury. Decreased levels may indicated central DI, psychogenic polydipsia, or nephrotic syndrome.
Serum somatotropin (growth hormone)	Measure of the hormone released by the pituitary gland to evaluate for disorders of growth Normal findings: less than 5 ng/mL	Increased levels may be indicative of gigantism or acromegaly. Decreased levels may be associated with dwarfism, hypopituitarism, or obesity.

UNIT 7 APPENDIX A

DIAGNOSTIC TESTS (Continued)

TEST	PURPOSE/ NORMAL FINDINGS	SIGNIFICANCE
		Levels may be increased by hypoglycemia, exercise, and stress as well as medications such as estrogen, dopamine, amphetamines, insulin, and levodopa. Levels may be decreased by phenothiazine and corticosteroid drugs.
Serum adrenocorticotropic hormone (ACTH or corticotropin)	Measurement of the amount of ACTH in serum, which is useful in identifying the basis of Cushing's syndrome or Addison's disease Normal findings (normal levels vary with a diurnal pattern): Morning, 8:00 AM—15 to 120 pg/mL Evening, 8:00 PM—less than 50 pg/mL	Elevated levels are found with Cushing's syndrome, ectopic ACTH-secreting sources (i.e., oat cell carcinoma), Addison's disease (primary adrenal insufficiency). Additional factors contributing to increased levels include hyperglycemia and stress. Decreased levels are found with pituitary insufficiency (secondary adrenal insufficiency), panhypopituitarism, adrenal cortical adenomas, and medications such as corticosteroids, amphetamines, estrogens, and ethanol.
PANCREAS (DIABETES)		
Fasting blood glucose ([FBG] fasting blood sugar [FBS])	Measurement of the body's ability to metabolize glucose Normal findings: 65 to 110 mg/dL	A FBG greater than 140 mg/dL on more than one occasion may be diagnostic for diabetes. Elevated FBG levels also may indicate Cushing's syndrome, acute stress, pancreatitis, chronic liver or renal disease, or pheochromocytoma. Decreased FBG levels may suggest cancer of the pancreatic islet cells, Addison's disease, starvation, or insulin overdose.
Two-hour postprandial blood glucose	Measurement of the glucose level after eating Normal findings: 65 to 139 mg/dL	After a meal in a non-diabetic person, blood glucose level is rarely elevated after 2 hours. Levels of 140 to 200 mg/dL may suggest glucose intolerance. Levels above 200 mg/dL are highly suggestive of diabetes. Levels also may be elevated with advanced cirrhosis, Cushing's syndrome, hyperthyroidism, or acromegaly. Levels may be decreased with hypopituitarism, Addison's disease, or islet cell adenomas.
Oral glucose tolerance test (OGTT)	Measurement of a person's ability to metabolize a large amount of oral glucose at 1/2, 1, 2, and 3 hours after ingestion Normal findings: FBG—70 to 110 mg/dL after 1/2 hour—110 to 170 mg/dL after 1 hour—120 to 170 mg/dL after 2 hours—70 to 120 mg/dL after 3 hours—70 to 120 mg/dL	All four levels must be within normal limits for the test to be considered normal. A diagnosis of diabetes is associated with at least two abnormal OGTT values. Decreased glucose tolerance may indicate diabetes, hyperthyroidism, Cushing's syndrome, central nervous system lesion, or pheochromocytoma. Increased glucose tolerance may indicate a pancreatic islet cell tumor, hypoparathyroidism, Addison's disease or liver disease. Smoking increases glucose levels. Drugs such as thiazide diuretics,corticosteroids, estrogen, pheonothiazines, and lithium may impair glucose tolerance.

(continued)

UNIT 7 APPENDIX A

DIAGNOSTIC TESTS (Continued)

TEST	PURPOSE/ NORMAL FINDINGS	SIGNIFICANCE
Glycosylated hemoglobin (HbA1c)	Measurement of blood glucose bound to hemoglobin reflecting average blood glucose levels (and overall control) over a 2- to 3-month period Normal findings (expressed as a percentage of total hemoglobin): Nondiabetic: 5.5 % to 8.5 % If diabetic: 7.5 % to 11.5 % (good control) 11.5 % to 15 % (moderate control) Greater than 15 % (poor control)	As a person with diabetes achieves optimal control, the values approach the nondiabetic range. Decreased levels also may be indicative of hemolytic anemia, abnormal blood loss, or chronic renal failure.
Serum insulin	Evaluation of the rate of insulin secretion from the islets of Langerhans B cell for use in determining insulinoma, abnormal lipid and carbohydrate metabolism, hypoglycemia from unknown origins, and in differentiating insulin resistance from non–insulin resistance in type 2 diabetes mellitus Normal findings: fasting levels—5 to 24 μ U/mL	Elevated levels are seen in obesity, insulinoma, Cushing's syndrome, pheochromocytoma, and acromegaly. Factors that may contribute to elevated levels include food intake and medications such as corticosteroids, estrogen, and levodopa. Decreased levels are seen in B cell failure in diabetes mellitus.
Serum glucagon	Evaluation of alpha cell function of the pancreatic islets of Langerhans for use in diagnosing suspected glucagonoma and supporting diagnosis of renal failure Normal findings: 30 to 200 pg/mL	Elevated levels are found with glucagonomas, renal failure or rejection of transplanted kidney, poorly controlled diabetes mellitus, pheochromocytoma, acute pancreatitis, and stress. Decreased levels are found with chronic pancreatitis and idiopathic glucagon deficiency.
Urine glucose	Evaluation of the kidneys' ability to reabsorb glucose in the proximal tubule Normal findings: Random specimen—negative 24-hour specimen—less than 0.3 g/24 hours	Glucosuria may occur after ingestion of a large meal or during emotional stress. Urine glucose measurement should be evaluated in light of blood glucose levels. Increased urine glucose levels may indicate diabetes, thyrotoxicosis, Cushing's syndrome, or renal tubular acidosis.
Urine ketones	Indirect measurement of carbohydrate metabolism reflecting the increased breakdown of fats Normal findings: negative	Ketonuria may indicate diabetes, starvation, prolonged vomiting, anorexia, or hypermetabolic states. Ketonuria is common in patients during acute illness in the absence of diabetes.

UNIT BIBLIOGRAPHY

Bardin, C. W. (1997). *Current therapy in endocrinology and metabolism.* St. Louis: Mosby.

Becker, K. D. et al. (1995). *Principles and practice of endocrinology and metabolism* (2nd ed.). Philadelphia: J.B. Lippincott.

Berne, R. M. & Levy, M. N. (1996). *Principles of physiology* (2nd ed.). Philadelphia: Mosby–Year Book.

Conn, P. M. & Melmed, S. (Eds). (1997). *Endocrinology: Basic and clinical principles.* Totowa, NJ: Humana Press.

Felig, P., Baxter, J. D., & Frohman, L. A. (Eds.) (1995). *Endocrinology and metabolism* (3rd ed.). New York: McGraw-Hill.

Frizzell, J. P. (1997). *The relationship between the physiologic and psychologic response to stress in patients with an acute myocardial infarction. A dissertation in nursing.* University of Pennsylvania.

Greenspan, F. S. & Strewler, G. J. (Eds.) (1997). *Basic and clinical endocrinology* (5th ed.). Stamford, CT: Appleton & Lange.

Loriaux, T. C. (1996). Endocrine assessment: Red flags for those on the front lines. *Nursing clinics of North America, 31*(4), 695–713.

McPhee, S. J., Lingappa, V. R., Ganong, W. F. & Lange, J. D. (Eds.) (1997). *Pathology of disease* (2nd ed.). Stamford, CT: Appleton & Lange.

Murray, R. K., Granner, K., Mayes, P. A., & Rodwell, V. W. (Eds.) (1996). *Harper's biochemistry* (24th ed.). Stamford, CT: Appleton & Lange.

Robin, N. I. (1996). *Endocrinology and metabolic disease.* New York: Parthenon.

Rusterholtz, A. (1996). Interpretation of diagnostic laboratory tests in selected endocrine disorders. *Nursing Clinics of North America, 31*(4), 715–724

Skelly, A. H. (1997). Endocrine disorders. *Lippincott's Primary Care Practice, 1*(5), 459–473.

Wilson, J. D., Foster, D. W., Kronenberg, H. M., & Larsen, P. R. (1998). *Williams textbook of endocrinology.* Philadelphia: W.B. Saunders.

Winger, J. M. & Hornick, T. (1996). Age-associated changes in the endocrine system. *Nursing Clinics of North America; 31*(4), 782–784.

ADRENAL GLAND DISORDERS

Baker, J. T. (1997). Adrenal disorders: A primary care approach. *Lippincott's Primary Care Practice, 1*(5), 527–535.

Burton, M. (1997). Pheochromocytoma. *American Journal of Nursing, 97*(11),57.

Clayton, L. H. & Dilley, K. B. (1998). Cushing's syndrome. *American Journal of Nursing, 98*(7), 40–41.

Cronin, C. C., Callaghan, N., Kearney, P. J., Murnaghan, D. J., & Shanahan, F. (1997). Addison disease in patients treated with glucocorticoid therapy. *Archives of Internal Medicine, 157*(4), 456–458.

Davis-Martin, S. (1996). Pearls for practice: Disorders of the adrenal glands. *Journal of the American Academy of Nursing Practitioners, 8*(7), 323–326.

Ganguly, A. (1998). Current concepts: Primary aldosteronism *New England Journal of Medicine: 339*(25), 1828–1834.

Gavaghan, M. (1997). Surgical treatment of pheochromocytomas. *AORN, 65*(6), 1043–1068.

Grinspoon, S. K. & Biller, B. M. K. (1994). Laboratory assessment of adrenal insufficiency. *Journal of Clinical Endocrinology and Metabolism, 79*(4), 931–932.

Gumowski, J. & Loughran, M. (1996). Diseases of the adrenal gland. *Nursing Clinics of North America, 3*(4), 747–767.

O'Donnel, M. (1997). Addisonian crisis. *American Journal of Nursing, 97*(3), 41.

Ram, C. V. S. (1996). Hypertension: When to suspect underlying pheochromocytoma or aldosteronism. *Consultant, 36*(1), 147–153.

Roberts, A. (1995). The adrenal glands. *Nursing Times, 91*(45), 34–37.

Roberts, A. (1995). The adrenal gland 2. *Nursing Times, 91*(50), 31–33.

Roberts, A. (1995). The adrenal gland 3. *Nursing Times, 92*(2), 31–33.

Streeten, D. H., Anderson, G. H., & Bonaventura, M. (1996). The potential for serious consequences from misinterpreting normal responses to the rapid adrenocorticotropin test. *Journal of Clinical Endocrinology and Metabolism, 81*(1), 285–290.

DIABETES

American Association of Diabetes Educators. (1998). *A core curriculum for diabetes educators* (2nd ed.).

American Diabetes Association. (1997). *Diabetes education goals.* Alexandria, VA: ADA.

American Diabetes Association. (1997). *Diabetes fact sheet.* Alexandria, VA: ADA.

American Diabetes Association. (1997). *Diabetes 1996: Vital statistics.* Alexandria, VA: ADA.

American Diabetes Association. (1998). Gestational diabetes mellitus (position statement). *Diabetes Care, 21*(Suppl 1), S60–S61.

American Diabetes Association. (1998). *Intensive diabetes management.* Alexandria, VA: ADA.

American Diabetes Association. (1998). *Medical management of pregnancy complicated by diabetes.* Alexandria, VA: ADA.

American Diabetes Association. (1998). *Physician's guide to insulin-dependent (type 1) diabetes: Diagnosis and treatment.* Alexandria, VA: ADA.

American Diabetes Association. (1998). *Physician's guide to non–insulin-dependent (type 2) diabetes: Diagnosis and treatment.* Alexandria, VA: ADA.

American Diabetes Association. (1995). *The health professional's guide to diabetes and exercise.* Alexandria, VA: ADA.

American Diabetes Association. (1998). Clinical practice recommendations. *Diabetes Care, 21* (Suppl. 1), 1–98.

American Diabetes Association. (1998). Screening for type 2 diabetes. *Diabetes Care, 21* (Suppl. 1), 520–522.

American Diabetes Association. (1998). Report of the Expert Committee on the Diagnosis and Classification of Diabetes Mellitus. *Diabetes Care, 21*(Suppl. 1).

American Diabetes Association. (1998). Economic consequences of diabetes mellitus in the U.S. in 1997. *Diabetes Care, 21*(2), 296–309.

Anderson, L., Janes, G., Zeimer, D., & Phillips, L. (1997). Diabetes in urban African Americans. Body image, satisfaction with size, and weight change attempts. *Diabetes Educator, 23*(3), 301–308.

Atkinson, M. A. & Maclaren, N. K. (1994). The pathogenesis of insulin dependent diabetes mellitus. *New England Journal of Medicine, 331*(21), 1428–1436.

Barnes, L. P. (1994). Gestational diabetes: Teaching aspects of self care. MCN: *American Journal of Maternal Child Nursing, 19*(3), 175.

Berry, R., Mohn, K. R., & Holzmeister, L. A. (1995). Monitoring diabetes therapy. *Home Healthcare Nurse, 13*(1), 39–42.

Bode, B., Steed, R., & Davidson, P. (1996). Reduction in severe hypoglycemia with long-term, continuous subcutaneous insulin infusion in type 1 diabetes. *Diabetes Care, 19*(4), 324–327.

Boland, E. & Savoye, M. (1997). Nutrition strategies for adolescents with insulin independent diabetes mellitus. *Lippincott's Primary Care Practice, 1*(3), 270–284.

Clark, C. M. & Lee, D. A. (1995). Prevention and treatment of the complications of diabetes mellitus. *New England Journal of Medicine, 332*(18), 1210–1217.

Centers for Disease Control and Prevention. (1997). *National diabetes fact sheet: National estimates and general information on diabetes in the United States.* Atlanta, GA: U.S. Department of Health and Human Services, Centers for Disease Control and Prevention.

CDC Diabetes Cost-Effectiveness Study Group. (1998). The cost-effectiveness of screening for type 2 diabetes. *Journal of the American Medical Association; 280,* 1757–1763.

Clement, S. (1995). Diabetes self management education. *Diabetes Care, 18*(8), 1204–1214.

Cryer, P. E., Fisher, J. N., & Shamoon, H. (1995). Hypoglycemia. *Diabetes Care, 17*(7), 734–755.

Dorgan, M., Bieke, J., Moretto, J. et al. (1995). Performing foot screening for diabetic patients. *American Journal of Nursing, 95*(11), 32–36.

Draso, J. & Peterson, A. (1996). Type II diabetes—exploring treatment options. *American Journal of Nursing 96*(11), 45–50.

The Expert Commitee on the Diagnosis and Classification of Diabetes Mellitus. (1997). The report of the Expert Commitee on the Diagnosis and Classification of Diabetes Mellitus. *Diabetes Care, 20*(7), 1183–1197.

Feldman, E. L., Stevens, M. J. & Greene, D. A. (1997). Pathogenesis of diabetic neuropathy. *Clinical Neuroscience, 4,* 365–370.

Fleming, D. R. (1999). Challenging traditional insulin injection practices. *American Journal of Nursing 99*(2), 72–74.

Fore, W. W. (1995). Non–insulin-dependent diabetes mellitus. The prevention of complications. *Medical Clinics of North America, 79*(2), 287–298.

Franz, M. J. & Bantle, J. P. (Eds.). (1999). *American Diabetes Association's guide to medical nutrition therapy for diabetes.* Alexandria, VA: ADA.

Freeland, B. S. (1998). Diabetic ketoacidosis. *American Journal of Nursing, 98*(8), 52.

Fujii, S. (1997). Advances in the understanding of diabetic vascular disease. *Journal of Cardiovascular Risk, 4*(2), 67–69.

Grinslade, S. & Buck, E. A. (1999). Diabetic ketoacidosis: Implications for the medical-surgical nurse. *MedSurg Nursing, 8*(1), 37–45.

Guay, A. T. (1998). Treatment of erectile dysfunction in men with diabetes. *Diabetes Spectrum, 11*(2), 101–111.

Halpin-Landry, J. E. & Goldsmith, S. (1999). Feet first—diabetes care. *American Journal of Nursing, 99*(2), 26–33.

Hernandes, D. (1998). Hospitalization can exacerbate devastating complications of type II diabetes, including retinopathy, neuropathy, and nephropathy. *American Journal of Nursing, 98*(6), 27–31.

Hoyson, P. M. (1995). Diabetes 2000: Oral medications. *RN, 58*(5), 34–40.

Inzucchi, S. E. et al. (1998). Efficacy and metabolic effects of metformin and troglitazone in type II diabetes mellitus. *New England Journal of Medicine, 338*(13), 867–872.

Janz, N. K. et al. (1995). Diabetes and pregnancy. Factors associated with seeking pre-conception care. *Diabetes Care, 18*(2), 157–165.

Joseph, D. H., & Patterson, B. (1994). Risk taking and the influence on metabolic control: A study of adult clients with diabetes. *Journal of Advanced Nursing, 19*(1), 77–84.

Joslin, E., Ronald, C., Kakn, M., & Weir, G. (1994). *Joslin's diabetes mellitus.* Philadelphia: Lea and Febiger.

Jones, T. L. (1994). From diabetic ketoacidosis to hyperglycemic hyperosmolar nonketotic syndrome: The spectrum of uncontrolled hyperglycemia in diabetes mellitus. *Critical Care Nursing Clinics of North America, 6*(4), 703–721.

Kitabchi, A. E., & Wall, B. M. (1995). Diabetic ketoacidosis. *Medical Clinics of North America, 79*(1), 9–37.

Klein, R. (1995). Hyperglycemia and microvascular disease in diabetes. *Diabetes Care, 18*(2), 258–268.

Kozak, G. P. et al. (1995). *Management of diabetic foot problems.* Philadelphia; W. R. Saunders.

Krug, L. M., Haire-Joshu, D., & Heady, S. A. (1994). Exercise habits and exercise relapse in persons with non–insulin-dependent diabetes mellitus. *Diabetes Educator, 17*(3), 185–187.

Lorber, D. (1995). Nonketotic hypertonicity in diabetes mellitus. *Medical Clinics of North America, 79*(1), 39–52.

Maffeo, R. (1900). Helping families cope with type I diabetes. *American Journal of Nursing, 96*(6), 36–39.

Marrero, D., Guare, J., Vandegriff, J., & Fineberg, N. (1997). Fear of hypoglycemia in the parents and adolescents with diabetes: Maladaptive or healthy response? *Diabetes Educator, 23*(3), 281–286.

McFarland, K. F. (1997). Type 2 diabetes: Stepped-care approach to patient management. *Geriatrics, 52*(10), 22–39.

Nathan, D. M. (1996). The pathophysiology of diabetic complications: How much does the glucose hypothesis explain? *Annals of Internal Medicine, 124*(1 pt 2), 86–89.

Niesen, K. M., & Rajan, M. J. (1994). Pregnancy complicated by diabetes mellitus, superimposed preeclampsia, and adult respiratory distress syndrome: A case study. *Critical Care Nursing Clinics of North America, 6*(4), 841–854.

Redman, B., & Fry, S. (1996). Ethical conflicts reported by registered nurse certified diabetes educators. *Diabetes Educator, 23*(3), 219–224.

Rendell, M. S. et al. (1999). Sildenafil for treatment of erectile dysfunction in men with diabetes. *Journal of the American Medical Association, 281*(5), 421–426.

Reynolds, H. R. (1998). Recipe for success. Medical nutrition therapy in diabetes care. *Advance for Nurse Practitioners, 6*(7), 46, 48–49, 64.

Sacks, D. B., & McDonald, J. M. (1996). The pathogenesis of type II diabetes mellitus. *American Journal of Clinical Pathology, 105,* 149–156.

Service, F. J. (1995). Hypoglycemia. *Medical Clinics of North America, 79*(1), 1–8.

Singer, I., Oster, J. R., & Fishman, L. M. (1997). The management of diabetes insipidus in adults. *Archives of Internal Medicine, 157,* 1293–1301.

Smitherman, K. O., & Peacock, J. E. Jr. (1995). Infectious emergencies in patients with diabetes mellitus. *Medical Clinics of North America, 79*(1), 53–77.

Spollett, G. (1997). Diet strategies in the treatment of non–insulin-dependent diabetes mellitus. *Lippincott's Primary Care Practice, 1*(3), 295.

Taub, L. E. M. (1998). The ADA's clinical practice recommendations in action. *American Journal of Nursing, 98*(10), 16B–16C, 16F.

Testa, M. A. & Simonson, D. C. (1998). Health economic benefits and quality of life during improved glycemic control in patients with type 2 diabetes mellitus. *Journal of the American Medical Association, 280*(17), 1490–1496.

Wang, C., & Fenske, M. (1996). Self-care of adults with non–insulin-dependent diabetes mellitus: Influence of family and friends. *Diabetes Educator, 22*(5), 465–470.

PARATHYROID GLAND DISORDERS

Elasy, T. A. & Skelly, A. H. (1997). Patient with hyperparathyroidism. *Lippincott's Primary Care Practice, 1*(5), 563–566.

Locker, F. G. (1996). Hormonal regulation of calcium homeostasis. *Nursing Clinics of North America, 31*(4), 797–803.

Lovell, C. L. (1997). Clinical consult. Obtaining accurate PTH readings. *ANNA Journal, 24*(2), 280–290.

PITUITARY GLAND DISORDERS

Counsell, C. M., Gilbert, M., & Snively, C. (1996). Challenging diagnosis. Management of the patient with a pituitary tumor resection. *Dimensions Critical Care Nursing, 15*(2), 75–81.

Mitchell, A., Steffenson, N., & Davenport, K. (1997). Hypopituitarism due to traumatic brain injury: A case study. *Critical Care Nursing, 17*(4), 34–51.

Romeo, J. H. (1996). Hyperfunction and hypofunction in the anterior pituitary. *Nursing Clinics of North America, 31*(4), 769–778.

Wierman, M. E. (ed). (1997). *Diseases of the pituitary: Diagnosis and treatment.* Totowa, NJ: Humana Press.

THYROID GLAND DISORDERS

American Association of Clinical Endocrinologists (AACE). (1996). *AACE clinical practice guidelines for evaluation and treatment of hyperthyroidism and hypothyroidism.* AACE.

Bauer, D. C. & Brown, A. N. (1996). Sensitive thyrotropin and free thyroxine testing in outpatients: Are both necessary? *Archives of Internal Medicine 156*(20), 2333–2337.

Braverman, L. E.(Ed). (1997). Diseases of the thyroid. Totowa, NJ: Humana Press.

Braverman, L. E., Dworkin, H. J. & MacIndoe, J. H. (1997). Thyroid disease: When to screen, when to treat. *Patient Care, 31*(6), 18–47.

Braverman, L. E. & Utiger, R. D. (1996). *Werner and Ingbar's the thyroid: A fundamental and clinical text* (7th ed.) Philadelphia: J. B. Lippincott.

Brent, G. A. (1994). The molecular basis of thyroid hormone action. *New England Journal of Medicine, 331*(13), 847–853.

Bunevicius, R., et al. (1999). Effects of thyroxine as compared with thyroxine plus triiodothyronine in patients with hypothyroidism. *New England Journal of Medicine, 11*(6), 424–429.

Danese, M. D., Powe, N. R., Sawin, C. T., & Ladenson, P. W. (1996). Screening for mild thyroid failure at the periodic health examination: A decision and cost-effectiveness analysis. *Journal of the American Medical Association, 276*(4), 285–292.

Falk, S. A. (Ed). (1997). *Thyroid disease: Endocrinology, surgery, nuclear medicine, and radiotherapy.* Philadelphia: Lippincott-Raven.

Gilkison, C. R. (1997). Thyrotoxicosis: Recognition and management. *Lippincott's Primary Care Practice, 1*(5), 485–498.

Heitman, B., & Irizarry, A. (1995). Hypothyroidism: Common complaints, perplexing diagnosis. *Nurse Practitioner, 20*(3), 540–560.

Hennessey, J. V. (1996). Diagnosis and management of thyrotoxicosis. *American Family Physician, 54*(4), 1315–1324.

Kaiser, F. E. (1995). Thyroid function tests: Use and interpretation. *Clinical Geriatric Medicine, 11*(2), 171–177.

Kennedy, J. W. & Caro, J. F. (1996). The ABCs of managing hyperthyroidism in the older patient. *Geriatrics, 51*(5), 22–32.

Lindsay, R. S. & Toft, A. D. (1997). Hypothyroidism. *Lancet, 347*(9049), 413–417.

Livolsi, V. A. (1994). The pathology of autoimmune thyroid disease: A review. *Thyroid: Official Journal of the American Thyroid Association, 4,* 333–339.

McKennis, A. & Waddington, C. (1997). Nursing interventions for potential complications after thyroidectomy. *ORL Head and Neck Nursing, 15*(1), 27–35.

Singer, P. A., Cooper, D. S., Levy, E. G., Ladenson, P. W., Braverman, L. E., Daniels, G., Greenspan, F.S., McDougall, I. R., & Nikolai, T. F. (1995). Treatment guidelines for patients with hyperthyroidism and hypothyroidism. *Journal of the American Medical Association, 273*(10), 808–812.

Streff, M. M. & Pachucki-Hyde, L. C. (1996). Management of the patient with thyroid disease. *Nursing Clinics of North America, 31*(4), 779–796.

ON-LINE RESOURCES

American Association of Clinical Endocrinologists *http://www.aace.com*

American Foundation of Thyroid Patients *http://thyroidfoundation.org*

American Thyroid Association *http://www.thyroid.org*

Cushing Support and Research Foundation *http://www.world.std.com/~csrf*

Endocrine Web, Inc. (with additional links to other sites) *http://www.endocrineweb.com*

Pituitary Tumore Network Assocation (PTNA) *http://www.pituitary.com*

DIABETES

American Association of Diabetes Educators *http://www.diabetesnet.com/aade.html*

American Diabetes Association *http://www.diabetes.org*

Diabetes Center *http://www.endocrineweb.com/diabetes*

Diabetes Monitor *http://mdcc.com*

Juvenile Diabetes Foundation International *http://www.jdfcure.com.*

National Institute of Diabetes and Digestive and Kidney Diseases(NIDDK) *http://www.niddk.nih.gov*

Net Health Diabetes.Com *http://diabetes.com*

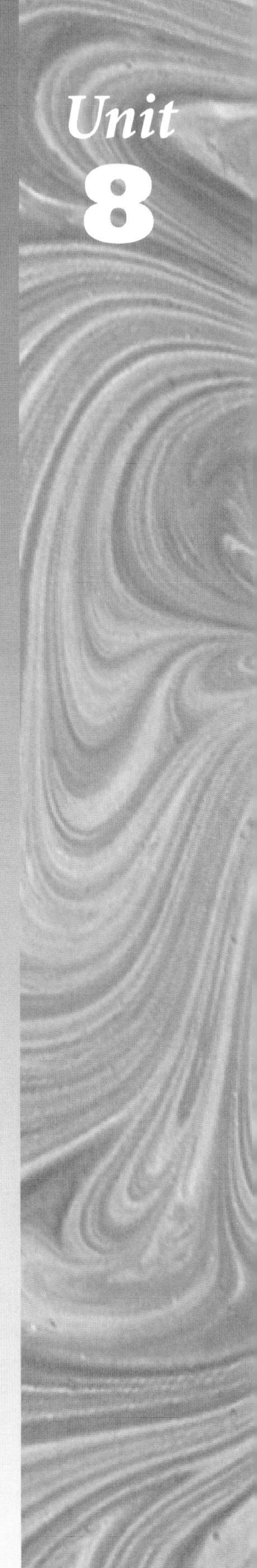

Digestion, Absorption, and Use of Food

FOCUS ON Gastrointestinal and Hepatobiliary Changes Through the Life Span

INFANCY (1–12 MONTHS):

Digestive system, relatively immature at birth, matures somewhat after age 2 to 3 months. Saliva secretion and stomach emptying time increase. By age 3 months, the stomach capacity increases to 150 mL. Amylase is deficient until about age 4 to 6 months. Adult levels of lipase are achieved at approximately age 4 to 5 months. Tooth eruption begins at about age 6 to 7 months. Peristalsis slows and stools become formed by 8 months. Solid foods are usually introduced after age 6 months. The liver is primarily immature throughout infancy. The ability to conjugate and secrete bilirubin occurs after the first few weeks of life. However, gluconeogenesis is relatively immature throughout the first year.

TODDLER AND PRESCHOOL AGE (1–5 YEARS):

Stomach size increases, and amounts of foods ingested at feeding increase. As growth rate decreases, the child may consume less food, possibly increasing the risk for nutritional problems, especially anemia. Stomach acidity increases gradually. Voluntary control of bowel function usually occurs during this time. All twenty deciduous teeth typically are present by age 3 years, with loss of these teeth beginning at the end of the preschool period.

SCHOOL AGE (6–12 YEARS):

Permanent teeth begin to erupt. Secretion, digestion, absorption, and stomach capacity increase with increased efficiency of excretion. Fewer stomach upsets are seen. Caloric needs are dependent on child's activity level and growth rate. Underweight and overweight are common problems.

ADOLESCENCE (13–19 YEARS):

Stomach capacity is mature with increased gastric acidity, active peristalsis, and normal adult liver function. Metabolic rate and nutritional needs increase. Malnutrition and obesity are common. Second molars appear at approximately age 13 years, with third molars appearing possibly as early as age 14 to 15 years.

YOUNG ADULT AND ADULT (20–45 YEARS):

Digestive organs usually function, with stomach capacity being 2000 to 3000 mL. Salivary ptyalin decreases after age 20 years. Digestive juices begin to decrease after age 30 years. Eruption of third molars usually occurs by age 21 years. Pregnancy and excessive dieting for weight loss may result in nutritional problems.

MIDDLE-AGED ADULT (46–64 YEARS):

Caloric needs decrease as metabolic needs begin to decline. Stress may lead to peptic ulcer disease or gastroesophageal reflux. A decrease in digestive juices also may cause some distress. Increased incidence of cholelithiasis is seen with a gradual decline in cholesterol absorption. Taste buds begin to atrophy with a greater loss of the sweet sensation. Saliva production decreases and esophageal emptying slows, with possible relaxation of the lower esophageal sphincter. Liver size begins to decrease.

LATE ADULTHOOD (65–100 + YEARS):

Oral mucosa atrophies and secretions decrease. Loss of nerve cells contributes to a decrease in intake. The gag reflex weakens. Dental disease may lead to impaired ability to chew food. Decreased peristalsis causes delayed stomach emptying. Gastric mucosa shrinks with a decline in hydrochloric acid, pepsin, lipase, and pancreatic enzymes. Bile becomes thicker, causing the gall bladder to empty more slowly. A general decrease in absorption of nutrients, such as fat, vitamins B_1 and B_{12}, calcium and iron, and drugs, occurs. Decreased intestinal motility, along with slowing and dulling of neural impulses, may lead to constipation. The liver's storage capacity decreases. Dilation and distention of the pancreatic ducts occur.

Chapter 25

Normal and Altered Function of the Gastrointestinal System

Denise A. Tucker

KEY TERMS

alimentary canal
chemoreceptive trigger zone
chief cells
chyme
crypts of Lieberkühn
diverticulum
duodenum
dysphagia
gastritis
gastroesophageal reflux
gingivitis
hiatal hernia
histamine
hypothalamus
ileum
intrinsic factor
jejunum
parietal cells
peristalsis
peritoneum
regurgitation
rugae
sphincter ani

The gastrointestinal tract is a basic tubular structure called the **alimentary canal**, which extends from the pharynx to the anus. Throughout this tubular structure, ingested food is processed, digested, and absorbed. The nutrients absorbed may be further processed by accessory organs, used for energy, or stored to be used later for energy. For digestion to occur, the vital functions of motility, secretion, and absorption must proceed in a regulated manner. Finally, by participating in the excretion of waste products, the gastrointestinal system helps to rid the body of unusable or toxic materials.

NORMAL STRUCTURE OF THE GASTROINTESTINAL TRACT

The gastrointestinal tract is a continuous structure beginning with the oral cavity and terminating with the anal sphincter, as shown in Figure 25-1. The gastrointestinal tract carries out the activities of ingestion, movement or passage of food, digestion, absorption, and removal of wastes or defecation.[34]

Oral or Buccal Cavity

The lips, tongue, cheeks, teeth, taste buds, and salivary glands prepare food for eventual absorption. Table 25-1 summarizes the oral structures and their participation in preparing food for digestion.

The submandibular, parotid, and sublingual salivary glands lie outside the oral cavity and pour their secretions into the mouth through ducts, as illustrated in Figure 25-2. The glands continuously secrete *saliva,* which contains large amounts of water and small amounts of *ptyalin, lysozyme*, sodium, potassium, chloride, bicarbonate, phosphates, urea, and a few other solutes. The average amounts of salivary secretion range from 1,000 to 1,500 mL/day.

Esophagus

During the process of swallowing, the pharynx actively moves food into the esophagus, while closing and sealing off the nasopharynx. The esophagus is a muscular tube lined with simple and compound mucous glands. It extends approximately 24 cm long and provides a passageway for food from the pharynx to the stomach.[11] An *upper esophageal sphincter (UES)* prevents food or fluid movement into the posterior pharynx and trachea. A sphincter is an opening that has an extra amount of muscle surrounding it.

About 5 cm above the esophageal entry to the stomach is a narrowed area called the *gastroesophageal, cardiac,* or *lower esophageal sphincter (LES)* (see Fig. 25-1). The gastroesophageal sphincter normally remains constricted but relaxes when a peristaltic wave is conducted

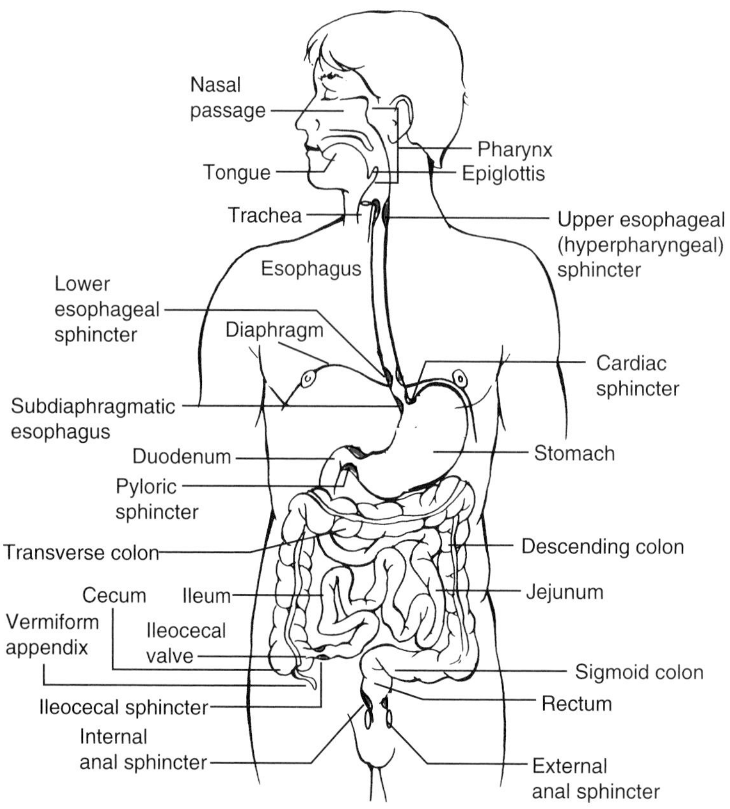

FIGURE 25-1. The digestive system.

TABLE 25-1

PARTICIPATION OF THE ORAL STRUCTURES IN DIGESTION

STRUCTURE	PROCESS
Teeth	Reduce food to sizes appropriate for swallowing; break down dense particles
Tongue	Places food in proper position for swallowing; mixes secretions to moisten food
Salivary glands	Moisten and lubricate foods in the mouth; add ptyalin enzyme for digestion of starches
Muscles of mastication, or chewing	Provide movement for the grinding of food to smaller particles; provide more surface area for the digestive enzymes to act

through it, allowing food to pass to the stomach. Normally the gastroesophageal sphincter prevents acid reflux into the esophagus. Table 25-2 summarizes the functions of the various sphincters along the esophageal passageway.

Stomach

The stomach is a pear-shaped, hollow, distensible organ whose parts consist of the (1) cardia, (2) fundus, (3) body, (4) antrum, and (5) pylorus. Figure 25-3 shows the positions of the greater and lesser curvatures of the stomach. The upper portion of the stomach is continuous with the esophagus and lies close to the diaphragm; the lower portion is continuous with the duodenum through the lower pyloric sphincter.

The interior lining of the stomach is composed of mucosal folds called **rugae**. Within the mucosal folds are glands that secrete gastric juices. The combination of food and gastric juice makes a semiliquid mass called **chyme**, which is propelled into the small intestine through the pyloric sphincter (see Fig. 25-3).

Peritoneum

The **peritoneum** is a serous membrane that lines the entire abdominal wall and envelops the abdominal viscera. The peritoneum consists of the *parietal* and

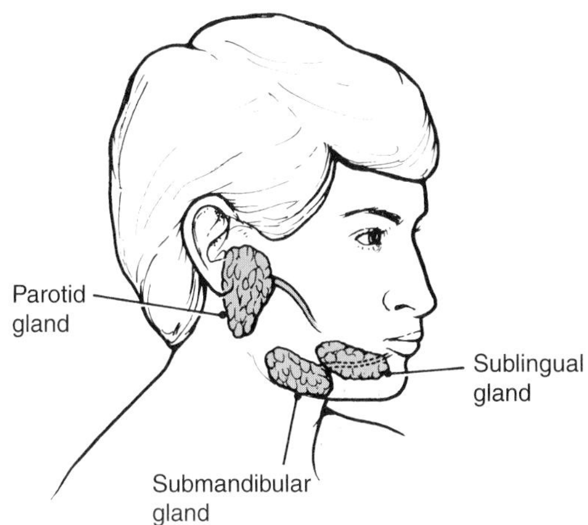

FIGURE 25-2. Salivary glands.

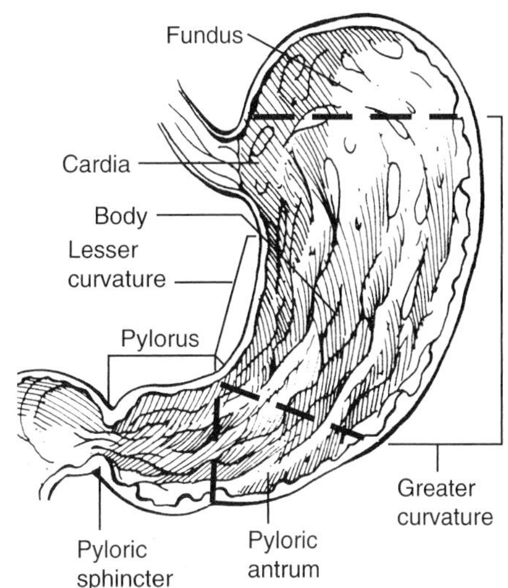

FIGURE 25-3. Segments of the stomach. Notice the greater and lesser curvatures.

visceral components. The parietal peritoneum lines the abdominal wall, and the visceral peritoneum envelops the abdominal viscera. The potential space between them is referred to as the *peritoneal cavity*. The peritoneum secretes a serous fluid that decreases the friction between the abdominal organs when they move against each other. It consists of various folds including the *mesentary*, *greater omentum*, and *lesser omentum*. The mesentary suspends the small intestine from the posterior abdominal wall. The greater omentum suspends from the greater curvature of the stomach and contains fat and lymph nodes. The lesser omentum suspends from the lesser curvature of the stomach and proximal duodenum and forms suspensory ligaments between the liver and stomach and the liver and duodenum.

TABLE 25-2

SPHINCTER FUNCTION

SPHINCTER	FUNCTION
Upper esophageal	Prevents expulsion of food into posterior pharynx
Lower esophageal	Transports food bolus from esophagus to stomach and prevents gastric reflux into upper esophagus
Pyloric	Coordinates organized emptying of stomach and prevents reflux of duodenal contents
Ileocecal	Prevents retrograde expulsion of intestinal contents
Anal	Inhibits expulsion of colonic contents unless voluntary relaxation is established

Small Intestine

The small intestine extends from the pylorus to the ileocecal valve. It is approximately 4 meters long. The small intestine is divided into sections: **duodenum**, **jejunum**, and **ileum**, as shown in Figure 25-1.

The intestinal wall is composed of four layers: mucosa, submucosa, muscularis, and serosa (Fig. 25-4). Figure 25-5 illustrates how the finger-like folds of the mucosa, called *villi*, project into the lumen of the interior of the intestines, increasing the absorptive surface by about 600 times. The **crypts of Lieberkühn** are pit-like structures that lie in grooves between the villi and are composed of absorptive cells and mucus-producing goblet cells. The absorptive cells are columnar and have a brush border on the luminal side. An intestinal epithelial cell lives about 5 days, after which it is shed into the intestinal secretions.[11]

Large Intestine

The large intestine begins with the end of the ileum at the ileocecal valve (see Fig. 25-1). The area of meeting is called the cecum. A small structure, called the *vermiform appendix*, extends from the cecum; it is a relatively nonfunctional pouch. The colon portion of the large intestine is subdivided into the ascending, transverse, descending, and sigmoid areas. The large intestine itself begins with the cecum, contains the colon, and terminates in the rectum and anal canal. The total length of the large intestine is approximately 1.5 meters.

The rectum is about 20 cm of the final descending portion of the large intestine and terminates in the anal

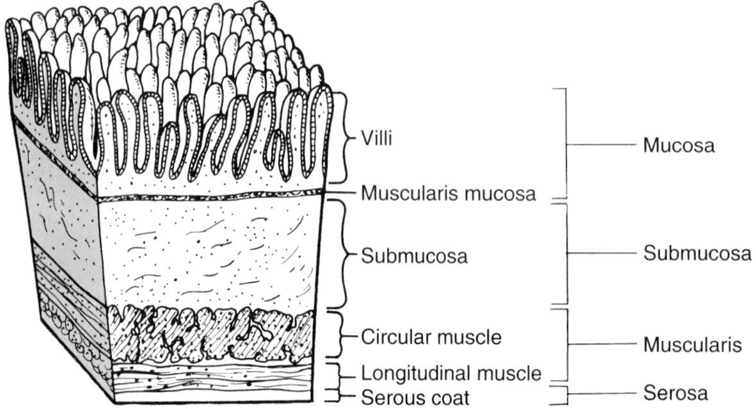

FIGURE 25-4. Layers of the intestinal wall.

canal. There is an internal anal sphincter 2 to 3 cm from the termination of the rectum and an external sphincter, the **sphincter ani**, which opens to the outside of the body.

The same four layers compose the wall of the large intestine as in the small intestine. However, the mucosal layer is thicker in the large intestine and contains no villi. The crypts of Lieberkühn are deeper and contain more goblet cells than those in the small intestine.

Blood Supply to the Gastrointestinal Tract

The gastrointestinal system blood supply is part of the *splanchic circulation*, which includes the gastrointestinal tract, liver, spleen, and pancreas. The arterial supply to this system is from the celiac, superior mesenteric, and inferior mesenteric arteries. The venous blood from the intestines, pancreas, and spleen drains directly into the portal vein and into the liver. From the liver it flows out to the vena cava and the general circulation.

The blood supply to the upper esophagus is from the inferior thyroid arteries; the middle part of the esophagus is supplied by segmental branches of the aorta, the inferior left bronchial artery, and esophageal branches of the thoracic aorta. The lower portion of the esophagus receives its blood supply from the esophageal branch of the left gastric and inferior phrenic arteries. Venous drainage from the esophagus is through the azygous and hemiazygous veins above the diaphragm and through the left gastric vein.

Nervous Supply to the Gastrointestinal Tract

The nervous supply to the gastrointestinal tract is through the intrinsic and the autonomic nervous systems. The intrinsic system begins in the esophagus and continues all the way to the anus. The layers involved in this system include the *myenteric* and the *submucosal plexuses.* These control the tone of the bowel, rhythmic contractions, and the velocity of excitation of the gut.

The gastrointestinal tract receives innervation from both components of the autonomic nervous system, the parasympathetic and the sympathetic systems. The parasympathetic innervation is supplied by (1) the cranial division through the vagus nerve and (2) the sacral division through the second, third, and fourth sacral cord segments. The cranial division provides extensive innervation to the esophagus and stomach and lesser innervation to the intestines. The sacral division supplies the lower large intestine, rectum, and anus. Generally, parasympathetic innervation increases activity of smooth muscle of the gastrointestinal tract and causes the various sphincters to relax.

The sympathetic nervous system innervation to all parts of the gastrointestinal tract is supplied from the T5–L2 spinal cord segments. Generally the sympathetic innervation inhibits the activity of smooth muscles of the gastrointestinal tract and causes the various sphincters to contract.

NORMAL FUNCTION OF THE GASTROINTESTINAL SYSTEM

Appetite, Hunger, and Satiety

The hunger and satiety centers, found in separate locations in the **hypothalamus**, drive nutritional status.[11] The hunger center responds to the concentration of glucose in the blood. A decrease in blood glucose intensifies the hunger response. Serum fat levels and amino acids tend to promote satiety, or satisfaction from hunger. Distention of the gastrointestinal tract suppresses the hunger signals, probably by the sensory signals transmitted by the vagus nerve. The appetite

FOCUS ON CELLULAR PHYSIOLOGY

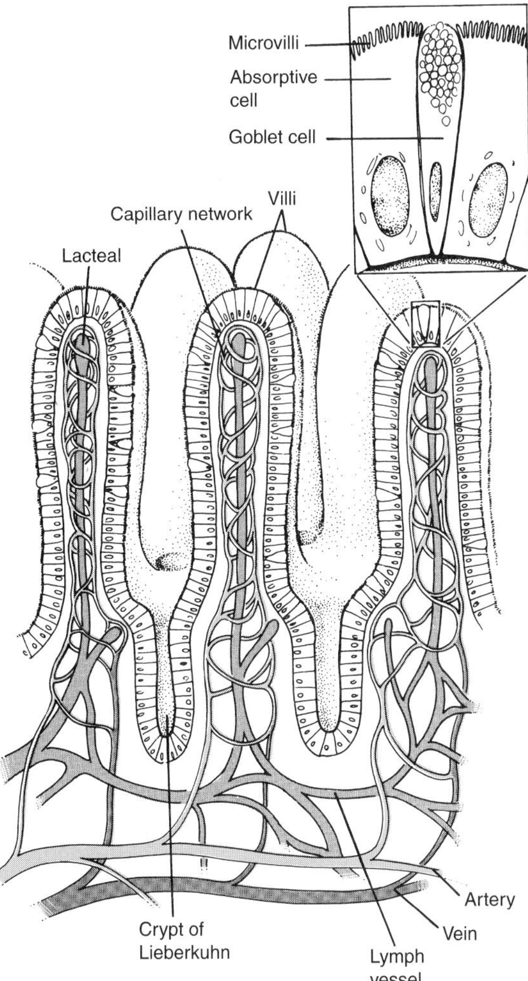

FIGURE 25-5. **Structure of the intestinal villi.**

center is more subtly controlled by the cortical areas and is stimulated by sight, touch, and smell.

Digestion of Food

Digestion takes substances in one form and breaks them down into molecules that are small enough to pass through the intestinal wall to the blood and lymphatic systems. This activity requires the coordination of chemical secretions and mechanical movements. The molecules may be moved by (1) simple diffusion, (2) active transport, or (3) facilitated diffusion. *Motility*, *secretion*, and *absorption* work together to make the process of digestion work.

ORAL SECRETIONS AND MOVEMENT OF FOOD TO THE STOMACH

The major digestive secretion of the salivary glands is the enzyme *ptyalin*, which breaks down from 30% to 40% of starches, beginning in the mouth and continuing in the stomach, until the digestive secretions of the stomach begin to alter the chyme.

Swallowing is the key event in the initiation of digestion because it increases esophageal peristaltic motion, decreases pressure in the lower esophagus, and initiates the gastroenteric reflex. The pharyngeal sphincter relaxes for 1 second or less, and the *primary peristaltic wave* is initiated, beginning in the pharynx and spreading to the esophagus.[11]

As food passes into the esophagus, peristalsis and pressure changes move it toward the stomach. **Peristalsis**, which occurs throughout the gastrointestinal tract, is a series of sequential muscular movements. The primary wave moves down the esophagus, and the wavelike movements of *secondary peristalsis* continue until all of the food is in the stomach.[11] As the food moves toward the lower esophageal or gastroesophageal sphincter, the wave of peristalsis causes the normally constricted area to relax, and the food moves into the stomach.

GASTRIC MOTILITY AND MOVEMENT OF FOOD THROUGH THE STOMACH

Gastric motility is governed by the peristaltic waves that occur every 15 to 25 seconds and mix ingested food with gastric secretions. The result of this movement and mixing is the thin, highly acidic liquid chyme. Chyme is moved into the small intestine mostly because of the higher pressure gradients in the stomach that exceed the duodenal pressure. The acidity and amount of chyme entering the duodenum help to regulate the duodenal and pancreatic secretions.

Gastric Secretion

The glands of the stomach secrete 1,500 to 3,000 mL of gastric juice per day. Secretory activity follows a regular daily pattern, with the least secretion occurring in the early morning. The amount of gastric secretion also varies with individual dietary habits, other stimuli that provoke secretions, and the strength of the inhibitory mechanisms.

Gastric juice is composed of secretions from four major cell types: (1) chief cells, (2) parietal cells, (3) mucus-producing cells, and (4) gastrin-producing cells (G cells). The **chief cells** secrete the proenzyme pepsinogen, which, when activated, digests proteins. The **parietal cells** secrete *hydrochloric acid*, which has a pH of about 0.8. It is thought that these cells also secrete the **intrinsic factor**, a glycoprotein that binds with vitamin B_{12} and makes it available for absorption in the small intestine.[11] *Mucus-producing cells* located in the gastric surface epithelium constantly secrete a thin mucus film. When stimulated, *gastrin cells* release gastrin into the blood.[11] Gastric juice also contains hydrochloric acid, pepsinogen, electrolytes, and bicarbonate; certain other enzymes are enumerated in Box 25-1.

Hydrochloric acid secretion is believed to relate to bicarbonate replenishment in the blood; the amount of bicarbonate entering the blood during the gastric secretory phase is directly proportional to the amount of acid secreted. Carbonic acid, formed by the reaction of carbon dioxide, water, and carbonic anhydrase, dissociates to bicarbonate and hydrogen. The hydrogen ion enters the parietal cell canaliculi by active transport, whereas bicarbonate is diffused back into the blood.[7,33] During digestion, the parietal cell takes carbon dioxide from the circulating blood. This elevates the venous pH after eating, which has been called the *postprandial alkaline tide.* The urine also becomes more alkaline.[10]

The surface of the gastric mucosa has a continuous layer of columnar epithelial cells that secrete large amounts of viscous, alkaline mucus, which coats the mucosa and creates a protective sheet. The epithelial lining of the stomach can reproduce itself in 36 to 48 hours. The amount of mucus secretion varies with vagal stimulation and irritation. The mucus lubricates the passage of food, absorbs pepsin, and washes away noxious substances. Failure to secrete mucus in adequate quantities to protect the underlying mucosa increases the susceptibility of the mucosa to the actions of hydrochloric acid and pepsin.[11]

FACTORS INFLUENCING GASTRIC SECRETION. Gastric secretion is also regulated by hormonal and chemical mechanisms. Distention of the stomach wall activates local neural reflexes to stimulate gastric secretion. The local reflexes elicit autonomic nervous system activity and cause the release of the hormone gastrin. This hormone is absorbed into the bloodstream and stimulates the gastric secretory glands to cause a marked increase in gastric acid secretion. Gastric secretion is thought to occur in three phases: *cephalic, gastric,* and *intestinal* (Fig. 25-6). Box 25-2 summarizes these three phases.

The best-known chemical stimulant of gastric secretion is **histamine**, which is released in response to injury by cells such as mast cells, basophils, and blood platelets. Although less potent than gastrin, histamine causes the parietal cells to secrete large amounts of gastric juice. Large amounts of endogenous histamine may be present in the gastric mucosa, and, during active secretion, small amounts are present in gastric juice and urine. Physical or emotional stress increases the release of histamine. Other factors that influence gastric secretions are summarized in Box 25-3.

BOX 25-1 ENZYME COMPONENTS OF GASTRIC JUICE

Pepsin
- Main proteolytic enzyme
- Secreted by chief cells in the form of pepsinogen
- Activated by HCl and previously activated pepsin
- Optimal function in pH of 2.0
- Inactive in pH of > 5

Gastric amylase
- Digestion of starch

Gastric lipase
- Acts on butterfat

Gastric urease
- Formed by bacteria that contaminate gastric mucosa
- Splits urea to produce ammonia

Gelatinase
- Liquefies proteoglycans in meats[11]

Carbonic anhydrase
- Present in epithelial and parietal cells
- Assists in formation of HCl

Lysozyme
- Carbohydrate-splitting enzyme

SECRETION AND ABSORPTION IN THE SMALL INTESTINE

The major nutrients are absorbed mostly in the small intestine, with the simpler substances usually being absorbed in the first portion of the small intestine. Substances that require greater hydrolysis and simplification are absorbed at later points in the small intestine. Table 25-3 identifies the specific absorption sites of major nutrients. In the small intestine, secretions are received from the pancreas and liver and supplemented by intestinal secretions. Secretions of the small intestine include enzymes, hormones, and mucus. These substances, listed in Tables 25-4 and 25-5, include secretions from the pancreas and liver. The major effects of all of the enzymes and hormones are detailed in the tables.

Biliary secretions include bile salts, lipids, water, electrolytes, and bilirubin. Of these, bilirubin is a waste product that gives color to the feces. Bile salts exert a detergent-like effect on fat and emulsify it. The pancreatic secretions contain enzymes and large amounts of bicarbonate and water. Formation of pancreatic and biliary secretions is discussed in Chapter 26.

The chyme that enters the duodenum is highly acidic because it was mixed with large amounts of hydrochloric acid in the stomach. All of the intestinal enzymes work best in an alkaline medium, which requires chyme to be neutralized and alkalinized. The amount of the alkaline pancreatic secretion is closely correlated with the pH of the chyme entering the small intestine.

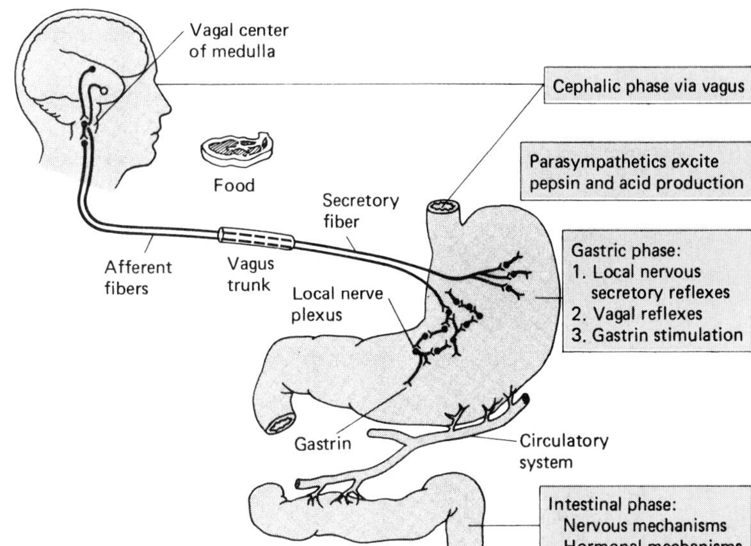

FIGURE 25-6. The phases of gastric secretion and their regulation. (Guyton, A. C. & Hall, J. E. [1996]. *Textbook of medical physiology* [9th ed.]. Philadelphia: W. B. Saunders.)

Chemical and mechanical digestion requires that food be changed into the forms that can be moved by absorption through the mucosal lining cells to the blood and lymph vessels. The diffusible forms include monosaccharides, amino acids, fatty acids, glycerol, and glycerides.[11] Figure 25-7 illustrates where materials are absorbed in the gastrointestinal system and notes that most nutrients are absorbed in the small intestine.

Carbohydrate, Protein, and Fat Absorption

Figure 25-8 illustrates the absorption of carbohydrates, proteins, and fats in the small intestine. Carbohy-

BOX 25-2

PHASES OF GASTRIC SECRETION

Cephalic phase
- Initiated by stimuli (sight, smell, thoughts of food)
- Prepares the stomach for food and digestion
- Hydrochloric acid and gastrin secreted[11]

Gastric phase
- Initiated by distention of the stomach from food
- Also triggered by mucosal exposure to secretagogues
- Gastrin released by acetylcholine stimulation
- Acid and pepsin secreted in response to gastrin
- Parasympathetic stimulation increases secretions
- Gastrin stimulates release of insulin and calcitonin
- Gastrin stimulates muscle contraction of the lower esophageal sphincter, small intestine, colon, and gallbladder
- Gastrin inhibits smooth muscle contraction of the pyloric, ileocecal, and Oddi sphincters

Intestinal phase
- Initiated as acidic chyme enters the small intestine
- May last for 8 to 10 hours while food remains in the duodenum
- Gastrin secretion increases
- Gastric secretion inhibited with partially digested proteins, acid, fat, or hypertonic solutions in the duodenum
- Enterogastric reflex initiated by intestinal distention of food, slowing the influence of the vagus nerve
- Stomach emptying delayed until some emptying occurs in the small intestine
- Intestinal hormones (secretin and cholecystokinin) oppose the stimulatory effects of gastrin
- The movement of chyme from the stomach to the small intestine is slowed to prevent excessive acid secretion, protecting the intestinal mucosa from injury[11]

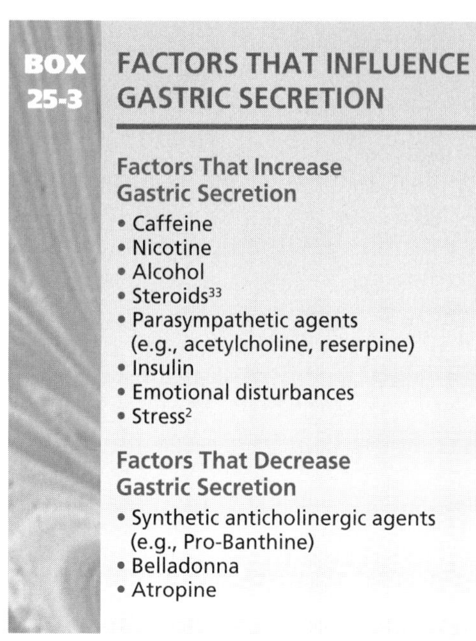

BOX 25-3

FACTORS THAT INFLUENCE GASTRIC SECRETION

Factors That Increase Gastric Secretion

- Caffeine
- Nicotine
- Alcohol
- Steroids[33]
- Parasympathetic agents (e.g., acetylcholine, reserpine)
- Insulin
- Emotional disturbances
- Stress[2]

Factors That Decrease Gastric Secretion

- Synthetic anticholinergic agents (e.g., Pro-Banthine)
- Belladonna
- Atropine

drates are ingested primarily as disaccharides, starches, and polysaccharides and absorbed by the small intestine. As a result of gastric pepsin and pancreatic enzymes, 70% of protein ingested in the diet is presented to the intestinal absorptive membrane in the form of small peptides, and 30% is in the form of amino acids. Many amino acids apparently need pyridoxine, a component of vitamin B_6, to aid in transport.

TABLE 25-3

PRINCIPAL SITES OF ABSORPTION

NUTRIENT	ABSORPTIVE SITE
Carbohydrates	Jejunum
Protein	Jejunum
Fat	Jejunum
Water	Jejunum; also duodenum, ileum, and colon
Fat-soluble vitamins—A, D, E, K	Duodenum
Vitamin B_{12}	Terminal ileum
Other water-soluble vitamins	Duodenum
Iron	Duodenum
Calcium	Duodenum
Sodium	Jejunum by passive diffusion; ileum and colon by active transport
Potassium	Jejunum and ileum
Magnesium	Distal ileum

Water and Electrolyte Absorption

About 8 L of water per day are absorbed from the small intestine into the portal blood entirely by diffusion.[11] Electrolytes cross the intestinal cell membrane by passing through its pores or by using a membrane carrier. Monovalent electrolytes, such as sodium, chloride, potassium, nitrate, and bicarbonate, are more easily absorbed than polyvalent electrolytes, such as calcium, magnesium, and sulfate.

Most iron is absorbed in its ferrous form in the duodenum, and an acid medium facilitates iron absorption. Vitamins are primarily absorbed in the proximal intestine, except for vitamin B_{12}, which forms a complex with the intrinsic factor and is absorbed in the ileum.

SECRETION, ABSORPTION, AND EXCRETION IN THE LARGE INTESTINE

The function of the large intestine (colon) is mainly to absorb water, but it also is vital in the synthesis of vitamin K and some B-complex vitamins and in the formation and excretion of feces. Water absorption regulates the consistency of the feces and provides for final water balance in the gastrointestinal system.

ALTERATIONS OF THE GASTROINTESTINAL SYSTEM

Alterations of the Oral Cavity

The gums, or gingiva, are subject to localized inflammatory diseases. **Gingivitis**, an inflammation of the borders surrounding the teeth, may result in pain, bleeding, and destruction of gingival tissue. When this inflammation spreads to the underlying tissues, bones, or roots of the teeth, it is called *periodontitis*. This destructive disease may result in purulent drainage, loss of teeth, spread to and infection of the surrounding lymph nodes, and sepsis.

Changes in the oral mucosa often reflect systemic changes in the body. For example, localized white lesions of the oral mucosa occur in a *Candida albicans* infection (thrush). Tumors of the oral mucosa are uncommon and are much like skin tumors, except that many of the oral growths are benign rather than malignant lesions.[5] The salivary glands may also develop benign or malignant tumorous growths.

Esophageal Alterations

ACHALASIA

Achalasia is a disorder of esophageal motility characterized by the inability of the cardiac sphincter of the stomach to relax (Figure 25-9A). It is caused by degeneration of the myenteric ganglion cells in the esophagus and alteration in vagal tone. Therefore, motility problems

TABLE 25-4

DIGESTIVE ENZYMES

ENZYME	SOURCE	SUBSTRATE	PRODUCTS	REMARKS
Ptyalin	Salivary glands	Starch	Smaller carbohydrates	
Pepsin	Chief cells of stomach mucosa	Protein (nonspecific)	Polypeptides	Activated by hydrochloric acid
Gastric lipase	Stomach mucosa	Triglycerides (lipids)	Glycerides and fatty acids	
Enterokinase	Duodenal mucosa	Trypsinogen	Trypsin	Activates or converts trypsinogen to trypsin; trypsinogen hydrolyzed to expose active site
Trypsin	Pancreas	Protein and polypeptides	Smaller polypeptides	Converts chymotrypsinogen to chymotrypsin
Chymotrypsin	Pancreas	Proteins and polypeptides (different specificity than trypsin)	Smaller polypeptides	
Nuclease	Pancreas	Nucleic acids	Nucleotides (base + sugar + PO_4)	
Carboxypeptidase	Pancreas	Polypeptides	Smaller polypeptides	Cleaves carboxy terminal end
Pancreatic lipase	Pancreas	Lipids, especially triglycerides	Glycerides, free fatty acids, glycerol	Very potent
Pancreatic amylase	Pancreas	Starch	2 disaccharide units = maltose	Very potent
Aminopeptidase	Intestinal glands	Polypeptides	Smaller peptides	
Dipeptidase	Intestine	Dipeptides	2 amino acids	
Maltase	Intestine	Maltose	2 glucose	
Lactase	Intestine	Lactose	1 glucose, 1 galactose	
Sucrase	Intestine	Sucrose	1 glucose, 1 fructose	
Nucleotidase	Intestine	Nucleotides	Nucleosides and phosphates (base + sugar)	
Nucleosidase	Intestine	Nucleosides	Base and sugar	
Intestinal lipase	Intestine	Fats	Glycerides, fatty acids, glycerol	

Note: Enzymes act on one another during and after digestion, but it is only after digestion (after their substrates are removed) that they have any marked effect on one another.

occur and food is retained within the area. Hypertrophy and dilatation of the lower esophagus occurs.[28]

This condition is progressive, becoming chronic. Clinical manifestations include dysphagia, weight loss, and regurgitation.[4] One third to one half of patients complain of retrosternal chest pain, often precipitated by eating.[4] Patients may induce vomiting to relieve feelings of discomfort after eating.[4] Lung changes and infections may occur from repeated episodes of nocturnal aspiration. Swallowing is often worsened by stress and anxiety.

Figure 25-9B illustrates the distended, nonemptying lower esophagus as a pouch that narrows into the esophagogastric junction. Although the LES does not open in response to swallowing, it may open slightly as food moves into the area to allow some contents to pass through.

ESOPHAGEAL DIVERTICULUM

An *esophageal diverticulum* is an outpouching of the esophagus at any level that can result in trapped food, **dysphagia**, and **regurgitation**. Esophageal diverticula occur mainly in the middle and lower thirds of the esophagus.[13] They may be due to congenital weakness or chronic inflammatory mediastinal diseases (such as tuberculosis or histoplasmosis) and may be associated with achalasia or high esophageal pressures generated by esophageal spasm or hypertensive LES.[13] In the pharyngeal portion of the esophagus, it is called *Zenker's*

TABLE 25-5

HORMONES OF DIGESTION

HORMONE	SOURCE	AGENTS THAT STIMULATE PRODUCTION	ACTION
Gastrin	Gastric mucosa (primarily pylorus)	Distention of stomach and some protein derivatives	Stimulates production of hydrochloric acid
Enterogastrone	Mucosa of small intestine and duodenum	Fats, sugars, or acids in intestine	Inhibits gastric secretion and mobility
Secretin	Duodenal mucosa	Polypeptides, acids, etc., in intestine (duodenum)	Stimulates pancreas to produce a watery, enzyme-poor juice, with high HCO_3^- content
Cholecystokinin	Duodenal mucosa	Fats in duodenum	Stimulates pancreas to produce enzyme-rich juice and stimulates gallbladder to contract and release bile

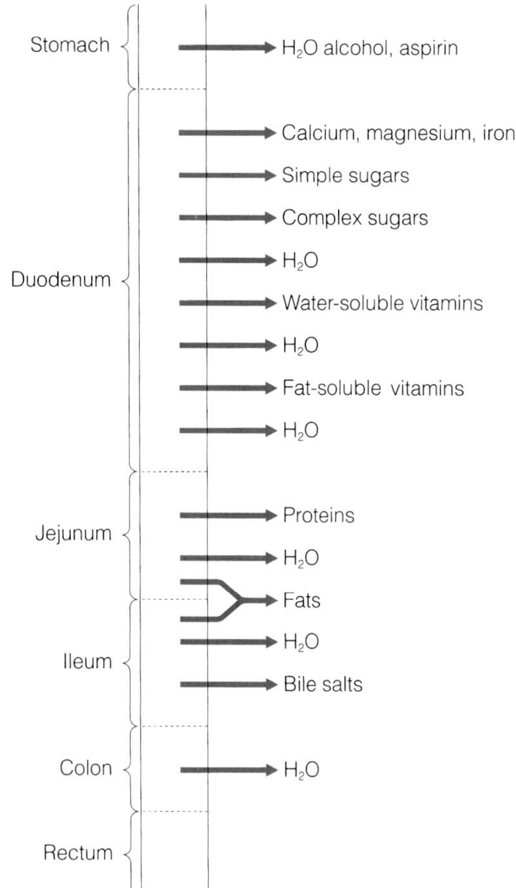

FIGURE 25-7. **Schematic representation of absorption of nutrients in the digestive tract.**

pouch or *diverticulum.* Symptoms include dysphagia and regurgitation or retention of food.[13]

GASTROESOPHAGEAL REFLUX DISEASE (GERD)

Gastroesophageal reflux is the movement of gastric contents into the esophagus. Normally, pressure on the LES prevents backflow of gastric contents from the esophageal mucosa. An incompetent LES is believed to be the primary cause of GERD and esophageal inflammation. Other causes include prolonged gastric intubation, ingestion of corrosive chemicals, uremia, infections, mucosal alterations, and systemic diseases such as systemic lupus erythematosus.[5] The most common clinical manifestations are heartburn (retrosternal burning pain radiating to the neck), acid regurgitation of stomach contents, and dysphagia.[17] GERD may induce laryngitis from the reflux of acid contents to the posterior larynx, and reflux-induced asthma from pulmonary aspiration of acid contents.[17]

ESOPHAGITIS

Esophagitis, inflammation of the esophageal mucosa, most often results from GERD due to prolonged vomiting or incompetent lower esophageal sphincter.[17] Reflux esophagitis causes mucosal damage from prolonged contact with the acidic gastric secretions.[30] Other causes of esophagitis may be associated with motility problems of the esophagus, infections, and ingestion of strong acids or alkali.

The manifestations of esophagitis are similar to GERD and often are precipitated by ingestion of fatty or spicy foods or alcohol. Obstruction due to perma-

FOCUS ON CELLULAR PHYSIOLOGY

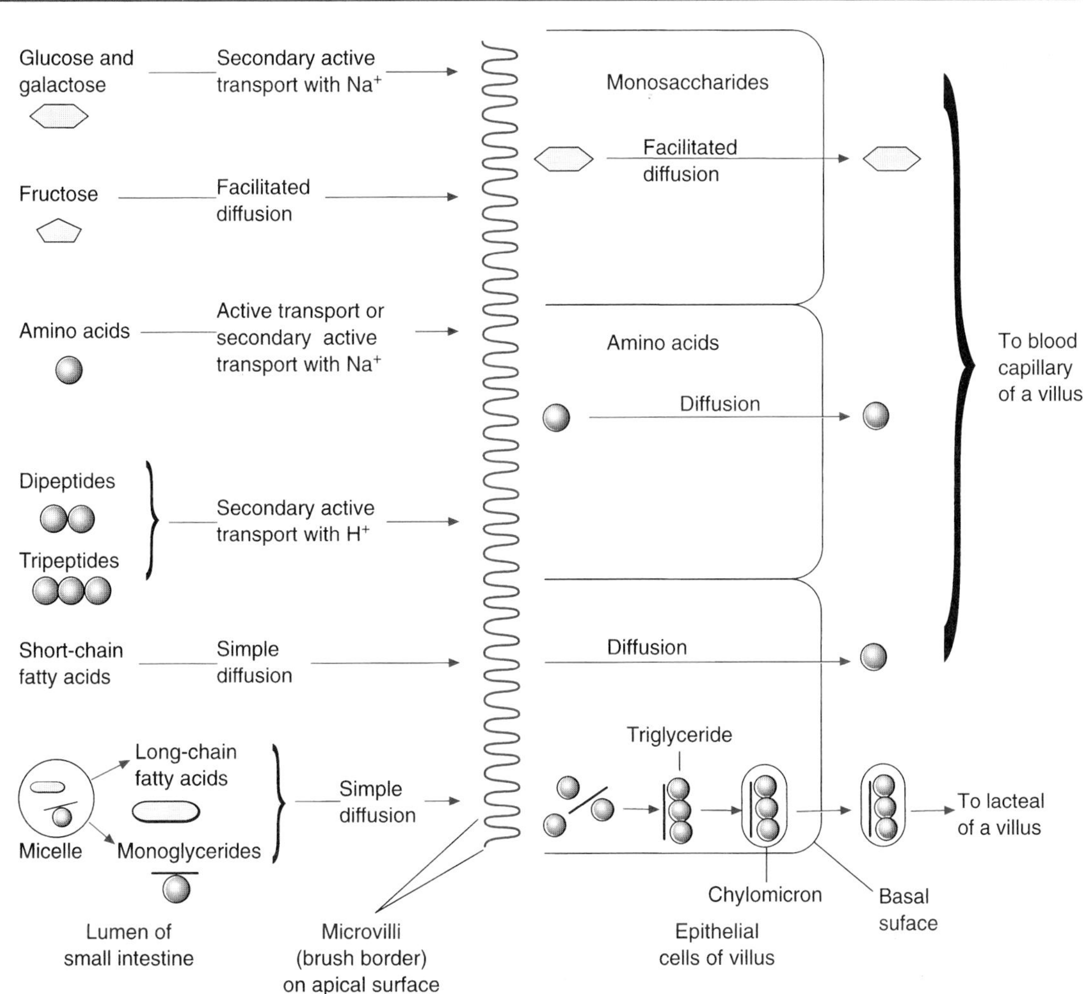

FIGURE 25-8. Absorption of digested nutrients in the small intestine. For simplicity, all digested foods are shown in the lumen of the small intestine, even though some nutrients are digested by brush border enzymes. (Tortora, G. & Grabowski, S. [1996]. *Principles of anatomy and physiology* [8th ed.]. New York: Harper Collins.)

nent strictures may develop, causing dysphagia. Mucosal irritation may cause bleeding, eventually producing an iron-deficiency anemia. Nocturnal reflux of stomach contents may lead to pulmonary aspiration.

HIATAL HERNIA

A **hiatal hernia** is a condition in which part of the stomach protrudes through the opening of the diaphragm. Hiatal hernias are typically acquired as persons age, either from the loss of elasticity of the phrenoesophageal membrane (causing the diaphragm juncture to widen) or increased intra-abdominal pressure (caused by obesity or straining while defecating).[19] They are common in erosive esophagitis and may be associated with gastric erosions, iron-deficiency anemia, or upper GI bleeding.[19]

This condition may be continuous or occur sporadically. Fewer than 10% of persons have the continuous type, called a rolling *paraesophageal hernia*, as shown in Figure 25-10A. The remainder have the sporadic type, or *sliding hernia*, which occurs with changes in position or increased peristalsis, as shown in Figure 25-10B. The stomach is forced through the opening of the diaphragm when the person reclines and moves back to its normal position when the person stands upright.

Most persons are asymptomatic.[19] Symptoms such as heartburn, gastric regurgitation, dysphagia, and in-

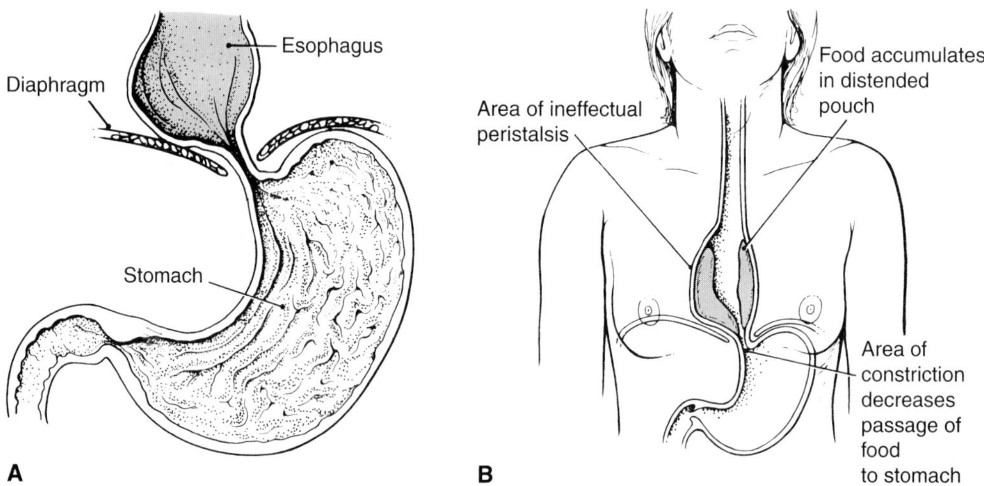

FIGURE 25-9. **A.** Location and appearance of achalatic esophagus. **B.** Nonemptying or poorly emptying lower esophagus resulting from achalasia.

digestion may occur and worsen when the person lies down after eating or with physical exertion and sudden changes in posture.

CANCER OF THE ESOPHAGUS

Esophageal cancers account for approximately 5% to 10% of gastrointestinal tract malignancies. Although relatively uncommon in the U.S., these malignancies have a very high mortality rate.[6,27] There is a strong correlation between cigarette smoking, excessive alcohol intake, and esophageal cancer, especially when smoking and alcohol consumption occur together.[27]

Squamous cell carcinoma is the most common morphologic form. Most tumors are located in the middle and lower one third of the esophagus. Adenocarcinomas of the esophagus, the second most common form, are most frequently found in the lower third of the esophagus and may arise from the gastric fundus.[28]

Clinical Manifestations

The person is typically asymptomatic early in the disease. By the time symptoms such as mild dysphagia appear, the malignancy is usually surgically unresectable. Postprandial regurgitation and weight loss occur later in the disease. Esophagoscopy with biopsy of the tumor mass generally reveals spread of the carcinoma to the lymph nodes. Prognosis is very poor; only about 3% survive 5 years.[5]

Alterations in the Stomach and Duodenum

GASTRITIS

Gastritis is a general term for an inflammation of the gastric mucosa. It may occur with excessive or completely absent gastric acid secretion. The classification into acute and chronic gastritis describes the onset and course of the disease.

Acute gastritis causes transient inflammation of the gastric mucosa, mucosal hemorrhages, and erosion into the mucosal lining. An *erosion* is a superficial mucosa defect of the stomach that does not penetrate the muscularis layer. It is frequently associated with alcohol or aspirin ingestion, smoking, and severely stressful conditions, such as trauma, burns, central nervous system (CNS) damage, chemotherapy, and radiation therapy.[8] Erosion of the gastric mucosa can result in massive hemorrhage. Generally, clinical manifestations of acute gastritis are variable and may range from anorexia, mild epigastric distress, and belching to severe epigastric pain, nausea and vomiting, and hematemesis.

Chronic gastritis may be associated with gastric mucosal atrophy, achlorhydria (lack of hydrochloric acid secretion), and peptic ulceration. The most common form of chronic gastritis is chronic atrophic gastritis. Chronic atrophic gastritis is associated with *Helicobacter pylori* infection. It occurs most often in the elderly. Clinical manifestations are vague, with chronic atrophic gastritis, and may include epigastric discomfort and anorexia.

STRESS ULCERS

Stress ulcers, or gastric erosions, occur after major insults to the body such as complications following major surgery, major trauma, burns, brain injury, stress, and ingestion of aspirin, NSAIDS, and alcohol.[18] Stress ulcers after brain injury are called *Cushing's ulcers*; those after burn injury are called *Curling's ulcers*.

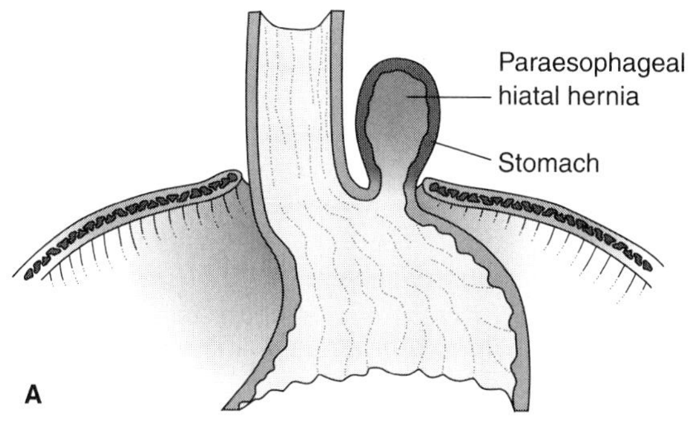

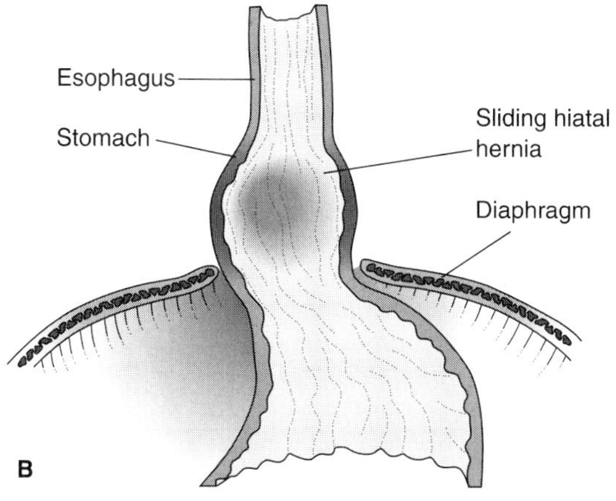

FIGURE 25-10. **Hiatal hernia comparison. A. Paraesophageal hiatal hernia. B. Sliding hiatal hernia. (Rubin, E. & Farber, J. L. [Eds.] [1999]. *Pathology* (3rd ed.). Philadelphia: Lippincott.)**

Stress ulcers are typically multiple and superficial and are present in large areas of the gastric mucosa, especially in the fundus. Erosions associated with stress ulcers permit damage by continual activation of pepsinogen. Gastric acid secretion is sometimes increased, and the erosions often localize in the acid-secreting portion of the stomach.

These ulcerations are usually attributed to poststress ischemia of the stomach mucosa, which causes a sympathetic vasoconstrictive action, disrupting the gastric mucosa. As shown in Flowchart 25-1, platelet-activating factor or prostaglandins may also promote gastric ulceration in ischemic injury. It is also postulated that there is enhanced back-diffusion of hydrogen ions due to increased sensitivity of the disrupted gastric mucosa to hydrochloric acid and pepsin.[28]

Clinical manifestations may be absent until a significant complication such as massive, painless gastric bleeding occurs after acute stress.

PEPTIC ULCER DISEASE

Peptic ulcer disease (PUD) is a common condition that results from an acid–pepsin imbalance. Ulcers develop when the aggressive proteolytic activities of the gastric secretions are greater than their normal protective abilities. An increase in acid and pepsin from any cause may produce ulcerations if the protective mechanisms are inadequate. Major factors that alter the mucosal barrier include (1) the failure to regenerate the mucous epithelium at a sufficient rate, (2) a decrease in quantity and quality of mucus, and (3) poor local mucosal blood flow.

Vascular occlusion of small nutrient vessels in the mucosa or submucosa may cause localized necrosis and subsequent ulcer formation. There is also evidence that *H. pylori* bacteria is a predisposing factor. Virtually all persons with active duodenal ulcer have *H. pylori*, and nearly 80% of persons with gastric ulcers have the organism; the incidence of recurrence declines when the organism is eradicated. However, many persons with the organism do not develop peptic ulcer disease.[25]

Zollinger-Ellison syndrome may also be a cause of severe peptic ulcer disease. Classic pathology with this syndrome includes (1) a gastrin-secreting tumor of the

FLOWCHART 25-1 **Effects of Platelet Activating Factor and Prostaglandins**

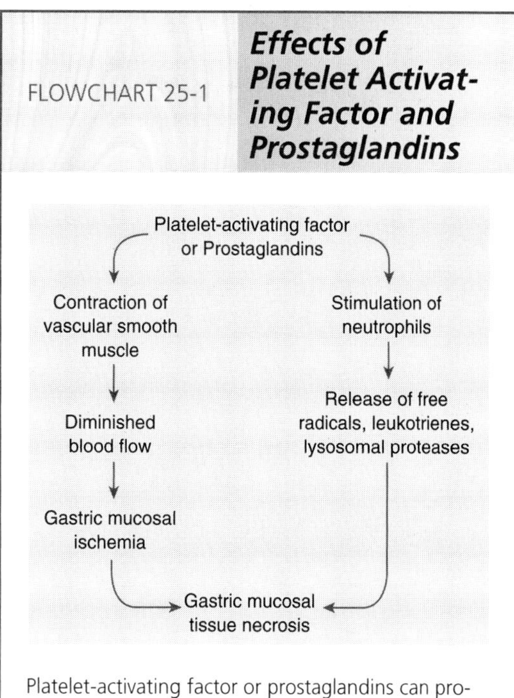

Platelet-activating factor or prostaglandins can promote gastric ulceration through ischemia or through the production of free radicals or other tissue toxic substances.

pancreas (gastrinoma), (2) peptic ulcers in uncharacteristic regions of the gastrointestinal tract, and (3) excessive gastric acid secretion. This syndrome may also be associated with multiple endocrine neoplasia syndrome, type I in some patients (see Chap. 24). Up to one third of these patients suffer acute complications such as perforation or pyloric obstructions.[20]

The two main types of peptic ulcer disease are gastric and duodenal ulcers (Fig. 25-11). The most common site for peptic ulcers is the pyloric region of the duodenum. Duodenal ulcers constitute 80% of all peptic ulcers. Lesions also occur in other regions of the stomach and are referred to as gastric ulcers. Table 25-6 contrasts gastric and duodenal ulcers.

Gastric Ulcers

The primary problem with gastric ulcers appears to be a disruption in the mucosal barrier. Gastric ulcers may be caused by a variety of ingested substances, including ulcerogenic drugs, tobacco, and alcohol. *H. pylori* and chronic bile reflux are also causative factors. Gastric ulcers are usually solitary and small, although occasionally multiple ulcerations may be evident. Figure 25-12 shows the classic ulcer that has a sharply punched-out appearance with a smooth, clean base and is surrounded by gastritis. The mucosa surrounding it is often edematous. Bleeding may occur if the ulceration erodes through a vessel. Malignant gastric ulcers exhibit a shaggy, necrotic base, as opposed to the smooth base of nonmalignant ulcers. Gastric ulcers transform into malignant tumors often enough to call them premalignant and to encourage frequent follow-up.

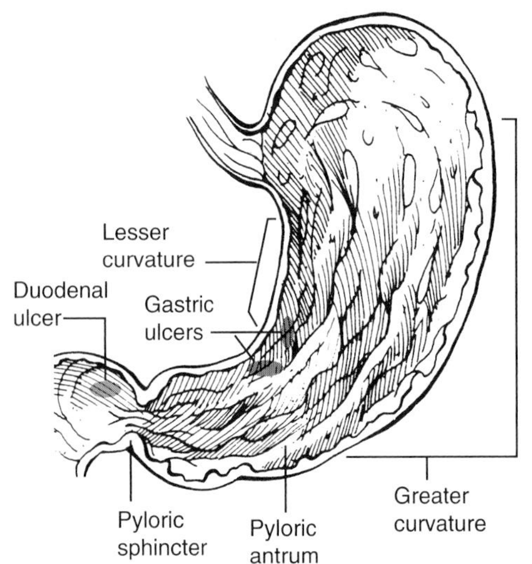

FIGURE 25-11. Common locations of gastric and duodenal ulcers.

Gastric ulcers can be diagnosed by barium swallow (upper gastrointestinal series) and direct endoscopy. Biopsy and routine cytologic studies can be performed with endoscopy. Benign ulcers frequently localize on the lesser curvature of the stomach and are usually smaller than malignant lesions. If there is associated achlorhydria, the ulcers are almost always malignant.

The most common symptom with gastric ulcer disease is epigastric pain. Healing and recurrence are common, with lack of healing or failure to decrease in size suggesting gastric malignancy.

Duodenal Ulcers

Numerous causes and predisposing factors in combination upset the balance between the protective mechanism and the acid–pepsin proteolytic action in the duodenal wall, resulting in duodenal ulcers. Ulcers occur in the presence of acid, but hyperacidity is not always a significant component. Persons with excess acid secretion may also have excess secretion of gastrin or gastrin-like substances from the duodenal wall as well as from the parietal cells. Duodenal ulcers occur predominantly among the type O blood group, supporting genetic transmission of the disease.[5] The genetic trait for hypersecretion of pepsinogen is autosomal dominant, and also may indicate a predisposition to duodenal ulcers.[5] Emotional factors that increase gastric secretions and influence the pathogenesis of duodenal ulcerations often precipitate the onset or recurrence of symptoms.[5] Figure 25-13 summarizes the gastric and duodenal factors implicated in the pathogenesis of duodenal peptic ulcers.

PATHOPHYSIOLOGY. Duodenal ulcers are usually deep, with a sharp line of demarcation from uninvolved tissue. Most of these ulcerations occur in the first portion of the duodenum, close to the pylorus. Disruption of the integrity of the mucosal wall caused by the acid–pepsin imbalance penetrates the entire thickness of the mucosal membrane, including the muscularis mucosa. Healing requires the formation of granulation tissue and scar. Secretory cellular functions are lost in the area of scarring. A typical duodenal ulcer is round or oval and indurated, with a funnel-shaped lesion that extends into the muscularis layer.

Acute ulcerations may develop on chronic ulcers, and perforations through the duodenal wall in active ulcers result in spilling of gastric or duodenal contents into the peritoneum and cause peritonitis. Erosion of an artery or a vein at the base of the lesion may cause a hemorrhage. The amount of bleeding depends on the vessel involved, and the effects are related to the rapidity and amount of blood loss. Scar formation may cause deformity, shortening, and stiffening of the duodenum, which may interfere with normal emptying of the stom-

TABLE 25-6

CONTRASTING GASTRIC AND DUODENAL ULCERS

CHARACTERISTIC	GASTRIC ULCERS	DUODENAL ULCERS
Location	Antral region and lesser curvature	Pyloric region
Incidence	Peak age 50–60 years; usually no family history	Peak age 30–45 years; higher incidence in blood type O; constitutes 80% of all peptic ulcers; usually family history present
Associated diseases	Increased with stress ulcers after major trauma or emotional stress	More common with alcoholic cirrhosis, hyperparathyroidism, COPD, renal failure, and chronic pancreatitis
Acid secretion	Normal to decreased	Increased
Helicobacter pylori	Present in 60–80%	Present in close to 100%
Pain	Food–pain pattern	Pain–food–relief pattern
Weight	Loss common	No loss
Complications	Hemorrhage, perforation, and obstruction	Hemorrhage, perforation, and obstruction

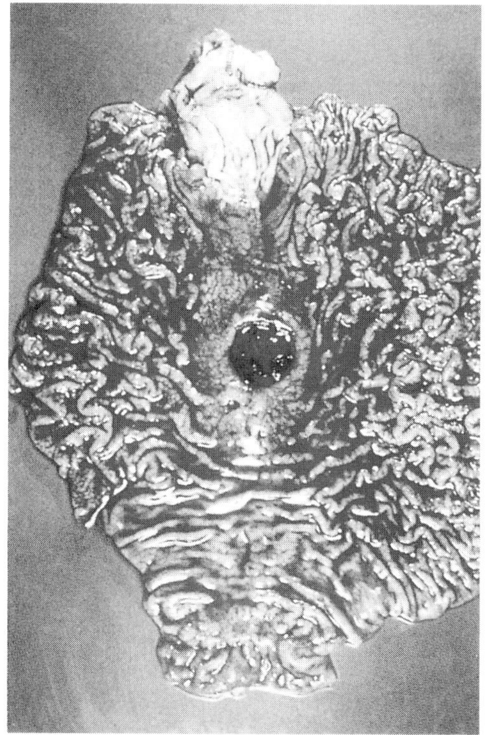

FIGURE 25-12. Gastric ulcer. The stomach has been opened to reveal a sharply demarcated, deep peptic ulcer on the lesser curvature. (Rubin, E. & Farber, J. L. [Eds.] [1999]. *Pathology* (3rd ed.). Philadelphia: Lippincott.)

ach. Actual obstruction may result from stenosis, spasm, edema, and inflammation.

CLINICAL MANIFESTATIONS. Clinical manifestations of duodenal ulcerations include a documented pattern of remissions and exacerbations over varying periods of time. An attack is frequently triggered by stress, and exacerbations are observed most frequently in the fall and spring. The characteristic pain of duodenal ulcer, noted in Table 25-6, typically follows a pain–food–relief pattern.[2] The pain mechanism in duodenal ulcers is thought to be related to irritation of exposed sensory nerve endings by hydrochloric acid. It may result from increased motility or spasm of the muscles at the ulcer site. In rare cases, no pain is described, and the ulcer is discovered when complications arise. Other gastrointestinal manifestations include heartburn and regurgitation of sour juice into the back of the mouth.

A reliable and accurate history of the character of pain may be supportive of duodenal ulcer. Radiologic and fluoroscopic examinations with barium swallow demonstrate ulcer craters, niches, and outlet deformities. Gastric endoscopy may reveal lesions too small or superficial to be seen on radiographs.

Complications of Peptic Ulcer Disease

Hemorrhage occurs in 15% to 20% of cases of peptic ulcer disease; approximately 25% of persons with gastric ulcers bleed. It may be manifested by *melena* (occult blood in the stools), *hematemesis* (vomiting of blood), and/or hemorrhagic shock.[2] Perforation of the

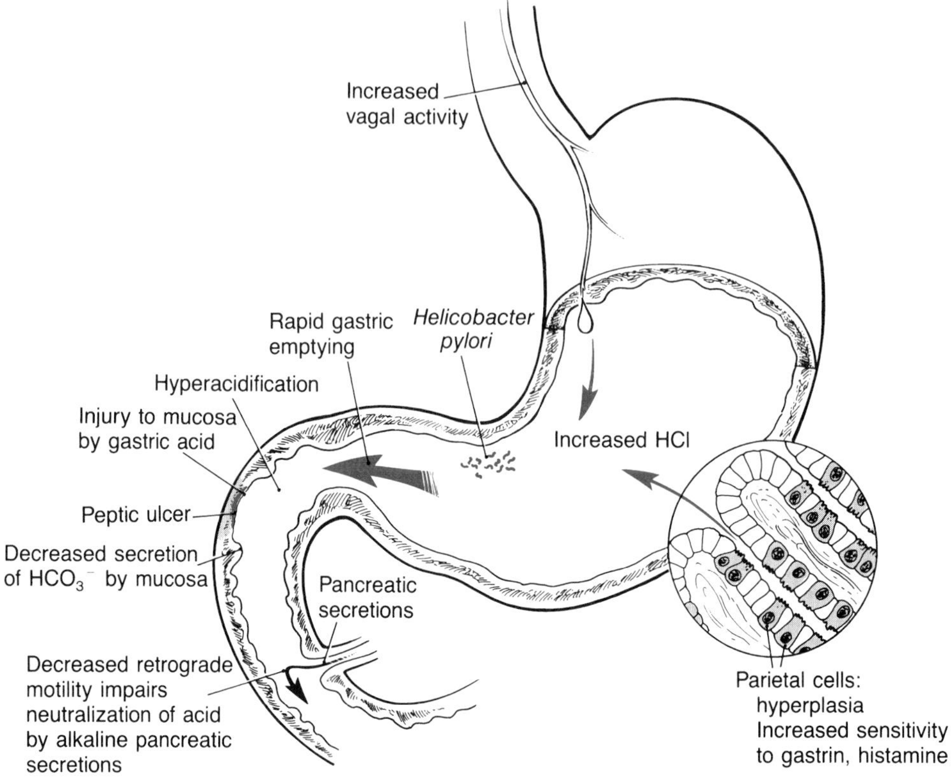

FIGURE 25-13. **Pathogenesis of duodenal peptic ulcers.**

wall may occur, most commonly in patients with duodenal ulcer disease, causing abdominal pain and peritonitis. However, the perforation of gastric ulcers carries a mortality rate between 10% to 40%.[28] Penetration of the ulcer into surrounding structures is relatively uncommon but may affect the pancreas, liver, and abdominal wall. Symptoms of penetration are those of damage to the affected area.

The inlet and outlet of the stomach may become obstructed; this is most common in the pyloric area. Obstruction may cause severe pain, vomiting, weight loss, and anorexia.

GASTRIC CARCINOMA

Of all malignancies of the stomach, 90% to 95% are classified as carcinomas. Survival rates are poor, with less than 5% to 15% of patients surviving for 5 years after diagnosis. With early diagnosis, however, the 5-year survival rate is over 90%.[12]

Environmental factors such as urban residence and diet have been identified as risk factors.[5] Nitrates that are used as food preservatives convert to nitrites in the body, which convert to potent carcinogens.[22,23] Genetic transmission is supported by an increased risk among families and the preponderance of occurrence in persons with blood type A. Gastric carcinoma also is associated with atrophic gastritis or polyps of the stomach.

Pathophysiology

Gastric carcinoma may arise anywhere on the mucosal surface. It begins as an *in situ* (localized) lesion that progresses to lesions called *early gastric carcinoma*, which are limited to the mucosa and submucosa. The lesions may spread through the gastric wall into nearby organs or spread within the gastric wall.[22] Ulceration may occur, with a shaggy, necrotic-appearing base. Carcinomatous masses may be polypoid or ulcerating in appearance (Fig. 25-14). Early metastasis or spread may be to lymph nodes in the region.

Clinical Manifestations

The clinical manifestations are often vague and non-specific, including early satiety, loss of appetite, weight loss, abdominal pain, vomiting, and change in bowel habits. Anemia and guaiac-positive stools may be discovered. Bleeding may result from vascular erosion as the tumor ulcerates. Pain in gastric carcinoma may mimic ulcer pain or be related to partial outlet obstruction. Massive hemorrhage may cause hemorrhagic shock.

FOCUS ON CELLULAR PATHOPHYSIOLOGY

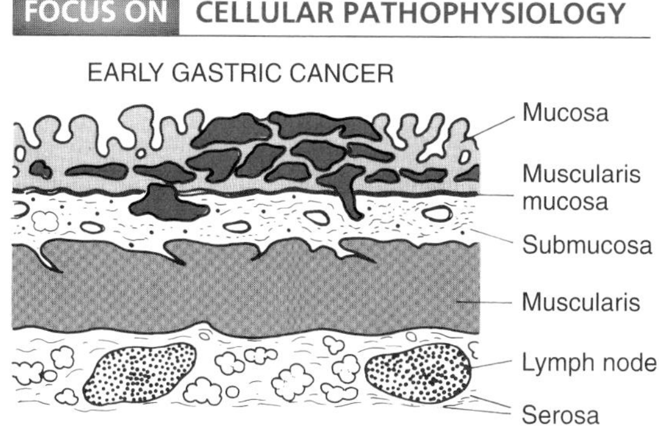

POLYPOID CARCINOMA

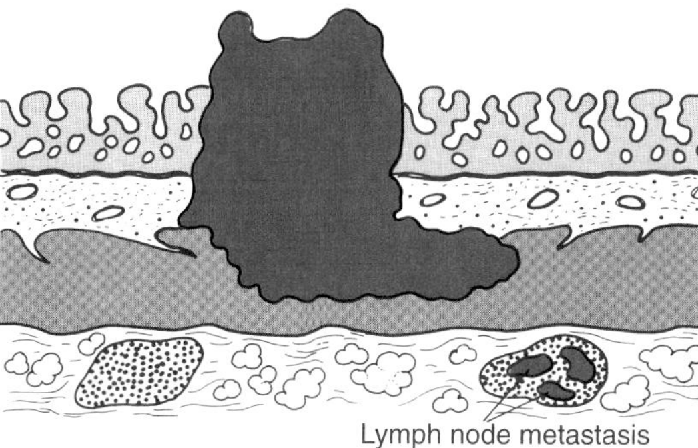

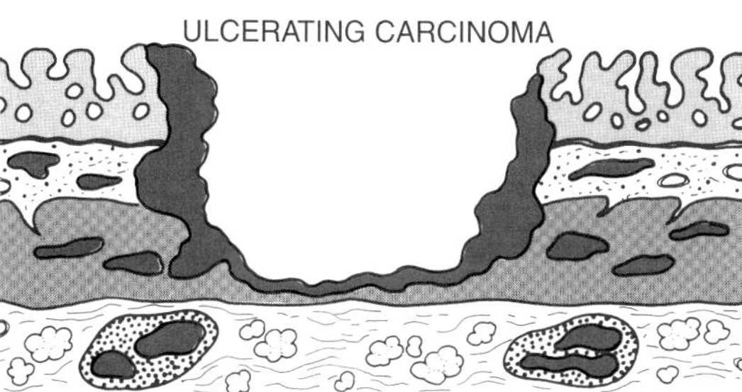

INFILTRATING CARCINOMA (LINITIS PLASTICA)

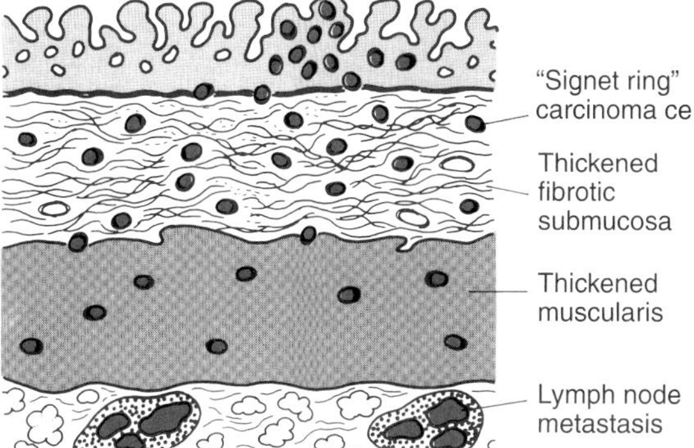

FIGURE 25-14. The major types of gastric cancer. (Rubin, E. & Farber, J. L. [1999]. *Pathology* [3rd ed.]. Philadelphia: Lippincott.)

The only definitive diagnostic test for gastric carcinoma is gastric biopsy, usually obtained through gastric endoscopy. Other studies may be helpful, such as barium swallow, blood work, and additional tests to demonstrate a mass in the gastric area.

Peritonitis

Peritonitis is an inflammation of the peritoneum. It may be caused by microorganisms or chemicals that have been introduced into the abdominal cavity. Most commonly, peritonitis is caused by the rupture of a diseased abdominal viscus such as an inflamed appendix or ulcerations anywhere in the gastrointestinal tract. Other causes may include rupture of the liver, spleen, ovarian cysts, and fallopian tubes. Bacterial organisms most often associated with peritonitis include *Escherichia coli*, *Bacteroides*, *Fusobacterium*, and various *Streptococcal* species.

Chemical peritonitis may be caused by substances such as pancreatic enzymes, hydrochloric acid, and blood that are released from the gastrointestinal tract into the peritoneal cavity. More rarely, foreign materials such as talc from surgical gloves may cause peritonitis.

Clinical manifestations of peritonitis are predominated by severe abdominal pain with rebound tenderness, abdominal rigidity, fever and chills, nausea and vomiting, rapid, shallow respirations, and dehydration. Severe peritonitis may be associated with paralytic ileus, septic shock, and heart failure.

Alterations in the Small Intestine

MALABSORPTION AND MALDIGESTION

Most nutrient absorption occurs in the small intestine. Any alteration of the integrity of the small bowel can result in malabsorption or maldigestion or both, whether the source is motor or mucosal. *Malabsorption* is a general term that refers to inadequate mucosal absorption of ingested nutrients and water. *Maldigestion* is a defect in chemical processes of the intraluminal digestion or at the brush border of the intestinal mucosa that results in the inability to absorb foodstuffs that have not been broken down adequately.

Virtually all nutrients are absorbed in the small intestine; thus, malabsorption syndromes are those affecting this area. Absorption of foodstuffs from the intestine consists of two phases: (1) luminal and (2) intestinal. The luminal phase consists of those processes that alter nutrients so that they can be absorbed. Examples of malabsorption dysfunction in the luminal phase include a deficiency in pancreatic enzyme secretion and inadequate biliary secretions. The intestinal phase includes those processes involved in transport of nutrients through the intestinal wall.[28] Abnormally functioning absorptive cells and microvilli, decreased absorptive area, and abnormal nutrient transport through the intestinal wall may all contribute to problems associated with absorption of nutrients in the intestinal phase.[19] Malabsorption may involve a single specific nutrient, such as vitamin B_{12}, or it may involve several or all major nutrient classes.

Causes of maldigestion include conditions such as decreased bile salts or decreased pancreatic enzymes. Hypersecretion of gastric acids, such as occurs with Zollinger-Ellison syndrome, can also contribute to maldigestion.

Clinical manifestations of malabsorption and maldigestion arise from inadequate absorption of foodstuffs or from secondary deficiencies that occur as a result of inadequate nutrient absorption. These may include weight loss, malnutrition, and the cachectic state.[28] Other manifestations may be steatorrhea, diarrhea, bloating and flatulence, and fluid and electrolyte imbalances.

VOMITING AND DIARRHEA

Because 3 to 6 L of gastrointestinal secretions fill the gastrointestinal lumen every day, excessive vomiting or diarrhea can lead to volume depletion and electrolyte abnormalities.[24] At high risk are elderly persons and young children, because they have less fluid in reserve and can suffer rapid depletion of fluid and electrolyte balance. Triggers of gastrointestinal losses include bacteria, viruses, drug reactions, toxins, and excessive use of laxatives and enemas.[15]

Emesis, or vomiting, is a complex reflex triggered by the CNS, which has a diffuse group of neurons located on the dorsal surface of the floor of the fourth ventricle called the **chemoreceptive trigger zone.** These neurons sense the presence of chemicals such as morphine or other stimuli in the blood and activate the vomiting center in the medulla. The vomiting center also can be directly activated by the stomach during gastrointestinal irritation by way of the sympathetic and vagal afferent neurons.[11] Figure 25-15 summarizes the physiology of the emesis response.

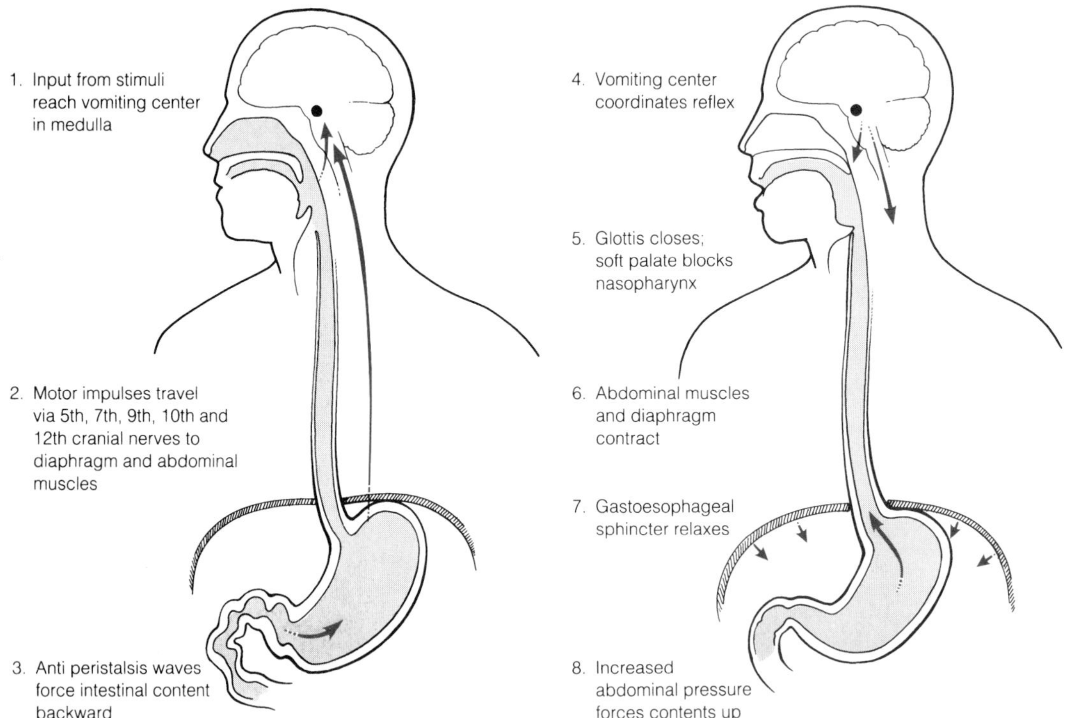
1. Input from stimuli reach vomiting center in medulla
2. Motor impulses travel via 5th, 7th, 9th, 10th and 12th cranial nerves to diaphragm and abdominal muscles
3. Anti peristalsis waves force intestinal content backward
4. Vomiting center coordinates reflex
5. Glottis closes; soft palate blocks nasopharynx
6. Abdominal muscles and diaphragm contract
7. Gastoesophageal sphincter relaxes
8. Increased abdominal pressure forces contents up

FIGURE 25-15. **Emesis response. Antiperistalsis is the first stage. Antiperistaltic waves travel backward from the intestine or stomach. Vomiting itself involves closure of the glottis, lifting of the soft palate to close the nares, and contraction of the diaphragm and abdominal muscles. The result of this is relaxation of the gastroesophageal sphincter, allowing expulsion of gastric contents through the esophagus.**

Varied conditions can stimulate the emesis response, and individuals are unique in their propensity for emesis. It may be associated with a pathologic condition, or it may be a response to stress, offensive odors, or other conditions of daily life (Box 25-4).

Diarrhea can be classified as *osmotic* or *secretory*.[26] Osmotic diarrhea occurs when there is a poorly absorbable solute in the alimentary tract. It contains large quantities of water and potassium. Copious osmotic diarrhea can lead to rapid fluid and potassium depletion. Secretory diarrhea results when the normal secretory processes are stimulated and electrolytes and water are not absorbed. Depletion of electrolytes, including sodium, bicarbonate, and potassium, occurs along with the water loss.[26] Rapid transit through the gastrointestinal tract typically occurs in diarrhea (Fig. 25-16).[26]

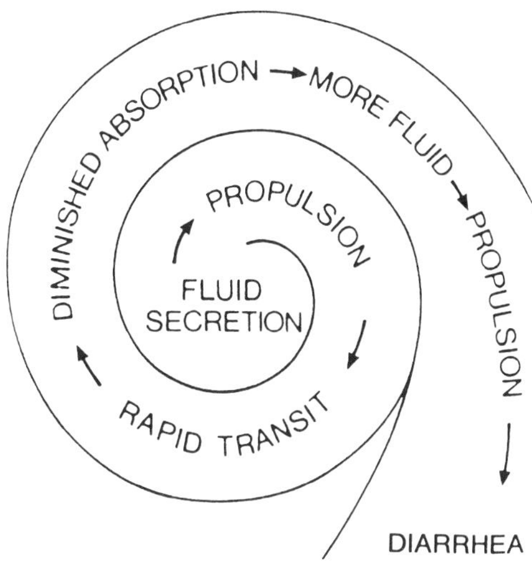

FIGURE 25-16. The diarrhea spiral. An increase in the amount of intraluminal fluid resulting from abnormalities in intestinal fluid and electrolyte transport initiate propulsive activity both by reflex and as a result of the same pathophysiologic processes that disturbed epithelial function. Rapid transit follows with decreased contact time and perhaps also with diminished surface area. This causes diminished absorption, more intralumenal fluid, more propulsion, and finally diarrhea. (Read, N. W. [1986]. Diarrhée motrice. *Clinical Gastroenterology, 15,* 657.)

ENTERITIS

Enteritis, or *gastroenteritis,* is an inflammatory process of the stomach or small intestine caused by viruses, bacteria, parasites, or allergic reactions. It may also be caused by the ingestion of contaminated food, especially food contaminated by staphylococci, which produce a toxin that reacts with the small intestine mucosa. Dysentery caused by bacteria affects the colon. The pathologic process has varying manifestations that result in abdominal cramping, diarrhea, and vomiting.

Eosinophilic enteritis is uncommon but may result from an allergy, as approximately half of these patients have an allergic history.[26] It is manifested by the accumulation of eosinophils in the gut wall. In general, enteritis causes inflammatory changes in the intestinal mucosa that return to normal when the precipitator is removed.

BOX 25-4 STIMULI FOR EMESIS RESPONSE

- Drugs
- Toxins
- Pregnancy
- Motion
- Alcohol consumption
- Radiation therapy
- Ketosis
- Pain
- Psychogenic conditions
- Infections
- Anesthesia
- Acute head injury
- Increased intracranial pressure
- Brain tumors
- Migraine headache
- Overdistention of gastrointestinal tract
- Obstruction of gastrointestinal tract
- Vestibular disease
- Fever

CELIAC ENTEROPATHY (NONTROPICAL SPRUE)

Celiac enteropathy is an intestinal disorder thought to be related to gluten intolerance. It occurs more often in women than in men, and the onset of symptoms usually occurs in young adulthood. Histopathologic changes in the absorptive surface occur in response to exposure to the protein gluten or its breakdown products, found mostly in wheat. A general malabsorption syndrome results. The mechanism underlying this reaction is unknown, but the data support a hypersensitivity reaction to gluten and its derivative, gliadin.[5]

Pathophysiology

Gluten proteins have been shown to have antigenic properties, and circulating antibodies to dietary gluten have been demonstrated in persons with active celiac enteropathy. The lamina propria of affected mucosa contains mononuclear leukocytes and plasma cells. In some cases, serum levels of IgA are elevated and levels of IgM are depressed.[5]

The intestinal villi are flattened or absent, and the epithelium is disorganized and consists of cuboidal rather than the normal columnar cells. The brush border is thickened, and the lamina propria is infiltrated with inflammatory cells. Cytoplasmic changes include membrane disruption and rounded mitochondria. All of these changes result in malabsorption, with impaired uptake and transport of nutrients.[28]

Clinical Manifestations

Clinical manifestations may include frequent, foul-smelling, steatorrheic stools with a fatty or greasy appearance. Loss of body weight and malabsorption of fat-soluble vitamins are common. Severe muscle wasting and hypoproteinemia may occur. The condition is most commonly diagnosed first in children who fail to thrive. When barley, wheat, rye, and oats are removed from the diet, a dramatic or delayed remission of symptoms occurs. There is restoration of the normal mucosal epithelium, and malabsorption decreases.

TROPICAL SPRUE

Tropical sprue differs in etiology from celiac enteropathy but is usually characterized by identical mucosal changes in the small intestine. It probably results from nutritional and bacterial alterations and occurs with the greatest frequency in certain tropical areas. It may be caused by *E. coli* bacteria. Symptoms may not arise for months or years after exposure.[5] Because the mucosal lesions result in malabsorption, the clinical picture closely resembles that of celiac enteropathy.

REGIONAL ENTERITIS: CROHN'S DISEASE

Crohn's disease is an idiopathic, chronic, inflammatory bowel disease that may affect any segment of the gastrointestinal tract, although it most commonly affects the terminal ileum or colon.[5] The frequency of this chronic inflammatory disease is equal in men and women, is higher in members of the Jewish race, and exhibits a familial predisposition. Onset is most common between the ages of 15 and 20, with a secondary peak between 55 and 60 years. It is much more common in the U.S., Britain, and Scandinavia than in Japan, Russia, and South America.[5] Crohn's disease and ulcerative colitis (discussed on page 744) have many etiologic similarities and commonly are grouped as *inflammatory bowel disease (IBD)*. The origins may be infectious, immunologic, psychosomatic, dietary, hormonal, or unknown. Viruses and specific bacteria, such as *Pseudomonas* and atypical mycobacteria, are possible causative factors. The immunologic features of the diseases may be a primary or secondary response to a vital organism.

Pathophysiology

Gross inspection of the affected bowel discloses shallow, longitudinal mucosal ulcers; long or short areas of stricture; and a cobblestone appearance of the mucosa. The cobblestone appearance results from interconnecting fissures that cut deeply into the intestinal wall and create islands of mucosa elevated by the existing transmural (full-wall thickness) inflammation and its accompanying edema.[9] Areas of involvement are localized and interrupted by areas of normal gut. Several segments of bowel are affected and often are separated by normal bowel. These segments are called *skip lesions* and produce chronic partial intestinal obstruction.[28] Fistulas to other parts of the gastrointestinal tract or other adjacent structures may be present.

Microscopically, all layers of the intestinal wall, particularly the submucosa, are edematous and infiltrated with aggregations of lymphocytes and macrophages.[5] Characteristic noncaseating granulomas, which have large mononuclear phagocytes and multinucleated giant cells, form in the bowel wall and often are present in the regional lymph nodes. Dilated lymphatic channels and lymphoid deposits occur at all levels of bowel involvement. The inflammatory changes cause functional disruption of the mucosa, producing malabsorption, especially of bile salts and vitamin B_{12}, which are normally absorbed in the jejunum and ileum. Fluid imbalances occur when large segments of the ileum are affected. The strictures and fistulas that occur with this disease predispose the intestine to bacterial overgrowth and abscess formation (Fig. 25-17). Bowel obstruction and peritonitis may result from the strictures and abscesses.

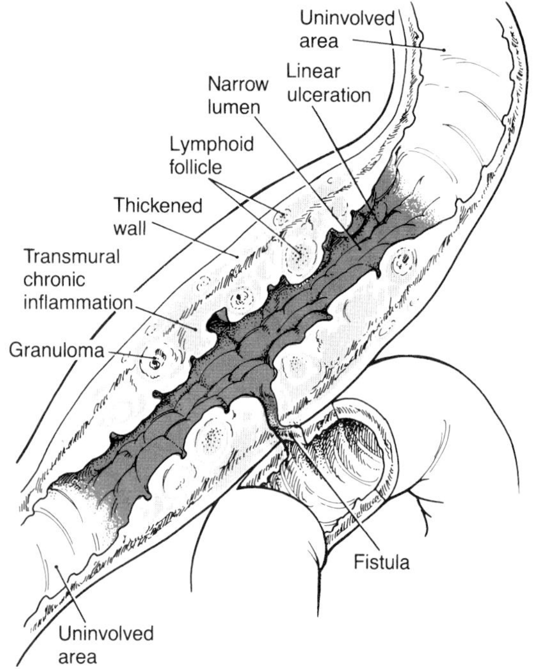

FIGURE 25-17. A schematic representation of the major features of Crohn's disease in the small intestine.

Clinical Manifestations

The clinical manifestations of Crohn's disease vary. Diarrhea is a dominant symptom and is often accompanied by fever and right lower quadrant or abdominal pain. The apparent linkage with stress and personality factors has been studied extensively, with depression and dependency being seen as typical personality traits. The symptoms usually begin with insidious onset of malaise and diarrhea. As the disease progresses, weight loss, occult blood in the feces, and nausea and vomiting occur. When involvement is diffuse, major features may be malabsorption and malnutrition. Intestinal obstruction and fistulas develop in 10% to 15% of cases, and peritonitis may result from rupture of the fistulous connection. A significant correlation of this disease with several autoimmune diseases and with adenocarcinoma of the small bowel exists. Chronic debilitation may finally require bowel resection.

Alterations in the Large Intestine

ADYNAMIC OR PARALYTIC ILEUS

An *ileus* is a functional obstruction of the bowel that may occur in the small or large intestine. It is often classified as physiologic or paralytic. Lack of propulsive peristalsis makes the bowel unable to move contents downward, which leads to absence of bowel sounds and bowel distention.

An ileus may be caused by the triggering of the sympathetic inhibitory reflex from noxious stimuli such as (1) anesthesia, (2) peritonitis, (3) appendicitis, (4) interruption of nerve supply, (5) abdominal injury or surgical manipulation, (6) intestinal ischemia, and (7) electrolyte (especially potassium) disturbances.[24] A true ileus can be described as *adynamic*, lacking propulsive motor activity.[28]

The result of ileus is distention of the bowel with gas and fluid. The process is similar to actual bowel obstruction. Colonic bacteria may contribute to the abdominal distention and cause marked alterations of fluid and electrolyte balance. Loss of potassium leads to further intestinal atony. Vomiting and hypotension can cause alteration in the acid-base balance. As fluid shifts to the intestinal area, central blood volume decreases and distention increases.[24] If there is associated mesenteric ischemia, necrosis and rupture of the bowel may occur, causing peritonitis. Clinical findings include abdominal distention, decreased or absent bowel sounds, and signs of dehydration and shock.

INTESTINAL ISCHEMIA AND INFARCTION

Intestinal ischemia occurs when tissue demand for oxygen exceeds the supply, and toxic metabolites accumulate. Ischemia is particularly prevalent in highly vascular systems, such as the mesentery, which supplies the intestines. Intestinal ischemia can result from any condition that interferes with blood supply to the mesentery. *Occlusive intestinal infarction* usually results from occlusion of the superior mesenteric artery by an embolus or a thrombus. It can also result from inferior mesenteric artery or venous thrombosis. *Nonocclusive intestinal infarction* may result from severe shock, in which blood is shunted away from the mesentery to other vital organs. *Chronic intestinal ischemia* may be produced by atherosclerosis of the superior mesenteric artery, which can produce abdominal angina, especially after eating. Ischemia may lead to patchy areas of infarction.

Clinical Manifestations

Symptoms of intestinal ischemia and infarction vary with the area affected and length of time of deprivation. Atherosclerotic ischemia may create an angina-like, cramping, abdominal pain that worsens after meals and then dissipates. Vasospasm and emboli produce an acute, severe abdominal pain with associated vomiting or diarrhea or both. Abdominal distention and tenderness are usually present. Bowel sounds may initially be loud and high-pitched (*borborygmi*) from an increase in rate and force of peristalsis. Hypotension may occur due to displacement of intravascular volume into the intestinal lumen.

If ischemia or infarction is prolonged, the epithelial cells in the intestinal villi detach from the basement membrane, causing loss of viable epithelial surface. This interferes with the absorption and processing of nutrients. The mucosal layer becomes necrotic and is shed into the stool as bloody diarrhea. Because the mucosal barrier is lost, intestinal bacteria can enter the bloodstream and cause bacteremia. Prolonged ischemia or infarction may also result in shock, peritonitis, or sepsis.

APPENDICITIS

Appendicitis is an inflammatory disease of the vermiform appendix. It is one of the most common causes of acute abdominal pain. Although the precise etiology of appendicitis is unknown, it is thought in many cases to result from obstruction of the appendix by fecal matter, tumors, or foreign bodies. The obstruction prevents drainage of the appendix and results in venous stasis and hypoxia of the tissue. Ulceration and microbial invasion eventually accompany the tissue hypoxia and result in gangrene and sometimes in perforation.

Clinical Manifestations

Clinical manifestations of appendicitis may evolve slowly and begin with right lower quadrant tenderness (McBurney's point) and epigastric discomfort that is attributable to indigestion. Some may experience periumbical pain, diarrhea, anorexia, nausea and vomiting, low-grade fever, and leukocytosis. In the elderly, appendicitis may manifest only as very mild discomfort until perforation is evident.

INTESTINAL OBSTRUCTION

Intestinal obstruction is blockage of the lumen of the bowel by an actual mechanical obstruction. Figure 25-18 illustrates some of the causes of intestinal obstruction.

Pathophysiology

After blockage occurs, gas and air are the primary bowel distenders, and distention occurs proximal to the area of blockage. As the process continues, gastric, biliary, and pancreatic secretions pool. Water, electrolytes, and serum proteins also begin to accumulate in the area. Pooling and bowel distention, shown in Figure 25-19, decrease the circulating blood volume due to a third-space shift. Bowel wall edema also interferes with the blood supply to the bowel tissue and depresses normal sodium transport in the mucosa.

Strangulation of a bowel segment may cause necrosis, perforation, and loss of fluid and blood into the inactive bowel. Impairment of blood supply leads at first to increased peristalsis and bacterial invasion of the tissue and finally causes necrosis and peritonitis when intestinal contents are released into the peritoneal cavity. Stasis of the intestinal contents provides an area for increased growth of organisms, with toxins being released into the tissues, further disrupting the intestinal cellular dynamics. Loss of fluids and electrolytes is a major problem and results in decreased systemic circulating fluid volume due to the shift from the vascular to the intestinal lumen.

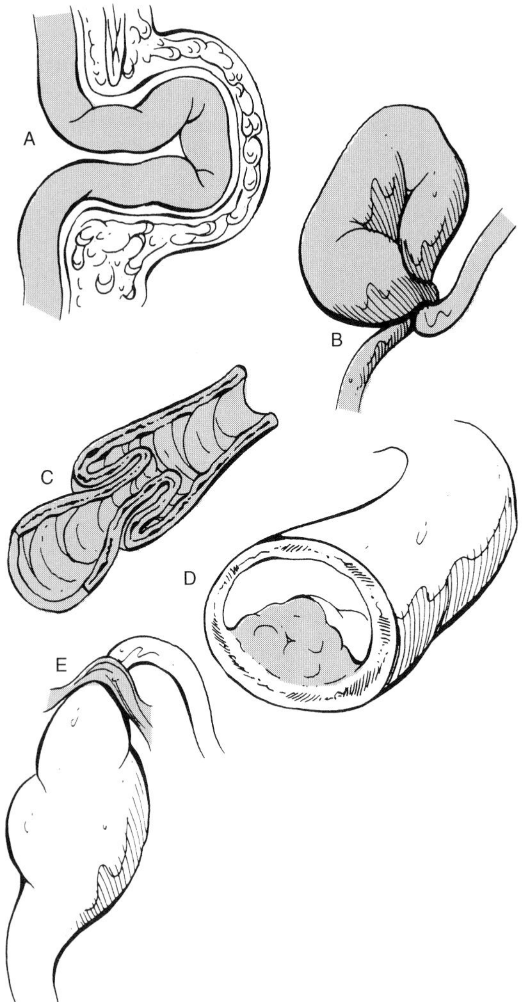

FIGURE 25-18. Major causes of actual intestinal obstruction. **A.** Hernia. **B.** Volvulus. **C.** Intussusception. **D.** Neoplasm. **E.** Adhesions.

Clinical Manifestations

Clinical manifestations include the acute onset of severe, cramping pain that correlates roughly to the area or level of obstruction. Pain may decrease in severity as distention of the bowel and abdomen increases, probably due to impaired motility in the edematous intestine. Increases in the rate and force of peristalsis cause borborygmi in the early period, but these may progress to a silent bowel as the condition persists. Vomiting is almost always present and may be bilious or feculent (having the appearance of feces), depending on the level of the obstruction. Diarrhea may occur if obstruction is not complete.

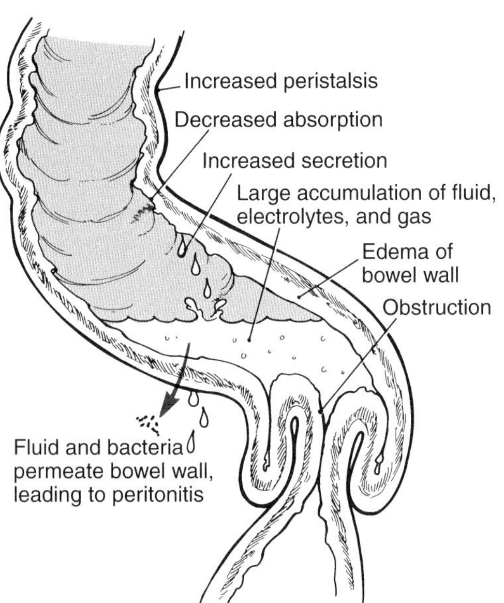

FIGURE 25-19. Pathophysiology of intestinal obstruction causing peritonitis.

Hypovolemic shock results with a shift of fluid greater than 10% of body weight. Septic shock may result from the release of intestinal gram-negative organisms into the vascular system or from contamination of the peritoneum when the bowel ruptures. Sepsis and hypovolemic shock produce a life-threatening clinical picture that must be treated aggressively.

Abdominal tenderness and rigidity and fever usually indicate peritonitis. Leukocytosis and elevation of serum amylase levels are also common. Distention of the bowel may be noted radiologically but is not conclusive evidence of the cause or exact level of obstruction.

HERNIAS

A *hernia* is a defect in the abdominal wall. It may occur in the scrotal or inguinal area or in the abdominal wall or diaphragm, as shown in Figure 25-20. Incisional hernias occur in an area weakened by surgical incision. Whatever the cause, the defect allows abdominal structures (e.g., peritoneum, fat, bowel, or bladder) to fill the area, producing a sac filled with the material. Abdominal contents usually move into the defect when abdominal pressure increases. If the bulging of the sac is intermittent, the hernia is called *reducible*. *Incarcerated hernias* contain trapped abdominal contents that are poorly drained by the venous circulation due to pressure at the neck of the orifice. *Strangulated hernias* cause necrosis of the abdominal contents due to lack of blood supply. Ischemia and necrosis of the bowel associated with these hernias reflect the clinical manifestations of intestinal obstruction.

MEGACOLON

Megacolon, or enlargement of the colon, may also be produced by any process that inhibits bowel evacuation. Among such processes are psychogenic megacolon, which results from ignoring the urge to defecate; some neurologic disorders; fecal impaction; and chronic depression. The clinical manifestations depend on the degree of aganglionosis or bowel distention. The person is often poorly nourished and anemic and rarely produces fecal material.

HIRSCHSPRUNG'S DISEASE

Hirschsprung's disease, also called *congenital megacolon*, is usually manifested in early infancy and is caused by congenital absence of parasympathetic ganglion cells in the submucosal and intramuscular plexuses of one or more segments of the colon. The entire colon and even parts of the small intestine are occasionally involved. When the colon is involved, the bowel becomes greatly dilated, with no peristaltic action in the aganglionic area.

Hirschsprung's disease is a congenital disorder with much higher frequency in boys than in girls. It is associated with other congenital conditions, such as *Down syndrome*. When manifested in early infancy, abdominal distention, constipation, and vomiting occur. Occasionally, this condition is diagnosed in young adults who describe a lifelong problem with constipation.

DIVERTICULAR DISEASE

Diverticula are multiple saclike protrusions of the mucosa along the gastrointestinal tract. Although the terms are loosely used, a *true diverticulum* has all layers of the bowel in its walls, whereas a *false diverticulum* occurs in a weak area of the muscularis of the bowel. False colonic diverticula are common and usually occur in the sigmoid colon.

An example of true diverticular disease is *Meckel's diverticulum*, which occurs in 1% to 2% of the population. Two thirds of affected persons are younger than 2 years of age. The diverticular sac, located 1 to 3 feet

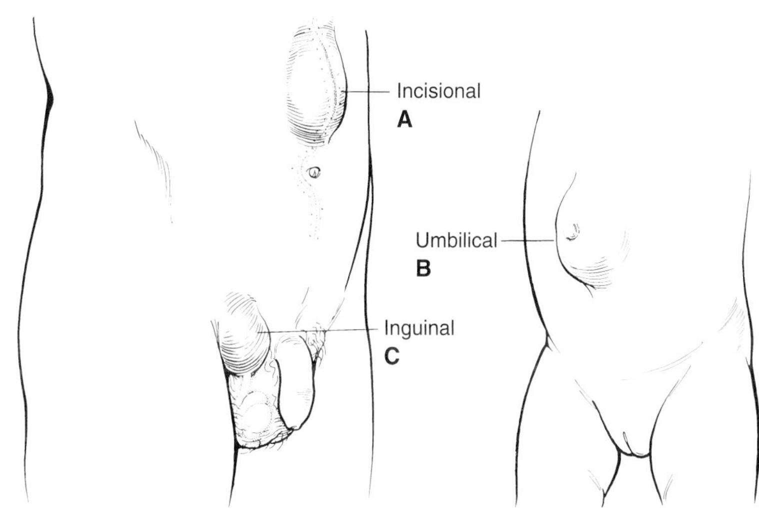

FIGURE 25-20. Types of hernia. **A.** Incisional hernia. **B.** Umbilical hernia. **C.** Inguinal hernia.

proximal to the ileocecal junction, is formed by the persistence of a mesenteric structure that normally closes in fetal life. It may be lined with ileal mucosa or contain other types of gastrointestinal mucosal cells. Meckel's diverticulum is usually asymptomatic, but it may cause symptoms that mimic acute appendicitis, Crohn's disease, or pelvic inflammatory disease. Gastrointestinal bleeding and intestinal obstruction may complicate the condition.[28]

Because of their frequency in elderly persons, diverticula are thought to be related to the blood supply or nutrition of the bowel in the elderly.[5] Lack of dietary fiber or roughage and decreased fecal bulk also have been correlated with this process.[28]

Diverticulosis refers to the presence of diverticula in the colon that are rarely symptomatic. *Diverticulitis* is inflammation in or around a diverticular sac that results in retention of undigested food and bacteria in the sac. This forms a hard mass called a *fecalith*.[28] Colonic obstruction, fistulas, and abscesses can result. Rupture of the infected material into the peritoneal cavity may lead to peritonitis.

The clinical manifestations of symptomatic diverticular disease vary. Eighty percent of affected persons have no symptoms. Constipation is reported frequently. Fibrosis in the area may develop and cause obstruction by adhesions. The complaint of lower left-sided abdominal pain may be associated with the signs of peritonitis, including guarding, fever, abdominal rigidity, and rebound tenderness. Radiographs and sigmoidoscopy may not indicate the extent of the problem.

HEMORRHOIDS

Hemorrhoids are dilatations of the venous plexus that surround the rectal and anal areas. These dilatations are very common and develop in susceptible persons due to persistently increased pressure in the hemorrhoidal venous plexus. Hemorrhoids are often related to other types of abnormalities, especially varicose veins. Predisposition may result from constipation or pregnancy. Bleeding hemorrhoids may be a dangerous outcome of portal hypertension (see Chapter 26).

The dilated venous sacs protrude into the anal and rectal canals, where they become exposed; thromboses, ulcerations, and bleeding then develop. Hemorrhoids may be painful and irritating. Bright red bleeding during defecation or with increased intra-abdominal pressure is common. Blood loss is usually insignificant, but chronic iron-deficiency anemia may result.[28]

ULCERATIVE COLITIS

Ulcerative colitis is primarily an inflammatory disease of the mucous membrane of the colon. The disease may be confined to the rectum, or it may affect segments of the colon or even the entire colon. The bowel fills with a bloody, mucoid secretion that produces a characteristic cramping pain, rectal urgency, and diarrhea.

The etiology of ulcerative colitis is unknown, but a genetic basis has been suggested because the disease occurs with increased frequency in some families. It occurs between ages 20 and 40, and it is much more common in whites than in other races.[14] Viruses, microorganisms, and autoimmunity have been implicated in this disease. The plasma serum in some persons with the disease has been shown to have an antibody to the colonic epithelial cells. Many of the etiologic factors of Crohn's disease are also common in ulcerative colitis.

Pathophysiology

Pathologically, ulcerative colitis usually begins in the rectal area and extends along the colon. Microscopic, inflammatory, ulcerated areas may be adjacent to healing areas, but the process is continuous, without the skip lesions characteristic of Crohn's disease.[5] In the *acute phase*, the colon mucosa is hyperemic and edematous and the usual secretions are absent. Small mucosal hemorrhages are evident, and abscesses form into small ulcerations. The mucosa tends to slough off and is lost in the feces. The ulcerations are confined to the mucosa and submucosa, and coalescence of the ulcers can denude large areas of the involved colon.[5] As the disease enters the *chronic phase*, the ulcerations become fibrotic and the bowel wall shortens and thickens.[28]

Clinical Manifestations

Clinical manifestations vary. The classic symptoms include cramping abdominal pain, bloody diarrhea, fever, and weight loss. Laboratory findings include anemia, leukocytosis, hypoalbuminemia, electrolyte imbalance, and increased serum alkaline phosphatase levels. Remissions and exacerbations are common and often can be directly related to major psychological stresses.[14] About 70% of affected persons have complete remissions between attacks, some of which may last for long periods. Approximately 20% have continuous symptoms without remission.[28] Despite their evident pathologic differences, ulcerative colitis and regional enteritis may be confused clinically; Table 25-7 shows the major differences between them.

Complications of ulcerative colitis include intestinal obstruction, dehydration, and major fluid and electrolyte imbalances. Malabsorption is common, and loss of blood in the stools may cause chronic iron-deficiency anemia. There is a significant relationship between ulcerative colitis and cancer of the colon. Ten percent to 15% of persons who have ul-

TABLE 25-7

MAJOR DIFFERENCES BETWEEN ULCERATIVE COLITIS AND CROHN'S DISEASE

LESION	CROHN'S DISEASE	ULCERATIVE COLITIS
MACROSCOPIC		
Thickened bowel wall	Typical	Uncommon
Luminal narrowing	Typical	Uncommon
"Skip" lesions	Common	Absent
Right colon predominance	Typical	Absent
Fissures and fistulas	Common	Absent
Circumscribed ulcers	Common	Absent
Confluent linear ulcers	Common	Absent
Pseudopolyps	Absent	Common
MICROSCOPIC		
Transmural inflammation	Typical	Uncommon
Submucosal fibrosis	Typical	Absent
Fissures	Typical	Rare
Granulomas	Common	Absent
Crypt abscesses	Uncommon	Typical

(Rubin, E. & Farber, J. L. [1999]. *Pathology* [3rd ed.]. Philadelphia: Lippincott.)

cerative colitis for more than 10 years will develop colon carcinoma.

POLYPS

A *polyp* in the large intestine is a benign growth that protrudes into the lumen. Polyps are divided into two major categories: (1) neoplastic (adenomatous and carcinomas) and (2) non-neoplastic (e.g., hyperplastic, inflammatory). *Adenomatous* polyps are thought to occur when cells deep within the crypts of the colonic mucosal glands proliferate outward from the crypt base, as shown in Figure 25-21.[16] Reproductive control is lost, so the cells continue to grow, forming the polyp. *Hyperplastic* polyps are raised lesions on the colonic mucosa from proliferation associated with many different entities.

Polyps are very common in the general population. They may be discovered by routine sigmoidoscopy or barium enema. They are most commonly less than 1 cm in diameter.[16] Although most are asymptomatic, they may cause symptoms by virtue of their protrusion into the bowel lumen; they may bleed, cause abdominal pain, or actually obstruct the intestine.[16]

The major clinical significance of hyperplastic polyps is that they have the potential to become neoplastic or adenomatous. Adenomatous polyps may be benign or malignant; it is difficult to determine the difference unless they have obviously invaded the surrounding mucosa. Smaller growths are called *tubular* or *glandular polyps*, and larger growths are called *villous adenomas*. Twenty-five percent to 50% of villous adenomas harbor carcinomas. These adenomas may be very large, up to 15 cm across.[28]

Some researchers believe that polyps develop through a series of stages from controlled hyperplasia to eventual carcinoma.[5] Polyps are usually surgically excised because they have such a close relationship with carcinoma of the colon.

COLORECTAL CARCINOMA

Colorectal carcinoma remains second only to lung cancer in causes of death from cancer in the United States. When colon and rectal cancer is detected and treated in early localized stages, there is a 5-year survival rate of 90.5%.[29] Factors that predispose a person to colorectal cancer are heredity, previous colorectal carcinomas, smoking, alcohol abuse, fat intake, inflammatory bowel disease, obesity, and polyposis of the colon.[29] It is common in both men and women; it occurs at all ages, but 90% occurs in persons older than 50 years of age, with the risk increasing sharply at the age of 40.[3] Prevalence is highest in northwest Europe and North America and lowest in South America, Africa, and Asia.

Investigations into causes of colorectal carcinoma have led to the study of animal fat in the diet, anaerobic bacteria of the large bowel, and fiber content of the

FOCUS ON CELLULAR PATHOPHYSIOLOGY

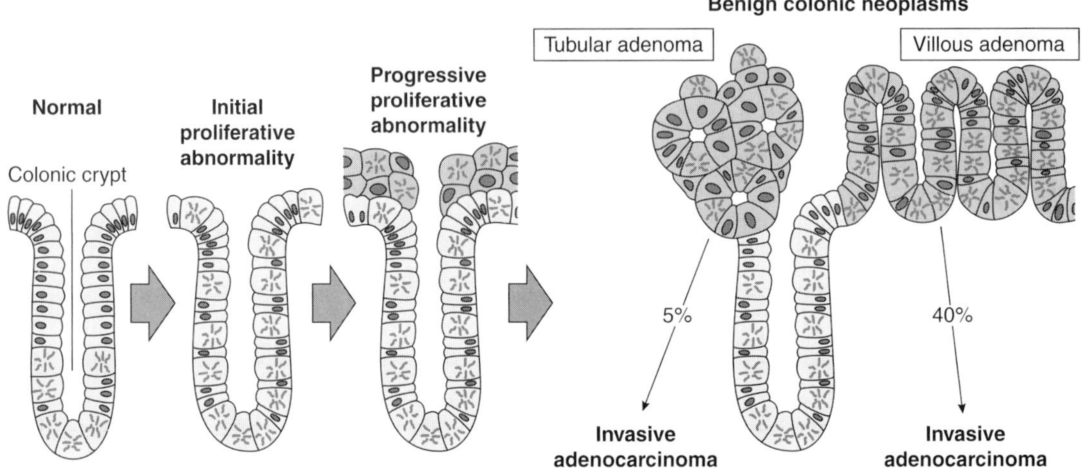

FIGURE 25-21. The histogenesis of adenomatous polyps of the colon. The initial proliferative abnormality of the colonic mucosa, the extension of the mitotic zone in the crypts, leads to the accumulation of mucosal cells. The formation of adenomas may reflect epithelial-mesenchymal interactions. (Rubin, E. & Farber, J. L. [1999], *Pathology* [3rd ed.]. Philadelphia: Lippincott.)

diet.[29] Each of these factors may partially explain the disease's geographic distribution. The fiber aspect is interesting in that increased bulk in the diet decreases the transit time and also the time of contact between food and bowel. In the average American diet, the transit time may be as much as 4 to 5 days compared with 30 to 35 hours in black Africans. Because the American diet is much lower in fiber than the black African diet, colonic cancer is much more prevalent in America.[5]

Pathophysiology

About 60% to 70% of these carcinomas arise in the rectum, rectosigmoid area, or sigmoid colon.[5] The type of growth depends on the area of origin. Left-sided carcinoma tends to grow around the bowel, encircling it and leading to early obstruction. On the right side, the tumors tend to be bulky, polypoid, fungating masses. The vast majority of these cancers are adenocarcinomas. Either type may penetrate the bowel and cause abscess, peritonitis, invasion of surrounding organs, or bleeding. These tumors tend to grow slowly, and they remain asymptomatic for long periods of time. Ninety-five percent of carcinomas of the colon are adenocarcinomas that secrete mucin, a substance that aids in extending the malignancy.[5] Metastasis may occur to the liver, lungs, bones, or lymphatic system.

Clinical Manifestations

Clinical manifestations depend on the location of the tumor. The person may have melena, diarrhea, and constipation; these are the most frequent manifestations of left-sided lesions. Right-sided tumors often cause weakness, malaise, and weight loss. Pain is rare with either type and, if present, may result from contractions of the bowel related to partial obstruction of the colon or nerve involvement. The tumor mass is often palpated on physical examination. Obstruction of the bowel may be the first sign of the disease. Metastasis is quite predictable, with invasion of the lymphatic channels, peritoneum, and venous channels producing the spread. The common sites of distant metastasis are the lungs, bones, and brain.[28] At the time of diagnosis, some extension of the tumor often has occurred, but because this malignancy grows slowly, it is considered to be highly curable with early diagnosis and surgical treatment.

Proctoscopy, barium enema, radionucleotide scanning, and determination of levels of tumor antigens help reveal the region and extent of involvement. Colon cancers produce a wide variety of tumor antigens, carcinoembryonic antigen (CEA) being the most well known. The test for CEA is positive in nearly all cases with widespread metastases.

The prognosis for colorectal carcinoma depends on the extent of bowel involvement, the presence or absence of spread, differentiation of the lesion, and the location of the lesion within the colon. Various classification systems exist for staging of colorectal cancer. The TNM classification system for staging colorectal cancer is delineated in Table 25-8, and the Dukes classification of the stages is shown in Figure 25-22.

TABLE 25-8

TNM CLINICAL CLASSIFICATION SYSTEM FOR STAGING COLORECTAL CANCER

PRIMARY TUMOR (T)

TX Minimum requirements to assess the primary tumor cannot be met
T0 No evidence of primary tumor
Tis Carcinoma in situ
T1 Tumor extends to the submucosa
T2 Tumor extends to the muscularis propria
T3 Tumor extends through the muscularis propria into the subserosa or into the subserosa or into nonperitonealized pericolic or perirectal tissues
T4 Tumor extends directly into other organs or tissues, or tumor perforates the visceral peritoneum of the specimen

REGIONAL LYMPH NODES (N)

NX Minimum requirements to assess the regional lymph nodes cannot be met
N0 No lymph node metastasis
N1 Metastatic tumor in 1–3 pericolic or perirectal lymph nodes
N2 Metastatic tumor in ≥4 pericolic or perirectal lymph nodes
N3 Metastatic to any lymph node along the course of a major named vascular trunk

DISTANT METASTASIS (M)

MX Minimum requirements to assess distant metastasis cannot be met
M0 No distant metastasis
M1 Distant metastasis present

STAGE GROUPINGS	TNM	DUKES CLASSIFICATION
Stage 0	T_{is}, N0, M0	
Stage I	T1, N0, M0	
	T2, N0, M0	A
Stage II	T2, N0, M0	
	T4, N0, M0	B
Stage III	Any T, N1, M0	
	Any T, N2, M0	C
	Any T, N3, M0	
Stage IV	Any T, Any N, M1	

(Meyers, M. A. [Ed.] [1998]. *Neoplasms of the digestive tract: Imaging, staging, and management.* Philadelphia: Lippincott-Raven, p. 308.)

FOCUS ON CELLULAR PATHOPHYSIOLOGY

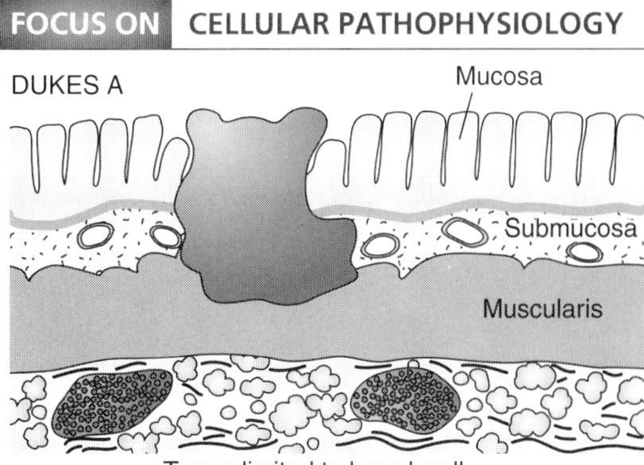

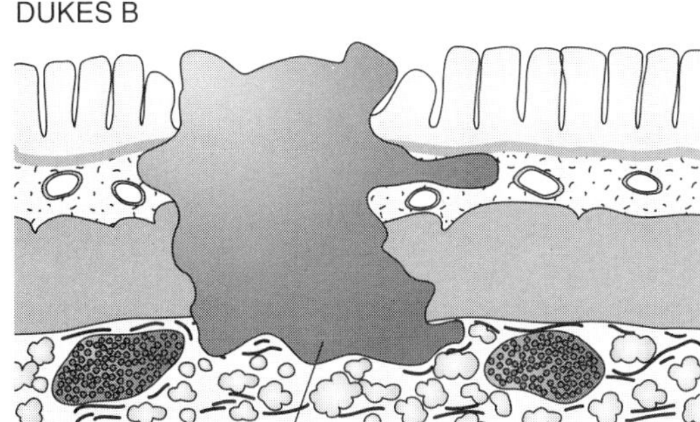

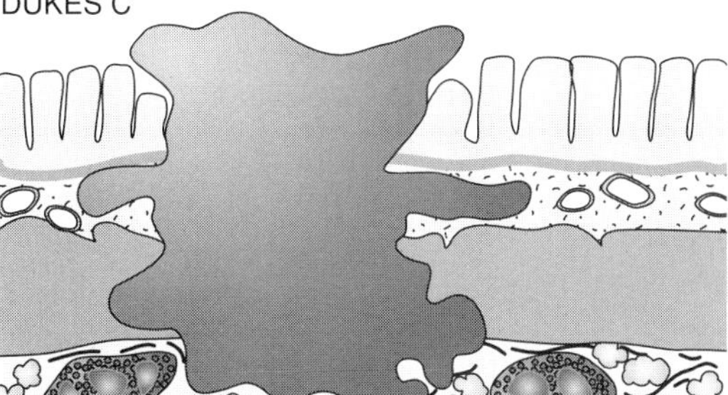

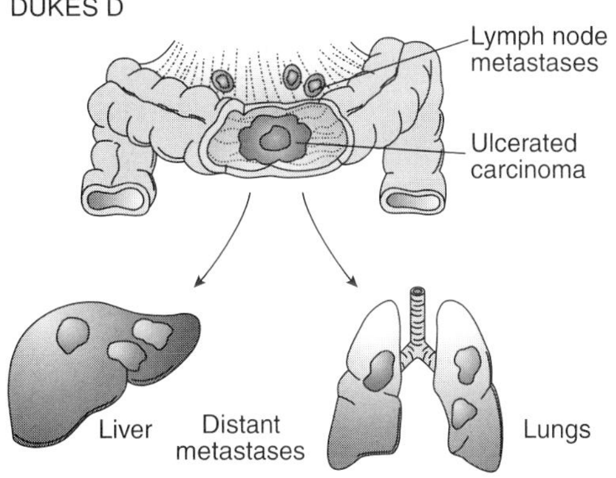

FIGURE 25-22. Dukes classification of the stages of carcinoma of the colon. (Source: Rubin, E. & Farber, J. L. [Eds.] [1999] *Pathology* [3rd ed.]. Philadelphia: Lippincott.)

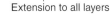

FOCUS ON THE CLIENT WITH COLON CANCER

Mr. F. is a 68-year-old Caucasian male who is undergoing evaluation for melena, diarrhea, and constipation. A questionable mass was palpated in the left lower quadrant by the examining physician. Proctoscopy revealed a polypoid lesion, which was biopsied; pathology reported carcinoma of the colon. Barium enema showed significant obstruction in the descending portion of the colon. CEA levels were tested and were shown to be 860 ng/mL (normal levels less than 2.5 ng/mL).

Questions

1. From the symptoms and diagnostic tests, what type of colon cancer does Mr. F. have?
2. What is the significance of the CEA levels?
3. When these cancers metastasize, what is the common route for the spread?
4. What are the risk factors for developing cancer of the colon? List at least four factors that may decrease the risk of this type of cancer.

REFERENCES

1. Axelrad, A. M., & Fleischer, D. E. (1998). Esophageal tumors. In M. Feldman, B. F. Scharschmidt, & M. H. Sleisenger (Eds.), *Sleisenger and Fordran's gastrointestinal and liver disease: Pathophysiology/diagnosis/management, vol. 1* (6th ed.). Philadelphia: Saunders.
2. Branch, M. S., Branzer, S. R., & Taylor, I. L. (1994). Peptic ulcer disease: Medical and surgical management. In G. Gitnick (Ed.), *Principles and practice of gastroenterology and hepatology* (2nd ed.). Norwalk, CT: Appleton & Lange.
3. Bresalier, R. S., & Kim, Y. S. (1998). Malignant neoplasms of the large intestine. In M. Feldman, B. F. Scharschmidt, & M. H. Sleisenger (Eds.), *Sleisenger and Fordran's gastrointestinal and liver disease: Pathophysiology/diagnosis/management, vol. 2* (6th ed.). Philadelphia: Saunders.
4. Clouse, R. E. & Diamant, N. E. (1998). Motor physiology and motor disorders of the esophagus. In M. Feldman, B. F. Scharschmidt, & M. H. Sleisenger (Eds.), *Sleisenger and Fordran's gastrointestinal and liver disease: Pathophysiology/diagnosis/management, vol. 1* (6th ed.). Philadelphia: Saunders.
5. Cotran, R. S., Kumar, V., & Robbins, S. L. (1994). *Robbins' pathologic basis of disease* (5th ed.). Philadelphia: Saunders.
6. DeVita, V. T., et al. (1993). *Cancer: Principles and practice of oncology* (4th ed.). Philadelphia: J. B. Lippincott.
7. Dharmsathaphorn, K. (1994). Transport of water and electrolytes in the gastrointestinal tract. In R. G. Narins, *Maxwell and Kleeman's clinical disorders of fluid and electrolyte balance* (5th ed.). New York: McGraw-Hill.
8. Eastwood, G. L. (1994). Gastritis and other gastric diseases. In J. H. Stein (Ed.), *Internal medicine* (4th ed.). St. Louis: C. V. Mosby.
9. Farmer, R. G. (1994). Crohn's disease. In G. Gitnick (Ed.), *Principles and practice of gastroenterology and hepatology* (2nd ed.). Norwalk, CT: Appleton & Lange.
10. Ganong, W. F. (1994). *Review of medical physiology* (16th ed.). Norwalk, CT: Appleton & Lange.
11. Guyton, A. C. & Hall, J. E. (1996). *Textbook of medical physiology* (9th ed.). Philadelphia: Saunders.
12. Hansson, L. E. (1997). Gastric cancer. In J. F. Johanson (Ed.), *Gastrointestinal diseases: Risk factors and prevention.* Philadelphia: Lippincott-Raven.
13. Harford, W. V. (1998). Diverticula of the hypopharynx and esophagus, the stomach, and the small bowel. In M. Feldman, B. F. Scharschmidt, & M. H. Sleisenger (Eds.), *Sleisenger and Fordran's gastrointestinal and liver disease: Pathophysiology/diagnosis/management, vol. 1* (6th ed.). Philadelphia: Saunders.
14. Harris, M. L. & Bayless, T. M. (1994). Ulcerative colitis. In G. Gitnick (Ed.), *Principles and practice of gastroenterology and hepatology* (2nd ed.). Norwalk, CT: Appleton & Lange.
15. Hasler, W. L. (1997). Approach to the patient with nausea and vomiting. In W. N. Kelley (Ed.), *Textbook of internal medicine, vol. 1* (3rd ed.). Philadelphia: Lippincott-Raven.
16. Itzkowitz, S. H. & Kim, Y. S. (1998). Colonic polyps and polyposis syndromes. In M. Feldman, B. F. Scharschmidt, & M. H. Sleisenger (Eds.), *Sleisenger and Fordran's gastrointestinal and liver disease: Pathophysiology/diagnosis/management, vol. 2* (6th ed.). Philadelphia: Saunders.
17. Kahrilas, P. J. (1998). Gastroesophageal reflux disease and its complications. In M. Feldman, B. F. Scharschmidt, & M. H. Sleisenger (Eds.), *Sleisenger and Fordran's gastrointestinal and liver disease: Pathophysiology/diagnosis/management, vol. 1* (6th ed.). Philadelphia: Saunders.
18. Laine, L. (1998). Acute and chronic gastrointestinal bleeding. In M. Feldman, B. F. Scharschmidt, & M. H. Sleisenger (Eds.), *Sleisenger and Fordran's gastrointestinal and liver disease: Pathophysiology/diagnosis/management, vol. 1* (6th ed.). Philadelphia: Saunders.
19. Long, J. D. & Orlando, R. C. (1998). Anatomy and developmental and acquired abnormalities of the esophagus. In M. Feldman, B. F. Scharschmidt, & M. H. Sleisenger (Eds.), *Sleisenger and Fordran's gastrointestinal and liver disease: Pathophysiology/diagnosis/management, vol. 1* (6th ed.). Philadelphia: Saunders.
20. McCarthy, D. M. (1994). Hypergastrinemic peptic ulcer disease. In G. Gitnick (Ed.), *Principles and practice of gastroenterology and hepatology* (2nd ed.). Norwalk, CT: Appleton & Lange.
21. McMinn, R. M. H., Hutchings, R. T., & Logan, B. M. (1998). *The concise handbook of human anatomy.* London: Manson Publishing.
22. MacDonald, W. C. (1994). Gastric tumors. In G. Gitnick (Ed.), *Principles and practice of gastroenterology and hepatology* (2nd ed.). Norwalk, CT: Appleton & Lange.
23. Mansfield, P. F. (1998). Management of gastric carcinoma. In M. A. Meyers (Ed.), *Neoplasms of the digestive tract: Imaging, staging, and management.* Philadelphia: Lippincott-Raven.
24. Metheny, N. (1996). *Fluid and electrolyte balance* (3rd ed.). Philadelphia: J. B. Lippincott.
25. Peterson, W. L., & Richardson, C.T. (1994). Peptic ulcer disease. In J. H. Stein (Ed.), *Internal medicine* (4th ed.). St. Louis: C. V. Mosby.

26. Powell, D. W. (1995). Approach to the patient with diarrhea. In T. Yamada (Ed.), *Textbook of gastroenterology, vol. 1* (2nd ed.). Philadelphia: J. B. Lippincott.
27. Roth, J. A., Putnam, Jr., J. B., Rich, T.A., & Forastiere, A. A. (1997). Cancer of the esophagus. In V. T. DeVita, Jr., S. Hellman, & S. A. Rosenberg (Eds.), *Cancer: Principles and practice of oncology, vol. 1* (5th ed.). Philadelphia: Lippincott-Raven.
28. Rubin, E. & Farber, J. L. (1999). *Pathology* (3rd ed.). Philadelphia: Lippincott.
29. Sandler, R. S. (1997). Colorectal cancer. In J. F. Johanson (Ed.), *Gastrointestinal diseases: Risk factors and prevention.* Philadelphia: Lippincott-Raven.
30. Schultze-Delrieu, K. S., & Summers, R. W. (1994). Esophageal diseases. In J. H. Stein (Ed.), *Internal medicine* (4th ed.). St. Louis: C. V. Mosby.
31. Shearman, D. J., & Finlayson, N. D. (1997). *Diseases of the gastrointestinal tract and liver* (3rd ed.). Edinburgh: Churchill Livingstone.
32. Sherlock, S. & Dooley, J. (1997). *Diseases of the liver and biliary system* (10th ed.). London: Blackwell Science.
33. Spiro, H. M. (1993). *Clinical gastroenterology* (4th ed.). New York: Macmillan.
34. Tortora, G. J., & Grabowski, S. R. (1993). *Principles of anatomy and physiology* (7th ed.). New York: Harper Collins.

Chapter

26

Normal and Altered Hepatobiliary and Pancreatic Exocrine Function

Denise A. Tucker

KEY TERMS

acinar cells
amylase
ascites
asterixis
biliary colic
bilirubin
cholecystokinin
cholestasis
cirrhosis
deamination
glucagon
gluconeogenesis
glycogen
glycogenesis
glycogenolysis
fulminant hepatic failure
hepatic encephalopathy
hepatitis
hepatocytes
jaundice
Kuppfer cells
lipase

The liver has a wide range of intricate metabolic functions. Its large, functional reserve accounts for the lack of clinical signs of dysfunction until approximately 90% of the organ is greatly diseased or damaged. This chapter includes a basic review of liver structure and function as well as the functions of the gallbladder and pancreas. Alterations in liver, gallbladder, and pancreas function are also discussed.

NORMAL HEPATOBILIARY AND PANCREATIC EXOCRINE FUNCTION

The Liver

STRUCTURE OF THE LIVER

The *liver* is a large, glandular organ weighing approximately 1.5 kg in the adult. It is composed of the right and left lobe (Fig. 26-1). The right lobe contains two lobes called the *quadrate* and *caudate* lobes. The lobes consist of many lobules that perform the functions of the liver. The lobules process many substances in the **hepatocytes**, the parenchymal cells of the liver. The venous blood supply, carried by a branch of the portal vein, carries highly concentrated foodstuffs, including fats, carbohydrates, and proteins that have been absorbed from the small intestine. The arterial blood supply provides high concentrations of oxygen for the metabolism of these substances. The lobules are composed of sinusoids, rows of cuboidal hepatocytes, bile capillaries, and branches of the hepatic artery and portal vein (Fig. 26-2). The sinusoids and surrounding hepatocytes process the raw materials delivered to the liver from the small intestine.

The sinusoids are lined with cells of the mononuclear phagocyte system, which are called **Kupffer cells**. The porous endothelial lining allows plasma proteins to pass from the sinusoid to a narrow space around the hepatocyte, called the *space of Disse.*[6] This space connects with the lymphatic system and allows drainage of plasma proteins and excess fluid.

Within the liver lobules are *canaliculi,* which hold the bile produced by the hepatocytes. A meshwork of bile ducts forms from the canaliculi and terminates eventually in the common bile duct, which empties into the duodenum during digestion. The gallbladder receives bile from the liver and then stores, concentrates, and releases it into the common bile duct under appropriate stimulation.

Blood Supply

Blood is supplied to the liver through divisions of the hepatic artery and portal vein, which pass through the complex sinusoidal network to form venules and veins. An admixture of venous and arterial blood is

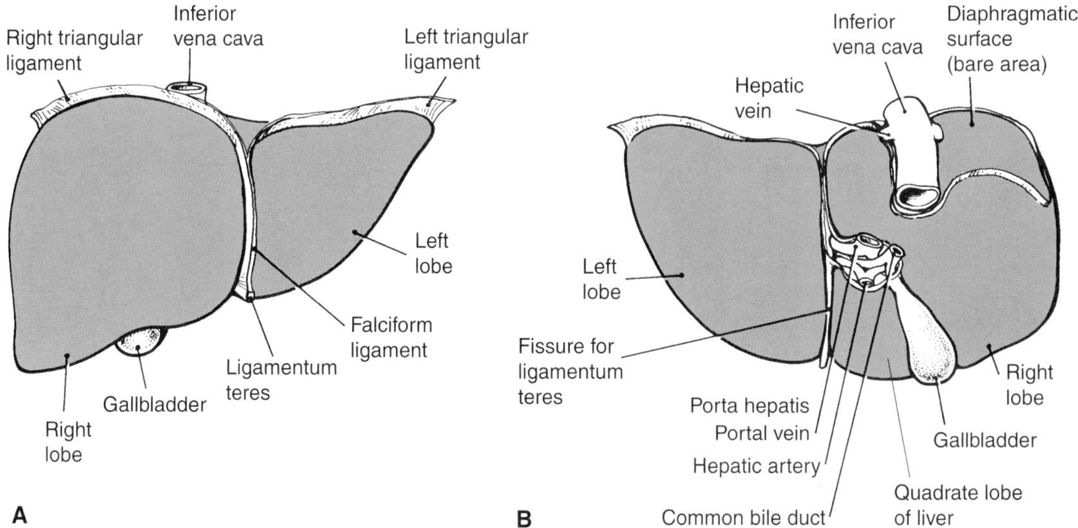

FIGURE 26-1. **A.** Anterior view of the liver. **B.** Posterior view of the liver. Note the location of the gall bladder.

carried into the sinusoids, which are the capillaries of the liver and provide both oxygen and nutrients to be processed. The venules and veins terminate in the hepatic vein, which empties into the inferior vena cava. The liver requires access to a large quantity of the circulation; about 30% of the cardiac output flows through the liver each minute, making this organ a large reservoir for blood. Even with its large volume and flow, the pressure in the portal system remains low. The liver can distend and increase its volume by a great margin before portal pressure increases.[2]

FOCUS ON CELLULAR PHYSIOLOGY

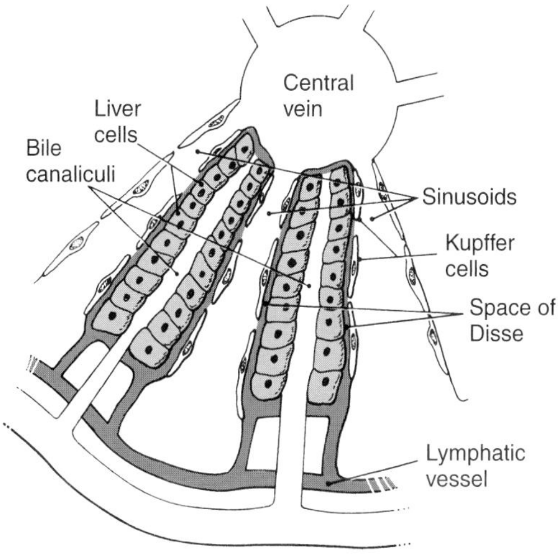

Central vein
Liver cells
Bile canaliculi
Sinusoids
Kupffer cells
Space of Disse
Lymphatic vessel

FIGURE 26-2. Schematic representation of part of a liver lobule showing Kupffer's cells and the space of Disse through which lymphatic material can flow.

FUNCTIONS OF THE LIVER

The liver performs a wide variety of vital, life-sustaining functions. The hepatocyte is responsible for maintaining these functions through its numerous organelles. The liver has over 500 functions. Some of the more significant functions are listed in Box 26-1.

Protein Synthesis and Metabolism

The liver is critical in protein metabolism through its deamination of amino acids, urea formation and ammonia removal, plasma protein formation, and interconversion among the different amino acids.[14] About 90% of all the plasma proteins are formed in the liver cells. Maximally, the liver can form 15 to 40 g of protein per day.[14] Unlike fats and carbohydrates, proteins are not stored, and the size of the amino acid pool is the result of the actual turnover of body proteins and

BOX 26-1 MAJOR FUNCTIONS OF THE LIVER

- Synthesis and metabolism of protein, carbohydrates, and fats
- Phagocytosis
- Biotransformation of foreign substances
- Production, metabolism, and excretion of bile
- Enzyme synthesis
- Biotransformation or inactivation of hormones
- Storage of vitamins and minerals

amino acids from exogenous or dietary sources. The role of dietary intake in maintenance of the amino acid pool is discussed in Chapter 7.

Synthesis of Amino Acids

The liver takes up amino acids from the nutrient-rich portal blood and converts them to various proteins. The amino acids are relatively strong acids that rarely accumulate in the bloodstream. Most amino acids are actively transported through the cell membranes and then converted into cellular proteins after an enzymatic reaction. These cellular proteins can be broken down rapidly to form amino acids that can be transported out of the cells to the bloodstream.[2] The amount of amino acids in blood remains fairly constant but may vary slightly with diet and the individual person. After the cells have reached their capacity for storing proteins, the excess amino acids can be degraded and used as energy or changed into fat or glycogen and stored.[14]

Amino Acid Metabolism

The liver is the major site of amino acid metabolism, and the process, called **deamination** of amino acids, results in the formation of ammonia. Deamination of amino acids is required before they can be used for energy or for conversion to fats or carbohydrates.[14] Large amounts of ammonia are formed from amino acids and also from bacterial action in the large bowel. The ammonia formed in the bowel is transported to the liver in the bloodstream. The liver normally removes 80% of ammonia as blood passes through the portal system.[30] The liver then converts the ammonia to urea, which is much less toxic to the central nervous system and is more readily excreted by the kidneys than is ammonia.

Synthesis and Metabolism of Plasma Proteins

Plasma proteins, mainly synthesized in the liver, are large molecules that circulate for the most part in the blood. The different types of plasma proteins, their functions and alterations are summarized in Table 26-1. Albumin, the most abundant plasma protein, is made in the liver. It serves many functions, including binding substances, such as bilirubin and barbiturates, in the plasma. Albumin is the principal protein necessary for maintaining *colloid osmotic pressure* (see page 161). It also binds hydrogen ions and alters serum pH.

When the amino acid levels in blood are decreased, the plasma proteins are split to make new amino acids to maintain equilibrium. Decreased levels of amino acids stimulate the liver to increase its production of plasma proteins. The concentration of plasma proteins normally remains at a constant ratio, with more albumin in plasma than globulin. The globulins consist of about 15% of plasma proteins and are the protein group to which antibodies produced by B lymphocytes belong.[14]

The liver also synthesizes most of the plasma proteins necessary to coagulate blood, including prothrombin and fibrinogen. For prothrombin formation, the liver uses vitamin K, the absorption of which depends on the production of bile. Fibrinogen is a large-molecule protein formed entirely by the liver and is part of the coagulation cascade.

TABLE 26-I

FUNCTION AND ALTERATIONS OF PLASMA PROTEINS

PLASMA PROTEIN	FUNCTION	ALTERATIONS
Albumin	Maintains plasma colloid osmotic pressure Binds molecules for transport	Hypoalbuminemia Decreased colloid osmotic pressure Systemic edema
Globulins	Production of antibodies Act with albumin to maintain colloid osmotic pressure	Decreased: Immunosuppression Chronic inflammation Nonspecific to liver disease
Fibrinogen	Assists with blood coagulation	Decreased: Disseminated intravascular coagulation Conditions causing fibrinolysis: hemorrhage, burns, poisoning, cirrhosis
Prothrombin	Assists with blood coagulation	Increased prothrombin time: Prothrombin deficiency Impaired vitamin K uptake Increased partial thromboplastin time: Bleeding disorders

Fat or Lipid Metabolism

The liver oxidizes fatty acids through beta oxidation in the mitochondria. This process provides energy for other cells through the formation of acetylcoenzyme A, which enters the citric acid cycle and releases large quantities of energy.[10] The liver also forms ketone bodies (acetoacetate, β-hydroxybutyrate, and acetone), which provide energy in certain conditions such as diabetes mellitus and starvation.

The liver synthesizes almost all of the fat from carbohydrates and protein. The fats are mostly in the form of triglycerides, which consist of three molecules of fatty acid and glycerol. Once formed these are transported to fat cells in the form of *very low-density lipoproteins (VLDL)*. When lipids are released from VLDL, their structure changes and they become *low-density lipoproteins (LDL)* and are returned to the liver. The LDL is the form of most of the total cholesterol of the plasma.[13] Cholesterol, synthesized in the liver, is used to form bile salts, which are important in the absorption of fats in the small intestine. Cholesterol is also used to form steroid hormones. Additionally, phospholipids, consisting of phosphoric acid and fatty acids are synthesized in the liver. Both cholesterol and phospholipids are used by the body to form cellular structures and membranes. *High-density lipoprotein (HDL)* is formed by the liver to scavenge excess cholesterol and triglycerides.

Carbohydrate Metabolism

Carbohydrate may be released by the liver in its usable form, glucose, after it has been stored in the form of **glycogen**. About 5% to 7% of normal liver weight is stored glycogen. When blood glucose increases above normal, **glycogenesis** is stimulated, which promotes more stored glycogen. Glycogenesis is the formation of glycogen from carbohydrate sources, especially glucose. Conversely, when the blood glucose level falls below normal, glycogenolysis is stimulated, which promotes the release of glucose into the blood to raise the blood glucose level. **Glycogenolysis** is the breakdown of glycogen into glucose.

The liver maintains normal blood glucose levels. After a high-carbohydrate meal, carbohydrates are delivered to the liver to be stored and released when the blood glucose level begins to drop. The pancreatic hormone **glucagon** initiates the release of glucose by the liver.

In the process called **gluconeogenesis**, the liver synthesizes glucose from noncarbohydrate substances, especially proteins. Glucose needs that cannot be met from glycogen stores or exogenous sources must be met through this process. Gluconeogenesis is critically important for cells that cannot use fat for metabolism—the blood cells and the cells of the kidney medulla. The cells of the central nervous system use glucose preferentially but can adapt to fatty acid oxidation in the form of ketones in 2 to 4 days. During fasting, such as between meals and during sleep, the carbon skeleton of amino acids is converted to glucose for energy.

Phagocytosis

The sinusoids of the liver are lined with Kupffer cells that act as *phagocytes* (cells that ingest microorganisms and other cellular debris). The portal vein, which circulates the venous blood from the intestine to the liver, carries a higher concentration of toxins and bacteria than other venous blood because these substances are absorbed when nutrients are absorbed from the intestine. The Kupffer cells, which probably originate in the bone marrow, can remove 99% of bacteria in portal venous blood.[14]

Biotransformation of Foreign Substances

Destruction, biotransformation, and inactivation of foreign substances are carried out in the hepatocytes, and substances are changed to acceptable forms for excretion. Many endocrine secretions and pharmacologic agents are inactivated in the liver. Some substances are conjugated in the same way as bilirubin, with glucuronic acid, whereas others may be inactivated by proteolysis, deamination, or oxidation. *Proteolysis* refers to the breakdown of proteins into simpler substances. Oxidative deamination causes the release of the amino radical.[10,30]

Bile Synthesis

Bile is formed by the liver and stored and concentrated by the gallbladder. The liver secretes 600 to 1,200 mL of bile per day. The hepatocytes make bile, which is a liquid material normally composed of bilirubin, plasma electrolytes, water, bile salts, bicarbonate, cholesterol, fatty acids, and lecithin.

Bile salts, formed by the liver with cholesterol precursors, function as detergents and break fat particles into smaller sizes. They aid in making fat more soluble by forming special complexes called *micelles*, which are soluble in the intestinal mucosa. The bile salts are also essential for the absorption of the fat-soluble vitamins A, D, E, and K.

Bilirubin Synthesis

Bilirubin is a waste product that is excreted from the body only in the form of *conjugated bilirubin*. Most bilirubin is released from the breakdown of red blood cells (RBCs) primarily in the spleen. The hemoglobin from RBCs breaks down into *heme* and *globin*. The globin portion is a protein that probably returns to the intracellular amino acid pool. The heme portion is broken down further into bilirubin and iron. The iron is either stored in the form of *ferritin* in the liver, spleen, and bone marrow or used to produce new hemoglobin.

Bilirubin undergoes several reactions and ends up being bound to albumin to be taken to the liver. It is called unconjugated, fat-soluble, or indirect bilirubin because it cannot be excreted in bile or through the kidneys. In the liver, it is converted on the smooth endoplasmic reticulum to a water-soluble form after combining with *glucuronic acid* through the interaction of the enzyme *glucuronyl transferase.*[14] In this water-soluble or conjugated form, it can be secreted into bile and excreted by the intestine or, in special circumstances, by the kidneys. In the intestine, the intestinal bacteria change the excreted bilirubin to *urobilinogen.* Some of this material is reabsorbed and reexcreted by the liver. Most of the bilirubin is converted to *stercobilinogen,* which is oxidized to *stercobilin* before being excreted in the feces.[14] Stercobilin and other bile pigments impart the brown color to the feces. Flowchart 26-1 outlines the process of hemoglobin degradation and the resulting fate of bilirubin.

FLOWCHART 26-1 **Fate of Hemoglobin**

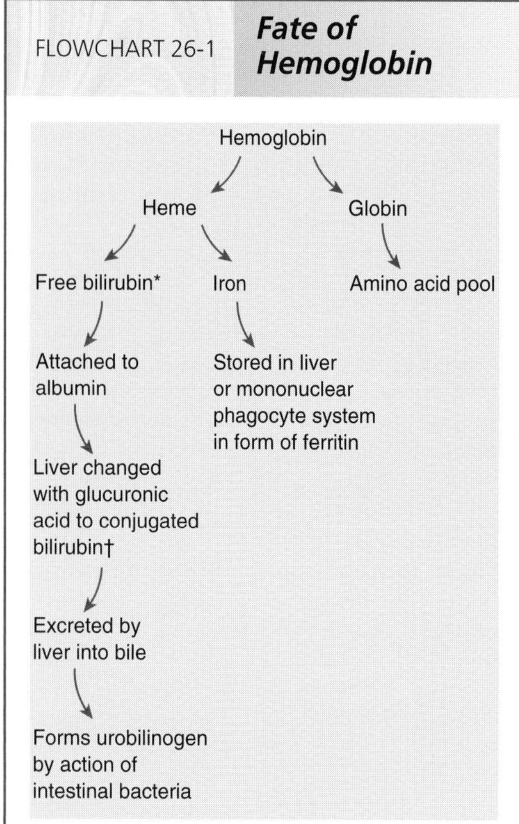

Free unconjugated, indirect bilirubin persists until the liver changes its form. This bilirubin is lipid soluble, water insoluble, and nonexcretable.* Conjugated, direct, or glucuronide bilirubin is the form after conjugation with glucuronic acid. Conjugated bilirubin is water soluble, fat insoluble, and excretable.†

DIAGNOSTIC LIVER TESTS: MAJOR LIVER FUNCTION TESTS

The major liver function tests provide an index of hepatic function and are helpful in establishing a differential diagnosis in intrahepatic and extrahepatic pathology. These tests are presented in Unit 9, Appendix A.

The Gallbladder

The *gallbladder* is a saclike organ attached to the inferior portion of the liver. As shown in Figure 26-3, it receives bile from the liver that has been diverted from the common bile duct. The liver secretes between 600 and 1,200 mL of bile each day, which flows continuously through the bile duct to the intestine. This flow is increased after meals.[14] The gallbladder is composed of folds and rugae and can enlarge to accommodate incoming bile.

The gallbladder empties its bile into the common bile duct on a stimulus from **cholecystokinin**, a hormone secreted by the duodenal mucosa, when fat-containing foods arrive in that area. The gallbladder is also stimulated by the autonomic nervous system. The parasympathetic division is the major mediator for contraction of the gallbladder, whereas stimulation of the sympathetic division causes relaxation of the organ.

The Exocrine Pancreas

The *pancreas* is a large organ that lies behind the stomach and extends between the spleen and the duodenum. As shown in Figure 26-3, it is composed of a head, a tail, and the area in between called the body. The pancreas contains acinar cells and the cells of the islets of Langerhans. The exocrine **acinar cells** secrete digestive juices, whereas the endocrine islet cells secrete hormones that are essential in glucose metabolism and are discussed in Chapters 23 and 24. The exocrine functions, or those related to digestion, involve the secretion of pancreatic juice into a system of ducts that empty into the pancreatic duct and, in turn, the ampulla of Vater.

SECRETION

Pancreatic juice is composed of an alkaline component and enzymes necessary for digesting proteins, fats, and carbohydrates. The alkaline component contains sufficient bicarbonate ion to give the pancreatic juice a pH of about 8. The pancreas normally secretes about 1,500 mL of fluid daily.[10] The enzymes are made by the acinar cells and stored until stimulated for release. These enzymes and their actions are presented in Table 26-2.

Nervous and Hormonal Regulation

Nervous stimulation of the pancreas is mainly through the vagus nerve, which transmits impulses to the

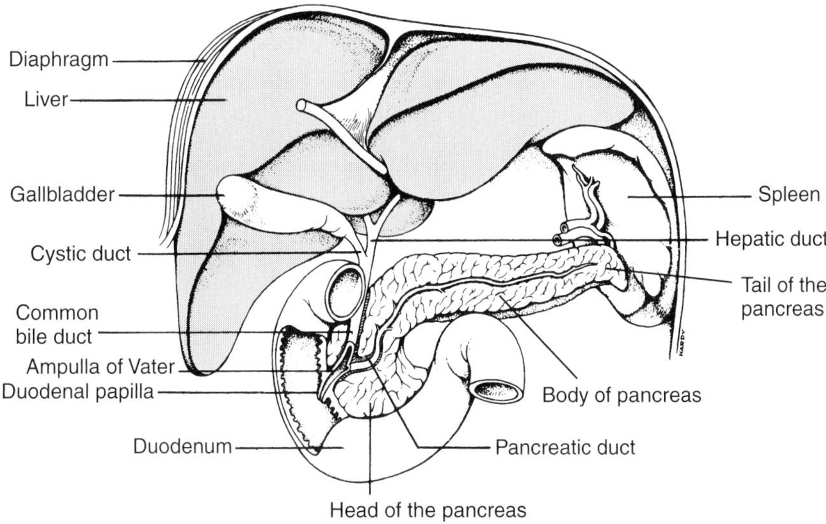

FIGURE 26-3. The liver and biliary system, including the gallbladder, bile ducts, and pancreas. (Chaffee, E.E. & Lytle, I.M. *Basic physiology and anatomy* [4th ed.]. Philadelphia: J.B. Lippincott.)

pancreas during the cephalic and gastric phases of digestion. This results in the secretion of enzymes by the acinar cells.

The hormonal mechanisms are mainly mediated through secretion of *cholecystokinin.* When chyme containing fat or amino acids comes into contact with the mucosal cells of the duodenum, the hormone is released, causing the pancreas to secrete large amounts of fluids with large amounts of bicarbonate and few or no enzymes. This alkaline secretion neutralizes the highly acidic gastric juice emptied into the duodenum from the stomach, stops the activity of gastrin, and provides an alkalinity of about pH 7, which is optimal for pancreatic enzyme activity. Cholecystokinin also is released from the intestinal mucosa in the presence of food, and it increases the secretion of pancreatic enzymes from the acinar cells. Distention of the intestinal wall by food is the apparent stimulus for the release of cholecystokinin.

PROTEIN, FAT, AND CARBOHYDRATE DIGESTION

Trypsinogen, a protein-splitting enzyme of the pancreatic juice, is converted to the active enzyme trypsin in an alkaline medium through the action of *enterokinase* in the duodenum. Trypsin then activates other trypsinogen molecules and triggers the conversion of chymotrypsinogen into chymotrypsin. These are enzymes that can split proteins into amino acids for absorption in the intestine. Two mechanisms prevent digestion of the pancreas by these enzymes:

1. Proteolytic enzymes are synthesized in a pro enzyme or inactive form.

TABLE 26-2

ENZYMES OF PANCREATIC SECRETION

ENZYME	ACTIVATOR	ACTION
Trypsin	Enterokinase	Proteolytic
Chymotrypsin	Trypsin	Proteolytic
Amylase		Breaks down starches to disaccharides and trisaccharides
Carboxypeptidase	Trypsin	Breaks down amino acids
Lipase		Breaks down triglycerides to fatty acids and monoglycerides

2. A trypsin inhibitor, stored in the cytoplasm of the cells surrounding the enzyme granules, prevents the activation of trypsin.

Pancreatic **lipase** works with the bile salts and helps to break down fats into fatty acids and glycerol.[14] Pancreatic **amylase** hydrolyzes starches, glycogen, and other carbohydrates into disaccharides.

ALTERATIONS IN HEPATOBILIARY AND PANCREATIC EXOCRINE FUNCTION

Liver Dysfunction

JAUNDICE

Excess bilirubin in the blood leads to the condition called **jaundice**. Clinical manifestation of jaundice, or *icterus*, are variable, depending on the etiology. Generally, a yellowish or greenish hue is tinting a person's skin. In adults, the degree of jaundice often correlates with the severity of liver dysfunction. Jaundice may not be detected until the serum bilirubin is increased from two and a half to three times above normal.[31] Because connective tissue has an affinity for bilirubin, the bilirubin may accumulate in unconjugated or conjugated form, depositing pigments in the skin, sclera, and all the tissues of the body. Additional clinical manifestations that may accompany jaundice include nausea, vomiting, abdominal pain, dark urine, and light-colored bowel movements.

Etiology and Pathophysiology

The major types of jaundice result from (1) impairment of uptake, conjugation, or secretion of bilirubin; (2) excessive destruction of RBCs; and (3) obstructive conditions.[7,31]

IMPAIRMENT OF UPTAKE, CONJUGATION, OR SECRETION OF BILIRUBIN. Decreased uptake and storage of bilirubin can be an *acquired* or *hereditary* problem. Acquired conditions are often due to specific drugs, such as rifamycin, that competitively inhibit uptake and storage of bilirubin.[33] Jaundice usually resolves within 3 days after discontinuing the agent.[20]

Immaturity and hereditary conditions can also cause bilirubin alterations. *Kernicterus* may result with the deposition of pigment in the basal ganglia of the brain, which causes brain damage. Kernicterus typically occurs in premature or newborn infants; the blood–brain barrier develops impermeability to bilirubin in early infancy. Some examples of impaired bilirubin uptake, conjugation, or secretion include:

NEONATAL JAUNDICE. This condition is caused by the deficiency of glucuronyl transferase, an enzyme necessary for the conjugation of bilirubin with glucuronic acid. This occurs often in premature infants. Phototherapy causes the isomerization of unconjugated bilirubin to a polarized compound, which can be excreted. Improvement usually occurs within days to weeks.

CRIGLER-NAJJAR SYNDROME. This rare autosomal recessive condition results when glucuronyl transferase activity is congenitally absent. The unconjugated bilirubin accumulates and crosses the blood–brain barrier; kernicterus may result.

GILBERT SYNDROME. This typically benign, familial condition occurs in up to 14% of the population, with a greater incidence among males.[24] It is probably the result of an autosomal dominant trait. Unconjugated bilirubin cannot be released from the albumin due to the lack of sufficient glucuronyl transferase.[24] When the stress response increases the metabolism of bilirubin and the need for conjugation, significant jaundice occurs.

DUBIN-JOHNSON SYNDROME. This is an uncommon benign, familial condition. Persons with this syndrome are unable to transport conjugated bilirubin in the bile for excretion. Therefore, they exhibit excessive conjugated hyperbilirubinemia.[7] Although the liver is grossly pigmented, persons are usually asymptomatic except for mild, intermittent jaundice.

EXCESSIVE DESTRUCTION OF RBCS. Excessive destruction of RBCs causes jaundice through hemolysis. Figure 26-4 shows the normal pathway for bilirubin conjugation and the change that can occur with increased destruction of the RBCs. The liver retains the capability to conjugate bilirubin, but it becomes overwhelmed with the free bilirubin and cannot conjugate all that is sent to it. Levels of either unconjugated or conjugated bilirubin or both may be elevated.

OBSTRUCTIVE JAUNDICE

Two major types of obstructive jaundice are: (1) *intrahepatic*, or failure of the hepatocytes to function (Fig. 26-5), and (2) *posthepatic*, which is an obstruction in the bile ducts, commonly resulting from cholestasis as an outcome of cholecystitis or cholelithiasis. **Cholestasis** is defined as biliary pigment that accumulates in the bile canaliculi and hepatocytes; as they become saturated, accumulation of these pigments occurs in the blood. The obstruction limits the excretion of bilirubin in the bile, and an excess of conjugated bilirubin accumulates.[7,18] Table 26-3 summarizes some causes of intrahepatic and posthepatic jaundice.

Hepatocellular failure often causes increased serum levels of unconjugated bilirubin because the hepatocytes cannot produce conjugated bilirubin. Extrahepatic obstruction causes increased levels of conjugated bilirubin with excretion of bilirubin in the urine. As the

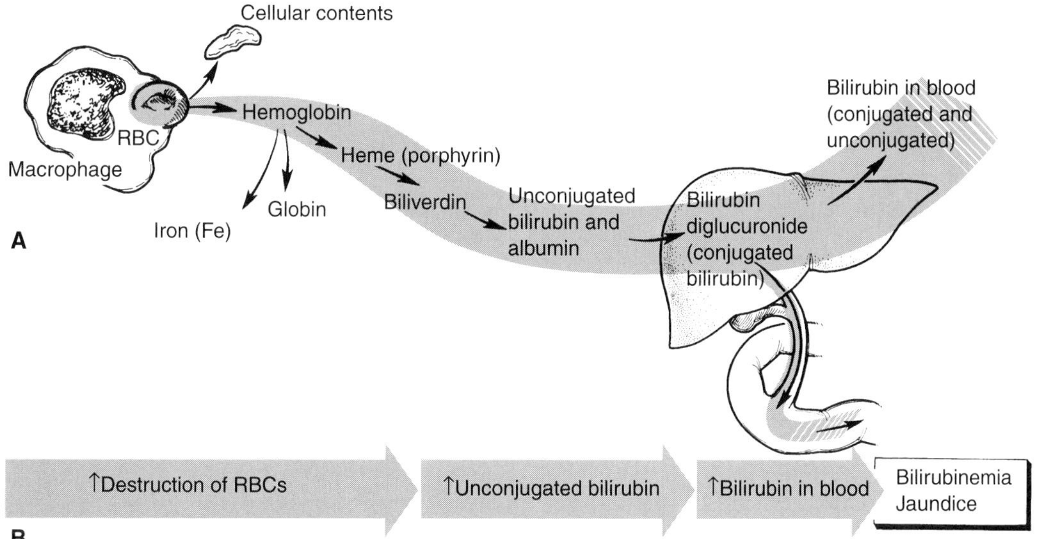

FIGURE 26-4. **A.** Normal process of conjugation of bilirubin by the liver, which promotes excretion through the bile. **B.** With increased destruction of red blood cells, large amounts of unconjugated bilirubin are released and the liver is unable to conjugate all that comes to it. Increased bilirubin in the blood results, which leads to bilirubinemia and jaundice.

liver becomes engorged with bilirubin, the activity of the hepatocytes diminishes, and the serum unconjugated and conjugated bilirubin levels increase. Determining whether jaundice is caused by conjugated or unconjugated bilirubin is important in establishing the source and sometimes the severity of the causative condition.

ASCITES

Ascites is the accumulation of fluid in the peritoneal cavity. Box 26-2 lists common causes of ascites. It usually results from increasing portal pressure, decreasing plasma protein levels, or both. Sodium retention as a result of aldosterone retention and excessive lymphatic

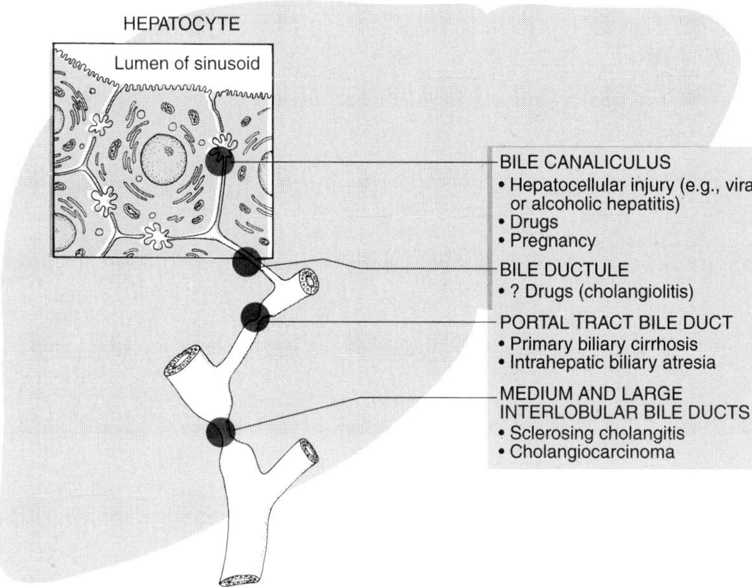

FIGURE 26-5. Sites of intrahepatic cholestasis. (Rubin, E. & Farber, J.L. [1999]. *Pathology* [3rd ed.]. Philadelphia: Lippincott-Raven.)

TABLE 26-3

OBSTRUCTIVE JAUNDICE

INTRAHEPATIC OBSTRUCTION	POSTHEPATIC OBSTRUCTION
Failure of Hepatocytes	**Results from Cholestasis**
• Hepatitis • Cirrhotic fibrosis • Hepatic scarring • Oral contraceptive agents • Chlorpropamide (Diabinese)	• Gallstones • Malignancies • Surgical obstruction of the ampulla of Vater • Congenital atresia of biliary tree (infants)[24]

flow may worsen the ascites. Generalized edema, or *anasarca*, results mostly from a decrease in the plasma colloid osmotic pressure generated from the decreased albumin levels, encouraging fluid exudation into all of the interstitial compartments. Figure 26-6 illustrates the factors that can contribute to the development of ascites.

PORTAL HYPERTENSION AND ESOPHAGEAL VARICES

Obstruction of blood flow through the liver results in increased pressure in the portal venous system. The term *portal hypertension* refers to high pressures in the portal vein and its tributaries, and the common cause of this condition is cirrhosis of the liver. Additional causes are listed in Box 26-3.

Meeting resistance in the portal vein, blood seeks collateral channels around the high-pressure areas or through the obstructed liver. Collateral channels provide a route for direct shunting of blood from the portal veins to the inferior vena cava, thus bypassing the liver. The shunted blood contains large amounts of ammonia that may precipitate onset of hepatic encephalopathy. The blood-borne bacteria absorbed from the small intestine and normally processed and biotransformed in the liver are also shunted directly into the systemic circulation. Toxic substances may bypass the liver without being metabolized and may accumulate in the body, adversely affecting the nervous system.

In the portal system, vessels most susceptible to the high pressure are the esophageal and the hemorrhoidal veins, as noted in Figure 26-7. The esophageal veins protrude into the lumen of the esophagus and become thin-walled varices that look like bulging bags on the inner surface of the esophagus. These vessels are fragile and very susceptible to hemorrhage.

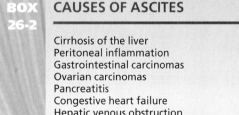

BOX 26-2

CAUSES OF ASCITES

Cirrhosis of the liver
Peritoneal inflammation
Gastrointestinal carcinomas
Ovarian carcinomas
Pancreatitis
Congestive heart failure
Hepatic venous obstruction
Nephrosis and peritoneal dialysis
Myxedema

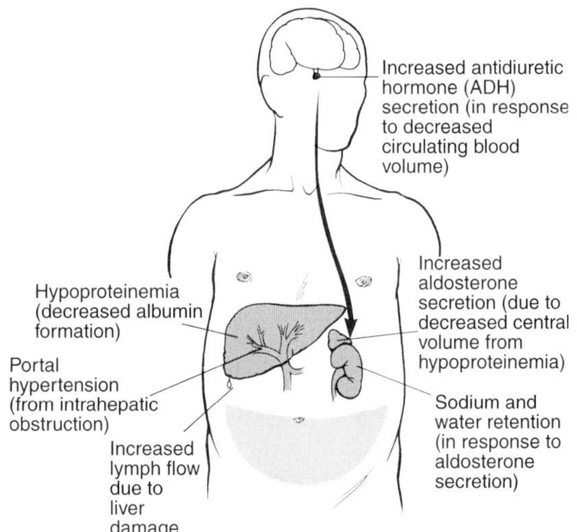

FIGURE 26-6. **Factors contributing to the development of ascites.**

BOX 26-3

CAUSES OF PORTAL HYPERTENSION

I. *Prehepatic*—Blockage occurs in blood flow to the liver
   Portal vein thrombosis
   Splenomegaly
   Arteriovenous fistula
II. *Intrahepatic*—Blockage occurs in blood flow within the liver
   Cirrhosis of the liver
   Fatty liver
   Biliary tuberculosis
   Idiopathic portal hypertension
III. *Posthepatic*—Increased pressure in the inferior vena cava blood return to the heart
   Severe right-side heart failure
   Constrictive pericarditis
   Hepatic veno-occlusive disease

Esophageal varices may hemorrhage for several reasons:

1. Most commonly, from a decrease in the formation of clotting factors or high portal pressure
2. Chemical breakdown of the variceal walls (as from alcohol)
3. Gastric acidity
4. Spasmodic vomiting
5. Rupture

Rupture of esophageal varices may result in exsanguination and death. Rectal hemorrhoids also may rupture and bleed under pressure, causing a massive amount of bright red bleeding from the rectum. Anything that can cause increased motility of the lower gastrointestinal tract can increase the risk of hemorrhage from this area.

Bleeding from esophageal varices, duodenal ulcers, or other sources may precipitate jaundice and production of ammonia due to the processing and

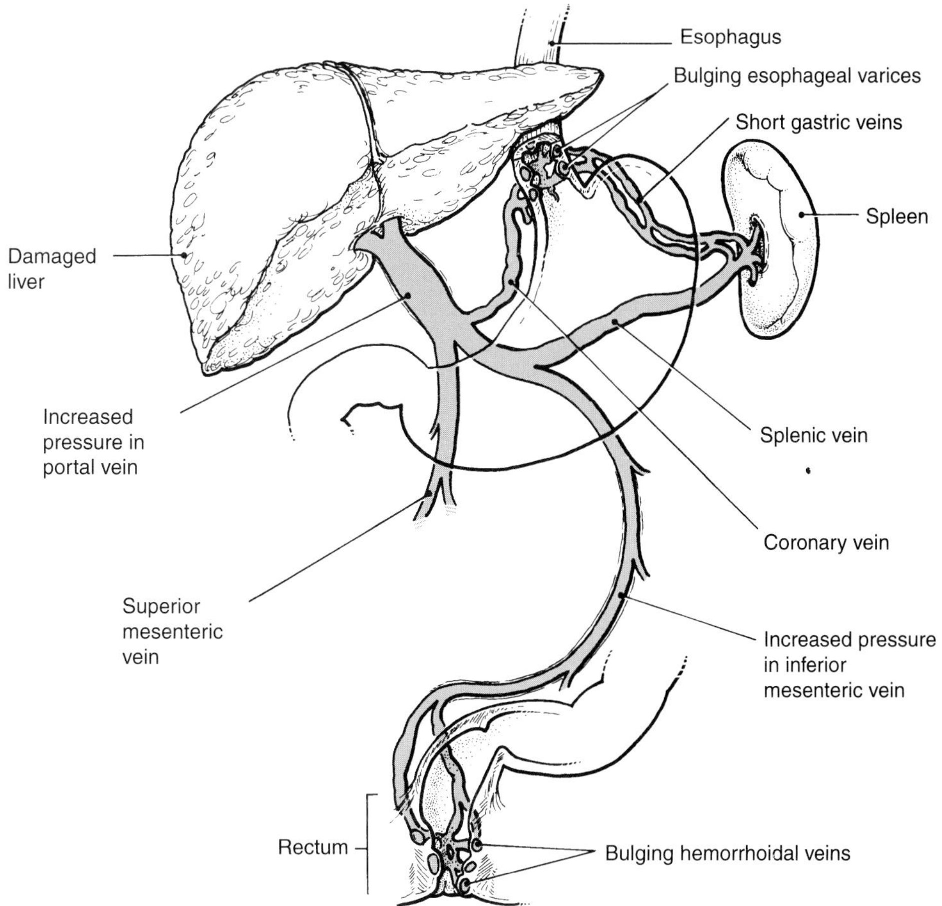

FIGURE 26-7. Appearance of esophageal varices and dilated hemorrhoidal veins resulting from portal hypertension.

absorption of products of the RBCs in the intestine. These developments may lead to increased risk of encephalopathy, which, with the bleeding event, is often life-threatening.

LIVER FAILURE

Liver failure refers to a variety of clinical manifestations that result from many types of liver disease. Cirrhosis and chronic active hepatitis are the most common causes of liver failure.[18] Chemicals and drugs, such as carbon tetrachloride and halothane, can cause massive liver necrosis. Reye's syndrome, fatty liver of alcoholism, and antibiotics, such as tetracycline, can cause functional insufficiency.[7]

Deficiency in clotting factors is one of the earliest signs of liver failure. Vitamin K deficiency may result from fat malabsorption. A decrease in the uptake of vitamin K into hepatocytes leads to defective synthesis of factors II (prothrombin), VII (proconvertin), IX (Christmas factor), and X (Stuart-Prower factor).[24] The major clotting dysfunction results from depressed production of prothrombin. The platelet count may be inadequate because of hypersplenism, which frequently occurs with liver failure. Hypersplenism results from congestion caused by the portal hypertension.[7] In liver failure, an increased risk of hemorrhage is always present, especially when associated with esophageal varices.

In liver failure, several other characteristic pathophysiologic changes occur. These changes include:

- Jaundice occurs from increased levels of conjugated and unconjugated bilirubin.
- Neurologic status changes occur from the hepatic encephalopathy, often leading to coma.
- Hypogonadism and gynecomastia may occur from the imbalance of androgen–estrogen levels.
- Palmar erythema results from vasodilation in hands and feet due to hyperestrogenism.
- Spider angiomas result from hyperestrogenism and clotting disturbances.
- Fetor hepaticus, the musty odor of the breath, is due to deficient methionine catabolism.
- Ascites and edema result from both portal hypertension and hypoalbuminemia.[7]

Fulminant Hepatic Failure

Fulminant hepatic failure refers to acute, rapidly developing liver dysfunction. The term is usually associated with the development of jaundice and encephalopathy within 4 weeks after an initiating event in a person who has experienced no previous liver disease. This event may include infections, drugs and toxins, ischemia, hypoxia, metabolic disorders, autoimmune conditions, and others.[34] A subacute process has been described, especially when the condition is drug or toxin induced, in which the manifestations of liver failure develop 8 to 20 weeks after exposure. Massive liver necrosis and destruction of lobules and even lobes of the liver result. The overall mortality rate is between 75% and 95%, with encephalopathy being the main cause of death.[25]

HEPATIC ENCEPHALOPATHY AND COMA

Hepatic encephalopathy refers to an alteration in the neurologic status in persons with significant liver disease because the liver can no longer remove neurotoxic metabolites from the blood. Its onset may be gradual, but more frequently it is precipitated by a major hemodynamic insult in an individual already suffering from cirrhosis of the liver. Conditions that may precipitate encephalopathy include (1) bleeding from esophageal varices; (2) ingestion of narcotics, barbiturates, or anesthetics; (3) excessive protein intake; (4) electrolyte imbalance; and (5) hemodynamic alterations, such as hypovolemia or shock. Anything that can increase the metabolic demands placed on the borderline liver can precipitate liver failure with resultant encephalopathy and coma.

Onset is noted when the liver is unable to metabolize nitrogenous products absorbed from the intestine. These nitrogenous products may include dietary protein or proteins released in gastrointestinal bleeding episodes. Serum ammonia levels are often elevated in encephalopathy, and other substances probably produce the clinical syndrome as well.[19,26]

The phases of hepatic encephalopathy vary in length (from days, weeks, and months) and may progress insidiously from one level to the next, ending in coma. Progression of encephalopathy begins with early behavioral changes and subtle impairment of intellectual abilities, and includes:

- Confusion
- Delusions
- Constructional apraxia and writing difficulty
- Diminished consciousness
- Hyperreflexia
- **Asterixis**, a "flapping tremor" that occurs with dorsiflexion of the wrist
- Violent, abusive behavior
- Electroencephalographic (EEG) changes

As the encephalopathy worsens, the patient becomes comatose, the asterixis disappears, and a Babinski sign appears. Persons exhibiting recurrent or progressive forms of this condition have distinctive changes in the brain tissue, with proliferation of the astrocytes and patchy cortical necrosis. When these changes occur, areas of permanent damage result.[7] In rapidly occurring liver failure, cerebral edema may be seen, which can cause uncal or cerebellar herniation.[24]

HEPATORENAL SYNDROME

Hepatorenal syndrome is a poorly understood renal failure associated with significant liver disease. In liver failure, the development of renal failure indicates a very poor prognosis; although they appear normal, the kidneys become functionally impaired. It is manifested by an elevated serum creatinine level and a decreasing urine output. Frequently it is precipitated by clinical deterioration, such as a gastrointestinal bleeding episode or the onset of hepatic coma.[7] Individuals suffering from hepatorenal syndrome generally have significant ascites.

DRUG-RELATED LIVER DAMAGE

Drug reactions are responsible for a number of toxic effects on the human body. Substances that are directly toxic to liver cells are called hepatotoxins. Alcohol, chlorpromazine, isoniazid, and halothane are examples of **hepatotoxins**.[22] Hepatotoxicity can result from formation of toxic metabolites as the liver is biotransforming the drug or from a drug metabolite converting an intracellular protein into an immunogenic molecule. The damage sustained depends on dosage and individual hypersensitivity. Table 26-4 indicates some mechanisms that cause drug-induced hepatotoxicity. Such damage may occur very quickly. Many drugs cause problems due only to hypersensitivity reactions, and these problems may not be manifested for weeks to months after initiating therapy. The pathology depends on the amount and location of injury.[7,34] Clinical manifestations may vary from asymptomatic to acute hepatitis to manifestations associated with fulminant hepatic failure. Generally, an elevation is observed in the liver enzyme studies.

REYE'S SYNDROME

Reye's syndrome is an acute illness that occurs most frequently in children between the ages of 6 months and 15 years.[7] The onset of symptoms begins about 3 to 5 days after a viral illness, such as varicella. In nearly every case, the viral fever has been treated with aspirin, which has led to the theory that there is a synergism between aspirin and viral infection.[24] The initial symptoms are vomiting, lethargy progressing to coma, and increased aminotransferases and serum ammonia levels.[7] Pathologically, there is massive infiltration of the liver parenchyma with fat (steatosis). Liver and brain mitochondria are swollen, and cerebral edema occurs in all cases.[7,24] The amount of cerebral edema corresponds to the severity of the neurologic dysfunction. Fatality rates vary from 10% to 40%, depending on early diagnosis and accurate reporting.[7] The incidence of Reye's syndrome is declining with education of adults to not treat febrile illness in children with aspirin.

CIRRHOSIS OF THE LIVER

Cirrhosis is a general term for a condition that destroys the normal structure of the liver lobules. The following changes occur:

- Destruction of liver parenchyma
- Separation of the lobules by fibrous tissue
- Formation of structurally abnormal nodules
- Resulting abnormal vascular architecture[7,24]

Cirrhosis is classified either according to its (1) causative agent or (2) the morphologic changes that result. The morphologic classification includes the micronodular type, which exhibits nodules less than 3 mm

TABLE 26-4

POSTULATED MECHANISMS OF DRUG-INDUCED HEPATIC INJURY

EFFECT	EXAMPLE
Alteration of the physical properties of membranes	Estrogens
Inhibition of membrane enzymes (eg, Na^+, K^+-ATPase)	Chlorpromazine metabolites
Interference with the hepatic uptake process	Rifampin
Impairment of cytoskeletal function	Chlorpromazine metabolites
Formation of insoluble complexes in bile	Chlorpromazine
Toxicity mediated by toxic intermediates:	
Electrophiles leading to covalent binding of proteins	Acetaminophen
Free radicals causing lipid peroxidation	Carbon tetrachloride
Redox cycling generating oxygen free radicals and protein thiol oxidation	Nitrofurantoin, menadione

ATPase, adenosine triphosphatase.
(Adapted from Bass, N. M., & Ockner, R. K. [1990]. Drug-induced liver disease. In D. Zakim & T. D. Boyer [Eds.] *Hepatology, a textbook of liver disease* [p.754]. Philadelphia: Saunders.)

in diameter, and the macronodular type, which exhibits grossly visible, coarse, irregular nodules encircled by bands of connective tissue.[24] The morphologic features of cirrhosis often depend on how long the condition has been present and how extensive the liver damage is. The major causes of cirrhosis are listed in Box 26-4.

Biliary Cirrhosis

Biliary cirrhosis may be due to an intrahepatic block that obstructs the excretion of bile or may occur secondary to obstruction of the bile ducts. The ultimate outcome differs with each type, and causes vary.

Primary intrahepatic stasis is caused by autoimmune destruction of interlobular bile ducts. This type occurs most often in women older than age 40 years, suggesting endocrine involvement. Specific and nonspecific immunologic abnormalities have been implicated based on the demonstration of antibodies and impaired T-lymphocyte function.[7]

Secondary biliary cirrhosis results from obstruction of the hepatic or common bile duct. With resulting stasis of bile in the liver, the following changes occur:

- Swollen and bile-stained liver
- Progressive fibrosis surrounding the hepatocytes and separating the lobules
- Parenchymal cell destruction
- Regenerative nodules resulting from a reaction of the interlobular bile ducts to increased amounts of bile
- Inflammation
- Injury and scarring close to interlobular bile ducts[7,24]

Jaundice may be severe with either type and is associated with bilirubinemia and clay-colored stools. Results of liver function tests are abnormal, with alkaline phosphatase and cholesterol levels often becoming markedly elevated. Serum triglycerides and low-density cholesterol levels are often elevated with this condition. Levels of conjugated and unconjugated bilirubin may rise. With increasing liver damage, the signs of hepatocellular failure may appear.

BOX 26-4

CAUSES OF CIRRHOSIS

Alcoholic liver disease
Chronic active hepatitis
Primary biliary cirrhosis
Extrahepatic biliary obstruction
Hemochromatosis
Wilson's disease
Cystic fibrosis
α_1-Antitrypsin deficiency
Glycogen storage disease, types III and IV
Galactosemia
Hereditary fructose intolerance
Tyrosinemia
Hereditary storage diseases: Gaucher's, Niemann-Pick, Wolman, mucopolysaccharidoses
Zellweger syndrome
Indian childhood cirrhosis

Rubin, E., & Farber, J. L. (1999). *Pathology* (3rd ed.). Philadelphia: Lippincott.

Alcoholic (Laënnec's) Cirrhosis

Laënnec's cirrhosis, also called *alcoholic liver disease,* is caused by chronic alcoholism, often following a pattern of fatty liver, alcoholic hepatitis, and, finally, alcoholic cirrhosis.[7] At least 10% of persons who are chronic alcoholics have some evidence of cirrhosis. Significant frequency of the disease is noted in highly civilized countries, among all economic classes, and in all races.

PATHOPHYSIOLOGY. Alcohol induces metabolic changes within the liver that lead to fat infiltration of the hepatocytes and scarring between the lobules. Alcoholic liver disease usually follows long-term ethanol ingestion of 40 to 80 g/d. Forty grams of ethanol is found in four 12-oz beers, 16 oz of wine, or 4 oz of 80-proof whiskey. In susceptible women, as little as 20 g/d over 10 years can produce alcoholic liver disease.[8] A close association between poor diet and long-term alcohol abuse is often found.

Alcoholic cirrhosis is the end result of progressive alcoholic liver disease. It usually progresses in stages as follows:

ALCOHOLIC STEATOSIS. As the liver increases its synthesis of triglycerides and fatty acids, a decrease in fatty acid oxidation and a decrease in the formation and release of lipoproteins cause a *fatty liver*, where hepatocytes are infiltrated by fat of lipid material.[7] Over time, the fatty cells become surrounded by fibrous tissue separating the liver lobules.[7] This stage may be asymptomatic or may be associated with malaise, anorexia, nausea, liver tenderness and enlargement, jaundice, or even sudden death.[7,22]

ALCOHOLIC HEPATITIS. During this stage, acute liver cell necrosis occurs. Inflammatory cell infiltrates and inclusions called *Mallory's bodies*, or alcoholic hyalin, may lead to fibrosis around the cells and veins.[7] The liver becomes enlarged, and hepatocytes degenerate and become infiltrated by leukocytes and lymphocytes. The inflammation decreases as the cirrhotic process progresses to the destruction of hepatocytes. Infiltrating fibroblasts and collagen formation lead to scar formation, causing inflammation and further damage to the liver parenchyma. The clinical picture of acute alcoholic hepatitis includes general debility (asthenia), jaundice, fever, abdominal pain, ascites, and loss of muscle mass.

ALCOHOLIC CIRRHOSIS. During this final stage, the liver capsule becomes firm. Regenerative nodules form, resulting in a hobnail appearance. As the pathology progresses, the liver shrinks in size and becomes finely nodular in appearance. The nodules are surrounded by evenly spaced, grayish connective tissue.[7,22] The liver pathology is usually associated with enlargement of the spleen.

CLINICAL MANIFESTATIONS. Clinically, alcoholic cirrhosis is insidious, causing abnormal liver function test results, fluid retention, ascites, esophageal varices, and many other manifestations (Fig. 26-8). Potential complications associated with alcoholic liver dysfunction include clotting disorders, cachexia, hepatorenal syndrome, hepatic encephalopathy, liver cancer, and gastrointestinal bleeding.[8] Alcoholic hepatitis typically recurs, leading to eventual liver failure. Fifty percent of persons with significant cirrhosis of the liver die of the disease within 5 years. However, disease progression may be slowed by abstinence from alcohol.[22] Death may be due to hepatic encephalopathy, liver failure, infection, gastrointestinal bleeding, or hepatocellular carcinoma, which appears in 3% to 6% of cases.[7]

CANCER OF THE LIVER

Tumors of the liver that cause functional impairment and hepatomegaly are almost always malignant. The rare benign tumors or tumor-like lesions are described as angiomas, adenomas, or nodular hyperplasias.

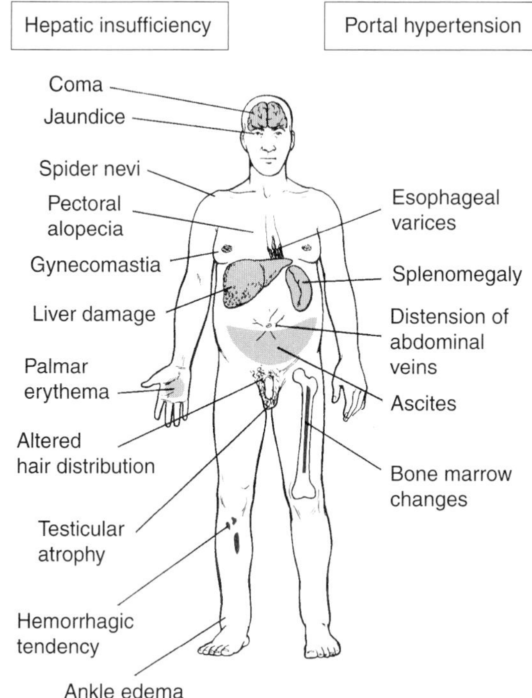

FIGURE 26-8. **Clinical effects of cirrhosis of the liver.**

Benign Hepatic Tumors

Most hepatocellular tumors are *adenomas* that occur in women and are related to oral contraceptive use. They cause a well-circumscribed, encapsulated mass that may have a diameter of 5 to 15 cm.[5] These tumors may be discovered as a result of complaints of abdominal pain or bleeding into the peritoneal cavity and do not recur after excision.[24] *Focal nodular hyperplasia*, thought to be a hamartomatous malformation, also occurs primarily in women of childbearing age. Although its etiology is unclear, it probably is not related to taking oral contraceptives for a long period of time.[5] Bile duct hamartomas and adenomas are small masses in the ductal structures. Usually they are asymptomatic.[7,24] Hemangiomas of the liver are common reddish purple lesions measuring about 2 to 4 cm. These may be congenital. They rarely are symptomatic but occur in up to 7% of routine autopsies.[24]

Primary Malignancies

Primary carcinoma of the liver is relatively rare and may arise within the hepatocytes or the biliary canaliculi, or it may be of mixed type. Hepatocellular carcinoma accounts for 80% to 90% of primary malignancies of the liver.[7]

ETIOLOGY AND PATHOPHYSIOLOGY. Primary liver tumors may be related to diet and other types of liver disease, especially hepatitis. In the United States, the prevalence of primary liver carcinoma is less than 3%. Some of the influences that may contribute to its occurrence are (1) carcinogenic agents in food, (2) cirrhosis of the liver, (3) viral infections of the liver, and (4) parasitic liver infections.[7] Hepatitis C antibodies are found in two thirds to three fourths of persons with primary hepatocellular carcinoma, making this viral infection an important risk factor for this malignancy.[24] Pathologically, the growth may be limited to one area, occur in numerous nodules, or occur as infiltrates on the surface of the liver.[5,17] The tumors may secrete different substances, especially bile products. Polycythemia, hypoglycemia, and hypercalcemia are very common and result from hormone production by the tumor.[24] Biliary obstruction with jaundice, portal hypertension with ascites, and different sorts of metabolic disturbances related to the functional impairment of hepatocytes may result. Hypoalbuminemia, hypoglycemia, and bleeding problems may occur. Usually the growth rate is rapid, and the tumor metastasizes early. Tumors of the liver are often inoperable. They often terminate in gastrointestinal hemorrhaging, liver failure, and death.

CLINICAL MANIFESTATIONS. Clinical manifestations include signs of debilitation, weight loss, and cachexia. Ninety-one percent suffer from abdominal pain, and from 50% to 90% exhibit hepatomegaly.[3] Early manifestations may resemble cirrhosis. Jaundice, ascites, and other signs of liver failure are often related to progression of the condition and frequently are seen in the terminal state.

The size and extent of the tumor as identified by computed tomography (CT) scans and magnetic resonance imaging can vary extensively.[3,15] Some lesions may be very small and are best viewed through angioportography.[3] Liver function tests reflect the degree of disruption of normal function. α-Fetoprotein can be used as a screening measure because its levels are often elevated above 4,000 ng/mL from a normal level of less than 10 ng/mL.

Metastatic Carcinoma

The liver is commonly the site of metastases of malignancies arising in other areas of the body. Persons with lung, colon, pancreatic, breast, and gastric carcinomas typically have metastases to the liver.[3] Physiologically, the liver is vulnerable to metastatic carcinoma because of the large volume of blood it receives each minute, the high nutrient level of its blood, and the large reserve of lymphatic drainage. Metastases usually involve large areas of the liver, causing disruption to its function. Results of liver function tests are frequently abnormal, especially alkaline phosphatase and serum enzymes. The level of carcinoembryonic antigen in the serum, which is elevated in many malignancies, is also elevated with many liver malignancies and metastases. Serum levels correlate to some extent with tumor size and degree of metastasis, and levels decrease markedly after successful treatment.

The clinical course depends on the rapidity of growth of the metastatic lesion and the site of the primary malignancy. The nutritional status of the affected person declines rapidly, with marked cachexia, muscle wasting, and hepatomegaly. Obstruction of bile flow may lead to jaundice, and all of the other dysfunctions of liver disease may be present, depending on the amount of liver involvement.

The prognosis for persons with liver metastasis is poor due to the lack of response to treatment and the impossibility of resecting the tumor surgically. The 5-year survival rate has been reported to be less than 5%.

VIRAL HEPATITIS

Hepatitis refers to inflammation and injury of the liver. It is a reaction of the liver to a variety of conditions, specifically viruses, drugs, and alcohol. *Viral hepatitis* is the term used for infection of the liver by viruses. Identification of the causative viruses is ongoing, but the agents of A, B, C, E, and D viruses account for about 95% of cases of acute viral hepatitis.[16] The viruses E and D are known as non-A, non-B hepatitis.[27] Table 26-5 contrasts the characteristics of various types of viral hepatitis.

Hepatitis A

Hepatitis A (HAV), formerly known as infectious hepatitis, results most frequently from fecal-oral contamination with the HAV, a single-stranded RNA virus. It frequently occurs in crowded, unsanitary living conditions, has no sex predilection, and is often epidemic in children or young adults.[27] This infection may also be transmitted by contaminated, inadequately cooked shellfish. Contaminated water has also been implicated as carrying the organism.

Children are usually *anicteric* (without jaundice); typical signs and symptoms are diarrhea, nausea, and malaise. Symptoms usually subside after 3 to 7 days. Adults, however, suffer a more severe course, usually with the onset of jaundice following a flulike syndrome (1–2 weeks).

The course is rather predictable, and typically progresses as follows:

- Exposure to infection
- Incubation period (2–6 weeks). No clinical signs are apparent.
- Prodromal phase. The person becomes symptomatic with anorexia, nausea, vomiting, and flulike symptoms. Fecal shedding of the virus occurs.[27]
- Icteric (jaundiced) phase. Jaundice, usually caused by conjugated hyperbilirubinemia (bilirubin above 2.5 mg/dL) appears, with dark urine and light stools (due to cholestasis).[7] Serum IgM and IgG levels rise. Alanine aminotransferase and aspartate aminotransferase levels also rise, indicating hepatocellular necrosis.[27] The icteric phase clears slowly.
- Recovery. Usually complete recovery of the liver parenchyma occurs.

A lifetime immunity probably results after the hepatitis A infection has run its course.[16] Serum IgG levels may remain elevated for decades, possibly for life.[27] In such areas as Costa Rica, where the disease is endemic, 90% of the population have anti-HAV antibodies by their teenage years.[7]

Hepatitis B

Hepatitis B (HBV), sometimes referred to as serum hepatitis, results most frequently from blood transfusion or needle virus contamination, but it also may be transmitted placentally and venereally. The fecal-oral route is relatively unimportant.[27] The HBV is a DNA virus that is present in all body fluids of an infected person.[27] It is estimated that there are more than 300 million persons chronically infected with HBV worldwide.[27] Box 26-5 lists populations at high risk for HBV. Hepatitis B vaccinations are available and are recommended for most health care workers.

Hepatitis B virus is a known carcinogen in humans, second only to tobacco.[27] The HBV also has been implicated in 60% to 90% of cases of hepatocellular carcinoma when it has reached a chronic carrier state.[16,24]

TABLE 26-5

CHARACTERISTICS OF VARIOUS TYPES OF VIRAL HEPATITIS

CHARACTERISTIC	Hepatitis A (HAV)	Hepatitis B (HBV)	Hepatitis C (HCV)	Hepatitis D (HDV)	Hepatitis E (HEV)
CAUSATIVE VIRUS	RNA virus	DNA virus	RNA virus;	Defective RNA virus; requires HBV coinfection	RNA virus
LABORATORY FINDINGS	Anti-HAV antibody: IgM signifies current infection and IgG signifies current or previous infection and immunity to HAV.	HBsAg present in both acute and chronic forms. Positive HBeAg signifies high infectivity in acute infection and during replication in chronic hepatitis. Elevated anti-HBc IgM reflects acute infection and elevated anti-HBc IgG reflects chronic hepatitis and carrier state. Anti-HBs signifies immunity to HBV.	Anti-HCV antibody	HDVAg in early infection; anti-HDV antibody later during infection and after infection	Anti-HEV antibody. IgM anti-HEV elevated early in the course; IgM anti-HEV elevated after IgM anti-HEV and continues to be elevated after the infection.
ONSET	Abrupt	Insidious	Insidious	Insidious	Abrupt
TRANSMISSION MODE	Fecal–oral	Blood and body fluids	Blood and body fluids	Blood and body fluids	Fecal–oral
INCUBATION PERIOD	15–50 d	45–180 d	14–160 d	30–180 d	15–60 d
CLINICAL MANIFESTATIONS	Manifestations are similar in all types of hepatitis and are variable for each case; they may range from asymptomatic to severe fulminant manifestations. Generally, common manifestations include flulike symptoms such as fatigue, malaise, nausea, fever and chills, diarrhea, anorexia, and abdominal pain, in addition to liver-specific symptoms such as jaundice, dark urine, and light-colored stools. Laboratory findings usually reveal elevated immunoglobulins, ALT, AST, and bilirubin during varying periods of the course of the disease.				
POSSIBLE SEQUELAE	Fulminant hepatitis (rare); cholestatic hepatitis	Chronic hepatitis Hepatocellular carcinoma Fulminant hepatitis (rare) Cirrhosis	Chronic hepatitis Cirrhosis Fulminant hepatitis (rare) Hepatocellular carcinoma	Chronic hepatitis Cirrhosis Fulminant hepatitis	Severe forms possible in pregnant women
CARRIER STATE	No	Yes	Yes	Yes	No
VACCINE	Immune globulin HAV vaccine	HBV vaccine	None	HBV vaccine	None

ALT, alanine aminotransferase; AST, asparate aminotransferase; DNA, deoxyribonucleic acid; RNA, ribonucleic acid

BOX 26-5

POPULATIONS AT RISK FOR HBV

- Exposure to needle contamination
  - Persons receiving many blood transfusions
  - Personnel and persons in renal dialysis units
  - Intravenous drug users
- Sexual partners of affected persons
- Male homosexuals
- Children with Down syndrome
- Persons taking immunosuppressive medications
- Families or other close contacts of any of the above

Clinical manifestations can occur up to 6 months after exposure. The HBV organism can be identified by the presence of the surface antigen, the hepatitis B surface antigen (HBsAg), previously called the *Australian antigen.* The HBsAg can be measured in the blood and persists through most of the infection. Its presence can be measured to establish the diagnosis of HBV infection.[16] The intact virion is known as the *Dane particle,* shown in Figure 26-9. The particle core is synthesized within the nucleus of the hepatocyte and is composed of HBV core, DNA, and antigen.[7] The core of the virus contains the core antigen, HBcAg, which is not found in the blood, but anti-HBc-IgM antibody is positive in the serum during acute infection and also in a "window period" when the HBsAg is negative.[16] The first viral antigen to appear is the HBsAg. Next, levels of DNA polymerase, HBV DNA, and HBeAg rise. These markers are indicative of the Dane particle, and precede the rise of serum transaminase levels. Once the serum transaminase levels peak, the Dane markers begin to clear the bloodstream and HBsAg levels start to decrease. Anti-HBs levels appear as the infection dissipates, and lifelong immunity to the infection results. When HBsAg clears from the serum, it indicates clearance of the virus.[27] In 10% of infected individuals, however, levels of HBsAg and Dane particle markers may remain in the system; these persons have chronic HBV infections.[27] Figure 26-10 shows typical serologic events in hepatitis B infection. Pathologically, HAV and HBV look much alike. Hepatocellular injury and necrosis are usually surrounded by inflammatory cells, mainly lymphocytes and macrophages. The regeneration of hepatocytes begins very early in the disease, and multinucleate hepatocytes, increased mitotic figures, and hepatocyte thickening indicate regeneration.[7] The necrotic pattern may be spotty, confluent (groups of hepatocytes), or massive when most of the liver is affected. The hepatocyte necrosis is probably related to T cell cytotoxicity against the HBV, which would explain why individuals with impairment of T cell function are more likely to have relatively mild necrosis, incomplete elimination of HBV, and often a chronic HBV infection.[27] In general, there is evidence of (1) liver cell injury and scarring, (2) regeneration of liver cells, and (3) proliferation of inflammatory cells, including Kupffer cells.

FOCUS ON CELLULAR PATHOPHYSIOLOGY

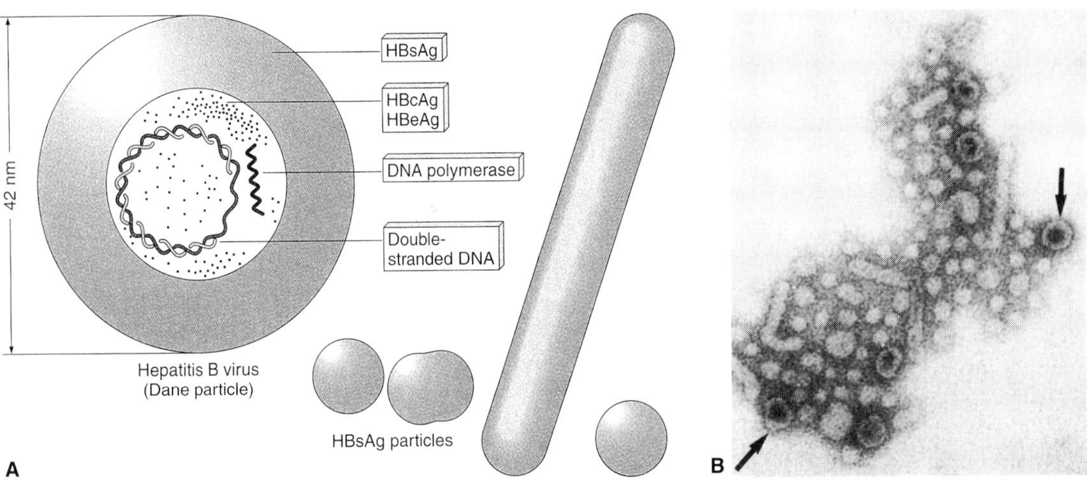

FIGURE 26-9. **(A)** Schematic representation of the hepatitis B virus (HBV) and serum particles associated with HBV infection. **(B)** Electron micrograph of particles from centrifuged serum in a case of hepatitis B. Rodlike and spherical particles containing HBsAg are evident. The complete virion, composed of the viral core and its surrounding envelope, is represented by Dane particles (*arrows*). (Rubin, E. & Farber, J. L. [1999]. *Pathology* [3rd ed.]. Philadelphia: Lippincott-Raven.)

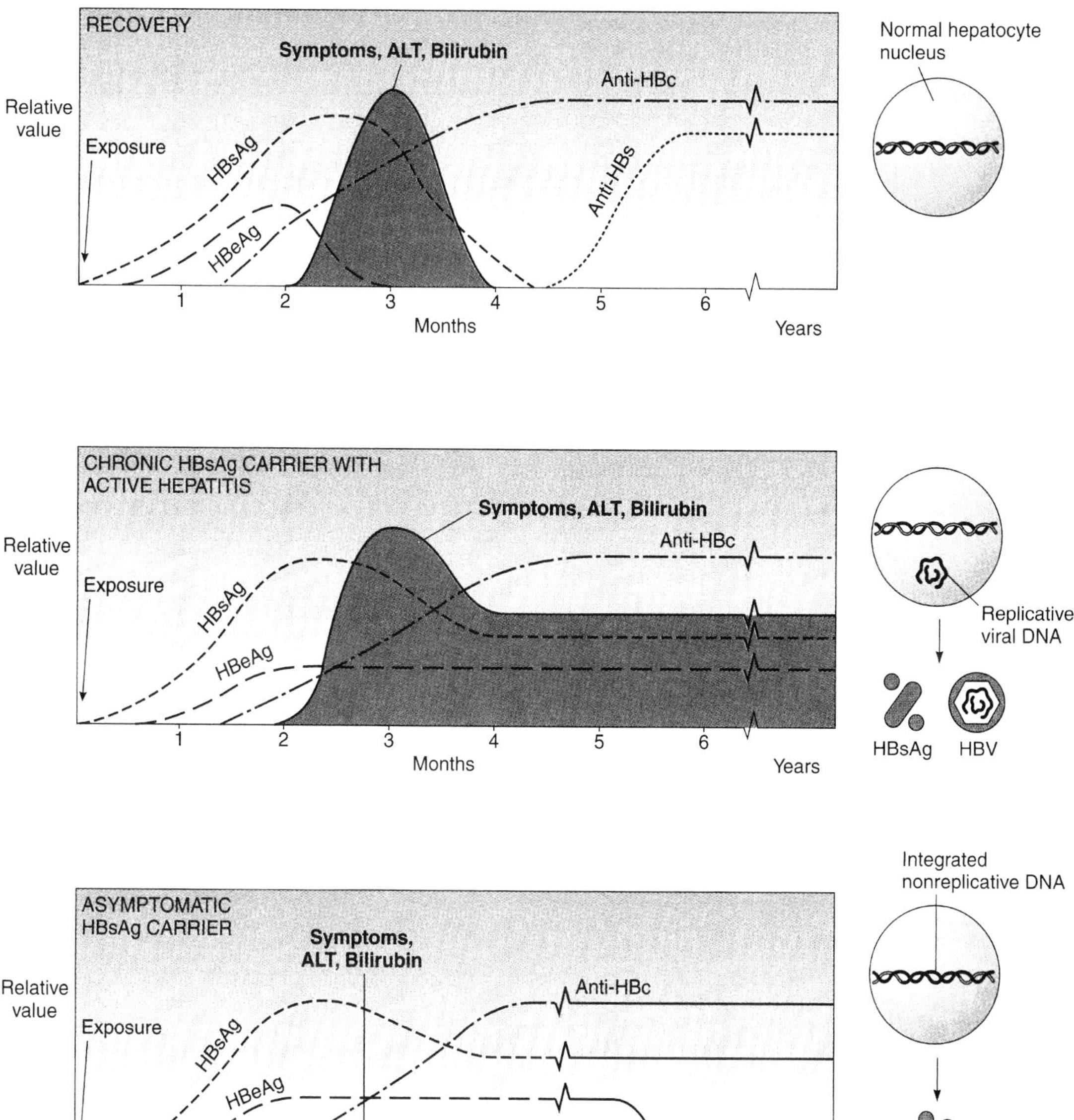

FIGURE 26-10. Typical serological events in three distinct outcomes of hepatitis B. (*Top panel*) In most cases, the appearance of anti-HBs ensures complete recovery. Viral DNA disappears from the nucleus of the hepatocyte. (*Middle panel*) In about 10% of cases of hepatitis B, HBs antigenemia is sustained for longer than 6 months, owing to the absence of anti-HBs. Patients in whom viral replication remains active, as evidenced by sustained high levels of HBeAg in the blood, develop active hepatitis. In such cases, the viral genome persists in the nucleus but is not integrated into host DNA. (*Lower panel*) Patients in whom active viral replication ceases or is attenuated, as reflected in the disappearance of HBeAg from the blood, become asymptomatic carriers. In these individuals fragments of the HBV genome are integrated into the host DNA, but episomal DNA is absent. (Rubin, E. & Farber, J. L. [1999]. *Pathology* [3rd ed.]. Philadelphia: Lippincott-Raven.)

The clinical syndrome of HBV is unpredictable and can include any of the following syndromes:

CARRIER STATE. "Healthy" carriers can transmit the disease even though they have no evidence of infection themselves. The serum in these individuals is chronically positive for HBsAg and often other markers, such as anti-HBc. Chronic carrier states are as high as 20% in some Asian populations.[27] Persons who are immunodeficient for any number of reasons are more likely to be carriers than are other persons. Children who receive the virus during childbirth are usually carriers.[7]

ACUTE, ICTERIC, OR NONICTERIC HEPATITIS. During the preicteric phase, anorexia, fever, chills, and fatigue occur.[27] Other liver symptoms, such as prolonged prothrombin time and hepatic tenderness, may be present. HBV is often not diagnosed due to lack of specific symptoms. Complete recovery and lifelong immunity is the rule for these persons.[24]

CHRONIC PERSISTENT OR CHRONIC ACTIVE HEPATITIS. Chronic persistent hepatitis is a smoldering infection that may not disrupt liver function severely. Nonspecific symptoms of anorexia and malaise may be noted with variable degrees of jaundice and hepatosplenomegaly.[24] Chronic active hepatitis progresses very rapidly to progressive liver damage, leading to cirrhosis, hepatic failure, and death.[7] Approximately 5% of HBV infections become chronic, and two thirds of these infections are chronic active hepatitis.[7,27]

FULMINANT HEPATITIS. This type progresses very rapidly from onset to fulminant liver failure and death in 2 to 3 weeks. It can result from other causative agents, but viral hepatitis accounts for 50% to 65% of all cases.[7]

Hepatitis Delta

The hepatitis delta virus (HDV) is produced by a defective RNA virus distinct from all others. Its onset is abrupt, with symptoms similar to HBV. The delta agent causes infection only in persons with active infection with HBV.[27] It is associated with more severe infection and a higher rate of fulminant hepatitis than HBV alone. When a person is infected with HBV, the HDV can replicate much more efficiently. Therefore, HDV becomes a superinfecting agent and may cause the exacerbation of previously stable chronic hepatitis B.[27] The replication of the HDV is limited to when the HBsAg is found in the sera and the organisms are cleared together.[24] It is transmitted parenterally. The diagnosis is often overlooked or called an exacerbation of chronic HBV. A chronic state may persist with the combination of HBV and HDV.

Hepatitis C

Hepatitis C (HCV), formerly called non-A, non-B hepatitis, is an RNA virus that may be transmitted through blood transfusions, through needle stick exposure, and perinatal transmission.[27] Intravenous drug abusers are at particular risk for HCV. In many persons infected with HCV, there is no identifiable source of infection.[24] Half the infected persons develop chronic hepatitis. This may persist as a continuing infection with elevated liver enzyme levels and minor symptoms, or it may become active and lead to cirrhosis, fulminant hepatitis, or hepatocellular carcinoma. Many chronic alcoholics with liver disease have antibodies to HCV, which may increase the liver injury in these persons.[24]

Hepatitis E

The main source of contamination for this non-A, non-B hepatitis is fecal contamination of water supply, especially in developing countries, such as India and southeast Asia. Its target population seems to be young adults and pregnant women. The disease has a fatality rate of 1% to 2%.[27] The clinical disease is similar to that of HAV except the course is usually more severe. No chronic or carrier state seems to exist, and the virus has been identified as a single-stranded RNA virus.[24]

Hepatitis F and G

Two new hepatitis viruses have been discovered; they have been tentatively designated hepatitis F and hepatitis G. They are non-ABCDE viruses, and are currently undergoing investigation for genetic coding, transmission, and treatment.[28]

Gallbladder Dysfunction

The most common disorders of the gallbladder are **cholecystitis** (inflammation) and **cholelithiasis** (gallstones). Cancer of the gallbladder is also a notable disorder.

CHOLECYSTITIS AND CHOLELITHIASIS

Inflammation of the gallbladder is the second most frequent cause of abdominal pain that requires abdominal surgery, the first being appendicitis. Dietary factors, including high fat intake, have long been associated with cholecystitis. Primary bacterial infection may cause cholecystitis, but in up to 80% of cases, obstructive stones in the bile duct are present. Therefore, it is thought that bacterial contamination either may be secondary to the stasis or may result from severe infection, such as septicemia. Pancreatic reflux may occur and cause irritation by contact of pancreatic enzymes with the mucosa of the bile duct.[1] Acute cholecystitis generally arises from obstruction of the cystic duct by gallstones and may cause complications with abscesses or perforation of the gallbladder. Chronic cholecystitis arises from repeated attacks of acute cholecystitis.

Cholelithiasis is a common disorder that refers to biliary tract stones, most of which form in the gallbladder itself. Their major constituents are *cholesterol* and *pigment,* and they often contain mixtures of components of bile. Stones composed primarily of cholesterol account for 80% of gallstones in the United States. Some predisposing factors include middle age, female sex, obesity, and possibly multiparity. Pregnancy, oral contraceptives, and estrogen therapy may be contributors.

Gallstones can intermittently obstruct the cystic duct. Obstruction of the duct is followed by acute cholecystitis that may be due to increased pressure and ischemia in the gallbladder or to chemical irritation of the organ caused by prolonged exposure to concentrated bile.

Clinical Manifestations

The clinical manifestations associated with cholecystitis and cholelithiasis vary from mild dyspepsia to recurrent pain, fever, and jaundice. The obstruction in the bile duct causes pain and blocks bile excretion. Visceral pain is precipitated by biliary contractions and is termed **biliary colic.** This pain is usually perceived as a steady, severe aching or pressure in the epigastrium.[1] The pain of cholecystitis may mimic myocardial infarction, peptic ulcer, or intestinal obstruction, among other conditions. Chronic cholecystitis is manifested by intolerance to fatty food, belching, nausea and vomiting, and pain after eating.

Stones of varying size may be visualized in the gallbladder by routine x-ray or abdominal ultrasonography.[1] The white blood cell count and serum alkaline phosphatase may be elevated. Bilirubin level is often increased, causing scleral and systemic jaundice.

CANCER OF THE GALLBLADDER

The most common form of cancer of the gallbladder is adenocarcinoma.[24] It is an aggressive cancer associated with a high rate of metastasis to the liver and surrounding lymph nodes. It usually presents in patients who have experienced longstanding cholecystitis and cholelithiasis. It is seen most often in the sixth or seventh decades, and women are affected more frequently than men. It may be found incidentally during a cholecystectomy, or it may produce clinical manifestations of biliary obstruction similar to cholelithiasis. However, by the time the tumor is symptomatic, it generally has metastasized extensively and carries a 5-year survival rate of less than 3%.[24]

Exocrine Pancreatic Dysfunction

ACUTE PANCREATITIS

Pancreatitis, or inflammation of the pancreas, is characterized by hemorrhage, necrosis, and suppuration of pancreatic parenchyma. Pathologic changes occur in varying degrees of severity and are caused by activation of proteolytic enzymes within the pancreas.

Acute pancreatitis occurs most frequently in middle life and more in women than in men. *Alcoholism* and *cholelithiasis* (gallstones) are responsible for 70% to 80% of cases in industrialized nations.[12] These and other factors associated with the etiology of pancreatitis are listed in Box 26-6.

Pathophysiology

The chemical and pathologic changes are the result of destructive effects of pancreatic enzymes. The precise mechanism that triggers the activation of enzymes and autodigestion is unknown. When the pancreas becomes damaged or when a duct is blocked, pancreatic secretions accumulate. It is hypothesized that the trypsin inhibitor is overwhelmed and the pancreatic enzymes become activated to cause acute pancreatitis.[14] Elastase exists in high concentrations in granules of acinous cells and is present in pancreatic secretions as an inactive precursor. When activated, hemorrhages occur as the elastic fibers of blood vessels and ducts dissolve. Trypsin causes prekallikrein to be converted to kallikrein, causing the release of bradykinin and kallidin (a plasma kinin); this further increases vasodilatation and vascular permeability. Phospholipase A acts on phospholipids, releasing compounds that have strong cytotoxic effects. Cell membranes and the ductal system are damaged, leading to necrosis. Leukocytic reactions appear around the areas of hemorrhage and necrosis. Secondary bacterial invasion may produce a suppurative necrosis or abscess. Milder lesions may be absorbed, or they may calcify or become fibrotic if severe. Flowchart 26-2 summarizes the pathogenesis of acute pancreatitis. Alcohol stimulates pancreatic secretions and also causes duodenal edema of the ampulla of Vater, obstructing flow of secretions. Long-term alcohol ingestion increases the protein concentration of secretions, which leads to the formation of protein plugs in the ducts and subsequent obstruction. Additionally, lysosomes and zymogen granules in the acini cells become fragile. Alcohol may increase pressure in the sphincter of Oddi or cause spasm.[12] Hyperlipidemia is associated with pancreatitis. Triglyceride by-products may induce pancreatitis. Toxic free fatty acids result from lipase acting on serum triglycerides, injuring the endothelial lining of small blood vessels in the pancreas. The injury leads to inflammation and thrombosis.[11] Hypercalcemia may cause the activation of trypsinogen, causing the subsequent development of acute pancreatitis. An association of pancreatitis with multiple myeloma, hyperparathyroidism, cardiac bypass, immobilization, and carcinomas has been observed.[11]

Clinical Manifestations

Abdominal pain and tenderness are present in approximately 95% of these patients. The pain may have no prodromal symptoms and often occurs after eating, ingesting alcohol, or vomiting.[12] It usually is severe and

BOX 26-6

FACTORS IN THE ETIOLOGY OF PANCREATITIS

Alcoholism
Biliary tract disease
Postoperative (abdominal, nonabdominal)
Postendoscopic retrograde cholangiopancreatography (ERCP)
Trauma (abdominal injury; intraoperative)
Metabolic (hyperlipidemia, uremia, renal failure, after renal transplantation, hypercalcemia, pregnancy, cystic fibrosis, kwashiorkor)
Vascular (shock, lupus erythematosus, thrombocytopenic purpura, polyarteritis, atheromatous embolism)
Drugs
- Association
  - Immunosuppressive—corticosteroids, L-asparaginase, azathioprine
  - Diuretics—thiazides, furosemide, ethacrynic acid
  - Estrogens, oral contraceptives
  - Antibodies—tetracyclines, sulfonamides
- Possible association
  - Acetaminophen
  - Isoniazid, rifampin
  - Propoxyphene
  - Valproic acid, procainamide
  - Anticoagulants

Infections (mumps, viral hepatitis, coxsackievirus, echovirus, *Ascaris, Mycoplasma*)
Mechanical (duct obstruction, duodenal obstruction)
Penetrating duodenal ulcer
Hereditary pancreatitis
Idiopathic

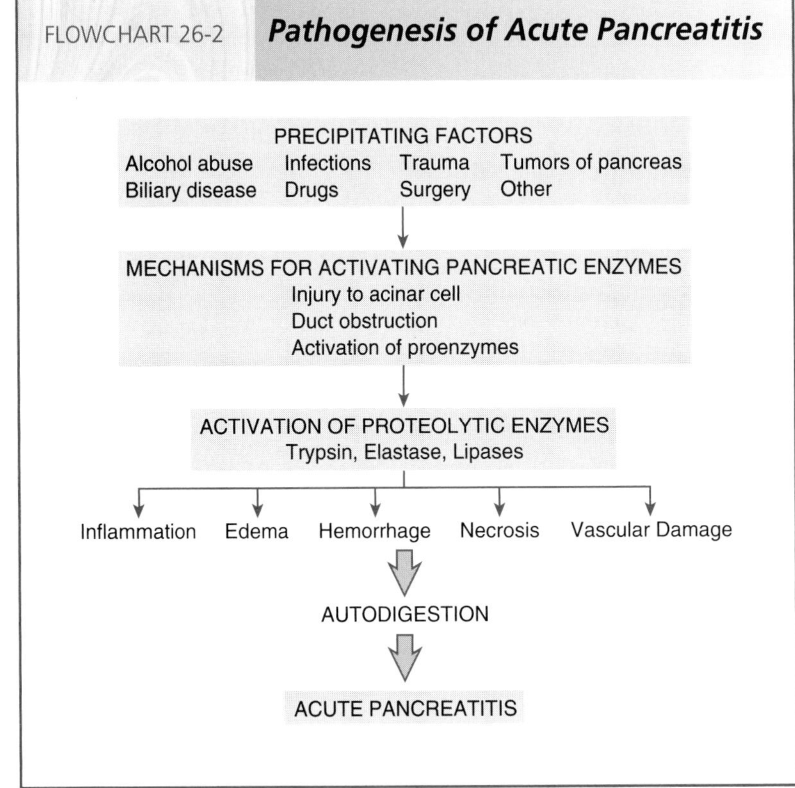

may reach full intensity in a matter of minutes or gradually over several hours; the pain may last for hours or days.[11] Pain is commonly localized in the epigastrium, frequently radiating to the back in over half of the patients.[12] Pancreatic pain usually is steady, boring, and penetrating. Affected persons are restless and anxious; they may seek relief by leaning or bending forward or flexing the knees against the chest.[12] The pain of pancreatitis is related to ductal swelling, extravasation of plasma and RBCs, and release of digested proteins and lipids into surrounding tissue. The pancreatic capsule is stretched by the edema, exudate, RBCs, and digestive products. These substances seep out of the gland into the mesentery, causing a peritonitis that stimulates the sensory nerves, causing intense pain in the back and flanks.

During an acute attack, the pain is generalized over the abdomen because of peritoneal irritation and release of kinins. Large doses of narcotics are avoided because they may induce spasm of the sphincter of Oddi, which aggravates the pancreatitis and increases pain. As pain increases with the spread of intraperitoneal and retroperitoneal inflammation, local or diffuse paralytic ileus may occur. Peripheral vascular collapse and shock may develop rapidly. The stretching of the gland may cause nausea and vomiting. Vomiting and abdominal distention also are related to intestinal hypomotility and chemical peritonitis.

The major findings of acute pancreatitis are increases in serum amylase and lipase from the leak of digestive enzymes. Serum amylase values usually exceed 200 Somogyi units; normal levels are 60 to 180 Somogyi units/dL. Serum lipase activity, most specific for acute pancreatitis, parallels that of serum amylase, and abnormal levels persist for a longer time. Normal serum lipase values are usually below 1.5 U/mL. The increased levels occur shortly after onset of the disease and may remain elevated for weeks. Leukocytosis with increased polymorphonuclear leukocytes and a shift to the left is frequent. The white blood cell counts are elevated, occasionally rising to 50,000/mm^3. The hematocrit may be elevated from loss of serum into the peritoneal spaces with resultant hemoconcentration. Hyperglycemia may occur due to increased glucagon, decreased insulin, and increased glucocorticoid and catecholamine levels. Levels of serum calcium and magnesium decrease. Hypocalcemia is an indicator of severe pancreatitis.

Other nonspecific findings include low-grade fever, hypotension, tachycardia, and shock. Bradykinin release causes peripheral vasodilatation and exudation of plasma into the retroperitoneal space. Fluid therefore accumulates in the small bowel from third-space shifting, causing a drop in blood pressure; hypovolemic shock may result with possible myocardial, renal, and cerebral ischemia. Mild jaundice may be present in patients who have biliary obstruction.[12] Swelling of the head of the pancreas impinges on the common bile duct, causing obstruction. If the bile duct is compressed by pseudocysts or stones, jaundice may be more severe. Bowel sounds usually are diminished. In severe necrotizing pancreatitis, discoloration of the flanks (*Turner's sign*) or around the umbilicus (*Cullen's sign*) may be noted. A pancreatic *pseudocyst* may be palpable in the upper abdomen. Pseudocysts are nonepithelium-lined cavities containing plasma, blood, pancreatic products, and inflammatory exudate, measuring 5 to 10 cm in diameter. They typically occur due to the destruction of tissue and obstruction in the ductal system. Pancreatic juice may collect and leak into the peritoneal cavity. Pseudocysts may impinge on neighboring structures, causing acute portal hypertension or jaundice. They also may rupture and cause generalized peritonitis. Box 26-7 lists additional complications of acute pancreatitis. The CT scan is the gold standard for diagnosis; in severe disease, it is virtually always abnormal.

CHRONIC PANCREATITIS

Manifestations of chronic pancreatitis are similar to those of acute pancreatitis except for their chronicity and recurrence. Alcohol abuse (70–80% of cases in Western countries) and malnutrition (worldwide) are the most common causes of chronic pancreatis. Nonalcoholic tropical pancreatitis and hereditary or familial pancreatitis are forms of chronic pancreatitis that are relatively rare.[21] Pancreatic insufficiency may ultimately result.

BOX 26-7 COMPLICATIONS OF ACUTE PANCREATITIS

- Hypovolemic shock
- Lactic acidosis
- Ileus
- Gastrointestinal bleeding
- Hyperlipidemia
- Pseudocysts
- Pancreatic abscess
- Fistulization
- Hypercoagulability
  Platelets, factor VIII, fibrinogen, and factor V are elevated.
- Pleural effusions
  Retroperitoneal transudation of fluid and increased secretion of amylase into the pleural cavity.
- Hypocalcemia
  Lipolysis of tissues causes release of free fatty acids, combining with calcium to form soaps.

Pathophysiology

In chronic pancreatitis, histologic changes remain even after the causative agent has been removed. The pathologic changes are characterized by the deposition of protein plugs in the pancreatic ductules. An inflammatory process begins, and fibrous tissue is deposited. Eventually intraductal calcification and marked parenchymal destruction are noted, with only a few islet cells and some acinar tissue remaining.

Clinical Manifestations

Exocrine pancreatic insufficiency is manifested by steatorrhea (excess fat in the stools), azotorrhea (excess nitrogenous material in the feces), and weight loss. Microscopically, the stool exhibits fat globules and striated meat fibers that indicate impaired digestion of fats and proteins. Abdominal pain is common and may be responsible for severe weight loss, malnutrition, and general debility. During early stages of the disease, the person may be asymptomatic between attacks.

The predominant complications of chronic pancreatitis that are associated with abdominal pain are pancreatic pseudocyst, stricture and obstruction of the common bile duct or pancreatic duct, and, occasionally, diabetes and carcinoma of the pancreas.

CANCER OF THE PANCREAS

Cancers of the pancreas occur mainly in the exocrine portion of the gland, and the most common site is the head of the pancreas.[32] They typically originate from the ductal epithelium.[32] Cancer of the pancreas is the fourth most common cause of death from cancer for men and the fifth most common for women in the United States.[4] Pancreatic cancers have a poor prognosis; 97% of the patients will die.[32] Smoking, alcohol intake, a history of pancreatitis, and consumption of meat and fat have been implicated as risk factors.[32] There is a higher incidence in African Americans and in men. Chemists and people exposed to industrial agents also are at higher risk for pancreatic cancer. Most tumors occur in people over age 60; they seldom occur before age 40.

Pathophysiology

Most carcinomas of the pancreas grow in well-differentiated glandular patterns, and over 80% are adenocarcinomas.[32] About 10% assume an adenosquamous pattern or an uncommon pattern of extreme anaplasia with giant cell formation. An uncommon type of pancreatic cancer, cystadenocarcinoma, originates from acinar cells; it is associated with a more favorable prognosis.[32] Acinar cell cancers are usually seen in the younger population.[32] Cancers of the pancreas progress insidiously, and most have metastasized before their discovery. Cancer cells may invade the stomach, duodenum, major blood vessels, the bile duct, colon, spleen, and kidney, as well as regional and distant lymph nodes.[32]

Clinical Manifestations

Clinical symptoms of cancer of the pancreas depend on its site of origin and manifestations of metastasis. Tumors of the head of the pancreas tend to obstruct the bile duct and duodenum and lead to early symptoms of obstructive jaundice, accompanied by pruritus and weight loss. Carcinoma of the body and tail are less easily recognized clinically and become apparent only when adjacent structures are involved or when metastatic dissemination produces symptoms.

Typical clinical manifestations relate to the compression on surrounding organs by the pancreas.[4] Dull epigastric abdominal pain that may radiate to the back, weight loss with anorexia, generalized malaise and weakness, and jaundice are among the few characteristic signs or symptoms that point to a diagnosis of pancreatic cancer.

Nausea, vomiting, weakness, fatigue, diarrhea, and dyspepsia also are fairly common. Vomiting may indicate gastric or duodenal encroachment or peritoneal metastasis. Hematemesis and melena indicate invasion of the tumor into duodenal or gastric organs that are vascular. About one fourth of persons with pancreatic cancer have a palpable abdominal mass when examined and often complain of both constipation and diarrhea. Emotional disturbances may be noted. Hyperglycemia and glucose intolerance may also occur from pancreatic cell dysfunction.[9] An abdominal bruit may be auscultated in the periumbilical area and left upper quadrant because of compression of the splenic artery by a tumor. Migratory superficial thrombophlebitis, also called Trousseau's syndrome, may be noted in cancer of the pancreas.[32] Laboratory studies provide clues to the presence of these cancers in their early stages. About 80% to 90% have elevated levels of *carcinoembryonic antigen.* Measurement of this antigen may be helpful in following the course of pancreatic cancer, with titers of greater than 20 mg/mL usually being associated with metastases. As with obstructive jaundice, serum bilirubin levels increase, stools become clay colored, and urine urobilinogen levels fall. Alkaline phosphatase levels are elevated.[4] Ultrasonography can assist in localizing tumors and differentiating them from cysts.

CYSTIC FIBROSIS

Cystic fibrosis (CF) is a multisystem disorder of infancy, adolescents, and young adults. CF has been clearly recognized as a disease entity only since the late 1930s. Historical notes tell of the midwife licking the forehead of the newborn to identify any salty taste. CF is characterized by alterations in the secretory process of the exocrine (mucous-producing) glands resulting in pulmonary disease, pancreatic insufficiency, and elevated sweat electrolytes.

Cystic fibrosis is a common inherited condition and the most fatal genetic disease in whites of European origin. The incidence is about 1/2,000 in white populations with a 1:25 carrier rate. Black and Oriental races are seldom affected. There is no difference in sex distribution. CF is transmitted by the autosomal recessive mode of inheritance. If both parents are carriers of the gene, there is a 25% chance that with each pregnancy that the child will have CF, a 50% chance that the child will carry the gene but not have the disease, and a 25% chance that the child will neither have CF nor carry the gene.[23] Chromosome number and structure are normal. Clinical manifestations are only evident in homozygotes. Carriers of the gene (heterozygotes) show no symptoms.

Pathophysiology

Cystic fibrosis results from a single mutation of a gene. The deletion of an amino acid accounts for most mutations and results in a protein (CF gene product) called the cystic fibrosis transmembrane conductance regulator (CFTR). CFTR molecules are normally found on the endoplasmic reticulum of cells lining ducts of exocrine organs, especially the lungs, pancreas, intestine, and sweat ducts of the skin. They function as regulators of ion and water channels through which electrolytes can pass. When CFTR-containing exocrine cells are sympathetically stimulated, mucus, electrolytes, and water are secreted into the duct openings. It is the combination of water and electrolytes that assists in hydration of exocrine secretions and mucus enabling them to move along the ducts and be released.[29] Because CFTR is inadequately synthesized, the thick, viscous secretions and protein plugs eventually ob-

FLOWCHART 26-3 **Pathogenesis of Cystic Fibrosis**

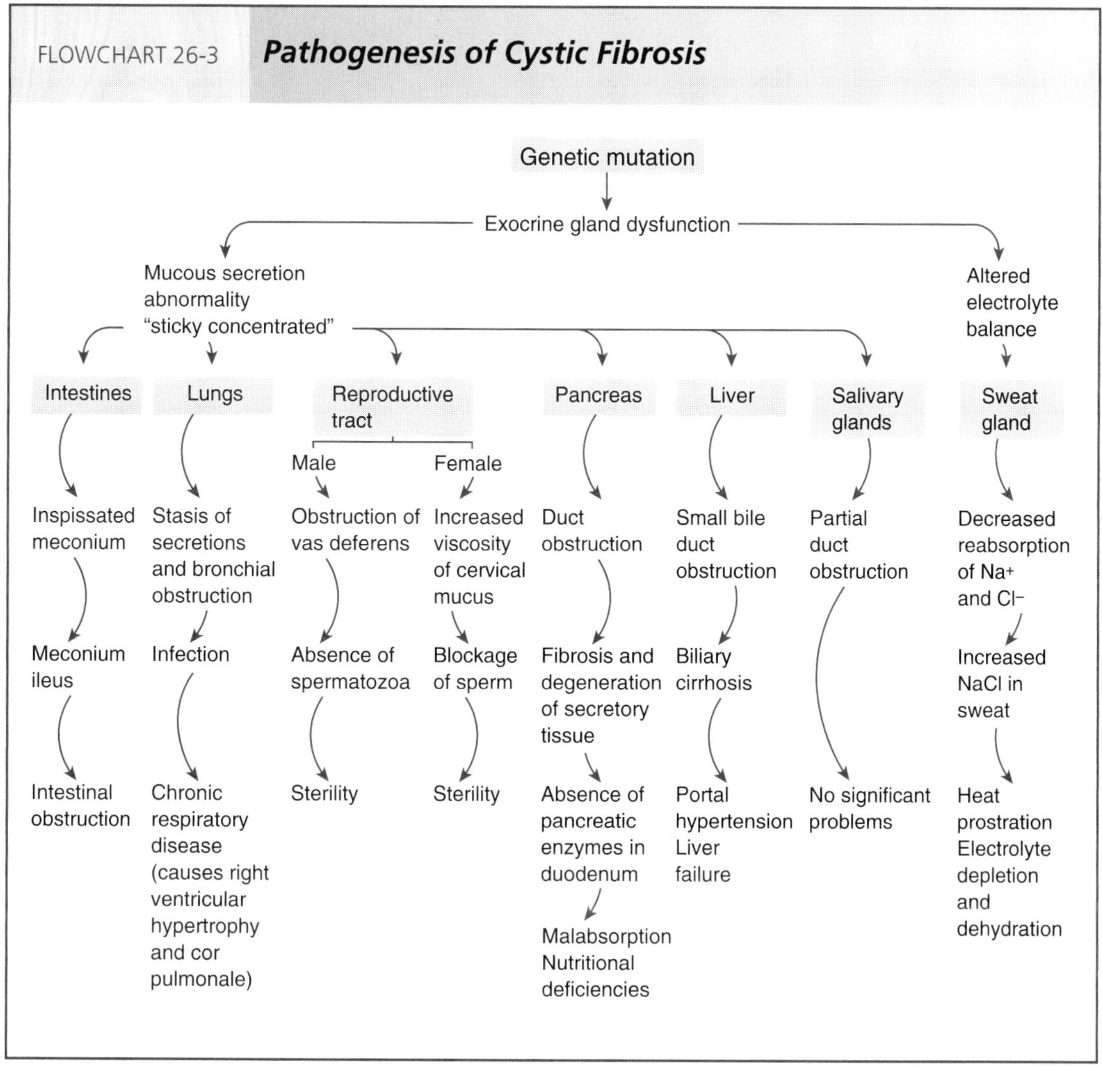

struct the ducts of exocrine organs, causing damage to acinar tissue, fibrosis and duct dilatation, and degeneration of the parenchyma. The ducts may be replaced by fat and fibrous tissue and converted into cysts. These changes in appearance are the bases for the designation fibrocystic disease of the pancreas. This alteration also affects chloride transport and is manifested by an increase in sodium chloride in sweat.[29] Pathologic changes begin during fetal life and frequently are severe enough by birth to prevent exocrine secretions from reaching the duodenum. Thick, heavy, dehydrated mucus obstructs the exocrine ducts, resulting in anatomic changes. Functional changes occur as a result of structural alterations.

Although the basic pathologic alterations in CF involve the pulmonary and digestive systems, many other parts of the body are affected. Flowchart 26-3 shows the multisystem effects of CF.

Clinical Manifestations

Clinical manifestations differ among children depending on disease progression and age of the child. Because CF affects several organ systems in varying degrees, it may be difficult to recognize. Most persons are diagnosed in early childhood because of symptoms related to the respiratory and gastrointestinal systems. As the child grows older, the impaired pancreatic function results in malabsorption of fats and the fat-soluble vitamins. The child has a good appetite but appears malnourished. Bleeding disorders may occurs as a result of vitamin K deficiency from malabsorption. In the classic case, the child is examined after several months of life because of respiratory symptoms, failure to thrive, and foul-smelling, bulky, greasy stools.

Newborn screening can be done by examination of a drop of dried neonatal blood for elevated levels of serum immunoreactive trypsinogen. However, there are significant false-positive and false-negative results. DNA mutation analysis can be done on dried blood.[23] Rarely, CF is diagnosed during adolescence or adulthood. Diagnosis is difficult because the sweat test is less reliable in these age groups than in younger ones. Persons affected with CF who have not had severe chest infections may have abdominal problems, diabetes, or liver disease.

FOCUS ON THE PERSON PRESENTING WITH ACUTE EPIGASTRIC PAIN

Mr. S., 55 years of age, comes to the emergency department (ED) of a large urban hospital. This is Mr. S.'s third admission to the ED within 3 years. He is complaining of severe epigastric pain radiating to his back. Nausea and vomiting are associated with the pain. He is disoriented when responding to the triage nurse.

Physical examination revealed poor skin turgor, and other signs of dehydration were evident. Slight jaundice, fever, tachycardia, orthopnea, midline tenderness, and guarding were present.

Mr. S. denies taking any medications. He is 5′10″ tall and weighs 245 lb. He admits to eating "mostly fast foods, like fried chicken" because he has very little time to prepare meals. He states he drinks socially but does not get intoxicated. However, he estimates that he has at least "two or three" drinks at night to help him sleep.

Mr. S. is employed as a painter. He lives alone but visits his sister frequently. His wife died 3 years ago from ovarian cancer. His only son lives over 500 miles away. Mr. S. had an oral cholecystectography 6 months ago, but results were normal.

Routine laboratory values:	WBC = 16,000/mm^3 (normal = 5,000–10,000/mm^3); all other values (CBC, electrolytes) within normal limits (WNL)
Serum glucose:	150 mg/dl (normal = 80–115 mg/dL)
Serum amylase:	640 IU/L (normal = 56–190 IU/L)
Urine amylase:	1240 IU/hr (normal = 3–35 IU/hr)
Serum lipase:	240 units/L (normal = 0–110 units/L)
Ultrasound of pancreas:	Head of pancreas enlarged and edematous
CT of abdomen:	Pancreas enlarged
ERCP:	Normal pancreatic duct

Radiograph revealed pleural effusion.

Questions

1. What are risk factors for the development of pancreatitis? In particular, what are Mr. S.'s risk factors?
2. What is the pathophysiologic basis for Mr. S.'s clinical manifestations of pancreatitis?
3. What triggers the autodigestive process that characterizes pancreatitis?
4. What is the major enzyme involved in activating the pathologic process?
5. What is a pancreatic pseudocyst? Differentiate between a pseudocyst and a pancreatic abscess.
6. Which of Mr. S.'s laboratory values would indicate a diagnosis of pancreatitis?

FOCUS ON THE CHILD WITH CYSTIC FIBROSIS

K., a blue-eyed, blond-haired female, age 14 months, is admitted to the pediatric unit with paroxysmal coughing and a respiratory infection. K. is the second child of a 32-year-old father and a 30-year-old mother. K. has a history of recurrent respiratory infections. She is pale and thin, especially her extremities. Her abdomen is distended and her mother reports that her stools are large, frothy in appearance, and foul smelling. She is in the 5th percentile for weight and the 10th percentile for height.

Both parents and older sister, age 4, are well. A maternal uncle died in his late twenties from pneumonia and heart failure secondary to cystic fibrosis. Physical examination revealed wheezing, rhonchi, tachypnea with a prolonged expiratory phase.

Diagnostic Evaluation

Chest radiograph revealed patchy atelectasis, hyperinflation, and air trapping.

Sweat electrolytes (iontophoresis):	Sodium = 90 mEq/L (normal < 70 mEq/L)
	Chloride = 70 mEq/L (normal < 50 mEq/L)
Secretin-pan creozymin test (duodenal aspirate):	Absence of trypsin
Fecal fat test 72-h:	Fat retention coefficient 80% (normal > 95%)
Oximetry readings:	88–92% in oxygen tent

Antibiotics and chest physiotherapy are ordered. The parents are instructed in pancreatic enzyme therapy. A high-protein diet with moderate fat and multiple vitamin supplements is ordered. Genetic testing and counseling are recommended.

Questions

1. What in K.'s history and clinical manifestations would explain why she has cystic fibrosis?
2. What is the genetic inheritance pattern? Could prenatal testing identify the disease prenatally? How?
3. Which two body systems are primarily affected and how?
4. What in the pathogenesis of cystic fibrosis leads to right ventricular hypertrophy development?
5. What pathophysiologic changes account for the appearance of K.'s stools?
6. Why would a sweat electrolyte test be ordered?
7. Why would a pancreatic enzyme test be ordered?
8. Why would a fat test be ordered?
9. How would genetic counseling benefit the family?

The pilocarpine iontophoresis sweat test is the simplest and most reliable diagnostic test for CF. Up to age 20, a level of more than 60 mEq/L of sweat chloride is diagnostic of CF. Values between 50 and 60 mEq/L are highly suggestive. The sweat test is repeated if results are questionable or if they are negative and clinical manifestations strongly suggest CF. Reliable sweat tests are difficult to obtain in the first 3 to 4 weeks of life because the sweat glands are not yet well developed functionally.

Chest x-rays reveal a slightly increased diameter of the upper chest, with overaerated lungs, widespread consolidation, and fibrotic changes. There may be areas of lobar or segmental collapse. Pulmonary function tests assist in evaluating the therapeutics and monitoring progress of the disease.

Changes in radiologic patterns of the small intestine are noted in CF as in other malabsorptive diseases. Fibrosis abnormalities also are evident in barium studies of the duodenum. In the female, cervical polyps may be detected on vaginal examination.

Pancreatic deficiency is noted on examination of duodenal contents for pancreatic enzyme (trypsin and chymotrypsin) activity. Trypsin is absent in about 80% of affected people. Chemical examination of feces reveals marked steatorrhea. Normal stools should not contain more than 4 g of fat per day. Stools of children with CF often contain 15 to 30 g/d.

REFERENCES

1. Apstein, M. D., & Carey, M. C. (1994). Biliary tract stones and associated diseases. In J. H. Stein (Ed.), *Internal medicine* (4th ed.). St. Louis: Mosby.
2. Arias, I. M., Boyer, J. L., Fausto, N., Jakoby, W. B., Schachter, D., & Shafritz, D. A. (1994). *The liver: Biology and pathobiology* (3rd ed.). New York: Raven Press.
3. Carr, B. I., Flickinger, J. C., & Lotze, M. T. (1997). Hepatobiliary cancers. In V. T. DeVita, Jr., S. Hellman, & S. A. Rosenberg (Eds.), *Cancer: Principles and practice of oncology* (5th ed.). Philadelphia: Lippincott-Raven.
4. Cello, J. P. (1998). Pancreatic cancer. In M. Feldman, B. F. Scharschmidt, & M. H. Sleisenger (Eds.), *Sleisenger & Fordran's gastrointestinal and liver disease: Pathophysiology/diagnosis/management* (6th ed., Vol. 1). Philadelphia: W. B. Saunders.
5. Chopra, S. (1994). Hepatic tumors. In J. H. Stein (Ed.), *Internal medicine* (4th ed.) St. Louis: Mosby.
6. Cormack, D. H. (1993). *Essential histology*. Philadelphia: Lippincott.

7. Cotran, R. S., Kumar, V., & Robbins, S. L. (1994). *Robbins' pathologic basis of disease* (5th ed.). Philadelphia: W. B. Saunders.
8. Crabb, D. W., & Lumeng, L. (1997). Alcoholic liver disease. In W. N. Kelley (Ed.), *Textbook of internal medicine* (3rd ed., Vol. 1). Philadelphia: Lippincott-Raven.
9. Evans, D. B., Abbruzzese, J. L., & Rich, T. A. (1997). Cancer of the pancreas. In V. T. DeVita, Jr., S. Hellman, & S. A. Rosenberg (Eds.), *Cancer: Principles and practice of oncology* (5th ed.). Philadelphia: Lippincott-Raven.
10. Ganong, W. F. (1994). *Review of medical physiology* (16th ed.). Los Altos, CA: Appleton-Lange.
11. Gorelick, F. S. (1995). Acute pancreatitis. In T. Yamada (Ed.), *Textbook of gastroenterology* (2nd ed., Vol. 2). Philadelphia: Lippincott.
12. Grendell, J. H. (1997). Pancreatitis. In W. N. Kelley et al. (Eds.), *Textbook of internal medicine* (3rd. ed., Vol. 1). Philadelphia: Lippincott-Raven.
13. Grundy, S. M. (1994). Disorders of lipids and lipoproteins. In J. Stein, et al. (Eds.), *Internal medicine* (4th ed.) St. Louis: Mosby, 1994.
14. Guyton, A. C., & Hall, J. E. (1996). *Textbook of medical physiology* (9th ed.). Philadelphia: Saunders.
15. Kang, E. H., & Brown, J. J. (1995). Magnetic resonance imaging. In T. Yamada (Ed.), *Textbook of gastroenterology* (2nd ed., Vol. 2). Philadelphia: Lippincott.
16. LaBreque, D. R. (1994). Acute and chronic hepatitis. In J. H. Stein et al. (Eds.), *Internal medicine* (4th ed.) St. Louis: Mosby.
17. Lotze, M. T., Flickinger, J. C., & Carr, B. I. (1993). Hepatobiliary neoplasms. In V. T. DeVita, S. Hellman, & S. A. Rosenberg (Eds.), *Cancer: Principles and practice of oncology* (4th ed.). Philadelphia: Lippincott.
18. Lucey, M. R. (1997). Approach to the patient with cirrhosis, portal hypertension, and end-stage liver disease. In W. N. Kelley (Ed.), *Textbook of internal medicine* (3rd ed., Vol. 1). Philadelphia: Lippincott.
19. Moseley, R. H. (1995). Approach to the patient with abnormal liver chemistries. In T. Yamada (Ed.), *Textbook of gastroenterology* (2nd ed., Vol. 1). Philadelphia: Lippincott.
20. Ostrow, J. D. (1994). Jaundice and disorders of bilirubin metabolism. In J. H. Stein (Ed.), *Internal medicine* (4th ed), St. Louis: Mosby.
21. Owyang, C., & Levitt, M. D. (1995). Chronic pancreatitis. In T. Yamada (Ed.), *Textbook of gastroenterology* (2nd ed., Vol 2). Philadelphia: Lippincott.
22. Reynolds, T. B., & Kanel, G. C. (1994). Alcoholic liver disease. In J. Stein, et al. (Eds), *Internal medicine* (4th ed.). St. Louis: Mosby.
23. Robinson, A., & Linden, M. (1993). *Clinical genetics handbook*. Boston: Blackwell Scientific.
24. Rubin, E., & Farber, J. L. (1999). *Pathology* (3rd ed.). Philadelphia: Lippincott.
25. Schenker, S., & Hoyumpa, A. M. (1994). Principal complications of liver failure. In J. H. Stein, et al. (Eds.), *Internal medicine* (4th ed.). St. Louis: Mosby.
26. Sherlock, S., & Dooley, J. (1997). *Diseases of the liver and biliary system* (10th ed.). London: Blackwell Science.
27. Shulman, S. T., Phair, J. P., & Sommers, H. M. (1997). *The biologic and clinical basis of infectious diseases* (5th ed.). Philadelphia: W. B. Saunders.
28. Sjogren, M. H. (1996). Serologic diagnosis of viral hepatitis. *Medical Clinics of North America, 80*(5), 929–956.
29. Spiro, H. M. (1993). *Clinical gastroenterology* (4th. ed.). New York: McGraw-Hill.
30. Tortora, G. J., & Grabowski, S. R. (1993). *Principles of anatomy and physiology* (7th ed.). New York: Harper Collins.
31. Van Dyke, R. W. (1997). Approach to the patient with jaundice. In W. N. Kelley (Ed.), *Textbook of internal medicine* (3rd ed., Vol. 1). Philadelphia: Lippincott-Raven.
32. Wanebo, H. J., & Vezeridis, M. P. (1996). Pancreatic carcinoma in perspective: A continuing challenge. *Cancer, 78*, 580–591.
33. Woodley, M. C., & Peters, M. G. (1995). Approach to the patient with jaundice. In T. Yamada (Ed.), *Textbook of gastroenterology* (2nd ed., vol. 1). Philadelphia: Lippincott.
34. Zimmerman, H. J. (1994). Drug- and toxin-induced liver disease. In J. H. Stein, et al. (Eds.), *Internal medicine* (4th ed.). St. Louis: Mosby.

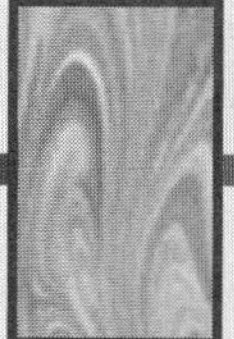

UNIT 8: CASE STUDY

The Person with Acute Gastrointestinal Bleeding

Introduction to the Patient

Mr. L. is a 40-year-old white male who arrived at the emergency department 2 days ago with complaints of bright-red gastrointestinal bleeding. He was admitted to the intensive care unit after blood work was drawn.

Present Illness

Mr. L. reports feeling weak and nauseated for the past 2 days. On the second day, he awoke in the middle of the night with nausea and weakness and vomited a large amount of bright red blood. This frightened him enough to call 911 and summon an ambulance to take him to the hospital.

Social History

Mr. L. is divorced from his second wife and has no children. He lives alone in a large urban center in the Midwest. He is an office manager for a major audiovisual sales and rental enterprise, typically working 6 days a week. He reports smoking two packs of cigarettes a day for the past 22 years and has a long history of alcohol abuse. At present, Mr. L. admits to "drinking an occasional cocktail on special occasions."

Past Medical History

Mr. L. states that he avoids going to his physician on a regular basis because "I don't like to hear bad news." He had been in good health until 2 years ago when he was diagnosed with cirrhosis of the liver. He was told to modify his diet and abstain from alcohol to improve his condition. In the past year, he has lost approximately 45 pounds.

Family History

Mr. L.'s parents have been in very good health. His father died at the age of 45 in an automobile accident. His mother, who is currently 73 years old, has a history of a hiatal hernia and diverticulosis. Otherwise, she is in excellent health and is living by herself in a nearby town. Mr. L. has no brothers or sisters.

Physical Examination

Mr. L. is 5 ft, 11 in tall and weighs 160 pounds. He is alert to person and place but is periodically confused to time. His vital signs are as follows: temperature—99.6°F; pulse—118; respirations—24; blood pressure—90/60. His skin is pale, cool, and jaundiced. Spider angiomas are visible on his face and trunk. Palmar erythema is noted on his hands.

Abdomen is distended and slightly tender. Bowel sounds are present in all four quadrants. Superficial abdominal vessels are visible on inspection. Percussion reveals enlarged areas of dullness in right upper quadrant. Hepatomegaly is noted. Tests for shifting dullness and fluid wave are positive. Urine is dark yellowish brown; stools are pale.

Diagnostic Tests

Serum bilirubin (total) 5.9 mg/dL
Serum ammonia: 200 ug/dL
Prothrombin time (PT): 25.5 seconds
Activated partial thromboplastin time (APPT): 58 seconds
Serum albumin: 2.0 g/dL
Serum AST: 112 IU/mL
Serum ALT: 51 IU/mL

CRITICAL THINKING QUESTIONS

1. Describe the effect of alcohol on the liver.
2. Explain what is the most probable source of Mr. L.'s gastrointestinal bleeding. Considering his past medical history, why would you expect the bleeding to be severe?
3. Relate the pathophysiology of cirrhosis to Mr. L.'s clinical picture and diagnostic test results.
4. Considering medications, nutritional therapy, and patient teaching, describe the possible treatment strategies that may be effective.
5. Based on Mr. L.'s clinical picture, for which potential complication is he most likely at risk? Support your conclusion.

Besides your pathophysiology text, you'll need a good pharmacology text, a gastroenterology text, a diagnostic/laboratory test text, a medical-surgical nursing text, and current research to complete this case study. Suggested references follow:

Chandrasoma, P. (1998). *Gastrointestinal pathology.* Norwalk, CT: Appleton & Lange.

Feldman, M., Scharschmidt, B., Sleisenger, M., & Zorab, R. (Eds.) (1997). *Sleisenger and Fordtran's gastrointestinal and liver disease: Pathophysiology, diagnosis, management* (6th ed.). Philadelphia: W.B. Saunders, 1997.

Fischbach, F. (1996). *A manual of laboratory and diagnostic tests* (5th ed.). Philadelphia: Lippincott-Raven Publishers.

Karch, A.M. (1999). *1999 Lippincott's nursing drug guide.* Philadelphia: Lippincott-Raven Publishers.

Kelley, W.N. (Ed.) (1997). *Textbook of internal medicine* (3rd ed.). Philadelphia: Lippincott-Raven.

Rubin, E. & Farber, J. (1999). *Pathophysiology* (3rd ed.). Philadelphia: Lippincott-Raven.

Smeltzer, S. & Bare, B. (2000). *Brunner and Suddarth's textbook of medical-surgical nursing* (9th ed.). Philadelphia: Lippincott Williams & Wilkins.

Yamada, T. (Ed.) (1999). *Textbook of gastroenterology* (3rd ed.). Philadelphia: Lippincott-Raven Publishers.

Website Resources:

Gastrointestinal Diseases *http:www.ohsu.edu/cliniweb/C6*

Gastrointestinal Pathology Index *http:www-medlib.med.utah.edu/WebPath/GIHTML/GIIDX.html*

Information on Specific Gastrointestinal Diseases *http://cpmcnet.columbia.edu/dept/gi/diseases.html*

Virtual Hospital: Gastrointestinal *http://www.vh.org/Providers/ProvidersOrgSys/OSGastrointestinal.html*

World Wide Web Sites of Interest to Gastroenterologists *http://www.gastro.org/links.html*

UNIT 8 APPENDIX A

DIAGNOSTIC TESTS

TEST	PURPOSE/NORMAL FINDINGS	SIGNIFICANCE
Stool analysis	Examination of the constituents of stool for abnormalities associated with gastrointestinal (GI) tract dysfunction and screen for possible colon cancer Normal findings: Appearance—soft, formed in amounts of 100 to 200 g/day with some fiber, vegetable skin, and seeds possible; variable odor with pH and diet	Paper towels and toilet tissue and drugs such as iron, magnesium, barium, tetracycline, and bismuth may interfere with the results of the analysis. Diarrheal stool with mucus and red blood cells may suggest large bowel cancer, amebiasis, cholera, typhus, or typhoid. Diarrheal stool with mucus and white blood cells may indicate ulcerative colitis, regional enteritis, salmonellosis, or intestinal tuberculosis. A bulky, frothy stool may suggest sprue or celiac disease. Narrow, ribbon-like stools may indicate spastic bowel, stricture, or partial obstruction. Foul odor is related to the breakdown of undigested protein and is produced by excessive carbohydrate metabolism. Sickly sweet odor is related to volatile fatty acid production and undigested lactose.
	pH—neutral to weakly alkaline (6.5 to 7.5)	pH is dependent on the fermentation of bacteria in the small intestine. When carbohydrate fermentation occurs, pH is acid. Protein breakdown results in an alkaline pH. Alkaline pH may suggest colitis or villous adenoma. Acidic pH may suggest fat or carbohydrate malabsorption or a disaccharide deficiency.
	Color—brown	Stool darkens on standing. Black stool color may be related to foods such as cherries or a very high intake of red meat or drugs such as iron, bismuth, or charcoal. Clay-colored stools may be a result of a high fat intake or a bile duct obstruction. Stool appearing dark red to tarry black may suggest a loss of approximately ¾ mL of blood from the upper gastrointestinal (UGI) tract.
	Blood—negative	Testing for occult blood aids in detecting GI tract disease, such as UGI bleeding or colon cancer. Stool positive for occult blood may suggest ulcerative colitis, diaphragmatic hernia, diverticulitis, ulcer, or gastric or colon cancer.
	Pus and mucus—negative	Mucus seen in stool is abnormal. Mucus accompanied by blood may suggest a tumor or inflammation of the rectal canal. Mucus along with blood and pus may suggest ulcerative colitis, acute diverticulitis, ulcerating cancer of the colon, or intestinal tuberculosis.

(continued)

UNIT 8 APPENDIX A

DIAGNOSTIC TESTS (Continued)

TEST	PURPOSE/NORMAL FINDINGS	SIGNIFICANCE
	Fat—up to 20% of total solids (fatty acids 0.60 g/24 hours)	This is the primary test for steatorrhea; specimen is collected over 48 to 72 hours. Increased fat may suggest nontropical sprue, celiac disease, cystic fibrosis (CF), enteritis, or chronic pancreatitis.
	White blood cells—negative	Increased white blood cells in stool may indicate a localized abscess, fistula of the sigmoid or anus, or chronic ulcerative colitis.
	Urobilinogen—125 to 400 Erhlich units/24 hours or 40 to 200 mg/24 hours	Increased levels may indicate hemolytic anemia. Decreased levels may indicate complete biliary obstruction, severe liver disease, or oral antibiotic therapy altering the normal flora of the GI tract.
	Trypsin—positive for small amounts	Young children have a greater amount of trypsin in stool than older children and adults. Decreased amounts may be associated with pancreatic deficiency, malabsorption syndromes, or CF.
Carcinoembryonic antigen (CEA)	Tumor marker involving immunoassay of a glycoprotein secreted onto the surface of the cells lining the GI tract, appearing during the latter half of fetal life; production is halted after birth Normal findings: 0 to 2.5 ng/mL (nonsmokers); up to 10 ng/mL (smokers)	Increased levels may be associated with cancer of the colon, pancreas, lung, stomach, ovary, bladder, thyroid, and breast (metastasis). It is also increased with inflammatory bowel disease, rectal polyps, active ulcerative colitis, pancreatitis, alcoholic cirrhosis, peptic ulcer disease, cholecystitis, chronic renal failure, bronchitis, and fibrocystic breast disease.
GASTROINTESTINAL (GI) TRACT		
Flat plate of the abdomen	Radiographic examination without the use of contrast medium to evaluate the structures of the abdominal cavity Normal findings: normal size, shape, and position of the abdominal structures	Cysts, tumors, or stones may be visualized. Abnormal fluid may indicate ascites. Abnormal gas distribution may suggest bowel perforation or obstruction. Displacement of the bowel may suggest an ovarian or uterine mass.
UGI series	Radiographic examination typically using a contrast medium to visualize the UGI organs (esophagus, stomach, duodenum, and upper jejunum), sphincters, and possibly the small bowel Normal findings: Normal stomach size, contour, motility, and peristaltic activity Absence of any anatomic or functional derangements	A double-contrast study involving a contrast medium and carbon dioxide-releasing tablets or a continuous infusion of a contrast medium and methylcellulose may be done to provide a more detailed picture. Displacement of gastric air bubble may suggest a mass external to the stomach. Perforation, gastric wall thickening, hiatal hernia, stenosis, congenital abnormalities, ulceration, or masses may be seen. Small bowel follow through may be ordered in conjunction with UGI to evaluate for small bowel diseases. Delays in small intestinal motility may be a result of drugs such as magnesium sulfate; increased motility may be related to fear, anxiety, or a high-fiber diet.

(continued)

UNIT 8 APPENDIX A

DIAGNOSTIC TESTS (Continued)

TEST	PURPOSE/NORMAL FINDINGS	SIGNIFICANCE
Lower GI series (barium enema [BE])	Radiographic examination using a contrast medium to visualize the position, filling, and movement through the colon Normal findings: normal position, contour, filling time, and patency	The colon must be completely cleared of stool for accurate visualization. Lesions, tumors, obstruction, fistula, inflammatory changes, stenosis, or polyps may be seen. If the patient has an active inflammatory bowel disease, barium enema is contraindicated. Instead, a water-soluble contrast study may be done.
Gastric analysis	Evaluation of gastric fluid components via a nasogastric tube inserted to estimate the secretory function of the gastric mucosa (samples taken every 15 minutes for 1 to 2 hours) Normal findings: pH—1.5 to 3.5 Fluid—clear to opalescent Absence of food, blood, drugs or bile Fasting total acid—15 to 50 mmol/L Basal acid output—0 to 5 mmol/L Maximal acid output (after stimulation)—10 to 20 mmol/L.	A cytologic examination of gastric washings may be done to identify acid-fast bacillus. Histamine or pentagastrin may be administered to stimulate gastric secretion. Decreased levels may indicate pernicious anemia, gastric malignancy, atrophic gastritis, or rheumatoid arthritis. Increased levels may indicate peptic ulcer disease, duodenal ulcer, or hyperplasia of the gastric cells of the antrum, or they may occur following a small intestine resection.
Endoscopy	Fiberscopic examination of the GI tract to visualize the UGI tract structures (esophagoscopy, gastroscopy, duodenoscopy, esophagogastroscopy, or esophagogastroduodenoscopy) or lower GI tract (anoscopy, proctoscopy, sigmoidoscopy), possibly the entire large intestine (colonoscopy) Normal findings: Appearance of tract normal Absence of irritation, ulceration, abnormal tissue, or bleeding	Polyps, tumors, ulceration, inflammation, or possible sites of hemorrhage may be seen. Tissue specimens may be obtained for biopsy. Esophagogastroduodenoscopy may reveal a hiatal hernia. Specific bowel cleansing measures are required prior to lower GI endoscopy.
Abdominal ultrasound	Use of sound waves to identify structures and organs of the abdominal cavity, including the liver, gall bladder, bile ducts, and pancreas Normal findings: normal pattern reflecting size and configuration of the structures	Fluid collections, masses, infection, or obstruction may be seen. Ultrasound also may identify ascites and variations in portal venous blood flow.
Abdominal computed tomography (CT) and magnetic resonance imaging (MRI)	Visualization of abnormalities not readily seen on routine x-rays by providing a three-dimensional view of the structures Normal findings: air appearing black; bone appearing white; soft tissue appearing gray; with shading corresponding to tissue density	Special contrast medium is usually administered prior to the test to allow differentiation of the bowel from other structures. Tumors, nodules, cysts, ascites, and abscesses may be seen.
Manometry	Evaluation of the function of the GI tract (esophagus, stomach, duodenum, and possibly the small intestine) function and response to therapeutic intervention by measuring motility and intraluminal pressures Normal findings: Pressure values normal Absence of acid reflux (with esophageal and/or gastroduodenal testing) Normal resting tone of internal anal sphincter and contractility of external anal sphincter (with anorectal testing)	Abnormal findings with esophageal and/or gastroduodenal manometry may reveal achalasia, esophageal spasm, or acid reflux. Anorectal manometry may be helpful in evaluating the cause of chronic constipation or fecal incontinence.

(continued)

UNIT 8 APPENDIX A

DIAGNOSTIC TESTS (Continued)

TEST	PURPOSE/NORMAL FINDINGS	SIGNIFICANCE
Radionuclide for gastric emptying	Evaluation to provide functional information about gastric emptying; using radiopharmaceutical substances mixed into ingested food and recorded in a photograph (scintigraph) by an imaging device showing the radioactive material in the stomach and small intestine Normal findings: some tracer-laced food usually evidenced through the stomach into the small bowel in 30 minutes.	Delayed gastric emptying is evidenced if timing of the gastric contents exceeds the normal values by two standard deviations. Too-rapid movement of food and fluid boluses may also occur (dumping syndrome). Delayed gastric emptying is more common than rapid gastric emptying and may be associated with mechanical problems (peptic ulcers and tumors) or functional problems (ineffective electromechanical activity associated with medications or conditions such as diabetes mellitus). Rapid gastric emptying is most often associated with dumping syndrome as a complication of a vagotomy for peptic ulcers. Other types of gastric surgeries may also cause dumping syndrome.
LIVER AND GALL BLADDER		
Serum alkaline phosphatase (ALP)	Measurement of the enzyme primarily of the bone, liver, and placenta; used as a tumor marker index of liver and bone disease Normal findings: 17 to 142 U/L	With liver disease, excretion of the enzyme is impaired secondary to an obstruction of the biliary tract. Increased levels may indicate obstructive jaundice, lesions of the liver, hepatocellular or biliary cirrhosis, or cholestatic hepatitis. Decreased levels may indicate hypothyroidism, malnutrition, or pernicious anemia.
Serum aspartate aminotransferase (AST[SGOT])	Measurement of the enzyme released after cellular injury or death found in metabolically active tissues; concentration typically decreased in the liver, heart, skeletal muscle, brain, pancreas, spleen, and lungs Normal findings: 5 to 35 U/L	Increased levels may be seen with acute myocardial infarction, hepatitis, active cirrhosis, hepatic necrosis, alcoholic hepatitis, infectious mononucleosis, pancreatitis, trauma, pulmonary embolism, malignant hyperthermia, or gangrene. Decreased levels may be seen with azotemia or chronic renal failure.
Serum alanine aminotransferase (ALT[SGPT])	Measurement of the enzyme found in high concentrations in the liver to identify possible liver disease Normal findings: 7 to 45 U/L	Moderately to highly elevated levels may be seen with hepatocellular disease. Mildly elevated levels may be seen with active cirrhosis or metastatic liver cancer and pancreatitis. Mildly to moderately elevated levels may be seen with obstructive jaundice or biliary obstruction. ALT is a less sensitive test to detect alcoholic liver disease than AST.
Serum lactic dehydrogenase (LDH)	Measurement of the enzyme widely distributed in tissues, including heart, kidney, skeletal muscle, brain, liver, and lungs, typically indicating cellular death Normal findings: 110 to 230 U/L	Increased levels may be seen with acute myocardial infarction, cirrhosis, acute viral hepatitis, pulmonary infarction, sickle cell disease, and hypothyroidism.

(continued)

UNIT 8 APPENDIX A

DIAGNOSTIC TESTS (Continued)

TEST	PURPOSE/NORMAL FINDINGS	SIGNIFICANCE
Serum bilirubin: direct (conjugated) and indirect (unconjugated)	Measurement of the product of hemoglobin breakdown removed by the liver and excreted in bile; two types—indirect (unconjugated), which is protein bound; and direct (conjugated), which circulates freely until reaching the liver and is then excreted into the bile Normal findings: Total—0.2 to 1.0 mg/dL Direct: 0.0 to 0.2 mg/dL Indirect—0.2 to 0.8 mg/dL	An increase in indirect bilirubin is more commonly associated with red blood cell hemolysis, whereas an increase in direct bilirubin is more commonly associated with hepatobiliary dysfunction. Increased levels accompanied by jaundice may indicate hepatocellular disease such as hepatitis, cirrhosis, or infectious mononucleosis; obstruction of the common bile duct or hepatic duct such as with stones or tumors; or hemolysis such as Rh incompatibility, pernicious anemia, sickle cell disease, or a transfusion reaction. Increased levels of direct bilirubin may suggest cancer of the head of the pancreas or choledocholithiasis.
Serum ammonia	Measurement of the end product of protein metabolism normally removed by the liver through the portal vein and converting it into urea for excretion by the kidneys Normal findings: 9 to 33 umol/L	Increased levels may indicate Reye's syndrome, liver disease, cirrhosis, hepatic coma, GI hemorrhage with liver disease, or GI infection with distention and stasis. Ammonia levels vary with protein intake. Exercise may increase ammonia levels.
Serum protein	Measurement of the proteins manufactured by the liver Normal findings: Total—6.0 to 8 g/dL Albumin—3.8 to 5.0 g/dL Alpha 1 globulin—0.1 to 0.3 g/dL Alpha 2 globulin—0.6 to 1.0 g/dL Beta globulin—0.7 to 1.4 g/dL Gamma globulin—0.7 to 1.6 g/dL	Increased total protein levels may be seen with liver disease, collagen disease, or chronic inflammation or infection. Decreased total protein levels may be seen with severe liver disease, alcoholism, renal disease, diarrhea associated with Crohn's disease or ulcerative colitis, severe hemorrhage, heart failure, or prolonged immobilization. Increased serum albumin levels may be seen with intravenous infusions or dehydration. Decreased serum albumin levels may be seen with liver disease, alcoholism, malabsorption syndromes, Crohn's disease, or starvation states. An increase in alpha-2 and beta globulins may indicate biliary cirrhosis or obstructive jaundice. An increase in gamma globulin may suggest chronic infection, hepatic disease, collagen disease, multiple myeloma, or leukemia.
Hepatitis A marker: Antibody (Anti-HAV)	Evaluation to detect active and past exposure to HAV Normal findings: negative	IgM anti-HAV is first to appear and is present in acute disease; IgG anti-HAV appears after the acute illness. IgM anti-HAV appears within a week after clinical manifestations and remains in the blood for several months. IgG anti-HAV appears about a month after the appearance of IgM and remains in the serum indefinitely. It indicates HAV immunity.

(continued)

UNIT 8 APPENDIX A

DIAGNOSTIC TESTS (Continued)

TEST	PURPOSE/NORMAL FINDINGS	SIGNIFICANCE
Hepatitis B markers: Surface antigen (HBsAg)	Evaluation to detect active infection, either acute or chronic HBV Normal findings: negative	HBsAg, the first antigen to appear in the blood, is detected in the blood about 2 weeks to 2 months before the onset of clinical manifestations. Titers peak during the first week of clinical manifestations and persist for 1 to 5 months. If present greater than 6 months, the individual has chronic HBV.
Surface antibody (HBsAb or Anti-HBs)	Evaluation to detect antibodies to HBV Normal findings: negative	This test indicates resolved infection and long-term immunity; HBsAb is present approximately 4 weeks after the HBsAg disappears. Surface antibody is the measure of immunity after immunization for HBV.
Core antibody (HBcAb or Anti-HBc)	Evaluation to detect acute and chronic HBV, HBV carriers, and individuals with prior HBV (HBcAg) does not circulate freely in the blood) Normal findings: negative	HBcAb (IgM) will be positive about 2 months after exposure. If HBcAb (IgG) is detected, the individual has recovered and is a useful marker of previous infection. Unlike HBsAb, it does not confer immunity.
HBe antigen (HBeAg)	Evaluation to detect acute or chronic HBV; its presence is indicative of maximal viral replication Normal findings: negative	HBeAg, the second antigen to appear in the blood of patients infected with HBV, is noted in the blood after HBsAg and before the onset of clinical manifestations. It usually disappears before HBsAg.
HBe antibody (HBeAg)	Evaluation to detect when acute infection is over Normal findings: negative	A positive finding indicates that infectivity is over. HBeAg may remain in the blood for over 2 years.
Hepatitis C markers: HCV RNA	Evaluation to detect acute or chronic infection Normal findings: negative	HCV RNA is detectable in blood about 1 month after exposure. In acute HCV, the HCV-RNA begins to disappear between 4 and 5 months after exposure. In chronic HCV, the HCV-RNA remains in the blood and the clinical manifestations wax and wane.
Antibody (Anti-HCV)	Evaluation to detect acute and chronic infection Normal findings: negative	Anti-HCV levels usually appear between 3 and 4 months after exposure. The appearance of anti-HCV is preceded by clinical manifestations of illness, including elevated ALT and bilirubin.
Hepatitis D markers: Antibody (Anti-HDV)	Evaluation to detect acute or chronic HDV Normal findings: negative	HDV occurs only with HBV infections. Anti-HDV is only indicated in individuals who are HBsAg positive.
Urine bilirubin	Measurement of the breakdown product of hemoglobin, which is transported to the liver and then excreted in the bile Normal findings: 0 to 0.2 mg/dL	Elevated urine bilirubin levels are an early indicator of hepatobiliary dysfunction, such as hepatitis, liver disease secondary to toxic exposure or infection, or obstructive biliary tract disease.

(continued)

UNIT 8 APPENDIX A

DIAGNOSTIC TESTS (Continued)

TEST	PURPOSE/NORMAL FINDINGS	SIGNIFICANCE
Urine urobilinogen	Measurement of the portion of bilirubin that is acted upon by bacterial enzymes and then carried to the liver for removal Normal findings: 0 to 4 mg/24 hours	Urobilinogen escaping removal by the liver is subsequently carried to the kidneys for excretion. Urobilinogen excretion is diurnal, peaking between 12 noon and 4 P.M. Increased levels may be associated with increased destruction of red blood cells; hemorrhage into tissues; or hepatic damage, such as biliary disease, cirrhosis, or acute hepatitis or cholangitis. Absent or decreased levels may be associated with cholelithiasis, severe inflammation of the bile ducts, or cancer of the head of the pancreas. Antibiotic altering the normal flora of the GI tract may cause low or absent levels.
Cholecystography	Radiographic evaluation of the gall bladder after oral ingestion or intravenous injection of contrast medium Normal findings: normal filling without shadows	This test largely has been replaced by ultrasound. Appearance of shadows may suggest stones. Inability to visualize the gall bladder may suggest gall bladder disease and need for repeat study. This test is not performed on patients with jaundice.
Ultrasound of the gall bladder and liver	Use of sound waves to visualize the gall bladder and liver for size, position, and configuration Normal findings: Size, position, and configuration normal Bile duct patent	Stones and dilation of bile duct are readily seen. Evidence of a thickened wall may suggest cholecystitis. Masses, such as tumors, cysts, or stones, may be detected.
T-tube cholangiography	Evaluation of the common bile duct using intravenous injection of contrast medium during or after gall bladder surgery to evaluate the patency of the common bile duct Normal findings: common bile duct open and patent	Obstruction from stenosis or stones may be seen.
Percutaneous transhepatic cholangiography (PTC)	Injection of contrast medium percutaneously into the liver and bile duct Normal findings: visualization of the liver and bile duct	Dilation of the biliary tree up to the point of obstruction may be seen. This test helps to differentiate jaundice secondary to liver disease from that due to biliary obstruction.
Endoscopic retrograde cholangiopancreatography	Endoscopic examination of the hepatobiliary system using a contrast medium instilled into the duodenal papilla or ampulla of Vater Normal findings: Duodenal papilla or ampulla of Vater, gall bladder, and pancreatic, hepatic, and common bile ducts normal	Stones, stenosis, or other abnormalities may be seen, suggesting possible biliary cirrhosis, cancer of the common bile duct, pancreatic cysts, or chronic pancreatitis.
Hepatobiliary (gall bladder) scan	Radionuclide imaging to visualize the gall bladder and evaluate patency of biliary tree Normal findings: Radioisotope excreted rapidly by the liver; transit time to biliary tree of 15 to 30 minutes Uptake positive with normal distribution	Ability to visualize the gall bladder rules out acute cholecystitis. Abnormalities of the biliary tree are revealed by irregular patterns of isotope concentration.

(continued)

UNIT 8 APPENDIX A

DIAGNOSTIC TESTS (Continued)

TEST	PURPOSE/NORMAL FINDINGS	SIGNIFICANCE
Liver scan	Radionuclide imaging of the liver to evaluate function, structure, and size Normal findings: normal shape, size, and position of liver within abdomen with normal function	This test aids in identifying the cause of jaundice. Abnormal patterns may suggest cirrhosis, hepatitis, trauma, abscess, ascites, or metastasis.
PANCREAS (EXOCRINE)		
Serum amylase	Measurement of the enzyme produced in the salivary gland, pancreas, liver, and fallopian tubes, responsible for changing starch to sugar Normal findings: 25 to 125 U/L (adults); 21 to 160 U/L (elderly adults)	Amylase and lipase levels are used to differentiate acute pancreatitis from other acute abdominal conditions. Highly elevated levels may be indicative of acute pancreatitis early on, usually within 3 to 6 hours after the onset of pain. Elevated levels also may be seen with acute exacerbation of chronic pancreatitis, perforated peptic ulcer, alcohol poisoning, acute cholecystitis, or intestinal strangulation. Decreased levels may be associated with pancreatic insufficiency, hepatitis, severe liver disease, advanced CF, or severe burns.
Serum lipase	Measurement of the enzyme produced primarily by the pancreas, responsible for changing fats to fatty acid and glycerol Normal findings: 10 to 14 U/L (adults); 18 to 180 U/L (adults over age 60)	Elevated levels may be seen with pancreatitis, but possibly not until 24 to 36 hours after the onset of illness; remain elevated for up to 2 weeks. Increased levels also are seen with cholecystitis, severe renal disease, strangulated bowel, or peritonitis.
Sweat test	Measurement of the concentration of sodium, chloride, and potassium in sweat following stimulation to diagnose CF Normal findings: Sodium—16 to 46 mmol/L Chloride—8 to 43 mmol/L Potassium—6 to 17 mmol/L In CF: Sodium—75 to 145 mmol/L Chloride—79 to 148 mmol/L Potassium—14 to 30 mmol/L	Sodium and chloride levels above 60 mmol/L in children or over 80 mmol/L in adolescents and adults are typically an indication of CF. Sodium and chloride levels between 40 to 60 mmol/L are considered borderline and require retesting. Increased levels of sweat electrolytes may also be seen with Addison's disease, congenital adrenal hyperplasia, G6PD, or glycogen storage deficiency.

UNIT BIBLIOGRAPHY

Abi-Hanna, P. (1997). Acute abdominal pain: A medical emergency in older patients. *Geriatrics, 52*(7), 72–72.

American Cancer Society. (1998). *Cancer facts and figures.* Atlanta: American Cancer Society.

Anand, A., Bashey, B., Mir, T., & Glatt, A. E. (1994). Epidemiology, clinical manifestations, and outcome of *Clostridium difficile*–associated diarrhea. *American Journal of Gastroenterology, 89,* 519–523.

Barkin, J.S. & Rogers, A. I. (Eds.) (1994). *Difficult decisions in digestive diseases.* St. Louis: Mosby–Year Book.

Butler, M. (1996). Preparing patients for endoscopic tests. *Practice Nurse, 11*(10), 707–708, 710, 712.

Cotran, R.S., Kumar, V., & Robbins, S. (1994). *Robbins' pathologic basis of disease* (5th ed.). Philadelphia: W.B. Saunders.

Dammel, T. (1997). Fecal occult blood testing. *Nursing, 27*(7), 44–45.

DeVita, V.T., Hellman, S., & Rosenberg, S.A. (1997). *Cancer: Principles and practice of oncology* (5th ed.). Philadelphia: J.B. Lippincott.

Dornschke, W. & Konturek, S.J. (1993). *The stomach: Physiology, pathophysiology, and treatment.* New York: Springer-Verlag.

Fauci, A.S., et al. (Eds.) (1997). *Harrison's principles of internal medicine* (14th ed.). New York: McGraw-Hill.

Feldman, M., Scharschmidt, B.F., & Sleisenger, M. H. (Eds.) (1998). *Sleisenger & Fortran's gastrointestinal and liver disease: pathophysiology/diagnosis/management, vols. 1 and 2* (6th ed.). Philadelphia: W.B. Saunders.

Grendell, J., et al. (Eds.) (1996). *Current diagnosis and treatment in gastroenterology.* Stamford, CT: Appleton & Lange.

Guyton, A.C. & Hall, J. E. (1996). *Textbook of medical physiology* (9th ed.). Philadelphia: W.B. Saunders.

Kelley, W.N., et al. (Eds.) (1997). *Textbook of internal medicine, vols. 1 and 2* (3rd ed.). Philadelphia: Lippincott-Raven.

Kirton, C. (1997). Assessing bowel sounds. *Nursing, 27*(3), 64.

McConnell, E. A. (1994). Managing nasoenteric decompression tube. *Nursing, 24*(3), 18.

Myers, M.A. (1998). *Neoplasms of the digestive tract: Imaging, staging, and management.* Philadelphia: Lippincott-Raven Publishers.

O'Hanlon-Nichols, T. (1998). Basic assessment series: Gastrointestinal system. *American Journal of Nursing, 98*(4), 48–53.

Parker, S.L., et al. (1997). Cancer statistics, 1997. *CA: A Cancer Journal for Clinicians, 47*(1), 5–27.

Peterson, W.L. & Lee, W.M. (1997). Gastroenterology and hepatology. *Journal of the American Medical Association, 277*(23), 1858–1860.

Richter, J., et al. (1994). *The functional gastrointestinal disorders.* Boston: Little, Brown.

Rubin, E. & Farber, J.L. (1999). *Pathology* (3rd ed.). Philadelphia: Lippincott Williams & Wilkins.

Rush, C. (1995). Gastrointestinal bleeding. *Nursing, 25*(8), 33.

Schmieding, N., Waldman, R., & Desaulles, C. (1997). Nasogastric tubes: Insertion, placement, and removal in adult patients. *Gastroenterology Nursing, 20*(1), 15–19.

Society of Gastroenterology Nurses and Associates. (1998). *Gastroenterology nursing: A core curriculum* (2nd ed.). St. Louis: Mosby–Year Book.

Stein, J. (Ed.) (1994). *Internal medicine* (4th ed.). St. Louis: C.V. Mosby.

Yamada, T., et al. (Eds.) (1995). *Textbook of gastroenterology, vols. 1 and 2* (2nd ed.). Philadelphia: Lippincott.

ORAL CONDITIONS

American Academy of Periodontology. (1996). Position paper: Epidemiology of periodontal diseases. *Journal of Periodontology, 67*(9), 935–945.

Kretzschmar, J.L. & Kretzschmar, D.P. (1996). Common oral conditions. *American Family Physician, 54*(1), 225–234.

Mandel, I.D. (1996). Caries prevention: Current strategies, new directions. *Journal of the American Dental Association, 127*(10), 1477–1488.

McEwen, D.R. & Sanchez, M.M. (1997). A guide to salivary gland disorders. *AORN Journal, 65*(3), 554–556.

ESOPHAGEAL CONDITIONS

Bhutani, M.S. Gastrointestinal uses of botulinum toxin. *American Journal of Gastroenterology, 92*(6), 929–933.

Bosset, J.F., et al. (1997). Chemoradiotherapy followed by surgery compared with surgery alone in squamous cell cancer of the esophagus. *New England Journal of Medicine, 337*(3), 161–167.

Eckardt, V.F., et al. (1997). Complications and their impact after pneumatic dilation for achalasias: Perspective long-term follow-up study. *Gastrointestinal Endoscopy, 45*(5), 349–353.

Eypasch, E., et al. (1997). Laparoscopic antireflux surgery for gastroesophageal reflux disease (GERD). Results of a consensus development conference held at the fourth international congress of the European Association of Endoscopic Surgery (EAES), Trondheim, Norway, June 21–24, 1996. *Surgical Endoscopy, 11*(5), 413–426.

Ilson, D.H. & Kelsen, D.P. (1996). Management of esophageal cancer. *Oncology (Huntingt), 10*(9), 1385–1396.

Larsen, R.R. (1997). Gastroesophageal reflux disease: Gaining control over heartburn. *Postgraduate Medicine, 101*(2), 181–182.

Paricha, P.J. & Kaltoo, A.N. (1997). Recent advances in the treatment of achalasia. *Gastrointestinal Endoscopy Clinics of North America, 7*(2), 191–206.

Stack, L.B. & Numter, D.W. Foreign bodies in the gastrointestinal tract. *Emergency Medicine Clinics of North America, 14*(3), 493–521.

Weant, C. (1995). Easing the pain of esophageal surgery. *RN,* 26–31.

ESOPHAGEAL VARICES

Baroncini, D., Milandri, G.L., Piemontese, A., et al. (1997). A prospective randomized trial of sclerotherapy versus ligation in the elective treatment of bleeding esophageal varices. *Endoscopy, 29,* 235–240.

Hartigan, P.M., Gebhard, R.L. & Gregory, P.B. (1997). Sclerotherapy for actively bleeding esophageal varices in male alcoholics with cirrhosis. *Gastrointestinal Endoscopy, 46*(1), 1–7.

Huston, C.J. (1996). Ruptured esophageal varices. *American Journal of Nursing, 96*(4), 43.

Jaffe, D.L., Chung, R.T. & Friedman, L.S. (1996). Management of portal hypertension and its complications. *Medical Clinics of North America, 80*(5), 1021–1032.

Laine, L. & Cook, D. (1995). Endoscopic ligation compared with sclerotherapy for the treatment of esophageal variceal bleeding. *Annals of Internal Medicine, 123*(4), 280–287.

Navarro, V.J. & Garcia-Tsao. (1995). Variceal hemorrhage. *Critical Care Clinics, 11*(2), 391–413.

Teran, J.C., Imperiale, T.F., Mullen, K.D., et al. (1997). Primary prophylaxis of variceal bleeding in cirrhosis: A cost-effective analysis. *Gastroenterology, 112*(2), 473–482.

Villaneuva, C., Balanzo, J., Novella, M.T., et al. (1996). Nadalol plus isosorbide mononitrate compared with sclerotherapy for the prevention of variceal rebleeding. *New England Journal of Medicine, 334,* 1624–1629.

GASTRIC CANCER

Jentschura, D., et al. (1997). Quality-of-life after curative surgery for gastric cancer: A comparison between total gastrectomy and subtotal gastric resection. *Hepatogastroenterology, 44*(16), 1137–1142.

Kirkwood, K.S. (1997). Prognostic indicators for cancer. Gastric cancer. *Surgical Oncology Clinics of North America, 6*(3), 495–514.

La Vecchia, C., et al. (1997). Diet diversity and gastric cancer. *International Journal of Cancer, 72*(2), 255–257.

Molloy, R.M. & Sonnenberg, A. (1997). Relation between gastric cancer and previous peptic ulcer disease. *Gut, 40*(2), 247–252.

Nakajima, T., et al. (1997). Combined intensive chemotherapy and radical surgery for incurable gastric cancer. *Annals of Surgical Oncology, 4*(3), 203–208.

Noda, M. (1997). Possibilities and limitation of endoscopic resection for early gastric cancer. *Endoscopy, 29*(5), 361–364.

Pectasides, D., et al. (1997). CEA, CA 19-9, and CA-50 in monitoring gastric carcinoma. *American Journal of Clinical Oncology, 20*(4), 348–353.

Schmieding, N.J. & Waldman, R.C. (1997). Gastric decompression in adult patients. *Clinical Nursing Research, 6*(2), 142–155.

Schmieding, N.J., et al. (1997). Nasogastric tubes: Insertion, placement, and removal in adult patients. *Gastroenterology Nursing, 20*(1), 15–19.

ULCER DISEASE

Brozenec, S.A. (1996). Ulcer therapy update. *RN, 59*(9), 48–50.

Fay, M. & Jaffe, P.E. (1996). Diagnostic and treatment guidelines for *Helicobacter pylori. Nursing Practice, 21*(7), 28–35.

Forbes, G.M. (1997). Review: *Helicobacter pylori.* Current issues and new directions. *Journal of Gastroenterology and Hepatology, 12*(6), 419–424.

Heslin, J. (1997). Peptic ulcer disease: Making a case against the prime suspect. *Nursing, 27*(1), 34–39.

Lazzaroni, M. (1997). Triple therapy with Ranitidine or Lansoprazole in the treatment of *Helicobacter pylori* associated with duodenal ulcer. *American Journal of Gastroenterology, 92*(4), 649–651.

NIH Consensus Conference. (1994). *Helicobacter pylori* peptic ulcer disease. NIH Consensus Development Panel on *Helicobacter pylori* in Peptic Ulcer Disease. *Journal of the American Medical Association, 271*(1), 65–69.

INTESTINAL DISORDERS

Borwell, B. (1996). Colostomies and their management. *Nursing Standard, 8*(11), 49–53.

Cerda, J., et al. (1997). Diverticulitis: Cure and management strategies. *Patient Care, 33,* 170–186.

Cerda, J., et al. (1996). Effective, compassionate management of IBS. *Patient Care, 30*(1), 131–136, 141–144.

Clayton, H.A., et al. (1997). Development of an ostomy competency. *MEDSURG Nursing, 6*(5), 256–269.

Collins, L. (1996). Laparoscopic extraperitoneal herniorrhaphy. *AORN Journal, 63*(6), 1089–1097.

Cox, J. (1995). Inflammatory bowel disease: Implications for the medical surgical nurse. *MEDSURG Nursing, 4*(6), 427–434.

Cumbie, B., et al. (1996). Action STAT, bowel obstruction. *Nursing, 26*(1), 33.

Doughty, D.B. (1994). What you need to know about inflammatory bowel disease. *American Journal of Nursing, 94*(7), 24–30.

Eckes, L., Norton, B. (1997). Ulcerative colitis: From medical management to ileal pouch anal anastomosis. *Gastroenterology Nursing, 20*(3), 91–100.

Epps, C. (1996). The delicate business of ostomy care. *RN, 59*(11), 32–37.

Gibson, P. (Ed.) (1997). Ulcerative colitis. *Clinical Gastroenterology, 11*(1).

Heitkemper, M., et al. (1995). Interventions for irritable bowel syndrome: A nursing model. *Gastroenterology Nursing, 18*(6), 224–230.

Kirsner, J. & Shorter, R. (1995). *Inflammatory bowel disease.* Philadelphia: Williams & Wilkins.

Martin, F. (1997). Ulcerative colitis: How to manage this chronic inflammatory disease and prevent systemic complication. *American Journal of Nursing, 97*(8), 38–39.

Mead, M. (1997). Diverticular disease. *Practice Nurse, 13*(2), 104–105.

Mead, M. (1996). Detecting appendicitis. *Practice Nurse, 11*(7), 486–487.

Mishkin, S. (1997). Dairy sensitivity, lactose malabsorption, and elimination diets in inflammatory bowel disease. *American Journal of Clinical Nutrition, 65*(2), 564–567.

Raskin, J. & Noed, H. (1995). *Colonoscopy: Principles and techniques.* New York: Igaku-Shoin.

Seaman, S. (1996). Basic ostomy management: Assessment and pouching. *Home Healthcare Nurse, 14*(5), 334–345.

COLON CANCER

Bond, J. (1997). Screening for colorectal cancer. *Hospital Practice, 32*(1), 59–78.

Cohen, L. (1996). Colorectal cancer: A primary care approach to screening. *Geriatrics, 51*(12), 45–49.

Hoebler, L., et al. (1997). *Cancer nursing, principles and practice: Colon and rectal cancer.* Boston: Jones and Bartlett.

Meisner, J. (1996). Caring for patients with colorectal cancer. *Nursing, 26*(11), 60–61.

Noe, C.A. & Barry, P.P. (1996). Healthy aging: Guidelines for cancer screening and immunizations. *Geriatrics, 51*(1), 75–77, 81–83.

Willian, N. (Ed.) (1996). *Colorectal cancer.* New York: Churchill Livinstone.

HEPATIC CONDITIONS

Evans, S.R.T. & Ascher, S.M. (Eds.) (1998). *Hepatobiliary and pancreatic surgery.* New York: Wiley-Liss.

Fabbri, A., Magrini, N., Bianchi, G., et al. (1996). Overview of randomized clinical trials of oral branched chain amino acid treatment in chronic hepatic encephalopathy. *Journal of Parenteral and Enteral Nutrition, 20*(2), 159–165.

Holstege, A., Schölmerich, J., & Hahn, E.G. (Eds.) (1995). *Portal hypertension.* Dordrecht: Kluwer Academic Publishers.

Kirsch, R., Robson, S., & Trey, C. (Eds.) (1995). *Diagnosis and management of liver disease.* London: Chapman and Hall Medical.

Klassen, L.W., Tuma, D., & Sorrell, M.F. (1995). Immune mechanisms of alcohol-induced liver disease. *Hepatology, 22*(2), 355–358.

Lee, W. & Williams, R. (Eds.). *Acute liver failure.* Cambridge, U.K.: Cambridge University Press.

Letizia, M. & Noonan, M.A. (1997). Drug-induced hepatic injury. *MEDSURG Nursing, 6*(3), 148–152.

Lieber, C.S. Medical disorders of alcoholism. *New England Journal of Medicine, 333*(16), 1058–1060.

Mahl, T.C. (1998). Approach to the patient with abnormal liver tests. *Lippincott's Primary Care Practice, 2*(4), 379–389.

Morgan, M.Y. (1995). The treatment of chronic hepatic encephalopathy. *Hepatogastroenterology, 38*(3), 377–382.

Moseley, R.H. (1996). Evaluation of abnormal liver function tests. *Medical Clinics of North America, 80*(5), 887–904.

National Institutes of Health, National Institute on Alcohol Abuse and Alcoholism. (1997). *Ninth special report to the U.S. Congress on alcohol and health.* Alexandria, VA: U.S. Department of Health and Human Services.

Pasha, T.M. & Lindor, K.D. (1996). Diagnosis and therapy of cholestatic liver disease. *Medical Clinics of North America, 80*(5), 995–1016.

Pitt, H.A., Carr-Locke, D.L., Ferrucci, J.T. (Eds.) (1995). *Hepatobiliary and pancreatic disease: The team approach to management.* Boston: Little, Brown.

Riordan, S.M. & Williams, R. (1997). Treatment of hepatic encephalopathy. *New England Journal of Medicine, 337*(7), 473–478.

Schenker, A., & Halff, G.A. (1995). Nutritional therapy in alcoholic liver disease. *Seminars in Liver Disease, 13*(2), 196–209.

Sherlock, S. (1995). Alcoholic liver disease. *Lancet, 345*(8944), 227–231.

Sherlock, S. & Dooley, J. (1997). *Diseases of the liver and biliary system* (10th ed.). London: Blackwell Science.

Schiff, E.R., Sorrell, M.F., & Maddray, W.C. (Eds.) (1998). *Schiff's diseases of the liver* (8th ed.). Philadelphia: Lippincott-Raven Publishers.

Siringo, S., Burroughs, A.K., Bolondi, L., et al. (1995). Peptic ulcer and its course in cirrhosis: An endoscopic and clinical prospective study. *Journal of Hepatology, 22*(6), 633–635.

Tibbs, C. & Williams, R. (1995). Viral causes and management of acute liver failure. *Journal of Hepatology, 22*(suppl 1), 68–73.

Zakim, D., & Boyer, T.D. (Eds.) (1996). *Hepatology: A textbook of liver disease* (3rd ed.). Philadelphia: W.B. Saunders.

HEPATITIS

Advisory Committee on Immunization Practices, American Academy of Pediatrics, American Academy of Family Physicians and the National Immunization Program, Centers for Disease Control and Prevention. (1995). Recommended childhood immunization schedule—United States. *MMWR, 43*(51 & 52), 959–960.

Allander, T., Gruber, A., Naghavi, M., et al. (1995). Frequent patient-to-patient transmission of hepatitis C virus in a hematology ward. *Lancet, 345*(8950), 603.

Czaja, A.J. (1996). Diagnosis and therapy of autoimmune liver disease. *Medical Clinics of North America, 80*(5), 973–991.

DeMedina, M. & Schiff, E.R. (1995). Hepatitis C: Diagnosis assays. *Seminars in Liver Disease, 15*(1), 33–40.

Fried, M.W. (1996). Therapy of chronic viral hepatitis. *Medical Clinics of North America, 80*(5), 957–972.

Herreid, J.A. (1995). Hepatitis C: Past, present, and future. *MEDSURG Nursing, 4*(3), 179–186.

Immunization Practices Advisory Committee. (1991). Hepatitis B virus: A comprehensive strategy for eliminating transmission in the United States. *MMWR, 40*(RR-13), 1–25.

Katkov, W.N. (1996). Hepatitis vaccines. *Medical Clinics of North America, 80*(5), 1189–1998.

Kowdley, K. (1996). Update on therapy for hepatobiliary diseases. *Nurse Practitioner, 21*(7), 78–88.

Scheig, R. (1998). Acute and chronic viral hepatitis. *Lippincott's Primary Care Practice, 2*(4), 390–397.

Sjogren, M. (1996). Serologic diagnosis of viral hepatitis. *Medical Clinics of North America, 80*(5), 929–953.

Strader, D.B. & Seeff, L.B. (1996). New hepatitis A vaccines and their role in prevention. *Drugs, 51*(3), 359–366.

LIVER CANCER

Dick, D., Regenstein, F., Blazek, J. & Farr, G. (1996). Liver transplantation for hepatocellular carcinoma: One center's experience, 1987–1994. *Journal of Transplant Coordination, 6*(3), 145–147.

Korpan, N.N. (1997). Hepatic cryosurgery for liver metastases. *Annals of Surgery, 225*(2), 193–201.

Leininger, S.M. (1997). Managing patients with cryosurgical ablation of the prostate and liver. *MEDSURG Nursing, 6*(6), 359–386.

Saini, S. (1997). Imaging of the hepatobiliary tract. *New England Journal of Medicine, 336*(26), 1889–1894.

Vauthey, J.N., et al. (1995). Factors affecting long-term outcome after hepatic resection for hepatocellular carcinoma. *American Journal of Surgery, 169*(1), 28–34.

Zuro, L.M. & Staren, E.D. (1996). Cryosurgical ablation of unresectable hepatic tumors. *AORN Journal, 64*(2), 231–248.

LIVER TRANSPLANTATION

Busuttil, R.W. & Klintmalm, G.B. (Eds.) (1996). *Transplantation of the liver.* Philadelphia: W.B. Saunders.

Cabello, C.C. & Tahan, H.A. (1998). Implementation of an interdisciplinary clinical pathway for patients after a liver transplant. *Nursing Care Management, 3*(6), 255–265.

Chappell, S.M. & Case, P. (1997). Anxiety in liver transplant patients. *MEDSURG Nursing, 6*(2), 98–103.

DeJong, W., Franz, H.G., Wolfe, S.M., et al. (1998). Requesting organ donation: An interview study of donor and nondonor families. *American Journal of Critical Care, 7*(1), 13–23.

Devlin, J., Wendon, J., Heaton, N., Tan, K., & Williams, R. (1995). Pretransplantation clinical status and outcome of emergency transplantation for acute liver failure. *Hepatology, 21*(4), 1018–1024.

Evans, R.W. (1997). Liver transplants and the decline in deaths from liver disease. *American Journal of Public Health, 87*(5), 868–869.

Hasse, J.M. (1997). Diet therapy for organ transplantation. *Nursing Clinics of North America, 32*(4), 863–879.

O'Connor, T.P., Lewis, W.D., & Jenkins, R.L. (1995). Biliary tract complications after liver transplantation. *Archives of Surgery, 130*(3), 312–317.

Rosen, H.R., Shackleton, C.R., & Martin, P. (1996). Indications for and timing of liver transplantation. *Medical Clinics of North America, 80*(5), 1069–1093.

Siminoff, L.A. (1997). Withdrawal of treatment and organ donation. *Critical Care Nursing Clinics of North America, 9*(1), 85–95.

Thomas, D.J. Returning to work after liver transplant: Experiencing the roadblocks. *Journal of Transplant Coordination, 6*(3), 134–138.

GALLBLADDER DISEASE

Attili, A., DeSantis, A., Capri, R., et al. (1995). The natural history of gallstones: The GREPCO experience. *Hepatology, 21*(3), 655.

Berci, G., & Cuschieri, A. (Eds.) (1997). *Bile duct and bile duct stones.* Philadelphia: W.B. Saunders.

Darzi, A., Grace, P.A., Pitt, H.A., & Bouchier-Hayes, D. (Eds.) (1995). *Techniques in the management of gallstone disease.* Osney Mead, Oxford: Blackwell Science.

Escarce, JJ, Chen, W., & Schwartz, J.S. (1995). Falling cholecystectomy thresholds since the introduction of laparoscopic cholecystectomy. *Journal of the American Medical Association, 273*(20), 1581–1585.

Schwesinger, W.H. & Diehl, A.K. (1996). Changing indications for laparoscopic cholecystectomy. *Surgical Clinics of North America, 76*(3), 493–502.

Shea, J.A., Healey, M.J., Berlin, J.A., et al. (1996). Mortality and complications associated with laparoscopic cholecystectomy: A meta-analysis. *Annals of Surgery, 224*(5), 609–620.

ON-LINE RESOURCES

American Cancer Society *http://www.cancer.org*

American Digestive Health Foundation *http://www.adhf.org*

American Gastroenterological Association *http://www.gastro.org*

American College of Gastroenterology *http://www.acg.gi.org*

Centers for Disease Control and Preventions *http://www.cdc.gov*

Combined Health Information Database (CHID) *http://chid.nih.gov*

Gastroenterology Web *http://cpmcnet.columabia.edu/dept/gi*

International Foundation for Functional Gastrointestinal Disorders *http://iffgd.org*

National Digestive Diseases Information Clearinghouse (NDDIC) *http://www.niddk.nih.gov/health/digest/nddic.htm*

National Institute of Diabetes and Digestive and Kidney Diseases (NIDDK), Digestive diseases *http://www.niddk.nih.gov/health/digest.htm*

Society of Gastroenterology Nurses & Associates, Inc *http://sgna.org*
United Ostomy Association *http://www.uoa.org*

ORAL CONDITIONS

American Dental Association *http://www.ada.org*
National Institute of Dental and Craniofacial Research National Institutes of Health *http://www.nidr.nih.gov*
National Oral Health Information Clearinghouse (NOHIC) *http://www.aerie.com/nohicweb*

ULCERS

Helicobactor pylori in Peptic Ulcer Disease, National Library of Medicine *http://www.nlm.nih.gov/nih/cdc/www94cvr.html*

INTESTINAL CONDITIONS

Celiac Disease Foundation *http://www.celiac.org*
Crohn's and Colitis Foundation of America *http://ccfa.org*
National Association for Colitis and Crohn's Disease *http://www.nacc.org.uk*

HEPATIC CONDITIONS

Al-Anon Family Group Headquarters *http://www.al-anon.alateen.org*
Alcoholics Anonymous (AA) World Services *http://www.alcoholics-anonymous.org.*
American Association for the Study of Liver Diseases *http://hkepar-sfgh.uscf.edu*
American Liver Foundation *http://www.gi.edu/alf/pubs.html*
Hepatitis Foundation International *http://www.hepfi.org.*
National Institute on Alcohol Abuse and Alcoholism *http://www.niaaa.nih.gov*
National Council on Alcoholism and Drug Dependence *http://www.ncadd.org*

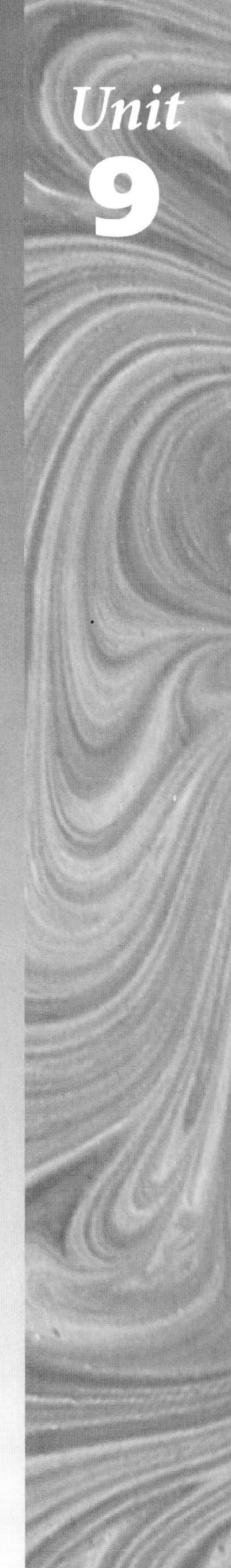

Musculoskeletal and Integumentary Functions

FOCUS ON Musculoskeletal Changes Through the Life Span

INFANT (1–12 MONTHS):

Increased growth and strength occurs from increase in size of existing muscle fibers. Bone calcification leads to bone growth and hardness. All bony structures undergo ossification after birth. A change in shape occurs as bones grow in length and width. Skin is functionally immature. Sweat gland development begins.

TODDLER AND PRESCHOOL AGE (1–5 YEARS):

Ossification slows but continues until early adulthood. Bone and joint shape changes lead to clumsiness early, with gradual correction later on. Muscles grow faster than bones; strength is related to the amount of muscle mass. The long bones contain red marrow, which produces blood cells. Skin becomes tougher and less susceptible to trauma with a gradual increase in sweating.

SCHOOL AGE (6–12 YEARS):

The long bones increase in length and size. Red marrow, gradually replaced by fatty tissue, is found only in the sternum, vertebrae, pelvic bones, and some skull and short-shafted bones. Girls begin to surpass boys in height and weight until the onset of puberty. Growing pains are common as the bones grow faster than adjacent muscles, stressing the muscles and ligaments. Posture becomes more adult-like, with increased muscle strength in the thoracic spine area. Muscle mass and strength gradually increase. Baby fat decreases. Skin structure becomes adult-like; sebum and eccrine sweat production remain low until puberty.

ADOLESCENCE (13–19 YEARS):

Maximal growth of muscle mass correlates with the growth of the skeletal system. Growth spurts and muscular strength vary, usually increasing in girls through age 15 years and in boys from ages 14 to 19 years. Muscle mass, closely related to androgen secretion, is twice as great in males than in females. Feet and hand elongation and body frame lengthening and broadening occur in both sexes. Females often stop growing within 3 years of menarche, whereas males often continue to grow during early adulthood. Sebaceous glands of the face, back, and chest become active. Acne may result. Eccrine glands are fully developed, and odorous sweating occurs.

YOUNG ADULT AND ADULT (20–45 YEARS):

Testosterone increases muscle mass and bone density. Muscle growth is due to an increase in size of muscle fibers. Peak muscular strength occurs around age 25 to 30 years. Legs of both sexes usually make up about half of the adult height. Peak bone mass occurs at approximately age 35 years, followed by bone loss (significantly greater for women than men). Skin has smooth turgor and taut appearance. Wrinkles begin at about age 25 to 30 years from decreased skin elasticity and decreased subcutaneous fat.

MIDDLE AGE ADULTS (46–64 YEARS):

After menopause, women experience a reduction in bone mass of 1% to 1.5% each year, significantly increasing the risk for osteoporosis. Male bone loss begins later, possibly not significant before age 70 years. Spinal vertebrae become compressed; cartilage between the vertebrae and hip joints loses water, becoming less elastic. Muscle mass decreases and muscle strength declines. Hair turns gray due to a decrease in tyrosinase necessary for melanin. Eye color fades and skin color begins to lighten. The epidermis thins. Loss of skin elasticity and subcutaneous fat lead to significant wrinkling, first at the eyes, mouth, and jaw line, and then the remainder of the body. Hair loss may occur due to genetic predisposition and decreased circulation to hair follicles.

LATE ADULTHOOD (65–100+ YEARS):

Bone loss, usually greater in females than males, occurs. By age 70 years, a woman's skeletal frame may have lost 30% or more of its calcium. An average loss of 1.2 cm in height for each 20 years of life occurs in both sexes. Vertebral collapse, collagen loss, and intervertebral disk atrophy cause spinal column compression. Posture becomes curved. Tendons shrink and harden. Bone and muscular strength and endurance are progressively lost. Flattening of the dermal–epidermal junction, reduced dermal thickness and vascularity, and elastin degeneration occur. Pigmented areas on the hands are common as melanocytes cluster together. Amounts of melanin in the hair continue to decrease. Skin becomes dry with decreased lubrication and turgor. The number and function of the sweat glands decrease. Nail growth slows and facial hair increases.

Chapter 27

Normal and Altered Functions of the Musculoskeletal System

Barbara Resnick / Reet Henze

KEY TERMS

actin
amphiarthroses
arthritis
atrophy
bursae
cancellous bone
cortical bone
cross-bridge
diaphysis
diarthroses
endosteum
epiphysis
hypertrophy
ligament
medullary bone
metaphysis
muscle fiber
myositis
myopathy
myosin
osteoblast
osteoclast
osteocyte
osteomyelitis
periosteum
red fiber
remodeling
sarcomere
sarcoplasmic reticulum
synarthroses
T-tubule
tendon
white fiber

Movement and the maintenance of an upright posture represents the action of the skeleton and muscle groups. There are 430 skeletal muscles in the body, found in pairs on the right and left side. Coordination of skeletal bones and muscles provides humans with functional abilities ranging from gross motor activities to fine, precise mobility. From the moment of conception, the human body is programmed to perform with coordination for many years. When alterations in musculoskeletal function occur, the entire body is affected.

NORMAL STRUCTURE OF SKELETAL MUSCLES

Skeletal or striated muscle forms the voluntary muscular system. Skeletal muscle is the predominant type of muscle in the human body and composes approximately 40% to 45% of the adult body weight. The superficial skeletal muscles are illustrated in Figure 27-1. Muscles are arranged in bundles encased in a sheath of connective tissue called *epimysium*, which is shown in Figure 27-2. The epimysium binds muscles to one another and to ligaments and bones.

Muscle Fibers

Striated muscle fibers differ from cardiac and visceral (smooth) muscle fibers (Fig. 27-3). Whereas striated and cardiac muscle (discussed in Chapter 15) have similar appearance, with the exception of the placement of the nucleus, smooth muscle lacks the characteristic striations. Smooth muscles, addressed in many areas of the book, are composed of many fibrils and divided into multiunit and visceral muscles. Multiunit smooth muscles are stimulated mainly by nerve signals such as those causing contraction of blood vessels. Visceral smooth muscles are arranged in contacting sheets or bundles, which allows them to contract as a group. This type of smooth muscle is found in many organs, including the gastrointestinal system as discussed in Chapter 25.

A single muscle is composed of many **muscle fibers** or *myofibers*. Muscle fibers are muscle cells consisting of bundles of long, multinucleated cells in which the oval-shaped nuclei are close to the cell membrane. Each muscle fiber is bound by a network of delicate tissue called *endomysium*. This tissue contains an extensive supply of capillaries and nerve fibers and provides

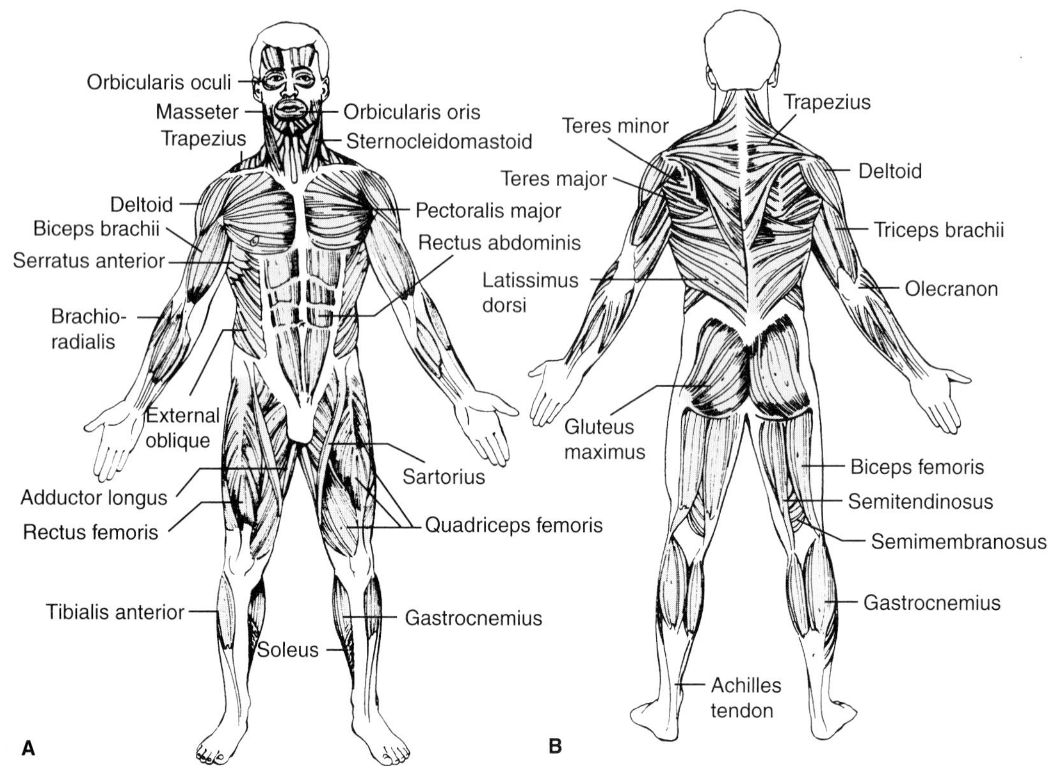

FIGURE 27-1. **A.** Anterior view of superficial muscles of the human body. **B.** Posterior view.

support for the blood vessels and nerves that are adjacent to the muscle fibers. Muscle cells have a reddish appearance due to the presence of the myoglobin pigment, an oxygen depot in muscles. The muscles that must maintain activity for periods of time usually contain more myoglobin than others.

Muscle fibers are arranged in bundles called *fascicles*, which are embedded in a web of connective tissue called the *perimysium* (see Fig. 27-2). Many fascicles constitute a single muscle, and these are encased in the epimysium, which tapers into the tendon that connects to the bone.

STRIATED MUSCLE FIBER TYPES

Muscles vary according to the work required of them. The speed of contraction is matched to the function endowed on the corresponding muscle. Eye muscles, for example, provide fine, precise movement and react swiftly, whereas large muscles, such as those necessary to maintain posture, react slowly. Muscle fibers have been classified into three basic types, each with different characteristics (Table 27-1):[5,25]

- *Slow-twitch* or *type I fibers*
- *Fast oxidative-glycolytic* or *type IIa fibers*
- *Fast glycolytic* or *type IIb fibers*

Slow-twitch, type I fibers are smaller and have more capillaries and mitochondria than do fast-twitch fibers. They are often called **red fibers** because they contain large quantities of myoglobin, an iron-containing protein similar to hemoglobin in red blood cells.[10] Slow-twitch fibers are lipid rich and glycogen poor and use mostly oxidative (aerobic) pathways for energy metabolism. They provide for muscular endurance activities.

Types IIa and IIb are both pale or **white fibers**, use slightly different energy sources, and are adapted for rapid and powerful muscle contractions as in sprinting and jumping.[18,25] Type IIa fibers are both lipid and glycogen rich and have fast contraction at times and good fatigue resistance, whereas Type IIb fibers are lipid poor and glycogen rich and have the fastest contraction times but poor resistance to fatigue. Type IIa fibers use glycolysis with high oxidative pathways; Type IIb fibers rely primarily on glycolysis and low oxidative pathways.

High oxidative pathways produce more adenosine triphosphate (ATP) than low oxidative or anaerobic pathways. However, the ATP production in oxidative metabolism is not as rapid as in anaerobic glycolysis. Although a specific type of muscle fibril predominates in various human muscles, they usually contain a combination of type I and type II fibers.

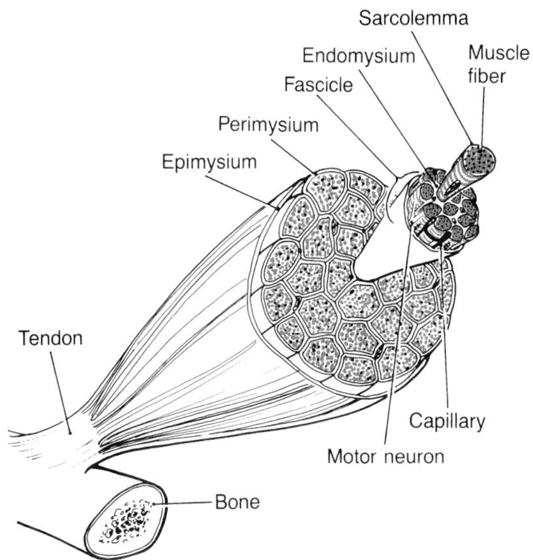

FIGURE 27-2. **Structures of skeletal muscle from muscle to bundle of fibers to single muscle fiber or cell.**

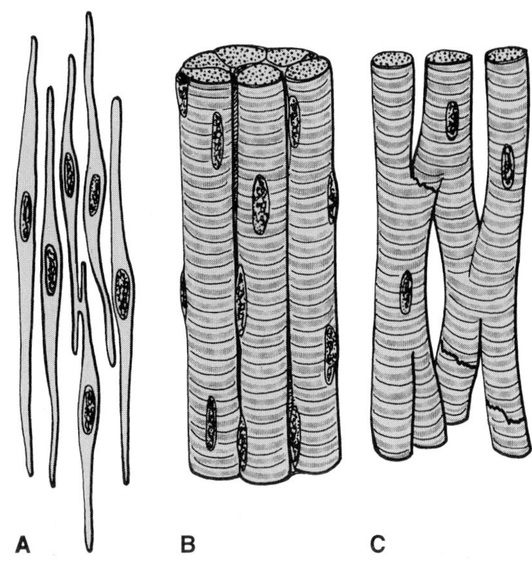

FIGURE 27-3. **A.** Appearance of smooth muscle fibers. **B.** Striated skeletal muscle shows characteristic multiple nuclei and alternating light and dark bands. **C.** Branched, striated, cardiac muscle fibers with a single nucleus and close approximation of cells through intercalated discs.

TABLE 27-1

MUSCLE FIBER TYPES

	TYPE I	TYPE IIA	TYPE IIB
MECHANICAL ASPECTS			
Time to peak tension	Slow	Faster	Fastest
Twitch tension	Low	Higher	Highest
Fatigue resistance	High	Lower	Lowest
Elasticity	Low	High	High
STRUCTURAL ASPECTS			
Motor neuron size	Small	Large	Large
Motor neuron conduction velocity	Slow	Fast	Fast
Motor neuron recruitment threshold	Low	High	High
Fiber diameter	Small	Larger	Largest
Sarcoplasmic reticulum development	Least	More	Most
Mitochondrial density	Highest	Less	Least
Capillary density	Very dense	Less	Poor
Myoglobin content	High	Moderate	Low
METABOLIC ASPECTS			
Phosphocreatine	Low	Higher	Highest
Glycogen	Low	High	High
Triglyceride	High	Moderate	Low
ATPase activity	Low	High	High
Glycolytic enzyme activity	Low	High	High
Oxidative enzyme activity	High	High	Low

(Dee, R., Hurst, L., Gruber, M., & Kottmeier, S. [1991]. *Principles of orthopedic practice.* New York: McGraw-Hill.)

MYOFIBRILS

Each muscle fiber contains thousands of contractile elements called *myofibrils*, which extend throughout the length of the muscle. The myofibrils are the contractile cells of the muscle. Figure 27-4 shows myofibril-repeating contractile units called **sarcomeres**, which are the functional units of skeletal and cardiac muscle and are composed of the proteins **actin** and **myosin**. Actin is a thin filament composed of two proteins, *troponin* and *tropomyosin*. Myosin filaments are thicker and have projections known as **cross-bridges** that extend outward toward the actin molecule. Actin and myosin overlap partially, causing the myofibril to exhibit striation, alternating light and dark bands when viewed under an electron microscope. The light bands containing only actin filaments are called *I bands*, and the dark bands containing myosin filaments and part of the actin filaments are called *A bands*. In the middle of the light band is a dark line called the *Z line*. The M line is a thickening of myosin filaments at midpoint in the A band. Figure 27-4 identifies the sarcomere between the Z lines.[10,30] During contraction the A band widens, the I band shrinks, and the H area disappears due to the effect of myosin pulling the actin filaments.[25]

MUSCLE HYPERTROPHY

Hypertrophy, the enlargement of individual muscle fibers, is an adaptive condition of the cells that results from an increased demand for work. Skeletal muscle cells cannot regenerate to adapt to a need for increased function; rather, they enlarge to meet the demand.[3] Nutrients such as ATP, creatine phosphate, and glycogen increase in concentration within the cell when there is need for increased work.

Most hypertrophy is considered to be adaptive in that it results when resistance is continually applied to the muscle walls. A weight lifter or athlete increases the workload through specific muscles that increase size and strength up to a physiologic limit.

Other Cellular Components

In addition to myofibrils, the muscle fiber also contains structural and chemical parts common to all cells. *Sarcoplasm* is the cytoplasm of the muscle cell that contains many of the following cellular components:

- *Mitochondria*, which provide energy for contraction
- **Sarcoplasmic reticulum** (SR), which is similar to the endoplasmic reticulum of other cells and functions to transport calcium into the sarcomere to initiate muscle contraction
- Transverse tubule system (**T-tubules**), which are closely aligned with the SR and extend across the sarcoplasm and communicate with the exterior of the muscle cell
- *Electrolytes* and *water*, which are present in large quantities of potassium, magnesium, and phosphates, together with enzymatic proteins, bicarbonate, sulfate, and small amounts of sodium, chloride, and calcium

Blood Supply to Muscles

Muscles are supplied with blood by arteries that penetrate the connective tissue coverings. These arteries branch out into tiny thin-walled vessels (capillaries), which carry an abundant supply of oxygen-rich blood to the muscles. Each muscle fiber is actually supplied with oxygen and glucose by several capillaries that surround the individual muscle cells.

Nerve Supply to Muscles

The nerve supply to large skeletal muscle fibers (extrafusal) stems through large A alpha fibers originating from alpha motor neurons. The nerve supply to small skeletal muscle fibers (intrafusal) in muscle spindles originates through A gamma fibers from small gamma motor neurons. Fibers from both large and small nerves transmit together from the spinal cord via the anterior horn (anterior motor neuron).[10] A single motor neuron may innervate many muscle fibers. All muscle fibers innervated by a single neuron constitute one *motor unit*,

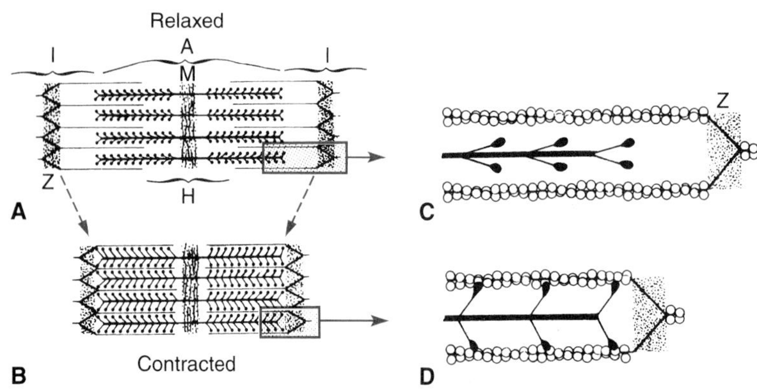

FIGURE 27-4. The components of a sarcomere that may be discerned as striations. The area indicated in **A** is shown in more detail in **C**, and the area indicated in **B** is shown in **D**. In **C**, the cross bridges on the thick filaments are not interacting with the actin in the thin filaments. In **D**, the interaction of the cross bridges with the actin is resulting in contraction. (Cormack, D. H. [1993]. *Essential histology.* Philadelphia: J. B. Lippincott.)

the functional unit of skeletal muscle. All muscle fibers in a single motor unit are of the same type and vary greatly in number, depending on the nature of the movement. Neuron fibers innervating muscles more resistant to fatigue and requiring less precise movement, such as those in the leg calf, innervate large numbers of muscle fibers. However, neurons innervating muscles that fatigue more easily and require more precise movement, such as those of the eye or hand, innervate far fewer muscle fibers.

Central control over the motor neurons is achieved by means of multiple descending direct and indirect pathways, including the principal efferent motor fibers of the corticospinal tract. The innervation from these usually comes through multiple spinal interneurons.

In its simplest form, neuronal innervation at the spinal level is the monosynaptic muscle stretch reflex. The afferent fiber to the dorsal horn from a muscle spindle synapses within the cord with an alpha motor fiber that returns innervation via the anterior horn to the same muscle spindle.

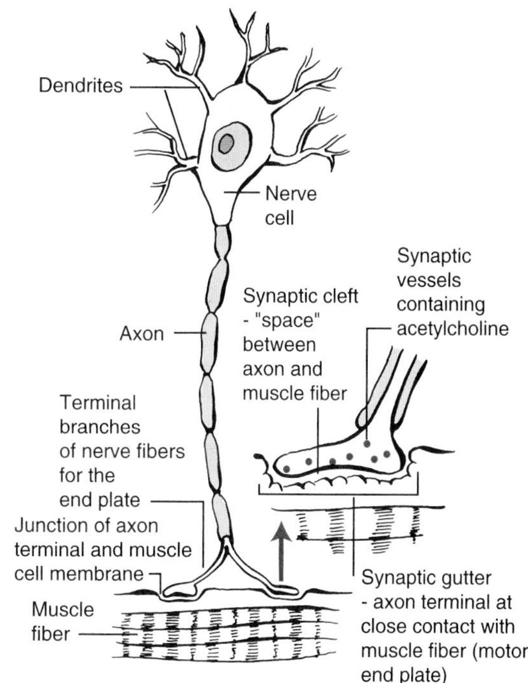

FIGURE 27-5. Myoneural or neuromuscular junction.

NEUROMUSCULAR JUNCTION

The junction between a motor nerve ending and a muscle fiber is called a *neuromuscular* or *myoneural junction* (Fig. 27-5). Each skeletal muscle fiber is contacted by at least one nerve ending. One motor nerve fiber can stimulate several muscle fibers at the same time. The axon terminals form flattened motor end plates on the surface of the muscle fibers.

The end branches of the motor neuron, known as axon terminals, gain access to the muscle fiber through the endomysium. At the junction between the muscle fiber and the motor neuron, the muscle fiber membrane forms a motor end plate.

NORMAL FUNCTION OF SKELETAL MUSCLE

Skeletal muscles function to produce skeletal movement; maintain posture and position; support soft tissues; shield internal organs from injury; provide control over swallowing; and help maintain body temperature. Muscle function is achieved through muscle contraction and relaxation. Other factors important to muscle function include movement of muscle groups, muscle tension, length–tension relationship, and tone. Measures of muscle function and metabolism are enumerated in the Appendix of this unit.

Muscle Contraction

MUSCLE ACTION POTENTIAL

For a skeletal muscle to contract, a stimulus must be initiated from the nervous system. The stimulus causes *acetylcholine* to be released into the synaptic cleft at the neuromuscular junction (see Fig. 27-5). Acetylcholine, an excitatory neurotransmitter, causes the muscle cell membrane to become permeable to cations in the cleft, allowing for the movement of sodium, potassium, and calcium through the ionic channels.[10] Sodium, however, is the primary cation that rushes into the muscle fiber, causing a rise in membrane potential or generation of end plate potential. The action potential thus generated passes down the sarcolemma, depolarizes the T-tubule system, and causes the release of calcium ions from the SR. The released calcium ions bind with troponin-tropomyosin, resulting in the sliding of actin onto myosin. This initiates the contractile phase.

SLIDING FILAMENT/CROSS BRIDGE THEORY

The sliding filament theory described by Huxley in 1954 (currently referred to as cross bridge theory) describes muscular contraction as the movement or sliding of actin onto myosin, which results in increased overlap of actin and myosin and shortening of the entire sarcomere unit.[3] Although the interaction of actin and myosin filaments generates tension, this interaction is regulated by the two proteins, troponin and tropomyosin. Actin and myosin have been shown to have a strong affinity for each other. The structure of myosin facilitates cross-linkages with actin, completing the system needed to perform the muscular contraction shown in Figure 27-4.

Pure actin filaments bind strongly with myosin when they are in the presence of magnesium ions and ATP, which exist in abundance in the myofibrils. When troponin and tropomyosin are added to the thin filaments, binding between actin and myosin is inhibited. When the muscle is at rest, troponin and tropomyosin cover the actin filaments so that they cannot bind with myosin. Initiation of the contractile process requires that troponin and tropomyosin be inhibited.

Calcium ions, released from the SR, bind to sites on troponin molecules. This binding causes the troponin molecule to change shape and pull on the tropomyosin strands, moving them to the side and uncovering the cross-bridge binding sites on the actin molecules.[30] Adenosine triphosphate interacts at the site, splits, and activates myosin. Myosin binds to actin, creating a cross-bridge that moves the thin (actin) filaments toward the center. The cross-bridge is broken by the binding on a new ATP molecule. Splitting of this molecule causes the binding to reform at a different place on the actin molecule. This power stroke pulls the actin on the myosin in a step-by-step process described by Huxley as a ratchet-like movement. The ATP is essential to provide energy for the cross-bridge movement and to break the myosin-actin connection, which allows the cross-bridge on myosin to return to its original position.

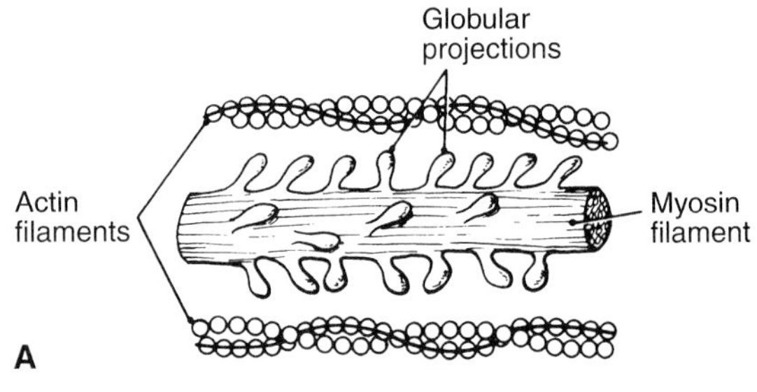

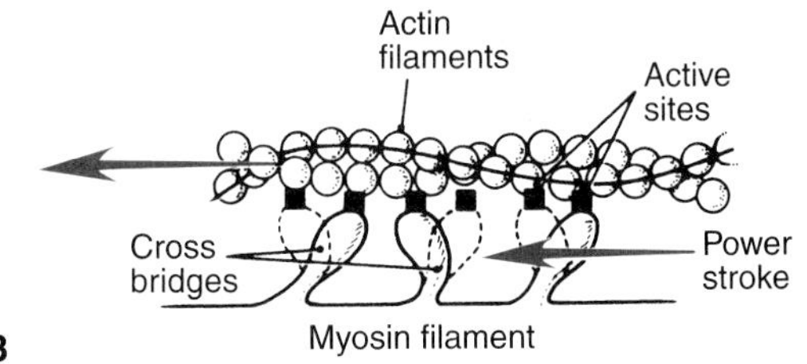

FIGURE 27-6. "Walk-along" mechanism for muscle contraction. **A.** The relationship between the myosin filament with its globular projections and the actin filaments. **B.** The hinges of the myosin filament attach to successive active sites on the actin filaments.

THE "WALK-ALONG" MECHANISM

The mechanism by which the cross-bridges on myosin interact with actin is not completely understood. Figure 27-6 identifies cross-bridges attaching to and disengaging from active sites on the actin filament in a "walk-along" fashion. The attachment causes dragging of the actin filament (sliding of actin on myosin). After this power stroke, the sites are disengaged and attach to the next active site, pulling the actin filament step by step toward the center of the myosin filament. Theoretically, the cross-bridges operate independently of each other, so that if more cross-bridges are in contact with the actin filament, the force of the contraction is greater.

METABOLIC REQUIREMENTS FOR MUSCLE CONTRACTION

Muscle contraction requires high amount of energy that is supplied through ATP. The small amount of ATP present in the muscle fiber is depleted quickly with muscle contraction. Therefore, energy must be manufactured rapidly when it is needed. Physiologic reactions provide for new ATP through phosphorylation of adenosine-diphosphate (ADP). These include:

- Conversion of high-energy stores from phosphocreatine (creatine phosphate). Muscle has a small store of creatine phosphate that can rapidly donate its phosphate ion to ADP to produce ATP and energy. This process occurs very rapidly, but the stores of creatine phosphate are rapidly depleted.
- Generation of ATP through anaerobic glycolysis. Anaerobic metabolism provides ATP when the cellular supply of oxygen is insufficient to produce enough to meet the energy requirements of the cell. In the muscular system, it is often used when the skeletal muscles are taxed, as in athletic exertion. Without adequate oxygen supply, pyruvate does not enter the citric acid cycle to yield carbon dioxide and water, but rather is reduced to lactic acid. This reduction to lactic acid produces energy that converts ADP into ATP. The net ATP formed is much less than with oxygen, but it allows the muscle cells to continue their activity for a short period of time.
- Oxidative metabolism of acetyl CoA (see p. 20). ATP is released when oxygen combines with various foodstuffs. As exercise is sustained, blood flow to the area is increased and a new steady state of muscle metabolism is achieved through the initiation of aerobic production of needed ATP. At rest, the skeletal muscle uses mostly fatty acids for energy production. During exercise the uptake of glucose and fat increases. It is estimated that 90% of carbon dioxide is produced through the use of consumed foodstuffs, with fat providing the greatest percentage for long-term muscle activity.[10]

MUSCLE RELAXATION

Calcium must be returned to the tubules of the SR so that troponin and tropomyosin can resume their inhibitory function. This is accomplished by an active calcium pump in the walls of the SR. This pump also can concentrate calcium within the tubules, creating a low level of calcium in the myofibrils. As calcium leaves troponin, it returns to its original configuration, which then allows tropomyosin strands to recover the actin-binding sites.[30] Without a communication between actin and myosin, the sarcomere unit extends and the muscle relaxes. Significant amounts of ATP are required to operate the calcium pump. Flowchart 27-1 summarizes the processes of muscle contraction and relaxation.

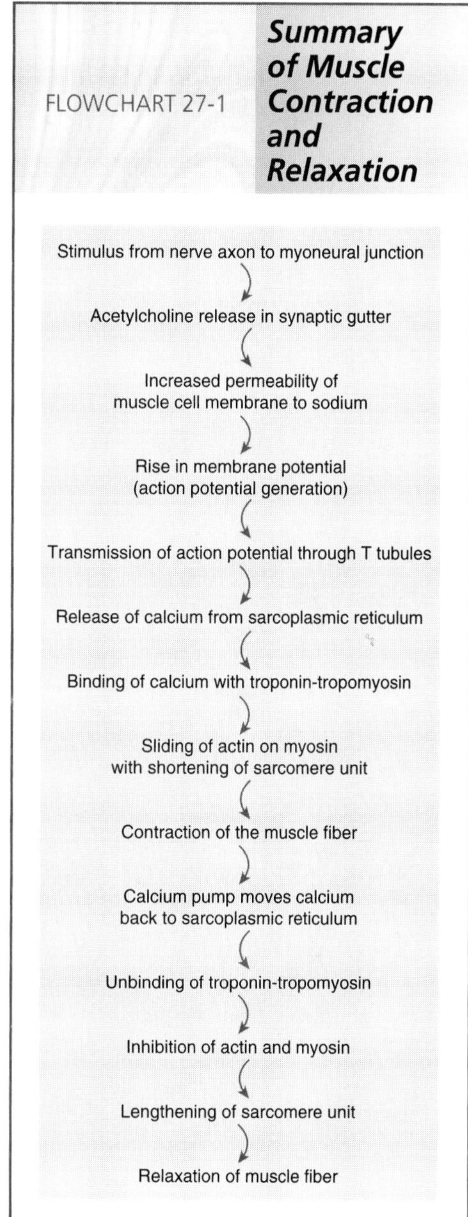

FLOWCHART 27-1
Summary of Muscle Contraction and Relaxation
Stimulus from nerve axon to myoneural junction
Acetylcholine release in synaptic gutter
Increased permeability of muscle cell membrane to sodium
Rise in membrane potential (action potential generation)
Transmission of action potential through T tubules
Release of calcium from sarcoplasmic reticulum
Binding of calcium with troponin-tropomyosin
Sliding of actin on myosin with shortening of sarcomere unit
Contraction of the muscle fiber
Calcium pump moves calcium back to sarcoplasmic reticulum
Unbinding of troponin-tropomyosin
Inhibition of actin and myosin
Lengthening of sarcomere unit
Relaxation of muscle fiber

Movement of Muscle Groups

Coordinated movement is associated with complex interneuronal innervation of muscle groups through motor reflex arcs producing contraction and relaxation. In movement, a prime muscle (agonist) contracts and the reciprocal muscle (antagonist) produces an opposite effect, relaxation. Muscles that have other muscles inserted into them are known as fixators. These muscles provide support for bones in movement.

Muscle Tension

The basic response of muscle to a single stimulus is a *twitch* (Fig. 27-7). When stimulated, the fiber develops tension rapidly and then relaxes. Tension can be increased by more rapid stimulation. The twitch tension for each higher stimulation rate increases in a steplike manner until *tetanus*, which is the full and complete contraction of the muscle.[9] Muscle tension can be altered by increasing the rate of stimulation. The force of muscle contraction can be increased by the incremental recruitment of additional motor units by the central nervous system.

Length–Tension Relationships

Muscle length varies with the type of muscle contractions. In *static* contractions the fiber length is constant, and in *dynamic* contractions the fiber lengthens. Static muscle action implies that no mechanical work is performed as force is developed without joint motion. This is referred to as an *isometric contraction*. With an isometric contraction, muscle tension equals the external load and muscle length is constant.

Dynamic muscle action implies that mechanical work is performed as force is developed through joint motion. Dynamic muscle action is either concentric or eccentric. In a concentric contraction, the muscle tension overcomes the external load and the muscle shortens. In an eccentric contraction, muscle tension does not overcome the external load and the muscle lengthens. Dynamic muscle action is also divided into isokinetic (maximal voluntary contraction), isoinertial (submaximal voluntary contraction), or isotonic (nonphysiologic).

Muscle Tone

Muscle tone is the term applied to the tautness of healthy muscle tissue at rest. Tone is maintained by spinal cord impulses and decreases as neuron excitability decreases or is lost. Additionally, tone is also affected by the activity from the muscle spindles. When tone is lost, the muscle is said to be flaccid. Increased excitability of the upper motor unit may cause spasticity or rigidity (see pp. 942–943).

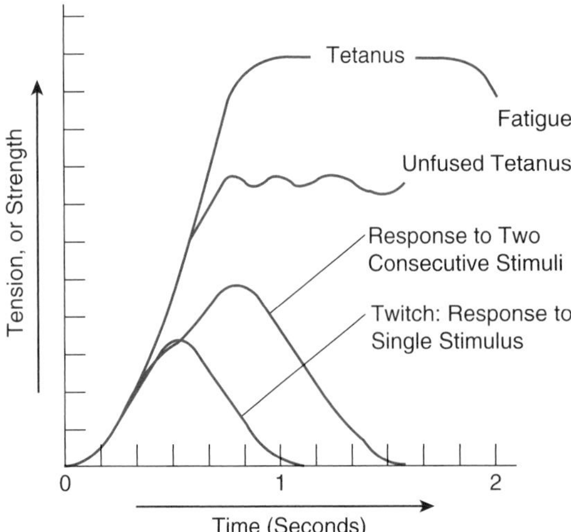

FIGURE 27-7. Muscle tension. The motor unit response to a single stimulus is a twitch. When a second stimulus to the same motor unit occurs before it completely relaxes from the first stimulus, the two summate so that the tension developed is greater than that produced by a single stimulus alone. If the stimuli are repeated, summation continues until the individual twitches are completely fused (tetanus). (Fox, E. L. et al. [1988]. *The physiological basis for exercise and sport* [5th ed.]. Dubuque, IA: Brown and Benchmark.)

NORMAL STRUCTURE OF BONES

Bone tissue has two structural forms: (1) **cortical** or compact (hard surface area), and (2) **cancellous** or spongy. Cortical bone is dense, highly calcified and less active metabolically. Cancellous bone is more active metabolically, light and porous, and contains bone marrow.

Figure 27-8 depicts the microscopic structural unit of compact bone. It consists of numerous, parallel, longitudinal canals (Haversian canals), which contain blood vessels and nerves. Around each canal are several concentric layers, or rings of *lamellae*. Connecting the Haversian canals with the lamellae are the canaliculi (minute canals) that carry oxygen and nutrients to the bone cells. Microscopic cavities called *lacunae* border the lamellae and contain osteocytes. Each canal with its contents and surrounding lamellae makes up a Haversian system or osteon (Figure 27-8*B*). Directly under the periosteum and surrounding the medullary cavity, several thicknesses of lamellae are laid down, surrounding the entire shaft with hard bone. The Haversian systems run parallel to each other and longitudinally, from metaphysis to metaphysis, and are connected transversely by tubes called Volkmann's canals. Blood vessels from the periosteum enter the bone and pass through these canals to enter and leave the Haversian system.

Cancellous bone, present in flat bones and in the ends of long bones, is a collection of *trabeculae*, or beams of bone, which gives it a spongy appearance (Fig. 27-9). The trabeculae add strength due to the many interlacing parts. The spaces between the trabeculae are filled with bone marrow. The red marrow actively participates in the formation of red blood cells and is present in the adult in the cancellous bone of the ribs, sternum, vertebrae, and pelvis. Red marrow is present in many bones in infants and is gradually converted to yellow marrow composed of fat cells. Most long bones of adults contain yellow marrow. The medullary cavity is simply a continuation of cancellous bone and is the central area filled with marrow, blood, and lymph vessels.

Periosteum and Endosteum

The outer and inner surfaces of bone are covered with specialized connective tissue. The dense, white, fibrous membrane wrapping the outside is called the **periosteum** and is composed of two layers. The outer, or fibrous, layer has relatively few cells and is made up of fibrous tissue. The inner layer of the periosteum is very vascular and has an osteogenic function. In addition to supplying a site of attachment for tendons and ligaments, the periosteum is richly supplied with nerves and blood vessels that are important in nourishing the bone. Lining the medullary cavity and Haversian canals as well as the spaces of spongy bone is a thin membrane called the **endosteum**. The cells of this membrane provide for growth and repair of bone tissue.

Bone Cells

Bone tissue consists of three types of cells: (1) **osteoblasts**, (2) **osteocytes**, and (3) **osteoclasts**. The primary role of osteoblasts is to synthesize osteoid, the nonmineralized portion of the bone matrix. Osteoid is a protein substance that becomes calcified to produce hard bone. Osteoblasts also help control the calcification of bone. Alkaline phosphatase, which is thought to aid in the mineralization process, is produced by osteoblasts.[9,22] Osteoblasts synthesize the organic components of bone matrix.[5] When the matrix surrounding the osteoblasts becomes calcified, the cells are called osteocytes. Osteocytes are the main cellular component of bone tissue and are encased in the lacunae. Osteoclasts are cells of monocyte-macrophage origin whose primary function is the resorption or removal of bone. The osteoclasts are the counterweights to osteoblasts. These cells produce acids that make the bone salts soluble and then digest the organic matrix.[5]

Nerve and Blood Supply to Bones

Because bone is a living tissue, nutrients must be supplied and waste material removed. Total bone blood

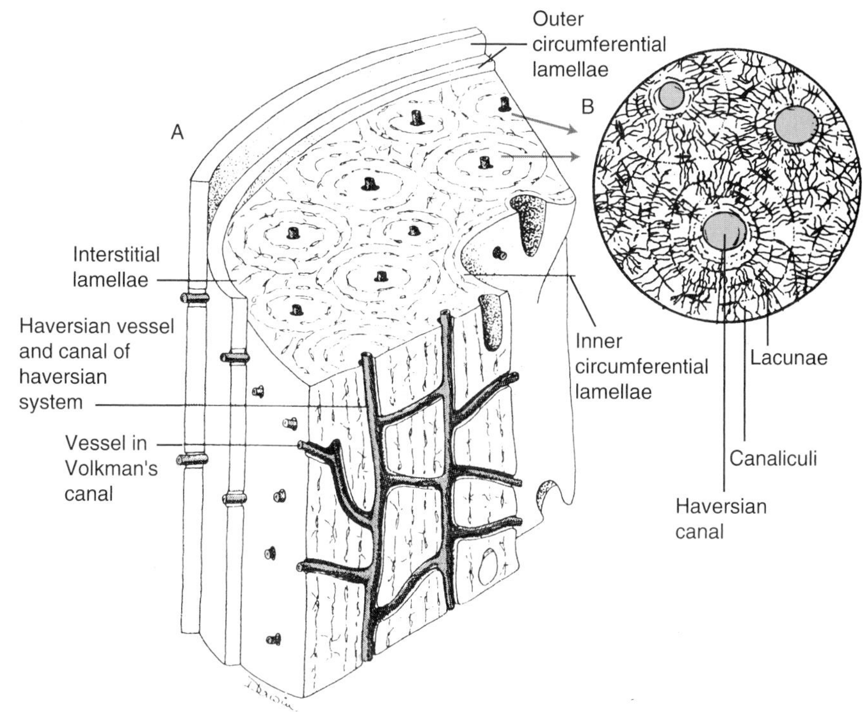

FIGURE 27-8. **A.** Compact bone organization in the cortex of a long bone. **B.** Enlarged structures of a Haversian system. (Modified from Cormack, D. H. [1993]. *Essential histology*. Philadelphia: J. B. Lippincott.)

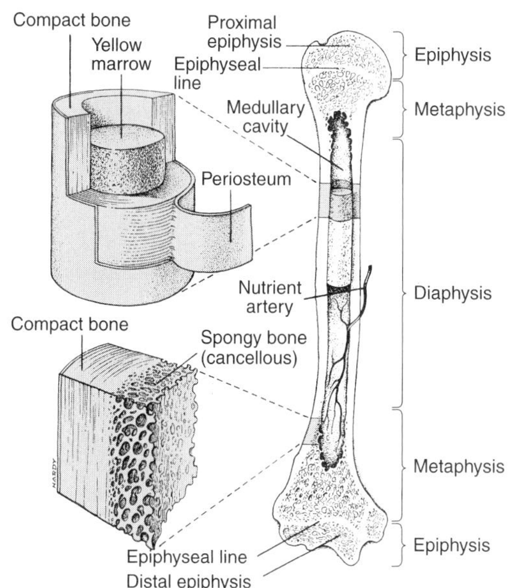

FIGURE 27-9. A long bone shown in longitudinal section.

flow has been estimated at 200 to 400 mL per minute. Small bones usually have a single artery and vein entering them, and large bones have several. The chief artery, which enters near the middle of the shaft of long bones, is called the principal nutrient artery. After piercing the shaft and reaching the medullary canal, it branches into ascending and descending branches and ends in sinusoidal capillaries. The artery and its branches supply the marrow and cortex, as well as the Haversian systems.

Nerve supply to bone is sparse and present mainly in the outer layer, the periosteum. It consists of both afferent (sensory) and sympathetic fibers, with the autonomic fibers controlling the dilatation of bone blood vessels.

Classification of Bones

Most commonly, bones are classified as long, short, flat, and irregular. Examples of the various types of bones are illustrated in the human skeleton in Figure 27-10.

LONG BONES

Long bones are the bones of the extremities and are elongated in shape. Figure 27-9 shows a long bone consisting of the following: (1) two **epiphyses,** or ends, which are knobby areas containing cancellous bone; (2) the **diaphysis**, which composes the shaft or long portion; and (3) the **metaphysis**, which contains the epiphyseal plate and newly formed bone. In the adult, the metaphysis and epiphysis are continuous.

SHORT BONES

Short bones, such as those in the wrist, are cube-shaped and consist of cancellous bone enclosed in a thin case of compact bone. These often are combined with other short bones.

FLAT BONES

The bones of the skull, ribs, scapulae, and sternum are examples of flat bones. Their function is largely protective. They consist of two plates of hard, compact bone covering a thin layer of cancellous bone. These bones, especially those of the ribs and sternum, are important sites for blood formation.

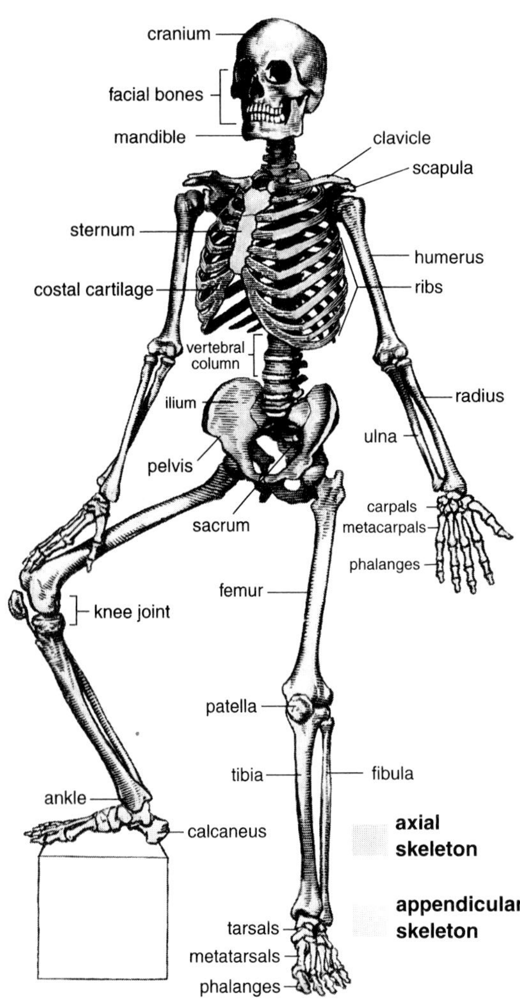

FIGURE 27-10. The human skeleton, showing the various major bones.

IRREGULAR BONES

Bones that are irregular in shape are similar in composition to the short bones. The vertebrae and the ossicles of the ears are examples of irregular bones.

NORMAL FUNCTION OF BONES

Bone has two basic functions: (1) to provide structural support to allow locomotion and protection of vital organs, and (2) to serve as a depot for calcium, phosphorus, magnesium, sodium, and carbonate. An essential role of bone is maintaining normal ion and buffer concentrations. Bone provides for the constant movement of calcium, phosphorus, and other minerals into and out of the bloodstream. Bone will be destroyed to maintain homeostasis of these elements.

Bone is a collagenous protein that is partially composed of complex calcium salts. The organic (nonmineralized) matrix of bone, the osteoid, is made up primarily of collagen (protein), some polysaccharides, and lipids. The salts, which consist of calcium carbonate ($CaCO_3$) and calcium phosphate ($Ca_3[PO_4]_2$), form a substance that is a hard crystalline salt. The matrix functions to supply *tensile strength* (resistance to being pulled apart), whereas the mineral deposits provide for *compressive strength* (resistance to being crumbled). This combination gives bone twice the energy-absorption capacity of an oak tree, and the same tensile strength as granite.

BONE GROWTH, REMODELING, AND FORMATION

Bone Growth

The epiphyses of a long bone are separated from the shaft by the *epiphyseal plate*, which is responsible for the longitudinal growth of bone. On the distal side of this plate, osteoblasts are constantly secreting the bone matrix, which immediately becomes ossified, increasing the length of the bone. At the same time, on the proximal side of the epiphyseal plate, new cartilage is being formed. During puberty, ossification exceeds cartilage formation. Gradually the cartilaginous epiphyseal plate becomes completely ossified, and linear bone growth ceases. Epiphyseal closure occurs about 3 years earlier in women than it does in men, in whom bone length ceases to increase after the age of 20.[9]

In the young adult, approximately one-sixth of total skeletal calcium is turned over every year, but when a person reaches the fourth or fifth decade of life, reabsorption begins to outpace formation. Thus, after age 40, approximately 0.5% to 1.0% of the total skeletal mass is lost yearly.

Bone Remodeling

Bone tissue is constantly being formed and older bone is reabsorbed. This process, known as bone **remodeling**, is facilitated by the osteoblasts and osteoclasts. Remodeling occurs on the bone surfaces in discrete packages called bone multicellular units (BMUs). The osteoblasts and osteoclasts work together in a synchronized fashion called coupling (Fig. 27-11). Remodeling occurs in 25% of trabecular bone and 33% of cortical bone each year. The entire remodeling process takes approximately 100 days.[11]

Bone Formation

During development and growth, bone formation can be occur by two pathways: (1) intramembranous and (2) endochondral ossification.

INTRAMEMBRANOUS OSSIFICATION

The swapping of the cartilaginous material with bone, begun in utero, continues until after puberty. Intramembranous ossification occurs in the flat bones of the face and skull. In the cartilaginous fetal structure, osteoblasts secrete organic material that calcifies; from this center of ossification, small bone spicules build up an interlacing network on which more bone is developed. Eventually, the osteoblasts are trapped in small spaces called lacunae and become osteocytes. The spongy bone developed is then covered by layers of compact bone.

ENDOCHONDRAL OSSIFICATION

The process by which the long bones of the body are formed is called endochondral ossification (Fig. 27-12). The "baby skeleton," which is cartilage, is transformed into bone by ossification, which begins in the center of the shaft (diaphysis) and in each end (epiphysis) of the bone. This formation spreads, and with it the destruction of cartilage, until only two thin strips are left at either end of the bone (the epiphyseal plate). These strips remain until bone growth and maturation are completed. As spongy bone is formed within, marrow is formed in the spaces and the marrow cavity develops in the center of the bone. The osteoblasts on the outside form layers of hard, compact bone. The perichondrium, which is the layer surrounding the early cartilage, becomes the periosteum. As more layers of compact bone are laid circumferentially, osteoclasts make the marrow (medullary cavity) larger to support the larger bone. The process has been described in zones, as illustrated in Figure 27-12. These are: (1) zone of resting cartilage, which functions to anchor the epiphyseal plate to the bone structure and provide blood supply to much of the calcifying cartilage; (2) zone of proliferating cartilage, which divides and supplies chondrocytes that are lost at the epiphyseal plate; (3) zone of maturing cartilage, in which chrondrocytes are filled with glycogen and lipid substances and secrete alkaline phosphatase, which facilitates the calcification of extracellular matrix; and (4) zone of calcifying cartilage, in which insoluble calcium salts become deposited and capillaries grow to provide adequate blood supply.[3]

FOCUS ON CELLULAR PHYSIOLOGY

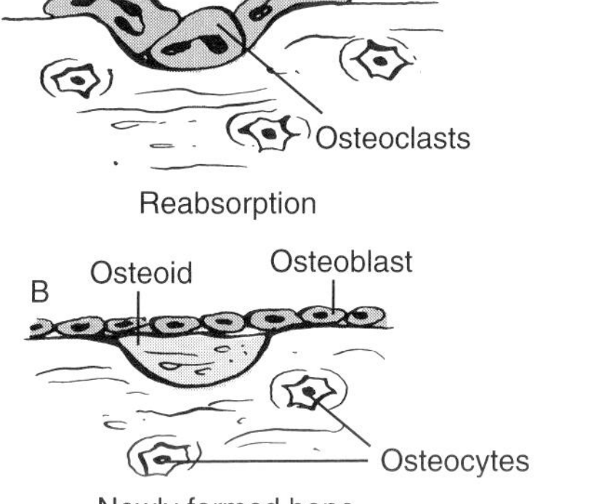

FIGURE 27-11. Bone remodeling. **A.** Osteoclasts are mobilized on the bone surfaces to reabsorb a pocket of bone. **B.** Osteoblasts lay down new bone in the pocket.

Factors Affecting Bone Growth and Formation

Bone growth and formation is influenced by such factors as calcium and phosphorus metabolism, hormones, weight bearing, diet, and environmental influences.

CALCIUM AND PHOSPHORUS

For new bone to form, adequate amounts of calcium and phosphorus must be present in the plasma and interstitial fluid that bathes the osteoblasts. These critical amounts are thought to be maintained, in part, by a partial membrane formed by osteoblasts. This membrane acts as a barrier between bone fluid and the extracellular fluid of the body. The osteoblasts connect with other osteocytes deep in the bone where calcium can move into and out of the cell. Calcium salts precipitate on the surface of collagen fibers at periodic intervals. These calcium salts become hydroxyapatite crystals, which provide the crystalline structure of bone mineralization.

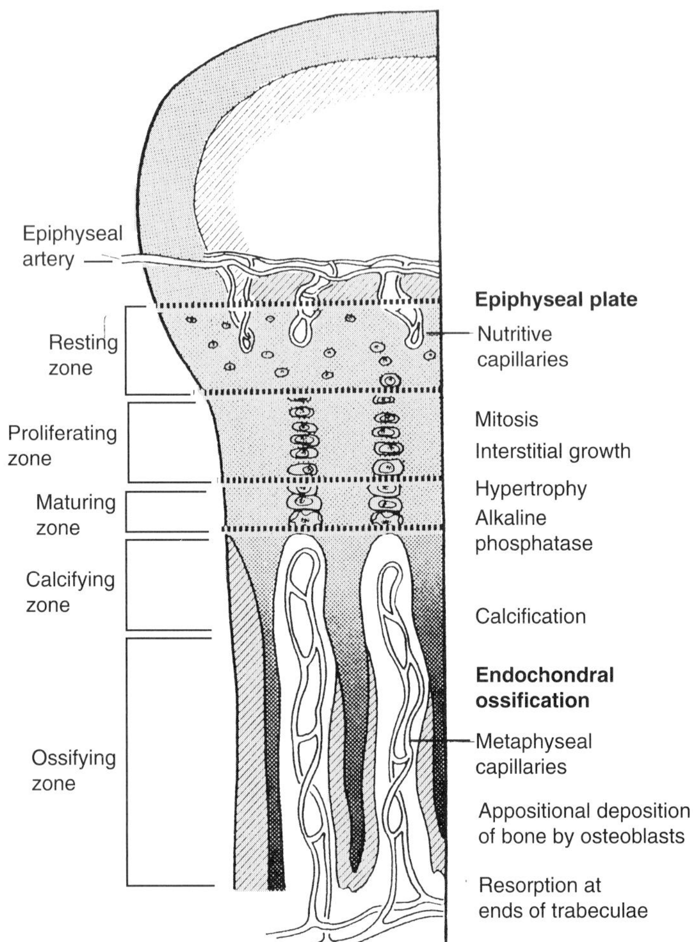

FIGURE 27-12. **The various parts of an epiphyseal plate showing the chief processes that occur in this region. (Cormack, D. H. [1993].** ***Essential histology.*** **Philadelphia: J. B. Lippincott.)**

With a normal diet, a person takes in approximately 1000 mg of calcium daily, of which 300 mg is absorbed by the intestines into the blood stream. From there it goes to the extracellular fluid, and some of it is returned to the intestinal tract through bile. A large amount of the daily calcium intake is excreted in the feces and, to a lesser extent, in urine.[11] Despite this large amount of calcium movement into and out of the body, the serum calcium level remains constant at about 10 mg/dL. The serum pH and albumin levels affect the amount of calcium in the blood, with about half of it being bound to serum albumin. This calcium can be released when the serum pH decreases.[20] The constancy of extracellular fluid calcium is dependent upon vitamin D, parathyroid hormone (PTH), and calcitonin (described below and in Chapter 23).

Phosphorus is a major component of bone and also is involved in many metabolic processes. Serum levels of phosphorus vary according to intake, blood pH, and other factors. Serum samples are accurate only if drawn in the fasting state.[11] Phosphorus is efficiently absorbed by the intestines, and its excretion is regulated by the proximal tubules of the kidney nephrons. If the renal capacity for excreting phosphorus is impaired, hyperphosphatemia results and there is an associated decrease in serum calcium levels (see p. 626).[20]

In the diet, calcium and phosphate are supplied mainly by milk and meats. Phosphate is absorbed with calcium. When calcium is absorbed in abundance, so is phosphate. Excess phosphate is excreted along with excess calcium in the feces and urine.

When the serum calcium ion concentration is high, production of PTH is curtailed. This results in a lowered serum calcium level. Conversely, when serum calcium levels are lowered, PTH secretion increases, which expands vitamin D activity and absorption of calcium in the intestinal tract. Parathyroid hormone promotes the formation of osteoclasts and retards the production of osteoblasts. The action of PTH is discussed further in Chapter 23.

VITAMIN D

Vitamin D and its metabolites are required for calcification of the bone matrix. Vitamin D is a steroid hormone that is taken in in the diet and is formed in the skin by the action of the ultraviolet rays of the sun. Vitamin D is designated as vitamins D_2 and D_3 according to their structural side chains, but they are metabolized identically and have equivalent biologic potencies.[11] For dietary vitamin D to be absorbed, bile must be present. Through a series of events in the liver and kidneys, vitamins D_2 and D_3 are converted to 1,25-dihydroxycholecalciferol (1,25[OH]$_2D_3$), which is the active form of the vitamin. Other metabolites are formed in the complex conversions that take place, but only 1,25(OH_2)D_3 is thought to have major physiologic action.[11] It affects serum calcium principally by controlling the absorption of calcium in the intestine. The feedback mechanism involves increased PTH, increased production of 1,25$(OH)_2D_3$, and increased calcium absorption from the ileum. Vitamin D also increases calcium reabsorption in the kidney nephrons.[10] Renal failure depresses the reabsorption of calcium by the kidneys as well as curtailing the production of 1,25$(OH)_2D_3$. In renal failure, vitamin D is virtually ineffective because of a decrease in the intestinal absorption of calcium.

THYROID AND PARATHYROID

The thyroid and parathyroid hormones are important regulators of proliferating cartilage. Parathyroid regulates the growth plate. Parathyroid hormone production increases when serum calcium levels drop, which increases 1,25-dihydroxycholecalciferol formation by the kidneys and leads to increased calcium absorption from the gut and from the bone. The role of PTH in calcium metabolism is discussed further on page 674. Lack of either calcium or active vitamin D over a period of time can alter bone formation and cause loss of bone mass.

Calcitonin is a thyroid hormone that is secreted in response to increased plasma calcium levels. Its immediate effect is to reduce bone reabsorption by decreasing osteoclast activity and increasing osteoblast activity. The effect of calcitonin is discussed further on page 656.

SEX HORMONES

Estrogen has an osteoblast-stimulating action. At puberty, a young girl has a rapid growth spurt before the epiphyseal plates close, which is attributed to estrogen. When growth plates close, girls stop growing; this occurs a few years, on average, before their male counterparts. Throughout the premenopausal period, estrogen promotes bone formation by increasing intestinal absorption of calcium and phosphorus and increasing calcitonin production. In the postmenopausal woman, osteoporosis can be caused by the lack of estrogen (see p. 819).

Testosterone in boys and men increases bone length and thickness and at the same time enhances epiphyseal closure. A decline in testosterone in the elderly man also can lead to osteoporosis.

GROWTH HORMONE

The anterior lobe of the pituitary gland secretes the growth hormone (GH, somatotropin), which stimulates linear increase in long bones by increasing cartilage formation, widening the epiphyseal plates, and increasing the amount of matrix laid down in the ends of the long bones. The role of growth hormone is further discussed on page 650, and abnormalities associated with altered GH secretion are discussed in Chapter 24.

WEIGHT BEARING

Muscles atrophy and bones demineralize when a limb is immobilized. Weightlessness experienced by astronauts has been noted to cause loss of bone calcium and bone weakness.[4] Physical compression stimulates osteoblastic deposition, probably by generating an electrical potential, which increases bone formation. Local skeletal mass increases in bones most used in physical exertions such as playing tennis, weight lifting, and dancing.[8,16]

OTHER FACTORS

Glucocorticoids inhibit bone growth by interfering with glucose utilization and energy production. Glucocorticoids cause an increase in protein breakdown in all tissues of the body. Because bone matrix is a protein product, an increase in steroids, as in Cushing's disease, can decrease matrix formation and weaken the bones, causing osteoporosis. Steroids also have the specific effect of depressing osteoblastic activity.[10] Two-thirds of the volume of bone is made up of osteoid organic material. Because all living tissues contain protein, anything that causes a decrease in protein in the body, such as starvation, retards bone formation and enhances bone loss. Lack of vitamins A and C also decreases the ground substance in bone and leads to decreased bone formation. Persons having long-term heparin therapy develop osteoporosis because heparin speeds up the breakdown of collagen.[22] Insulin increases the ability of the collagen matrix to produce osteoblasts. A summary of factors affecting bone growth is presented in Figure 27-13.

NORMAL STRUCTURE AND FUNCTION OF CARTILAGE

Cartilage is rigid connective tissue classified into three types: (1) hyaline cartilage, (2) elastic cartilage, and (3) fibrocartilage.

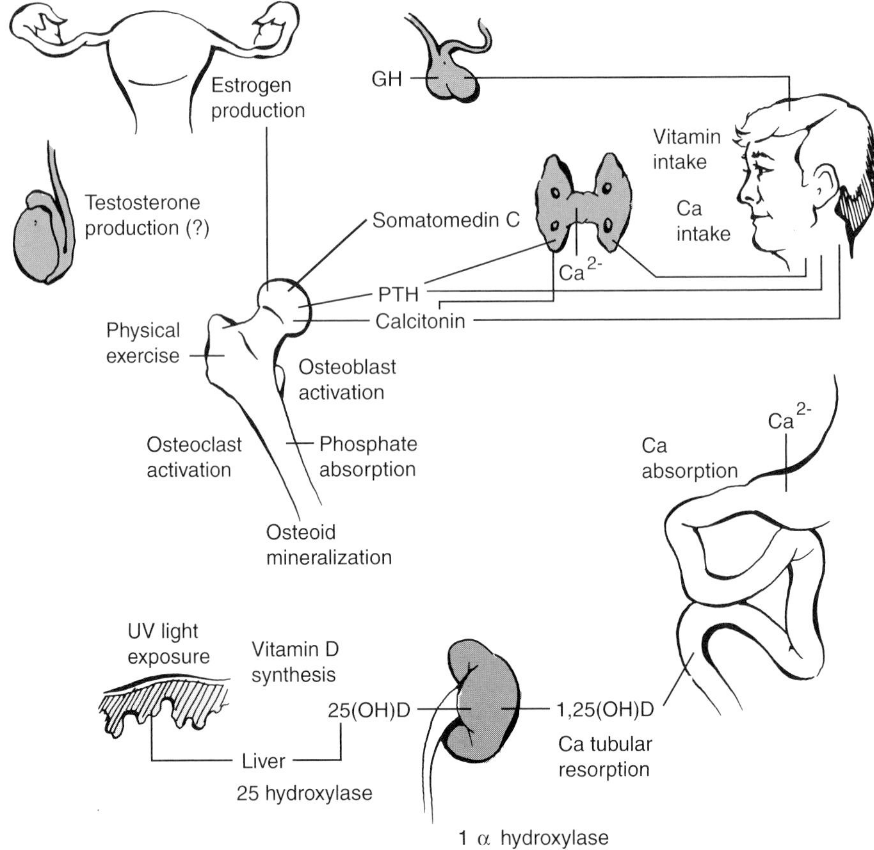

FIGURE 27-13. Factors that impact bone growth. (Dipiro, R., Yee, G., Matzke, G., Wells, B., & Posey, L. [1997]. *Pharmacotherapy: A physiological approach.* Stamford, CT: Appleton & Lange.)

Hyaline cartilage is the most common type of cartilage. It is found in most joints (articular cartilage), the epiphyseal plate, nose, and trachea. *Elastic cartilage* is found in the ear, larynx, and epiglottis. It is more flexible than hyaline cartilage. *Fibrocartilage* is found between vertebral disks, pelvic joints, and at areas of tendon and bone attachment. It is the most rigid form of cartilage. The discussion here focuses on hyaline or articular cartilage.

Articular cartilage is composed of cartilage cells (chondrocytes) and a matrix of collagen, water, and proteoglycans (macromolecules comprising proteins, carbohydrates, and hyaluric acid). Chondrocytes synthesize as well as digest collagen. The collagen fibers are arranged in an organized manner that makes the cartilage more resistant to stress and breakdown. Under normal conditions, a collagen level is maintained by the chondrocytes through balanaced secretion of catabolic enzymes and enzymes that inhibit the degradation. Collagen renewal and remodeling is continuous and is under the influence of cytokines. Water and proteoglycans are critical in reducing friction and providing elasticity in the cartilage. Cartilage lacks blood vessels, lymph drainage, and nerve endings; therefore, it does not generate pain and requires long periods for healing after injury. It receives nourishment into its matrix through diffusion from surrounding capillaries. The function of articular cartilage is to provide for shock absorption, reduce friction, and distribute weight bearing.

NORMAL STRUCTURE AND FUNCTION OF JOINTS

Joints are articulations that allow for movement of various body parts. Almost all of the bones of the body are joined to one another in one way or another. Some permit a range of motion, whereas some allow no movement. Joints are classified in several ways, but the most common grouping is according to the degree of movement they permit, as follows:

- **Synarthroses,** immovable
- **Amphiarthroses,** somewhat movable
- **Diarthroses,** freely movable

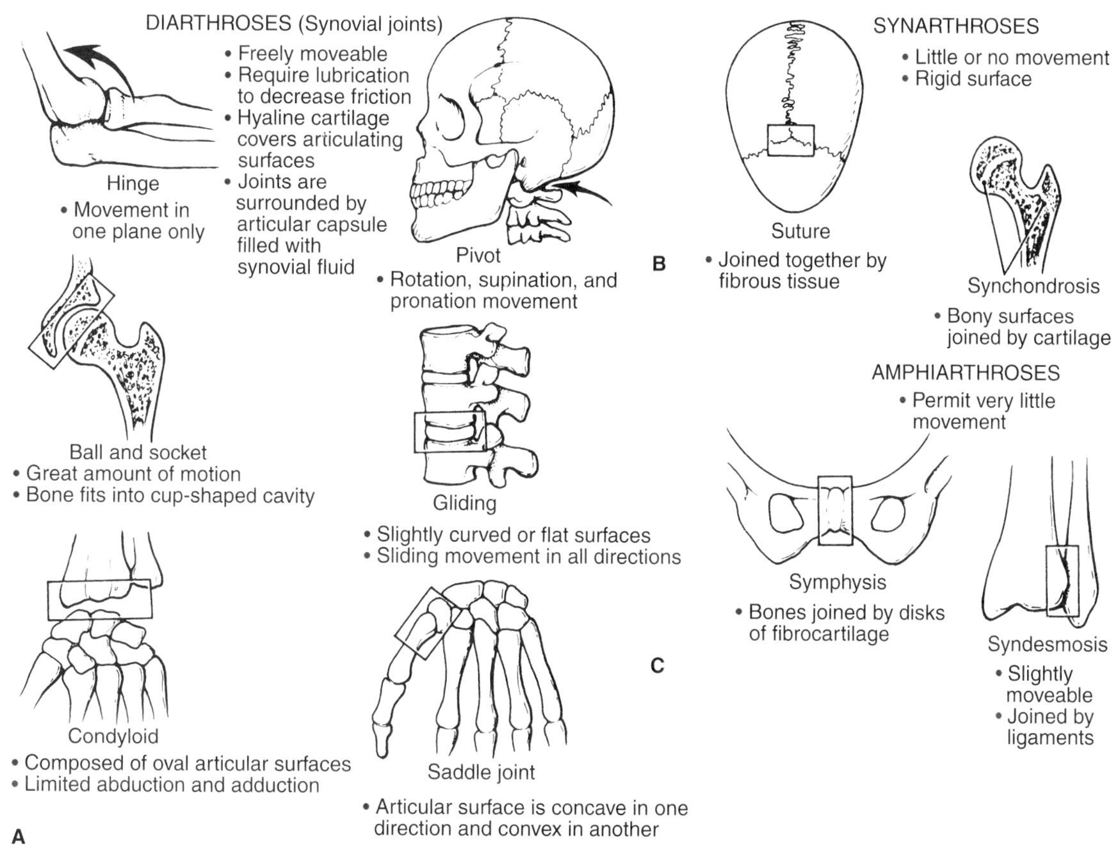

FIGURE 27-14. Types of joints based on degree of movement.

Figure 27-14 illustrates the structure of joints based on their movement. Joints may also be classified according to the material that connects them, such as (1) cartilaginous, (2) fibrous, and (3) synovial.

Cartilaginous Joints

Cartilaginous joints have only slight movement and are encased with hyaline cartilage and supported by ligaments. They unite cartilage with bones. Two types of cartilaginous joints are (1) *synchondrosis* and (2) *symphysis.* Synchondrosis joints, such as in sternochondral joints (uniting ribs and sternum), are covered entirely by hyaline cartilage. Symphysis joints, such as the pubic symphysis, have a fibrocartilage connecting the bones. These joints provide for some shock absorption and slight flexibility in times of physical stress.

Fibrous Joints

Fibrous joints have a rigid surface, are joined by fibrous connective tissue, and provide stability. An example of fibrous joints is the cranial bone connections. Cranial bones are joined together by fibrous tissue and interlocking projections and indentations. Cranial bone joints are an example of a **synarthrosis** joint. These joints are not completed at birth and contain gaps (fontanelles), which provide slight flexibility in the birth process. The gaps normally close by 18 months.

Synovial Joints

The synovial joint is structured to allow movement in one or more directions between two or more major segments of the human skeleton under either weight-bearing or non–weight-bearing conditions. The joint provides a low friction articulation to enable movement of the body with minimal effort.

Joint mobility is provided by movement of the cartilaginous surfaces on one another. Each joint has unique load and positional requirements, which are reflected in the individual design of the joint. The range of motion possible at joints is restrained by opposition of soft tissue, by limitations in the articular surface, and by muscles.

Synovial joints, illustrated in Figure 27-15, are encased in an articular capsule, and the articulating surfaces of the joint are covered by a white, slick, hyaline

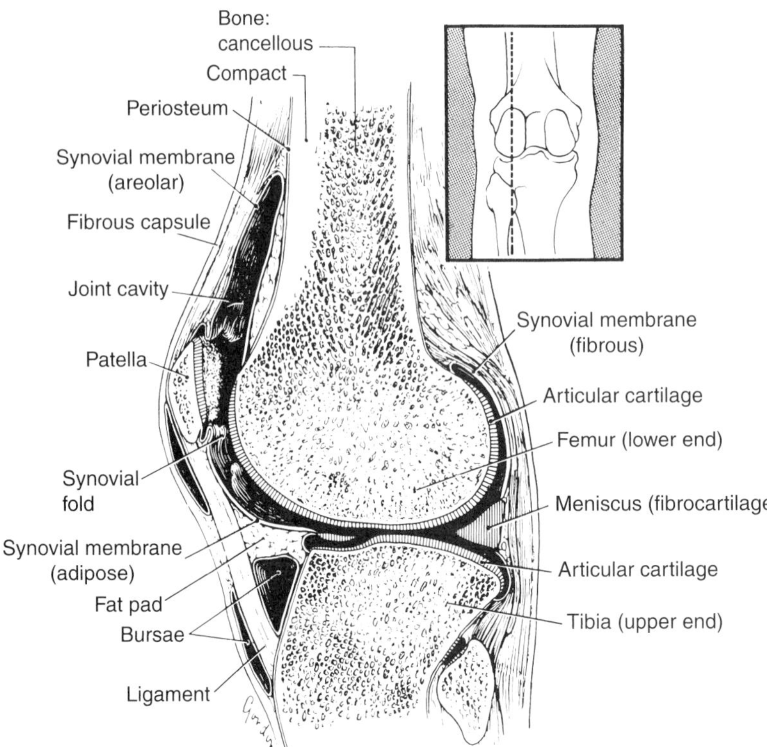

FIGURE 27-15. Diagram of a knee joint cut in the sagittal plane indicated in the inset. (Cormack, D. H. [1993]. *Essential histology*. Philadelphia: J. B. Lippincott.)

cartilage. The joint capsule consists of an outer fibrous layer called the *fibrous capsule* and an inner layer called the *synovial membrane*. The inner layer of the capsule is a slippery, smooth membrane, whereas the outer layer is a tough, fibrous membrane. This inner, or synovial, membrane is rich in capillaries and cells and is composed of secreting and phagocytic cells. The secretory cells produce *synovial fluid*, which contains water, glucose, and protein. Synovial fluid is like interstitial fluid except that it contains large quantities of mucopolysaccharides, which accounts for its viscosity and lubricating qualities.[3] The chief function of this fluid is to lubricate and supply nutrients to the cartilage. The excess protein it contains is returned to the blood by way of the lymphatic system that drains the area. Synovial joints are supplied with sensory nerves that sense pain when there is an accumulation of inflammatory cells in the synovial tissues.

Ligaments may be incorporated into the capsule or separated from it by **bursae,** small, flat cavities filled with synovial fluid. The chief function of bursae is to reduce friction between moving parts.

The synovial joints permit a variety of motion and are classified according to the shape of the articulation and the motion they facilitate. Movements of joints may be classified as (1) *gliding*, producing some bone displacement; (2) *angular*, in which the angle between bones is changed; and (3) *rotating*, or twisting of a body part.

LIGAMENTS AND TENDONS

Ligaments and **tendons** constitute the connective tissue that hold the body together. There are two types of ligaments: (1) those that connect viscera to one another and (2) those that connect one bone to another.[3] Tendons always connect voluntary muscle to another structure. Ligaments are composed of distinct bands of connective tissue: (1) yellow ligaments, which are elastic (vertebral column) and allow for stretching; and (2) white ligaments, such as those in the knee, which do not stretch and provide for stability.

Tendons are actual extensions of muscles, as illustrated in Figure 27-2, that attach muscle to bones or to other tissues. The thick, collagenous tissue has fibers that run in one direction so that it can withstand a great deal of pull. These parallel bundles give tendons a glistening, shiny, white appearance. When part of broad and flat muscles, they have the same general appearance; similarly, when they are part of a long slender muscle, they are cordlike. The long, hard, cordlike tendons running into the hands and feet have been termed *leaders*. Tendons that cross bones or other tendons are lubricated by a slippery solution similar to synovial fluid that contains hyaluronic acid.[3] Tendons receive sensory fibers from muscle nerves, nearby deep nerves, and overlying superficial nerves. Blood supply to tendons is scarce, and it is for this reason that injured tendons heal slowly.

ALTERED FUNCTION ASSOCIATED WITH SKELETAL MUSCLES

Common Alterations in Muscles

Myofibers have a very limited ability to regenerate following injury; therefore, muscular problems are very common. These problems result from overuse, especially following an extended layoff from exercise. A temporary soreness is often described, which may result from small tears in the muscle tissue, muscle spasms, and overstretching of the muscle.[18] The soreness is often delayed in onset (1 to 3 days) and usually goes away with rest and moderate usage. Other muscle alterations or problems include cramps, strain, injury, and others described below.

WEAKNESS

Weakness usually is a subjective phenomenon and relates to loss of strength in one or more muscle groups. It may be subjective in nature but is objective when the muscular power is actually decreased on tests of muscular function. This problem is a component of many disorders and is characteristic in chronic illnesses, especially diabetes mellitus. It may reflect primary muscle disease, or it may reflect the underlying disease. Any condition of decreased cardiac output and chronic infectious disease may lead to generalized weakness. Weakness in one limb may be an indicator of multiple sclerosis.

CRAMPS

Any step in the sequence of events leading to a muscle contraction (motor neuron activity, membrane excitability, contraction coupling) can result in a cramp. Cramps are involuntary spasms of specific muscle groups in which the muscles become taut and painful. They may occur in the calf, thigh, hip, or any other major muscle group. Visible fasciculations may also occur before and after cramps. Cramps are frequent occurrences in the skeletal muscles. They may be idiopathic or associated with motor system disease, metabolic disease (e.g, uremia), tetanus, and electrolyte depletion, especially of sodium, potassium, and calcium. Muscle cramps are often reported at night or during rest and may be due to lowered blood sugar levels at night. Dehydration also may cause cramping, especially if associated with sodium depletion.

STRAIN

Muscle strains are the result of excessive stretch or tension on the muscle, resulting in local muscle damage such as tearing or rupture. Frequently strained muscles are those that are used in the control of regulation of motion promoted by other muscle groups. Strains usually occur during activities that demand speed, acceleration and deceleration, and changes of direction. Often strains also involve the tendon. Repeated excessive stretching of muscles can result in chronic muscle strain. Muscle strains may also result from penetrating injury with knives or guns and result in muscle rupture. Hemorrhage may occur into the muscle, which produces an inflammatory response in the muscle and the tissue around it. Clinical manifestations reveal pain, inflammation, erythema, ecchymosis, and warmth to touch. Muscle cells regenerate, and healing usually occurs without complications.

TWITCHES, FASCICULATIONS, AND FIBRILLATIONS

Various reactions may result from spontaneous discharge of motor units or single muscle fibers. Twitches occurring at rest may be idiopathic or associated with hyperkalemia, motor neuron disease, and peripheral neuropathies.

Fasciculations are involuntary contractions of a single motor unit. They may occur in healthy persons and cause visible dimpling or twitching of the skin. Fasciculations may occur rhythmically, starting and stopping for no apparent reason. Those that occur during contraction of a muscle indicate excessive irritation and can occur years after poliomyelitis or a degenerative nervous system disease. The molecular pathogenesis is not fully understood but is likely related to hypersensitivity of the neuronal membrane to acetylcholine. Continuous fascicluations, called myokymia, of unknown etiology may involve all of the voluntary muscles. Fasciculation is often confused with fibrillation, which results from the contraction of single muscle fibers. Fibrillation is not visible and is noted on electromyography.[30] It occurs when the motor unit of the axon is destroyed. The fibers contract rhythmically, often up to 3 to 10 times per second. As denervation continues, the muscle fibers atrophy and fibrillation stops.[10]

TETANY

Tetany, a spasmodic condition of muscles, most frequently results from hypocalcemia that can be associated with vitamin D deficiency. Other causes include alkalosis or hypoparathyroidism (see Chapter 24). Hyperventilation may also precipitate tetany by lowering the serum carbon dioxide level, which reduces the level of ionized calcium. Tetany is probably due to unstable depolarization of the distal segments of the motor nerves. Neurons become more excitable with decreased serum calcium levels and, therefore, generate action potentials spontaneously, resulting in tetanic muscle contractions. Additional clinical manifestations include muscle twitching, cramping, and sharp flexion of the wrist and ankle (carpopedal spasm or tetany). Seizures and laryngeal stridor may be observed in some cases.

MYOCLONUS AND TICS

Myoclonus is a sudden, unexpected contraction of a single muscle or group of muscles that involves the limbs more than the trunk. This disorder has many causes, from idiopathic benign (sleep) jerks to central nervous system disease.

Tics differ from myoclonus in that they are sudden, behavior-related, repetitive movements that may be a form of learned behavior or occur as a part of Tourette's syndrome. In the latter, tics may be accompanied by involuntary vocalizations.

ATROPHY

Atrophy refers to a decrease in muscle mass due to diminution in size of the myofibrils. Atrophic muscles can result from such diverse factors as aging, immobilization, chronic ischemia, malnutrition, and denervation.[4,16] Currently it is believed that the most prominent mechanism in the loss of muscle fiber bulk with age is anterior horn cell changes causing denervation within the muscle. Muscle atrophy can occur very rapidly, with significant wasting occurring within a few days when the muscle is immobilized in a shortened position. Disuse atrophy denotes wasting of muscle tissue due to lack of muscle stress such as occurs with atrophic changes after a bone fracture and treatment with casting.

More muscle weight is lost in the initial days after injury or disuse than in subsequent days. Bedrest, for example, results in 1.0% to 1.5% loss of muscle mass per day. With loss of weight and mass, there is also a loss of force and endurance, and biochemical changes that result in a decrease in energy supply and an increase in levels of lactic acid.

Denervation causes atrophic muscular changes that become irreversible. Loss of normal neural stimulation and reduction of muscle tone seem to be the major factors in these changes, rather than lack of weight bearing. If a muscle cell is reinnervated within 3 to 4 months, full function can be restored. After this time, some of the muscle fibers become permanently atrophied, and after 2 years muscle function is rarely restored.

Atrophy of muscle tissue may also occur in malnutrition or in wasting diseases such as cancer and cirrhosis of the liver. The muscle does not receive adequate nutrition, and consequently protein wasting occurs.

Widespread muscular atrophy is a consequence of aging and relates to reduction of muscle fiber size and number. Muscle strength decreases, on the average 25% after the age of 60 years, and the amount of work the muscle can perform decreases even more.[9,21]

Disease Processes Associated With Skeletal Muscles

Disease processes associated with skeletal muscles include muscular dystrophies, myasthenia gravis, myopathies, fibromyalgia-fibrositis, polymyalgia rheumatica, and rhabdomyosarcoma. Multiple sclerosis (MS) and amyotrophic lateral sclerosis (ALS or Lou Gehrig's disease) cause muscle weakness and paralysis. However, these diseases originate in the central nervous system and are discussed in Chapter 33.

MUSCULAR DYSTROPHIES

The *muscular dystrophies* are genetically determined, progressive diseases of specific muscle groups. They are characterized by progressive weakness of the voluntary muscles, usually the proximal muscles, in a symmetric pattern.[19,25] The syndromes can be classified mainly by the distribution of involved muscles, pattern of inheritance, age of onset, and speed of progression (Table 27-2).[4] Several members of the same family may be affected, with males predominating and females carrying the genetic abnormality. Muscle fiber atrophy, necrosis, regeneration, and fibrosis are components of variable frequency, depending on the type of muscular dystrophy exhibited.

Rapidly Progressive Muscular Dystrophy

Duchenne muscular dystrophy (DMD) is a rapidly progressive, severe, X-linked muscle disorder that occurs almost exclusively in males. Recent advances in molecular biology have identified the defective gene on the short arm of the X chromosome.[4,19] The affected gene fails to direct the production of dystrophin, a protein normally found adjacent to the sarcolemmal membranes in myocytes and thought to affect muscle fiber contraction.[4] Muscle fibers that do not have dystrophin may lack the normal interaction between the sarcolemma and the extracellular matrix.[25]

Pathologic changes include degeneration of muscle fibers, progressive fibrosis, and an attempt at regeneration by the muscle fibers.[25] As the disease progresses, there is almost complete loss of skeletal muscle fibers, which become replaced by fat and connective tissue.[4,25] Clinical manifestations associated with DMD are characterized by early development of motor difficulties, inability to walk, symmetric weakness of the arms, and enlargement of the muscles of the calves. Intellectual impairment is common. The disease characteristically begins with lower extremity weakness that progresses upward and finally affects the head and chest muscles. The characteristic *pseudohypertrophy* of calf muscles is

TABLE 27-2

MANIFESTATIONS OF SELECTED MUSCULAR DYSTROPHIES

TYPE OF MUSCULAR DYSTROPHY	MUSCLE INVOLVEMENT	ONSET	PROGRESSION	INHERITANCE	OTHER CHARACTERISTICS
Duchenne's (pseudo-hypertrophic)	Generalized with pelvic girdle and shoulders most involved	Usually by age 5	Rapid	X-linked recessive	Pseudohypertrophy, cardiac involvement, mental retardation, death by adulthood
Becker's	Generalized	Age 5 to 15	Slow	X-linked recessive	Cardiac involvement is rare; nearly normal life span possible in some cases
Facio-scapulo-humeral	Face, neck, shoulders	10 to 30 years	Slow	Autosomal dominant	Inflammatory infiltrates may be present in muscle
Limb-girdle	Shoulder and pelvic musculature	10 to 30 years	Usually slow	Varies	Weakness in proximal muscles of the upper and lower extremities

due to infiltration of the fibers with fatty deposits and connective tissue. The muscle becomes significantly weakened. Weakness of the back muscles results in lordosis. Respiratory or cardiac failure often causes death, with death usually occurring before the age of 20.

Slowly Progressive Forms of Muscular Dystrophy

More slowly progressive forms of muscular dystrophy, such as *Becker's*, *limb-girdle*, and *facioscapulo-humeral*, generally have a later onset and may differ somewhat in the pattern of muscle involvement and inheritance. Though Becker's muscular dystrophy is similar to DMD, it has a later onset and is less common and less severe than DMD. Most individuals live well into adulthood. Becker's muscular dystrophy shows identifiable dystrophin, which reflects mutations that allow synthesis of some dystrophin.[6] The limb-girdle and fascioscapulohumeral forms of the disease are inherited in the autosomal recessive and autosomal dominant pattern, respectively. They have an onset at about 10 to 30 years and involve weakness of different muscle groups and variable rates of progression. Other forms of muscular dystrophy have been described but are rare.

Clinical Manifestations

Clinical manifestations in most persons with any form of muscular dystrophy will reveal muscle weakness, elevated levels of creatine phosphokinase (CPK), lactic dehydrogenase (LDH), glutamic transaminase, and glucose phosphate isomerase. These enzymes normally are present in the muscles, and their elevated levels here indicate abnormal muscle plasma membranes.[4] Electromyography (described in the unit Appendix) reveals weak electrical currents present in the muscle cell. Muscle biopsies are abnormal due to the presence of fatty tissue deposits in the cell.

MYASTHENIA GRAVIS

Myasthenia gravis is a disease related to the inability of the neuromuscular junctions to transmit nerve impulses to the muscle cells effectively and is discussed on page 1009. This disease is probably autoimmune in causation and is mostly seen in females, with onset of muscle weakness especially of the ocular, head, and neck muscles.

MYOSITIS

Myositis refers to inflammation of muscle tissue. It may result from various conditions, including trauma and infections. Myositis may also be associated with malignancies or connective tissue diseases such as scleroderma, lupus erythematosus, and Sjögren's syndrome. It also accompanies systemic inflammatory myopathies (discussed below). The clinical manifestations vary with the conditions associated with myositis but generally include muscle tenderness and weakness.

MYOPATHIES

The term **myopathy** refers to primary disorders of the muscle. Myopathies may be of autoimmune origin, inherited, or secondary to other conditions. They are associated with decreased functioning muscle cells, weakness, and decreased muscle bulk and strength.

Inflammatory Myopathies

Polymyositis and dermatomyositis are examples of inflammatory myopathies. These are rare inflammatory myopathies of autoimmune or viral origin.[24,29] The presence of autoantibodies supports the autoimmune bases of these myopathies.[25] The triggering mechanism for the immune-mediated muscle inflammation may be viral in origin. The onset is usually evident in adulthood, with proximal limb and neck weakness associated with muscle pain. Muscle necrosis is patchy, and inflammation becomes chronic. In dermatomyositis, cutaneous manifestations of papules, erythematous patches over the joints, and erythema of the face and neck are associated with the muscle weakness and joint pain.[29] The progression of weakness in both polymyositis and dermatomyositis often affects the heart and pulmonary systems. Other clinical manifestations include elevation of the transaminases and myoglobinuria in those who have lost considerable muscle mass.[24,29]

Inherited Myopathies

Inherited myopathies include metabolic myopathies, mitochondrial myopathies, and congenital myopathies. These diverse myopathies affect muscle tone and produce muscle weakness, often in infants. Examples of *inherited metabolic myopathies* include glycogen storage disease and lipid metabolism abnormalities.[12] In the inherited *McArdle's syndrome*, an abnormality in the glycolytic pathways for the production of energy results from deficiencies of the muscle enzyme, phosphorylase. Lipid metabolism abnormality myopathies result from carnitine or carnitine palmitoyltransferase deficiency, leading to accumulation of lipid droplets in the muscle.

The *mitochondrial myopathies* exhibit varying pathologies of the mitochondria, including point mutations, deletions, and duplications, and a wide range of effects such as muscle weakness and varying dysfunctions of the eyes, heart, kidney, brain, and other organs. An example of mitochondrial deletion myopathy is *Kerns-Sayer syndrome*. In this condition the individual most often presents with visual defects, cerebellar ataxia, and cardiac manifestations.

Examples of *congenital myopathies* include central core disease, nemaline myopathy, and central nuclear myopathy. The pathologic basis of congenital myopathies is various abnormalities within the muscle cells. The congenital myopathies have varying inheritance patterns and often present in the form of a "floppy infant" with reduced reflexes and decreased muscle bulk as well as other associated developmental diseases.[4]

Acquired Myopathies

Acquired myopathies may have metabolic or toxic etiology. They are associated with decreased functioning muscle cells, weakness, and decreased muscle bulk and strength.

Acquired metabolic myopathies are often secondary to disorders of the endocrine system, such as thyrotoxic myopathy or hyperparathyroidism. Many endocrine dysfunctions can cause weakness and fatigue, although they usually respond to appropriate endocrine management.[19] Nutritional and vitamin deficiency may lead to myopathy, especially protein deficiency and lack of vitamins D and E.

Toxic myopathies are related to certain drugs and chemicals. Focal, localized myopathies are related to the injection of narcotic analgesics, especially pentazocine and meperidine.[19] Penicillamine, cimetidine, procainamide, and other drugs have been shown to produce weakness, myositis, and even muscle fiber necrosis. In most cases the mechanism of toxicity to the muscles is poorly understood.[19] Corticosteroid therapy causes steroid-induced muscle weakness due to type II muscle fiber atrophy. Differentiating it from the initial condition being treated with corticosteroids can be difficult.

Excessive alcohol usage can produce a severe *rhabdomyolysis* (breakdown of striated muscle), which can affect the skeletal and heart muscle.[4] Scattered areas of muscle necrosis surrounded by macrophages are typical pathologic findings associated with rhabdomyolysis. Renal failure may result when there is significant elevation of the myoglobin in the urine.

FIBROMYALGIA-FIBROSITIS

Fibromyalgia-fibrositis syndrome is a common condition of diffuse musculoskeletal pain without evidence of arthritis. The etiology is largely unknown but is theorized to be associated with affective disorders, sleep disturbances, or endocrine imbalances. It occurs predominantly in women of childbearing age with the following clinical manifestations: (1) musculoskeletal pain, (2) stiffness, (3) anxiety and depression, and (4) easy fatigability. The muscle stiffness tends to improve with movement. Muscle biopsies are inconclusive, but decreased ATP and creatine phosphate in areas of described tenderness have been noted. The most commonly related feature is a disturbance of stage 4 (non-REM) sleep.

POLYMYALGIA RHEUMATICA

Polymyalgia rheumatica may be mistaken for a polymyositis or dermatomyositis and is a disease of the older adult. It is associated with inflammation of large arteries and is a condition of unknown etiology.

Clinical manifestations reveal painful morning stiffness, predominantly affecting the upper proximal limbs. Pain increases with movement, and stiffness increases with rest. Muscle weakness is most commonly due to pain and disuse.[27] Other manifestations may include weight loss, depression, and localized temporal artery tenderness (temporal arteritis).

RHABDOMYOSARCOMA

Rhabdomyosarcoma is an uncommon malignant tumor of striated muscle. It occurs most commonly in children and adolescents and may affect the striated muscles of the extremities, head, or neck. This type of sarcoma is very invasive, with extremely anaplastic cells.[4] Five-year survival is 30% to 40%. It is diagnosed by the presence of a characteristic rhabdomyoblast cell. Clinical manifestations vary in accordance with the involved body region.

ALTERED FUNCTION ASSOCIATED WITH BONES

Fractures

Fractures are most commonly defined as breaks in continuity of bone. They may have associated extensive soft tissue damage with hemorrhage into muscles and joints, dislocation and rupture of tendons, nerve damage, and disruption of blood supply. In general, soft tissue damage is greatest when a direct force is applied over the area, but is usually decreased when the force that breaks the bone is applied distal to the fracture.

ETIOLOGY

Fractures are ruptures of living tissue and normally are the result of trauma or, less commonly, stress and fatigue (stress fracture) or an underlying disease (pathologic fracture). Table 27-3 lists the types of fractures and the associated pathology. These relate primarily to the long bones but may also occur in other types of bones.

Fractures occur when a force (energy) is imposed on a bone that is greater than it can absorb. Fractures can be described by the type of break line and are illustrated in Figure 27-16.

TABLE 27-3
TYPES OF FRACTURES AND ASSOCIATED PATHOLOGY

TYPE OF FRACTURE	ASSOCIATED PATHOLOGY
Simple (closed)	Fracture contained within intact skin
Compound (open)	Fracture associated with break in overlying skin
Complete	Complete disruption of continuity of the bone
Incomplete	Portion of the bone remains intact
Comminuted	Fracture associated with three or more fragments
Impaction	One fragment of bone is embedded in another
Depressed	Inward-driven fracture such as those associated with skull fractures
Pathologic	Associated with disease that impairs bone remodeling: infection, osteoporosis, metabolic disorders, or cancer
Avulsion	Bone fragment torn off main part of bone by severe twisting or pulling by a tendon or ligament
Compression	Crushed bone such as those commonly seen in spinal cord fractures
Stress	Minute fracture associated with fatigue; a reaction of the bone to accumulated repetitive submaximal stresses

PATHOPHYSIOLOGY AND HEALING OF FRACTURES

Immediately after a fracture the inflammatory response is initiated, and there is pain, swelling, erythema, and warmth. This persists for 24 to 72 hours. As inflammation abates, the repair process can begin. Initially following the fracture, blood vessels and periosteum rupture and blood seeps into the fracture site. This is called the *fracture hematoma*, which develops within 48 to 72 hours after injury. This hematoma surrounding the fracture site provides a loose fibrin mesh from which fibroblasts and capillary buds form a granulation tissue that replaces the blood clot. Bone necrosis occurs at the ends of the site of the fracture.[5] Osteoblasts and chondroblasts become active in forming new bone and cartilage, which within a week are dispersed throughout the soft tissue callus. This temporary bony union is called a *provisional* or *primary union* or *procallus*.[5] The procallus creates a balloon or collar over the fracture site and extends well past it. As healing continues, a bridging external callus is formed. New bone spicules proliferate as mineral salts are laid down. The late medullary callus appears to be responsible for the slow growth of new bone across a fracture gap. As the gap in fractured bone is bridged and fracture fragments become united, mature bone begins to replace the callus.[8] The excess callus already laid down is reabsorbed by the osteoclasts. The fracture site becomes firm in about 3 to 4 months, and radiographs show united bone. The pathology and healing sequence of events associated with a fracture are illustrated in Figure 27-17. If aligned correctly, simple fractures resume an almost normal appearance within 1 year. Various factors within the host influence healing of fractures; these are listed in Box 27-1.

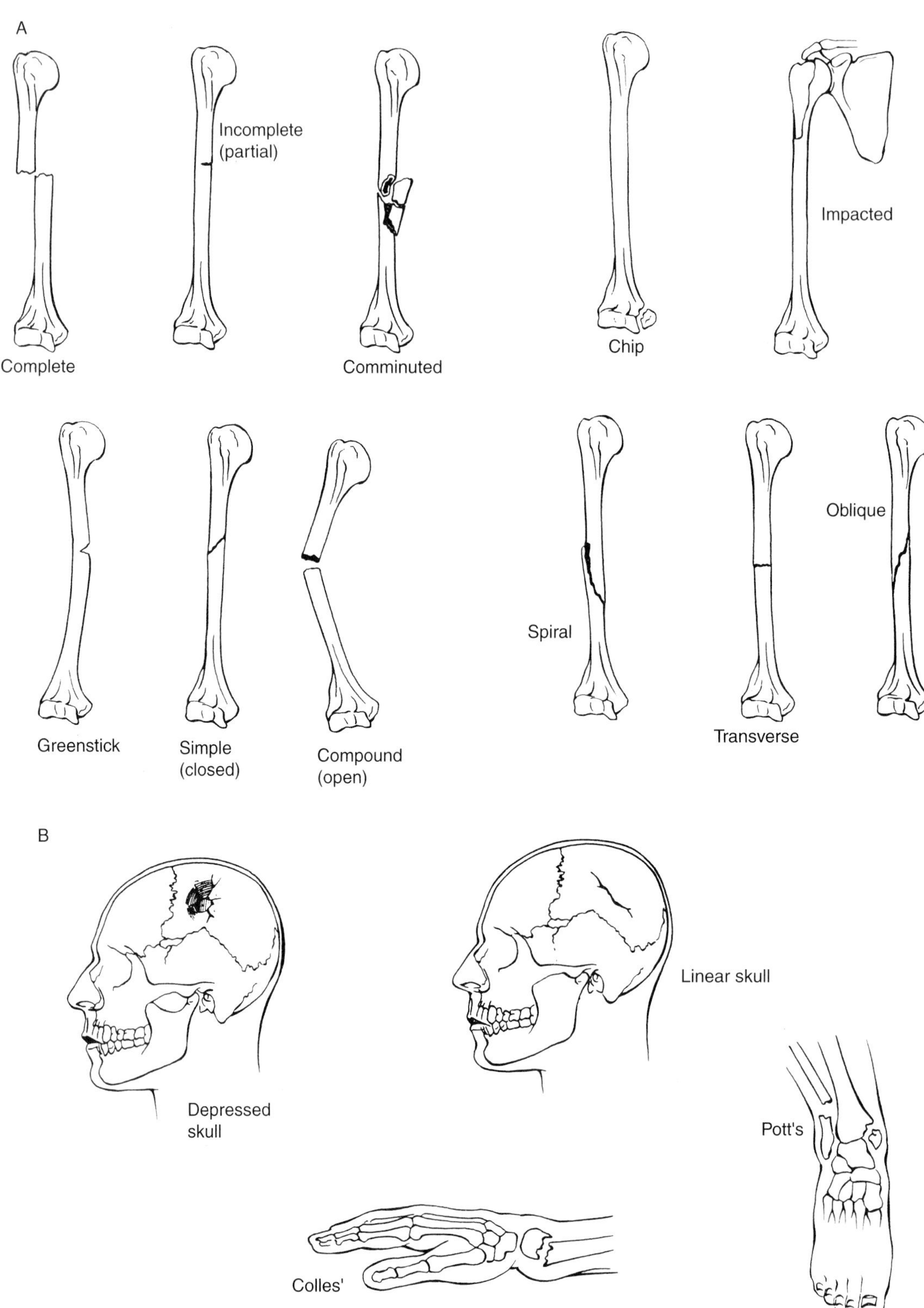

FIGURE 27-16. **A.** Fractures associated with long bones. **B.** Fractures near joints and in skull.

FOCUS ON CELLULAR PHYSIOLOGY

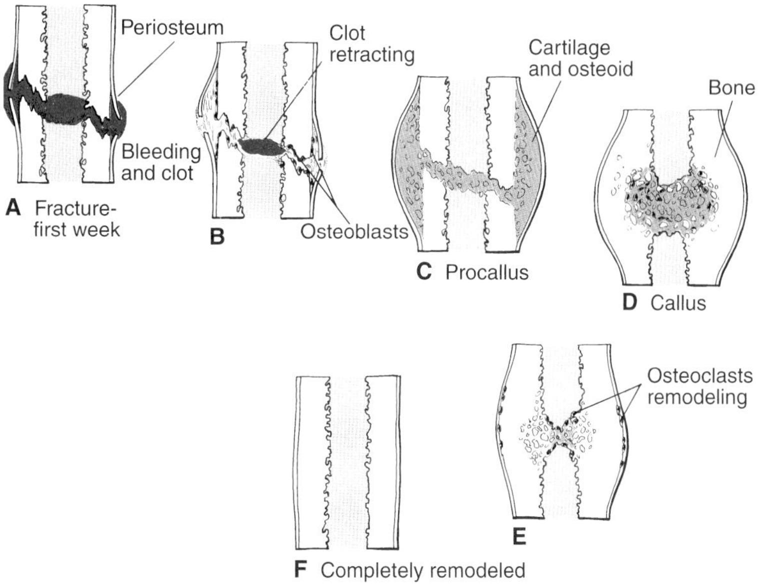

FIGURE 27-17. Healing of a fracture. **A.** Immediately after fracture, blood seeps into the area and a hematoma forms. **B.** After 1 week, osteoblasts begin to form as clot retracts. **C.** After about 3 weeks, a procallus begins to form and stabilize the fracture. **D.** From 6 to 12 weeks, a callus forms with bone cells. **E.** In 3 to 4 months, osteoclasts begin to remodel the fracture site. **F.** With normal apposition, the bone will be completely remodeled in 12 months.

CLINICAL MANIFESTATIONS OF FRACTURES

Common findings associated with fractures include: (1) local swelling, (2) loss of function or abnormal movement of the affected part, and (3) deformities such as angulation, shortening, or rotation of the part. *Crepitation*, a grating sound, may be produced by bone fragments rubbing together. Pain or local tenderness is normally present. It is not uncommon, however, for local shock to cause complete anesthesia and flaccidity of the area for a period of a few minutes to a half-hour after a fracture. This is due to a temporary loss of nerve function at the site of the fracture. Associated vascular injury causes swelling, pallor, pain or numbness, and pulselessness. When the sharp, burning pain becomes a deep, throbbing sensation, tissue anoxia is suspected.

BOX 27-1 FACTORS THAT IMPACT BONE HEALING

- Infection
- Co-morbid medical conditions: diabetes, cancer, COPD, heart disease
- Ischemia
- Estrogen/androgen deficiency
- Vitamin deficiency
- Starvation
- Steroid use
- Bone positioning: movement of bone fragments or distraction (poor bone end contact)
- Interposition of soft tissue over one or both bone fragments
- Heparin
- Excess parathyroid level

COMPLICATIONS ASSOCIATED WITH BONE FRACTURES

Infection

Compound fractures open internal structures to various microorganisms; therefore, infection becomes the major complication of bone healing. The open area is a rich culture medium for infection and osteomyelitis in the tissues. Osteomyelitis retards healing by destroying newly forming bone and interrupting its blood supply (see below).

Alterations in Bone Union

Alterations in bone union may be a *delayed union*, a *nonunion*, or a *malunion*. Delayed union is a term used to denote an increased healing time. Although each person heals at a different pace, the average time needed to completely heal a fracture is generally consistent. A delayed union normally results from a breakdown in the early stages of healing, which occurs from inadequate immobilization, breakdown in hematoma formation, or poor alignment. Infection at the fracture site delays union, usually until the infectious process is stopped.

Nonunion occurs when the fragments fail to unite over a 5-month period. This is due to a variety of factors, including age, health, degree of trauma, underlying disease, and especially infection and movement. Infection causes continuous bleeding and breakdown of osteoid matrix. Movement at the fracture site causes repeated bleeding episodes and decalcification at the fragment ends. It may cause the fracture gap to increase to such an extent that the ends no longer touch, leading to a permanent nonunion.

Malunion is union of the fragments in an abnormal position that may modify function.

Fat Embolism Syndrome

Fat embolism syndrome is a rare complication of fracture of the long bone or pelvis, generally following severe trauma or bone surgery. Fat globules are released into circulation from the stores in the fractured bones. The fat globules attract platelets, which become part of the microembolus and deplete the circulating platelets. The pathophysiology of fat embolism syndrome results from fat microemboli lodging in and occluding small vessels in various organs, most commonly in the lungs and brain. Injury to the vasculature results from the fatty acids released by the fat globules.

The clinical picture, although not clearly understood, involves the onset of adult respiratory distress syndrome (ARDS) 24 to 72 hours after the traumatic event. Activation of coagulation and the resultant disseminated intravascular coagulation (DIC) often complicates the picture. It is not known if DIC is directly related to the fat embolism. Cerebral edema is associated with microembolic fat in the brain circulation.[4] The patient experiences chest pain and sudden respiratory difficulty. A low-grade fever, mental confusion, thrombocytopenia, petechiae, and fat globules in the urine may be associated with fat embolism syndrome.

Nerve Damage

Some fracture may cause injuries to adjacent nerves. Bone fragments may rupture and compress nerves that may also be damaged by dislocation or direct trauma. The axillary nerve may be damaged by fractures or dislocations around the shoulder or by penetrating wounds and direct blows. The axillary nerve emerges at the level of the humerus head and winds around the neck of the humerus. It supplies the deltoid and teres minor muscles. The deltoid muscle is used as an abductor for the shoulder; therefore, inability to abduct the shoulder indicates damage to the axillary nerve.

The radial nerve is commonly injured in spiral fractures of the humerus. It may be completely severed, impaled on a fractured fragment, or entrapped between the fragments. It is primarily a motor nerve that innervates the biceps, supinates the forearm, and extends the wrist, fingers, and thumb; therefore, injury usually results in inability to extend the elbow or supinate the forearm. A typical wrist drop occurs that includes inability to extend the fingers. Complete return of function can be expected in most persons with temporary nerve damage.

Compartment Syndromes

The compartments of the leg and forearm are composed of bones, muscles, nerves, and other associated structures encapsulated by the fascia and the skin, thus making a closed space (Fig. 27-18). When injury occurs, the pressure builds within the compartment due to bleeding and soft tissue reaction. When the swelling reaches a point at which the fascia permits no further outward enlargement, the increasing pressure is directed inward and compresses blood vessels and other components of the compartment. When tissue pressure increases to equal the diastolic pressure, the microcirculation ceases, although the peripheral pulse is unchanged. Within 30 minutes, damage to nerves begins;

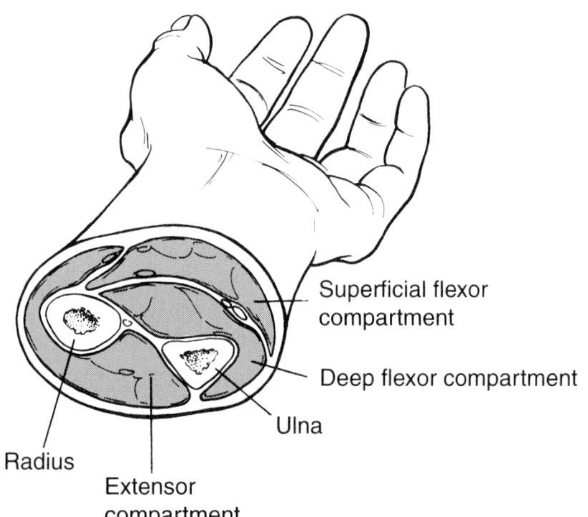

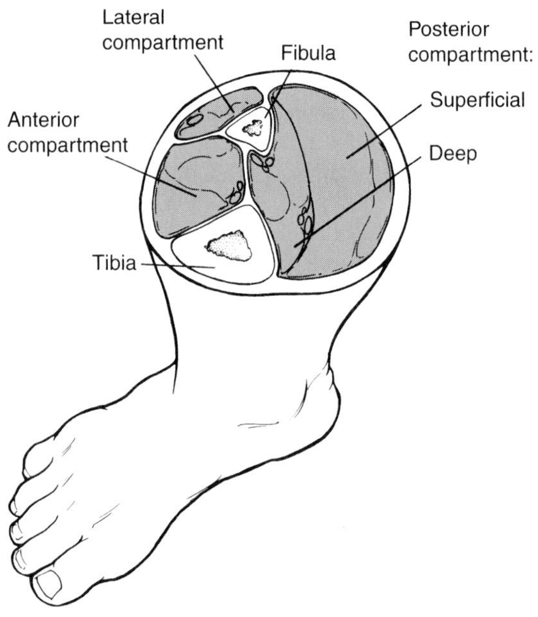

FIGURE 27-18. Compartments of the lower leg and forearm.

if swelling is allowed to persist for 12 hours, irreversible functional loss occurs. Muscles require an abundant blood supply, and when the microcirculation is severely compromised they become ischemic, with necrosis occurring in 2 to 4 hours and becoming irreversible in 12 hours.

Compartmental syndromes are uncommon complications of fractures and affect primarily the forearm and tibia. They are generally referred to as *Volkmann's ischemia* or *anterior tibial compartmental syndromes.* Volkmann's ischemia (volar compartmental syndrome) usually is related to the common supracondylar fracture of the humerus in children. Fracture of the tibia is common in anterior compartmental syndrome. Compartmental syndromes may also result from a cast that is placed too tight.

Anterior compartmental syndrome is heralded by pain in the anterior aspect of the tibia, paresthesia over the distribution of the deep peroneal nerve, and pain on passive dorsiflexion of the toes. The area appears swollen and blisters may develop on the skin. If the syndrome is allowed to proceed unchecked, paralysis, anesthesia, contractures, foot drop, and gangrene may develop, which in turn may lead to loss of the limb.

Volkmann's ischemia produces a disturbing contracture if untreated. Pain is the predominant symptom; it is referred to the palmar area and is exacerbated on passive extension of fingers. Some degree of sensory loss in the fingers occurs in the early stages. Contractures (clawlike deformities of the hand), wrist drop, and paralysis then result.

Idiopathic Alterations in Bone

PAGET'S DISEASE

First described in 1877 by Sir James Paget, this disease of chronic bone inflammation causes softening and bowing of long bones. The disease is rare in persons under 40 years of age, and men and women are equally affected. The frequency of the disease has ranged statistically from 3% to 4% of the population over the age of 50.[6]

Etiology

The possible causes are many, but no exact etiology has been defined. Paget himself thought it was due to a chronic infection, and he called the disease osteitis deformans. Viral causation has been investigated, and antigens identical to the respiratory syncytial virus (RSV) and the measles virus have been identified.[4,6] The disease occurs late in life, which allows for a long period of latency. Other etiologic possibilities include hormonal dysfunction, autoimmune states, vascular disorders, and neoplastic disease.

Pathophysiology

The pathologic feature of Paget's disease is an increase in osteoclastic bone reabsorption with a compensatory increase in bone formation, a phenomenon that can occur in different stages in the same person and even in the same bone. The histologic features are usually described in phases:

OSTEOLYTIC OR DESTRUCTIVE PHASE. This initial phase is marked by extensive reabsorption of existing bone, with the presence of numerous multinucleated osteoclasts.[5,6]

MIXED OR ACTIVE PHASE. This next phase occurs when the osteoclasts destroy the ordered lamellar bone, and osteoblasts respond to the destruction by rapid disposition of vascular connective tissue and remodeled lamellar bone. During this phase, the area appears to be highly vascular, with cement lines forming at sites where the lamellae are erratically joined, giving a mosaic appearance that may completely replace the preexisting bone.[4]

OSTEOBLASTIC OR SCLEROTIC PHASE. This last phase occurs when bone formation outstrips reabsorption, with lamellar bone as the predominant ingredient. Bone size and thickness are increased primarily in the head, femurs, humeri, and scapulae. This bone is soft, poorly mineralized, and subject to fractures. In individuals with widespread disease, almost every bone may be affected.[11]

Clinical Manifestations

The clinical manifestations progress slowly, and bone deformities can be considered part of the normal aging process. The condition is usually polyostotic (affecting more than one bone). The long bones of the legs become bowed and the pelvis misshapen. The thorax shortens, causing a loss of height. The bones of the skull are often affected, leading to symptoms of vertigo, headache, progressive deafness due to compression of the eighth nerve, and spinal stenosis. In the early stages of disease, pain in the affected bones may be experienced. Increased vascularity of the rebuilding bone, together with cutaneous vasodilatation, can produce warmth over affected bone, requiring an increase in cardiac output. Alkaline phosphatase elevations generally correlate with the extent of the process.[11] Radiolucency with areas of density (lytic areas and areas of increased calcification) are evident on bone roentgenographs.

VON RECKLINGHAUSEN'S DISEASE

Osteitis fibrosa cystica, or von Recklinghausen's disease of the bone, is characterized by progressive resorption and destruction of bone brought about by long-standing *hyperparathyroidism*. Parathyroid hormone excretion causes calcium and phosphorus to be removed from bone. Hyperplasia or neoplasia of the parathyroid glands may cause a hypersecretion of this hormone and thus demineralization of bone. Secondary hyperparathyroidism, as in chronic renal insufficiency, leads to decreased conversion of vitamin D to its active form in the kidneys and decreased absorption of calcium in the intestine. The low serum calcium level stimulates PTH secretion (see p. 172).

In the early stages of both primary and secondary hyperparathyroidism, changes in bone resemble osteomalacia or osteoporosis. With advanced disease, there is osteoclastic resorption of bone, which is replaced by fibrous tissue in the marrow spaces. The cancellous and cortical bones undergo thinning, with resultant deformities. In focal areas of bone resorption, large, fibrous scars develop, yielding minute to very large cysts, called brown tumors. These nonmalignant granulomas receive their brownish color from degeneration and hemorrhage into the site. Because of earlier diagnosis and treatment, only 10% to 15% of persons with primary hyperparathyroidism have significant skeletal changes.[4] Secondary hyperparathyroidism due to renal failure (discussed in Chapter 22) causes only a part of the syndrome of *renal osteodystrophy*, which also includes osteomalacia and osteosclerosis.

OSTEONECROSIS

Osteonecrosis (generalized death of bone tissue) is synonymous with *avascular necrosis*, *aseptic necrosis*, and *ischemic necrosis* of bone.[1,5] It has been identified as one of the most common causes of hip pain and incapacity. Box 27-2 lists the traumatic and nontraumatic causes of osteonecrosis.

Osteonecrosis in the Adult

Necrosis of femoral and humeral heads is secondary to various systemic diseases that affect blood supply to the bone. Pathologically, the lesions occur primarily in subcortical areas of long bones that have a narrower capillary circulation than other bones. The initial cause appears to be ischemia, which can be produced by obstruction or compression of the microcirculation.[4] A history of alcoholism has been reported in 10% to 39% of cases. Traumatic osteonecrosis usually occurs with impaired blood supply to femoral or humeral heads. Nontraumatic osteonecrosis occurs most frequently in persons treated with glucocorticoids, especially those with systemic lupus erythematosus and renal transplants.[1] The most common symptom is pain on active motion. Pain at rest and at night is also very common. Limitation of motion also occurs as the disease progresses. Radiographic abnormalities may develop from several months to 5 years after pain is described.[1]

BOX 27-2 FACTORS ASSOCIATED WITH OSTEONECROSIS

Traumatic

Subcapital hip fracture
Fracture or dislocation of the hip

Nontraumatic

Idiopathic
Systemic steriod treatment
Gaucher's disease
Hemoglobinopathies
Irradiation
Dysbaric osteonecrosis
Alcoholism
Hematologic neoplasms
Hyperlipoproteinemia
Pregnancy
Organ transplantation
Systemic lupus erythematosus
Chronic kidney failure
Gout
Pancreatitis
Venous occlusion
AIDS

Legg-Calvé-Perthes Disease

Legg-Calvé-Perthes disease is an example of osteonecrosis in the femoral head in children. The pathology is brought about by avascular necrosis in the area that causes the bone of the epiphysis to soften and die (Fig. 27-19). The onset of the condition appears to be growth related. Until ages 3 and 4 the predominant blood supply to the femoral head comes across the growth plate from the metaphysis of the femur, with other supply from the lateral epiphyseal vessels. At about 4 years of age, the growth plate begins to block the metaphyseal blood supply, and full development of the ligament artery supply to the femoral head is reached when a child is 7 or 8 years old. This leaves a period of time when the blood supply to the femoral head is dependent on the lateral epiphyseal vessels.

Precipitating causes of avascular necrosis may be trauma, infections, or inflammation. In the 2- to 4-year course of the disease, three stages occur: (1) necrosis, (2) removal of dead bone, and (3) reossification. These stages may occur simultaneously within the same bone. Children may complain of aching pain and limited motion early in the disease, but later processes remain painless.

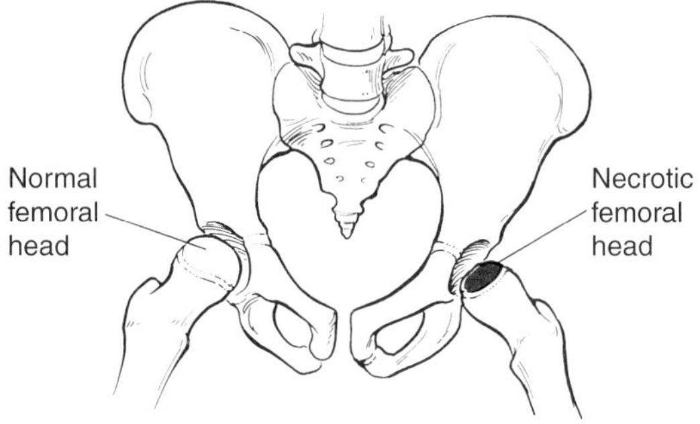

FIGURE 27-19. Legg-Calvé-Perthes disease. Flattened femoral head is the result of necrosis. Left femoral head is normal.

OSGOOD-SCHLATTER DISEASE

Osgood-Schlatter disease is considered a traction *apophysitis* (inflammation of a bone outgrowth) that results from an abnormal position of the patella.[31] This condition causes a deficiency in the vascularization of the tibial tuberosity. The quadriceps muscle in the affected leg has to make a stronger contraction to achieve the same function as the muscle in the nonaffected leg. This increase in the pulling force is likely an etiologic factor in this traction apophysitis. Also, in Osgood-Schlatter disease the patella is positioned too low, part of the tibial tuberosity loosens, and an avulsion fracture can occur. This disorder is seen mostly in boys between the ages of 10 to 15 and causes pain and swelling during sports or after trauma.[31]

Bone Alterations Associated With Metabolic and Nutritional Causes

OSTEOPOROSIS

Osteoporosis is defined as a universal gradual decrease in bone mass (*osteopenia*) in a patient whereby the skeleton is compromised and fractures occur easily. Over time, bone resorption is greater than bone formation. Bone loss occurs both in the matrix and the minerals. The World Health Organization (WHO) defines low bone mass as bone density that is 1 to 2.5 standard deviations less than the normal premenopausal value.[32] Osteoporosis is identified by bone densities more than 2.5 standard deviations less than the normal premenopausal value. Severe osteoporosis is identified as bone densities more than 2.5 standard deviations less than the normal premenopausal value plus a history of fractures.[32]

Osteoporosis is a heterogeneous disease process involving a number of etiologic and pathogenic factors (Box 27-3).[22] Three categories of osteoporosis have been established: *Type I—postmenopausal*; *Type II—senile*; and *Type III—secondary* (Table 27-4).

Type I, or postmenopausal osteoporosis, affects primarily trabecular bone in women within the first 15 to 20 years following menopause. Estrogen deficiency is associated with an increase in bone reabsorption without an increase in bone formation. The precise mechanism of estrogen effect is unclear. However, there are estrogen receptors on osteoblasts that may be stimulated directly by the presence of estrogen. Estrogen also inhibits interleuken 6 (IL-6) stimulation of osteoclastic activity, thus reducing bone resorption.[9]

Type II, or senile osteoporosis, affects men and women over the age of 70 years. Cortical and trabecular bone density values show a proportionate loss. Maximal bone mineral content of cortical bone occurs in men and women in the second to fourth decade of life, followed by a slow decline. Women have less bone mass at skeletal maturity, requiring less bone to be lost before the threshold for fractures is reached. Women lose cortical bone at a rate of 3% per decade until menopause; the rate then accelerates to about 9% per decade until it returns to normal 10 to 20 years after menopause. Men lose bone at the rate of 3% to 4% per decade throughout life.

Type III osteoporosis is secondary to other diseases or medications and can occur in either sex at any age. Specifically, heparin, excessive thyroid replacement, glucocorticoids, anticonvulsants, and cyclosporine have been associated with low bone density and fractures. The usual presentation of osteoporosis is one of shortened stature, kyphosis (see below), lordosis (see below), or fractures. Fractures commonly involve the

BOX 27-3 FACTORS ASSOCIATED WITH OSTEOPOROSIS

Genetic
White/Asian
Known family history
Small frame

Lifestyle
Nicotine use
Inactivity
Nulliparity
Early natural menopause
Late menarche

Nutritional Factors
Low calcium intake
Excessive alcohol use
High animal protein intake

Health Problems
Thyrotoxicosis
Cushing's syndrome
Insulin-dependent diabetes
Altered gastrointestinal absorption
Rheumatoid arthritis
Hemolytic anemia
Anorexia nervosa
Impaired hepatobiliary function

Drugs
Thyroid replacement
Glucocorticoid drugs
Anticoagulants (heparin)
Chronic lithium therapy
Chemotherapy
Anticonvulsant treatment
Extended tetracycline use
Diuretics producing calciuria
Phenothiazine derivatives
Cyclosporin
Aluminum-containing antacids

TABLE 27-4

CLASSIFICATION OF OSTEOPOROTIC TYPES

	TYPE I POST-MENOPAUSE	TYPE II SENILE	TYPE III SECONDARY
Age	55–70	75–90	Any age
Years past menopause	5–15	25–40	Any age
Sex ration F:M	20:1	2:1	1:1
Fracture site	Spine	Spine, hip, pelvis, humerus	Spine, hip
Bone loss			
Trabecular	++++	++	+++
Cortical	+	++	+++
Contributing factors			
Menopause	+++	++	++
Age	+	+++	++
Biochemistry			
PTH	Decrease	Increase	Increase/decrease
$1,25(OH)_2D_3$	Decrease	Decrease	Increase/decrease
Calcium	Decrease	Decrease	Decrease
Response to PTH	Increase	Unchanged	Unknown

distal forearm (Colles' fracture), head of the femur, and vertebrae.

OSTEOMALACIA/RICKETS

Osteomalacia is a condition of abnormal mineralization of bone, commonly caused by lack of vitamin D. In the United States, the incidence of osteomalacia is low as vitamin D is supplemented in foods and absorbed via sunlight. In the infant or growing child, osteomalacia is called *rickets*. It affects the child's growth due to defective calcification of the epiphyseal cartilage.

Etiology and Pathophysiology

The etiology of osteomalacia and rickets is summarized in Box 27-4. Mineral deficiency can result from either a decrease in calcium absorption or an increase in phosphorus loss through the kidneys. In chronic renal failure, the kidneys are unable to activate vitamin D and excrete phosphate. Hyperparathyroidism that may accompany chronic renal failure increases bone reabsorption of calcium. In elderly individuals, low dietary intake of calcium and vitamin D, decreased sun exposure, and altered kidney and liver function, combined with intestinal malabsorption, can decrease bone mineralization and lead to osteomalacia.

Clinical Manifestations

Clinical manifestations result from the lack of mineralization, which makes the bones soft and bow and break easily. Because bone formation in the growing child is most accelerated at the ends of the long bones, the epiphyseal tissue in rickets is soft,

BOX 27-4

ETIOLOGY OF OSTEOMALACIA AND RICKETS

Abnormalities in Vitamin D

Nutritional deficiency
Lack of sunlight exposure
Absorption abnormalities
Chronic renal failure
Aging
Biliary cirrhosis
Hypoparathyroidism
Pseudohypoparathyroidism
Anticonvulsant drugs
Nephrotic syndrome

Phosphate Deficiency

Nutritional deficiency
Neonatal rickets
Excess aluminum hydroxide ingestion
Impaired reabsorption
Primary and secondary hypoparathyroidism

Defects in Mineralization

Enzyme deficiency
Chronic renal failure
Fluoride
Aluminum or iron intoxication

with the normally sharp, narrow line of ossification replaced by a wide, irregular zone of soft, gray tissue. Bowed legs (genu varum) and deformities of the costochondral junction (rachitic rosary) and thorax (pigeon breast), together with defective tooth enamel, are evidence of rickets. In the adult, osteomalacia is displayed by mineral changes and pain in the lumbar vertebrae, pelvic girdle, and long bones of the lower limbs.[25] Fractures occur with only minor trauma. Over time, the mineralization defect leads to decreased bone matrix and a hybrid state of osteomalacia-osteoporosis evolves.[4] Deformities can also occur in adults when the muscles and tendons change the shape of the softened bone.

Infectious Disease of Bone

Osteomyelitis is an infectious process of the bone and its marrow. It may progress from acute to chronic forms. The term **osteomyelitis** usually refers to infection caused by pyogenic organisms, but it can also refer to granulomatous infections such as tuberculosis and to viral or fungal infections.

ACUTE OSTEOMYELITIS

Acute osteomyelitis manifests with acute systemic involvement and malaise. It can progress to chronic osteomyelitis if not identified and treated promptly.

Etiology and Pathophysiology

The infecting organism causing acute osteomyelitis in most cases is hemolytic *Staphylococcus aureus*, although streptococci, *E. coli*, coliform bacteria, pneumococci, gonococci, or any bacterial or fungal agent may be involved. Immune-suppressed or debilitated patients are at greater risk and may develop infections due to *Salmonella, Pseudomonas, Hemophilus influenzae*, and group B streptococci.[14] The organism may reach the bone by (1) hematogenous spread from systemic infections associated with other organs, (2) a primary bone infection, (3) an extension of soft tissue infection adjacent to bone, or (4) a penetrating wound or open fracture.[5,25] The infecting organism enters the bone through the nutrient or metaphyseal vessels and moves into the medullary canal. Vascularity increases and causes edema. Polymorphonuclear leukocytes accumulate in the involved area. In a few days, thrombosis of local vessels occurs, resulting in ischemia and death of portions of bone. The pus in this confined space is under pressure and is pushed out through Volkmann's canals to the surface of the bone (Fig. 27-20). It can also spread subperiosteally and enter the bone at another level or burst out into the surrounding tissue.

In infants, before the epiphyseal cartilage seals off the metaphysis, spread can go directly to the joint and cause a suppurative arthritis. In older persons, if joint involvement occurs, it does so through subperiosteal spread. Necrotic bone (*sequestrum*) is separated from viable tissue, and granulation tissue forms beneath the area of dead bone and infection. New bone forms from the elevated periosteum. This bone, called the *involucrum*, envelopes the granulation tissue and sequestrum. Small sinuses permit the pus to escape.[25]

Clinical Manifestations

The person with acute osteomyelitis appears acutely ill with fever, chills, malaise, increased ESR, and variable degrees of leukocytosis. If the osteomyelitis is in a limb, it becomes very painful. The pain is often described as a constant throbbing. Redness and swelling usually occur over the site, and sensitivity to the touch is characteristic. Radiologic evidence is noted after about 10 days and reflects bone destruction. In the early stages of osteomyelitis the MRI will show intraosseous and extraosseous changes before changes are seen on routine x-ray films. Blood cultures may or may not be positive for the causative organism; massive antibiotic therapy usually arrests the disease. With vertebral osteomyelitis, blood cultures are usually negative and needle biopsy of infected bone is necessary.[14]

CHRONIC OSTEOMYELITIS

Chronic osteomyelitis is associated with nonresolving acute osteomyelitis. Granulation tissue below the infection becomes scar tissue and forms an impenetrable area around the infection. The localized area of suppuration is called *Brodie's abscess*.[24] A new area of bone develops to isolate the area further. The process is characterized by chronically draining sinuses with organisms that are resistant to antibiotic therapy. Localized manifestations of chronic osteomyelitis include pain, swelling, redness, and warmth.

TUBERCULOSIS

Tuberculosis is a chronic granulomatous infection caused by *Mycobacterium tuberculosis*. The organism spreads through the body through lymphatic or hematogenous routes (see p. 228). Involvement of bone and joints is due to hematogenous spread, with the spine the most common site. Other sites of spread include the knee, hip, ankle, wrist, sacroiliac joint, pubic symphysis, and small bones of the hands and feet. The infection causes destruction of bone tissue and caseous necrosis that may enter the joint cavities or occur under the skin as an abscess with draining sinuses. Tubercular skeletal lesions usually do not wall themselves off, so invasion of joints and intervertebral disks may cause many deformities. Tuberculosis of the spine, called *Pott's disease*, most frequently occurs in children and can lead to kyphosis, scoliosis, or the hunchback deformity.

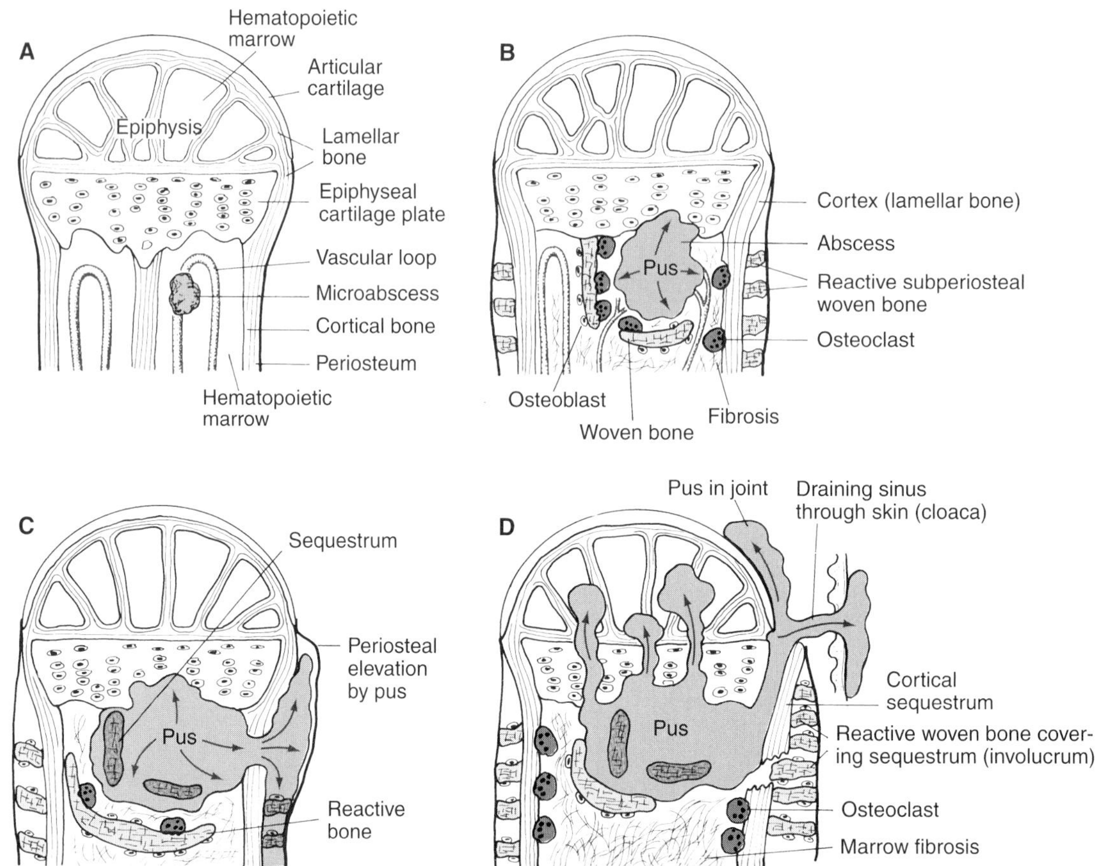

FIGURE 27-20. **Pathogenesis of hematogenous osteomyelitis. A. The epiphysis, metaphysis, and epiphyseal plate are normal. A small, septic microabscess is forming at the capillary loop. B. The expansion of the septic focus stimulates resorption of adjacent bony trabeculae. Woven bone begins to surround this focus. The abscess expands into the cartilage and stimulates reactive bone formation by the periosteum. C. The abscess, which continues to expand through the cortex into the subperiosteal tissue, shears off the perforating arteries that supply the cortex with blood, thereby leading to necrosis of the cortex. D. The extension of this process into the joint space, the epiphysis, and the skin produces a draining sinus. The necrotic bone is called a sequestrum. The viable bone surrounding a sequestrum is termed the involucrum. (Rubin, E. & Farber, J. L. [1999].** ***Pathology*** **[3rd ed.]. Philadelphia: Lippincott Williams & Wilkins.)**

The onset of skeletal tuberculosis, in contrast to acute pyogenic osteomyelitis, is insidious, beginning with a vague description of pain. Swelling and stiffness may also be present in earlier stages of the disease. With progressive disease, atrophy, deformities, and dysfunction become evident if joints are involved. Infections may drain to the skin via subcutaneous tracts from the bone. Complications of tuberculosis of the spine include paraplegia and meningitis.

SYPHILIS

Congenital or acquired syphilis of the bone is rare in the United States. In congenital syphilis, the spirochetes are delivered through the fetal bloodstream to the bones, where they inhibit osteogenesis. The epiphyseal plate is severely damaged and may actually be separated from the metaphysis. Bone syphilis is marked by endarteritis and periarteritis, and reactive bone forms from viable surrounding periosteum. Granulation tissue between the periosteum and cortical bone is laid down. In the tibia, a resulting "saber-shin" deformity gives a curved appearance to the anterior portion of the bone.[25] Acquired syphilis may also cause epiphysitis (inflammation of the epiphysis) or periosteitis (inflammation of the periosteum). Syphilitic lesions may appear within the medullary canal. The skull and vertebrae, as well as the long bones, can be affected in acquired syphilis.

Alterations in Skeletal Structure

ABNORMAL SPINAL CURVATURES

Abnormal spinal curvatures give significant clues for underlying musculoskeletal disorders. The following are alterations in normal curvature of the spine.

Scoliosis

Scoliosis is a lateral curvature of the spine resulting from varying factors. Scoliosis may be classified as *nonstructural* or *structural.* Nonstructural scoliosis has no anatomic abnormality and usually results from pain or poor posture. Structural scoliosis involves anatomic abnormalities in the spine, bones, or muscles and includes congenital, neuromuscular, and idiopathic scoliosis (Table 27-5). It may be associated with another disease such as polio or cerebral palsy. Most commonly, scoliosis is an idiopathic disorder.

Traditionally, idiopathic scoliosis has been divided into three categories according to the age of onset: infantile (0–3 years), juvenile (4–10 years), and adolescent (10 years or above). It is estimated that over 1 million Americans have some degree of scoliosis, and girls are affected eight times more often than boys. Scoliosis is most frequent in the early adolescent years.

The curvatures are classified according to location and consist of a primary, fixed curve with compensatory curves above and below (Fig. 27-21*A*). The deformity occurs slowly and is accelerated by the preadolescent growth spurt. The shoulder blade protrudes, the level of the iliac crests becomes unequal, and the curvature appears to be exaggerated when the individual bends over (Fig. 27-21*B*).[28] In general, the younger the age when the curvature is noticed and the higher up in the thorax it occurs, the poorer the prognosis. Severe scoliosis can affect the heart and lungs by restrictive action. It may be markedly improved by surgical procedures.

TABLE 27-5

TYPE OF SCOLIOSIS AND ASSOCIATED ETIOLOGY

TYPE OF SCOLIOSIS	ETIOLOGY
STRUCTURAL	Associated with identifiable problems in the structure of the vertebral column or its ligaments and muscles
Congenital	Faulty embryonic development of spinal column; frequently associated with other congenital malformations
Neuromuscular	Faulty muscle control and support for the vertebral column; associated with conditions such as cerebral palsy and muscular dystrophy
Idiopathic	No identifiable pathologic basis; genetic link has been speculated
NONSTRUCTURAL	No identifiable structural problems evident with the vertebral column and its supporting muscles and ligaments; most often is associated with poor posture, which may result from varying causes such as fatigue, malnutrition, and inactivity

Other Abnormal Spinal Curvatures

Various other curvatures of the spine may result from conditions affecting the spine. These include:

- *List,* which is a lateral tilt of the spine from the T1 level (Fig. 27-22). It may result from a herniated disk or a painful spasm of the muscles along the spine.[28]
- *Gibbus,* which is an angular deformity noted with a collapsed vertebra (Fig. 27-23). Multiple causes include metastatic malignancy of the spine and tuberculosis.[28]
- *Flattening of the lumbar curve,* which is an abnormal finding indicative of a herniated lumbar disk or ankylosing spondylitis.[28] The normal curve in the lumbar area becomes straight, as shown in Figure 27-24.
- *Lordosis,* which is an accentuation of the normal lumbar curve (Fig. 27-25*C*) often resulting from obesity or pregnancy as a compensation for the protuberant abdomen.[28]

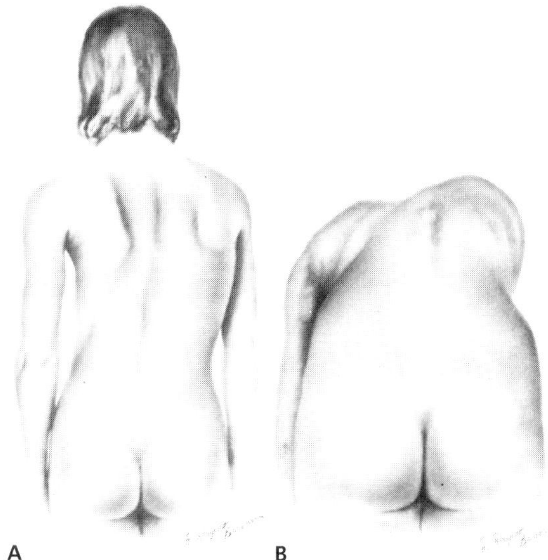

FIGURE 27-21. **A.** Scoliosis of the spine with a thoracic primary curve and compensatory curve in the lumbar spine. **B.** The rotary deformity of scoliosis produces a hump or "razor back" deformity. This deviation is best demonstrated by asking the client to bend at the waist.

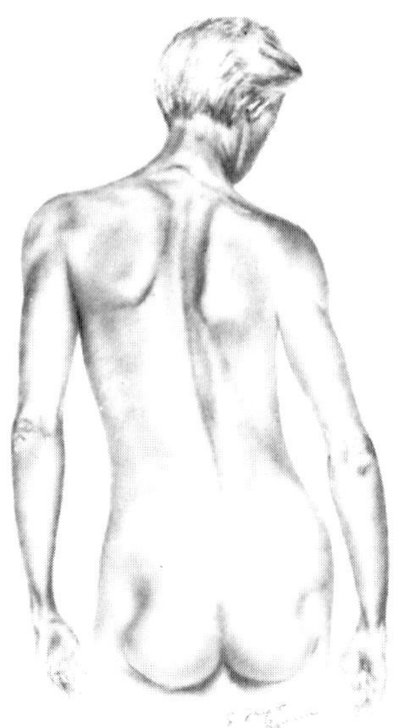

FIGURE 27-22. List is a lateral tilt of the spine. When a plumb line dropped from the spinous process of T1 falls to one side of the gluteal cleft, a list is present. Causes include a herniated disc and painful spasms of the paravertebral muscles. Scoliosis is inherent in a list but has not been fully compensated for by a spinal deviation in the opposite direction.

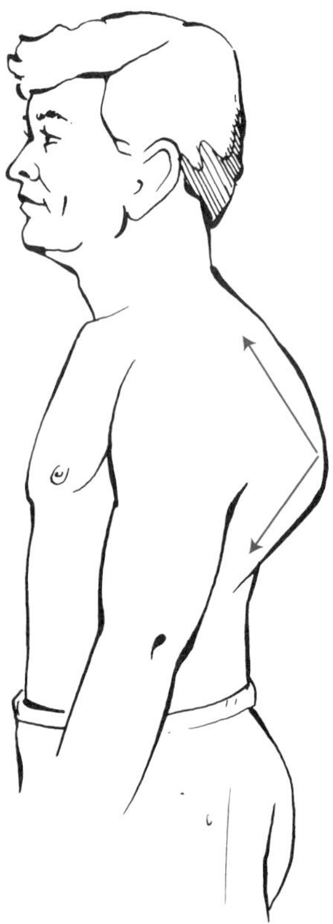

FIGURE 27-23. Gibbus is a very pronounced convex angular curvature of the spine (extreme kyphosis). It is often associated with collapsed vertebral bodies.

- *Kyphosis,* which appears as a rounded thoracic convexity, especially in elderly women (Fig. 27-25*B*).[28] It is caused by vertebral collapse and may be the first indication of osteoporosis in the elderly person. It may be accompanied by pain in the vertebral area and radiologic signs of osteoporosis.

CLUBFOOT (TALIPES)

Clubfoot deformities, the most frequent of the orthopedic congenital deformities of the lower extremities, occur with greatest frequency in boys. Two thirds of the cases are unilateral. Clubfoot may be caused by genetic and environmental factors. Generally, the talus points downward and the foot is adducted. The clinical varieties are *easy* and *resistant,* with the easy cases responding to strapping and stretching alone and the resistant cases requiring surgical intervention.

CONGENITAL DISLOCATION OF THE HIP

Congenital dislocation of the hip is probably caused by a combination of genetic and environmental factors. Genetic factors are linked to both joint laxity and acetabular dysplasia. Also, just prior to delivery of a full-term infant, the pregnant woman secretes a ligament-relaxing hormone that crosses the placental barrier and enhances joint laxity. This accounts for the relative rarity of hip dislocation in premature infants. Other environmental factors include intrauterine malposition, breech presentation during delivery, and, in some cultures, swaddling of neonates.

Pathologically, the acetabulum is defective and the femoral head is completely out of the joint, located posterior and superior to the acetabulum. Most frequently, this is a unilateral occurrence. Asymmetric groin skin creases are seen on examination, and the affected leg is shorter than the other. The leg cannot abduct completely. When it is extended and flexed at the hip, a click called *Ortolani's click* may be felt or heard. Because the femoral head must be in correct alignment with the acetabulum for the bones and joint to grow and develop normally, early detection is necessary.

Bone Tumors

Tumors in the skeletal system can be either primary or secondary. Primary lesions can be benign or malignant. Of these, benign tumors are much more common and usually are self-limiting. Malignant tumors of the bone, although rare, are devastating and often fatal.

Benign bone tumors are usually slow-growing, noninvasive, and well-localized. Adolescents or young adults are usually affected most frequently, and the tumor growth stops when the skeletal system reaches maturity. Because of their noninvasive characteristics,

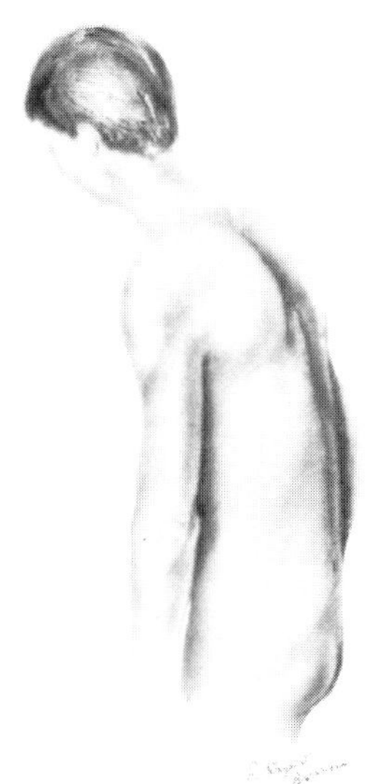

FIGURE 27-24. Flattening of the lumbar curve, muscle spasm in the lumbar area, and decreased spinal mobility suggest the possibility of a herniated lumbar disk or, especially in men, ankylosing spondylitis.

benign tumors cause little or no pain and are often discovered secondarily to another complaint or a pathologic fracture.

Malignant neoplasms grow rapidly, spread and invade irregularly, and cause pain. Classic signs are constant or intermittent pain, usually worse at night; an unexplained swelling over a bone; and a feeling of warmth of the skin over the bone, with prominent veins. Adolescents and young adults are most commonly affected. These tumors metastasize to other parts of the body and are usually fatal without early diagnosis and treatment.

Secondary tumors of the skeletal system are usually metastatic from primary sites in the breasts, lungs, kidneys, or other body systems. As the primary lesion grows and invades surrounding tissue, clumps of cancerous tissues are carried by the blood and lymphatic system to the bone, where they continue to grow and cause destruction.

CLASSIFICATION OF BONE TUMORS

Primary bone neoplasm may be classified according to the skeletal tissue from which it arises: osseous, cartilage, or marrow. Tumors in each of these categories

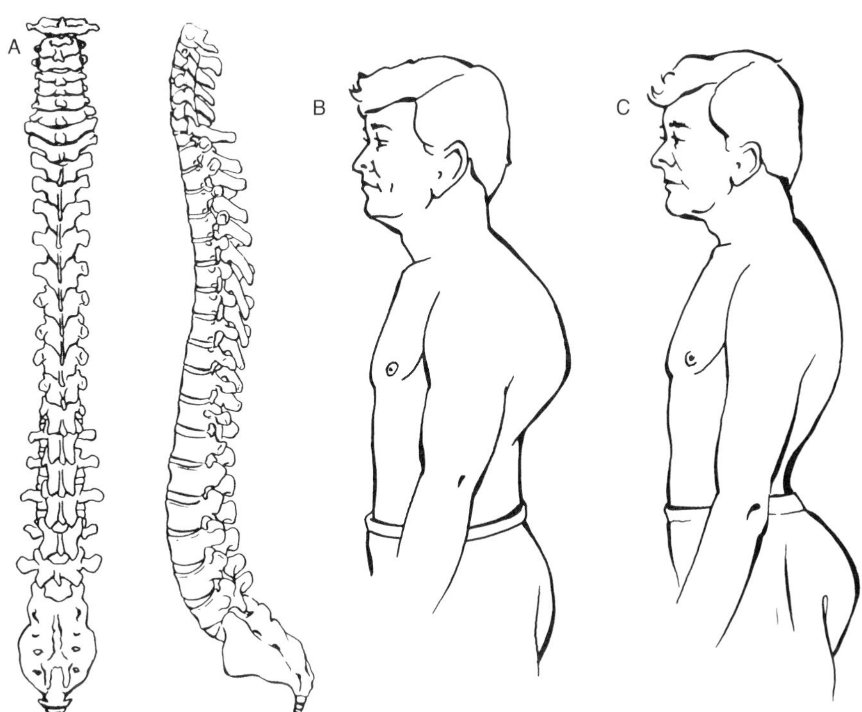

FIGURE 27-25. **A.** The normal orientation of the lumbar spine is that of mild lordosis. Exaggerated lordosis may predispose the patient to mechanical back pain. **B.** Kyphosis. **C.** Lordosis that develops to compensate for the protuberant abdomen of pregnancy or marked obesity. It may also compensate for kyphosis and flexion deformities of the hips. A deep midline furrow may be seen between the lumbar paravertebral muscles.

may be benign or malignant. Other bone tumors, such as giant-cell tumors, do not have these origins. This section discusses the more common benign and malignant tumors. These are grouped as *osteogenic* (bone-forming), *chondrogenic* (tumors of cartilage origin), those of *unknown origin*, and *hematopoietic malignancies.*[5]

Osteogenic Tumors

FIBROUS DYSPLASIA. Fibrous dysplasia is a benign pathologic condition that affects skeletal development. It is characterized by replacement of cancellous bone by fibrous tissue, and it can affect one bone (monostotic) or many bones (polyostotic). Monostotic forms account for about 70% of cases and usually affect the ribs, femur, tibia, maxilla, mandible, or humerus.[4] The condition may be asymptomatic, or disfigurement from bony distortion may be seen. In the polyostotic form, the craniofacial bones are affected most frequently, but crippling deformities also may be associated.

The fibrous lesion begins in the medullary canal and spreads to the cortex, with cancellous bone and marrow replaced by yellow-gray, fibrous tissue. The cortex is thin, and bowing deformities and fractures are common. If the disease occurs in the monostotic form, the lesion grows slowly, but eventually deformity occurs unless the mass is surgically removed.

If the polyostotic form of the disease is accompanied by extraskeletal signs and endocrine pathology, it is called *Albright's syndrome.* Albright's syndrome is differentiated by precocious puberty in girls, café-au-lait pigmentation of the skin over the bone involvement, and predominant unilateral bone deformity, especially of the skull and long bones.[4] When the facial bones are affected, asymmetry of the face with distortions of the nose, jaw, and even severe displacement of an eye may occur. Although fibrous dysplasia has no proven genetic links, multisystem involvement of the polyostotic form does suggest some basic genetic defect. Many endocrine associations have been identified, including hyperthyroidism, Cushing's syndrome, acromegaly, and hyperparathyroidism.[4]

OSTEOMAS. Compact osteoma is a benign tumor composed of dense bone with a well-circumscribed edge. It frequently arises in the cortical surface of bone of the skull and paranasal sinuses. Symptoms are caused from impingement of the tumor on the brain or sinuses. The tumors cause the face to become unfortunately distorted.[4] Osteoid osteoma most commonly affects the femur and tibia, but it can grow in any bone in the body except the skull. It is usually located in the diaphysis of long bones. It occurs predominantly in boys and young men between the ages of 5 and 25. The tumor consists of a well-rounded, central nidus that is sharply demarcated from a surrounding zone of bone. The nidus may range from a few millimeters to a centimeter and consists of osteoid tissue and trabeculae. The tissue is reddish-gray and is granular to the touch. The main clinical manifestation is increasingly severe, localized pain in a lower limb.[5]

OSTEOBLASTOMA. Benign osteoblastoma is a rare benign tumor that is sometimes confused with osteoid osteoma or even giant-cell tumors. It occurs most frequently in boys and young men, usually in the first three decades of life. Its most common site is the spinal cord. Pain is a cardinal symptom, usually due to the pressure on adjacent structures, such as the spinal cord or nerve roots. It seems to be less severe than that caused by an osteoid osteoma and may be referred to a site distant from the tumor. Other symptoms depend on the location of the tumor and include weakness or even paraplegia. There is no characteristic radiographic appearance. In some cases, one may see bone destruction that is more or less demarcated from normal bone. Surgical removal usually relieves compression on the spinal column and nerve root. When the tumor is in a long bone, it may take on the appearance of an osteoid osteoma with a sclerotic border, except that the nidus may be many times longer.

OSTEOSARCOMA. The most prevalent malignant tumor of osteoid origin is osteogenic sarcoma or *osteosarcoma*, in which tumor cells proliferate osteoid or immature bone. Osteosarcoma is the most common and most fatal primary bone tumor, often affecting people between the ages of 10 and 20 years.[25] It occurs more often in young men than in young women, usually during periods of rapid skeletal growth. It usually arises near the end of a long bone, especially around the knee. Irradiation and oncogenic viruses have been explored in its etiology.[25] When this lesion does occur in later years of life, it is usually related to Paget's disease or prior radiation treatment. To be classified as a true osteogenic sarcoma, an osteoid substance must be produced. The tumor may show a predominance of elements, with osteoid, chondroid, or fibromatoid differentiation. Bizarre pleomorphic cells with abundant mitoses or multinucleated giant cells are characteristic.[5,25]

Osteosarcomas usually occur in long tubular bones, but the skull, maxilla, spinal column, and clavicles, as well as other bones, are also affected. The femurs, tibia, and ulnae are the most frequent sites (Fig. 27-26). After the age of 25, its frequency in flat and long bones is nearly equal.[22] The tumor usually is a localized swelling with tenderness associated with a large mass. Pain may or may not be present. Sometimes the tumor is found on incidental radiographic examination of an injury. It tends to recur within 1 to 2 years.

Chondrogenic Tumors

Benign chondrogenic tumors include osteochondroma, enchondroma, and chondroblastoma. Chondrosarcoma is a malignant tumor of the cartilage. Many

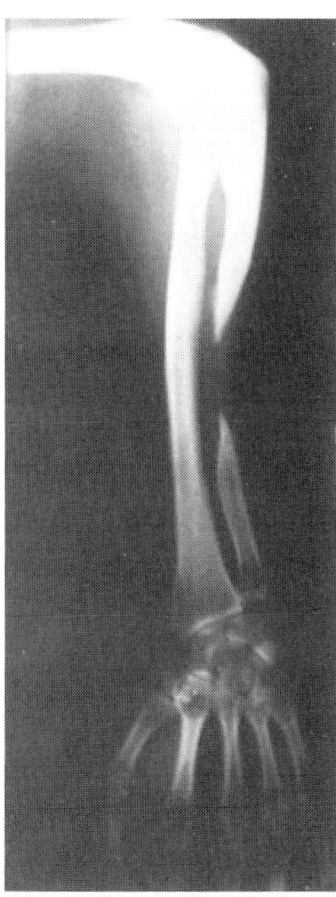

FIGURE 27-26. **Osteogenic sarcoma. Note the complete destruction of the ulna.**

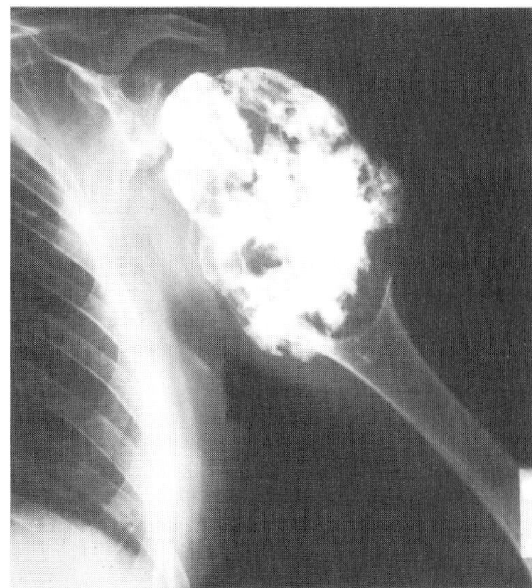

FIGURE 27-27. **Osteochondroma of the proximal right humerus is unusually large; shows cartilaginous and osteoid matrix being laid down.**

of these tumors are asymptomatic and are only discovered accidentally because of an injury to the area.

OSTEOCHONDROMAS. Osteochondromas form a long mass produced by progressive endochondral ossification of a growing cartilaginous cap. The tumor is basically osseous and protrudes from the cortex of the bone with or without a stalk. The caps are usually cauliflower-shaped and occur mainly in persons between the first and second decades of life (Fig. 27-27). The growth of the tumor parallels that of the adolescent, and once the epiphyses have closed, it normally stops. Multiple osteochondromas may occur when more than one bone is affected, with each growth having the same characteristics as the single osteochondroma.

Osteochondromas rarely undergo malignant change to osteosarcomas. This transformation may occur if there are multiple tumors or occasionally after surgical removal of an osteochondroma. The most common site for the tumorous mass is the metaphyseal region of long bones, specifically the femur and tibia, but it can affect any bone that develops by endochondral ossification.

ENCHONDROMA. Enchondroma is a hyaline cartilage tumor within the medullary cavity that is encapsulated by an intact cortex. It is the most common intraosseous cartilage tumor and most frequently affects the small tubular bones of the hands and feet, but it may affect the ribs, sternum, spine, and long bones of persons between 20 and 50 years of age. The tumor usually affects the phalanges of the hand, producing a central area of rarefaction (decreasing density and weight). Normally discovered during treatment of a fracture after a trivial injury, the tumor appears radiographically as a well-defined, translucent area with the cortex intact and areas of calcification.

BENIGN CHONDROBLASTOMAS. Benign chondroblastomas closely resemble giant-cell tumors and affect mainly persons under the age of 20 years or before epiphyseal closure, whereas giant-cell tumors are rare under the age of 20 years. Histologically, chondroblastomas differ from giant-cell tumors in that they contain foci of calcification, trabeculae of osteoid tissue, well-developed bone, and well-defined areas of cartilaginous matrix. Chondroblastomas are virtually always benign, localized lesions that do not recur and do not invade.

Localized pain may be experienced and is often referred to the adjacent joint region. Wasting of muscle mass, due to disuse caused by pain and limping, may also be observed.

Radiographically, an area of central bone destruction is clearly demarcated by surrounding normal bone. There may be margins of increased bone density with mottled areas of calcification within the lesion. The tumor almost always involves the epiphysis and frequently the adjacent metaphysis, which are also seen on the films.[4]

CHONDROSARCOMA. Chondrosarcoma is a malignant bone tumor of cartilaginous origin. It can arise from benign chondrogenic origins, as described earlier, or may develop spontaneously. The tumor occurs more frequently in men than in women and is primarily a condition of adulthood and old age. It rarely metastasizes until it has grown to a large size.[15] Chondrosarcomas usually originate in the trunk and the upper ends of the femur and humerus. Points of attachments of muscle to bone at the knee, pelvis, shoulder, and hip are prevalent. Any bone of the body can be affected. Physical symptoms may include pain, swelling, and a palpable mass due to the active invasive growth of the tumor. Tumors located in the trunk and long bones may be evidenced only by pain, which makes radiographic findings important. These usually include mottled areas of calcification and areas of osseous destruction. Even when treated with wide resection, recurrence has been encountered even after 10 years. Metastases may occur many years after initial diagnosis and treatment.[15]

Tumors of Undetermined Origin

EWING'S SARCOMA. Ewing's sarcoma, although rare, is one of the most lethal bone tumors. Approximately 90% of people affected are under age 30, with the greatest number of tumors occurring in the second decade of life. They affect men more than women by a 2 to 1 margin.[25] The long tubular bones are most commonly involved, with the innominate bones of the pelvis, ribs, scapula, and sternum following in that order, and then virtually any other bone in the body.

Ewing's sarcoma, like many other invasive tumors, results in pain, a tender mass, and venous distention. Some individuals may have anemia, temperature elevation, and sometimes leukocytosis.[2] This tumor generally has its origin in the medullary canal, growing outward and creating a lytic area on radiographs. Ewing's sarcoma is composed of nondistinctive, small, round cells that are not easily identified.[7] Some spicules of bone may be seen, but this is reactive bone and not part of the neoplasm. Elevation of the periosteum is typical, followed by periosteal bone formation, which creates what is known as an onion-skin appearance, seen radiologically.[4,5]

GIANT-CELL TUMORS. Giant-cell tumors are poorly understood, apparently malignant, distinct neoplasms. Cases of seemingly benign giant-cell tumors have been reported to undergo malignant transformation. For this reason, a histomorphic grading system has been developed, with grade I being benign, grade II being borderline, and grade III being frankly malignant.[15] Unfortunately, this system is not always accurate, as one part of the tumor may appear benign while another part may appear malignant. Giant-cell tumors generally affect individuals between 20 and 55 years of age; peak occurrence is in the third decade of life. They affect women somewhat more frequently than men.[15] Most giant-cell tumors arise in the epiphyses of long bones, with over one-half of the lesions close to the knee in the distal femur and proximal tibia; other sites include the sacrum, vertebrae, humerus, and radius.[15]

Giant-cell tumors usually begin forming within cancellous bone. As they grow and invade, the cortex may be thinned or even broken, but new reactive bone generally preserves the cortex. The expansion of the tumor in the epiphyses classically forms a clublike deformity. Radiographs reveal a somewhat translucent area at the ends of the long bones, with a thin cortex (Fig. 27-28). Other clinical manifestations may include pain and pathologic fractures.

Hematogenic Neoplasias

Hematogenic neoplasias or malignancies arise from the stem cells in the bone marrow and cause skeletal and extraskeletal manifestations. Common bone marrow hematogenic neoplasias are the leukemias and multiple myeloma. The proliferation of cells in the bone marrow in leukemia may present with bone pain and many varied systemic manifestations (discussed in Chapter 13). Likewise, multiple myeloma involves extraosseous sites and manifestations. The skeletal effects of this condition are discussed here.

MULTIPLE MYELOMA. Multiple myeloma is a plasma cell cancer and is the most common primary neoplasm of the bone. The affected bone marrow is composed of plasma cells showing variable degrees of differentiation The incidence of multiple myeloma is 2 to 3 per 100,000. It is a disease of older adults and often presents with signs and symptoms of bone marrow failure, hypercalcemia, and renal failure.

Multiple myeloma affects women and men equally, rarely occurs before the age of 50, and has its peak frequency in the fifth and sixth decades. It has a predilection for the vertebral column, but the ribs, skull, pelvis, and virtually any bone in the body may be affected.

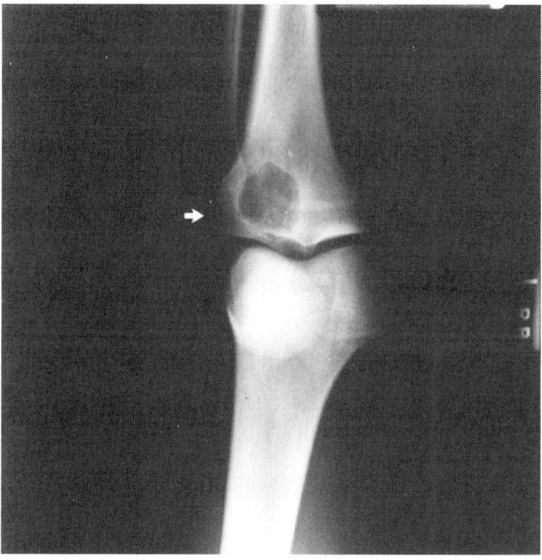

FIGURE 27-28. Giant-cell tumor of the tibia (*arrow*).

Multiple myeloma appears radiographically as multifocal destructive bone lesions throughout the skeletal system, producing what appear to be rounded, punched-out areas.[4] These areas may measure up to 5 cm, with no surrounding zone of sclerosis. Various cytokines, especially interleukin 6, seem to generate myeloma cells and mediate the formation of the bone lesions. The bone lesions usually begin in the **medullary bone** and invade into the cancellous bone.

The individual has a history of pain that is often referred to the spinal column. Pathologic fractures of the vertebrae are common. When the myeloma lesion grows, it may result in compression of vertebral bodies or nerve roots and cause various neurologic symptoms. Weakness, loss of weight, hemorrhagic disorders, and renal involvement are also associated with multiple myeloma. Hypercalcemia, hyperuricemia, and the presence of Bence-Jones proteins in the urine are frequently noted.[25]

Metastatic Bone Disease

Metastatic cancer is the most common bone tumor in patients over the age of 40. The hallmark of metastatic bone disease is pain, and approximately 10% of cancer patients present with bony involvement as the first sign of disease. Radiographic x-rays may be normal initially, but a bone scan will demonstrate an increased uptake early on. The most common sites of involvement are the spine (thoracic and then lumbar), pelvis, femur, and ribs. Laboratory data may show hypercalcemia, reflecting accelerated bone reabsorption.

ALTERED FUNCTION ASSOCIATED WITH JOINTS

Joints allow the body to be mobile; therefore, alterations in joints (arthropathies) impact mobility. The synovial joints are most affected by alterations. Alterations involve traumatic joint injury or dislocation or various joint disease processes. Frequently the cartilage, ligaments, and tendons are involved.

Joint Injuries

The support structures, tendons and ligaments, of the joint may be injured. The extent of injury may vary greatly, from mild, self-limiting sprains and tendinitis to avulsion and rupture of the structures. Dislocation and subluxation may be associated with traumatic injuries and degenerative joint conditions.

SPRAINS

Sprains refer to injury to a single or multiple joint ligaments. They are associated most commonly with trauma and result from extending the joint beyond its normal range. Although they may occur in any joint, the most common joints involved are the ankle, knee, and wrist. Sprains are classified according to the amount of ligament damage: (1) First-degree sprains involve only a few ligament fibers and produce a mild inflammatory response. (2) Second-degree sprains involve more fibers as well as some surrounding blood vessels. Therefore, hemorrhage and hematoma formation accompany the more extensive inflammatory response. (3) Third-degree sprains involve complete tearing of the ligament from its bony attachment (avulsion). (4) Fourth-degree sprains involve complete tearing of the ligament as well as fracture of the bone at the ligament attachment (avulsion fracture). Muscles and tendons may be injured in association with ligaments.

Clinical Manifestations

Clinical manifestations vary with severity of the sprain. The inflammatory response develops rapidly after injury and accounts for many of the manifestations, which include pain, swelling, heat, and joint immobility. Additionally, ecchymosis, joint instability, deformity, *dislocation* (complete displacement of the joint articular surfaces) and *subluxation* (partial displacement of the joint articular surfaces) may be present in more severe cases. Mild sprains usually heal within a few weeks; severe sprains require more extensive intervention and rehabilitation. Most individuals with sprains experience a favorable outcome with recovery of good joint function.

TENDINITIS

Tendinitis, an inflammation of the tendons, may be associated with traumatic injuries or may result from overuse in daily activities or sports activities. Tendinitis may also be associated with inflammatory arthropathies such as rheumatoid arthritis. Tendinitis frequently involves the region where the tendon attaches to the bone; it is then known as *epicondylitis.*

Traumatic tendinitis may be accompanied by tendon strains and contusions that have been caused by overstretching and tearing. Achilles tendinitis, a common traumatic tendinitis, results from a rapid, unexpected plantar heperflexion. Overuse tendinitis results from excessive pressure on the tendon and frequently involves tendons of the wrist, elbow, shoulder, and knee. It commonly results in athletes who have not trained properly, either with improper technique or through training too much, too soon, or too long. An example of overuse tendinitis is tendinitis secondary to rotator cuff impingement. The impingement may also cause bursitis (see below) if the bursa is involved. Sometimes referred to as an *impingement syndrome,* it results from repetitive overhead motion. Soft tissue is compressed within the subacromial space between the head of the humerus and the coracoacromial arch. The soft tissue compression is aggravated by swelling, excessive acromium overhang, or mineral deposition, all which narrow the subacromial space. Impingement of the rotator cuff may affect elderly individuals with acromioclavicular joint arthritis or younger individuals engaged in athletic activities who have developed impingement of the subacromial tissues as a result of excessive movement of the humerus on the glenoid labrum.

Clinical Manifestations

Clinical manifestations with traumatic tendinitis may reveal a sudden, audible "pop" or "snap" and a sense of sudden, forceful hitting or kicking. The pain may not be significant for a few hours after the injury, usually peaking the following day. The pain is localized and is associated with swelling, possibly ecchymosis, and limited joint mobility. The manifestations of overuse tendinitis may persist for several weeks and range from mild discomfort in the involved tendons with activity without functional impairment to continuous pain in the involved tendon region and significant impairment of activity. The individual with rotator cuff impingement usually presents with a history of several weeks of shoulder pain that continues to be aggravated by activity.

TENOSYNOVITIS

Tenosynovitis is an inflammation of the tendon sheath and the enclosed tendon. It primarily affects the wrists, shoulders, and ankles. This condition is thought to be related to use, and occupational stresses, such as typing and heavy labor, may precipitate it. Synovial fluid and fibrin constituents within the tendon sheath may cause adhesions. These inflammations cause extreme pain on movement and may exhibit heat and redness or inflammation. Bacterial invasion by pyrogens and tuberculosis also have been implicated as causes of tenosynovitis.

BURSITIS

Bursae are enclosed sacs containing a small amount of fluid that lubricates and cushions joints. Inflammation of a bursa—bursitis—is common and may be caused by unusual use of a part, trauma, infection, or rheumatoid arthritis. The inflammation results in an excessive production of fluid in the sac, which becomes distended and presses on sensory nerve endings, causing pain. Commonly affected bursae are (1) the prepatellar bursa, caused by kneeling (housemaid's knee or nun's knee); (2) the olecranon bursa, subject to the repeated trauma of leaning on one's elbows (bartender's elbow); (3) the bursa located on the plantar aspect of the heel, which is subjected to repeated pressure (postman's heel); and (4) the bursa of the metatarsophalangeal joint of the great toe (bunion).

Joint Diseases

Diseases of the joint (arthropathies) may be classified in various ways. They may be primary to the joint (arthritis) or secondary to a systemic problem (gout), inflammatory (rheumatoid arthritis) or noninflammatory (osteoarthritis), or involve cyst (Baker's cyst) or tumor formation (sarcomas).

ARTHRITIS

The most frequent joint diseases are the arthritides, which affect 1 out of every 20 to 30 Americans and constitute a financial and health problem of considerable magnitude.[4] **Arthritis** simply means inflammation of a joint, and it occurs in many forms. Degenerative joint disease or trauma often is related to an increased incidence of *osteoarthritis.* Metabolic disturbances may cause *gouty arthritis,* or it may be associated with conditions such as psoriasis or bursitis. *Suppurative arthritis* implies an infection of the joint with pyogenic organisms; *tuberculous arthritis* is inflammation secondary to tuberculosis. Autoimmune conditions produce many types of arthritis, the most crippling of which is *rheumatoid arthritis.*

Rheumatoid Arthritis

Rheumatoid arthritis (RA) is the most common systemic inflammatory disease, characterized by symmetric joint involvement. RA has a prevalence rate of 2% to 3%, with no racial predilections.[4] The disease, which often occurs between the ages of 20 to 50, is more common in women than in men, with a ratio of 6:1 for those between 15 and 45 years of age; however, the incidence is equal between men and women in other age groups.

ETIOLOGY. It is believed that there is a genetic predisposition, as a majority of patients with RA have the major histocompatibility genes associated with the HLA-DR halotypes (DR4 and DR1). Genetic factors also indicate that there is an increased frequency of the disease in close relatives.[33] Although no specific microorganisms have been identified in joints of individuals with RA, it is theorized that viruses such as Epstein-Barr virus (EBV) or others play a role in the initiation of the disease in genetically susceptible individuals. Despite the lack of an identifiable virus, the preponderance of evidence supports an autoimmune causation, with both cellular and humoral factors associated. Increased physical or emotional stress has always been recognized as a precipitator of acute exacerbations, but the mechanisms of the stress interaction are unknown.

PATHOPHYSIOLOGY. The disease process usually begins with joint infection and migration of lymphocytes to the inflammatory site. Synovial lymphocytes produce IgG, which is targeted as foreign, and the production of IgG and IgM anti-immunoglobulins results. These anti-immunoglobulins represent the rheumatoid factor (RF) and bind with the Fc fragment of IgG. The resulting complex activates complement, which amplifies the immune response by encouraging chemotaxis, phagocytosis, and the release of lymphokines by mononuclear cells. These substances cause joint destruction.

Joint destruction is a major pathologic feature of RA and may affect any synovial membrane in the body. Joint inflammation with effusion is accompanied by capsular and periarticular soft tissue inflammation, causing swelling, redness, and painful motion of the joint. Joint motion causes bleeding within the cavity. Clots of fibrin and newly formed granulation tissue fill the joint space. Proliferative synovitis persists, and the synovium becomes a thickened, hyperemic, densely cellular granulation tissue called a *pannus*. Over time, pannus invades and erodes surrounding cartilage and underlying bone, causing fibrous fusion (ankylosis) of the joint.[25,33] Local degenerated muscle is gradually replaced by fibrous tissue, and the involved bones may show osteoporosis.

Rheumatoid nodules, which are present in about one-fourth of persons affected, are areas of fibrinoid necrosis surrounded by macrophages, lymphocytes, and plasma cells. They may be found in various locations throughout the body but tend to form more in areas of pressure. The nodules may arise in the pericardium, heart valves, lung parenchyma, and skin and present unique pathologic features of the organ dysfunction.

The synovial fluid aspirated from the RA-affected joint is thin and cloudy and has elevated protein and polymorphonuclear cell levels. See the unit Appendix for a description of normal synovial fluid findings.

CLINICAL MANIFESTATIONS. The patient with RA manifests insidious or acute joint pain with systemic symptoms. These may include general achiness, depression, fatigue, low-grade fever, anorexia, malaise, weakness, and weight loss. The joints may be tender, painful, swollen, red, and stiff. If multiple joints are involved, the pattern of involvement is usually symmetric. Joints most typically involved are the small joints of the hands and feet; proximal interphalangeal, metacarpophalangeal, and metatarsophalangeal joints; and wrists, elbows, knees, and ankles. Hand deformities are characteristic of RA and reveal ulnar deviation and subluxation of the metacarpophalangeal joints (Fig. 27-29). *Swan neck* (flexion of the distal interphalangeal joint and hyperextension of the proximal interphalangeal joint) and *boutonnière* (fixed flexion of the proximal interphalangeal joint and hyperextension of the distal interphalangeal joint) deformities are also common in the joints. The patient complains of morning stiffness lasting longer than 1 hour, nocturnal pain, pain at rest, and decreased range of motion.

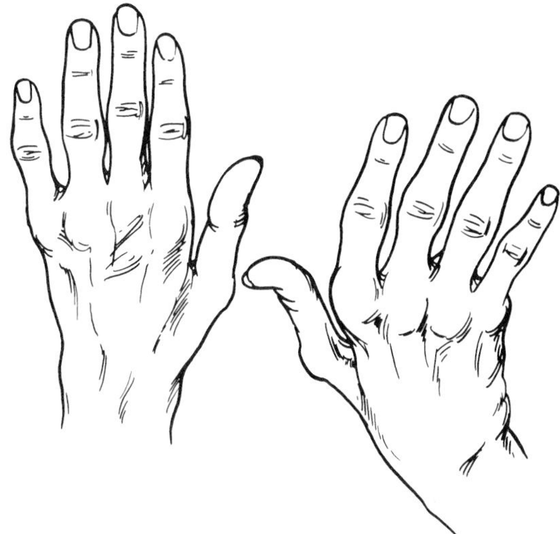

FIGURE 27-29. Ulnar deviation and subluxation of the metacarpophalangeal joints have occurred in the patient's right hand. These joints also appear swollen. Muscle atrophy has developed in the dorsal musculature of both hands.

Although RF is not diagnostic for RA, it is demonstrated in about 80% of individuals with RA. Other inflammatory and noninflammatory conditions may also manifest RF. Seropositive RA patients do tend to have a more aggressive course of their illness, and the presence of high titers frequently correlates with severe and unremitting disease.[25] Criteria (manifestations) developed by the American College of Rheumatology for the diagnosis of RA are presented in Table 27-6. At least four of these must be present for at least 6 weeks.

Juvenile Rheumatoid Arthritis

A variant of rheumatoid arthritis is *juvenile rheumatoid arthritis* (JRA). The onset of JRA in persons aged 16 years or younger is usually more abrupt than the adult form. It characteristically presents with systemic manifestations such as chills, high fever, leukocytosis, skin rash, and hepatomegaly. Other systemic manifestations that may be present include inflammation of the iris (uveitis), pericarditis, myocarditis, and glomerulonephritis. Although joint pathology is similar to the adult form, JRA has a tendency to involve a single joint (monarticular), usually a large joint. The rheumatoid nodules and rheumatoid factor commonly are not present. If the disease appears before the closure of epiphyseal growth plate, growth retardation may occur. Fortunately, over one-half of these young persons have a complete remission. Permanent deformities are more common in those with an acute febrile onset, multiple joint involvement, and a positive RF.[26,33]

TABLE 27-6

CRITERIA FOR RHEUMATOID ARTHRITIS

CRITERIA	DEFINITION
Morning stiffness	Morning stiffness in and around the joints lasting at least 1 hour before maximal improvement
Arthritis of three or more joint areas	At least three joint areas have simultaneously had soft tissue swelling or fluid (not bony overgrowth alone) observed by a physician. The 14 possible joint areas are (right or left): PIP, MCP, wrist, elbow, knee, ankle, and MTP joints
Arthritis of hand joints	At least one joint area swollen as above in wrist, MCP, or PIP joint
Symmetric arthritis	Simultaneous involvement of the same joint areas (as in 2) on both sides of the body (bilateral involvement of PIP, MCP, or MTP joints is acceptable without absolute symmetry)
Rheumatoid nodules	Subcutaneous nodules, over bony prominences, or extensor surfaces, or in juxta-articular regions, observed by a physician
Serum rheumatoid factor	Demonstration of abnormal amounts of serum "rheumatoid factor" by any method that has been positive in less than 5% of normal control subjects
Radiographic changes	Radiographic changes typical of RA on posterior-anterior hand and wrist x-rays, which must include erosions or unequivocal bony decalcification localized to or most marked adjacent to the involved joints (osteoarthritis changes alone do not qualify)

(American College of Rheumatology. 1987 Criteria for classification of rheumatoid arthritis.)

Osteoarthritis

Osteoarthritis (OA) is the most common degenerative noninflammatory joint disease. It affects both men and women equally. Risk factors include increasing age, previous joint injury, congenital and developmental abnormalities, hereditary factors, decreased bone density, and obesity. OA may be classified in two categories: (1) primary and (2) secondary. *Primary osteoarthritis* is a disease of unknown etiology, whereas *secondary osteoarthritis* has a known underlying cause such as injury, infection, or metabolic disorder.[2]

Pathophysiology. OA joint disease is characterized by destruction of articular cartilage and subchondral bone with cyst and osteophyte formation.[25] Degenerative changes are also found in the joint capsule, synovial membrane, ligaments, and muscles and tendons that surround the affected joint.[17] Joints have a limited way in which to respond to the compressive forces in day-to-day living. In osteoarthritis, the matrix in the articular cartilage is depleted, thus "unmasking" the basic collagen structure. Normally, the matrix spreads compression stress hydrostatically, but with its depletion the collagen fibers may rupture, causing flaking, fissuring, and eroding of the articular cartilage. The exposed subchondral bone may form cracks and allow synovial fluid into the marrow, forming subchondrial cysts.

The bone immediately under the affected area shows proliferation of fibroblasts and new bone formation. Periosteal bone growth also increases at the joint margins and at the site of ligament or tendon attachments, developing into bone spurs or ridges called *osteophytes*. The synovial capsule decreases in size, and movement is limited. Osteoporosis is not a direct component of the disease, but because of age considerations it may also be seen.

Clinical Manifestations. Narrowing joint space or cyst formation may be apparent on radiographs. Osteoarthritis generally affects joints of the fingers and those that are weight bearing, especially the spine, knees, hips, and shoulders. Pain and stiffness occur after joint use and are relieved by rest early in the course of the disease. Later, pain occurs with motion or rest.[2] Spurs may be formed on the distal interphalangeal joints (*Heberden's nodes*) and on the proximal interphalangeal joints (*Bouchard's nodes*) of the fingers. Flexor and lateral deviations of the fingers are common, especially in the elderly individual. Box 27-5 summarizes the clinical manifestations in the individual with OA.

Ankylosing Spondylitis

Ankylosing spondylitis is an arthritic condition that is classified as one of a group of seronegative spondylarthritides. Box 27-6 lists the conditions that are placed in this classification. The disease is only slightly

BOX 27-5

CLINICAL PRESENTATION OF OSTEOARTHRITIS

Age

Usually elderly

Sex

Age <45 more common in men
>45 more common in women (hands)

Symptoms

Pain
Deep, aching
Pain on motion
Early in disease—pain with use
Late in disease—pain at rest
Stiffness
Rarely exceeds 15 min; related to weather
Localized to involved joints
Limited joint motion
Instability of weight-bearing joints
Crepitus, crackling

Signs/Physical Examination

Monoarticular or oligoarticular; asymmetrical involvement
Joints frequently involved
Hands—DIP, PIP, first carpometacarpal joint
Foot—first metatarsophalangeal
Hips, knees, cervical spine, lumbar spine
Observations on joint examination
Bony proliferation or occasional synovitis
Local tenderness
Crepitus
Muscle atrophy
Limited motion with passive/active movement
Effusions
Characteristics of synovial fluid
High viscosity
Mild leukocytosis (<2000 WBC:mm^3)

Laboratory Values

No specific test
ESR, hematologic survey, chemistry survey are normal
No systemic manifestations

Key: DIP, distal interphalangeal; PIP, proximal interphalangeal; ESR, erythrocyte sedimentation rate.
(Dipiro, R., Yee, G., Matzke, G., Wells, B. & Posey, L. [1997]. *Pharmacotherapy: A physiological approach.* Stamford, CT: Appleton & Lange.)

more prevalent in men than in women, and the symptoms in men are more severe. The peak age range is from 20 to 40 years.[4] Ankylosing spondylitis is characterized by inflammation of the spine and can lead to fusion of these joints. Destruction of cartilage and bone results in fibrous and bony ankylosing of the spine, giving the patient the typical stiff or "poker" spine. Mobility of the spine is usually decreased symmetrically but does improve somewhat with exercise. Discomfort is insidious in onset and often is described as morning stiffness.[12] If peripheral joints are affected early in the disease, joint replacement procedures may become necessary. An elevated ESR is characteristic, but evidence of immune complex formation is found less frequently than in rheumatoid disease.[12]

BOX 27-6

SERONEGATIVE SPONDYLARTHROPATHIES

Ankylosing spondylitis
Reiter's syndrome
Psoriatic arthropathy
Intestinal arthropathy
Juvenile ankylosing spondylitis
Reactive arthropathy

GOUT

Gout is associated with an inborn error of uric acid (an end product of purine synthesis) metabolism that leads to the accumulation of monosodium urate crystals in joints and tissues. Gout is used as a general term for a group of diseases with one or more of the following manifestations: (1) increased serum urate concentration; (2) recurrent attacks of acute arthritis with urate crystals in synovial fluid; (3) aggregated deposits of urate in joints, leading to crippling and deformity; (4) renal disease; and (5) uric acid nephrolithiasis.[8] The prevalence of gout in the United States has been estimated at 275 per 100,000. Urate concentrations and risk of gout increase with age, male gender, alcohol use, hypertension, and obesity.[7] A variant of classic gout is *pseudogout*, which is associated with deposits of calcium pyrophosphate-dihydrate crystals in connective tissue. It is associated with aging, joint trauma, and a variety of metabolic diseases such as hyperparathyroidism, hypothyroidism, and Wilson's disease. It has manifestations similar to hyperuricemic gout.

Etiology

Gout is generally classified as primary or secondary. *Primary gout* is a genetic disorder in which the exact defect of uric acid metabolism is unknown in the vast majority of cases. Ninety percent of all gout is primary, with men most frequently affected.[25] *Secondary gout* occurs whenever some superimposed condition either increases the production of uric acid or decreases its excretion.[6] Diseases characterized by rapid breakdown of cells (e.g., leukemia), hemolytic anemia, cytolytic agents, and drugs that decrease excretion of urates (e.g., thiazides and mercurial diuretics) have all been implicated in secondary gout.

Pathophysiology

Normally, individuals produce 600 to 800 mg of uric acid daily, and excrete less than 600 mg in the urine and the remainder through the gastrointestinal tract. Gout is a *hyperuricemic syndrome* that can result from overproduction of uric acid, retention of uric acid due to renal malfunction, or both.[2] Although the precise error of purine metabolism is unknown, overproduction is thought to be related to two enzyme abnormalities in the purine synthesis pathways: (1) the increase in the activity of phosphoribosyl pyrophosphate, and (2) deficiency of hypoxanthine-guanine phosphoribosyl transferase.[4,25] Hyperuricemia at an excessive point results in the formation of insoluble monosodium urate crystals, which are deposited throughout the connective tissues. These crystals also precipitate in the joints and cause painful inflammation. Small masses of urate crystals called *tophi* accumulate over time (Fig. 27-30). These are infiltrated with lymphocytes, plasma cells, and macrophages and cause inflammation in the surrounding tissue. Tophi may clump together and form large plaque-like encrustations that invade the articular surface and underlying bone, causing deformities.

Clinical Manifestations

Gout is described in four clinical phases: (1) asymptomatic hyperuricemia, (2) acute gouty arthritis, (3) intercritical gout, and (4) chronic tophaceous gout.[28] In *asymptomatic hyperuricemia*, the serum urate level is elevated even though there are no symptoms. In *acute gouty arthritis*, there is a sudden onset of severe pain in the great toe or occasionally the heel, ankle, wrist, fingers, elbows, or instep. When the monosodium urate crystals are deposited in the synovial fluids they can rapidly lyse neutrophils, which release lysosomal enzymes and contribute to the inflammatory process. The affected joint becomes hot, red, and tender. The pain becomes intense and intolerable. It may be associated with chills, fever, and an elevated white blood count and resolve spontaneously or with treatment. Untreated, these attacks last for 3 to 14 days. The intervals between attacks are called *intercritical gout*. Crystal deposition persists during this phase. In the fourth phase, *chronic tophaceous gout*, tophi occur in many locations, even in the aorta and heart valves. Deforming arthritis is common and can involve any joint.[7] Tophi may accumulate in any area but are most commonly observed in the periphery of the body, including the helix of the ear, the hands, and in the metatarsophalangeal joint of the big toe. The lower temperatures in the periphery may contribute to precipitation of urate crystals in tissues. Less commonly, urate crystals may be deposited in the kidney and form uric acid stones.

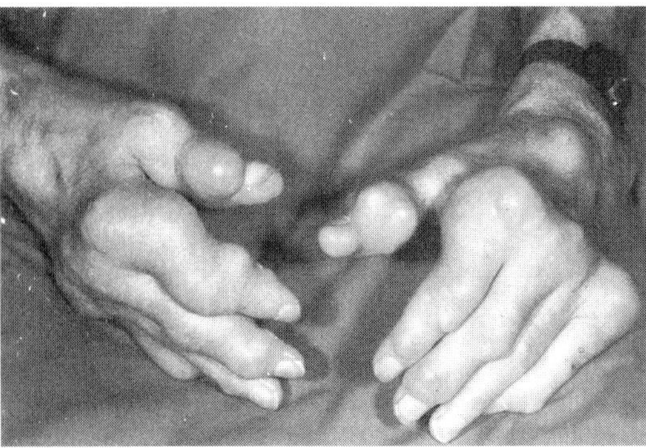

FIGURE 27-30. Gouty tophi projecting from fingers. (Rubin, E. & Farber, J. L. [1999]. *Pathology* [3rd ed.]. Philadelphia: Lippincott Williams & Wilkins.)

BAKER'S CYST

Baker's cyst is a firm, cystic mass along the medial border of the popliteal space. It occurs mostly in children, especially boys, and is believed to be caused by fluid distention of the bursal sac associated with local muscles. In adults these cysts tend to be associated with internal derangement of the knee. Some cysts communicate directly with the joint cavity. Swelling is usually the only clinical manifestation.

TUMORS OF JOINTS

Tumors of joints are uncommon, but they may occur on the tendon sheath, the bursae, and around the joints. They are classified as sarcomas of the synovial lining. Primitive mesenchymal cells, rather than synovial membrane cells, form the primary tumor. A gray-white mass invades along muscle and fascial planes, and although the tumor is slow-growing, it can metastasize to the lungs, bones, and brain. Clinical manifestations vary with specific tumors and may include joint pain and swelling and difficulty with movement.

FIBROMATOSIS

Fibromatoses are nodular collections of fibroblasts or myoblasts surrounded by collagen. They may be found on the hand (palmar fibromatosis), the foot (plantar fibromatosis), or the penis. Palmar fibromatosis denotes chronic hyperplasia of the fascia in the palm of the hand, leading to fibrosis and a deformity called *Dupuytren's contracture*. Usually bilateral, this condition is most frequent in Caucasians, and the risks increase with age. Heredity is believed to be a major factor in causation. Myofibroblasts are responsible for the contractures of the palmar fascia. The fingers, most often the ring and little fingers, contract into a fixed, flexed position.

Plantar fibromatosis is similar to palmar fibromatosis, but it usually does not cause contractures. Nodular masses of fibrocytes arise from the plantar fascia, usually on the medial side of the foot. Trauma is thought to be the cause.

Penile fibromatosis (Peyronie's disease) is discussed in Chapter 36.

HEREDITARY ALTERATIONS IN CONNECTIVE TISSUE

Osteogenesis Imperfecta

Osteogenesis imperfecta includes a group of hereditary disorders in which defective connective tissue formation leads to extremely fragile bones. The disorders have various levels of severity of bone, eye, ear, dental, and cardiovascular involvement. Different types are described, some of autosomal dominant inheritance and some of autosomal recessive.[23] The bones of the skull and face may be poorly ossified, with numerous fractures occurring in the long bones. The skeletal aspect of this condition is a hereditary form of osteoporosis. Some types have few fractures but exhibit any combination of blue sclerae, deafness, short stature, joint dislocation, and opalescent teeth.[20] In severe cases, death of the infant during childbirth may occur due to trauma to the brain, which is relatively unprotected by the soft, membranous skull.

FOCUS ON THE PERSON WITH GOUT

P. J. is a 72-year-old retired farmer. He complains of acute pain in his right great toe. He states that it has been sore for the past couple of days, but this morning it is more painful. The pain was so intense that he could not put on his usual shoes. On examination the toe appears red, swollen, and is warm and very tender to touch.

P. J. is about 40 pounds overweight and has a history of hypertension. He and his wife have recently been instructed on the importance of a healthy diet and exercise. P. J. was also prescribed a diuretic to help control his blood pressure.

The physician suspects that P. J. may have gout. He orders a radiograph of the great toe and a variety of laboratory tests, including a uric acid level, which returns at 13 mg/dL. The WBC is 11,000 per microliter. Other laboratory work is in the normal range. The radiograph reveals soft tissue swelling and increased density around the first metatarsophalangeal joint.

Questions

1. Discuss the risk factors and etiology of gout (primary and secondary).
2. What risk factors does P. J. present for gout?
3. Describe the stages of gout. From the above findings, which of the stages is P. J. in?
4. Discuss the pathophysiology of gout. What are tophi, and what are the most common sites for them?
5. Delineate the common clinical manifestations associated with acute gout.

Marfan Syndrome

Marfan syndrome is an autosomal-dominant disorder characterized by abnormal body proportions. The basic pathologic mechanism is a mutation in the fibrillin-1 (FBN1) gene coding on the long arm of chromosome 15.[25] Fibrillin is a connective tissue protein found in many body tissues. Clinical manifestations in affected individuals include long arms, long digits (arachnodactly), thoracic deformity such as pectus excavatum, curvature of the thoracic spine, and hyperextensibility of the joints.[13] Associated connective tissue defects result in abnormalities in many organs, including dilatation and dissection of the aorta along with aortic insufficiency. Cardiovascular abnormalities are the most common cause of death.

REFERENCES

1. Alacron, G. (1997). Osteonecrosis. In J. H. Klippel, C. M. Weyand & R. Wortman (Eds.), *Primer on the rheumatic diseases* (11th ed.). Atlanta: Longstreet Press.
2. Boh, L. (1997). Osteoarthritis. In R. Dipiro, G. Yee, G, Matzke, B. Wells, & L. Posey (Eds.), *Pharmacotherapy: Physiological approach*. Stamford, CT: Appleton & Lange.
3. Cormack, D. H. (1993). *Essential histology*. Philadelphia: J. B. Lippincott.
4. Cotran, R. S., Kumar, V., Collins, T., & Robbins, S. L. (1998). *Robbins' pathologic basis of disease* (6th ed.). Philadelphia: W. B. Saunders.
5. Dee, R., Hurst, L., Gruber, M., & Kottmeier, S. (1997). *Principles of orthopedic practice*. New York: McGraw-Hill.
6. Drezner, M. K., McGuire, J. L. & Marks, S. C. (1997). Metabolic bone disease. In W. N. Kelley (Ed.), *Textbook of internal medicine* (3rd ed.). Philadelphia: Lippincott.
7. Edwards, N. (1997). Clinical features of gout. In J. H. Klippel, C. M. Weyand & R. Wortman (Eds.), *Primer on the rheumatic diseases* (11th ed.). Atlanta: Longstreet Press.
8. Fox, I. H. (1997). Crystal-induced synovitis. In W. N. Kelley (Ed.), *Textbook of internal medicine* (3rd ed.). Philadelphia: Lippincott.
9. Ganong, W. (1997). *Review of medical physiology* (17th ed.). Norwalk, CT: Appleton & Lange.
10. Guyton, A. C. & Hall, J. E. (1996). *Textbook of medical physiology* (9th ed.). Philadelphia: W.B. Saunders.
11. Holick, M. F., Krane, S. M., & Potts, J. T. (1997). Calcium, phosphorus and bone metabolism: Calcium-regulating hormones. In A.S Fauci et al. (Eds.), *Harrison's principles of internal medicine* (14th ed.). New York: McGraw-Hill.
12. Khan, M. (1997). Ankylosing spondylitis and the spondylarthropathies. In J. H. Klippel, C. M. Weyand & R. Wortman (Eds.), *Primer on the rheumatic diseases* (11th ed.). Atlanta: Longstreet Press.

13. Lindsay, J., Debakey, M. E., & Beall, A. C. (1994). Diagnosis and treatment of diseases of the aorta. In R. C. Schlant & R. W. Alexander, *Hurst's the heart* (8th ed.). New York: McGraw-Hill.
14. Mader, J. T. (1994). Osteomyelitis. In J. Stein (ed.), *Internal medicine* (4th ed.). St. Louis: C.V. Mosby.
15. Malawer, M. M., Link, M. P. & Donaldson, S. S. (1993). Sarcomas of bone. In V. T. DeVita, S. Hellman, & S. A. Rosenberg, *Cancer: Principles and practice of oncology* (4th ed.). Philadelphia: J. B. Lippincott.
16. Malone, T., McPoil, T., & Nitz, A. (1996). *Orthopedic and sports physical therapy*. St Louis: Mosby–Year Book.
17. Marks, R. & Cantin, D. (1997). Symptomatic osteoarthritis of the knee: The efficacy of physiotherapy. *Physiotherapy, 83*, 306–311.
18. McArdle, W. D., Katch, F. I. & Katch, V. L. (1996). *Exercise physiology: Energy, nutrition, and human performance* (4th ed.). Philadelphia: Lea and Febiger.
19. Mendell, J. R., Griggs, R. C. & Ptacek, L. J. (1997). Hereditary myopathies. In H. A. Fauci et al. (Eds.), *Harrison's principles of internal medicine* (14th ed.). New York: McGraw-Hill.
20. Narins, R. G. et al. (1994). The metabolic acidosis. In R. C. Narins (Ed.), *Clinical disorders of fluid and electrolyte metabolism* (5th ed.). New York: McGraw-Hill.
21. Norton, M., Anderson, G., & Pope, M. (1997). *Musculoskeletal disorders in the workplace.* St Louis: Mosby.
22. O'Connell, M. & Bauwens, S. (1997). Osteoporosis and osteomalacia. In R. Dipiro, G. Yee, G. Matzke, B. Wells, & L. Posey (Eds.), *Pharmacotherapy: A physiological approach.* Stamford, CT: Appleton & Lange.
23. Pyeritz, R. E. (1997). Heritable disorders of connective tissue. In J. H. Klippel, C. M. Weyand & R. Wortman (Eds.), *Primer on the rheumatic diseases* (11th ed.). Atlanta: Longstreet Press.
24. Reichlin, M. (1997). Polymyositis and dermatomyositis. In J. H. Klippel, C. M. Weyand & R. Wortman (Eds.), *Primer on the rheumatic diseases* (11th ed.). Atlanta: Longstreet Press.
25. Rubin, E. & Farber, J. L. (1999). *Pathology* (3rd ed.). Philadelphia: Lippincott.
26. Schuna, A. & Walbrandt, D. (1997). Rheumatoid arthritis and the seronegative spondyloarthropathies. In R. Dipiro, G. Yee, G. Matzke, B. Wells, & L. Posey (Eds.), *Pharmacotherapy: A physiological approach.* Stamford, CT: Appleton & Lange.
27. Scott, D. (1998). Arthritis in the elderly. In R. Dallis, H. Fillit, & J. Brocklehurst, *Geriatric medicine and gerontology.* London: Harcourt Brace.
28. Seidel, H., Ball, J., Dains, J., & Benedict, G. (1999). *Mosby's guide to physical examination* (4th ed). St Louis: Mosby.
29. Tandan, R. (1998). Dermatomyositis and polymyositis. In A. S. Fauci et al. (Eds.), *Harrison's principles of internal medicine* (14th ed.). New York: McGraw-Hill.
30. Tortora, G. & Grabowski, S. (1993). *Principles of anatomy and physiology* (7th ed.). New York: Harper Collins.
31. Winkel, D. (1997). *Diagnosis and treatment of the lower extremities.* Gaithersburg, MD: Aspen.
32. WHO Study Group (1994). *Assessment of fracture risk and its application to screening for postmenopausal osteoporosis.* Geneva: World Health Organization.
33. Zvaifler, N. J. (1994). Rheumatoid arthritis. In J. Stein (Ed.), *Internal medicine* (4th ed.). St. Louis: Mosby.

Chapter 28

Normal and Altered Functions of the Skin

Janice Allwood / Kim Curry

KEY TERMS

basal cell carcinoma
carbuncles
decubitus ulcers
dermatitis
dermis
eczema
electrothermal burns
epidermis
eponychium
eschar
eumelanin
exfoliation
folliculitis
furuncles
hair shaft
hemangioma
herald patch
impetigo
keratinization
keratocanthoma
lunula
malignant melanoma
melanin
melanocytes
perifolliculitis
pheomelanin
pilosebaceous ducts
pityriasis rosea
psoriasis
seborrheic keratosis
squamous cell carcinoma
staphylococcal scalded skin syndrome (SSSS)
striae gravidarum
subcutaneous tissue
toxic epidermal necrolysis syndrome (TENS)
urticaria
verrucae
zone of coagulation
zone of hyperemia
zone of stasis

The skin is the largest organ of the body. The skin and its component parts, including hair, nails, glands, and nerve supply, make up the integumentary system. This system plays a primary role in regulating body temperature and fluid balance, as well as preventing microbial invasion. The skin serves as a membranous barrier to the body's environment and has a consistency ranging from the thick, tough, outer covering of the body to the thin, delicate mucous membranes of the mouth, nose, and eyelids. The skin is both pliable and durable and allows for mobility and protection. At the same time it is one of the most sensitive organs of the body, capable of transmitting a variety of sensations, such as fine touch, pain, temperature, and pressure.[34]

The skin functions as a barrier against pathogenic organisms and a protectant against trauma from environmental forces. It is waterproof but can regulate body temperature through sweating. It protects the body from excessive ultraviolet light through production of the pigment **melanin**. After injury, skin has the capacity to regenerate, thus facilitating the healing process. The skin also gives an indication of the nutritional and metabolic health of a person through color, texture, and alterations in continuity.[26]

Common alterations in skin integrity include inflammatory conditions, infections, neoplasms, and traumatic alterations in skin integrity such as burns and decubitus ulcers. Skin diseases have characteristic features called primary lesions. These lesions can be obscured by secondary lesions that result from the evolutionary process of the skin disease, treatment, scratching, or infection.[16] The usual response of the skin to injury is to generate the inflammatory response. Sources of injury to the skin include bacteria, viruses, temperature extremes, and chemical or mechanical irritants. Inflammation alters the surrounding blood vessels and adjacent tissues and causes redness or erythema. An irritant causes injury to the site, which results in a vascular reaction with fluid exudation and edema. Pressure from the edema or chemical irritation from the release of various mediator substances causes pain due to irritation of the nerve fibers in that area.

STRUCTURE AND FUNCTION

The skin is composed of three major layers; from the surface inward, these layers are the **epidermis**, **dermis**, and **subcutaneous tissues**. The layers of the skin are depicted in Figure 28-1. Major functions of the skin are listed in Box 28-1.

Epidermis

The main layers, or *strata,* of the epidermis, from the dermis to the surface, are the (1) stratum germinativum, (2) stratum spinosum, (3) stratum granulosum, (4) stratum lucidum (present only on the palms of the hands and soles of the feet), and (5) stratum corneum. The functions of these layers are summarized on Table 28-1 and further described below.

BASAL LAYER (STRATUM GERMINATIVUM)

This layer is one cell thick and lies in contact with the dermis. Within the basal layer are basal cells. These cells are attached to a basement membrane connecting the epidermis to the dermis. Interlocking extensions, or processes, are present in varying numbers throughout the skin, attaching the epidermis to the dermis. Areas such as the eyelids have few of these processes, whereas nipples have a complex system of ridges, and fingertips have parallel ridges that form cavernous valleys and tunnels.[9] The highly individualized patterns of fingerprints are the result of these valleys. In the nor-

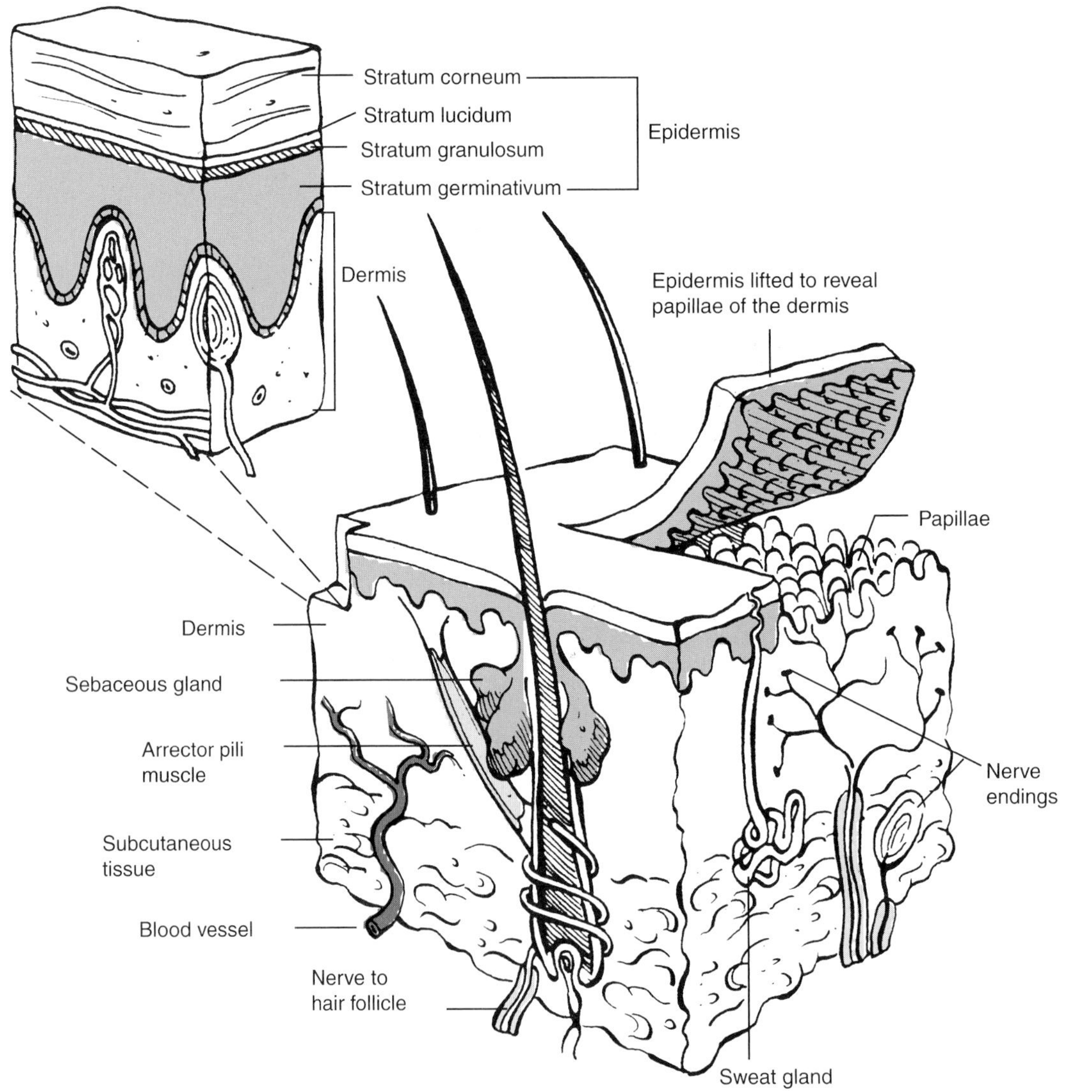

FIGURE 28-1. Three-dimensional view of the skin.

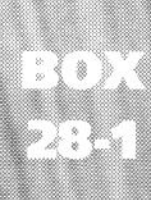

BOX 28-1

MAJOR FUNCTIONS OF THE SKIN

- Protect against the external environment
- Maintain and regenerate skin layers
- Defend against foreign substances
- Preserve the internal fluid environment
- Excrete wastes
- Regulate body temperature
- Produce vitamin D
- Provide sensation
- Provide cosmetic identity

mal epidermis, mitosis of new basal cells is limited to the basal layer. Throughout the basal layer are dispersed melanocytes, which form melanin and are responsible for pigmentation of the skin. These cells are wedged between the basal cells.

SPINOUS LAYER (STRATUM SPINOSUM)

This layer lies directly above the basal layer. As newly formed skin cells migrate up through the spinous layer, they acquire a polygonal shape. Bridges hold the cells together. As the cells move toward the surface they begin to flatten.

GRANULAR LAYER (STRATUM GRANULOSUM)

This layer is from two to four cells thick and lies directly above the stratum spinosum. While in this layer, the skin cells continue to mature into the squames, or scale-like cells of the epidermis.

STRATUM LUCIDUM

This layer is only found in the thick epidermis, such as in the palms of the hands and soles of the feet. The cells in this layer are dead and are little more than cell membranes containing prekeratin filaments and protein.[16] This layer provides for toughness and friction.

KERATIN LAYER (STRATUM CORNEUM)

This outermost layer of the skin varies in thickness from 0.02 mm on the forearm to 0.5 mm or more on the soles of the feet. The cells of this layer are flat and without nuclei. Keratin is a tough, fibrous protein that resists chemical change. This layer shields the body from environmental damage and maintains the internal milieu. The skin has the lowest water permeability of any biologic membrane. This low permeability

TABLE 28-1

LAYERS AND FUNCTIONS OF THE SKIN

LAYER	COMPONENT	FUNCTION
Epidermis	Stratum corneum	Contains squamous cells (flattened keratin cells) Protects body from harmful substances Prevents water loss
	Stratum lucidum	Provides toughness Protects from friction
	Stratum granulosum	Shapes keratin cells
	Stratum spinosum	Shapes keratin cells
	Stratum germinativum (basal layer)	Forms keratin cells Connects epidermis and dermis Contains melanocytes and basal cells
	Basement membrane	Connects epidermis to dermis
Dermis	Papillary dermis	Provides nourishment to epidermis Contains sensory nerve receptors
	Reticular layer	Provides strength and toughness of skin
Subcutaneous	Adipose layer	Heat insulation Shock absorption Calorie reserve depot

retards water loss and prevents most toxic agents from entering the body, although some substances are readily absorbed. The horny keratin cells (keratinocytes) are shed continuously, making way for new cells.

CELLULAR COMPONENTS OF THE EPIDERMIS

Epidermal cells include keratinocytes, which form the protective barrier of the skin, and melanocytes, which synthesize melanin and give the skin its color. The epidermis contains carbohydrates and various enzymes that influence skin cell activity. The epidermis also contains glucose, which diffuses easily into the cells, the amount depending on the serum glucose levels. Eighty percent to 90% of the energy in epidermal cells is derived from adenosine triphosphate (ATP), which is generated through respiration and glycolysis. The ability to harness these energy sources is especially important during wound healing.

Life Cycle of Epidermal Cells

The life cycle of epidermal cells involves three phases: (1) mitosis, (2) keratinization, and (3) exfoliation. Epidermal cells are continuously formed in the basal or germinative layer at a rate commensurate with the constant loss. New cells move from the basal layer to the stratum corneum in a random fashion that is influenced by the rate of keratinization and by the time that each cell left the basal layer. Transit time from basal layer to surface is anywhere from 12 to 25 days.[34]

MITOSIS. Mitosis is the first phase of the epidermal cell life cycle. This phase occurs in the basal layer of the skin. The rate of mitosis is affected by sleep cycles and hormonal changes. Mitosis seems to occur at a greater rate during periods when the body is at rest or asleep.

Hormonal influences in skin cell mitosis include:

- Male sex hormones (androgens) cause the growth of hair in the typical masculine locations: over the pubis, on the face, on the chest, and on other locations of the body. Androgens aid in the formation of hair follicles and sebaceous glands.
- Female sex hormones (estrogens) aid in the formation of the vaginal epithelium and provide for skin softness.
- Adrenaline may inhibit mitosis. Adrenaline levels are increased during times of wakefulness.

KERATINIZATION. The second phase in the epidermal cell life cycle is **keratinization**. As the epidermal cell from the basal layer moves toward the surface, it loses its ability to undergo mitosis. Instead, it begins to synthesize proteins, keratin, and membrane-coating granules. The cell finally loses its nucleus and cellular organelles, becomes part of the keratin layer, and is shed.

EXFOLIATION. At the end of keratinization, cornified cells are cemented together in varying thicknesses. **Exfoliation**, which is the last phase in the life of an epidermal cell, occurs as those cells at the surface are shed.

Skin Pigmentation

Skin color is determined by **melanocytes**, which originate in the basal layer of the epidermis and in hair follicles. The main function of melanocytes is to synthesize pigment granules, or melanosomes. The main component of melanosomes is melanin, which provides the pigment for skin color. The melanocytes appear in the basal layer of the epidermis as clear cells before they begin to produce melanin.[16]

Melanocytes produce and disperse melanin to keratinocytes and hair cells.[25,30] The amount of melanin determines skin color. In light-skinned persons, melanin is present primarily in the basal layer of the epidermis. In dark- or black-skinned persons, it is present throughout the epidermis, including the outermost horny layer. Melanogenesis increases after exposure to ultraviolet light or x-rays. After exposure, the melanocytes in the basal layer increase activity, become larger, develop longer dendrites, and produce more melanin. They may multiply after exposure to ultraviolet light.[13] Melanin acts as a protective screen to protect the deep layers of the epidermis and the dermis from too much solar ultraviolet radiation. Protection from ultraviolet light exposure should begin at birth to prevent skin damage.[33]

Skin pigmentation is controlled by genes and hormones. Genes regulate the number and shape of melanocytes in the epidermis and hair follicles. Estrogen, progesterone, and melanocyte-stimulating hormone contribute to increased pigmentation in various areas of the body during pregnancy.[30]

Vitamin D Synthesis

Vitamin D is an essential fat-soluble vitamin that, when activated, aids in the absorption of calcium and phosphate in the intestine. The activated form of vitamin D (1,25-dihydroxycholecalciferol) is commonly referred to as vitamin D hormone. It improves mineralization of bone by increasing plasma calcium and phosphate concentrations to support the formation of bone.[27]

Vitamin D hormone is not a single compound but is a family of compounds, the two most important of which are vitamin D_2 and D_3. Vitamin D_2 is the plant-derived form of Vitamin D. Vitamin D_3 is produced in the skin when it is exposed to ultraviolet irradiation. The skin cells contain 7-dehydrocholesterol in the epidermis. Ultraviolet light penetrates the epidermis and causes 7-dehydrocholesterol to undergo photolysis to form previtamin D, which within a few hours isomerizes to form vitamin D_3. Vitamin D_3 is then transported in the blood bound to serum protein. It is converted in two steps, first by the liver and then the kidneys, to vitamin D hormone and may then be stored in the liver and in body fat.[27]

Dermis

The dermis, or *corium*, as illustrated in Figure 28-1, lies between the epidermis and subcutaneous tissues. It consists of a matrix of loose connective tissue. The dermis is traversed by blood vessels, nerves, and lymphatics and is penetrated by epidermal appendages. The mass of the dermis accounts for 15% to 20% of total body weight.[13] The dermis provides the main protection of the body from external injury. Its flexibility allows joint movement and localized stretching but resists tearing, shearing, and local pressure. The dermis also provides the necessary base on which the epidermis receives nutrients and grows.

LAYERS OF THE DERMIS

The two main layers of the dermis are (1) the finely textured papillary dermis and (2) the deeper, thicker, coarsely textured reticular layer. The combined layers of the dermis vary in thickness. They are thinnest over the eyelids and thickest over the back.[13] The upper layer of the dermis is the papillary layer. This layer lies directly beneath the epidermis and serves to nourish the living cells of the epidermis. The reticular layer lies beneath the papillary layer and extends to the subcutaneous tissue. This layer is responsible for the strength and toughness of the skin. Sensory nerve endings, hair follicles, and sweat and sebaceous glands are present in the reticular layer.

CELLULAR COMPONENTS OF THE DERMIS

Three major types of cells are present in the dermis: (1) fibroblasts, (2) macrophages, and (3) mast cells. *Fibroblasts* are the most abundant. Connective tissue is developed from these cells. *Macrophages* help rid the dermis of foreign substances and cell residue. They participate in the immune response and are vital to wound healing, inflammation, tissue reabsorption, and recycling of tissue components. *Mast cells* are present in perivascular connective tissue. Their cytoplasm is filled with large metachromatic granules. These cells degranulate and release the substance histamine under certain physical and chemical conditions, such as injury, infection, or exposure to allergens. Histamine increases capillary permeability, allowing antibodies and white blood cells to move to the site of injury, where they destroy foreign substances.

CHANGES IN THE STRUCTURE OF THE DERMIS

Fibers in the dermis made up of elastin and collagen provide the strength and flexibility of the skin. When skin is at rest, the protective collagen network within the dermis is slack. When exposed to tension, the skin "gives" until the slack is taken up. Skin kept taut for long periods of time becomes fatigued, and stretching results. This is exhibited by stretch marks or **striae gravidarum** (pinkish white or gray lines seen where skin has been stretched by pregnancy, obesity, or tumor), which are irreversible. The skin also becomes thinner when compressed under force and wells up around the source of compression. Pressure damage may occur from long duration of pressure and distribution of force. Most damage is a result of long duration of pressure, but severe point pressure can also injure the cutaneous tissues.

Subcutaneous Tissues

The third major layer of skin is the subcutaneous tissue. This layer is connected to the muscles. It is loose-textured, white, and fibrous. Fat and slender elastic fibers are intermingled. Subcutaneous papillae jut into the dermis. These papillae are larger and more dispersed than dermal papillae. It is through subcutaneous papillae that blood vessels and nerves enter the upper layers of skin.

The subcutaneous tissue layer contains blood and lymph vessels, roots of hair follicles, secretory portions of sweat glands, cutaneous and sensory nerve endings, and fat. Subcutaneous fat varies in amount throughout the body and is absent in the eyelids, penis, scrotum, nipples, and areolae. The unequal fat distribution between males and females is partially a result of hormonal influence. Strands or sheets of white, fibrous, connective tissue support the fat tissue. Subcutaneous tissue is a heat insulator, shock absorber, and calorie-reserve depot.

Blood Supply and Nervous Control

Blood supply to the skin varies in different parts of the body, depending on such factors as the type of skin perfused, thickness of the skin's layers, and types and numbers of skin appendages. Common to skin throughout the body are a deep subdermal arterial plexus, or network of blood vessels, and a superficial subpapillary plexus. The number of blood vessels is greater than necessary to meet the biologic needs of the skin tissues. The vessels have two functions: (1) to provide oxygen and nutrients to skin cells, together with removing wastes, and (2) to aid in thermal regulation.

Figure 28-2 illustrates that the blood vessels are arranged in a three-dimensional network consisting of the two plexuses (deep and superficial) and the vessels that connect them. The deep plexus is joined to larger vessels in the subcutaneous layer and lies in the lower portion of the dermis. The superficial plexus lies beneath the papillary dermis. A network of capillaries reaches up into the dermal papilla to nourish the upper layers of skin.

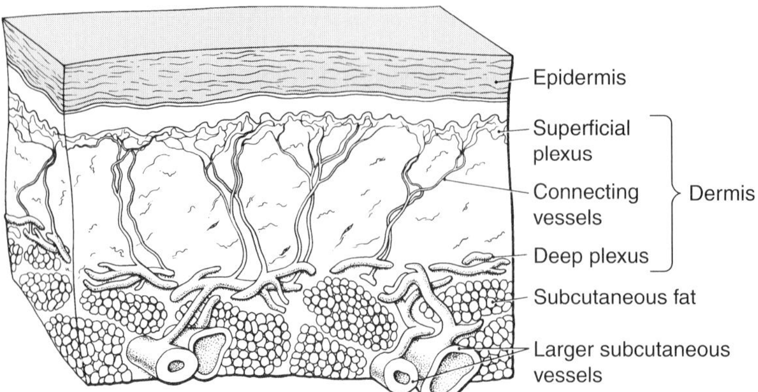

FIGURE 28-2. **Blood vessels of the subcutaneous tissues.**

In addition to the deep and superficial arterial plexuses, a second route of blood flow is through arteriovenous shunts located in the upper part of the reticular dermis. These shunts are important in regulating heat. They are present throughout the skin but are particularly prevalent in the pads and nail beds of fingers and toes, soles and palms, ears, and center of the face. The shunts enable blood to bypass the capillaries and increase blood flow. The plexuses and arteriovenous shunts are controlled by the sympathetic nervous system and constrict and dilate in response to various chemical agents, such as epinephrine and histamine. Vasodilation causes the skin to become hot and red, whereas vasoconstriction causes it to become cold, often with a pale or bluish hue.[25]

The skin is a major sensory organ. Dermal nerve endings receive stimuli from touch, pressure, temperature, pain, and itch. Nerve endings are most numerous on the palms, soles, fingers, and mucocutaneous areas of the lips, glans penis, and clitoris.

Temperature, pain, pressure, and itch are perceived by nerves ending in the dermal papilla and surrounding hair follicles. Examples of these nerve endings are on page 883. Sensory nerves arise from the spinal cord, return by way of the dorsal root ganglia, and receive sensations of temperature, pain, and itch on the unmyelinated nerve ends. Autonomic nerves to the skin are motor nerves. Branches of nerves from the sympathetic nervous system innervate blood vessels, arrectores pilorum muscles, and eccrine and apocrine glands.

Epidermal Appendages

The sweat glands, sebaceous glands, and hair compose the epidermal appendages. As illustrated in Figure 28-1, these extend through the three layers of the skin. The types and functions of the glands are summarized in Table 28-2. The nails protect the ends of the fingers and toes and are specialized epithelial cells.

TABLE 28-2

SWEAT AND SEBACEOUS GLANDS

TYPE OF GLAND	LOCATION	FUNCTION
Eccrine sweat glands	All over body Numerous in thick skin Extended from dermis to epidermis	Regulate body temperature Respond to emotional distress Respond to physiologic stimuli
Apocrine sweat glands	Axillae	Respond to hormonal influences
	Nipples, breasts Anogenital region External ear canal Eyelids	Respond to emotional distress
Sebaceous glands	All over body except palms of hands, dorsum, and soles of feet	Produce sebum to lubricate hair and skin

SWEAT GLANDS

There are two types of sweat glands: (1) eccrine and (2) apocrine.

Eccrine Sweat Glands

The eccrine sweat glands are present all over the body and are most numerous in thick skin. They open to the surface epidermis and descend through the dermis to just above the subcutaneous layer of the skin. These glands are especially prominent on the soles of the feet, palms of the hand, and axillae.

Eccrine glands produce sweat to aid in regulating body temperature. Control of sweating is located in the hypothalamus, which responds to changes in body temperature.[27] Not all eccrine glands function all of the time, but they respond promptly to heat stress. The amount of sweat produced depends on the amount of heat to which the person is exposed. Two to 3 liters of sweat per hour may be produced in an adult exposed to extreme heat conditions. Eccrine sweat is a colorless and odorless hypotonic solution that is 99% water and 1% solutes, such as sodium chloride, potassium, urea, protein, lipids, amino acids, calcium, phosphorus, and iron.

The eccrine units, together with the cutaneous blood vessel network, participate in regulatory heat exchange. The sweat glands cool the surface of the skin with the liquid sweat, which evaporates, causing further cooling. The cutaneous vessels dilate or constrict to dissipate or conserve body heat. The control seat for this process is in the hypothalamus, the neural thermostat.

The hypothalamus is stimulated by changes in surface and blood temperatures. An increase in body temperature of 0.5°C causes the hypothalamus to send a message by way of cholinergic fibers of the sympathetic nervous system to the sweat glands, which pour sweat onto the body surface, causing cooling when it evaporates.[30]

Heat is the primary stimulus to eccrine sweat production, but other physiologic stimuli can stimulate sweating. Gustatory sweating occurs on the face and scalp after eating spicy foods. Emotional stress causes sweating on the palms, soles, axillae, and forehead that may extend to the whole body. Pain, nausea, or vomiting also may cause localized or generalized sweating.

Apocrine Sweat Glands

Apocrine gland ducts empty into the pilosebaceous follicle above the entrance of sebaceous gland ducts. The coiled secretory gland is located in the lower dermis or subcutaneous tissues. The straight duct empties into the hair follicle.

Apocrine sweat has a milky color and contains protein and carbohydrates. In the duct, the sweat is sterile and odorless. Only after reaching the surface, where it contacts bacteria, does it assume an odor. Excretion may be stimulated by emotional stress or hormones, such as epinephrine. The function of apocrine sweat glands is unknown in humans. In animals, the secretion attracts members of the opposite sex.

SEBACEOUS GLANDS

Sebaceous glands arise as epithelial buds from the outer root sheath of the hair follicle. The glands are present throughout the body, except in the palms of the hands and soles and dorsa of the feet. Because these glands develop as buds from the hair root sheath, they are usually associated with hair follicles but are found in some hairless skin, such as that of the nipples, prepuce, labia, and glans penis. Sebaceous glands are largest where hair is sparse or absent, such as on the forehead, nose, chest, and back.

The germ cells in the sebaceous glands discharge their contents of lipid and cell debris into the sebaceous duct as sebum. Other components of sebum include phospholipids, esterified cholesterol, triglycerides, and waxes. Sebum is then evacuated to the follicle and to the surface. Sebum produces oily skin; it lubricates the hair and skin and prevents drying.

HAIR

Human beings are covered with hair in all areas except the palms, soles, dorsum of digits, lips, glans penis, labia, and nipples. Hair is needed to screen the nasal passages and protect the scalp and eyes from sun and sweat.

Hair Types

There are several types of hair. Primary hair, or lanugo, is present on the human fetus and infant. These same fine hairs may be noted on the adult as vellus hairs. An example is the bald man who has fine vellus hair on his scalp. Adult hair is coarse and pigmented. This type of hair is most developed on the scalp, the beard and chest areas in men, and pubic and axillary areas in both genders.

Morphologically, hair is divided into three types: straight, wavy, and woolly, depending on the angle of the hair follicles. Straight hair is found in native Americans, Chinese, and the Mongol races and is coarse.[9] Wavy hair is found in many ethnic groups, whereas woolly hair is found typically in black races.[13]

Hair Color

The color of hair depends on the amount and distribution of melanin within it. The pigments of the melanin are black, brown, and yellow. The brown and black melanins are called **eumelanin**, and the yellow is called **pheomelanin**. The amounts produced are genetically controlled. It is thought that hair becomes gray when the melanocytes of the bulbs of the hair follicles fail to make tyrosinase.[34]

Hair Formation

Hair originates in the hair follicle, illustrated in Figure 28-3, and the two may be considered one structure. The hair bulb lies at the lower end of the follicle and encloses an ovoid, vascular papilla of connective tissue. The matrix cells of the bulb surround the papilla as it juts upward into the bulb. When the hair and inner sheath reach the external root sheath, the inner sheath disintegrates and the outer sheath begins to cornify. As the hair reaches the surface opening of the follicle, it is called a **hair shaft** and is a dead, cornified structure extending out from the follicle.

Attached to the hair follicle is the arrectores pilorum, a smooth muscle attached to the connective tissue hair sheath and inserted in the dermal papilla. Contraction of this muscle erects hair, squeezes out sebum, and creates gooseflesh in response to sensory input such as changes in room temperature or emotional state.

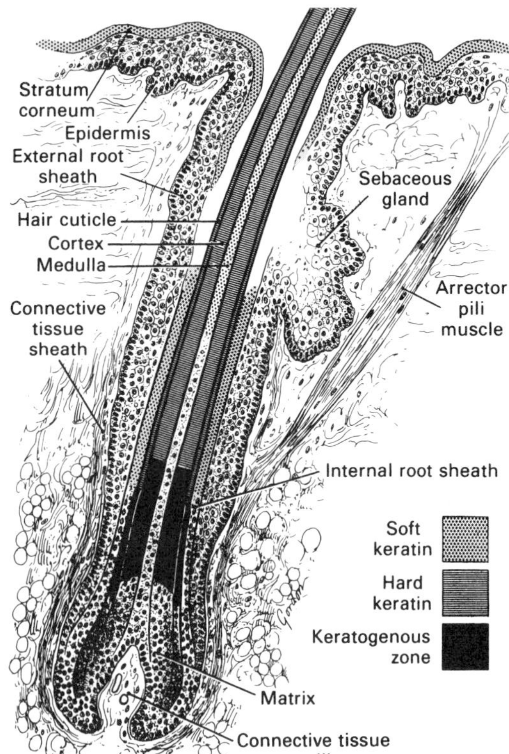

FIGURE 28-3. Parts of a hair follicle and location of sebaceous gland. (Cormack, D. H. [1993] *Essential histology*. Philadelphia: J. B. Lippincott.)

Hair Growth

The growth of hair occurs in cycles: *anagen*, growing; *catagen*, involuting; and *telogen*, resting. Each hair follicle operates independently; therefore, each hair may be in a different phase of the cycle from its neighbor.[17] The life cycle of hair through the three stages varies in different parts of the body. Scalp hair, which is in anagen from 3 to 10 years, in catagen for 3 weeks, and in telogen for 3 months, has the longest growth period of any hair on the body. The longer the growing period, the longer the hair. The phases of the hair cycle may be influenced by illness, which may change growing-phase hairs into resting-phase hairs that can be more easily lost or shed.[9]

In addition to cyclical growth, hair growth can be influenced by other factors such as overall health and hormonal changes within the body. For example, pubic and axillary hair develop during puberty in response to sex hormones.

NAILS

The nails are composed of specialized layers of epithelial cells and are protective coverings at the ends of the fingers and toes. The structure of a nail is illustrated in Figure 28-4. The rectangular nail plates on the dorsal surfaces of the ends of fingers and toes are composed of closely welded cells of cornified epithelium. They are semitransparent and allow the pink of the vascular nail bed to show. Each nail plate is surrounded by a fold of skin called the nail bed. The nail plate rests on top of the nail bed, where fibers attach the nail to the periosteum of the distal phalanx of each digit. The nail bed is abundant with blood vessels and sensory nerve endings. The distal edge of the nail is freely movable. The proximal edge is attached firmly at the base of the nail. The **lunula** is a white, half-moon-shaped area at the base of the nail and is the most actively growing portion of the nail. The epithelium in this area of the nail is thick, and the cells here become keratinized with harder keratin than that present in the hair or the epidermis. The soft cuticle that forms over the proximal nail plate is called the **eponychium**.

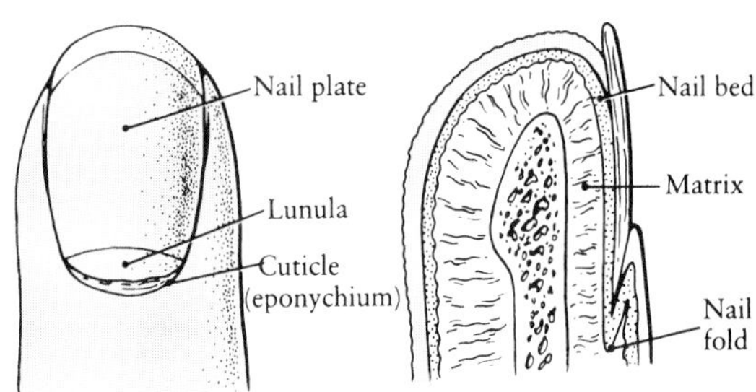

FIGURE 28-4. Structure of the nail in cross-section of a finger.

ABNORMAL CONDITIONS OF THE SKIN

Lesions, or abnormal changes in the appearance of the skin, can result from a wide variety of causative factors. Important aspects for determining the pathophysiology of skin disease include the following: (1) characteristics of the lesion (Table 28-3), (2) distribution/configuration of lesions (Table 28-4 presents descriptive terms), (3) length of time present and recurrence, (4) medications taken, both systemic and topical, (5) family history of disease, and 6) environmental or personal exposure to hazardous material. Table 28-3 lists the basic nomenclature used to describe lesions. Figure 28-5 shows the appearance of various lesions. Description of a lesion may require a combination of these terms. The following sections of this chapter will discuss common inflammations, infections, tumors, and traumatic alterations of the skin.

TABLE 28-3

CHARACTERISTICS AND NOMENCLATURE OF SKIN LESIONS

LESION	DESCRIPTION
Blister	Fluid-filled vesicle or bulla
Bulla	Blister larger than 1.0 cm
Comedo	Plugged and dilated pore, called blackhead or whitehead
Crust	Dried exudate over a damaged epithelium; may be associated with vesicle, bullae, or pustules
Cyst	Semisolid or fluid-filled mass, encapsulated in deeper layers of skin
Desquamation	Shedding or loss of debris on skin surface
Erosion	Loss of epidermis; may be associated with vesicles, bullae, or pustules
Excoriation	Epidermal erosion usually caused by scratching
Fissure	Crack in the epidermis usually extending into the dermis
Macule	Flat area of skin with discoloration, less than 5 mm in diameter
Nodule	Solid, elevated lesion or mass, 5 mm to 5 cm in diameter
Papule	Solid, elevated lesion less than 5 mm in diameter
Plaque	Raised, flattened lesion greater than 5 mm in diameter
Pustule	Papule containing purulent exudate
Scale	Skin debris on the surface of the epidermis
Tumor	Solid mass, larger than 5 cm in diameter; usually extends to dermis
Ulceration	Loss of epidermis, extending into dermis or deeper
Urticarial	Raised wheal-like lesion
Vesicle	Small fluid-filled lesion, less than 1 cm in diameter
Wheal	Transient, irregular pink elevation with surrounding edema

TABLE 28-4

DISTRIBUTION/CONFIGURATION OF SKIN LESIONS

TERM	DEFINITION
Annular	Circular
Confluent	Lesions run together
Discrete	Separate lesions
Grouped	Clusters of lesions
Linear	Line, i.e., scar
Zosteriform	Along nerve root

Inflammations

When skin cells are injured, an inflammatory response is initiated. This is usually caused by physical agents such as heat, cold, radiation, or mechanical trauma. Inflammation is often incorrectly used as a synonym for infection. Inflammation is always present with infection; however, infection is not always present with inflammation. An inflammation of the skin typically includes a reddened appearance and often involves swelling of the skin.

URTICARIA

Urticaria is a vascular reaction, also referred to as hives or wheals. It is an erythematous or white, nonpitting, edematous plaque that changes in size and shape during the few hours or days that the lesion exists. These hives result from localized capillary vasodilation, followed by transudation of protein-rich fluid into the surrounding tissue. They resolve when these fluids are slowly reabsorbed. A reddened halo often surrounds the raised hive or wheal.[16] Urticaric lesions are usually pruritic and may cause a stinging sensation.

Acute urticaria can be defined as a cutaneous vascular reaction that evolves over a short period, from days to several weeks, and usually has a detectable cause. It resolves completely. Urticaria lasting longer than 6 weeks is classified as chronic urticaria. It may persist for years; it also may go away and then recur. The underlying cause of chronic urticaria is usually unknown. The etiologies of both types of urticaria are numerous and are summarized in Table 28-5.

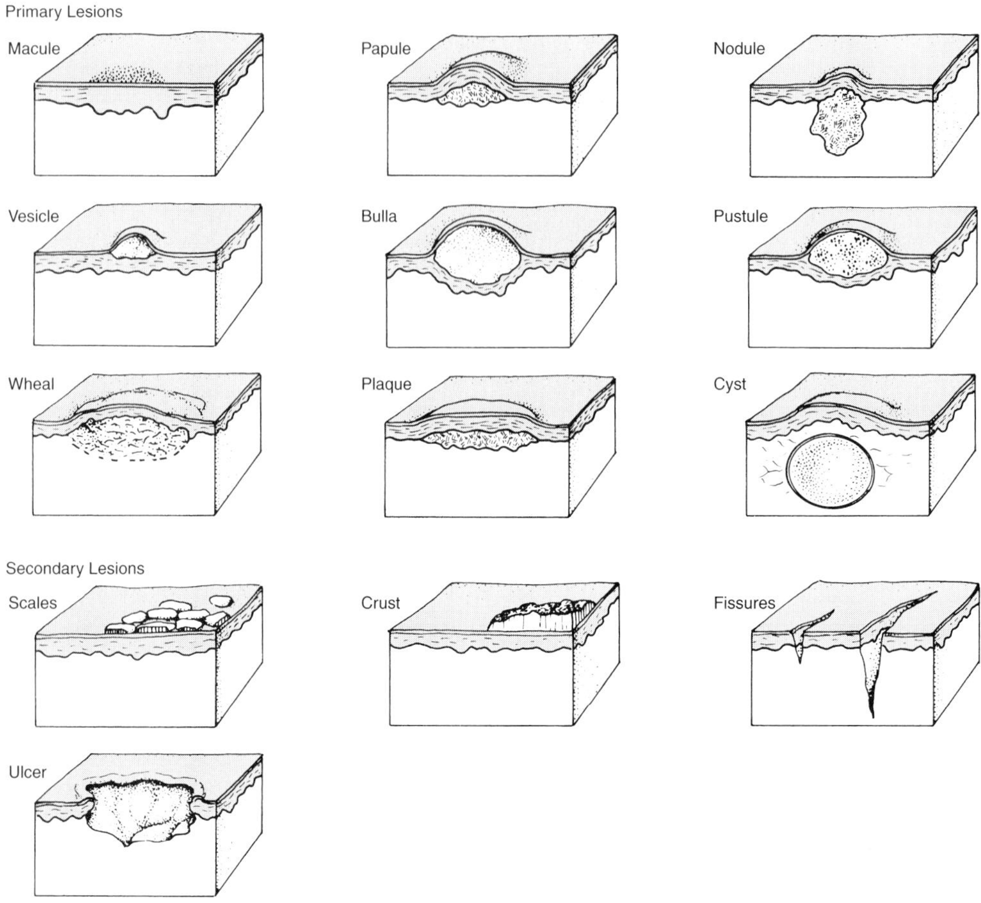

FIGURE 28-5. Types of skin lesions. (Smeltzer, S.C, & Bare, B.G. [1996]. *Brunner and Suddarth's textbook of medical-surgical nursing* [8th ed.]. Philadelphia: Lippincott.)

ANGIOEDEMA

Angioedema is a reaction that involves edema not only of the superficial skin but also of the subcutaneous tissues in response to allergens or environmental changes. Angioedema can be described as giant wheals, or raised, itching lesions. Inflammatory involvement often includes the mucous membranes. It can cause many physical symptoms, including severe respiratory distress if the larynx is affected.

CHRONIC DRY SKIN

Dry skin in itself is a noninflammatory condition, but it can become reddened when it persists unrelieved. This common defect of chronic dry skin, which occurs often in the aging process, involves loss of water, electrolytes, and skin lipids. It occurs often in dry and cold climates, and environmental conditions aggravate the condition if it previously existed. This dehydration causes drying of the surface keratin and consists of roughened, flaky skin with or without pruritus. Itching and inflammatory changes can be superimposed.[16]

ACNE

Acne vulgaris is a common, chronic inflammatory disease of the sebaceous glands and hair follicles of the skin, also known as the **pilosebaceous ducts**. It is pictured in Figure 28-6. The exact cause of acne is unknown, but it may be due to either increased activity of the sebaceous glands or inability of the material secreted to escape through a narrow opening.

Pathophysiology

Acne results from two pathophysiologic factors: (1) accumulation of sebum, the fatty secretion liberated by the breakdown of sebaceous cells, and (2) irritation of the area around the hair follicle, leading to a **perifolliculitis**. The resulting inflammation is precipitated by the combination of sebum, bacteria, and subsequent release of fatty acids. The release of fatty acids is caused by the hydrolytic action of the lipases,

TABLE 28-5

ETIOLOGIES OF URTICARIA

CATEGORY	EXAMPLES
Foods	Fish, shellfish, nuts, eggs, chocolate, strawberries, tomatoes, port, cow's milk cheese, wheat, yeast
Food additives	Salicylates, dyes such as tartrazine, benzoates, penicillin. Aspartame (NutraSweet) probably does not cause hives. Sulfites.
Drugs	Penicillin, aspirin, sulfonamides, and drugs that cause a non-immunologic release of histamine (e.g., morphine, codeine, polymyxin, dextran, curare, quinine)
Infections	Chronic bacterial infections (e.g., sinus, dental, chest, gallbladder, urinary tract), *Campylobacter enteritis,* fungal infections (dermatophytosis, candidiasis), viral infections (hepatitis B prodromal reaction, infections mononucleosis, coxsackie), protozoal and helminthic infections (intestinal worms, malaria)
Inhalants	Pollens, mold spores, animal danders, house dust, aerosols, volatile chemicals
Internal disease	Serum sickness, systemic lupus erythematosus, hyperthyroidism, autoimmune thyroid disease, carcinomas, lymphomas, juvenile rheumatoid arthritis (Still's disease), leukocytoclastic vasculitis, polycythemia vera (ache urticaria—urticarial papule surmounted by a vesicle), rheumatic fever, some blood transfusion reactions
Physical stimuli (the physical urticarias)	Dermographism, pressure urticaria, cholinergic urticaria, exercise-induced anaphylactic syndrome, solar urticaria, cold urticaria, heat vibratory, water (aquagenic)
Nonimmunologic contact urticaria	Plants (nettles), animals (caterpillars, jellyfish), medications (cinnamic aldehyde, compound 48/80, dimethyl sulfoxide)
Immunologic or uncertain mechanism contact urticaria	Ammonium persulfate used in hair bleaches, chemicals, foods, textiles, wood, saliva, cosmetics, perfumes, bacitracin
Skin diseases	Urticaria pigmentosa (mastocytosis), dermatitis herpetiformis, pemphigoid, amyloidosis
Hormones	Pregnancy, premenstrual flare-ups (progesterone)
Genetic, autosomal dominant (all rare)	Hereditary angioedema, cholinergic urticaria with progressive nerve deafness, amyloidosis of the kidney, familial cold urticaria, vibratory urticaria

which are furnished by the bacteria on the sebum itself. The inflammatory reaction and resulting edema probably cause the sebaceous follicle to perforate its wall and develop perifolliculitis. The development of acne depends on several factors, including heredity, use of oil-based cosmetics or skin treatments, ingestion of drugs (e.g., steroids, androgens), and the presence of bacteria. Hormones influence sebaceous gland secretion. Psychological situations of increased stress that enhances secretion of adrenal androgens results in increased secretion of sebaceous glands and subsequent acne.

Clinical Manifestations

Acne lesions are located in the areas of predominant pilosebaceous glands—the face, chest, back, neck, and upper arms. The early, noninflammatory lesions are of two types, white (closed) and black comedones. The white comedo occurs in a closed excretory duct that has a very small, possibly microscopic, opening that prevents drainage. This lesion may lead to an inflammatory process and give rise to a papule or pustule. The black comedo (blackhead) is a widely dilated follicle filled with oxidized melanin that plugs an excretory duct of the skin.[28] Both types of lesions obstruct the emptying of sebum to the surface and may develop into small papules, pustules, nodules, or cysts. Most pustules and cysts eventually open, drain, and heal. If severe, these lesions may result in scarring. Black comedones are less likely to result in inflammation.[16] The prevalence of acne is increased during adolescence and early adulthood, but it is usually self-limited.

ACUTE ECZEMATOUS DERMATITIS

Dermatitis and **eczema** are words that are often used interchangeably. They constitute the superficial inflammatory diseases of the skin. There are five major classifications of eczematous dermatitis: contact dermatitis (Fig. 28-7), drug-related eczematous dermatitis, photoeczematous dermatitis, primary irritant

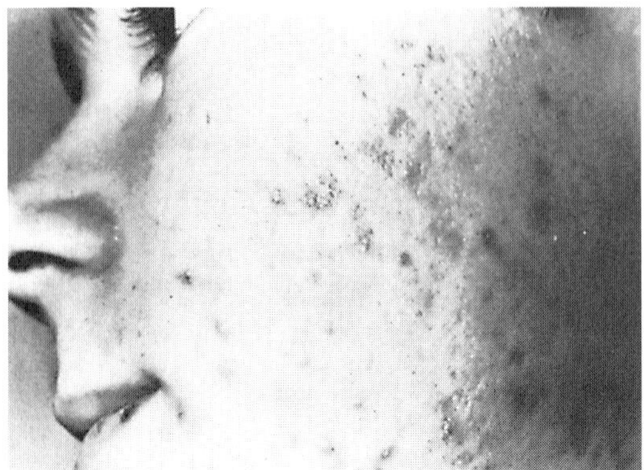

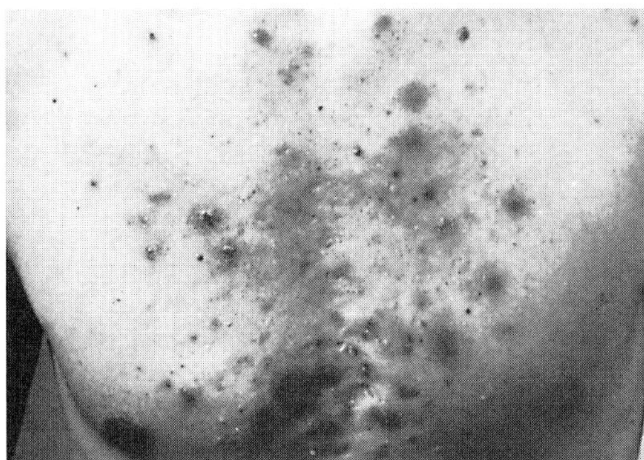

FIGURE 28-6. Acne of the face and chest. (Sauer, G. C. [1996]. *Manual of skin diseases* [7th ed.]. Philadelphia: J. B. Lippincott.)

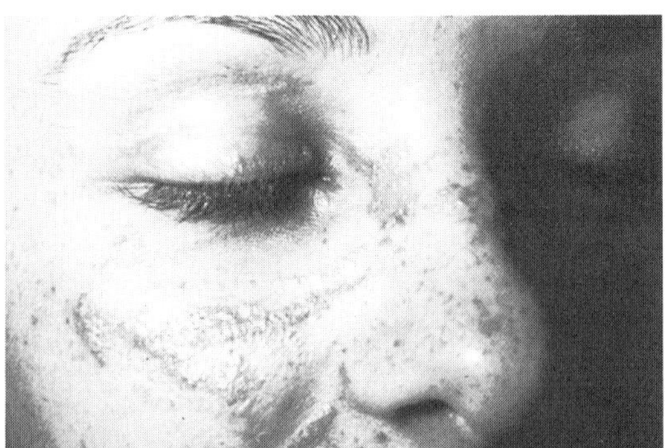

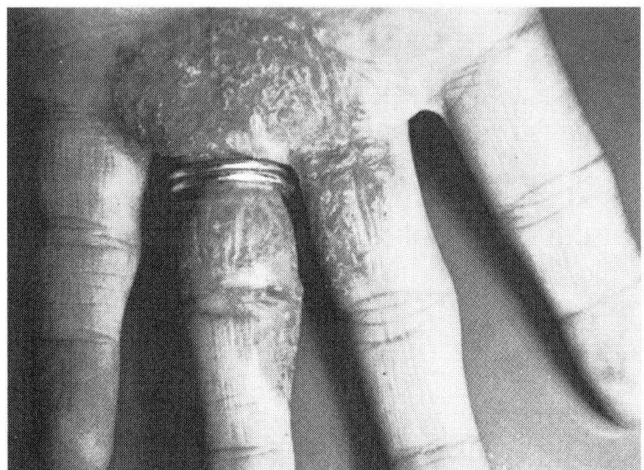

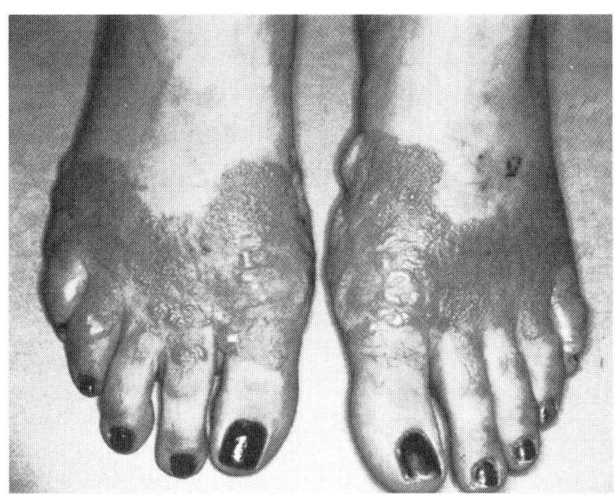

FIGURE 28-7. Contact dermatitis. (Sauer, G. C. [1996]. *Manual of skin diseases* [7th ed.]. Philadelphia: J. B. Lippincott.)

dermatitis, and atopic dermatitis. The cause or pathogenesis and clinical features for each classification are identified in Table 28-6.

Infections

Infections of the skin involve invasion of skin tissues and cells by microorganisms such as viruses, bacteria, or fungi.

VIRAL INFECTIONS OF THE SKIN

Most common viral infections involving the skin are summarized in Table 28-7. Characteristics of herpes zoster and simplex vary significantly and are further highlighted in Figure 28-8. Warts, also caused by viral infections, are discussed below.

Warts, or **verrucae**, are caused by localized viral infections of the skin or mucous membranes by one of over 60 different types of DNA containing human papilloma-viruses (HPV). There are three main types: verruca vulgaris (common wart), verruca plantaris (plantar wart), and condyloma acuminatum (venereal wart). The etiology of warts is not clearly understood, but they can be transmitted by contact from person to person. They are benign lesions and frequently occur at sites of injury or along a break in the skin.

The following are variations of warts:

- *Verruca vulgaris*, common warts, are typically single or multiple, raised, well-circumscribed, flesh-colored, dome-shaped growth with a rough surface. They can occur anywhere but are most often present on the hands.
- *Verruca plantaris* differs from the common wart by its location and the effect that pressure has on the le-

TABLE 28-6

CLASSIFICATION OF ECZEMATOUS DERMATITIS

TYPE	CAUSE OR PATHOGENESIS	CLINICAL FEATURES
Contact dermatitis	*80% non-allergic or irritant:* Topically applied chemicals/ detergents *20% allergic:* Pathogenesis: delayed hypersensitivity	Marked itching or burning or both; requires antecedent exposure. Chronic: skin thickening
Atopic dermatitis (eczema)	Unknown, may be heritable	Erythematous plaques in flexural areas; family history of eczema, hay fever, or asthma
Drug-related eczematous dermatitis	Systemically administered antigens or haptens (e.g., penicillin)	Eruption occurs with administration of drug; remits when drug is discontinued
Photoeczematous eruption	Ultraviolet light	Occurs on sun-exposed skin; phototesting may help in diagnosis
Primary irritant dermatitis	Repeated trauma (rubbing)	Localized to site of trauma

sion. The wart tends to grow on the soles of the feet, and pain is frequent due to the irritation of walking. As a result, the wart tends to grow inward.

- *Condylomata acuminata* are lesions established primarily in warm, moist anogenital areas. Also known as venereal warts, they may or may not stem from sexual contact. They are large, pinkish or purplish projections with a rough surface.

BACTERIAL INFECTIONS OF THE SKIN

Impetigo

Impetigo is an acute bacterial infection occurring frequently in children and often in persons in ill health. Causative organisms include group A beta-hemolytic streptococci and coagulase-positive staphylococci. Impetigo is autoinoculable and can be transmitted among humans. Influencing factors include poor hygiene, tropical climates, and improper sanitation. Impetigo occurs superficially on the skin as serous and purulent vesicles that later rupture and form a golden crust. A common location for lesions is the face, but they may involve the extremities or buttocks.[14] A serious complication is glomerulonephritis, which may not be prevented by antibiotic treatment.

Folliculitis

Folliculitis is a bacterial infection of the skin that originates within the hair follicle. Staphylococci are the usual causative organisms. Predisposing factors include poor hygiene and maceration. Immunosuppressed persons or those with diabetes mellitus have a greater incidence of severe outbreaks of this condition.[14] Folliculitis appears as a pustule located at the opening of the hair follicle, predominantly on the scalp and extremities. The basic lesion is a reddened macule or papule surrounding the hair follicle. Folliculitis can extend into the hair bulb and the deeper skin layers if not treated promptly.

Furuncles and Carbuncles

Furuncles, also known as boils, frequently develop from a preceding staphylococcal folliculitis and are usually located in body areas containing hair follicles. Irritation, maceration, and lack of good hygiene are predisposing factors in their development. The lesions are nodules that are usually tender and red. They frequently remain tense for days and produce throbbing pain and severe tenderness. These nodules become fluctuant with abscess formation, which later drains a necrotic plug and purulent drainage.[14] **Carbuncles** are large staphylococcal abscesses that are similar to that of a furuncle and are composed of several adjacent furuncles. The etiology of carbuncles is the same as that for furuncles. Carbuncles appear as a cluster of furuncles and may be quite painful. They are often located on the back or neck area or in skin folds (intertriginous areas).

FUNGAL DISEASES OF THE SKIN

Fungal diseases of the skin can be classified in three groups: superficial, intermediate, and deep. The superficial diseases result in ringworm (tinea capitis), athlete's foot (tinea pedis), "jock itch" (tinea cruris), and tinea versicolor. Table 28-8 highlights the location and specific clinical manifestations of each of these superficial

(text continues on page 852)

TABLE 28-7

SUMMARY OF VIRAL INFECTIONS OF THE SKIN

VIRAL INFECTION	ETIOLOGY	INCUBATION PERIOD	EPIDEMIOLOGY	NATURE OF RASH	OTHER SIGNS AND SYMPTOMS
Herpes simplex	HSV (Herpes-viridae) Types 1 and 2	Lesions last approximately 7–14 days	Childhood: usually HSV-1 with oropharyngeal entry Adults: usually HSV-2 with sexual transmission Neonatal: usually HSV-2 acquired during vaginal delivery; life threatening in newborns	Clear fluid-filled vesicles, in clusters on erythematous base, progressive to crusted lesions	Pain, visceral involvement
Varicella (chicken-pox)	VZV (Herpes-viridae)	10–20 days from exposure to appearance of vesicles	Epidermis: fall–spring preschool and school-aged children most often infected; close-contact transmission	Vesicular lesions on erythematous base, progressing to pustular, then crusted lesions; distribution usually on face, scalp, trunk, and arms	Mild fever, malaise, pruritus, anorexia, listlessness
Herpes zoster (Shingles)	VZV Latent form after primary varicella infection	Pain usually precedes lesions by 1–2 days, vesicles crust and clear in about 3 weeks	Most often occurs in elderly population, but can occur in any age group	Papules, vesicles, pustules on an inflammatory base in a dermatomal distribution (see Fig. 28-8)	Burning pain and tenderness
Erythema infectiosum (fifth disease)	Parvo virus	4–14 days	Outbreaks in elementary and junior high schools; household spread common; the virus may cause illness in people of all ages, from fetus to elderly	Macular erythemic rash, symmetric; intensely red, flushed "slapped cheeks" appearance; spreads to arms, trunk, buttocks and thighs	Low-grade fever in 15–30% of patients, prodromal headache, URI symptoms
Roseola (sixth disease) Exanthum Subitum	Human herpesvirus 6	Approximately 9 days, usually spring and summer	Highest attack rate in children 6–24 months of age; rare under 3 months or after 4 years	Rash immediately, follows defervescence, erythematous maculopapular rash on trunk, spreads to face and legs (lacy looking)	Fever, seizures, adenopathy, respiratory signs and symptoms, mild diarrhea, pharyngitis

TABLE 28-7

SUMMARY OF VIRAL INFECTIONS OF THE SKIN (Continued)

VIRAL INFECTION	ETIOLOGY	INCUBATION PERIOD	EPIDEMIOLOGY	NATURE OF RASH	OTHER SIGNS AND SYMPTOMS
Rubeola (measles)	Paramyxovirus	10–15 days, usually winter and spring	Highly contagious childhood illness, spread by respiratory droplet aerosols produced by sneezing or cough	Maculopapular rash appears first along hairline, on neck and behind the ears, spreads rapidly over face and proceeds downward; may be hemorrhagic or purpuric	High fever, chills photophobia, cough, conjunctivitis; pathognomic enanthem—Koplik's spots (blue/white spots) on buccal mucosa before rash erupts
Rubella (German measles)	Togaviridal range	14–21 days	Peak incidence in late winter/ early spring; affects children under 10 years, occasional cases in young adults; very serious in pregnant women, especially in first trimester, transmission results in fetal anomalies	Maculopapular, nonconfluent, erythematous eruption evolves over 12–24 hours and lasts 3–5 days; begins on face and progresses downward	Adenopathy, fever, low-grade
Molluscum contagiosum	Poxviridae; molluscipoxvirus genus	Estimated to be between 2 weeks and 6 months	Has become a common infection in patients and acquired immunodeficiency syndrome; spread through contact with infected persons, contaminated objects and through inoculation; affects school-aged children; has been associated with contact sports Adults: sexual transmission	Pearly, umbilicated, dome-shaped papules with a smooth glistening surface, often confused with vesicles; in children lesions occur on face, trunk; and extremities; in young adults lesions occur in genital area and adjacent skin; self limiting in immunocompetent patients	Surrounding dermatitis, eyelid lesions may be associated with 2-hour conjunctivitis

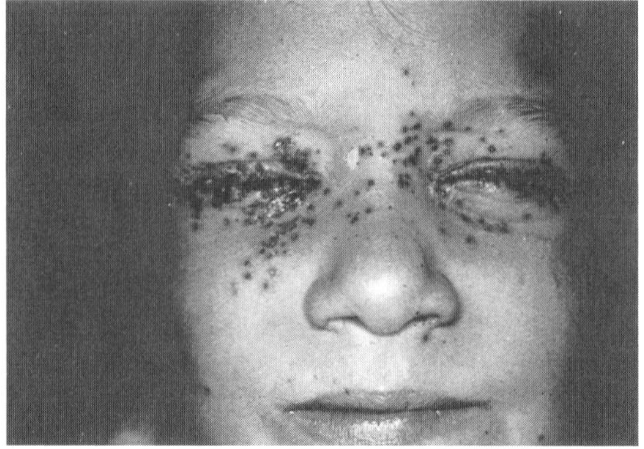

(**A**) Primary herpes simplex around the eyes in a 5-year-old child

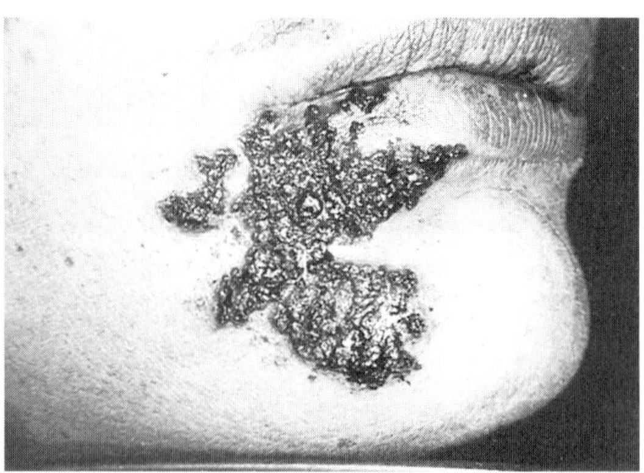

(**B**) Recurrent herpes simplex on chin with secondary bacterial infection

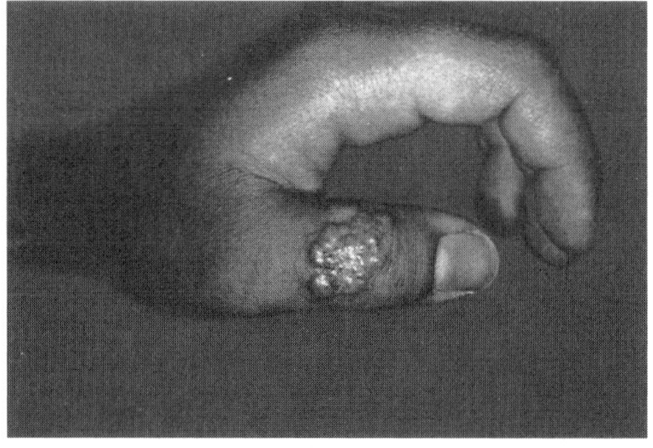

(**C**) Recurrent herpes simplex on a thumb

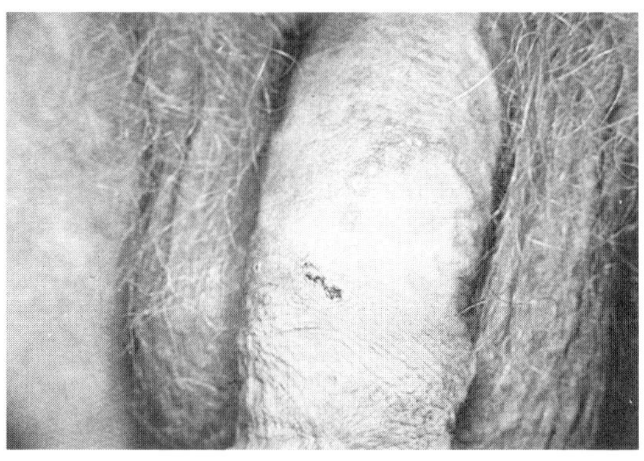

(**D**) Recurrent herpes simplex on the penis

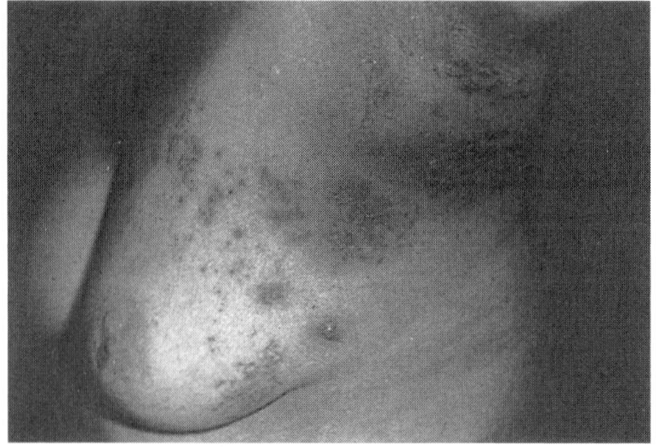

(**E**) Herpes zoster of left breast area

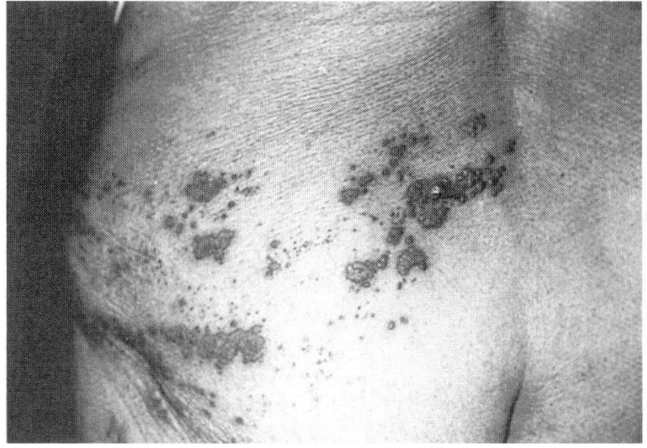

(**F**) Hemorrhagic zoster of the left hip area

FIGURE 28-8. Herpes simplex and zoster. (Sauer, G. C. [1996] *Manual of skin diseases* [7th ed.]. Philadelphia: J. B. Lippincott.)

fungal diseases of the skin. Dermatophytes (fungal parasites) are responsible for most skin, nail, and hair fungal infections. There is evidence that genetic susceptibility may predispose a patient to dermatophyte infection. Clinical manifestations common to all superficial fungal infections include itching; presence of vesicles within a raised, red border; and scaling of the skin. Moisture, heat, and maceration are predisposing factors for growth; consequently, lesions appear in areas between toes, the axillae, nails, and groin.

Intermediate fungal diseases invade both the superficial and deeper tissues. Moniliasis caused by *Candida*

TABLE 28-8

SUPERFICIAL FUNGAL INFECTIONS

CLINICAL NAME	COMMON NAME	LOCATION	SPECIFIC CLINICAL MANIFESTATIONS
Tinea capitis	Ringworm of the scalp	Scalp	Raised red or white areas, hair loss
Tinea corporis	Ringworm of the body	Body, trunk, and extremities	Well-demarcated annular lesions with raised red borders
Tinea pedis	Athlete's foot	Feet	Inflamed skin of toe webbing and soles of feet with skin flaking and exfoliation
Tinea cruris	Jock itch	Genital area	Bright-red, raised lesions of groin, scrotum, or anal area
Tinea versicolor	(NONE)	Trunk, extremities	Yellow or tan patches on body
Onychomycosis	Nail fungus	Fingernails, toenails	Thickened, flaking nail with inflamed paronychium

albicans is an example. Pregnancy, oral contraceptives, antibiotic therapy, diabetes or other endocrine disorders, skin maceration, steroid therapy, or any immunocompromised state may allow the yeast to become pathogenic and produce deep invasion.

Deep fungal infections invade deeper structures of living tissue such as muscle and bone and include diseases such as sporotrichosis, candidiasis, histoplasmosis, and aspergillosis.

Scaling Disorders of the Skin

PSORIASIS

Psoriasis is a chronic, genetically determined disease of epidermal proliferation. Psoriasis infects persons of all ages, affecting 1.5% to 2.0% of the population in Western countries. The precise etiology is not known, but genetic and environmental factors are important in its development. It is viewed as a chronic disease with much diversity in its location, severity, and frequency. Exacerbating factors include local trauma, overexposure to the sun, infection, stress, physical illness, and several drugs.[14] Psoriasis may be associated with arthritis. Alcohol abuse, smoking, and lack of exercise have been considered as risk factors for psoriasis.[12] It is pictured in Figure 28-9. The increased cell turnover rate and production of immature cells result in the classic features of sharply marginated erythematous plaques covered by silvery white, loosely adherent scales.[14] Psoriasis is often distributed over the knees, elbows, scalp, and lumbosacral skin. When involved, the nails show pitting and dimpling. A serious but rare condition known as *pustular psoriasis* also can occur, causing sterile pustules, high fever, elevated white blood cell count, electrolyte imbalance, and malaise. This condition can be fatal.

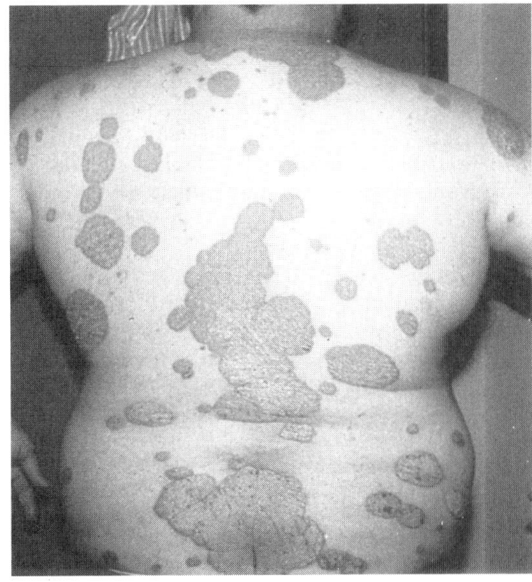

FIGURE 28-9. A patient with psoriasis shows large, confluent, sharply demarcated, erythematous plaques on the trunk. (Rubin, E., & Farber, J. L. [1999]. *Pathology* [3rd ed.]. Philadelphia: Lippincott Williams & Wilkins.)

PITYRIASIS ROSEA

Pityriasis rosea is a common, acute disease of the skin, usually affecting adolescents and young adults. Its course is self-limited and is thought to be infectious, possibly caused by a virus. The etiology is unknown.

Clinical manifestations often arise after a prodrome of malaise, fatigue, and headache. The first lesion, known as the **herald patch**, is a single, oval, ringlike plaque, usually seen on the trunk (Figure 28-10). This lesion is later followed by lesions that are usually flat, erythematous patches covered by fine scales that resemble the primary plaque but are smaller. Lesions are often pruritic. Distribution is commonly on the neck, trunk, and arms.

Skin Tumors

Skin tumors, like all tumors, are of two basic categories, benign and malignant. Benign tumors are slow growing, and growth may stop entirely. Malignant lesions show disorganization and abnormalities. They may grow rapidly and infiltrate surrounding tissues. Metastasis may occur, depending on the origin of the tumor. The occurrence of both benign and malignant skin tumors is correlated with sunlight exposure. Two types of ultraviolet (UV) rays may cause cellular genetic damage and therefore cause the growth and replication of abnormal skin cells. UVA rays penetrate deeply. They cause tanning and wrinkling but are less strongly associated with the development of skin lesions. UVB rays have a shallow penetration and are most significantly implicated in the development of skin cancers.

BENIGN TUMORS

Seborrheic Keratosis

Seborrheic keratosis is the most common benign epithelial tumor in the elderly. These lesions are hereditary and usually do not appear until around 30 years of age.[14] A strong predisposing factor is prolonged exposure to the sun. Figure 28-11 shows the skin lesion is slightly raised, light brown, and sharply demarcated; pigmentation may deepen and the skin may become thick. Early lesions are usually small (1.0–3.0 mm) and are a barely elevated papule with or without pigment. Late lesions resemble a plaque with a warty surface and have a "stuck on, greasy" appearance. These are usually nodules from 1.0 to 6.0 cm in diameter.[14] Locations include the trunk, shoulders, face, and scalp. Malignant transformation is uncommon.

Hemangioma

A **hemangioma** is an idiopathic, benign tumor of newly formed blood vessels. There are many different types. A *strawberry hemangioma* frequently appears as a dome-shaped, fully red, soft lesion with sharply demarcated edges. It tends to grow slowly and usually regresses completely.

The *nevus flammeus* (ordinary birthmark) is a congenital vascular malformation that occurs in approximately one third of all infants as a light pink to dark purple patch on the nape of the neck and tends to regress spontaneously.[14] The *port wine stain* is usually on the face and unilateral. Port wine stains do not regress spontaneously and tend to grow with the child and can cause significant cosmetic disfigurement. *Cavernous hemangiomas* are deep, vascular malformations that may occur in both the skin and subcutaneous tissues. The features of the lesions depend on their extent, varying from round to flat and from bright red to deep purple.

Keratoacanthoma

Keratoacanthoma is a firm, raised nodule with a central keratin plug, often occurring on the face. It is typically seen on sun-exposed skin of persons over 50 years of age.[14] It resembles squamous cell carcinoma

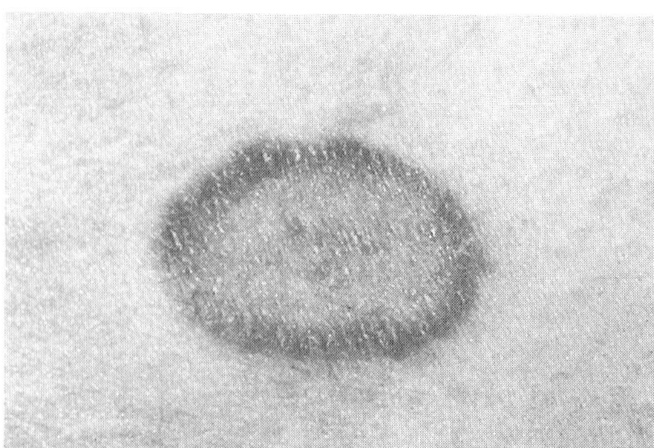

FIGURE 28-10. The herald patch of pityriasis rosea. (© Dr. H. C. Robinson/SPL/Science Source/Photo Researchers.)

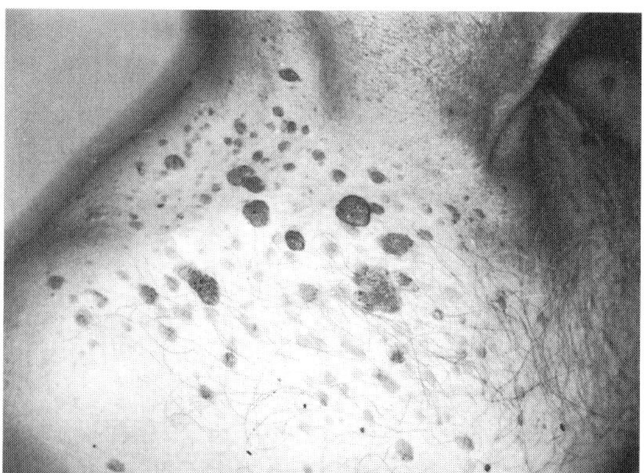

FIGURE 28-11. Seborrheic keratoses on the neck. (Sauer, G. C. [1996]. *Manual of skin diseases* [7th ed.]. Philadelphia: Lippincott-Raven.)

in appearance; however, keratocanthomas usually subside spontaneously.

Actinic or Solar Keratosis

Actinic keratoses (AKs) are the most common premalignant lesions. Lesions are sharply demarcated, rough, red, yellow to brown, or gray (Fig. 28-12). AKs are better recognized by palpation than by inspection. At high risk for developing this condition are fair-skinned persons whose skin easily burns with sun exposure. Induration or inflammation suggest possible development into malignancy.[16] Age of onset is related to the amount of sun exposure. AKs sometimes undergo remission if sunlight exposure is reduced.

Leukoplakia, actinic keratosis of the mucous membranes, is a common premalignant lesion, occurring most often in elderly women. This lesion is usually caused by exposure to chemical or mechanical irritants such as cigarette smoking or intraoral smokeless tobacco. It appears as a whitish patch on the mucosa of the oral cavity that cannot be rubbed off.[14]

MALIGNANT DISORDERS

Malignant disorders of the skin include basal cell carcinoma, squamous cell carcinoma, and malignant melanoma.

Basal Cell Carcinoma

Basal cell carcinoma is the most common type of skin cancer and occurs almost exclusively in whites. Most basal cell carcinomas arise from the epidermis and hair follicles on the head and neck. They tend to occur mainly in older persons, and most lesions appear with cumulative, prolonged exposure to the sun.[10] Persons who have had radiation therapy for breast, lung, or other types of internal malignancies have an increased risk. These common tumors are slow growing; although they rarely metastasize, treatment is necessary because they are capable of significant local destruction and disfigurement.

Characteristically, the carcinoma has a smooth surface with a pearly border, often with ulceration of its center (Fig. 28-13). Usually, numerous localized groups of dilated, small blood vessels are visible.[10]

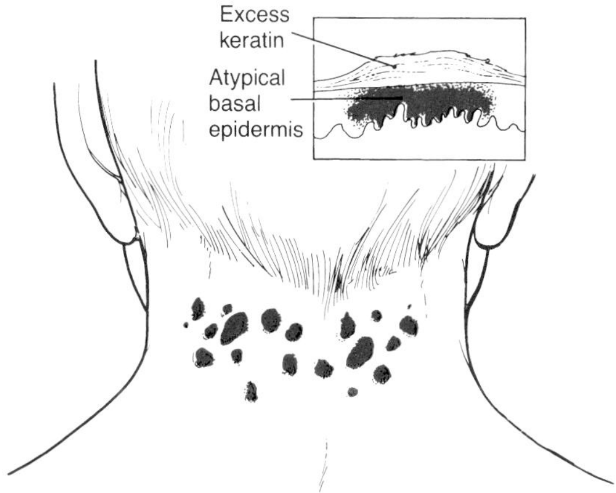

FIGURE 28-12. Actinic keratoses are often seen on the back of the neck.

Squamous Cell Carcinoma

Squamous cell carcinoma is a malignant lesion that can affect both the skin and mucous membranes. It most frequently occurs in sun-damaged areas of the body or areas exposed to irradiation or burns. The squamous cell carcinoma may also arise in scars, chronic ulcers, fistulas, and sinuses. Scars from burns may serve as an initiator, or co-carcinogen, in the production of these malignancies.[10] Characteristically, the carcinoma appears as a rough, hyperkeratotic nodule with an indurated base. It may ulcerate and can metastasize.

Malignant Melanoma

Malignant melanoma is a cancer arising from the melanin-producing cells. It is associated with a high risk for invasion and metastasis. Risk of developing some forms of the disease is increased with exposure to the sun. The worldwide frequency of this malignancy is rising more rapidly than any other cancer except lung cancer in women. The at-risk populations are all male or female persons with fair complexions that are more likely to sunburn than to tan after even brief exposure to sun, and persons with a family history of melanoma.[21] Melanoma occurs most frequently in young and middle-aged adults.

The most common location in men is the trunk and in women the legs.[3,21] The tumors exhibit variable colors and irregular borders and surfaces. Tumors may be brown or black with shades of red, white, or blue. Growth of melanoma lesions is generally rapid. Figure 28-14 shows a classic example of malignant melanoma.

The precursor lesions to melanomas are the congenital nevus and the dysplastic nevus. The congenital nevus rarely becomes malignant if it is small (less than 1.5 cm in diameter). Large congenital nevi (larger than 20 cm in diameter) have a 5% to 20% risk of becoming malignant.[31] All suspicious nevi should be inspected regularly, and self-examination should be taught. Dysplastic nevi are usually larger lesions of various colors with irregular borders and sometimes a central papule. These often appear late in childhood or adolescence but may appear after the age of 35. When these develop in fair-skinned persons, they will more likely develop into melanoma than will the congenital nevi.

Melanomas are of various types, with the most common being the *superficial spreading melanoma.* This melanoma usually arises within a nevus. Other types are described and compared in Table 28-9. Staging systems allow for grouping tumors for prognostic

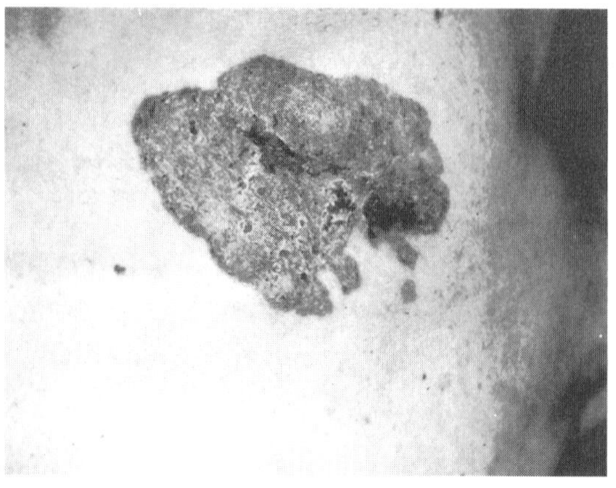

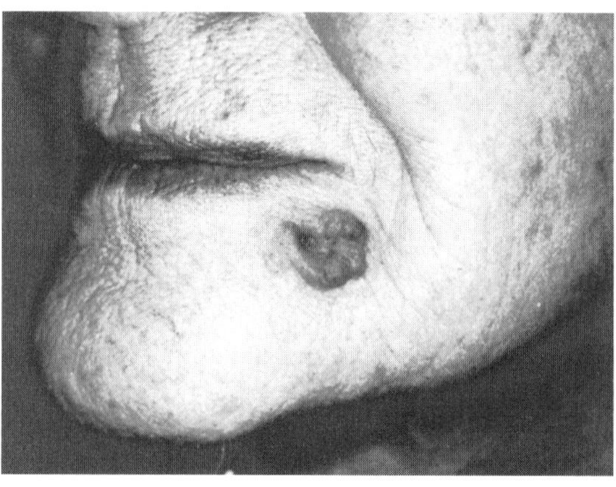

A B

FIGURE 28-13. **A.** A large superficial basal cell carcinoma on the back. **B.** Basal cell carcinoma on the chin. (Sauer, G. C. [1996]. *Manual of skin diseases* [7th ed.]. Philadelphia: Lippincott-Raven.)

and treatment purposes. Prognosis depends on the stage of the malignant melanoma at diagnosis. Most melanomas are highly invasive and spread rapidly to the lymphatic system, followed by metastasis to any organ of the body. Table 28-10 displays the four-stage classification system, the most widely used system for staging melanoma. Melanoma invasiveness is guided by "Clark's levels," shown in Box 28-2.

Traumatic Alterations in the Skin

BURNS

Burns are suffered by approximately 2 million persons annually, of which 60,000 persons require hospitalization and 6,000 die.[15] Burn injuries occur in every age group and both sexes. When they occur, they involve not only the skin tissue but also all of the systems of the body. The depth of thermal injuries depends on the burning agent, temperature, and length of exposure to the heat. Flames, scalds, chemicals, and electricity are the major causes of burns. No matter what the cause of burn injury, the local and systemic pathophysiologic alterations are similar.[2] Electrical and chemical burns have unique clinical considerations and are specifically discussed later in this chapter. The equilibrium point for skin is approximately 44°C (111.2°F). This temperature can be tolerated for up to 6 hours without burning. The rate of skin destruction doubles with each degree rise, so that at 70°C (158°F), fleeting exposure will produce total epidermal necrosis.[23]

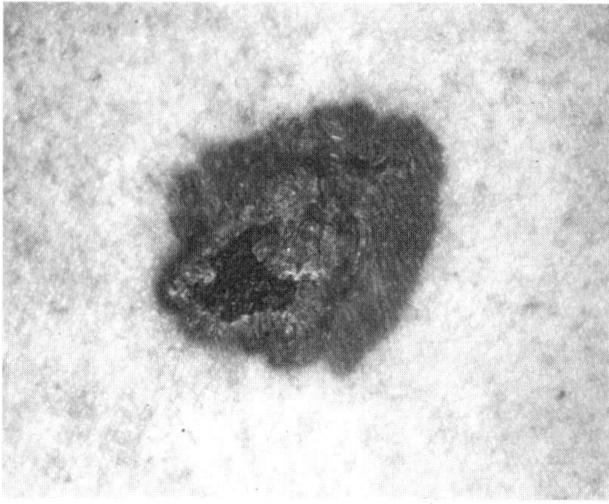

FIGURE 28-14. Malignant melanoma in a nevus present since birth on the scapular area. (Sauer, G. C. [1996]. *Manual of skin diseases* [7th ed.]. Philadelphia: Lippincott-Raven.)

Burns are classified as (1) superficial partial thickness, (2) deep partial thickness, and (3) full thickness. These are described further in Table 28-11. The depth of injury is often difficult to assess in the initial postburn period due to the changing hemodynamics. The classic rule of nines illustrated in Figure 28-15 has been a standard for estimating total body surface area burned.

A major burn injury is the ultimate trauma and is typically an unexpected injury that profoundly affects all major body systems. The extent of injury is directly related to (1) the depth and (2) body surface area involvement of the burn.

Localized Manifestations of Burn Injury

The most obvious body system affected is the integumentary system (although these effects are not usually the most life threatening). The functions of the skin (i.e., providing a protective barrier, regulating body temperature, and indicating nutritional and metabolic health) must be considered when a burn injury has occurred. All of these functions are altered. When

TABLE 28-9

COMPARISON OF CLINICAL FEATURES OF CUTANEOUS MELANOMA

TYPES OF MELANOMA	FREQUENCY (%)	DURATION BEFORE DIAGNOSIS (YR)	MEAN AGE AT DIAGNOSIS (YR)	SITE	CLINICAL FEATURES
TYPES WITH RADIAL GROWTH PHASES					
Superficial spreading melanoma	70	1–7	Mid-40s	Any site; lower legs in females, back in both sexes	Raised border on palpation or inspection; pinks, whites, grays, and blues in brown lesion
Acral lentiginous melanoma (including subungual melanoma)	10	1–10	60s	Sole, palms, mucous membranes, subungual	Flat, irregular border; predominantly dark brown to black
Lentigo maligna melanoma	5	5–50	70s	Nose, cheeks, temples	Highly irregular border with areas of regression; brown-tan macular lesion with variation in pigment pattern; may be amelanotic
TYPES WITH NO RADIAL GROWTH PHASE					
Nodular melanoma	15	Months	Mid-to-late-40s	Any site	Nodule arises in apparently normal skin or in a nevus; brown to brown-black; may have bluish hues; may be amelanotic

(Modified from Langley, R. G. B., Fitzpatrick, T. B., & Sober, A. J. [1998]. *Clinical characteristics in malignant melanoma.* St. Louis: Quality Medical Publishing.)

skin is burned, many localized changes occur. There is significant thrombosis of all vessels and microvasculature in the skin as well as inflammation at the site. The capillary walls are leaking due to the release of vasodilator substances from the inflammatory response. This results in edema—fluid loss from the vasculature into the tissues. Large amounts of fluid are also lost from the burn wound itself due to the loss of the water vapor barrier of the keratin layer of the skin.

There are three zones of burn injury. The central area is called the **zone of coagulation** and is composed of nonviable tissue. Coagulated nonviable tissue is called burn **eschar**. Surrounding this is the **zone of stasis**. This is the area that is significantly affected in the first 24 to 48 hours post-burn. During this acute period, ischemia and hypoperfusion may prevail, combining this zone with the zone of coagulation. Surrounding the zone of stasis is the **zone of hyperemia**, which contains viable tissue.[8,19] The melanocytes in the epidermis do not regenerate well, and in deep burns the skin color usually does not return. As blood vessels are damaged from the thermal injury, color changes occur in the burn. In sunburn, the vessels in the subpapillary and papillary plexuses dilate, causing reddening. In a severe burn, coagulation of vessels causes the area to lose redness and become whiter, with the vessels themselves coagulating into blackened lines in the wound.

The dermis, composed of collagen fibers, elastin, and mast cells, is damaged when exposed to high degrees of heat. The epidermal appendages, if intact, contain epidermal cells in the external sheaths of the hair

TABLE 28-10

FOUR-STAGE CLASSIFICATION SYSTEM FOR MELANOMA

CLASSIFICATION	DESCRIPTION
PRIMARY TUMOR (pT)	
pTX	Primary tumor cannot be assessed
pTO	No evidence of primary tumor
pTis	Melanoma in situ (atypical melanotic hyperplasia, severe melanotic dysplasia), not an invasive lesion (Clark's level I)
pT1	Tumor 0.75 mm or less in thickness and invades the papillary dermis (Clark's level II)
pT2	Tumors more than 0.75 mm but not more than 1.5 mm in thickness and/or invades the papillary-reticular interface (Clark's level III)
pT3	Tumor more than 1.5 mm but not more than 4 mm in thickness and/or invades the reticular dermis (Clark's level IV)
pT3a	Tumor more than 1.5 mm but not more than 3 mm in thickness
pT3b	Tumor more than 3 mm but not more than 4 mm in thickness
pT4	Tumor more than 4 mm in thickness and/or invades the subcutaneous tissue (Clark's level V) and/or satellite(s) within 2 cm of the primary tumor
pT4a	Tumor more than 4 mm in thickness and/or invades the subcutaneous tissue
pT4b	Satellite(s) within 2 cm of primary tumor
LYMPH NODE (N)	
NX	Regional lymph nodes cannot be assessed
NO	No regional lymph node metastasis
N1	Metastasis 3 cm or less in greatest dimension in any regional lymph node(s)
N2	Metastasis more than 3 cm in greatest dimension in any regional lymph node(s) and/or in-transit metastasis
N2a	Metastasis more than 3 cc in greatest dimension in any regional lymph node(s)
N2b	In-transit metastasis
N2c	Both (N2a and N2b)
DISTANT METASTASIS (M)	
MX	Presence of distant metastasis cannot be assessed
MO	No distant metastasis
M1	Distant metastasis
M1a	Metastasis in skin or subcutaneous tissue or lymph node(s) beyond the regional lymph nodes
M1b	Visceral metastasis

STAGE GROUPING

Stage	1A	pT1	NO	MO
	1B	pT2	NO	MO
Stage	II	pT3	NO	MO
	IIB	pT4	NO	MO
Stage	III	Any pT	N1,N2	MO
Stage	IV	Any pT	Any N	M1

(Anderson, R. G. [1995]. Skin tumor II: Melanoma. *Selected Readings in Plastic Surgery, 8*(7).)

BOX 28-2

CLARK'S LEVELS TUMOR INVASION: MELANOMA

Level I: In situ. All the tumor cells are above the basement membrane—i.e., the tumor is confined entirely to the epidermis.

Level II: Papillary dermis level. Tumor cells have broken through the basement membrane and extend into the papillary dermis, but have not reached the reticular dermis for the most part. Only an occasional cell or small nest of cells may extend to the reticular dermis.

Level III: Papillary-reticular dermis level. Tumor cells are widely impinging upon, but not invading, the reticular dermis.

Level IV: Reticular dermis level. Melanoma cells have invaded the reticular dermis, and tumor cells can be seen between collagen bundles.

Level V: Subcutaneous level. Tumor has invaded the subcutaneous tissue.

follicles. Glands can grow out and form new epithelium. When the burn extends to the subcutaneous tissues, the collagen fibers that normally anchor the dermis to the subcutaneous layer now hold the leathery burn eschar in place. This burn eschar harbors bacteria, which can produce burn wound infections. Risks of infection due to the loss of the protective function of the skin are a major concern in burns.

Systemic Manifestations of Burn Injury

Many changes occur throughout the body as a result of burn injury. Fluid loss is tremendous in the initial post-burn phase, and the sympathetic nervous system attempts to compensate by activating catecholamines, causing tachycardia and vasoconstriction. This temporary compensation allows for blood pressure maintenance; however, organ and tissue perfusion is not maintained.[4] Tissue hypoxia to vital organs may result, causing a shift to anaerobic metabolism. Acidosis and irreversible damage can occur.

EDEMA. The capillaries lose protein-rich fluid through their abnormally permeable walls into the surrounding tissues, creating the most characteristic feature of the burn wound, edema. After burn injury, colloids (plasma proteins such as albumins and globulins) also leak out of the damaged capillaries and into the interstitial spaces. The loss of protein-rich fluid decreases the intracapillary colloid osmotic pressure, causing fluid to shift into the tissues. There is also an accompanying rise in intracapillary pressure as a result of capillary dilatation and increased blood flow of the inflammatory process. The amount of fluid loss into the tissues is correlated with the severity of the burn. The more severe the burn, the more protein is lost. Capillary permeability also increases in tissues around the burn and other areas of the body.

Edema can be displaced by pressure, move to dependent areas, and spread beyond the burn. The rate of edema formation depends on the temperature of the injuring heat source, duration of exposure, area of the burn, and time since injury. It is difficult to ascertain fluid loss by the amount of visible edema, because such loss occurs deep in the wound beneath it and in the vulnerable third spaces, such as the peritoneal cavity and the lungs. The leathery eschar does not expand with edema pressure, and large amounts of fluid collect beneath it, putting pressure on underlying tissues and causing ischemia as previously described.

Studies show that fluid losses occur rapidly in the period immediately after the burn and decline in about 48 hours.[14] The rate of loss slows when the capillary endothelium returns to its normal state, when the tissue pressure is in balance with capillary hydrostatic pressure, or when capillary stasis occurs. In minor uncomplicated burns, edema is chiefly reabsorbed by the lymphatic system; this takes approximately as long as it took the edema to form. Lymphatics also drain larger burns, but this process may take weeks.

FLUID AND ELECTROLYTE IMBALANCE. Water and electrolytes shift back and forth across normal capillary walls. Burn injury alters the shifts by increasing capillary permeability, causing protein loss and altered colloid osmotic pressure. Potassium is released from severely injured cells, causing elevated serum potassium levels and cardiac dysrhythmias. Sodium level may increase in burn tissue, taking water with it. When the victim begins diuresis after approximately 48 hours, potassium and sodium are excreted.

RESPIRATORY SYSTEM ALTERATIONS. The respiratory system is often altered by burn injury, by inhalation injury, and by therapy. Respiratory tissues are irritated by gases from burning materials, such as carbon monoxide, and cause inflammation of the linings of the trachea and larynx, blocking the airway. The mucosal surface of the upper airways efficiently humidifies and normalizes the temperature of inspired gas, making it impossible to produce a thermal injury to the lower respiratory system.[5] The lower respiratory tract, however, can suffer significant damage from the chemical products of combustion. Altered circulation may lead to inadequate pulmonary circulation. Hypoxia may result from the decreased amount of oxygen circulating. Aspiration pneumonia may develop from vomiting episodes. Tra-

TABLE 28-11

DEPTH OF BURN

	SUPERFICIAL PARTIAL THICKNESS (FIRST DEGREE)	PARTIAL THICKNESS (SECOND DEGREE)	DEEP DERMAL PARTIAL THICKNESS (SECOND DEGREE)	FULL THICKNESS (THIRD DEGREE)
Possible sources	Sunburn, ultra-violet exposure	Brief exposure to flash flame and liquid spills	Hot liquids or solids, flash flame, direct flame, intense radiant energy	Prolonged contact with flames, hot liquids, hot objects; steam; chemicals; electric current
Injury	Minimal epithelial damage	Epidermis; minimal damage to dermis	Entire epidermis and varying levels of dermis; intact epidermal lined appendages (hair, sweat)	Epidermis, dermis, epidermal appendages; portion of subcutaneous fat; possible involvement of connective tissue, muscle, bone
Appearance	Red, dry, tender, slightly erythematous, painful	Moist, bright pink or mottled red, blisters, intact blanching, intact tactile and pain sensors	Pale, waxy, absent blanching, mostly dry; sensitive to pressure but not pinprick	Dry, leathery, insensate, avascular; pale yellow to brown to charred; thrombosed vessels
Healing time	Approximately 5 days no scarring	Within 21 days with minimal scarring	Prolonged healing period; unstable epithelium, late hypertrophic scarring, marked contracture formation; possible conversion to full thickness; no benefit from skin grafting	Destruction of entire epidermis and dermis leaving no residual epidermal cells to repopulate. Will not epithelialize and can only heal by wound contraction or skin grafting

(Allwood, J. S. [1995]. The primary care management of burns. *Nurse Practitioner, 20*(8), 74–87.)

cheal or laryngeal obstruction may result from edema in the head and neck region, causing pressure against the trachea and larynx. Edema under tight eschar in burns of the torso restricts chest movements, which may lead to restrictive respiratory problems. Adult respiratory distress syndrome is an ominous complication of burn injury that frequently results after inhalation injury, shock, or severe hypoxia. Finally, pulmonary emboli are always a danger as a result of changes in the vasculature, sepsis, and immobilization.

Physical findings that may raise suspicions of inhalation injury include singed facial or nasal hairs, a history of being burned in a closed space, dyspnea, dysphonia, carbonaceous sputum, and reddened or dark pharynx.

INCREASED METABOLIC RATE. Profound increases in metabolic rates are not uncommon in burn patients. Stimulation of the sympathetic nervous system and activation of the stress response result in release of stress hormones. These hormones lead the patient into a catabolic state. A negative nitrogen balance state results from the breakdown of proteins and the loss of large amounts of nitrogen through the burn wound. This negative nitrogen balance state and overall catabolic state result in a loss of lean body mass and a decreased ability to respond to stress. Subsequently, these patients require aggressive nutritional support.[11,20]

Other Systemic Dysfunctions. Gastric dilatation and paralytic ileus may appear early after burn injury. These conditions are neurologic in origin, may be secondary to fear or pain, or may occur as a result of hypovolemia or sepsis.[7] Liver dysfunction often occurs with burn injury. Factors that contribute to liver dysfunction include bacterial infection, lack of proper nutrition, drugs, anesthesia, blood transfusions leading to viral or serum hepatitis, and hepatic hypoxemia.

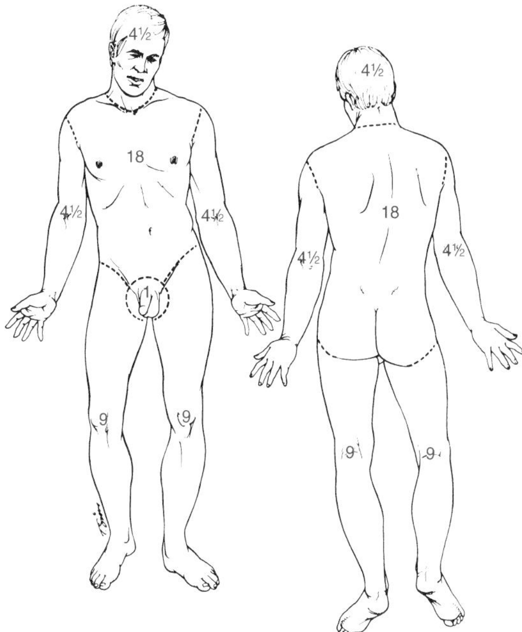

FIGURE 28-15. **The rule of nines. Each arm is 9%; the head, 9%; the torso and abdomen, 18%; the back, 18%; and each leg, 18%.**

Hepatic hypoxemia seems to result from a decrease in circulating fluid volume. The necrosis that results is usually minimal and focal, of a fatty nature, and reversible.

The kidney changes that occur may be permanent or temporary. Temporary kidney changes are manifested by oliguria, which results from a decreased glomerular filtration rate from the decreased circulating blood volume. Blood urea nitrogen and creatinine levels are elevated, and the level of antidiuretic hormone may be increased. Tubular damage may occur when the kidney is presented with an increased amount of protein breakdown products from the burn. If there is a history of kidney disorder or if the person does not receive adequate fluid resuscitative treatment, permanent damage may occur. Hematuria may be present as a result of damaged red blood cells.

Electrical Burn Injuries

The injury in electrical burns may be one or more of three types: (1) contact wounds, (2) electrothermal burns (flash or arc burns), and (3) flame burns. Contact wounds, often referred to as entry and exit wounds, may be small or large and usually appear as an ischemic, yellow-white, coagulated area. These may be charred, dry, and painless, with generally well-defined edges. However, the extent of damage may be far greater than is evident on the surface. Necrosis of subcutaneous tissues and muscle from arterial thrombi may occur, or lack of thrombosis may cause hemorrhaging. Damage may be due to heat from the passage of current or due to the action of the current itself.[35]

Electrothermal burns are from the heat of the current passing near, but not through, the skin. The depth of the wound depends on the closeness to the electrical source. These are mainly associated with high-voltage current. The electricity arc leaping from the high current has a temperature of 2,500°C. Flame burns occur when heat from an electrical current ignites clothing.

The tetanic contractions that lock the victim to the electric source may cause fractures and dislocations of joints. Cataracts often develop months to years after an electrical injury. Abdominal injury may occur as a result of electrical trauma to the abdomen. The extent of injury is difficult to determine initially. Abdominal symptoms may not arise until days after the injury. Renal involvement seems to be more prevalent in electrical than in thermal injury. The damage may be caused by the initial electric shock, direct current damage to the kidneys or kidney vessels, abnormal protein breakdown in the damaged tissue, or a combination of all three.[31]

Various lesions occur as a result of electrical burns. Six factors determine the extent of these injuries: (1) type of current (direct or alternating), (2) voltage of current, (3) resistance of body tissues, (4) value of current flowing through the tissues, (5) pathway of the current through the body, and (6) duration of the contact with the electrical source.

TYPE AND VOLTAGE OF CURRENT. Direct current does not produce the same contraction of muscle as alternating current, and low-voltage direct current is not as dangerous as alternating current. High-voltage direct current, however, is often fatal. Low voltage means less than 500 volts; high voltage is greater than 500 volts.

Alternating current produces tetanic muscle contraction at low voltages, which prevents the victim from releasing contact with the circuit. These low-voltage currents often result in ventricular fibrillation.[18] Low-voltage injuries most often occur in the home and are likely to involve children and infants. The usual source of current is a household plug; a curious child may stick a small object into the outlet. High-voltage injury commonly occurs in adults working with electric lines or equipment. These injuries have a high mortality, often due to cardiac asystole.

BODY RESISTANCE. The body tissues offer varying degrees of resistance to electrical current. The resistance of tissues, in order of least to greatest, is as follows: nerves, blood, muscles, skin, tendons, fat, and bone. Skin resistance varies from person to person. The epidermis is nonvascular and offers high resistance when it is dry, but moisture decreases resistance and enhances the flow of current. The dermis offers low resistance because it is highly vascular.

Thin skin is less resistant than thick skin, making the palms and soles most resistant. Usually, the greater the skin resistance, the greater the local burn, and the less the skin resistance, the more the internal injury. Current in contact with the skin eventually causes blistering. Blisters are moist and conduct current through the skin along the tissues of least resistance—blood vessels and nerves. Vessel walls are damaged and thrombi occur, often at a site far from the site of the electrical injury, making it difficult to evaluate the full extent of damage at the initial evaluation. Progressive tissue necrosis can occur for 12 to 14 days after the injury.[23]

BODY SYSTEM MANIFESTATIONS. Electric current may flow through the heart, producing ventricular fibrillation and often immediate death. High-voltage current often travels to the respiratory center of the brain, causing respiratory arrest and death.[23] Neurologic complications are the most common results of electrical injury and include varying levels of unconsciousness and spinal cord injuries. In burned extremities, peripheral neuropathies are common.[18] More recently, psychological sequelae have been found to be a common problem after electrical injury.

THE VALUE OF THE CURRENT. The value of the alternating current flowing through the body determines the resulting injury. Contact with a circuit produces muscle contraction, which may be severe enough to prevent the victim from releasing himself or herself from the source of current. If cardiac or respiratory arrest does not occur and the victim remains conscious, he or she may report ringing in the ears, deafness for a time, or visual disturbances such as flashes and brilliant luminous spots. The pathway through the body is also important in determining the extent of injury. The longer the contact, the greater the amount of damage.

Chemical Burn Injuries

Chemical burns result from exposure to acids or alkaline chemicals. Most lethal burns result from military conflict and industrial accidents. The severity of a chemical burn is often underestimated on first examination. Several chemical injuries that have distinct pathophysiology and appearance are summarized in Table 28-12.

Complications of all types of burn wounds include infection, contractures from scarring, renal failure, ulcers, liver failure, pneumonia, urinary tract infection, and acidosis. The frequency of complications increases with the severity of the burn.

TABLE 28-12

CHEMICAL BURNS: PATHOPHYSIOLOGY AND APPEARANCE

CHEMICAL	PATHOPHYSIOLOGY	APPEARANCE
ACID BURNS		
Sulfuric Nitric Hydrochloric Trichloroacetic Phenol Hydrofluoric	Exothermic reaction; cell dehydration; protein precipitation	Gray, yellow; brown, black; soft to leathery eschar
ALKALI BURNS		
Potassium hydroxide Sodium hydroxide Lime	Exothermic reaction; cellular dehydration; saponification of fat; protein precipitation	Erythema and blister; soapy, thick eschar; painful
Ammonia	Same as above, plus laryngeal and pulmonary edema	Gray, yellow; brown, black; soft leathery texture
Phosphorus	Thermal effect; melts at body temperature; runs and ignites at 34°C	Gray blue green; glows in dark; depressed, leathery eschar

(Modified from Arndt, K. [1989]. *Manual of dermatologic therapeutics* [4th ed.]. Boston: Little, Brown.)

TOXIC EPIDERMAL NECROLYSIS

The development of **toxic epidermal necrolysis syndrome (TENS)** is a life-threatening medical emergency with a mortality incidence of 30% to 50%. Drug reactions remain the most common precipitating factor. Common offending drugs are antibiotics, anticonvulsants, NSAIDS, and allopurinol. Viral, bacterial, and fungal infections also have been associated with TENS. Less common associations have included neoplasms, vaccines, and radiotherapy.[11,14]

TENS is characterized by distinctive and widespread skin sloughing. Burning, itching, fever, nausea, lethargy, malaise, photophobia, and arthralgia have all been reported as common manifestations. Areas of affected skin develop large, flaccid bullae, which slough with minor trauma. Mucous membrane involvement is also a prominent feature.[11]

TENS may be confused with other dermatologic conditions. The **staphylococcal scalded skin syndrome (SSSS)** may present with similar features but, due to its different etiology, requires different treatment. Accurate distinction between the two may be made by obtaining appropriate histologic specimens to distinguish the level of cutaneous split. TENS results in necrolysis of the entire epidermis at the epidermal/dermal junction, whereas SSSS is within the epidermis only.[14]

Mucous membrane involvement contributes significantly to the morbidity of TENS. The eyes, respiratory mucosa, genitourinary system, and entire gastrointestinal system may exhibit exfoliation. In these situations, hemorrhage, fever, sepsis, and fluid imbalances make this relatively rare condition extremely fatal.

DECUBITUS ULCERS (PRESSURE SORES)

Decubitus ulcers, derived from the Latin word *decumbo* meaning "lying down," are sores on the skin derived from prolonged pressure.[29] Persons at risk for pressure sores have conditions that alter mobility, including individuals with spinal cord injuries, the ill elderly who are incontinent, or persons who are bed- or wheelchair-bound. Numerous studies have also linked pressure sores with malnutrition.[6] Decubitus ulcers are significant health problems because they increase the length of hospitalization, health care costs, and the chances of death.

Etiology

Four crucial factors play a role in decubitus formation: (1) pressure, (2) shearing forces, (3) friction, and (4) moisture. Moisture can be caused by fecal matter, urine, or perspiration, which can macerate the skin and make it more vulnerable to pressure-sore formation. Pressure is the most crucial factor, and these ulcers are accurately called pressure sores.

Pathophysiology

Compression that exceeds the mean skin capillary pressure of approximately 25 mm Hg will occlude the blood vessels so that surrounding tissues become anoxic and cannot survive. The amount of damage is directly related to the extent and duration of pressure. Individuals at risk are unable to sustain pressures as high as healthy individuals. Repositioning every 1 to 2 hours can prevent ischemia and ulcer formation. Secondary bacterial infections can complicate a very small open ulcer by extending to underlying structures such as the bone to produce osteomyelitis or the bloodstream to produce septicemia. Infection can also impair or prevent healing.

Clinical Manifestations

Pressure sores are often described using a three-color concept for wounds—red, yellow, and black. *Red* refers to the color of healthy granulation tissue and indicates that normal healing is occurring. *Yellow* is the color of suppurative exudate that results from microorganisms in the wound. The presence of this pus interferes with the normal healing process. *Black* is the color of necrotic tissue. The dead tissue, also referred to as eschar, becomes a focus of infection and more tissue loss. The black wound requires debridement, antibiotic therapy, and moist dressings.

Box 28-3 illustrates the AHCPR guidelines for staging pressure sores.

BOX 28-3 AHCPR GUIDELINES FOR STAGING PRESSURE SORES

Stage I: Norblanchable erythema of intact skin, the heralding lesion of skin ulceration. In individuals with darker skin, discoloration of the skin, warmth, edema, induration, or hardness may also be indicators.

Stage II: Partial thickness skin loss involving epidermis, dermis, or both. The ulcer is superficial and presents clinically as an abrasion, blister, or shallow crater.

Stage III: Full thickness skin loss involving damage to or necrosis of subcutaneous tissue that may extend down to, but not through, underlying fascia. The ulcer presents clinically as a deep crater with or without undermining of adjacent tissue.

Stage IV: Full thickness skin loss with extensive destruction, tissue necrosis, or damage to muscle, bone, or supporting structures (e.g., tendon, joint capsule). Undermining and sinus tracts also may be associated with Stage IV pressure ulcers.

OTHER TRAUMAS

Other traumas to the skin include blunt wounds, abrasions (scrapes), incised wounds (such as an incision), puncture wounds, and lacerations (cuts). An abrasion is a superficial open wound in which the outer surface layers of skin are scraped off. Nerve endings are exposed and bleeding is minimal. The wound often contains foreign matter that may initiate an inflammatory response. This type of wound normally heals spontaneously. An incision is a clean, straight-edged wound that goes through all layers of skin; it bleeds freely and heals cleanly when sutured. Puncture or stab wounds are deeper than they are wide and are caused by such objects as knives, pins, needles, and spikes. Underlying structures may be damaged, with concealed blood loss. A laceration is a cut or tear of tissues, which is unlikely to heal without treatment.

In all traumatic skin wounds, tissue viability is crucial and depends on circulation of blood to the area. Wounds with tissue loss (i.e., from deep abrasions or avulsion) not only have to undergo the normal stages of wound healing, but actual wound closure requires epithelial migration and wound contraction. Epithelialization is a very slow process and is often insufficient for timely wound closure. Furthermore, epithelialization occurs without an accompanying dermal layer and is therefore more vulnerable to injury and severe contraction.

FOCUS ON THE PERSON WITH CRITICAL BURN INJURY

A 32-year-old, 80-kg male was brought in to the local emergency room by paramedics. He was found in smoldering clothing and unconscious where he apparently fell asleep while smoking in bed. He has burns to his face and anterior neck; bilateral legs and arms circumferentially; and anterior chest. Carbon particles are present around the nose and mouth. The family was contacted and state that he has no significant medical history and no known allergies.

Questions

1. Based on the history of the event, what would be the most life-threatening issue in the immediate post burn phase?
2. Using the Rule of Nines, calculate this patient's body surface area burn.
3. Discuss whether this patient meets American Burn Association Criteria for transfer to a burn center.
4. What would be the correct fluid resuscitation needs for this patient in the first 24 hours post-burn?
5. What is the most frequent error in fluid resuscitation?

REFERENCES

1. Achauer, B. M., Brody, G. S., Frank, D. H., et al. (1991). *Everyday wounds: A guide for the primary care physician.* Arlington Heights, IL: Plastic Surgery Educational Foundation.
2. Allwood, J. S. (1995). The primary care management of burns. *Nurse Practitioner, 20*(8), 74–87.
3. Anderson, R. G. (1995). Skin tumor II: Melanoma. *Selected Readings in Plastic Surgery, 8*(7), 1–38.
4. Arturson, G. (1996). Cardiovascular system. In J. A. D. Settle (Ed.), *Principles and practice of burns management.* New York: Churchill Livingstone.
5. Beeley, J. M., & Clark, R. J. (1996). Respiratory problems in fire victims. J. A. D. Settle (Ed.), *Principles and practice of burns management.* New York: Churchill Livingstone.
6. Bergstrom, N., Bennett, M. A., Carlson, C. E., et al. (1994). *Treatment of pressure ulcers. Clinical practice guideline No. 15* (AHCPR Publication. No. 95-0652). Rockville, MD: U.S. Department of Health and Human Services. Public Health Service, Agency for Healthcare Policy and Research.
7. Burgess, M. D. (1991). Initial management of a patient with extensive burn injury. *Critical Care Nursing Clinics of North America, 3*(2), 165.
8. Byers, J. F., & Flynn, M. B. (1996). Acute burn injury: A case report. *Critical Care Nurse,* 16(4), 55–65.
9. Cormack, D. H. (1993). *Essential histology.* Philadelphia: J. B. Lippincott.
10. Cottell, W. I. (1995). Skin tumors I: Basal cell carcinoma and squamous cell carcinoma. *Selected Readings in Plastic Surgery, 8*(6), 1–32.
11. Cruse, C. W., & Krizek, T. J. (1996). *Manual of burn care.* Tampa, FL: Tampa Bay Regional Burn Center and University of South Florda, Department of Surgery, College of Medicine.
12. Farber, E. M., & Raychaudhuri, S. P. (1997). Concept of total care: A third dimension in the treatment of psoriasis. *Cutis, 59*(1), 35–39.
13. Fitzpatrick, T. B., et al. (1993). *Dermatology in general medicine* (4th ed.). New York: McGraw-Hill.
14. Fitzpatrick, T. B., Johnson, R. A., Wolff, K., et al. (1997). *Color atlas and synopsis of clinical dermatology* (3rd ed.). New York: McGraw-Hill.
15. Gillespie, R. W., Dimick, A. R., Gillespi, P. W., et al. (1993). *Advanced burn life support provider's manual.* Lincoln, NE: National Burn Institute.
16. Habif, T. P. (1996). *Clinical dermatology* (3rd ed.). St. Louis: Mosby-Year Book.
17. Harrist, T. J., & Clark, W. H. (1994). The skin. In E. Rubin & J. L. Farber (Eds.), *Pathology* (2nd ed.). Philadelphia: J. B. Lippincott.
18. Heimbach, D. M. (1992). Electrical injury. In W. N. Kelley (Ed.), *Textbook of internal medicine* (2nd ed.). Philadelphia: J. B. Lippincott.
19. Hunt, J. L., Purdue, G. F., Rohrich, R.J., et al. (1997). Acute burns, burn surgery, and post burn reconstruction. *Selected Readings in Plastic Surgery, 7*(12), 1–41.
20. Laitung, G. (1996). Nutrition. In J. A. D. Settle (Ed.), *Principles and practice of burns management.* New York: Churchill Livingstone.
21. Langley, R. G. B., Fitzpatrick, T. B., & Sober, A. F. (1998). Clinical characteristics. In C.M. Balch (ed.), *Cutaneous melanoma* (3rd ed.). St. Louis: Quality Medical Publishing.
22. Lewis, E. J., Lam, M., & Crutchfield, C. E. (1997). An update on molluscum contagiosum. *Cutis, 60*(1), 29–34.
23. Munster, A. M., & Ciccone, T. G. (1985). Burns. In F. J. Dagher (Ed.), *Cutaneous wounds.* Mt. Kisco, NY: Futura.
24. Murphy, G. F., & Mihm, M. C. (1994). The skin. In R. Cotran, V. Kumar, & S. Robbins (Eds.), *Robbin's pathologic basis of disease* (5th ed.). Philadelphia: W. B. Saunders.

25. Noble, J. (Ed.) (1996). *Textbook of primary care medicine* (2nd ed.). St. Louis: Mosby-Year Book.
26. Padgett-Coehlo, D. (1997). Skin, hair and nails examination. *Health assessment: A learning package.* http://www.sou.edu/nursing/health/skin.htm.
27. Rhoades, R., & Pflanzer, R. (1996). *Human physiology* (36th ed.). Orlando, FL: Harcourt Brace College Publishers.
28. Sauer, G. C. (1991). *Manual of Skin diseases* (6th ed.). Philadelphia: J.B. Lippincott.
29. Sebern, M. (1987). Home-team strategies for treating pressure sores. *Nursing 87, 17*(4), 50.
30. Seidel, H. M., Ball, J. W., Dains, J. E., & Denedict, G. W. (1995). *Mosby's guide to physical examination* (3rd ed.). St. Louis: Mosby-Year Book.
31. Stadelmann, W. K., Rappaport, D. P., Soong, S., et al. (1998). Predictive factors that influence melanoma outcomes. In *Cutaneous melanoma* (3rd ed.). St. Louis: Quality Medical Publishing.
32. Stevens, D. L., & Mandell, G. L. (1995) *Atlas of infectious diseases, Vol. II.* Philadelphia: Current Medicine.
33. Tierney, L. M., McPhee, S. J., & Papadakis, M. A. (Eds.) (1997). *Current medical diagnosis and treatment* (36th ed.). Stanford, CT: Appleton & Lange.
34. Tortora, G., & Grabowski, S. (1993). *Principles of anatomy and physiology* (7th ed.). New York: Harper Collins.
35. Wallace, J. (1991). Electrical injuries. In J. Wilson et al. (Eds.), *Harrison's principles of internal medicine* (12th ed.). New York: McGraw-Hill.

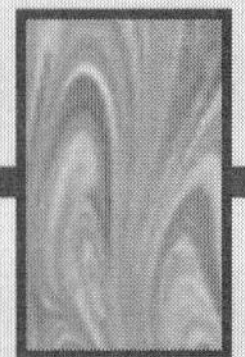

UNIT 9: CASE STUDY

The Person with Severe Joint Pain

Introduction to the Patient

Mrs. L. is an 83-year-old female who is referred to the clinic by her primary care physician in another state for chronic management of severe joint pain and assistance with activities of daily living due to disabling pain and joint disfigurement from arthritis.

Present Illness

Mrs. L. has been relatively healthy and still perceives herself to be healthy with the exception of the constant pain that she is suffering. She states that her hands, knees, and ankles are very painful now and she rarely gets relief. Morning stiffness and pain seem to get better by noon. She is wearing a splint on her left wrist, stating, "I wear it almost all the time. Sometimes it helps." She has noticed an increased difficulty with walking and finds it almost impossible to do tasks such as peeling potatoes and cutting bread due to the painful hand and wrist joints. Her primary care physician has prescribed a variety of medications over the years. Currently, she is taking prednisone 10 mg every day and methotrexate 2.5 mg four times a week for her arthritis. She states that she occasionally takes acetaminophen but that "it really doesn't help that much."

She reports that she tires by early afternoon and usually takes a 1- or 2-hour nap every day. She has lost about 15 pounds in the last year. She is 5 ft, 5 in tall (formerly 5 ft, 8 in tall at age 50) and weighs 128 pounds.

Social History

Mrs. L., a widow for the past 10 years, lives alone in a small two-story home. Up until 2 months ago, she did volunteer work at a local children's hospital 3 days a week. "Now I have trouble just going down the stairs." One daughter lives nearby, who brings her meals about once a day and takes her to the grocery store. Her other two children live approximately 100 miles away in neighboring states.

Past Medical History

Mrs. L.'s medical record reveals that she started having signs of joint stiffness and occasional joint pain when she first arose in the mornings when she was in her mid-fifties. In the early stages, the pain would disappear and often would not be noticeable for months. She had a positive rheumatoid factor many years ago, and the primary care physician diagnosed her with rheumatoid arthritis.

Her medical record also reveals that she has significant osteoporosis. Previously, she had knee aspirations for a ruptured Baker's cyst. Two weeks ago, she had a cortisone injection into her right knee for acute bursitis.

Mrs. L. had an abdominal hysterectomy at age 53 for intrauterine fibroids. She also reports a history of occasional "heart palpitations," mild heart failure for which she takes digoxin 0.25 mg per day, and hypertension for which she takes captopril 50 mg twice a day. At age 68, she suffered a Colles' fracture.

Family History

Mrs. L. is the middle child of three children. Her sister, age 85, is alive and in good health. Her brother, age 79, is alive with a history of angina and mild arthritis. Mrs. L.'s father died of throat cancer at age 72. Her mother, who had mild arthritis, died of a stroke at age 74.

Physical Examination

Mrs. L. appears in moderate discomfort as evidenced by her slowness and difficulty in ambulating and the painful grimacing on her face. She is alert and oriented × 3. Her vital signs are as follows: temperature—99.4°F; pulse—104; respirations—18; blood pressure—182/96. PERRLA with pupils approximately 5 mm in size bilaterally. Carotid pulsations are equal without bruits. Slight decrease in range of motion is noted at neck. Lungs are clear to auscultation. S3 heart sound is present without murmurs, rubs, or gallops. Abdomen is soft, nontender, with slight splenomegaly. Kyphosis with prominent hump and pain in upper spine are present. Skin is unremarkable except for slightly irritated, reddened area under splint.

Extremities exhibit weak symmetric grasp, pain, and swelling. Slight redness of proximal interphalangeal (PIP), metacarpophalangeal (MCP), and wrist joints is present. Metatarsophalangeal (MTP), ankle, knee, and hip also are painful. Nodules are noted around elbows.

Diagnostic Tests

Radiographs: loss of articular cartilage and narrowing of joint spaces of knees, feet, and hands
Ulnar deviation of fingers
Red blood cell count: 3.76^6/μL
MCV: 81 μm^3

MCHC: 34 g/dL
White blood cell count: 11,000/mm^3
Erythrocyte sedimentation rate: 57 mm/hour
Rheumatoid factor: 33 IU
Synovial fluid analysis: volume—57 mL; color—mildly turbid, pale yellow; white blood cells—11,000 cells/mm^3 with great majority being polymorphonuclear leukocytes; decreased viscosity

CRITICAL THINKING QUESTIONS

1. Propose some hypotheses about the etiological basis of rheumatoid arthritis.
2. (a) Describe the pathophysiology of rheumatoid arthritis and the associated osteoporosis that Mrs. L. exhibits. (b) What type of anemia is exhibited? (c) Interpret the synovial fluid finds. (d) Relate Mrs. L.'s development of Baker's cyst and bursitis to the pathophysiology of rheumatoid arthritis.
3. Explain the rationale for using methotrexate and prednisone as treatment for Mrs. L.'s rheumatoid arthritis.
4. Suggest possible medication that might be ordered to help manage Mrs. L.'s osteoporosis.
5. One of the nursing diagnoses identified for Mrs. L. is "Risk for impaired skin integrity related to decreased mobility and use of splint." Suggest possible nursing interventions to minimize her risk.

Besides your pathophysiology text, you'll need a good pharmacology text, a rheumatology text, a diagnostic/laboratory test text, a medical-surgical nursing text, and current research to complete this case study. Suggested references follow:

Cornell, S. (1997). New directions in rheumatoid arthritis. *Advanced Nurse Practice, 5*(3), 61–64.

Cotran, R. S., Kumar, V. & Robbins, S. L. (1998) *Robbin's pathologic basis of disease* (6th ed.). Philadelphia: W. B. Saunders.

Fischbach, F. (1996). *Manual of laboratory and diagnostic tests,* (5th ed.). Philadelphia: Lippincott-Raven.

Karch, A. M. (1999). *1999 Lippincott's nursing drug guide.* Philadelphia: Lippincott-Raven.

Kipple, J. H., Weyand, C. M. & Wortman, R. (Eds.) (1997). *Primer on rheumatic diseases* (11 th ed.). Atlanta, G. A.: Longstreet Press.

Drug, B. (1997). Rheumatoid arthritis and osteoarthritis. A basis comparison. *Orthopedic Nursing, 16*(5), 73–75.

Smeltzer, S. & Bare, B. (2000). *Brunner and Suddarth's textbook of medical-surgical nursing* (9th ed.). Philadelphia: Lippincott Williams & Wilkins.

Website Resources:

Arthritis Foundation *http://www.arthritis.org*

Arthritis Information and Resources *http://pslgroup.com/ARTHRITIS.HTM#Disease*

Focus on. . . . Rheumatoid Arthritis *http://pharminfo.com/pubs/msb/rheumart.html*

Mayo Clinic: Rheumatoid Arthritis *http://www.mayhealth.org/mayo/9809/htm/rheu.htm*

Osteoporosis Information and Resources *http://www.pslgroup.com/OSTEOPOROSIS.HTM*

UNIT 9 APPENDIX A

DIAGNOSTIC TESTS

TEST	PURPOSE/NORMAL FINDINGS	SIGNIFICANCE
MUSCULOSKELETAL		
Serum calcium	Measurement of the total amount of calcium stored in the skeleton and teeth, which act in maintaining calcium levels in the blood Normal findings: 9 to 11 mg/dL	Increased calcium levels may indicate hyperparathyroidism, Paget's disease, vitamin D intoxication, immobility, sarcoidosis, tumor. Decreased calcium levels may indicate hypoparathyroidism, vitamin D deficiency.
Serum alkaline phosphatase	Measurement of the enzyme, primarily of the bone, liver, and placenta used as a tumor marker index of liver and bone disease Normal findings: 17 to 142 U/L	Increased alkaline phosphatase levels may indicate hyperparathyroidism, tumor, Paget's disease, or vitamin D deficiency. It is also elevated during fracture healing.
Erythrocyte sedimentation rate (ESR)	Measurement of the rate of erythrocyte clumping as an indication of plasma proteins Normal findings: 0 to 15 mm/hour (males) 0 to 20 mm/hour (females) Slight increase in both sexes after the age of 50 years	Elevation may suggest inflammation or neoplasms.
Serum phosphorus	Measurement of the body's total phosphorus content, which is combined with calcium in the bone Normal findings: 2.5 to 4.5 mg/dL	Increased levels indicate tumor, vitamin D intoxication, immobility, or hypoparathyroidism. Decreased levels may indicate vitamin D deficiency or hyperparathyroidism.
Rheumatoid factor	Measurement of an abnormal antibody associated with connective tissue disease Normal findings: less than 30 IU/mL	Screening test for antibodies (IgM, IgG, or IgA) found in the sera of persons with rheumatoid arthritis, SLE, scleroderma, infectious mononucleosis, tuberculosis, leukemia, old age, and other conditions.
Urine calcium	24-hour urine specimen to evaluate body calcium Normal finding: 100–300 mg/day (normal diet) 50–150 mg/day (low calcium diet)	The amount of calcium excreted varies with the amount of calcium ingested in the diet. Increased levels may suggest hyperparathyroidism, Paget's disease, renal tubular acidosis, vitamin D intoxication, diabetes, or thyrotoxicosis. Increased urine calcium levels almost always are associated with increased serum calcium levels. Decreased levels may suggest hypoparathyroidism, vitamin D deficiency, pre-eclampsia, acute nephrosis, or metastatic prostate cancer. Corticosteroids, immobilization, or excessive milk intake may falsely elevate urine calcium levels. Thiazide diuretics or antacids may falsely depress urine calcium level.
Bone and joint X-rays (anterior-posterior and lateral)	Evaluation of the structure of the bone or joint and surrounding tissues Normal findings: normal osseous and soft tissue	Two views orthogonal to each other should be done with proper immobilization to ensure accuracy. Abnormalities may be indicative of fracture, degenerative joint disease, or tumor.
Arthrography	Radiographic evaluation of joint capsule using a contrast medium Normal findings: normal filling of the encapsulated joint structure, joint space, bursae, menisci, ligaments, and articular cartilage	The knee is the joint most commonly evaluated with this test. This test may reveal arthritis, dislocation, ligament tears, synovial changes, or joint space narrowing.

UNIT 9 APPENDIX A

DIAGNOSTIC TESTS (Continued)

TEST	PURPOSE/NORMAL FINDINGS	SIGNIFICANCE
Myelography	Radiographic evaluation of the spinal subarachnoid space using a contrast medium to reveal the spinal cord, nerve roots, and distortions of the dura; the "gold standard" for measuring neural compression Normal findings: lumbar and/or cervical subarachnoid space without filling defects	This test measures the ability of the cerebrospinal fluid to flow around extradural lesions. Extradural masses show up as filling defects in the contrast. A distortion in the subarachnoid space may indicate ruptured intervertebral disk, compression and stenosis of the spinal cord, level of intravertebral tumor, or spinal canal obstruction.
Ultrasound	Use of high-frequency sound waves to visualize bone and soft tissue structures Normal findings: bone cortex appears as a bright, "echogenic" line	This test can identify trauma, soft tissue tumors, infection, pediatric disorders, bone mineral density, degree of fracture healing, or cysts. Any discontinuity represents a fracture.
Computed tomography (CT) and magnetic resonance imaging (MRI)	Visualization of abnormalities not normally seen with routine x-rays Normal findings: bone appears white; soft tissue appears gray with shading correlating to tissue density	This test can identify abnormalities in bone, blood vessels, intra- and periarticular anatomy, and muscles.
Bone scan	Radionuclide imaging of the bone using radioisotopes Normal findings: areas with equal concentration of isotope uptake	Tracer uptake is a reflection of bone turnover (osteoblastic activity). This test is used primarily to evaluate metastatic disease, with lesions appearing 3 to 6 months earlier than seen on x-ray. Increased bone production results in increased uptake ("hot spots"). Decreased uptake is indicative of decreased blood flow ("cold spot").
Electromyography	Evaluation of electrical potential of muscles and nerves to determine function of the motor end plate, using needles inserted into selected muscles with responses recorded on an oscilloscope Normal findings: Brief interval of depolarization Normal muscle silent at rest Minimal voluntary contraction eliciting a single motor unit action potential Increasing voluntary contraction generating a full interference pattern with asynchronous discharge of many muscle fibers	An unstable muscle membrane is indicative of tumor, electrolyte imbalance, or upper motor neuron lesion. When the axons innervate fewer than normal numbers of muscle fibers, and there is small amplitude and short duration during voluntary contraction, a myopathy is possible. This test helps to differentiate among disorders of the nerve, neuromuscular junction, and muscle.
Bone mineral density (BMD) using dual-energy x-ray absorptiometry	Qualitative measure of bone density Normal findings: within 1 standard deviation of the young adult reference mean	Low bone mass is suggested when the BMD is −1.0 to −2.0 deviations below the young adult reference mean. Osteoporosis usually is present when the BMD is −2.5 or more below the young adult reference mean. Bone density measurements vary with sex and race. African-American men have the densest bone, followed by African-American women and white men, then white women, and finally other ethnic groups. Density decreases with age.
Synovial fluid analysis	Examination of aspirated (arthrocentesis) synovial joint fluid for examination Normal findings: clear, pale, straw-colored fluid; scanty amount with few cells	Cloudy, milky, or dark yellow fluid with numerous inflammatory cells, such as white blood cells or complement, suggests an inflammatory condition.

(continued)

UNIT 9 APPENDIX A

DIAGNOSTIC TESTS

TEST	PURPOSE/NORMAL FINDINGS	SIGNIFICANCE
		Immune complexes may be present in rheumatoid arthritis. Decreased viscosity is also seen in some inflammatory conditions. Hemarthrosis may indicate trauma, rheumatoid arthritis, other inflammatory conditions, or joint disorders. Fat globules may be present in intra-articular fractures. Crystals may be found in gout and pseudogout.
INTEGUMENTARY		
Skin biopsy	Evaluation of tissue specimen obtained by excision or skin punch to determine histology Normal findings: absence of abnormal or malignant cells	Skin biopsy may reveal malignancy or determine an exact diagnosis of the skin lesion.
Skin culture	Examination of skin scrapings or fluid of vesicular lesions to identify pathologic organisms Normal findings: organisms present but in low numbers	Staphylococci, streptococci (group A), and *Corynebacterium haemolytica* are the most common bacteria associated with skin infections.
Skin tests	Evaluation of the immune response to a specific disease, organism, or allergen Normal findings: negative	A positive reaction indicates a lack of immunity to a specific disease or sensitivity to an allergen. Three methods may be used: scratch test (positive reaction seen as swelling or redness at site within 30 minutes); patch test (positive reaction evidenced as swelling or reddened skin at the patch site within a specified period of time); or intradermal test (positive reaction evidenced as reddened, inflamed area at injection site within a specified period of time). Inadvertent injection of substance into the subcutaneous tissue may yield a false negative result.
Immunofluorescence (IF)	Evaluation of tissue via biopsy using dye to identify the site of the immune reaction Normal findings: negative	Direct IF testing identifies autoantibodies to the skin. Indirect IF test identifies antibodies in the patient's serum.

UNIT BIBLIOGRAPHY

Barry, G. (Ed.) (1997). *Body systems review: Nervous, skin, connective tissue, musculoskeletal* (2nd ed.) Philadelphia: Lippincott-Raven.

Cotran, R., Kumar, V., & Robbins, S. L. (1998). *Robbins' pathologic basis of disease* (6th ed.). Philadelphia: W. B. Saunders.

DeVita, V. T., Hellman, S., & Rosenberg, S. A. (1997). *Cancer: Principles and practice of oncology* (5th ed.). Philadelphia: Lippincott-Raven.

Fauci, A. S. et al. (Eds.) (1997). *Harrison's principles of internal medicine* (12th ed.). New York: McGraw-Hill.

Govan, A. D. T., Macfarland, P. S. & Callander, R. (1995). *Pathology/Illustrated* (4th ed.). New York: Churchill Livingstone.

Guyton, A. & Hall, J. (1995). *Textbook of medical physiology* (9th ed.). Philadelphia: W. B. Saunders.

Kelley, W. N. (1997). *Textbook of internal medicine* (3rd ed.). Philadelphia: Lippincott-Raven.

Rubin, E. & Farber, J. L. (1999). *Pathology* (3rd ed.). Philadelphia: Lippincott-Raven.

Tallis, R., Fillit, H., & Brocklehurst, J. (1998). *Geriatric medicine and gerontology.* London: Churchill Livingstone—Harcourt Brace.

MUSCULOSKELETAL

Agency for Health Care Policy and Research. (1994). *Acute low back problems in adults.* Clinical Practice Guidelines. Quick Reference Guide Number 14. Rockville, MD: USHHS, PHS, AHCPR, AHPR Pub. No. 95-0643.

Barrett, D. (1994). *Essential basic sciences for orthopaedics.* Boston: Butterworth-Heineman.

Blue, C. (1996). Preventing back injury among nurses. *Orthopedic Nursing, 15*(6), 9–20.

Bucholz, R. (1996). *Orthopaedic decision making* (2nd ed.). St. Louis. Mosby.

Davis, A. (1996). Primary care management of chronic musculoskeletal pain. *Nurse Practitioner; 21*(8), 72–82,89

Dee, R., Hurst, L., Gruber, M., & Kottmeier, S. (1997). *Principles of orthopedic practice.* New York: McGraw-Hill.

Doheny, M. et al. (1995). Reducing orthopaedic hazards of the computer work environment. *Orthopedic Nursing, 14*(1), 7.

Emery, A. E. H. (1993). *Duchenne muscular dystrophy* (2nd ed.). Oxford: Oxford University Press.

Fitzpatrick, T. B., Johnson, R. A., Wolff, K., et al. (1997). *Color atlas and synopsis of clinical dermatology* (3rd ed.). New York: McGraw-Hill.

Gallegos, S. & Michalec, D. (1996). Neurological assessment of the orthopaedic patient. *Orthopedic Nursing, 15*(5), 23–29.

Gardner, D. L. (1992). *Pathological basis of connective tissue diseases.* Philadelphia: Lea and Febiger.

Gould, J. A., & Davies, C. J. (1996). *Orthopaedic and sports physical therapy* (3rd ed). St. Louis: Mosby.

Hertling, D. (1995). *Management of common musculoskeletal disorders: Physical therapy principles and methods* (3rd ed.). Philadelphia: J. B. Lippincott.

Jones, A. (1997). Primary care of acute low back pain. *Nurse Practitioner, 22*(7), 50–52, 61–63, 66;68.

Magee, D. J. (1997). *Orthopedic physical assessment* (3rd ed.). Philadelphia: W. B. Saunders.

Maher, A. B. et al. (1998). *Orthopaedic nursing* (2nd ed.). Philadelphia: W. B. Saunders.

Malone, T. (1997). *Orthopedic and sports physical therapy* (3rd ed.). St. Louis: Mosby.

Mercer, W. (1996). *Mercer's orthopaedic surgery.* London: Oxford University Press.

Mourad, L. (1995). *Orthopaedic nursing.* Albany, NY: Delmar.

Neal, C. (1997). The assessment of knowledge and application of proper body mechanics in the workplace. *Orthopedic Nursing 16*(1), 66–69.

Newman, R. J. (1992). *Orthogeriatrics: Comprehensive orthopaedic care for the elderly patient.* Boston: Butterworth-Heineman.

Nichol, D. (1995). Understanding the principles of traction. *Nursing Standard, 9*(46), 25–28.

Novy, C. & Jagmin, M. (1997). Pain management in the elderly orthopaedic patient. *Orthopedic Nursing, 16*(1), 51–57.

Norton, M., Anderson, G., & Pope, M. (1997). *Musculoskeletal disorders in the workplace.* St. Louis: Mosby–Year-Book.

Paletta, J. (1997). Nursing care of sports-related injuries. *Orthopedic Nursing, 16*(6), 43–46.

Patel, P. & Lauerman, W. (1997). The use of magnetic resonance imaging in the diagnosis of lumbar disc disease. *Orthopedic Nursing, 16*(1), 59–65.

Piasecki, P. (1996). Nursing care of the patient with metastatic bone disease. *Orthopedic Nursing, 15*(4), 25–33.

Ross, D. (1996). Chronic compartment syndrome. *Orthopedic Nursing, 15*(3), 23–27.

Salmond, S. W. et al. (Ed.). (1996). *Core curriculum for orthopaedic nursing* (3rd ed.). Pitman, NJ: National Association of Orthopaedic Nurses.

Schwappach, J. et al. (1997). Orthopedics. *JAMA, 277*(23), 1883–1884.

Simon, R. & Koenigsknecht, S. (1995). *Emergency orthopedics: The extremities* (3rd ed.) Norwalk, CT: Appleton & Lange.

Mercier, L. et al. (1995). *Practical orthopedics* (4th ed.). St. Louis: Mosby–Year Book.

Woessner, J. F. & Howell, D. S. (1993). *Joint cartilage degradation: Basis and clinical aspects.* New York: M. Dekker.

FRACTURES

Brown, C. et al. (1996). Surgical treatment of patients with open tibial fractures. *AORN Journal, 63*(5), 875–881, 885–896.

Paton, D. F. (1995). *Fractures and orthopaedics* (2nd ed.). New York: Churchill Livingstone.

Sims, M. & Saleh, M. (1996). Protocols for the care of external fixation pin sites. *Professional Nurse, 11*(4), 261–264.

Zavotsky, K. E. & Banavage, A. (1995). Management of the patient with complex orthopaedic fractures. *Orthopedic Nursing, 14*(5), 53–54, 56–57.

JOINT DISORDERS (ARTHRITIS)

Ailinger, R. L., & Dear, M. R. (1997). An examination of the self-care needs of clients with rheumatoid arthritis: *Rehabilitation Nursing, 22*(3), 135–140.

Allaire, S. H., Anderson, J. J. & Meenan, R. F. (1996). Reducing work disability associated with rheumatoid arthritis: Identification of additional risk factors and persons likely to benefit from intervention. *Arthritis Care Research, 9*(5), 349–357.

Allaire, S. H. (1996). Gender and disability associated with arthritis: Difference and issues. *Arthritis Care Research, 9*(6), 435–440.

Altizer, L. (1995). Total hip arthroplasty. *Orthopedic Nursing, 14*(4), 7–18.

Anders, R. & Ornellas, E. (1997). Acute management of patient with hip fracture. *Orthopedic Nursing, 16*(2), 31–46.

Bradley, C. & Kozak, C. (1995). Nursing care and management of the elderly hip fractured patient. *Journal of Gerontologic Nursing, 21*(8), 15–22.

Barrows, S. (1995). Easing your patient's joint replacement *Nursing 95, 25*(5), 32C–32D, 32F.

Beckles, S. Community assessment of a patient following hip replacement. *British Journal of Nursing, 5*(20), 1241–1246.

Bautch, J. C., Malone, D. G. & Vailas, A. C. (1997). Effects of exercise on knee joints with osteoarthritis: A pilot study of biologic markers. *Arthritis Care Research, 10*(1), 48–55.

Brown, F. (1996). Anterior cruciate ligament reconstruction as an outpatient procedure. *Orthopedic Nursing, 15*(1), 15–20.

Burma, M. R., Rachow, J. W. Kolluri, S. & Saag, K. G. (1996). Methotrexate patient education: A quality improvement study. *Arthritis Care Research, 9*(3), 216–222.

Carlisle, D. (1996). Fresh look at rehabillitation of hip-replacement patients. Elderly care counts. *Nursing Times, 92*(44), 32–33.

Cash, J. M. & Wilder, R. L. (1995). Refractory rheumatoid arthritis. Therapeutic options. *Rheumatic Diseases Clinics of North Americas 21*(1), 1–18.

Cicuttini, F. M. & Spector, T. D. (1995). Osteoarthritis in the aged. *Drugs & Aging* 6(5), 409–420.

Crutchfield, J. et al. (1996). Preoperative and postoperative pain in total knee replacement patients. *Orthopedic Nursing, 15*(2), 65–72.

Dowdy, S. W., et al. (1996). Gender and psychological well-being of persons with rheumatoid arthritis. *Arthritis Care Research, 9*(6), 449–456.

Farhey, Y. & Hess, E. V. (1997). Mixed connective tissue disease. *Arthritis Care Research, 10*(5), 333–342.

Gammon, J. & Mulholland, C. (1996). Effect of preparatory information prior to elective total hip replacement on psychological coping outcomes. *Journal of Advanced Nursing, 24*(2), 303–308. 15.

Gerber, L. H. & Hicks, J. E. (1995). Surgical and rehabilitation options in the treatment of the rheumatoid arthritis patient resistant to pharmacologic agents. *Rheumatic Disease Clinics of North America, 21*(1), 19–39.

Katz, P. P. & Criswell, L. A. (1996). Differences in symptom reports between men and women with rheumatoid arthritis. *Arthritis Care Research, 9*(6), 441–448.

Kelley, W. N. (1996). *Textbook of rheumatology* (5th ed). Philadelphia: W.B. Saunders.

Kirwan, J. R. & Lim, K. K. T. (1996). Low dose corticosteroids in early rheumatoid arthritis: Can these drugs slow disease progression? *Drugs & Aging, 8*(3), 157–161.

Klippel, J. H., Weyand, C. M. & Wortman, R. (Eds.) (1997). *Primer on the rheumatic diseases* (11th ed.). Atlanta: Longstreet Press.

Knight, R. & Pellegrini, V. Jr. (1996). Bladder management after total joint arthroplasty. *Journal of Arthroplasty, 11*(8), 882–888.

Krug, B. (1997). Rheumatoid arthritis and osteoarthritis: A basic comparison. *Orthopedic Nursing, 16*(5), 73–75.

Lin, P. et al. (1997). Comparing the effectiveness of different educational programs for patients with total knee arthroplasty. *Orthopedic Nursing, 16*(5), 43–49.

Marks, R. & Cantin, D. (1997). Symptomatic osteoarthritis of the knee: The efficacy of physiotherapy. *Physiotherapy, 83*, 306–311.

Meyers, S. et al. (1996). Inpatient cost of primary total joint arthroplasty. *Journal of Arthroplasty, 11*(3), 281–285.

Oddis, C. V. (1996). New perspectives on osteoarthritis. *American Journal of Medicine, 100*(52A), 2A-105–155.

O'Brien, S. et al. (1996). A study of the factors in hip replacement dislocation. Part 1. *Nursing Standard, 11*(7), 33–38.

O'Brien, S. et al. (1996). A study of the factors in hip replacement dislocation. Part 2. *Nursing Standard, 11*(8), 39–42.

Pannush, R. S. & Arend, W. P. (1997). Emerging role of biologic therapies for treatment of rheumatic disease. *JAMA, 277*(23), 1899–1900.

Pigg, J. S. (1997). Case management of the patient with arthritis. *Orthopedic Nursing*, 33–40.

Polisson, R. (1996). Nonsteroidal anti-inflammatory drugs: Practical and theoretical considerations in their selection. *American Journal of Medicine, 100*(Suppl. 2A), 2A-31S–2A-36S.

Ross, C. (1997). A comparison of osteoarthritis and rheumatoid arthritis: Diagnosis and treatment. *Nurse Practitioner, 22*(9), 20–41.

Schilke, J. et al. (1996). Effects of muscle-strength training on the functional status of patients with osteoarhtritis of the knee joint. *Nursing Research, 45*(2), 68–72.

Simms, R. W. (1996). Fibromyalgia syndrome: Current concepts in pathophysiology, clinical features, and management. *Arthritis Care Research, 9*(4), 315–328.

Wegener, S. T. (ed.) (1996). *Clinical care in the rheumatic diseases.* Atlanta: American College of Rheumatology.

Williamson, V. (1997). Clinical pathways for a patient with a total joint replacement. *Orthopedic Nursing*, 41–45.

OSTEOPOROSIS

Hooker, R. (1998). Management of estabilished osteoporosis. *Lippincott's Primary Care Practitioner, 2*(1), 32–37.

Kessenich, C. (1997). Obtaining a diagnosis of postmenopausal osteoporosis. *Lippincott's Primary Care Practitioner, 1*(5), 474–484.

Kessenich, C. (1996). Update on pharmacolgic therapies for osteoporosis. *Nurse Practitioner, 21*(8), 19–24.

Linsey, R. (1996). The menopause and osteoporosis. *Obstetrics and Gynecology, 87*(27), 16S–19S.

Silverman, S. L. et al. (1997). Effect of bone density information on decisions about hormone replacement therapy: A randomized trial. *Obstetrics and Gynecology, 89*(3), 321–325.

Thomas, T. (1997). Lifestyle risk factors for osteoporosis. *MEDSURG Nursing, 6*(5), 275–277, 287.

WHO Study Group. (1994). *Assessment of fracture risk and its application to screening for postmenopausal osteoporosis.* Geneva: World health Organization.

INTEGUMENTARY

Arndt, K. A., Wintroub, B. U., Robinson, J. K. & LeBoit, P. E. (1997). *Primary care dermatology.* Philadelphia: W.B. Saunders.

Bryant, R. L. (1995). Preventative foot care program: A nursing perspective. *Ostomy/Wound Management, 41*(4), 28–34.

Demis, D. J. (Ed.) (1998). *Clinical dermatology.* Philadelphia: Lippincott-Raven.

Fitzpatrick, T. B. et al. (1997). *Color atlas and synopsis of clinical dermatology* (3rd ed.). New York: McGraw-Hill.

Freedberg, I. M. (ed.) (1998). *Fitzpatrick's dermatology in general medicine.* New York: McGraw-Hill.

Habif, T. P. (1996). *Clinical dermatology* (3rd ed.). St. Louis: Mosby–Year Book.

Helm, K. & Marks, J. (1998). *Atlas of differential diagnosis in dermatology.* New York: Churchill Livingstone.

Kerstein, M. D., Nicol, N. H., Ruszkowski, A. M., & Moore, J. A. (1995). Contact dermatitis and the role of patch testing in its diagnosis and management. *Dermatology Nursing,* Supplement.

Lookingbill, D. P. & Marks, J. P. (1993). *Principles of dermatology* (2nd ed.). Philadelphia: W.B. Saunders.

McMichael, A. J. (1996). Successful aging in the elderly dermatology patient. *Journal of Geriatric Dermatology, 4*(4), 132–136.

Noble, S. L. Fórbes, R. C. & Stamm, P. L. (1998). Diagnosis and management of common tinea infections. *American Family Physician, 58*(1), 163–174, 177–178.

Rasmussen, J. E. (1995). Erythema multiforme, Stenvens-Johnson syndrome, and toxic epidermal necrolysis. *Dermatology Nursing, 7*(1), 37–43.

Ruszkowski, A. M. Nicol, N. H., & Mooree, J. A. (1995). Patch testing basics: Patient selection, application techniques, and guidelines for interpretation. *Dermatology Nursing,* Supplement.

Sheretz, E. E., & Byers, S. V. (1997). Common patch test allergens: General guidelines For avoidance. *Dermatology Nursing, 9*(2), 122–126.

Talarico, L. D. (1998). Aging skin: Best approaches to common problems. *Patient Care Nurse Practitioner, 1*(5), 28–40.

Wolkenstein, P. E., Roujeau, J. C., & Revuz, J. (1998). Drug-induced toxic epidermal necrolysis. *Clinical Dermatology, 16*(3), 399–408.

PSORIASIS

Farber, E. M., & Raychaudhuri, S. P. (1997). Concept of total care: A third dimension in the treatment of psoriasis. *Cutis, 59*(1).

Laffrey, S. C., Bailey, B. J., & Craig, K. K. (1996). Social support and health promotion outcomes of adults with psoriasis. *Dermatology Nursing, 8*(2), 109–112, 117–119.

SKIN CANCER

Anderson, R. G. (1995). Skin tumor II: Melanoma. *Selected Readings in Plastic Surgery, 8*(7).

Centers for Disease Control (1998). Sun-protection behaviors used by adults for their children—US 1997. *MMWR, 47*(23), 48–52.

Cottell, W. I. (1995). Skin Tumors I: Basal cell carcenoma and squarous cell carcinoma. *Selected Readings in Plastic Surgery, 8*(6).

Requena, L. & Sangueza, O. P. (1998). Cutaneous vascular proliferations, part III: Malignant neoplasms, other cutaneous neoplasms with significant vascular component and disorders erroneously considered as vascular neoplasms. *Journal of the American Academy of Dermatology, 38*(2, Pt. I), 143–175.

Wachsmuth, R. C. (1998). The atypical mole syndrome and predisposition to melanoma. *New England Journal of Medicine, 339*(5),348–349.

Weinstock, M. A., & Rossi, J. S. (1998). The Rhode Island Sun Smart Project: A scientific approach to skin cancer prevention. *Clinical Dermatology, 16*(4), 411–413.

PRESSURE ULCERS

Agency for Health Care Policy and Research. (1992). *Pressure ulcers in adults: Prediction and prevention.* Clinical Practice Guideline No. 3. Rockville, MD: U.S. Department of Health and Human Services. Public Health Service, Agency for Healthcare Policy and Research. AHCPR Publication No. 92-0047.

Agency for Health Care Policy and Research. (1994). *Treat ment of pressure ulcers.* Clinical Practice Guideline No. 15. Rockville, MD: U.S. Department of Health and Human Services. Public Health Service, Agency for Healthcare Policy and Research. AHCPR Publication No. 95-0652.

Krastnen, D., & Kane, D. (1997). *Chronic wounds.* Wayne, PA: Health Management Publications. Murphy, J. I. (Ed.) Nurse Practitioner Prescribing Reference. New York, NY, Prescribing Reference, Inc. Summer 1998.

Phillips, T. J. (1996). Leg ulcer management. *Dermatology Nursing, 8*(5), 333–340.

BURNS

Allwood, J. S. (1995). The primary care management of burns. *Nurse Practitioner, 20*(80), 74–87.

Byers, J. F., & Flynn, M. B. (1996). Acute burn injury: A case report. *Critical Care Nurse, 16*(4), 55–65.

Cruse, C. W., & Krizek, T. J. (1996). *Manual of burn care.* Tampa, FL: Tampa Bay Regional Burn Center and University of South Florda, Department of Surgery, College of Medicine.

Gillespie, R. W., Dimick, A. R., Gillespi, P. W., et al. (1993). *Advanced burn life support provider's manual.* Nebraska: National Burn Institute.

Munster, A. M. (1993). *Severe burns: A family guide to medical and emotional recovery.* Baltimore: John Hopkins.

Richard, R. (1994). *Burn care and rehabilitation: Principles and practice.* Philadelphia: F.A. Davis.

Settle, J. A. D. (Ed.) (1996). *Principles and practice of burns management.* New York: Churchill Livingstone.

ON-LINE RESOURCES

MUSCULOSKELETAL

American College of Rheumatology (ACR) *http://www.rheumatology.org*

The Arthritis Foundation *http//:www.arthritis.org*

Fibromyalgia Network *http://fmnetnews.com*

Fibromyalgia patient information *http://www.rheumatology.org/patients/factsheet/fibromya.htm*

Fibromyalgia Association (USA) *http://www.w2.com/fibrol.html*

Fibromyalgia and Chronic Fatigue Syndrome Center *http://www.coloradohealthnet.org/ffibro/fibro_center.htm*

Muscular Dystrophy Association *http://www.mdause.org*

Myasthenia Gravis Foundation of America (MGFA) *http://www.myasthenia.com*

Myasthenia gravis Web Forum *http://neuro-www.mgh.harvard.edu/forum/myastheniagravismenu.html*

National Institutes of Health Consensus Development Conference Statement *http://text.nlm.nih.gov/nih/cdc/www/43.html*

National Institute of Arthritis and Musculoskeletal and Skin Diseases National Institutes of Health *http://www.nih.gov/niams/*

National Association of Orthopaedic Nurses (NAON) *http://naon.inurse.com*

Osteoarthritis *http://www.ama. assn.org/insight/spec_com/arthriti.htm*

Osteoporosis information and resources *http://www.pstgroup.com/OSTEOPOROSIS.HTM*

INTEGUMENTARY

American Academy of Dermatology *http://www.aad.org*

Padgett-Coehlo, Deborah (1997). Skin, hair and nails examination. Health assessment: A learning package. *http://www.son.edu/nursing/health/skin.htm*

National Psorias is Foundation *http://www.psoriasis.org*

Skin Cancer Foundation *http://www.skincancer.org*

Unit
10

Neural Control

FOCUS ON Neurologic Changes Through the Life Span

INFANT (1–12 MONTHS):

Vital functions, unstable at birth, stabilize within the first few months. Cerebellar function improves to allow movement and equilibrium. The cerebral cortex develops rapidly, with increased sensory perception, motor functioning, speech, and understanding. Myelin continues to form around nerve sheaths, accounting for coordination of voluntary movement in the later parts of this stage.

TODDLER AND PRESCHOOL AGE (1–5 YEARS):

Myelinization becomes nearly complete by age 2 years. Differences between the sexes are noted. In general, language ability is more developed in girls, whereas coordination for activities is more developed in boys. Fine motor coordination begins to develop with toilet training, walking, jumping, dressing, eye–hand coordination, puzzles, and other more complex activities. Ninety percent of myelinization occurs by age 5 years.

SCHOOL AGE (6–12 YEARS):

Brain achieves adult size by age 12 years. Neuromuscular coordination becomes complete, with improved transmission of nerve impulses, increased reaction time and coordination, and skilled movements. By age 12 years, eye–hand coordination is equal to that of adults. A rapid increase in cognition and perception occurs.

ADOLESCENCE (13–19 YEARS):

Nerve conduction is maximal. Brain wave activity stabilizes with some increase in myelinization and reticular formation.

YOUNG ADULT/ADULT (20–45 YEARS):

Final myelinization occurs by age 25 years. Brain, which receives maximal (30%) cardiac output, is very active metabolically. No regenerative potential for neurons is present. Brain weight begins to decline about 1 gm per year after age 30 years.

MIDDLE-AGED ADULT (46–64 YEARS):

A gradual loss of neurons occurs without a decrease in cognition. Nerve conduction speed decreases about 5%. Voice changes occur that are probably due to changing levels of estrogen and testosterone.

LATE ADULTHOOD (65–100+ YEARS):

Neuron loss continues with associated decrease in cerebral blood flow. Reaction times slow due to decreased levels of neurotransmitters. Gait and balance are affected with decreased proprioception. Sleep patterns are altered. Brain weight, mainly in the cerebral cortex, may decrease up to 10%.

Chapter

29

Normal Structure and Function of the Nervous System

Reet Henze

KEY TERMS

action potential
afferent neuron
association neuron
autonomic nervous system
brain barriers
convergence
corticospinal tract
dendrites
dermatome
diencephalon
divergence
efferent neuron
extrapyramidal tract
facilitation
falx cerebri
ganglia
meninges
mesencephalon
myotome
neuron
neurofibrils
neuroglia
neurotransmitter
nuclei
prosencephalon
pyramidal tract
reflex arc
reticular formation
rhombencephalon
sensory receptors
somatic efferent system
synapse
telencephalon
tentorium cerebelli
visceral efferent system

Humans interact with the environment through the nervous system, perceiving and responding to the stimuli that continually affect them. A complex system of connections and interconnections of nerve cells provides for perception, interim processing, and response. In addition, characteristics that endow humans with the ability to think, feel, reason, and remember evolve from the interacting neuronal networks of the brain.

The nervous system is composed of central and peripheral components. The fundamental structure in each is the neuron. The neuron and groups of neurons communicate within the environment of the central and peripheral nervous systems.

THE NEURON

The **neuron**, shown in Figure 29-1, is the structural and functional unit of nerve tissue. Neurons have distinctive cellular shapes. Unlike other cells, mature neurons lack centrosomes and are incapable of mitosis. Subsequently, neurons are unable to reproduce themselves. If the cell body dies, the entire neuron dies. Under certain circumstances it is possible for the axons of peripheral nerves to regenerate if the cell body is preserved.[5,15]

Neuron Structure

The structural components of a neuron include the cell body, dendrites, and axons. The cell body, also known as the perikaryon, contains the nucleus and nucleolus and is the metabolic center of the neuron. It receives transmissions from other neurons directly or via its dentrites and axons of other neurons. **Dendrites** are long, complex branching structures that evolve from the cell body. Axons (nerve fibers) are singular cytoplasmic tubes that extend from the cell body and provide the structure for action potentials. The axon originates from the axon hillock of the cell body and transmits signals from the cell body to various parts of the nervous system. Axons, therefore, differ from dendrites, which carry transmissions to the cell. Some axons are myelinated, whereas others have no myelin sheath.

Myelin is a fatty layer that surrounds the nerve fiber and helps increase conduction of nerve impulses. Myelin gives the axon its characteristic white color and provides protective, nutritive, and conductive functions for the axon. The myelin is interrupted by periodic gaps known as the *nodes of Ranvier*. Axon collaterals or fibers may emerge from these gaps. Exchange of metabolites

FOCUS ON CELLULAR PHYSIOLOGY

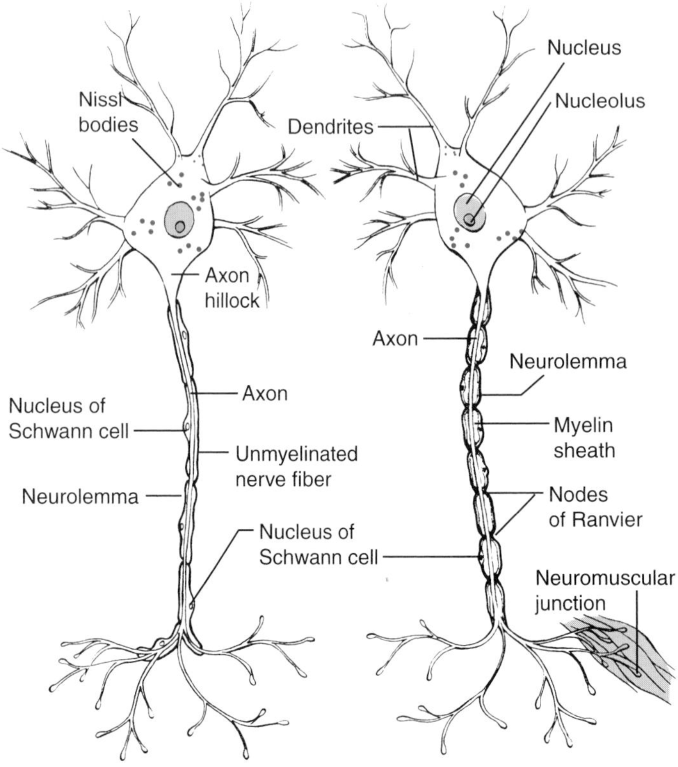

FIGURE 29-1. **Typical efferent neurons: unmyelinated fiber (left), myelinated fiber (right).**

takes place between the axon and the extracellular environment at the nodes. The nodes of Ranvier are present in both central and peripheral nervous system neurons. However, they are much easier to identify in the peripheral nervous system. Schwann cells located along the peripheral axons produce the lipoprotein myelin sheath of numerous concentric wrappings around the central core axon (Fig. 29-2). Unmyelinated fibers also contain Schwann cells but lack the concentric wrappings.

The outermost thin layer of myelin of the myelinated fibers is known as the *neurolemma* or *endonurium* of the axon. This neurolemma also enwraps the unmyelinated axon. However, in the myelinated fibers within the spinal cord and brain, the neurolemma is absent.

Morphologically, neurons are identified according to projections arising from the cell body as (1) unipolar, (2) bipolar, or (3) multipolar. A unipolar neuron consists of one projection, an axon that usually extends in two directions. A bipolar neuron consists of one axon and one dendrite. The multipolar neuron, most prevalent in the nervous system, consists of one major projection from the cell body, the axon, and generally multiple complex branchings (dendrites) (Fig. 29-3).

Functionally, neurons also are classified as *sensory, motor,* or *association* neurons.

- Sensory (**afferent**) neurons relay messages about the internal and external environment to the central nervous system (CNS).
- Motor and secretory (**efferent**) neurons transmit messages from the CNS to the periphery.
- **Association** (internuncial or interneurons) neurons relay messages from one neuron to another within the brain and spinal cord.

Clusters of neurons within the CNS are called **nuclei** (gray matter); examples of nuclei include those in the thalamus and basal ganglia. Groups of neurons outside the CNS are known as **ganglia**; examples are the dorsal root ganglia and the autonomic nervous system ganglia.

PERIPHERAL AXONAL DEGENERATION AND REGENERATION

An injured neuron may regenerate as long as its cell body remains relatively unharmed. However, serious damage to the cell body results in death of the entire neuron. A crushed or severed axon of a peripheral nerve fiber triggers certain cellular changes within a few hours of injury. Changes in the axon distal (portion of axon cut off from the cell body) to the injury are referred to as *wallerian degeneration* and are particularly dramatic

FOCUS ON CELLULAR PHYSIOLOGY

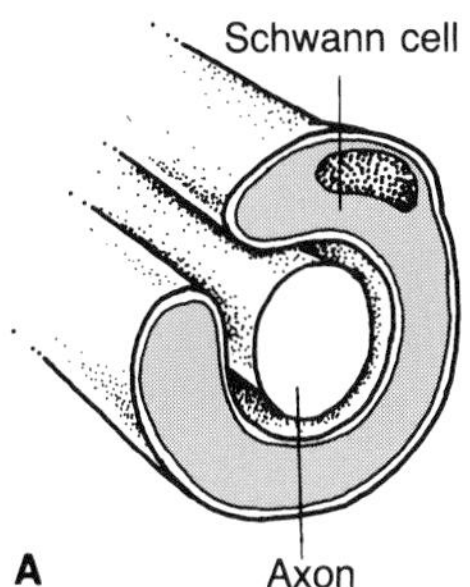

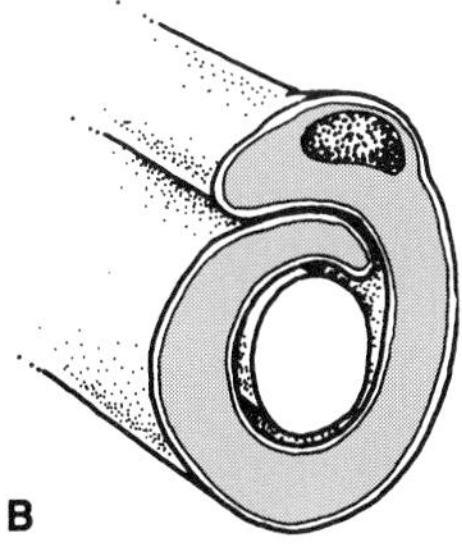

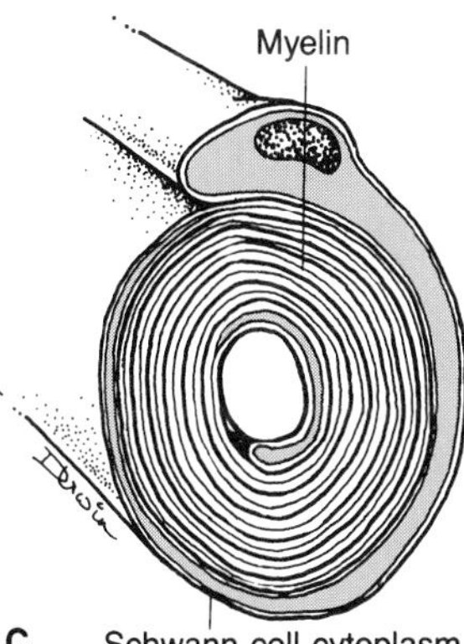

FIGURE 29-2. Three consecutive stages in the myelination of a segment of an axon by a Schwann cell of the peripheral nervous system. The Schwann cell adheres to its surrounding basement membrane (**A**) and its inner margin grows around the axon (**B**, **C**). (Cormack, D. H. [1993]. *Essential histology.* Philadelphia: J. B. Lippincott.)

because that portion has been severed from the metabolic control of the cell body.[1,5] Initially, the distal portion swells due to influx of sodium and water. The terminal neurofilaments hypertrophy and Schwann cells proliferate. Mitochondrial damage results from uncontrolled calcium influx. The myelin sheath shrinks and retracts at the nodes of Ranvier, where the remaining nerve fiber becomes exposed. The axon gradually disappears, and myelin disintegrates into fragments that are phagocytized by the Schwann cells and tissue macrophages.[14]

Changes also occur proximal to the injury in both the axon and the cell body (*retrograde degeneration*). Degenerative changes similar to those in the distal portion of the axon occur for a few millimeters at the proximal portion from the injury. The extent of cellular change is related to the location of the injury along the axon. An axon injury near the cell body produces greater changes in the cell than an injury that is more distant.

Cellular cytoplasm swells, displacing the nucleus toward the cell wall. In response, cellular metabolic activity, protein synthesis, and mitochondrial activity increase. Injured **neurofibrils** (delicate threads projecting into the axon from the cell body) attempt to grow back into their original placements and begin sprouting from the proximal portion of the injured axon within 7 to 14 days after injury. If the fibrils are successful in finding their way into the neurolemma, which generally remains intact, they generally grow at a rate of 1.5 mm per day.[5,14] The remaining Schwann cells form a sheet of myelin around the restored neurofibril, and the nodes of Ranvier are reformed as the nerve regenerates. Early surgical repair of severed peripheral nerves facilitates nerve regeneration. Regeneration of injured nerves in the CNS is more difficult due to glial scarring, which frequently inhibits new fibrils from reaching their destinations.

SYNAPSE

Information concerning the environment is relayed through a succession of neurons in contact with one another. The area of contact between the neurons is called the **synapse.** The terminal portion of the presynaptic axon, the *bouton* or *knob*, may synapse with the cell body (axosomatic), dendrites (axodendritic), axons of other nerve cells (axoaxonic), or effector cells of muscles or glands (Fig. 29-4). This presynaptic bouton is divided from the postsynaptic membrane by a narrow space of about 200 to 300 angstroms (A), known as the *synaptic cleft.* The presynaptic bouton contains stored particles of a transmitter substance that is released at the synapse in response to a stimulus to excite or inhibit the postsynaptic or effector neuron. Mitochondria in the presynaptic bouton provide the ATP for synthesizing the released substance that is continually regenerated.

Neuron Function

The neuron has the capability to generate and conduct electrochemical impulses. The cellular, cytoplasmic, and metabolic activities that maintain cell life are sim-

FOCUS ON CELLULAR PHYSIOLOGY

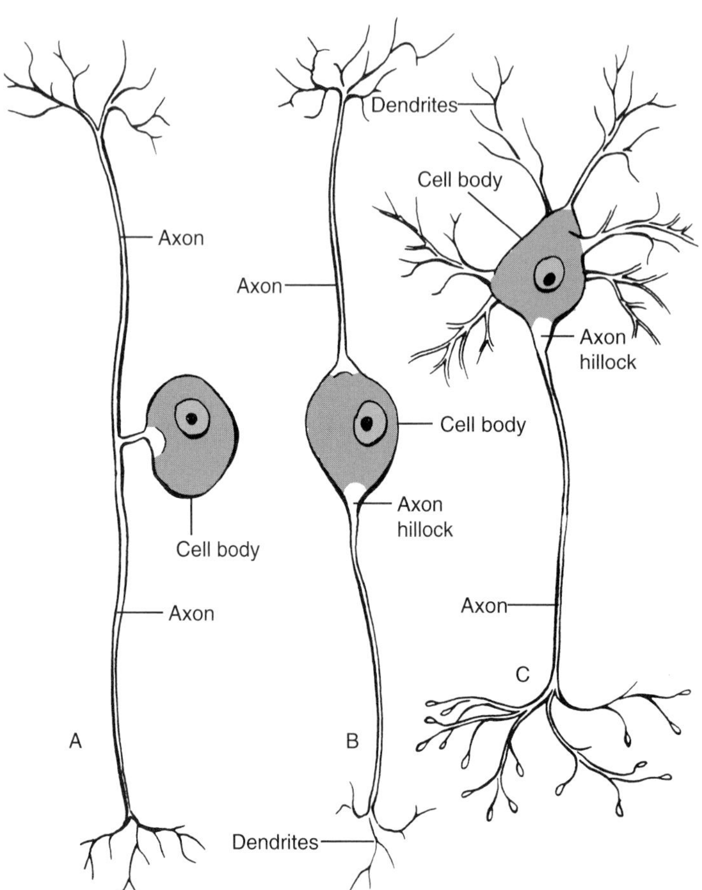

FIGURE 29-3. **The three basic shapes of neurons. A.** Unipolar; **B.** bipolar; **C.** multipolar.

ilar to those of other cells. Neurons are distinct with their structural synapses allowing them to conduct impulses from one to another.

NEURONAL CONDUCTION

Conduction of neuronal impulses depends on membrane potentials. Membrane potentials are generated because of a disparity between cations and anions at the semipermeable and selectively permeable nerve cell membrane. Specific proteins at the cell membrane allow the movement of ions and facilitate the nerve cell potential and impulse propagation. These proteins include cell membrane pumps and channels. Pumps maintain appropriate ion concentrations in the cell side of the membrane by actively moving ions against concentration gradients. Channel proteins provide selective paths for specific ions to diffuse across the cell membrane. When the neuron is resting, its membrane potential results because of an excess of negative charges inside and positive charges outside. The resting membrane potential is maintained by the sodium-potassium pump.

Action Potential

Unique to nerve, muscle, and gland cells is the change that can occur in a resting cell membrane potential when the cells are stimulated by electrical, chemical, or mechanical means. These stimuli can produce a sudden increase in cell membrane permeability to sodium, which results in a very brief, positive potential within the cell. The sequence of physiochemical events that results in an alteration in the resting potential lasts a few milliseconds and is called the **action potential.** The events of the action potential are described in Chapter 1.

Conduction Velocity in Nerve Fibers

The velocity of nerve conduction is influenced by the myelinization and diameter of the axon. Myelin acts as an effective insulator and inhibits electrochemical conduction along the full segment of the membrane. This selectivity facilitates an increase in conduction velocity. As the current passes over the myelin and through the extracellular fluid, it enters the nodes of Ranvier at 1-mm to 2-mm intervals, where the membrane is permeable to the ions. Figure 29-5 shows cur-

FOCUS ON CELLULAR PHYSIOLOGY

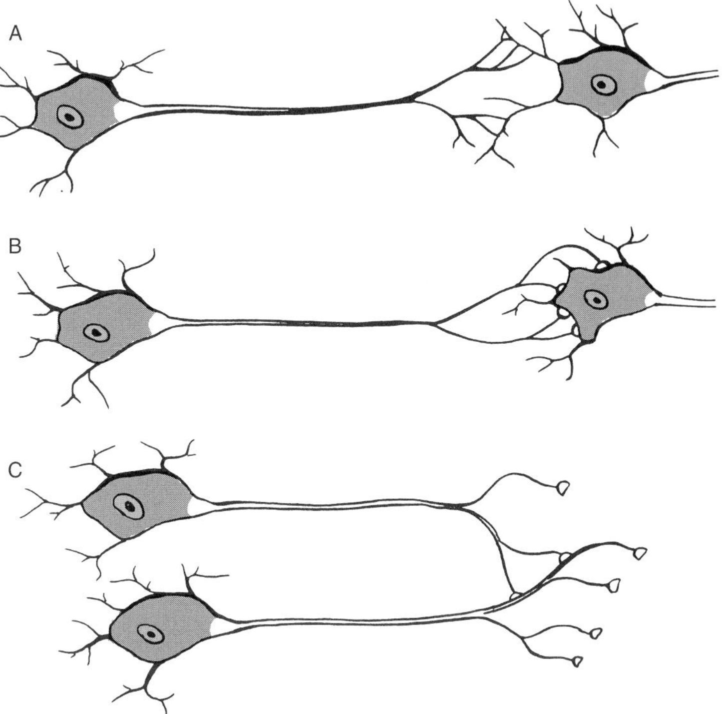

FIGURE 29-4. **Different types of synapses. A. Axodendritic; B. axosomatic; C. axoaxonic.**

rent propagation in myelinated fibers, which is known as *saltatory conduction,* implying a leaping or hopping phenomenon.

The myelin sheath enhances the velocity of current conduction as capacitance is reduced, which results in reduced numbers of charges propagating the length of the fiber. The large myelinated fibers transmit impulses at approximately 100 m/second.[13] In contrast, small unmyelinated fibers may conduct impulses as slow as 0.5 m/second.[13] Figure 29-5 shows that the wave of action potential leaks out and dissipates with distance in an unmyelinated fiber, whereas the myelinated fiber retains the action potential current longer.

The diameter of the fiber is an additional important factor contributing to nerve conduction velocity. Velocity is increased in large-diameter nerve fibers due to lower internal resistance and a quicker depolarization time.

SYNAPTIC TRANSMISSION

Conduction of impulses through synapses is unidirectional, occurring only through terminal boutons of presynaptic membranes to postsynaptic membranes. Impulses at the synapse can be transmitted through chemical or electrical means. Chemical synapses, by far the most common, involve the release of a chemical substance (**neurotransmitter**) in response to a stimulus. This substance has an excitatory or inhibitory effect on the postsynaptic cell membrane. The electrical synapse, fused synapses very rare in the CNS, are found only in a few neural circuits such as the inferior olive and oculomotor nuclei.[5] Electrical synapses propagate uninterrupted impulses. The discussion here is limited to chemical synapses.

A very low level of spontaneously released neurotransmitter substances occurs from the terminal bouton in the resting synapse.[5] This causes spontaneous mini-depolarizations at the synapse. When an action potential spreads to the presynaptic bouton, as shown in the neuromuscular junction in Figure 29-6, depolarization of the membrane triggers release of the transmitter substance. It is thought that the trigger release at the terminal bouton requires calcium ions. This theory is supported by observations that low extracellular calcium levels result in diminished amounts of transmitter substance being released.[14] The neurotransmitter substance then attaches to the postsynaptic receptor sites, and the postsynaptic membrane potential is modified. The neurotransmitter substance not taken up by the postsynaptic receptors may be (1) taken up by the presynaptic bouton and stored,

FOCUS ON CELLULAR PHYSIOLOGY

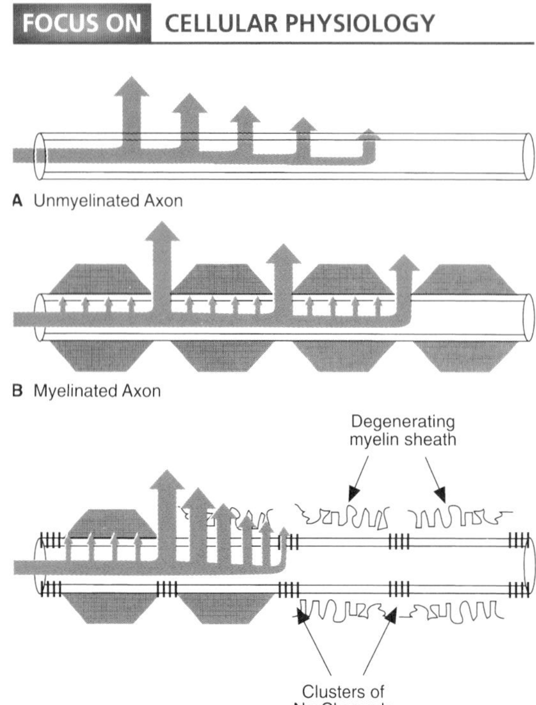

FIGURE 29-5. Excitatory current spreads over a greater distance in a myelinated axon than an equivalent-diameter unmyelinated axon. **A.** The wave of excitatory positive current that spreads down an unmyelinated axon ahead of an advancing action potential leaks out of the axon and dissipates with distance. **B.** The insulating properties of myelin retard this leakage and allow more current to be available at greater distances to depolarize and excite the membrane at the nodes of Ranvier. **C.** Degeneration of the myelin sheath short-circuits this insulation and shunts excitatory current to the extracellular space by means of K channels unmasked by the demyelination. As a consequence, insufficient charge is available to excite enough nodal Na channels to threshold levels, and action potential conduction can fail. (Conn, P. M. [1995]. *Neuroscience in medicine.* Philadelphia: J. B. Lippincott.)

(2) inactivated at the synaptic cleft or at the postsynaptic membrane by enzymes, or (3) lost through extracellular diffusion.[6,14]

The threshold for stimulation of an action potential is lowest on the axon hillock, whereas the thresholds of the cell body and dendrites are considerably higher. Therefore, action potentials initiated in most neurons originate in the axon hillock.

Presynaptic release of an excitatory neurotransmitter substance can initiate a depolarizing response in the postsynaptic membrane that is referred to as the *excitatory postsynaptic potential (EPSP)*.[5,6] The EPSP is the result of an increase in the permeability of the postsynaptic membrane to sodium, potassium, chloride, and calcium ions. Sodium ions flow in across the membrane and decrease the negativity of the postsynaptic cell, producing a threshold voltage change.[5] Many active terminals discharging spontaneously are required to elicit an action potential, a phenomenon known as *spatial summation*.[5] Thus, the amplitude of the EPSP depends on the number of activated synapses; if sufficient numbers are firing, an action potential results.

Some synapses involve inhibitory transmitters such as glycine and gamma-aminobutyric acid (GABA). These produce limited permeability to chloride, increasing the negativity of the already negative postsynaptic cell, and a state of hyperpolarization. This is called an *inhibitory postsynaptic potential (IPSP)*.[8,12] The permeability change is very brief because active

FOCUS ON CELLULAR PHYSIOLOGY

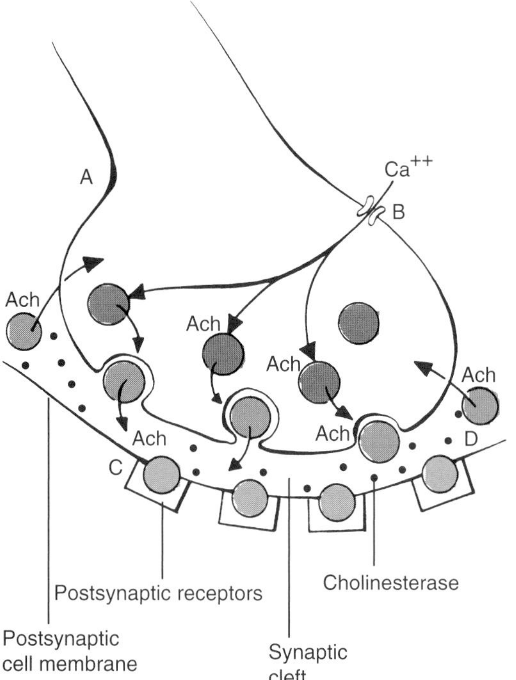

FIGURE 29-6. Summary of cholinergic synaptic transmission at neuromuscular junction. **A.** Presynaptic bouton containing acetylcholine (Ach) vesicles. **B.** Action potential causes Ca^{++} to enter presynaptic bouton and fuse with Ach vesicle, resulting in release of Ach into the synaptic cleft, **C.** Ach binds with post-synaptic receptors, causing depolarization of the post-synaptic membrane. **D.** Cholinesterase hydrolyzes some synaptic Ach, while some Ach is returned intact to presynaptic bouton for reuse.

transport of chloride out of the cell restores resting potential rapidly. During the IPSP, the cell is less excitable because the membrane potential is more negative. Increased excitatory activity is needed to reach the threshold level.

In addition to the IPSP, another form of inhibition, called *presynaptic inhibition*, occurs throughout the nervous system. Although concentrated in the peripheral afferent fibers, this type of inhibition occurs at the presynaptic bouton. No change takes place in the postsynaptic membrane. An inhibitory terminal bouton acts on the presynaptic bouton by releasing a neurotransmitter that partially depolarizes the presynaptic terminal. This greatly reduces the voltage of the action potential and thus reduces the excitability in the membrane. It is thought that presynaptic inhibition provides a control mechanism for sensory inflow, so that less important input is eliminated, allowing major signals to be relayed more clearly to the CNS.

Facilitation

Many presynaptic terminals converge on each postsynaptic neuron. A certain number of action potentials must be transmitted simultaneously for a sufficient amount of neurotransmitter to be released to produce an action potential in the postsynaptic membrane. If an insufficient amount of a neurotransmitter is released, the postsynaptic membrane is excitatory, although not to threshold level. Termed **facilitation,** the action potential is above resting potential but below threshold value. The neuron is very receptive to a stimulus that can activate it with ease.

Divergence and Convergence

Extremely complex networks of neurons exist in the nervous system. Extensive interactions among neurons are mediated through highly organized circuit connections. Neurons divide and subdivide into many collateral branches that synapse with various numbers of other neurons. This presynaptic division is known as **divergence.** For example, the fibers of afferent neurons entering the spinal cord generally divide and subdivide into collateral branches that supply terminal boutons to many other postsynaptic spinal neurons. As a result, no one fiber contributes to an action potential but, rather, many fibers cooperatively produce the innervation. The repetitive subdivision strengthens the afferent information, which is made available to various parts of the CNS through the process of divergence. Similarly, most postsynaptic neurons receive terminal boutons from many presynaptic fibers. This postsynaptic anatomic phenomenon is known as **convergence**. Many axons may converge on a single neuron, and the EPSP is dependent on sufficient amplitude of the active boutons converging upon it.

Neurochemical Transmitter Function

Presynaptic bouton vesicles store specific chemical substances, called neurotransmitters, that, when released into the synaptic cleft, either excite or inhibit other cells. Some transmitter substances are present only in the specific parts of the nervous system, whereas others are widely dispersed. Table 29-1 lists a few of the neurochemical transmitters that have been identified. Since the identification of the first neurotransmitter in 1921, more than 40 have been identified.[11] It is expected that many more will be identified in the future. It has been difficult to pinpoint these substances because of the complex structure of the nervous system fibers.

Substances are considered to be neurochemical transmitters if they have the following general characteristics: (1) they must be present in the presynaptic bouton and contain an enzyme in the presynaptic bouton for its synthesis, (2) they are released by the presynaptic bouton on stimulation, (3) they produce excitation or inhibition in the postsynaptic cell, (4) they have receptors present on the surface of cells responsive to it, and (5) they have demonstrated a mechanism that diminishes the effects of the transmitter.[7]

ACETYLCHOLINE. Acetylcholine (Ach) is a well-established neurotransmitter whose activity at the neuromuscular junction is well understood. The terminal bouton of cholinergic nerve fibers contains vesicles, each of which holds about 10,000 molecules of acetylcholine. A vesicle fuses with the presynaptic membrane and results in the release of acetylcholine, a process known as *exocytosis.*[8] It is thought that the fusion of the vesicle to the presynaptic membrane is brought about by a sudden, transient increase in the concentration of calcium ions in the terminal bouton. The exact mechanism of the calcium activity in exocytosis is unknown. When the fused vesicle has discharged its acetylcholine at the presynaptic membrane, some of the unused Ach is reclaimed by the bouton and restored for future use. The synthesis of acetylcholine occurs in the bouton in the following manner:[8,11,15]

$$\text{Acetylcoenzyme A(acetate)} + \text{Choline} \xrightarrow{\text{Choline acetyltransferase}} \text{Acetylcholine}$$

The acetylcholine that diffuses across the synaptic cleft binds with an acetylcholine receptor on the postsynaptic membrane. This receptor is a channel protein that, in the presence of acetylcholine, lowers its energy state to an open conformation, allowing passage of sodium and potassium ions. Thus, a postsynaptic potential or voltage change is produced.

TABLE 29-1

NEUROTRANSMITTERS: SOURCE AND ACTION

NAME	SECRETION SOURCE	ACTION
AMINES		
Acetylcholine (Ach) First neurotransmitter identified	Neurons in many areas of brain Large pyramidal cells (motor cortex)	Usually excitatory Inhibitory effect on some of parasympathetic nervous system (*e.g.*, heart by vagus)
Chief transmitter of parasympathetic nervous system (NS)	Some cells of basal ganglia Motor neurons that innervate skeletal muscles Preganglionic neurons of autonomic NS Postganglionic neurons of parasympathetic NS Postganglionic neurons of sympathetic NS	
Serotonin (5-HT) Controls body heat, hunger, behavior, and sleep	Nuclei originating in the median raphe of brain stem and projecting to many areas (especially the dorsal horns of the spinal cord and hypothalamus)	Inhibitor of pain pathway cord; helps to control mood and sleep
CATECHOLAMINES		
Dopamine (DA) Affects control of behavior and fine movement	Neurons on the substantia nigra; many neurons of the substantia nigra send fibers to the basal ganglia that are involved in coordination of skeletal muscle activity	Usually inhibitory
Norepinephrine (NE) Chief transmitter of sympathetic nervous system	Many neurons whose cell bodies are located: In brain stem and hypothalamus (controlling overall activity and mood)	Usually excitatory, although sometimes inhibitory
	Most postganglionic neurons of sympathetic NS	Some excitatory and some inhibitory
AMINO ACIDS		
Gamma-aminobutyric acid (GABA)	Nerve terminals of the spinal cord, cerebellum, basal ganglia, and some cortical areas	Inhibitory
Glutamic acid	Presynaptic terminals in many sensory pathways; cerebellum mossy fibers	Excitatory
Glycine	Synapses in spinal cord	Inhibitory
Substance P	Pain fiber terminals in the dorsal horns of the spinal cord; also, the basal ganglia and hypothalamus	Excitatory
POLYPEPTIDES		
Enkephalin	Nerve terminals in the spinal cord, brain stem, thalamus, and hypothalamus	Excitatory to systems that inhibit pain; binds to the same receptors in the CNS that bind opiate drugs
Endorphin	Pituitary gland and areas of the brain	Binds to opiate receptors in the brain and pituitary gland; excitatory to systems that inhibit pain

NS = nervous system; ANS = autonomic nervous system; CNS = central nervous system.
(Hickey, J. V. [1997]. *The clinical practice of neurological and neurosurgical nursing* [4th ed.]. Philadelphia: Lippincott.)

The chemically gated postsynaptic potentials differ from action potentials of neurons. Their amplitude is smaller, their duration is longer, and they are graded in accordance with the amount of transmitter released.

Within 2 or 3 msec of its release into the synaptic cleft, after it has depolarized the postsynaptic membrane, acetylcholine is hydrolyzed by the enzyme acetylcholinesterase in the following manner:[15]

Acetylcholinesterase
↓
Acetylcholine → Choline + acetate

Insights into neurotransmitters and their inhibiting enzymes have been gained through the use of various pharmacologic agents that act on or compete with these substances. For example, the muscle relaxant curare competes with acetylcholine for receptor sites at the postsynaptic membrane.[5,15] Thus, acetylcholine cannot bring about the membrane permeability for depolarization. Some drugs, such as nicotine, simulate acetylcholine action. Neostigmine and physostigmine inactivate the enzymatic action of acetylcholinesterase. Elevated magnesium levels inhibit acetylcholine release by competing with the calcium ions that are necessary for release of acetylcholine.[5]

NOREPINEPHRINE. Norepinephrine is the transmitter substance at all postganglionic sympathetic fibers, except those innervating sweat glands and skeletal muscle vasculature. This substance is formed through a series of steps catalyzed by enzymes. The process begins with the active transport of tyrosine from the circulation into the nerve terminals as follows:[11,15]

Tyrosine
↓ tyrosine hydroxylase
Dopa
↓ dopa-decarboxylase
Dopamine
↓ dopamine beta-hydroxylase
Norepinephrine

A nerve impulse initiates the release of norepinephrine into the cleft. Norepinephrine activity at the post-synaptic receptor is terminated primarily through its uptake into the terminal bouton. In addition, a small amount of norepinephrine is inactivated by the activity of intraneural MAO and extraneural catechol-*O*-methyltransferase. An additional small amount escapes the terminal bouton uptake and enters the systemic circulation, where it is metabolized by the liver into vanillylmandelic acid (VMA) and excreted in the urine.[11,15] Disease states exhibiting increased production of catecholamines characteristically show increased VMA urinary excretion. Minute amounts of released norepinephrine, which escape uptake and metabolic breakdown in the liver, appear unchanged in the urine.

NEUROGLIA

The supporting structure for the neurons of the CNS is provided by the **neuroglia**. Neuroglia are the counterpart cells to the Schwann cells in the peripheral nervous system (PNS). Considerably more numerous than neurons, neuroglia protect, nourish, and support the neurons. Different types of neuroglial cells and their functions are highlighted in Figure 29-7. They include:

- Astrocytes
- Oligodendroglia
- Microglia
- Ependymal cells

SENSORY RECEPTORS

Sensory receptors are specialized nerve cells that respond to specific information from the internal and external environments. These receptors typically respond to specific types of stimulation. Classifications of sensory receptors and their stimulating modalities are shown in Table 29-2.

Sensory Receptor Structure

Figure 29-8 shows that specific receptors exhibit a wide range of morphologic and sensitivity differences. Some have free nerve endings with coils, spirals, and branching networks; may be present throughout the body; and detect pain, cold, warmth, and crude touch. Other receptor cells are encased in variously shaped capsules and detect tissue deformation.

Sensory Receptor Function

Information sensed by the receptors is transmitted by spinal or cranial nerves to specific areas of the CNS for interpretation. Various forms of natural energy from the environment are converted into action potentials in neurons. This transduction of energy is common to all receptors.

SENSORY RECEPTOR STIMULATION

Each receptor cell has adapted to respond to one specific type or modality of stimulus at a lower threshold than other receptors. This response in receptors is referred to as *labeled line stimulus*.[12] It remains the same no matter how the receptor is stimulated. The specific point where the nerve terminates in the CNS determines the interpretation given to that stimulation.

When a constant stimulus is applied to a receptor, the frequency of action potentials initiated in the sensory nerve decreases. This phenomenon is known as *adaptation*.[11,12] There is a wide variation in sensory

FOCUS ON CELLULAR PHYSIOLOGY

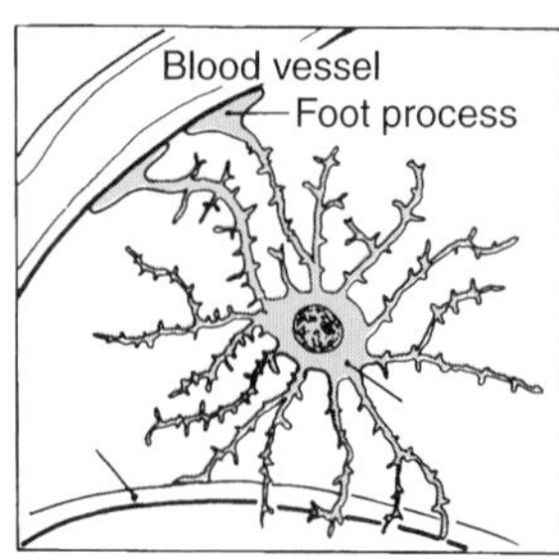

Astrocytes
(star-shaped cells)
- Function in metabolism of neurotransmitters
- Function in formation of blood-brain barrier
- Provide a supporting network in brain and vasculature
- Proliferate at site of nervous system injury[14]

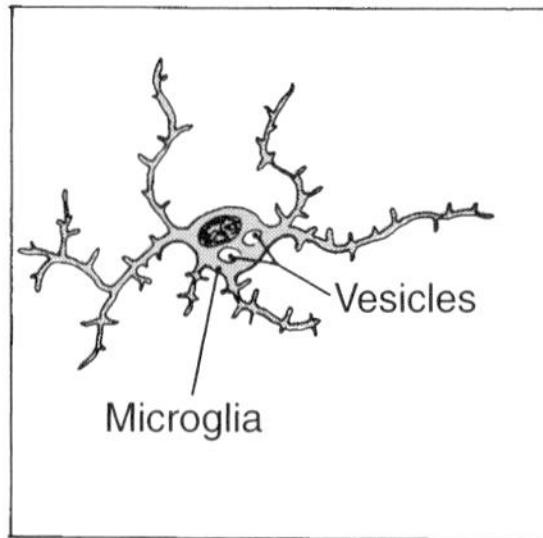

Microglia
(small glial cells)
- Function in phago-cytosis and clearing injured areas of CNS
- May migrate from one site to another

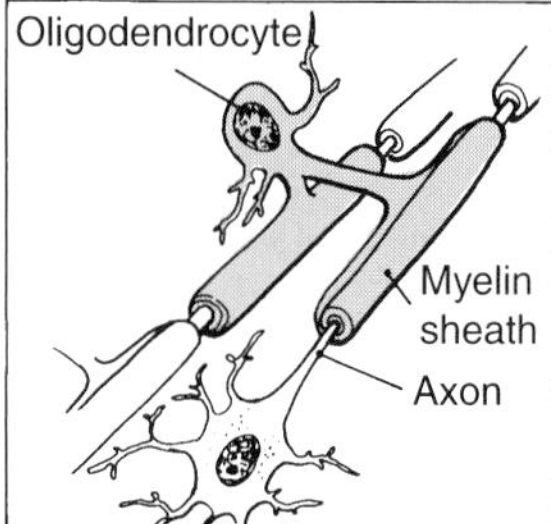

Oligodendrocytes
- Provide support
- Produce myelin sheaths in the CNS axons

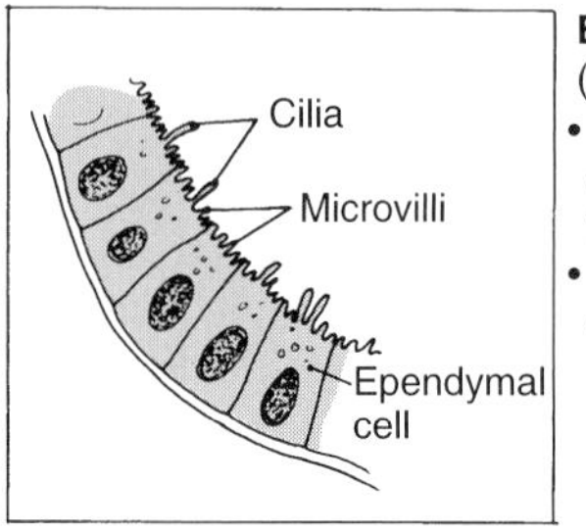

Ependymal cells
(epithelial cells)
- Form continuous epithelial lining for ventricles
- Assist in circulation of cerebrospinal fluid

FIGURE 29-7. Types of neuroglial cells.

organ adaptation. For example, the pressure applied to a pacinian corpuscle, which is found in connective tissue throughout the body, results in a receptor potential that adapts rapidly. The fast-adapting receptors are called *phasic* receptors. In contrast, the muscle spindles and receptors for pain adapt very slowly. These receptors are known as *tonic* receptors.

Receptor Potential

Specific receptors convert modalities of sensation into electrical energy and action potentials through graded receptor potentials (also known as generator potentials). The receptor potentials are not an all-or-nothing event like the action potentials of neurons. Rather, the magnitude is dependent on the intensity of the stimulus. As the magnitude of the stimulus is increased, the receptor potential increases.

Receptor potentials are stationary, producing a local flow of current that spreads electrically to surrounding cell areas as a result of a change in membrane permeability and movement of ions caused by a stimulus. This movement of ions spreads to the *nerve terminal* (the part of the nerve fiber in contact with the receptor) and becomes an action potential at the first node of Ranvier.[11]

The mechanisms that generate receptor potentials vary with receptors. For example, deformation (stimulation causing change in shape) generates receptor potential in the pacinian corpuscles, and chemicals initiate receptor potentials in the rods and cones of the eyes. Because most receptor terminals are minute in size and difficult to study, less information is available about their activity than about that of the action potentials.

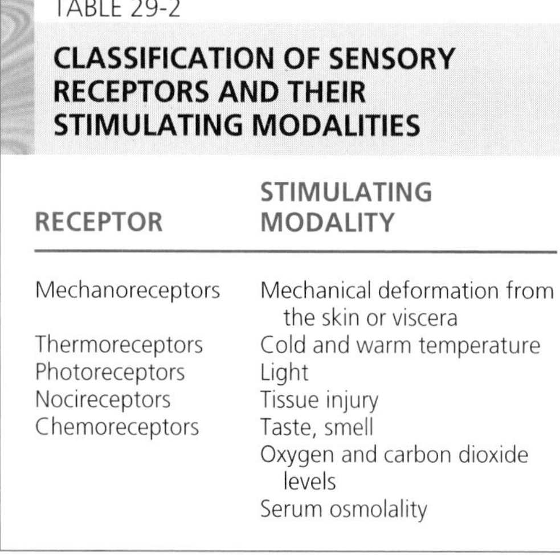

TABLE 29-2

CLASSIFICATION OF SENSORY RECEPTORS AND THEIR STIMULATING MODALITIES

RECEPTOR	STIMULATING MODALITY
Mechanoreceptors	Mechanical deformation from the skin or viscera
Thermoreceptors	Cold and warm temperature
Photoreceptors	Light
Nocireceptors	Tissue injury
Chemoreceptors	Taste, smell
	Oxygen and carbon dioxide levels
	Serum osmolality

THE CENTRAL NERVOUS SYSTEM

Three distinct regions in the CNS that are based on the embryonic brain are (1) the **rhombencephalon** or *hindbrain*, (2) the **mesencephalon** or *midbrain*, and (3) the **prosencephalon** or *forebrain* (Fig. 29-9). The

FOCUS ON CELLULAR PHYSIOLOGY

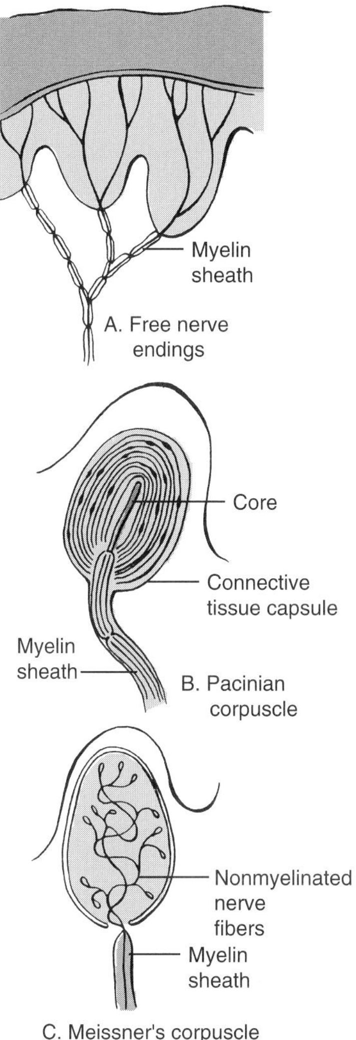

FIGURE 29-8. **Sensory receptors.**

most sophisticated activities and complex subdividing occur in the prosencephalon, which includes the cerebral hemispheres, basal ganglia, and olfactory tract. This portion of the brain is subdivided into (1) the **telencephalon** or *endbrain* and (2) the "deep inside" component of the prosencephalon, the **diencephalon**. Visual pathways traverse the prosencephalon and terminate in the optic nerves of the retinae at the inferior surface of the forebrain (see Chap. 34). The mesencephalon connects the forebrain with the hindbrain. Below the mesencephalon is the rhombencephalon, which is subdivided into the *metencephalon* and the *myelencephalon*. Box 29-1 lists the major structures in each of these regions of the brain. Extending from the rhombencephalon inferiorly is the spinal cord.

Central Nervous System Structure

The CNS structure is organized in an ascending hierarchical manner. The spinal cord, a more rudimentary structure, is addressed first. Structures necessary for reflex activity and nervous system processing from and to higher centers are encased in this region. The next level structures in the rhombencephalon and mesencephalon contain centers vital for life as well as a region for nerve tracts between higher and lower areas of the CNS. The prosencephalon houses structures for many activities, including neuroendocrine and motor control, as well as functions that provide for the high-order mental processing in human beings.

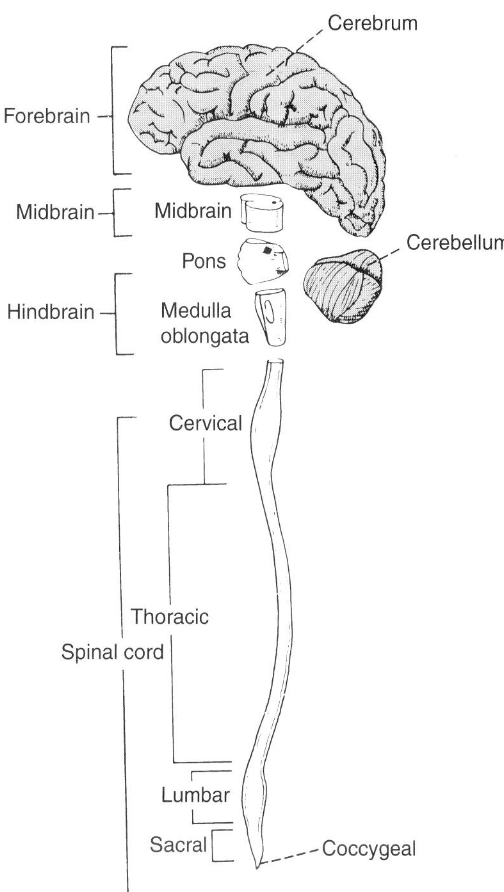

FIGURE 29-9. **The brain develops from three regions: hindbrain, midbrain, and forebrain. (Snell, R. S. [1995]. *Clinical neuroanatomy for medical students* [4th ed.]. Philadelphia: Lippincott-Raven.)**

BOX 29-1

ORGANIZATION OF THE CENTRAL NERVOUS SYSTEM

Prosencephalon (Forebrain)

Telencephalon

Cerebral cortex
Cerebral hemispheres
Basal ganglia
Rhinencephalon (limbic system)

Diencephalon

Epithalamus
Thalamus
Hypothalamus
Subthalamus

Mesencephalon (Midbrain)

Cerebral peduncles

Corpora quadrigeminas

Superior colliculus
Inferior colliculus

Tegmentum

Rhombencephalon (Hindbrain)

Metencephalon

Pons
Cerebellum

Mylencephalon

Medulla oblongata

Spinal Cord

SPINAL CORD

The spinal cord, which is encased in the vertebral canal and protected by the vertebral column, is approximately 42 to 45 cm long in the adult and is segmented into cervical, thoracic, lumbar, and sacral sections. The vertebral column consists of 24 movable vertebrae: 7 cervical, 12 thoracic, and 5 lumbar, and the fused 5 sacral and 4 coccygeal vertebrae. *Intravertebral disks* separate each of the vertebrae. The central cartilaginous portion of the intervertebral disk is known as the *nucleus pulposus* and the outer fibrous capsule as the *anulus fibrosus.*

Thirty-one pairs of spinal nerves exit the vertebral column through the intervertebral foramin. The cervical spinal nerves exit the vertebral column above the corresponding vertebral body, named for that vertebra. The C8 spinal nerve has no corresponding vertebral body because it exits between C7 and T1. From this point the spinal nerves are named for the vertebral body directly above its exit area.

The spinal cord is approximately 25 cm shorter than the vertebral canal, ending at the level of the first or second lumbar vertebra in the adult. It emerges from the base of the skull, the foramen magnum, and continues to the coccyx, where it ends in a tapered cone called the *conus medullaris.* A thin filamentous connective tissue called the *filum terminale* extends from the conus. Together, the lumbosacral nerve roots project from the conus and are called the *cauda equina.*[10] The spinal cord enlarges at the lower cervical segments and again at the lower lumbar segments. These enlargements denote the origins of the *brachial* and *lumbar plexuses*, respectively. These are regions of nerve interconnections before they emerge to innervate skin and muscles in various parts of the body. These, as well as other plexuses and the nerves constituting them, are identified in Box 29-2.

The cell bodies of fibers innervating peripheral structures are located in the inner, butterfly-shaped, gray portion of the spinal cord, and the ascending and descending projection nerve fibers form the outer white area. The spinal cord is divided into a symmetrical right and left section, with each section containing anterior, lateral, and posterior columns (ventral and dorsal are terms used interchangeably in the nervous system with anterior and posterior, respectively). These columns run the entire length of the cord. Major ascending and descending tracts (groups of neurons transmitting similar information) and their transmissions are shown in Figure 29-10. A small opening in the middle of the spinal cord, the central canal, is lined by ependymal cells and contains cerebrospinal fluid (CSF).

The afferent (sensory) spinal nerves enter the cord at the posterior horn (somatic sensory and visceral), and efferent nerves emerge at the anterior horn (motor and autonomic). The cell bodies of efferent motor fibers are located in the anterior horn, and the cell bodies of the afferent sensory fibers are situated outside the spinal cord in the posterior root ganglion. Contact between the afferent and efferent fibers is made within the spinal cord through interneurons.

The spinal cord cross-section of the gray matter is divided into ten lamina, or cell layers, according to cell characteristics (Fig. 29-11).

BOX 29-2

NERVE PLEXUSES

Cervical plexus: C1–C4
  Innervates neck and shoulder muscles
Brachial plexus: C5–T1
  Innervates upper extremities
Lumbar plexus: L1–L4
  Innervates lower extremities
Sacral plexus: L5–S4
  Innervates muscles of the perineum and toe flexion

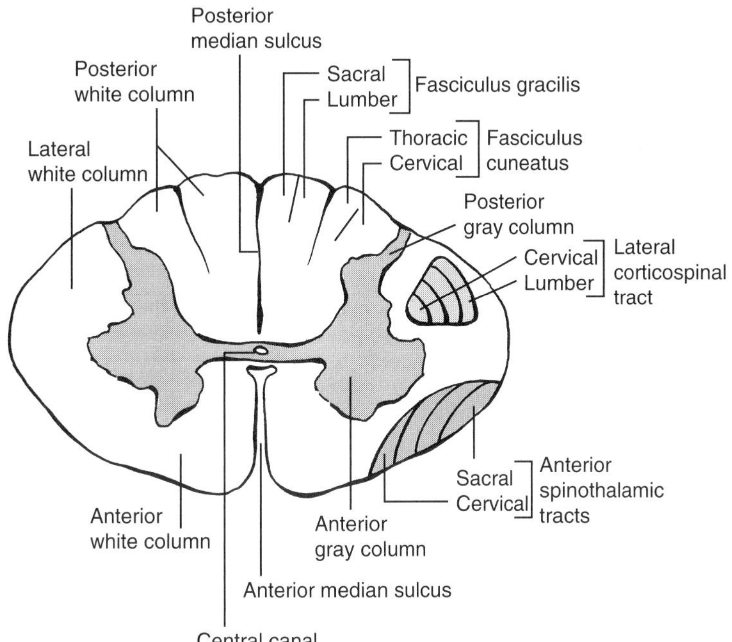

FIGURE 29-10. **Segmental organization in the spinal cord. (Modified from Waxman, S. G. & deGroot, J. [1995]. *Correlative neuroanatomy.* Norwalk, CT: Appleton & Lange.)**

RHOMBENCEPHALON (HINDBRAIN)

The major components of this region are the medulla oblongata, pons, cerebellum, and fourth ventricle; they are pictured in Figure 29-12.

Medulla Oblongata

The medulla extends directly from the cervical spinal cord at the level of the foramen magnum and lies below the pons and fourth ventricle. The medulla is subdivided into three distinct sections: (1) anterior, (2) lateral, and (3) posterior. Fissures and sulci provide landmarks that distinguish these divisions. The anterior portion contains two prominent ridges known as the *pyramids* that contain the *descending pyramidal tract.* These fibers project from the primary motor and somasthetic cortical areas and cross from one side to the other (pyramidal decussation) at the lower medulla before entering the spinal cord (Fig. 29-13*A*). By far, the majority of these fibers decussate here and descend as the *lateral corticospinal* tract. The fibers from the motor cortex that remain uncrossed descend into the spinal cord as the *anterior corticospinal* tract. Injury anywhere along the corticospinal tract above the decussation results in voluntary motor deficits of the contralateral extremities.

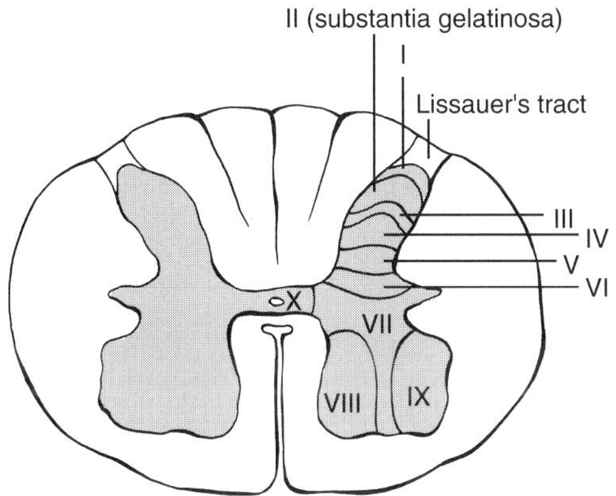

FIGURE 29-11. **Rexed's laminae of the spinal cord gray matter.**

The *olive*, a prominent mass, is located in the lateral section of the medulla. This structure gives rise to the *inferior olivary nuclear complex*, which is important in controlling movement, postural change, locomotion, and equilibrium through an interconnecting network of fibers among the cerebral cortex, spinal cord, and cerebellum. This region contains nuclei for four cranial nerves: XVII (hypoglossal), XI (spinal accessory), X (vagus), and IX (glossopharyngeal).

The posterior portion of the medulla forms a portion of the floor of the fourth ventricle. The ascending *medial lemniscus* tract arises here from the crossed-over *fasciculi cuneatus* and *gracilis fibers*, as shown in Figure 29-13*B*.

Pons

The pons is continuous with the medulla and midbrain, separated by the pontine sulcus from the medulla and the superior pontine sulcus from the midbrain. The pons lies anterior to the cerebellum and is divided into

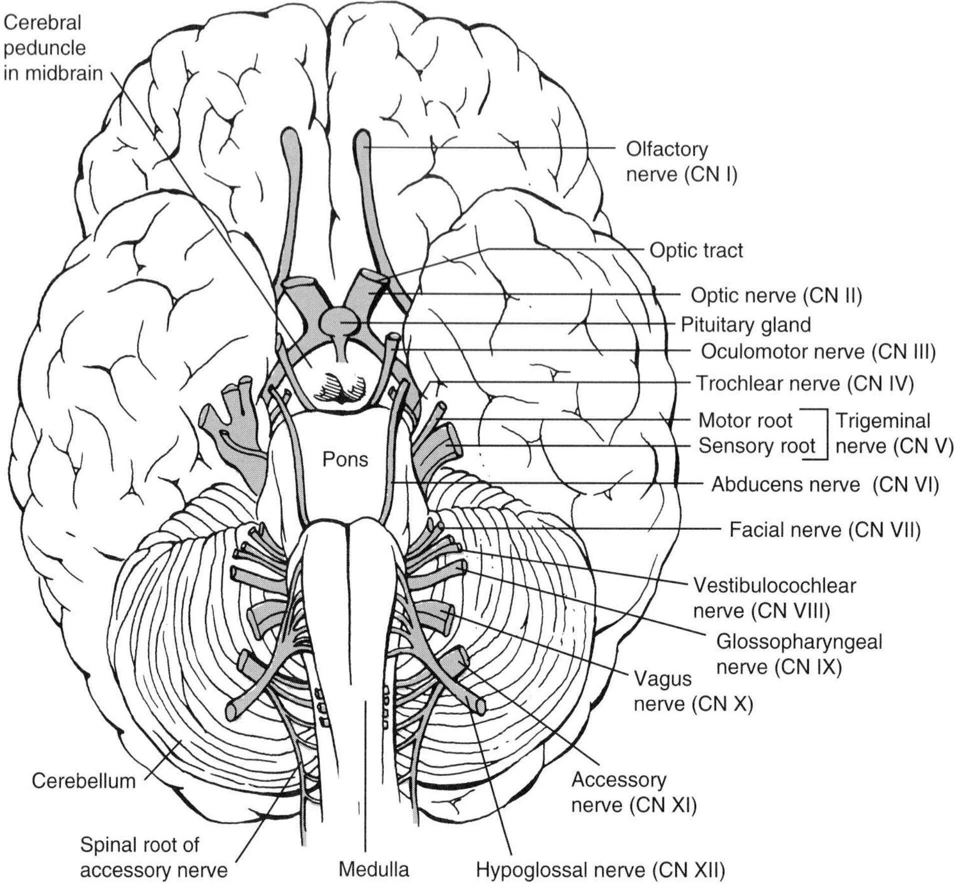

FIGURE 29-12. Ventral view of the brain stem showing cranial nerves and other structures.

two parts: (1) a dorsal portion, the pontine tegmentum, and (2) a ventral portion, the pons proper.[4] The dorsal portion is continuous with the medullary reticular formation and, together with the medulla, forms the floor and lateral wall of the fourth ventricle. This portion also contains important ascending and descending tracts and nuclei for cranial nerves V (trigeminal), VI (abducens), VII (facial), and VIII (auditory or vestibulocochlear). The *raphe nuclei* are partially encased in the pons and partially in the medulla.

The ventral portion of the pons consists of a large mass of orderly longitudinal and transverse fiber bundles that are interspersed with many pontine nuclei. The longitudinal fiber bundles traversing through this portion of the pons are the corticospinal, corticopontine, and corticobulbar. The transverse fibers arise from the pontine nuclei and cross to the opposite side to form the middle cerebellar peduncle.

Cerebellum

The cerebellum, the largest structure of the hindbrain, lies in the posterior cranial fossa. It is separated from the cerebrum by the tentorium cerebelli, which is an extension of the thickened dura mater. Thick fiber bundles called the (1) superior, (2) middle, and (3) inferior cerebellar peduncles connect the cerebellum to the midbrain, pons, and medulla, respectively. The cerebellar structures are divided into two major lateral hemispheres and an intermediary section, the vermis (Figure 29-14). Fissures divide the hemispheres into three principal lobes: (1) the *archicerebellum* (flocculonodular lobe), (2) the *paleocerebellum* (anterior lobe), and (3) the *neocerebellum* (posterior lobe).

Fourth Ventricle

The fourth ventricle, located anterior to the cerebellum and posterior to the pons, contains openings that allow the CSF to flow from the brain into the subarachnoid space. The fourth ventricle opens into the subarachnoid space through a single median opening and two lateral apertures.[13] Superiorly the fourth ventricle is continuous with the third ventricle through the cerebral aqueduct of the midbrain. The central canal of the medulla oblongata provides its inferior outflow to the

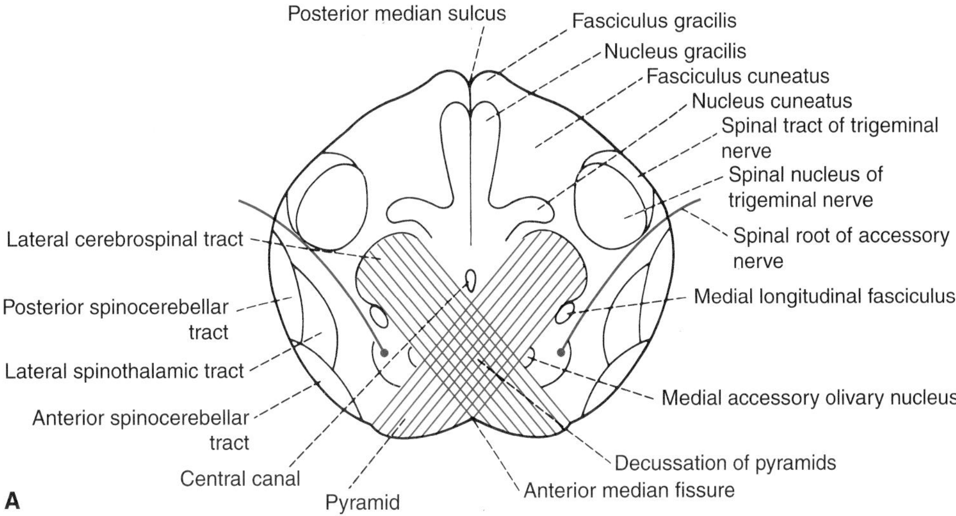

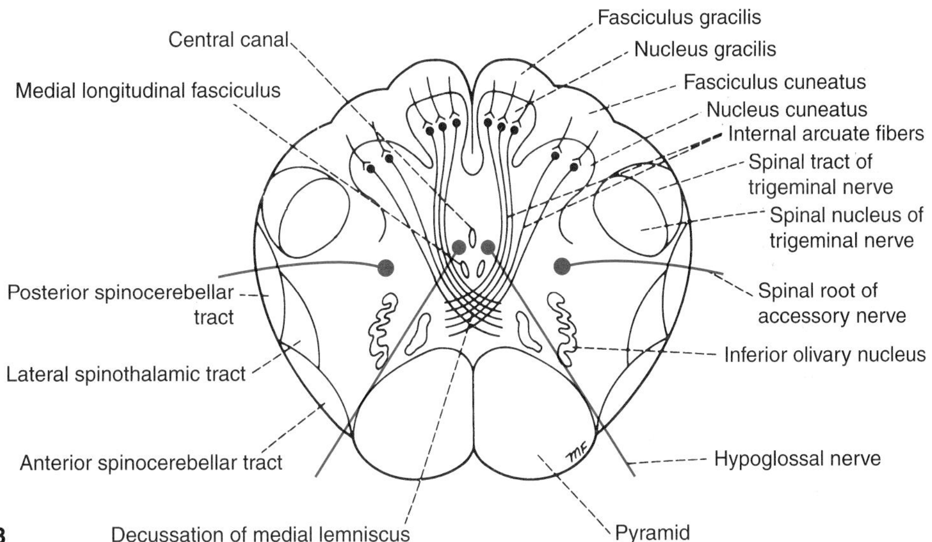

FIGURE 29-13. **Transverse sections of the medulla oblongota. A. Level of decussation of the pyramids. B. Level of decussation of the medial lemnisci. (Snell, R. S. [1997]. *Clinical neuroanatomy for medical students.* Philadelphia: Lippincott-Raven.)**

spinal cord. The fourth ventricle is lined with ependyma (ciliated epithelial cells) and, along with other ventricles, contains the *choroid plexus*, a CSF-producing structure.

MESENCEPHALON (MIDBRAIN)

The midbrain extends from the pons and projects briefly between the two cerebral hemispheres, connecting the lower centers with the diencephalon. The nuclei for third and fourth cranial nerves originate in this region. The *cerebral aqueduct* (aqueduct of Sylvius), a small channel between the third and fourth ventricles, lies in the midbrain. The midbrain *tegmentum* is located ventral to the cerebral aqueduct and is continuous with the pontine tegmentum. The reticular formation in this region contains the *substantia nigra* (a large, pigmented mass containing neurotransmitters, particularly dopamine) and the *red nucleus*. The *superior colliculus*, a relay center for the optic system, and the *inferior colliculus*, which relays information concerning auditory impulses, are also contained in this area. The superior and inferior colliculi together are referred to as the *corpora quadrigemina* and compose the tectum. The *crus cerebri* is a mass on the ventral surface of the midbrain that comprises the motor fibers, corticospinal, corticobulbar, and corticopontine tracts.[13]

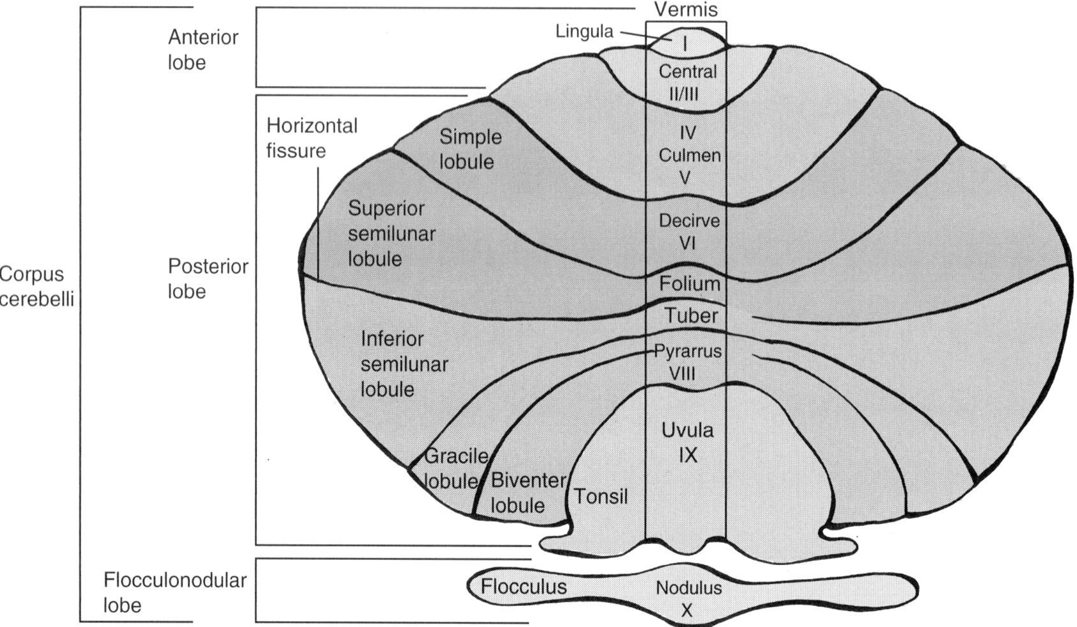

FIGURE 29-14. Schematic of the flattened cerebellum, showing the fissures, lobes, and lobules of the human cerebellum. The Roman numerals designate the ten lobules of the vermis. (Conn, P. M. [1995]. *Neuroscience in medicine.* Philadelphia: J. B. Lippincott.)

PROSENCEPHALON (FOREBRAIN)

The forebrain consists of the structures of the diencephalon and the telencephalon. The diencephalon arises from the midbrain and is considered to be a part of the forebrain. It lies between the cerebral hemispheres and encases the third ventricle. Included in the diencephalon are the epithalamus, thalamus, hypothalamus, and subthalamus. The telencephalon comprises the basal ganglia, limbic system, cerebral hemispheres, and cerebral cortex.

Thalamus

The thalamus, the largest portion of the diencephalon, consists of groups of nuclei in the third ventricle. Internal medullary lamina divide the thalamus into three sections: anterior, medial, and lateral. Intralaminal thalamic nuclei serve as an area for sensory data relay.

The reticular activating system continues its upward projection to the thalamic nuclei. From the thalamic nuclei, fibers diffuse to all areas of the cerebral cortex. This system, known as the *diffuse thalamocortical system,* is also referred to as the nonspecific thalamocortical system. The diffuse thalamocortical system activates the first two layers of the cerebral cortex. The paleospinothalamic pathway terminates in the diffuse thalamacortical system. Lateral and medial geniculate bodies are contained in the posterior end of the thalamus. Axons of the optic tract synapse in the lateral geniculate body and project posteriorly to terminate in the visual cortex.[13]

Hypothalamus

The hypothalamus lies below the thalamus and forms part of the walls and floor of the third ventricle. It consists of a group of nuclei with specific functions and is divided into the anterior and posterior portions. It is connected to the pituitary gland via the pituitary stalk, providing a route for neuroendocrine control. The hypothalamus is a focal structure in the limbic system.

Epithalamus and Subthalamus

The epithalamus is located in the region above the thalamus and contains the roof of the third ventricle. It consists of the pineal gland, habenular nuclei, and posterior commissure. The subthalamus is found between the midbrain tegmentum and dorsal thalamus.

Basal Ganglia

The basal ganglia, shown in Figure 29-15, are masses of gray matter situated deep within the cerebral hemispheres. Variation exists among neuroscientists in the terminology used to describe the basal ganglia. However, commonly they are subdivided into the corpus

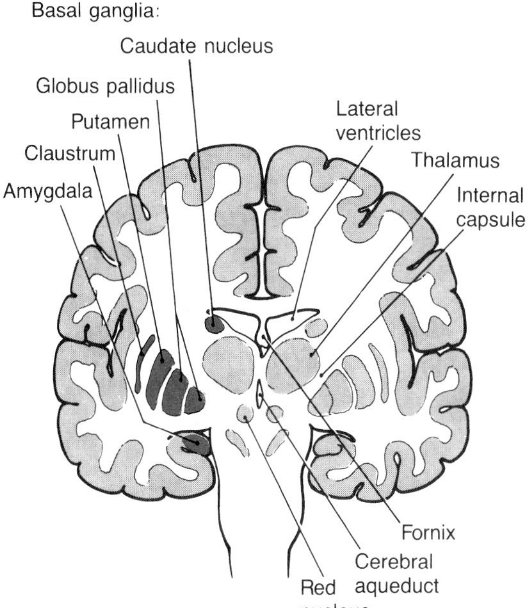

FIGURE 29-15. **Coronal section of brain showing basal ganglia.**

striatum, lenticular nuclei, and substantia nigra and include (1) the *caudate nucleus,* (2) the *putamen*, and (3) the *globus pallidus.* These nuclear masses have complex interconnections with the subthalamic nucleus and the *substantia nigra*, which are considered part of the basal ganglia system. The claustrum and amygdaloid body, considered by some authors to be part of the basal ganglia, are not directly involved in motor control.

Limbic System

The limbic system consists of a group of interconnecting structures that are important in emotion, memory, and behavior. Structures of this system are illustrated in Figure 29-16.

Cerebrum

Anatomically, the highest and largest portion of the brain, the cerebrum, is thought to be phylogenetically related to the thalamus because of its closely associated structure and function. All areas of the cerebral cortex (surface area of the cerebrum) have afferent and efferent fibers interconnecting with specific areas of the thalamus. As previously noted, this relationship is affirmed through the diffuse thalamocortical system.

The gray matter of the cerebral cortex consists of six layers: molecular, external granular, external pyramidal, internal granular, internal pyramidal, and multiform cellular. The most numerous cells are the pyramidal and stellate (Fig. 29-17). *Pyramidal cells* are projection cells; they have pyramid-shaped bodies with axons that extend into the subcortical white matter. The *stellate cells* are interneurons that have a star-shaped body with short axons and dendrites that remain in the cortex. The cells are organized into (1) horizontal layers according to cell type and (2) vertical columns according to functional units of cells.

The white matter of the cerebral hemispheres is composed of three types of myelinated nerve fibers: (1) projection, (2) transverse, and (3) association. *Projection fibers* connect the cerebral cortex with lower centers of the brain and spinal cord; *transverse fibers* or commissures connect areas of the two cerebral hemispheres; and *association fibers* provide interconnections within the same cerebral hemisphere.[13] Convergence of cortical afferent and efferent fibers occurs in the *internal capsule* located adjacent to the thalamus and basal ganglia. The cerebral surface appears as a series of convolutions (*gyri*) and grooves (*sulci*) that are instrumental in identifying the structural and functional geography of the cortex (Fig. 29-18).

The deeper grooves, called *fissures*, assist in establishing the major cerebral regional divisions: (1) the frontal (extending from the central sulcus [fissure of Rolando] forward and from the lateral fissure [fissure of Sylvius] upward); (2) the parietal (lying between the central sulcus and parieto-occipital fissure); (3) the temporal (extending down from the lateral fissure and posteriorly to the parieto-occipital fissure), and (4) the occipital lobes (lying posterior to the parietal lobe; divided from the cerebellum by the parieto-occipital fissure). Similarly, the two cerebral hemispheres are distinguished from each other by the deep *longitudinal fissure.* The cerebral hemispheres, which exhibit contralateral body control, are divided by a continuation of the dura mater known as the **falx cerebri**, which projects into the longitudinal cerebral fissure. Directly inferior to the longitudinal cerebral fissure, the fibers of the corpus callosum join the hemispheres. In the great majority of the population, the left hemisphere is dominant in the language and speech functions and the right hemisphere dominates in visual-motor tasks.[9]

VENTRICULAR SYSTEM. The ventricular system of the brain consists of four interconnecting cavities—two lateral ventricles and a third and fourth ventricle (Fig. 29-19). The ventricles are lined with ependymal cells, which provide a protective barrier between the CSF and the brain. The ciliated cuboidal epithelium of the choroid plexus is derived from the ependyma and is important in CSF formation. Cerebrospinal fluid is manufactured, circulated, and absorbed in the ventricles.

SKULL. The brain, weighing approximately 3 pounds in the adult, is encased within the skull, a nonflexible structure composed of several fused bones. The three depressions in the base of the skull, as illustrated in Figure 29-20, are the following:

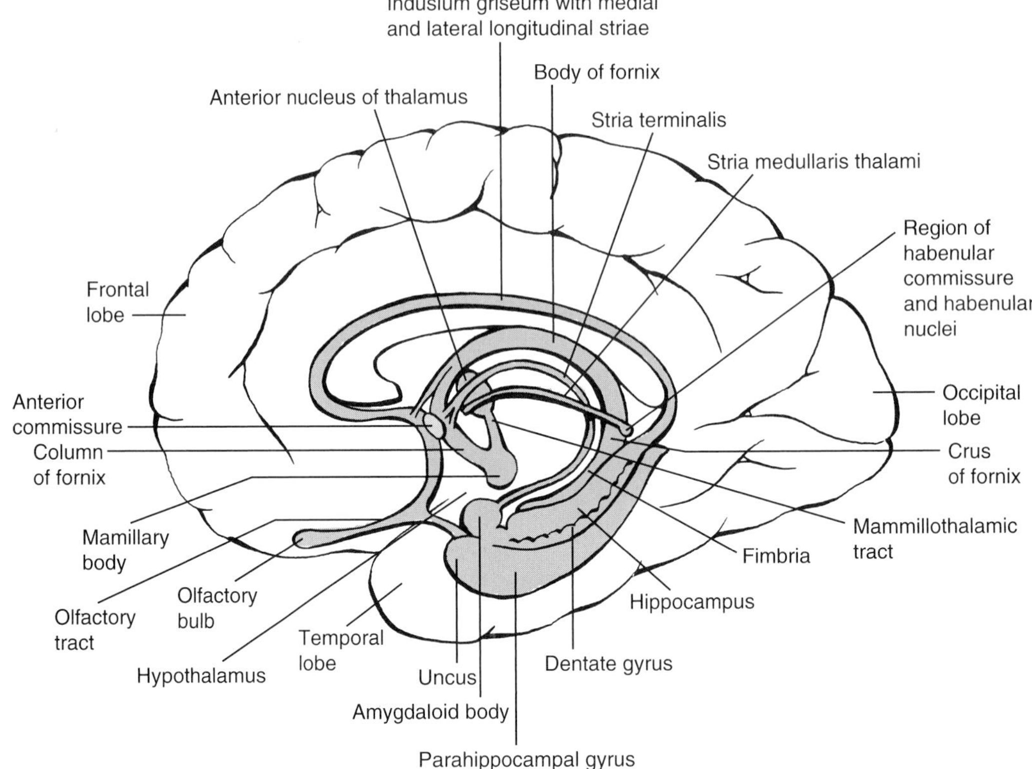

FIGURE 29-16. **Structures that form the limbic system. (Snell, R. S. [1997].** ***Clinical neuroanatomy for medical students.*** **Philadelphia: Lippincott-Raven.)**

- *Anterior fossa,* which encases the frontal lobes
- *Middle fossa,* which encases the lower portion of the diencephelaon and the temporal lobes
- *Posterior fossa,* which houses the brain stem and cerebellum

A major opening, the *foramen magnum,* is at the base of the skull and allows information to be processed between higher and lower centers. At birth, openings within the skull, known as the *fontanelles,* can be noted. These generally close by 18 months of age.

MENINGES

The brain and spinal cord are protected by three connective tissue membranes—the dura, arachnoid, and pia mater, collectively called the **meninges** (Fig. 29-21). The *dura mater* is a thick, tough, nonelastic fibrous membrane composed of the endosteal (inner surface of the skull) and meningeal layers (the dura mater proper) lying directly below the skull. The extension of the dura between the cerebral hemispheres is known as the falx cerebri. Between the cerebrum and cerebellum it is known as the **tentorium cerebelli**; between the lateral lobes of the cerebellum as the *falx cerebelli*; and above the sella turcica as *diaphragma sellae.* The *epidural space* lies between the inner surface of the skull and the dura mater. The space between the dura and arachnoid is known as the *subdural space.* A network of small blood vessels traverses this space.

The *arachnoid mater* is a delicate spider web–like covering. Below this layer, CSF is contained and absorbed. The area below the arachnoid membrane containing the CSF is known as the *subarachnoid space.* The arachnoid layer projects small extensions called *arachnoid villi* into the dura mater responsible for reabsorbing CSF into the blood. Larger blood vessels lie in the subarachnoid space and branch into smaller vessels that pass through the pia mater as they enter the brain tissue.

The *pia mater* is a fragile, lacelike connective tissue covering directly adherent on the surface of the brain and spinal cord. It encases surface and penetrating blood vessels. A layer of the dura mater, together with the arachnoid and pia mater, extends through the foramen magnum and lines the vertebral column.

FOCUS ON CELLULAR PHYSIOLOGY

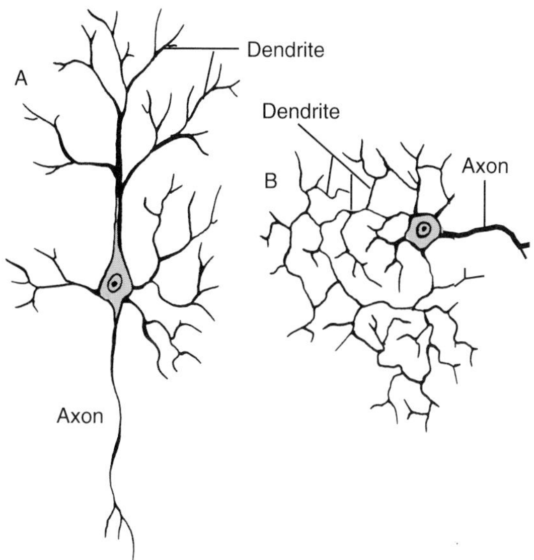

FIGURE 29-17. **Cells of the cerebral cortex. A. Pyramidal cell. B. Stellate (granule).** (Westmoreland, et al. [1994]. *Medical neurosciences: An approach to anatomy, pathology, and physiology by systems and levels.* Boston: Little, Brown.)

ARTERIAL AND VENOUS CIRCULATION

The brain receives its blood supply from two distinct systems: (1) the anterior system from the internal carotid arteries and (2) the posterior system through the vertebral arteries (Fig. 29-22). As the internal carotid arteries, which originate from the aorta on the left and common carotid on the right, ascend into the brain, they eventually branch into the anterior and middle cerebral arteries. The vertebral arteries, originating from the subclavian arteries, ascend and become the basilar artery at the pons level. The basilar artery terminates in the right and left posterior cerebral arteries, which supply the posterior regions of the cerebrum. The anterior and posterior cerebral arteries are joined by smaller communicating arteries and form a ring known as the *circle of Willis.* The blood supply to both cerebral hemispheres is identical. Although anomalies are common, for the most part they are clinically insignificant. The venous system drains the blood from the cerebrum and cerebellum through deep veins and dural sinuses that ultimately empty into the internal jugular veins.

Central Nervous System Function

The CNS functions to correlate and integrate information from various internal and external sources. Neural networks serve to provide functions from simple reflex responses to high-level mental processing.

RETICULAR FORMATION

The **reticular formation** (RF) is a diffuse system of neurons that evolves from the core regions of the medulla and midbrain and extends to the autonomic centers of the brain stem and spinal cord. Some fibers continue on from the thalamus to the cortex and are part of the *diffuse thalamocortical system.* The RF is composed of a myriad of complex, intertwining multisynaptic networks, receiving and sending signals within various levels in the nervous system.[3] The component of the RF that is important in modulating wakefulness, arousal, and conscious perception of the environment is the reticular activating system (RAS). These fibers receive sensory stimulation from a variety of somatosensory systems, which allows for focused attention and provides for generalized arousal and alertness as well. The cerebral cortex and midbrain RAS are important in maintaining consciousness. Other components of the RF are important in regulating endocrine, cardiovascular, and respiratory function and influencing sensory modalities, skeletal muscle tone, and somatic reflexes.

SPINAL CORD PROCESSING

The spinal cord is responsible for transmitting more complex signals from and to higher centers by way of the major ascending and descending tracts (Table 29-3). The lamina of the gray areas are important areas of synaptic connection and neural transmission to other areas in the CNS and are identified in Table 29-4. The spinal cord responds spontaneously to sensory information with automatic motor responses called *reflexes.*

Reflex Arc

The reflex is a fundamental component of the nervous system and, in its simplest form, occurs at the spinal cord level. A stimulus from the external environment may produce an immediate stereotypical reflex response from the CNS. For a reflex response to occur, the following mechanisms must be functional: an afferent neuron with its receptor, an area for the synapse transmission to occur (one or more central neurons), and an efferent neuron with its effector organ. The impulse passes from receptor to effector and commands a quick organ response. This simple chain of neuronal activity is known as a **reflex arc** and, at its most elemental level, is a *monosynaptic reflex* consisting of only one synapse and two neurons. It does not require input from higher levels of the CNS. Most reflexes result from many more synaptic interconnections and are referred to as *polysynaptic reflexes* (Fig. 29-23). The reflex activity encountered at higher levels in the CNS is considerably more complex.

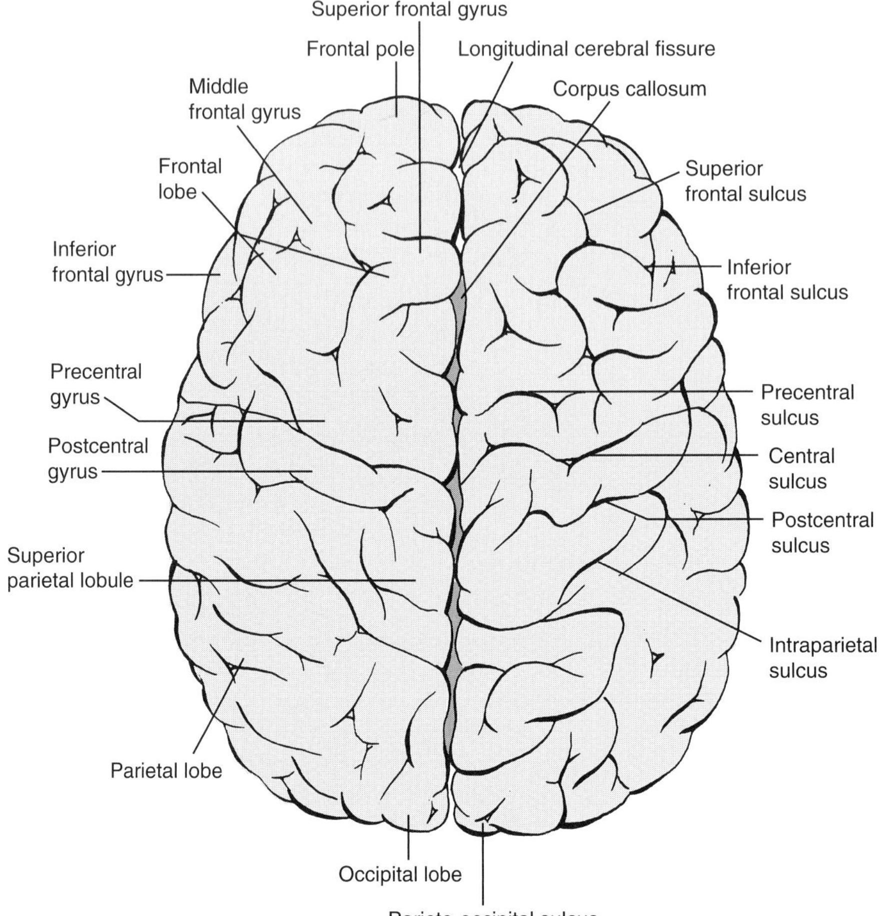

FIGURE 29-18. **Superior view of the cerebral hemispheres. (Snell, R. S. [1997].** ***Clinical neuroanatomy for medical students.*** **Philadelphia: Lippincott-Raven.)**

RHOMBENCEPHALON (LOW-BRAIN) PROCESSING

The next level of processing in the CNS takes place in the rhombencephalon. The processing encountered at this level occurs at the unconscious level and influences such vital activities as respiratory, cardiac, and vasomotor control.

Cardiac and vasomotor control evolve from the RF of the medulla oblongata. Respirations are controlled by the medullary center in coordination with the pneumotaxic center in the pons. The medial lemniscus is a major ascending brainstem tract that carries discriminative tactile information, pressure sensation, proprioception, and vibration sensation to the sensory thalamic nucleus. Lesions in the medial lemniscus result in contralateral sensory deficits.

The neurons from raphe nuclei secrete serotonin and are important in modulating pain and sleep/wakefulness cycles. The pons regulates rhythmic respirations through its pneumotaxic center from the superior cerebellar peduncle. The ventral portion of the pons is an important relay center between the cerebral cortex and the opposite cerebellar hemisphere in providing smooth, coordinated movements.

Cerebellar Processing

Transmission to and from the cerebellum is through nerve tracts at the cerebellar peduncles. The cerebellum exerts ipsilateral limb control: the right side of the cerebellum influences limbs on the right side of the body, and the left side of the cerebellum influences limbs on the left side of the body.[15] Additionally, each of the three principal lobes plays important roles in influencing movement (Table 29-5).

The cerebellum processes and transmits information through signals it receives from the motor cortex of the cerebrum by way of the *corticocerebellar* pathway and from various sensory receptors by way of the *anterior* and *posterior spinocerebellar* tracts. Other significant tracts relaying this information to the cerebellum include the *spinoreticular* tract by the reticular area of the brainstem and the *spino-olivary tract* by the inferior

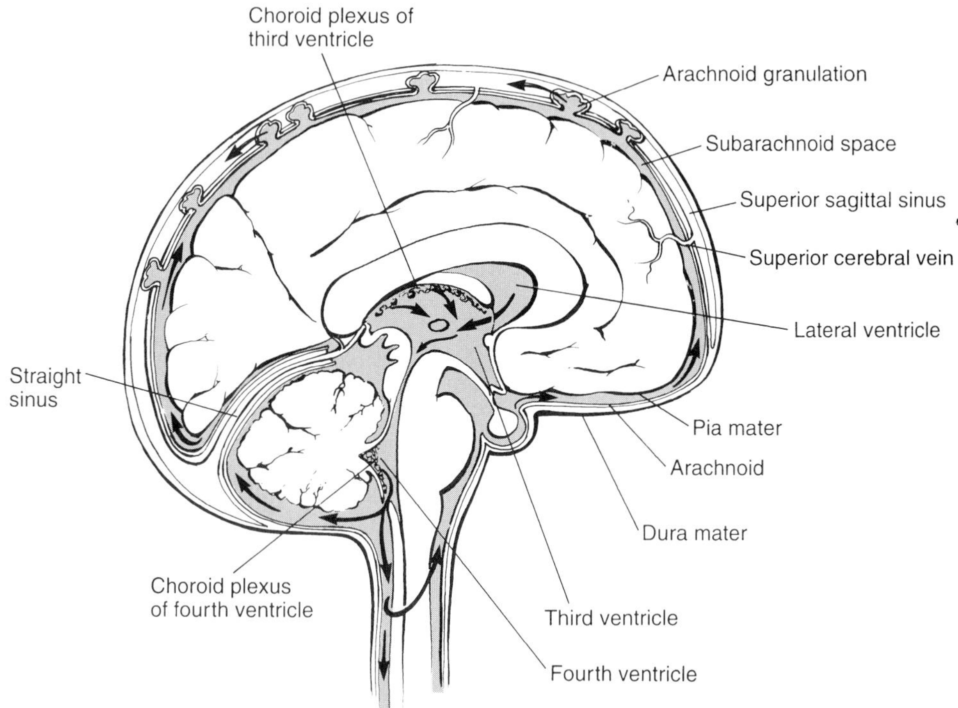

FIGURE 29-19. Cerebrospinal fluid (CSF) is formed and secreted by the choroid plexuses in the lateral, third, and fourth ventricles. The great vascularity of the plexuses imparts a reddish cast to these tissues. In adult humans, the total weight of the choroid plexus in the four ventricles is 2 to 3 g. Choroidal tissue is not present in the subarachnoid CSF space that surrounds the brain hemispheres and spinal cord. (Conn, P. M. [1995]. *Neuroscience in medicine.* Philadelphia: J. B. Lippincott.)

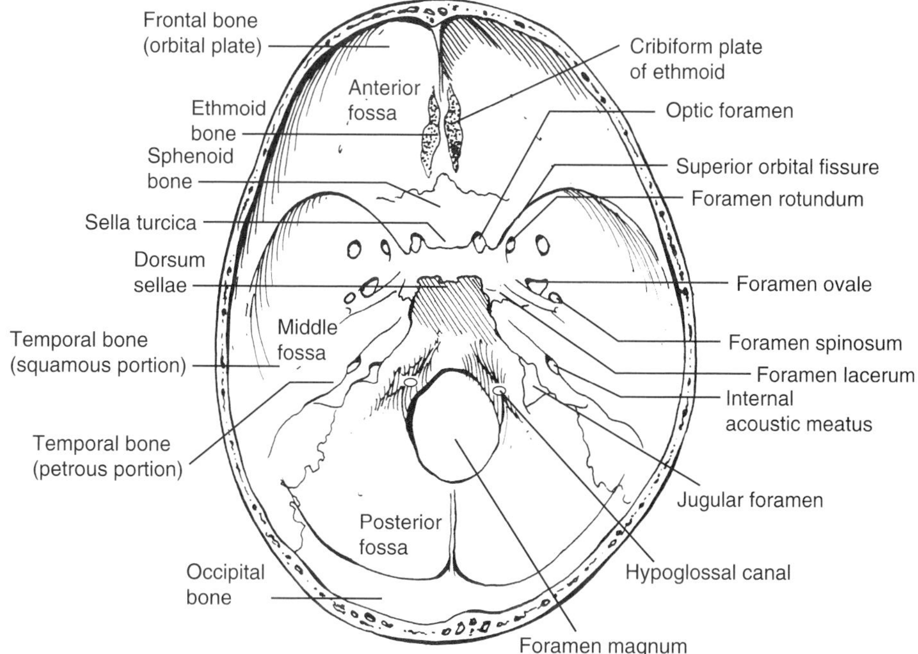

FIGURE 29-20. Base of the skull with major bones and foramina. (Westmoreland, B. F. et al. [1994]. *Medical neurosciences: An approach to anatomy, pathology, and physiology by systems and levels.* Boston: Little, Brown.)

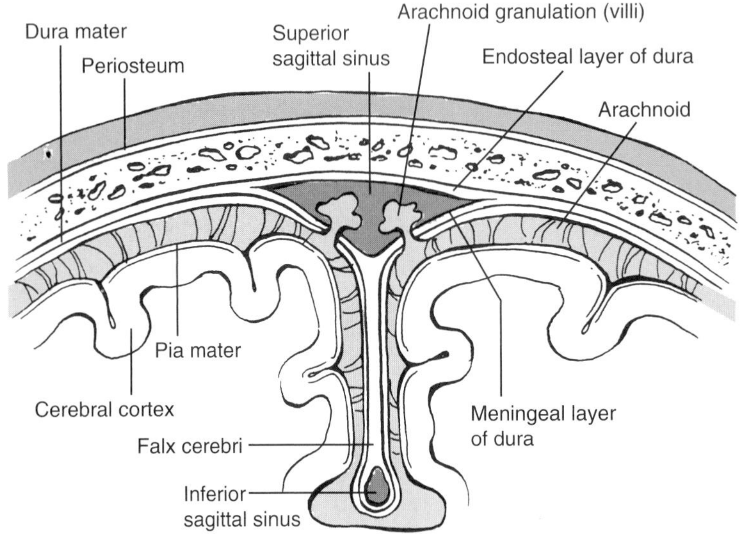

FIGURE 29-21. The cranial meninges.

olivary nucleus. Fiber-efferent tracts originate in various cerebellar nuclei and transmit information to the cerebral motor cortex, basal ganglia, red nucleus, RF, and vestibular nuclei.[10] Because the pathways from the cerebral cortex to the cerebellum are not direct descending motor tracts, disruption of cerebellar function does not hinder voluntary movement, although movement no longer is smooth and coordinated. Disruption of cerebellar function can result in ataxia, intention tremor, adiadochokinesia (inability to perform rapid alternating movements), dysmetria (inability to judge distances when reaching out toward an object), hypotonia, tremor, and asthenia.

(*text continues on page 901*)

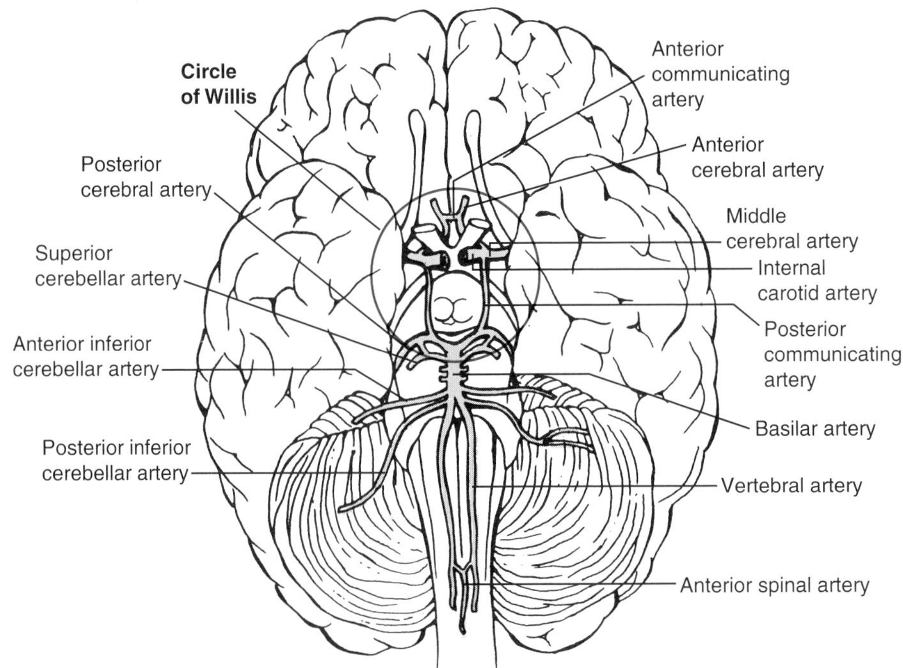

FIGURE 29-22. The arterial supply to the brain.

TABLE 29-3

MAJOR SPINAL CORD TRACTS

NAME	ORIGIN	TERMINATION	CROSSED	FUNCTION	DYSFUNCTION
ASCENDING TRACTS					
Fasciculus gracilis	Spinal cord at sacral and lumbar level	Medulla → thalamus → cerebral cortex (sensory strip)	Yes	Conscious proprioception, fine touch,* and vibration sense from lower body	Lower body Astereognosis Loss of vibration sense Loss of two-point discrimination Loss of proprioception
Fasciculus cuneatus	Spinal cord at thoracic and cervical levels	Medulla → thalamus → cerebral cortex (sensory strip)	Yes	Conscious proprioception, fine touch,* and vibration sense from upper body	Upper body Astereognosis Loss of vibration sense Loss of two-point discrimination Loss of proprioception
Posterior spinocerebellar	Posterior horn	Cerebellum	No	Conduction of sensory impulses from muscle spindles and tendon organs of the trunk and lower limbs from one side of the body to the same side of cerebellum for the subconscious proprioception necessary for coordinated muscular contractions	Ipsilateral uncoordinated postural movement
Anterior spinocerebellar	Posterior horn	Cerebellum	Some	Conduction of sensory impulses from muscle spindles and tendon organs of the upper and lower limbs from both sides of the body to the cerebellum for the subconscious proprioception necessary for coordinated muscular contractions	Ipsilateral uncoordinated postural movements
Lateral spinothalamic	Posterior horn	Thalamus → cerebral cortex	Yes	Interpretation of pain and temperature	Loss of pain and temperature sensation contralaterally below the level of the lesion
Anterior spinothalamic	Posterior horn	Thalamus → cerebral cortex	Yes	Conduction of sensory impulses for pressure and crude touch† from extremities and trunk	Because one branch of the first neuron immediately synapses with a second, which ascends ipsilaterally for many levels; cord injury rarely results in complete loss of pressure and crude touch sensation
DESCENDING TRACTS					
Lateral corticospinal	Motor cortex (area 4) → internal capsule → midbrain → pons → medulla	Anterior horn; all spinal levels in laminae IV through VII and IX	80%–90% cross at the medulla	Controls voluntary muscle activity	Voluntary muscle paresis/paralysis

(continued)

TABLE 29-3

MAJOR SPINAL CORD TRACTS (Continued)

NAME	ORIGIN	TERMINATION	CROSSED	FUNCTION	DYSFUNCTION
Anterior corticospinal	Motor cortex (area 4) → internal capsule → midbrain → medulla → anterior funiculus of the cervical and upper thoracic levels	Anterior horn (at each level of cord, axons cross to other side)	Not at medulla; synapse with cells of lamina VIII	Controls voluntary muscle activity	Voluntary muscle paresis/paralysis
Corticobulbar	Areas 4, 6 and 8 of cortex → internal capsule → brain stem	Brain stem; connects with cranial nerves V, VII, IX, X, XI, and XII	Yes	Controls voluntary head movement and facial expression	Because of bilateral innervation, facial expression is usually not affected
Rubrospinal	Midbrain (red nucleus)	Anterior horn	Yes	Facilities flexor alpha and gamma motor neurons and inhibits extensor motor neurons; also influences muscle tone and posture, particularly of the arms	Altered muscle tone and posture
Reticulospinals Pontine reticulospinal Medullary reticulospinal	Reticular formation (brain stem)	Anterior horn	No	Facilitates extensor motor neurons, particularly of the legs; input to gamma motor neurons	Altered muscle tone and posture
Vestibulospinal	Reticular formation (brain stem)	Anterior horn	No	Conveys autonomic information from higher levels to preganglionic autonomic nervous system neurons to influence sweating, pupillary dilatation, and circulation	Altered muscle tone and sweat gland activity
Lateral vestibulospinal			No	Facilitates extensor alpha motor neurons and inhibits flexors	Altered muscle tone and postural equilibrium
Medial vestibulospinal			No	Inhibits fibers to upper cervical alpha motor neurons; influences extraocular movements and visual reflexes	Altered muscle tone and equilibrium in response to head movement

* Fine touch is the ability to identify various (e.g., a key) that are placed in the hand while the eyes are closed.
†Crude touch refers to light touch, and may be tested with a wisp of cotton placed in the hand while the eyes are closed.
(Hickey, J. V. [1997]. *The clinical practice of neurological and neurosurgical nursing* [4th ed.]. Philadelphia: Lippincott.)

TABLE 29-4

SPINAL CORD LAMINA AND THEIR FUNCTIONS

LAMINA	FUNCTIONS
I	Receives nociceptive stimuli and transmits to contralateral spinothalamic tract, other spinal cord segments, reticular formation, and thalamus. Substance P found in high concentrations.
II	Receives nociceptive stimuli from unmyelinated C fibers and transmits to other regions. Known as substantia gelatinosa. Rich in substance P.
III	Receives position and light touch sense through mechanoreceptors. Known as nucleus proprius.
IV	Same as Lamina III. Gives rise to spinothalamic tract.
V	Receives nociceptive and mechanicoreceptive stimuli from reticulospinal tract and lamina IV.
VI	Receives mechanical sensations from skin and joints.
VII	Contains nucleus dorsalis, which gives rise to posterior spinocerebellear and intermediolateral column. Preganglionic sympathetic fibers project from here via anterior roots and white rami communicantes to the sympathetic ganglia. Receives information from the corticospinal and reticulospinal tracts.
VIII	Contains medial and lateral motor neuron columns.
IX	Same as Lamina VIII.
X	Small neurons surrounding the central canal.

MESENCEPHALON (MIDBRAIN) PROCESSING

The midbrain is a major motor and sensory fiber pathway between the higher and lower centers. The substantia nigra supports motor function through its connections with the thalamus, corpus striatum, and superior colliculus.[4] The red nucleus influences movement; it receives crossed fibers from the cerebellum and projects fibers to the thalamus and contralateral spinal cord.[15]

PROSENCEPHALON (FOREBRAIN) PROCESSING

The major functions of the diencephalon are summarized in Table 29-6. Olfactory impulses are relayed through the epithalamus, and visual reflexes are associated with certain fibers in the posterior commissure. The subthalamus serves as an important extrapyramidal motor connecting center.

THALAMIC PROCESSING. The thalamus is a major center for processing sensations and relaying them to the cerebral cortex. Input from all sensoria, except that for olfaction, is processed here. Numerous afferent nerve tracts from lower levels transmit information to the specific relay nuclei of the thalamus.

HYPOTHALAMIC PROCESSING. Major processing of internal stimuli evoking the autonomic nervous system is concentrated in the hypothalamus. The limbic system, in concert with the hypothalamus, performs an important role in overall behavior, emotions, and memory.[14] Because vital autonomic functions are processed here, destruction of the hypothalamus results in death. The majority of the hypothalamic activity occurs at an unconscious level, but excessive stimulation may evoke a conscious response. Responses to emotions of fear, anger, and excitement—reflected by increased pulse and respiratory rates, increased gastric acidity, and sweating—are communicated from the hypothalamus. Prolonged stimulation of the hypothalamus may result in hypertension or ulcers. The hypothalamus controls the anterior pituitary hormone production through its releasing and inhibiting factors.

BASAL GANGLIA PROCESSING. The basal ganglia play an important role in motor control and information processing in the extrapyramidal system. Figure 29-24 shows that basal ganglia transmissions involve neurotransmitters and occur through a series of loops including (1) striatum to globus pallidus to the thalamus to cortex to striatum, (2) striatum to substantia nigra to striatum, and (3) globus pallidus to subthalamus to globus pallidus.[15] Generally, glutamate and acetylcholine act as excitatory neurotransmitters and dopamine and GABA act as inhibitory neurotransmitters.[11,15] Lesions in the basal ganglia result in an overactive facilitory area and underactive inhibitory area, causing body rigidity. Gross intentional movement that is performed without conscious thought is regulated by the basal ganglia. Disorders of the basal ganglia produce abnormalities in movement and muscle tone.

CEREBRAL PROCESSING. The cerebral cortex maintains the highest level of information processing in the human. Some functional areas are localized; others are more general and widely dispersed. Brodman is credited with mapping specific functional areas on the cerebral cortex (identified in Fig. 29-25). Over 100 of these areas have been identified.

The significant localized functional areas include the primary motor projection and somatosensory projection areas. The motor projection area is located on the anterior wall of the central sulcus and adjacent to the precentral gyrus. The fibers from this area initiate skeletal muscle movements of the contralateral body and modulate the ascending systems in the thalamus, brain stem, and spinal cord. The disproportionate

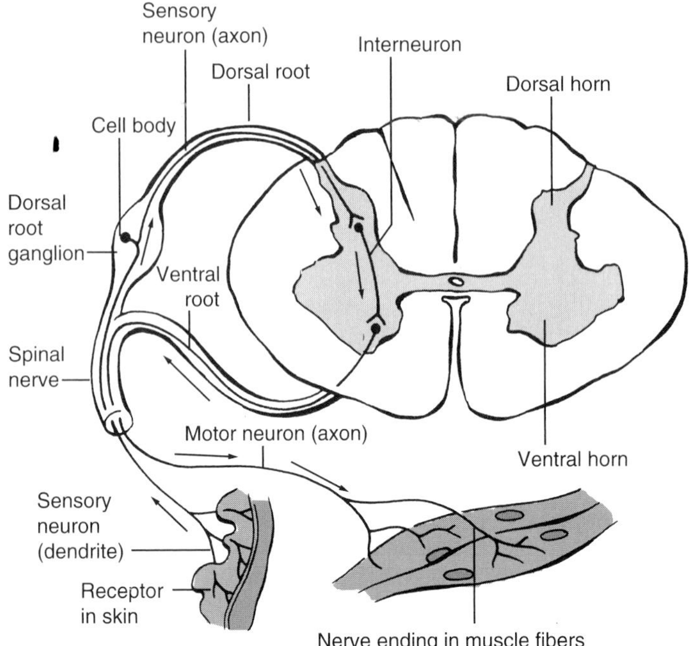

FIGURE 29-23. **Reflex arc showing the pathway of impulses and cross section of the spinal cord.**

space representation of control of body parts on the motor cortex is illustrated on the motor homunculus (a proportional pictorial representation of the human motor and sensory functions on the cerebral cortex) in Figure 29-26A. The sensory projection area (somesthetic area) is located on the postcentral gyrus and receives input from the thalamus-projected sensations of the contralateral side of the body. The sensory homunculus is depicted in Figure 29-26B.

TABLE 29-5

FUNCTION OF THE CEREBELLAR LOBES

CEREBELLAR LOBE	FUNCTION
Archicerebellum (flocculonodular lobe)	Coordinates head and eye movements
Paleocerebellum (anterior lobe)	Receives proprioceptive and interoceptive input and helps maintain equilibrium, and coordinates automatic movements as well as maintains muscle tone
Neocerebellum (posterior lobe)	Coordinates ipsilateral voluntary movement and has extensive connections to cerebral cortex

Other rather well-localized functions processed in the cortex include visual, hearing, olfaction, and somatic interpretations. The mental and intellectual activities in humans are processed and interpreted in widely dispersed association areas of the cortex. Table 29-7 presents the major functions of the lobes of the cerebral hemispheres.

CEREBROSPINAL FLUID

Cerebrospinal fluid circulates in the subarachnoid space around the brain and spinal cord and provides an important supportive and protective mechanism for the CNS. Together with support from blood vessels, nerve roots, and fine fibrous arachnoid trabeculae, the brain and spinal cord are directly encased within the subarachnoid CSF and receive buoyancy from it that prevents the vessels and nerve roots from stretching in response to movements. Table 29-8 summarizes this and other roles of the CSF in the CNS.

Formation and Absorption of Cerebrospinal Fluid

The CSF is produced, circulated, and reabsorbed continuously. Its principal formation site is in the *choroid plexus* of the lateral ventricle, with most of the remainder being formed in the third and fourth ventricles. The choroid plexus is a network of capillary tufts surrounded by cuboidal epithelium. The CSF is produced through (1) filtration, (2) diffusion, and (3) active transport from the blood. Sodium ions are actively trans-

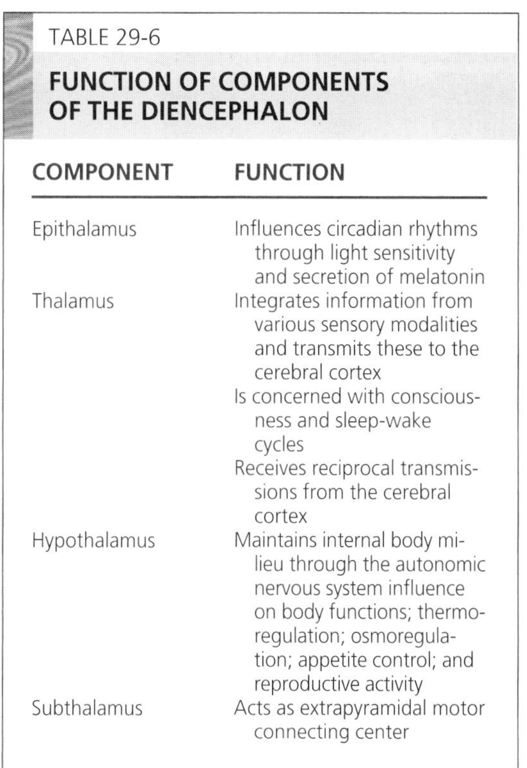

TABLE 29-6

FUNCTION OF COMPONENTS OF THE DIENCEPHALON

COMPONENT	FUNCTION
Epithalamus	Influences circadian rhythms through light sensitivity and secretion of melatonin
Thalamus	Integrates information from various sensory modalities and transmits these to the cerebral cortex Is concerned with consciousness and sleep-wake cycles Receives reciprocal transmissions from the cerebral cortex
Hypothalamus	Maintains internal body milieu through the autonomic nervous system influence on body functions; thermoregulation; osmoregulation; appetite control; and reproductive activity
Subthalamus	Acts as extrapyramidal motor connecting center

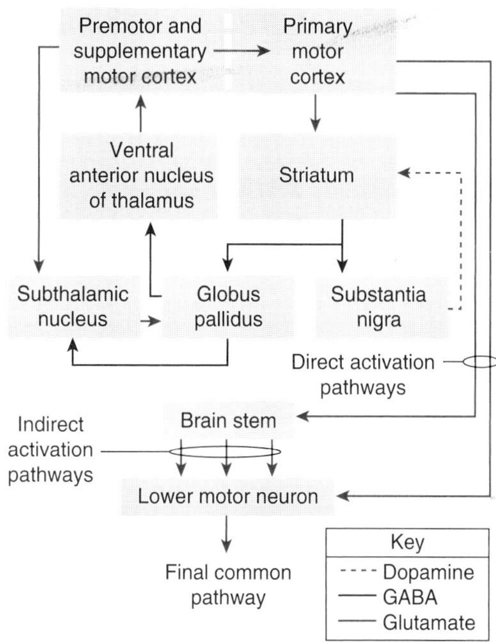

FIGURE 29-24. **Basal ganglia pathways. The major outflow pathway is from the globus pallidus to the cortex via nucleus ventralis anterior in the thalamus. (Westmoreland, B. F. et al. [1994].** ***Medical neurosciences: An approach to anatomy, pathology, and physiology by systems and levels.*** **Boston: Little, Brown.)**

ported across the epithelial cells into CSF from blood; this results in a greater osmotic force in the CSF. Therefore, to maintain osmotic equilibrium, water passively follows the ions. Thus, water is extracted from the capillaries and is responsible for the secretory (filtration) function of the choroid plexus. Facilitated diffusion allows transportation of glucose in both directions.[11] A second lesser source of CSF is from the ependymal cells lining the ventricles and meningeal blood vessels.

In the adult human, approximately 500 mL of fluid is produced per 24 hours, and approximately 125 mL is circulating at any given time. Wide fluctuations may occur in the amount produced during any given 24-hour period (see Appendix in this unit).

The CSF is reabsorbed into the venous circulation through *arachnoid villi,* granulations that project from the cerebral subarachnoid space into the venous sinuses. The CSF is passively absorbed because its hydrostatic pressure is greater than that of venous blood in the venous sinuses. Certain particles, such as red blood cells and creatinine, pass unimpeded through the arachnoid villi.

Circulation of Cerebrospinal Fluid

CSF arrives in the third ventricle from the lateral ventricles through the interventricular foramen. It flows on to the fourth ventricle through the cerebral aqueduct, and then goes on to the subarachnoid cisterns through the foramina of Magendie and Luschka. As the fluid flows over the cerebral hemispheres, it passes into the sagittal sinus for rapid reabsorption through the arachnoid villi.

Interference along the pathway of the flow of CSF results in ventricular enlargement and a condition known as *hydrocephalus.* If CSF flows freely between the ventricles and lumbar subarachnoid space, it is *communicating hydrocephalus* and a problem exists with reabsorption of CSF. Blockage within the ventricular system that prevents free flow of CSF from one or more ventricles results in *noncommunicating hydrocephalus.* Ventricular dilation results in both types and leads to increased intracranial pressure (see Chap. 31).

BRAIN BARRIERS

Brain cell function is dependent on a closely controlled environment. Not all circulating substances in the blood pass freely to the brain or CSF. This occurs either because their molecules are too large or the molecules they bind with are too large to cross the CNS membranes. Substances pass into the brain from the blood through capillaries to the extracellular space of the brain, or through the choroid plexus into the CSF, from which small amounts are passed into the brain. **Brain barriers** exist between (1) the blood and brain,

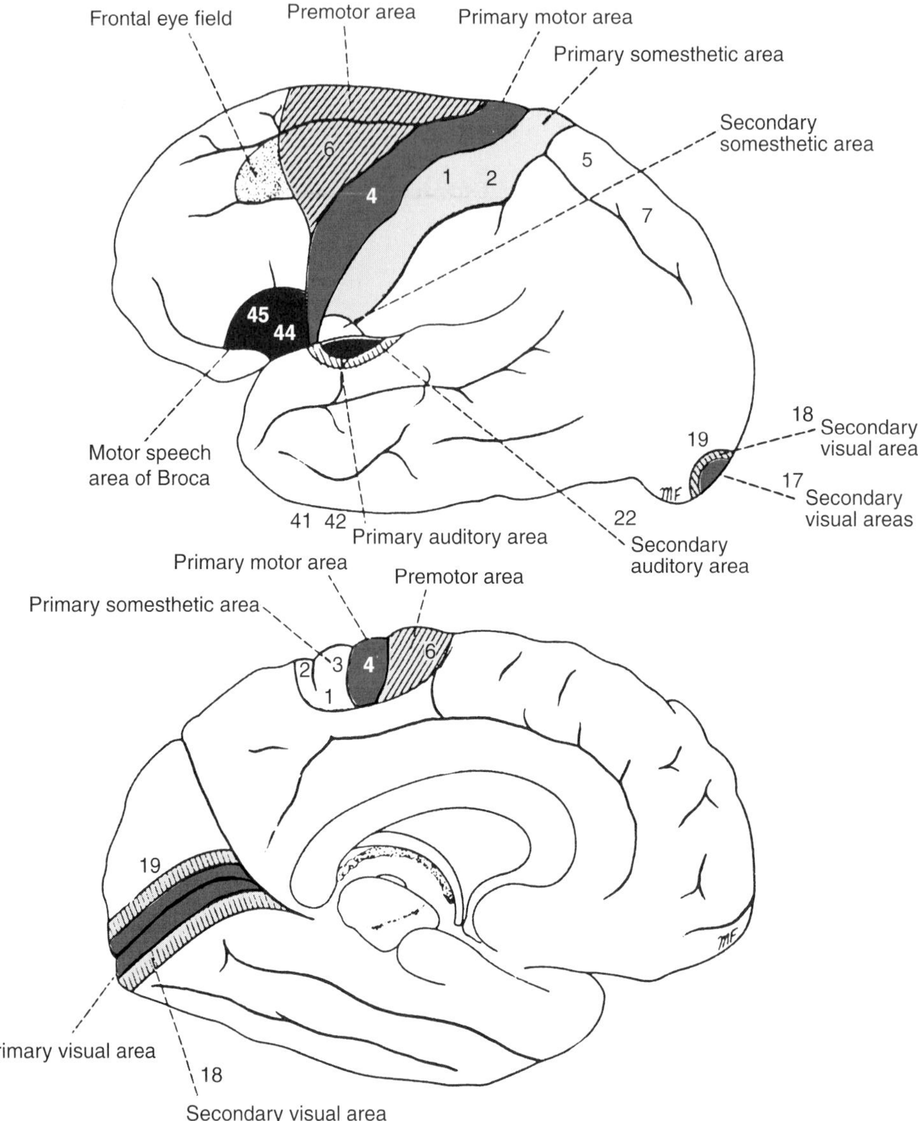

FIGURE 29-25. **Functional localization of the cerebral cortex based on Brodmann's cytoarchitectonic map. A. Lateral view of the left cerebral hemisphere. B. Medial view of the left cerebral hemisphere. (Snell, R. S. [1997].** ***Clinical neuroanatomy for medical students.*** **Philadelphia: Lippincott-Raven.)**

and (2) the blood and CSF. The components are described in Box 29-3 and pictured in Figure 29-27. Barriers protect the brain by inhibiting potentially toxic substances from entering. However, they facilitate the entry of substances essential for its metabolism.

The membranes and cells separating the various cerebral compartments, in essence, are responsible for the entrance and exit of materials to and from the CSF and brain. The choroid plexus and the brain parenchyma (except the hypothalamus) provide the barriers to free movement of substances into the brain. The rate of diffusion across the cerebral membranes and cells is affected by molecular size, charge, and lipid solubility. Small molecules and lipid-soluble substances penetrate more readily than large molecules and water-soluble compounds. Plasma proteins are excluded from the CNS because of their large molecular size. Nonionized substances pass more readily into the brain and CSF than ionized substances. Substances such as water, glucose, oxygen, carbon dioxide, and most lipid-soluble substances pass to the brain readily through the capillary system that maintains a constant environment for

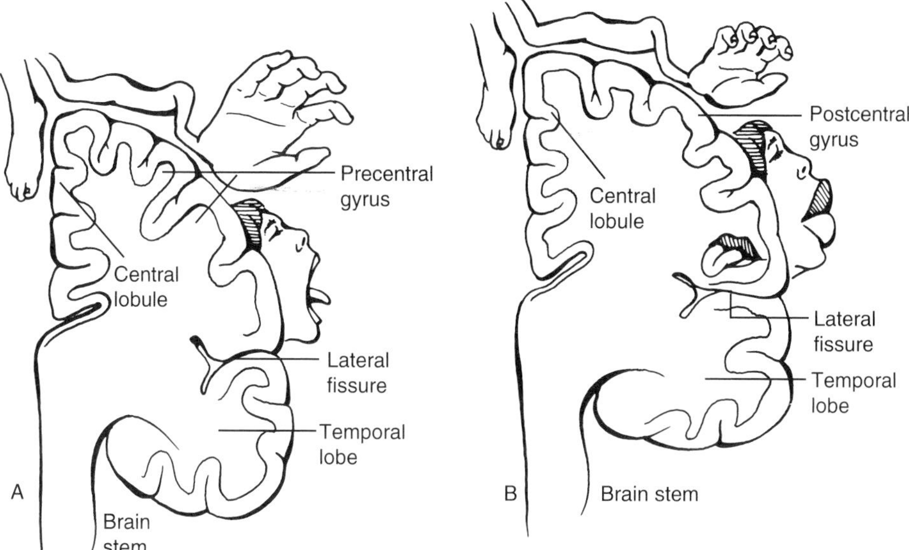

FIGURE 29-26. **A.** Motor homunculus showing location of motor control for various body parts on precentral gyrus. **B.** Sensory homunculus showing location of sensory representation of body parts on post-central gyrus.

the CNS neurons. Certain drugs penetrate the barrier with more ease than others. This is important in the treatment of CNS infections because certain antibiotics, such as chlortetracyclines and penicillin, have very limited access to the brain. Others, such as erythromycin and sulfadiazine, enter readily. Because proteins are not readily available for binding, drugs generally do not accumulate in the CSF.

Radiotherapy, infections, trauma, and tumors interrupt the brain-barrier systems and allow transport of materials that normally are not readily accorded entrance.

AUTOREGULATION AND CEREBRAL BLOOD FLOW

The healthy brain has the ability to maintain a fairly constant blood flow, approximately 50 mL/100 gm/minute or 15% of the cardiac output, even within widely fluctuating physiological conditions. Normal

TABLE 29-7

MAJOR FUNCTIONS OF THE CEREBRAL LOBES

LOBE	BRODMAN'S AREAS	MAJOR FUNCTIONS
Frontal	4 (primary motor area) 6 (premotor area) 8 (frontal eye field)	Voluntary motor control of contralateral body
	44, 45 (Broca's speech area)	Motor speech
	Frontal association areas	Integration of multiple sensory modalities
Parietal	3,1,2 (primary somesthetic area) 5,7 (sensory association areas)	Processing of somatosensory and visual information
	Wernicke's area in dominant hemisphere	Sensory (receptive) speech
Occipital	17 (primary visual area) 18, 19 (visual association areas)	Visuospatial processing, movement, and color discrimination
Temporal	41 (primary auditory cortex)	Sound localization
	42 (associative auditory area)	Memory
	Wernicke's area in posterior region of temporal lobe and overlaps to parietal lobe	Smell interpretation Sensory (receptive) speech

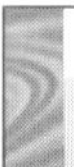

TABLE 29-8
ROLES OF CEREBROSPINAL FLUID IN SERVING THE BRAIN

CEREBROSPINAL FLUID (CSF) FUNCTIONS	EXAMPLES
Buoyancy effect	Because brain weight is effectively reduced by more than 95%, shearing and tearing forces on neural tissue are greatly minimized.
Intracranial volume adjustment	CSF volume can be adjusted, increasing or decreasing acutely in response to blood volume changes or chronically in response to tissue atrophy or tumor growth.
Micronutrient transport	Nucleosides, pyrimidines, vitamin C, and other nutrients are transported by the choroid plexus to CSF and eventually to brain cells.
Protein and peptide supply	Macromolecules like transthyretin, insulin-like growth factor, and thyroxine are transported by the choroid plexus into CSF for carriage to target cells in brain.
Source of osmolytes for brain volume regulation	In acute hypernatremia there is bulk flow of CSF with osmolytes, from ventricles to surrounding tissue. This promotes water retention by shrunken brain, i.e., to restore volume.
Buffer reservoir	When brain interstitial fluid concentrations of H^+, K^+, and glucose are altered, the ventricular fluid can help to buffer the extracellular fluid changes.
Sink or drainage action	Anion metabolites of neurotransmitters, protein products of catabolism or tissue breakdown, and xenobiotic substances are cleared from the central nervous system by active transporters in the choroid plexus or by bulk CSF drainage pathways to venous blood and the lymphatics.
Immune system mediation	Cells adjacent to ventricles have antigen-presenting capabilities. Some CSF protein drains into cervical lymphatics, with the potential for inducing antibody reactions.
Information transfer	Neurotransmitter agents like amino acids and peptides may be transported by CSF over distances to bind to receptors in the parasynaptic mode.
Drug delivery	Some drugs do not readily cross blood-brain barrier but can be transported into the CSF by endogenous proteins in choroid plexus epithelial membranes.

(Conn, P. M. [1995]. *Neuroscience in medicine.* Philadelphia: J. B. Lippincott.)

BOX 29-3
BRAIN BARRIERS

Blood–Brain Barrier
Composed of endothelial cells with tight junctions, a continuous basement membrane surrounding the endothelial cells, and foot processes of astrocytes adhering to the outer surfaces of the capillary wall. No fenestrations exist between adjacent endothelial cells. Substances must be transported through the endothelial cells by active transport, endocytosis or exocytosis, making this a highly selective barrier.

Blood–CSF Barrier
Barrier in the choroid epithelium produced by a continuous basement membrane outside the endothelial cell, pale cells, and tight-junctioned epithelial cells of the choroid.

cerebral blood flow (CBF) is provided when the cerebral perfusion pressure (CPP) is maintained between 60 and 130 mm Hg. The CPP commonly ranges around 80 to 90 mm Hg. Cerebral perfusion pressure is determined by subtracting the intracranial pressure (ICP) from the mean systemic arterial pressure (MSAP): CPP = MSAP − ICP.

Autoregulatory mechanisms in the healthy brain maintain the relatively constant blood flow through metabolic and pressure autoregulatory mechanisms. The metabolic autoregulatory mechanism operates in response to increases in carbon dioxide tension and decreases in oxygen tension. Carbon dioxide is the most potent cerebral vessel vasodilator. When increased, CBF increases, allowing for removal of excess carbon dioxide and restoration of oxygen levels toward normal. Hypercapnea and hypoxia have significant effects on the vessel diameter and, thus, on the intrinsic control of the cerebral blood flow. Likewise, the pH level affects cerebral arteries. Increased hydrogen ion concentrations have a powerful dilating effect on the cerebral vessels.

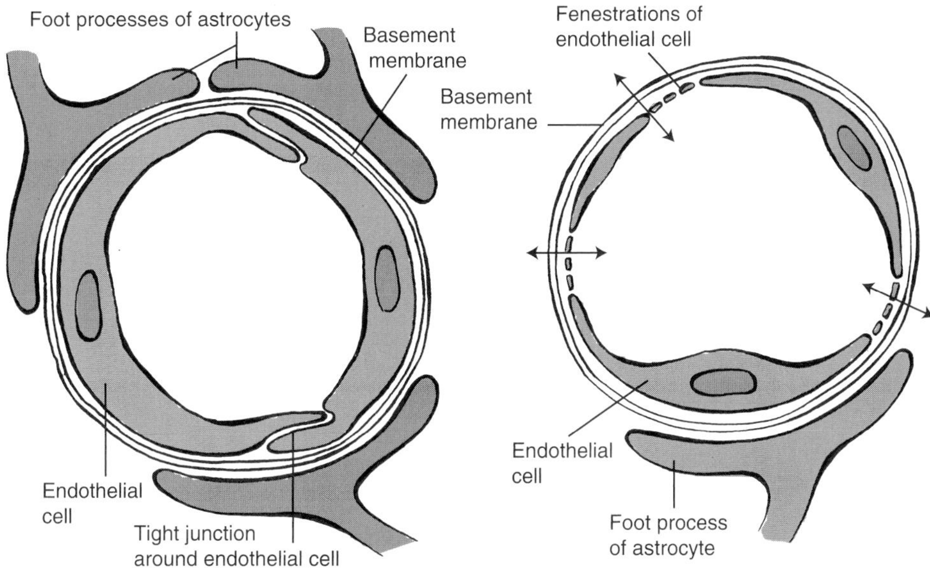

FIGURE 29-27. **Blood–brain barrier. A.** Intact blood–brain barrier. **B.** Absence of blood–brain barrier. Note the presence of fenestrations in endothelial cells. (Adapted from Snell, R. S. [1997]. *Clinical neuroanatomy for medical students.* Philadelphia: Lippincott-Raven.)

Pressure autoregulation responds to vessel resistance resulting from changes in intracranial pressure and systemic blood pressure. As a result of this mechanism, a relatively constant blood flow is maintained in the presence of wide fluctuations in systemic arterial blood pressure. Cerebral vessels constrict in response to increased systemic arterial pressure and dilate when the systemic pressure decreases. A mean systemic arterial blood pressure below 60 mm Hg results in decreased cerebral perfusion. Pressure autoregulation is maintained in the healthy brain when ICP is below 30 mm Hg, MAP is between 60 to 160 mm Hg, and CPP ranges from 50 to 150 mm Hg. Autoregulation ceases when the CPP is less than 40 mm Hg. When the ICP increases significantly and equals the MAP, CPP becomes zero. Marked reduction of CBF occurs when intracranial pressure rises rapidly to about 35 mm Hg.

Other factors that affect cerebral blood flow include cerebral outflow, blood viscosity, and cardiac output. Impedance in cerebral outflow may result in increased intracranial pressure and compromise autoregulation. Increases in blood viscosity decrease CBF, and decreased blood viscosity increases CBF. Cerebral blood flow is reduced when cardiac output is decreased by one third.

THE PERIPHERAL NERVOUS SYSTEM

The peripheral nervous system encompasses nerve tissue outside the brain and spinal cord. It is composed of spinal and cranial nerves and numerous groups of cell bodies called ganglia or plexuses. Functionally the peripheral nervous system is divided into the *somatic* and **autonomic nervous systems.** The somatic nervous system supplies skeletal muscles, tendons, and skin; the autonomic nervous system supplies the viscera, smooth muscles, and glands.

Peripheral Nervous System Structure

SPINAL NERVES

The peripheral nervous system consists of 31 pairs of spinal nerves. Every spinal nerve contains two roots, a *dorsal (afferent)* root, which carries nerve transmissions to the CNS, and a *ventral (efferent)* root, which carries nerve transmissions away from the CNS. The somatic afferent nerve cells lie within the dorsal root ganglia and convey sensory information to the CNS through the dorsal root to the dorsal gray column. The somatic efferent cell bodies lie within the ventral gray column of the spinal cord and conduct through ventral roots of all spinal nerves primarily to the skeletal muscle. Visceral afferent transmission is from visceral receptors via afferent pathways to the CNS. Efferent visceral transmission is through preganglionic and postganglionic neurons to effector organs. The arrangement of afferent and efferent somatic and visceral spinal nerves is illustrated in Figure 29-28.

Most spinal nerves are myelinated and segmented by the nodes of Ranvier. Each segment of the myelinated nerve contains one Schwann cell. A single nerve consists of bundles of fibers. Sensory ganglia (posterior root ganglia) are enlargements of cell bodies found on the posterior root of each spinal nerve. A network of spinal nerves branch and join neighboring nerves in complex plexuses in the cervical, bracheal, lumbar, and sacral regions.

Spinal nerves are mixed nerves since they transmit both afferent and efferent somatic and visceral impulses. The somatic impulses convey sensory and motor information associated with body wall, joints, tendons, and voluntary striated muscles. Visceral impulses convey sensory and autonomic information associated with organs of the body.

CRANIAL NERVES

The peripheral nervous system also consists of 12 pairs of cranial nerves. Ten pairs of the cranial nerve nuclei are contained in the brainstem. The remaining two pairs, the olfactory and optic nerves, arise from the olfactory nasal mucosa and ganglion cells in the retina, respectively. Some cranial nerves have only sensory components, some only motor components, and others contain both (mixed). Their names and general functions are presented in Table 29-9, and alterations in function are described in Chapter 31.

Peripheral Nervous System Function

AFFERENT DIVISION FUNCTION

The afferent (sensory) division of the peripheral nervous system detects, transmits, and processes environmental information from internal and external sources through a variety of specific receptors. The *somatic afferent* fibers carry impulses from receptors in the skin, skeletal muscles, joints, and tendons to the CNS. The *visceral afferent* fibers carry impulses from the viscera to the CNS.

The receptors of afferent fibers transmit to the CNS by numerous converging fibers through peripheral nerves. As a result of the convergence of neurons, injury to a nerve fiber does not result in clearly defined sensory deficits. Rather, the area that responds in an altered manner is vaguely defined.

The area of the skin supplied by a single spinal nerve transmitting to a dorsal root ganglion and spinal cord segment is called a **dermatome**. Dermatomes perceive cutaneous sensation and have been arranged to correspond to the spinal cord segments; they are detailed in Figure 29-29. A rather loose topographic division of these segments includes the 8 cervical, 12 thoracic, 5 lumbar, and 5 sacral cord regions. Considerable overlapping exists between the dermatomes. Generally, sensory deficits are identified when more than a single spinal nerve is interrupted.

Afferent transmission from the periphery to the primary sensory area in the cortex occurs by a chain of three neurons and two synapses. Figure 29-30 shows the first afferent fibers (#1) entering the spinal cord by way of the dorsal roots to the dorsal root ganglia, which contains its cell body, and then continuing to the posterior column. The first synapse is with the second neu-

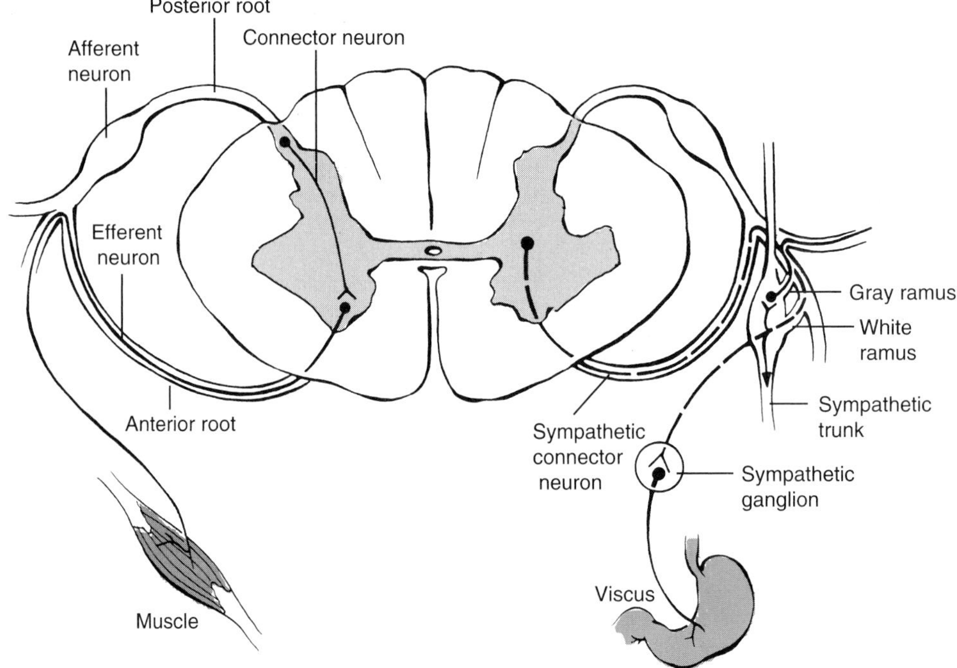

FIGURE 29-28. The general arrangement of the somatic part of the nervous system **(left)** and the autonomic nervous system **(right)**. (Redrawn from Snell, R. [1997]. *Clinical neuroanatomy for medical students* [4th ed.]. Philadelphia: Lippincott-Raven.)

TABLE 29-9

CRANIAL NERVES

NUMBER	ANATOMIC LOCATION	NAME AND TYPE OF NERVE	GENERAL FUNCTION
I	Cerebral hemispheres	Olfactory (sensory)	Sense of smell
II	Diencephalon	Optic (sensory)	Vision
III	Midbrain	Oculomotor (motor)	Motor control for four eye muscles and upper eyelid elevator; pupillary constriction and accommodation
IV	Midbrain	Trochlear (motor)	Movement of eye down and medially
V	Pons	Trigeminal (mixed)	Facial sensation perception over entire face; mastication; blink reflex (motor component)
VI	Pons	Abducens (motor)	Movement of eye laterally
VII	Pons	Facial (mixed)	Facial expression; blink reflex (sensory component); taste sensation from anterior portion of the tongue; salivation
VIII	Pons	Vestibulochochlear (sensory)	Equilibrium and hearing
IX	Medulla	Glossopharyngeal (mixed)	Salivation; movement and sensation of pharynx; taste sensation of posterior tongue; carotid baroreceptor sensations
X	Medulla	Vagus (mixed)	Swallowing; pharyngeal control; phonation; parasympathetic innervation to thoracic and abdominal viscera
XI	Medulla	Spinal accessory (motor)	Head and shoulder movement
XII	Medulla	Hypoglossal (motor)	Movement of tongue

ron (#2) in the posterior gray column, either shortly after entering and becoming the lateral spinothalamic tract, or higher in the column in the brain stem where it becomes the anterior or ventral spinothalamic tract. The second synapse is with the third neuron (#3) in the anteriolateral nucleus of the thalamus, and the third neuron projects from this area to the cerebral cortex.

The major tracts that transmit sensory information are described in Table 29-3, earlier in the chapter. Fibers that transmit pain and temperature are anatomically related, cross over, and ascend through the *lateral spinothalamic tract* to the posterior ventral nucleus of the thalamus. Many of the fibers from receptors that are sensitive to touch, proprioception, and pressure are contained in the *ventral spinothalamic tracts.* From here, they proceed to the somesthetic postcentral gyrus. Impulses from muscles, tendons, ligaments, and joints (proprioceptive fibers) disperse in a variety of tracts. Some simply cross the cord to the anterior horn (stretch reflex). Others synapse with the posterior gray column and ascend the spinocerebellar tracts to the cerebellum. Yet others ascend by way of the posterior white columns, decussate at the medial lemniscus, and continue to the posterior ventral nucleus of the thalamus. The ascent from this region continues to the sensory cortex at the postcentral gyrus.

The postcentral gyrus contains the somesthetic projection area. The body areas that contain more sensory receptors are accorded a larger area on the surface of the sensory cortex. As shown in the sensory homunculus in Figure 29-26B, the face and fingers, which are rich with receptors, occupy a larger neuronal area in the cortex than does the large body area of the trunk with its comparatively smaller receptor population.

An important component of the afferent division is the thalamus, primarily because almost all sensory

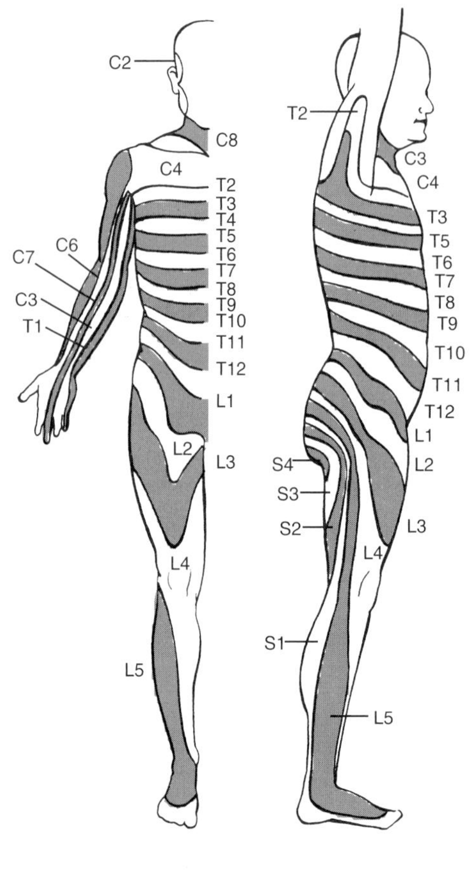

Dorsal Root	Dermatome
C2	Back of head
C3	Neck
C4	Shoulder, Upper chest
C5	Lateral part of shoulder and upper arm
C6	Thumb, index finger, medial (radial) part of lower arm
C7	Middle finger and middle part of lower and upper arm
C8	Little finger, ring finger and lower lateral (ulnar) side of arm
T1 and T2	Inner aspect of arm hand on ulnar side
T3	Upper chest and axilla
T4	Nipple line
T7 and T8	Lower edge of rib cage
T10	Umbilical area
T11-L1	Lower abdomen, groin
L2	Upper anterior thigh and upper and lateral buttock
L3	Anterior lower thigh
L4	Anterior and medial lower leg
L5	Lateral (outer) aspect of lower leg and top of foot
S1	Sole of foot, last two small toes
S2	Posterior medial buttock and posterior upper and lower leg
S3	Lower buttock and posterior upper medial thigh
S4 and S5	Perirectal and genital areas

FIGURE 29-29. A dermatome is the area of skin supplied by axons from a single dorsal root ganglion. (Conn, P. M. [1995]. *Neuroscience in medicine.* Philadelphia: J. B. Lippincott.)

systems convey impulses to its specific nuclei through either the dorsal column or anterolateral tracts. Together with the thalamus, the cortex is concerned with conscious perception of sensory stimuli that occur distantly from it. The thalamus provides perception of touch and pressure, whereas more complex discrimination sensations, such as texture, size, and weight of objects, are interpreted by the cortex.

EFFERENT DIVISION FUNCTION

Both voluntary and involuntary body activities that are initiated by the efferent (motor) division are transmitted in response to the stimuli the CNS has received from the afferent division. Efferent responses are transmitted through the upper and lower motor neurons through (1) the general **visceral efferent system**, which includes preganglionic and postganglionic transmissions to smooth muscles, cardiac muscle, and glands by way of the autonomic nervous system, or (2) the general **somatic efferent system**, which transmits impulses to the striated skeletal muscles, tendons, and joints from alpha and gamma motor neurons in lamina IX. Skeletal muscle innervation by a specific spinal root motor axon is called a **myotome**.

Both efferent and afferent fibers transmit concurrently in most peripheral nerves. Therefore, injury to a nerve could result in both sensory and motor deficits. The efferent fibers receive impulses from simple spinal reflex circuits or more complex descending pathways from higher centers. Significant higher centers important in relaying efferent responses to the periphery include the precentral gyrus where the corticospinal tract originates, basal ganglia, brainstem, and cerebellum. The fibers that transmit from these areas do so through two principal tracts: pyramidal and extrapyramidal. The nerve tracts in the efferent motor system are summarized in Table 29-3, earlier in the chapter.

FOCUS ON CELLULAR PHYSIOLOGY

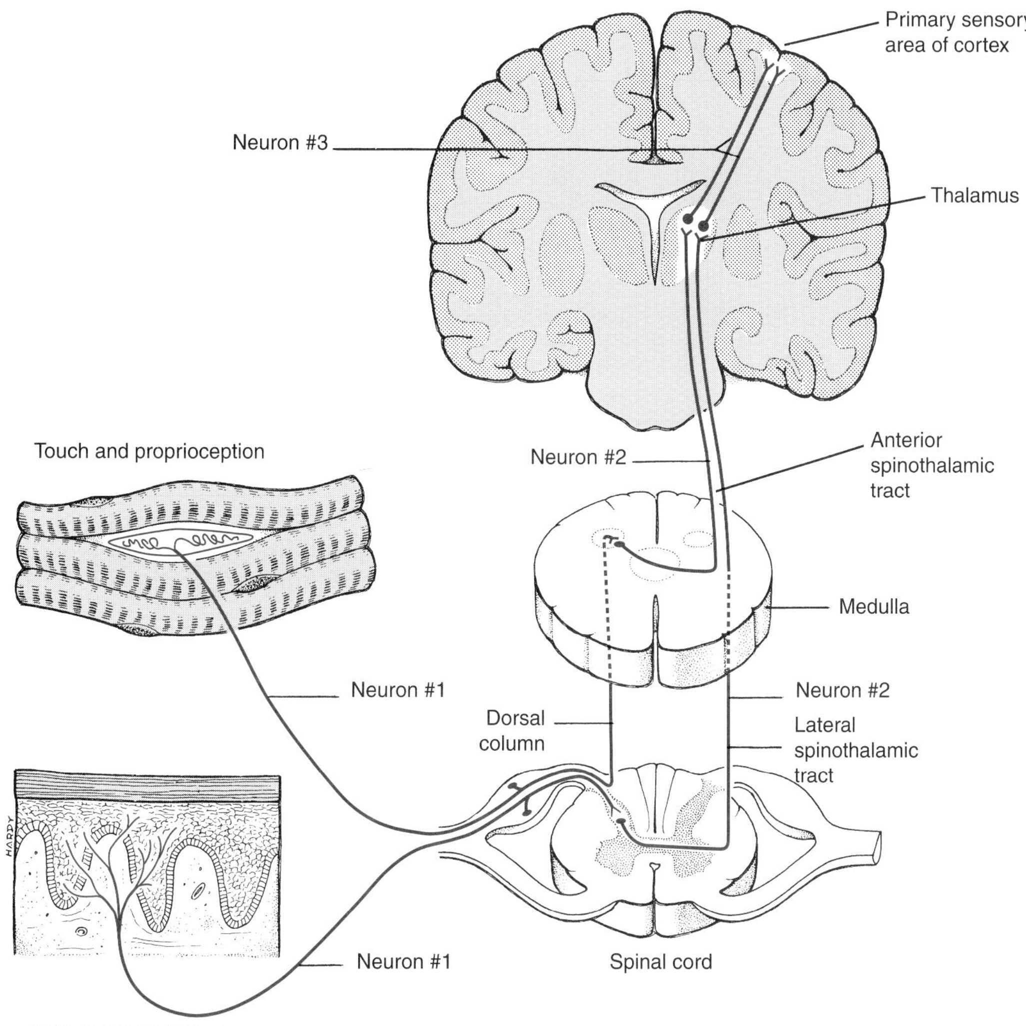

FIGURE 29-30. **Representation of the touch-pressure pathways (Neuron #1) ascending in the dorsal column to the medulla, where they synapse with second-order neurons (Neuron #2) that cross to the opposite side (decussate) and ascend in the interior or lateral spinothalamic tract to the thalamus. Third-order neurons (Neuron #3) connect the thalamus with the cerebral cortex. (Adapted from Hudak, C. M. & Gallo, B. M. [1998].** ***Critical care nursing*** **[7th ed.]. Philadelphia: Lippincott.)**

Pyramidal and Extrapyramidal Tracts

The **pyramidal tract (corticospinal tracts)** is composed of a three-neuron chain. Both the lateral corticospinal and ventral corticospinal tracts originate in the sensorimotor cortex (precentral gyrus, Brodman's area 4) of the cerebral cortex. The tracts transmit, uninterrupted, in a descending manner through the basal ganglia and brainstem. The area where they join other projection fibers, between the basal ganglia and the thalamus, is known as the *internal capsule*. Most of the fibers decussate and project through a structure known as the *pyramid* in the medulla. The crossed fibers then continue to descend as the lateral corticospinal tract and terminate in the ventral horn of the gray matter at specific spinal cord levels. A few fibers continue to descend without decussation by way of the ventral corticospinal tract and cross near the level of their termination in the ventral horn (Fig. 29-31).

The fibers (the first two neurons in the three-neuron chain) of the pyramidal tract are contained in the CNS and compose the *upper motor neurons*. The pyramidal fibers synapse with segmental anterior horn cells (motor neurons), which, in turn, synapse with peripheral efferent fibers (the third neuron in the three-

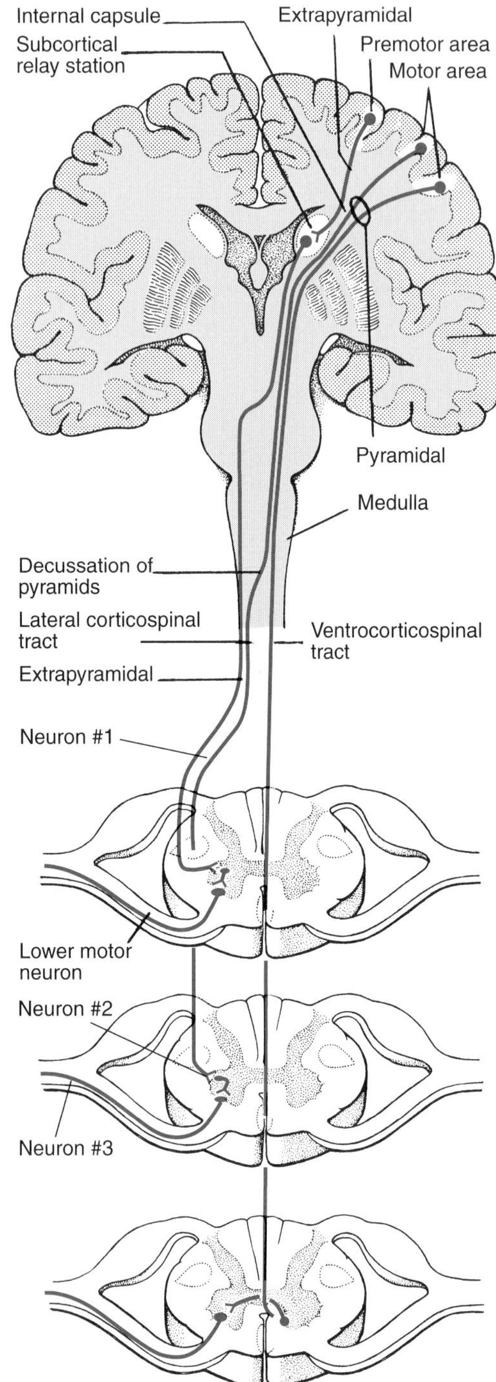

FIGURE 29-31. Descending motor pathways showing the crossed lateral corticospinal tract and the uncrossed ventral corticospinal tract. (Adapted from Hudak, C. M. & Gallo, B. M. [1998]. *Critical care nursing* [7th ed.]. Philadelphia: Lippincott.)

neuron chain) innervating specific muscles, tendons, and joints. The neurons innervating skeletal muscle are known as the *lower motor neurons*. Upper and lower motor neurons are further discussed in Chapter 31.

The *corticobulbar* fibers are homologous to the corticospinal tract and connect with interneurons of the efferent cranial nerve nuclei. The lower facial muscles are innervated by contralateral corticobulbar fibers, whereas all other cranial nerve nuclei receive innervation from both cerebral cortices.[10,13] The remaining efferent fibers that do not traverse the pyramid in the brainstem are part of the **extrapyramidal tracts**. Unlike the pyramidal tract, the extrapyramidal tracts do not continue to the cord uninterrupted. The system is more complex, less directed, and highly interconnected and is considered by some authors to be a functional, rather than an anatomic, entity.[4,13] Many of the fibers descend from the cortex directly to specific areas in the basal ganglia and brainstem, whereas others make intermediate synapses. Several extrapyramidal tracts originate in the brainstem and are named for their site of origin. Examples of these include the:

- *Vestibulospinal tract* from the lateral vestibular nucleus in the medulla
- *Rubrospinal tract* from the red nucleus in the midbrain
- *Tectospinal tract* from the roof (superior colliculus) of the midbrain
- *Reticulospinal tracts* from the reticular formation in the pons and medulla

The majority of the extrapyramidal fibers decussate with the reticulospinal tract. In addition to the named tracts, other important fibers of the extrapyramidal system originate in the cerebellum and the vestibular apparatus.

The pyramidal tract processes information regarding voluntary movement dealing with precise and specific activities of muscles, whereas the extrapyramidal tracts provide the "supporting" type of movement that accompanies the more precise movements afforded by the pyramidal tract. For example, the gross movements necessary to engage in the activity of writing are influenced by the extrapyramidal tracts. Included here are such movements as might be necessary for proper body positioning, particularly of the upper arm and shoulder. The more precise movement of holding the pencil effectively is controlled by the corticospinal tract.

THE AUTONOMIC NERVOUS SYSTEM

The autonomic nervous system, also referred to as the general visceral efferent system, maintains the internal environment in a relatively steady state. Though it is outside the CNS, it is influenced by the CNS and is distinct from the peripheral nervous system.

Autonomic Nervous System Structure

The autonomic nervous system consists of two functionally distinct divisions: (1) sympathetic and (2) parasympathetic (Fig. 29-32). Many visceral effector organs have a dual nerve supply, one from each division. The sympathetic division assists the body into action during physiologic and psychologic stress by supportive activities, such as increasing heart and respiratory rates and mobilizing glucose from glycogen stores to supply the skeletal muscles with additional energy. The parasympathetic division provides a counterbalance for the sympathetic division.

AUTONOMIC NERVE FIBERS

Autonomic fibers differ from somatic efferent fibers in that they consist of a double-neuron chain from the spinal cord to the visceral effectors, whereas the somatic efferents transmit through one neuron from the spinal cord. Visceral efferent fibers transmit in spinal nerves and in several cranial nerves. Visceral efferent innervation frequently accompanies somatic efferent activity. For example, a jogger receives innervation from the somatic efferent fibers to provide the skeletal muscle responses required in jogging. Simultaneously, the somatic efferent system innervates the cardiac and smooth muscle. The somatic efferent responses can be observed readily, whereas the visceral efferent responses are less obvious.

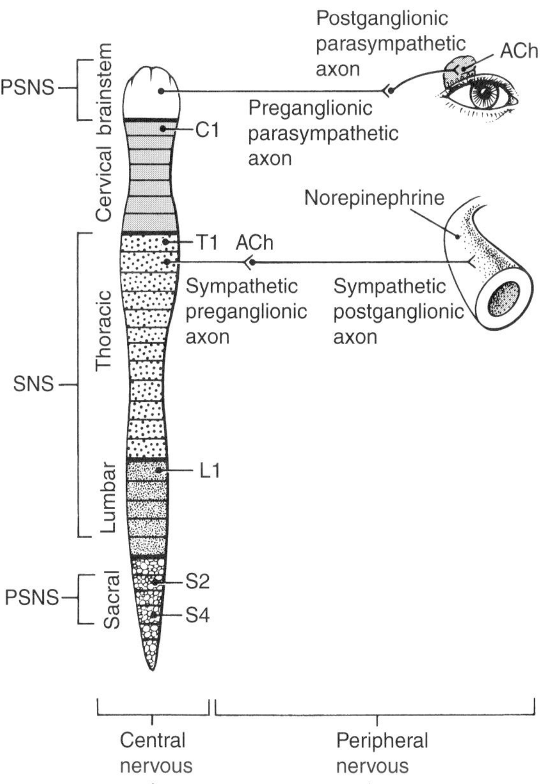

FIGURE 29-32. Schematic overview of the origins of sympathetic (SNS) and parasympathetic (PSNS) nervous systems with corresponding major transmitter substances at the synapses: acetylcholine (ACh) and norepinephrine (noradrenalin).

In addition to the autonomic efferent fibers, afferent fibers from the viscera transmit directly through the sympathetic ganglia and join the spinal nerves through the white rami communicantes. From this point they may become part of a segmental reflex or may continue their transmission to higher centers in the brain.[12]

AUTONOMIC GANGLIA

Nerve cells of both divisions group outside the CNS in structures known as *autonomic ganglia*. Neurons in this system are referred to as:

- *Preganglionic neurons* when the cell fibers terminate with a synapse at the ganglia and retain the cell body within the CNS
- *Postganglionic neurons* when the nerve cell bodies are in the ganglia and axons extend to the organs and glands

The sympathetic system, pictured in Figure 29-33, has a chain or trunk of paired ganglia extending the full length on either side of the spinal cord. These are referred to as *paravertebral ganglia* and are connected on each side by nerve trunks and referred to as the right and left *sympathetic chains* or *sympathetic trunks.* In addition to the paired ganglia, single ganglia exist surrounding the abdominal aorta and its larger branches, where preganglionic neurons terminate without synapsing in the sympathetic chain. These are known as *collateral (prevertebral) ganglia* and include the celiac and superior and inferior mesenteric ganglia.

Autonomic Nervous System Function

Autonomic fibers project innervations, which are activated involuntarily from the CNS to smooth muscles, cardiac muscle, and glands to regulate activities related to (1) respiration, (2) cardiovascular function, (3) digestion, (3) excretion, (4) body temperature, and (5) sexual function. Centers in the hypothalamus, brainstem, and spinal cord transmit reflex responses via autonomic fibers to visceral organs.

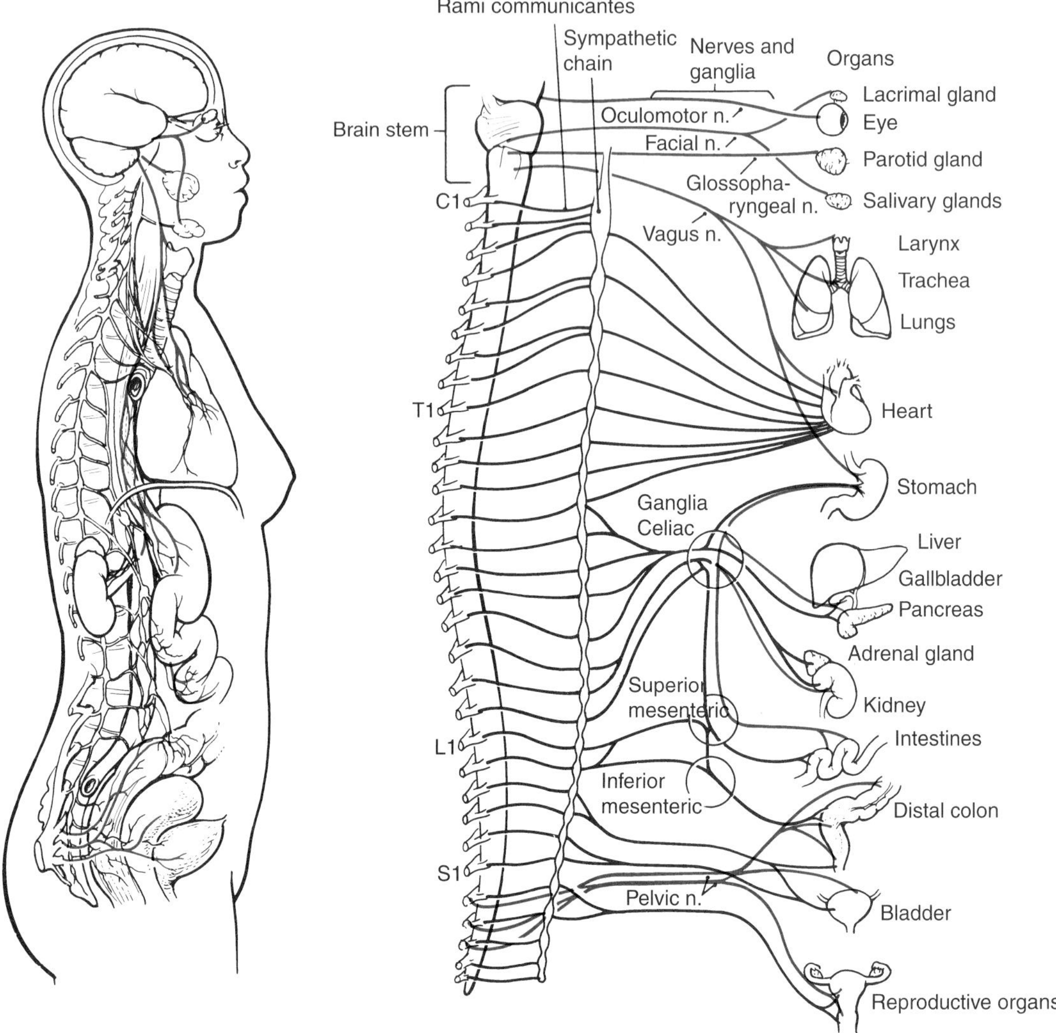

FIGURE 29-33. **Anatomy of the autonomic nervous system. (Memmler, R. L., Cohen, B. J. & Wood, D. L. [1995].** ***The human body in health and disease*** **[8th ed.]. Philadelphia: J. B. Lippincott.)**

SYMPATHETIC DIVISION (THORACOLUMBAR) FUNCTION

The cell bodies of the short preganglionic sympathetic neurons arise from the sympathetic motoneurons of the intermediolateral horns of the spinal cord between the first thoracic and second lumbar vertebrae. The fibers of these neurons pass through the intervertebral foramina in conjunction with respective spinal nerves. Shortly, the sympathetic fibers (preganglionic) depart from the spinal nerve and enter a sympa-thetic chain through the white rami communicans (Fig. 29-28). They may synapse here immediately with a postganglic neuron or pass directly through the sympathetic chain to synapse with a single sympathetic ganglion, or pass up or down the sympathetic chain and synapse at a different level.

Some postganglionic sympathetic fibers, after having synapsed in the sympathetic chain, pass back into the spinal nerve through the gray rami communicans and accompany the spinal nerve to innervate blood vessels, sweat glands, and piloerector muscles in the skin.

PARASYMPATHETIC DIVISION (CRANIOSACRAL) FUNCTION

The autonomic fibers identified in Figure 29-33 as arising from the cranial (brainstem) and sacral portions of the CNS compose the parasympathetic nervous system. Somatic efferent fibers in the cranial region arise in conjunction with the (1) oculomotor (CN III), (2) facial (CN VII), (3) glossopharyngeal (CN IX), and

(4) vagus (CN X) nerves. The vagus nerve transmits the majority of the parasympathetic impulses through its wide distribution in the thoracic and abdominal viscera. The remaining cranial nerves innervate organs of the head. The sacral fibers arise from the anterior roots of the second, third, and fourth sacral spinal nerves and innervate pelvic organs and the colon. Most of the preganglionic fibers transmit without interruption to the organs they innervate, where they synapse with the parasympathetic ganglia that are located in the area of the effector organ. In contrast to the sympathetic fibers, the parasympathetic preganglionic fibers are long and the postganglionic fibers are short.

POSTGANGLIONIC NEURONAL TRANSMISSION IN THE AUTONOMIC NERVOUS SYSTEM

Chemical mediation is necessary for neuronal transmission between neurons and between neurons and their effector organs. Excitation results from chemical release of neurotransmitter substances between preganglionic and postganglionic neurons and their effectors in the autonomic nervous system. The neurotransmitter substance released at the preganglionic neurons in both the sympathetic and parasympathetic nervous systems is acetylcholine (Ach). Acetylcholine continues to be the neurotransmitter substance from the parasympathetic postganglionic neurons. Because of the secretion of Ach, these fibers are known as *cholinergic* and their receptors are *cholinoceptive*. The primary transmitter substance secreted by the postganglionic fibers of the sympathetic nervous system is norepinephrine (NE). The fibers are referred to as *adrenergic* and terminate on *adrenoceptive* receptors. Adrenoceptive receptors on end organs are separated into alpha (α) and beta (β) adrenergic receptors, based on their responses to certain neurotransmitters or drugs. In general, stimulation of alpha receptors is associated with an excitatory sympathetic nervous system response, and stimulation of beta receptors is associated with an inhibitory sympathetic response.[12,13,15] Adrenoreceptors are further subdivided into receptor subtypes alpha-1, alpha-2, beta-1, and beta-2. The responsiveness of these receptors and other autonomic nervous system receptors is summarized in Table 29-10.

STIMULATION AND INHIBITION OF THE AUTONOMIC NERVOUS SYSTEM

The actions of the sympathetic and parasympathetic nervous systems on specific receptor organs are summarized in Table 29-11. The dual actions are a cooperative effort to maintain a constant internal environment in response to the ever-changing external world.

TABLE 29-10

RECEPTOR RESPONSES TO AUTONOMIC NERVOUS SYSTEM STIMULATION

RECEPTOR	LOCATION	RESPONSE TO STIMULATION
ADRENERGIC		
alpha-1	Wide dispersion; predominately in precapillary sphincters of smooth muscles of blood vessels	Vasoconstriction
alpha-2	Brain; preganglionic neurons	Suppression of norepinephrine
beta-1	Heart	Increased heart rate; lipolysis
beta-2	Smooth muscle of bronchi and blood vessels	Bronchoconstriction Vasodilaton
CHOLINERGIC		
Muscarinic	Central nervous system, heart, smooth muscle of viscera, and glands	Generally inhibitory except for stimulation of glandular secretion
Nicotinic	Skeletal neuromuscular junction and autonomic ganglia	Excitatory effect at the skeletal neuromuscular junction and autonomic ganglia
OTHER		
Dopaminergic D-1	Kidney blood vessels Regions of the brain	Vasodilation
Dopaminergic D-2	Caudate nucleus and other regions of the brain	Inhibition of sympathetic ganglion action: inhibition of prolactin secretion and prolactin release from striatum

TABLE 29-11

EFFECT OF AUTONOMIC STIMULATION ON EFFECTOR ORGANS

ORGAN	SNS ORGAN RECEPTOR	SYMPATHETIC STIMULATION	PARASYMPATHETIC STIMULATION
EYE			
Radial muscle of iris	α_1	Contraction (mydriasis)	
Sphincter muscle of iris			Cholinergic (miosis)
Ciliary muscle	β_2	Relaxation for far vision	Contraction for near vision
HEART			
SA node	β_1	Increased rate	Decreased rate
Atria	β_1	Increased contractility	Decreased contractility
Ventricles	β_1	Increased contractility	
AV node	β_1	Increased automaticity and conduction	Decreased automaticity and conduction
Coronary arterioles	α_1, β_2	Constriction; vasodilation	Constriction
SKIN			
Sweat glands	α_1	Localized secretion	Generalized secretion
Pilomotor muscles	α_1	Contraction	
LUNGS			
Bronchial muscle	β_2	Bronchodilation	Bronchoconstriction
Bronchial secretions	α_1, β_2	Decreased; increased	Increased
INTESTINES			
Motility	α_1, α_2, β_2	Decreased	Increased
Sphincters	α_1	Contraction	Relaxation
LIVER	α_1, β_2	Glycogenolysis	Glycogen synthesis
GALL BLADDER	β_2	Relaxation	Contraction
PANCREAS			
Acini cells	α	Decreased secretion	Secretion
Islet cells	α_2, β_2	Inhibition of insulin and glucagon secretion; stimulation of insulin and glucagon secretion	Increased insulin and glucagon secretion
SALIVARY GLANDS	α_1	Thick secretions	Profuse thin secretions
FAT CELLS	α_2, β_1	Inhibition of lipolysis; stimulation of lipolysis	
BLADDER			
Detrusor muscle	β_2	Relaxation	Contraction
Trigone	α_1	Contraction	Relaxation
PENIS	α_1	Ejaculation	Erection
BASAL METABOLISM		Increased	
ADRENAL MEDULLA		Secretion of epinephrine and norepinephrine	
MENTATION		Increased	

SNS, sympathetic nervous system; SA, sinoatrial; AV, atrioventricular; α, alpha receptors; β, beta receptors
(Modified from Ganong, W. F. [1995]. *Review of medical physiology* [17th ed.]. Norwalk, CT: Appleton-Lange.)

General responses of the sympathetic nervous system are activated under emergency situations to make internal adjustments that facilitate an appropriate response by the body. For example, in response to stressful exercise, the cardiovascular system is stimulated by the sympathetic system to increase cardiac output by increasing heart rate and force, thus providing additional perfusion to skeletal muscle, brain, and liver, while simultaneously reducing the blood supply to the viscera. The parasympathetic system, in contrast, promotes activities that maintain body function from day to day, including digestion and elimination.

The visceral effectors that receive stimulation from both the sympathetic and parasympathetic systems generally receive antagonistic stimulation. An example of this is the effect on bronchial secretions. Sympathetic stimulation decreases bronchial secretions; parasympathetic stimulation increases them. In another example, the sympathetic system dilates the pupils, whereas the parasympathetic system constricts them. The dual system does not function consistently in a cooperative balance since some organs receive innervation primarily from only one system. Examples include the smooth muscles of the skin, hair, sweat glands, and cutaneous blood vessels, which are primarily innervated from the sympathetic system. Although most organs and viscera receive innervation from both the sympathetic and parasympathetic systems, one of these generally has an inhibitory effect and the other an excitatory effect. There is no consistent rule of thumb for guidance as to which system stimulates and which inhibits.

REFERENCES

1. Adams, D. A., Victor, M., & Hopper, A. H. (1998). *Principles of neurology* (6th ed.). New York: McGraw-Hill.
2. Affifi, A., & Bergman, R. A. (1997). *Functional neuroanatomy.* New York: McGraw-Hill.
3. Aminoff, M., Greenberg, D. A., & Simon, R. P. (1997). *Clinical neurology* (3rd ed.). Stamford, CT: Appleton & Lange.
4. Carpenter, M., & Sutin, J. (1983). *Human neuroanatomy* (8th ed.). Baltimore: Williams & Wilkins.
5. Conn, P. M. (1995). *Neuroscience in medicine.* Philadelphia: J. B. Lippincott.
6. Fischbach, G. (1992). Mind and brain. *Scientific American, 267,* 50–53.
7. Fluharty, S. (1994). Synaptic transmission. In T. Alan, P. Molinoff, & A. Winokur (Eds.), *Biological bases of brain function and disease.* New York: Raven Press.
8. Ganong, W. F. (1995). *Review of medical physiology* (17th ed.). Norwalk, CT: Appleton & Lange.
9. Gazzaniga, M. S. (1998). The split brain revisited. *Scientific American, 279*(1), 50–55.
10. Gilman, S., & Newman, S. (1997). *Manter and Gatz's essentials of clinical neuroanatomy and neurophysiology* (9th ed.). Philadelphia: F.A. Davis.
11. Guyton, A. C. (1998). *Textbook of medical physiology* (8th ed.). Philadelphia: W.B. Saunders.
12. Snell, R. S. (1995). *Clinical anatomy for medical students* (5th ed.). Boston: Little, Brown.
13. Snell, R. S. (1997). *Clinical neuroanatomy for medical students* (4th ed.). Philadelphia: Lippincott-Raven.
14. Waxman, S., & deGroot, S. (1995). *Correlative neuroanatomy and functional neurology* (22nd ed.). Norwalk, CT: Appleton & Lange.
15. Westmoreland, B. F., Benarroch, E. E., Daube, J. R., Reagan, T. J., & Sandok, B. A. (1994). *Medical neurosciences: An approach to anatomy and pathology by systems and levels* (3rd ed.). Boston: Little, Brown.

Chapter

30

Neurobiology of Psychotic, Anxiety, and Mood Disorders

Joan E. Zuckerman

KEY TERMS

agoraphobia
alogia
anticipation
avolition
benzodiazepines
bipolar disorder
compliance
compulsions
delusions
depression
gliosis
hallucinations
hypomania
hypothalamic–pituitary–adrenal axis
mania
manic-depression
major depression
morbidity
neuroleptics
obsessions
phobia
relapse
selective serotonin reuptake inhibitors
trinucleotide repeat amplifications
unipolar disorder

Psychotic, anxiety, and mood disorders affect over 22% of the population during any given year, with 9% of individuals demonstrating significant dysfunction.[40] The emotional and economic costs of these psychiatric illnesses, along with their increased mortality and **morbidity**, are striking. These disorders have been the subject of intense study in an attempt to understand how genetic and environmental factors may be involved in their etiology. In the 1990s, during the "Decade of the Brain," exciting new findings have occurred, with many significant research studies published and controversial new pathophysiologic theories proposed. A better understanding of neurophysiology and new technology is providing a better "window into the brain." However, many questions about normal and pathologic brain function remain unanswered.

Various approaches have been used to understand the pathophysiology of neurobiologic disorders. Genetic studies have focused on the heritability of disorders in monozygotic (identical) and dizygotic (nonidentical) twins; such studies help reveal the relative contribution of genes and environment in the transmission of disorders. Other studies have examined the risk of disease for first-degree relatives (parents, siblings, and children) of those affected within a single family.[43] The emergence of genetic engineering and human genome mapping has led investigators in search of susceptibility genes on specific chromosomes, exploring whether altered forms of specific candidate genes are present. Pharmacologic challenge studies have been designed, using a specific neurochemical or physiologic system to better understand its role in the disorder. The synthesis and metabolism of neurotransmitters and their postsynaptic receptors have been examined for alterations. Early studies searched post-mortem brain samples for signs of pathologic changes; currently, sophisticated neuroimaging techniques are being used to search for anatomic and functional defects.

In the United States, these illnesses generally are diagnosed on the basis of specific signs and symptoms, which are evaluated by focused, standardized, and well-validated questionnaires, rather than physiologic and anatomic alterations. These illnesses are categorized according to specific diagnostic criteria, which have co-evolved along with the field of neuropsychiatry over the past 25 years.[1] However, because of the heterogeneity of clinical manifestations of these disorders, the classification schemes are complex and detailed.

THE BIOLOGY OF MAJOR NEUROTRANSMITTERS

The disorders presented in this chapter have all been associated with alterations in the functioning of neurotransmitter (NT) systems in the central nervous system (CNS). Initially, the discovery of neurochemical alterations led to proposals that deficits or excesses of single neurotransmitters were responsible for the various disorders. Now, it is realized that the regulation of the activity of different neuronal pathways and their interactions is more complex than initially thought. Functional changes in more than one neurotransmitter system are thought to contribute to each of these disorders. The most important neurotransmitters are (1) dopamine (DA), (2) norepinephrine (NE), (3) gamma-aminobutyric acid (GABA), and (4) serotonin (5-HT).

Dopamine

The cell bodies of DA-releasing neurons are located in specific areas of the brain, the substantia nigra and the ventral tegmental areas of the midbrain (Fig. 30-1). Bundles of axons from these neurons (pathways or tracts) project to various areas of the brain. The *mesocortical* and *mesolimbic* pathways originate from the ventral tegmentum area and innervate the prefrontal cortex (medial frontal lobe) and the medial limbic structures (amygdala and hippocampus), respectively. These pathways are thought to be involved in cognition, abstract thinking, and mental planning. The *nigrostriatal* pathway originates in the substantia nigra and projects to the caudate nucleus and putamen (in the basal ganglia), located deep in the cerebral hemispheres. This pathway is thought to play a role in voluntary movement. Degeneration of this pathway is observed in Parkinson's disease. The last pathway, the tuberoinfundibular pathway, links part of the mesolimbic pathway with the hypothalamus, which in turn directs the activity of the pituitary. Dysfunction of this pathway may contribute to the neuroendocrine abnormalities seen in some studies of schizophrenics.[30]

Norepinephrine

Norepinephrine (NE) is the major NT released at sympathetic postganglionic fibers and by the adrenal medulla. The activity of this system is increased during stress when the sympathetic fight or flight response is activated. NE is also released in the CNS by neurons whose cell bodies are located in the locus ceruleus (LC) in the pons. This nucleus sends ascending axons to the hypothalamus, thalamus, hippocampus, and diffusely throughout the cerebral cortex. Electrical stimulation of the LC produces increased arousal. It is proposed that hyperactivity of the LC may occur in anxiety dis-

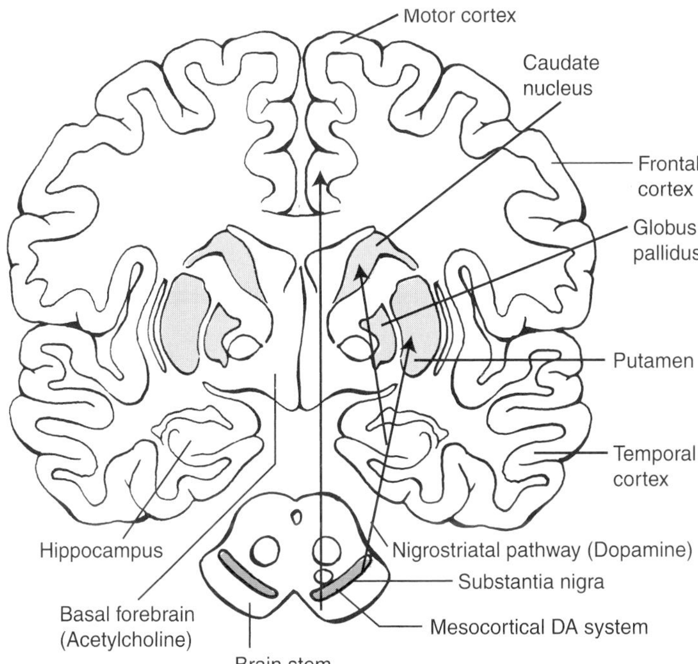

FIGURE 30-1. Selected neurotransmitter pathways in the human brain. (Modified from Joyce, J. & Hurtig, H. [1994]. Neurodegenerative disorders. In A. Frazer, P. Molinoff, & A. Winokur [Eds.], *Biological basis of brain function and disease.* New York: Raven Press.)

orders. Alterations in noradrenergic function (functions mediated by norepinephrine) may also occur in mood disorders. Inhibition of presynaptic reuptake of NE, for example with antidepressant medications, increases NE's effect.

Serotonin

Many of the cell bodies of neurons releasing serotonin (5-HT or 5-hydroxytryptamine) are located in the raphe nuclei in the brainstem and project to almost every part of the CNS, including the cerebellum, cerebral cortex, hypothalamus, limbic system, and basal ganglia. Inhibition of the presynaptic reuptake of 5-HT, such as with antidepressants and **selective serotonin reuptake inhibitors** (SSRIs) used for the treatment of anxiety and depression, increase 5-HT's effectiveness at the postsynaptic receptor.

Gamma-aminobutyric Acid (GABA)

Gamma-aminobutyric acid (GABA), an amino acid, is the major inhibitory neurotransmitter in the CNS. Its primary role appears to be to slow increased activity in other neuronal pathways. A deficiency of this NT may lead to the increased neural excitation associated with epilepsy. The GABA system is also thought to be involved in anxiety disorders. GABA receptors are concentrated in two brain areas: (1) the limbic system, which controls emotional behavior, and (2) the locus ceruleus, which controls arousal. The $GABA_A$ receptor acts by opening postsynaptic Cl^- channels, leading to hyperpolarization and inhibition of the postsynaptic neuron. There is a separate but adjacent receptor site near the $GABA_A$ receptor, which binds a class of drugs called **benzodiazepines**. These drugs act as allosteric agonists (producing an enhanced response). When a benzodiazepine binds to its receptor, an increase in the affinity for GABA occurs at the $GABA_A$ receptor, leading to greater Cl^- influx. Thus, a benzodiazepine increases the action of GABA, calming brain activity and producing sedation, anticonvulsive effects, muscle relaxation, and a lessening of anxiety.

PSYCHOTIC DISORDERS

Psychotic behavior has been described for centuries, but the criteria that currently help health care professionals diagnose psychotic disorders were developed only in the 1970s. The perception of reality, communication, and the ability to form and maintain interpersonal relationships are all altered. These disorders are characterized by (1) hallucinations, (2) delusions, (3) disorganized speech, and (4) catatonic behavior. Psychotic illnesses include schizophrenia, schizophreniform disorder, schizoaffective disorder, brief psychotic disorder, delusional disorder, and shared psychotic disorder. Psychosis can also result as a complication of a medical condition or be induced by chemicals. Schizophrenia represents the most commonly encountered and the most studied of the psychotic disorders.

Schizophrenia

Schizophrenia affects less than 1% of the population of the U.S. but accounts for 22% of the costs of all mental illnesses.[57] It was first described in the medical literature in the late 1800s by Emil Kraeplin, a physician who termed the disorder "dementia praecox." In the early 1900s, Eugen Bleuler renamed the disorder schizophrenia, meaning "split minds," and recognized that there were excessive and decreased behaviors leading to various subtypes of the disorder. Current criteria for the diagnosis of schizophrenia take into account the significant variability in clinical manifestations and separate these manifestations into "positive" and "negative" categories. Many people mistakenly believe that multiple personalities are part of this disorder.

Schizophrenia is a chronic and deteriorating illness for many of those afflicted. The emotional and economic impact of this disease is immense; after disease onset, work, social relationships, and self-care are all compromised. A significant proportion of patients are chronically affected and are never able to function fully in society. Schizophrenic patients occupy 20% to 25% of all the beds available in psychiatric in-patient care facilities and account for 40% of all long-term hospital stays.[46] The economic costs of this disorder are estimated at $73 billion annually, based on the expense of treatment and on lost wages.[3]

The majority of cases of schizophrenia are diagnosed between the ages of 15 and 45 years of age; 75% of schizophrenia patients become ill between the ages of 15 and 30.[24] For men, the mean age for the first acute episode is 21.4 years; for women, it is 26.8 years.[3] This difference has been hypothesized to occur due to estrogen levels exerting a protective effect and delaying onset of the disorder.[24] One consequence of this age difference at onset is that more women have the opportunity to marry and start a family. There is a less common late-onset form, which is diagnosed when a patient is older and appears to have a different spectrum of clinical manifestations.

Cognition, the process of knowing, is severely impaired in schizophrenia. Those affected do not recognize that their ideas and associations between concepts are different from those of others. These individuals also experience problems with the processing of other types of information and with operations including memory, attention, concentration, speech, decision making, and thought content.

Schizophrenia is generally regarded to be a heterogeneous disease, in which several etiologies lead to a similar set of signs and symptoms. Researchers have been searching for a set of shared pathophysiologic changes that unite the different subsets of this disorder. This is a challenging task, and to date no consistent single biochemical or morphologic alteration has been found.

ETIOLOGY AND PATHOPHYSIOLOGY

Recent research has revealed a number of alterations in neuropsychological testing, brain imaging studies (MRI, PET, SPECT), chromosome structure, neurophysiology, and neurotransmitter biology. It has been speculated that schizophrenia arises as a result of abnormal brain development influenced by genetic and environmental factors. This increasingly popular "neurodevelopmental hypothesis" proposes that adverse prenatal, perinatal, or very early postnatal events cause functional and anatomic alterations early in development, possibly making an individual more susceptible to environmental and/or endogenous triggers that subsequently induce schizophrenia.

GENETICS. There is a 1% lifetime risk of developing schizophrenia in the general population. However, in families with a history of the disease, the risk is much greater. Family, twin, and adoption epidemiologic studies have been performed to assess disease heritability.

Monozygotic (identical) twins share 100% of their genes, whereas dizygotic (non-identical or fraternal) twins share 50% of their genes. If one monozygotic twin has schizophrenia, the second twin has a 53% chance of schizophrenia. Since the chance of schizophrenia for an second identical twin is not 100%, there must be environmental factors that modify the risk. Studies of dizygotic twins also suggest heritability of susceptibility genes since the incidence of a second nonidentical twin having it is 15%. Having one or both parents with schizophrenia also increases one's risk (15% or 35%, respectively).[29,58,68]

Children of schizophrenics who are raised by adoptive parents in a different environment still retain their higher chance of having the disease, suggesting that in utero or genetic factors are strong determinants of the disease. However, there are many cases of "sporadic" schizophrenia where there is no apparent family history. It is unknown if these cases are the manifestation of a environmentally related developmental disturbance or are due to the rare expression of a lower genetic risk. Data from twin studies have led investigators to estimate that genetic transmission accounts for about 65% of the cases of schizophrenia.[33]

Studies of families with a history of schizophrenia have attempted to identify chromosomes that may be linked to disease risk and have suggested that loci on chromosomes 6, 8, and 22 may be involved in determining susceptibility.[32,49] Other studies have unsuccessfully attempted to document alterations in one or more specific neurotransmitter receptor proteins, neurotransmitter catabolic enzymes, or candidate proteins and genes that have been hypothesized to be involved in the disease. Thus, there are no consistent biologic or genetic markers identified with the disorder.

It was recently discovered that some heritable diseases show a decreased age of onset and increase in severity over successive generations. This phenomenon, called **anticipation**, is due to a mutation that leads to multiple trinucleotide segments of a gene (**trinucleotide repeat amplifications**) being introduced into DNA whenever it is replicated. These areas of repeated DNA increase with each generation. Several neurodegenerative diseases (fragile X syndrome, myotonic dystrophy, and spinocerebellar ataxia) are thought to arise in this manner, leading investigators to examine whether this occurs in schizophrenia. This phenomenon may help explain risk differences in identical twins and the variability of gene expression. Although some repeat sequences were found in selected family studies, no consistent association between age of onset and size of the repeated DNA has been found.[30,32]

PREGNANCY AND BIRTH COMPLICATIONS. A relationship between obstetric complications such as hypoxia, preeclampsia, and prolonged labor, all postulated to lead to developmental alterations, and the incidence of sporadic cases of schizophrenia (cases in which there is no clear family history of the disorder) has been proposed.[12] Some studies suggest that mothers of schizophrenic patients have a 21% to 40% greater incidence of obstetric complications as compared with normal control subjects, whereas other studies have shown no such association.[12,29] Alternatively, it has been proposed that preexisting developmental damage may actually cause the pregnancy and birth complications.[58] The risk of schizophrenia from obstetric complications is thought to be relatively minor in comparison to genetic factors.[66]

SEASONAL BIRTH AND VIRAL HYPOTHESES. As part of retrospective epidemiologic studies after influenza epidemics, several studies have demonstrated that maternal and fetal exposure to the influenza virus during the second trimester leads to a slightly increased rate of schizophrenia.[28] Before this period of development, neurons have formed but have not yet made specific connections. Infection may disrupt the ability of these neurons to make the proper connections, causing a developmental disorder that manifests itself later.

A seasonal influence on the incidence of schizophrenia also has been shown, with a 5% increase in schizophrenic births occurring during the late winter to early spring months. The basis for this finding is not understood, but some have hypothesized that there could be a link to exposure to an infectious agent.[29,58,66]

DOPAMINE HYPOTHESIS. Over the last 30 years, investigators have recognized that dopaminergic pathways are implicated in schizophrenia. Drugs that increase dopamine release or turnover (such as amphetamine and cocaine) are known to cause psychotic symptoms. The classic drugs used for schizophrenia (**neuroleptics** or antipsychotic drugs) are potent dopamine antagonists, specifically competing with dopamine for binding at one of the dopamine receptor subtypes (D_2). The efficacy of these drugs is directly related to their affinity as competitive antagonists at this receptor. These drugs can also reverse amphetamine-induced psychosis in humans. These findings led to the hypothesis that excessive dopamine neurotransmission was the central, dominant change in the disorder. However, studies of dopamine and its metabolites in brain tissue, CSF, and serum have not yielded consistent evidence for this hypothesis.[27,66] Modifications of this theory were subsequently proposed, suggesting that the activity of specific dopaminergic tracts was altered.

The dopaminergic mesocortical pathway is thought to be involved with planning, judgment, motivation, cognition, and abstract thinking. The mesolimbic pathways are associated with memory and emotion. In schizophrenia, the mesolimbic neurons could be overactive, causing the positive symptoms, while the mesocortical neurons could be less active, inducing the negative symptoms.[17] This hypothesis fits with the reduced frontal lobe glucose utilization seen in PET imaging studies, but it does not satisfactorily account for the various alterations in brain morphology and biochemistry.

Recently, more complicated hypotheses have been proposed, involving many other neurotransmitters and receptor subtypes. It is now clear that a simple alteration in the concentration of one neurotransmitter, such as dopamine, or of one receptor subtype is unlikely; alternatively, multiple neurotransmitters and different neuronal pathways are probably involved.

INVOLVEMENT OF OTHER NEUROTRANSMITTERS. Serotonin (5-HT or 5-hydroxytryptamine) has long been implicated in the pathogenesis of schizophrenia. Animal studies demonstrate that serotonin can modulate dopaminergic neurons and/or dopamine receptor function. LSD, a serotonin receptor agonist, can produce a psychosis similar to that seen in schizophrenia. It is significant that many of the newer, atypical antipsychotic agents such as risperidone and clozapine are antagonists at the 5-HT_2 receptor and appear to have greater efficacy at treating both the negative symptoms and refractory patients than do the classic neuroleptics. These results have intensified efforts to understand the role of serotonin and its many receptor subtypes in the pathogenesis of the disorder.[61]

Abnormal glutamate transmission has long been suspected in schizophrenia. PCP (phencyclidine or angel dust) blocks a subtype of glutamate receptors (the NMDA receptor) in the brain and induces a psychosis that shows both positive and negative symptoms. Numerous studies show increased orbito- and pre-frontal cortex glutamate receptors in schizophrenics.[66] Additional studies are needed to understand the interactions between these different transmitter systems.

STRUCTURAL AND FUNCTIONAL NEUROANATOMIC CHANGES. Postmortem studies were first performed in the late 1800s in an effort to determine whether schizophrenics had a demonstrable neuroanatomic defect. Over the years, these studies have consistently shown enlarged lateral and third ventricles and widening of sulci (especially in the frontal lobes) in schizophrenic brains. New technology, such as computed tomography (CT) and magnetic resonance imaging (MRI), has corroborated these findings. Figure 30-2 compares an MRI of the ventricles and sulci of a normal person in a control group (A) and two patients with schizophrenia (B) and (C); there appears to be a loss of neural tissue. Many imaging studies show a reduction of the volume of the frontal lobes, temporal lobes, and thalamus.[13,27] Similar changes have been noted in the brains of childhood-onset schizophrenics, who generally experience chronic schizophrenia as adults.[12] These abnormalities are not restricted to schizophrenia; ventricular size is also increased in neurodegenerative diseases. However, in contrast to these disorders, necrosis or **gliosis** (inflammation of glial cells) is not seen in brain tissue of schizophrenics, implying that an acute or prolonged inflammatory event has not taken place.[27] Reductions in prefrontal cortical thickness have been noted as well.[70] These morphologic changes may either remain stable or progress over time, and their severity may be correlated with prognosis.[23,70]

Functional imaging techniques, such as photon emission tomography (PET), single photon emission computed tomography (SPECT), and proton magnetic resonance spectroscopic imaging (MRSI), have revealed abnormalities in the frontal lobes, temporal lobes, and basal ganglia.[12] Many studies have shown decreased cerebral blood flow (CBF) and hypometabolism in the dorsolateral frontal cortex when patients are asked to perform various cognitive tasks. Increased CBF or metabolism in the left temporal lobe has also been observed.[12] Many investigators relate the frontal lobe changes to the manifestation of negative symptoms, whereas the increased temporal lobe activity may be related to the expression of positive symptoms.[14,38]

NEUROLOGIC AND NEUROPSYCHOLOGICAL CHANGES. Schizophrenics show a higher than expected rate of abnormalities during neurologic exams. Non-schizophrenic siblings also show abnormalities, but of a lesser severity.[26] A recent study suggests that familial and sporadic schizophrenics vary in the pattern of abnormalities, suggesting that the etiology is different for these two patient groups.[22]

Patients with schizophrenia also show deficits in attention, memory, adaptation to the environment, and cognitive functions, all of which involve the

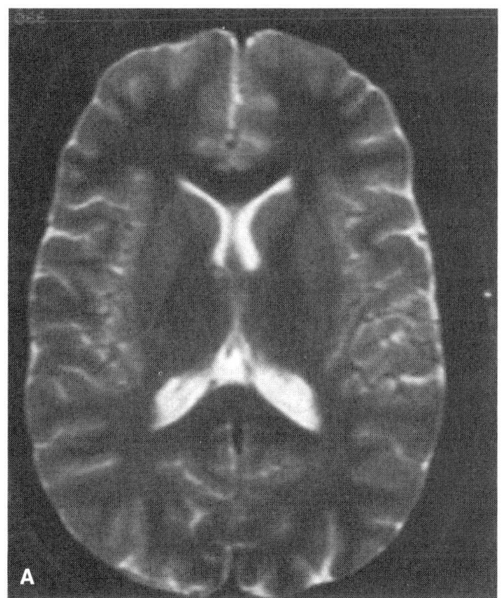

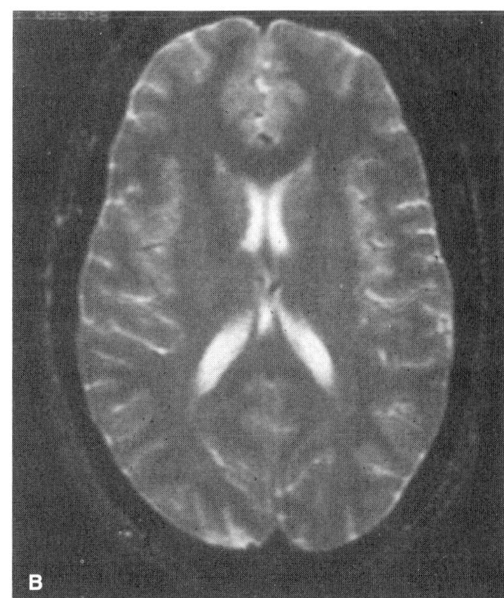

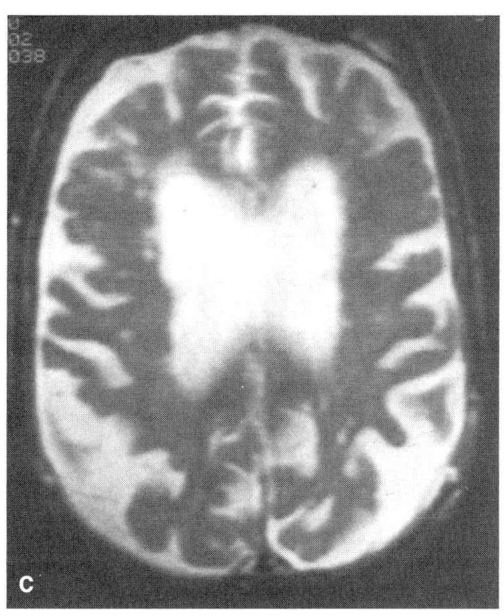

FIGURE 30-2. **A.** MRI of normal control. Note that the CSF in ventricles and sulci (white) is barely visible. **B,C.** MRI of two patients with schizophrenia. Note the greater prominence of CSF in **B** and marked prominence in **C.** (Gur, R. [1994]. Schizophrenia. In A. Frazer, P. Molinoff, & A. Winokur [Eds.], *Biological basis of brain function and disease.* New York: Raven Press.)

frontal and temporal lobes. It has been proposed that connections between the frontal cortex and the basal ganglia, thalamus, and reticular formation are altered, with a concomitant imbalance in major neurotransmitter systems.[27]

CLINICAL MANIFESTATIONS

Schizophrenia is characterized by significant alterations in personality, distorted thinking, bizarre delusions, altered perceptions, inappropriate emotional responses, and withdrawal from emotional contact. Clinical manifestations are classified as being "positive" or "negative" (Table 30-1). Schizophrenia presents a complex clinical picture because the signs and symptoms vary in different individuals.

In many cases, a gradual alteration in behavior is noted by family and friends when a person is approaching or in his or her early twenties. This strange behavior, associated with social withdrawal, delusions, and hallucinations, may at first be dismissed as "growing pains." The changes may be brief and vague at first, but eventually the symptoms and associated behavior disrupt normal social function. Commonly, the initial

TABLE 30-1

CLASSIFICATION OF SYMPTOMS OF SCHIZOPHRENIA

POSITIVE SYMPTOMS (EXCESSIVE OR DISTORTED FUNCTIONING)	
Delusions:	Usually implausible, erroneous beliefs involving a misinterpretation of perceptions or experiences; these are clearly not appropriate to the observer (For example: a person may feel followed or persecuted or may believe that an advertisement or newspaper article is specifically directed at him or her.)
Hallucinations:	Altered sensory input, usual auditory, received by the person but not perceptible by others (For example: a person may hear one or two voices commenting on or judging his or her thoughts or behavior.)
Disorganized thinking:	Demonstrated by questions that elicit irrelevant or incoherent answers that impair communication (For example: a person may constantly "go off on a limb" and never give an adequate or direct answer to questions.)
Grossly disorganized or catatonic behavior:	Inappropriate behavior, ranging from silliness to agitation or decreased reactivity to surroundings (For example: a person may shout or swear unpredictably or maintain a rigid posture.)
NEGATIVE SYMPTOMS (DECREASE OR LOSS OF FUNCTIONING)	
Affective flattening:	Decrease in range and intensity of emotional expression (For example: during interactions, person demonstrates an unresponsive facial expression and poor eye contact)
Poverty of speech (alogia):	Limited spontaneous speech or brief and succinct replies to questioning
Avolition:	Inability to initiate and persist in goal-directed activities (For example: a person may sit quietly and silently in the midst of a room full of active people.)

A diagnosis of schizophrenia requires that two symptoms from the above list (one or two of the four positive symptoms and/or a negative symptom) be manifested.

(Reprinted with permission from *Diagnostic and statistical manual of mental disorders* [4th ed.]. Copyright 1994, American Psychiatric Association.)

evaluation occurs while the patient is in an agitated, anxious, or aggressive state. The individual does not realize that he or she needs treatment and believes that the delusions and hallucinations are real. A diagnosis of schizophrenia is made if a person exhibits a combination of positive and negative symptoms for 1 month in duration and shows signs of a disturbance dating back for at least 6 months. The individual must also demonstrate significant social or occupational dysfunction. The disorder has a variable course that may last for decades and either fluctuate or, more rarely, go into remission and disappear.

Co-morbidity

Many studies have attempted to analyze the long-term prognosis of individuals with schizophrenia; these studies generally agree that a significant number of patients will exhibit a long-term disability. Clinical depression is not uncommon, with approximately 20% to 50% of patients attempting suicide and 10 % actually committing suicide.[73]

Other psychiatric disorders occur at a higher-than-expected rate in the relatives of schizophrenics. For example, the risk for schizotypal personality disorder is five times greater among first-degree relatives (siblings, parents, children) of schizophrenics than for a control population.[29] However, studies suggest that the risk for all types of psychiatric illness is not increased.

Relapse (acute episodes or exacerbations) commonly recur in most patients. More than 50% of patients have a greater number of acute relapses and show a progressive deterioration in personality and decreased ability to function.[58]

The traditional antipsychotic drugs (neuroleptic drugs such as haloperidol and chlorpromazine) can induce movement disorders with Parkinson-like symptoms, sedation, and a "wooden" subjective experience, possibly compromising patient **compliance** and thus leading to relapses when the patient decides to go off medication. The newer "atypical" antipsychotic drugs (risperidone, remoxipride, and clozapine) have fewer side effects than the classical neuroleptics and appear to decrease the number of relapses, leading to less disability overall. There may also be a greater degree of improvement in negative symptoms and significant efficacy noted in patients resistant to the classical neuroleptics.[2]

ANXIETY DISORDERS

Anxiety, a common emotion, is a subjective experience unable to be observed directly. When present, however, it can lead to physiologic and psychological dysfunction. An anxiety disorder is diagnosed when a person's functioning or interaction with others is affected. Anxiety disorders include panic disorder (PD), generalized anxiety disorder (GAD), obsessive-compulsive disorder (OCD), phobias, and post-traumatic stress disorder (PTSD). These disorders are summarized in Table 30-2.

It has been estimated that 25% of the population will suffer from an anxiety disorder at some point in life.[44] Individuals with anxiety disorders experience anxiety in particular situations or in response to specific triggers, resulting in a variety of physiologic, emotional, cognitive, and behavioral manifestations. These include fear, apprehension, nervousness, panic, restlessness, tension, agitation, trembling, fainting, headaches, sweating, and blood pressure and heart rate changes.

Panic Disorder

Panic disorder (PD) is the most studied of the anxiety disorders and appears to be a very common psychiatric illness, with a lifetime prevalence of approximately 2%. Around the world, panic disorder occurs reproducibly at similar rates and about two to three times more often in women than men.[72] The age of onset is typically in the late teens to early thirties and often follows 6 months or more after a major stressful event.

ETIOLOGY AND PATHOPHYSIOLOGY

Evidence exists for a number of different neurochemical, endocrine, morphologic, and physiologic alterations in PD. Because the panic attack can be elicited reproducibly in many patients, studies have been designed to provoke a panic attack while stimulating or provoking a specific biochemical or neurochemical pathway or system to understand its role in the pathophysiology of the disease process. Multiple neurotransmitter systems and multiple neuroanatomic sites appear to be involved.[28]

GENETICS. Although limited, twin studies show a higher than anticipated rate of PD and agoraphobia in monozygotic (identical) than dizygotic (nonidentical) twins (31% versus 4%, respectively), suggesting a genetic basis for the disorder.[67] Patients report secondary cases of PD in 12% to 15% of first-degree relatives (parents, siblings, children), in contrast to a 2% rate in the general population.[16] However, so far studies aimed at linking the disorder to a specific chromosome or gene alteration have proved unsuccessful.

SUFFOCATION HYPOTHESIS. Abnormalities in respiratory function have been hypothesized to be the cause of PD. Exposure to certain substances (panicogenic agents such as sodium bicarbonate, sodium lactate, and carbon dioxide) can elicit a panic attack in a significant number of people with the disorder but to a much lesser degree, or not at all, in control subjects. These substances are hypothesized to increase CO_2 and decrease the pH of the CSF, thus activating medullary chemoreceptors. This activation might occur more readily in hypersensitive individuals. The effects of suffocation are mimicked by triggering a "false suffocation alarm,"[36] resulting in hyperventilation and panic. Indeed, almost all patients with PD complain of shortness of breath or dyspnea during attacks. The antidepressants used for therapy of spontaneous panic attacks can also prevent these "artificial" attacks. This hypothesis has gained recognition and support over the last several years as more research studies have been performed.

ALTERED NORADRENERGIC RESPONSE. Panic attacks are associated with signs and symptoms suggesting an increase in the activity of the sympathetic nervous system. However, no consistent peripheral noradrenergic alterations have been found. Attention has turned to the role of central noradrenergic neurons using yohimbine, an α_2-adrenergic antagonist, to elicit a panic attack in 60% to 70% of PD patients.[15] These findings led investigators to propose that a supersensitivity of presynaptic α_2-adrenergic receptors exists in patients with PD.

A major brain stem nucleus, the locus ceruleus (LC), located in the pons, contains half of all brainstem noradrenergic neurons. Its widespread ascending axonal branches terminate in the dorsal thalamus, hypothalamus, cerebellum, basal forebrain, and hippocampus.[59] The LC responds to sensory input with a burst of activity, as demonstrated when the LC of monkeys is electrically stimulated, resulting in increased fear and anxiety. The LC neurons may act as an "alarm system," notifying the higher brain centers of adverse or sudden sensory stimuli. Thus, hyperactivity of this system could cause PD.[39]

SEROTONIN INVOLVEMENT. Serotonin has long been thought to play a role in the transmission of anxious and fearful behaviors. Pharmacologic challenge studies with 5-HT precursors and receptor agonists have pro-

TABLE 30-2

DIAGNOSTIC CLASSIFICATION OF ANXIETY DISORDERS

DISORDER	SPECIFIC CHARACTERISTICS
Panic disorder (PD) with agoraphobia	Recurrent panic attacks are present, with at least one of the attacks followed by a month of worry about additional attacks or a significant change in behavior related to the attack. Agoraphobia is the fear of being in open spaces, in crowds, standing in a line, etc. The person fears that he or she may have a panic attack and may not be able to escape the situation.
Panic disorder without agoraphobia	As above but without agoraphobia.
Specific phobia	A marked and persistent fear that is excessive or unreasonable occurs with the presence or anticipation of exposure to a specific object or situation.
Social phobia (SP)	Marked and persistent fear is brought on by social or performance situations. The person feels that he will embarrass himself or herself or do something wrong in front of a large group of people. There may also be a fear of being harshly judged.
Obsessive-compulsive disorder (OCD)	Obsessions or compulsions (activities that are excessive and interfere with a person's normal routine) must be present. The person feels as if the body is acting independent of the will, but he or she also realizes that these actions are self-induced and extreme.
Generalized anxiety disorder (GAD)	General worry about a number of events or activities *occurs* which lasts for a majority of days within a 6 month period. To be diagnosed, one has at least three of the following symptoms: restlessness or being on edge, difficulty concentrating or blanking out, irritability, muscle tension, sleep disturbance.
Post-traumatic stress disorder (PTSD)	Exposure to a traumatic event was experienced in which death or serious injury occurred or was threatened. The person responded to this threat with horror, intense fear, or helplessness. Over time, the traumatic event is re-experienced and the person becomes emotionally numbed.
Acute stress disorder	This is similar to PTSD, sharing some of the same symptoms but occurring as an acute response after a traumatic event. Symptoms last for at least 2 days and do not persist longer than a month. The person experiences a sense of detachment, reduced awareness of his or her surroundings, and has difficulty recalling specific details of the event.

(Reprinted with permission from *Diagnostic and statistical manual of mental disorders* [4th ed]. Copyright 1994, American Psychiatric Association.)

duced equivocal findings.[15] It is very difficult to selectively examine portions of the serotonin system and its role in PD because there are multiple receptor families and subtypes (14 to date) and many of these can be present simultaneously on the same neuron. The demonstrated therapeutic efficacy of serotonin reuptake inhibitors (SSRIs) strongly suggests a role for serotonin dysfunction in the disorder. These drugs can block both spontaneous and induced panic attacks by blocking the reuptake of serotonin into the presynaptic neuron. As a result, serotonin remains in the synaptic cleft for a longer time, thus exerting a greater postsynaptic effect. SSRIs may allow serotonergic neurons to increase their inhibitory effects on noradrenergic neurons in the LC.[15]

GABA. GABA receptors are concentrated in two brain areas: (1) the limbic system, which controls emotional behavior, and (2) the LC. The $GABA_A$ receptor acts by opening Cl^- channels, which leads to hyperpolarization and inhibition of the postsynaptic neuron.

High doses of benzodiazepines, which bind near the GABA receptor and increase GABA's inhibitory activity, can block panic attacks. It has been proposed that patients with PD may have an intrinsic benzodiazepine receptor subsensitivity or a deficiency of an endogenous chemical that binds at the benzodiazepine receptor.[15,39]

NEUROPEPTIDES. Corticotropin-releasing hormone (CRH), a neuropeptide released from the hypothalamus, triggers the anterior pituitary to release adrenocorticotrophic hormone (ACTH), which in turn triggers the adrenal cortex to release cortisol. This pathway, the **hypothalamic–pituitary–adrenal axis** (HPA), is activated by physiologic and emotional stressors, causing cortisol to be released. CRH can also act as a neurotransmitter, with high levels of receptors in the forebrain (in the frontal cortex, amygdala, and hippocampus) as well as the brain stem (in the LC). It may moderate the endocrine, autonomic, and behavioral responses to stress. A disruption in functional connections between CRH and the noradrenergic system in the LC may cause PD.[15]

Another neuropeptide, cholecystokinin (CCK), with high concentrations and high-affinity receptors found in the cerebral cortex, amygdala, and the hippocampus, has also been implicated in the etiology of panic disorders. It is postulated that PD may result from an increased production of CCK or receptor hypersensitivity. CCK agonists induce severe anxiety or panic attacks in laboratory animals and normal control subjects. Persons with panic disorders appear to be more sensitive to these drugs. These effects also are blocked by CCK antagonists.[8,9] PD may indeed occur as a result of increased CCK since CCK agonists increase PD and antagonists decrease it.

NEUROANATOMIC CHANGES. Evidence of structural abnormalities with MRI has been found in regions near the right temporal lobe in some lactate-sensitive PD patients. Overall, the results were variable but were viewed as providing support for a role of the limbic system in the disorder.[21,28] A decrease in hippocampal perfusion and glucose utilization as compared with normal controls has been shown with PET and SPECT studies.[21]

CLINICAL MANIFESTATIONS

Panic normally occurs in individuals when they are placed in a life-threatening situation. However, people with PD experience a very rapid onset of panic in response to situations that they perceive as life threatening but that actually are not. They experience intense fear, discomfort, or dread accompanied by physical and behavioral signs of increased sympathetic nervous system activity. These attacks recur and patients feel that they must flee from where they are or they will suffocate, "lose their mind," or die as a result of the attack. The experience is overwhelming, and further attacks are feared by the individual. Approximately one-third of patients also are diagnosed with **agoraphobia**, which is the fear of being alone or in a public or open space when one of these attacks occurs. This fear may lead to reclusive behavior and reluctance to leave home.

Panic disorder can be devastating for the patient, leading to subsequent job loss, loss of financial independence, excessive use of medical facilities, and additional psychiatric disorders (depression, suicidal behavior). To be diagnosed with PD, four attacks must occur within a 4-week period or one or more attacks must have been followed by a prolonged period in which there is persistent fear of having another attack.[1]

The manifestations of panic attacks last between 10 and 30 minutes. However, the increased anxiety associated with these attacks can last for hours. During the panic attack, patients can experience a number of different symptoms, as summarized in Box 30-1. Arrhythmias, asthmatic symptoms, and diarrhea also may be reported.[5] Individuals may be suspected of having a myocardial infarction because of the similarity of signs and symptoms. Extensive testing for coronary artery disease, endocrine disturbances, inflammatory bowel disorder, neurologic disorders, and asthma is commonly performed due to the varied clinical manifestations.[15,31] Misdiagnosis is common. Patients may report an average of 12 to 14 different symptoms, pos-

BOX 30-1 CRITERIA FOR DIAGNOSIS OF A PANIC ATTACK

Patient experiences a period of intense fear in which at least four of the following symptoms appear suddenly and reach a peak within 10 minutes:

- Palpatations, rapid heart rate, "pounding" heart
- Trembling or shaking
- Sensation of smothering, shortness of breath, or gasping for air
- Feeling of choking
- Chest pain or discomfort
- Nausea or gastrointestinal distress
- Dizziness, lightheadedness, feeling faint
- Feelings of unreality or of personal detachment
- Fear of going crazy or of losing control
- Fear of dying
- Paresthesias (numbness or tingling sensations)
- Chills or hot flashes, diaphoresis

(Adapted with permission from American Psychiatric Association. [1994]. *Diagnostic and statistical manual of mental disorders* [4th ed.]. Washington, DC: American Psychiatric Press.)

sibly visit as many as 10 physicians, and be in the healthcare system for 10 years before a correct diagnosis of PD is made.[5]

CO-MORBIDITY. Panic disorder is a chronic illness. Although follow-up studies show that patients improve during therapy with antidepressants or benzodiazepines, many remain symptomatic.[54] People with PD are more likely to develop another type of anxiety disorder such as agoraphobia or social phobia or to suffer from major depression in their lifetime.[15,72] Patients with agoraphobia generally present with more severe symptoms, have a more chronic disease course, and show a more limited response to therapy.[54]

Generalized Anxiety Disorder (GAD)

GAD is characterized by unrealistic and excessive daily worry about any number of different situations or occurrences. The intensity, duration, or frequency of worry is out of proportion with the likelihood or impact of the feared event. Worry about everyday, routine issues is common, and the focus of this worry may shift from one issue to another. This disorder has a lifetime prevalence of 4% to 6%, so it is about three times more common than PD.[10] Women are twice as likely to be diagnosed with this disorder as men. The onset of the disorder can occur at any age; thus, unlike PD, it is also diagnosed in young children and the elderly.

ETIOLOGY AND PATHOPHYSIOLOGY

GAD has been the subject of fewer epidemiologic and research studies than has PD; thus, fewer definitive findings are available. Some neurochemical similarities to PD have been noted.

GENETICS. Evidence for genetic transmission of GAD is not conclusive; one twin study was negative, whereas a familial study showed an increased rate of GAD in first-degree relatives of patients. However, the incidence of other anxiety disorders was not increased in these family members.[15]

NEUROTRANSMITTER INVOLVEMENT. Noradrenergic dysfunction has been implicated with GAD, but research findings do not indicate that it plays a primary role.[11,15] Serotonin and the GABA/benzodiazepine systems are believed to play a major role because patients respond to treatment with SSRIs and benzodiazepines. Few studies have been performed to examine neuropeptide dysfunction. As in PD, they are believed to be involved in the pathophysiology.

NEUROANATOMIC CHANGES. Researchers have noted conflicting results regarding alterations in brain metabolism and regional blood flow. GAD has been associated with a reduction in metabolic rate of the basal ganglia and temporal lobes, suggesting involvement of limbic structures. However, situations involving either increased stress or decreased stress were both associated with increases in basal ganglia activity and decreased temporal and occipital activity.[28] Further studies are needed to address this paradoxical finding.

CLINICAL MANIFESTATIONS

The onset of GAD is gradual, and many patients remember being worried and anxious as children. These individuals report constant worry that is difficult to control and affects their ability to complete tasks. Along with anxiety or worry, three or more of the following symptoms must be present for a diagnosis of GAD: restlessness, fatigue, difficulty concentrating, irritability, muscle tension (causing trembling, twitching, or soreness), and difficulty falling or staying asleep. Somatic symptoms may also be reported, including cold, clammy hands, dry mouth, diaphoresis, nausea or vomiting, urinary frequency, and trouble swallowing.[1] Considered a chronic disorder, GAD is diagnosed if symptoms persist for most of the days within a 6-month period.

CO-MORBIDITY. Most patients with chronic GAD have an additional psychiatric disorder. Social phobia, simple phobia, depression, and panic disorder are the most common.[10]

Obsessive-Compulsive Disorder

Obsessive-compulsive disorder (OCD) is the fourth most commonly diagnosed psychiatric disorder, three to four times more common than PD. Its actual incidence may be even greater, given that it is often underdiagnosed and untreated because it is kept a secret by many of those affected. During one's lifetime, the chance of developing this disorder is estimated at 2.5%.[48]

Unlike other anxiety disorders, males and females overall are affected equally. However, an early-onset form associated with a tic disorder called Giles de la Tourette's syndrome occurs more commonly in young males. A later-onset form not associated with tics more commonly affects women.[48] As many as 80% of all cases of OCD are thought to arise during childhood and adolescence, suggesting a neurodevelopmental basis for the disorder.[60]

ETIOLOGY AND PATHOPHYSIOLOGY

The etiology of OCD appears to differ from the other anxiety disorders. Specific corticostriatal pathways and the limbic system have been implicated. The serotonin neurotransmitter system has remained the focus of many pharmacologic and biochemical investigations.

GENETICS. Both genetic and environmental factors are associated with OCD. The disease appears to be heterogeneous, with different subpopulations. Some forms do appear to be familial. Twin studies have been limited but show a higher-than-anticipated rate of OCD in monozygotic (identical) than dizygotic (nonidentical) twins (53%–87% versus 22%–47%, respectively), suggesting that genetic factors may play an important role. A significantly higher rate of OCD and milder OCD-like syndromes has been found in first-degree relatives of some patients. Tic disorders (Tourette's syndrome) are also more common in these relatives, suggesting that some forms of OCD share the same etiology with tic disorders. Some cases of OCD arise without a family history of either OCD or tics, suggesting that environmental factors may be primarily involved in this subgroup of patients.[48]

NEUROTRANSMITTER INVOLVEMENT. Although it is unlikely that an alteration in one neurotransmitter system is primarily responsible for the disorder, evidence implicates serotonin in the pathophysiology of OCD. Some patients with OCD experience anxiety and exacerbation of their OCD symptoms if given a 5-HT receptor agonist.[53,75] This response can be completely blocked by administration of a serotonin antagonist. In most patients, agents that have serotonin effects (such as SSRIs) relieve the symptoms of the disorder.

Some investigators suggest that dopaminergic pathways may also be involved since dopamine agonists may induce stereotypic and repetitive behaviors in both animals and in humans. Some brain imaging studies implicate the ventral prefrontal cortex and striatum in the disorder; many serotonergic and dopaminergic neurons connect these structures.[60]

AUTOIMMUNE RESPONSE. Recently a subgroup of children with OCD and/or tic disorders showed the onset of their symptoms following streptococcal infection. Exacerbations could be triggered by reinfection or pharyngitis. Antineuronal antibodies have been found in some children with OCD and in children diagnosed with Sydenham's chorea, a variant of rheumatic fever associated with the development of OCD symptoms. These studies suggest that early-onset OCD may belong to a new class of pediatric autoimmune neuropsychiatric disorders.[65]

NEUROANATOMIC CHANGES. A consistent brain lesion has not been identified. However, some studies suggest a smaller caudate nucleus (part of the corpus striatum.). Another portion of the striatum, the putamen, also shows a reduction in size in both Tourette's and pediatric OCD patients.[60]

An increased metabolic rate in the striatum and the orbitofrontal region of the brain in patients with OCD has been demonstrated with functional imaging. A significant decrease in activity occurred when patients responded to either pharmacologic treatment or behavioral therapy.[6] Hyperactivity in these regions could cause the behavioral alterations seen in OCD. Further support for this hypothesis comes from follow-up studies of treatment-refractory patients who received ventromedial frontal lobotomy in the early 1970s. All subjects showed and have maintained an improvement in symptoms; subjects with frontostriatal surgery were the most improved. It is postulated that lobotomy decreased OCD-related hyperactivity.[25] Thus, several lines of evidence point to hyperactivity in the orbitofrontal cortex and the caudate nucleus as the fundamental alteration in the disorder.[48,60]

CLINICAL MANIFESTATIONS

OCD is characterized by recurring thoughts or impulses (**obsessions**) that are intrusive and cause anxiety. These obsessions lead one to perform **compulsions**, which are time-consuming and repetitive behaviors or mental activities in response to the obsession. These behaviors become rituals and are performed to reduce the distress or prevent the development of a dreaded situation.

The obsessions or compulsions are either time consuming, requiring more than 1 hour per day, or they significantly interfere with normal functioning. Typical compulsions can include activities such as repetitive handwashing, arranging or counting items, and checking items. They also can be restricted to mental acts such as praying or counting. Obsessions about contamination are the most common, accompanied by cleaning and washing compulsions.[48] OCD patients realize that these thoughts or activities are unreasonable and hide them from others.

This disorder is characterized by an inability to properly assess risk, the presence of extreme self-doubt, and a need for certainty or perfection.[55] These patients fear that they will harm someone or something if their compulsions are not performed. For example, a patient who dreads causing a house fire may repeatedly check that the stove is turned off; this compulsion to repeatedly check may make him or her unable to leave the house.

CO-MORBIDITY. Major depression commonly occurs in up to 50% of OCD patients. Other types of anxiety disorders such as phobias or PD also occur. Up to 50% of patients with Tourette's syndrome have OCD, but much fewer patients with OCD (5%–7%) have Tourette's.[1]

Phobias

Phobias are excessive, unreasonable fears that lead a person to avoid specific situations or exposure to certain items. High levels of anxiety or fear are experienced immediately if exposure occurs. There are two major types of phobia: social phobia (SP) and specific phobias. In social phobia, fear results when an individual feels that he or she may be scrutinized by others or may be embarrassed in front of others. For example, activities such as public speaking or eating are feared and avoided by some patients. Social phobia is estimated to affect 13% of all adults at some time in their life.[4] SP begins in the late childhood to early adolescence and usually becomes a chronic disorder.

Specific phobias occur in response to a specific object or situation. For example, some individuals fear snakes, heights, air travel, darkness, or thunderstorms.[1] Many specific phobias may only mildly interfere with a patient's life since the phobia is restricted to a single situation or object, which the patient learns to avoid. Specific phobias may be triggered by traumatic events (animal attack or entrapment in an enclosed space), by unexpected panic attacks when exposed to a feared object or situation, or after observation of others undergoing trauma or fearing an object or situation.[1] Many childhood-onset specific phobias remit spontaneously as a child matures.[15] The incidence of specific phobias is much higher in woman than in men.

ETIOLOGY AND PATHOPHYSIOLOGY

Limited and sometimes conflicting data are available regarding the pathophysiology of phobias. These disorders share some similarities with PD, namely the ability of panicogenic agents to induce a panic attack in these patients, and several differences, including the demonstrated efficacy of different behavioral therapies.

GENETICS. A specific phobia may aggregate in families. First-degree relatives of persons with animal phobias are likely to have animal phobias, which may be directed towards another type of animal. Fears of blood and injury also show a strong familial aggregation. Social phobia also shows familial transmission, occurring more frequently among first-degree relatives of those affected as compared with the general population.[1]

NEUROTRANSMITTER INVOLVEMENT. Social phobia is hypothesized to involve catecholamines because beta-blockers have been effective in treating performance anxiety. Limited studies have addressed this. However, no abnormalities have been noted in catecholamine function and turnover.[28]

Serotonin also may play a role since some patients with social phobia respond to SSRIs. Panicogenic agents such as lactate or CO_2 inhalation can induce mild panic attacks in phobic patients. These responses are much weaker than in patients with PD but greater than those induced in control subjects.[28] Thus, there may be neurochemical similarities between phobias and PD.

CLINICAL MANIFESTATIONS

When placed in a social phobic situation, patients report tachycardia, diaphoresis, trembling, tremor, and blushing, all suggestive of adrenergic overactivity. Many patients with specific phobias also have PD with agoraphobia and experience panic attacks.

COMORBIDITY. In some situations, patients experiencing phobias may also exhibit depressive episodes and anxiety. Alcohol abuse and suicidal ideations have been identified in some phobic patients. A small percentage of schizophrenic patients experience phobias, particularly social phobia.

Post-traumatic Stress Disorder

Post-traumatic stress disorder (PTSD) is characterized by specific symptoms that occur following traumatic events. These events may include sexual abuse, burn injury, violent assault, military combat, and being a prisoner of war or a survivor of a natural disaster. Currently, only a small percentage of those exposed to trauma actually develop PTSD. The prevalence of PTSD in the general population is estimated at 7.8%.[35]

ETIOLOGY AND PATHOPHYSIOLOGY

The most common causes of PTSD in men are combat and witnessing death or severe injury, whereas in women it is most commonly associated with rape and sexual molestation.[35] Many studies have focused on the roles of noradrenergic system since this system is believed to play a role in anxiety and the stress response. The HPA has been studied intensively since it plays an important role in the modulation of stress, with activation causing the release of cortisol.

PERIPHERAL SYMPATHETIC NERVOUS SYSTEM INVOLVEMENT. Resting heart rate and blood pressure are elevated in PTSD. Exposure to traumatic stimuli causes greater increases in heart rate as compared with controls or patients with GAD,[15] suggestive of noradrenergic hyperactivity.

NEUROTRANSMITTERS. Much indirect evidence exists suggesting an alteration in the serotonin system. Aggression and suicidal actions, associated with low serotonin activity, are also seen in PTSD. Additionally, SSRIs, which increase the effectiveness of endogenous serotonin, can help control the intrusive memories and avoidance behaviors seen in PTSD.[15] As in PD, the efficacy of SSRIs may result from the increased inhibitory effect of serotonin on noradrenergic neurons in the LC.[18]

NEUROENDOCRINE ALTERATIONS. Neurohormones such as cortisol, epinephrine, norepinephrine, and endogenous opioids are released in response to stress. Figure 30-3 shows the anatomic and functional relationships of the elements of the HPA. A number of abnormalities in this system have been found in PTSD and are summarized in Box 30-2.

Since stress is normally associated with high levels of cortisol release, plasma and urinary cortisol levels

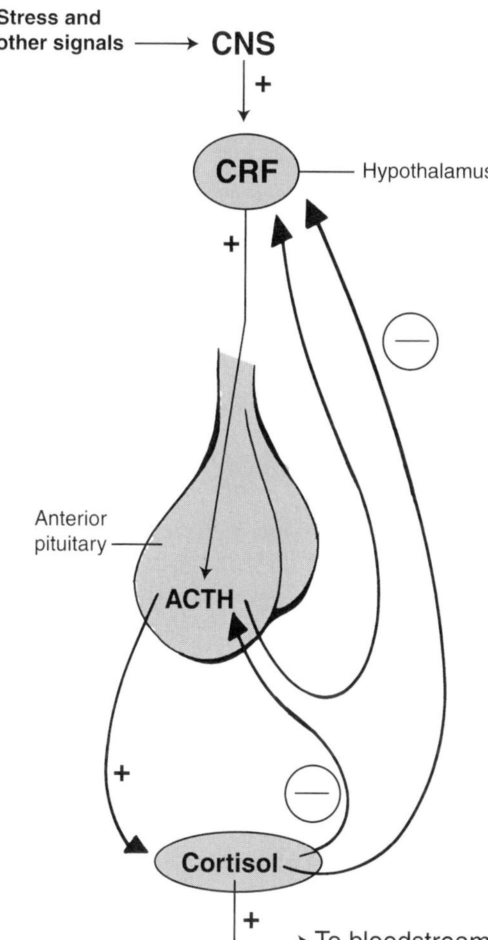

FIGURE 30-3. Anatomical and functional relationships between the components of the hypothalamic-pituitary axis. Stress and other signals cause activation of the HPA, leading to the release of cortisol (+ *arrows*). Excessive levels of cortisol and ACTH through a negative feedback system cause the inhibitions of secretion from the anterior pituitary gland and/or hypothalamus (– *arrows*).

were presumed to be elevated in PTSD. Instead, most studies have shown decreased levels.[75] It has been proposed that the lower cortisol baseline may be a result of the disorder or actually represent a predisposing risk factor.[69] To exert its biologic actions, cortisol must bind to glucocorticoid receptors. In PTSD, the number of receptors is increased. Receptor up-regulation then may be a consequence of the decreased cortisol. Alternatively, the receptor increase could be secondarily influencing cortisol secretion.[75]

Other functional studies of the HPA have revealed abnormal responses to administered dexamethasone. Normally, exogenous dexamethasone suppresses cortisol secretion via a negative feedback mechanism. In PTSD, the cortisol suppression is much greater than normal. Dexamethasone administration also leads to a decrease in the number of cytosolic glucocorticoid receptors because some of these receptors bind the steroid and shuttle it into the nucleus. In PTSD, there are even fewer cytosolic glucocorticoid receptors remaining after dexamethasone, indicating a more effective shuttling mechanism leading to greater biologic activity. All these changes in HPA function suggest adaptations to chronic stress. Chronic increases in corticotropin-releasing hormone may lead to enhanced negative feedback of the HPA, possibly providing a protective effect for the body.[69,74]

BOX 30-2 ALTERATIONS IN THE HYPOTHALAMIC-PITUITARY-ADRENAL AXIS ASSOCIATED WITH PTSD

- Decreased cortisol levels
- Increased cytoplasmic glucocorticoid receptors
- Exaggerated suppression of cortisol by exogenous dexamethasone
- Greater depletion of cytoplasmic glucocorticoid receptors by exogenous dexamethasone

NEUROANATOMIC CHANGES. Experimental animals exposed to stress or high levels of glucocorticoids show hippocampal shrinking, leading researchers to specifically examine the hippocampus of patients with PTSD. Reduced hippocampal volume has been repeatedly observed, suggesting a loss of neurons. Additionally, the degree of hippocampal shrinkage has been correlated with the severity of PTSD. The cause of this lesion is unknown.[74]

CLINICAL MANIFESTATIONS

Patients with PTSD re-experience the trauma through intrusive memories, nightmares, and flashbacks. Sleep disturbances are common. Patients with PTSD exhibit exaggerated startle responses to loud noises and heightened physiologic arousal in response to sounds, images, and thoughts associated with the trauma. There are signs of autonomic hyperactivity, including diaphoresis and increased heart rate. Patients react physiologically and psychologically to cues that remind them of the traumatic event. Many patients also experience irritability, depression, and aggression.[1]

CO-MORBIDITY. Major depression is commonly associated with PTSD, with 70% of patients experiencing it during their lifetime. OCD and PD also occur, but to a lesser extent (in 5% and 12% of patients, respectively).[18]

MOOD DISORDERS

Mood fluctuations are a part of everyday existence and occur normally as one reacts to an ever-changing environment. Disorders of mood are diagnosed when a mood persists or recurs and causes disruption of one's personality and ability to function. Two major mood extremes are recognized: **mania** (exaggerated elation or irritability) and **depression** (exaggerated sadness or grief). Those affected by mood disorders may demonstrate mainly depressive symptoms and are said to have **unipolar disorder** (or **major depression**). Others may show periods of mania followed by depression and are diagnosed as having **bipolar disorder** (or **manic-depression**).

Major depression (MD) and bipolar disorder appear to share some similarities as well as demonstrate major differences in neurobiology and pathophysiology. Other types of mood disorders include dysthymic disorder, a chronic but less severe depressive disorder, and cyclothymic disorder, characterized by many cycles of brief and/or less severe depression alternating with mild mania (**hypomania**). Mood disorders may also occur as a result of a general medical condition or due to substance abuse.[1]

Major Depression

Major depression is the most common neuropsychiatric disorder. The lifetime rates vary widely for different countries. One's culture appears to play a role in determining how major depressive episodes are manifested. In the U.S., the risk for major depression is three times greater for women than men. The mean age of onset for both genders is estimated to be 25 years.[71] Epidemiologic studies suggest that the age of onset appears to be decreasing.[1] Episodes of MD commonly occur after severe psychological stress has been experienced. Possible factors that increase one's risk of developing major depression are highlighted in Box 30-3.

MD is also a problem for children and the elderly. In children, it is a serious illness with chronic effects and a high recurrence rate. Its incidence has increased since the 1950s. Depression in older adults is also significant, especially for those in institutional settings or those who are ill or disabled. The overall 1-year prevalence of major depression in persons aged 65 or older who are not institutionalized or hospitalized is approximately 1%. MD has the highest incidence for those in nursing homes (12%), with less severe but still clinically significant depression occurring in an additional 30% to 35%.[62] There are several subtypes of depression; among these are postpartum depression, which has an acute onset after childbirth, and seasonal affective disorder (SAD), which is a recurring depression lasting from fall through the winter months.

BOX 30-3 RISK FACTORS FOR AFFECTIVE DISORDERS

- Prior episode of depression
- Family history
- Lack of support system
- Stressful event (laid off, fired, divorce, death of loved one)
- Substance abuse
- Pre-existing medical illness
- Premature parental loss

ETIOLOGY AND PATHOPHYSIOLOGY

No single biochemical dysfunction model that has been proposed adequately accounts for the variety of physiologic and biochemical alterations that occur during mood disorders. Aggregation of mood disorders in families suggests inheritance of susceptibility genes. Several neuroendocrine and functional brain abnormalities detected in patients with MD and BP have led to several hypotheses.

GENETICS. Danish twin studies show a high heritability of MD. If one monozygotic twin has MD, the second twin has a 54% chance of MD.[7] Since the chance of MD for the second identical twin is not 100%, there must also be environmental factors involved that modify the genetic risk. If a dizygotic twin has MD, the second twin has a 24% chance of MD.[56] Linkage of the disorder to a specific chromosomes or to an alteration in a specific proteins has been proposed but not reproducibly verified.

VIRAL INFECTION. A recent small epidemiologic study found a relationship between second-trimester exposure to influenza and an increased risk of MD.[42] This suggests that major depression may, in some individuals, be induced as a result of a developmental disorder.

NEUROENDOCRINE DISTURBANCES. Hormone dysfunction in MD had been suspected for some time; the signs and symptoms of decreased appetite, weight loss, insomnia, and GI disorders suggested dysfunction of two separate parts of the neuroendocrine system, specifically the HPA and the hypothalamic–pituitary–thyroid axis (HPT).

Various studies point to hypersecretion of CRF, ACTH, and cortisol in most MD patients.[51] A summary of the alterations of the HPA and HPT in depression is shown in Box 30-4. These findings are very different from the HPA alterations documented for PTSD.

BOX 30-4 NEUROENDOCRINE ALTERATIONS IN DEPRESSION

Hypothalamic–Pituitary–Adrenal Axis (HPA)

- Increased cortisol levels during depression
- Increased cytoplasmic glucocorticoid receptors
- Non-suppression of cortisol or ACTH by exogenous dexamethasone
- Greater depletion of cytoplasmic glucocorticoid receptors by exogenous dexamethasone

Hypothalamic–Pituitary–Thyroid Axis (HPT)

- Increased TRH in the CSF of depressed patients
- Down-regulation of pituitary TRH receptors

NEUROTRANSMITTER INVOLVEMENT. Nearly 30 years ago it was hypothesized that decreased NE in the brain led to depressive disorders and that an increase in catecholamine levels was associated with mania. Evidence of a decreased level of a metabolite of NE in the CSF of depressed patients, an up- regulation of post-synaptic receptors in the brains of suicide victims, and an elevation of urinary catecholamine metabolites during mania supports this view. Recently, the efficacy of using SSRIs for major depression has shifted attention to the role of 5-HT. A central deficit of this neurotransmitter has also been postulated in the pathogenesis of mood disorders. Studies have found a decreased level of a 5-HT metabolite and up- regulation of post-synaptic 5-HT$_2$ receptors in depressed patients.[50]

NEUROANATOMIC CHANGES. The most reproducible anatomic finding in MD has been hyperintensities in deep subcortical white matter in the frontal and frontal/parietal regions of both hemispheres. These changes are also found in BD but are not specific for mood disorders. These changes are permanent and stable over time. It is not known whether these lesions represent a risk factor predisposing one to mood disorders or are a consequence of mood disorders. Frontal cortex, cerebellar, and basal ganglia volume reductions in MD have also been noted.[63] Functional imaging studies have shown regional decreases in CBF and metabolism in the basal ganglia and frontal lobes.[50]

CLINICAL MANIFESTATIONS

A depressive episode is characterized by specific criteria, summarized in Box 30-5. Additionally, these individuals exhibit a sad, forlorn facial expression and stooped

BOX 30-5 CLINICAL MANIFESTATIONS DURING MANIC AND DEPRESSIVE PHASES

Manic Episode

Characterized by the presence of an excessive, elated mood, which must last for at least 1 week and include at least three of the following symptoms:

- Inflated self-esteem or grandiosity; may include delusions; possibly non-realistic plans to obtain wealth or considering self an expert in an area for which he has no background
- Decreased need for sleep; may go for days without sleep or require very little
- Non-stop, loud, rapid and/or confusing speech pattern
- Flight of ideas; thoughts pass faster than can be articulated
- Distractibility; less ability to filter out non-important sensory stimuli
- Increased involvement in goal-directed activities
- Excessive involvement in pleasurable activities

Depressive Episode

Characterized by a depressed mood or loss of interest or pleasure in life activities, which lasts for at least 2 weeks and includes four of the following symptoms:

- Change in appetite, weight, sleep, or psychomotor activity
- Decreased energy
- Feelings of worthlessness or guilt
- Difficulty with decision-making, concentration, or planning
- Attempted suicide or recurrent thoughts of death and suicide

(Adapted with permission from American Psychiatric Association. [1994]. *Diagnostic and statistical manual of mental disorders* [4th ed.]. Washington, DC: American Psychiatric Press.)

posture. Anhedonia, the inability to experience pleasure from activities previously pleasurable, develops early on in the course of depression. Individuals with depressive episodes have very low self-esteem and view the future as bleak and dismal.

CO-MORBIDITY. Mood disorders commonly occur with other types of neuropsychiatric illness such as anxiety and psychosis. Patients with major depression have an almost three-fold higher risk of drug abuse or dependence, a nine-fold higher risk of PD, and a five-fold higher risk of OCD as compared with individuals without major depression.[71] Over 50% of patients who have experienced even a single major depressive episode will eventually have another, and 20% to 40% of these patients will be resistant to treatment and experience chronic, recurring episodes.[1,45] Up to 15% of patients with major depression die as a result of suicide.[1]

Bipolar Disorder

Bipolar disorder (BD) occurs much less frequently than major depression, affecting men and women equally. The mean age of onset is 18 years, which is significantly earlier than for MD. Two major types of BD have been identified: BD I is distinguished by cycles of major depression and severe mania; BD II is characterized by cycles of major depression and much less severe mania (hypomania).[1] Additional subgroups have been proposed based on the frequency of mood disorders; one of these, rapid-cycling BD, is associated with four or more affective episodes per year. Rapid-cycling BD is three times more common in women as in men.[41]

ETIOLOGY AND PATHOPHYSIOLOGY

Like MD, no single model has been found to explain BD.

GENETICS. Danish twin studies demonstrate an even higher degree of heritability of BD than major depression. If one monozygotic twin has BD, the second twin has a 79% chance of BD.[7] Since the chance of BD for the second identical twin is not 100%, environmental factors must also be involved, as for all neurobiologic disorders showing heritability. If a dizygotic twin has BD, the second twin has a 19% chance of BD.[56] Familial aggregation of BP also occurs. First-degree relatives of patients with BD are reported to be over 24 times more likely to develop BD than the relatives of control subjects.[50]

Decreasing age of onset and increasing episode frequency in BD suggests that trinucleotide repeat amplification might be occurring. This suggests a molecular basis for BD.[47]

To date, no clear, reproducible link of BD to a specific genetic marker has occurred. Several recent genetic screening studies of families with a history of BD have suggested the presence of susceptibility genes on chromosomes 21, 18, 16, and 5.[56] Chromosome 18 findings have generated the most interest and the most controversy, with various researchers replicating or refuting the association.[20,37]

VIRAL INFECTION. A recent small epidemiologic study found a relationship between second-trimester exposure to influenza and a trend towards increased risk of BD.[1]

NEUROENDOCRINE DISTURBANCES. Alterations in the HPA and HPT have been found in BD. In contrast with the usual findings of hyperthyroidism in MD, many patients with BD have evidence of hypothyroidism, with a higher prevalence of this abnormality in the rapid-cycling subtype. Many of these patients respond to exogenous thyroid hormone.[50]

NEUROANATOMIC CHANGES. In BD, an increase in the volumes of the lateral and third ventricles also has been reported. In functional imaging studies, regional, rather than generalized, reductions in CBF and metabolism have been detected, specifically in the frontal

FOCUS ON THE PERSON WITH A REPETITIVE BEHAVIOR

S. E. is a 35-year-old computer programmer who drives about 15 miles to and from work each day. He has been leaving earlier and earlier in the morning in order to get to work on time and has requested special work projects that he can complete at home. One night, his wife becomes concerned when he arrives home hours later than expected. When questioned, he admits that he has been driving home during the entire period of time but had to keep stopping to check if he hit anyone. His wife learns that any time S.'s car hits a pothole or bump, he has to stop, check under the wheels and car, and ask bystanders if they saw anyone near his car or hit by his car. If a policeman is near, he will ask if anyone in the area has been taken to the hospital.

Questions

1. What general group of disorders best fit this case?
2. What is the probable diagnosis for S.?
3. What specific types of behavior led to your diagnosis? How would you classify these types of behavior?
4. What is S.'s prognosis?

FOCUS ON THE PERSON WITH A BEHAVIOR CHANGE

F. C. is a 20-year-old who recently dropped out of college and now works in a sporting goods store. His coworkers at the store notice that F.'s appearance has changed; he is often distracted, and he is having difficulty interacting with customers. He keeps scraps of paper in a shoebox that he always carries with him. When questioned by his coworkers, he mumbles that he is being followed by different strangers and has been told to document this whenever it happens. He knows that this is valuable evidence and he always carries it with him.

Questions

1. What is the probable diagnosis for F.?
2. What specific types of behavior led to your diagnosis? How would you classify these types of behavior?
3. What is F.'s prognosis?

FOCUS ON THE PERSON WITH HEALTH CONCERNS

M. W. is a 30-year-old with two children. Her mother died of a heart ailment when she was a child. In the last 2 months, M. has experienced several episodes of tension and irritability, followed by dizziness, a pounding heart, and a tightness in her chest. She fears that she will die during one of these attacks and has been rushed to the emergency room twice. During these hospitalizations, a number of diagnostic tests were run and all were normal. M. is sure she has undiagnosed cardiac disease and will suffer the same fate as her mother.

Questions

1. What is the probable diagnosis for M.?
2. What specific types of behavior led to your diagnosis? How would you classify these types of behavior?
3. Why are her laboratory results normal?

FOCUS ON THE PERSON WITH SOCIAL FEAR

D. D. is a 38-year-old quality control specialist who has been working at a food processing plant for the last 16 years. The company has just been sold and D. has been laid off. She has remained at home during the past 5 weeks, watching television and feeling unable to move. She has been sleeping more than normal and takes a daily afternoon nap. She has not seen any of her friends during this period; she thinks she won't be able to control her emotions in front of them. She doesn't think that she will be able to get another job.

Questions

1. What is the probable diagnosis for D.?
2. What specific types of behavior led to your diagnosis? How would you classify these types of behavior?

lobes. A recent PET study has found decreased activity in a specific area of the prefrontal cortex in both familial unipolar and familial bipolar depression. This same region was activated during episodes of mania. A subsequent MRI study showed a significant reduction in volume of this region of the brain as compared with control subjects. This anatomic abnormality persisted during remission and during antidepressant drug treatment.[19] Structural and functional changes in the frontal lobes are thought to be associated with functional deficits in pathways linking the prefrontal, limbic system, and basal ganglia, affecting emotional behavior and the response to stress and leading to mood disorders.[19,52,64]

CLINICAL MANIFESTATIONS

A manic episode is characterized by specific criteria, summarized in Box 30-5. Additionally, these individuals exhibit poor control of their impulses and have unrealistic appraisal of their abilities.

REFERENCES

1. American Psychiatric Association (1994). *Diagnostic and statistical manual of mental disorders* (4th ed.). Washington, DC: American Psychiatric Press.
2. Andersson, C., Chakos, M., Mailman, R., & Liberman, J. (1998). Emerging roles for novel antipsychotic medications in the treatment of schizophrenia. *Psychiatric Clinics of North America, 21,* 151–179.
3. Andreason, N. C. & Black, D. W. (1995). *Introductory textbook of psychiatry* (2nd ed.). Washington, DC: American Psychiatric Press.
4. Antony, M. M. (1997). Assessment and treatment of social phobia. *Canadian Journal of Psychiatry, 42,* 826–834.
5. Ballenger, J. C. (1997). Panic disorder in the medical setting. *Journal of Clinical Psychiatry, 58*(suppl. 2), 13–17.
6. Baxter, L. R., Schwartz, J. M., Bergman, K. S., Szuba, M. P., Guze, B. H., Mazziotta, J. C., Alazraki, A., Selin, C. E., Ferng, H-K., Munford, P., & Phelps, M. E. (1992). Caudate glucose metabolic rate changes with both drug and behavior therapy for obsessive-compulsive disorder. *Archives of General Psychiatry, 49,* 681–689.
7. Bertelesen, A., Harvald, B., & Hayge, M. (1977). A Danish twin study of manic-depressive disorders. *British Journal of Psychiatry, 130,* 220–354.
8. Bradwejn, J., Koszycki, D., Payeur, R., Bourin, M., & Bothwick, H. (1992). Replication of the action of cholecystokinin tetrapeptide in panic disorder: Clinical and behavioral findings. *American Journal of Psychiatry, 149,* 962–964.
9. Bradwejn, J. & Koszycki, D. (1994). The cholecystokinin hypothesis of anxiety and panic disorder. *Annals of the NY Academy of Science, 713,* 273–282.
10. Brawman-Mintzer, O., & Lydiard, R. B. (1996). Generalized anxiety disorder: Issues in epidemiology. *Journal of Clinical Psychiatry, 57*(suppl. 7), 3–8.
11. Brawman-Mintzer, O., & Lydiard, R. B. (1997). Biological basis of generalized anxiety disorder. *Journal of Clinical Psychiatry, 58*(suppl. 3), 16–25.
12. Buckley, P. F. (1998). The clinical stigmata of aberrant neurodevelopment in schizophrenia. *Journal of Nervous and Mental Diseases, 186*(2), 79–86.
13. Buckley, P. F. (1998). Structural brain imaging in schizophrenia. *Psychiatric Clinics of North America, 21*(1), 77–91.
14. Busatto, G. F., & Kerwin, R. W. (1997). Schizophrenia, psychosis and the basal ganglia. *Psychiatric Clinics of North America, 20*(4), 897–909.
15. Charney, D. S., Nagy, L. M., Bremner, J. D., Goddard, A. W., Yehuda, R., & Southwick, S. M. (1996). Neurobiological mechanisms of human anxiety. In B. S. Fogel, R. B. Schiffer, & S. M. Rao (Eds.), *Neuropsychiatry.* Baltimore: Williams & Wilkins.
16. Crowe, R. R., Noyes, R., Pauls, D. L., & Slymen, D. (1983). A family study of panic disorder. *Archives of General Psychiatry, 40,* 1065–1069.
17. Davis, K. L., Kahn, R. S., Ko, G., & Davidson, M. (1991). Dopamine in schizophrenia: A review and reconceptualization. *American Journal of Psychiatry, 148,* 1474–1486.
18. Davis, L. L., Suris, A., Lambert, M. T., Heimberg, C., & Petty, F. (1997). Post-traumatic stress disorder and serotonin: New

directions for research and treatment. *Journal of Psychiatry and Neuroscience, 22*(5), 318–326.

19. Drevets, W. C., Price, J. L., Simpson, J. R., Todd, R. D., Reich, T., Vannier, M., & Raichle, M. E. (1997). Subgenual prefrontal cortex abnormalities in mood disorders. *Nature, 386,* 824–827.
20. Gershon, E. S., Badner, J. A., Goldin, L. R., Sanders, A. R., Cravchik, A., & Detera-Wadleigh, S. D. (1998). Closing in on genes for manic-depressive illness and schizophrenia. *Neuropsychopharmacology, 18*(4), 233–242.
21. Goddard, A. W., & Charney, D. S. (1997). Toward an integrated neurobiology of panic disorder. *Journal of Clinical Psychiatry, 58*(suppl. 2), 4–11.
22. Griffiths, T. D., Sigmundsson, T., Takei, N., Rowe, D., & Murray, R. M. (1998). Neurological abnormalities in familial and sporadic schizophrenia. *Brain, 121,* 191–203.
23. Gur, R. E., Cowell, P., Turetsky, B. I., Gallacher, F., Cannon, T., Bilker, W., & Gur, R. C. (1998). A follow-up magnetic resonance imaging study of schizophrenia: Relationship of neuroanatomical changes to clinical and behavioral measures. *Archives of General Psychiatry, 55,* 145–152.
24. Hafner, H., van der Heiden, W., Behrens, S., Gattaz, W. F., Hambrecht, M., Loffer, W., Maurer, K., Munk-Jørgensen, P., Novotny, B., Riecher-Rossler, A., & Stein, A. (1998). Causes and consequences of the gender difference in age at onset of schizophrenia. *Schizophrenia Bulletin, 24*(1), 99–113.
25. Irle, E., Exner, C., Thielen, K., Weniger, G., & Ruther, E. (1998). Obsessive-compulsive disorder and ventromedial frontal lesions: Clinical and neurophysiological findings. *American Journal of Psychiatry, 155*(2), 255–263.
26. Ismail, B., Cantor-Graae, E., & McNeil, T. F. (1998). Neurological abnormalities in schizophrenia patients and their siblings. *American Journal of Psychiatry, 155*(1), 84–89.
27. Jeste, D. V., Galasko, D., Corey-Bloom, J., Walens, S., & Granholm, E. (1996). Neuropsychiatric aspects of the schizophrenias. In B. S. Fogel, R. B. Schiffer, & S. M. Rao (Eds.), *Neuropsychiatry.* Baltimore: Williams & Wilkins.
28. Johnson, M. R., & Lydiard, R. B. (1995). The neurobiology of anxiety disorders. *Psychiatric Clinics of North America, 18*(4), 681–725.
29. Jones, P., & Cannon, M. (1998). The new epidemiology of schizophrenia. *Psychiatric Clinics of North America, 21*(1), 1–25.
30. Kandel, E. R. (1992). Disorders of thought: Schizophrenia. In E. R. Kandel, J. H. Schwartz, & T. M. Jessell (Eds.), *Principles of neural science* (3rd ed.). East Norwalk, CT: Appleton & Lange.
31. Kanton, W. (1996). Panic disorder: Relationship to high medical utilization, unexplained medical symptoms, and medical costs. *Journal of Clinical Psychiatry, 57*(suppl. 10), 11–18.
32. Karayiorgou, M., & Gogos, G. A. (1997). A turning point in schizophrenia genetics. *Neuron, 18,* 967–979.
33. Kendler, K. S. (1983). Overview: A current perspective on twin studies of schizophrenia. *American Journal of Psychiatry, 140,* 1413–1425.
34. Kendler, K. S., McGuire, M., Gruenberg, A. M., O'Hare, A., Spellman. M., & Walsh, D. (1993). The Roscommon family study. I. Methods, diagnosis of probands, and risk of schizophrenia in relatives. *Archives of General Psychiatry, 50,* 527–540.
35. Kessler, R., Sonnega, A., Bromet, E., & Nelson, C. B. (1995). Posttraumatic stress disorder in the National Comorbidity Survey. *Archives of General Psychiatry, 52,* 1048–1060.
36. Klein, D. F. (1993). False suffocation alarms, spontaneous panics and related conditions: An integrative hypothesis. *Archives of General Psychiatry, 50,* 306–317.
37. Knowles, J. A., Rao, P. A., Cox-Matise, T., Loth, J. E., de Jesus, G. M., Levine, L., Das, K., Penchazadeh, G. K., Alexander, J. R., Lerer, B., Endicott, J., Ott, J., Gilliam, T. C., & Baron, M. (1998). No evidence for significant linkage between bipolar affective disorder and chromosome 18 pericentromeric markers in a large series of multiplex extended pedigrees. *American Journal of Human Genetics, 62,* 916–924.
38. Kotrla, K. (1997). Functional neuroimaging in psychiatry. In S. C. Yudofsky & R. E. Hales (Eds.), *The American Psychiatric Press textbook of neuropsychiatry* (3rd ed.). Washington, DC: American Psychiatric Press.
39. Krystal, J. H., Niehoff-Deutsch, D., & Charney, D. S. (1996). The biological basis of panic disorder. *Journal of Clinical Psychiatry, 57*(suppl. 10), 23–31.
40. Kupfer, D. J. (1995). Introduction to clinical neuropsychopharmacology. In F. E. Bloom & D. J. Kupfer, *Psychopharmacology: The fourth generation of progress.* New York: Raven Press.
41. Leibenluft, E. (1997). Issues in the treatment of women with bipolar illness. *Journal of Clinical Psychiatry, 58*(suppl. 15), 5–11.
42. Machon, R. A., Mednick, S. A., & Huttunen, M. O. (1997). Adult major affective disorder after prenatal exposure to an influenza epidemic. *Archives of General Psychiatry, 54,* 322–328.
43. Malaspina, D., van Kammen, M., Johnson, J., & Kaufmann, C. A. (1997). Epidemiologic and genetic aspects of neuropsychiatric disorders. In S. C. Yudofsky & R. E. Hales, *The American Psychiatric Press textbook of neuropsychiatry* (3rd ed.). Washington, DC: American Psychiatric Press.
44. Mavissakalian, M. R. & Prien, R. F. (1966). *Long-term treatments of anxiety disorders.* Washington, DC: American Psychiatric Press.
45. Mayberg, H. S., Mahurin, R. K., & Brannan, S. K. (1997). Neuropsychiatric aspects of mood and affective disorders. In S. C. Yudofsky & R. E. Hales, *The American Psychiatric Press textbook of neuropsychiatry* (3rd ed.). Washington, DC: American Psychiatric Press.
46. Meise, U. & Fleischhacker, W. W. (1997). Perspectives on treatment needs in schizophrenia. *British Journal of Psychiatry, 168*(suppl. 29), 9–16.
47. Mendlewicz, J., Lindbald, K., Souery, D., Mahieu, B., Nylander, P. O., De Bruyn, A., Zander, C., Engstrom, C. Adolfsson, R., Van Broeckhoven, C., Schalling, M., & Lipp, O. (1997). Expanded trinucleotide CAG repeats in families with bipolar affective disorder. *Biological Psychiatry, 42,* 1115–1122.
48. Miguel, E. C., Rauch, S. L., & Jenike, M. A. (1997). Obsessive-compulsive disorder. *Psychiatric Clinics of North America, 20*(4), 863–883.
49. Mowry, B. J., Nancarrow, D. J., & Levinson, D. F. (1997). The molecular genetics of schizophrenia: An update. *Australia and New Zealand Journal of Psychiatry, 31,* 704–713.
50. Nathan, K. I., Musselman, D. L., Schatzberg, A. F., & Nemeroff, C. B. (1995). Biology of mood disorders In A. F. Schatzberg & C. B. Nemeroff, (Eds.), *The American Psychiatric Press textbook of psychopharmacology.* Washington, DC: American Psychiatric Press.
51. Nemeroff, C. B. (1998). The neurobiology of depression. *Scientific American, 278*(6), 42–49.
52. Norris, S. D., Krishnan, R. R., & Ahearn, E. (1997). Structural changes in the brain of patients with bipolar affective disorder by MRI: A review of the literature. *Progress in Neuro-psychopharmacology and Biological Psychiatry, 21,* 1323–1337.
53. Pigott, T. A., Hill, J. L., & Grady, T. A. (1993). A comparison of the effects of oral versus intravenous mCPP administration in OCD patients and the effect of metergoline prior to IV mCPP. *Biological Psychiatry, 33,* 3–14.
54. Pollack, M. H., & Smoller, J. W. (1995). The longitudinal course and outcome of panic disorder. *Psychiatric Clinics of North America, 18*(4), 785–801.

55. Rasmussen, S. A., & Eisen, J. L. (1992). The epidemiology and differential diagnosis of obsessive compulsive disorder. *Journal of Clinical Psychiatry, 53*(suppl. 4), 4–10.
56. Reus, V. I. & Freimer, N. B. (1997). Behavioral genetics '97. Understanding the genetic basis of mood disorders: Where do we stand? *American Journal of Human Genetics, 60*, 1283–1288.
57. Rice, D. P., & Miller, L. S. (1996). The economic burden of schizophrenia: Conceptual and methodological issues and cost estimates. In M. Moscarelli, A. Rupp, & N. Sartorius (Eds.), *Schizophrenia, Vol. 1: Handbook of mental health economics and health policy.* New York: John Wiley and Sons.
58. Roberts, G., Leigh, W., Nigel P., & Weinberger, D. R. (1993). Schizophrenia. In *Neuropsychiatric disorders.* London: Wolfe Publishing.
59. Role, L. W., & Kelly, J. P. (1992). The brain stem: Cranial nerve nuclei and the monaminergic systems. In E. R. Kandel, J. H. Schwartz, & T. M. Jessell (Eds.), *Principles of neural science* (3rd ed.). East Norwalk, CT: Appleton & Lange.
60. Rosenberg, D. R., & Keshavan, M. S. (1998). Toward a neurodevelopmental model of obsessive-compulsive disorder. *Biological Psychiatry, 43*, 623–640.
61. Roth, B. L., & Meltzer, H. Y. (1995). The role of serotonin in schizophrenia. In F. E. Bloom & D. J. Kupfer (Eds.), *Psychopharmacology: The fourth generation of progress.* New York: Raven Press.
62. Saltzman, C., Schneider, L. S., & Alexopoulos, G. S. (1995). In F. E. Bloom & D. J. Kupfer, D. J. (Eds.), *Psychopharmacology: The fourth generation of progress.* New York: Raven Press.
63. Soares, J. C., & Mann, J. J. (1997). The anatomy of mood disorders: A review of structural neuroimaging studies. *Biological Psychiatry, 41*, 86–106.
64. Soares, J. C., & Mann, J. J. (1997). The functional anatomy of mood disorders. *Journal of Psychiatric Research, 31*(4), 393–432.
65. Swedo, S. E., Leonard, H. L., Garvey, M., Mittleman, B., Allen, A. J., Perlmutter, S., Lougee, L., Dow, S., Zamkoff, J., & Dubbert, B. K. (1998). Pediatric autoimmune neuropsychiatric disorders associated with streptococcal infections: Clinical descriptions of the first 50 cases. *American Journal of Psychiatry, 155*(2), 264–271.
66. Tamminga, C. A. (1997). Neuropsychiatric aspects of schizophrenia. In S. C. Yudofsky & R. E. Hales (Eds.), *The American Psychiatric Press textbook of neuropsychiatry* (3rd ed.). Washington, DC: American Psychiatric Press.
67. Torgersen, S. (1983). Genetic factors in anxiety disorder. *Archives of General Psychiatry, 40*, 1085–1089.
68. Tsuang, M. T., Gilbertson, M. W., & Farone S. V. (1991). The genetics of schizophrenia: Current knowledge and future directions. *Schizophrenia Research, 4*, 157–171.
69. van der Kolk, B. A. (1997). The psychobiology of posttraumatic stress disorder. *Journal of Clinical Psychiatry, 58*(suppl. 9), 16–24.
70. Weickert, C. S., & Kleinman, J. E. (1998). The neuroanatomy and neurochemistry of schizophrenia. *Psychiatric Clinics of North America, 21*(1), 57–75.
71. Weissman, M. W., Bland, R. C., Canino, G. J., Faravelli, C., Greenwald, S., Hwu, H-G., Joyce, P. R., Karam, E. G., Lee, C-K., Lellouch, J., Lepine, J-P., Newman, S. C., Oakley-Browne, M. A., Rubio-Stipec, M., Wells, J. E., Wickramaratne, P. J., Wittchen, H-U., & Yeh, E-K. (1996). The cross-national epidemiology of major depression and bipolar disorder. *Archives of General Psychiatry, 54*, 305–309.
72. Weissman, M. W., Bland, R. C., Canino, G. J., Faravelli, C., Greenwald, S., Hwu, H-G., Joyce, P. R., Karam, E. G., Lee, C-K., Lellouch, J., Lepine, J-P., Newman, S. C., Oakley-Browne, M. A., Rubio-Stipec, M., Wells, J. E., Wickramaratne, P. J., Wittchen, H-U., & Yeh, E-K. (1997). The cross-national epidemiology of major panic disorder. *Archives of General Psychiatry, 54*, 305–309.
73. Winokur, G. & Tsuang, M. (1975). Suicide in mania, depression and schizophrenia. *American Journal of Psychiatry, 132*, 650–651.
74. Yehuda, R. (1997). Sensitization of the hypothalamic-pituitary-adrenal axis in posttraumatic stress disorder. *Annals of the NY Academy of Science, 821*, 57–75.
75. Zohar, J., Insel, T. R., Zohar-Kadouch, R. C., Hill, J. L., & Murphy, D. L. (1988). Serotoninergic responsivity in obsessive-compulsive disorder: Effects of chronic clomipramine treatment. *Archives of General Psychiatry, 45*, 167–172.

Chapter 31

Traumatic and Vascular Injuries of the Central Nervous System

Reet Henze

KEY TERMS

agnosia
anisocoria
anosmia
anterior cord syndrome
aphasia
apraxia
arteriovenous malformation
autonomic dysreflexia
Broca's aphasia
Brown-Sèquard syndrome
central cord syndrome
coma
concussion
contusion
cytoxic edema
decerebrate posturing
decorticate posturing
elastance
epidural hematoma
epilepsy
generalized seizure
global aphasia
hemorrhagic stroke
hemiparesis
interstitial edema
intracerebral hematoma
ischemic edema
ischemic stroke
lower motor neuron lesion
oculocephalic reflex
oculovestibular reflex
paraplegia
partial seizure
primary brain injury
quadriplegia
secondary brain injury
spinal shock
subarachnoid hemorrhage
subdural hematoma
transient ischemic attack (TIA)
uncal herniation
upper motor neuron lesion
vasogenic edema
Wernicke's aphasia

Traumatic brain and cerebrovascular injuries of the nervous system may result in significant brain disruption and alteration in the level of consciousness. Clinical manifestations such as altered motor, pupillary, and respiratory responses commonly accompany the varying levels of consciousness associated with traumatic and cerebrovascular injuries.

Traumatic brain injuries may result in varying types of impairments, depending on the mechanism and force of injury and the region of the brain most significantly involved. Diffuse axonal injury, contusions, and traumatic vascular injuries are examples of common traumatic brain injuries. Additionally, individuals suffering from traumatic head injuries frequently have accompanying secondary injuries such as cerebral edema, hypoxia, and increased intracranial pressure. Individuals suffering from cerebrovascular disease experience similar secondary injuries.

Nontraumatic cerebrovascular injuries such as strokes may present deficits similar to those associated with traumatic brain injury. The major effects of stroke result from disruption of blood flow to a region of the brain. The magnitude of the deficits is reflected by the size and region of the vascular disruption. Changes may occur in the level of consciousness, pupil and eye responses, speech patterns, and various sensory and motor functions.

Injuries to the cranial nerves frequently accompany traumatic head injuries. Mass effect, which acts like a compressing lesion, sometimes associated with cerebral hematomas or cerebral edema, may also lead to injury to the cranial nerves. Cranial nerve injuries are reflected in varying deficits associated with pupillary function, eye movement, motor and sensory function of the face, swallowing, and tongue sensation and movement.

Spinal cord injury may accompany traumatic brain injury or occur alone. Various complete or incomplete spinal cord injuries result in significant deficits that reflect the region and level of the cord involved. Recovery from spinal cord injury, particularly high spinal cord injury, is a long and frequently complicated process.

Seizures may accompany many neurologic conditions, including traumatic brain injury and cerebrovascular injury.

COMA

Coma refers to a disruption of the conscious state in which wakefulness and awareness are lacking. It is used here as a general term, because the disorders discussed may produce varying alterations in the level of consciousness (LOC). LOC may range widely from an alert state to deep coma. A person with a normal LOC is awake, aware, and interacting appropriately with the environment when not engaged in normal sleep. However, subtle changes in consciousness, which can occur slowly or progress very rapidly over a short period of time to a totally unresponsive state (coma), reflect underlying brain pathology.

General responses to one's surroundings provide valuable information about brain function. However, interpretation of these responses may be highly subjective. Some less precise terms frequently used to describe variations in LOC are presented in Table 31-1. To provide an objective evaluation of a person's LOC, a tool such as the Glasgow Coma Scale (GCS) may be used to communicate alterations in consciousness (Table 31-2). This tool numerically rates a patient's response in three categories: eye opening, best motor response, and verbal response. When totaled, the score ranges from 3 to 15. A person with a GCS of 8 is usually considered to be in a coma. This individual would not open eyes in response to verbal stimuli, at best would respond to pain with weak flexion, and utter incomprehensible sounds in response to pain.

Etiology

Disruption of the conscious state occurs when structures necessary for consciousness suffer physiologic or structural injury. Coma is commonly viewed from an etiologic basis of (1) structural or (2) metabolic/toxic origin and, uncommonly, from (3) psychogenic causes. In addition to the etiologic basis, each of these can be distinguished by some unique clinical manifestations. These are summarized in Table 31-3.

Coma also may be further associated with lesions and disorders involving structures above the tentorium (supratentorial) and those involving structures below the tentorium (infratentorial). Figure 31-1 identifies the tentorium and shows the areas above the tentorium, such as the cerebral hemispheres and diencephalon, and those below the tentorium, such as the pons, cerebellum, and medulla.

TABLE 31-1

TERMS USED TO DESCRIBE LEVEL OF CONSCIOUSNESS

LEVEL OF CONSCIOUSNESS	CLINICAL FINDINGS
Alert	Oriented to time, place, person. Appropriate interaction with environment.
Confusion	Inattentive and disoriented.
Lethargy	Somnolent, drowsy, sluggish response to verbal stimuli. Occasional disorientation.
Obtundation	Repeated verbal or tactile stimulation needed for responsiveness; then slow response to stimuli. Sleep state if undisturbed.
Stupor	Vigorous stimuli necessary to evoke a response, then potentially able to give brief responses to questions. Some spontaneous movement present.
Coma	Unarousable unresponsiveness.
Light/semi-coma	Reflexive motor response to noxious stimuli.
Deep coma	No reflexive response to vigorous noxious stimulation. Flaccid motor response.

SUPRATENTORIAL COMA

Supratentorial lesions/disorders are those found above the tentorium cerebelli in one or both cerebral hemispheres and deep diencephalic structures. Typically, isolated, small lesions of the cerebral hemispheres above the level of the tentorium are not sufficient to cause coma as long as the ascending reticular formation (RF) and its connections to the cortex are intact. However, with progressively larger hemispheric lesions in regions above the tentorium, behavior becomes dulled, increasingly deteriorating until maximum obliteration of the cortex occurs and no content of consciousness is preserved.

Supratentorial hemispheric lesions produce coma by enlarging sufficiently to cross midline structures, compressing the opposite hemisphere, or by causing caudal compression of the diencephalon and midbrain. If hemispheric compression occurs, herniations of the diencephalon or uncus through the tentorial notch (transtentorial herniation) may result, causing

TABLE 31-2

GLASGOW COMA SCALE

CRITERIA	PATIENT RESPONSE	SCORE ASSIGNED
Eye opening	Opens eyes spontaneously	4
	Opens eyes to speech command	3
	Opens eyes to noxious stimuli	2
	Does not open eyes	1
Best motor response	Follows commands	6
	Pushes noxious stimulus away	5
	Withdraws from noxious stimulus	4
	Abnormal flexion (decorticate response)	3
	Abnormal extension (decerebrate response)	2
	No motor response to noxious stimuli	1
Verbal response	Oriented and converses	5
	Converses but is confused and disoriented	4
	Articulates inappropriate words	3
	Incomprehensible sounds	2
	No sound	1

Note: Scores range from 3 to 15. Generally an individual whose score is 8 or less is considered to be in a coma.

vascular obstruction and accentuating the already present ischemia. Similarly, cerebrospinal fluid (CSF) circulation is blocked with transtentorial herniations, causing an increase in intracranial pressure (ICP). Additionally, brainstem hemorrhages and ischemia, thought to be caused by the midbrain and pons stretching the medial branches of the basilar artery, usually accompany transtentorial herniation. Herniation syndromes are discussed further on page 951.

INFRATENTORIAL COMA

Infratentorial lesions/disorders are those that arise below the tentorium cerebelli and involve structures that normally activate both cerebral hemispheres. These include problems of the brain stem, reticular activating system, thalamus, hypothalamus, and cerebellum.[13] The brain stem may be injured by strokes, neoplasms, aneurysms, hematomas, infectious processes, and head trauma.

If the cerebellum and midbrain herniate upward through the tentorial notch, the mesencephalic tegmentum (see Fig. 31-1) of the brain stem may be compressed. This compression results in tissue distortion and vascular obstruction, ischemia, and eventual coma. If the cerebellar tonsils herniate through the foramen magnum, downward compression of the brain stem may occur, causing compression and ischemia of the medulla and subsequent circulatory and respiratory aberrations.[22]

Clinical Manifestations

Clinical manifestations of coma showing alteration in function are reflective of the level and extent of underlying brain pathology and depth of the coma. These include alterations in motor responses, respiratory patterns, pupillary responses, and eye movements.

MOTOR RESPONSES

Limb movement provides a means of identifying asymmetry of function in the nervous system. Lesions at certain levels within the central nervous system (CNS) result in specific types of motor responses that are readily observable clinically and support the region of the pathology.

Purposeful motor responses to noxious stimuli reflect the relative integrity of the sensory and corticospinal pathways. Abnormal motor responses are stereotyped patterns commonly indicating the level or region of damage. **Decorticate** and **decerebrate posturing** are examples of abnormal involuntary motor responses indicative of significant neurologic damage

TABLE 31-3

ETIOLOGIC BASIS AND CLINICAL MANIFESTATIONS OF COMA

TYPE OF COMA	ETIOLOGY	CLINICAL MANIFESTATIONS
Structural	Physical damage to the brain (both cerebral cortices, one cerebral cortex and brainstem, or brainstem only) by trauma, tumors, infections, hemorrhage, contusions, and edema Brain expansion and possible herniation with compression of vital structures and subsequent secondary damage to structures necessary for consciousness	• Commonly asymmetric dysfunction • Focal signs possibly reflecting region of the brain involved. • Poor eyelid tone with deep coma
Metabolic/toxic	Ingestion of exogenous nervous system poisons such as certain sedative drugs and alcohol or endogenous (disease) processes such as renal failure, DKA, electrolyte imbalance, acidosis, liver failure, hypoxia, hypoglycemia, hypercapnea	• Usually symmetric body dysfunction • Poor eyelid tone with deep coma
Psychogenic	Psychogenic origin, including fainting, hysteria, and catatonia	• Good eyelid tone • Active resistance to eyelid opening

below the cerebral cortex. These are illustrated and described in Figure 31-2.

Decorticate Posturing

Decorticate posturing denotes supratentorial dysfunction commonly observed when corticospinal pathways are interrupted by lesions of the internal capsule or cerebral hemisphere. The upper extremities exhibit a flexion response, whereas the lower extremities exhibit an extension response. The arms are adducted and in rigid flexion, with the hands rotated internally and the fingers flexed.

Decerebrate Posturing

Decerebrate posturing is seen in persons with extensive brain stem damage to the midpontine level and large cerebral lesions that compress the lower thalamus and midbrain. Severe metabolic disorders, such as hypoglycemia, hepatic coma, and certain drug intoxications, which may diminish brain stem function, can induce a decerebrate response. Both upper and lower extremities exhibit characteristic extension responses.

The decerebrate individual exhibits *opisthotonos* (head extended, body arched) posturing with clenched teeth and arms rigidly extended, adducted, and hyperpronated. The legs are stiffly extended and feet are plantar flexed. The extent of the decerebrate response correlates with the severity of the pathology. Wavering back and forth between decorticate and decerebrate is seen occasionally, a reflection of the physiologic changes occurring.

Decerebrate responses of the upper extremities accompanied by flaccidity of the lower extremities indicate more extensive brain stem damage extending even beyond the pons level. In certain persons, asymmetry of abnormal responses and normal responses may reflect underlying cerebral pathology. For example, a person may exhibit a unilateral decorticate response or a decorticate response on one side and decerebrate on the other side.

Hemiplegia

Hemiplegia refers to a unilaterally absent motor response, which indicates a disruption in the contralateral corticospinal pathway. Hyperreflexia and the presence of the Babinski sign provide additional evidence for structural lesions of the CNS as the origin of the coma. Certain metabolic abnormalities, such as hypoglycemia and uremia, may cause the same signs. How-

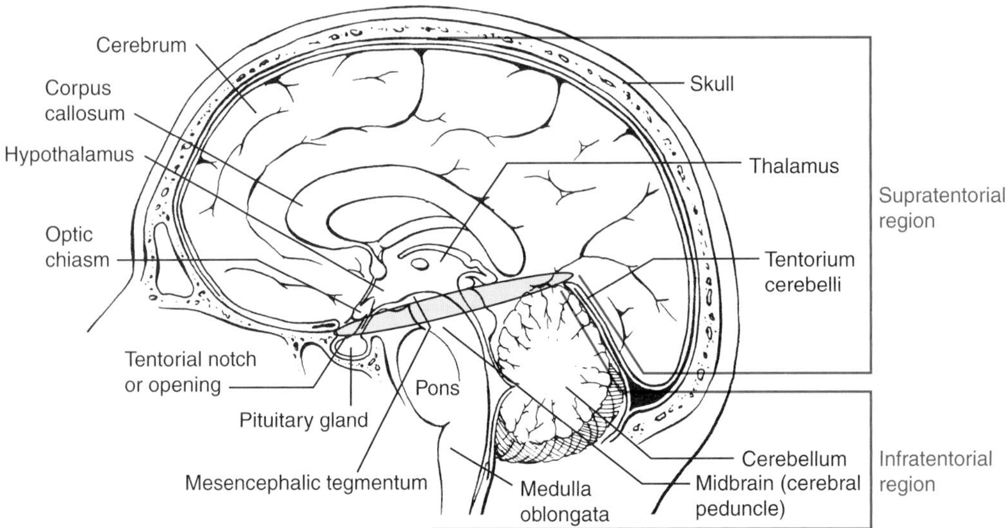

FIGURE 31-1. Supratentorial and infratentorial regions of the brain in relation to the tentorium cerebelli.

ever, these conditions can be quickly confirmed or ruled out by laboratory studies.

Paralysis

Paralysis, the loss of voluntary movement, is relatively common with injury and diseases of the nervous system. Lesions involving the corticobulbar and corticospinal tracts result in contralateral spastic paralysis and are referred to as **upper motor neuron lesions** (Fig. 31-3*A*). Lesions in motor cranial nerves, whose cell bodies are in the brainstem nuclei, and spinal nerves, whose cell bodies are in the anterior horn of the spinal cord, result in an ipsilateral flaccid paralysis and are referred to as **lower motor neuron lesions** (Fig. 31-3*B*). Table 31-4 compares the characteristics of upper and lower motor neuron lesions.

PUPILLARY RESPONSES

The close anatomic relationship of fibers that control pupillary reactions and consciousness provides a valuable guide to the location of the pathologic processes causing coma. Other origins of coma also may be assessed by the pupillary responses because metabolic aberrations leave little effect on the pupils, whereas certain structural pathology produces distinct changes.

Pupillary responses are regulated by a balance between sympathetic and parasympathetic nervous systems, producing a pupillary opening appropriate to the prevailing environment. *Mydriasis* (dilation) is produced by the sympathetic nervous system, and *miosis* (constriction) by the parasympathetic nervous system. The sympathetic innervation arrives by a more complex route that originates in the hypothalamus, traverses the brainstem, and travels along with the internal carotid artery into the skull where it reaches the eye through the filaments of the ophthalmic artery and a division of the fifth nerve. The parasympathetic impulses arrive through the third cranial nerve in the midbrain.

Pupils normally are at midposition and conjugate (symmetrically positioned) at rest. In coma, eyes may exhibit slow, random, roving movements that may be conjugate or dysconjugate. These movements cannot be mimicked voluntarily, hence they provide valuable information. Pupil responses with damage to specific areas of the brain are identified in Figure 31-4 and produce the following characteristic responses:

- *Midbrain lesions* result in fixed pupils that are not reactive to light but do fluctuate in size. These lesions generally impinge on both the sympathetic and parasympathetic eye pathways. Lesions affecting the midbrain most commonly result from transtentorial herniation. Other causes include neoplasms and vascular abnormalities affecting the midbrain.
- *Pontine lesions* interfere with descending sympathetic pathways producing bilateral small pupils. Generally, pupils react to light, but this may be difficult to discern without a magnifying glass.
- *Oculomotor (third cranial nerve) paralysis* may be observed if the lesion compresses the temporal uncus sufficiently to cause herniation and the resultant third nerve compression against the tentorium. Initially, a unilateral, dilated, nonreactive pupil **(aniso-**

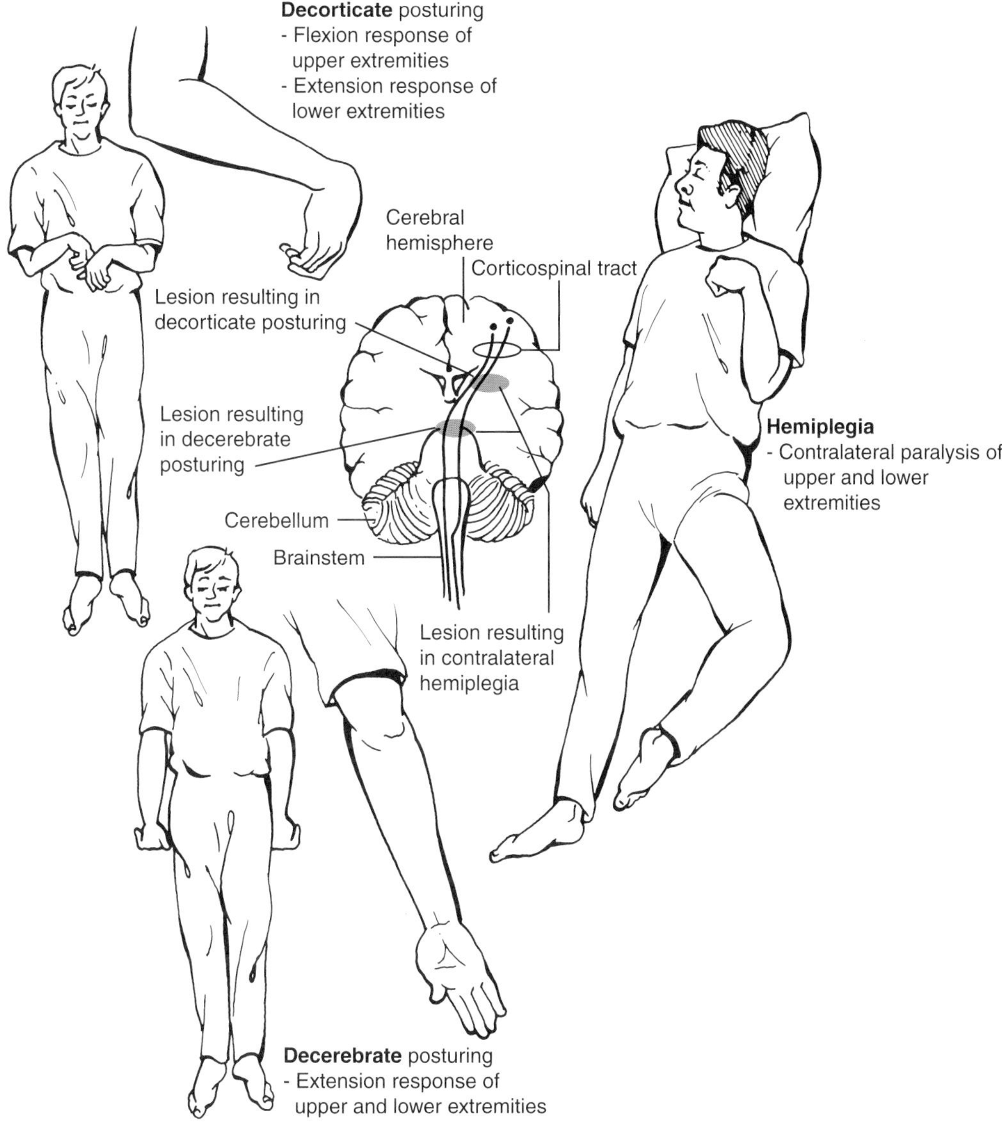

FIGURE 31-2. Abnormal motor responses with lesions at various areas of the brain.

coria [two pupils of unequal diameter]) is observed, possibly progressing to bilateral involvement as the lesion expands.

- *Horner's syndrome,* which involves compression of sympathetic fibers, either centrally between the hypothalamus and spinal cord or peripherally at the superior cervical ganglion, cervical sympathetic chain, or along the carotid artery, results in ipsilateral pupillary constriction, ptosis (drooping eyelids), and anhidrosis (absence of sweat) of the face. The pupillary light reflex remains intact with hypothalamic damage. The combinations of symptoms indicating Horner's syndrome with central involvement are significant because they may lead to progressive neurologic deterioration, resulting in transtentorial herniation.

Other conditions causing coma may affect pupillary response. Severe hypoxia, usually secondary to severely diminished cardiac output, results in dilated, nonreactive pupils. In rare cases, a tight constriction may be observed. Metabolically produced coma generally results in pupils that are reactive until the terminal stage, thus providing significant data for determining the underlying problem.

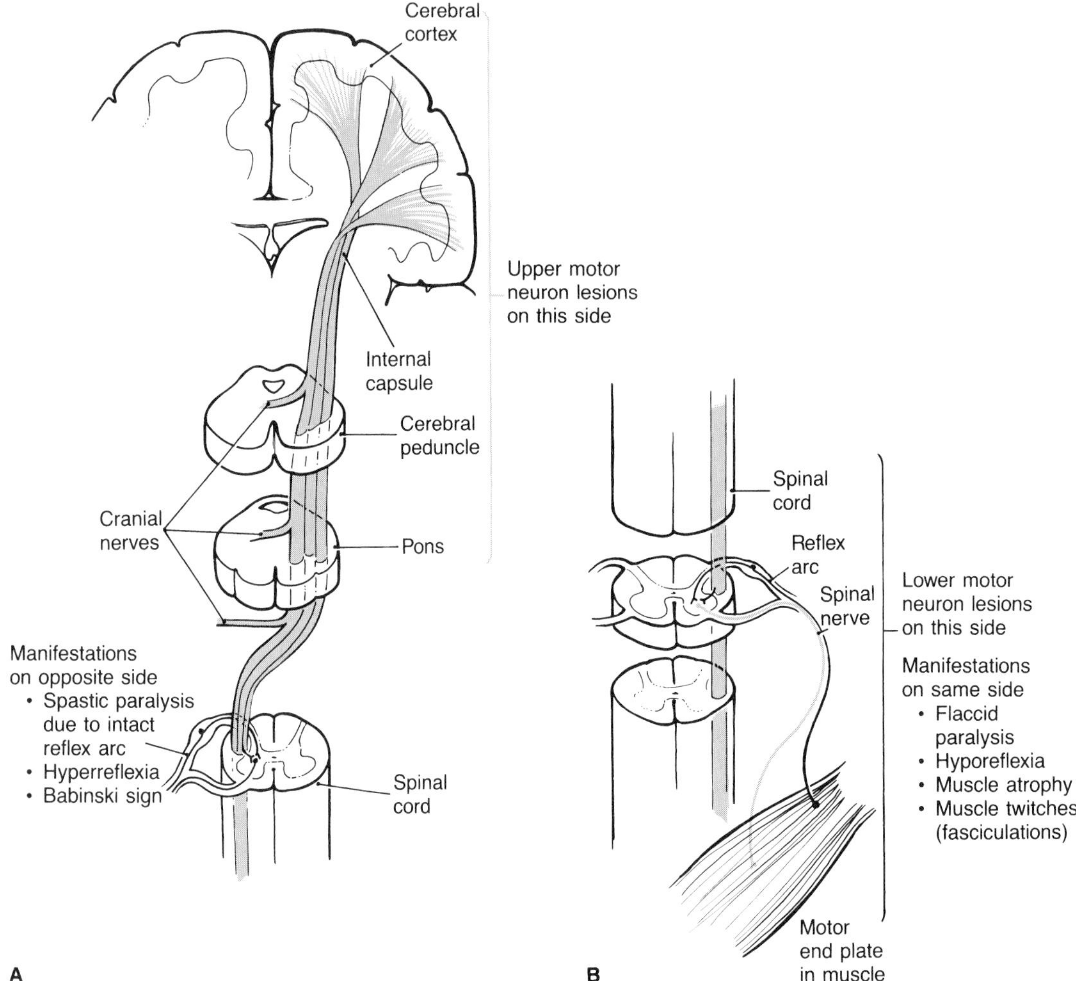

FIGURE 31-3. **A.** Effect of upper motor neuron lesions. **B.** Effect of lower motor neuron lesions.

Drugs also may affect pupils, but these effects vary depending on the drug. Heroin, morphine, and other opiates produce pupils characteristic of pontine lesions. That is, pupils become pinpoint and difficult to assess for light reactivity. Cocaine dilates pupils by interfering with norepinephrine absorption by nerve endings. Epinephrine also dilates pupils. Ingestion of large amounts of atropine and scopolamine results in dilated, nonreactive pupils, possibly giving a false impression of a structural lesion. Other drugs that produce pupillary dilation are phenylephrine hydrochloride (Neo-Synephrine), hydroxyamphetamine, phenylephrine, and cyclopentolate.

EYE/BRAIN STEM REFLEXES

Vestibulo-ocular reflex pathways occupy areas controlling consciousness and, therefore, provide a useful assessment guide of the unconscious individual. The **oculocephalic reflex** (doll's eye response) is assessed by briskly rotating the head from side to side with eyelids held open. In the positive (normal) response, eyes deviate conjugatively (in unison) in the direction opposite to the head deviation. As the neck is extended, the eyes deviate to a downward gaze; as it is flexed, the eyes deviate to an upward gaze. The presence of the doll's eye response indicates that the oculocephalic reflex arc is intact.

The oculocephalic reflex is tested in individuals whose voluntary eye responses cannot be tested due to coma. Absence of the doll's eye response, in which the eyes remain midline and move with the head, indicates serious brain stem dysfunction. An abnormal response, in which the eyes rove or move in opposite directions, indicates a lesser degree of brain stem dysfunction than absence of the response. The oculocephalic reflex may also be absent in severe metabolic disturbances.

TABLE 31-4

CHARACTERISTICS OF UPPER AND LOWER MOTOR NEURON LESIONS

	CHARACTERISTICS
Lower motor neuron lesions	Interruption of the reflex arc, which provides the muscle with tone Atony and soft, hypotonic, unresponsive muscles Inability to elicit voluntary activity and reflex action when the final common pathway of the lower motor neuron is severed Absent deep tendon reflexes Normal or absent plantar reflex Muscle atrophy and fasiculations
Upper motor neuron lesions	Intact reflex arc with loss of voluntary movement control Paralysis involving pyramidal tract and its collaterals and other descending tracts that influence lower motor neurons Muscle hard, very sensitive to stretch, and hypertonic with resultant spastic paralysis Positive Babinski sign Increased deep tendon reflexes after initial areflexia Less degree of muscle atrophy than with lower motor neuron lesions

Oculovestibular reflex (cold caloric test) is obtained by introducing cold water slowly into the intact, patent ear canal. A normal response is present and reflected by an intermittent conjugate tonic nystagmus deviation of the eyes to the side of the irrigated ear, implying intact brain stem function. Disconjugate eye movement is abnormal and indicates some degree of brain stem dysfunction, whereas no response reflects little or no brain stem function. Like the oculocephalic reflex, the oculovestibular reflex is also absent in some severe metabolic problems. The reflex arc for both the oculocephalic and oculovestibular responses includes the vestibulocochlear (CN VIII) as the afferent limb and the oculomotor (CN III) and abducens (CN VI) as the efferent limb.

RESPIRATORY PATTERNS

Neurologic influences on respiration occur in various regions of the brain, making respiratory patterns a significant assessment finding. Figure 31-4 shows specific respiratory patterns produced by lesions in various areas in the brain, which are described as the following:

- *Central neurogenic hyperventilation* is deep, rapid breathing generally indicating dysfunction in the brain stem tegmentum between the midbrain and pons. It accompanies traumatic brain injury and intracranial hypertension. Arterial blood gases reveal respiratory alkalosis as evidenced by low carbon dioxide tension and high pH.
- *Apneustic* breathing consists of a prolonged inspiratory phase followed by an expiratory pause. This pattern reflects pontine-level damage, most generally pontine infarctions secondary to basilar artery occlusions.
- *Ataxic* breathing, which results from lesions in the reticular activating system (RAS) of the dorsomedial portion of the medulla, is characteristically a very irregular breathing pattern with irregularly inter-

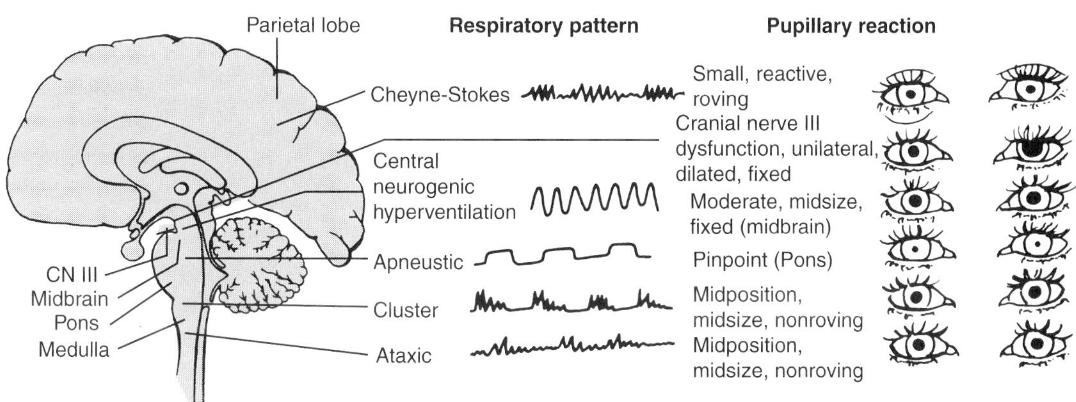

FIGURE 31-4. Level of lesion/injury and associated respiratory and pupillary responses.

spersed pauses. Minimal depression, either with mild sedation or sleep, may lead to apnea because the respiratory center is rather hyposensitive. Generally, individuals with ataxic respirations who are apneic secondary to depressant drugs or sleep respond to verbal commands to resume breathing. In severe medullary compression or lesions, ataxic breathing is viewed as a preterminal event.

- *Cheyne-Stokes* respiration, which consist of a regular crescendo-decrescendo pattern alternating with periods of apnea, reflects bilateral hemispheric dysfunction with an essentially intact brain stem. The hemispheric disturbances resulting in Cheyne-Stokes respiration are generally deep within the brain, involving the basal ganglia and internal capsule. This respiratory pattern also accompanies disturbances of metabolic origin affecting similar cerebral regions, such as with heart failure. An increased sensitivity to carbon dioxide levels leads to hyperpnea (increased respiratory rate). Blood carbon dioxide level falls to below the stimulatory level, resulting in a period of apnea. During the apneic period, the carbon dioxide again accumulates to the respiratory threshold level, and the cyclic hyperpnea and apnea continue.
- *Cluster* breathing, such as *Biot's* breathing, is an irregular pattern of cluster breaths interspersed with varying periods of apnea. It may result from damage in the high medulla or low pons region. Lesions in the low brainstem also may lead to frequent yawning and hiccups. The underlying mechanism for this is not clearly understood.
- *Posthyperventilation apnea* is observed occasionally with diffuse, bilateral hemispheric disease. Respirations cease when the pCO_2 levels have dropped after a period of hyperventilation and return when the pCO_2 levels are normalizing.

HEAD INJURY

Typically, head injury and subsequent injury to the brain and possibly the cranial nerves is associated with trauma, with a great majority resulting from automobile crashes. Injury to the brain also may result from nontraumatic causes involving a disruption in cerebral blood flow.

The cranial vault affords protection to the brain with the hair, skin, bone, meninges, and CSF. When force is applied, these protective encasements absorb energy that would normally be transmitted to the cranial contents. When the force exceeds absorption capacity, it is transmitted to the brain and tissue damage results. This traumatic head injury usually correlates with the amount of force applied to the cranial contents. Neck injuries are always assumed to be present with traumatic head injuries until ruled out.

Traumatic head injuries with no obvious external damage but with an intact skull are referred to as *closed head injuries*. Closed head injuries commonly result from sudden acceleration-deceleration accidents (Fig. 31-5). Initially the head hits against a relatively stationary object and results in brain injury at the site of impact (*coup* injury). The cranial contents then shift to the opposite side of the impact within the rigid skull; this is referred to as the *contrecoup* injury and may lead to contusions and lacerations as the semisolid brain moves over rough projections within the cranial cavity. In addition, the cerebrum may rotate with trauma, resulting in damage to the upper midbrain and areas of the frontal, temporal, and occipital lobes.

In contrast, *open head injuries* may reveal penetration of the scalp, skull, meninges, or brain tissue. Open head injuries are usually associated with skull fractures and may result in communication with the environment. In some skull fractures, bony fragments may be

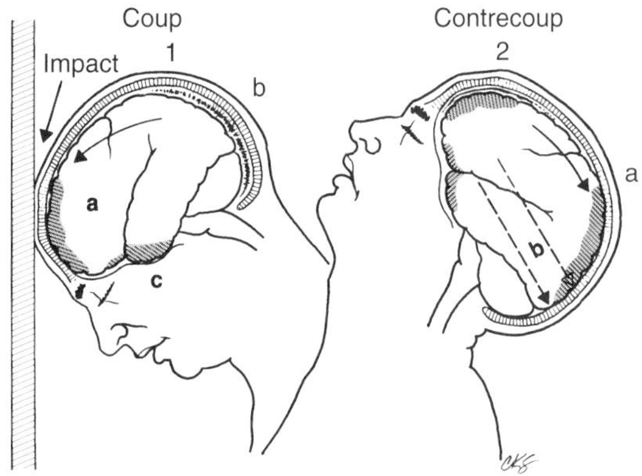

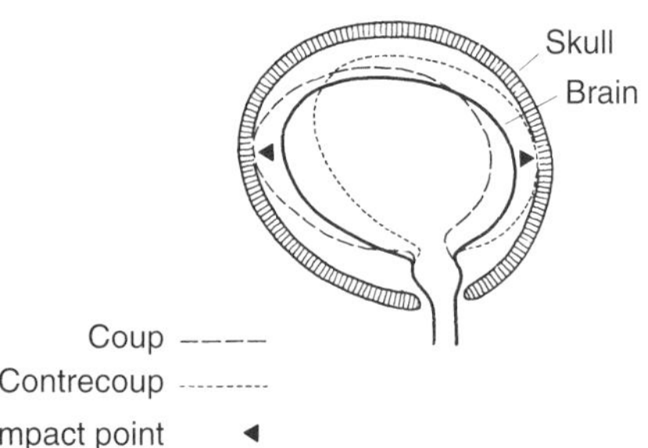

FIGURE 31-5. Coup and contrecoup head injury after blunt trauma. 1. Coup injury: impact against object; a. site of impact and direct trauma to brain; b. shearing of subdural veins; c. trauma to base of brain. 2. Contrecoup injury: impact within skull; a. site of impact from brain hitting opposite side of skull; b. shearing forces throughout brain. These injuries occur in one continuous motion—the head strikes the wall (coup), then rebounds (contrecoup). (Hudak, C. & Gallo, B.) [1997]. *Critical care nursing: A holistic approach* [6th ed.]. Philadelphia: Lippincott.)

driven into the brain tissue, resulting in meningeal tears, escape of CSF, and frequently underlying hematomas. The risk of infection is very high because of the exposure of the brain to the environment.

Skull Fractures

Skull fractures may be classified as one of the following:

- *Linear* fractures: simple line fractures without displacement or communication with cranial contents
- Comminuted fractures: multiple linear fractures with the same characteristics
- *Depressed* skull fractures: fractures driven toward the dura resulting in possible displacement of the cranial tissue by bone fragments; decreased volume of the cranial cavity, possibly producing herniation syndromes; venous return possibly impeded, resulting in secondary hemorrhages
- *Basilar* skull fractures: fractures involving the base of the skull at either the anterior, middle, or posterior fossa or combinations of the three regions

PATHOPHYSIOLOGY

A skull fracture results from a blow to the head leading to one or a combination of the types of skull fractures described above. Skull fractures may not be problematic unless outside communication with the brain results and the cranial contents or bone fragments are driven into the neural tissue. These injuries indicate that a major blow to the head has occurred and that a potentially severe injury has been incurred by the brain.

CLINICAL MANIFESTATIONS

Skull fractures may present without signs and symptoms, reflecting the underlying brain trauma only. With more severe skull fractures, discontinuity and displacement of the bone structure may be exhibited. Associated facial fractures may reveal motor-sensory dysfunction. Injuries also may occur to the cranial nerves.

Basilar skull fractures present some characteristic clinical signs. Fractures of the anterior and middle fossae in association with severe head trauma are more common than those of the posterior fossa. Persons with *anterior fossa basilar skull* fractures may exhibit periorbital ecchymosis (raccoon eyes), cranial nerve injury reflecting **anosmia** (loss of smell due to first cranial nerve involvement), and pupil abnormalities (second and third cranial nerve involvement). The presence of CSF rhinorrhea (CSF leakage from the nose) strongly suggests an anterior fossa basilar skull fracture. The signs of *middle fossa basilar skull fractures* include CSF otorrhea (CSF leakage from the ear), hemotympanium (blood accumulation at the tympanic membrane), ecchymosis over the mastoid bone (Battle's sign), and facial paralysis (seventh cranial nerve injury). Involvement of the *posterior fossa basilar skull* may be indicated by signs of medullary dysfunction such as cardiovascular and respiratory failure.

Primary Traumatic Brain Injury

The effect of trauma to the head may be a structural injury directly resulting from the trauma. This is termed **primary brain injury**. Primary injuries include direct injury to the (1) neurons and their axons, (2) glial cells, and (3) blood vessels.

DIFFUSE AXONAL INJURY (DAI)

Diffuse axonal injury (DAI) is associated with significant acceleration-deceleration and rotational forces that result in shearing and stretching of the neuronal axons.[14] This diagnosis encompasses severe head injury that results in loss of consciousness that is not attributable to expanding cerebral lesions, such as those associated with cerebral hematomas. Although generally DAI results in severe brain injury, its least severe presentation is the concussion.

PATHOPHYSIOLOGY. Axonal shearing and stretching results in microscopic hemorrhages throughout the brain, primarily within the deep structures of the brain and the frontal and temporal lobe axons. The cellular changes associated with DAI reflect chromatolysis (cell swelling, nuclear relocation, and dissolution of Nissl bodies).

CLINICAL MANIFESTATIONS. Clinical manifestations vary with severity of the injury, although commonly the patient is unconscious, in a deep coma, with flexor or extensor responses. Patients suffering from mild DAI present with a GCS of 13 to 15; those who have experienced moderate DAI present with a GCS of 9 to 12; and those with severe DAI present with a GCS of less than 8.

CONCUSSION

A **concussion** is caused by sudden movement of the brain resulting in a diffuse but transient and reversible injury to the brain. The word concussion means to "shake violently." Damage may occur in many areas, and the extent of involvement is very variable, ranging from very mild dysfunction to severe involvement characterized by neurologic dysfunction, unconsciousness, and death. Involvement of the brain stem reticular formation and certain subcortical areas may result in prolonged unconsciousness. Relatively minor concussions from mild blows cause a temporary physiologic disruption of the reticular formation, possibly leading to transient loss of consciousness. If present, the period of unconsciousness ranges from seconds in mild cases to as long as a few hours or more in severe cases.

Pathophysiology. Usually no permanent structural injury is sustained, and the effect of the concussion is reversible when neuronal function returns. However, certain biochemical changes have been associated with concussions in laboratory animals. These include depletion of mitochondrial adenosine triphosphate (ATP), disruption of the blood–brain barrier in the impact area, an increase in the relative sodium level in the brain, and elevated acetylcholine and lactate levels in more severe concussions.[1] The loss of consciousness is thought to be associated with (1) abrupt pressure changes in the areas responsible for consciousness, (2) sudden depolarization or hyperpolarization of neurons, (3) ischemia, and (4) neuronal structural distortion resulting in transient changes in function.[24]

Clinical Manifestations. Typically the patient experiences a brief, immediate loss of consciousness. The individual also exhibits a brief loss of respiration, areflexia, hypotension, and bradycardia. These usually normalize within a few seconds even though the person may remain unconscious for a longer period. Once consciousness returns, the individual is amnesic to the precipitating event and may appear confused for a short period. The memory loss associated with events prior to the time of injury is referred to as *retrograde amnesia*; the loss associated to events after the time of injury is noted as *antegrade amnesia*. Those individuals suffering from both retrograde and antegrade amnesia are said to have *traumatic amnesia*. The length of unconsciousness and amnesia is generally proportional to the severity of the concussion. The longer the period of unconsciousness and amnesia, the more severe the injury.

Generally, further deterioration does not result from the concussion after the initial impact, and neurologic signs return to normal rapidly. However, headaches and dizziness, which often accompany concussions, may persist for a long time after the injury. Some individuals also continue to experience problems with attention, anxiety, irritability, memory, judgment, and concentration. These symptoms are collectively referred to as the *postconcussion syndrome*.

CONTUSION

Contusion, bruising of the brain, occurs as a result of blunt trauma in closed head injuries. Focal brain tissue destruction occurs at the area of the blow (*coup area*) or at the opposite side of the blow (*contrecoup area*). Concussions frequently accompany contusions. The cerebral hemispheres, particularly the basal anterior portions of the frontal and temporal lobes, and the posterior portions of the occipital lobe are frequently involved because these areas slide over bony irregularities of the base of the skull. Blows to the back of the head may result in contrecoup injuries to the frontal and temporal lobes. A variety of neurologic abnormalities may result from bruising of the cerebral hemispheres (hemispheric contusions), even though consciousness may be retained. In contrast, brain stem contusions result in loss of consciousness from tissue injury to the brain stem reticular formation. The period of unconsciousness may range from hours to a lifetime.

Pathophysiology. Small petechial hemorrhages are common in areas of contusion. Cerebral lacerations also may be associated with contusions and result in hematomas of varying sizes. The blow to the head results in petechial hemorrhage, leading to visible bruising. The injured area swells and becomes visibly red and then progressively purple due to venous obstruction, local edema, tissue infarction, and necrosis. With large hemorrhages or clusters of small hemorrhages, ICP increases. Regional hypoxia and acidosis occur in the contused area, producing hyperemia and further contributing to increased ICP. Cerebral oxygen consumption is reduced in contused tissue and cerebral lactate production is greatly increased, probably due to increased regional hypoxia and the resultant anaerobic metabolism.

Clinical Manifestations. Clinical findings depend on the region of the brain involved and the extent of tissue injury. Wide variations are seen in the LOC, motor responses, pupil responses, and vital signs. Electroencephalographic (EEG) recordings directly over an area of contusion reveal progressive abnormalities with the appearance of high-amplitude theta and delta waves. Computed tomography (CT) or magnetic resonance imaging (MRI) findings support the diagnosis of brain contusion, showing changes in tissue density and possible displacement of the surrounding structures.

Contusions may be partially reversible, depending on the severity of the blow and the amount of tissue injury. When blood flow and oxygenation to the contused area are re-established, some neuronal recovery may result.

TRAUMATIC VASCULAR INJURIES

Traumatic vascular brain injuries may result in hemorrhage into the cranial vault from epidural, subdural, subarachnoid, and intracerebral vascular sources. These sources of hemorrhage are commonly associated with cerebral contusions and other brain injuries. Individuals who are lucid for a period of time after trauma and then begin to deteriorate neurologically are, in all probability, suffering from cerebrovascular injury and bleeding into the cranial contents. Bleeding into the rigid cranium results in increased ICP, manifested by its localized or generalized effects on the brain.

Epidural Hematoma

Epidural hematoma or hemorrhage, a serious sequelae of head injuries, generally is associated with arterial bleeding into the extradural space. The blood accumulates between the skull and dura (Fig. 31-6). Less commonly, it arises from the dural venous sinuses. Epidural hematomas can occur in various regions of the brain. Those occurring in the lateral brain tend to be most acute, running a course more rapid than other, more slowly developing epidural hematomas in the frontal and occipital areas (Fig. 31-7). Most commonly, injury to the middle meningeal artery in the parietotemporal area results in epidural bleeds. This bleed is frequently accompanied by linear skull fractures at the temporal region over the middle meningeal artery.

Pathophysiology and Clinical Manifestations. The individual with a parietotemporal epidural hematoma follows a somewhat predictable clinical course. After the initial blow to the head, a brief period of unconsciousness frequently occurs, reflecting the concussive effects of head injury. Typically, a lucid interval of varying length follows; this may vary from 10 to 15 minutes to hours and, rarely, days. During this period, the patient often complains of a severe headache. Progressive loss of consciousness and deterioration in neurologic signs follow as a result of the expanding lesion and extrusion of the medial portion of the temporal lobe through the tentorial opening. Temporal lobe **(uncal) herniation** compresses the brain stem, producing the distinct clinical manifestations of intracranial hypertension.

Deterioration in the level of consciousness results from the compression of the brain stem reticular formation as the temporal lobe herniates on its upper portion. Respirations, initially deep and labored, later become shallow and irregular. Contralateral motor deficiencies result due to compression of the corticospinal tracts that pass through the brain stem. Distinct ipsilateral pupillary dilation can be observed because the third cranial nerve is compressed. Seizures may occur at any time during this progressive course. Without surgical intervention, continual bleeding leads to progressive neurologic degeneration, evidenced by bilateral pupillary dilation, bilateral decerebrate response, increased systemic blood pressure, decreased pulse, and profound coma with irregular respiratory patterns. The CT scan identifies any abnormal masses and structural shifts within the cranium.

Subdural Hematoma

Subdural hematomas, the most commonly encountered meningeal hemorrhage, result from an accumulation of blood in the subdural space (between the dura mater and arachnoid mater). They may occur in the acute, subacute, and chronic forms and may be unilateral or bilateral. The different forms of subdural hematomas are contrasted in Table 31-5.

Subdural hematomas are usually associated with torn connecting veins in the cerebral cortex. Rarely, bleeding may be from arterial origins. Acute subdural hematomas constitute a surgical emergency requiring prompt treatment.

Subacute subdural hematomas have an improved prognosis because the venous bleeding tends to be slower than in the acute form. The presence of suba-

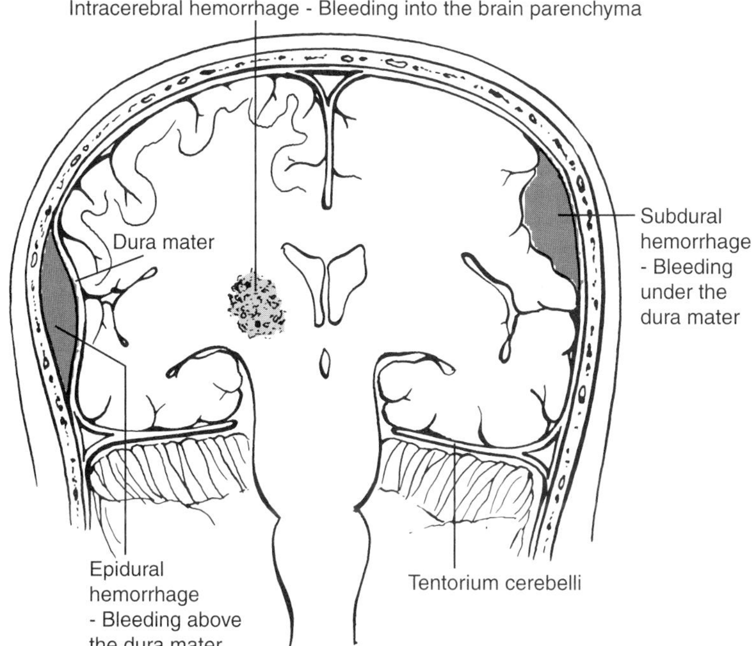

FIGURE 31-6. Types of traumatic vascular injuries.

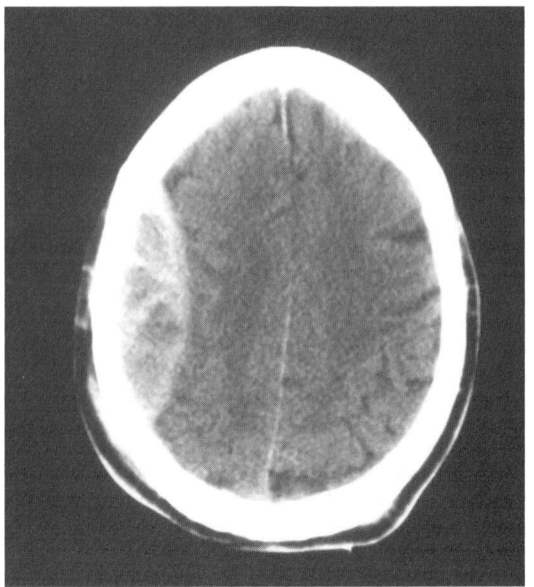

FIGURE 31-7. Epidural hematoma in right temporal region.

cute subdural hematomas is established by the clinical signs and evidence of masses and tissue shifting seen on MRI, CT, or roentgenograms.

Chronic subdural hematomas may be identified by the xanthochromic (yellow appearance) and relatively low protein content of the CSF. Tomographic scans, radiographs, and arteriography reveal the visible mass and altered blood flow in the area, confirming the hematoma.

Subdural Hygroma

Subdural hygroma, an excessive collection of fluid under the dura mater, most commonly results from trauma. Subsequent tearing of the arachnoid allows CSF to escape into the subdural space. Due to the vascularity of the arachnoid, some vessels are generally damaged, also allowing CSF to mix with blood in the subdural space. This mixing produces a high-osmotic fluid that continues to pull fluid into the subdural space, slowly expanding it in size.

Evidence of fluid obtained through a burr hole skull opening confirms the hygroma. Developing signs and

TABLE 31-5

CONTRASTING ACUTE, SUBACUTE AND CHRONIC SUBDURAL HEMATOMAS

HEMATOMA	TYPE OF INJURY	ONSET OF SYMPTOMS FROM TIME OF INJURY	CLINICAL MANIFESTATIONS
Acute subdural hematoma	Severe head injury, frequently associated with brain laceration and contusion	Shortly after injury, usually within 48 hours	Rapid deterioration to drowsiness, agitation, stupor, and coma. Signs of brain stem compression may be evident, i.e., unilateral pupil dilation and contralateral hemiparesis.
Subacute subdural hematoma	Moderate head injuries, which may be associated with cerebral contusions	Usually 2 days to 2 weeks after injury	Lucid period after injury that degenerates slowly to drowsiness, stupor, and coma. Periods of fluctuating neurologic signs that lead to increased intracranial pressure may be present.
Chronic subdural hematoma	Slow bleeding from a mild injury; most common in infants, elderly, demented, or alcoholic individuals on long-term anticoagulation	Usually weeks to several months after injury	Dull headache, slowness in thinking, apathy, drowsiness, confusion, contralateral hemiparesis, and progressive neurologic changes such as papilledema, homonymous hemianopia, aphasia, waxing and waning of level of consciousness.

symptoms of subdural hygromas after trauma are very similar to those of chronic subdural hematomas.

Intracerebral Hematoma

Intracerebral hematoma refers to a traumatic or spontaneous disruption of cerebral vessels within the brain parenchyma resulting in neurologic deficits, depending on the location and amount of bleeding. The shearing forces resulting from brain movement within the skull frequently lead to vessel laceration and hemorrhage into the parenchyma. Common sites of intracerebral bleeding are the frontal and temporal lobes. Those intracerebral hematomas associated with trauma constitute a small percentage of all intracerebral hematomas. The majority of these occur as a result of hypertension and are discussed on page 956.

Individuals with intracerebral bleeding may be unresponsive immediately or experience a lucid period before lapsing into a coma. Motor deficits may be present, and decorticate or decerebrate responses may occur. CT scanning or cerebral arteriography identifies the bleeding site. The CSF pressure may be elevated, and the fluid may appear red or xanthochromic (yellow or straw-colored from hemoglobin breakdown).

Secondary Traumatic Brain Injury

Traumatic head injury may result in a primary brain injury, but a **secondary brain injury** also may occur from the body's response to the primary injury. Secondary injuries include (1) cerebral edema, (2) hemorrhage, and (3) hypoxia.

CEREBRAL EDEMA

Cerebral edema, a common and serious sequela of traumatic and nontraumatic head injury, results when the total water content in the brain parenchyma becomes excessive. Cerebral edema may also occur with intracranial surgery, brain tumors, hemorrhage, hypoxemia, infarctions, and infections.

As cerebral edema increases within the nonflexible skull, clinical signs indicate increased ICP and decreased cerebral blood flow. If edema progresses, neurologic function continues to deteriorate due to intracranial shifts or herniations.

The morphologic changes in the edematous brain as seen at surgery or autopsy are characteristic and striking. The brain appears heavy and boggy. The gyri have lost their normal triangular appearance and the sulci have been obliterated. Brain sections reveal flattened ventricles and an indiscernible subarachnoid space.[18] Four types of cerebral edema have been identified: (1) **vasogenic**, (2) **cytotoxic**, (3) **ischemic,** and (4) **interstitial**. Their etiologic basis and pathophysiology are described in Table 31-6.

CEREBRAL HYPOXIA

Cerebral hypoxia is a common sequela of traumatic brain injuries as well as many other neurologic problems, including infarctions, hemorrhage, infections, and tumors. Systemic problems (especially cardiovascular and respiratory) may also lead to cerebral hypoxia. Cerebral hypoxia can result in ischemic cell damage and cessation of oxidative metabolism, resulting in complex pathologic changes (Flowchart 31-1).

Considerable variation seems to exist in the irreversible damage that occurs to neurons with hypoxia. Areas of the brain that appear to be particularly susceptible to hypoxia (e.g., the hippocampus) contain large numbers of glutamate receptors, and those that seem more resistant to damage (e.g., gyrus granule cells) contain higher levels of calcium-binding proteins.[9]

INCREASED INTRACRANIAL PRESSURE (ICP)

Increased ICP refers to ICP greater than 15 mm Hg. Head injuries may lead to increased ICP when compensatory mechanisms are exhausted due to expanding brain volume, increased blood volume, or increased accumulation of CSF. Without treatment, the increased pressure may compromise neurologic function and life itself. In addition to trauma, increased ICP accompanies many other neurologic problems and conditions, such as tumors, infections, and bleeds.

PATHOPHYSIOLOGY. In the adult, normal ICP is less than 15 mm Hg. The skull affords a nonflexible encasement around the brain tissue (which makes up 80% of the cranial contents) and extracellular fluid, which is primarily blood and CSF (each making up approximately 10% of the cranial contents). Although total intracranial volume varies slightly in the healthy brain, ICP remains relatively constant. Transient increases are normal and are associated with activities such as coughing, sneezing, and straining. Small increases in volume of one of the cranial components are compensated for normally by a decrease in the volume of another (*Monro-Kellie hypothesis*). For example, intracranial CSF may be shifted to the subarachnoid space of the spine, and the vascular bed of the brain may be reduced by shifting the blood to areas of less resistance.[13]

A measure of stiffness of the brain is known as **elastance** and indicates the brain's tolerance for increases in volume. Elastance is described by the formula $E = P/V$ (E = elastance; P = pressure; and V = volume). If elastance is low, then there is volume reserve. High elastance indicates a stiff or tight brain.

Intracranial compliance, the ability of the cranial contents to adapt to changes in volume, is determined by the volume and rate of displacement of intracranial tissue, blood, and CSF. Compliance (C) is the reciprocal of elastance and can be described by the following formula: $C = V/P$.

TABLE 31-6

TYPES OF CEREBRAL EDEMA

TYPE OF EDEMA	ETIOLOGICAL BASIS	PATHOPHYSIOLOGY
Vasogenic	• Associated with damage to or dysfunction in cerebral blood vessels • Primarily occurring in the white matter as a result of trauma, surgery, infections, contusions, inflammatory processes, neoplasms, and hematomas	Increased permeability of the vascular membranes and widening of the junctions between the cells occurs (breakdown of the blood–brain barrier). Plasma proteins and water from the blood pass into the extracellular spaces of the brain and cause interstitial edema.
Cytotoxic	• Associated with conditions that cause cerebral hypoxia such as certain intoxications, metabolic disorders, and water overload • Primarily affecting the gray matter	The adenosine triphosphate (ATP)–dependent sodium pump is not able to remove accumulating intracellular sodium. Accumulated intracellular sodium pulls water into the cell, waste products of anaerobic metabolism accumulate, and the cell becomes dysfunctional.
Ischemic	• Associated with large hemispheric strokes and peaks 24–96 hours after a stroke	Ischemia causes release of cellular lysosomal substances, which contribute to cell injury, necrosis, and death. Initially this is a cytotoxic edema, which later becomes vasogenic.
Interstitial edema	• Associated with a noncommunicating hydrocephalus	Fluid accumulates in the cerebral ventricles and in the white matter around the ventricles. Total water volume increases in the brain.

During the period of compensation when the volume/pressure curve is increasing slowly, relatively large increases in intracranial volume can be tolerated without significant ICP changes (adequate compliance, low elastance).[10] Figure 31-8 shows that when a small margin of compensation within the cranium is exhausted, small increases in volume result in large rises in ICP (decreased compliance, high elastance). Without intervention, decompensation and death ensue.

CLINICAL MANIFESTATIONS. When present, clinical indicators of increased ICP include headache, recurrent vomiting, decreased LOC, papilledema, pupillary dilation, peripheral motor changes, and respiratory irregularities. The headache associated with increased ICP is thought to occur as a result of traction on the pain-sensitive structures by the increased brain bulk. Increasing pressure on the vagal motor centers in the fourth ventricle stimulates recurrent vomiting. The changes in the LOC result from compression of the reticular formation of the brain stem and decreased perfusion to the brain. Papilledema and pupillary changes result from increased ICP on the optic nerve and the interference in normal nerve transmission. Motor changes occur secondary to compression of the voluntary motor transmission tracts. Respiratory irregularities result primarily from pressure on the brain stem.

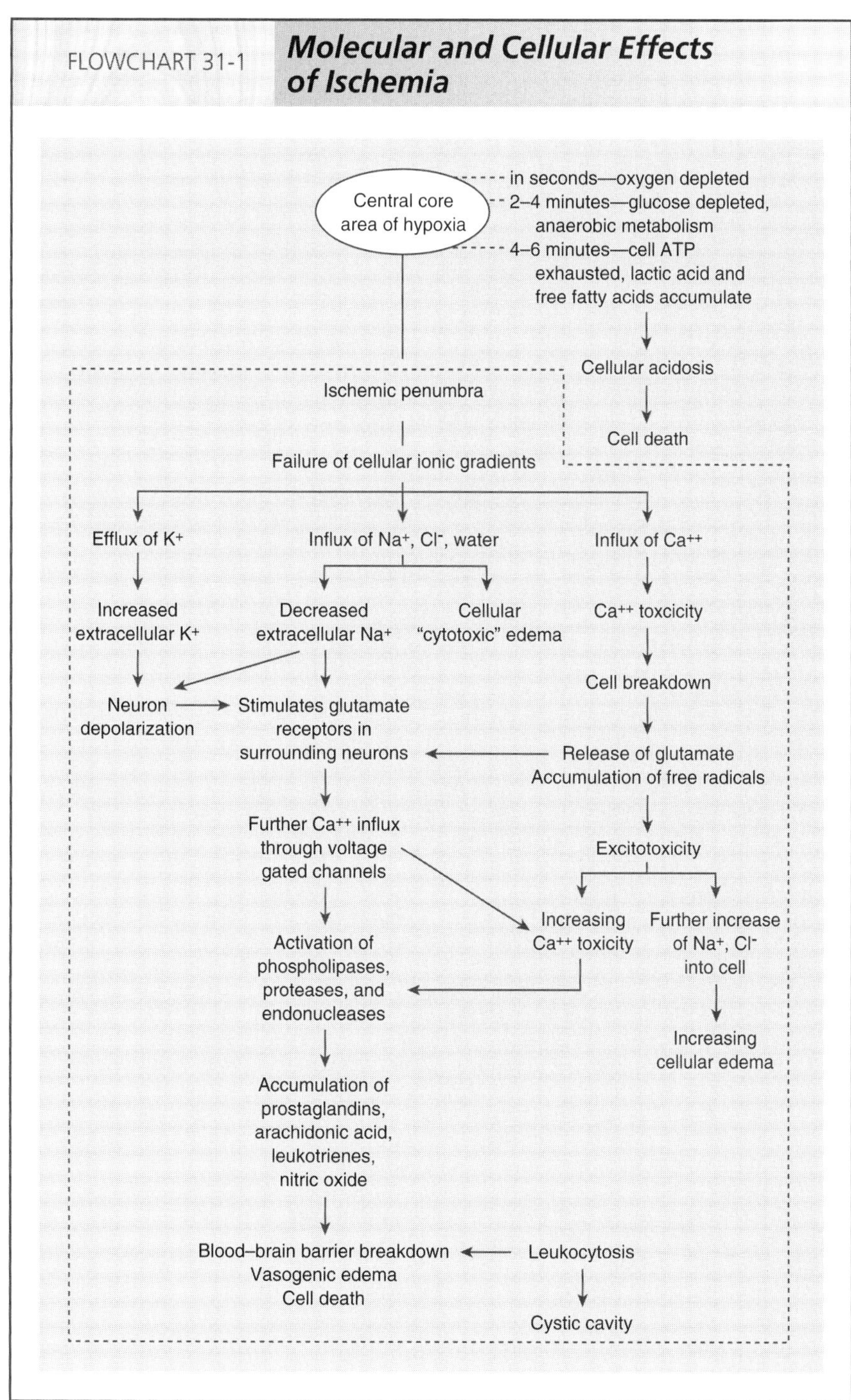

Decreasing pulse, elevated systolic pressure, and widening pulse pressure (Cushing's response) are compensatory mechanisms in an attempt to maintain cerebral blood flow. Generally, when clinical signs indicating brain stem involvement (hypertension, bradycardia, irregular respirations) are present, the individual has experienced some intracranial shifting (herniation). Brain shifts that can occur with expanding cerebral pathology include (1) cingulate herniation, (2) transcalvarial herniation, (3) central herniation, (4) uncal herniation, and (5) cerebellar foramen magnum herniation. Herniation syndromes are summarized in

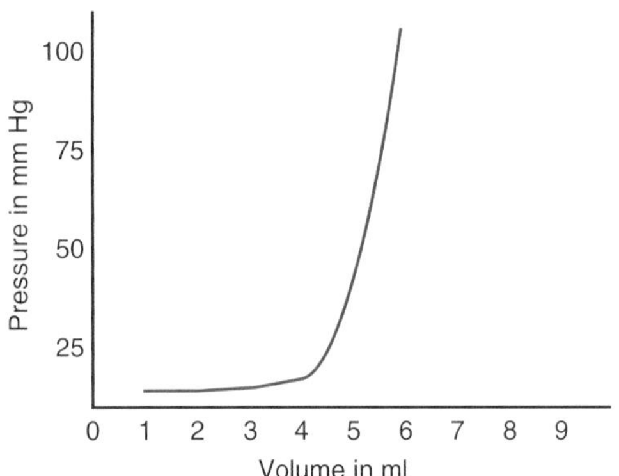

FIGURE 31-8. **Volume and pressure relationship. If the volume continues to expand in a capacity-limited skull, the intracranial pressure increases rapidly.**

Figure 31-9 and Table 31-7. When herniation occurs, the patient has reached a state of decompensation and has a poor prognosis for recovery.

Nontraumatic Vascular Brain Injury

Disruption of cerebral blood flow from nontraumatic causes, either sudden or over time, causes cerebrovascular brain injury and various neurologic dysfunctions. Because the brain has no oxygen reserve, it does not tolerate anoxia. Therefore, permanent cell damage can occur rapidly when blood flow is disrupted. Brief periods of hypoxia generally result in reversible neurologic deficits, whereas those lasting longer can lead to permanent neurologic deficits and cerebral infarction.

Neurologic impairments that result from nontraumatic disruption of the blood supply to an area of the brain are known as brain attacks, cerebrovascular accidents (CVAs), or strokes. Strokes are the third leading cause of death (after heart disease and cancer) in the United States, accounting for approximately 150,000 deaths annually. Certain risk factors have been associated with stroke. Although some are not modifiable, many are (Box 31-1). Major disabilities frequently remain in those who survive the initial stroke assault. Paresis, aphasia, agnosia, and apraxia are among common associated impairments.

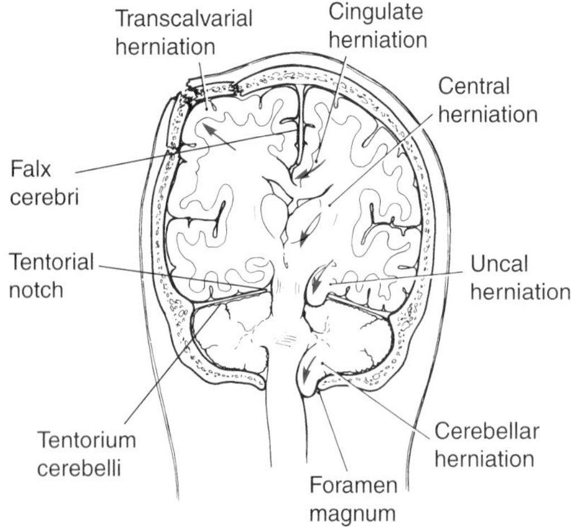

FIGURE 31-9. **Major types of intracranial herniations.**

ETIOLOGY

Nontraumatic disruption of cerebral blood flow in cerebrovascular disease may result from occlusion of cerebral arteries or hemorrhage. Occlusive or ischemic strokes, which account for 84% of strokes, result from thrombosis or embolism. Hemorrhagic strokes, accounting for 16% of strokes, result from intracerebral (parenchymal) or subarachnoid bleeding. Warning signs of impending stroke may or may not be present. Whatever the cause, ischemia and eventual necrosis of the brain parenchyma may result.

CLASSIFICATION OF STROKES

Strokes are classified according to etiology, onset, and duration. The major types of strokes include ischemic and hemorrhagic strokes. The characteristics of each and subclassifications are summarized in Table 31-8.

The course of strokes varies, depending on the etiology. A stroke is said to be completed when the blood supply has been cut off to a portion of the brain and permanent neurologic alterations follow. *Progressing* or *evolving stroke*, usually seen with occlusive disease, progresses over hours or days, finally resulting in permanent deficits. Strokes that last from a few minutes to a few hours with resolution of any neurologic deficits are referred to as **transient ischemic attacks (TIAs)**.

Transient Ischemic Attacks

Transient ischemic attacks result in a temporary episode of neurologic dysfunction from a diminished blood supply to a specific area of the brain, generally from thrombotic origins secondary to atherosclerosis (atheroma). Transient ischemic attacks usually last no longer than 15 minutes, although some patients may exhibit signs up to 24 hours.[25] Persons experiencing a TIA have a significant risk for major strokes at a later time.

Virtually any cerebral artery may be involved, and symptoms vary according to the area of involvement (Fig. 31-10). Minor focal deficits or major deficits resulting in complete loss of consciousness may be present. Since the same diseased vessel is usually involved, the recurring TIA symptoms are similar with each episode. Common findings with TIAs include transient episodes of contralateral weakness of the face, arms, and legs (**hemiparesis**), as well as sensory deficits (hemiparesthesias) and visual impairments. Involvement of

TABLE 31-7

HERNIATION SYNDROMES

TYPE OF HERNIATION SYNDROME	DESCRIPTION OF HERNIATION	ETIOLOGIC BASIS	PATHOPHYSIOLOGY	CLINICAL MANIFESTATIONS
Cingulate herniation	Compression of the cingulate gyrus under the falx cerebri	Expanding cerebral mass	Internal cerebral vein displacement leading to ischemia and edema	Varying signs of increased intracranial pressure, depending on the extent of brain tissue displacement
Transcalverial herniation	Brain tissue extruding through an unstable fractured skull	Open head injuries	Brain tissue injury and ischemia resulting in cerebral edema and increased brain mass	Varying signs of increased intracranial pressure
Central herniation	Pressure exerted centrally; downward displacement occurring through the tentorial notch, encroaching on the diencephalon and midbrain; be possibly preceded by cingulate and uncal herniation	Most commonly associated with diffuse increased intracranial pressure such as diffuse axonal injury and Reye's syndrome and, to a lesser extent, supratentorial lesions	Compression of structures passing through the tentorial notch (corticospinal tract, cranial nerves, reticular activating system) resulting in injury to these structures and the lower brain stem structures controlling respiratory, cardiac and vasomotor functions	Initially, subtle changes in the level of consciousness, which, with unchecked herniation, continue to coma Papilledema, changes in visual acuity; and pupil size, large, fixed pupils observed terminally Babinski response, extremity rigidity with progression to decortication or decerebration and flaccidity with continuing herniation
Uncal herniation	Crowding in the medial part of the temporal lobe (uncus and hippocampal gyrus), resulting in slippage of the uncus into the tentorial opening	Lesions in the lateral middle fossa or medial part of one temporal lobe	Compression of the third nerve, corticospinal tracts, and reticular activating system Possible displacement of the diencephalon and midbrain to the opposite side	Unilateral, ipsilateral dilated pupil, ptosis, paralysis of extraocular muscles, contralateral hemiparesis or hemiplegia, decorticate or decerebrate posturing to flaccidity, respiratory and cardiovascular irregularities Terminal signs similar to central herniation
Cerebellar foramen magnum herniation	One or more cerebellar tonsils herniating through the foramen magnum	Expanding lesions of the cerebellum	Compression of the brain stem, especially the medulla. Centers for vital function are encroached	Rapidly expanding lesions resulting in loss of consciousness, abnormal respiratory patterns, paralysis of extraocular muscles, hemiparesis, hemiplegia, decorticate, and decerebrate posturing to flaccidity with progression Cranial nerve dysfunction and vasomotor, cardiac, and respiratory arrest

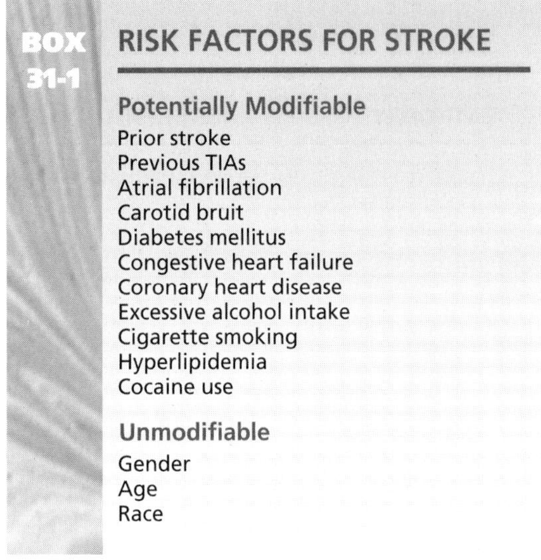

BOX 31-1

RISK FACTORS FOR STROKE

Potentially Modifiable

Prior stroke
Previous TIAs
Atrial fibrillation
Carotid bruit
Diabetes mellitus
Congestive heart failure
Coronary heart disease
Excessive alcohol intake
Cigarette smoking
Hyperlipidemia
Cocaine use

Unmodifiable

Gender
Age
Race

the ophthalmic artery results in unilateral visual symptoms, known as *amaurosis fugax*. In this condition, the individual loses sight in one eye for 2 to 3 minutes as a result of a transient ischemia of the retina.

Angiography reveals the location of the pathologic process in the cerebral arteries. Radiopaque substances are injected to outline the cerebral vasculature, identifying areas of narrowing or disease.

Ischemic Strokes

Ischemic stroke results from thrombosis formation and emboli in the cerebral vessels. The effects of occlusion vary with its extent of involvement, time, and location. In addition, the collateral vessels available to divert the remaining circulation affect the blood flow to a specific area of the brain. Obstruction of the flow to any region rapidly results in cellular ischemia and potentially irreversible necrosis and cerebral infarction.

CELLULAR AND MOLECULAR EFFECT OF ISCHEMIC STROKES. Whether the ischemic stroke results from a thrombus or embolus, oxygen is depleted within 10 seconds of cessation of blood flow to the central ischemic core area. Irreversible neuron damage occurs here within 2 to 4 minutes.[20] The area surrounding the central ischemic core, called the *ischemic penumbra*, remains potentially viable for longer periods. Current research is focusing on a means to protect and salvage this tissue. It has been observed that neurons die in the ischemic penumbra area as a result of excessive stimulation of glutamate receptors.[18] Glutamate, an excitatory neurotransmitter, is normally closely regulated by sodium reuptake systems in neurons and glia. These systems are no longer functional with ischemia.

The most devastating events occur in the central core area of blood-deprived tissue where cell viability is short lived. Mitochondria can no longer produce ATP,

TABLE 31-8

MAJOR TYPES OF STROKES

TYPE OF STROKE	ETIOLOGY	WARNING SIGNS	ONSET	COURSE
ISCHEMIC				
Thrombotic	Atherosclerosis of large cerebral arteries	TIA often	During sleep or upon awakening	Sudden or stuttering progression over minutes to hours
Embolic	Myocardial infarction, CHF, valvular disease, atrial fibrillation	TIA occasionally	Sudden during activity	Sudden, singular event attaining maximum deficits within minutes of onset
HEMORRHAGIC				
Parenchymal	Hypertension	Headache	During activity	Sudden event with progressive worsening of deficits over 15–30 minutes
Subarachnoid	Ruptured cerebral aneurysm or arteriovenous malformation (AVM)	Headache	During activity	Single event with rapid deterioration of function

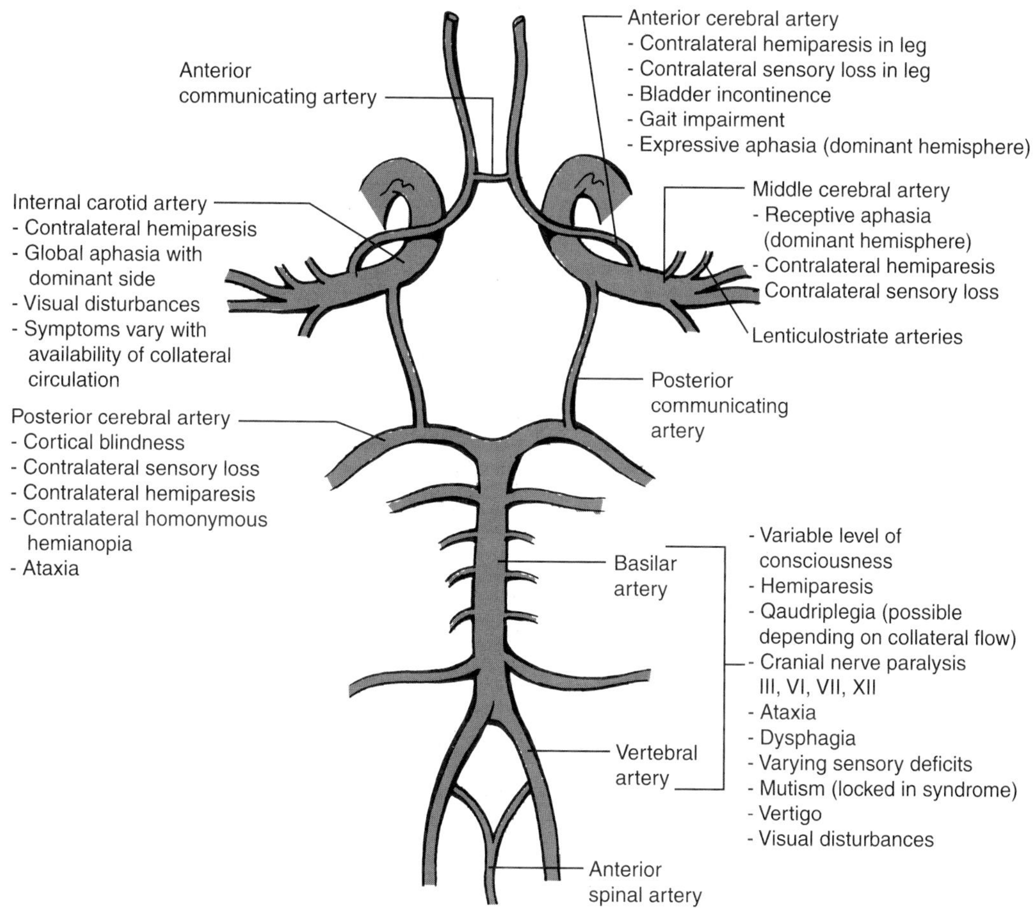

FIGURE 31-10. **Clinical manifestations of occlusion of major cerebral arteries at the circle of Willis. Variation is seen when adequate collateral circulation is present.**

the energy for cellular processes. Anaerobic glucose metabolism and accumulation of lactate (lactic acid) result.

Ionic gradients are disrupted, resulting in cellular influx of sodium, chloride, calcium, and water. The loss of the transmembrane sodium gradient inhibits glutamate uptake.[18] Destructive processes occur with the accumulation of glutamate and other ionic substances, resulting in the cell-damaging process known as *excitotoxicity*. However, the primary culprit in excitotoxicity is glutamate.[17,18,24]

Glutamate accumulation stimulates glutamate receptors in the surrounding neurons to allow calcium and sodium into the cell, resulting in neuron depolarization and influx of yet more calcium through voltage-gated channels.[18] Excessive intracellular calcium produces severe cellular damage, including the activation of cellular substances such as prostaglandin, arachidonic acid, cytokines, and leukotrienes, all of which can destroy cell membranes, cytoskeleton, and DNA.[9]

Free radicals are associated with hypoxic neuron damage and breakdown. Free radicals, molecules with unpaired electrons, are produced through many metabolic processes but primarily in the mitochondria, where they are produced as a result of the oxidative processes generating ATP. Free radicals also contribute to increases in intracellular calcium levels by damaging the proteins involved in calcium regulation.[17] Elevated intracellular calcium stimulates further production of free radicals and accumulation of nitiric oxide (NO), also contributing to cellular breakdown. The cascade of biochemical and molecular events occurring with hypoxia is depicted in Flowchart 31-1.

After about 24 hours, liquefaction (the change to a liquid by action of hydrolytic enzymes) of the ischemic area becomes evident. Demyelination and loss of glial tissue results. Edema peaks about 3 days after the occlusion.[9] Liquefactive necrosis and invasion by leukocytes is evident by the fourth day after occlusion.[8] Scar tissue forms at the margins of the necrotic area. Gliosis (proliferation of glial cells) around the area is characteristic and is followed by polymorphonuclear leukocyte (PMN) exudation, leading to removal of the necrotic debris. The necrotic tissue is removed by scavenger cells and replaced by cystic scar tissue.

THROMBOTIC STROKES. Atherosclerotic thrombosis is the leading cause of strokes. The thrombus occludes the blood vessel, greatly reducing the blood flow. The most common areas of thrombus formation are those where atheromatous plaques have already resulted in narrowing of the vessels, most commonly at curves and bifurcations. Sites frequently affected include the internal carotid artery in the region of the carotid sinus, the junction of the vertebral and basilar arteries, the bifurcation of the middle cerebral artery, the posterior cerebral artery in the area of the cerebral peduncle, and the anterior cerebral artery in the area of the corpus collosum.[7]

Wide variations may be observed in clinical signs resulting from disruption of blood flow to specific regions of the brain. Occlusion of major cerebral arteries (identified in Figure 31-10) manifests the clinical findings. The resulting obstruction to blood flow leads to infarction in the area distal to the obstructed affected artery. Obstructions proximal to the circle of Willis are better tolerated than those distal because collateral circulation from the circle may be able to compensate for the obstruction. Those obstructions distal to the circle of Willis result in end artery obstruction and infarction.

The course of cerebral thrombosis usually exhibits periods of progression and periods of improvement. Progression is indicated by increasing neurologic deficits. When the stroke progresses, the pattern is apparently due to spread of the thrombus and is called a *thrombotic stroke in evolution*. The thrombosis leads to a cerebral infarction. Symptoms such as headache, vertigo, mental confusion, aphasia, and focal neurologic signs often begin or are noted in the early morning, occurring weeks to months before the stroke is completed.

Recovery is variable, depending on the location and amount of intracerebral damage. For example, improvement in function in an affected leg usually is recovered prior to arm and hand function, which may not return at all.

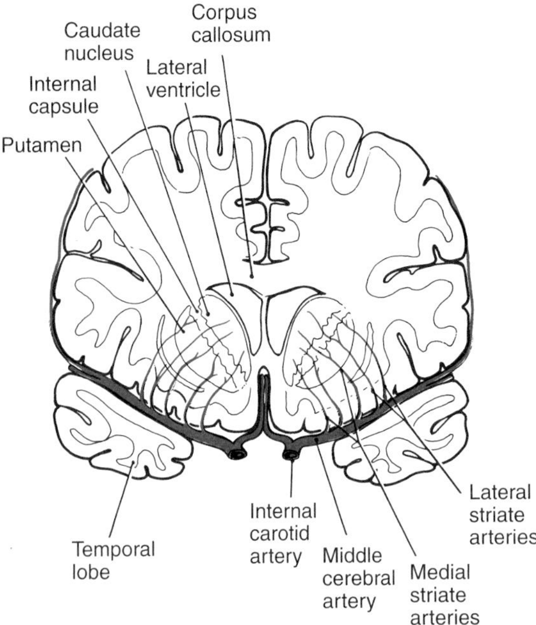

FIGURE 31-11. Coronal section of cerebral hemispheres, showing striate arterial supply from the middle cerebral artery. (Snell, R. S. [1997]. *Clinical neuroanatomy for medical students* [4th ed.]. Philadelphia: Lippincott-Raven.)

EMBOLIC STROKES. Cerebral embolism is second only to thrombosis as a cause of stroke. The main source of emboli is the heart.[19] Heart conditions that predispose an individual to cerebral embolization include atrial fibrillation, bacterial endocarditis, rheumatic endocarditis and the valvular diseases that may follow it, and congenital heart disease.[7] Less common sources of emboli include fat, air, or tumor cell emboli. The embolus frequently lodges in the middle cerebral artery, a direct continuation of the carotid artery. Massive brain infarction occurs when a large embolus lodges in a major cerebral vessel. Frequently, however, large thrombi break into smaller ones that travel to occlude more distal branches.

The onset of embolic infarction is sudden and the effect is immediate. Although usually without warning signs, some persons do experience TIAs. The clinical features depend on the artery affected and the amount and location of brain infarction.

Hemorrhagic Strokes

Hemorrhagic stroke resulting from intracranial hemorrhage is the third leading cause of strokes. Hemorrhage may occur in vessels deep within the parenchyma or close to the surface of the brain. Clinical manifestations may reflect focal involvement with localized hematomas or diffuse signs when blood extravasates throughout the subarachnoid space. Extravasated blood from any ruptured vessel is irritating to brain tissue, possibly leading to vasospasm and edema in the surrounding area.

Intracerebral Hemorrhage

Hypertension is the major cause of spontaneous bleeding into the brain parenchyma. Continued significantly elevated blood pressure weakens the vessel and eventually causes its rupture. It is thought that microaneurysms called *Charcot-Buchard aneurysms* form at bifurcations of small intracerebral arteries, probably as a result of the sustained hypertension.[3,4] A common location of small arterial hemorrhage is the penetrating branches of the middle cerebral artery, the striate arteries (Fig. 31-11). The severity of the hemorrhage is related to the amount of extravasated blood and the region of the brain affected. Intracerebral hemorrhages generally tend to occur deep within the brain substance (Fig. 31-12*A*). The most common areas of bleeding in the brain secondary to hypertension are the putamen and the adjacent internal capsule; these areas account for about 50% of cases.[1] Other potential areas include the caudate nucleus; thalamus; central white matter of the temporal, parietal, and frontal lobes; cerebellum; and pons.

In large bleeds, the extravasation of blood forms a circular type mass that disrupts and compresses surrounding brain tissue, resulting in infarction and tissue necrosis. These hemorrhages may displace midline structures that can compress vital centers, lead to coma and, eventually, death. Commonly, blood seeps into the ventricular system (Fig. 31-12*B*). Analysis of CSF reflects the presence of blood in the great majority of those who have suffered large hemorrhages. Intracerebral hemorrhages may also be small, single bleeds or have several foci. Some may reflect no obvious neurologic deficits, whereas a large number of small hemorrhages in the parenchyma may result in severe neurologic impairment.

Intracerebral bleeds occur abruptly and the symptoms evolve rapidly. Headache and nausea are warning signs. Other symptoms relate to the region of the brain involved. The blood in the parenchyma causes extensive neuronal destruction, with the central area of hemorrhage often surrounded by small hemorrhages. The blood is treated like foreign material and eventually is broken down, phagocytized by macrophages, and removed from the area. The remaining area is eventually filled with connective tissue and new capillaries.

Subarachnoid Hemorrhage

Subarachnoid hemorrhage (SAH) refers to bleeding into the subarachnoid space. Figure 31-13 shows the diffuse nature of subarachnoid hemorrhages. These may occur spontaneously with a disruption in the vascular integrity; accompany cerebral trauma, tumors, atherosclerosis, or infections (mycotic aneurysms); or, most commonly, result from congenital malformations of cerebrovascular beds, such as arteriovenous malformations or cerebral aneurysms (berry aneurysms). These may be single or occur as multiple developmental defects in the media (muscle layer) of vessels.

PATHOPHYSIOLOGY. Bleeding into the subarachnoid space originates from arterial sources. The blood mixes freely with the circulating CSF, irritating the contacting CNS structures. Arterial spasm (vasospasm), one complication of subarachnoid hemorrhage, may lead to brain infarction.

CLINICAL MANIFESTATIONS. The clinical manifestations in subarachnoid hemorrhage are generalized and in many situations do not focus in the area of involvement. Therefore, they are not significant in localizing

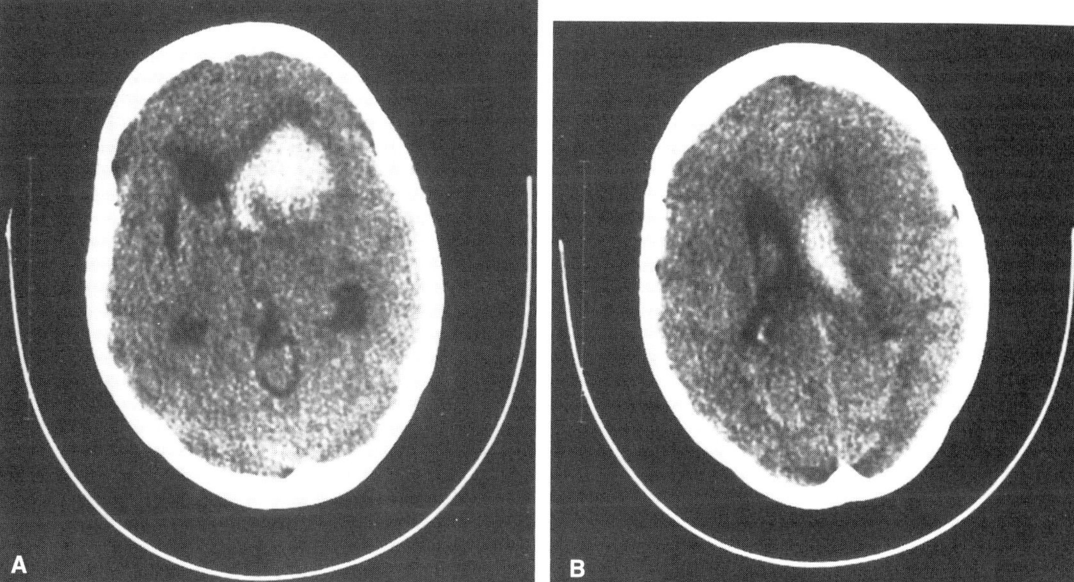

FIGURE 31-12. **A.** CT scan showing a large right hemispheric intracerebral bleed. **B.** Same bleed showing intraventricular involvement.

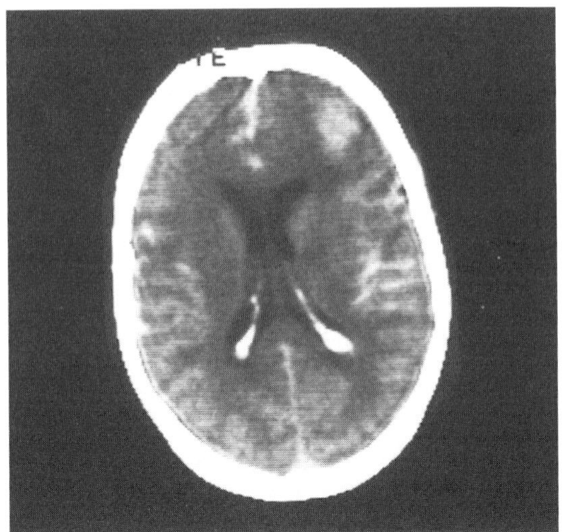

FIGURE 31-13. Subarachnoid bleeding (light diffuse areas throughout brain).

the site of hemorrhage. Clinical manifestations of subarachnoid hemorrhage are summarized in Box 31-2. On examination, the spinal fluid is grossly bloody with increased pressure, monocytes, and protein. Xanthochromia is noted within a few hours and persists for about 20 to 30 days. Cerebral angiography and CT scan may show the area of involvement and identify the subarachnoid hemorrhage by its diffuse involvement throughout the brain.

Aneurysms

Aneurysm refers to a localized dilation in the wall of a blood vessel. The etiology of cerebral aneurysms is related mainly to developmental defects, which account for 95% of aneurysms that rupture.[10] These defects involve a weakness in the middle layer (tunica media) of the vessel, resulting in a saccular out-pouching at the weakened area. Referred to as *saccular* or *berry* aneurysms, they can vary from one to several centimeters in size and generally have a well-defined neck that originates most often near bifurcations in the anterior vessels of the circle of Willis (Fig. 31-14).

Cerebral aneurysms can remain silent for many years, often going undetected throughout life and only being discovered on routine postmortem examination. They become evident during life when they rupture or compress adjacent nerve tissue, causing focal cerebral disturbances. Berry aneurysms have the highest frequency of rupture in persons between 30 and 60 years of age, affecting both sexes equally. Of individuals with developmental cerebral aneurysms, about one fifth demonstrate numerous aneurysms.

Less common than developmental aneurysms are those associated with atherosclerotic degenerative changes of the cerebral vasculature. These are known as *fusiform aneurysms* and result from a weakening of the tunica media secondary to degenerative atherosclerotic processes. The arteries become thin and fibrous, apparently as a result of long-term hypertension. Although fusiform aneurysms of cerebral arteries may occur in some younger individuals, they generally affect those over the age of 50 years.

CLINICAL MANIFESTATIONS. When an aneurysm ruptures, bleeding into the subarachnoid space occurs. The signs and symptoms may be localized from the pressure exerted on surrounding tissue. When present, focal signs are related to the region of the brain involved and may include visual defects, cranial nerve paralysis, hemiparesis, and focal seizures. Generalized signs reflect meningeal irritation and include photophobia, fever, malaise, vomiting, abnormal mentation with disorientation, and nuchal rigidity. If conscious, the person complains of a severe headache of a different nature from any experienced previously. Transitory unconsciousness or extended coma may accompany bleeding from ruptured aneurysms. Initial and prolonged coma generally indicates an unfavorable outcome.

Neurologic findings after a ruptured cerebral aneurysm are commonly categorized according to the severity of neurologic deficits, using the Hunt and Hess Clinical Grading Scale system as follows:[11]

- Grade I—Alert and oriented, mild headache, minimal nuchal rigidity, no neurologic deficits
- Grade II—Alert and oriented, moderate to severe headache, signs of meningeal irritation, no neurologic deficits except cranial nerve palsies.
- Grade III—Drowsy and confused, minimal focal neurologic deficits, signs of meningeal irritation
- Grade IV—Stuporous and unresponsive, major neurologic deficits may be present, mild decerebrate rigidity
- Grade V—Coma and decerebrate rigidity, moribund appearance

BOX 31-2

CLINICAL MANIFESTATIONS OF SUBARACHNOID HEMORRHAGE

Severe headache
Visual disturbances (photophobia, diplopia, visual deterioration)
Fever
Malaise
Vomiting
Nuchal rigidity
Alteration in mentation and disorientation
Possible loss of consciousness

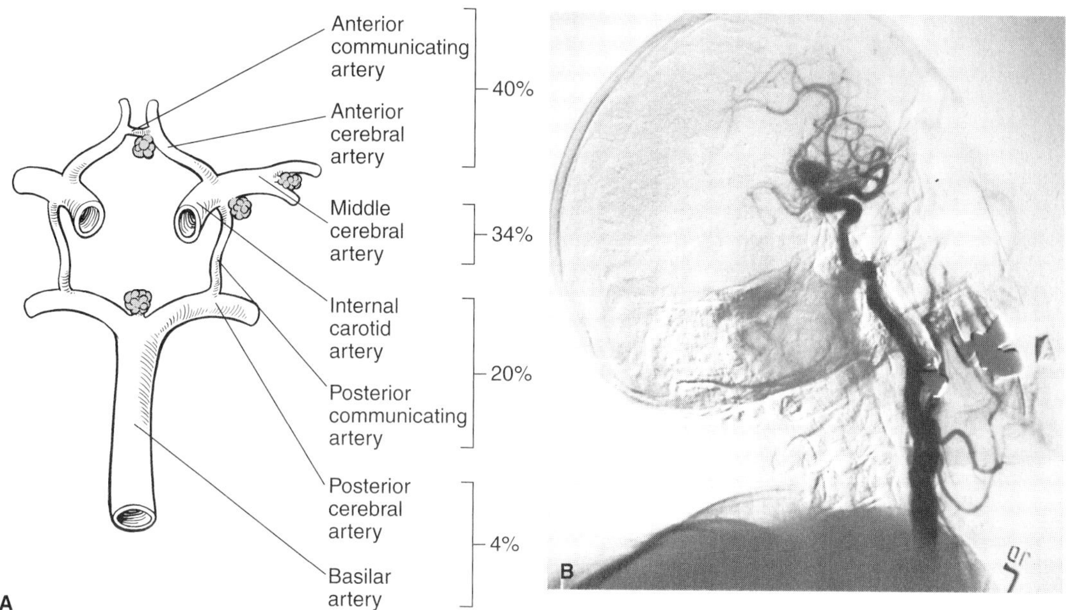

FIGURE 31-14. **A.** Common sites for berry aneurysms in the circle of Willis. **B.** Arteriogram showing cerebral aneurysm involving the anterior communicating artery.

After rupture, the aneurysm decreases in size and a fibrin clot forms over the site of the rupture.

COMPLICATIONS. Following rupture, the individual is at risk for rebleeding and vasospasm. The greatest risk of a recurrence of bleeding occurs during the first 24 hours after the initial bleed. Recurrent bleeding in cerebral aneurysms increases mortality risk considerably.

Vasospasm, a luminal narrowing of blood vessels surrounding a ruptured cerebral aneurysm, accounts for 50% of the morbidity and mortality of individuals who survive the initial bleed.[16] Vasospasm has been shown to develop 3 to 12 days after hemorrhage, with its highest incidence occurring 4 to 8 days after the bleed.[5,15]

With vasospasm, the vessel lumen narrows, the amount of blood flow decreases, and the velocity of the blood flow increases. These events may lead to cerebral ischemia and infarction and clinically evident neurologic deficits. These deficits appear insidiously as the amount of cerebral blood flow is decreased and are reflected as changes in the LOC, speech, headache, and orientation in concert with focal motor deficits.

The precise cause of vasospasm is unknown, but it is thought to be related to the release of certain intrinsic chemicals associated with lysis of the clot. These include calcium ions from lysed red blood cells, oxygen free radicals from tissue damage, and oxyhemoglobin, which in turn induce lipid peroxidation.[5] Other vasoactive substances associated with inflammation, such as serotonin, prostaglandins, catecholamines, histamine, and angiotensin, are speculated to contribute to vasospasm.[5,16]

Arteriovenous Malformations (AVM)

Arteriovenous malformations, vascular malformations, are much less common than cerebral aneurysms and usually result from developmental defects of the cerebral veins and arteries in localized regions of the brain.[14] These defects have very few distinguishing characteristics associated with their location since the changes in blood flow associated with AVMs may cause symptoms remote from the AVM.

Veins in the vascular malformations appear to connect to the arteries without an intermediate capillary bed (Fig. 31-15). The vessel walls are very thin and dilated (due to high blood flow) and lack the normal structure of arteries and veins. Although most common on the surface of the cerebral hemispheres, they may appear deeper within the cerebral lobes, brain stem, or spinal cord. Because they lack the intermediary capillary bed, they do not supply the brain with blood.

Although many AVMs are present from birth, they may not become evident until young adulthood or later. Their presence in adulthood is manifested by a clinical triad of symptoms: (1) headaches, (2) hemorrhage, and (3) seizures. Focal neurologic deficits are presumed to be secondary to ischemia from vascular "steal" (shunting of blood from better-perfused areas to the area of low intra-arterial pressure surrounding the AVM). Therefore, hypoperfusion ischemia separate from the AVM results and is manifested through neurologic deficits. Headaches may be the initial symptom presented by the patient. Their location varies, though patients frequently complain of occipital headaches,

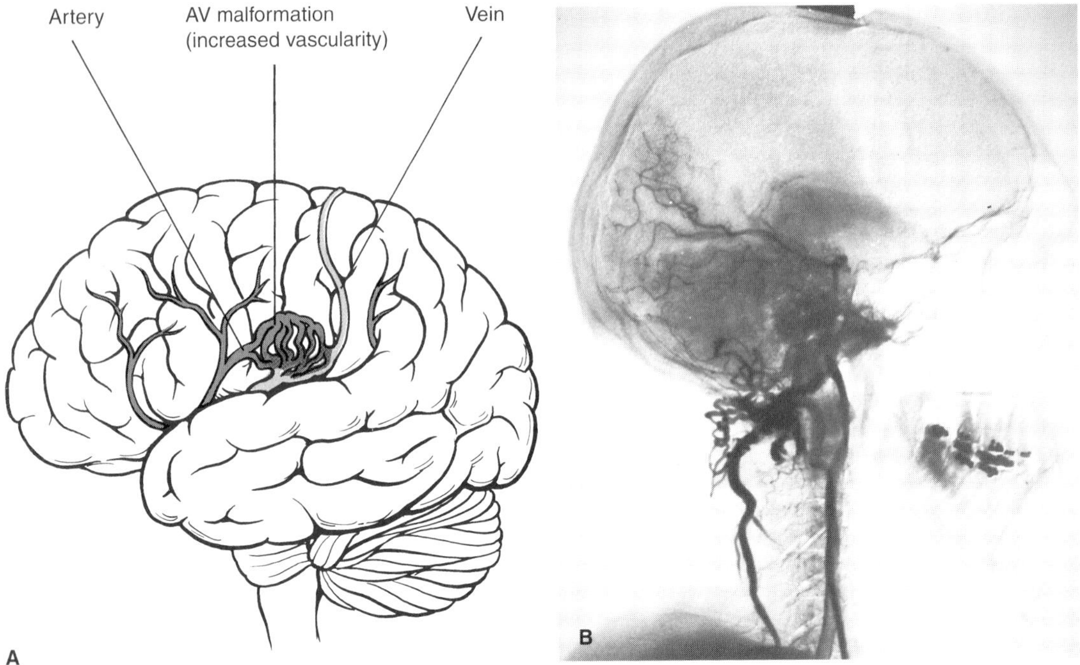

FIGURE 31-15. **A.** Appearance of superficial arteriovenous malformation. Vessels are dilated and tortuous. **B.** Arteriogram showing an arteriovenous malformation that is fed by the vertebral artery and drains into superficial veins and internal jugular vein.

describing them as similar to migraine headaches. The headache is thought to be associated with arterial engorgement and meningeal compression by the AVM.[11] A bruit may be audible over the area of the malformation.

Hemorrhage has been reported in 42% to 71% of patients who have AVMs.[11] As the very thin walls of these vessels become engorged, the vessels are particularly vulnerable to rupture and hemorrhage. Hemorrhage most commonly occurs into the subarachnoid space; therefore, the symptoms are similar to those observed with ruptured cerebral aneurysms. In addition, specific findings reflect the region of the brain that is involved. Seizures, which occur in about 70% of persons having AVMs, are associated mostly with large, superficial, supratentorial AVMs.[11] CT scan, which often detects AVMs first, reveals the tortuous vessels, which may have become calcified with time.

Traumatic Injury to Cranial Nerves

Persons who have suffered a head injury may experience partial or total loss of function of cranial nerves. Any brain injury may be accompanied by cranial nerve dysfunction; however, persons who have experienced brain stem injury are particularly susceptible to cranial nerve injury. Table 31-9 summarizes cranial nerve injuries that may accompany traumatic head injuries.

SPINAL INJURY

Spinal injuries can be traumatic or nontraumatic. Traumatic spinal injuries result when excessive force is exerted on the spinal cord. Any region of the cord may be involved, and the associated clinical manifestations reflect the deficits at the level of injury. Nontraumatic spinal injuries may also occur in some situations with no identifiable history of trauma.

Spinal Cord Injury

Traumatic spinal cord injuries (SCIs) are increasing due to the extensive use of the automobile and increased time spent in recreation and sports activities. Traumatic spinal cord injury affects the male population more frequently than females.

The extent and level of SCI vary widely. For example, whiplash, an injury to the cervical spine or its supporting structures, occurs in acceleration injuries and may result in very minor discomfort from the mild hyperextension type of cord injury. Total quadriplegia may result from serious spinal cord damage associated with severe fracture dislocations of the cervical vertebral column. Traumatic injury to the spinal cord can occur

TABLE 31-9

CRANIAL NERVE INJURIES

CRANIAL NERVE	FUNCTION	MECHANISM OF INJURY	RESULTING DEFICIT
CN I olfactory	Smell	Damage of nerve filaments with anterior fossa basilar skull fractures	**Anosmia** (loss of smell)
CN II Optic	Vision	Injury to retina and/or visual pathways, to blood vessels supplying them, to occipital area; most commonly associated with fracture of frontal skull	Varying patterns of visual loss
CN III, IV, VI Oculomotor Trochlear Abducens	III—Innervation of levator palperae superious muscle (eyelid elevation), superior and inferior recti, inferior oblique, minor rectus, and constrictor muscle of eye IV—Innervation of superior oblique muscle VI—Innervation of superior, inferior and medial rectus muscles	Compression of CN III at cerebral peduncle Injury to midbrain and pons Brain stem hemorrhage or injury	Ptosis, anisocoria, decreased light reflex response Paralysis of extraocular movements (EOMs) Diplopia
CN V Trigeminal	Sensation over entire face Innervation of muscles of mastication	Compression fracture of supraorbital area Laceration of infraorbital area Extracranial portions most often involved in traumatic injuries	Paresthesias, hyperesthesias, and neurologic pain of forehead and scalp Anesthesia of cheek and upper lip
CN VII Facial	Motor control of face muscles of expression and taste sensation in anterior two-thirds of tongue	Fracture of petrous porous portion of temporal bone and basilar skull fracture	Facial paralysis
CN VIII Vestibulocochlear	Hearing, balance, and equilibrium	Skull fracture and hemorrhage extending through the middle ear	Hearing impairment, vertigo, nausea, and vomiting
CNN IX, X Glossopharyngeal Vagus	IX—Innervation of muscles of the pharynx, mediates sensation from posterior one third of tongue, sensations of tonsils, pharynx, carotid sinuses and bodies	Injury to lower brain stem, fracture of posterior fossa, and vascular injury to vessels supplying these nerves	Dysphagia Diminished or absent gag reflex Autonomic disequilibrium
XI Accessory	Innervation of sternocleidomastoid and trapezius muscles	Low brain stem injury Posterior fossa basilar skull fracture	Weakness of sternocleidomastoid and trapezius muscles
XII Hypoglossal	Innervation of muscles of tongue	Same as CN XI	Unilateral tongue weakness

at any level, although the areas most frequently damaged are the lower cervical spine, particularly the C-5–C-6 region (Fig. 31-16) and the upper thoracic spine. Usually there is an associated vertebral column injury with spinal cord injury.

ETIOLOGY

Common mechanisms of SCI from traumatic impact include (1) hyperextension, (2) hyperflexion injuries, frequently accompanied by (3) rotational movement, (4) vertical compression, or (5) lateral flexion.[1,21] Penetrating injuries, such as missile trauma or stab wounds, are commonplace. The resultant spinal cord damage may be transient or permanent, depending on the extent of parenchymal damage. Primary and secondary injuries similar to those occurring to the brain can also occur to the spinal cord, including concussion, contusion, hemorrhage, laceration, ischemia, and edema.

Associated vertebral injuries may lead to spinal cord damage in subluxation (incomplete), compression fractures, and fracture dislocations, and other vertebral injuries. The extent of cord damage in vertebral injuries is related to the degree of bony encroachment or compression on the cord. Severe injuries result in partial or complete functional transection of the spinal cord. These make the individual susceptible to immobility, muscle atrophy, bone demineralization, infections, thrombus formation, and skin breakdown.

PATHOPHYSIOLOGY

Experimentally induced SCI in laboratory animals has provided insight into the structural changes occurring at varying times after injury. A force strong enough to result in irreversible total paraplegia causes severe ischemia, edema, and hemorrhage within a few hours, which then lead to massive necrosis and, finally, parenchymal and vessel destruction.

Immediately after cord injury, ischemic events similar to those described for traumatic brain injury and focal hemorrhages begin in the gray matter. The gray matter rapidly increases in size until the entire gray matter is hemorrhagic and necrotic, eventually forming a cystic cavity surrounded by glial scarring. Hemorrhages occurring in the white matter proximal to the gray matter do not fuse but are associated with massive edema that envelops all of the white matter. The cord edema frequently spreads to involve surrounding segments. It has been speculated that norepinephrine, which is released in large amounts by the traumatized cord, contributes to the hemorrhagic necrosis caused through direct physical damage.[10] The lesion, the area of injury, is progressive for several hours. After the injury, the hemorrhage into the gray matter is present within 15 minutes, and disintegration of the myelin sheath and axonal shrinkage occur within 1 to 4 hours.[2,10]

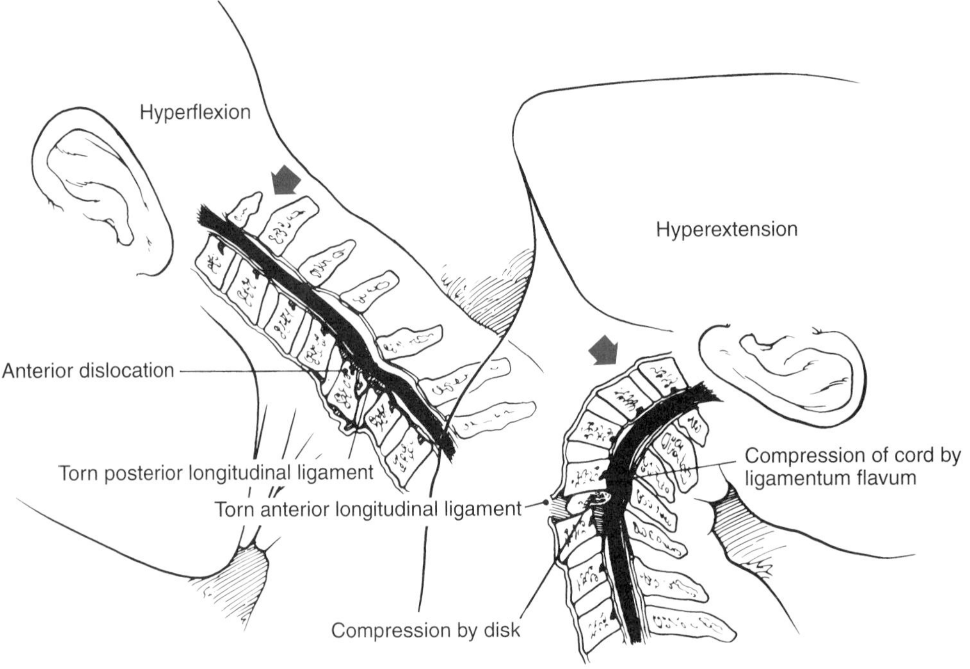

FIGURE 31-16. Mechanisms of spinal injury. (Kenner, C. V., Guzetta, C. E. & Dossey, B. M. [1992]. *Critical care nursing* [3rd ed.]. Philadelphia: J. B. Lippincott.)

CLINICAL MANIFESTATIONS

Clinical manifestations of spinal cord injuries are reflective of the level of injury on the vertical plane and the region of cord involvement on the horizontal plane. Figure 31-17*A* shows the loss of motor and sensory function below the level of the lesion in complete spinal cord transection.

Complete Cord Syndromes

In complete cord syndromes, all motor and sensory function is lost below the level of the lesion.

CERVICAL CORD INJURY. Significant cervical cord injuries render the individual quadraplegic. Clinical manifestations of the cervical level injured vary.

- Injuries at the fourth cervical spine (C-4) and above may be fatal because innervation of the diaphragm and intercostal muscles may be obliterated by the injury, and the individual dies from respiratory failure if not supported immediately with artificial ventilations. High cervical cord transection results in **quadriplegia**.
- Patients with fifth cervical cord (C-5) injuries have full innervation of the sternocleidomastoid, trapezius, and other muscles; therefore, neck, shoulder, and scapula movement is retained.
- Patients with sixth cervical segment (C-6) injuries have function of the shoulder and elbow and partial function of the wrist. Complete innervation of the rotator muscles of the shoulder is retained, and partial innervation is transmitted to the serratus, pectoralis major, and latissimus dorsi muscles. The wrist muscles and the biceps retain innervation, allowing for elbow and wrist flexion.
- Patients with injuries at the seventh (C-7) and eighth (C-8) cord segments exhibit additional elbow, wrist, and hand function. Innervation is intact to the triceps and common and long finger extensors, enabling elbow extension and flexion, and functional, although weak, finger extension and flexion.

THORACIC CORD INJURY. Significant injuries to the region of the thoracic cord result in **paraplegia**. Specific clinical manifestations vary based on the thoracic level injured.

- Patients with high thoracic injury, of the first thoracic cord segment (T-1), retain full innervation of upper-extremity musculature. Respiratory compromise results from incomplete intercostal innervation of the respiratory muscles.
- Patients with injuries at the sixth thoracic segment (T-6) have an increased respiratory reserve as intercostal innervation is intact.
- Patients with 12th thoracic segment (T-12) lesions have partial innervation to the lower extremities and may, in fact, regain ambulation when supported by long-leg braces and assisted by crutches.
- Patients with low lumbar and sacral cord lesions have full innervation to the upper extremities and trunk, hip flexors and extensors, knee extensors, and ankle movement. Therefore, these individuals are able to ambulate with minimal supportive devices.

Incomplete Cord Injuries (Cord Syndromes)

Whereas complete cord lesions result in loss of all motor and sensory function below the level of the lesion, partial lesions produce varying injuries with unique clinical manifestations.

CENTRAL CORD SYNDROME. **Central cord syndrome** (Fig. 31-17*B*) results from lesions or injury to the central part of the cord, usually as a result of hyperextension injuries secondary to trauma of the cervical cord. To a lesser extent, it is also associated with disruption in cervical cord blood supply and degenerative processes of the spine. Central cord syndrome symptoms vary with the extent of trauma and edema and the specific

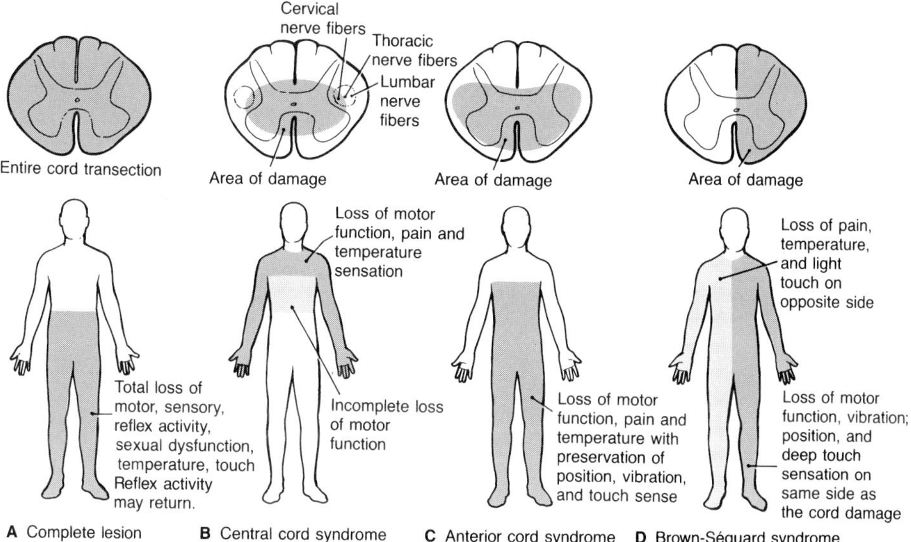

FIGURE 31-17. Spinal cord syndromes.

location. Motor weakness occurs in both upper and lower extremities. However, the upper extremities exhibit a greater motor weakness because more damage occurs to the centrally located cervical tracts supplying the upper extremities. Loss of pain and temperature sensation varies, although greater losses occur in the upper extremities.

ANTERIOR CORD SYNDROME. With **anterior cord syndrome**, damage occurs to the anterior portion of the spinal cord. Anterior cord syndrome injuries occur as a result of forward dislocation or subluxation of vertebrae, acute intravertebral herniations, flexion injuries, and conditions that compress arteries supplying the anterior spinal cord.[23] This relatively rare injury is usually seen in individuals over the age of 40. With anterior cord syndrome, motor function, touch, pain, and temperature sensation below the level of the injury is abolished (Fig. 31-17*C*). The senses of vibration, touch, and position are retained. The spinothalamic and corticospinal tracts project through this area of the cord and therefore, produce clinical findings associated with disruption of these tracts.

BROWN-SÈQUARD SYNDROME. **Brown-Sèquard syndrome** results from injury to one side of the spinal cord, possibly the result of a transverse hemisection secondary to stab or missile injury, trauma resulting in fracture-dislocation of a spinous process, or an acute herniated intervertebral disk (Fig. 31-17*D*). The clinical findings reveal ipsilateral paralysis and loss of proprioception, touch, and vibratory sense, in conjunction with contralateral loss of pain and temperature sensation below the level of the lesion. Horner's syndrome may accompany Brown-Sèquard cord injuries at or above the T-1 level. This is supported by findings of ptosis, pupillary constriction, and anhidrosis on the affected side. In Horner's syndrome, the preganglionic sympathetic neurons are involved at the level of injury.[6,24]

Spinal Cord Recovery After Injury

Significant spinal cord injuries such as cord transections result in immediate loss of all voluntary movement from the segments below the injury. The skin and other tissues become permanently anesthetized. Initially, with spinal shock, reflex activity is abolished; however, reflexes eventually return and may become hyperactive. Recovery after spinal cord injury can be viewed through stages of (1) spinal shock, (2) return of flexion-extension reflexes, and (3) return of autonomic reflexes.

SPINAL SHOCK. The rapid depression of cord reflex activity after high cord injury (above T-6) is referred to as **spinal shock**. It results from the interruption of neural pathways with the remainder of the CNS. Spinal shock is most dramatically associated with complete cord transections; in lesser injuries it may not be as severe or may even be absent.

Although the exact mechanism causing spinal shock and recovery of reflexes is still elusive, it has been speculated that the excitatory effects of alpha and gamma motor neurons from higher centers on other spinal motor neurons are lost due to disruption of the descending pathways. Therefore, inhibitory spinal internuncial neurons become disinhibited, resulting in reduced resting excitability and diminished reflexes. Considerable variability of the duration of spinal shock exists in humans. Some reflexes may reappear as early as 2 or 3 days after injury, whereas others may not return for 6 weeks or longer. The earliest indicator of resolution of spinal shock is the return of perianal reflexes. Spinal shock is more pronounced in the cord segments surrounding the lesion, and recovery of reflexes generally occurs there last.

In addition to areflexia in spinal shock, clinical signs include unopposed parasympathetic autonomic deficits, reflected in hypotension from loss of vasomotor tone; bradycardia, associated with reflex vagal stimulation; and loss of sweating, piloerection, and body temperature control below the area of injury. The body tends to assume the temperature of the environment (*poikilothermia*). Because of depressed vasoconstrictive action below the level of the lesion, individuals are susceptible to severe postural hypotension. Bowel and bladder reflexes from the sacrum are inhibited, and control over their functions is temporarily lost during spinal shock. Loss of sensation and flaccid paralysis occur below the transection site. Considerable variation exists with individual functional capacity after cord injury; therefore, variation is observed in the extent of spinal shock.

FLEXION-EXTENSION REFLEXES. The return of stretch and flexion reflexes after severe cord injury is first noted in response to noxious stimulation. An example of this response is the dorsiflexion of the great toe (Babinski's sign) in response to stimulation of the sole of the foot. Complications such as infection and malnutrition may delay the return of the flexor responses. As the flexor reflex recovers, it gradually becomes excited more readily from wider areas of the skin.

As recovery progresses after cord injury, flexor reflexes are interspersed with extensor spasms, ultimately progressing to predominantly extensor activity. Individuals with partial cord transection generally exhibit strong extensor spasticity. However, this seldom occurs with complete transection.

AUTONOMIC REFLEXES. The autonomic spinal reflexes include those that control reflexive action of vasomotor activity, diaphoresis, and emptying of the bladder and rectum. Vasomotor reflexes are abolished below the level of transection during spinal shock. With time, tonic autonomic activity returns and wide fluctuations in arterial pressure diminish. Temperature control by the skin is essentially abolished for a time after spinal transection as autonomic innervation for sweating is suppressed.

Reflex emptying of the bladder and rectum does occur in individuals with spinal transections after a period of initial atony and increased sphincter tone. Dilation of the bladder with urine eventually overcomes sphincter resistance and overflow incontinence occurs. With progression of time, spontaneous, brief contractions of the bladder evolve into larger contractions that are accompanied by bladder sphincter opening and brief micturition. Thus, small amounts of urine are voided with varying amounts of residual urine retained. Sensory stimuli such as tapping on the abdomen, anal stimulation, or stroking the inner aspect of the upper thigh may be used to precipitate micturition.

AUTONOMIC DYSREFLEXIA OR AUTONOMIC HYPERREFLEXIA. **Autonomic dysreflexia** is an exaggerated autonomic response involving a cluster of symptoms in which many spinal cord autonomic responses discharge simultaneously and excessively. This syndrome occurs in persons with high spinal cord injuries above the level of the sixth or seventh thoracic cord segment.[10] Its occurrence is highly unpredictable, possibly arising unexpectedly years after the injury.

The symptoms, a result of afferent sensory transmission blockage at the level of the lesion, occur in response to specific noxious stimuli, appear quickly, and may lead to life-threatening conditions, such as severe hypertension, seizures, cerebral hemorrhage, and myocardial infarction.[1,12] Precipitating factors leading to autonomic dysreflexia most commonly include bladder and bowel distention or manipulation. Other triggering stimuli may include pressure ulcers, spasticity, stimulation of pain receptors, pressure on the penis, and strong uterine contractions.[12]

A large portion of the sympathetic nervous system is being stimulated by sensory receptors. Visceral or noxious agents stimulate sensory receptors, which transmit to the spinal cord and ascend the posterior columns and spinothalamic tracts.

As the impulses ascend the cord, they reflexively stimulate the neurons of the sympathetic nervous system in the lateral horn of the cord. Since the modulating effects from higher centers are blocked, the sympathetic reflex activity continues unabated, causing arteriolar spasm and vasoconstriction of the skin and pelvic viscera.[12] As a result, the individual may experience a pounding headache, blurred vision, and severe hypertension that may rise as high as 300 mm Hg systolic.

The increased blood pressure distends the carotid sinus and aortic arch baroreceptors, which in turn stimulate the vagus nerve to decrease the heart rate and dilate the skin vessels above the level of the lesion in an attempt to lower the blood pressure. The dilated vessels produce flushing and profuse diaphoresis above the level of injury.

Because the impulses from higher centers are blocked to the lower body, the vessels there remain vasoconstricted and the individual exhibits *cutes anserina* (goose flesh) and pale skin below the lesion. Other symptoms include restlessness, nasal congestion, and nausea. The events and clinical manifestations of autonomic dysreflexia are summarized in Figure 31-18.

Intervertebral Disk Herniation

Intervertebral disks, fibrocartilagenous bodies positioned between the vertebrae of the spinal column, are composed of a central portion, the semigelatinous *nucleus pulposus*, surrounded by fibrous rings, the *annulus fibrosus*. The nucleus pulposus serves as a transport medium between the disk and surrounding capillaries and as a shock absorber for the vertebral column. In addition to encasing the nucleus pulposus, the annulus fibrosus also serves as a vertebral shock absorber and allows for vertebral motion. Intervertebral disks and vertebral bodies are joined by longitudinal ligaments anteriorly and posteriorly within the vertebral canal.

Approximately 50% of the cases of herniation or rupture of the nucleus pulposus of the intervertebral disk are caused by minor or major trauma. In other cases, however, the onset is acute with no history of serious trauma. Sudden straining of the back in an unusual position and lifting while bending forward are frequently reported to be associated with disk herniation. The most common injury occurs in the lumbosacral intervertebral disks (L-4–L-5 and L-5–S-1), which reflects a clinical picture of sciatica. Herniations of the cervical disks occur occasionally, whereas those in the thoracic region are rare.

Herniation of the nucleus pulposus produces pain, sensory loss, and paralysis from pressure on the spinal nerve roots or on the spinal cord (Fig. 31-19).

Symptoms of herniated disk are similar to those of other conditions, including spinal cord tumors, syringomyelia, spinal arthritis, and other degenerative disk conditions. Radiologic findings supportive of a herniated disk show loss of normal curvature of the spine, scoliosis, and narrowing of intervertebral spaces.

LUMBOSACRAL HERNIATIONS

The vast majority of the lumbosacral herniations occur between the fourth or fifth lumbar and first sacral interspaces. Sciatic symptoms associated with a lumbosacral herniation include pain in the lower back radiating down the posterior surface of one or both legs. The pain occurs as a result of posterolateral displacement of the disk and compression on the pain sensory pathways of the cord or sensory part of the compressed nerve. In unilateral involvement, scoliosis oc-

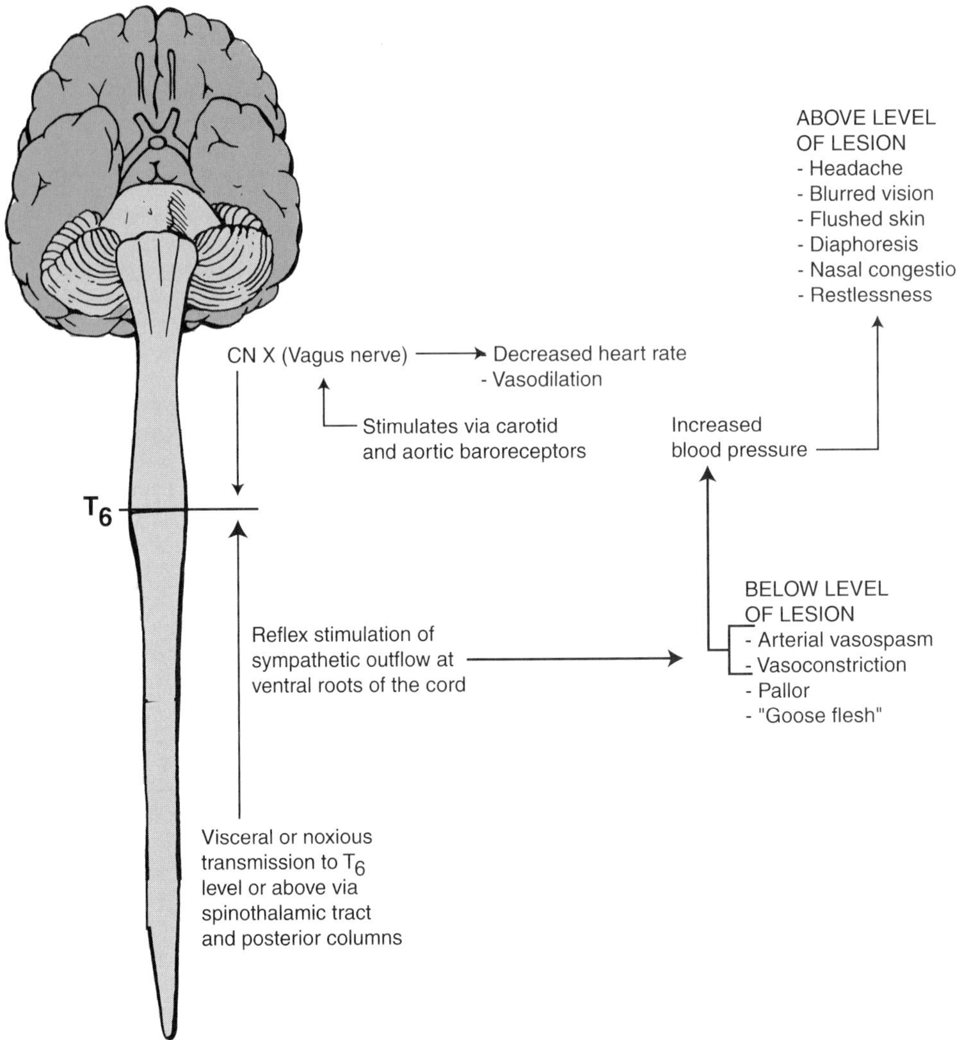

FIGURE 31-18. **Autonomic dysreflexia showing mass sympathetic stimulation below the level of lesion with resulting findings below the level of lesion. Counterbalancing stimuli from above the level of lesion are blocked. Resulting manifestations above the level of lesion are identified.**

curs toward the side opposite the sciatic pain, and movement of the lumbar spine is limited. Paresthesias in the leg or foot are common. Tenderness is experienced on palpation along the course of the sciatic nerve. Motor weakness occurs in a small percentage of cases. Hypoesthesia to touch or pinprick is present in about one-half of cases. A decreased or absent ankle reflex is common with herniation of the lumbosacral disk. Coughing, sneezing, or straining may produce radiation of pain along the course of the sciatic nerve. Generally, symptoms are unilateral; however, with large central protrusions, they may be bilateral.

CERVICAL HERNIATIONS

Herniation of the cervical disks occurs most commonly at the level of the fifth through seventh cervical roots. Displacement of the disk in this region causes neck stiffness and shoulder pain radiating down the arm into the hand. Paresthesias may accompany the pain. Weakness and atrophy of the bi-

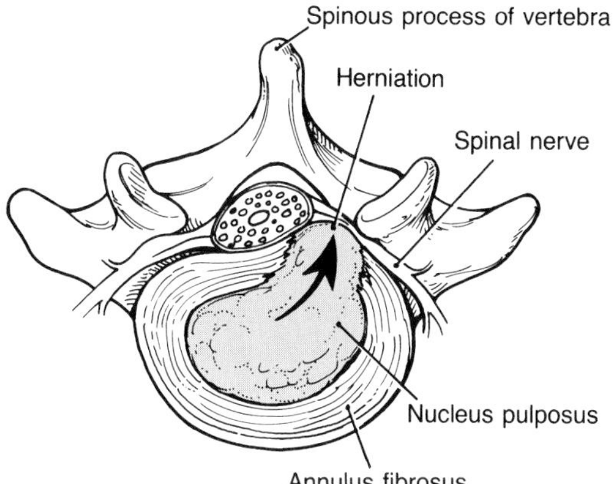

FIGURE 31-19. **Herniated disk with the nucleus pulposus in the spinal root.**

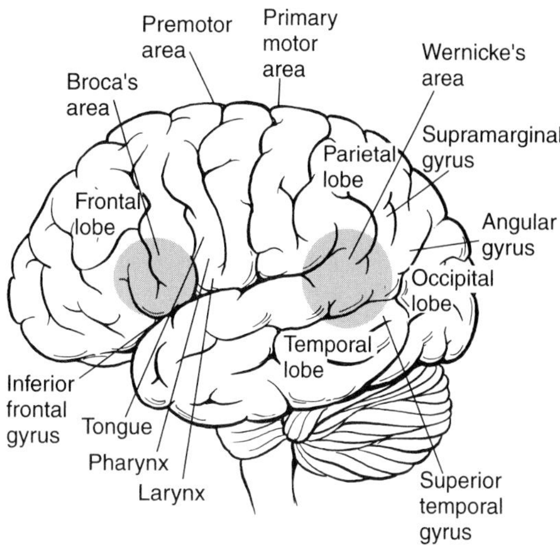

FIGURE 31-20. **Location of language centers in the brain.**

ceps and diminution of the biceps reflex may be present with sixth cervical root damage. Paresthesias and sensory loss in the index finger, weakness of the triceps muscle, and loss of triceps reflex are indicative of involvement of the seventh cervical root. Eighth cervical root compression reflects forearm pain along the medial side, as well as sensory loss along the medial cutaneous nerve of the forearm and ulnar nerve distribution in the hand.

HIGHER CORTICAL LEVEL INJURY

Many neurologic deficits in higher nervous system function can be associated with traumatic, cerebrovascular, and other neurologic disorders. These include deficits in language and problems with comprehension and recognition of oneself, others, and one's surroundings. Seizures reflect a brain disorder that manifests chaotic electrical activity, frequently as a result of underlying injury or disease.

Aphasia

Aphasia is the loss of neurologic capacity for language. Language is a function primarily of the dominant (left) cerebral hemisphere. Figure 31-20 shows the approximate location of the speech centers in the brain. The ability to produce language depends on the normal function and integrity of the primary receptive area in the temporal lobe and the expressive areas in the inferior part of the frontal lobe of the dominant hemisphere. To speak, one must initially formulate the thought to be expressed, choose appropriate words, and then control the motor activity of the muscles of phonation and articulation. Simultaneously, accurate recording of visual and auditory stimuli is necessary before the significance of the words used can be appreciated. Language and speech may become impaired in many ways. Regardless of the cause, the results are generally similar when the brain is damaged.

The ability either to comprehend and integrate *receptive language* or to formulate and use *expressive language*, or both, are impaired. The receptive language modalities are

- Reading, which requires visual integration and comprehension of the printed word
- Listening, which necessitates auditory integration and comprehension of the verbal word

The expressive language modalities are

- Writing, which requires visual-motor formulation and use of the printed word
- Speaking, which requires oral-motor formulation and the use of verbal words

The aphasic individual usually has some impairment of all language modalities.

ETIOLOGY

Aphasia is usually caused by organic brain disease resulting from a lesion in the left cerebral hemisphere. This hemisphere is considered to be dominant in the reception and expression of language in most individuals. Infrequently, aphasia has occurred in right-sided lesions associated with right-handed individuals; however, their right-handedness has sometimes been forced or induced. In left-handed persons, lesions of the left or right hemisphere may cause aphasia, but more frequently the left hemisphere.

Vascular disturbances are the most common cause of aphasia. When certain portions of the cortex and subcortical association pathways of the dominant hemisphere are altered by lack of blood supply (loss of oxygen or hemorrhage to the brain tissue), speech patterns become altered, limited, or destroyed, depending on the magnitude of the pathology. Infarction, caused by thrombotic or embolic occlusion of the middle cerebral artery or the left internal carotid artery, is implicated in the majority of cases of aphasia. Both spoken and written language are impaired. Transient ischemic attacks and migraine headache may trigger transitory language disorders.

Trauma and space-occupying lesions, such as intracerebral hemorrhage, intracranial tumors, and infections, also may cause aphasia. Left hemisphere aphasia results from damage to a specific region of the brain, the first and second temporal gyri, the insula, and the posterior part of the third convolution. Visual and auditory impulses reach the cerebral cortex posteriorly through the occipital lobe and anteroinferiorly through the temporal lobe. Many cortical areas and association pathways are concerned in the integration of the function of speech.

Many combinations of vascular, neoplastic, and traumatic causes and locations of lesions lead to different language patterns. Classifications have been developed to define prominent characteristics, to localize position and size of cerebral lesions, and to assess the language deficit pattern in each category of aphasia. The primary types of speech disorders are: (1) Wernicke's (receptive) aphasia, which causes disturbances of all language activities except articulation; (2) Broca's (expressive) aphasia, involving disturbances in spoken and written language with dysarthria (disorder of articulation); (3) global aphasia, involving both Wernicke's and Broca's aphasia; and (4) selective disorders of receptive and expressive activities of spoken or written language.

Wernicke's Aphasia

Wernicke's aphasia (receptive or sensory aphasia) is an impairment in comprehension of speech and includes central, receptive, cortical, sensory, auditory, semantic, and conduction aphasia. It is also referred to as fluent aphasia. The posterior one third of the superior temporal gyrus of the dominant hemisphere is called *Wernicke's area.*[23] This area, known as the general interpretative area that influences the understanding and interpretation of word symbols, is of major importance because most intellectual functions of the brain are processed here. Association fibers provide the connection between various areas of the cerebral hemispheres and the cortex, allowing coordination of widely separated hemispheric areas. Here they provide a connection between Wernicke's area and the surrounding areas to coordinate many interpretative functions.

Lesions in surrounding areas, particularly in the posterior half of the dominant hemisphere, angular gyrus, and supramarginal gyrus, also influence speech function through association fibers, and injury to these areas produces problems with word meanings.

Affected persons have fluent, spontaneous speech with normal rhythm and articulation, but comprehension, repetition, and naming are impaired. They appear confused and lack insight into their deficit. Speech appears devoid of meaning despite the fluency and spontaneity. Expression is hindered by difficulty in choosing words to speak and to write. Repetition, reading aloud, and writing from dictation are deranged. Understanding of spoken language is disturbed. The speech of others is heard, but the words are not comprehended. Speech lacks content and contains much meaningless expression; likewise, written words lack meaning. Box 31-3 summarizes major findings associated with Wernicke's aphasia.

A common pathologic finding in Wernicke's aphasia is the occlusion of the inferior or posterior branches of the middle cerebral artery in the dominant hemisphere. Infarction of the superior temporal gyrus results, leading to significant deficits in language interpretation.

Broca's Aphasia

Broca's aphasia is a disorder of motor or expressive language resulting from lesions located in the posterior part of the inferior frontal gyrus. The person may have extremely limited speech or be unable to utter a word. It is also referred to as nonfluent aphasia because the speech is generally slow and poorly articulated. Small words are frequently omitted from sentences. Simultaneously, the person fully comprehends the spoken word and obeys commands. Efforts to speak are frustrated by an inability to find appropriate words. Box 31-3 summarizes manifestations associated with Broca's aphasia.

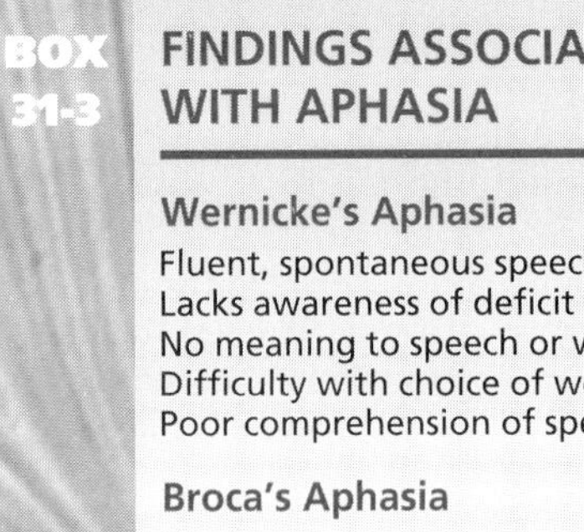

BOX 31-3 **FINDINGS ASSOCIATED WITH APHASIA**

Wernicke's Aphasia

Fluent, spontaneous speech
Lacks awareness of deficit
No meaning to speech or written word
Difficulty with choice of words
Poor comprehension of speech

Broca's Aphasia

Nonfluent, hesitating speech
Difficulty with articulation of words
Obeys commands
Comprehension of speech
Awareness of deficit

Agraphia (inability to write) coexists with aphasia and can be more severe in some individuals. *Agrammatism* (inability to arrange words in grammatical sequence or to form an intelligent sentence), when present in spoken language, is also present in written language. Unlike those suffering with Wernicke's aphasia, these individuals are aware of the problem and frequently suffer from feelings of frustration and depression.

Global Aphasia

Global aphasia is caused by large lesions involving both Broca's and Wernicke's areas of the dominant hemisphere. Commonly, the lesion is an occlusion of the left internal carotid artery or middle cerebral artery. Blood supply to the language areas of the brain is supplied almost exclusively through the middle cerebral artery.

As the term implies, global aphasia affects all aspects of speech. Individuals with global aphasia generally have right hemiplegia and are unable to comprehend or speak. At best, they may be able to utter an occasional isolated word or well-known cliché. They are unable to repeat what is said to them and are unable to read and write. Prognosis for recovery generally is poor.

Selective Disorders of Language

The pure disorders of receptive and expressive language include anarthria, agraphia, alexia, and word-deafness. In *anarthria*, reading aloud and voluntary speech repetition are disturbed, whereas understanding of spoken and written language and writing remains normal. It usually appears as a sequela to Broca's aphasia.

In *agraphia*, all forms of writing are defective. The lesion may be located in the posterior part of the second frontal gyrus. *Alexia* severely impairs reading of words, but reading of letters is less obstructed. Language activities may be normal except for the recognition of written symbols.

Apraxia

Apraxia is the inability to carry out a voluntary, purposeful motor skill despite the conductive systems being intact, indicating cerebral cortical integrative impairment. The person is able to perform individual movements involved with executing a certain act but cannot execute the total act. There is no paralysis, ataxia, abnormal movement, or sensory loss.

To execute a skilled movement, one must use a logical routine. First, the command is received at the primary auditory cortex and relayed to the auditory association areas for comprehension. Information then is relayed by the association fibers to the motor association areas in the premotor cortex of the dominant hemisphere. From the dominant premotor cortex, information is conveyed to the premotor and motor cortices of the nondominant hemisphere to enable the nondominant hand to perform the learned skilled movement.

If a person cannot carry out motor activities that were previously performed without difficulty, he or she is said to have *ideomotor apraxia*. Introducing an object will improve ideomotor apraxia. For example, a person may not be able to brush his or her teeth on command, but if a toothbrush is handed to him or her, the commanded activity is able to be performed. Ideomotor apraxia is caused by lesions to the corpus collosum, Broca's areas, and arcuate fasiculus. *Ideational apraxia* involves difficulty with conception of movements. The person may have difficulty performing an activity at all or in sequencing the activity. Introduction of objects does not improve ideational apraxia. Ideational apraxias result from tempero-parietal-occipital lesions.

Apraxia of the lips and tongue is fairly common. It may occur with lesions of the left supramarginal gyrus or the left motor association cortex, and frequently accompanies apraxia of the limbs. Apraxia of the limbs may be classified as limbic-kinetic, dressing, or constructional. These and other types of apraxias are defined in Table 31-10.

Gerstmann's Syndrome

Lesions of the left (dominant) parietal lobe, particularly of the supramarginal and angular gyrus areas, may produce one or more of a complex of symptoms known as Gerstmann's syndrome (bilateral asomatognosia). It includes right-left disorientation, that is, the inability to distinguish right from left. Finger agnosia is exhibited by failure to recognize one's fingers in the presence of intact sensation and is associated with constructional apraxia. Acalculia (inability to solve mathematical problems) and dyslexia (inability to read) are common when the lesion involves the angular gyrus of the dominant hemisphere.

Agnosia

The process of recognizing the significance of sensory stimuli is known as *gnosia*. **Agnosia**, therefore, is the impairment of recognition caused by lesions of the association areas of the cerebral cortex, even though the primary sensory pathway is intact. Perception occurs when sensory data originating at sensory receptors are forwarded by peripheral and spinal pathways to the primary sensory cortex for analysis and sorting. These data are dispatched to the association areas that contain the memory banks for higher-order interpretation. There they are translated into codes and symbols of language.

TABLE 31-10

APRAXIAS

APRAXIA	MANIFESTATIONS	AREA OF LESION
Ideational	Inability to grasp the idea required in executing a motor activity	Large areas of the cerebral cortex, corpus collosum, Broca's area, and arcuate fasiculus
Idiomotor	Inability to perform the motor act required to perform an activity	Dominant hemisphere, temporal, parietal, and occipital lobes
Limb-kinetic	Inability to execute fine motor activity in a single limb	Premotor cortex
Dressing	Inability to dress/groom oneself correctly; May be unilateral, frequently involving left side	Nondominant parietal lobe
Constructional	Inability to construct objects accurately due to disruption of spatial relationships	Right or left parietal lobe
Gait	Inability to walk in a smooth, coordinated manner; gait is short and shuffling in manner	Frontal lobe and basal ganglia
Facial	Inability to produce facial movements when commanded	Dominant hemisphere

Types of agnosia include: (1) visual agnosia, an inability to recognize objects seen; (2) tactile agnosia, an inability to identify objects by touch; and (3) auditory agnosia, an inability to recognize sounds even though auditory sensation is intact. The individual recognizes objects by one sense, yet does not recognize the same object by another sensory modality. A person with visual agnosia may not recognize a safety pin just by looking at it but can name it instantaneously if it is placed in the hand. Conversely, an individual with tactile agnosia visually identifies the safety pin that he or she was unable to recognize when it was placed in the hand.

VISUAL AGNOSIA

Visual agnosia is caused by a lesion of the visual association areas in the parieto-temporal or corpus collosum region. Lesions limited to these areas do not cause blindness; rather, objects are clearly seen but are not recognized or identified. Visual agnosia is characterized by an inability to recognize any object or shape by sight, although it can be recognized through other senses, such as touch or smell. Categories include agnosia for objects, colors, and loss of recognition of familiar faces (*prosopagnosia*).

Persons suffering from object agnosia are unable to recognize objects visually. Those with color agnosia are unable to recognize colors, a defect that may be confined to one half of the visual field (called *hemiagnosia* for colors). Prosopagnosia renders the person unable to recognize faces, sometimes even his or her own face in the mirror. The individual is unable to recognize a familiar face but can identify a person once that person starts to speak. Lesions causing prosopagnosia arise from the temporal and occipital lobes.

TACTILE AGNOSIA

Normal tactile recognition is the ability to identify an object by feeling, without the help of other sensory information. Feeling movements provide impressions until the object is identified. Lesions of the parietal lobe posterior to the somesthetic area produce tactile agnosia, or the inability to identify objects by touch and feeling, often called *astereognosis*. Some previously acquired factual information is lost from the brain's memory stores. Therefore, one cannot compare present sensory phenomena with past experience.

AUDITORY AGNOSIA

Auditory agnosia is the inability to recognize sounds. The auditory sensation is intact, but the difficulty lies in separating them from the sensory aphasias. The first temporal convolution and part of the second temporal convolution of the dominant hemisphere are considered important for auditory recognition.

From the descriptive point of view, auditory agnosia is the inability to recognize familiar concrete sounds, such as animal noises, a sounding bell, or the ticking of a clock (agnosia for nonlinguistic sounds). Other auditory perceptual disorders include verbal agnosia (the inability to recognize spoken language), sensory amusia (the inability to recognize music), and congenital auditory agnosia (primary retardation of speech development, usually associated with mental retardation).

UNILATERAL NEGLECT

Unilateral neglect is the failure to respond to stimuli in the body regions contralateral to a hemisphereic lesion. Humans build images of their bodies from sensory impulses from the special senses (skin, muscles, bones, and joints) that provide information about relationships with the body and the external environment. This concept of body image is stored in the association areas of the parietal lobes. Therefore, in unilateral neglect lesions of the nondominant (usually right side) parietal lobe, particularly the inferior parietal lobe, create abnormalities in concepts of body image whereby the individual may not respond to tactile, visual, or auditory stimuli.

Lack of awareness of the left side of the body is inhibited despite intact cortical and primary sensation. Lack of awareness of the hemiparesis is observed, such as when the individual bumps into objects on the neglected visual field side and fails to care for the neglected side of the body. Although unilateral neglect is observed primarily with parietal lesions, it may also be present with lesions of other regions of the cerebral hemispheres.

Seizure Disorders

Seizures (**epilepsy**) are characterized by sudden, excessive discharges of electrical energy in neurons. These electrical discharges, called brain waves, are recorded in cycles per second or hertz (Hz) by electroencephalogram (EEG). Normal brain waves are illustrated in Figure 31-21.

Seizures are common; there is a 6% chance of having a seizure in a person's lifetime.[9] The incidence is highest in the very young and very old. Seizures originate from diverse causes, including congenital, metabolic, toxic, degenerative, genetic, infectious, neoplastic, and traumatic, as well as from unknown causes.

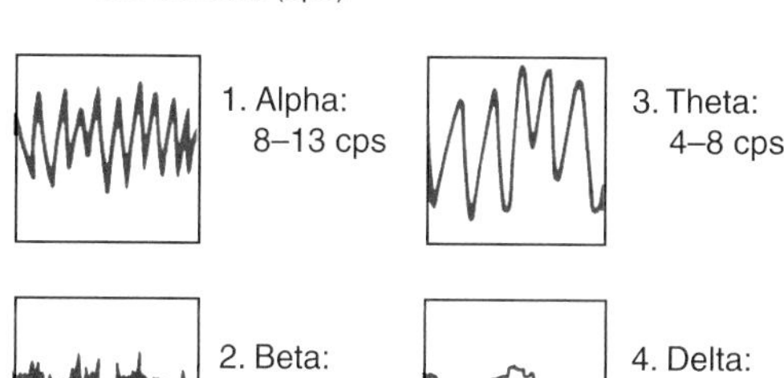

FIGURE 31-21. Frequencies of brain waves.

PATHOPHYSIOLOGY

Seizures may be linked with (1) increased local excitability (epileptogenic focus), (2) reduced inhibition, or (3) a combination of both. Some neurons in focal lesions have been identified as hypersensitive and remain in a state of partial depolarization. Increased permeability of their cytoplasmic membranes makes them susceptible to activation by hyperthermia, hypoglycemia, hyponatremia, hypoxia, trauma, infections, and repeated sensory stimulation. Reduced inhibition may be caused by impairment of the inhibitory interneurons.

When the intensity of a seizure has progressed sufficiently, it may spread to adjacent cortical, thalamic, brain stem nuclei, and other regions of the brain. Excitement feeds back from the thalamus to the primary focus and to other parts of the brain. This process is evidenced by the high-frequency discharge shown on EEG. Within the process, a diencephalocortical inhibition intermittently interrupts the discharge and converts the *tonic phase* (muscle contraction) to the *clonic phase* (alternating contraction and relaxation). The discharges become less and less frequent until they cease.

Severe seizures may cause systemic hypoxia with accompanying acidosis from accumulation of lactic acid, resulting from respiratory spasms, airway blockage, and excessive muscular activity that accompanies seizures. An extremely severe prolonged seizure can cause respiratory arrest or cardiac standstill. Metabolic needs increase markedly during a seizure, causing increased cerebral blood flow, glycolysis, and increased oxygen consumption.

CLASSIFICATION OF SEIZURES

Seizures have been classified according to the location of the focus, etiologic basis, and clinical features. The International Classification System adopted worldwide is based on clinical features and associated EEG findings in generalized and partial seizures (Box 31-4). **Generalized seizures** have bilaterally symmetric epileptigenic foci originating within deep subcortical diencephalic structures, whereas **partial seizures** usually begin in a cortical focus but may also arise from subcortical structures. Seizures may be *primary* or *idiopathic* if their origin is unknown, or *secondary* or *symptomatic* if a definitive origin is determined.

Partial Seizures

Partial seizures arise from a focal area and progress in a manner consistent to the area of irritation. They are characterized by specific, repeated patterns of activity and are of two general types: (1) *simple* or *elementary*, in which consciousness remains unimpaired, and (2) *complex*, in which there is an accompanying al-

INTERNATIONAL CLASSIFICATION OF PARTIAL AND GENERALIZED SEIZURES

I. Partial seizures (focal origin)
   A. Simple (unimpaired consciousness)
      1. Motor (Jacksonian)
      2. Sensory (visual, auditory, olfactory, gustatory, vertiginous)
      3. Autonomic
   B. Complex (impaired consciousness)
      1. Temporal lobe (psychomotor)
   C. Secondary generalization
      1. Simple or complex
II. Generalized seizures (bilateral symmetric, without focal onset)
   A. Tonic-clonic (grand mal)
   B. Absence (petit mal)
      1. Simple
      2. Complex
   C. Myoclonic
   D. Infantile spasms
   E. Atonic
   F. Lennox-Gastaut syndrome

teration in consciousness. Partial seizures may have a motor, sensory, or varied complex focus.

FOCAL MOTOR SEIZURES (JACKSONIAN SEIZURES). Focal motor seizures usually originate in the premotor cortex and cause involuntary movements of the contralateral limbs. The seizure may remain in a localized region or spread to the adjacent regions and the clinical manifestations change accordingly. Focal seizures may be associated with glial scarring, brain masses, and cerebral edema.

Typically, the convulsive movement begins in the distal portion of an extremity and progresses medially. For example, a seizure starting in the foot may move up the leg, down the arm, and to the face, or it may begin in the hand, spread to the face, and then to the leg. This is called *jacksonian march*. The seizure begins with a tonic contraction and rapidly progresses to a clonic movement. Aphasia may be present if the dominant hemisphere is involved. The episode usually lasts 20 to 30 seconds without loss of consciousness. It may spread to the opposite hemisphere and result in loss of consciousness, thus becoming a generalized seizure. Stationary focal seizures are more frequent in young children, whereas the jacksonian march appears most often in adolescents and adults.

FOCAL SENSORY SEIZURES. A lesion in the postcentral or precentral convolution of the sensory cortex in the parietal lobe provokes focal sensory seizures. Any sensory modality may be involved. A simple, uniform, tactile, auditory, or visual experience with complaints of abnormal sensations such as numbness, tingling, pins-and-needles sensation, coldness, or a sensation of water running over a portion of the body may be described. This type of seizure usually begins in the lips, fingers, and toes and remains localized or progresses to adjacent body parts. If the lesion is in the sensory association area, the experience is more complex and may be visual or auditory. If visual, sensations of light, darkness, or color may be experienced. If auditory, the person may complain of buzzing, roaring in the ears, or hearing voices or words. Consciousness and memory are preserved.

COMPLEX PARTIAL SEIZURES. Complex partial seizures, also known as psychomotor seizures, result from abnormalities in the temporal lobe, the medial surface of the hemispheres, the limbic system, and the frontal lobe. Complex partial seizures constitute approximately 40% of all seizures occurring most frequently in the second to fourth decades, although they may be manifested in adolescence. They may be related to previous significant childhood febrile seizures, birth, or traumatic head injury. It is believed that following these events, there is injury to some neurons. The surrounding neurons send out axons to reinnervate the region, and the new neuron circuitry is thought to be hyperexcitable.[9]

Complex partial seizures are characterized by slow, paroxysmal waves in either the anterior or posterior leads of the EEG. Seizures may begin with an olfactory aura such as an unpleasant smell or unusual taste. The person may exhibit bizarre behavior and exaggerated emotionality. Episodic fluctuations in attitude, attention, behavior, or memory occur. The individual seems to interact in a purposeful, although inappropriate, manner. The person may experience hallucinations or perceptual illusions or perceive strange objects or people as familiar (*deja vu*) and familiar objects and people as strange (*jamais vu*).

Although appearing to be in a dreamy state, possibly mumbling a few words, and being unresponsive to verbal stimulation, the individual mechanically performs tasks while the seizure is progressing (automatic behavior or automatisms). Automatisms, when present, include chewing, smacking, licking of the lips, and clapping of the hands. Less frequently, the head and eyes may turn to one side, or tonic spasms of the limbs may occur. Because of the nature of complex seizures, affected persons are frequently thought to have psychiatric disturbances. Usually, seizures last from seconds to minutes, but some may continue for hours; others may progress to tonic, tonic-clonic, or other forms of generalized seizures.

SECONDARY GENERALIZATION SEIZURES. Secondary generalized (symptomatic) seizures are caused by some metabolic or structural underlying disorder. Metabolic disturbances can result from conditions such as renal failure, hypoglycemia, hypoxia, hyponatremia, hypernatremia, hypercalcemia, hepatic failure, and withdrawal of drugs. Meningitis and encephalitis in children lead to strong convulsive tendencies. After recovery, there may be residual recurrent generalized, focal, or psychomotor seizures. Many structural lesions are caused by disorders in cerebral blood supply, intracranial tumors, trauma, and infections and result in scarring of areas of the brain. These can produce various types of seizure activity.

Generalized Seizures

Generalized seizures involve both cerebral hemispheres and commonly result in a variable period of loss of consciousness. Anterograde (immediately before the seizure) and retrograde (after the seizure) amnesia frequently accompanies the loss of consciousness. The most common forms of generalized seizures are petit mal (absence) and grand mal (tonic-clonic). Generalized seizures also include myoclonic and atonic types.

TONIC-CLONIC SEIZURES (GRAND MAL). Electrical disruption with grand mal seizures originates anywhere in the forebrain and usually involves the whole forebrain. For several hours preceding the seizure, vague prodromal sensations, such as epigastric distress, muscular twitching, or other unnatural sensations, may occur. Commonly, a brief aura, an indication of an impending seizure consisting of a specific movement or unnatural sensation, is the last thing the individual remembers before losing consciousness.

After the aura, if present, the individual abruptly loses consciousness, falls to the ground, and suffers generalized tonic contractions, followed by clonic contractions of all muscles. Muscle contraction in the tonic phase lasts for a few seconds. During the tonic phase the entire body becomes rigid with the arms and legs extended. The jaws become clenched, the head may be retracted, and the eyeballs are rolled backward. As air is forced through the closed vocal cords, the diaphragm contracts and a loud cry may be heard. Breathing usually ceases during this time.

In the clonic phases, movements become jerky as muscle groups contract and relax. The arms and legs contract and relax forcibly. Breathing becomes noisy and stertorous, and profuse perspiration is noted. Excessive salivation and loss of bladder or bowel sphincter control may also occur. The epileptic discharge on EEG shows generalized recurring spike discharges in the tonic phase and nonfocal high-frequency, high-amplitude spike-and-wave discharges in the clonic phase.[24]

Contractions become slower, sometimes irregular, and then stop. The entire seizure usually lasts 1 to 2 minutes and usually is followed by a period of unconsciousness (postictal period). Spasms of the tongue and jaw may cause biting injuries to the tongue or cheeks. Unconsciousness for the entire seizure is characteristic and may continue up to ½-hour after the episode. As consciousness is regained, the individual is often confused, fatigued, and drowsy and complains of muscle soreness. The individual has no memory of the seizure but usually remembers the aura. In the early part of the postictal period, there may be reflex signs characteristic of upper motor neuron disorder. Paralysis may follow the attack for a short time and is described as postconvulsive (*postictal*), or Todd's paralysis.

FEBRILE SEIZURES. *Febrile general tonic-clonic seizures*, common in children between the ages of 3 months and 5 years, are predominantly seen in children between the ages of 6 months and 3 years of age experiencing an episode of a usually benign viral illness. These seizures are generalized and of short duration. Seizures lasting less than 5 minutes usually do not recur during the illness. Those lasting longer than 10 minutes can be associated with secondary problems such as meningitis or encephalitis and should be investigated by thorough neurologic evaluation. In general, there is a high familial tendency for febrile seizures, and these children may go on to experience epilepsy from non-febrile seizures in later life.

ABSENCE SEIZURES (PETIT MAL). The term *absence seizure* is used because the person, although present physically, is absent with respect to higher cortical functions during the episode. The majority of such persons have normal intelligence and have no significant abnormal physical findings on neurologic examination. Onset is usually about the age of 5 years, and attacks are most prevalent in childhood. Absence seizures decrease after puberty.

Petit mal seizures may be characterized by a loss of awareness (simple) or may be accompanied by automatisms (complex), such as flicking of the eyelids, twitching of facial muscles, or staring into space while general postural tone is preserved. They may be precipitated by seeing bright or flashing lights or hearing loud noises, and may be preceded by hyperventilation. Attacks may recur numerous times during the day, possibly lasting from 5 to 10 seconds, after which consciousness is abruptly restored and the interrupted activity is promptly resumed. Memory may be defective only through the seizure. These seizures exhibit a characteristic spike-and-wave pattern with 3 Hz on the EEG. As the person reaches adolescence, their frequency decreases and the individual may develop other types of seizures, usually tonic-clonic.

STATUS EPILEPTICUS. Tonic clonic or absence seizures that follow one another without restoration of consciousness are called *status epilepticus*. Common precipitating factors include abrupt cessation of anticonvulsant medication and alcohol withdrawal. This disorder is life threatening and produces greatly accelerated neuronal metabolic rate, hypoxia, acidosis, hyperthermia, and alterations in cerebral blood flow. Damage occurs to the cerebral cortex, hippocampus, and cerebellum, along with other metabolic derangements.

MYOCLONIC SEIZURES. Individuals with myoclonic seizures have sudden, rapid flexion of the limbs and trunk singularly or repeatedly, generally with a momentary loss of consciousness. Loud sounds or bright lights may precipitate the episodes. Intentional movement worsens them. These disorders occur with greatest frequency in childhood but may continue after puberty. Bilateral, synchronous 3-Hz discharges are noted on EEG during each episode.

Myoclonic spasms occurring in infancy, called *massive spasms*, are first noted at 6 to 9 months of age and continue to age 2 or 3 years. There is usually associated

FOCUS ON THE PERSON WITH TRAUMATIC BRAIN INJURY

C. S. is a previously healthy 37-year-old maintenance worker who was in a head-on car accident while on his way home from his sister's birthday celebration. He was the unrestrained driver in a small truck and had no passengers. C.'s truck was severely damaged and required extensive manipulation to get C. extricated. At the scene, the paramedics found him somewhat dazed but responding appropriately to questions. He had bruises and lacerations about his face and scalp that were bleeding quite profusely. Paramedics noted an area of indented, broken glass on the truck windshield, which they surmised could have been hit by C.'s head. C. complained of head, neck, and leg pain at the scene.

First vital signs obtained by the paramedics were blood pressure 152/94, pulse 124, respirations 32. Airway, breathing, and circulation were adequate. Other assessments at the scene were as follows:

Level of consciousness—responding slowly, knows own name, uncertain of own address, asks "What happened?"
Glasgow Coma Scale score = 13.

Motor activity—moves all extremities, diminished strength, equal handgrasp.

Head—bleeding from head and scalp lacerations, possible depressed region on high forehead.

Pupils—pupils equal and react to light, 6 cm.

Extremities—compound fracture of right thigh, moderate amount of blood noted in seat of truck around right thigh.

After C. was transported to the local trauma center, the following physical assessment was made on admission:

Level of consciousness—anxious, agitated; knows own name, asks repetitively what happened to him; responds appropriately to command. Glasgow Coma Scale score = 14.

Sensory—complaining of head, neck, leg pain; demanding a pain killer.

Vital signs—blood pressure 148/96, pulse 128, respirations 34.

Pupils—pupils equal and react to light, 5 cm.

Head—multiple bleeding cuts on face and scalp; depressed area on high forehead, bruising around eyes and behind the ears.

Thirty minutes after arrival, the following observations were recorded:

Level of consciousness—difficult to arouse.

Pupils—right pupil 4 cm, reactive to light; left pupil 8 cm, nonreactive.

Motor activity—moving right extremities less than left extremities: right handgrasp much weaker than left; bilateral decortication noted with noxious stimulation.

Vital signs—blood pressure 174/104, pulse 88, respirations 22; respirations appear in clusters interspersed with short periods of apnea. Glasgow Coma Scale score = 7.

Questions

1. What is the apparent mechanism of injury experienced? Based on this, discuss the neurological injuries that could be anticipated with C.
2. What are primary and secondary brain injuries? What primary and secondary injuries threaten C.?
3. What is a brain concussion, and what are its presenting signs and symptoms? Which of these, if any, are evident in C.? What long-term changes in function and behavior may be anticipated?
4. Discuss the pathological basis and clinical findings of a brain contusion. How is a brain contusion diagnosed? Given the information regarding C., is it possible to identify a contused brain with him?
5. After controlling for the immediate life-threatening injuries and problems, what are the major concerns in managing C.'s neurologic injuries early after injury? What assessments and interventions should be employed in preventing and minimizing these?
6. What is the significance of the bruising around C.'s eyes and behind his ears? What other signs would you look for with this type of injury? What are the potential hazards associated with this type of injury?
7. Discuss the pathological significance of the changes in C.'s level of consciousness, pupillary responses, motor responses, and vital signs. What interventions are required?
8. C. has a possible depressed skull fracture. Describe the physical findings associated with depressed skull fractures and the potential hazards to the patient.

See Appendix A for discussion.

retardation of psychomotor development. The spasms may be related to other conditions, such as phenylketonuria, perinatal brain damage, pyridoxine deficiency, or tuberous sclerosis.

Myoclonic spasms may be generalized or multifocal and tend to disappear with growth. However, other seizure patterns may emerge. In adults, myoclonic seizures may accompany dementia in conditions such as Creutzfeldt-Jacob disease and certain acute conditions, such as acute viral encephalitis. A benign form of myoclonus, associated with sudden myoclonic jerks when falling asleep or awakening, has been described.

ATONIC SEIZURES. In these seizures, persons experience sudden loss of consciousness and fall to the ground without contraction or motion. Muscle tone is lost briefly, but stance is resumed almost immediately. A history of infantile spasms and mental retardation is often present.

INFANTILE SPASMS. Characteristically, infantile spasms affect children in the 3-month to 2-year-old age group. These seizures may be associated with an unknown metabolic disturbance (*primary infantile spasms*) or caused by a variety of known degenerative, structural birth injuries or developmental conditions such as amino acid abnormalities, phenylketonuria, and tuberous sclerosis (*secondary infantile spasms*). The seizures are characterized by flexor spasms of the extremities and frequently are associated with mental retardation.

LENNOX-GASTAUT SYNDROME. Lennox-Gastaut seizures have their onset in childhood, usually between the ages of 2 and 6 years. They may recur spontaneously or with subsequent infections and febrile illnesses, but often they follow infantile spasms. Lennox-Gastaut syndrome is very difficult to treat and may continue to adulthood. These seizures may be compounded by combinations of atonic and ataxic spells, minor partial seizures, tonic seizures, and atypical petit mal and temporal lobe seizures. They are associated with a distinctive slow spike-and-wave EEG pattern. Mental retardation is a common finding.

FOCUS ON THE PERSON WITH TRAUMATIC SPINAL CORD INJURY

J. is a 47-year-old female who, along with her husband, joined the annual summer cross-country motorcycle trek with the Smithfield Motorcycle Club. One day, shortly after getting on the road again, J. was pulling out to pass an automobile when a truck in the third lane pulled over into J.'s lane and into her motorcycle. Immediately after crashing and hitting the pavement, J. attempted to get up, but she instantly fell to the ground and lay motionless. A policeman who happened to be following closely behind the motorcycle group stopped and activated the emergency medical system.

Findings on admission to the emergency room of the local hospital were as follows:

Level of consciousness—alert, oriented, highly anxious, complaining of severe neck pain.
Vital signs—blood pressure 92/48, temperature 97.8°F, pulse 62, respirations 28 and shallow.
Motor and sensory activity—no movement or sensation in lower extremities, flaccid paralysis: exhibits gross arm movements; shoulders seem elevated.
Chest—diminished breath sounds in bases, decreased chest expansion, increased abdominal excursion with breathing.
Extremities—warm to touch; right lower leg is deformed; multiple abrasions and bruises on arms and legs.
Abdomen—no bowel sounds.

The following interventions were done: 1) neck and spine immobilization; 2) large-bore intravenous needle inserted in left antecubital area; 3) magnetic resonance imaging, showing fracture-dislocation at C4–C5; 4) X-ray studies, showing fractured right fibula (cast applied); 5) peritoneal tap (negative); 6) Gardner-Wells tongs with 35-lb weights. Ten days after admission, J. had a cervical fusion operation.

Two months after her discharge to the Rehabilitation Hospital, J. complained of a severe headache and dizziness. Her blood pressure was 287/126, pulse 62, respirations 32 and shallow.

Questions

1. Discuss the pathophysiological basis and associated clinical findings in terms of respiratory function or dysfunction with J.'s spinal cord injury.
2. What are potential early postinjury hazards for J.?
3. Discuss the pathological basis of spinal shock. What clinical findings with Josephine support a diagnosis of spinal shock?
4. What bowel or bladder changes are anticipated with J. early after injury? What interventions are necessary?
5. J. is prone to a lifetime of physical hazards based on her injury. Discuss these.
6. What most likely happened to J. at the Rehabilitation Hospital during her hypertensive episode? What could have caused this, and what is its pathological basis? What rapid interventions may be employed? What are the major hazards associated with this condition?

See Appendix A for discussion.

REFERENCES

1. Adams, R., & Victor, M. (1998). *Principles of neurology* (6th ed.). New York: McGraw-Hill.
2. Aisen, M. (1993). Differential diagnosis of spinal cord disease. In L. Barclay (Ed.), *Clinical geriatric neurology*. Philadelphia: Lea and Febiger.
3. Aminoff, M., Greenberg, D. A., & Simon, R. P. (1996). *Clinical neurology*. Stamford, CT: Appleton & Lange.
4. Baltuch, G. H., Bogousslavsky, J., & Tribolet, N. (1997). Hypertensive intracranial hemorrhage: Epidemiology and pathophysiology. In H. H. Batjer (Editor-in-chief), *Cerebrovascular disease*. Philadelphia: Lippincott-Raven.
5. Bell, T., LaGrange, K. M., Maier, C. M. & Steinberg, G. K. (1992). Transcranial Doppler: Correlation of blood velocity measurement with clinical status in subarachnoid hemorrhage. *Journal of of Neuroscience Nursing, 24,* 4.
6. Biller, J. (1997). *Practical neurology*. Philadelphia: Lippincott-Raven.
7. Caplan, L. R. (1994). Cerebrovascular disease (stroke). In J. Stein (Ed.), *Internal medicine* (4th ed.). St. Louis: C. V. Mosby.
8. Chandrasoma, P. & Taylor, C. R. (1995). *Concise pathology* (2nd ed.). Norwalk, CT: Appleton & Lange.
9. Collins, R. (1997). *Neurology*. Philadelphia: W. B. Saunders.
10. DeGirolami, U., Frosch, M. P. & Anthony, D. C. (1994). The central nervous system. In R. Cotran, V. Kumar, & S. Robbins, *Robbins' pathologic basis of disease* (5th ed.). Philadelphia: W.B. Saunders.
11. Fischer, W. S. (1997). Intracranial vascular malformations: Clinical presentations. In H. H. Batjer (Editor-in-chief), *Cerebrovascular disease*. Philadelphia: Lippincott-Raven.
12. Guttierrez, P., Vulpe, M., & Young, R. (1994). Spinal cord injury. In J. Stein (Ed.), *Internal medicine* (4th ed.). St. Louis: Mosby.
13. Guyton, A. (1996). *Textbook of medical physiology* (9th ed.). Philadelphia: W.B. Saunders.
14. Hickey, J. V. (1997). *The clinical practice of neurological nursing* (4th ed.). Philadelphia: Lippincott-Raven.
15. Ho, H. W., Chandler, J., & Batjer, H. H. (1997). Intracranial aneurysm: Clinical manifestation. In H. H. Batjer (Editor-in-chief), *Cerebrovascular disease*. Philadelphia: Lippincott-Raven.
16. Macdonald, R. L. & Weir, B. (1997). Cerebral vasospasm: Prevention and treatment. In H. H. Batjer (Editor-in-chief), *Cerebrovascular disease*. Philadelphia: Lippincott-Raven.
17. Mattson, M., & Mark, R. (1996). Excitotoxcicity and excitoprotection In vitro. In B. K. Siesjo & T. Wieloch (Eds.), *Advances in neurology (vol. 71): Cellular and molecular mechanisms of ischemic brain damage*. Philadelphia: Lippincott-Raven.
18. McPhee, S. J., Lingappa, V. R., Ganong, W. F., & Lange, J. D. (1997). *Pathophysiology of disease: An introduction to clinical medicine*. Stamford, CT: Appleton & Lange.
19. Mergner, W. J. & Trump, B. F. (1994). Hemodynamic disorders. In E. Rubin & J. L. Farber, *Pathology* (2nd ed.). Philadelphia: J. B. Lippincott.
20. Richard, T. S. (1997). Cerebral resuscitation after global brain ischemia: Linking research to practice. *AACN Clinical Issues, 8*(2), 171–181.
21. Rubin, E. & Faber, J. L. (1999). *Pathology* (3rd ed.). Philadelphia: Lippincott Williams & Wilkins.
22. Tortora, G. & Grabowski, S. (1988). *Principles of anatomy and physiology* (8th ed.). Reading, MA: Addison-Wesley.
23. Waxman, S. & deGroot, J. (1995). *Correlative neuroanatomy*. Norwalk, CT: Appleton & Lange.
24. Westmoreland, B. F., Benarroch, E. E., Daube, J. R., Reagan, T. J., & Sandok, B. A. (1994). *Medical neurosciences: An approach to anatomy, pathology, and physiology by systems and levels* (3rd ed.). Boston: Little, Brown.
25. Wiebers, D. O., Feigein, V. & Brown, R. D. (1997). *Handbook of stroke*. Philadelphia: Lippincott-Raven.

Chapter 32

Tumors and Infections of the Central Nervous System

Gretchen McDaniel

KEY TERMS

astrocytoma
cerebral neuroblastoma
chordoma
craniopharyngioma (Rathke's pouch tumor)
dermoid
empyema
encephalitis
ependeymoma
extramedullary intradural tumor
ganglioglioma
germinoma
glioblastoma
hemangioblastoma
intramedullary intradural tumor
mass effect
medulloblastoma
meningioma
neurofibroma
neurilemmoma (schwannoma)
oligodendroglioma
pituitary adenoma
prion disease
teratoma

Tumors, both benign and malignant, and infections of the central nervous system (CNS) result in varying alterations and clinical manifestations. In either case, the aggressiveness of the tumor or infective agent plays a significant role in the patient presentation, course of illness, and eventual outcome.

This chapter discusses the major classifications of tumors: the gliomas; tumors of neuronal, embryonic, and meningeal origins; and others, including those that metastasize from other regions of the body. Those from glial tissue origins are the most common CNS neoplasms, followed by meningeal neoplasms. Some tumors, such as craniopharyngiomas and pituitary adenomas, grow in specific areas and reflect unique clinical manifestations. Others, such as the gliomas, may occur in any CNS parenchymal region and reflect manifestations of that area.

Although CNS tumors may be benign or malignant, certain benign tumors such as well-differentiated astrocytomas infiltrate the parenchyma and eventually cause death. Therefore, the distinction between benign and malignant nature of tumors becomes less significant in the CNS than in other regions of the body.

Many infective processes may be associated with CNS dysfunction. The CNS may be invaded by various viruses, bacteria, fungi, protozoa, and parasites. Organisms may gain access to the CNS through hematogenous spread from other regions in the body, direct implantation during CNS procedures, or through extension from infected sinuses or the peripheral nervous system. Many microorganisms prefer to localize in specific CNS areas such as in the meninges, white matter, or motor neurons, causing neuronal and supporting tissue destruction. The pathologic effects and manifestations of various microorganism colonizations in the CNS are discussed in this chapter.

TUMORS

Tumors of the CNS include both benign and malignant neoplasms of the brain and spinal cord. They can arise from the glial cells, blood vessels, connective tissue, meninges, pituitary gland, and pineal gland (Fig. 32-1). Primary CNS neoplasms account for 2% of all cancers and 20% of cancers in children under the age of 15.[7] The CNS is also a common site for metastasis from primary cancers, such as pulmonary and breast cancers.

The location, size, and invasive quality of CNS neoplasms are responsible for neurologic symptoms. The destruction and displacement of surrounding tissue caused by an intracranial tumor is shown in Figure 32-2.

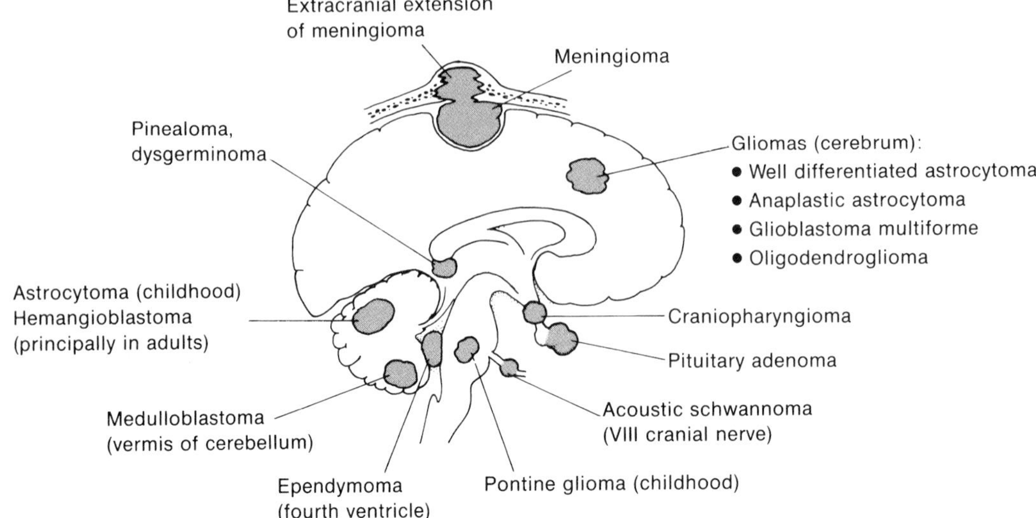

FIGURE 32-1. The distribution of common intracranial tumors. (Rubin, E., & Farber, J. L. [1999]. *Pathology* [3rd ed.]. Philadelphia; Lippincott.)

Pathophysiology

INTRACRANIAL TUMORS

Brain tumors are classified as benign or malignant based on their cellular histology and morphology. An overview of intracranial tumor types and distinguishing features is presented in Table 32-1. All tumors of the brain are potentially harmful because of their location near vital structures and the critical amount of **mass effect** (compression of surrounding tissue structures) that eventually destroys neuronal function.[4]

Within the confined space of the skull, a growing tumor alters the normally stable volume of the brain, blood, and CSF, leading to focal disturbances and increased intracranial pressure. Intracranial tumor growth can produce any of the following alterations:

- Compression of brain tissue and invasion of brain parenchyma, causing destruction of neural tissue
- Decreased blood circulation to an extent leading to necrosis of brain tissue
- Compression, infiltration of neural tissue, and decreased blood supply, possibly leading to altered neural excitability and seizures

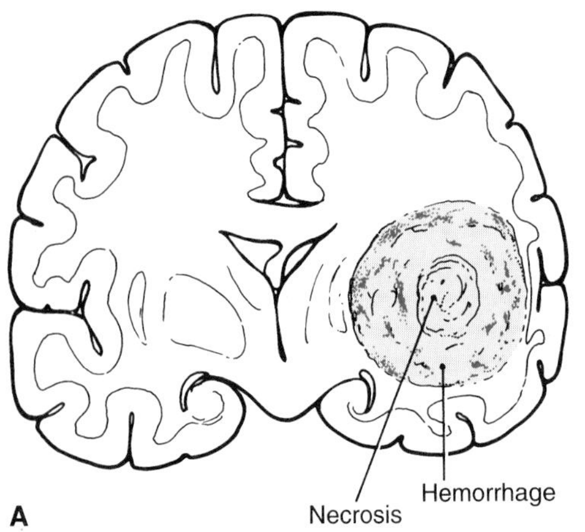

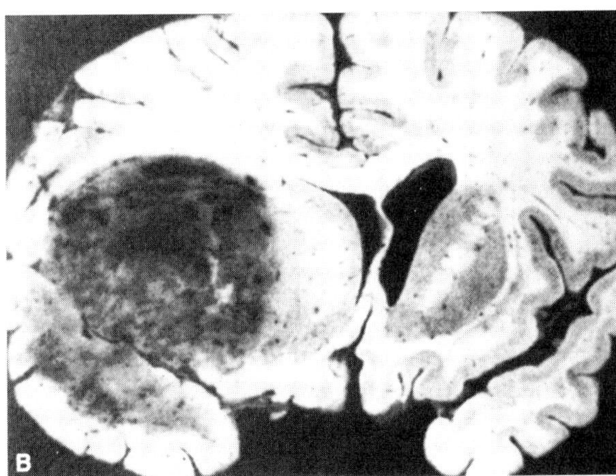

FIGURE 32-2. **A.** Glioblastoma showing well-defined tumor with surrounding inflammation and necrosis and hemorrhage within the tumor. **B.** Large glioblastoma with edema in the left insula and displacement of cerebral midline structures. (Adams, J., & Graham, D. [1994]. *An introduction to neuropathology* [2nd ed.]. London: Churchill-Livingstone.)

TABLE 32-1

AN OVERVIEW OF TUMOR TYPES AND DISTINGUISHING FEATURES

TUMOR TYPE	ORIGIN OF CELLS	COMMON LOCATIONS	AGE GROUPS	GROWTH CHARACTERISTICS	COMMENTS
Astrocytoma	Astrocytes				
Pilocytic		Cerebellum	Children	Slow-growing	Wide variety of growth patterns from benign to malignant. Treatment based on most aggressive cells.
Brain stem gliomas		Brain stem	Children	Mixed	
Grade I Grade II		Cerebral hemispheres	Adults	Slow-growing	
Grade III (anaplastic)	Astrocytes	Cerebral hemispheres	Adults	Rapidly growing	
Grade IV (glioblastoma)					
Oligodendroglioma	Oligodendrocytes	Cerebral hemispheres	Men 35–40	Two types; slow- and fast-growing; may spread via cerebral spinal fluid	May be cystic or have calcifications.
Ependymomas	Ependymal cells	Lining of ventricles, fourth ventricle most common	Children and teenagers	Slow, but there is a rapid-growing variant	Location may make resection difficult, may obstruct CSF flow.
Primitive neural ectodermal tumors (medulloblastoma)	Primitive undifferentiated cells	Cerebellum	Young children boys > girls	Rapid growth, seed in cerebral spinal fluid	Causes hydrocephalus by CSF obstruction, vomiting most common symptom.
Germ cell tumors	Embryonal, endodermal and cells similar to those found in testes and ovaries	Pineal hypothalamic regions	Men > women 10–20	Rapid growth, may seed via cerebral spinal fluid	May metastasize or regrow after surgical resection, may obstruct CSF flow.
Lymphomas	Lymphocytes	Cerebral hemispheres, leptomeninges	Adults	Variety of growth patterns	Can be isolated tumor or infiltrative, multiple lesions. Common in HIV and organ transplant patients.
Papillomas	Choroid plexus	Within ventricles	Children and young adults	Slow-growing but highly vascular	Obstructs CSF, producing hydrocephalus. Location may make resection difficult.
Meningiomas	Arachnoid granulations	Lining of dura: convexity or base of brain, cavernous sinus, sphenoid ridge	Adults, women > men	Majority are slow-growing, some have rapid growth, highly vascular	Headache or seizure often first symptom.
Sarcomas	Connective tissue, dura, leptomeninges	Dura over cerebral hemispheres	Rare	Slow or rapid growth	Fibrosarcoma most common.

(continued)

TABLE 32-1

AN OVERVIEW OF TUMOR TYPES AND DISTINGUISHING FEATURES (Continued)

TUMOR TYPE	ORIGIN OF CELLS	COMMON LOCATIONS	AGE GROUPS	GROWTH CHARACTERISTICS	COMMENTS
Pituitary tumors	Pituitary gland	Underneath brain in sella turcica	20–45	Slow-growing	May cause increase or decrease in hormonal secretion.
Acoustic neuromas	Nerve sheath	Cranial nerve VIII, but also found on V, VII, and XII	Women > men middle-age adults	Slow-growing	Loss of hearing is usually first symptom, may be bilateral.
Hemangioblastomas	Blood vessels	Cerebellum, medulla	40–60	Slow-growing	May be solid or have cystic nodule.
Craniopharyngioma	Squamous nest cells	Suprasellar region, midline	30–40, also seen in children	Slow-growing	Can reduce vision owing to pressure on optic chiasm.

CSF = cerebrospinal fluid.
(Bronstein, K. [1995]. Epidemiology and classification of brain tumors. *Critical Care Nursing Clinics of North America, 7*(1): 80.)

- Elevation of capillary pressure, due to compression of venules in the area adjacent to the tumor, is thought to be the basis for localized vasogenic cerebral edema (Fig. 32-3) that frequently surrounds the tumor. Compression of the vascular capillary wall by the tumor damages the capillary and allows vascular fluid to escape into the interstitium.
- Displacement of CSF from the subarachnoid space and ventricles through the foramen magnum to the spinal subarachnoid space and also through the optic foramen to the perioptic subarachnoid space, impairing venous drainage from the optic nerve head and retina (manifested by papilledema or choked disk)
- Obstruction of CSF circulation from the lateral ventricles to the subarachnoid space, with resultant hydrocephalus secondary to growth of the mass

Rapid development of any of these situations causes a life-threatening increase in intracranial pressure. Compensatory mechanisms include (1) decreased parenchymal cell numbers, (2) decreased intracellular fluid contents, (3) decreased CSF volume, and (4) decreased intracranial blood volume. These compensatory mechanisms may take days or months to be effective and thus are not useful with rapidly developing intracranial pressure.[19] Untreated increased intracranial pressure (ICP) may cause brain herniation (see Chapter 31).

INTRASPINAL TUMORS

Intraspinal tumors are classified according to (1) their location in relation to the dura and spinal cord and (2) their histologic type. Thus, two groups are generally considered: (1) *extradural*, those arising from the extradural space or vertebral bodies, and (2) *intradural*, further subdivided as **extramedullary** (those arising from the blood vessels, meninges, or nerve roots) or **intramedullary** (those tumors arising from within the substance of the spinal cord itself). Extramedullary tumors are more common than intramedullary tumors.

Alterations occurring as a result of intraspinal tumors are largely due to (1) compression of the spinal cord, (2) interference with circulation, and (3) pressure on veins or arteries. Ischemia of cord segments and edema below the level of compression occur. Extradural spinal tumors usually result from extraneural metastases, particularly from the breast or lung. These cause rapid compression of the spinal cord. Hemorrhage due to the metastases and possible vertebral column collapse add to the compressive effects of extradural tumors.

Generally benign, extramedullary tumors are of two types: (1) neurofibromas and (2) meningiomas. **Neurofibromas** grow in the nerve root and often form an hourglass-like expansion that extends into the extradural space. **Meningiomas** grow from the arachnoid membrane. These tumors are commonly present in the posterolateral aspect of the cord. They often result in Brown-Séquard syndrome, due to the compressive damage to one half of the spinal cord (see Chapter 31).

Intramedullary tumors are histologically the same as intracranial tumors. These lesions damage neurons and sensory fibers that cross each other in the center of the cord. There is a frequent association between intramedullary tumors and syringomyelia.[1]

FOCUS ON CELLULAR PATHOPHYSIOLOGY

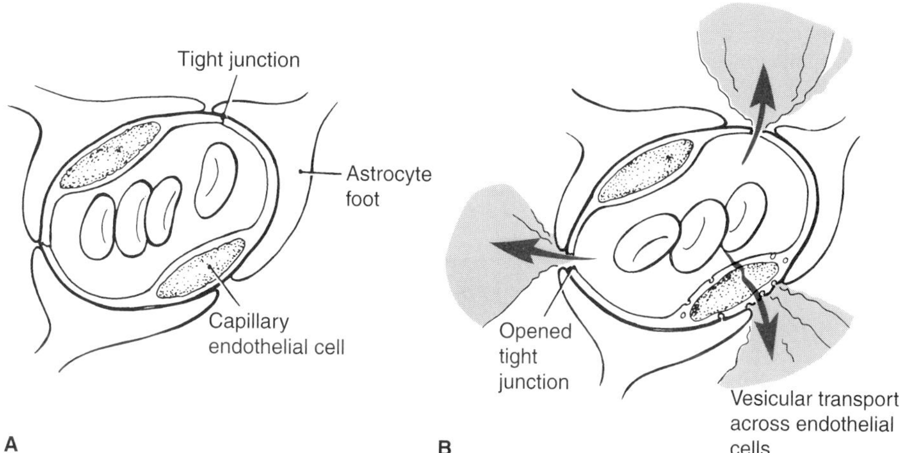

FIGURE 32-3. Development of cerebral edema as a response to tumor presence. **A.** Normal. **B.** Vasogenic edema.

Clinical Manifestations

INTRACRANIAL TUMORS

The symptoms produced by intracranial tumors are variable and depend on characteristics of the neoplasm, invasive qualities, location, and rate of growth. Lumbar puncture, rarely indicated but performed to examine the CSF only if there is no evidence of increased ICP, usually reveals a normal CSF glucose, an elevated protein level in 70% of patients, and tumor cells in 30% of cases.[16]

Cerebral angiography detects displacement of vessels from their normal position due to tumor growth and also provides information concerning the vasculature of the tumor.

Somatosensory evoked potentials (SSEPs), a neurodiagnostic test, helps to localize sensory deficits because brain tumors may cause delays in sensory pathway conduction from brain tissue compression and abnormal vascularization.[11] These and additional tests are described in the Appendix of this unit.

Because intracranial tumors eventually give rise to an increase in intracranial pressure, three symptoms are common: headache, vomiting, and papilledema.

HEADACHE. Headache is a common symptom of intracranial tumors. Early in the course of tumor growth, headache is thought to result from local displacement and traction of pain-sensitive structures within the skull—cranial nerves, arteries, veins, and venous sinuses. As the tumor grows, the pain is reflective of generalized increased ICP.

In general, the headache provides little information about the tumor's location. The headache, usually temporary, may be severe, dull or sharp, and intermittent. Generally most severe on awakening, it tends to improve throughout the day, being aggravated by stooping, coughing, or straining to have a bowel movement.

VOMITING. Vomiting, associated with intracranial tumors—particularly those of the posterior fossa—is a result of stimulation of the emetic center in the medulla. Vomiting associated with tumors is frequently projectile and not necessarily preceded by nausea. Although often occurring before breakfast, vomiting typically is not related to the ingestion of food.

PAPILLEDEMA. Papilledema, possibly absent in the early stages of tumor growth, occurs as ICP increases. However, in some persons, papilledema does not develop even when the ICP becomes greatly elevated. Hemorrhages may be noted around the optic disk in association with papilledema. Complaints of blurred vision and halos around lights with enlargement of a blind spot and fleeting moments of dimmed vision (amaurosis fugax) may be elicited.

LOCAL EFFECTS. Local effects of intracranial tumors occur due to irritation, destruction, or compression of neural tissue in the location of the tumor. Generally, *supratentorial* lesions give rise to paralysis, seizures, memory loss, visual field defects, and impairment in consciousness. *Infratentorial* lesions give rise to cranial nerve dysfunction and ataxia. Tumor location and associated symptoms are presented in Table 32-2.

INTRASPINAL TUMORS

Clinical manifestations associated with spinal cord tumors depend on the type of lesion and the level at which the lesion occurs. A soft, slow-growing mass causes gradual compression of the spinal cord with gradually increasing neurologic signs. Malignant and metastatic tumors cause rapid compression of the spinal cord and destruction of the neural tissue. Extradural tumors usually result from metastasis from primary tumor sites. Extramedullary lesions are usually benign and involve the periphery of the cord early in their growth. Intramedullary tumors tend to be histologically more benign, are slow growing, and have a more benign course than similar intracranial tumors. Symptoms associated with these spinal cord tumors are presented in Table 32-3.

Compression by spinal cord tumors typically includes the following levels: foramen magnum, cervical region (C5, C6, C7, and C8), thoracic region, lumbar region, and sacral region. A summary of musculoskeletal signs and symptoms associated with these lesions is presented in Table 32-4.

Gliomas

The glial cells, which include astrocytes, oligodendroglia, and ependymal cells, provide support and protection for nerve cells. Gliomas, as a group, are the most common primary brain tumors, constituting 40% to 60% of primary brain tumors in adults.[3,13,19] The tumors are named and classified according to cell type as **astrocytomas, oligodendrogliomas**, and **ependymomas**. Gliomas, infiltrating by nature, may invade any area of the CNS; also, they may spread from one area of the brain or spinal cord to another.

ASTROCYTOMAS

PATHOPHYSIOLOGY. Astrocytomas develop from astrocytes. These spider-shaped or star-shaped cells, frequently associated with various-sized cysts, infiltrate brain tissue. Their invasive nature usually makes surgical removal difficult. An exception is the pilocytic astrocytoma, which grows in the cerebellum and optic nerve and has a good prognosis after removal.[5]

Astrocytomas have varying degrees of malignancy. They are graded from I to IV, with grade I being composed of slower-growing, well-differentiated cells and

TABLE 32-2

INTRACRANIAL TUMOR LOCATION AND ASSOCIATED SYMPTOMS

PRINCIPAL SYMPTOMS	TUMOR LOCATION	PRINCIPAL SYMPTOMS	TUMOR LOCATION
"Dementia"/ personality change	Frontal lobe		
		Laterizing signs	Cerebral hemisphere
	Corpus callosum		
		Headache, gait ataxia	Bifrontal/corpus callosum
	Multiple sites		Posterior fossa
			Leptomeningeal
Headaches, vomiting, papilledema	Frontal lobe		
	Temporal lobe (nondominant)		
		Headache, cranial neuropathy	Subfrontal
	Intraventricular (third, lateral)		Cerebellopontine angle
			Sellar/suprasellar
	Posterior fossa		Parasellar
	Leptomeningeal		Brain stem
		Seizures	Cerebral hemisphere
		Parinaud syndrome	Pineal region
	Clivus/base of skull		
Headache, endocrinopathy	Sellar/suprasellar		

(Modified from Kelley, W. N. [Ed.] [1997]. *Textbook of internal medicine* [3rd ed.]. Philadelphia: Lippincott-Raven.)

grade IV being composed of fast-growing, highly undifferentiated cells. Well-differentiated tumors may grow slowly for many years. Over time, they become more undifferentiated and are then classified as **glioblastomas**. Gross inspection usually reveals poorly defined, gray-white, infiltrative masses that enlarge and distort underlying CNS tissue. There is increasing evidence that fibroblast growth factor is linked to increased proliferation and invasiveness of astrocytoma cells.[15]

Clinical Manifestations. The initial symptom frequently is a focal or generalized seizure. Headaches, mental disturbances, and signs of increased ICP may develop several years later.

GLIOBLASTOMA MULTIFORME

Glioblastoma multiforme tumors are extremely malignant, highly vascular tumors that arise from undifferentiated astrocytomas. They are also referred to as Grade III and IV astrocytomas. Their appearance on gross inspection varies according to the region of the brain in which they arise, the degree of necrosis, and the presence of hemorrhage. Glioblastomas grow very rapidly, are invasive, and are resistant to various combinations of treatment. Tissue necrosis and brain edema are characteristic; thus, prognosis is poor.

OLIGODENDROGLIOMAS

Oligodendrogliomas arise from oligodendroglia. The frontal lobe is the most common site for this tumor (40% to 70% of patients).[2] Gross examination usually reveals well-defined, gray, globular masses possibly containing cystic foci, calcifications, and hemorrhagic areas.[18] These tumors, like astrocytomas, generally grow slowly. On occasion, however, rapid growth occurs, imitating glioblastomas. Histologic examination aids in differentiating oligodendrogliomas from glioblastomas.

TABLE 32-3

CLINICAL MANIFESTATIONS OF SPINAL CORD TUMORS

TUMOR LOCATION	CLINICAL MANIFESTATION	DESCRIPTION
Extradural (often result from primary site metastasis)	Local, dull pain	Intensification with movements of the spinal cord; later, spinal cord compression leading to severe pain.
	Loss of joint position sense, vibration sense; spastic weakness below level of lesion	Result of spinal cord compression
Intradural Extramedullary (usually benign)	Pain in back, along spinal roots, medullary referred pain	Pain worse at night (due to recumbency), aggravated by movements or straining (Valsalva maneuver); shooting or burning over peripheral areas (not influenced by Valsalva maneuver)
	Sensory loss	Associated with posteriorly situated tumors, sensory loss first below the level of the lesion; numbness, tingling
	Motor dysfunction	Associated with anterior cord compression
	Brown-Séquard syndrome	Associated with lateral cord compression; ipsilateral motor weakness, deep sensory loss; contralateral loss of pain and temperature perception below lesion
Intramedullary (usually benign, slow growing)	Dull, aching pain	Area of lesion
	Dissociated sensory loss	Bilateral loss of pain and temperature sense; however, touch, motion, position, and vibration usually preserved

Oligodendrogliomas also have a tendency to form focal calcification.

EPENDYMOMAS

Ependymal cells line the ventricular walls and form the central canal in the spinal cord. Ependymomas occur more frequently in children and adolescents than in adults.[1] Generally, cranial ependymomas appear as fairly well-defined masses that grow by expansion.[5] Ependymomas tend to form small canals (rosettes) within the tumor. The tumor cells also align themselves around blood vessels (pseudorosettes). Those that arise from ependymal cells lining the walls of the ventricular system fill and obstruct the ventricles and invade adjacent tissue, possibly obstructing CSF passage, which leads to the development of hydrocephalus. The most common site of ependymomas is the fourth ventricle.

Ependymomas that arise within the spinal cord represent a large percentage of intraspinal gliomas. Symptoms are related to the spinal level at which they occur. The location of these tumors often makes them inaccessible to surgical removal.

Tumors of Neuronal Origin

CEREBRAL NEUROBLASTOMAS

Cerebral neuroblastomas arise in precursor cells of neurons. Gross examination reveals well-defined, gray, granular masses that may contain areas of necrosis, hemorrhage, and cysts.[5] Neuroblastomas, although rare, usually occur during the first decade of life. Their growth rate is rapid, and commonly they recur after surgery.

GANGLIOGLIOMAS

Gangliogliomas are very rare tumors composed of a mixture of mature-appearing neurons and neuroglial tissue. Gross inspection reveals well-defined masses with granular surfaces. Calcifications and small cysts may be present within the mass. These tumors are most common in children and young adults.

TABLE 32-4
MUSCULOSKELETAL SYMPTOMS ASSOCIATED WITH LEVELS OF SPINAL CORD LESIONS

LEVEL	CLINICAL MANIFESTATIONS			
	Pain Location	Sensory Loss	Motor Loss	Weakness and Atrophy
Foramen magnum	Suboccipital			Head and neck weakness
Cervical	Lower neck, arm, shoulder tip, medial scapula, radial forearm	Deltoid, radial side of hand, index finger, thumb	Biceps	Biceps, shoulder abductors
	Lower neck, medial scapula, forearm, ulnar hand, fourth and fifth fingers	Middle, index fingers, ulnar hand, fourth and fifth fingers	Triceps	Triceps, hand muscles
Thoracic	Across the chest and abdomen	Lower extremity	Abdominal	Intercostal muscles
Lumbar	Low back, thigh, lateral leg, foot dorsum, great toe	Anterior, lateral leg and thigh, medial foot dorsum	Quadriceps	Quadriceps, ankle dorsiflexors and evertors, toe extensors
Sacral	Low back, posterior thigh and leg, heel, lateral foot	Posterior leg, heel, lateral foot	Achilles	Dorsi- and plantar flexion of ankle

Tumors of Embryonic Origin

Medulloblastomas arise predominantly from primitive cells in the cerebellum with the potential to develop along neuronal or neuroglial lines. Gross inspection generally reveals fairly well-demarcated, gray-white masses with indistinct edges.[5] Medulloblastomas occur almost exclusively in children, affecting more boys than girls, although in rare situations they have been found in adults up to the sixth decade of life. They are highly malignant, grow rapidly, and infiltrate throughout the subarachnoid space with resultant widespread meningeal foci. The CSF pathways become blocked, producing signs of increased ICP. Increasing ataxia, headaches, and forceful vomiting are common.

Tumors of the Meninges

MENINGIOMAS

Meningiomas, pictured in Figure 32-4, are primary tumors arising from the meninges, possibly involving the arachnoid cells, fibroblasts, and blood vessels. They are most common in females, generally occurring in older age and accounting for 15% of all primary intracranial tumors.[1,9] Often, gross inspection tends to reveal tough, gray-white, irregular to round, lobular masses.[5] Meningiomas, which are quite vascular, are seen readily on radioisotope scans. They are usually well-circumscribed, encapsulated, and press into surrounding tissue. The tumors may penetrate adjacent bone, but widespread infiltration of surrounding nervous tissue is not common.

CLINICAL MANIFESTATIONS. Most of these tumors are benign and grow slowly so that initial symptoms may

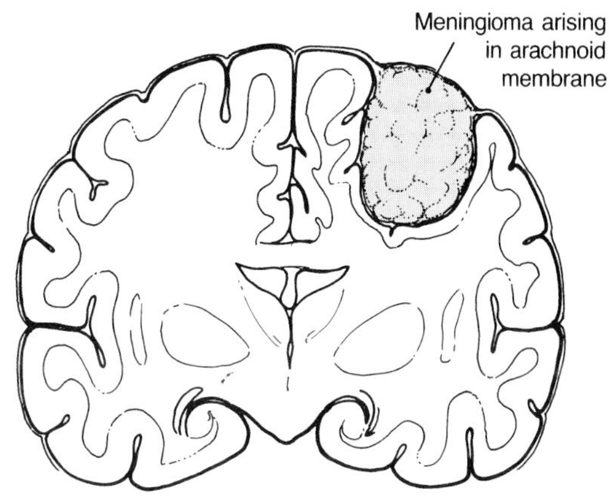

FIGURE 32-4. Meningioma. A tumor that arises from the arachnoid indents the underlying cortex.

be overlooked. As they continue to grow, symptoms include seizures, headache, visual impairment, hemiparesis, and aphasia.

Tumors of the Pituitary Gland

Pituitary adenomas are a special group of nervous system tumors that produce neurologic signs and symptoms because of the pressure exerted on the hypothalamus, optic chiasm, third ventricle, and medial temporal lobe. These tumors arise from the three cell types in the anterior pituitary: (1) basophil cells, (2) eosinophil cells, and (3) chromophobe cells.

Although usually classified according to cell type, it is more accurate to identify these tumors as hormone secreting (functioning) or nonsecreting (nonfunctioning). They usually contain a predominant cell type, however, and the chromophobe cells give rise to these tumors most frequently.

The initial symptoms are hormonal disturbances or visual field defects. The endocrine effects are discussed in Chapter 24.

HORMONE-SECRETING PITUITARY ADENOMAS

PROLACTIN-SECRETING PITUITARY ADENOMAS. Approximately 60% to 70% of the pituitary secreting adenomas in both males and females are prolactin-secreting tumors. Serum prolactin levels are increased (hyperprolactinemia), and amenorrhea in females and impotence in males may be evident. Additional manifestations are those associated with larger tumors, such as headaches and visual abnormalities. Hyperprolactinemia is discussed further in Chapter 24.

ADRENOCORTICOTROPIC HORMONE (ACTH)–PRODUCING PITUITARY ADENOMAS. Adrenocorticotropic hormone (ACTH)–producing pituitary adenomas, primarily composed of basophil cells, are usually so small that adjacent tissue is not compressed. They have powerful effects, however, due to hypersecretion of ACTH, which is one of several mechanisms that produce Cushing's syndrome. Symptoms of Cushing's syndrome include weakness, emotional lability, moon face, obesity of the torso, hypertension, salt and water retention, diabetes mellitus, glycosuria, osteoporosis, skin striae over the abdomen, hirsutism, and amenorrhea (see Chapter 24).

GROWTH HORMONE–PRODUCING PITUITARY ADENOMAS. Pituitary adenomas that cause an increase in the output of growth hormone result in gigantism and acromegaly (discussed in Chapter 24). These tumors, primarily composed of acidophilic cells, are small and rather slow growing. However, they may grow to such size that they press on the optic chiasm, causing complete or partial bitemporal hemianopsia or other visual disturbances.

NONSECRETING PITUITARY ADENOMAS

Nonsecreting pituitary adenomas, the most common pituitary tumors, are composed primarily of chromophobe cells. Although these cells have no known special function, tumors arising from them are rather large and produce symptoms by compressing the pituitary gland, optic chiasm, hypothalamus, and adjacent brain tissue. These tumors usually produce hypopituitarism, which is discussed in Chapter 24.

Tumors of the Cranial and Peripheral Nerves and Nerve Roots

Three types of cells within the nerve sheaths of the cranial nerves, peripheral nerves, cauda equina, and nerve roots may give rise to tumors. These cells include (1) Schwann cells, (2) perineural cells, and (3) fibroblasts in the epineurium and endoneurium. Although the three cells are similar morphologically, Schwann cells are generally the primary source of tumors. Two major types of tumors arise in this area: neurolemmomas (schwannomas) and neurofibromas.

NEURILEMMOMAS

Neurilemmomas (schwannomas), tumors that arise from the Schwann cells, occur on any of the nerves or nerve roots on the same nerve or throughout the body. They often involve the vestibulocochlear division of the acoustic (eighth) nerve (*acoustic neuroma*), most frequently at the cerebellopontile angle, or where the acoustic nerve enters the internal auditory meatus. Bilateral involvement of the acoustic nerve occurs in von Recklinghausen's neurofibromatosis, type 2.

CLINICAL MANIFESTATIONS. Acoustic neuromas produce clinical manifestations based on their position or disruption in function. Manifestations may include impaired hearing; tinnitus; vertigo; balance and coordination difficulties; ataxia; loss of caloric vestibular reactivity with horizontal nystagmus; palsies of the third, fifth, and seventh cranial nerves; and signs of increased ICP as the normal flow of CSF is obstructed.

NEUROFIBROMAS

Neurofibromas arise primarily from Schwann cells and fibroblasts. Gross examination reveals multiple encapsulated tumors with enlargement of the affected nerve or nerve root. Numerous tumors are often present, especially when associated with the hereditary disease, von Recklinghausen's neurofibromatosis.

Primary Lymphoma and Blood Vessel Tumors

Hemangioblastomas are neoplasms made up of an aggregation of blood vessels, possibly appearing as cysts. These arise most commonly in the cerebellum but may occur in the cerebrum. Clinical manifestations include ataxia, dizziness, and signs of increased ICP. Because erythropoietin is often secreted from these tumors, polycythemia may be exhibited. When a cerebellar hemangioblastoma occurs in association with cysts of the kidneys and pancreas and angiomatosis of the retinae, the disease is known as *von Hippel-Lindau syndrome*, an autosomal-dominant inherited disorder.

Other Tumors and Tumor-Like Lesions

DERMOIDS

Dermoids, congenital cystic tumors, may occur anywhere in the CNS but frequently arise in the ventricular system. They may obstruct the third ventricle, the aqueduct of Sylvius, or the fourth ventricle. Dermoids contain skin appendages and are often accompanied by overlying bone and skin defects.

CRANIOPHARYNGIOMAS (RATHKE'S POUCH TUMORS)

Craniopharyngiomas (Rathke's pouch tumors) are tumors derived from Rathke's pouch, a pouch in the embryonic membrane that develops into the anterior lobe of the pituitary. This tumor, most often located above the sella turcica, is encapsulated, growing as a solid mass or more frequently as a cyst. The cyst often contains thick, brown, oily fluid, often with some degree of calcification. Rupture of the cystic fluid into the subarachnoid space may cause recurrent bouts of "sterile" meningitis or, in some cases, bacterial meningitis. As the craniopharyngioma grows, pressure is applied to the pituitary gland and the optic chiasm. Erosion of the sella wall may occur. Clinical manifestations, most commonly occurring in children and young adults, reflect signs and symptoms of pituitary hypofunction, hydrocephalus, visual disturbances, and diabetes insipidus.

Germ Cell Tumors

Germinomas are the most common germ-cell (early stage of cell development) tumors usually found in the pineal and hypothalamic region. **Teratomas**, which are more common in children, are rare germ-cell tumors found in the pineal region. As a result of embryonic displacement of cells and tissue to areas where they are not usually found, the more differentiated teratomas may contain cartilage and bone.

Chordomas

Chordomas are congenital, malignant tumors that are derived from remnants of the primitive notochord. They are jelly-like, gray-pink growths that grow near the sella turcica, at the base of the brain, or at the cervical or sacrococcygeal areas. These tumors erode the bone and invade the dura. Symptoms, which usually develop within the first 10 years of life, depend on the size and location of the lesion. More common manifestations include paralysis of the extraocular eye muscles and pharyngeal swallowing muscles and loss of vision.

Metastatic Tumors

Metastases most commonly occur from primary sites in the lungs and breast, but neoplasms of the gastrointestinal and genitourinary tracts, bone, thyroid gland, and nasal sinuses can also metastasize to the brain and spinal cord. Metastatic tumors are generally solid, circumscribed masses that are surrounded by vasogenic edema. They may be solitary tumors or multiple small masses scattered throughout the CNS. Clinical manifestations vary with the location, size, and number of lesions.

INFECTIONS

Central nervous system tissue is not immune to viral, bacterial, or other infections. Initially, the infection usually arises in another region of the body. The organism then gains access to the CNS in several ways: (1) by spread from adjacent structures—nasal sinuses, skull, middle ear; (2) by entrance through penetrating wounds; and (3) through the bloodstream. Once infectious organisms enter the CNS, they can spread rapidly by way of the CSF, leading to widespread, devastating results. As noted in Figure 32-5, there are six potential sites for CNS infections: (1) bone, (2) extradural space, (3) subdural space, (4) subarachnoid space, (5) intracerebral, and (6) intraventricular.

Evidence of the infective organism, together with changes in pressure, glucose, and protein levels of the CSF, are highly suggestive of a CNS infection. Magnetic resonance imaging may provide evidence of focal inflammatory disease. The CNS alterations and clinical manifestations vary according to the type of infection.

Viral Infections

Viruses may gain access to the body orally, through the respiratory system, by animal or mosquito bites, or across the placenta to the fetus. Once inside the body, they make their way to the CNS through the hematogenous route by the cerebral capillaries and the choroid plexus. Other entry routes include the peripheral nerves and possibly, by penetration of the olfactory mucosa.[2]

Within the CNS, viruses apparently affect specific, susceptible cells, producing widely variable pathologic

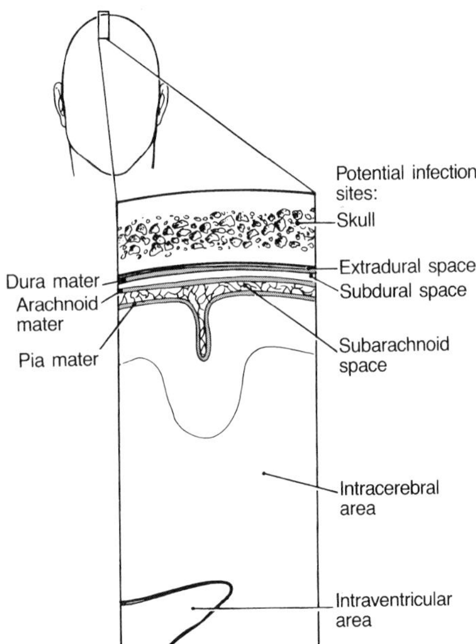

FIGURE 32-5. **Six potential sites for CNS infections: Bone (skull), extradural space, subdural space, subarachnoid space, intracerebral area, intraventricular area.**

effects. Damage to the CNS may result from several mechanisms:

- Direct viral invasion of cells with subsequent lysis (acute encephalitis)
- Selective lysis with resulting demyelination (progressive multifocal leukoencephalopathy)
- Immune responses to viral antigens (acute disseminated encephalomyelitis)
- Cellular destruction without apparent inflammatory or immune response (in some cases)

Viruses may also remain latent in cells for months or years until circumstances trigger acute infections.

BOX 32-1 CAUSES OF VIRAL ENCEPHALITIS AND VIRUS-RELATED ACUTE ENCEPHALOPATHIES

- Viral encephalitis
  - Sporadic
    - Mumps
    - Herpes simplex viruses
    - Lymphocytic choriomeningitis virus
    - Cytomegalovirus
    - Epstein-Barr virus
    - Adenovirus
    - Rabies
  - Epidemic
    - Arboviruses (St. Louis, Eastern, Western, California, Venezuelan equine, Colorado tick fever)
    - Enteroviruses (coxsackievirus and echoviruses)
- Postinfectious encephalomyelitis
  - Measles
    - Varicella
    - Mumps
    - Rubella
    - Influenza
  - Vital infections in immunocompromised patients
    - Cytomegalovirus
    - Herpes simplex viruses
    - Enteroviruses
    - Adenoviruses
    - Measles
    - JC virus (progressive multifocal leukoencephalopathy)
    - Human immunodeficiency viruses (HIV)
  - Virus-associated encephalopathy
    - Reye syndrome

(Weiner, L. P. [1993]. Viral encephalitis. In R.T. Johnson [Ed.], *Current therapy in neurologic disease.* Philadelphia: B.C. Decker.

ACUTE ENCEPHALITIS

Encephalitis is a general term that encompasses infections of the brain parenchyma. Viruses are the most common cause; however, encephalitis also may be caused by bacteria, rickettsia, parasites, and fungi. A variety of causes of viral encephalitis and virus-related acute encephalopathies is presented in Box 32-1.

Although a wide range of symptoms may be present, the specific signs and symptoms depend on the causative organism. Common clinical manifestations include (1) headache, (2) high fever, (3) confusion, (4) convulsions, and (5) restlessness that progresses to stupor and coma. Focal CNS impairment, such as hemiparesis, asymmetry of tendon reflexes, Babinski's sign, involuntary movements, ataxia, and difficulty in speaking or understanding, also may be present. Brainstem involvement may be manifested by facial weakness or ocular palsies. Analysis of CSF usually reveals increased numbers of lymphocytes, normal to slightly increased pressure, slightly increased protein, normal glucose, and normal chloride levels.[16] A comatose state may persist for days, weeks, or months after the acute infection. Residual effects are possible and may include behavior and personality changes, mental deterioration, parkinsonism, paralysis, and persistent seizures.

ARTHROPOD-BORNE (ARBO) VIRUS ENCEPHALITIS. This large group of viruses commonly causes encephalitis. The organisms seem to occur in certain geographic locations and during certain seasons, especially summer and early fall when mosquitoes are biting. Except for tick-borne arboviruses, all of these viruses involve vertebrate hosts with mosquito vectors. The principal site of infection is the brain.[20] Types of ARBO viral encephalitis are described in Table 32-5.

Clinical manifestations among the different arboviruses are similar. However, they may vary with the age of the afflicted individual; for example, the onset of fever and convulsions is most abrupt in children.

HERPES SIMPLEX. Herpes simplex virus (HSV), a very serious and common form of encephalitis, may produce illness in any age group. This type of encephalitis has been reported in all parts of the world.

PATHOPHYSIOLOGY. Most frequently, the disease is associated with type I HSV, which is also the common cause of oral mucosal lesions. The virus may be introduced from a primary lip infection to the brainstem by the trigeminal nerve. Type II HSV causes genital infection and, when present in the mother, produces acute encephalitis in the neonate, acquired during passage through an infected birth canal.[2]

Alterations in the CNS are more common in the medial and inferior portions of the temporal lobes and orbital gyri of the frontal lobes. The lesions, shown in Figure 32-6, include hemorrhagic necrosis, inflammation, and perivascular infiltrates.

CLINICAL MANIFESTATIONS. Clinical manifestations include acute onset with headache, fever, convulsions, confusion, stupor, and coma, in addition to focal disturbances related to lesions in specific portions of the temporal and frontal lobes. The CSF reveals an increased pressure, increased protein level, increased number of lymphocytes, and the presence of red cells due to the hemorrhagic nature of the lesions. Serologic tests and brain biopsy confirm a diagnosis of herpes simplex encephalitis.

RABIES. Clinical cases of rabies in humans are rare, but once the disease is established, it is almost always fatal. This dreaded viral disease can affect anyone who has sustained a bite through the skin by a rabid animal (usually dogs, cats, bats, foxes, raccoons, or skunks). Its incubation period varies from 14 days to 3 months. Survival of inoculated victims depends on specific post-exposure prophylaxis.

PATHOPHYSIOLOGY. The virus makes its way from the wound to the CNS through the peripheral nerves, producing degenerative changes in these neurons. Alterations in the CNS include brain edema, neuron degeneration, and vascular congestion. Inflammatory reactions seem to be greatest in the basal nuclei, midbrain, and medulla. The spinal cord, sympathetic ganglia, and dorsal root ganglia may also be involved. *Negri bodies*, which are oval-shaped, eosinophilic, cytoplasmic inclusions, are a characteristic histologic feature of rabies.

CLINICAL MANIFESTATIONS. Clinical manifestations occur in stages, beginning with generalized malaise, apathy, fever, and headache. These general symptoms, together with pain and numbness in the area of the wound, are diagnostic of the illness in its early stage. Within 24 to 72 hours after the general symptoms, there is an excitement phase marked by extreme

TABLE 32-5

TYPES OF ARBO VIRUS ENCEPHALITIS

ARBO VIRUS TYPE	LOCATION	AREA OF INVOLVEMENT	CLINICAL MANIFESTATIONS
Eastern equine encephalitis	Eastern states	Extensively wide destruction of cerebral cortex and white matter	Rarely seen (1 to 19 cases yearly); survivors have residual effects including blindness, deafness, mental retardation, emotional disorders, and hemiplegia; large number of polymorphonuclear leukocytes in CS
Western equine encephalitis	Western region	Upper spinal cord and large portions of the brain	Fever, stupor, dizziness, confusion, and headache; sequela of postencephalitic Parkinsonism
St. Louis encephalitis	Central and Western states	Brain and spinal cord with prominent meningeal involvement	Fever, athetosis, drowsiness, or stupor; tremors and seizures (more common)
California encephalitis	Northern Midwest and Northeastern states	Diffuse areas of microscopic hemispheric injury and necrosis	Insidious onset with headache, fever, vomiting, mental confusion, and seizures; stupor deteriorating to coma; residual effects including learning difficulties, emotional lability, and seizures

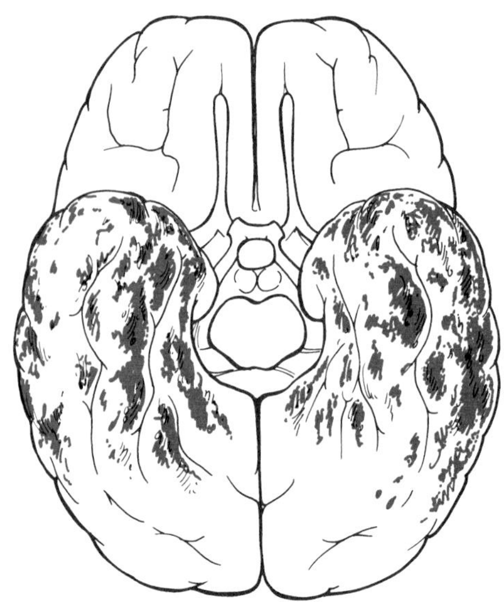

FIGURE 32-6. **Herpes simplex encephalitis. The temporal lobes are preferentially involved by a hemorrhagic, necrotizing inflammation. (Adams, J. & Graham, D., [1994]. *An introduction to neuropathology* [2nd ed.]. London: Churchill-Livingstone.)**

fear, violent spasms of the larynx with swallowing leading to hydrophobia, and dysphagia leading to salivating with frothing from the mouth. Heightened sensitivity to external stimuli can produce localized twitching and generalized seizures. Facial numbness, dysarthria, hallucinations, and a confusional psychosis accompany this phase, which lasts approximately 2 to 7 days. Finally, alternating periods of stupor and mania, high fever, flaccid paralysis, coma, and respiratory failure follow. Death usually occurs from cardiopulmonary arrest.

PRION DISEASE

Prion disease is a group of encephalitis-inducing diseases with slow onset and a long latent period. True prion disease, which includes subacute sclerosing panencephalitis (SSPE), progressive multifocal leukoencephalopathy (PML), and progressive rubella panencephalitis, is caused by known conventional viruses such as the measles virus. A second type, unconventional agent infections (spongiform), which include Creutzfeldt-Jakob (C-J) disease and kuru, are caused by yet-unidentified agents that have some resemblance to viruses but do not produce an immune reaction in the host.[1] Unlike the acute encephalitis, the prion diseases go through a long latent period, lasting from months to years, before symptoms are manifested. Once symptoms have appeared, these diseases tend to progress at a slower pace.

SUBACUTE SCLEROSING PANENCEPHALITIS. This illness usually occurs in children and is related to a prior infection by the measles virus. Granular regions, areas of focal destruction, and proliferation of neuroglial cells are present in the CNS.

CLINICAL MANIFESTATIONS. The illness occurs in stages over several years: (1) initially, personality changes occur; (2) intellectual deterioration, seizures, ataxia, and visual disturbances follow; and (3) rigidity, progressive unresponsiveness, and signs of autonomic dysfunction cause death within a few months or 1 to 3 years. The CSF reveals increased protein, increased gamma globulin fraction, and high levels of measles antibody. There is also evidence of measles antigen in neurons and glial cells. Bursts of high-voltage and sharp waves are noted on EEG examination.

PROGRESSIVE MULTIFOCAL LEUKOENCEPHALOPATHY (PML). This condition most often occurs in middle-aged persons who have a chronic debilitating disease such as rheumatoid arthritis, acquired immune deficiency syndrome (AIDS), or neoplastic disease, or in those who are receiving immunosuppressive therapy. Opportunistic viruses, such as C-J virus or simian virus 40 (SV-40), cause CNS alterations, including widespread demyelinization of white matter, particularly of the cerebral hemispheres, brainstem, cerebellum, and, rarely, the spinal cord.

CLINICAL MANIFESTATIONS. Symptoms of PML include hemiparesis, visual field defects, aphasia, ataxia, dysarthria, confusion, and eventually coma. The CSF usually remains normal. Computerized axial tomography reveals the lesions.[2] Death occurs within 3 to 20 months after onset of symptoms.

PROGRESSIVE RUBELLA PANENCEPHALITIS. This type of encephalitis, associated with rubella either of congenital or childhood origin, appears after a long latent period and continues on a progressive course. Progressive rubella panencephalitis seems to affect the white matter primarily, destroying nerve cells and attracting lymphocytes and mononuclear cells.

CLINICAL MANIFESTATIONS. Initially, subtle changes in behavior and intellectual performance are noted. Seizures arise in association with progressive mental deterioration, motor incoordination, and spasticity; mutism, quadriplegia, and ophthalmoplegia mark the terminal stages of the disease.

SUBACUTE SPONGIFORM ENCEPHALOPATHY (CREUTZFELDT-JAKOB DISEASE, TRANSMISSIBLE VIRAL DEMENTIA). This rare, rapidly progressive disease, which usually occurs in late middle age, produces CNS alterations, primarily in the cerebral and cerebellar cortices and occasionally in the basal ganglia. Alterations include neural degeneration, gliosis, and a spongelike condition in affected areas.

Clinical Manifestations. The early clinical manifestations include personality changes, memory loss, visual abnormalities (distortions of shape, decreased visual acuity), and delirium. These symptoms are followed rapidly by dementia, myoclonic contractions, dysarthria, and ataxia. Eventually, stupor and coma occur even though myoclonic contractions continue. Although serologic studies and CSF are normal, the EEG shows an associated, distinctive pattern of diffuse nonspecific slowing, which changes to sharp waves or spikes on an increasingly flat background.[2] Death usually occurs within 1 to 2 years after the onset of symptoms.

Kuru. *Kuru*, the first slow viral infection documented in humans, occurs in the Fore natives of Papua, New Guinea. The disease is associated with the tribe's cannibalism. Although the CNS alterations are similar to those associated with subacute spongiform encephalopathy, in kuru the spongelike conditions are more prominent in the corpus striatum and cerebellum.[17]

Clinical Manifestations. Clinical manifestations include progressive cerebellar ataxia, shivering tremors, abnormal extraocular movement, incontinence, progression to complete immobility, and dementia in the terminal stage. After the onset of symptoms, death usually occurs within 3 to 6 months.

HUMAN IMMUNODEFICIENCY VIRUS-TYPE 1

All parts of the CNS may be involved in the course of human immunodeficiency virus–type 1 (HIV-1). One or more neurologic syndromes have been reported in approximately 40% of persons who have AIDS.[4] Neurologic complaints are the initial symptoms in 10% of all patients with AIDS. Nervous system involvement may result from primary HIV infection, secondary to opportunistic processes (immunosuppression), or both. The major neurologic complications associated with HIV-1 infection are presented in Table 32-6.

TABLE 32-6

MAJOR NEUROLOGIC COMPLICATIONS OF HIV-1 INFECTION

DIRECT EFFECTS OF HIV-1	OPPORTUNISTIC PROCESSES
Acute aseptic meningitis	Cryptococcal meningitis*
Chronic pleocytosis	Toxoplasmosis*
HIV-1 encephalopathy*	CMV retinitis/encephalitis*
Vacuolar myelopathy	Other CNS opportunistic infections*
Predominantly sensory neuropathy	Herpes group radiculitis
Inflammatory demyelinating polyneuropathy	Progressive multifocal leukoencephalopathy*
Mononeuritis multiplex	Primary CNS lymphoma*
Myopathy	Systemic lymphoma*
	Neurosyphilis

* AIDS-defining condition.
AIDS, acquired immunodeficiency syndrome; *CNS*, central nervous system; *CMV*, cytomegalovirus; *HIV*, human immunodeficiency virus.
(McArthur, J. [1993]. Neurologic diseases associated with HIV-1 infection. In R. T. Johnson [Ed.], *Current therapy in neurologic disease* [4th ed.]. Philadelphia: B.C. Decker.)

Direct Neurologic Effects of HIV-1

Persons initially infected with the HIV-1 virus may develop *acute aseptic meningitis* as a result of CNS response to viral invasion. A mild lymphocytosis and modest CSF protein elevation may occur.[1] Clinical manifestations include headache, cranial neuropathies, and symptoms associated with meningeal irritation and transient encephalopathies.

HIV-1 encephalopathy and encephalitis have been described as the most common neurologic pathologies associated with AIDS. One third of patients with AIDS develop these conditions early in the course of the disease, whereas two thirds develop them late in the illness.[2] Also known as *AIDS dementia complex*, HIV encephalopathy occurs as a result of direct HIV invasion of the CNS through infected macrophages or through the blood–brain barrier by endothelial cells. Computerized tomography scans or MRI reveals mild to moderate brain atrophy and white matter changes (Fig. 32-7). Examination of CSF reveals mononuclear pleocytosis (increased cells) and elevated protein.

Many microscopic changes have been described in HIV dementia. Recommended neuropathology terminology for HIV-associated CNS disease based on these microscopic changes is presented Table 32-7.

The correlation between pathologic changes and the clinical features of progressive dementia in AIDS remains somewhat unclear,[14] and the clinical manifestations differ depending on the person's age. In adults, clinical manifestations *typically* include progressive dementia with memory loss, disorientation, intellectual impairment, mood changes, psychotic behavior, leg weakness, seizures, and headache. In infants and children, manifestations include developmental delays, cognitive deterioration, microencephaly, and corticospinal tract signs such as spasticity and weakness.

HIV-1 Associated Opportunistic Processes of the CNS

Opportunistic processes involving the CNS that affect patients with AIDS reflect the underlying immune defi-

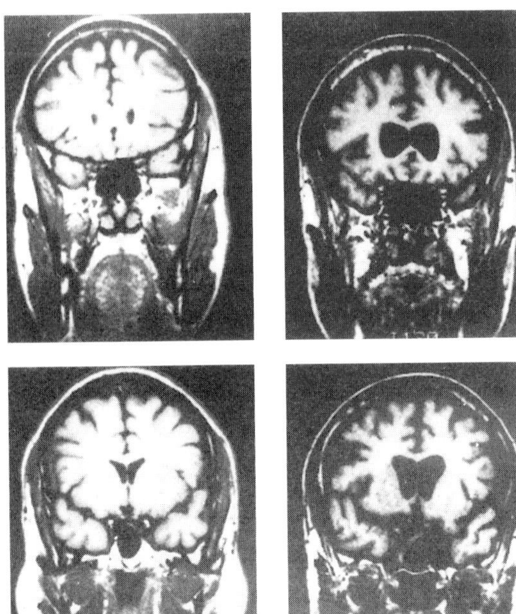

FIGURE 32-7. Atrophy in HIV dementia: MRI. Patient with severe HIV dementia showing central and cortical atrophy on the right, with age-matched control on the left. (Appel. S. [1994] *Current neurology.* St. Louis: Mosby.)

ciency produced by HIV and destruction of CD4 lymphocytes by this virus. During the course of the AIDS illness, many opportunistic processes may occur concurrently with one another, thus complicating diagnosis and treatment. HIV-1 opportunistic processes include:

- Cerebral toxoplasmosis, the most common and treatable intracranial focal complication, is caused by the obligate intracellular protozoan *Toxoplasma gondii.* Multiple inflammatory and necrotic abscesses are produced throughout the cerebral hemispheres, especially in the basal ganglia. These abscesses are present on CT and MRI studies. Cerebrospinal fluid reveals elevated protein, decreased glucose levels, and pleocytosis.
- *Cryptococcus neoformans,* a yeast, is the most frequent fungal infection affecting the CNS in AIDS patients. Clinical manifestations are typical of meningitis and include headache, neck stiffness, fever, altered mentation, and nausea. Actual culture isolation of the cryptococci may be found in CSF.
- Cytomegalovirus (CMV) and human papovavirus can produce encephalitis in AIDS patients. Cytomegalovirus may cause infection in the retina and visual loss in 20% of patients with AIDS.[14]
- Herpes zoster and neurosyphilis also affect the CNS. Herpes zoster radiculitis occurs in 5% to 10% of patients with AIDS.[1] Although neurosyphilis is not strictly an opportunistic infection, it has been suggested that the course of syphilis is accelerated in patients with AIDS.[14] Also, there appears to be an increase in frequency of syphilitic meningitis and meningovascular syphilis in patients with AIDS.

ASEPTIC MENINGITIS COMPLEX (BENIGN VIRAL MENINGITIS)

Aseptic meningitis complex refers to disorders with evidence of meningeal irritation but without evidence of pyogenic organisms, parasites, or fungi in CSF. However, lymphocytes are commonly present. A virus is believed to be the cause. Viruses such as mumps, herpes

TABLE 32-7

RECOMMENDED TERMINOLOGY FOR HIV-ASSOCIATED CNS DISEASE

NEW NAME	OLD NAME	DEFINITION
HIV encephalitis	Giant cell encephalitis, multinucleated cell encephalitis, subacute encephalitis	Multiple disseminated foci of microglia, macrophages, MNGCs. If MNGCs not present. HIV antigen or nucleic acids demonstrated by immunocytochemistry or in situ hybridization
HIV leukoencephalopathy	Diffuse myelin pallor, progressive diffuse leukoencephalopathy	Diffuse damage to white matter with myelin loss, reactive astrogliosis, macrophages and MNGCs, or detectable HIV antigen or nucleic acids
Diffuse poliodystrophy	Subacute encephalitis	Diffuse reactive astrogliosis and microglial activation involving cerebral gray matter. NOTE: This term designates diffuse pathology of cortical and subcortical gray matter structures that may underlie neuronal loss or changes in synaptic or dendritic anatomy
Vacuolar myelopathy	Vacuolar myelopathy	Multiple areas of spinal cord involved by vacuolar myelin changes with intravacuole macrophages

CNS, central nervous system: *HIV,* human immunodeficiency virus: *MNGC,* multinucleated giant cells.
(McArthur, J., & Harrison, M. [1994]. HIV-associated dementia. In Appel. S. [Ed.] *Current neurology.* St. Louis: Mosby.)

simplex, coxsackievirus, lymphocytic choriomeningitis virus, and ECHO virus have been found in over one third of individuals with aseptic meningitis complex.

CLINICAL MANIFESTATIONS. Clinical manifestations are mild and include headache, fever, and signs of meningeal irritation. Most individuals recover from these illnesses without significant residual effects.

CONGENITALLY ACQUIRED VIRUSES

Viruses are capable of crossing the placenta to reach the fetus, especially during the first trimester of pregnancy. They often produce devastating effects on the fetus. Although it is possible for many types of viruses to infect the fetus, the most common ones are rubella and cytomegalovirus (CMV).

RUBELLA. Congenital rubella often occurs during the first 10 weeks of gestation. The virus invades the brain of the fetus and contributes to the establishment of severe mental retardation, seizures, and motor defects. Other manifestations may include low birth weight, abnormally small eyeballs, pigmentary retinal degeneration, glaucoma, cloudy cornea, cataracts, neurocochlear deafness, enlarged liver and spleen, jaundice, and patent ductus arteriosus or intraventricular septal defects.[2] These severe effects are preventable by ensuring that women receive the rubella vaccine prior to becoming pregnant.

CYTOMEGALOVIRUS. Cytomegaloviruses usually infect the fetus early in the first trimester of pregnancy, possibly producing cerebral malformation. Later in the pregnancy, CMV may produce inflammatory necrosis in various parts of the fetal brain. Nervous system effects of this infection may include mental defects, convulsions, microcephaly, and often hydrocephalus. Other manifestations include an enlarged liver and spleen, jaundice, melena, hematemesis, and petechiae.[2] Because the infection is not apparent in pregnant women, CMV infection in a fetus cannot be determined until birth (and in some cases, several years later).

MYELITIS

POLIOMYELITIS. Since the advent of the Salk vaccine in 1955 and the oral Sabin vaccine in 1958, cases of paralytic poliomyelitis are uncommon. Approximately 15 cases are reported each year in the United States.[2] Although the synonym for poliomyelitis is *infantile paralysis*, the disease occurs in all age groups throughout the world. Its peak frequency is during the summer months.

PATHOPHYSIOLOGY. The human intestinal tract is the main viral reservoir for the poliomyelitis virus, a ribonucleic acid (RNA) virus. Infection occurs through the fecal–oral route. Incubation lasts from 1 to 3 weeks. The virus then penetrates intestinal walls, invades the bloodstream, and is carried throughout the body.

In the CNS, nerve cells are destroyed. Cellular infiltration, edema, and severe inflammatory processes that produce tissue necrosis and hemorrhages also occur. Although the entire CNS may be involved, the predominant site of alterations is the anterior horn of the spinal cord.

CLINICAL MANIFESTATIONS. The majority of persons infected with the virus experience no symptoms or only a vague illness, because of the failure of the virus to invade the CNS. Even after CNS invasion, however, clinical effects range from a mild, nonparalytic form of the disease to a severe, paralytic form. This variation in symptoms is related to the severity of the inflammatory response and to the degree to which nerve cells are injured.

Examination of CSF usually shows no evidence of the virus during the clinical disease. However, protein levels are elevated, glucose level is normal, and the number of lymphocytes is increased.

Nonparalytic poliomyelitis produces general symptoms of fever, headache, listlessness, anorexia, nausea, vomiting, sore throat, and aching muscles. At this point, the disease may be resolved. With increasing irritability, restlessness, muscle tenderness and spasms, neck and back pain, and neck stiffness, in addition to Kernig's and Brudzinski's signs, the paralytic form of the disease is often imminent.

Paralytic poliomyelitis is often divided into three types: (1) spinal, (2) bulbar, and (3) encephalitic. This division is used primarily for description since these types are often combined during the course of the disease.

- *Spinal* involvement may include muscle weakness with fasciculations, diminished reflexes accompanied by progressive abdominal and limb muscle weakness, eventual paralysis (the level varying among different age groups), and muscle atrophy.
- *Bulbar* involvement impairs the ability to swallow, disturbs respiration and vasomotor control, and progressively slows respirations. Cyanosis and hypertension may occur, followed by hypotension and circulatory collapse. With accompanying phrenic and intercostal muscle paralysis, mortality is as high as 75%.[2]
- *Encephalitic* involvement (of the high brainstem and hypothalamus) produces restlessness, confusion, and anxiety initially, progressing to stupor and coma.[2]

HERPES ZOSTER (SHINGLES). Herpes zoster infection, caused by the varicella zoster virus, occurs most commonly in adulthood, particularly with advancing age, and in persons with underlying systemic diseases, such as the leukemias or lymphomas. Although its development is not completely understood, herpes zoster infection is believed to represent a reactivation of varicella virus infection that persists in the nerve ganglia after a primary infection with chickenpox. Herpes zoster is not communicable, except possibly to people who have not had chickenpox.[2] Individuals who have herpes zoster infection usually have a past history of chickenpox. Nervous system alterations include congested, edematous, and hemorrhagic dorsal root ganglion. There is also disintegration of ganglion cells.

Clinical Manifestations. Painful, vesicular skin eruptions, which harbor varicella zoster virus, are associated with involvement of the corresponding dorsal root ganglion or gasserian ganglion. The most frequently involved dermatomes are T-5 to T-10; however, any dermatome may be involved. In some cases, accompanying sensory loss and motor palsies occur. Although most individuals recover, the process is often slow and painful. The pain may persist for months or even years, causing much despair for the person.

POSTINFECTIOUS/POSTVACCINAL DISEASES

Acute disseminated (postinfectious) encephalomyelitis, acute inflammatory polyradiculoneuropathy (Guillain-Barré syndrome, discussed in Chapter 33) and Reye's syndrome (discussed in Chapter 26) often occur during or shortly after viral infections. Although rare, they may occur after vaccinations for smallpox, rabies, or typhoid. These conditions often require individual susceptibility to the virus or viral effects.

Acute Disseminated (Postinfectious) Encephalomyelitis. Postinfectious encephalomyelitis, developing 2 to 4 days after a rash, is thought to be an autoimmune response to myelin, which is triggered by a virus.[5] Demyelination occurs in the region of the brainstem and spinal cord. In addition, the meninges are infiltrated by inflammatory cells. Clinical manifestations include headaches, neck stiffness, lethargy, and eventually coma. Ten to 20% of affected persons die in the acute phase of the illness.[2] Neurologic residual effects are severe in those who survive.

Bacterial Infections

PYOGENIC INFECTIONS

The brain or its coverings can be infected by pyogenic (pus-forming) microorganisms, most commonly those that are normally harbored in the nasopharynx of the general population. Bacteria enter the CNS, spreading from adjacent cranial structures through the bloodstream. In a few cases, the infection is iatrogenic, for example, from a lumbar puncture or contaminated scalpel. Determining the exact entry route of the organism frequently is difficult. Once within the CNS, the effects of pyogenic microorganisms may be disastrous.

Bacterial Meningitis (Leptomeningitis)

The leptomeninges and subarachnoid space are primary targets for invasion by pyogenic microorganisms. Once an infection enters any part of the subarachnoid space, it spreads quickly throughout CSF pathways in the brain and spinal cord. Thus, an inflammatory reaction occurs in the pia and arachnoid mater and in the ventricles.

Etiology. Any microorganisms entering the body may cause meningitis. However, some bacteria are more prominent and seem to be more prevalent in certain age groups. For example, pneumococcus organisms are commonly cultured in very young patients and in adults over 40 years of age, often related to a prior infection in the lungs, nasal sinuses, and heart valves. *Escherichia coli* is common in the neonatal period. *Hemophilus influenzae* is seen in infants and young children, commonly following ear and upper respiratory infections. *Neisseria meningitidis* is seen in adolescents and young adults.

Pathophysiology. Meningococcal infections develop more rapidly and distinctly than other forms of meningitis, occurring as a singular event or in epidemics where overcrowding exists. The organism is spread by droplet infection from those harboring the meningococcus in their nasal passages.

With the various bacterial infections, swelling and congestion of the brain and spinal cord occur. Exudate collects within the subarachnoid space (Fig. 32-8). In severe cases, inflammatory cells can occlude vessels that penetrate the brain, resulting in areas of necrosis.

Clinical Manifestations. Disease onset is heralded by a distinctive petechial or purpuric rash. Other clinical manifestations include fever, headache, pain with eye movement, photophobia, neck and back stiffness, positive Kernig's and Brudzinski's signs, generalized convulsions, drowsiness, and confusion. Focal signs may be observed with some bacterial infections as a result of occlusion of vessels and regional brain necrosis.[18] Stupor, followed by coma and death, may occur without prompt and adequate treatment. The CSF reveals elevated protein, decreased glucose and chloride

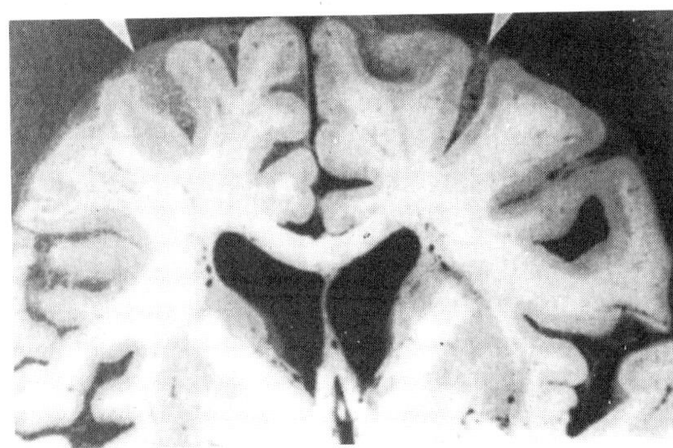

FIGURE 32-8. Acute meningitis. There is a thick layer of pus in the subarachnoid space (*arrows*). (Adams, J. & Graham, D. [1994]. *An introduction to neuropathology* [2nd ed.]. London: Churchill-Livingstone.)

levels, elevated pressure (above 180 mm of water), and the presence of large numbers of leukocytes.

After any bacterial meningitis, a disastrous event (Waterhouse-Friderichsen syndrome) may occur. This is most commonly associated with *fulminant meningococcemia.* This condition is manifested by overwhelming bacteremia, adrenocortical necrosis, and vasomotor collapse.

Because of destruction or fibrotic thickening of the meningeal framework, residual effects such as optic arachnoiditis, meningomyelitis, and chronic meningoencephalitis with hydrocephalus are possible.[12]

Brain Abscess

Approximately one half of all brain abscesses are secondary to infection in the nasal cavity, middle ear, and mastoid cells. The remaining cases are due to a primary focus of infection elsewhere in the body, particularly the lungs or pleura, heart, and distal bones. Streptococci, staphylococci, and pneumococci are often the causative organisms. A small proportion (about 10%) of cases result from infection being introduced through compound skull fractures or intracranial operations.[2]

PATHOPHYSIOLOGY. An abscess forms when an inflammation, caused by an invading organism, liquefies and white blood cells begin to accumulate. A fibrous capsule forms to contain the pus. As the abscess expands, nerve tissue is compressed and destroyed. Figure 32-9 depicts the chronic inflammation (inset) and edema surrounding the abscess and a secondary abscess that may form from the primary abscess.

CLINICAL MANIFESTATIONS. The most frequent initial clinical manifestation is headache, with other symptoms being similar to those produced by growing masses within the brain. Notably, the increased intracranial pressure and focal complaints related to the location of the abscess are important. A brain abscess also can rupture and lead to other complications, such as sinus thrombosis, ventriculitis, or meningitis. The CSF associated with brain abscesses reveals a normal glucose level, increased protein level, and increased white cell count. The CSF pressure is often moderately elevated early in the abscess formation and markedly elevated in the later stages. If the abscess ruptures into the subarachnoid space or ventricles, organisms can be cultured from the CSF.

Subdural Empyema

Empyema refers to pus in a body cavity. Thus, subdural empyema is a suppurative process in the subdural space, usually occurring between the dura's inner surface and the arachnoid's outer surface. The most common causative organisms are streptococci or bacteroides, and less often *Staphylococcus aureus, E. coli,* and pseudomonas.[2]

PATHOPHYSIOLOGY. Infective organisms usually travel to the subdural space by spread from thrombophlebitis or by erosion through bone or dura from the frontal sinuses, ethmoid sinuses, middle ear, or mastoid cells. Exudate is present on the undersurface of the dura. As the empyema grows, pressure is applied to the underlying cerebral hemisphere. Thrombophlebitis of cerebral veins near the subdural empyema can contribute to ischemic necrosis of the cortex.

CLINICAL MANIFESTATIONS. Many affected persons have a history of chronic mastoiditis or sinusitis. If the infection has spread to the subdural space, clinical manifestations may include fever, general malaise, a localized headache that becomes generalized, associated vomiting, and neck stiffness. As the empyema enlarges, focal neurologic signs, lethargy, and coma develop. The CSF reveals elevated pressure, increased protein and normal glucose levels, and an increased number of lymphocytes.

TUBERCULOUS INFECTIONS

Tuberculous meningitis and tuberculomas of the brain and spinal cord are usually secondary to a tuberculous focus in another part of the body. With the recent resurgence of tuberculosis, the frequency of tuberculous meningitis and tuberculomas of the brain and cord may also be increased.

Tuberculous Meningitis

Tuberculous meningitis is caused by *Mycobacterium tuberculosis.* It occurs primarily in young children in areas of high tuberculosis prevalence and most commonly in the elderly as a result of reactivation of dormant organisms in low-frequency areas. This condition has a slower onset and more chronic course than pyogenic meningitis.

PATHOPHYSIOLOGY. The base of the brain and the spinal cord become compressed by shaggy, necrotic, fibrinous, yellow exudate. There may also be large areas of caseation (crumbly cheese-like necrosis) and tiny tubercles around the blood vessels.[2]

CLINICAL MANIFESTATIONS. Clinical manifestations depend on the chronicity of the disease and the extent of pathologic processes. Due to the slow onset of this illness, neurologic damage may be present before the patient comes in for evaluation. In general, adults have headache, fever, lethargy, confusion, neck stiffness, positive Kernig's and Brudzinski's signs, weight loss, and night sweats. Young children frequently experience vomiting, irritability, and seizures.

The CSF reveals increased pressure, elevated protein, and decreased glucose levels (but not as low as values observed in pyogenic meningitis). Polymorphonuclear leukocytes and lymphocytes also may be seen, and tubercle bacilli may be recovered from CSF.

FOCUS ON CELLULAR PATHOPHYSIOLOGY

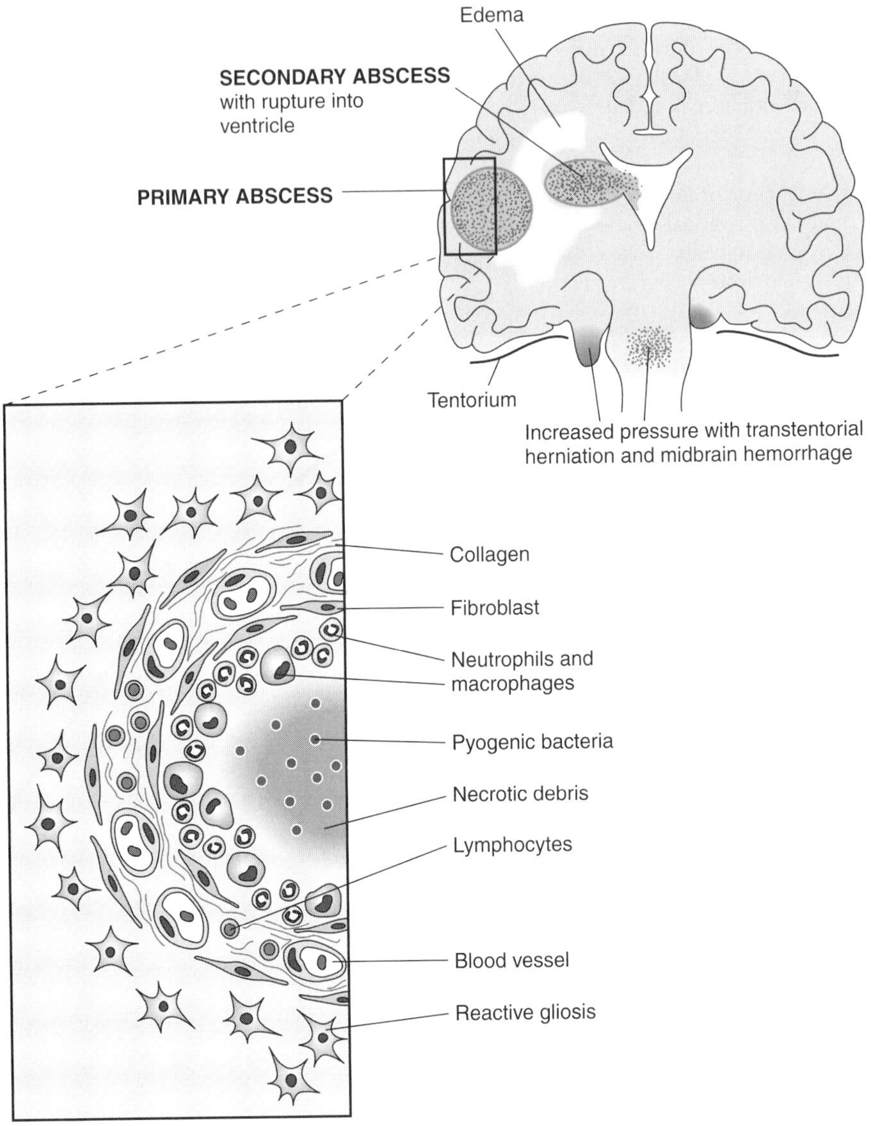

FIGURE 32-9. Brain abscess and its complications. A cerebral abscess may cause death through the production of secondary abscess with intraventricular rupture; alternatively, death may result from transtentorial herniation. (Rubin, E., & Farber J. L. [1999]. *Pathology* [3rd ed.]. Philadelphia: Lippincott.)

Long-term effects, such as recurrent seizures, retarded intellectual development, mental disturbances, visual disturbances, deafness, and hemiparesis may follow.

Tuberculomas of the Brain and Spinal Cord

Tuberculomas (tuberculous granulation masses), although rare in the United States, constitute from 5% to 30% of all intracranial space-occupying lesions in underdeveloped countries.[2] Tuberculomas may be single or multiple and contain a core of caseation necrosis surrounded by a fibrous capsule. Tuberculomas of the brain and spinal cord have been known to calcify while still small, before any neurologic changes have occurred.

Within the brain and spinal cord, they produce neurologic effects similar to those of other expanding intracranial and intraspinal lesions. Increased protein levels and a small number of lymphocytes are found in the CSF.

Tuberculous infection may affect the spinal cord in a number of ways, causing spinal block. Evidence of spinal root disease may be the result of inflammatory meningeal exudate invasion of the underlying parenchyma. Compression by an epidural mass of granulation tissue produces spinal symptoms such as pain and varying motor-sensory deficits, including Pott's paraplegia, a paraplegia from epidural cord compression.[2]

NEUROSYPHILIS

Treponema pallidum, a spirochete, is a spiral, motile organism that causes syphilis. Once this organism is introduced into the body, it usually invades the CNS within 3 to 18 months. Neurosyphilis is progressive in the large majority of individuals and includes several stages: asymptomatic neurosyphilis, meningovascular syphilis, general paresis, and tabes dorsalis. The frequency of neurosyphilis (tertiary stage of syphilis) has decreased in the last several decades due to prompt diagnosis and treatment of early syphilis. The overall frequency of syphilis is increasing, however, particularly in young persons.

Meningitis is the initial event, but the severity of symptoms varies among the different stages, with the patient possibly remaining asymptomatic for several years. Symptoms associated with the stages of neurosyphilis are presented in Table 32-8.

The CSF is the most accurate, sensitive indicator that an active neurosyphilitic infection is present. Changes in CSF include positive serologic tests such as the Venereal Disease Research Laboratory (VDRL) slide test, Kolmer test, fluorescent treponemal antibody absorption test, and treponema immobilization test; increased protein level; increased lymphocytes, plasma cells, and mononuclear cells.

LYME DISEASE

Lyme disease, caused by the spirochete *Borrelia burgdorferi* transmitted to humans by the ixodid deer tick, is the most common vector-borne disease in the United States. Its frequency is increasing, with an increase in incidence in the United States from 226 cases in 1980 to over 7000 cases in 1989 to 1990.[8] This increase is thought to be due to the resurgence of the deer population, the spread of tick vectors to new areas, and the spreading of suburban populations into once-rural areas.[10] The disease typically occurs in warmer months between May and August, and 25% to 50% of cases are reported in children less than 16 years of age.[8]

A multisystem disease with neurologic manifestations occurs in 10% to 15% of cases after an interval of 1 to 6 months. Neurologic involvement is manifested as meningitis, meningoencephalitis with severe headache, cranial nerve palsies (especially CN VII), polyradiculoneuropathy, mononeuropathy multiplex, a neuropathy resembling Guillain-Barré syndrome, or myelopathy. Late neurologic manifestations include a multiple sclerosis–like syndrome.[8] Serologic studies reveal IgG antibodies to *Borrelia*.

TABLE 32-8

MANIFESTATIONS ASSOCIATED WITH THE STAGES OF NEUROSYPHILIS

NEUROSYPHILIS STAGE	PHYSIOLOGIC CONSEQUENCE AND MANIFESTATIONS
Asymptomatic (initial)	Usually no physical signs or symptoms of meningitis Positive CSF and serologic test results
Meningovascular (6 to 7 years)	CNS alterations including infiltration of meninges and blood vessels with plasma cells and lymphocytes; inflammation of arteries, fibrosis Symptoms similar to low-grade meningitis, cerebrovascular accident, or mental derangement
General paresis (15 to 20 years)	Diffuse destruction of cortical neurons; proliferation of astrocytes; plasma cell and lymphocyte accumulation around blood vessels Progressive mental deterioration, memory loss, behavioral changes progressing to severe dementia; progressive physical deterioration including dysarthria, tremor of tongue and hands, myoclonic jerks, muscular hypotonia, hyperactive tendon reflexes, Babinski sign, seizures, Argyll Robertson pupils
Tabes dorsalis (many years after onset of infection)	Degeneration of the posterior columns, fibrosis around posterior roots, destruction of proprioceptive fibers in the radicular nerves General paresis Physical symptoms including ataxia, lightning pains, urinary incontinence, epigastric pain with vomiting, Argyll Robertson pupils, Charcot joints, absence of vibration sense and deep tendon reflexes, positive Romberg sign

DISORDERS DUE TO BACTERIAL EXOTOXINS

Bacterial exotoxins can have powerful effects on the CNS. The major diseases produced by these toxins include tetanus, diphtheria, and botulism, which can result in life-threatening motor problems.

TETANUS. *Clostridium tetani*, an anaerobic, spore-forming bacilli, produces tetanus. It occurs following contamination of penetrating wounds with the organism or of the newborn's umbilical cord by the organism's spores.

Clostridium produces two exotoxins: a tetanolysin and a tetanospasmin. Neurotoxic effects are produced by tetanospasmin. Most of the toxin enters the peripheral endings of motor neurons from the bloodstream, travels up the fibers to the spinal cord and brainstem, and crosses the synaptic cleft to the inhibitory neurons, preventing the release of glycine, a neuromuscular transmitter acting as an inhibitor, secreted mainly in the synapses of the spinal cord. Tetanospasmin has an affinity for the sympathetic nervous system, the medullary centers, the anterior horn cells of the spinal cord, and the motor end plates in skeletal muscle. It produces uninhibited motor responses leading to the typical muscle spasm.

The incubation period varies from several days to several months. Some patients develop symptoms 1 to 2 days after contamination and within 2 weeks after wound contamination. The initial manifestation is usually difficulty opening the jaw (*trismus*)—thus, the synonym *lockjaw.* There is generalized muscle stiffness with eventual muscle spasms (tetanic seizures or convulsions). These convulsions are very painful and can occur spontaneously or in response to the slightest stimuli. Facial spasms produce a characteristic sardonic smile (*risus sardonicus*). Contractions of back muscles produce a forward arching of the back (opisthotonos). Spasms of glottal, laryngeal, and respiratory muscles cause difficulty in breathing and frequently lead to death due to asphyxia. Since the toxin is not able to cross the blood–brain barrier, the patient's mental status is unaffected.[5]

DIPHTHERIA. *Corynebacterium diphtheriae* is the causative organism for diphtheria, an acute infection. Although open wounds in any part of the body can provide entry for this organism, the usual portal of entry is the oral cavity. During the incubation period of 1 to 7 days, the organism becomes established and proliferates at the site of implantation, usually the throat and trachea. The bacteria produce an exotoxin that is absorbed by the blood and carried to the CNS and heart. Early general manifestations of the disease include fever, sore throat, chills, and malaise. Local neurologic manifestations occur within 5 to 12 days of the onset of symptoms and include vomiting, dysphagia, possible cranial nerve involvement, and nasal voice quality due to palatal paralysis. Blurred vision and loss of accommodation secondary to ciliary body paralysis occur in the second or third week. Between the fifth and sixth weeks, weakness and paralysis of the extremities may occur. Most neurologic disturbances disappear slowly. Individuals usually improve completely if respiratory obstruction or cardiac failure does not supervene.

BOTULISM. *Clostridium botulinum* can contaminate and produce exotoxins in food, such as fruits, vegetables, and meats that are kept unrefrigerated for long periods of time. When ingested, the toxin, which resists gastric digestion, is absorbed by the blood and then travels to the nervous system. The botulinus toxin, acting only on the presynaptic endings of neuromuscular junctions and autonomic ganglia, prevents the release of acetylcholine. Symptoms resembling those of myasthenia gravis, a descending form of paralysis from the cranial nerves downward, occur. Clinical manifestations occur within 12 to 36 hours after ingestion of the contaminated food.[2] Neural symptoms may or may not be preceded by nausea and vomiting. The individual may develop cranial nerve palsies, blurred vision, diplopia, ptosis, strabismus, hoarseness, dysarthria, dysphagia, vertigo, deafness, constipation, and progressive muscle weakness. Deep tendon reflexes may be absent. Sensation remains intact, and the person is conscious throughout the illness. Paralysis of respiratory muscles and respiratory infections may lead to death in approximately 15% of cases.[5]

Fungal Infections

Although less common than bacteria and viruses, fungi can infect the CNS with effects similar to those of bacterial infections. However, CNS fungal infections are more difficult to treat.

ETIOLOGY

Fungal infections may produce brain abscesses, meningitis, meningoencephalitis, and thrombophlebitis of vessels within the CNS. Like other infections, fungal infections of the CNS are usually secondary to a primary source of infection elsewhere in the body. In addition, they may be a complication of another disease process, such as cancer, or related to immunosuppressant drugs.

Many types of fungi may invade the CNS. The most common infections are candidiasis, cryptococcosis, coccidioidomycosis, and mucormycosis.

PATHOPHYSIOLOGY

Fungi usually spread to the CNS by the bloodstream. Once in the CNS, they cause an inflammatory reaction, and a purulent exudate involves the meninges.

In some cases, invasion of vessel walls results in vasculitis and thrombosis with subsequent nervous tissue infarction. The process develops slowly over days or weeks.

CLINICAL MANIFESTATIONS

Clinical manifestations are similar to those of tuberculous meningitis. In addition, hydrocephalus is a frequent related complication. CNS symptoms associated with the different types of fungal infections are presented in Table 32-9. The CSF reveals elevated pressure, increased protein and decreased glucose levels, moderate pleocytosis (increased number of lymphocytes), and often the isolation of the infective organism.

Protozoal Infections

MALARIA

Plasmodium vivax produces the most common form of malaria. This organism does not actually invade brain tissue, but the parasitized red blood cells block microcirculation, leading to tissue hypoxia and ischemic necrosis. The vessel blockage within the brain leads to glial necrosis, which causes drowsiness, confusion, and seizures.

Plasmodium falciparum produces a more severe form of malaria. The parasite fills capillaries. Durck's nodes (small foci of necrosis surrounded by glia) are present in brain tissue. Clinical manifestations include focal neurologic signs, headache, seizures, aphasia, cerebellar ataxia, hemiplegia, hemianopsia, and eventually coma. The CSF contains white blood cells and reveals elevated pressure.

TOXOPLASMOSIS

Toxoplasma gondii produces an infection that is either acquired, by eating raw beef or by contact with cat feces, or congenital. Rarely does acquired toxoplasmosis produce clinical effects. However, when it does, the white and gray matter contain necrotic lesions that harbor *T. gondii*, and clinical manifestations are similar to those of meningoencephalitis. Acquired toxoplasmosis is observed rather frequently in persons with AIDS.

Congenital toxoplasmosis causes widespread destruction of the neonatal brain. Fever, rash, seizures, and an enlarged liver and spleen may be present at birth. Slow psychomotor development becomes evident early in life. In some cases clinical manifestations of the illness, including hydrocephalus, retardation, cerebral calcification, and chorioretinitis, are not present for days, weeks, or months.

AMEBIASIS

Infection with amoebae usually involves the *Naegleria* genus, possibly occurring after swimming in lakes or

TABLE 32-9

CNS SYMPTOMS ASSOCIATED WITH SELECTED FUNGAL INFECTIONS

INFECTION	PHYSIOLOGIC CONSEQUENCES
Candidiasis (*Candida albicans*)	Normally present in gastrointestinal tract
	No problems unless the host is immunocompromised or breach or protective barriers to infection
	Lymphocytes found in CSF. CNS symptoms appearing as meningitis
	Candida in the eye possibly affecting the retina leading to blindness
Cryptococcosis (torulosis) (*Cryptococcus neoformans*)	Most frequent cause of CNS fungal infection; usually secondary to respiratory infection
	Cysts and granulomas in the cortex, deep white matter, and basal ganglia
	Symptoms similar to meningitis or encephalitis
Coccidioidomycosis (*Coccidioides immitis*)	Common in Southwestern United States
	Involvement of meninges and CSF; possibly becoming a chronic, diffuse granulomatous disease spreading throughout the body
	Mild, flulike symptoms initially CNS symptoms similar to tuberculous meningitis
Mucormycosis (*Murcorales*, opportunistic infection)	Nasal sinuses as primary site of invasion, spreading to periorbital tissue and cranial vault
	Nervous tissue infarctions occurring due to vascular occlusion
	Physical symptoms dependent on areas of infarction

ponds. A prevalence of cases is found in the southeastern United States.

The CNS alterations include abscesses in the cortex and purulent exudate involving the meninges. The disease is rapidly progressive, with symptoms of nausea, vomiting, fever, neck stiffness, focal neurologic signs, seizures, and eventually coma. The CSF findings are similar to those of bacterial meningitis.

TRYPANOSOMIASIS

Several strains of *Trypanosoma brucei* produce African sleeping sickness, transmitted by the tsetse fly. Two epidemiologic patterns are described: Rhodesian (East African) and Gambian (Middle and West African). The Rhodesian type is more severe, with intercurrent infections and myocarditis as the dominating manifestations. Within 2 years after infection with the Gambian form, trypanosomes produce meningoencephalitis, with thickening of the meninges and cerebral edema. Symptoms range from somnolence to convulsions and coma.

Trypanosoma cruzi produces Chagas' disease, found primarily in Central and South America and rarely in North America. The organism is transmitted by biting bugs, commonly called assassin bugs. Chagas' disease can be acute or chronic. The acute form, prevalent in children, produces fever, an enlarged liver and spleen, myocardial involvement with heart failure, and eventually involvement of the lungs, meninges, and brain. Months or years after an acute attack, the chronic form may develop, with subsequent meningoencephalitis.

TRICHINOSIS

Trichinella spiralis enters the body when raw or insufficiently cooked pork is eaten. Within 2 to 3 days, early symptoms of the disease become apparent from the invasion of muscle by larvae. Mild gastroenteritis, muscle weakness, and tenderness are seen. Three to 6 weeks after ingestion, larvae invade the nervous system. Lymphocytic and mononuclear infiltration of the meninges, as well as focal gliosis, occur. Symptoms of CNS involvement include headache, confusion, neck stiffness, seizures, and occasionally coma. Although trichinosis is usually not fatal, seizures and neurologic deficits may continue indefinitely.

Parasitic Infections

CYSTICERCOSIS

Cysticercosis, most common in South American countries, results from ingestion of encysted eggs of the pork tapeworm, *Taenia solium*. The larvae spread throughout the body and develop cysts in any body tissue. Within the brain, these cysts produce symptoms similar to those of brain tumors. Jacksonian seizures are common.

ECHINOCOCCOSIS (HYDATID DISEASE)

Echinococcosis is caused by the ingestion of larvae of the canine tapeworm, *Echinococcus granulosus*. The larvae invade the liver, lungs, bones, and, less frequently, the brain. The larvae, at first microscopic, become encysted. However, within 5 or more years, the cysts may grow to massive sizes of 10 cm or more.[6] Thus, within the brain symptoms are similar to those associated with brain tumors.

Rickettsial Infections

Rickettsial infections, relatively rare in the United States, are caused by obligate intracellular parasites that multiply only within living cells of susceptible hosts. An animal reservoir and an insect vector (ticks, fleas, lice, mites, and humans) are involved in the organism's cycle. However, epidemic typhus involves only a cycle with lice and humans.

FOCUS ON THE PERSON WITH A BRAIN TUMOR

Mrs. M. is a 35-year-old teacher who is married and has one child. She has enjoyed good health except for having a tonsillectomy at age 8. Mrs. M. began experiencing early morning headaches about 6 months before her initial visit to her family physician. Episodes of nausea and vomiting prompted Mrs. M.'s visit. During her check-up, Mrs. M. stated that she thought she was losing her mind because her husband had been noticing a difficulty in her ability to name objects and had complained about her irritability and mood swings. Also, she had noticed ringing in her right ear. Mrs. M. was scheduled for further neurologic testing. While awaiting the tests, she had a seizure.

Mrs. M. was given a detailed neurologic examination that revealed the presence of papilledema. Also, neuroimaging studies were performed. The results of a computed axial tomography scan revealed a poorly demarcated mass causing expansion of the right temporal lobe. Magnetic resonance imaging confirmed these results and additionally revealed the presence of cerebral edema. Eventually Mrs. M. was diagnosed with astrocytoma.

Questions

1. What type of brain tumor is an astrocytoma?
2. Isn't Mrs. M. too young to have an astrocytoma?
3. Describe the symptoms of a brain tumor that Mrs. M. is exhibiting.
4. Why are computed tomography and magnetic resonance imaging useful techniques for diagnosis of a brain tumor?
5. What is the treatment and prognosis for Mrs. M.?

See Appendix A for discussion.

Major rickettsial diseases include epidemic (primary) typhus, louse-borne; murine (endemic) typhus, flea-borne; scrub typhus or tsutsugamushi fever, mite-borne; Rocky Mountain spotted fever, tick-borne; and Q fever, tick-borne and airborne. Within the CNS, rickettsial diseases can produce lesions in the gray and white matter. Focal gliosis, together with mononuclear leukocytes, produce characteristic typhus nodules.

CLINICAL MANIFESTATIONS

All the rickettsial diseases except Q fever have similar pathologic and clinical effects. A 3- to 18-day incubation period is followed by the abrupt onset of high fever, chills, headache, and weakness, followed by a generalized macular rash. During the second week after the onset of fever, the CNS becomes involved, producing apathy, dullness, intermittent episodes of delirium, and eventually stupor and coma. Occasionally, in untreated cases, there are focal neurologic manifestations and optic neuritis. The CSF may be completely normal. Q fever, not accompanied by a rash, produces symptoms similar to those of a low-grade meningitis.

REFERENCES

1. Adams, J., & Graham, D. (1994). *An introduction to neuropathology* (2nd ed.). London: Churchill Livingstone.
2. Adams, R., & Victor, M. (1997). *Principles of neurology* (6th ed.). New York: McGraw-Hill.
3. Barker, F., & Israel, M. (1997). Brain tumors: Epidemiology, molecular and cellular abnormalities. In J. Bertino (Editor in chief), *Encyclopedia of cancer, vol. 1*. San Diego: Academic Press.
4. Bronstein, K. (1995). Epidemiology and classification of brain tumors. *Critical Care Nursing Clinics of North America, 7*, 1.
5. Cotran, R. S., Kumar, V., & Robbins, S. L. (1994). *Robbins' pathologic basis of disease* (5th ed.). Philadelphia: W.B. Saunders.
6. Dohrmann, G., & Rubin, J. (1997). Ultrasonic characteristics of brain tumors. In P. Kornblith & M. Walker (Eds.), *Advances in neuro-oncology II*. Armonk, NY: Futura.
7. Ellison, D., Love, S., Chimelli, L., Harding, B., Lowe, J., Roberts, G., & Vinters, H. (1998). *Neuropathology: A reference text of CNS pathology*. London: Mosby.
8. Guberman, A. (1994). *An introduction to clinical neurology*. Boston: Little, Brown.
9. Inskip, P., Linet, M., & Heineman, E. (1995). Etiology of brain tumors in adults. *Epidemiologic Reviews, 17*, 2.
10. Jacobs, R. (1994). Infectious diseases: Spirochetal. In L. Tierney, S. McPhee, & M. Papadakis (Eds.), *Current medical diagnosis and treatment* (23rd ed.). Norwalk, CT: Appleton & Lange.
11. Kaye, A. (1997). *Essential neurosurgery* (2nd ed.). New York: Churchill Livingstone.
12. Koroshetz, W., & Swartz, M. (1998). Chronic and recurrent meningitis. In S. Fauci, E. Braunwald, K. Isselbacher, J. Wilson, J. Martin, D. Kasper, S. Hauser, & D. Longo (Eds.), *Harrison's principles of internal medicine*. New York: McGraw-Hill.
13. Laws, E., & Thapar, K. (1993). Brain tumors. *CA: A Cancer Journal for Clinicians, 43*, 5.
14. McArthur, J., & Harrison, M. (1994). HIV-associated dementia. In S. Appel (Ed.), *Current neurology*. St. Louis: Mosby.
15. Morrison, R., Yamada, S., & Yu, Y. (1997). Fibroblast growth factors in astrocytomas. In P. Kornblith & M. Walker (Eds.), *Advances in neuro-oncology II*. Armonk, NY: Futura.
16. Ravel, R. (1995). *Clinical laboratory medicine: Application of laboratory data* (6th ed.). St. Louis: Mosby.
17. Sagar, S., & Israel, M. (1998). Tumors of the nervous system. In S. Fauci, E. Braunwald, K. Isselbacher, J. Wilson, J. Martin, D. Kasper, S. Hauser, & D. Longo (Eds.), *Harrison's principles of internal medicine*. New York: McGraw-Hill.
18. Scheld, W. (1998). Bacterial meningitis, brain abscess, and other suppurative intracranial infections. In S. Fauci, E. Braunwald, K. Isselbacher, J. Wilson, J. Martin, D. Kasper, S. Hauser, & D. Longo (Eds.), *Harrison's principles of internal medicine*. New York: McGraw-Hill.
19. Schwartz, S. I. (Ed.) (1994). *Principles of surgery* (6th ed.). New York: McGraw-Hill.
20. Tyler, K. (1998). Aseptic meningitis, viral encephalitis, and prion diseases. In S. Fauci, E. Braunwald, K. Isselbacher, J. Wilson, J. Martin, D. Kasper, S. Hauser, & D. Longo (Eds.), *Harrison's principles of internal medicine*. New York: McGraw-Hill.

Chapter 33

Chronic and Degenerative Alterations in the Nervous System

Julie Tackenberg / Reet Henze

KEY TERMS

Arnold-Chiari malformation
athetosis
bradykinesia
bradyphrenia
bulbar palsy
chorea
dementia
hydrocephalus
Lewy bodies
meningocele
myelin sheath
myelomeningocele
neurofibrillary tangles (NFTs)
neuritic or senile plaque
Pick bodies
pseudotumor cerebri
syringomyelocele
syringomyelia
syrinx

Discussing chronic and degenerative disorders according to their functional presentation helps to focus on the underlying pathologic processes, even though it does not give much evidence to their precise nature. The location of the changes in the nervous system determines the clinical manifestations regardless of whether the lesion that interrupts the generation or transmission of nerve impulses is developmental, infectious, degenerative, vascular, neoplastic, or traumatic.

The selected degenerative and chronic disorders in this chapter share many similar clinical manifestations because they cause structural or chemical alterations in common locations in the nervous system. Many of these neurologic problems have a long and difficult course without significant recovery. However, progress has been made in recent years in better understanding the genetic, cellular, and molecular basis of some common degenerative neurologic conditions.

DEVELOPMENTAL OR CONGENITAL DISORDERS

Despite the intricacies of human function, the embryonic origin of the human central nervous system (CNS) is a simple tubular structure. Human embryonic development has been characterized as developing in 23 stages, with each stage having a typical duration. Developmental disorders occur when there is interference with the sequence, components, or duration of these stages leading to failure of mature size or function during embryoyogenesis. Abnormal development of neural tissue can occur as early as 16 days' gestation and as late as 80 days' gestation. The *exact* cause of developmental disorders is unknown. However, many mechanisms are suspected, including infection, folate deficiency, prenatal drug use, trauma, and toxic factors.[15,19] Congenital abnormalities are those conditions present at birth and related to genetic factors.

Spina Bifida

Spina bifida, meaning "open spine,"[28] is a developmental disorder of the vertebral arches. The incidence of spina bifida is 1 to 3 in 1000 live births, depending on the genetics of the population.[18]

PATHOPHYSIOLOGY

During embryoyogenesis, the vertebral arch fails to close completely, leaving a gap in the bony protection of the spinal cord. The bony defect, identifiable by radiography or palpation, may be marked by dimpling of the skin or wisps of hair on the skin surface. If there is only a vertebral defect, it is called *spina bifida occulta* because there are no neurologic deficits to signal its presence. Most cases of spina bifida occulta are innocuous. This type of spina bifida can be found in 15% of the general population on x-ray.[18,34]

In more complex situations, spina bifida is associated with a defect in the closure of the neural tube. The most common terms reflective of spinal cord involvement include:

- **Syringomyelocele:** the dilated portion of the spinal cord protruding through the bony defect, devoid of spinal cord tissue but containing cerebrospinal fluid (CSF)
- **Meningocele:** a sac that contains the meninges and CSF
- **Myelomeningocele:** a sac that contains the meninges and portions of the spinal cord (most common defect associated with spina bifida)

Figure 33-1 identifies the different types of spina bifida. Incomplete skin covering and leakage of CSF may be present with any of these defects. When cord protrusion is involved, 78% occur in the lumbar area, 10% in the sacral area, and 11% in the cervical/thoracic vertebrae.[18,28,39]

CLINICAL MANIFESTATIONS

Clinical manifestations vary with the level and degree of cord involvement. If the sac is a meningocele, the infant may show no signs of neurologic deficit. The extent of neurologic deficit is dependent on the size and level of the lesion. If the defect occurs in the lumbosacral area, flaccid paralysis of the lower limbs and absence of sensation below the level of the lesion are usually present. Bowel and bladder sphincter control also is affected. However, if the tip of the conus terminalis is intact, some external bowel sphincter control may be present due to an intact reflex arc.[18,28,43] The frequency of accompanying mental retardation with severe spina bifida is high.

Radiographic studies indicate the level and degree of bony and cord malformations. Prenatally, amniocentesis and ultrasonography may reveal the bony defect.

Arnold-Chiari Malformations

First identified in 1891, an **Arnold Chiari malformation** (ACM) is a cerebellar deformity associated with hydrocephalus. The cerebellum and brain stem are displaced downward through the foramen magnum.

PATHOPHYSIOLOGY

This defect has four morphologic classifications that remain valid today. However, the use of the term Arnold-Chiari malformation has become associated primarily with type I or type II malformations.[1] Many of the morphologic findings associated with type I and type II ACMs are presented in Figure 33-2.

CHIARI TYPE I. Chiari type I involves a conical elongation of the cerebellar tonsils and neighboring cerebellar hemispheres through the foramen magnum into the vertebral canal without displacement of the fourth ventricle. Although there is no association with myelomeningocele, two thirds of patients with type I ACM are found to have syringomyelia.

CHIARI TYPE II. Chiari type II involves herniation of the cerebellar tonsils, combined with deformities of the medulla. It is a deformity found in infants with meningomylocele and hydrocephalus. In 90% of infants with ACM, thinning to complete erosion of the cranial vault can be found, as well as shallow posterior fossae and a shortened and fenestrated falx.[6,18] Herniation of the cerebellar tissue may extend down as far as the upper dorsal vertebral segments. Often the vermis,

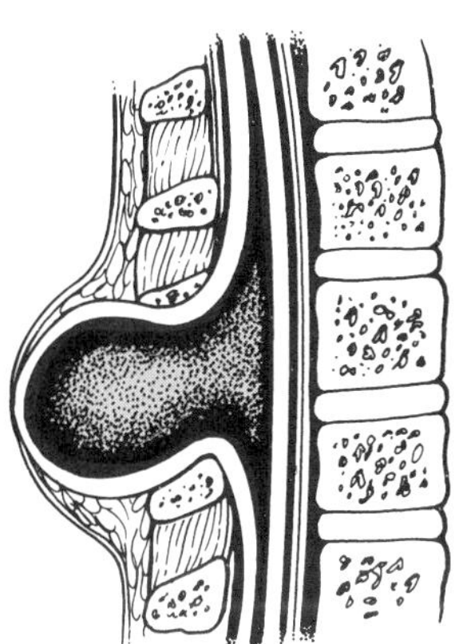

A Syringomyelocele (sac with CSF only)

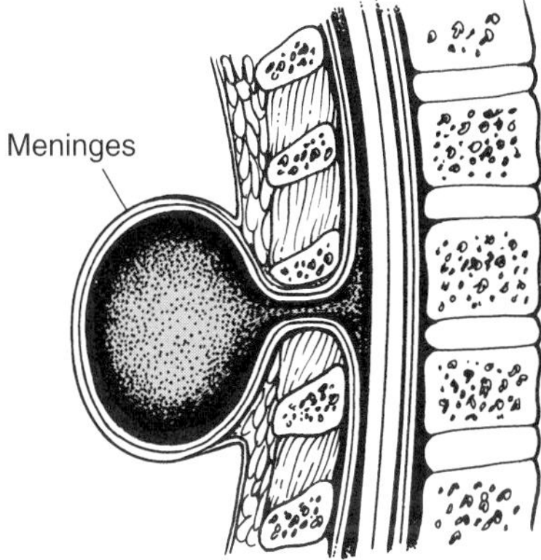

B Meningocele (sac contains meninges)

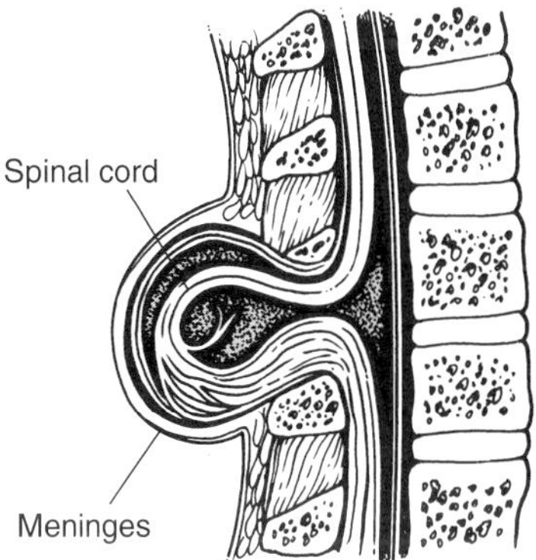

C Myelomeningocele (sac contains meninges and spinal cord tissue)

FIGURE 33-1. Types of spina bifida and associated spinal cord involvement.

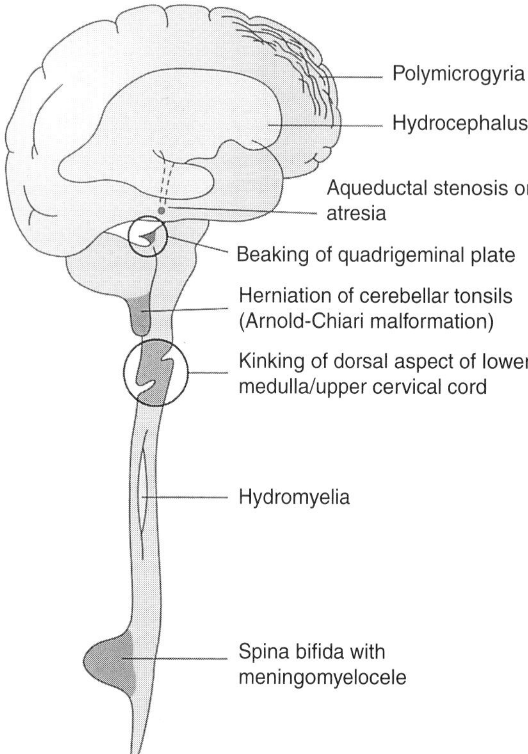

FIGURE 33-2. Arnold-Chiari malformation and associated lesions. (Rubin, E. & Farber, J. [1999]. *Pathology* [3rd ed.]. Philadelphia: Lippincott.)

associated with the choroid plexus, becomes bound to the medulla by meningeal adhesions. The entire brain stem, especially the medulla and fourth ventricle, become elongated, kinked, and displaced. The foramen magnum is enlarged and the tentorium is poorly developed. In 50% of patients, the lower medulla forms a kink just above the cervical cord.[6,18,39] Spina bifida, with meningomyelocele more dominant than meningocele, invariably accompanies Chiari type II.

Conflicting theories exist about how type II develops. The earliest theories suggested that pressure from a ruptured fourth ventricle provided pressure from above, forcing the hindbrain downward. The concept of a spinal cord tethered to the myelomeningocele placing downward traction on the brainstem is another explanation.[17] Most recently, all the neurologic defects are considered secondary to the skeletal anomalies of the shallow posterior fossa.

CHIARI TYPE III. Chiari type III, which is rare, consists of a high cervical or occipitocervical meningomyelocele with cerebeller herniation.[1] Lumbar spina bifida is often associated with this malformation.

CHIARI TYPE IV. Chiari type IV manifests as cerebeller hypoplasia.[1]

CLINICAL MANIFESTATIONS

Clinical manifestations of ACM depend on the age and development of the child. Infants generally demonstrate signs and symptoms of brainstem dysfunction associated with type II ACM and the problems associated with hydrocephalus. Children and adolescents have cervical spinal cord or cerebellar dysfunction associated more directly with type I ACM.[1] The clinical manifestations are summarized in Table 33-1. These patterns of manifestations are not mutually exclusive, however.

Syringomyelia

Syringomyelia refers to a tubular cavitation (**syrinx**) of the spinal cord.[5,12] A syrinx, usually found in gray matter of the cord, often extends over more than one segment of the spinal cord.

Most commonly found in adults, occasionally syringomyelia is encountered in infants. The incidence is 8.4 in 100,000, with symptoms beginning in the second or third to fifth decades. ACM type I is common in 90% of persons with idiopathic syringomyelia.[6,18] It is also highly associated with hydrocephalus, tumors, infections, and infarction in the CNS.

The course of the disease varies with patterns of progression, remission, or static symptoms. Although the etiology is controversial, the most common theories include (1) maldevelopment, (2) neoplasms, (3) inflammatory conditions, and (4) trauma.

PATHOPHYSIOLOGY

The syrinx causes enlargement of the affected spinal cord, which alters the normal flow of CSF. Figure 33-3 shows the syrinx in the spinal cord.

A syrinx found in the medulla is known as a *syringobulbia*. These clefts may contain aspects of the lateral medullar and reticular formation and the hypoglossal nerve. Cavitations are rarely found above the medulla. Largest in the cervical area, the cavity frequently extends across the cord, involving the posterior parts of the ventral horns, and across the midline behind the central canal. In the thoracic areas the cavity is generally unilateral, invading the posterior horns. The syrinx is filled with a clear fluid similar in content to CSF or yellow with a high protein content.

CLINICAL MANIFESTATIONS

Syringomyelia is characterized by the onset of progressive motor symptoms in the second or third decade. Two patterns of onset are noted to exist: (1) slowly progressive symptomology and (2) sudden onset with rapid initial increase of symptoms, which then taper.

TABLE 33-1

MANIFESTATIONS OF ARNOLD-CHIARI MALFORMATIONS

AGE	TYPE OF MALFORMATION	MALFORMATIONS	CLINICAL MANIFESTATIONS
Infants	Type II Chiari	1. Downward displacement of cerebellum 2. Elongated and kinked medulla oblongata 3. Fourth ventricle foramina displaced to below the foramen magnum 4. Pressure on cranial nerves from displacement of above structures 5. Aqueductal stenosis 6. Flattening of the base of the skull 7. Hydrocephalus 8. Meningomyelocele	Manifestations may be a combination of any of the following: Involvement of lower CNs manifesting as facial asymmetry, sternocleido-mastoid muscle weakness, laryngeal stridor, and tongue fasciculations Ocular palsies, visual-perceptual abnormalities Deafness Spinal deformities, i.e., scoliosis and kyphosis Dysfunction of the medullary respiratory center Vocal cord paralysis and obstructive apnea, ventilatory insensitivity to marked hypercapnia Increased intracranial pressure Seizures
Children, adolescents, and adults	Type I Chiari	Similar to above without the meningomyelocele Syringomyelia and hydromyelia (expansion in central canal) possible	Manifestations possibly not evident until adulthood and may be a combination of the following: Varying cranial nerve dysfunction Medullary dysfunction Cerebellar signs such as ataxia, uncoordination Symptoms of increased intracranial pressure Neck pain and occipital headaches Upper extremity weakness, loss of fine motor control, and sensory loss Increased DTRs in upper extremities

CNs = cranial nerves; DTRs = deep tendon reflexes.

Symptoms may cease to progress at any time. Unless associated with life-threatening bulbar symptoms, the disease is not life threatening.

Because pain and temperature fibers cross immediately in the cord and relay through the dorsal horns, analgesia and thermoanesthesia with preservation of tactile sensation are characteristics of early syringomyelia. Pain is the most frequent presenting symptom. Accompanying these early signs are weakness and wasting of hands and arm. Scoliosis and smaller breast and chest development are found on the side of the cavitation.[18] If the syrinx spreads anteriorly, signs of lower motor neuron damage with small-muscle atrophy occur. Signs and symptoms develop asymmetrically at first, possibly progressing to complete paralysis from cord compression.

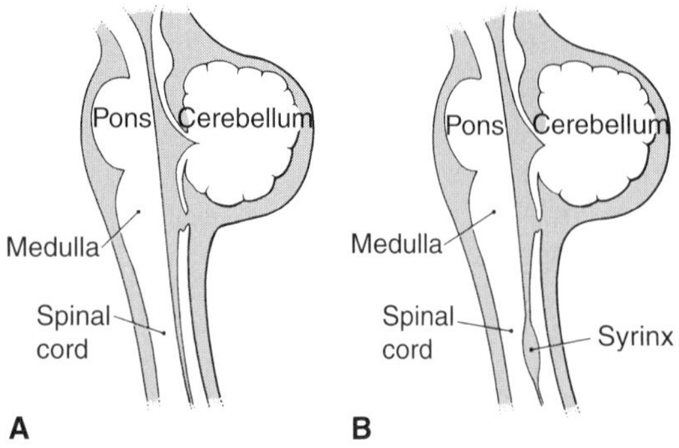

FIGURE 33-3. Syringomyelia. **A.** Normal. **B.** Presence of a syrinx in the spinal cord.

Physical examination reveals the pattern of cord interruption. A lumbar puncture (LP) reveals fluid similar to CSF. Radiographic studies (CT/MRI) will show evidence of lesions and associated structural changes.

Hydrocephalus

The term **hydrocephalus** refers to an increased quantity of CSF within the ventricular system of the cerebrum, resulting in increased intracranial pressure and ventricular enlargement. Generally, the lateral ventricles are involved. Forms of hydrocephalus include (1) obstructive/non-communicating, (2) communicating, (3) ex vacuo, and (4) hypersecretory.

A condition that commonly occurs in young, obese women, **pseudotumor cerebri** is related to hydrocephalus and associated with increased intracranial pressure of unknown origin developing over a period of weeks or months. The incidence of this disorder is 1 in 100,000 in the general population and 19 in 100,000 in obese young women[1] with a female-to-male ratio of 8 : 1.[9,12] In children, obesity is not a consistent finding, and the disorder does not appear to be predominant in one sex.

ETIOLOGY

The most common cause of hydrocephalus is *obstruction*, indicating that the free flow of CSF from the lateral ventricles into the subarachnoid space is impeded. Figure 33-4 shows areas that may cause obstruction of CSF flow, possibly as the result of lesions in the foramen magnum, the third ventricle, the aqueduct of Sylvius, the fourth ventricle, or the foramina of Magendie and Luschka. Lesions causing obstruction may result from abnormalities of the cerebellar tonsils, trauma, infection, or tumor.

Communicating or *malresorptive* hydrocephalus results when CSF flows freely from the ventricles into the subarachnoid space but is not resorbed there.[40] The resorptive problem lies within the subarachnoid space, either obstructing flow around the cistern ambiens or at the arachnoid villi. This type of hydrocephalus is associated with post-meningitic or post-hemorrhagic states.

Hydrocephalus ex vacuo is also referred to as atrophic or compensatory hydrocephalus.[16,17] This condition is commonly found in patients with severe head injury, vascular disease, multi-infarct dementia, or other forms of degenerative brain disorders.[16,18] *Hypersecretory* hydrocephalus, associated with excessive production of CSF, is rare. In these instances, papillomas of the choroid plexus have been found.[17,18]

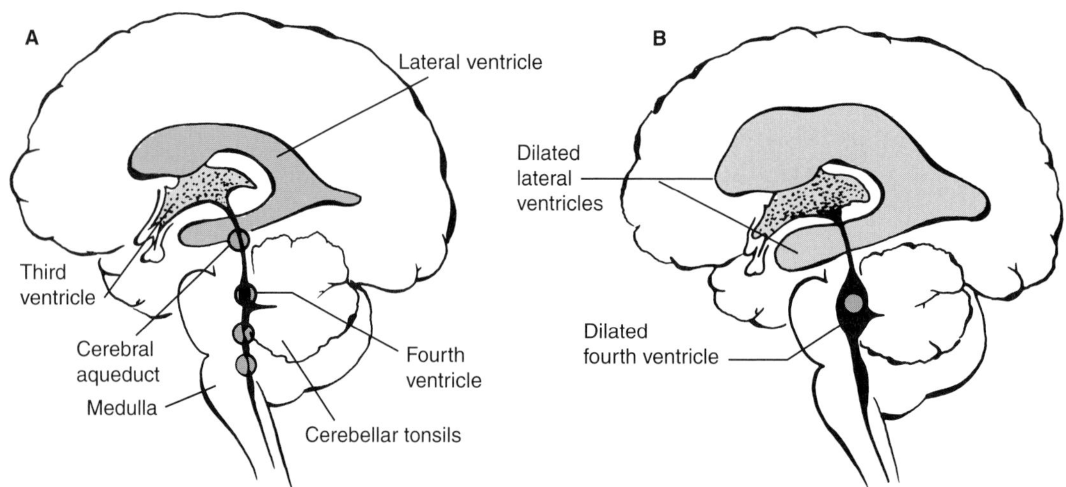

FIGURE 33-4. **A.** Schematic representation of areas of possible obstruction to flow of CSF. **B.** Resulting ventricular enlargement.

CLINICAL MANIFESTATIONS

Clinical manifestations of hydrocephalus depend on the age and rapidity of onset as well as its etiology and success of treatment. A newborn infant who exhibits a grossly enlarged head, widely separated cranial sutures, and protruding eyes usually has irreversible signs of prolonged increased intracranial pressure such as blindness from optic atrophy, paralysis, and mental retardation. In other infants, rapidly increasing head circumference, feeding problems, irritability, delayed motor skills, high-pitched cry, and turned down ("setting sun") eyes are signs of progressive hydrocephalus. Figure 33-5 shows ventricular changes with setting sun eyes. Because cerebral expansion is permitted by the open sutures and fontanels in infancy, classic signs of increasing intracranial pressure, such as headache, vomiting, and altered vital signs, usually are minimal or absent. In older children or adults whose cranial sutures have closed, headaches and vomiting are often early signs and develop with smaller volumes of trapped CSF.

Cranial Malformations

Congenital variations in brain size may result in abnormally small (*microcephaly*) or abnormally large (*megalencephaly*) brain volume. Genetic and environmental influences have been linked to congenital brain size abnormalities. Abnormally small brains are far more common than abnormally large brains, and the discussion here will be limited to these.

ETIOLOGY AND PATHOPHYSIOLOGY

Microcephaly vera, or small head, is a genetic defect resulting from arrested brain growth. Two types of inheritance, autosomal recessive or sex-linked gene, results in premature suture closure of the skull.[1,12,18] Other etiologies recently coming to the forefront include microencephaly associated with fetal alcohol syndrome and human immunodeficiency virus 1 (HIV-1) infections in utero.[12]

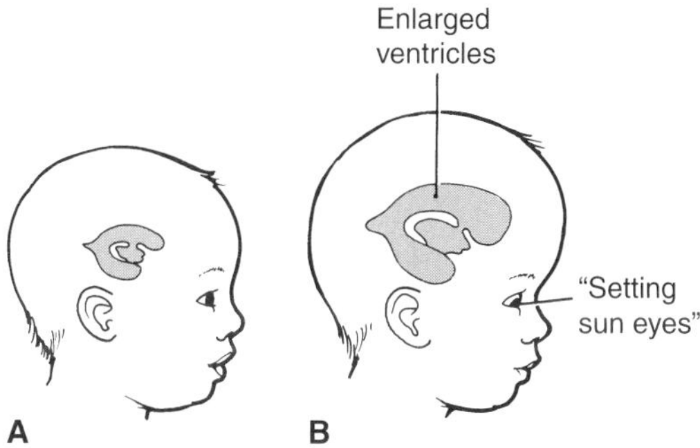

FIGURE 33-5. **A.** Normal cephalic shape. **B.** Hydrocephalus with characteristic "setting sun" eyes.

Microcephaly is often associated with mental retardation, cerebral palsy, and seizure activity. The cerebral cortex is grossly abnormal. It is thick and deficient in neurons, with reduced sulci.[1] In some cases a cerebellar hypoplasia accompanies the cerebral abnormalities.

Craniostenosis, early closure and ossification of one or more of the sutures in the skull, occurs before brain growth is arrested. Skull growth is inhibited in a direct 90-degree angle to the closed sutures.[12,18,39]

CLINICAL MANIFESTATIONS

Microcephaly results in severe mental retardation. Neurologic deficits range from decerebration and complete unresponsiveness to autistic behaviors, mild motor impairment, educable mental retardation, or mild hyperkinesias.

With craniostenosis, the manifestations depend on which sutures close, the duration of the process, and the ability of the other sutures to compensate by expansion.

Cerebral Palsy

The term *cerebral palsy* (CP) includes a wide variety of non-progressive brain disorders that occur during intrauterine life, delivery, or early infancy. Cerebral palsy, by definition, is a syndrome of motor disabilities possibly accompanied by mental retardation, seizures, or both.

ETIOLOGY AND PATHOPHYSIOLOGY

Causes of CP are many and include cerebral developmental disorders such as microcephaly, intracranial hemorrhage, cerebral anoxia, and toxins such as excessive bilirubin. Prenatal factors include infection with rubella, nutritional deficiency, and blood factor incompatibility. Asphyxia may produce CP prenatally or during labor or delivery. Intrapartally, CP may be related to anesthesia or various metabolic disturbances. Development of CP after birth is relatively uncommon but may occur after CNS infections, asphyxia, or head trauma.[4,12,43]

CLINICAL MANIFESTATIONS

Table 33-2 summarizes the different types of cerebral palsies and their manifestations.

DISORDERS OF PROGRESSIVE WEAKNESS OR PARALYSIS

Progressive weakness and paralysis indicate involvement of the pyramidal system of the brain, spinal cord, or the final common pathway between the cord and the

TABLE 33-2

TYPES AND CLINICAL MANIFESTATIONS OF CEREBRAL PALSIES

TYPE	OCCURRENCE	CLINICAL MANIFESTATIONS
Spastic	50%	Upper motor neuron motor dysfunction (pyramidal tract involvement) predominated by spasticity. Great variability in intellectual ability but impairment is common.
Diplegia		Bilateral involvement of the extremities. Lower extremities affected predominantly. Delayed sitting, standing, and walking. Walking may be awkward, often with crossing of the legs (scissors gait). Lower legs may be splayed outward and feet flexed.
Quadriplegia		All four extremities involved. The individual is non-ambulatory and attains little or no speech or sphincter control.
Hemiplegia		One side of the body involved. It is the most common form of spastic CP.
Dyskinetic/athetoid	20%	Slow, writhing movement of the extremities, neck, trunk and face. Intellectual impairment may be present.
Ataxic	5%	Wide-based ataxic gate, imbalance, and incoordination predominate. Poor performance of rapid, repetitive movements.
Mixed	25%	Combination of various forms of CP, reflecting any combination of clinical manifestations. Most common mixed CP is a combination of spastic and athetoid forms.

muscle. These disorders may be idiopathic or may result from dietary deficiencies, autoimmune dysfunction, genetic defects, or infectious diseases. If the reflex arc remains intact, the usual sign is *spastic paresis or paralysis* with normal or hyperactive deep tendon reflexes. If the lower motor neuron or final common pathway is interrupted, the result is *flaccid paralysis* with diminished or absent reflexes. With damage throughout the motor system, spasticity is present until the final common pathway is interrupted, then flaccidity and atrophy of the muscles predominate. Motor neuron problems are discussed further in Chapter 31.

Myasthenia Gravis

Myasthenia gravis (MG) is a chronic autoimmune disorder involving the destruction of the acetycholine (Ach) receptors at the postsynaptic membrane of the neuromuscular junction.[29] It is found in 5 to 10 of 100,000 persons.[41] The number of receptor sites is reduced, and nerve impulse transmission to voluntary muscles is impaired.

ETIOLOGY AND PATHOPHYSIOLOGY

The triggering mechanism for this autoimmune disease continues to be elusive. It is postulated that the circulating Ach-receptor antibodies link themselves to receptor sites in the voluntary muscle, damaging and blocking the activity of the receptors (Fig. 33-6).

The postsynaptic membrane abnormalities result in muscles that are less responsive to nerve impulses. Muscle contractions become less effective with each succeeding nerve impulse. Myasthenic mothers may pass the antibodies to their infant through the placenta. These infants may experience spontaneous recovery from the myasthenic symptoms within 1 to 3 months, or the muscular impairment may persist throughout their lifetime. Hyperplasia of the thymus is frequently associated with MG, and approximately 12% of persons have a benign thymic tumor.[12,29] In some cases, aggregates of lymphyocytes are present in the muscles and other organs.

CLINICAL MANIFESTATIONS

Myasthenia gravis has a common onset in young adults and is variable but progressive in nature, with patterns of remission and exacerbations. It is characterized by activity-induced abnormal muscle fatigability. Initial symptoms commonly include drooping of eyelids (ptosis) and development of a nasal voice and slurred speech due to dysfunction of the jaw, tongue, face, and palate muscles. Weakness of the proximal portion of the extremities may be noted simultaneously. Because several primary muscle disorders cause a

FOCUS ON CELLULAR PATHOPHYSIOLOGY

ANTIBODY BLOCKS NATURAL CHEMICAL TRANSMISSION (Myasthenia gravis)

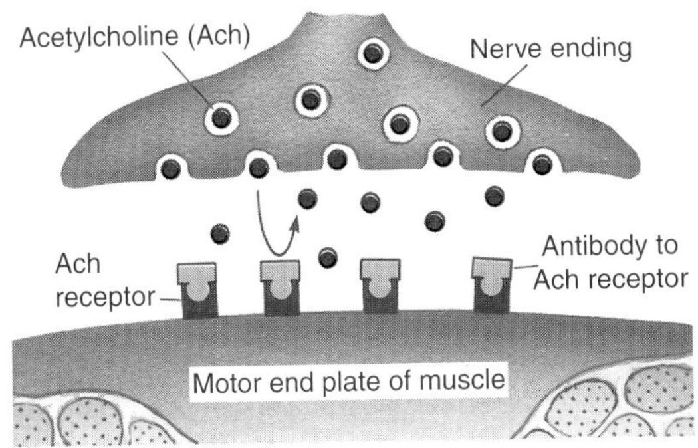

FIGURE 33-6. Inhibition of synaptic transmission of Ach in myasthenia gravis leads to profound muscle weakness. (Rubin, E. & Farber, J. L. [1999]. *Pathology* [3rd ed.]. Philadelphia: Lippincott.)

similar clinical picture, administration of an anticholinesterase agent followed by immediate, although temporary, relief of the motor symptoms confirms the diagnosis.

Symptoms worsen throughout the day, with some degree of recovery with rest or use of medications. Over a period of time, muscles atrophy secondary to their lack of response and use. Subsequently, the person becomes susceptible to secondary complications such as pneumonia. Reflexes may remain normal or reflect fatigue, decreasing with repeated testing. Sensory alterations are not present.

Myasthenia crisis, a severe exacerbation of the disease, is characterized by extreme muscle weakness, respiratory insufficiency, and great difficulty in swallowing. These symptoms are associated with insufficient drug therapy. *Cholinergic crisis involves* clinical signs of excessive drug activity, which also produce voluntary muscle weakness mimicking the symptoms of the disease itself. Additional differential signs include nausea, vomiting, gastrointestinal irritability, bradycardia, diarrhea, pallor, miosis, and excessive salivation.

Electrodiagnostic studies show slowing of nerve conduction in most affected persons. Rapid, although intermittent, relief of symptoms with an intravenous administration of edrophonium may also provide help in confirming the disease.

Guillain-Barré Syndrome

Guillain-Barré syndrome (GBS) is an acute neurologic disorder, considered here because some of its basic pathology resembles other chronic conditions.

ETIOLOGY AND PATHOPHYSIOLOGY

Guillain-Barré syndrome is an acute polyneuritis thought to be caused by an allergic response or some type of hypersensitivity reaction. The onset usually occurs a few days or weeks after a febrile illness, vaccination, injury, or surgery. Guillain-Barré syndrome has no predilection for age, ethnic group, sex, or race; if an infectious cause (most often respiratory or gastrointestinal) can be demonstrated, it usually is viral. The syndrome also has occurred after immunizations.

Evidence from laboratory models identifies the existence of an IgM antimyelin antibody that initiates the myelin destruction process.[1] However, the specific triggering mechanism for the disturbance in the human immune response remains elusive. Lymphocytes become sensitized and begin to destroy myelin.[11]

Inflammation with cellular infiltration, an early finding in GBS, contributes to demyelination and degeneration of the **myelin sheath** and axon. Degeneration occurs in the segmental peripheral nerves and the anterior and posterior spinal nerve roots. Lymphocytes and macrophages infiltrate the myelin sheath initially. Later, if disease progression continues, the axon itself is involved.[11,38] Myelin swells and obliterates the nodes of Ranvier (Fig. 33-7). High levels of soluable interleukin (IL-2) receptors and IL-2 itself have been found in the serum of patients during the acute phase of GBS.[1]

CLINICAL MANIFESTATIONS

Initially, general bilateral weakness begins in the lower extremities and progresses symmetrically in an ascending direction. Eventually the trunk, upper extremities, and cranial nerves may be affected. Accompanying symptoms include paresthesias and possibly pain in the back and neck.[31] Complete flaccid paralysis may or may not occur. Maximum manifestations of the disease occur in about 1 to 2 weeks, although the rate of spread varies.

In severe cases, total paralysis develops rapidly, requiring ventilatory support. Sensory involvement is usually less profound than the motor involvement, although the paresthesias can be quite painful and difficult to manage. Proprioceptive and vibratory alterations are the most common sensory dysfunctions. Autonomic dysfunction may occur in advanced cases and is reflected by diaphoresis, urinary retention, and unstable heart rate and blood pressure.

Reflexes are normally diminished or lost but occasionally remain intact. A finding of elevated CSF protein without increased cells (albuminocytic dissociation) a few days after the onset of the illness is seen.

Multiple Sclerosis

Multiple sclerosis (MS) is a relatively common chronic and progressive, inflammatory, demyelinating disease of the CNS. Estimated to affect 250,000 to 350,000 peo-

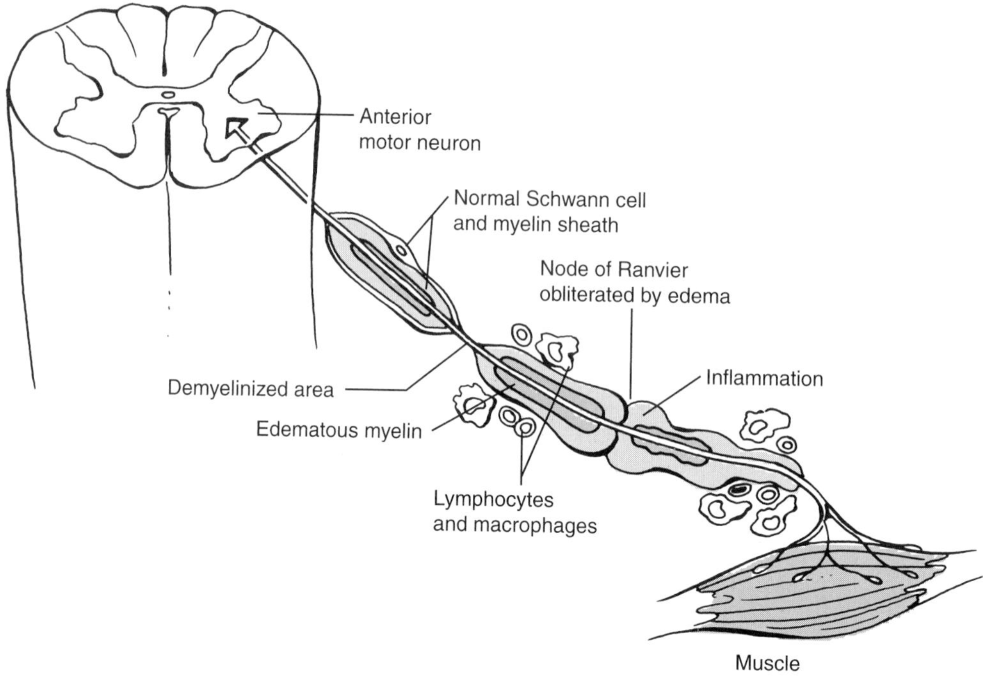

FIGURE 33-7. **Pathologic changes in peripheral nerve associated with Guillain-Barré syndrome.**

ple in the United States,[4,20,21] MS results in diverse manifestations of neurologic alteration, depending on the areas involved.

ETIOLOGY

The basic cause or causes of MS is unknown. It probably is an autoimmune disorder influenced by a genetic susceptibility.[10] The possibility that a latent viral infection precipitates the disease has been investigated without success.

Dietary deficiencies and acute viral infections also have been studied as causative agents. Stress and trauma seem to play a role in precipitating the onset of MS or in exacerbating the symptoms. MS is most common in colder climates, the incidence increasing as the geographical distance from the equator in Europe and Northern America increases.[20] The onset usually occurs between the ages of 20 and 40 years. Women have a higher incidence than men.[12,20]

The incidence of MS is much higher in people of European origin and much lower among Orientals, Africans, and Native Americans.[2,12] The incidence in first-degree relatives is 30 to 40 times higher than the average risk of 0.1% in the normal population, leading to speculation that exposure to a pathogenetic agent or inherited susceptibility to the disease may be in-[illegible][20,21] If one of a set of identical twins has MS, there is a 50% chance that the other will develop some evidence of MS.[11]

An association also has been documented between MS and HLA antigens of chromosome 6, which participate in regulation of immune function. The severity of the disease seems to be associated with a constellation of particular genes. A3, B7, and DR2 are present more often in women or in more benign cases. A1, B8, and DR3 occur more often in men with severe disease.[20]

In individuals with MS, support for the immune theory is evidenced by the following findings: (1) elevation of helper/inducer T-cells in CSF at the onset of the exacerbation, (2) decrease of T-suppressor cells in the blood immediately before and during an exacerbation, (3) immunocompetent cells within plaques, and (4) intrathecal antibody production.

PATHOPHYSIOLOGY

The hallmark of MS pathology is plaque formation that occurs randomly, but predominantly throughout the white matter of the CNS. The plaque lesions vary in size and their pathologic findings. Plaque formation and destruction of the myelin sheath slows, blocks, or distorts transmission of nerve impulses.[27]

Areas more commonly involved include optic nerves and areas around the ventricles.[1] Other areas frequently involved include the cervical spinal cord (related to head movement) and the area between the thoracic and lumbar spine (back motion).[20]

Opening of the blood-brain barrier has been demonstrated in the early stages of plaque development. The openings persist for approximately 6 weeks and seem to precede the development of plaques.[20]

An inflammatory reaction also is part of the pathogenesis of MS. Inflammation is found around the plaques themselves and also within surrounding normal-appearing tissue, contributing to early acute symptoms. During the course of the disease, some of the myelinated fibers may regenerate, and associated symptoms may disappear. Gliosis eventually occurs in the lesions; scar tissue replaces myelin and may replace the axons themselves, leading to permanent disability. From this gliosis comes the term *sclerosis*, meaning induration or scarring. In time, oligodendrocytes disappear and astrocytes proliferate at the plaque sites.[7,22]

CLINICAL MANIFESTATIONS

The disease often begins rather suddenly with focal symptoms such as limb weakness (40%), sensory symptoms (20–30%), visual disturbance (25%), or brain stem symptoms (10–15%), or various combinations of these.[8] Initial symptoms may be transient and often are followed by complete or nearly complete recovery as the myelin is replaced. Periods of remission are common. Later, alterations become permanent, with remissions and exacerbations limited to new symptoms superimposed on a baseline of disability. This permanence in symptoms is caused by gradual disruption and finally destruction of the nerve cells themselves.[2]

Clinical manifestations relate to the region of the brain most directly affected by the lesions (Table 33-3). Emotional changes may range from emotional lability to sustained euphoria or severe depression.[2,10,21]

Brain stem lesions produce symptoms of cranial nerve dysfunction. The optic, oculomotor, trochlear, and abducens nerves and the vestibular branch of the auditory nerve are especially common sites of damage.

The classic triad described by Charcot in 1868, which occurs late in the disease, includes (1) nystagmus, (2) intention tremor, and (3) speech disorders.[2] Spastic paraplegia, incontinence, dementia, and extreme emotional lability also are typical of the late stages of MS.

TABLE 33-3

CLINICAL MANIFESTATIONS OF MS ASSOCIATED WITH CNS AREAS INVOLVED

FUNCTIONAL AREA	AREAS OF CNS INVOLVED	ASSOCIATED MANIFESTATIONS
Sensory system	Sensory tracts in the brain stem and spinal cord Posterior columns of the spinal cord	Paresthesias (tingling, numbness), loss of touch, vibration, proprioception senses
	Lateral spinothalamic tracts	Paroxysmal sensory symptoms of short duration, (e.g., Lhermette's sign occurs as a shocklike sensation that shoots down the spinal cord in response to flexion of the neck)
Motor system	Pyramidal tract	Asymmetric spastic weakness of limbs (hemiparesis, paraparesis, monoparesis) Babinski's sign, hyperactive DTRs, absent abdominal reflexes
Cerebellar system	Cerebellum and corticospinal tracts	Gait ataxia, hypotonia, intention tremor of hands, head tremor, nystagmus, dysarthria, imbalance, uncoordinated voluntary movements Slurred, uncoordinated articulation Heaviness or sensation of tiredness in one or more extremities
Visual system	Optic nerve, optic tract, and optic radiations, CN nuclei in brainstem	Diplopia, central scotoma, blurred vision, blindness, nystagmus, and hemianopia
Bladder	Corticospinal tract	Hesitancy, urgency, frequency, incontinence, and retention
Cerebral white matter	Frontal lobe of cerebrum	Alterations in mood, depression, euphoria, cognitive dysfunction, and loss of memory

CN = cranial nerves; MS = multiple sclerosis; CNS = central nervous system.

Studies of antibodies in the blood or CSF often show gamma-globulin abnormalities in patients with established MS. The most consistent CSF finding is the presence of increased amounts of oligoclonal bands of immunoglobulin G (normally less than 5 mg/dL).[11]

Amyotrophic Lateral Sclerosis

Amyotrophic lateral sclerosis (ALS, or Lou Gehrig disease) is a primary neurologic disease of the motor neurons of the cerebral cortex, brain stem, and spinal cord. The disease leads to progressive weakness and muscle wasting and death, usually within 5 years of diagnosis.[8] The onset of ALS usually occurs after age 50, and the disease is twice as prevalent in men as in women. It is a noninflammatory disease of the upper and lower motor neurons, with demyelination secondary to axon degeneration.

ETIOLOGY AND PATHOPHYSIOLOGY

The hallmark of ALS pathology is the loss of motor neurons in the (1) cortex, (2) brain stem, and (3) spinal cord. The basis for this neuron loss remains elusive.

Although the cause of ALS is unknown, premature aging of nerve cells as a result of some environmental or genetic factor, nutritional deficiencies, heavy-metal poisoning, an autoimmune response, metabolic defects, and even a dormant virus have all been identified as possible causes. Familial autosomal dominant patterns account for 5% to 10% of total cases, and the gene is located on chromosome 21q.[12,41] Glutamate transport, found to be abnormal in ALS patients, is proposed as possibly leading to excitotoxicity of motor neurons.[8]

CLINICAL MANIFESTATIONS

Loss of the motor cells in the cerebral cortex can result in signs of upper motor neuron damage, with weakness or spastic paralysis and hyperactive reflexes. Respiratory muscles are weakened, eventually becoming paralyzed. Eye movements and continence are normally preserved. Muscle involvement is asymmetrically distributed, especially in the lower limbs. Damage to cranial nerves in the medulla produces signs of bulbar palsy of either the spastic or flaccid type. **Bulbar palsy** refers to weakness or paralysis of the muscles supplied by the motor cranial nerves. Commonly, upper and lower motor neuron damage is mixed in ALS. Lower motor signs predominate in the upper extremities, and upper motor signs predominate in the lower extremities. When reflexes are interrupted, muscles atrophy secondary to denervation and loss of muscle tone. In these areas, diminished reflexes or flaccid paralysis occurs. Muscle atrophy often is present in the upper [illegible]nd tongue.

Degeneration may occur anywhere within the pyramidal system, in the anterior motor cells of the spinal cord, or in the ventral nerve roots. It is most severe in the cervical cord and characteristically does not affect peripheral nerves.

A common early sign of brain stem involvement may be muscle *fasciculations* of the tongue. Fasciculations, which also may be seen in the hands or upper limbs, are small local muscle contractions that occur if a muscle is tapped or moved passively. Slurred speech and weakness of the palate and facial muscles may also occur with brain stem involvement. Swallowing eventually is affected, and speech may become unintelligible.

Weakness and clumsiness are first noted in the distal portions of the upper limbs, and wasting of the muscles of the hand is characteristic. Sexual dysfunction, such as impotence, is an early sign; bowel and bladder sphincters usually are not affected until late in the disease. Characteristically, there is no sensory alteration in ALS, and intellectual function is retained until death. Paralysis of the trunk and respiratory muscles occurs late in the course of the disease if bulbar palsy does not cause death first. Biopsy of muscle and electromyography show denervation atrophy.

DISORDERS OF ABNORMAL MOVEMENTS

Abnormal movements often indicate alterations in the extrapyramidal motor system. Because this system is not clearly understood, the relationship of the pathology and structural alterations to the clinical manifestations is not clear. Abnormal movements often result from alterations and reflect a disturbance in the balance between the excitatory and inhibitory neurotransmitters in the basal ganglia. The major neurotransmitters involved include dopamine, Ach, and gamma-aminobutyric acid (GABA). The basal ganglia most often affected are the four structures that make up the corpus striatum: caudate, putamen, globus pallidus, and claustrum. In some disorders, such as early parkinsonism, conscious effort can temporarily suppress these movements, but typically they return if the person relaxes or is distracted.

Parkinson's Disease

Parkinson's disease (PD), also known as paralysis agitans or idiopathic parkinsonism, is a common, chronic degenerative disease of the late-middle-aged and elderly populations. Prevalence ranges from 100 to 200 in 100,000 inhabitants. In most studies, PD is slightly more common in men than women.[26]

ETIOLOGY

The cause of idiopathic Parkinson's disease is still unknown. Parkinson-like manifestations are also associated with certain known factors such as certain drugs, episodes of cerebral anoxia, carbon monoxide poisoning, repeated head trauma, and illicit designer drug use (1-methyl-4-phenyl-1,2,3,6-tetrahydropyridine, or MPTP).

Proposed theories for idiopathic PD include (1) advanced age, (2) genetic factors, and (3) endogenous/exogenous factors toxic to dopaminergic cells.

PATHOPHYSIOLOGY

Parkinson disease is an extrapyramidal disorder of the basal ganglia. The subthalamic nucleus and substantia nigra, together with the basal ganglia and the motor neurons of the spine, form the extrapyramidal system (see Chapter 29). The extrapyramidal motor system helps to maintain an upright posture, muscle tone, and coordination. It regulates some of the automatic movements in expressions and walking that produce smooth motion.[6]

Dopamine is a neurotransmitter that is found in dopamine-containing cells in the midbrain and the hypothalamus. One of the most significant dopamine-containing tracts, the nigrostriatal pathway, has its origin in the brain stem in the pars compacta (pigmented cells) of the substantia nigra and projects to the striatum (putamen and caudate nucleus) of the basal ganglia.

Dopamine and Ach are important in controlling complex movements. Dopamine acts as an inhibitory transmitter, and Ach acts as an excitatory transmitter. Coordinated voluntary motor activity occurs as a result of a balance between the excitatory cholinergic and inhibitory dopaminergic secretions.

Significant pathologic findings associated with PD include (1) depigmentation and cell loss from the substantia nigra and (2) the presence of **Lewy bodies** (spherical cytoplasmic eosinophilic inclusions) in the nigral neurons. Although Lewy bodies are not specific to PD, their presence is a precondition.[26]

For yet unknown reasons, pigmented cells of the substantia nigra in PD die slowly and progressively, eventually resulting in degeneration of the nigrostriatal pathway. The loss of these neurons results in significant depletion of dopamine to the corpus striatum and is the predominant basis for the clinical manifestations of PD. Other neurotransmitters noted to be reduced in PD include L-tyrosine hydoxylase (TH), which limits the rate of dopamine synthesis, L-dopa-decarboxylase, serotonin, and GABA.[26] The clinical importance of depletion of these neurotransmitters is much less than that of dopamine depletion.

CLINICAL MANIFESTATIONS

Major clinical manifestations in PD reflect alterations in movement. Other manifestations are associated with alterations in cognition, autonomic nervous system function, and neuroendocrine function.

With dopamine depletion in Parkinson disease, the classic triad of parkinsonism appears: (1) tremors, (2) rigidity, and (3) **bradykinesia** (slow movement). The striatal cells, under the predominance of Ach, initiate action potentials more rapidly because the counterbalance of dopamine is decreased or absent. This results in the absence of the modifying effect of the basal ganglia on pyramidal and extrapyramidal motor activity, causing significant alterations in movement.

The clinical manifestations of PD are summarized in Box 33-1. The tremors associated with PD appear insidiously and early in the disease process. Commonly they occur during rest in the hands first and then progress to involve the ankles, head, or mouth.[3]

Because the basal ganglia influences hypothalamic function, autonomic nervous system (ANS) manifestations are also present in PD. Neuroendocrine manifestations may result from hypersecretion of hormone-releasing factors influencing the anterior pituitary and lead to increased secretion of androgen.

Depression and **bradyphrenia** (slowness in thinking without intellectual impairment) is commonly observed in PD. Dementia develops in approximately 30% of patients.[26] It is unclear if this dementia is due to PD alone or to the varying co-morbidities, such as Alzheimer's disease or multi-infarct dementia, that accompany PD or the diffuse presence of Lewy bodies.[14,39]

Huntington's Disease

Huntington's disease, or Huntington's chorea, first described in 1872, is an autosomal dominant inherited disorder characterized by a progressive degeneration of the cerebral cortex and basal ganglia, particularly the caudate nucleus and putamen. This relatively uncommon inherited disease has its onset of symptoms between 35 and 50 years of age.[15,16] A genetic marker has been traced to a defect on chromosome 4. This gene encodes an abnormal protein mutation that consists of an expanded and unstable trinucleotide (CAG) repeat, which remains latent for several decades.[32] It seems that if the allele is inherited from the affected father, the expression of the disease is earlier than if inherited from the mother.[32]

ETIOLOGY AND PATHOPHYSIOLOGY

In Huntington's chorea, the neurotransmitter GABA, believed to be an inhibitory transmitter whose major function is inhibition of target pathways, is markedly reduced in the involved areas of the brain.[25,37] Ach also

BOX 33-1

CLINICAL MANIFESTATIONS ASSOCIATED WITH PARKINSON'S DISEASE

Motor Manifestations

Tremors
Rigidity
Bradykinesia
Diminished automatic movements (e.g., infrequent blinking, loss of arm swing with walking)
Quiet, monotonous speech
Small writing that leads to an indecipherable trail
Small, shuffling steps that pick up speed as the person travels
Jerky or spastic movements of both extensor and flexor muscles
Difficulty in initiating voluntary acts (akinesia)
Slow and clumsy movements

Cognitive and Affective Manifestations

Deterioration in memory and problem solving
Dementia in some patients
Masklike facial expression

Autonomic Nervous System Manifestations

Heat intolerance
Excessive salivation
Abnormal diaphoresis
Constipation
Bladder problems
Dysphagia

Neuroendocrine Manifestations

Hypersecretion by sebaceous glands, leading to oily skin and seborrheic dermatitis

seems to be reduced, resulting in an imbalance among the three transmitters-GABA, Ach, and dopamine. If dopamine predominates, chorea results, indicating heightened dopamine sensitivity of the striated receptors.[15]

Chorea denotes random, brief, dancelike, abrupt, jerking movements involving the eyes, face, torso, and limbs as a result of overactivity of dopaminergic neurons. If chorea is the major motor symptom, degenerative lesions are especially common in the caudate. In those occasional persons in whom rigidity and tremors predominate, lesions seem to be more likely in the putamen. In many cases of Huntington's chorea, lesions are common throughout the corpus striatum and the thalamus.[36]

Examination of the brain reveals significant atrophy of the frontal lobes and enlargement and changes in structure of the lateral ventricles (Fig. 33-8). The number of neurons in the caudate and putamen is significantly reduced.[32]

CLINICAL MANIFESTATIONS

On average, the initial manifestations of HD present around age 40, with about 5% of patients showing symptoms before age 20 and 5% after 60.[32] In addition to the dramatic rapid *choreiform movements*, there is progressive deterioration of higher intellectual functions, such as memory and judgment, to the point of severe dementia and death. **Athetosis**, movements that are more writhing and slower than choreiform movements, may also be present. When noted together they are called *choreoatheoid* movements, commonly in the face, neck, trunk, and arms. Cognitive and emotional impairments precede abnormal motor manifestations. Dementia develops that is characterized by impulsiveness, paranoia, neurosis, emotional outbursts, loss of judgment and memory, irritability or apathy, delusions or hallucinations, and suicidal tendencies. The

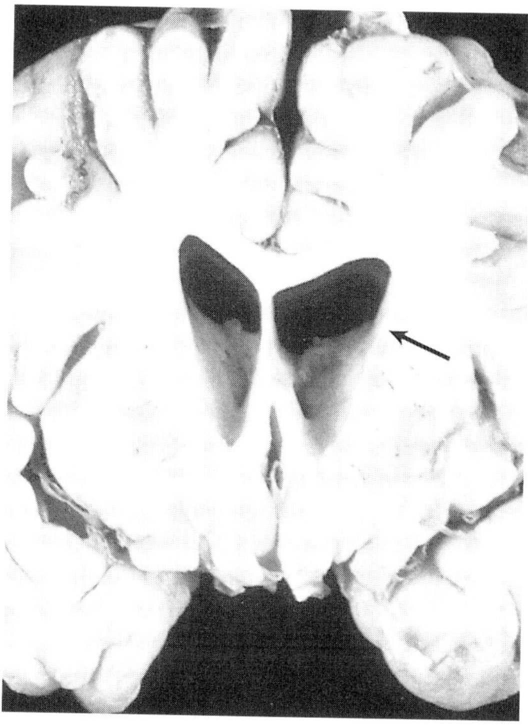

FIGURE 33-8. Huntington's disease. The caudate nuclei (*arrow*) are markedly atrophic, thereby imparting a concave rather than a normal convex curvature to the lateral walls of the ventricles. (Rubin, E. & Farber, J. [1999]. *Pathology* [3rd ed.]. Philadelphia: Lippincott.)

dementia seems to result from atrophy of the cerebral cortex, especially over the frontal and parietal lobes.

DISORDERS OF COGNITION

The term **dementia** refers to an organically caused syndrome of cognitive impairment characterized by decreasing quality of judgment, loss of abstract thinking and reasoning, diminished memory, and emotional changes. Among the elderly, dementing illnesses are among the leading causes of morbidity and mortality. Consensus about its clinical pattern of development is lacking, making diagnosis difficult. There are many variations on the clinical picture of dementia, but there is no theory for the cause or pathophysiology for most of these diseases.[4]

The prevalence of reported dementia increases sharply between the ages of 75 and 90. Population studies demonstrate a doubling of the prevalence for every 5 years after age 75 to an incidence of 32% to 47% in those 85 and older.[13] Some, but not all, researchers have found a higher frequency in women than men.[13] Although there are many causes of dementia, most cases can be categorized as one of the following: (1) Alzheimer's disease, (2) atherosclerotic disease, or (3) diffuse Lewy body disease. Alzheimer's disease accounts for 60% to 75% of dementias, atherosclerotic 15% to 20%, and Lewy body disease an additional 10%.[13,30]

Previously, dementia was thought to be the norm for aging persons because non-demented elderly persons typically demonstrate some of the same structural changes noted with dementia (neurofibrillary tangles and plaques). However, these abnormalities generally are not found in the posterior, pre/post anterior lobe, or primary sensory regions in unaffected individuals and therefore do not produce the dementia symptoms.

Alzheimer's Disease

Alzheimer's disease (AD) is a common, insidious, and slowly progressive cerebral degeneration characterized by dementia. It may be sporadic or have a familial tendency. Although AD commonly presents in individuals over 65, it does have an early onset in a very small subset of individuals who get the disease. In addition to advanced age, other risk factors for AD include head trauma, family history, and the presence of the risk gene, apoE4.

ETIOLOGY

The cause of AD remains unknown. Extensive research has been conducted in an attempt to better understand this devastating disease, and a variety of theories have been proposed for its etiologic basis (Table 33-4).

Links have been made to the genetic basis of AD in some patients. In a majority of the patients diagnosed with AD, the epsilon 4 allele of apolipoprotein E (apoE4) on the long arm of chromosome 19 has been identified as a risk factor for late-onset forms of AD.[23,42] ApoE4 is a protein synthesized and secreted by astrocytes and macrophages that enhances binding of lipoproteins.[24] It is also thought to be instrumental in lipid mobilization in the developing nervous system and in repair of peripheral nerves after injury. In AD apoE4 enhances plaque deposition.[8,24]

The absence of the ApoE4 genotype does not exclude the presence of AD and has, in fact, been associated with a more aggressive form of the disease.[35] The presence of the ApoE4 genotype in AD patients is associated with a less aggressive form of AD.[35]

PATHOPHYSIOLOGY

Pathologic changes noted in this disease are most prominent in the hippocampus, entorhinal cortex, association cortex, and basal forebrain.[24] Figure 33-9 shows the enlargement of the ventricular system associated with AD. Characteristic degenerative changes result in a decreased number of functioning neurons, which leads to deterioration in cognition, memory, and other thought processes.

Molecular Neuropathology in Alzheimer's Disease

The hallmarks of molecular neuropathology in AD are neurofibrillary tangles (NFTs) and neuritic plaques (NPs). Although these are present in normal aging brains, their numbers are few and they do not present the dramatic clinical manifestations observed in AD.

Microscopically, **neurofibrillary tangles (NFTs)** appear as bundles and strands through the cytoplasm, which displace the nucleus and other cellular organelles. They are composed of paired helical filaments formed by excessive phosphorylation of tau proteins. Though tau protein is a normal constituent of the axon cytoskeleton, in AD it is abnormally phosphorylated into an abnormal protein that no longer provides stability to the cell structures.[9,19] Figure 33-10 shows the flamelike appearance of NFTs. Not unique to AD, NFTs are also found in other degenerative diseases. In AD they tend to appear mostly in the hippocampus and temporal and parietal cortices, sparing the primary motor and sensory areas until late in the disease.[19]

Neuritic or senile plaques (NPs) are clusters of coalesced, degenerated neurons, dendrites, and axons surrounding a central dense core of amyloid (amyloid beta-peptide). Reactive astrocytes and microglia are also evident in the area of NPs. The amyloid beta-peptide is an abnormal protein complex generated by

TABLE 33-4

PROPOSED ETIOLOGIES FOR ALZHEIMER'S DISEASE

PROPOSED ETIOLOGY	MAJOR TENET OF ETIOLOGY	BASIS FOR PROPOSED ETIOLOGY
Slow virus	An unknown, unconventional virus with a very long incubation period infects the individual and causes progressive pathology of the brain.	A slow virus has been identified in two other dementias (kuru and Creutzfeldt-Jakob disease) with pathologic changes similar to Alzheimer's disease.
Acetylcholine (Ach) deficiency	Reduced levels of Ach in the brain provide the basis for manifestations of Alzheimer's disease.	Ach levels in the cerebral cortex and hippocampus in Alzheimer's patients is dramatically lower than in healthy individuals. Pharmacologic agents interfering with Ach levels in the brain produce temporary interference with cognition in healthy individuals.
Excessive aluminum in the brain	Excessive aluminum in the brains of Alzheimer's patients contributes to the pathophysiology of AD.	Aluminum has been shown to induce neurofibrillary tangles in animal brains.
Autoimmune processes	Alzheimer's patients have developed antibodies against their own brain tissue.	Increased circulating interleukin 1 (IL-6) in AD patients supports immune activation.[36]
Accumulation of amyloid beta-peptide fragments	Amyloid-bearing neuritic plaques cause degeneration of surrounding neurons and interfere with cognition.	Amyloid beta-peptide plaques have been found in brains of persons with AD.
Genetic transmission	AD results from multiple complex genetic components that program progressive pathologic deterioration of AD.	The precursor of the amyloid beta-peptide is encoded on chromosome 21. Individuals with Down syndrome, a condition associated with chromosome 21, develop AD around the fourth decade. Genetic mutations associated with familial AD are located on chromosomes 1, 14, and 21.
Neurofibrillary tangles (NFTs)	Accumulation of NFTs results in neuronal destruction.	NFTs are found in the hippocampus and cortical areas of the brains of AD patients.
Head trauma	Head trauma may initiate secretion of $ApoE_4$ and other reactants.[8]	ApoE4 accelerates amyloid production.

proteolysis of a transmembrane glycoprotein called *amyloid precursor protein (APP)*, which is encoded on chromosome 21.[10,24] Genetic evidence for the role of APP in AD is supported by the fact that almost all patients with trisomy 21 (Down syndrome) develop degenerative changes similar to AD, indicating that the extra gene provides for additional APP for conversion into amyloid beta peptide.[24]

Neuritic plaques are unique to normal aging, Down syndrome, and AD. Some believe that their numbers correlate directly with the degree of brain dysfunction,[19] whereas others believe there is little evidence for a correlation between the number of plaques and the severity of AD.[24] As noted earlier, amyloid deposition is enhanced by the presence of ApoE4 gene.[23] The accu-·lation pattern of amyloid beta-peptide in the AD linked to areas of the cerebral cortex associated ·on. In addition to the amyloid accumula-NPs, amyloid of the same chemical composition also accumulates in cerebral blood vessels in AD patients.[10] This interferes with nutrient exchange and disrupts the blood–brain barrier.

Finally, there is a marked reduction in the production of neurotransmitters, particularly Ach. Choline acetyltransferase (ChAT) levels have been reported to be significantly decreased in AD patients.[19] ChAT is necessary for the production of Ach. There seems to be a correlation between the degree of dementia and the loss of Ach in the brain.[30]

CLINICAL MANIFESTATIONS

Early symptoms are insidious and include loss of memory, carelessness about personal appearance, emotional disturbances that progress with time to complete disorientation, severe deterioration in speech, incontinence, and stereotyped, repetitive movements. Depression in the early course of the disease is common

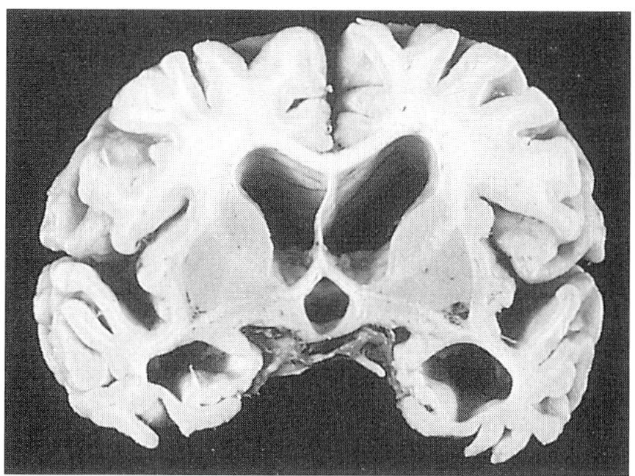

FIGURE 33-9. **Alzheimer's disease. Severe atrophy of the hippocampus causes the fissures to gape and the ventricles to enlarge (hydrocephalus ex vacuo). (Rubin, E. & Farber, J. [1999]. *Pathology* [3rd ed.]. Philadelphia: Lippincott.)**

as the person recognizes the cognitive decline that is occurring.

The clinical manifestations have been divided into three overlapping stages of the disease and are noted in Table 33-5. Progression to severe dementia is relentless and occurs over a period of years. Although the rate of progression varies, the average lifespan after diagnosis is about 8 years. Terminally, the person loses all cognitive and much of the motor ability.[13]

At present there is no in vivo diagnostic test that is definitive for AD. It is defined by the severe memory loss and the presence of NFTs and NPs. Typically, CT or MRI will show medial temporal lobe atrophy.

Arteriosclerotic Dementia

Arteriosclerotic dementia, the second most common cause of dementia after Alzheimer's disease, usually refers to dementia resulting from multiple infarctions over a period of months or years.[8,24] The infarctions may involve major cerebral blood vessels, but more commonly they involve small penetrating arterioles in the white matter. This type of dementia is frequently associated with hypertension and diabetes mellitus.

Vascular dementias associated with arteriosclerotic process can be classified into three generally accepted categories: (1) multi-infarct dementia, (2) lacunar disease, and (3) Binswanger's disease.

MULTI-INFARCT DEMENTIA

Multi-infarct dementia is associated with multiple strokes that progressively destroy brain parenchyma. Usually progressive, signs and symptoms evolve from an abrupt beginning, indicating ongoing vascular events. Clinical manifestations reveal progressive mental and physical neurologic deficits.

LACUNAR INFARCTIONS

Small subcortical cerebral infarctions are referred to as *lacunar infarctions.* These commonly involve lenticulostriatal arterioles and other deep penetrating small arterioles in the region of the basal ganglia and thalamus. Pseudobulbar palsy with slow dysarthric speech and emotional lability frequently accompany lacunar infarctions.[24] Cognitive processing is disturbed. Focal neurologic deficits such as hemiparesis, aphasia, and sensory losses may also be present.

BINSWANGER'S DISEASE

In some cases there is involvement of the deep penetrating vessels in white matter and regions around the ventricles, while the cortex and basal ganglia are spared.[24] These pathologic findings associated with *Binswanger's disease* are identified as coalesced is-

FOCUS ON CELLULAR PATHOPHYSIOLOGY

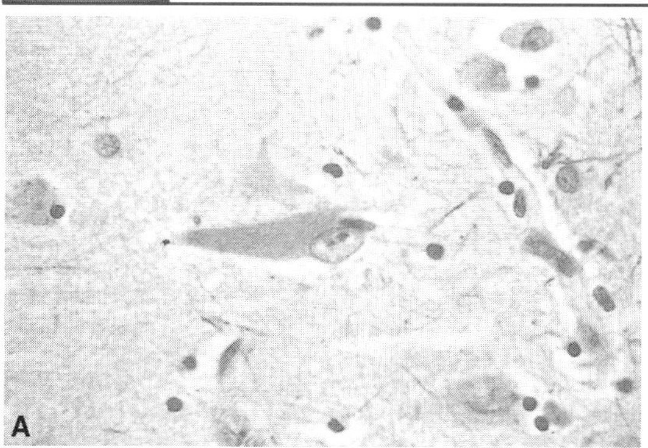

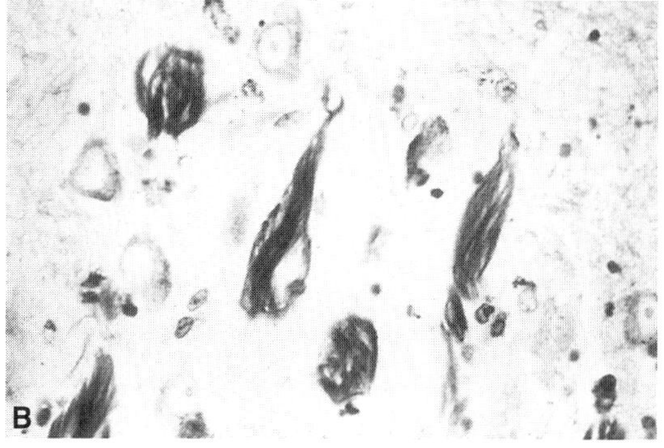

FIGURE 33-10. Alzheimer's disease. **A.** The cytoplasm of a neuron is distended by neurofibrillary tangles. **B.** A silver stain of A demonstrates the fibrillary character of the cytoplasmic inclusions. (Rubin, E. & Farber, J. [1999]. *Pathology* [3rd ed.]. Philadelphia: Lippincott.)

TABLE 33-5

CLINICAL MANIFESTATIONS IN STAGES OF ALZHEIMER'S DISEASE

EARLY STAGE (2–4 YEARS)	MIDDLE STAGE (2–10 YEARS)	FINAL STAGE (1–2 YEARS)
Subtle memory changes Mood and personality changes—often angered and/or depressed Poor judgment Difficulty in making decisions Problems with paying bills Quick to anger Poor work performance Self-doubt Decreased ability to concentrate Some loss of ability to use correct terms or words Careless in actions or appearance Uncharacteristic behavior or use of words (swearing) Disinterest in environment and events Asking same questions and making same statements repeatedly	Dramatic decline in memory Paces aimlessly—increased restlessness, especially at night Hides things, more paranoid Seems thoughtless and self-centered Inappropriate behavior, especially in crowded, noisy places Loss of perceptive powers and cannot follow conversation Difficulty using objects, reading, writing, and speaking Difficulty finding things and locations in own home Inability to comprehend television or radio Mumbles, makes up own words or language Walks with unsteady gait, head down, shoulders bent, shuffles Becomes wary of water, personal hygiene declines Unable to recognize people Inappropriate sexual behavior Needs reminding to perform activities of daily living Sundowning—late afternoon/evening anxiety	Unable to communicate in words Unable to recognize self or others Unaware of environment, bizarre/unpredictable behavior Forgets how to eat, bathe, swallow, walk, sit and eventually becomes bedridden Urine and bowel incontinence Dehydrated and constipated Inability to express pain or describe things happening to self Lost all the time Misidentifies people, objects, rooms Increased delusions and hallucinations Falls/loses balance often Seizures Susceptible to frequent illnesses such as pneumonia, which is frequently the cause of death Emaciated

(Summarized from the Alzheimer's Association.)

chemic or infarcted lesions on MRI scans. The clinical presentation of Binswanger's disease has considerable overlap with Alzheimer's disease and other vascular-associated dementias. A history of stroke risk factors and clinical presentations of strokelike episodes that may have reflected subtle neurologic deficits aid in differentiation.

Pick's Disease

Pick's disease (PD) is a degenerative neurologic disease generally occurring in the fourth and fifth decades. Thought to be transmitted by an autosomal dominant gene, it affects women more than men and may occur in families.[4] Because of the region of the brain involved, it is categorized as a frontal lobe dementia.

PATHOPHYSIOLOGY

Neuronal degeneration occurs, with atrophy of the frontal lobe most distinctly. The first three cortical lay- of the frontal lobe are most severely involved, and re so dramatically atrophied that they give this brain the appearance of a dried walnut. bes also are involved, but to a lesser degree.

Microscopically, the neurons contain paired helical filaments (PHFs) known as **Pick bodies.** Pick bodies are formed by hyperphosphorylated tau protein known as PHFtau.[22] The hyperphosphorylated tau in Pick's disease has been formed through a biochemical pathway that is similar to Alzheimer's hyperphosphorylated tau; however, its molecular structure is unique and distinct to PD.[22] The accumulation of hyperphosphorylated tau eventually compromises the viability of neurons in the frontal and temporal regions of the brain.

CLINICAL MANIFESTATIONS

In contrast to AD and Huntington's chorea, the initial manifestations of PD reflect personality changes that elude the person's awareness. The behavioral deterioration is evidenced by disinterest in surroundings, irritability, forgetfulness, confusion, cognitive sluggishness, apathy, and dementia. As the disease progresses there is difficulty with finding the right words and language deterioration to echolalia (parrot-like repetition of words), stereotyped words and phrases, incomprehensible jargon, and, finally, mutism. Motor deterioration begins with gait disturbances, weakness, and

FOCUS ON THE PERSON WITH PROGRESSIVE MUSCLE WEAKNESS

P. M. is a 63-year-old male who comes for evaluation of complaints of increasing muscle weakness and difficulty ambulating over the past several months. He reports that his left leg seems to drag when he walks and "sometimes, it even hits the other leg." "I feel like a clumsy oaf." He also states that he's noticed that he doesn't have as much strength in his hands as he did before. "Sometimes I can't even open a jar of pickles." Patient is right handed.

Examination reveals fasciculations of the tongue and in the hands and weakness of the muscles of the palate and face. Muscle weakness and wasting is noted in his right hand and left leg. Sensory and cognitive function intact. Testing with anticholinesterase agent negative; no improvement in symptoms is seen. Muscle biopsy and electromyography reveal loss of motor neurons and atrophy. A diagnosis of amyotrophic lateral sclerosis (ALS) is made.

Questions

1. Explain how P. M. fits the typical clinical presentation of a patient with ALS based on incidence and pathophysiology.
2. Describe the possible causes associated with ALS.
3. Explain how P. M. was evaluated for fasciculations of his hands.
4. Discuss the possible additional manifestations that may occur as P. M.'s condition progresses.

rigidity and progresses to flexion contractions and paraplegia.

Computed tomography scans show lobar atrophy in advanced cases, but the electroencephalogram is often normal until very late in the course of the disease. PET scans show a decreased blood flow and decreased metabolism in the frontal lobes even before the atrophy becomes visible by CT or MRI.[8]

REFERENCES

1. Adams, R., & Victor, M. (1998). *Principles of neurology* (6th ed.). New York: McGraw-Hill.
2. Antel, J. P., & Arnasan, B. G. (1997). Demyelinating diseases. In A. Fauci et al. (Eds.), *Harrison's principles of internal medicine* (14th ed.). New York: McGraw-Hill.
3. Barker, E., & Hobdell, R. (1994). Neuromuscular disorders. In E. Barker, *Neuroscience nursing*. St. Louis: Mosby.
4. Beal, M. F., Richardson, E. P., & Martin, J. B. (1997). Degenerative diseases of the nervous system. In A. Fauci et al. (Eds.), *Harrison's principles of internal medicine* (14th ed.). New York: McGraw-Hill.
5. Buettner, U. W. & Caplan, L. R. (1996). Syringomyelia and syringobulbia. In *Neurological disorders: Course and treatment*. San Diego, CA: Academic Press.
6. Bunting, L. & Fitzsimmons, B. (1994). Degenerative disorders. In E. Barker, *Neuroscience nursing*. St. Louis: Mosby.
7. Chandrasoma, P. & Taylor, C. R. (1998). *Concise pathology* (3rd ed.). Norwalk, CT: Appleton & Lange.
8. Collins, R. (1997). *Neurology*. Philadelphia: W.B. Saunders.
9. Corbet, J. J. & Wullner, U. (1996). Pseudotumor cerebri. In *Neurologic disorders: Course and treatment*. San Diego, CA: Academic Press.
10. Dawson, D. (1994). Demyelinating diseases. In J. Stein (Ed.), *Internal medicine* (4th ed.). St. Louis: Mosby.
11. De Girolami, U. D., Anthony, D. C., & Forsch, M. P. (1994). Peripheral nerve and skeletal muscle. In R. Cotran, V. Kumar, & S. Robbins, *Robbins' pathologic basis of disease* (5th ed.). Philadelphia: W.B. Saunders.
12. De Girolami, U. D., Frosch, M. P., & Anthony, D. C. (1994). The central nervous system. In R. Cotran, V. Kumar, & S. Robbins, *Robbins' pathologic basis of disease* (5th ed.). Philadelphia: W.B. Saunders.
13. Esiri, M. M., Bradley, T. H., Beyreuther, K., & Masters, C. L. (1997). Aging and dementia. In D. I. Graham & P. L. Lantos (Eds.), *Greenfield's pathology*. London: Oxford University Press.
14. Folstein, M. F., & Ross, C. (1997). Cognitive impairment in the elderly. In W. N. Kelley (Ed.), *Textbook of internal medicine* (3rd ed.). Philadelphia: J. B. Lippincott.
15. Gasser, T. & Harding, A. E. (1996). Huntington's disease and Sydenham's chorea. In *Neurological disorders: Course and treatment*. San Diego, CA: Academic Press.
16. Govan, A. D. T., Macfarlane, P. S., & Callander, R. (1995). *Pathology illustrated* (4th ed.). New York: Churchill Livingstone.
17. Guazzo, E. P. & Bahr, M. (1996). Hydrocephalus. In *Neurological disorders: Care and treatment*. San Diego, CA: Academic Press.
18. Harding, B., & Copp, A. J. (1997). Malformations. In D. I. Graham & P. L. Lantos (Eds.), *Greenfield's pathology*. London: Oxford University Press.
19. Joyce, J. N. & Hurtig, H. I. (1994). Neurodegenerative disorders. In A. Frazer, P. Molinoff, & A. Winokur, *Biological basis of brain function and disease*. New York: Raven Press.
20. Kesselring, J. (Ed.) (1997). *Multiple sclerosis*. London: Cambridge University Press.
21. Lazar, R. B. (1998). *Principles of neurologic rehabilitation*. New York: McGraw-Hill.
22. Lieberman, A. P., Trojanowski, J., Lee, V., Ding, X., Morrison, D., & Grossman, M. (1998). Cognitive, neuroimaging, and pathlogical studies in a patient with Pick's disease. *Annals of Neurology, 43,* 259–263.
23. Mayeux, R., Saunders, A. M., Shea, S., Mirra, S., Evans, D., Roses, A. Hyman, B., Crain, B., Tang, M., & Phelps, C. (1998). Utility of apolipoprotein E genotype in the diagnosis of Alzheimer's disease. Alzheimer's Disease Centers Consortium on apolipotrotein E and Alzheimer's disease. *New England Journal of Medicine, 338,* 506–511.
24. McPhee, S. J., Lingappa, V. R., Gangong, W. F., & Lange, J. D. (1997). *Pathology of disease: An introduction to clinical medicine*. Stamford, CT: Appleton & Lange.
25. Mueller, F., Duchgans, J., & Jankovic, J. (1996). Dyskinesias. In *Neurological disorders: Course and treatment*. San Diego, CA: Academic Press.
26. Oertel, W. H., & Quinn, N. P. (1996). Parkinsonism. In *Neurologic disorders: Course and treatment*. San Diego, CA: Academic Press.
27. Prineas, J. W. (1997). Demyelinating diseases. In D. I. Graham & P. L. Lantos (Eds.), *Greenfield's pathology*. London: Oxford University Press.
28. Rekate, H. L. (1991). *Comprehensive management of spina bifida*. Boston: CRC Press.
29. Rodnitzky, R. L. (1995). Clinical correlation: Myasthenia gravis. In P. M. Conn, *Neuroscience in medicine*. Philadelphia: J. B. Lippincott.

30. Rodnitzky, R. L. (1995). Clinical correlation: Dementia and abnormalities of cognition. In P. M. Conn, *Neuroscience in medicine*. Philadelphia: J. B. Lippincott.
31. Rodnitzky, R. L. (1995). Clinical correlation: Peripheral neuropathy. In P. M. Conn, *Neuroscience in medicine*. Philadelphia: J. B. Lippincott.
32. Rubin, E. & Faber, J. L. (1999). *Pathology* (3rd ed.). Philadelphia: Lippincott.
33. Singh, V. K. & Guthikonda, P. (1997). Circulating cytokines in Alzheimer's disease. *Journal of Psychiatric Research, 31,* 657–660.
34. Smithells, D. (1992). Prevention of spina bifida and hydrocephalus. In C.M. Bannister & B. Tew (Eds.), *Current concepts of spina bifida and hydrocephalus*. New York: MacKeith Press.
35. Stern, Y., Brandt, J., Albert, M., Jacobs, D., et al. (1997). The absence of an apolipoprotein e4 allele is associated with a more aggressive form of Alzheimer's disease. *Annals of Neurology, 41,* 615–620.
36. Sudarsky, L. R. (1994). Parkinsonism and movement disorders. In J. Stein (Ed.), *Internal medicine* (4th ed.). St. Louis: Mosby.
37. Sundberg, D. K. (1995). Chemical messenger systems. In P. M. Conn, (Ed.), *Neuroscience in medicine*. Philadelphia: J. B. Lippincott.
38. Thomas, P. K., Landon, D. N., & King, R. H. M. (1997). Disease of the peripheral nerves. In D. I. Graham & P. L. Lantos (Eds.), *Greenfield's pathology*. London: Oxford University Press.
39. Vogel, F. S., & Bouldin, T. W. (1994). The nervous system. In E. Rubin & J. L. Farber, *Pathology* (2nd ed.). Philadelphia: J. B. Lippincott.
40. Welch, K., & Lorenzo, A. V. (1992). The pathology of hydrocephalus. In C. M. Bannister & B. Tew (Eds.). *Current concepts in spina bifida and hydrocephalus*. New York: MacKeith Press.
41. Weller, R. O., Cumming, W. J. K., & Mahon, M. (1997). Diseases of the muscle. In D. I. Graham & P. L. Lantos (Eds.), *Greenfield's pathology*. London: Oxford University Press.
42. Welsh-Bohmer, K., Gearing, M., Saunders, A., Roses, A., & Mirra, S. (1998). Apolipoprotein E genotypes in a neuropathological series from the consortium to establish a registry for Alzheimer's disease. *Annals of Neurology, 42,* 319–325.
43. Wong, D. L. & Whaley, L. F. (1998). *Whaley's and Wong's nursing care of infants and children* (6th ed.). St. Louis: Mosby.

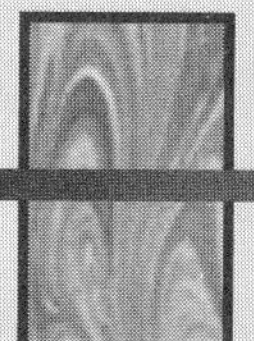

UNIT 10: CASE STUDY

The Person Experiencing Neurologic Deficits

Introduction to the Patient

Mr. O. is a 59-year-old African-American male who is brought to the emergency department by ambulance. He is awake and mumbling incoherently. His wife is by his side.

Present Illness

Mrs. O. states that her husband awakened this morning complaining of a headache. He was in the bathroom shaving when she heard a thump coming from there. She ran to the bathroom, finding Mr. O. on the floor, trying to talk. She stated, "He was trying to tell me something, but I couldn't understand him." She was unable to get him up, noting that his right arm and leg seemed very weak and his pajamas were wet with urine. She immediately called 911 to take him to the hospital. "This happened so fast. It's been less than an hour since he fell."

Social History

Mr. O., married to his wife for almost 30 years, is employed as a marketing executive for a national department store chain. According to Mrs. O., he spends most of his work time in his office, but travels to other cities in the United States on business about 1 week per month. She reports that he smokes about 1½ packs of cigarettes a day. They enjoy going out to dinner at least once a week when he usually has one to two martinis with dinner. "He always orders steak and baked potato with butter and sour cream."

Past Medical History

Mrs. O. states that her husband hasn't seen a doctor for the last 3 years. "He always says that he's fine and doesn't have the time. The last time he saw the doctor, his blood pressure was a little high." She also reports that he has never been diagnosed with hypertension or heart disease but that occasionally he does complain of some "palpitations." Mrs. O. denies any history of Mr. O.'s recreational drug use. "The only medicine he takes is ibuprofen and only once in a while for a headache."

Family History

Mr. O. is the youngest of four children. He has two sisters, ages 65 and 63 years. Both are alive and well, but one sister has diabetes and high blood pressure. His brother, age 61 years, has had two heart attacks. Mr. O.'s father died at age 55 years from a heart attack. His mother, now age 86 years, alive and fairly well for her age, has a history of diabetes and arthritis.

Physical Examination

Mr. O. appears awake and alert but somewhat anxious. He seems to understand when spoken to, responding to yes/no questions by nodding his head and obeying simple commands. However, his speech is unintelligible. Glasgow coma scale score is 12. His vital signs are as follows: temperature—98.8°F; pulse—124; respirations—22; blood pressure—180/96. Mrs. O. states that Mr. O. is 5 ft, 9 in tall and weighs 230 pounds. Skin is pale, warm, and dry.

Examination of the head and neck reveals pupils 4 mm in size; PERRLA and equal carotid pulsations. A grade 3 bruit is auscultated in left carotid. Visible drooping noted on the right side of his mouth.

Chest is clear to auscultation. Heart rate elevated and slightly irregular. S1 and S2 are present. No murmurs, rubs, or gallops noted. His abdomen is soft and nontender with active bowel sounds. Some urinary incontinence noted. Extremities are warm to touch with quick capillary refill; pulse +2/4 in all extremities.

Neurologic examination reveals that the patient is alert and awake with right-sided hemiplegia. +5 muscle strength is noted on left side; +1 on right. Sensation to pin prick is intact on left side but absent on right side. Deep tendon reflexes are +2 on the left and +1 to 0 on the right. No papilledema or microaneurysms are noted on ophthalmoscopic examination. Cranial nerves grossly intact.

Diagnostic Tests

Complete blood count: WBC—7000/mm^3; hemoglobin—14.1; hematocrit—40
Serum electrolytes: sodium—142 mEq/L; chloride—99 mEq/L; potassium—4.6 mEq/L
Coagulation studies: PT—13.0 secs; APTT—36 secs; INR—1.5
Platelets: 250,000/mm^3
Urinalysis: normal
CT (non-contrast): normal; no evidence of hemorrhage
ECG: atrial fibrillation
Echocardiogram (done a few days after admission): slightly dilated left ventricle with normal contractility

CRITICAL THINKING QUESTIONS

1. Correlate possible risk factors for stroke with Mr. O.'s history and physical examination.
2. Hypothesize about which cerebral artery(ies) is (are) most likely involved.
3. Describe the pathophysiologic basis for Mr. O.'s aphasia.
4. Discuss the criteria necessary to determine if Mr. O. is a candidate for recombinant tissue plasminogen activator (r-TPA) therapy.
5. Elaborate on the pros and cons of anticoagulant and antiplatelet therapy on discharge. Include areas that need to be addressed in patient teaching.

Besides your pathophysiology text, you'll need a good pharmacology text, a neurology text, a diagnostic/laboratory test text, a medical-surgical nursing text, and current research to complete this case study. Suggested references follow:

Adams, H. (1998). Treating ischemic stroke as an emergency. *Archives of Neurology, 55,* 457–461.

Adams, H. P. et al. (1996). Guidelines for thrombolytic therapy for acute stroke: A supplement to the guidelines for the management of patients with acute ischemic stroke. *Stroke, 27*(9), 1711–1718.

Fischbach, F. (1996). a *Manual of laboratory and diagnostic tests,* (5th ed.). Philadelphia: Lippincott-Raven.

Furlan, A. & Kanoti, G. (1997). When is thrombolysis justified in patients with acute ischemic stroke? *Stroke, 28*(1), 214–218.

Hickey, J. V. (1997). *Clinical practice of neurological nursing* (4th ed.). Philadelphia: Lippincott-Raven.

Karch, A. M. (1999). *1999 Lippincott's nursing drug guide.* Philadelphia: Lippincott-Raven.

Neurology Standard Subcommittee. (1996). Practice advisory: Thrombolytic therapy for acute ischemic stroke-summary statement. *Neurology, 47,* 835–839.

Schneck, M. J. (1998). Acute stroke: An aggressive approach to intervention and prevention. *Hospital Medicine, 34*(1), 11–12, 17–20, 25–26, 28.

Smeltzer, S. & Bare, B. (2000). *Brunner and Suddarth's textbook of medical-surgical nursing* (9th ed.). Philadelphia: Lippincott Williams & Wilkins.

Wiebers, D. O., Feigein, V. & Brown, R. D. (1997). *Handbook of stroke.* Philadelphia: Lippincott-Raven.

Website resources:

Neurology *http://www.medmatrix.org/SPages/Neurology.asp*

American Stroke Association *http://www.amhrt.org/Stroke/index.html*

National Stroke Association *http://www.stroke.org/*

Stroke Information Guide *http://www.ninds.nih.gov/*

Mayo Clinic Division of Cerebrovascular Research *http://www.mayo.edu/cerebro/research/*

Atrial Fibrillation *http://www.americanheart.org/Heart_and_Stroke_A_Z_Guide/afib.hmtl*

Aspirin in Heart Attack and Stroke Prevention *http://www.americanheart.org/Heart_and_Stroke_A_Z_Guide/aspirin.html*

UNIT 10 APPENDIX A

DIAGNOSTIC TESTS

TEST	PURPOSE/NORMAL FINDINGS	SIGNIFICANCE
Electroencephalography (EEG)	Graphic representation of the electrical activity of the brain vial electrodes placed on the scalp Normal findings: normal brain wave pattern, frequency, amplitude, and characteristics	Alpha waves have frequencies of 8 to 13 cycles per second (cps), are perceived in healthy adults in the occipital and parietal regions, and are present in a resting person whose eyes are closed. Beta waves have frequencies of about 13 cps, are recorded from the frontal lobe, and represent the activity of the motor cortex. Theta waves have frequencies of 4 to 7 cps and are recorded in the parietal and frontotemporal region of the brain. Delta waves have frequencies of less than 4 cps and are commonly observed in deep sleep in children. Changes in EEG waves may indicate organic brain pathology. EEG, if recorded between seizure activity, may be normal in patients with generalized seizures, but abnormalities may be induced by hyperventilation or sleep. Sedatives and stimulants should be avoided for 24 to 48 hours prior to the EEG to prevent interference in wave patterns or masking of abnormalities. Hypoglycemia also may affect the EEG waveform.
Lumbar puncture for CSF analysis	Evaluation of CSF after needle inserted into the lumbar subarachnoid space Normal findings: Appearance: clear, colorless, odorless Pressure: 50 to 180 mm H_20 Specific gravity: 1.006 to 1.008 Red blood cells (RBCs): 0 Leukocytes: 0 to 5/mm^3 Protein: 20–45 mg/dL Glucose 40–80 mg/dL (60–75% of serum glucose) Chloride: 120–130 mEq/L Sodium: 140 mEq/L Potassium: 3.0 mEq/L Bicarbonate: 23.6 mEq/L	Yellowish (xanthochromia) fluid may be observed with disintegrating red blood cells from hemorrhage or high protein count. Cloudiness may be seen with increased protein levels, infection, and increased white blood cells. Pink, blood-tinged, or bloody fluid may indicate cerebral contusion, laceration, or subarachnoid hemorrhage (SAH). Bloody CSF may also indicate a traumatic tap. Pressure may be decreased with dehydration or blockage in the subarachnoid space. Elevated pressure may be seen with brain tumors, abscesses, hydrocephalus, edema, or cerebral hematomas. An elevated leukocyte count may indicate infections, CNS tumors, or multiple sclerosis. Increased neutrophils are associated with bacterial infection; increased lymphocytes are associated with viral infections. Elevated protein levels may indicate infections, brain tumors, Guillain-Barré syndrome, demyelinating diseases, or meningeal hemorrhage. Decreased glucose may be seen with infections, such as meningitis, SAH, tuberculosis, or tumors. Elevated glucose is associated with diabetes mellitus.

UNIT 10 APPENDIX A

DIAGNOSTIC TESTS (Continued)

TEST	PURPOSE/NORMAL FINDINGS	SIGNIFICANCE
Evoked potentials	EEG recording using specialized electrode placement to evaluate conduction times in the peripheral nervous system and determine specific afferent nerve pathways (auditory [see Unit 11], visual [see Unit 11], and sensory [somatosensory] pathways) Normal findings: neural conduction without delay	Abnormal somatosensory evoked potentials may be seen with spinal cord lesions, CVA, or multiple sclerosis.
Radiographs (x-ray films)	Evaluation of the skull, spinal cord, and surrounding tissues Normal findings: normal appearance of the skull and spinal cord structures	Abnormalities may reveal fractures, displacement, or compression of the bones of the skull and vertebral column. Pineal gland shift may be visualized with brain displacement.
Myelography	Radiographic evaluation of subarachnoid space after injection of contrast medium Normal findings: spinal cord and nerve roots clearly outlined; absence of distortion in the dura	Abnormalities may suggest ruptured intervertebral disk, intervertebral tumor, spinal canal obstruction, avulsion of the nerve roots, or compression and stenosis of the spinal cord.
Computed tomography (CT scan)	Specialized radiographic cross-sectional view of bone and soft tissue structures of the brain and spinal cord, distinguishing white matter from gray matter and identifying ventricles and sulci Normal findings: Absence of tumors, fracture, or other abnormalities Low-density tissues black High-density tissues gray	CT may be used in conjunction with contrast myelography or angiography to visualize details of vascular or tissue structure. A wide variety of cranial and spinal abnormalities, such as intracranial hemorrhages, infarctions, neoplasms, abscesses, hydrocephalus, intracranial shifts, and spinal cord compressions, may be visualized. Increased tissue density pattern may be seen with meningiomas, astrocytomas, aneurysm, degenerated or infected tissue, intracerebral hemorrhage, or hematoma. Decreased tissue density patterns may be seen with infarction, tumor necrosis, degenerative changes, or edema.
Magnetic resonance imaging (MRI)	Evaluation of soft tissues, fluid, and bony structures of the nervous system by viewing successive layers of the brain in any plane within a powerful magnetic field Normal findings: absence of abnormalities	A variety of abnormalities in bone, tissue, and vascular tissue of the CNS may be visualized.
Cerebral angiography	Radiographic evaluation of cerebrovascular system after injection of a contrast medium into a major artery Normal findings: vessels patent and normal in structure without evidence of narrowing	This test may identify vascular lesions—aneurysms, arteriovenous malformations, vasospasm, vascular tumors, or occlusions of vessels.
Digital subtraction angiography	Combination of radiography after injection of contrast medium and computerized subtraction to visualize vascular structures of the CNS Normal findings: normal carotid and vertebral arterial system	Contrast medium is usually injected through a peripheral vessel. DSA may reveal aneurysms, arteriovenous malformations, tumors, or hematomas of the CNS.
Echoencephalography	Evaluation of brain structures in response to ultrasonic signals displayed as echo pulsations on an oscilloscope	This test may visualize shifts of midline structures associated with trauma, cerebrovascular alterations, or space-occupying lesions.

(continued)

UNIT 10 APPENDIX A

DIAGNOSTIC TESTS

TEST	PURPOSE/NORMAL FINDINGS	SIGNIFICANCE
	Normal findings: Midline structure position normal Distance from midline to lateral or third ventricular wall normal	Dilation of ventricles may indicate hydrocephalus.
Transcranial Doppler sonography	Ultrasonic evaluation of cranial blood flow to detect changes in lumen size or flow Normal findings: blood flow velocity within normal limits	This test is useful in detecting vasospasm. Increased velocity may indicate arterial narrowing if there is a corresponding low velocity in collateral arteries.
Carotid duplex scan	Evaluation of the major arteries supplying the brain to evaluate cerebrovascular blood flow Normal findings: Common carotid, internal carotid, and external carotid without occlusion or stenosis Blood flow normal	This test may be used to evaluate ischemia, dizziness, hemiparesis, paresthesia, or speech and visual problems. Abnormalities may reveal plaques, tumors, occlusions, or aneurysms.
Brain scan	Evaluation of radionuclide uptake by brain tissue Normal findings: absence of uptake	Radionuclide substances accumulate in abnormal areas such tumors, abscesses, and subdural hematomas. These regions would emit gamma rays, which are measured by a special scanner.
Positron emission tomography (PET scan)	Visualization of normal brain-processing information by measuring gamma rays that are emitted as a radioactive substance is metabolized Normal findings: Normal pattern of tissue metabolism based on use of oxygen, glucose, fatty acids, and protein synthesis Blood flow and tissue perfusion normal	Abnormalities of cerebral vessels and tumors may reveal the physiologic basis for aberrant behavior. Focal areas associated with acute epilepsy may be evidenced as areas of increased tissue metabolism.
Single photon computed emission tomography (SPECT)	Evaluation of blood perfusion in regions of the brain by measuring commercially prepared injected radioactive tracers with a rotating gamma camera Normal findings: same as PET scan	Abnormal cerebral blood perfusion may be demonstrated in dementia, cerebrovascular disease, and cerebral trauma.

UNIT BIBLIOGRAPHY

Adams, R., & Victor, M. (1998). *Principles of neurology* (6th ed.). New York: McGraw-Hill.

Affifi, A. & Bergman, R. A. (1997). *Functional neuroanatomy.* New York: McGraw-Hill.

Aminoff, M., Greenberg, D. A., & Simon, R. P. (1997). *Clinical neurology* (3rd ed.). Stamford, CT: Appleton & Lange.

Conn, P. M. (1995). *Neuroscience in medicine.* Philadelphia: J. B. Lippincott.

Barker, E. (1994). *Neuroscience nursing.* St. Louis: Mosby.

Buettner, U. W. & Caplan, L. R. (1996). Syringomyelia and syringobulbia. In *Neurological disorders: Course and treatment.* San Diego, CA: Academic Press.

Chandrasoma, P. & Taylor, C. R. (1998). *Concise pathology* (3rd ed.). Norwalk, CT: Appleton & Lange.

Collins, R. (1997) *Neurology.* Philadelphia: W.B. Saunders.

Fauci, A. S. et al. (Eds.) (1997). *Harrison's principles of internal medicine* (14th ed.). New York: McGraw-Hill.

Frazer, A., Molinoff, P. & Winokur, A. (1994). *Biological basis of brain function and disease.* New York: Raven Press.

Gazzaniga, M. S. (1998). The split brain revisited. *Scientific American, 279*(1), 50–55.

Gilman, S., & Newman, S. (1997). *Manter and Gatz's essentials of clinical neuroanatomy and neurophysiology* (9th ed.). Philadelphia: F.A. Davis.

Graham, D. I. & Lantos. P. L.(Eds.) (1997). *Greenfield's pathology.* London: Oxford University Press.

Kesselring, J. (Ed.) (1997). *Multiple sclerosis.* London: Cambridge University Press.

Lazar, R. B. (1998). *Principles of neurologic rehabilitation.* New York: McGraw-Hill.

Rubin, E. & Faber, J. L. (1999). Pathology (3rd ed.). Philadelphia: Lippincott-Raven.

Waxman, S. & deGroot, S. (1997). *Correlative neuroanatomy and functional neurology* (22nd ed.). Norwalk, CT: Appleton & Lange.

Welsh-Bohmer, K., Gearing, M., Saunders, A, Roses, A., & Mirra, S. (1998). Apolipoprotein E genotypes in a neuropathological series from the consortium to establish a registry for Alzheimer's disease. *Annals of Neurology, 42,* 319–325.

ALZHEIMER'S DISEASE AND DEMENTIAS

Lieberman, A. P., Trojanowski, J., Lee, V., Ding, X., Morrison, D., & Grossman, M. (1998). Cognitive, neuroimaging, and pathological studies in a patient with Pick's disease. *Annals of Neurology, 43,* 259–263.

Mayeux, R., Saunders, A. M., Shea, S., Mirra, S., Evans, D., Roses, A. Hyman, B., Crain, B., Tang, M., & Phelps, C. (1998). Utility of apolipoprotein E genotype in the diagnosis of Alzheimer's disease. Alzheimer's disease centers consortium on apolipoprotein E and Alzheimer's disease. *New England Journal of Medicine, 338,* 506–511.

Singh, V. K. & Guthikonda, P. (1997). Circulating cytokines in Alzheimer's disease. *Journal of Psychiatric Research, 31,* 657–660.

Stern, Y., Brandt, J., Albert, M., Jacobs, D., et al. (1991). The absence of an apolipoprotein E4 allele is associated with a more aggressive form of Alzheimer's disease. *Annals of Neurology, 41,* 615–620.

CENTRAL NERVOUS SYSTEM INJURY

Barker, E. (1995). Don't dismiss whiplash. *RN, 58*(11), 26–31.

Criss, E. (1995). Back to back: Assessment of spinal trauma. *Journal of Emergency Medical Services, 20*(4), 46–57.

Darvovic, G. (1997). Assessing pupillary responses. *Nursing, 27*(2), 49.

Ditunno, J. F. Jr., Graziani, V., & Tesslen, A. (1997). Neurological assessment in spinal cord injury. *Advances in Neurology, 72,* 325–333.

Juarez, V. J. & Lyons, M. (1995). Interrater reliability of the Glasgow Coma Scale. *Journal of Neuroscience Nursing, 27*(5), 283–286.

McDonald, J. W. (1999). Repairing the damaged spinal cord. *Scientific American, 281*(3), 64–73.

Souder, E., Saykin, A. & Alavi, A. (1995). Multi-modal assessment in Alzheimer's disease: ADL in relation to PET, MRI and neuropsychology. *Journal of Gerontologic Nursing, 21* (9), 1–13.

Wooten, C. (1996). The trauma top 10: The top 10 ways to detect deteriorating central neurological status. *Journal of Trauma Nursing 3*(1), 25–27.

BRAIN TUMOR

Bronstein, K. (1995). Epidemiology and classification of brain tumors. *Critical Care Nursing Clinics of North America, 7,* 1.

Kornblith, P. & Walker, M. (Eds.) (1997). *Advances in Neurooncology II.* Armonk, NY: Futura.

Ellison, D., Love, S. Chimelli, L., Harding, B., Lowe, J., Roberts, G., & Vinters, H. (1998). *Neuropathology: A reference text of CNS pathology.* London: Mosby.

CEREBROVASCULAR DISEASE

Adams, H. (1998). Treating ischemic stroke as an emergency. *Archives of Neurology, 55,* 457–461.

Batjer, H. H. (Editor-in-chief) (1997). *Cerebrovascular disease.* Philadelphia: Lippincott-Raven.

Furlan, A. & Kanoti, G. (1997). When is thrombolysis justified in patients with acute ischemic stroke? *Stroke: A Journal of Cerebral Circulation, 28*(1), 214–218.

Hickey, J. V. (1997). *The clinical practice of neurological nursing* (4th ed.). Philadelphia: Lippincott-Raven.

Schneck, M. J. (1998). Acute stroke: An aggressive approach to intervention and prevention. *Hospital Medicine, 34*(1), 11–12, 17–20, 25–26, 28.

Siesjo, B. K. & Wieloch, T. (Eds.) (1996). *Advances in neurology (vol. 71): Cellular and molecular mechanisms of ischemic brain damage.* Philadelphia: Lippincott-Raven.

Richard, T. S. (1997). Cerebral resuscitation after global brain ischemia: Linking research to practice. *AACN Clinical Issues, 8*(2), 171–181.

Wiebers, D. O., Feigein, V. & Brown, R. D. (1997). *Handbook of stroke.* Philadelphia: Lippincott-Raven.

EPILEPSY

Brown, T. & Holmes, G. (1997). *Handbook of epilepsy.* Philadelphia: Lippincott-Raven.

Engel, J. & Pedley, T. A. (1997). *Epilepsy: A comprehensive textbook.* Philadelphia: Lippincott-Raven.

French, J., Divhter, M, & Leppik, L.(1997). *Antiepileptic drug development (Advances in neurology, vol. 76).* Philadelphia: Lippincott-Raven.

PARKINSON'S DISEASE

Bajaj, N. P., Shaw, C., Warner, T. & Ray, C. (1998). The genetics of Parkinson's disease and parkinsonian syndromes. *Journal of Neurology; 245* (10), 625–633.

Gilb, D. J., Oliver, E., & Gilman, S. (1999). Diagnostic criteria for Parkinson disease. *Archives of Neurology, 56*(1), 33–39.

AMYOTROPHIC LATERAL SCLEROSIS

Milonas, I.(1998). Amytrophic lateral sclerosis: An introduction. *Journal of Neurology, 245* (Suppl.), 2, S1–S3.

Mitsumoto, H., Chad, D. A., Pioro, E. P., & Gilman, S. (Eds.) (1998). Amytrophic lateral *sclerosis (Contemporary neurology series, No. 49).* London: Oxford University Press.

GUILLAIN BARRÉ

Bonduelle, M. (1998). Guillain Barré syndrome. *Archives of Neurology, 55*(11), 1483–1484.

Pemberton, L. (1998). Guillain Barré syndrome. *Nursing Times, 94*(46), 50–53.

MULTIPLE SCLEROSIS

Paty, D. W., & Ebers, G. (1997). *Multiple sclerosis.* Philadelphia: F.A. Davis.

Raine, C., McFarland, H., & Tourtellotte, W. (1997). *Multiple sclerosis: Clinical and pathogenetic basis.* Philadelphia: Lippincott-Raven.

Russell, W. E. & Russell, W. C. (1997). *Molecular biology of multiple sclerosis.* New York: John Wiley.

MENTAL HEALTH AND ILLNESS

American Psychiatric Association. (1994). *Diagnostic and statistical manual of mental disorders* (4th ed.). Washington, DC: American Psychiatric Press.

Andreason, N. C. & Black, D. W. (1995). *Introductory textbook of psychiatry* (2nd ed.). Washington, DC: American Psychiatric Press.

Fogel, B. S., Schiffer, R. B., & Rao, S. M. (Eds.) (1996). Neuropsychiatry. Baltimore: Williams & Wilkins.

Schatzberg, A. F., & Nemeroff, C. B. (Eds.) (1995). The American Psychiatric Press Textbook of Psychopharmacology. Washington, D.C.: American Psychiatric Press, Inc.

Yudofsky, S. C. & Hales, R. E. (Eds.) (1997). The American Psychiatric Press Textbook of Neuropsychiatry (3rd Edition). Washington, DC: American Psychiatric Press, Inc.

SCHIZOPHRENIA

Andersson, C., Chakos, M., Mailman, R., & Liberman, J. (1998). Emerging roles for novel antipsychotic medications in the treatment of schizophrenia. *Psychiatric Clinics of North America, 21,* 151–179.

Buckley, P. F. (1998). The clinical stigmata of aberrant neurodevelopment in schizophrenia. *Journal of Nervous and Mental Diseases, 186*(2), 79–86.

Buckley, P. F. (1998). Structural brain imaging in schizophrenia. *Psychiatric Clinics of North America, 21*(1), 77–91.

Busatto, G. F., & Kerwin, R. W. (1997) Schizophrenia, psychosis and the basal ganglia. *Psychiatric Clinics of North America, 20*(4), 897–909.

Jones, P., & Cannon, M. (1998). The new epidemiology of schizophrenia. *Psychiatric Clinics of North America, 21*(1), 1–25.

Weickert, C. S., & Kleinman, J. E. (1998). The neuroanatomy and neurochemistry of schizophrenia. *Psychiatric Clinics of North America, 21*(1), 57–75.

PANIC DISORDERS

Ballenger, J. C. (1997). Panic disorder in the medical setting. *Journal of Clinical Psychiatry,* 58(Suppl. 2), 13–17.

Goddard, A. W., & Charney, D. S. (1997). Toward an integrated neurobiology of panic disorder. *Journal of Clinical Psychiatry,* 58(Suppl. 2), 4–11.

Pollack, M. H., & Smoller, J. W. (1995). The longitudinal course and outcome of panic disorder. *Psychiatric Clinics of North America, 18* (4), 785–801.

ANXIETY DISORDERS

Brawman-Mintzer, O., & Lydiard, R. B. (1996). Generalized anxiety disorder: Issues in epidemiology. *Journal of Clinical Psychiatry, 57*(Suppl. 7), 3–8.

Brawman-Mintzer, O., & Lydiard, R. B. (1997). Biological basis of generalized anxiety disorder. *Journal of Clinical Psychiatry, 58*(Suppl. 3), 16–25.

Johnson, M. R., & Lydiard, R. B. (1995). The neurobiology of anxiety disorders. *Psychiatric Clinics of North America, 18*(4), 681–725.

POST-TRAUMATIC STRESS DISORDER

Davis, L. L., Suris, A., Lambert, M. T., Heimberg, C., & Petty, F. (1997). Post-traumatic stress disorder and serotonin: New directions for research and treatment. *Journal of Psychiatry and Neurosciences, 22*(5), 318–326.

Kessler, R., Sonnega, A., Bromet, E., & Nelson, C. B. (1995). Posttraumatic stress disorder in the National Comorbidity Survey. *Archives of General Psychiatry, 52,* 1048–1060.

Van der Kolk, B. A. (1997). The psychobiology of posttraumatic stress disorder. *Journal of Clinical Psychiatry, 58*(Suppl. 9), 16–24.

OBSESSIVE-COMPULSIVE DISORDERS

Irle, E., Exner, C., Thielen, K., Weniger, G., & Ruther, E. (1998). Obsessive-compulsive disorder and ventromedial frontal lesions: Clinical and neurophysiological findings. *American Journal of Psychiatry; 155*(2), 255–263.

Miguel, E. C., Rauch, S. L., & Jenike, M. A. (1997). Obsessive-compulsive disorder. *Psychiatric Clinics of North America,* 20(4), 863–883.

MOOD DISORDERS

Nemeroff, C. B. (1998). The neurobiology of depression. *Scientific American, 278*(6), 42–49.

Reus, V. I. & Freimer, N. B. (1997). Behavioral genetics '97. Understanding the genetic basis of mood disorders: Where do we stand? *American Journal of Human Genetics, 60,* 1283–1288.

ON-LINE RESOURCES

American Academy of Clinical Neurophysiology *http://www.presenter.com/~dtjorneh*
American Academy of Neurology *http://www.aan.org*
American Brain Tumor Association *http://abta.org*
American Neurological Association *http://aneuroa.org*
Brain Disorders Network *http://brainnet.org*
Brain Facts and Figures *http://www.u.washington.edu/~chudler/facts.html*
Brain Injury Association *http://biausa.org*
Brain Web *http://www.bic.mni.mcgill.ca*
Decade of the Brain (Library of Congress) *http://lcweb.loc.gov/loc/brain*
Human Brain Project (NIH) *http://www-hbp.scripps.edu/ Home.html*
Hydrocephalus Association Homepage *http://neurosurgery.mgh.harvard.edu/ha*
National Institute of Neurological Disorders and Stroke *http://www.ninds.nih.gov/healinfo/nindspub.htm*
Neuroscience Net *http://neuroscience.com*
Neurosciences on the Web *http://neuroguide.com*

CEREBROVASCULAR ACCIDENT

National Stroke Organization *http://www.stroke.org*

EPILEPSY

American Epilepsy Society *http://aesnet.org*
Epilepsy Foundation of America *http://efa.org*

SPINAL CORD TRAUMA

American Spine Injury Association (ASIA) *http://www.asia-spinalinjury.org*
National Spinal Cord Injury Association *http://www.trader.com*

ALZHEIMER'S DISEASE AND DEMENTIAS

Alzheimer Association *http://www.alz.org*
Alzheimer's Disease Education and Referral Center (ADEAR) *http://alzheimers.org*
National Aging Information Center (NAIC) *http://www.aoa.dhhs.gov/naic/Notes/alzheimerdisease.html*
National Family of Caregivers Association *http://www.nfcacares.org*
Pick's Disease Support Group *http://psdg.org.uk*

PARKINSON'S DISEASE

National Parkinson Foundation *http://parkinson.org*

AMYOTROPHIC LATERAL SCLEROSIS

ALS/Motor Neuron Diseases Societies and Foundations International *http://http1.brunel.ac.uk:8080/~hssrsdn/alsig/als_socs.txt*
Amyotrophic Lateral Sclerosis Association *http://www.alsa.org*

GUILLAIN BARRÉ SYNDROME

Guillain Barré Syndrome Foundation International *http://www.webmast.com*

HUNTINGTON'S DISEASE

Huntington's Disease Society of America *http://hdsa.org*

MULTIPLE SCLEROSIS

Multiple Sclerosis Association of America *http://www.msaa.org*
Multiple Sclerosis Foundation, Inc. *http://www.msfacts.org*
National Multiple Sclerosis Society *http://nmss.org*

MYASTHENIA GRAVIS

Myasthenia Gravis Foundation of America *http://www.myasthenia.org*

CEREBRAL PALSY

United Cerebral Palsy Association *http://www.ucpa.org*

MENTAL HEALTH AND ILLNESS

American Psychiatric Association (APA) *http://psych.org*

American Psychological Association (APA) *http://www.apa.org*

Anxiety Disorders Association of America (ADAA) *http://www.adaa.org*

Anxiety, Panic, and Phobic Disorders *http://mhsource.com/disorders/anxiety.html*

International Society for Traumatic Stress Studies *http://www.istss.com*

National Alliance for Research on Schizophrenia and Depression *http://mhsource.com*

National Alliance for the Mentally Ill (NAMI) *http://www.nami.org*

National Center for Post Traumatic Stress Disorders *http://www.dartmouth.edu*

National Depressive and Manic-Depressive Association (NDMDA) *http://www.ndmda.org*

National Institute of Mental Health (NIMH) *http://nimh.nih.gov*

National Mental Health Association (NMHA) *http://nmha.org*

Obsessive Compulsive Disorder *http://ocdresource.com*

Panic Disorders *http://brainnet.org/panicdis.htm*

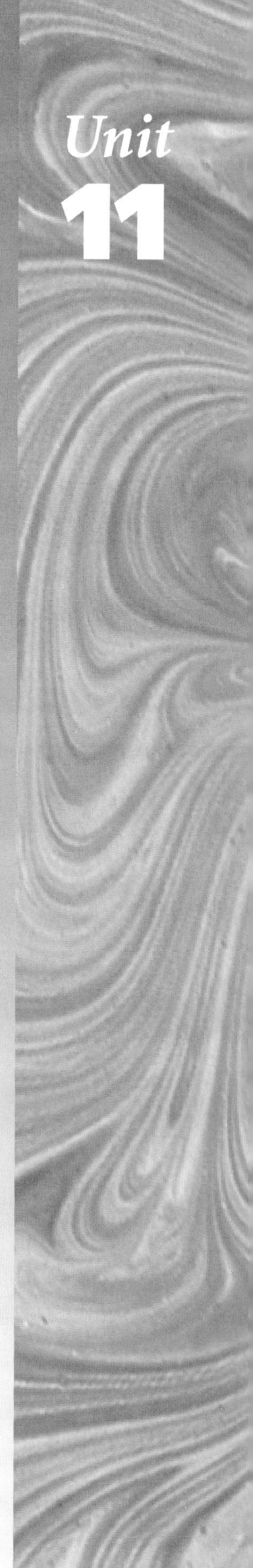

Specialized Sensory Experiences

FOCUS ON Changes Associated with the Special Senses and Pain Through the Life Span

INFANT (1–12 MONTHS):

Coordination of stimuli for various sense organs begins by age 3 months. Eyes fix on midline object by age 1 month. Visual acuity is approximately 20/100 at age 1 month. Strabismus present until age 6 weeks. Binocular vision develops after age 6 weeks. Depth perception develops by age 7 to 9 months. Ability to localize sound at level of the ear develops by age 2 months and in any direction by 12 months. Cerebellum function improves to allow equilibrium. Taste preferences develop around age 7 months. Sense of smell is evidenced shortly after birth. Ability to sense pain is evidenced by body movements, crying, and facial expression. Stimulus for the cause of pain is not recognized prior to the pain experience.

TODDLER AND PRESCHOOL AGE (1–5 YEARS):

Binocular vision is well developed. Visual acuity of 20/20 is achieved (although acuity of 20/40 is acceptable in the toddler age group). Hyperopia may be present because depth of eye globe is insufficient to allow light rays to focus on retina. Hearing, smell, and taste continue to develop, become increasingly refined, coordinated, and associated with other experiences as child explores and investigates the environment. Specific food likes and dislikes are established. Ability to balance on alternate feet with eyes closed is achieved by age 5 years. Intense emotional upset and physical resistance are seen with any actual or perceived painful experience from age 1 to 3 years. By age 3, the child is usually able to communicate information about pain.

SCHOOL AGE (6–12 YEARS):

Eye globe achieves adult size by age 10 years. Visual changes are common. Hyperopia diminishes at about age 5 years (if it remains, child needs referral for corrective lenses.) Myopia occurs in approximately 10% of this age group. Increase in tonsillar and adenoid tissues may result in obstruction of eustachian tube and possible temporary conductive hearing loss. Variety of food tastes are tried and acquired. Verbal ability to communicate information about pain including intensity, location, and description is evidenced.

ADOLESCENT (13–19 YEARS):

Visual and auditory capabilities peak. Myopia, if present, plateaus. Risk for possible cochlear damage is seen due to widespread use of portable radios and cassette and compact disk players among this age group. Adult pain control mechanisms are used. Reaction to pain typically involves issues of self-control.

YOUNG ADULT/ADULT (20–45 YEARS):

Eye lens becomes thicker. Presbyopia usually begins after age 40 years. Hearing acuity declines after age 20 years. Responses to pain vary.

MIDDLE AGED ADULT (46–64 YEARS):

Eye lens becomes less elastic and accommodation is lost. Perception of certain tones, especially high-pitched sounds, decreases from gradual degeneration of auditory nerve and bone (presbycusis). Number and function of taste buds and olfactory cells begin to decline. Possible decline in ability to sense pain may begin due to gradual loss of neurons and sensory receptors and lowered nerve conduction velocity.

LATE ADULTHOOD (65–100+ YEARS):

Changes in middle age continue and progress. Visual field narrows, resulting in increased difficulty with peripheral vision. Pupils become less sensitive to light. Differentiation of color perception involving blues, greens, and violets becomes more difficult. Depth perception is distorted. Dark and light adaptation is prolonged. Intraocular fluid reabsorption is less efficient. Lacrimal secretions are reduced. Corneal reflex slows. Presbycusis continues, affecting middle and lower frequencies. Tympanic membrane undergoes sclerosis and atrophy. Cerumen increases in amount and becomes hardened. Vestibular structures degenerate. Taste and smell become less acute. Pain threshold increases. Vibratory sense at the ankle decreases after age 70.

Chapter 34

Normal and Altered Function of the Special Senses

Reet Henze

KEY TERMS

ageusia	hypogeusia
astigmatism	myopia
cataract	near point
emmetropia	optic disc
glaucoma	presbyopia
hemianopia	refraction
hyperopia	vertigo

The special senses of vision, hearing, taste, and smell assist individuals to interact with their environment. They provide human beings with the means to perceive the environment and respond in ways that support adaptation and, at times, even survival. When the receptors of the eyes, ears, tongue, and nose are stimulated, messages are transmitted to specific regions of the cerebral cortex for processing. Alterations in the function of these senses, particularly vision and hearing, can result in physiologic, psychological, sociologic, and economic difficulties.

VISION

Normal Structure

The structures of the eye are integrated with central nervous system structures of vision, which include the optic nerve and chiasm, the optic tracts, and radiations.

EYE

The eye is a complex peripheral structure that transmits vision signals to the visual area of the occipital lobe of the cerebral cortex. It is protected by the external structures of the eyelids, conjunctiva, and lacrimal glands. The eye nestles in the orbit, a cone-shaped cavity with fragile walls composed of the frontal, maxillary, zygomatic, sphenoid, ethmoid, lacrimal, and palatine bones. The thinness of the orbital wall makes this area particularly susceptible to fractures. The eyeball occupies the anterior portion of the orbital cavity.

The eye is composed of three layers: (1) sclera, (2) choroid, and (3) retina. Its principal structures are identified in Figure 34-1.

The area of the orbit not occupied by the eyeball is filled with fascia, fat, nerves, blood vessels, muscle, and the lacrimal gland. Six extrinsic muscles, most of which arise from the apex of the orbit and insert into the scleral lining, allow for the movement and rotation of the eyeball. These are the (1) superior rectus, (2) inferior rectus, (3) medial rectus, (4) lateral rectus, (5) superior oblique, and (6) inferior oblique muscles. Innervation for these muscles arrives from the third, fourth, and sixth cranial nerves.

Sclera

The *sclera,* the outermost layer of the eyeball, is composed of dense fibrous tissue and forms a white, opaque membrane around the eyeball except at the cornea. Here it becomes transparent, allowing light rays to enter the eye to stimulate the rods and cones.

Choroid

The middle layer of the eyeball is the *choroid*, a highly vascular and pigmented area responsible for nutrient exchange. This layer is continuous with the ciliary muscle and iris, a circular muscular disk. The ciliary muscle facilitates light and accommodation reflexes. The iris, the colored portion of the eye, has a central opening, the pupil, which is responsible for controlling the amount of light entering the eye by changes in its size. The ciliary

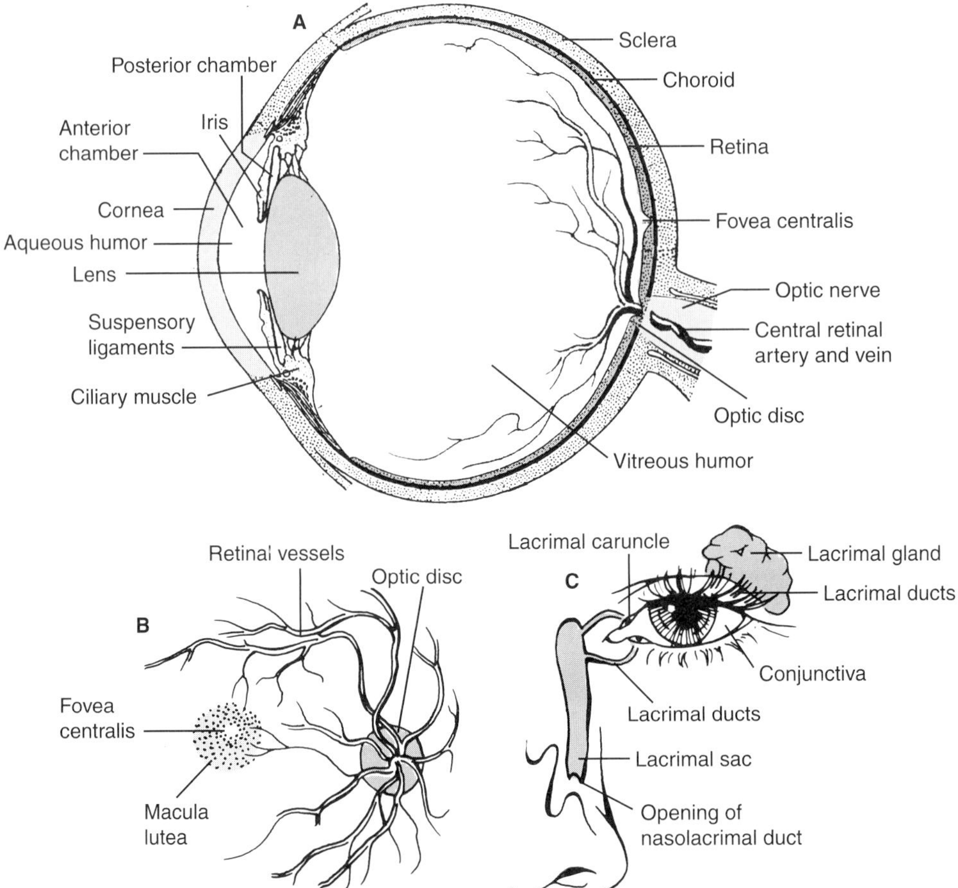

FIGURE 34-1. **A.** Structures of the eyeball. **B.** Structures of the optic disc, including the macular region. **C.** The lacrimal apparatus.

muscle and iris are innervated by the third cranial nerve and the superior cervical ganglion.

Retina

The third and innermost layer of the eyeball, the *retina,* consists of two parts: (1) the outer pigmented layer attached to the choroid and (2) the inner sensory layer, consisting of a series of synaptic nervous tissue. The retina is formed by numerous layers of interconnecting cells, fibers, and ganglia. The dendrites of the ganglion cells synapse with bipolar cell axons in the inner plexiform layer, and their axons converge to enter the optic nerve.

The retina contains specialized receptors called rods and cones. The cones mediate daylight vision, allowing perception of detail and color of objects. The rods mediate night vision, allowing visualization of outlines of objects without revealing color or detail. The rods, however, are very sensitive to movement of objects in the visual field.

The *macula lutea,* a yellowish spot near the center of the retina, encompasses a small depression in its center called the *fovea centralis* (Fig. 34-1*B*). The fovea centralis is composed of tightly packed cones that connect individually to the optic nerve, whereas in other parts of the retina they share fibers with many other rods and cones. The pigmented layer of the retina is the outermost layer, which decreases light reflection.

Medial to the fovea centralis is the **optic disc** (physiologic blind spot) where the optic nerve exits from the eyeball. Increased intraocular pressure is reflected in the optic disc by its cupped shape (i.e., the disc appears to be pushed backward). In contrast, increased intracranial pressure produces the opposite effect, an optic disc that is pushed inward, called a *choked disc* or papilledema. The retina receives its blood supply from the central artery, a branch of the ophthalmic artery.

Lens

The *crystalline lens* is a transparent biconvex structure attached to the ciliary muscle by ligaments. Contraction or relaxation of the ciliary muscle causes the lens to change its thickness, bending the rays of light (**refraction**). This change in shape allows light rays to be projected properly on the retina.

Cavities

The eye consists of two cavities, the anterior and posterior cavities. The anterior cavity contains an anterior and posterior chamber. Both chambers are filled with *aqueous humor*. The anterior chamber is a fluid-filled space posterior to the cornea and anterior to the iris and lens. Along with the posterior chamber, which is bounded by the iris, ciliary muscle, and lens, constant pressure in the eyeball is maintained. Normal *intraocular pressure* is between 10 and 22 mm Hg, with the most common pressure being 15 or 16 mm Hg. The posterior cavity, the space behind the lens, is filled with *vitreous humor*, a soft and gelatinous fluid that helps maintain the shape of the eyeball.

Visual Pathways

The ganglionic cell axons of the retina emerge from the optic disk as the optic nerve. Axons from the nasal half of each eye cross in the optic chiasm and terminate in the opposite occipital lobe. Axons from the temporal half of each eye do not cross but terminate on their respective sides in the superior colliculi and lateral geniculate nuclei of the thalamus.[5] Those fibers terminating in the lateral geniculate body seem to be associated with visual perception, and those terminating in the superior colliculus excite reflex activity.[9] The fibers from the lateral geniculate body emerge as the optic radiations and continue to the striate cortex in the occipital lobe.

Normal Function

IMAGE FORMATION

The refractive surfaces of the cornea and lens initiate the mechanism for image formation. These surfaces, along with the aqueous and vitreous humor, provide varying densities for the light to pass through, thus accounting for the refractive phenomenon.

If a light ray passes into a denser medium, it is bent toward the perpendicular and the speed of transmission is slowed. A less dense medium bends the light ray away from the perpendicular and speeds its transmission. The degree of light impediment, or the power of a substance to bend light, is its *refractive index*. Light strikes the cornea at different angles and is bent in different amounts depending on the curvature and refractive indexes of the interposed structures. Refraction of light occurs at the corneal interface, aqueous humor, and crystalline lens. Light then is projected on the retina in an inverted and reverted manner that is perceived by the brain as upright.

ACCOMMODATION

Accommodation is the ability of the crystalline lens to vary its refractive power through relaxation or contraction of the ciliary muscle. This allows clear vision to be maintained when changing vision from distant to near objects. For distance vision, the ciliary muscle relaxes and the lens is more flattened. The ciliary muscle contracts to increase the curvature of the lens for viewing of objects closer to the eye. The increased curvature of the lens increases its power, shortens the focal length, and focuses near objects on the retina. This is the process of *accommodation*. The closest point at which a person can clearly focus on an object is called the **near point**. Ocular convergence (upward turning of the eyes to view near objects), which ensures that images recorded are focused on the macular area at the fovea centralis, and pupillary constriction (miosis) are associated with the accommodation reflex.[10]

As a person ages, the near point recedes. Progressive age also reduces the efficiency of accommodation because of the loss of elasticity of the lens. The eye may remain focused almost permanently on a constant distance. This deterioration is known as **presbyopia**.

PUPILLARY APERTURE RESPONSE

The pupillary aperture in the human eye can vary from 1.5 to 8.0 mm in diameter. In normal eyes, the aperture is a reflex response to change in light intensity.

The iris controls the amount of light that enters the eye through the action of its two sets of smooth muscles: the sphincter and dilator muscles. *Miosis* (constriction) is accomplished through the contraction of the sphincter muscle, and *mydriasis* (dilation) is facilitated through the contraction of the dilator muscle. Pupils constrict in response to increased light intensities and dilate in response to decreased light intensities (*pupillary light reflex*). If illumination enters only one eye, both pupils constrict. This simultaneous constriction of the contralateral eye is referred to as the *consensual light reflex*. Photoreceptors of the retina, including rods and cones, are receptors for the light reflex.

The pupillary light reflex and miosis of accommodation are not identical mechanisms, possibly occurring independently of each other. For example, the *Argyll Robertson pupil* may occur as a complication of syphilis. In this phenomenon, the pupil remains constricted and unresponsive to light but does respond to the accommodation mechanism.[8]

VISUAL STIMULI INTERPRETATION

In the retina, the rods and cones contain pigments responsible for visual interpretation. In the rods, *rhodopsin*, a light-sensitive protein and aldehyde of vitamin A compound, breaks down when light reaches it. Less is known about the pigments in the cones. Reflection densitometry has demonstrated the presence of pigments in the foveal region that peak in the blue, green, and red parts of the spectrum. Although the cone pigments are similar to rhodopsin in composition, they vary, allowing absorption of a variety of colors to different extents and resulting in color-dependent nerve impulses. These impulses are interpreted by the visual cortex as color sensations.

Light passes through the layers of the retina to reach the light-sensitive portion of the rods and cones deep in the retina (Fig. 34-2). Light energy is absorbed by the pigment, rhodopsin, or visual purple. This initial activity produces the generator potential.

Once the generator potential is created, synaptic depolarization occurs in the ganglionic cells, stimulating all-or-nothing threshold spikes that are propagated along their axons to the lateral geniculate body. Three types of responses are observed in ganglionic cells. One fires only in response to a light stimulus on the retina and is known as the "on fiber"; another discharges only in response to light off and is known as the "off fiber." The third, most numerous type responds to both light on and off and is called the "on-off fiber."

The horizontal cells, important in detecting visual contrasts and color differentiations, transmit inhibitory impulses laterally from rods and cones to bipolar cells. In response to stimulation from bipolar cells and possibly from the rods and cones, amacrine cells exert a transient inhibitory effect on the ganglionic cells. Amacrine cell inhibition seems to enhance the contrast experienced in visual images.

Color Vision

The differentiation of wavelengths of the visible spectrum allows the human eye to detect color in the environment. The precise mechanism that is responsible for color detection has been sought by researchers throughout the past century. Most of the investigation seems to be based on the *trichromatic theory or Young-Hemholtz theory*, which assumes that there are three variations in cones, each containing a different photochemical substance. One type of cone is responsible for red color, another for blue, and the third for green.[6] *Erythrolabe*, a pigment identified in the fovea, absorbs light in the red part of the spectrum. *Chlorolabe* is a pigment that absorbs light in the green part of the spectrum in the fovea. A third cone pigment, *iodopsin*, a violet-sensitive substance isolated from the retina of chickens, is also thought to exist in the human eye cones. Additionally, a pigment receptor for blue substances has also been identified.

Each of these cones gives rise to a distinct impulse that travels to the visual cortex of the occipital lobe. Red, blue, and green are colors that may produce any

FOCUS ON CELLULAR PHYSIOLOGY

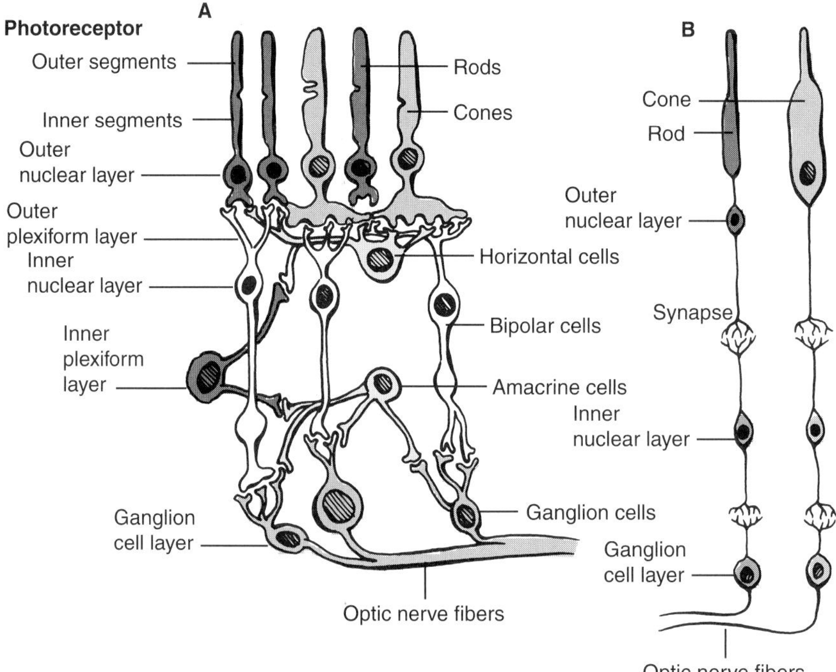

FIGURE 34-2. **A.** Constituent neurons of the neural retina. **B.** An expanded view of the rods and cones. (Adapted from Cormack, D. H. [1993]. *Essential histology*. Philadelphia: Lippincott.)

color in the spectrum by correct proportionate mixture. If all of the cones are stimulated equally, the sensation of white results. In contrast, if no stimulation of three types of cones occurs, black is experienced. Other colors are perceived as a result of the combined stimulation of the three types of cones to varying degrees.

Dark Adaptation

The eyes are said to be *dark adapted* after a period of time in darkness. This decline in visual threshold is at its maximum after approximately 30 minutes in the dark environment. On return to the light environment, the uncomfortable brightness requires the eyes to adapt to light again. This adaptation takes about 5 minutes and is called *light adaptation.*

Dark adaptation occurs, in part, as rhodopsin stores are rebuilt in the rods and some similar, yet unknown, process occurs in the cones.[6] Only the periphery of the retina of the human eye is sensitive to light in the dark-adapted eye. Therefore, the sensitivity to darkness is much greater in the rods than the cones. Rods are not exclusively responsible for dark adaptation, however. Because of the presence of both rods and cones, dark adaptation takes place in two stages. First, a small increase in sensitivity occurs, which is accomplished in about 7 minutes and is attributed to dark adaptation of cones. After this, a less rapid but quantitatively greater adaptation occurs in rods.[2]

Alterations in External Structures of the Eye

Alterations in the external structures of the eye are primarily related to inflammation and infections of the eyelid, conjunctiva, and lacrimal gland.

INFLAMMATION AND INFECTIONS OF THE EYELID

Common conditions associated with the eyelid include blephritis, hordeolum, and chalazion. *Blephritis* is a common inflammatory process of the eyelid caused by seborrheic dermatitis or *Staphylococcus* infection. A *hordeolum* (sty) is a localized suppurative infection originating in the sebaceous glands of the eyelid. These conditions commonly appear as acute, red, and painful localized masses of the eyelid.

A *chalazion* is a localized infection originating in the meibomian or oil-secreting glands of the eyelid. This condition commonly appears as a painless localized mass on the eyelid.

CONJUNCTIVITIS

Conjunctivitis is an inflammation of the conjunctiva. The conjunctiva, a thin, transparent mucous membrane, lines the posterior surface of the eyelids and anterior surface of the sclera. Conjunctivitis may be caused by bacteria, viruses, allergies, or chemical irritants. Bacterial conjunctivitis commonly is caused by *Staphylococcus* or *Haemophilus* organisms. Viral conjunctivitis is frequently associated with adenovirus. Both bacterial and viral conjunctivitis are highly contagious. They are characterized by keratitis (inflammation of the cornea), hyperemic conjunctival blood vessels (*pink eye*), and a mucopurulent, serous, or fibrinous drainage. The drainage may cause the eyelids to stick together.

Trachoma is an acute or chronic, mildly contagious conjunctivitis that is caused by the *Chlamydia trachomatis* organism. It is associated with poor sanitary conditions and is the leading cause of blindness in the world.

Allergic conjunctivitis is associated with a variety of allergens. Pollens are common allergens producing the inflammatory response in the conjunctiva.

LACRIMAL GLAND ALTERATIONS

Lacrimal glands produce tears. Tear production may become diminished (dry eyes) with aging or with certain conditions such as Sjögren disease (keratoconjunctivitis sicca). Sjögren disease may occur as a primary condition or in association with autoimmune diseases such as rheumatoid arthritis, scleroderma, and systemic lupus erythematosus (SLE). In this condition, the lacrimal glands are infiltrated by lymphocytes, eventually becoming fibrotic and unable to produce tears. The lack of tears leads to drying, inflammation, and ulceration of the corneal epithelium.

Alterations in Vision

Disturbances in vision may be manifested by various pathologic mechanisms within the eyeball or in its pathways. Commonly these include color vision defects, refraction defects, visual field defects, and visual acuity disturbances such as glaucoma and cataracts.

COLOR VISION DEFICITS

Many forms of color vision defects or color blindness exist, but the most common variety is the inability to distinguish between red and green. Color blindness may be (1) hereditary, (2) congenital, or (3) acquired. The most common modality is inheritance to the male through the x-linked recessive gene. Congenital color vision defects also tend to be red-green defects with intact yellow-blue vision. A variety of color defects may be acquired.[1] Acquired visual defects may involve partial loss, such as in a quadrant or half of the visual field.

REFRACTION DEFECTS

Deficits in refraction, the most common visual alteration, involve irregularities of the cornea. Causes of the irregularities include abnormal corneal curvature, lens focusing power, and the length of the eye. Box 34-1 describes refractive alterations: **emmetropia, myopia, hyperopia**, and **astigmatism**.

BOX 34-1

ALTERATIONS IN REFRACTION

Emmetropia (normal refraction)

- Relaxed eye is capable of clearly focusing distant parallel light rays on the retina.
- Nearby vision requires contraction of the ciliary muscle to bring the object to focus.
- Defects of vision are present if the light rays converge either in front of or behind the retina or if the eyeball is abnormally shaped.

Myopia (nearsightedness)

- Parallel light rays are focused in front of the retina as a result of increased anteroposterior diameter of the eyeball.
- Myopic persons cannot focus on a distant object sharply.
- As the individual moves closer to the object, the rays become more focused and the focal point eventually falls on the retina.

Hyperopia (farsightedness)

- Eyeball is abnormally short.
- Parallel light rays are focused beyond the retina in the relaxed eye.
- Focus on distant objects through the mechanism of accommodation occurs.
- Images become blurred and accommodation can no longer compensate as objects move closer to the eye.
- The near point in persons with hyperopia is abnormally distant.

Astigmatism (defect of the curvature of the cornea and lens producing refractive errors)

- Parallel light rays are imperfectly focused on the retina.
- Light striking peripheral areas is bent at different angles and not focused on a single point on the retina.

VISUAL FIELD DEFECTS

Visual field defects occur as a result of lesions in the visual pathway or disturbances in the eye. Normally, a person's visual field extends approximately 90 degrees to the temporal side, 60 degrees to the nasal side, and 130 degrees vertically. Visual field defects such as **hemianopia** (blindness for one-half of field of vision in one or both eyes) occur as a result of lesions in the visual pathway. Figure 34-3 highlights the type of field defect resulting from lesions at specific areas of the visual pathway.

AMAUROSIS FUGAX. Visual defects may also result from vascular insufficiency. *Amaurosis fugax*, a condition involving recurrent, transient episodes of partial blindness, usually is associated with atherosclerotic lesions of the carotid arteries that have dislodged and occluded the arteries supplying the eye. This condition usually involves one eye and reflects ipsilateral carotid artery insufficiency caused by plaque accumulation.

INCREASED INTRAOCULAR PRESSURE

Glaucoma

Glaucoma is associated with (1) increased intraocular pressure and (2) loss in the visual field. Glaucoma is described as (1) chronic simple (open angle) or (2) acute (closed angle or narrow angle). The angle refers to the area in which the iris meets the cornea in the anterior chamber.

ETIOLOGY. Several underlying conditions, such as infections, tumors, hemorrhage, and trauma, can result in increased intraocular pressure. However, the most common cause is the blockage or stenosis of aqueous outflow channels.[6,7] *Chronic simple glaucoma* is thought to have a hereditary basis and is a common cause of blindness.

PATHOPHYSIOLOGY. Normally, the aqueous humor, which is produced by the ciliary epithelium, flows from the posterior chamber of the eye through the pupil into the anterior chamber. Aqueous humor then leaves the anterior chamber and returns to the venous system by passing through the trabecular mesh of the anterior chamber into the *Canal of Schlemm.* A balance between production and absorption of aqueous humor maintains normal intraocular pressure (8–21 mm Hg). In chronic simple glaucoma, although the anterior chamber angle is open, an obstruction exists to the flow of aqueous humor through the trabecular mesh. Acute glaucoma occurs if an obstruction, either complete or partial, in the flow of aqueous humor is produced by closure of the anterior chamber angle. This may result from an anteroposterior thickening of the lens or a forward movement of the lens that causes the iris to press against the lens capsule and thereby prevent outflow of aqueous humor (Fig. 34-4).

CLINICAL MANIFESTATIONS. Chronic simple glaucoma may be asymptomatic for years, only being revealed after the patient experiences peripheral vision loss, difficulty with dark adaptation, blurring of vision, halos around lights, and difficulty focusing on near objects.

With acute glaucoma, complete closure of the angle occurs and intraocular pressure increases, presenting a dramatic clinical picture of severe eye pain, blurred or

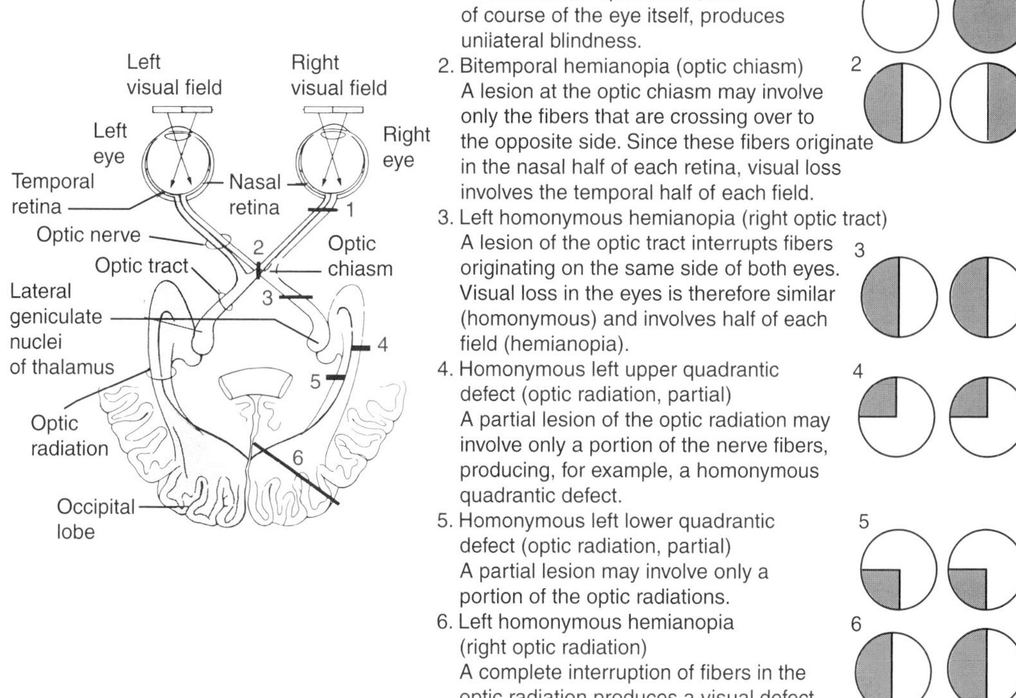

Left
visual field
Right
visual field
Left
eye
Right
eye
Temporal
retina
Nasal
retina
Optic nerve
Optic tract
Optic
chiasm
Lateral
geniculate
nuclei
of thalamus
Optic
radiation
Occipital
lobe
1
2
3
4
5
6
1. Blind right eye (right optic nerve)
A lesion of the optic nerve,and
of course of the eye itself, produces
uniiateral blindness.
2. Bitemporal hemianopia (optic chiasm)
A lesion at the optic chiasm may involve
only the fibers that are crossing over to
the opposite side. Since these fibers originate
in the nasal half of each retina, visual loss
involves the temporal half of each field.
3. Left homonymous hemianopia (right optic tract)
A lesion of the optic tract interrupts fibers
originating on the same side of both eyes.
Visual loss in the eyes is therefore similar
(homonymous) and involves half of each
field (hemianopia).
4. Homonymous left upper quadrantic
defect (optic radiation, partial)
A partial lesion of the optic radiation may
involve only a portion of the nerve fibers,
producing, for example, a homonymous
quadrantic defect.
5. Homonymous left lower quadrantic
defect (optic radiation, partial)
A partial lesion may involve only a
portion of the optic radiations.
6. Left homonymous hemianopia
(right optic radiation)
A complete interruption of fibers in the
optic radiation produces a visual defect
similar to that produced by a lesion
of the optic tract.
Left
Right

FIGURE 34-3. **Visual pathways and visual field defects resulting from lesions at various areas along the pathways. (Adapted from Bickley, L., & Hoekelman, R. [1998].** ***Bates' guide to physical examination and history taking*** **[7th ed.]. Philadelphia: Lippincott-Raven.)**

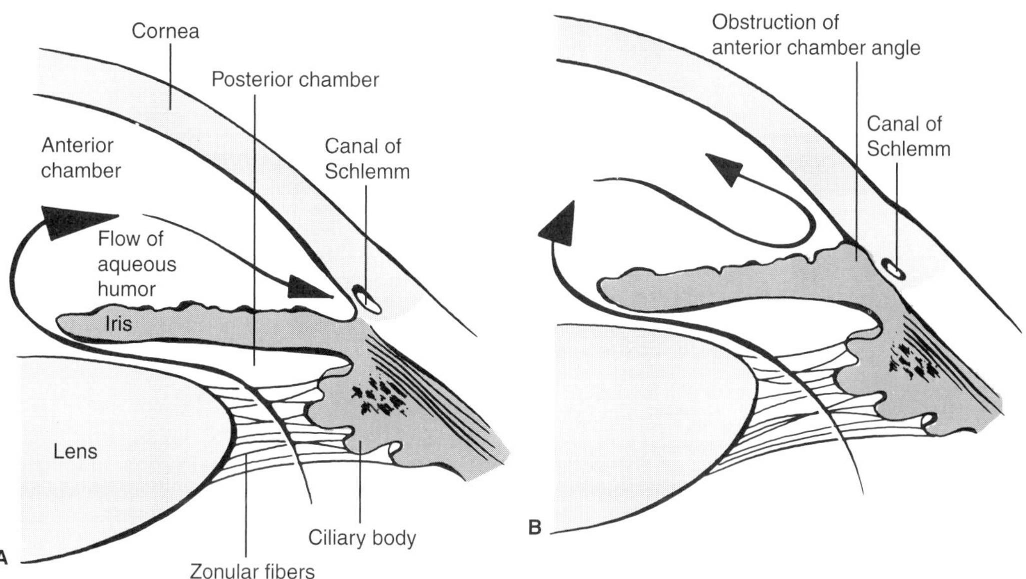

FIGURE 34-4. **A.** Normal flow of aqueous humor. **B.** Obstruction of flow in acute glaucoma.

cloudy vision, halos around lights, a hard red eye with a cloudy cornea, and nausea and vomiting. Intraocular pressure is elevated.

ALTERATIONS IN VISUAL ACUITY

Decreased visual acuity, the inability to see objects in sharp detail, is associated with a variety of changes in the eye or its neural pathways, including trauma, lesions, drug therapies, and nutritional deficiencies. Another common pathologic change in the eye that results in disturbances in visual acuity is cataract formation.

Cataracts

Cataracts are associated with clouding of the lens and loss of visual acuity. They may result from trauma to the eye, elevated glucose levels in the aqueous humor (diabetes mellitus), irradiation to the lens, viruses, chemicals, infections, and amino acid or vitamin deficiencies. Occasionally cataracts are congenital, but more commonly they are associated with advancing age (*senile cataracts*). Also, they have been associated with certain disease processes of the skin, skeleton, and nervous system and with certain chromosomal abnormalities.

PATHOPHYSIOLOGY. Early in the course of this condition, the cells in the lens degenerate. This results in an increase in the water content in the cells. With progression, the entire lens becomes involved. The cellular debris from the lens escapes through the degenerated lens capsule into the aqueous humor. The debris is phagocytized by macrophages and may also contribute to obstruction of aqueous humor outflow.

CLINICAL MANIFESTATIONS. Cataracts produce decreased visual acuity and visual abnormalities as a result of decreased light transmission and optical aberrations such as spots or halos in the visual field.[6] Manifestations of glaucoma become apparent with obstruction of the aqueous humor outflow.

HEARING

Hearing is mediated through the ear, a mechanoreceptor sensitive to rapid changes in pressure that are transmitted to its fluid medium. The hearing function is transmitted through the cochlear branch of the vestibulocochlear nerve (eighth cranial nerve). In addition to hearing, ear receptors also mediate a sense of position and equilibrium through the vestibular component of the eighth cranial nerve.

Normal Structure

EAR

The ear, in essence, is a mechanical transducer. The ear is anatomically segmented into outer, middle, and inner areas (Fig. 34-5).

Outer Ear

The outer or external ear consists of the auricle and external auditory canal. The external auditory canal is an S-shaped, 3-cm tube that is supplied with ceruminous and sebaceous glands and hair follicles. The canal is lined with squamous epithelium. Cartilage and bone provide support and maintain its patency. The canal also has resonance properties because sound waves are reflected from the tympanic membrane, possibly enhancing or dampening incoming waves.

Middle Ear

The middle ear is separated from the outer ear distally by the tympanic membrane (eardrum). It is also bounded medially by the oval and round windows, small openings in the wall of the middle and inner ear responsible for transmitting vibrations to the inner ear.

The eardrum is fibrous tissue that vibrates freely with all audible sound frequencies, transmitting them to the three auditory ossicles of the middle ear: the *malleus* (attached to the tympanic membrane), *incus* (attached to the malleus and stapes), and *stapes* (attached to the oval window).

The middle ear with its three ossicles is situated in an air cavity of the temporal bone. It communicates with the nasopharynx by means of the auditory or eustachian tube. The mucous membrane that lines the middle ear extends to line the pharynx and the air cells of the mastoid. The tympanic membrane, innervated by the fifth cranial nerve, and stapes muscles of the middle ear, innervated by the seventh cranial nerve, prevent the bones from transmitting excessive vibrations by pulling on them to decrease contact with the tympanic membrane and oval window.

Inner Ear

The inner ear, encased in the temporal bone, mediates sound-induced nerve impulses, position orientation, and balance. It is composed of two labyrinths, one within the other. The outer labyrinth is bony and is separated from the inner membranous one by perilymph fluid. It contains the cochlea, the vestibule, and the three semicircular canals. The membranous labyrinth, which lies within the bony labyrinth, contains fluid called *endolymph*. The anterior portion of the membranous labyrinth contains the cochlea, which receives the sound waves from the oval window.

The cochlea, a small, shell-shaped structure, is divided into three chambers: the *scala vestibuli*, *scala tympani*, and *cochlear duct*. Posteriorly, the cochlea opens into the osseous vestibule, which, in turn, extends to the three semicircular canals. Figure 34-5*B* illustrates the components of the membranous labyrinth. The *organ of Corti*, located on the basilar membrane within the cochlea, contains the receptor cells of hearing.

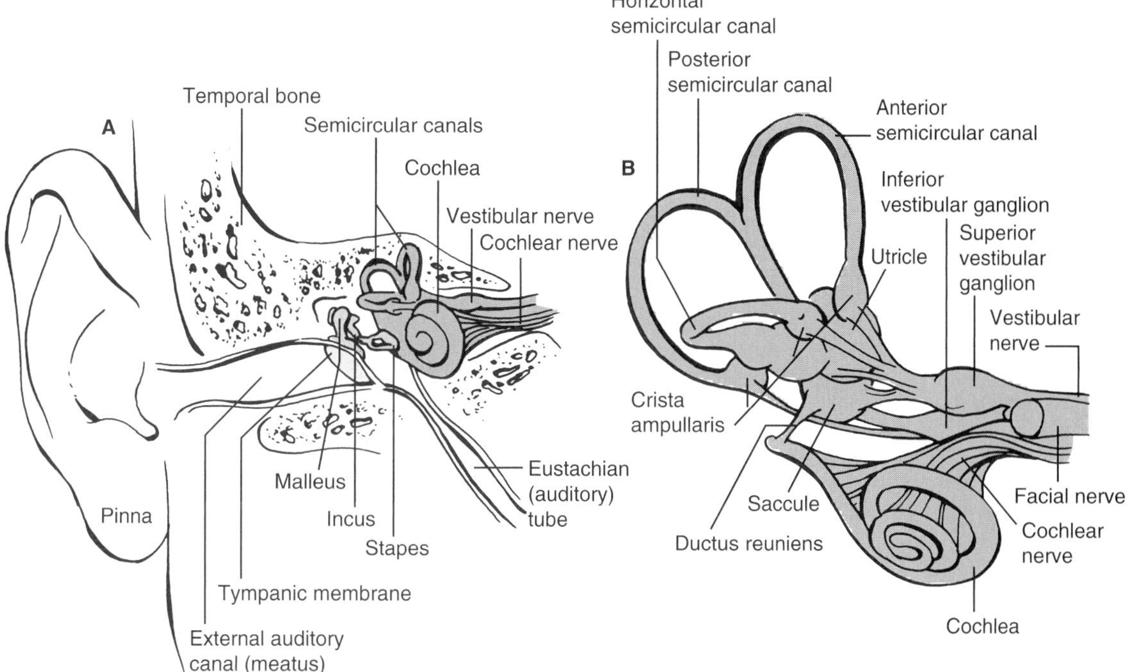

FIGURE 34-5. **A.** Structures of the ear, including the external, middle, and inner ear. **B.** Components of the membranous labyrinth, including the three semicircular canals (horizontal, anterior, and posterior), the otolith organs (saccule and utricle), and the cochlea. The spiral-shaped cochlea winds around a central bony modiolus.

VESTIBULAR SYSTEM. The vestibular system of the inner ear is responsible for maintaining position and a sense of equilibrium. The *utricle*, *saccule*, and *semicircular canals* function together to maintain equilibrium. These structures are housed in a bony labyrinth, which contains a membranous labyrinth composed of the semicircular canals and the two chambers: the utricle and the saccule. Within the utricle and saccule are *maculae* that provide sensory areas to detect the relation of the head to gravitational pull and other forces. Within the semicircular canals, *endolymph* flows and stimulates the sensory nerve fibers that join up with the vestibular nerve. Fluid flow in the opposite direction inhibits these sensory nerve fibers.

The vestibular portion of the eighth cranial nerve has its peripheral endings on the hair cells of the maculae of the utricle and saccule and on the cristae in the ampullae of the three semicircular canals. The maculae of the utricle and saccule record linear acceleration and static phenomena; the semicircular canals record angular acceleration.[3] Recent evidence implies that the utricle is more related to the semicircular canals' vestibular functions and the saccule has a closer association with hearing.

Hearing Pathways

The axons of bipolar neurons from the cochlea enter the pons and divide into the dorsal and ventral cochlear nuclei. Second-order neurons cross here and ascend by the lateral lemniscus to the inferior colliculus. From there, they transmit to the medial geniculate body and on to the auditory cortex in the temporal lobe by the auditory radiations. The auditory cortex allows a person to recognize tone patterns, analyze characteristics of sound, and localize sound. In the auditory cortex, low-frequency tones are recognized anteriorly and high-frequency tones posteriorly. Neurons throughout the auditory cortex respond to onset, duration, and direction of stimulus.

The auditory association area lies inferior to the primary auditory center in the temporal lobe and is thought to associate auditory information with other sensations, as well as different sound frequencies with each other. Lesions in this area prevent a person from comprehending the meaning of sounds heard; words can be heard but not understood. The origin (location) of sound is determined by the pattern of the sound's arrival to the two ears. One ear receives information before the other, and the ear that is closer to the sound source receives a louder sound.

Normal Function

SOUND CONDUCTION

The outer ear funnels sound waves conducted through the air to the tympanic membrane, causing it to vibrate. These vibrations are carried through the middle ear to the oval window, subsequently causing the footplate of the stapes to vibrate. The vibrations cause the perilymph to vibrate, subsequently stimulating the receptor cells of hearing within the cochlea. Under certain circumstances, sound may also be conducted through bone. If a vibrating tuning fork is placed on a bony protuberance of the skull, the individual will hear sound. This occurs because vibrations of the skull cause fluid vibrations in the cochlea, stimulating the receptor cells of hearing.

The receptor cells of hearing are hair cells that generate nerve impulses in response to sound vibrations from the oscillations of the oval window. Impulses that stimulate the dendrites of the cochlear division of the acoustic nerve are transmitted to the hearing center in the temporal lobe of the cortex. The various frequencies of sound generate different patterns of vibrations and allow sounds to be differentiated from one another. Subjective interpretation of the frequency of sound waves results in the recognition of *pitch*.

Sound at various frequencies is converted into nerve impulses through the cochlear component of the acoustic (eighth cranial) nerve. These impulses then are transmitted into the central nervous system for interpretation. Sound is conducted through air, ossicles, and fluid and is measured in number of vibrations per second, which is recorded as *cycles per second (cps)* or *Hertz (Hz)*. The human ear is able to perceive frequencies to 20,000 Hz. Aging reduces the number of frequencies perceived. The greatest sensitivity of the human ear is in the range of 1,000 to 4,000 Hz.

The amplitude of vibrations affects the perception of loudness at a constant frequency. A greater amplitude produces greater loudness. However, this does not hold true if two sounds of different frequency are contrasted simultaneously because auditory sensitivity is a function of frequency. Frequency and amplitude are both significant in determining the perception of loudness if there are two or more simultaneous sounds.

VESTIBULAR FUNCTION

Position and Equilibrium

The vestibular system maintains position and equilibrium via impulse transmission by way of the vestibular branch of the vestibulocochlear nerve. The ganglion cells of the vestibular division of the eighth cranial nerve are located in the internal auditory meatus, and the dendrites end in the specialized epithelium of the hair cells. The axons pass back to the upper medulla, accompanied by the cochlear nerve. On entering the medulla, the fibers pass directly to the cerebellum and go to connect with the nuclei of the third, fourth, and sixth cranial nerves and the upper cervical and accessory nerves. This connection results in vestibular influence on movement of the neck, eyes, and head.

A close interrelation exists between the vestibular nerves and the cerebellum. The maculae of the utricle and saccule provide vestibular input to the cerebellum. The cerebellum, in turn, provides the brain stem vestibular and reticular nuclei feedback from various muscles. The influence of this two-way communication results in coordination of the muscles of the neck and the coordination required for posture.

Two vestibulospinal tracts arise from the vestibular nuclei. The lateral tract, from the lateral vestibular nucleus, extends to the sacral level of the cord. The medial tract from the medial vestibular nucleus extends through the cervical level. Impulses descending in these tracts assist in local myotactic (muscle-stretching) reflexes, reinforcing the tonus of the extensor muscles of the trunk and limbs. This reinforcement produces the extra force needed to support the body against gravity and to maintain an upright posture.

Communication between the vestibular nuclei and the cerebral nuclei is not established but may exist because vertigo and dizziness have resulted from cortical stimulation of posterior aspects of the temporal lobe.

Alterations in Hearing

HEARING LOSS

Hearing loss, or deafness, is the most common pathologic process associated with hearing alteration. It can result from disorders of the central hearing mechanisms or the peripheral pathways. There are several different types of hearing loss:

- Conduction hearing loss—peripheral hearing loss involving impairment of sound transmission in the external and middle ear
- Sensorineural hearing loss—hearing loss resulting from impairment of the neural pathway
- Mixed hearing loss—hearing problems involving both conductive and sensorineural impairments with a resultant reduction in sensitivity and sound discrimination in varying degrees

TABLE 34-1

CONTRASTING CONDUCTION AND SENSORINEURAL HEARING LOSS

	CONDUCTION HEARING LOSS (CONDUCTION DEAFNESS)	SENSORINEURAL HEARING LOSS (SENSORINEURAL DEAFNESS)
Cause	Defect in conductive system resulting from obstruction of the external canal by: • Cerumen • Foreign objects • Tumor • Damage to tympanic membrane • Congenital malformations • Other disease processes	Defect in auditory pathway at the organ of Corti, cochlear nerve, or cochlear muscle from pathology of: • Cochlear hair cells • Aging process • Infections • Persistent exposure to loud noise • Disease processes in the auditory nerve pathway • Long-term antibiotic therapy with mycins
Resultant hearing impairment	Impaired mechanisms for transmitting sound into the cochlea, tympanic membrane, or ossicle chain	Normal sound transmission Impaired perception of sound acuity and speech discrimination
Other characteristics	Loudness of sounds affected Sound localized in deaf ear Possible hearing restored with use of hearing aid	Constant high-pitched ringing in ears experienced Loss usually permanent

- Central hearing loss—hearing loss associated with lesions involving the cochlear nuclei and their connectiveness in the brain

Table 34-1 highlights the differences between conduction and sensorineural hearing loss.

Alterations in Vestibular Function

Disorders of coordination may originate from the vestibular system through disruption of the labyrinthine and righting reflexes. Lesions can occur in the labyrinths, in the vestibular nerve, or in vestibular pathways within the brain stem, cerebrum, or cerebellum. Vertigo and labyrinthine ataxia are examples of equilibrium disorders of the vestibular system.

VERTIGO

Vertigo is a disturbance of equilibrium that results in sensations of whirling, rotation, weakness, lightheadedness, or faintness. Posture is maintained by the normal interaction of several structures: labyrinths, eyes, muscles, joints, and higher neural centers. The causes of vertigo are multitudinous and include disorders of the labyrinth, vestibular nerve, vestibular nuclei, cerebellum, brain stem, eyes, and cerebral cortex. There are several types of vertigo: *acute paroxysmal, chronic,* and *benign positional.* The differences between the three types of vertigo are described in Box 34-2.

Clinical Manifestations

Attacks of vertigo can be disabling because the person may be thrown to the ground in reaction to false clues of movement. Nausea, vomiting, pallor, nystagmus, sweating, hypotension, excessive salivation, and

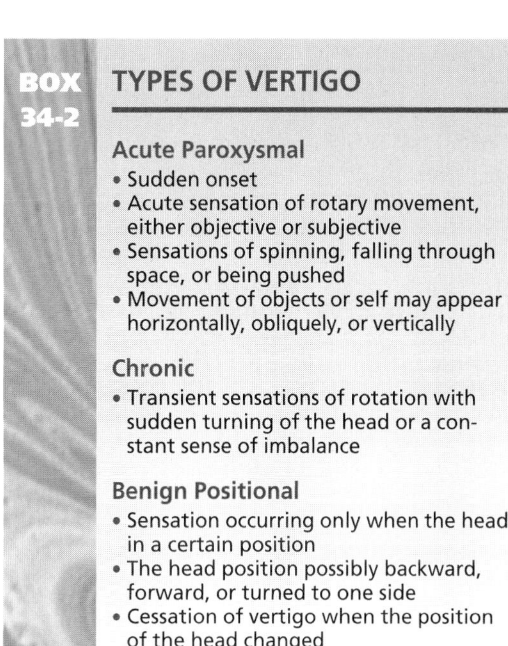

BOX 34-2 **TYPES OF VERTIGO**

Acute Paroxysmal
- Sudden onset
- Acute sensation of rotary movement, either objective or subjective
- Sensations of spinning, falling through space, or being pushed
- Movement of objects or self may appear horizontally, obliquely, or vertically

Chronic
- Transient sensations of rotation with sudden turning of the head or a constant sense of imbalance

Benign Positional
- Sensation occurring only when the head in a certain position
- The head position possibly backward, forward, or turned to one side
- Cessation of vertigo when the position of the head changed

difficulty with walking may accompany acute attacks of vertigo.

The vestibular nuclei seem to work by comparing signals from both labyrinths. If a labyrinth is destroyed, the other side overcompensates for the missing input. Rapid destruction of one labyrinth causes vertigo, nystagmus, and, occasionally, temporary nausea and vomiting. Bilateral destruction of the labyrinths does not cause nystagmus or vertigo, but rather a disturbance with equilibrium.

LABYRINTHINE ATAXIA

Labyrinthine ataxia, a striking vestibular disease, is characterized by disturbances of equilibrium in standing and walking. However, isolated limb movements are not affected.

Causes of ataxia include degenerative, demyelinating, or inflammatory lesions and lesions in the thalamus and subthalamic region near the main cerebellar and sensory pathways. The most common mixed ataxias are the cerebellar and vestibular forms and the posterior column and cerebellar forms.

Labyrinthine ataxia shares many common features of cerebellar ataxia, such as the broad-based, staggering gait, the tendency to lean over backward or to one side, and the deviation from direction of gait. However, unlike cerebellar ataxia, labyrinthine ataxia is associated with nystagmus and vertigo. In multiple sclerosis, symptoms of ataxia are mainly of the cerebellar and vestibular forms.

TASTE

Normal Structure

TASTE BUDS

Taste buds are the organs of taste. These oval structures, most numerous in the fungiform papillae of the tongue, are also present in the palate, pharynx, and epiglottis.[4,6] Microvilli project from the buds to the surface and come into contact with the substances dissolved in the fluids of the mouth. This contact is thought to be the basis for the generator potentials.

Innervation for the taste buds arrives from their base through small myelinated fibers. Each taste bud is innervated by several nerve fibers, and each nerve fiber receives innervation from several taste buds. The life span of a taste bud is unknown in humans. As buds degenerate, new buds are formed and innervated. The total number of taste buds diminishes with aging, accounting for the diminished sense of taste in elderly persons.

Normal Function

TASTE SENSATION

The sense of taste is a specialized function that is concerned with identification of food. The four primary taste sensations are sweet, sour, bitter, and salty. The other, more complex sensations that human beings perceive are combinations of the primary sensations together with the olfactory sensation. Even though the tip of the tongue perceives all four tastes, specific areas of the tongue are more sensitive to particular sensations, as shown in Figure 34-6.

Innervation from the taste buds to the central nervous system is through the seventh, ninth, and tenth cranial nerves. All three of these nerves terminate in the medulla oblongata and form the *tractus solitarius*. From this region, second-order neurons transmit to the thalamus and then on to the post-central gyrus of the cerebral cortex, where taste sensation shares projection sites with other somatic sensations.

Alterations in Taste Sensation

The sense of taste may be diminished (**hypogeusia**) or absent (**ageusia**) secondary to other underlying problems, such as dryness of the tongue, irradiation of the head, respiratory infections, and aging. Alterations in taste are associated with heavy smoking and may accompany Bell's palsy. Lesions of the thalamus and partial lobe may result in impairment or loss of taste on the opposite side of the tongue, and parietal lobe seizures may be heralded by an aura of a specific taste. Certain medications can alter the interpretation of taste.

Idiopathic hypogeusia is a syndrome associated with hyposmia (diminished smell), dysosmia (impaired smell), and dysgeusia (perversion of taste), in conjunction with diminished taste acuity. The smell and taste of food are most unpleasant for people with this syndrome. They often experience weight loss, depression, and anxiety. One identified cause of this syndrome is depression of zinc content in the parotid saliva.[1]

SMELL

In human beings, the sense of smell is closely associated physiologically with the sense of taste. Many foods are perceived partially by both senses, as their receptors are chemoreceptors that are stimulated by substances in the nose and mouth.

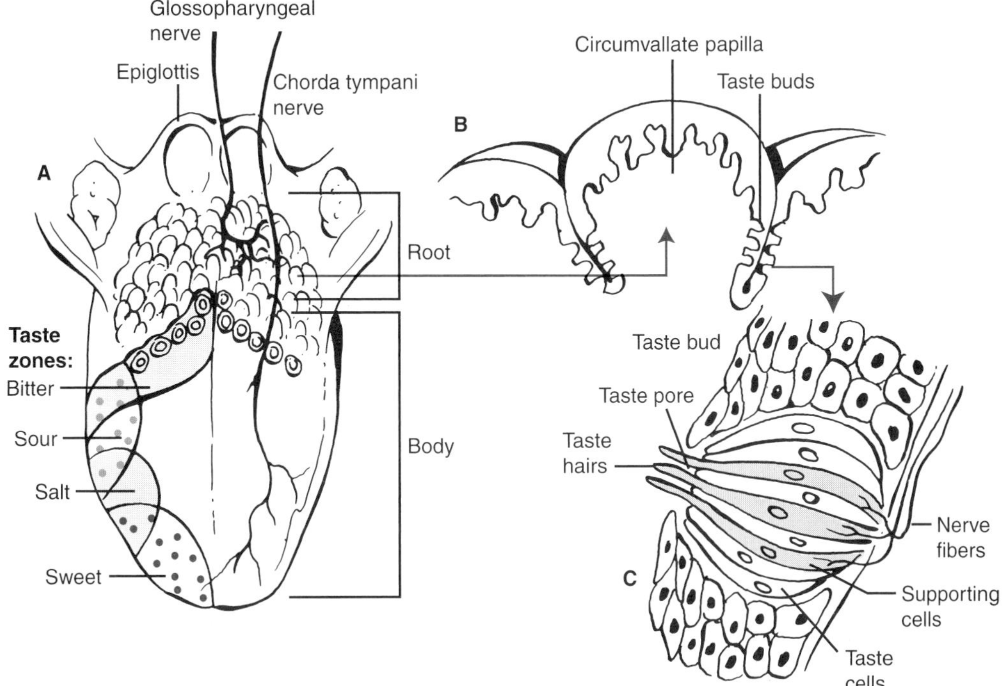

FIGURE 34-6. Peripheral sensory apparatus for taste sensation. **A.** Dorsal surface of the tongue showing areas for perception of sweet, sour, bitter, and salt tastes, and innervation of taste buds by the glossopharyngeal nerve and chorda tympani nerve. **B.** Microscopic appearance of the circumvallate papilla. **C.** Microscopic appearance of a taste bud.

Normal Structure

OLFACTORY CELLS

The receptor cells of olfaction, the bipolar *olfactory cells*, are located in the olfactory mucous membrane. Unlike other nerve cells, the olfactory cells are continuously dying and being replaced by newly generated ones. Peripherally, these cells have dendrites that terminate on the surface of the mucosa of the nasal cavity and project a group of cilia. The axons of the olfactory neurons pass through the *cribriform plate* of the ethmoid bone and enter the olfactory bulb.

Normal Function

ODOR DISCRIMINATION AND DIFFERENTIATION

Olfactory receptors are stimulated by volatile lipids and water-soluble substances that are inhaled into the mucosa of the nasal cavity. Little is known about the excitatory process of the individual receptor cells, although researchers have elicited several potentials in response to different odors. Conduction to the prepyriform cortex and frontal cortex through the thalamus causes the perception of odor and the sensation of smell.[9]

Although the physiologic basis for odor discrimination and differentiation is still unknown, physiologists have proposed the existence of primary odors that excite specific cells. It is believed that the odor molecules fit into specifically shaped receptor sites on the surface of the olfactory microvilli membranes. Other attempts to explain odor discrimination link physical properties of the stimulant with molecular vibrations. The limbic system connections probably account for emotional and memory-related responses to odors.[9]

Alterations in Smell

Smell disturbances may be caused by a variety of conditions including upper respiratory infections, sinusitis, allergies, facial injuries, tumors, and exposure to smoke and other pollutants. Alterations in smell are associated with disruption or damage of the cells in the olfactory bulb and nasal lining. Box 34-3 describes three of the most common smell disturbances: (1) *anosmia*, (2) *hyposmia*, and (3) *dysosmia*.

BOX 34-3

SMELL DISTURBANCES

Anosmia (loss of smell)

- Most frequently occurring smell disturbance
- Associated disorders such as hypertrophy of nasal mucosa, sinusitis, upper respiratory infections, and allergies

Hyposomia (reduced sense of smell)

- Most frequently associated with heavy smoking
- Possibly occurring with facial injuries involving the cribriform plate and certain tumors involving the olfactory groove
- Olfactory hallucinations and delusions possible with certain mental illnesses and temporal lobe disorders
- Possibly preceding seizures arising from the uncal region (specific smells)

Dysosmia (distortion of smell)

- Also known as parosmia
- Possibly resulting from local nasopharyngeal conditions, such as partial injuries
- Possibly occurring with aging, resulting from a decreased number of cells in the olfactory bulb and nasal lining
- Long-standing exposure to smoke or other pollutants contributing to diminution of sense

FOCUS ON THE PERSON WITH VISUAL DIFFICULTY

R. M. is a 72-year-old male with a history of diabetes mellitus who comes to the health care provider's office complaining of a change in his vision. He states that over the past few years, "Things seem to be getting hazy, especially in bright light." An avid golfer for the past 40 years, R. M. now reports having to wear a hat with a visor to cut down on the glare. He denies any complaints of eye pain. Further examination and testing reveal absence of the red reflex and some lens opacity in both eyes. A diagnosis of bilateral cataracts is made.

Questions

1. Propose possible factors associated with R. M.'s development of cataracts.
2. Explain the pathophysiologic events involved with cataract formation.

R. M. is treated surgically. Approximately 24 hours after surgery, he complains of severe eye pain, seeing halos around lights, and nausea and vomiting. Intraocular pressure is increased. A diagnosis of acute glaucoma is made.

3. Describe the physiologic mechanism for maintaining intraocular pressure within the normal range.
4. Suggest a possible explanation for R. M.'s new condition based on his previous history.

REFERENCES

1. Adams, R., Victor, M. & Ropper, A. (1997). *Principles of neurology* (6th ed.). New York: McGraw-Hill.
2. Celesia, G. & DeMarco, P. (1994). Anatomy and physiology of the visual system. *Journal of Clinical Neurophysiology, 11*(5), 482–492.
3. Ganong, W. (1997). *Review of medical physiology* (18th ed.). Norwalk, CT: Appleton & Lange.
4. Gartner, L. (1994). Oral anatomy and tissue types. *Seminars in Dermatology, 13*(2), 68–73.
5. Gilman, S. & Newman, S. (1996). *Manter and Gatz's essentials of clinical neuroanatomy and neurophysiology* (9th ed.). Philadelphia: F. A. Davis.
6. Guyton, A. & Hall, J. (1996). *Textbook of medical physiology* (9th ed.). Philadelphia: W. B. Saunders.
7. Hejtmanik, J. (1995). Vision. In P. Conn, *Neuroscience in medicine*. Philadelphia: Lippincott.
8. Parent, A. (1996). *Carpenter's human anatomy* (9th ed.). Baltimore: Williams & Wilkins.
9. Tortora, G. & Grabowski, S. (1996). *Principles of anatomy and physiology* (8th ed.). Reading, MA: Addison-Wesley.
10. Walton, J. (1995). *Brain's diseases of the nervous system* (10th ed.). Oxford: Oxford University Press.

Chapter

35

Pain

Kay Sackett / Christine A. Cannon

KEY TERMS

A-delta fiber
acute pain
algesic agent
allodynia
bradykinin
C-fiber
chronic pain
cutaneous pain
deep somatic pain
endorphins
enkephalins
fast pain
modulation
neurogenic pain
nociception
nociceptor
opioid system
pain threshold
pain tolerance
perception
perceptual dominance
prostaglandins
psychogenic pain
referred pain
slow pain
somatogenic pain
substance P
suffering
transduction
transmission
visceral pain

The complex sensation of pain is a unique experience that results from the interplay of biologic, cognitive, emotional, social, and cultural factors. Pain is defined as "an unpleasant sensory and emotional experience associated with actual or potential tissue damage or described in terms of such damage" by the International Association for the Study of Pain (IASP).[21] It is a subjective symptom of an unpleasant sensation that is uniquely experienced. Many factors influence the perception of pain and its associated thoughts, feelings, and behaviors. **Suffering**, the emotional anguish experienced in pain, reflects the interactions between physiologic, psychological, and social functioning.

THE PAIN EXPERIENCE

Pain is a common symptom associated with many acute and chronic illnesses. Although a protective mechanism for attracting a person's attention and responses to control it, pain often lingers beyond its usefulness, with unpleasant and destructive consequences. The prevalence of chronic pain is widespread, estimated to affect 25% to 30% of people living in industrialized countries and resulting in huge economic impacts.

At a more personal level, pain is a major problem that is often not well controlled despite major pharmacologic and nonpharmacologic advances. Inadequacies in pain assessment along with client and health care provider biases and misinformation regarding opioid addiction, new drug delivery modes, complementary therapies, and related areas exist. Often, the biopsychosocial impact of pain is not assessed or addressed using multidisciplinary and multimodal approaches. More professional help to mobilize intrapersonal coping strategies and interpersonal support is needed to control pain and needless suffering.[1,2]

The Study of Pain

The study of pain is often organized around classifications of pain by its origin as **somatogenic** (known physiologic cause) or **psychogenic** (no physiologic cause). Somatogenic pain is often referred to as *nociceptive* (cutaneous, deep somatic, or visceral origins of pain) and/or *neurogenic* (pain originating from within an altered nervous system). Often, the pain experience is studied based on its duration and nature as **acute pain** (a functional physiologic response to injury, often lasting less than 6 months) or **chronic pain** (pain that continues beyond the normal time of healing, often more than 6 months in duration).[29] Recently, it has been suggested that pain be studied on the basis of its physiologic mechanisms. Pain symptoms (constituting a syndrome such as low back pain) would be understood in terms of their underlying cellular and tissue pain mechanisms. The outcomes of this mechanism-based approach to understanding pain include the identification of pharmacologic, surgical, and physical therapy interventions targeted to specific mechanisms.[30]

Theories of Pain

Several theories related to pain are described, including the Specificity, Intensity, Pattern, and Gate Control theories. The Melzack-Casey conceptual model of pain and Loesser's multifaceted model of the components of pain are two of several models that focus on the psychological and behavioral factors in pain. Each of the theories adds to the understanding of pain mechanisms that are not understood by one theory alone.

THE SPECIFICITY THEORY

The *specificity theory* describes four types of cutaneous sensation—touch, warmth, cold, and pain—each resulting from the stimulation of specific skin receptor sites and specific neural pathways dedicated to one of the four sensations. When specific pain neurons are stimulated, the pain sensation is transmitted along specific pain fibers. According to this theory, nociceptor neurons synapse in the *substantia gelatinosa*, cross to the opposite side of the cord, and ascend the specific pain pathways of the spinothalamic tract to the thalamus and the pain receptor areas of the cerebral cortex. The specificity theory focuses on the direct relationship between the pain stimulus and perception, but does not account for adaptation to pain and the psychosocial factors that modulate it.[20]

THE INTENSITY THEORY

The *intensity theory* states that pain is the result of excessive stimulation of sensory receptors. Disorders or processes that produce pain are thought to create an intense summation of non-noxious stimuli. This theory does not explain the existence of intense stimuli not perceived as pain.[20]

THE PATTERN THEORY

The *pattern theory* states that nonspecific receptors transmit specific patterns (characterized by the length of the pain sensation, the amount of involved tissue, and the summation of impulses) from the skin to the spinal cord that are perceived as pain. Pattern theory takes into account components of the intensity theory, stating that pain may occur with intense stimulation of the sensory receptors regardless of receptor type or pathway. The neuromatrix theory proposed by Melzack holds that sensations are imprinted in the brain. Sensory inputs may trigger a pattern of sensation from the neuromatrix (a proposed network of neurons looping between the thalamus and the cortex and the cortex and the limbic system). However, the sensation pattern may occur without the sensory trigger. This pattern type theory helps to explain the existence of phantom pain, discomfort perceived as originating from a paralyzed or amputated limb.

THE GATE CONTROL THEORY

The *gate control theory* (1965) of Melzack and Wall proposes that pain is transmitted from the skin to cells of the substantia gelatinosa in the dorsal horn via the small-diameter **A-delta** and **C-fibers**, where interconnections between other sensory pathways exist. Stimulation of the large-diameter, fast, myelinated A-beta and A-alpha fibers closes the "gate" composed of the cells of the substantia gelatinosa, restricting the transmission of the impulse to the central nervous system (CNS) and diminishing the perception of pain. Large-fiber stimulation may be provided through massage, scratching or rubbing the skin, or electrical stimulation as in the use of *transcutaneous electrical nerve stimulation (TENS)*. Thus, concurrent firing of pain and touch paths reduces the transmission and perception of the pain impulses, while the touch impulses are transmitted and perceived. An increase in small-fiber activity inhibits the substantia gelatinosa cells, "opening the gate" and increasing pain transmission and perception.

The substantia gelatinosa acts as a gate-control system to modulate (inhibit) the flow of nerve impulses from peripheral fibers to the CNS (Fig. 35-1). In addition, central trigger cells (T cells) act as a CNS control to stimulate selective brain processes that influence the gate-control system. If T cell activity is inhibited, pain impulses are not transmitted to the brain because the gate is closed. The T cells activate neural mechanisms in the brain that are responsible for pain perception and response. These transmitters partly regulate the release of **substance P**, the peptide that conveys pain information. Pain modulation is also partly controlled by the neurotransmitters enkephalin and serotonin. If pain signals are persistent, the fraction of impulses allowed to pass through the various gates gradually declines. It is thought that descending efferent impulses from the brain may close, partially open, or completely open the gate. This theory continues to be referred to as the basis for pain management involving massage and electrical stimulation and in the development of additional theories and models.[20]

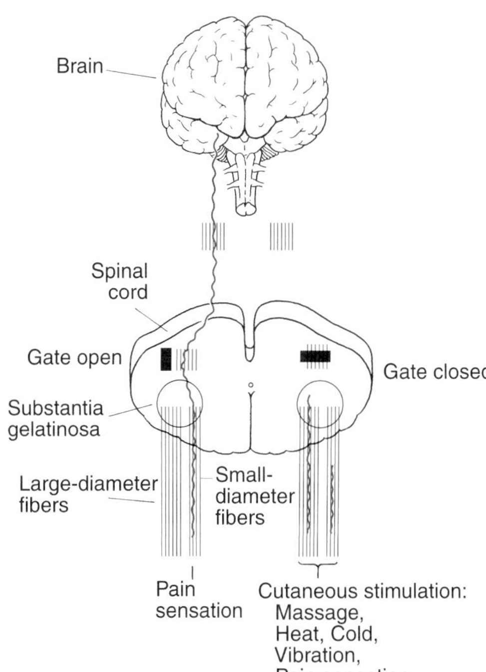

FIGURE 35-1. Gate control theory of pain. (Hudak, C. M., Gallo, B., & Morton, P. G. [1998]. *Critical care nursing* [7th ed.]. Philadelphia: Lippincott-Raven.)

THE MELZACK-CASEY CONCEPTUAL MODEL OF PAIN

The *Melzack-Casey conceptual model* of pain suggests that there are three major psychological dimensions of pain: sensory-discriminative, motivational-affective, and cognitive-evaluative. The interactions between the sensory discriminative information (from the thalamus and somatosensory cortex), the affective and motivational features of pain (from the reticular formation), and cognitive functioning can produce descending inhibitory influences that alter pain input to the dorsal horn. Ultimately, modifications of sensory pain experience and motivational-affective dimensions may occur. Pain is localized and identified by its characteristics, evaluated by past experiences, and undergoes further cognitive processing, suggesting the powerful role of psychological functioning in determining the quality and intensity of pain. The complex sensory, motivational, and cognitive interactions determine motor activities and behaviors associated with the pain experience.[26]

OTHER MODELS

Other models, such as Loeser's multifaceted model of the components of pain, focus on the interactions between nociceptive processes that cause pain and the perception and recognition of the sensation. Pain triggers the emotional response to the sensation, suffering, which results in observable pain behaviors. The multidimensional models of pain and the recognition of motivational, affective, and environmental factors that influence pain behaviors provide the basis for approaching pain management in a comprehensive, multimodal way employing multidisciplinary expertise.[18]

NOCICEPTION

Often pain is studied, diagnosed, and treated based on whether the origin of the pain lies outside the nervous system (nociceptive) or within the nervous system (neurogenic or neuropathic).

Often, pain is caused by tissue-damaging ("noxious") chemical, thermal, or mechanical agents that stimulate a specialized group of sensory receptors called **nociceptors**. Information from the nociceptors travels along afferent pathways to the spinal cord, where autonomic and motor reflexes are stimulated, and to various parts of the brain, where the information is perceived as pain. **Nociception** refers to the activation of pain fibers and the subsequent responses to noxious stimuli. It involves the processes of pain **transduction** (conversion of noxious stimuli into electrical impulses), **transmission** (spread of impulses through sensory nervous system), **modulation** (modifications of the pain transmission), and **perception** (development of the subjective, sensory, and emotional pain experience).[10]

Etiology

NOCICEPTIVE STIMULI

Tissue injury, inflammation, and cell death caused by mechanical, thermal, or electrical damage and chemical stimulation of the free nerve endings results in pain perception. Major causes of nociception include trauma, surgery, burns, infection, and exposure to toxins. A variety of noxious mechanisms in many inherited disorders and acquired diseases stimulate nociception.[26] Cancer pain is often caused by the side effects of treatment, including the toxicities of radiation and chemotherapy and the result of surgery and invasive procedures. Tumor progression can lead to diffuse bone pain, nerve compression, or neuropathies. When tubular structures such as intestines or ureters are compressed, a build-up of contents under pressure leads to distention and pain. Inflammation and infection cause pain as tumors grow into the lungs and pneumonia occurs. Pain results when blood and lymph vessels are compressed. Vascular inflammation or occlusion is another source of pain in cancer. Sudden reduction of blood flow to tissues results in acute ischemic pain. In the end stage of cancer, cell death increases, with tissue necrosis creating severe pain.[12]

Another common example of a disease that causes both acute and chronic pain is atherosclerosis. Acute pain results from embolic or thrombotic arterial occlusion and infarction. Chronic pain is due to tissue ischemia, when oxygen demands outweigh oxygen supplied by the coronary or peripheral circulations. Ischemic pain of the myocardium is called *angina pectoris*. Chronic arterial peripheral vascular disease causes the episodic pain of *intermittent claudication* with walking. Obstruction of arterial flow leads to tissue necrosis and, often, gangrene.

Nociception is triggered by the release of pain-producing biochemical agents in the extracellular fluid that surrounds the nociceptors during cell injury, inflammation, and disease. These pain-producing substances (also called **algesic** or algogenic agents) include potassium, hydrogen, serotonin, and histamine, prostaglandin from the tissues, and bradykinin from the blood plasma. Substance P, released from the nerve terminals, sensitizes nociceptors. Substance P causes the release of histamine and serotonin from platelets and mast cells, which contributes significantly to capillary vasodilation and permeability associated with inflammation. Inflammation further produces **bradykinin** and **prostaglandins** (from actions of the enzyme cyclooxygenase on cell membrane–derived arachidonic acid). Prostaglandin E_2 sensitizes the nociceptors to the stimulating influence of bradykinin. Bradykinin seems to be a particularly potent pain stimulator. These substances then cause nociceptors' threshold for pain to be lowered.[2,3,18,26] Box 35-1 lists common nociceptive stimuli. Unlike other sensory receptors, pain receptors adapt very little, if at all, and may even increase in excitation with continued stimulation.

POPULATIONS AT RISK

In addition to people affected by common chronic diseases such as cancer, atherosclerosis, and AIDS, certain groups are at risk for pain related to injury. These include those who work in physically strenuous jobs or in jobs that require prolonged periods of sitting in front of a computer monitor and/or using repetitive movements. Low back pain, neck pain, and carpal tunnel disease are major painful occupational health hazards. People who do not practice good sitting or standing postures and are less physically fit risk neuromuscular and skeletal health problems and thus are more prone to injury.

People having surgery, particularly of the spine, abdomen, chest, and joints, are at risk for severe pain. Iatrogenically induced pain often accompanies invasive treatment or monitoring procedures. The incidence of postoperative pain due to undertreatment in adults and children is high despite major advances in analgesics and their administration.

Finally, stage of life influences the risk for specific kinds of pain. In infants, pain cannot be verbally described; thus, procedures (such as circumcisions) may be performed with no or inadequate analgesia. In premature neonates, the descending pain control aspect of nociception is not complete; therefore, pain goes unrelieved, with cardiovascular and neurologic consequences possibly jeopardizing the premature infant's recovery. With cognitive development during childhood, levels of pain are better discriminated and pain thresholds increase. Types of age-related pain include the colic of early infancy, otitis media of early childhood, migraine headaches of adolescence, and menstruation-associated pain in adolescent girls. Young adulthood is characterized by risks of trauma-related and child-bearing pain. The elderly are at risk for the pain of arthritis, osteoporosis, cancer, and atherosclerosis. Changes in drug metabolism in older adulthood influence the level of pain experienced.

BOX 35-1

COMMON NOCICEPTIVE STIMULI

- Algesic substances surrounding nociceptors
- Distention and contraction of hollow organs
- Stretching of organ capsule
- Muscle ischemia
- Compression of ligaments and vessels

(Adapted from Raj, P. P. [1996]. Pain mechanisms. In P. P. Raj, *Pain medicine: A comprehensive review.* St. Louis: Mosby.)

Physiology

TRANSDUCTION BY PERIPHERAL MECHANISMS

Free nerve endings of A-delta and C afferent pain fibers are unevenly distributed in the skin, muscle, the pulp of the teeth, the arteries, the periosteum, the meninges, and some internal organs (predominantly in the abdomen, pelvis, and thorax). Some nociceptors (nerve endings) found in the skin, mucous membranes, and walls of body cavities are *unimodal*, meaning that they respond only to one type of stimuli. These receptors are sensitive to mechanical agents. The majority of free nerve endings distributed in the skin and deep tissues are *polymodal*, meaning that they respond to more than one type of stimulation. These are stimulated by thermal, chemical, electrical, and mechanical agents. A-delta and C fibers located in the viscera may be stimulated by inflammation, disease, ischemia, distention, and isometric contraction. Stimulation of free nerve endings of the afferent nerve fibers by algesic substances released at the site of cell injury or inflammation creates electrical impulses. This first component of the pain phenomena, the conversion of noxious stimuli into electrical impulses with depolarization of the nerve membrane, is called transduction.[26]

AFFERENT TRANSMISSION OF PAIN

Transmission of the pain impulse includes several steps. Initially, the pain impulses travel to the dorsal horn of the spinal cord through two types of nerve fibers: the small-diameter, lightly myelinated A-delta fibers and the unmyelinated C fibers. When stimulated, A-delta fibers elicit a rapid response or **fast pain**. These fibers transmit well-localized, sharp, stinging, or pinprick-type pain sensation elicited by either mechanical or thermal stimuli. A-delta fibers connect with secondary neurons mostly on laminae I, II, and V (neural groupings in the dorsal horn).

The C nerve fibers are smaller, unmyelinated fibers that connect with second-order neurons in lamina I and II. (Lamina II includes the substantia gelatinosa, an area in which modulation of pain occurs.) When stimulated, C fibers elicit a response within 1 second. Considered a **slow pain** response, it is most frequently caused by chemical rather than thermal or mechanical stimuli. A slow pain response is less well localized and is described as a dull, aching, or burning sensation.

Thus, there is a two-pronged response to pain: first an acute response immediately transmitted through fast pain pathways that allows the individual to withdraw from the pain, and then the lingering pain transmitted through slow pathways that continues or worsens over time.[7]

Transmission, the second component of the pain process, continues with the synapse of the afferent neurons with other neurons in the dorsal horn. The cell bodies of the A-delta and C fibers are located in the dorsal root ganglia and their axons continue into the spinal cord, where they synapse with second-order neurons in laminae I, II, and III. Substance P and calcitonin-gene-related peptide are thought to relay the pain message across the synapse. Some afferent fibers travel deep into the cord and cross to the opposite side, whereas others send branches for short distances up and down the cord.[7,26] Pain transmission ascends the spinal cord through the pathways of the *spinothalamic tract* (*STT*) (also known as the *neospinothalamic tract*) and the *spinoreticulothalamic tract* (*SRT*) (the *paleospinothalamic tract*) to the brain. The cell bodies of neurons in the STT are located mainly in lamina I, with the neuronal axons ascending via the anterolateral columns of the spinal cord to the thalamus. Pain perception occurs as the STT axons reach the thalamus. Sensory aspects are provided by neural connections to the cerebral cortex (the primary somesthetic cortex where discrimination as to location and intensity occurs, and the somesthetic association cortex where pain perception and meaning is provided).

The STT carries pain impulses perceived as sharp, pricking, or stinging.[26] Figure 35-2 depicts the primary pain pathways.

The SRT transmits arousal and the affective components of pain. Information travels through the small, unmyelinated C fibers to the dorsal horn. Many of the cell bodies of SRT neurons terminate in laminae I and II of the dorsal horn. A majority of these neurons synapse with interneurons before crossing to the opposite side of the cord and ascending to the medulla via the anterolateral pathway. These neurons make multiple synaptic connections in the reticular formation, mesencephalon, and thalamus. From the thalamus, axons travel to the cerebral cortex, limbic system (involved with emotional, motivational, and affective aspects of pain), and basal ganglia. The SRT carries dull, aching, or burning pain that lingers after the initial sharp pain abates.[23,26]

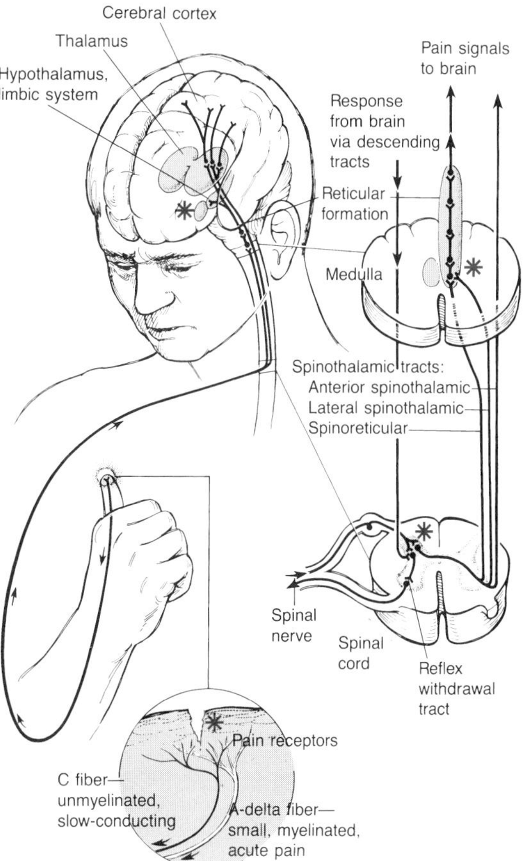

FIGURE 35-2. Neural pathways of pain and fibers transmitting pain.

MODULATION

Modulation is described as the modification of the sensory experience leading to restraint of nociception. Modulation occurs with the activation of descending inhibitory processes involving neurons originating in the cerebral cortex and brainstem. Pathways descend in the spinal cord, terminating in laminae I through VII.

Additional modulation and control of afferent pain input involves the stimulation of the endogenous pain control system of the brain, which includes the *periaqueductal gray (PAG) region* of the mesencephalon and upper pons, the *raphe magnus nucleus*, and the *pain inhibitory complex* in the dorsal horn of the spinal cord, as shown in Figure 35-3. Information from the cortex, limbic system, and thalamus provides input to the endogenous pain control system. Pathways extend from the PAG to laminae I, II, and IV, where afferent input enters the spinal cord. Serotonin from the mesencephalon and pons, norepinephrine from the pons, and endorphins found in the brain and spinal cord inhibit the pain experience by decreasing the release of nociceptive neurotransmitters.[18,19]

Endorphins and Enkephalins

Endorphins play a major role in modulation of pain transmission, affecting afferent nociceptive impulses and descending responses. Endorphins, including the **enkephalins** named beta-endorphin, met-enkephalin and leu-enkephalin, are naturally occurring, morphine-like polypeptides that provide analgesia (**opioid system**). It is speculated that enkephalins inhibit specific presynaptic receptors that secrete substance P, thereby inhibiting both type A-delta and type C pain fibers.[11] It is thought that, in stress, analgesia may be induced with the release of pituitary opioids and endorphins. Sympathetic activity in stress has been associated with the adrenal production of endogenous opioids. Chronic pain may be associated with deficient levels of endogenous opioids.[16]

The central pain control structures also include multiple areas that contain opiate receptors. Mu and sigma receptors are more concentrated in the brain than the spinal cord. Mu receptors, also present in the periphery, may have greater attraction for opioids than kappa (concentrated in spinal cord), sigma, or delta receptors. Opioids, endogenous and exogenous, vary in their affinity for specific receptor sites.[11]

FOCUS ON CELLULAR PHYSIOLOGY

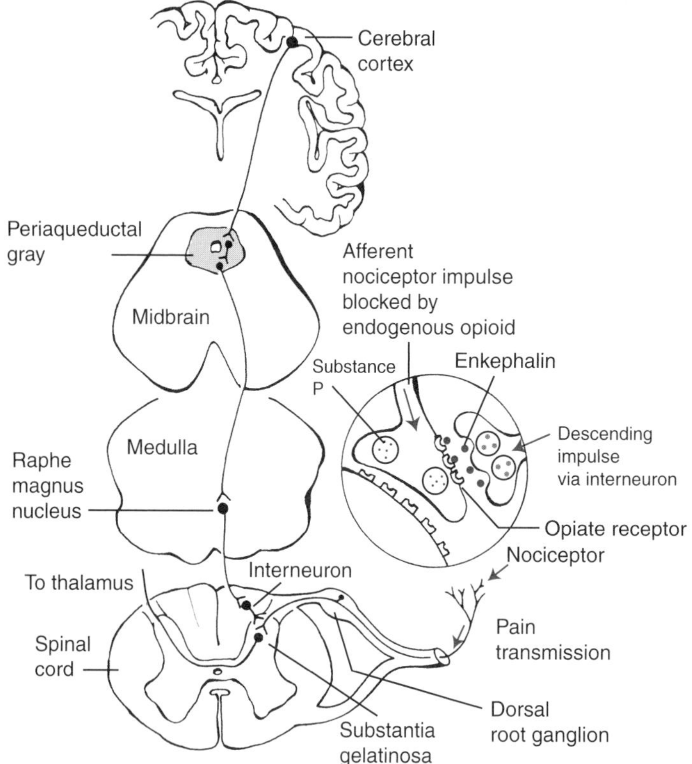

FIGURE 35-3. Endogenous pain control system.

PERCEPTION

Pain perception is the end result of the neural activity of pain transduction, transmission, and modulation. Pain becomes a conscious experience at this point. No predictable direct relationship between the intensity of pain and one's perception or response exists because this relationship between the perception of pain and nociception is not completely understood. The perception and localization of pain is thought to take place within the cortical structures in the somatosensory cortex and the limbic system. The reticular system and limbic system are thought to be responsible for alerting, arousing, and motivating behaviors. The limbic system influences emotional and behavioral responses to pain. The medulla and hypothalamus are involved with cardiovascular responses and fight-or-flight responses.[10] Three important concepts associated with pain perception are pain threshold, perceptual dominance, and pain tolerance.

PAIN THRESHOLD. The **pain threshold** is the point at which a stimulus is perceived as pain. The pain threshold does not differ significantly from person to person or within one person over time. For example, the temperature at which water is felt to "burn" the skin is fairly consistent among people and over time.

PERCEPTUAL DOMINANCE. One factor that may change the pain threshold for one area of pain is the coexistence of another area of more intense pain, termed **perceptual dominance.** Perceptual dominance leads to an increase in the pain threshold for one location, while the pain is more intense from the more dominant location. When pain is relieved from the dominant location, the pain threshold is lowered at the other location.

PAIN TOLERANCE. **Pain tolerance** is the duration or intensity of pain that one will endure before initiating a response to the pain. Pain tolerance varies widely among people and is influenced by physical and mental health, roles, and individual, social, and cultural expectations. Repeated pain experiences, anxiety, fatigue, and sleep deprivation lower tolerance, whereas medications, relaxation, alcohol, and distraction may increase tolerance.

Clinical Manifestations

Nociceptive pain varies by source of pain. It is subcategorized as cutaneous, deep somatic, or visceral in origin. Table 35-1 compares the subcategories of nociceptive pain. Additionally, pain is often categorized by its pattern of duration as acute or chronic, each with very different clinical pictures.

CUTANEOUS PAIN

Cutaneous pain, or superficial somatic pain from skin or mucous membrane injury (such as a paper cut or insect bite), is easily located due to the abundance of sensory receptors in the skin. A-delta myelinated fibers perceive a sharp pain when noxious thermal or mechanical stimulation occurs. When thermal, chemical, or mechanical stimuli activate the unmyelinated C fibers, the cutaneous pain is felt as a long-lasting, burning pain.[7]

TABLE 35-1
CHARACTERISTICS OF NOCICEPTIVE PAIN TYPES

PAIN TYPE	SOURCE	QUALITY	EXAMPLES
Cutaneous	Skin Mucous membranes Superficial subcutaneous tissues	Sharp pain and/or burning quality Easily localized and distributed along dermatomes (or close to dermatome)	Paper cut Insect bite
Deep somatic	Deep body structures: periosteum, muscles, tendons, joints, blood vessels	*Chronic pain:* Dull aching pain with sharp pain on movement More diffuse than cutaneous pain Possible radiation of pain *Acute pain:* Sharp, burning, throbbing, localized	Sprained ankle Fracture Peripheral vascular disease with ischemia Arthritis
Visceral	Soft organs in the thorax, abdomen, or pelvis	Deep, dull, vague Poorly defined, difficult to locate Radiation away from affected organ Autonomic nervous system responses, such as nausea, vomiting, pallor	Chest pain due to myocardial infarction Biliary and renal colic Appendicitis Cholecystitis Pancreatitis

DEEP SOMATIC PAIN

Deep somatic pain originates from muscles, bones, joints, and other connective tissue due to mechanical trauma or a build-up of chemicals, such as potassium or lactic acid. Deep somatic nociception is characterized by dull, aching pain that may be more diffuse than cutaneous pain. Sudden trauma such as a sprain creates sharp, burning, throbbing, and well-localized pain, whereas chronic pain such as that experienced in arthritis is dull and aching, punctuated by sharp pain with joint movement. Deep somatic pain occurs along segments similar to dermatomes (see Chapter 29) and is subject to being referred to an area beyond the area of injury or inflammation.[10]

VISCERAL PAIN

Visceral pain arises from internal organs, possibly being felt on the skin or in a location distant from its nociceptive site. The visceral pain receptors are located in the capsules of solid organs (such as the Glisson's capsule of the liver) and in the smooth muscle layers of hollow organs (such as the myocardium of the heart). Visceral pain is transmitted through small C fibers. The stimuli that produce visceral pain are different from the stimuli for cutaneous pain and also vary by organ. For example, distention, contraction against obstruction, and traction are the stimuli for intestinal pain, whereas compression is a noxious stimulus for organs such as the testes. The myocardial nociceptors respond to the effects of ischemia.[7] Visceral pain tends to be dull or burning and is usually accompanied by intense autonomic vasovagal stimulation, causing diaphoresis, nausea and vomiting, and a fall in blood pressure. The pain is diffuse or poorly localized and may be referred to a myotome or dermatome a distance away from the source of pain. For example, the visceral pressure of myocardial ischemia may be felt in the epigastric area, neck, jaw, and over the inner aspect of the left arm.

Visceral pain from pathology in upper abdominal organs is often poorly localized, leading to mistakes in differentiating the heartburn of gastroesophageal reflux disease or the colic of cholelithiasis from myocardial ischemia. Reflex muscle spasm is common with intense and persistent visceral nociception. Over time, the spasm and other reflex autonomic responses may generate pain in the absence of the initial visceral nociception.[10]

Referred pain is pain that is felt a distance away from the site of the noxious stimulation. The location of the referred pain falls within the same spinal segment as the actual site of injury. Referred pain is often visceral. Figure 35-4 illustrates areas of referred pain. Many cutaneous and visceral pain impulses are transmitted on the same ascending neurons, causing the origins of the pain impulses to be indistinguishable by the brain. Often the nature of the visceral pain is altered so that even though it is transmitted through the slow pain C fibers, it is referred as sharp, burning, often severe pain to other areas on the skin.[13]

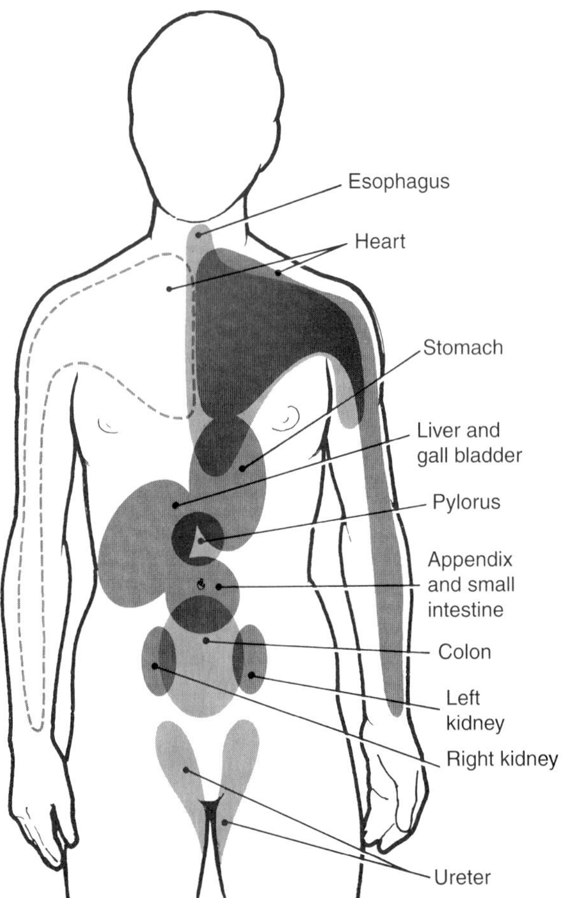

FIGURE 35-4. Typical areas of referred pain from visceral organs.

ACUTE PAIN

Acute pain is characterized by its transitory nature—its sudden onset and limited duration for the time of ongoing physiologic injury. Acute pain is commonly associated with surgery, diagnostic procedures, burns, and trauma. Usually easily localized, it responds to treatment. Acute pain resolves as healing occurs in a predictable time frame.

Physiologic responses to acute pain are associated with neuroendocrine changes associated with stress. Occasionally, acute pain may cause a fall in blood pressure and diaphoresis if vagal stimulation occurs. When the sympathetic nervous system is stimulated in acute pain, selective vasoconstriction leads to cold hands and feet and rises in blood pressure. Increased cardiac output results from increased stroke volume and tachycardia. Increased metabolic rate and oxygen consumption may increase respiratory rate. Decreased gastrointestinal and urinary tract tone lead to decreasing stomach emptying and urinary retention, respectively. Increased muscle tone often leads to muscle spasm.[10] Behavioral responses to pain often include grimacing, guarding, and verbal expressions of pain.

Acute anxiety often occurs with acute pain and/or its anticipation. Acute pain mobilizes the person experiencing it to take immediate actions to relieve the pain. Anxiety and fear contribute to neuroendocrine responses associated with stress.

CHRONIC PAIN

Chronic pain is often prolonged beyond 6 months and less defined in its source and course. Chronic pain has been described in a variety of ways that reflect its complexity and impact on quality of life. Chronic nonmalignant pain is associated with conditions other than cancer, whereas chronic malignant pain is associated with cancer. Low back pain and headache pain are the two most common types of chronic nonmalignant pain.[4]

Chronic pain may have no identifiable pathophysiology and no purpose. Pain threshold is thought to be low due to a deficiency in serotonin and endorphin levels. Physiologic adaptation to pain causes the heart rate and blood pressure to fall within the normal ranges.[18,23] The hypothalamus and pituitary gland overseeing the release of hormones may be influenced by the stress of chronic pain. Pain is associated with the release of cortisol, antidiuretic hormone, aldosterone, renin, catecholamines, growth hormone, and glucagon. Insulin and testosterone secretion is decreased. As a result of these hormonal alterations, clinical manifestations found in pain may include hyperglycemia, hypernatremia, hypokalemia, water retention, and others.[10]

Chronic pain interferes with many facets of everyday life, from sleeping and eating to maintaining one's self-esteem, job, relationships, financial security, and an acceptable quality of life. The chronic pain experience is one of the body and the mind. More than one-half of people with chronic pain experience depression and/or anxiety disorders, both of which can intensify pain and suffering. Chronic pain is often associated with frustration, a sense of hopelessness, and helplessness that may lead to depression. Problems associated with increased or decreased eating, sleeping, and preoccupation with pain are common. Occasionally, depression is manifested as chronic pain. Depressive and anxiety disorders often lead to the misinterpretation of normal body functioning.[27]

NEUROGENIC PAIN

Nociceptive pain is caused by direct injury and/or inflammation to superficial and deep somatic or visceral tissues in those with normal, intact nervous systems. In contrast, neuropathic or **neurogenic pain** is due to altered nervous system functioning associated with neural injury, causing neuropathies or problems such as phantom limb pain or postherpetic neuralgia.

Etiology

Neurogenic pain stimuli are hard to identify. The cutting, crushing, and/or compression of the nervous system due to trauma, surgery, tumor growth, chemotherapy, or radiation may cause neurogenic pain. The nervous system damage may lead to pain related to spontaneous discharges of the nerve, spontaneous dorsal root activity, or degeneration of modulatory mechanisms. In neurogenic pain, there is no nociceptor activation, no classic pain pathway transmission, and no passage through opioid-sensitive synapses.

Clinical Manifestations

Because it is different from fast pain sensations, the cutting, burning, tingling, shooting, or electric-like neurogenic pain is difficult to describe. The pain is not easily localized, often being felt in unexpected areas. Neurogenic pain is characterized by **allodynia**, pain due to a stimulus that normally does not cause pain, such as a light touch. Often pain may have both nociceptive and neuropathic components.[18]

PSYCHOGENIC PAIN

Somatogenic pain, regardless of the type, is pain with a defined physical cause such as disease or trauma, whereas psychogenic pain has no known physical cause. Two types of psychogenic pain are described in DSM-IV. Pain Disorder Associated with Psychological Factors is diagnosed in cases in which psychological factors are assessed to play a major part in the onset, severity, exacerbation, or maintenance of the pain. The DSM-IV diagnosis Pain Disorder Associated with Both Psychological Factors and a General Medical Condition is characterized by pain onset, severity, exacerbation, or maintenance due to nociceptive and psychogenic factors.[3] It is important not to initially label all pain without an apparent physical cause as psychogenic. On the other hand, the client should not be subjected to a continuous and potentially dangerous quest to find a physical cause for all pain complaints.[20]

DISORDERS OF PAIN

Postoperative Pain

Despite the increasing availability of effective pain management options, postoperative pain remains unnecessarily experienced. Poor understanding of pain assessment on the part of physicians and nurses, combined with wide variations in pain perception and expression by clients, interferes with adequate care planning. Misinformation regarding the incidence of postoperative narcotic addiction may prevent physicians from prescribing needed medications in adequate dosages.[19]

ETIOLOGY AND PHYSIOLOGY

The source of postoperative pain is the injury-induced release of chemical mediators that occurs with the acute inflammatory response. Bradykinin, substance P, and prostaglandins are released from the injured cells. Pain stimuli sensitize pain receptors so that once the brief period of injury is over, long-standing changes in the neurons maintain the pain postoperatively. Prevention of intraoperative pain transmission may reduce postoperative pain perception.[14]

CLINICAL MANIFESTATIONS

The clinical manifestations of postoperative pain vary. The intensity of pain depends on (1) the type of surgery (increased with abdominal, chest, spine, and joint surgery), (2) the psychological makeup (increased with anxiety, fear, uncertainty and helplessness) of the client, (3) the extent of preoperative preparation for anesthesia and surgery (increased intensity if no or little preparation), (4) the amount of intraoperative trauma, (5) the skill and expertise of the surgeon, (6) the presence of serious complications (increased with pneumonia, paralytic ileus, thrombophlebitis), and (7) the quality of postoperative care.[4]

Atelectasis, the most common complication after surgery, is most frequently the result of postoperative pain. Atelectasis results from the inhibition of breathing and the spasm of abdominal and thoracic muscles following abdominal or chest surgery. When alveoli collapse, inflation becomes increasingly difficult.[17] Pain limits deep breathing, coughing, and mobility, increasing the risk of other common postoperative complications, such as pneumonia and thrombophlebitis.

Pain increases anxiety and anxiety increases pain, creating a cycle of stress with muscle spasm and sympathetic stimulation. As a result, tachycardia and hypertension occur. Oxygen needs are increased, and sleep deprivation is common. Muscle tissue breakdown, suppression of the immune function, and delayed healing may occur. These effects and complications contribute to increased lengths of postoperative hospital stays.[17]

Low Back Pain (LBP)

Low back pain (LBP) is a common type of pain for which medical help is sought. Although often acute and related to sudden injury, it can become a chronic, lifelong problem with costs in physical, mental, social, and economic well-being.

ETIOLOGY AND PATHOPHYSIOLOGY

The most common cause of LBP is postural change associated with primary or secondary injury to supporting muscles and ligaments. Inadequate abdominal muscle tone transfers weight bearing from the anterior to the posterior structures of the spine, causing muscle spasm and LBP. Over time, postural discomfort gives way to herniated disks and myofascial pain.[5]

LBP also may be evidenced with many disorders due to pathology of muscles, tendons, joints, bones, disks, blood vessels, and lower abdominal organs. The nociceptive pain mechanism in many of the disorders involves injury such as tearing, rupture, or compression; acute and chronic inflammation with the production of pain-causing chemicals; and diseases or disorders associated with infection, calcification, bone loss, and degeneration. Table 35-2 lists many of the causes of low back pain and the physiologic changes responsible for pain.

The common denominator in many of the causes of LBP is the mechanism of inflammation—due to mechanical compression of the nerve root, irritation, abnormal contact between bone and nerve root, poor posture, or swelling. Nerves that are inflamed, swollen, or scarred exhibit electrical instability with low thresholds for depolarization, altered vascular permeability (leading to edema around the nerve fibers), sensitivity to mechanical stimulation, and increased impulse transmission.[6]

CLINICAL MANIFESTATIONS

The history, physical examination, and diagnostic test data are reviewed to elicit the cause. In many cases of acute injury, such as strain, sprain, or fracture, healing occurs with rest, support, and pain control. When underlying chronic conditions such as osteoporosis, osteoarthritis, or degenerative disc disease are present, low back pain remains a chronic problem. The various physiologic, psychological, social, and occupa-

TABLE 35-2

MULTIPLE ETIOLOGIES OF LOW BACK PAIN (LBP)

DISORDER	POSSIBLE ETIOLOGY
MUSCULOTENDINOUS DISORDERS	
Acute musculotendinous strains	Muscle tears, hemorrhage, inflammation
Acute lumbosacral sprains	Tears of supporting ligaments of spine
Fibromyalgia syndrome	Possible muscle changes
Myofascial pain syndrome	Pain of unknown pathophysiology
ARTICULAR DISORDERS	
Ankylosing spondylitis	Spinal inflammation, ligament calcification
Rheumatoid arthritis	Multiple joint inflammation
Reiter's spondyloarthropathy	Joint, conjunctival, urethral inflammation
Psoriatic arthritis	Joint inflammation, psoriasis
ARTERIAL DISORDERS	
Osteoarthritis of spine	Spinal degeneration, nerve impingement
Diffuse idiopathic skeletal hyperostosis	Calcification, osteophytes
Lumbar spondylosis	Degenerative osteoarthritis
Degenerative disk disorder	Bulging of disks
Facet syndrome	Degenerative osteoarthritis, hypermobility
Spondylolisthesis	Subluxation of vertebral body
Scoliosis	Curvature of spine
LBP WITH NEURAL IMPINGEMENT	
Herniated disk	Nerve root compression
Lumbar spondylosis with spinal stenosis	Degeneration, spinal cord compression
Piriformis syndrome	Compression neuropathy
Epidural abscess, hematoma	Infection, pressure on spinal cord
BONE	
Osteoporosis with compression fracture	Degeneration, trauma
Osteomalacia	Loss of bone mineral to bone mass
Paget's disease of bone	Bone resorption, irregular new bone form
Osteomyelitis of vertebra	Vertebral infection
Spinal column tumors	Tumor growth
Multiple myeloma	Tumor of bone marrow, bone destruction
VASCULAR	
Abdominal aortic aneurysm	Pressure of mass
PELVIC/RETROPERITONEAL	
Endometriosis	Growth, change in endometrial tissue—colon
Prostatitis	Inflammation, infection

(Johnson, E. R. & Ugalde, V. [1998]. Low back pain: Diagnosis and management. In M. E. Gershwin & M. E. Hamilton [Eds.], *The pain management handbook*. Totowa, NJ: Humana Press.)

tional effects of low back pain make its assessment challenging.

LBP may be associated with nervous, muscular, skeletal, and vascular system dysfunction and result in problems with walking, bending, and activities of daily living. Structural or postural abnormalities, muscle spasm, or scars may be noted on inspection. Range-of-motion restriction or provocation of leg pain with flexion of the lumbar spine or back pain with rotation or extension of the spine may be noted. Tension of the nerve roots may be indicated by radicular pain on coughing or sneezing or by the reproduction of leg or buttock pain with straight leg raising. When leg pain occurs in the symptomatic leg with straight leg raising of the normal leg, a prolapsed disk may be the cause. Sciatic pain may be elicited by dorsiflexion of the foot. Muscle wasting and diminished strength may be seen with flexion of the hips (L1, L2 roots), knees (L5, S1, S2 roots), and ankles (plantar S1 root; dorsiflexion L4, L5 roots) and with extension of the knees (L3, L4 roots) and big toes (L5, S1 roots). Patellar reflexes and ankle reflexes indicate intact L3/L4 and S1/S2 nerve roots, respectively. Sensation to cotton wool or pinprick may indicate locations deficient in touch or hyperalgesia.[12]

The "red flags" requiring immediate attention in persons suffering with low back pain include: (1) progressive neurologic deficits (with central disk herniation), (2) onset of bowel or bladder control problems, (3) back pain that increases in the supine position, (4) fever and chills along with LBP, and (5) a history of cancer, recent intravenous drug use, or immunosuppression.[27] Because of the poor correlation between diagnostic imaging results and symptoms, a large number of people with LBP are not given a definitive diagnosis.

A psychosocial evaluation may help to uncover the interdependence between the pain and sense of individual, marital, and family functioning and sense of well-being. Pain changes the functioning of the family system, and the family system can have a positive or negative impact on the pain experience.

If LBP is considered psychogenic, specific characteristics described by Hackett and Bouckoms are seen.[15] The mnemonic "MADISON" is used to identify these findings (Box 35-2).

Headache

Headaches are common phenomena that may result from stimuli inside or outside of the cranium.

MIGRAINE HEADACHES

In the United States, 18% of females and 6% of males report migraine headaches.[24]

Etiology and Pathophysiology

Migraine headaches are caused by vasodilatation of the dura mater. One vascular theory proposes that the vasodilatation results from arterial spasm in the brain stem and the production of vasoconstricting serotonin (by the aggregation of platelets). An aura may occur from reductions in cerebral blood and oxygen supply. Homeostatic changes occur that will counteract the vasoconstriction and cause the vasodilatation—experienced as a headache. Another neurologic theory involves the trigeminal innervation of the CNS. The ophthalmic branch of the trigeminal nerve receives a pain signal from the dura mater and the blood vessels. The pain impulse travels to the thalamus. Substance P and/or calcitonin-gene-related peptide are released from the nerve fibers, causing cerebral vasodilatation and inflammation of the dura mater. The inflammation triggers the migraine pain, and the aura ends with the increase in blood flow.[24]

Migraine triggers vary among people who get this type of headache. Environmental triggers include emotional upset, excess or lack of sleep, changes in estrogen levels during the menstrual cycle, air pollution (including smoke, perfume, pesticides, and other airborne substances), and dietary factors (red wine, beer, chocolate, MSG, caffeine, and skipping meals). Severe, long, and frequent migraines have been associated with ovulation, the menstrual cycle, and pregnancy.[9]

Clinical Manifestations

Migraine headaches are of two different types: (1) classic and (2) common. *Classic* migraine headaches are preceded by an aura (seeing a flashing light or zigzag lines or a temporary loss of vision) within 30 minutes of the headache. Weakness in the extremities, tingling of the face or hands, and confusion may occur along with other transient sensory or motor symptoms before the headache begins. The headache is usually described as pulsating, throbbing, or pounding pain that starts on one side of the head (forehead, temple, ear, eye) and then spreads to the other side over 24 to 48 hours. The headache is often accompanied by nausea, vomiting, photophobia, and phonophobia.[22]

Common migraine headaches are characterized by the absence of an aura. Sufferers may have confusion, mood changes, fatigue, or fluid retention before the headache. The headache may be located either unilaterally or bilaterally in the frontal or temporal areas of the head. Diarrhea, nausea, vomiting, and increased urination may occur over the 3 to 4 days of the attack.[22]

TENSION-TYPE HEADACHES

Tension-type headaches are very common, occurring in 68% of all men and 88% of women. The frequency of tension headaches decreases with aging.

BOX 35-2 PSYCHOGENIC LOW BACK PAIN CHARACTERISTICS

M ultiplicity of pain
A uthenticity—efforts to prove symptoms are real
D enial of stress or problems that could account for problem
I nterpersonal variability—symptoms change with different audiences
S ingularity—their pain is the worst ever
O nly effective medical help is from your kind, intelligent care
N othing in the past has helped

(Hackett, T. P. & Bouckoms, A. [1987]. The pain patient: Evaluation and treatment. In T. P. Hackett & N. H. Cassem [Eds.] *Massachusetts General Hospital handbook of general hospital psychiatry* [2nd ed.]. Littleton, MA: PSG Publishing.)

Etiology and Pathophysiology

Stress, eyestrain, frustration, or poor posture may trigger episodic tension headaches and chronic tension headaches. These triggers cause muscular contraction in the neck, face, and scalp. Muscle spasm with resultant extracranial vasoconstriction may stimulate the pain receptors in the brain, leading to headache.[28]

Clinical Manifestations

Both episodic and chronic tension headaches produce bilateral, mild- to moderate-intensity, constricting or pressing pain in the occipital, frontal, temporal or upper neck areas. The pain is most common on awakening or shortly after and changes in severity during the episode. Episodic tension-type headaches typically occur less than 15 days per month, lasting from 30 minutes to 7 days each time; phonophobia or photophobia may occur. Chronic tension-type headaches occur more than 15 days per month; nausea, photophobia, or phonophobia may be associated.[25]

CLUSTER HEADACHES

Cluster headaches, most common in men and often beginning in the late twenties, occur most frequently in a series during a 2- to 3-month period in spring or fall every 1 to 2 years. Episodic cluster headaches occur very easily and are followed by a headache-free period, whereas chronic cluster headaches continue without remission or with only a brief break of less than 14 days.[25]

Pathophysiology

The underlying changes thought to produce cluster headaches involve the biologic clock and the neurotransmitter serotonin. Two small cell groups in the anterior hypothalamus called the suprachiasmatic nuclei (SCN) generate the 24-hour circadian rhythm. The SCN has a visual pathway linked to the retina to allow it to receive the light and dark stimuli needed for rhythm generation. The SCN is also connected with the pain-modulating midbrain (which releases serotonin). When serotonin release is altered or fluctuates, the circadian rhythm is disrupted, potentially causing cluster headaches and illnesses related to hormonal, body temperature, and other circadian-regulated activities. The exact pathophysiologic mechanisms in cluster headaches are under study. Research and the use of blood flow studies have discounted the role of vascular dilatation in causing cluster headaches.[25]

Clinical Manifestations

The pain of cluster headaches is described as unilateral, burning, and/or stabbing, located behind or around the eye and radiating to the temple, jaw, chin, or teeth. Histamine release causes nasal congestion, lacrimation, and facial flushing.[8] During spring and fall, cluster headaches can occur as multiple attacks each day—most often at night, when the severity of the pain interrupts sleep.

FOCUS ON THE PERSON WITH LOW BACK PAIN

J. J. is a 42-year-old nurse, wife, and mother of three children, ages 10 to 15. Seven years ago, while reaching for a box of patient teaching materials, J. J. twisted at the waist and felt excruciating pain in her low back and down her right leg. At the time of the injury, she broke out in a sweat and felt as if she was going to "pass out." The sharp pain shooting down her right leg was accompanied by severe spasm of her back muscles, making it difficult to move, sit, or bend. Leg and low back edema accompanied the continuing drilling pain.

In the days following her injury, the pain remained severe despite rest, ibuprofen, and diazepam. Following a series of diagnostic tests, it was determined that J. J. had herniated L4–L5 and L5–S1. She was hospitalized, placed in traction, and given pain medication. A diskectomy was performed at the sites of herniation. Within a year after surgery, sciatic pain continued related to additional herniation and the presence of scar tissue. Over the last 3 years, low back pain has increased. J. J. had to change her job and home responsibilities to manage her pain and to prevent increasing spasm. She used hydrotherapy for relaxation, exercise, and massage. Work responsibilities provided diversion from the chronic pain. Pain control with long-acting oxycodone (Oxycontin) (with immediate-acting oxycodone for breakthrough pain) enabled J. J. to remain functional and maintain social relationships with her family and friends—until now. The severe aching pain and its effects were threatening even the most basic activities of living. J. J. was left feeling helpless, tired, and hopeless.

Questions

1. Describe the alterations in cellular, tissue, organ, and system functioning that occurred at the time of injury.
2. Discuss the pathophysiologic mechanisms underlying J. J.'s chronic pain.
3. Explain how the endogenous opioid system modulates pain. What might be a possible explanation for this system not providing significant pain modulation in J. J.'s case?
4. Using the gate control theory of pain, explain how transelectrical nerve stimulation (TENS) may be used to relieve J. J.'s pain.

REFERENCES

1. Agency for Health Care Policy and Research (AHCPR) (1992). *Clinical practice guideline: Acute pain management: Operative or medical procedures and trauma.* Rockville, MD: U.S. Department of Health and Human Services.
2. Agency for Health Care Policy and Research (AHCPR) (1994). *Clinical practice health guideline: Management of cancer pain.* Rockville, MD: U.S. Department of Health and Human Services.
3. American Psychological Association. (1994). *Diagnostic and statistical manual of mental disorders* (4th ed.). Washington, DC: American Psychological Association.
4. Bonica, J. (1990). *The management of pain* (2nd ed.). Philadelphia: Lea & Febiger.
5. Caillet, R. (1977). Low back pain. In R. Caillet (Ed.), *Soft tissue pain and disability.* Philadelphia: F. A. Davis.
6. Calder, T. M. & Rowlingson, J. C. (1996). Low back pain. In P. P. Raj, *Pain medicine: A comprehensive review.* St. Louis: Mosby.
7. Cleland, C. & Gebhart, G. (1997). Principles of nociception and pain. *In Expert pain management.* Springhouse, PA: Springhouse Corporation.
8. Cluster headache symptoms, *http://www.bhs.berkeley.k12.ca.us/departments/Science/anatom*, 1998.
9. Environmental trigger, *http://www.bhs.berkeley.k12.ca.us/departments/Science/anatom*, 1998.
10. Fine, P. G. & Ashburn, M. A. (1998). Functional neuroanatomy and nociception. In M. A. Ashburn & L. J. Rice, *The management of pain.* New York: Churchill Livingstone.
11. Ganong, W. (1997). *Review of medical physiology* (18th ed.). Norwalk, CT: Appleton & Lange.
12. Grady, K. M. & Severn, A. M. (1997). *Key topics in chronic pain.* Oxford, UK: BIOS Scientific Publishers.
13. Gupta, R. & Staats, P. S. (1997). Diagnostic tools in the management of pain. In *Expert pain management.* Springhouse, PA: Springhouse Corporation.
14. Hacobian, A. & Warfield, C. A. (1997). Management of acute pain. In *Expert pain management.* Springhouse, PA: Springhouse Corporation.
15. Hackett T. P. & Bouckoms, A. (1987). The pain patient: Evaluation and treatment. In T. P. Hackett & N. H. Cassem (Eds.), *Massachusetts General Hospital handbook of general hospital psychiatry* (2nd ed.). Littleton, MA: PSG Publishing.
16. Hejtmanik, J. (1995). Vision. In P. Conn, *Neuroscience In medicine.* Philadelphia: Lippincott.
17. Hough, A. The management of postoperative pain. In P. E. Wells, V. Frampton, & D. Bowsher (Eds.), *Pain management by physical therapy* (2nd ed.). Oxford, UK: Butterworth-Heinemann.
18. Kingdon, R. T., Stanley, K. J. & Kizior, R. J. (1998). *Handbook for pain management.* Philadelphia: W.B. Saunders.
19. Lavies, N. (1992). Identification of patient, medical and nursing staff attitudes to postoperative opioid analgesia. *Pain, 48,* 313–319.
20. Melzack, R. & Wall, P. (1965). Pain mechanisms: A new theory. *Science, 15,* 971–979.
21. Merskey, H. & Bogduk, N. (1994). *Classification of chronic pain: Descriptions of chronic pain syndromes and definitions of pain terms* (2nd ed.). Seattle: IASP Press.
22. Migraine headache symptoms, *http://www.bhs.berkeley.k12.ca.us/departments/Science/anatom*, 1998.
23. Nowak, T. & Handford, A. (1994). *Essentials of pathophysiology.* Dubuque, IA: Wm. C. Brown Publishers.
24. Parent, A. (1996). *Carpenter's human anatomy* (9th ed.). Baltimore: Williams & Wilkins.
25. Pathology of cluster headache, *http://www.bhs.berkeley.k12.ca.us/departments/Science/anatom*, 1998.
26. Raj, P. P. (1996). Pain mechanisms. In P. P. Raj, *Pain medicine: A comprehensive review.* St. Louis: Mosby.
27. Richeimer, S. H. (1998). The assessment of the patient with pain. In M. E. Gershwin & M. E. Hamilton (Eds.), *The pain management handbook.* Totowa, NJ: Humana Press.
28. Tension-type headache symptoms, *http://www.bhs.berkeley.k12.ca.us/departments/Science/anatom*, 1998.
29. Verhaak, P., Kerssens, J., Dekker, J., Sorbi, M., & Bensing, J. (1998). Prevalence of chronic benign pain disorder among adults: A review of the literature. *Pain, 77,* 231–239.
30. Woolf, C. J. (1998). Towards a mechanism-based classification of pain? *Pain, 77,* 227–229.

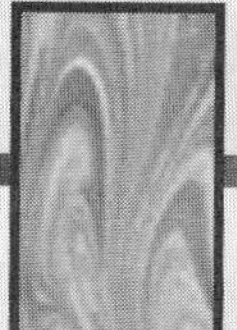

UNIT 11: CASE STUDY

The Patient Presenting With a Headache

Introduction to the Patient

A. B. is a 28-year-old white female who has sought medical attention complaining of a severe throbbing headache since arising this morning, approximately 12 hours ago. She also reports seeing flashes of lights immediately prior to the onset of the headache.

Present Illness

Ms. B. awoke this morning feeling fine. Shortly after arising, she remembers seeing flashes of light. She also noticed some numbness and tingling in her hands and weakness in her legs. Approximately ½ hour later, the headache began, initially located at the right temporal area but now beginning to spread to the other side. She describes the headache as "pounding and throbbing" and "the most severe headache" she's ever had. She also reports some nausea, vomiting, sensitivity to light, and a feeling of spinning. A. B. has taken acetaminophen, 2 tabs (1 gm) orally every 4 hours without relief.

Social History

Ms. B. is married with two young children, ages 4 and 6 years. She works full time as a nursing assistant in a long-term care facility and is currently enrolled in a nursing program, part-time, attending classes two evenings a week and on Saturdays. Her husband is a self-employed carpenter who helps out with child care and meal preparation. Ms. B. states that her husband "brought home Chinese food for dinner last night." She denies any history of tobacco or recreational drug use but does engage in social drinking. She reports having had two glasses of red wine last night with dinner after returning home from her classes. A. B. drinks decaffeinated beverages, stating, "I don't want to be up all night."

Past Medical History

Ms. B. states that she is in fairly good health with only one or two colds over the past year. She reports a history of headaches for many years, similar to this episode. Usually she takes acetaminophen every 4 hours with relief. The headaches typically disappear in approximately 24 hours. She states that she has studied about headaches recently in her nursing course and decided that it would be prudent to "check this out."

A. B. denies any menstrual or urinary tract problems. Her menstrual cycles are regular, occurring every 29 days without complaints of dysmenorrhea. Her last menstrual period was 6 days ago. She takes no prescription medications at present. Currently, she is taking only acetaminophen for her headache relief.

Family History

Ms. B. is the youngest of three children. She has one brother and one sister. Both are alive and well. Her mother and grandmother have a history of migraine headaches. Ms. B.'s husband and children are relatively well, except for the occasional cold or sore throat.

Physical Examination

A. B. is a thin woman who appears pale, diaphoretic, and very irritable, stating, "This pain is terrible." She is oriented to person, place, and time. Her vital signs are as follows: temperature—98.4°F; pulse—100 and regular; respirations—24; blood pressure—140/86. Lungs are clear to auscultation. Skin pale, cool, and damp. Scalp tender bilaterally at both temples. Temporal pulses palpable and bounding. During the examination, she complains of nausea and vomits approximately 75 ccs of yellowish-brown liquid material. Eyes swollen, reddened, and tearing; stating that "the light hurts her eyes."

Neurologic assessment within normal limits except for complaints of slight tingling in hands, which has improved since the headache began. PERRLA. Nuchal rigidity is absent. Fundoscopic examination reveals a normal optic disc and retinal vessels without evidence of hemorrhage or exudates.

Diagnostic Tests

Skull x-ray and computed tomography within normal limits; complete blood count, urinalysis, and serum electrolyte levels normal.

CRITICAL THINKING QUESTIONS

1. Analyze the case study for features that might lead you to suspect migraine headache.
2. Propose possible events that may have triggered Ms. B.'s headache.
3. Create a chart highlighting the major pharmacologic agents used for treating this acute attack and

for preventing future attacks. Include drug name, indication and action, drug dosage and route, possible adverse effects, and nursing implications.

4. Identify the priorities of care for A. B. and suggest possible measures to address these priorities.
5. Develop a patient teaching checklist for A. B. to reduce the risk of future attacks.

Besides your pathophysiology text, you'll need a good pharmacology text, a neurology text, a pain management text, and current research to complete this case study. Suggested references follow:

Genzen, J. R. (1998). The internet and migraine: Headache resources for patients and physicians. *Headache, 38*(4), 312–314.

Hickey, J. (1997). *Neurological and neurosurgical nursing* (4th ed). Philadelphia: Lippincott-Raven.

Karch, A. M. (1999). *1999 Lippincott's nursing drug guide.* Philadelphia: Lippincott-Raven.

McCaffery, M. (1999). *Pain: Clinical manual* (2nd ed.). St. Louis: Mosby–Year Book.

Sherman, R. A. (1998). Initial exploration of pursuing electromagnetic fields for treatment of migraine. *Headache, 38*(3), 208–213.

Smeltzer, S. & Bare, B. (2000). *Brunner and Suddarth's textbook of medical-surgical nursing* (9th ed.). Philadelphia: Lippincott Williams & Wilkins.

Smith, R. (1997). Diagnosing headache. *Hospital Medicine, 33*(7), 26–28, 33–34, 36, 38, 41–42.

Smith, R. (1997). Treating headache. *Hospital Medicine, 33*(9), 13–16, 21–22, 24, 27–28.

Wilson, J. R., Foresman, B. H., Gamber, R. G., & Wright, T. (1998). Hyperbaric oxygen in the treatment of migraine with aura. *Headache, 38*(2), 112–115.

Website resources:

American Council for Headache Education *http://www.achenet.org*

Migraine: What it is and where we are in understanding it

http://www.ion.bpmf.ac/uk~headache/migraine.html

How to identify and eliminate migraine triggers *http://www.perlhealth.com/chap_14.htm*

JAMA Migraine Information Center *http://www.ama-assn.org/special/migraine/migraine.htm*

UNIT 11 APPENDIX A

DIAGNOSTIC TESTS

TEST	PURPOSE/ NORMAL FINDINGS	SIGNIFICANCE
EYE		
Visual acuity	The standard and routine method for determining clarity of the cornea, lens, and vitreous humor and function of the visual pathways form the retina to the brain Eye chart placed at a distance of 20 feet from patient; with both eyes open and one eye covered, each line of chart read until print can no longer be distinguished Acuity expressed as ratio of 20 (relates to distance person with normal vision can see from a distance of 20 feet) to the number of the line read (relates to what the patient can see from a distance of 20 feet) Normal visual acuity: 20/20	Acuity less than 20/20 when corrected with glasses requires patient referral to ophthalmologist. Normal visual acuity does not ensure a disease-free visual system. Myopia is present when the bottom number is larger than the top number; the larger the bottom number, the poorer the vision. Acuity of 20/200 is considered the boundary of legal blindness.
Ophthalmoscopy	Direct inspection of the structures posterior to the iris, providing a detailed view of the internal eye Normal findings: • Red reflex normally easily visible, round with regular borders • Optic disc round to oval with sharp, defined borders; nasal edge possibly blurred • Normally creamy yellow-orange to pink in color, approximately 1.5 mm in diameter • Physiologic cup is slightly depressed and lighter in color than disc; ring or crescents possible around border of disc • Retinal vessels (four sets of each-arterioles and venules) seen passing through optic disc • Arterioles bright red, becoming progressively smaller in diameter as they move away from optic disc • Venules appearing darker red and larger than arterioles, becoming progressively smaller in diameter as they move away from the disc • Retina variable in color from light red-orange to dark brown or gray, depending on the patient's skin color • Anterior chamber translucent	Room should be darkened to help with pupil dilation. Eye drops may be necessary to dilate pupils. Black spots against the background of the red reflex indicate cataracts. Swollen optic disc, blurred margins, hyperemic-appearing with more visible and numerous disc vessels and lack of physiologic cup indicates papilledema, possibly resulting from hypertension or increased intracranial pressure. Enlarged physiologic cup (more than ½ the disc's diameter) with pale background and obscured or displaced retinal vessels signifies glaucoma. White optic disc with lack of vessels suggests optic atrophy caused by death of optic nerve fibers. Widening of arterioles and a copper coloring is seen with hypertension early on. Thickening with opaque or silver-colored arterioles suggests long-standing hypertension. Arterial wall nicking, tapering, and banking may be seen with hypertension or arteriosclerosis. Soft or hard exudate appearing as light-colored spots on retinal background may indicate diabetes or hypertension. Red spots or streaks on the retinal background may suggest hemorrhage and microaneurysms. Hyphema secondary to trauma may occur as red blood cells settle in the lower half of the anterior chamber. A cloudy appearance in front of the iris secondary to hypopyon (accumulation of

(continued)

UNIT 11 APPENDIX A

DIAGNOSTIC TESTS (Continued)

TEST	PURPOSE/ NORMAL FINDINGS	SIGNIFICANCE
	• Macula, darker area one disc diameter in size, located to the temporal side of the optic disc • Fovea appearing as "starlike" light reflex	white blood cells in the anterior chamber) is indicative of an inflammatory reaction. Clumping pigmentation suggests detached retina or retinal injury.
Tonometry	Technique for measuring intraocular pressure (IOP) using calibrated instruments that indent or flatten the corneal apex Normal pressure range for each eye: 8 to 21 mm Hg recorded as a fraction (right eye pressure/left eye pressure)	Increased IOP is the cardinal sign of glaucoma.
Slit lamp examination	Test to illuminate and examine in detail the anterior segment of the eye (including eyelids, eyelashes, conjunctiva, sclera, cornea, tear film, anterior chamber, iris, lens, and vitreous) under magnification Fluorescein stain necessary if corneal or conjunctival abnormalities suspected Normal findings: fluids and tissues appearing translucent or nearly translucent	Early-stage lens opacities may suggest cataracts. Absorption of stain is increased in areas with surface defects, such as corneal abrasions and ulcers, iritis, and conjunctivitis.
Visual evoked response	Test of visual pathway function, measuring the change in the eye's electrical potential Electrical response in the visual cortex of the occiput from visual stimulation recorded by electrodes placed on the vertex and occipital lobes. Normal findings: first major positive peak ([absolute latency]) P 100) ranging from 89–114 milliseconds (msec)	Abnormalities suggest lesions of the optic nerve, optic tract, or visual cortex.
Fluorescein angiography	Photographs of fundus taken in rapid succession after intravenous injection of contrast medium (fluorescein) to allow visualization of the microvascular structures of the retina and choroid, including blood vessel appearance and retinal circulation Normal findings: • Filling phase: 12 to 15 seconds • Choroidal flush: evidenced as evenly mottled appearance • Arterial phase: evidenced with filling of the arteries • Arteriovenous phase: evidenced with complete arterial and capillary filling and beginning of venous filling • Venous phase: evidenced by arterial emptying with venous filling and emptying • Recirculation phase: 30–60 minutes after injection of dye; dye barely detectable in vessels • No leakage from retinal vessels	Abnormalities indicate retinal vascular disorders. Abnormalities of filling phase suggest microaneurysms, arteriovenous shunts, or neovascularization. Delayed or absent flow through arteries is possible evidence of arterial occlusion. Vessel dilation or leakage is possible with venous occlusion. Increased vascular tortuosity and areas of nonperfusion may suggest hypertensive retinopathy. Leakage of dye with hard yellow exudate may indicate aneurysm or capillary hemangioma. Vascular leakage in disc area suggests papilledema.

UNIT 11 APPENDIX A

DIAGNOSTIC TESTS (Continued)

TEST	PURPOSE/ NORMAL FINDINGS	SIGNIFICANCE
Orbital imaging (CT or MRI)	Visualization of abnormalities not readily seen on routine x-ray; providing a three-dimensional image of orbital structures, including ocular muscles and optic nerve, with or without use of contrast medium Normal findings: • Marked contrast of dense orbital bone • Clearly defined optic nerve and lateral rectus muscle • Optic canals equal in size	Orbital enlargement, indentation of orbital walls, bone density, or inability to identify orbital structures suggests intra- or extra-orbital space-occupying lesions. Irregular density areas indicate infiltrative lesions. Clearly defined masses of consistent density suggest encapsulated tumors. Thickening of optic tract suggests gliomas, meningiomas, or secondary tumors. Irregularity in bone structure may indicate fracture.
Ocular ultrasonography	Measurement of high-frequency sound wave transmission through the eye as the waves are reflected from the ocular structures • A scan: echoes converted to waveforms with crests denoting the positions of different structures; helps to differentiate benign and malignant tumors and monitor congenital glaucoma • B scan: echoes converted into dots forming a cross-sectional image of ocular structures; helps to identify structures that may be blocked by hemorrhage, cataract, or other opacities Normal findings: • Characteristic image formation of optic nerve and posterior lens capsule • Smooth, concave, curved appearance of posterior eye wall • No echoes evidenced by lens or vitreous	Degree of density of image denotes hemorrhage in vitreous. Dense sheetlike echo on B scan suggests retinal detachment. Size, shape, location, and texture of tumors can be identified.
EAR		
Otoscopy	Direct visualization of external auditory canal and tympanic membrane Normal findings: • Small amount of odorless cerumen varying in color (yellow, orange, red, brown, gray, or black) and consistency (soft, moist, dry, flaky, or hard) • Canal walls pink and smooth without nodules	Foul-smelling, sticky, yellow discharge suggests otitis externa or impacted foreign body. Bloody, purulent discharge may indicate otitis media if the tympanic membrane has ruptured. Bloody or watery drainage may indicate cerebrospinal fluid secondary to trauma. Reddened, swollen canals suggest otitis externa.
	• Tympanic membrane slightly concave, smooth, intact; appears pearly, gray, shiny, and translucent without bulging or retraction • Light reflection at 5 and 7 o'clock in right and left ear, respectively • Landmarks clearly visible • Fluttering of center of tympanic membrane with Valsalva maneuver	Red, bulging membrane suggests acute otitis media. Yellowish, bulging membrane with bubbles implies serous otitis media. Whit spots suggest scarring from infection. Diminished or absent light reflex is typical of otitis media. Increase prominence of landmarks may suggest obstructed eustachian tube.

(continued)

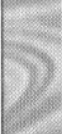

UNIT 11 APPENDIX A

DIAGNOSTIC TESTS (Continued)

TEST	PURPOSE/ NORMAL FINDINGS	SIGNIFICANCE
		Diminished or absent landmarks may suggest chronic otitis media. Decreased mobility is seen with areas involving healed perforations. Absent mobility suggests pus or fluid in middle ear or a blocked eustachian tube.
Pure tone audiometry	Measurement of the lowest intensity levels at which a person can hear sounds through earphones or bone conduction vibrator Normal finding: average intensity heard of 0–25 dB	Soundproof room is necessary for accurate results. Normal results do not ensure absence of pathology. Levels of 26 to 40 dB indicate mild hearing loss. Levels of 41 to 55 dB indicate moderate hearing loss. Levels of 56 to 70 dB indicate moderately severe hearing loss. Levels of 71 to 90 dB indicate severe hearing loss. Levels of 91 or more dB indicate profound hearing loss.
Tympanography	Measurement of the flow of sound into the ear and responses to change in air pressure in a sealed ear canal as an indication of middle ear muscle reflex function and compliance of tympanic membrane Normal findings: middle ear pressure range of ± 100daPa with a smooth symmetric waveform shape	Flat tympanogram reflects no changes in response to air pressure, suggesting fluid in middle ear, perforated eardrum, or impacted cerumen. Increased amplitude of the waveform suggests an eardrum abnormality or discontinuity of the ossicles. Decreased amplitude may indicate fixation of the ossicles or serous otitis media.
Electronystagmography (ENG)	Graphic recording and measurement of changes in the electrical potential resulting from eye movements in response to specific stimuli (such as looking at different objects, opening and closing eyes, changing positions, or instillation of air or warm or cold water) to evaluate the vestibulo-ocular reflex Normal findings: • Vestibulo-ocular reflex normal • Expected nystagmus accompanying head movement	Abnormal results are classified as indicating a peripheral, central, or undetermined lesion. • Peripheral lesion may involve the end organ or vestibular branch of the 8th cranial nerve. • Central lesion may involve the brain stem, cerebellum, cerebrum, or any of the communicating structures.
Auditory brain stem response (ABR)	Objective measure of hearing that evaluates the response of the 8th cranial nerve and ascending auditory pathways through electrophysiologic potentials produced from sound stimulation Normal findings (first 5 waveforms measured in milliseconds at a sound stimulation rate of 11 clicks/second): average range • Wave I: 1.7 msec • Wave II: 2.8 msec • Wave III: 3.9 msec • Wave IV: 5.1 msec • Wave V: 5.7 msec	Abnormal ABRs suggest possible acoustic neuroma, cerebrovascular accident, multiple sclerosis, or a lesion affecting any portion of the nerve or brain stem.

UNIT BIBLIOGRAPHY

Adams, R., Victor, M. & Ropper, A. (1997). *Principles of neurology* (6th ed.). New York: McGraw-Hill.

Bartoshuk, L. (1989). The functions of taste and olfaction. *Annals of the New York Academy of Science, 575,* 353–361.

Fauci, A. S., et al. (Eds.)(1997). *Harrison's principles of internal medicine* (14th ed.). New York: McGraw-Hill.

Gilman, S. & Newman, S. (1996). *Manter and Gatz's essentials of clinical neuroanatomy and neurophysiology* (9th ed.). Philadelphia: F.A. Davis.

Guyton, A, & Hall, J. (1996). *Textbook of medical physiology* (9th ed.). Philadelphia: W.B. Saunders.

Parent, A. (1996). *Carpenter's human anatomy* (9th ed.). Baltimore: Williams & Wilkins.

Rubin, E., & Farber, J. L. (1999). *Pathology* (3rd ed.). Philadelphia: Lippincott Willliams & Wilkins.

EYE

Albert D. M., & Jakobiec F. A., (Eds.)(1994). *Principles and practice of ophthalmology: Clinical practice,* vols. 1–5. Philadelphia: W.B. Saunders.

Boyd-Monk, H., & Steinmetz, C. G. (1987). *Nursing care of the eye.* Norwalk, CT Appleton & Lange.

Brow, A. J., Tripathi, R. C., & Tripathi, B. J. (1997). *Wolff's anatomy of the eye and orbit.* London: Chapman & Hall Medical.

Corn, B., & Koenig, A. (Eds.)(1996). *Foundations of low Vision.* New York: AFB Press, American Foundation for the Blind.

Cullom, Jr., R. D., & Chang, B. (1999). *The Wills eye manual: Office and emergency room diagnosis and treatment of eye disease* (3rd ed.) Philadelphia: Lippincott Williams & Wilkins.

Fishkind, W. J. (1998). A better way to assess cataract patients. *Review of Ophthalmology, 5*(3), 59–66.

Glaucoma Research Foundation (1996). *Understanding and living with glaucoma: A reference guide for people with glaucoma and their families.* San Francisco, CA: Glaucoma Research Foundation.

Goldblum, K. (1997). *Core curriculum for ophthalmic nursing.* Dubuque, IA: Kendall/Hunt.

Kanski, J. J. (1994). *Clinical ophthalmology.* Oxford: Butterworth-Heinemann Ltd.

Kanski, J., McAllister, J., & Salmon, J. (1996). *Glaucoma: A color manual of diagnosis and treatment.* Oxford: Butterworth-Heinemann Ltd.

Leibowitz, H. M., & Waring, III, G. O. (1998). *Corneal disorders: Clinical diagnosis and management.* Philadelphia: W.B. Saunders.

Margolis, S., & Schachat, A. P. (1998). *Vision disorders.* The Johns Hopkins White Papers. New York: Medletter Associates, Inc.

Moore, J. E., Graves, W., & Patterson, J. B.(Eds.) (1997). *Foundations of rehabilitation counseling with persons who are blind or visually impaired.* New York: AFB Press, American Foundation for the Blind

Orticio, L. (1994). Do perceptions of blindness affect care? *Journal of Ophthalmic Nursing and Technology, 13*(4), 172–179.

Ritch, R., Shields, M., & Krupin, T. (1996). *The glaucomas: Clinical science, vols.* 1–111. Salem, MA: Mosby.

Rootman, J., & Chang, K. W. (1998). *Diseases of the orbit.* Philadelphia: Lippincott, Raven.

Scientific American. (1998). *Sciences vision: The mechanics of sight.*

Shields, G. (1998). *Textbook of glaucoma.* Baltimore: Williams & Wilkins.

Snell, R. S., & Lemp, M. A. (1998). *Clinical anatomy of the eye* (2nd ed.). Melbourne, Australia: Blackwell Science.

Varma, R. (1997). *Essentials of eye care: The Johns Hopkins Wilmer handbook.* Philadelphia: Lippincott-Raven.

Vaughn, D. G., Asbury, T., & Riorda-Eva, P. (Eds.)(1995). *General ophthalmology.* Stamford, CT: Appleton & Lange.

Wright, K. (Ed)(1997). *Textbook of ophthalmology.* Baltimore: Williams & Wilkins.

EAR

Blitzer, A. et al. (Eds.) (1998). *Office-based surgery in otolaryngology.* New York: Thieme Medical Publishers.

Cohen, H. Rubin, A. M. & Gombash, L. (1992). The team approach to treatment of the dizzy patient. *Archives of Physical Medicine and Rehabilitation, 73*(8), 703–708.

Cummings, C. W. et al. (1998). *Otolaryngology—head and neck surgery.* St. Louis: C.V. Mosby.

Meyerhoff, W. L. & Rice, D. H. (1992). *Otolaryngology—head and neck surgery.* Philadelphia: W.B. Saunders.

National Institutes of Health (1991). *NIH Consensus Development Conference Statement. Acoustic neuroma.* Dec 11–13, 9(4).

Paparella, M. M. et al. (1991). *Otolaryngology, vol. 2: Otology and neuro-otology.* Philadelphia: W.B. Saunders.

Pollock, K. J. (1995). Meniere's disease: A review of the problem. *ORL—Head and Neck Nursing, 13*(2),10–13.

Siglen, B. A. & Schuring, L. T. (1993). *Ear, nose, and throat disorders—Mosby's Clinical Nursing Series.* St. Louis: C.V. Mosby.

Society of Otorhinolaryngology—Head and Neck Nurses, Inc. (1994). *Nursing practice guidelines for care of the otorhinolaryngology—head and neck patient.* New Smyrna Beach, FL: Author.

PAIN

Agency for Health Care Policy and Research (AHCPR). (1992). *Clinical practice guideline: Acute pain management: Operative or medical procedures and trauma.* Rockville, MD: U.S. Department of Health and Human Services.

American Pain Society (1999). *Principles of analgesic use in the treatment of acute pain and chronic cancer pain: A concise guide to medical practice* (4th ed.). Skokie, IL: Author.

Ashburn, M. A. & Rice, L. J. (1998). *The management of pain.* New York: Churchill Livingstone.

Faucett, J. A., & Levine, J. D. (1991). The contribution of interpersonal conflict to chronic pain in the presence or absence of organic pathology. *Pain, 44,* 35–43, 130–141.

Ferrell, B. R. (Ed.)(1996). *Suffering.* Boston: Jones & Bartlett.

Gagliese, L., & Melzack, R. (1997). Chronic pain in elderly people. *Pain, 70*(1), 3–14.

Gershwin, M. E. & Hamilton, M. E. (Eds.)(1998). *The pain management handbook.* Totowa, NJ: Humana Press.

Kingdon, R. T., Stanley, K. J. & Kizior, R. J. (1998). *Handbook for pain management.* Philadelphia: W.B. Saunders.

McCaffery, M., & Beebe, A. (1998). *Pain: Clinical manual for nursing practice* (2nd ed.). St. Louis: C.V. Mosby.

Melzack, R.(1975). The McGill Pain Questionnaire: Major properties and scoring methods. *Pain, 1,* 277–299.

Melzack, R. & Wall, P. (1965). Pain mechanisms: A new theory. *Science, 150,* 971–979.

Merskey, H. & Bogduk, N. (1994). *Classification of chronic pain: Descriptions of chronic pain syndromes and definitions of pain terms* (2nd ed.). Seattle: IASP Press.

Moreau, D. (Ed.) (1997). *Expert pain management.* Springhouse, PA: Springhouse Corporation.

Page, G., & Ben-Eliyahu, S. (1998). *Pain kills: Animal models and neuro-immunological links.* Seattle: IASP Press.

Puntillo, K. A. (1991). *Pain in the critically ill: assessment and management.* Gaithersburg, MD: Aspen Publishers.

Puntillo, K. A., & Weiss, S. J. (1994). Pain: Its mediators and associated morbidity in critically ill cardiovascular surgical clients. *Nursing Research, 43,* 31–36.

Raj, P. P. (1996). *Pain medicine: A comprehensive review.* St. Louis: Mosby.

Ready, L. B., & Edwards, W. T. (Eds.) (1992). *Management of acute pain: A practical guide.* Seattle, WA: International Association for the Study of Pain.

Sellick, S. M., & Zaza, C. (1998). Critical review of 5 nonpharmacologic strategies for managing cancer pain. *Cancer Prevention & Control, 2*(1), 7–14.

Siddall, P. J., & Cousins, M.J. (1997). Neurobiology of pain. *International Anesthesiology Clinics, 35*(2), 1–26.

Verhaak, P., Kerssens, J., Dekker, J., Sorbi, M., & Bensing, J. (1998). Prevalence of chronic benign pain disorder among adults: A review of the literature. *Pain, 77,* 231–239.

Wall, P. D., & Melzack, R. (Eds.) (1994). *Textbook of pain* (3rd ed.). New York: Churchill Livingstone.

Willis, W. D., & Westlund, K. N. (1997). Neuroanatomy of the pain system and of the pathways that modulate pain. *Journal of Clinical Neurophysiology, 14*(1), 2–31.

Woolf, C. J. (1998). Towards a mechanism-based classification of pain? *Pain,* 77, 227–229.

ON-LINE RESOURCES

EYE AND VISION

American Academy of Ophthalmology *http://www.eyenet.org*
American Optometric Association *http://www.aoanet.org*
American Council of the Blind *http://www.acb.org*
American Foundation for the Blind *http://www.afb.org*
Eye Bank Association of America *http://www.restoresight.org*
(The) Foundation Fighting Blindness *http://www.blindness.org*
The Glaucoma Foundation *http://www.glaucoma-foundation.org/info*
Glaucoma Research Foundation *http://www.glaucoma.org*
Lighthouse International *http://www.lighthouse.org*
Lions Clubs International *http://www.lionsclubs.org*
National Association for Visually Handicapped *http://www.navh.org*
National Federation of the Blind *http://www.nfb.org*
Low Vision Gateway *http://www.lowvision.org*
National Eye Institute, National Institutes of Health *http://www.nei.nih.gov*

EAR AND HEARING

Acoustic Neuroma Association *http://ANAusa.org*
Alexander Graham Bell Association for the Deaf, Inc. *http://www.agbell.org/index.html*
American Academy of Audiology *http://www.audiology.com/*
American Board of Facial Plastic & Reconstructive Surgery *http://www.abfprs.org*
American Academy of Otolaryngology—Head and Neck Surgery *http://www.entnet.org*
American Speech-Language-Hearing Association *http://www.sha.org*
American Tinnitus Association *http://www.ata.org*
National Institute on Deafness and Other Communication Disorders, National Institutes of Health *http://www.nih.gov/nided*
Society of Otorhinolaryngology and Head—Neck Nurses, Inc. *http://www.entnet.org/sohn*
Vestibular Disorders Association *http://www.teleport.com/~veda/*

PAIN

American Pain Society *http://www.wmpainsoc.org*
Cluster Headache Symptoms *http://www.bhs.berkeley.k12.ca.us/departments/Science/anatom,* 1998
International Association for the Study of Pain. IASP Pain Terminology *http://www.halcyon.com/iasp/terms-p.html,* 1998.
Migraine Headache Symptoms *http://www.bhs.berkeley.k12.ca.us/departments/Science/anatom,* 1998.
Pathology of Migraine *http://www.bhs.berkeley.kl2.ca.us/departments/Science/anatom,* 1998.
Pathology of Cluster Headache *http://www. bhs.berkeley.kl2.ca.us/departments/Science/anatom,* 1998.
Pathology of Tension-Type Headache *http://www.bhs.berkeley.k12.ca.us/departments/Science/anatom,* 1998.
Relieving the Cluster Headache *http://www.bhs.berkeley.kl2.ca.us/departments/Science/anatom,* 1998.

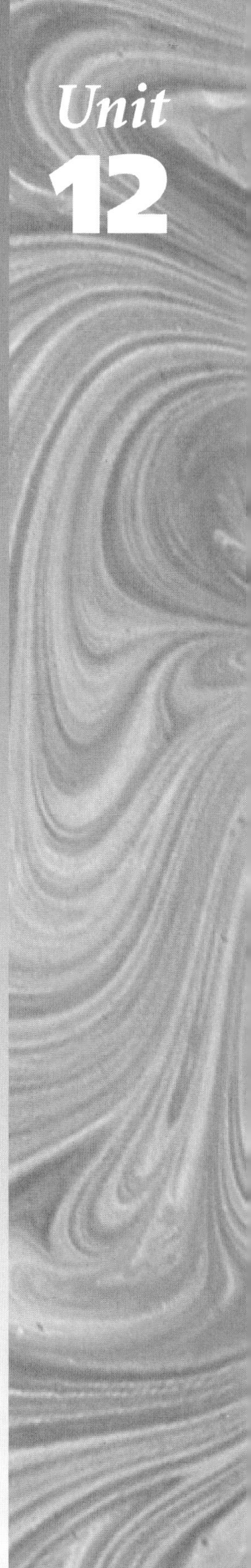

Reproduction

FOCUS ON Male and Female Reproductive Changes Through the Life-Span

INFANT (1–12 MONTHS):

Temporary breast engorgement may be evident due to fetal estrogen stimulation, usually disappearing within a few days to 2 months. In male newborns, the scrotum is edematous and rugated. The penis is approximately 2 cm in length. In females, the vulva may be swollen and pseudomenstruation (mucous vaginal discharge) may be present during the first week of life secondary to the effect of maternal hormones. These disappear once maternal hormones are cleared from the infant's system.

TODDLER AND PRESCHOOL AGE (1–5 YEARS):

Sexual organs remain small in both sexes. Sexual curiosity is common, especially during toilet training.

SCHOOL AGE (6–12 YEARS):

Growth spurt occurs, often heralding changes in the reproductive system. Preliminary characteristics of sexual maturity begin. Subcutaneous fat deposits increase and beginning growth of body hair occurs. Sebaceous glands become active. Secretion of sex hormones gradually increases. In females, breast tissue begins to develop with enlargement of areolar diameter. Vaginal secretions change from alkaline to acidic, and vaginal flow changes to lactic acid–producing bacilli. Vaginal epithelium thickens. Pubic hair may form in some girls as early as age 8 years, beginning on the labia and spreading to the mons. Menarche typically occurs around age 12 years but may occur as early as 8 or 9 years.

ADOLESCENCE (13–19 YEARS):

Development of secondary sex characteristics becomes complete. In boys, testicles enlarge and the scrotum becomes textured. Pubic hair develops, initially light and downy on the sides, later becoming darker, thicker, and curly and spreading across the pubis and pubic area, and eventually to the inner thighs. Penis increases in size and length. Axillary and facial hair develop with facial hair growing and extending to the anterior neck. Voice deepens. Spermatogenesis and seminal emissions begin. With the onset of testicular function, androgen levels increase in males as compared with females. Sexual drive is high. In females, breast enlargement continues with projection of areola and papilla, eventually leading to protrusion of nipple with areola no longer projecting separately from the rest of breast tissue. Pubic hair grows initially along the labia, then spreading to the pubis to form a triangle, increasing in quantity and denseness and becoming curly, eventually abundant, and possibly extending to the medial portion of the thighs.

YOUNG ADULT AND ADULT (20–45 YEARS):

Sexual drive is high throughout young adulthood, then gradually declines. Patterns of sexual behavior develop and sexual activity is at its peak. In females, menstrual patterns vary. Premenstrual syndrome is common due to hormonal shifts. Female reproductive function peaks during this time.

MIDDLE-AGED ADULT (46–64 YEARS):

Males experience less frequent orgasms, and greater direct stimulation is needed for an erection. The testes gradually decrease in size. Prostate enlarges. Testosterone secretion slowly decreases. In females, estrogen and progesterone secretion decrease, leading to menopause (average age of onset is 50 years).

LATE ADULTHOOD (65–100+ YEARS):

In males, fewer visible sperm are seen, possibly with defects. Sexual act requires more time to attain an erection; refractory period is longer. Prostatic hyperplasia occurs. In females, the vaginal wall thickens and vaginal secretions decrease and become more alkaline. Vulva and external genitalia decrease in size. The ovaries, fallopian tubes, and endometrium atrophy. Labia flatten. Often a decrease in sexual desire and performance are related to decreased lubrication.

Chapter

36

Normal and Altered Male Reproductive Function

Susan P. Gauthier

KEY TERMS

androgen
balanitis
balanoposthitis
benign prostatic hyperplasia (BPH)
cryptorchidism
diethylstilbestrol
dihydrotestosterone (DHT)
epididymitis
epispadias
hydrocele
hypospadias
impotence
infertility
monorchidism
orchitis
paraphimosis
penile carcinoma
Peyronie's disease
phimosis
priapism
prostate cancer
prostate-specific antigen
prostatitis
spermatogenesis
sterility
testicular cancer
testosterone
torsion
varicocele

The male reproductive system has evolved to achieve the goal of delivering sperm to the vagina of the female for the purpose of propagating the species. In order to achieve this goal, sperm must be manufactured, stored, and then released within the female. Although a male individual can survive quite well with a nonfunctional reproductive system, survival of the human species depends on proper functioning of the reproductive systems of both sexes. In addition to the normal functioning reproductive structures, emotional and psychological responses in the reproductive process play a key role in sexual satisfaction.

NORMAL MALE REPRODUCTIVE STRUCTURE

The male reproductive system comprises the structures illustrated in Figure 35-1. These can be classified as (1) essential, (2) accessory, and (3) supportive components. The testes (sing. testis) are the *essential*, functional organs of the male reproductive system. *Accessory* organs consist of a system of ducts, glands, and the penis, which store, nourish, and eject sperm. The duct system includes the seminiferous tubules, epididymis, vas deferens, ejaculatory ducts, and urethra. Glands, which add fluid and nutrients to the sperm, include the seminal vesicles, prostate gland, and bulbourethral (Cowper's) glands. The penis is the male organ of copulation. *Supporting structures* of the male reproductive system that provide structural and protective functions include the scrotum and spermatic cords.

Penis and Urethra

The *penis* is a long, cylinder-like structure covered by a loose layer of skin. It has a dual function of urine elimination and ejection of seminal fluid during copulation. The penis consists of the body and the glans. As Figures 36-1 and 36-2 illustrate, the body contains three compartments of erectile tissue: (1) two corpora cavernosa and (2) one corpus spongiosum. The two *corpora cavernosa* are large and run parallel to each other on the dorsal aspect of the penis. The *corpus spongiosum* is located on the ventral side of the penis and contains the urethra. Distally, the corpus spongiosum expands to form the glans penis. In the uncircumcised male, a fold of loose skin, the prepuce (foreskin), covers the glans. The erectile tissue is spongelike and contains large venous sinuses interspersed with arteries and veins. Sexual stimulation

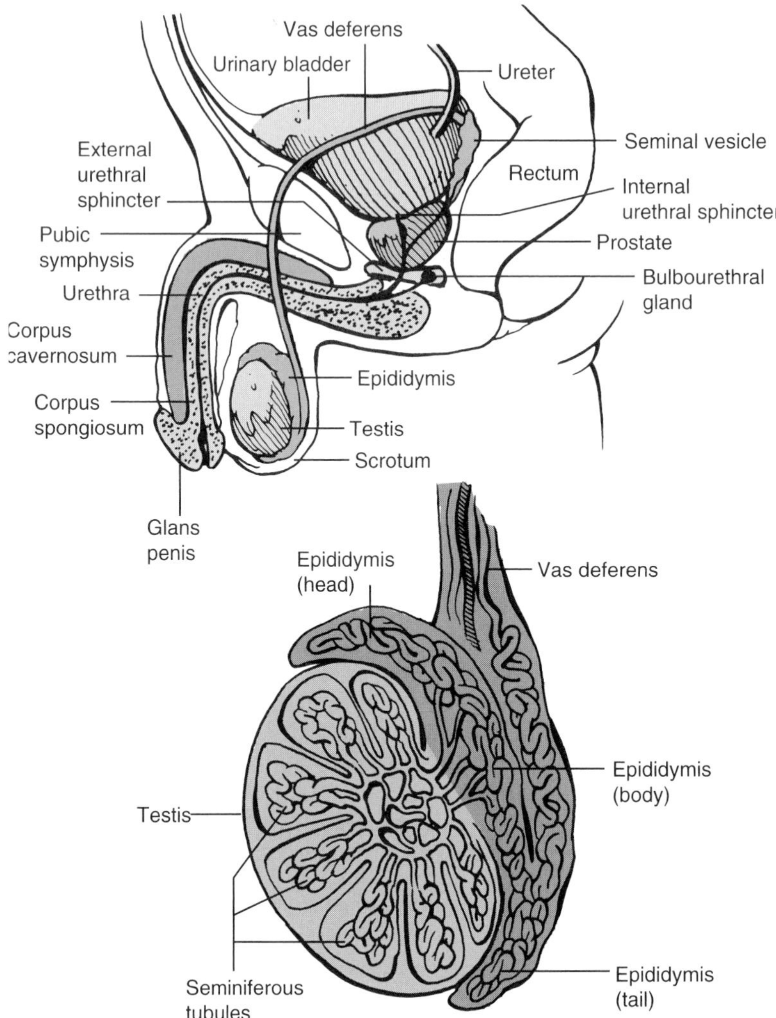

FIGURE 36-1. **A.** Structures of the male reproductive system **B.** Gross structures of the testes.

results in erection of the penis. The penis contains the urethra, a passageway that provides a route for elimination of urine. It is composed of the terminal portion of the seminal fluid passageway and is about 18 to 20 cm long. During the sex act, when the sperm and seminal fluid are forced through the ejaculatory duct, sphincters at the base of the bladder contract, preventing expulsion of urine.

Testes

The paired gonads, or *testes* (sing. testis), are essential structures that generate spermatozoa, the male sex cells and synthesize male sex hormones. As seen in Figure 36-1, they are small, oval-shaped organs suspended in the two sacs of the scrotum. Each testis is encapsulated by a tough, fibrous membrane, the tunica albuginea, extensions of which project inward as septa to divide the testis into lobules. Each lobule contains a long, coiled *seminiferous tubule* (shown in Figure 36-1*B*), which is the site of spermatogenesis. The *interstitial (Leydig) cells* (shown in Figure 36-3) are dispersed in the areas between seminiferous tubules. These cells secrete **androgens**, or male sex hormones, the major one being testosterone.

The *spermatic cord* is composed of the vas deferens and extends from the inguinal ring of the abdomen, through the inguinal canal, to the testes. As Figure 36-1*B* shows, it contains arteries, veins, lymphatic vessels, nerves, and the vas deferens. The spermatic cord and attached testis are surrounded by connective tissue and the tunicavaginalis, a thin, serous covering acquired from the peritoneum when the testis descended into the scrotum during development.

GENITAL DUCTS SYSTEM

The genital duct system is responsible for storing and providing an emission route for the sperm and the associated secretions. This system consists of the epididymis, vas deferens, and ejaculatory ducts.

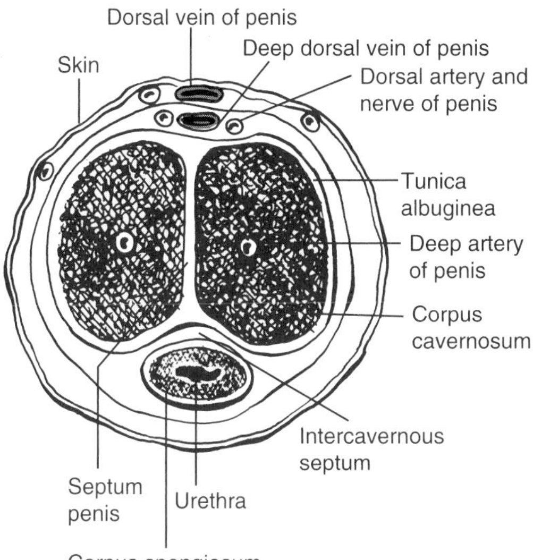

FIGURE 36-2. Penis. Cross-section of penile shaft showing blood vessels, erectile compartments, and supporting elements.

Every day millions of sperm are released into the lumen of the seminiferous tubules. They then travel to the *epididymis*, a long, tortuous genital duct that rests atop each testis and lies between the testis and vas deferens. Sperm are stored in the epididymis for up to 2 weeks, during which they develop the power of motility and become capable of fertilizing an ovum.

FOCUS ON CELLULAR PHYSIOLOGY

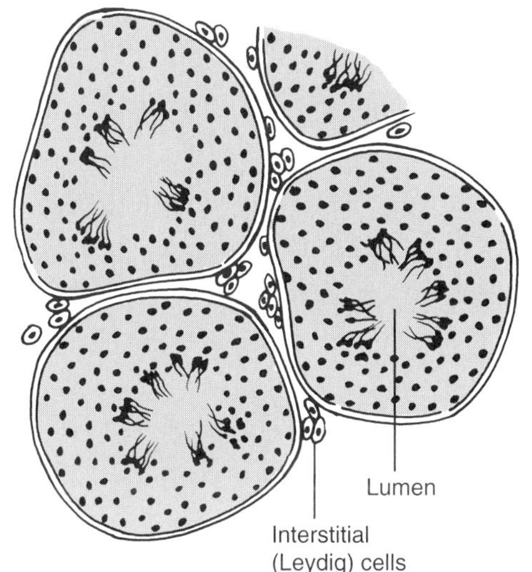

FIGURE 36-3. Seminiferous tubule in cross-section with nests of interstitial cells located between tubules.

The *vas (ductus) deferens* is a straight, fibromuscular tube that ascends from the epididymis into the abdomen, where it loops over the ureter and passes to the posterior aspect of the bladder. Here the vas enlarges into the ampulla and joins with the duct from the seminal vesicle to form an ejaculatory duct. The vas deferens stores most of the sperm. When stimulated, smooth muscles in the walls of the vas produce peristaltic contractions that propel stored sperm into the ejaculatory duct.

The *ejaculatory ducts* are two short tubes about 2 cm in length, formed by union of the ampullae of the vas deferens and ducts of the seminal vesicles. The ejaculatory ducts descend through the prostate gland and terminate in the prostatic urethra, where sperm and secretions from the seminal vesicles and prostate are emitted.

Glands

The glands add fluid, increase the bulk of the sperm, provide nutrients to the sperm, and aid in the fertilization of the ovum. The *seminal vesicles*, shown in Figure 36-4, are two saclike glands about 5 cm long located at the posterior base of the bladder. They produce a viscous, alkaline, yellowish fluid that makes up about 60% of the total seminal fluid volume. Fluid from the seminal vesicles is rich in fructose, an energy source for sperm. This fluid also contains citric acid, coagulation proteins, and prostaglandins, the function of which remains unknown.[4] Stimulation of the seminal vesicles causes them to contract, expelling their contents into the ejaculatory ducts.

The *prostate gland* is a walnut-sized gland, normally weighing about 20 g, located just below the bladder, surrounding the ejaculatory ducts and urethra (see Fig. 36-4). It is divided into five lobes and is enclosed by a tough, fibrous capsule. The normal prostate gland can

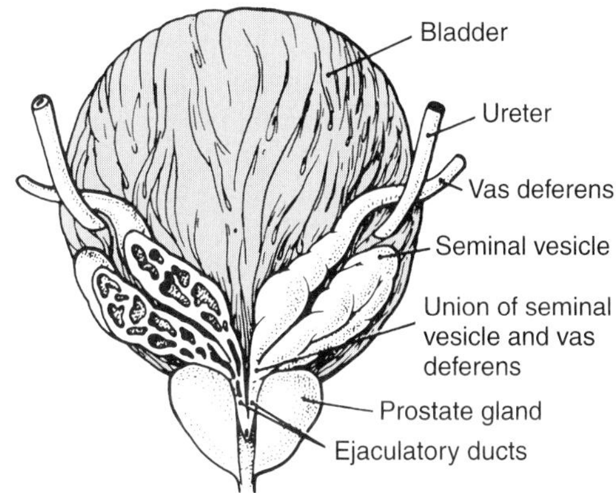

FIGURE 36-4. Male reproductive glands and ducts. Posterior view of the two vas deferens, seminal vesicles, and ejaculatory ducts as they meet to enter the prostate gland.

also be divided into different structural and functional zones. This becomes important in assessing for benign versus malignant prostatic enlargement.

The prostate gland secretes a thin, milky-colored, alkaline fluid that serves to liquefy seminal fluid and promote sperm motility as well as protect sperm from the acidic fluids of the male urethra and female vagina. In addition, the prostate gland secretes prostate-specific antigen (PSA), which can be used in assessment of prostatic function, and acid phosphatase (PAP), the function of which is unknown.[17]

The *bulbourethral (Cowper) glands* are two pea-sized glands located just below the prostate gland. On sexual stimulation, these glands secrete a clear, viscous, alkaline fluid that coats the internal urethra, neutralizes the pH, and lubricates the tip of the penis in preparation for intercourse.

Scrotum

The *scrotum* is a loose pouch suspended in the perineal area between the penis and anus. It has two lateral compartments, each of which houses a testis. The scrotum functions to protect and support the testes. In the mature male, the scrotum is covered with sparse hair and is darker than adjacent skin. It is sensitive to touch, temperature, pain, and pressure. Smooth muscle, known as the *dartos*, and a thin skeletal muscle called the *cremaster* contract when cold to draw the testes close to the body. When warm, the muscles relax, allowing the testes to drop away from the body. This mechanism permits the testes to maintain a temperature of 95°F (35°C), the ideal temperature for spermatogenesis.

Blood Supply and Neural Control

Arterial blood supply to the penis arrives via the internal pudendal arteries from the anterior division of the hypogastric artery. The pudendal arteries further divide into the deep cavernous artery, uretheral artery, and bulbar artery. Venous blood drains from numerous veins of the penis into the retropubic venous plexus.

Neural control is provided by both the sympathetic and parasympathetic nervous systems. The parasympathetic nerves transmit from the sacral spinal cord through pelvic nerves and, in response to sexual stimulation, effect erection and secretion of mucus. Sympathetic innervation arrives from L1 and L2 cord regions through the hypogastric and pelvic sympathetic plexuses to stimulate emission and ejaculation.

NORMAL MALE FUNCTION OF THE REPRODUCTIVE SYSTEM

The male reproductive system serves three primary functions:

- **Spermatogenesis**, the process of sperm production
- Procreation, the process by which sperm are transported and deposited into the female
- Hormonal regulation, a process that monitors and controls male reproduction

Spermatogenesis

The seminiferous tubules of the newborn male's testes contain primitive sex cells called *spermatogonia* that are arranged in several layers on the outer border of the seminiferous tubules. At puberty, spermatogenesis begins in all the tubules as a result of stimulation by the anterior pituitary gonadotropic hormones. Located in the walls of the seminiferous tubules, large *Sertoli (nurse) cells* envelop the developing gametes and secrete nutrients for them as they undergo meiosis and mature into sperm. The entire process of spermatogenesis is shown in Figure 36-5.

During spermatogenesis, *meiosis*, or reduction division, occurs. The spermatogonia are stem cells containing 46 chromosomes that divide by mitosis to produce two daughter cells. One remains a stem cell. The other becomes a progenitor spermatogonium, destined to develop into a sperm. This spermatogonium divides by mitosis to form two *primary spermatocytes*, each with 46 chromosomes. The primary spermatocytes then complete the first meiotic division, producing two *secondary spermatocytes*, each of which contains 23 chromosomes (1N). The secondary spermatocytes subsequently undergo the second meiotic division to produce four *spermatids*, each with 23 chromosomes, 22 autosomes, and one sex chromosome (X or Y).

As illustrated in Figure 36-5, during spermatozoa production each cell loses most of its cytoplasm and elongates into a sperm, which consists of a head, middle piece, and tail. The head comprises the nucleus with its enclosed 23 chromosomes and the overlying *acrosome*, which contains several proteolytic enzymes necessary to digest the outer cell layers of the ovum. The sperm head of a single sperm penetrates and fertilizes the ovum. The middle piece of the sperm is packed with mitochondria, which use fructose from seminal fluid to provide ATP necessary for the lashing motions of the sperm tail that result in locomotion.

Male fertility depends on the quantity of semen ejaculated, the number of sperm per milliliter, and the morphology and motility of the sperm. Normally, seminal fluid ejaculated with each coitus has a volume of 1.5 to 5 mL and contains approximately 50 to 250 million sperm per milliliter.

The Male Sex Act

Procreation through the male sex act includes the entire process in which sperm are transported and deposited into the female vagina. It includes erection, emission, and ejaculation (Flowchart 36-1).

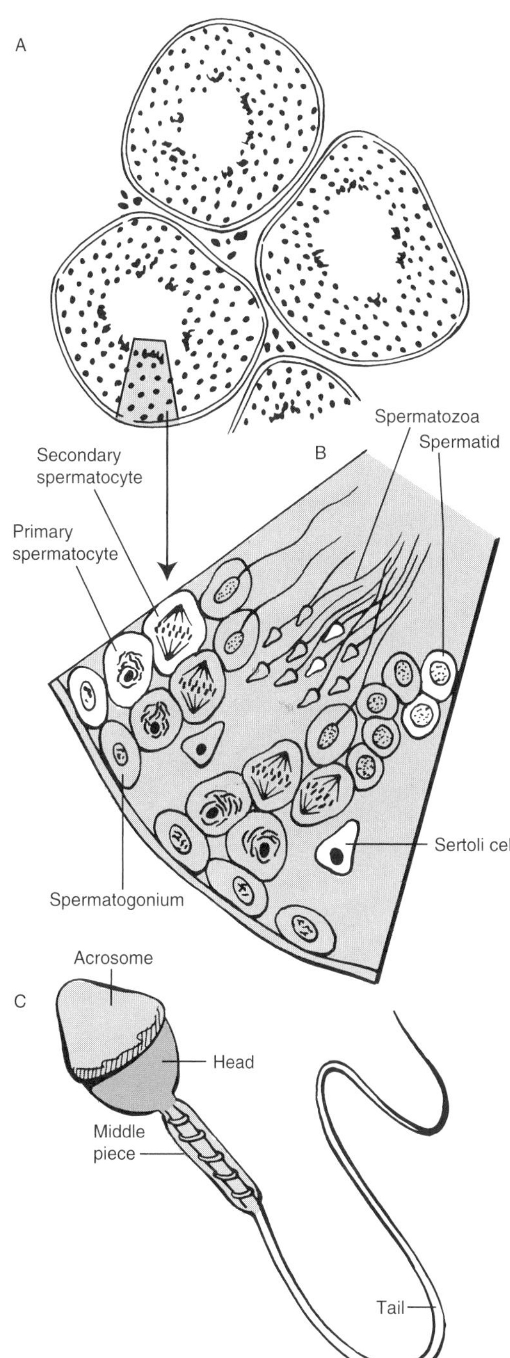

FIGURE 36-5. Spermatogenesis. **A**. Several loops of seminiferous tubules in cross-section. **B**. Wall of seminiferous tubule enlarged to show cells undergoing meiosis and developing into sperm with the Sertoli cells as support. Interstitial cells under basement membrane secrete testosterone. **C**. A mature sperm.

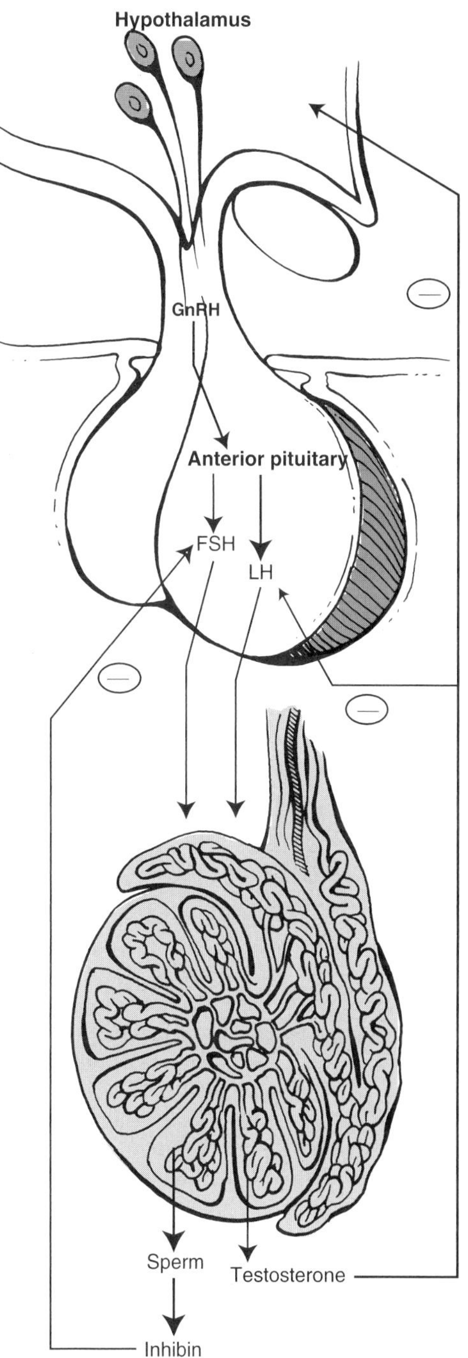

FIGURE 36-6. The hypothalamic-pituitary-testes axis. GnRH secreted by the hypothalamus reaches the pituitary gland by way of a portal blood system and causes the release of LH and FSH from the pituitary gland. LH acts on interstitial cells in the testes causing them to secrete testosterone and then increased testosterone levels provide a negative feedback to both the hypothalamus (to reduce GnRH) as well as the pituitary gland (to reduce LH). FSH acts on germ cells in the testes to enhance spermatogenesis, producing more sperm and a protein called inhibin, which provides a negative feedback to the pituitary gland to reduce FSH (but not LH).

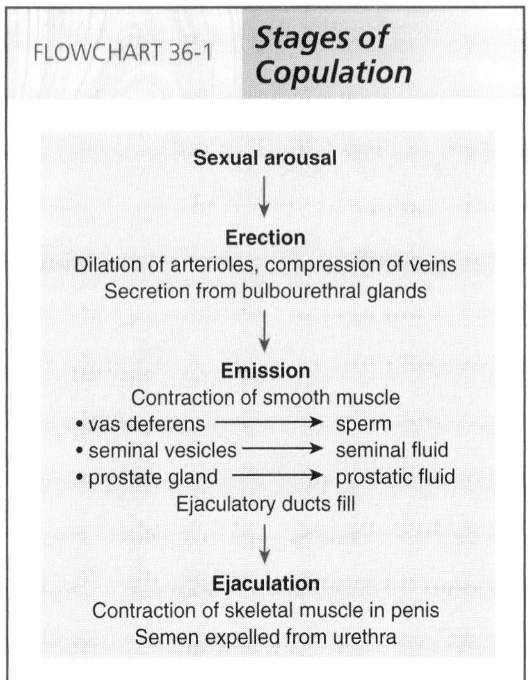

FLOWCHART 36-1
Stages of Copulation
Sexual arousal
Erection
Dilation of arterioles, compression of veins
Secretion from bulbourethral glands
Emission
Contraction of smooth muscle
• vas deferens → sperm
• seminal vesicles → seminal fluid
• prostate gland → prostatic fluid
Ejaculatory ducts fill
Ejaculation
Contraction of skeletal muscle in penis
Semen expelled from urethra

Erection occurs first, as the male is sexually aroused. The penis is normally flaccid because arterioles that supply its vascular spaces are constricted. Sexual arousal causes arterioles to dilate, allowing much more blood to enter the cavernous spaces. As these spaces distend with blood, venous vessels are compressed. Blood is trapped, under great pressure, in the vascular spaces of the erectile tissue, producing a hard, elongated penis capable of insertion into the female vagina. Also, during this early stage of the male sexual response, nervous stimulation results in discharge of lubricating fluid, primarily from the bulbourethral glands into the urethra.

Emission is initiated when impulses are emitted by reflex centers in the spinal cord to the smooth muscle of the genital ducts, producing contractions that force sperm from the vas deferens, and seminal fluid from the seminal vesicles and prostate gland, into the ejaculatory ducts.

Ejaculation immediately follows emission, as filling of the ejaculatory ducts initiates nervous impulses that cause contractions of skeletal muscle at the base of the penis. During these contractions a sphincter at the base of the bladder constricts, preventing expulsion of urine. Then, seminal fluid is expelled through the external urethral orifice. The contractions of ejaculation are part of the male *orgasm*, which includes all sensations, physical and psychological, associated with the abrupt ending of sexual stimulation.

Hormonal Regulation

The function of the male reproductive system is under a complex negative feedback control mechanism that involves the hypothalamus, anterior pituitary gland, and testes (see Fig. 36-6). The male sex hormone, **testosterone**, is secreted by the testes and is essential for both primary and secondary sexual characteristics.

During primary sexual development, the influence of testosterone on male sex characteristics begins as early as the second month of embryonic life when placental hCG stimulates production of small amounts of testosterone, which steers the undifferentiated gonads, ducts, and external genitalia to develop into the testes, ducts, glands, penis, and scrotum. Without this initial dose of male hormone, the undifferentiated genitalia develop along the female pathway.

During childhood, virtually no testosterone is produced until puberty, at which time secretion rapidly increases. After puberty and continuing until maturity at about age 20, testosterone orchestrates secondary sexual development, including enlargement of the penis, scrotum, and testes; initiation of spermatogeneses; and virilization of other body tissues. Since testosterone also stimulates protein anabolism, it promotes bone and muscle growth, increasing size and strength; hair growth on the face, axillae, and chest; and thickening of cartilage in the larynx, deepening the voice. Testosterone affects metabolism and tends to increase basal metabolic rate (BMR). It also affects fluid and electrolyte balance by promoting retention of sodium, potassium, calcium, and water. High levels of testosterone inhibit secretion of gonadotropin by the anterior pituitary gland.

Flowchart 36-2 shows the fate of secreted testosterone. Testosterone circulates in the bloodstream for

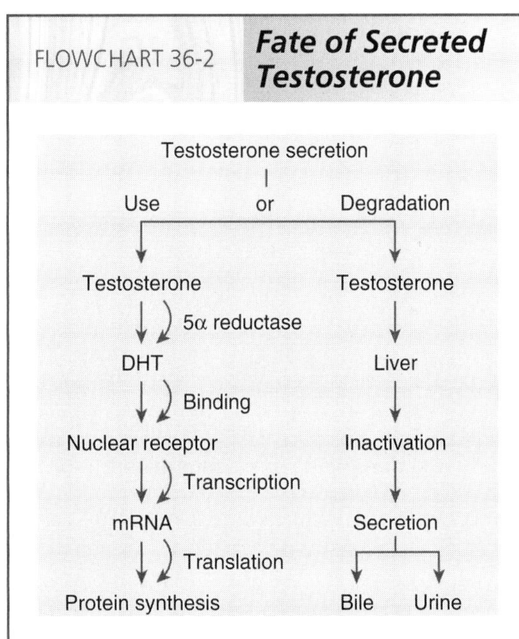

only 15 to 30 minutes before it is either fixed in tissues to perform its functions or is degraded by the liver. After testosterone enters cells, it is converted to **dihydrotestosterone** (DHT), which then binds to nuclear receptors, promoting messenger ribonucleic acid (mRNA) synthesis and, in turn, cellular protein production.

The *hypothalamus* ultimately controls testicular function through the controlled release of GnRH (gonadotropic releasing hormone). As Figure 36-6 shows, when GnRH is secreted by the hypothalamus it travels to the *pituitary gland*, stimulating the release of two *gonadotropic* hormones, follicle-stimulating hormone (FSH) and luteinizing hormone (LH).

When LH levels increase, interstitial (Leydig) cells in the testis are stimulated to increase testosterone secretion. A rise in the blood level of testosterone provides negative feedback to the hypothalamus and anterior pituitary, thus reducing the levels of GnRH and LH. When FSH levels increase and testosterone levels are adequate, the development of spermatogonia into mature sperm proceeds. Without FSH spermatogenesis does not occur, and without testosterone sperm do not mature. As sperm production is increased, Sertoli cells release *inhibin*, a hormone that feeds back to the pituitary gland, modulating FSH production, without affecting LH production. Stress and emotions affect secretory function of the hypothalamus and usually decrease secretion of GnRH.

ALTERATIONS IN MALE REPRODUCTIVE FUNCTION

Alterations in male function may be disturbing if they represent a threat to reproductive function, sexual satisfaction, and a man's self-image. Alterations can occur in any reproductive organ at any age. What follows is an overview of conditions that alter male reproductive function. Processes responsible for these alterations include congenital anomalies, trauma, inflammation, and neoplasia.

Penis

Alterations in the penis and penile function can be congenital or acquired. They include the following conditions:

HYPOSPADIAS AND EPISPADIAS

These are both congenital anomalies. At about 7 to 8 weeks' gestation, the embryo develops a genital tubercle and two genital swellings. In the male fetus, the genital tubercle develops into the penis and the two genital swellings develop into the urethral and scrotal folds, which merge and fuse. This fusion closes the urethra in the penis and forms the scrotum. Failure of these folds to fuse on the ventral side results in the congenital anomaly of **hypospadias** in which the urethral orifice is located on the underside of the penis. The orifice may be only slightly off center or located anywhere on the ventral side of the penis or on the perineum (Fig. 36-7). The foreskin on the ventral side commonly is absent, but sphincters are usually functional.

Epispadias is a rare congenital anomaly in which the urinary meatus opens on the dorsal surface of the penis rather than in the center of the glans (see Fig. 36-7). The urethral opening may be found just behind the glans, or it may extend the length of the penis if associated with exstrophy of the bladder. Sphincters are usually defective, so surgical repair is aimed at providing urinary continence and future sexual function.

PHIMOSIS AND PARAPHIMOSIS

Both of these conditions occur only in the uncircumcised male and are compared in Figure 36-8. **Phimosis** is a condition in which the prepuce is too narrow or stenosed to retract easily over the glans penis. In the most severe cases, urinary flow may be obstructed, causing a ballooning of the prepuce during urination (see Fig. 36-8). Phimosis is frequently congenital, but it may follow infection or injury. If untreated, this condition increases risk of secondary infection, scarring, and perhaps cancer because *smegma*, a secretion of sebaceous glands, accumulates under the prepuce and cannot be cleaned away. Forcible retraction of the foreskin may lead to **paraphimosis**, in which the foreskin is

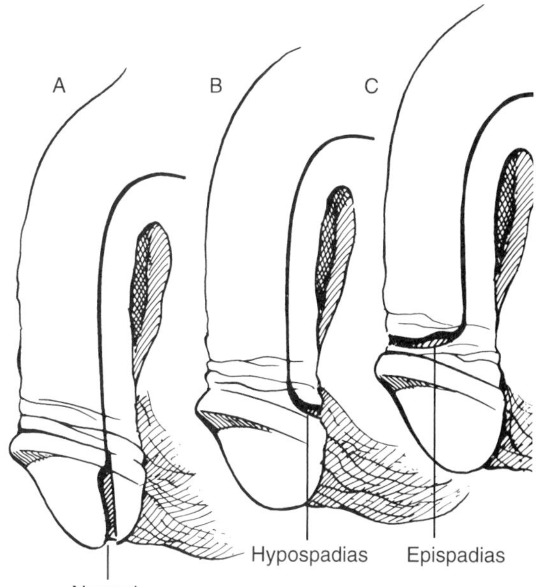

FIGURE 36-7. Congenital anomalies of the male genitalia. **A.** Normal newborn penis: urethral opening is in the center of the glans. **B.** Hypospadia: urethral opening is located on the ventral surface of the penis. **C.** Epispadias: urethral opening is located on the dorsal surface of the penis.

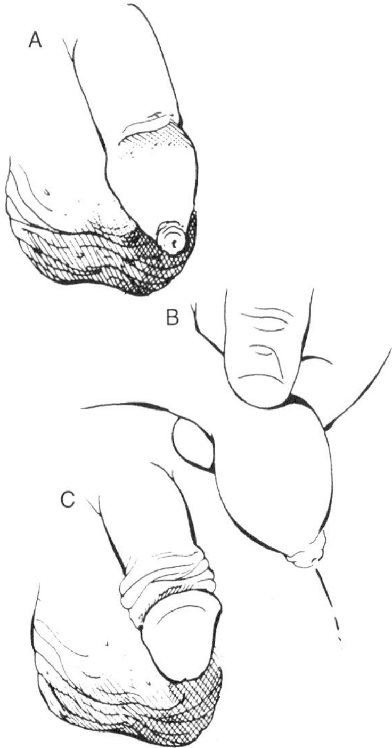

FIGURE 36-8. Phimosis and paraphimosis. **A.** Phimosis: opening in prepuce is too small to allow retraction over glans. **B.** Phimosis during urination: resistance to urine flow causes ballooning of foreskin. **C.** Paraphimosis: retracted prepuce cannot be withdrawn to its normal position.

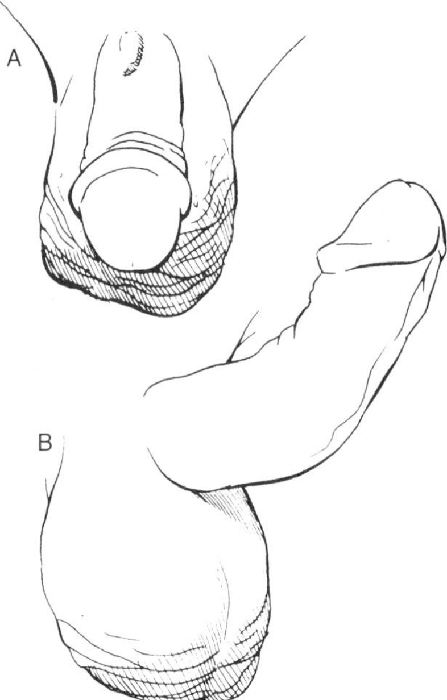

FIGURE 36-9. Peyronie's disease. **A.** Hard, nontender plaques can be palpated just below the skin, usually on the dorsal side of the penis. **B.** During erection the penis is curved and usually painful.

retracted and trapped behind the glans, causing constriction and impaired blood flow that lead to edema and pain of the glans penis. If the foreskin fails to return to its normal location, either through manual correction or surgical repair, necrosis of the glans may result.

BALANITIS AND BALANOPOSTHITIS

Balanitis is an inflammation of the glans penis, and **balanoposthitis** is an inflammation of the glans and overlying prepuce (foreskin). They are mostly seen in uncircumcised males who exercise poor hygiene or with sexually transmitted infections. Clinical manifestations include redness, swelling, pain, foul odor, and purulent drainage. Infection may cause adhesions and scarring. Culture and sensitivity tests are performed to diagnose the infective organism and initiate appropriate antibiotic therapy.

PEYRONIE'S DISEASE

Peyronie's disease, shown in Figure 36-9, is a condition of unknown etiology characterized by the formation of fibrous plaques on the dorsal side of the penis. The condition is found primarily in middle-aged and older men. During erection, there is abnormal penile curvature and pain. There may be urinary obstruction. Peyronie's disease is often associated with Dupuytren contracture, a flexion contracture of the fingers.

PRIAPISM

Priapism refers to an abnormally prolonged penile erection in the absence of sexual stimulation. The condition is extremely painful and may last from several hours to days. The cause is unknown in most cases. However, it has been associated with drugs, infection, leukemia, and sickle cell anemia.[10]

IMPOTENCE

Impotence is the inability to achieve an erection. Erection occurs as a result of an adequate penile blood supply, normal nervous system and hormonal actions, and appropriate psychological and social responses. Abnormalities associated with any of these factors, as well as ingestion of certain medications, can lead to impotence.

Arterial blood supply to the penis can be disrupted by atherosclerotic disease in the larger arteries and by conditions such as diabetes mellitus in the smaller vessels.[8] Neural disruption may occur as a result of surgical intervention, such as that associated with radical prostatectomy, or through systemic disease such as diabetic neuropathy. Decreased testosterone levels have a lesser impact on impotence than problems associated with blood supply and nervous system functioning.[8] Psychological problems seem to be a common underlying cause for impotence, but their underlying mechanisms are poorly understood.

Medications have been implicated in causing impotence in some males. These medications include spironolactone and cimetidine, which are known to act as antiandrogens. Other groups of medications known to cause impotence in some males are certain diuretics, antihypertensives, antidepressants, and antihistamines. The mechanism causing impaired erection with the use of these medications is largely unknown.

TABLE 36-1

STAGING OF PENILE CARCINOMA*

STAGE	DESCRIPTION
I	Tumor limited to glans or prepuce
II	Tumor invasion into penile shaft or corpora
III	Inguinal lymph node involvement but operable
IV	Tumor invading adjacent structures, inoperable lymph node involvement, or distant metastasis

* Jackson staging system.

PENILE CARCINOMA

Primary squamous cell carcinoma of the penis is a rare neoplasm in the United States. It usually is seen in uncircumcised males over 60 years of age. Risk factors include poor hygiene and infection with human papilloma virus (HPV), especially types 16, 18 and 33.[20] Early circumcision almost entirely eliminates the future development of this neoplasm.

Squamous cell carcinoma primarily affects the prepuce and glans, rarely the shaft. Early lesions are superficial and may appear as a subtle red macule or small, gray, crusted papule, although there is no single appearance that is typical. The lesion gradually enlarges, with more advanced tumors becoming nodular. They may have irregular borders, look edematous, and have central ulcerations. Regional spread to lymph nodes is rapid owing to the numerous lymphatic channels in the erectile tissue. See Table 36-1 for the staging of penile cancer.

Testes and Scrotum

Alterations in the testes can be congenital or acquired. Acquired conditions may be traumatic, inflammatory, or neoplastic. These conditions are discussed below:

CRYPTORCHIDISM

During fetal development, the testes form in the abdomen and normally descend through the inguinal canal into the scrotum during the last trimester of pregnancy. Incomplete descent results in **cryptorchidism**. As seen in Figure 36-10, a testis may remain in the abdomen or be arrested in the inguinal canal or high in the scrotum. This is the most common congenital testicular condition. Although present in about 3% of all newborns at birth, most testes descend by age 1 year.[5] It is usually unilateral (**monorchidism**) but is bilateral in 25% of cases. The cause of cryptorchidism is unknown, but endocrine, neural, and mechanical factors are thought to be responsible.[5] It is necessary to surgically correct the condition early, preferably at 1 year of age, in order to avoid future sterility and/or testicular cancer.

HYDROCELE

A **hydrocele**, shown in Figure 36-11*A*, is an accumulation of clear or straw-colored fluid within the tunica vaginalis sac that encloses the testis. It is the most common cause of scrotal enlargement. In the neonate, it results from late closure of the tunica vaginalis. In older individuals it frequently develops without a known cause, but it may follow epididymitis, orchitis, injury, or neoplasm. The condition may be asymptomatic or may cause pain or tension in the scrotum. Transillumination may be present with hydrocele, whereas this is not the case with solid testicular masses.

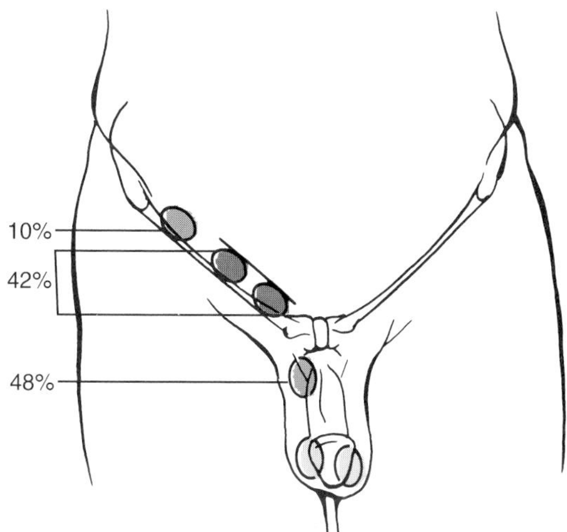

FIGURE 36-10. Cryptorchidism: undescended testis (or testes) can rest in the abdominal cavity, inguinal canal, or high in the scrotum. Numbers are approximate percentages for a particular location.

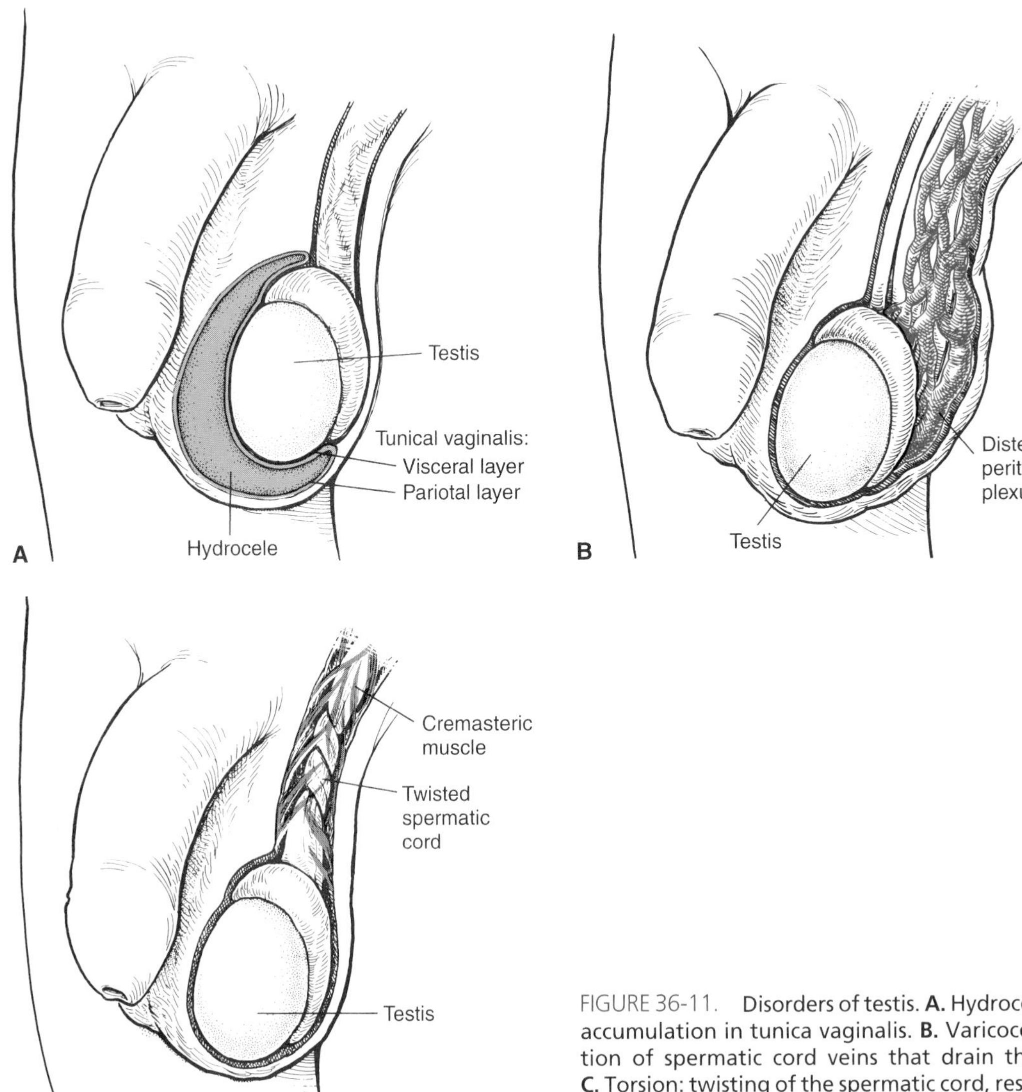

FIGURE 36-11. Disorders of testis. **A.** Hydrocele: fluid accumulation in tunica vaginalis. **B.** Varicocele: dilation of spermatic cord veins that drain the testis. **C.** Torsion: twisting of the spermatic cord, resulting in reduced blood flow.

VARICOCELE

As seen in Figure 36-11*B*, a **varicocele** is an abnormal dilation of the internal spermatic veins above the testis due to incompetent or congenitally absent spermatic vein valves. Because of anatomic differences between the left and right testicular blood vessels, it is almost always found on the left side. Occurrence on the right side is strongly suggestive of a tumor obstructing a vein above the scrotum. Palpation reveals dilated and tortuous veins, often described as a "bag of worms." The primary clinical concern relates to the potential for infertility. Because venous engorgement may interfere with blood flow, sperm number and/or motility may be decreased. The condition is usually asymptomatic, but there may be complaints of a dragging sensation or dull pain in the scrotum.

ORCHITIS

Inflammation of the testes, or **orchitis**, may be bilateral or unilateral. It is usually due to an ascending bacterial infection of the urogenital tract, but organisms may be acquired by lymphatic spread. Infection caused by ascending bacteria are usually due to *Staphylococcus*, *Streptococcus*, *Escherichia coli*, *Klebsiella pneumoniae*, and *Pseudomonas aeruginosa*. Orchitis can be a complication of mumps, because the mumps virus is excreted in urine. This primarily affects adults and occurs in about 20% of men with mumps.

Clinical manifestations of orchitis include severe testicular pain, swelling, chills, and fever. On examination, the testis appears swollen and is tender; the scrotum is swollen and red. Complications, including hydrocele and abscess, may result in sterility or impotence.

TORSION

As seen in Figure 36-11*C*, **torsion** is a twisting of the spermatic cord that results from rotation of the spermatic cord and testis within the tunica vaginalis. With winding of the spermatic cord, blood entry to the testis is compromised, and venous obstruction results in vascular engorgement, sometimes with extravasation of blood into the scrotal sac. If blood flow is completely blocked, germ cells in the testes are destroyed within a few hours. Torsion is an infrequent cause of testicular enlargement that primarily occurs during adolescence after vigorous physical exercise, although it may occur spontaneously. The first symptom usually is sudden onset of severe pain in the testicular area. It is unrelieved by rest or scrotal support and may radiate into the groin. Other manifestations include testicular tenderness, scrotal edema, and perhaps nausea and vomiting. Untreated torsion of the testis may result in infarction, atrophy, abscess, or infertility.

TESTICULAR CANCER

Testicular cancer is not a common neoplasm, but it strikes a young population. In 1998 there were an estimated 7,600 new cases and 400 deaths due to testicular cancer.[2] The exact cause of testicular cancer remains unknown. According to the American Cancer Society, risk factors for testicular cancer include:[2]

- *Age:* Although testicular cancer can occur at any age, it is most prevalent between the ages of 15 and 40.
- *Cryptorchidism:* About 14% of cases occur in males with a history of undescended testicle; of these, 25% occurred in the normally descended testicle. It has been proposed that a single, unknown factor may be responsible for both cryptorchidism and testicular neoplasia.[14]
- *Genetics:* Risk is increased for first-degree relatives, such as a brother. The incidence in white males is four times greater than in African-American males, and in the past 2 decades the incidence has doubled in white males.
- *Environmental factors:* Non-seminoma tumors are more frequent among miners and workers in the oil, gas, utility, and leather industries, as well as among janitors and food processors.
- *HIV infection:* Especially during the AIDS stage, this imparts increased risk.
- *History of testicular cancer:* Cancer in one testis increases the risk of its development in the other.

Malignant neoplasms of the testis can arise from germ (sperm precursor) cells or from stromal (supporting) elements. Most (90%–95%) testicular cancers are of germ cell origin, which includes seminoma and the non-seminoma tumors (Table 36-2).

Seminoma is the most common of the testicular malignancies. Seminomas are well-differentiated neoplasms that appear as gray-white, fleshy masses. They remain localized until late in the course of the disease, when metastasis occurs to retroperitoneal nodes. The tumor marker beta human chorionic gonadotropin (βhCG) is elevated in about 10% of cases.

Embryonal carcinoma cells are poorly differentiated, forming sheets of primitive epithelial tissue. This highly malignant neoplasm forms a gross tumor that is soft, solid, and friable. The tumor marker α-fetoprotein (α-FP) is frequently elevated in embryonal carcinoma, and βhCG may be as well. Metastasis to the lymph nodes, lungs, liver, and bones is frequent.

Teratomas are composed of cells that show somatic differentiation, forming tissues normally derived from the primary germ layers (ectoderm, mesoderm, endoderm) of the embryo. In *mature* teratomas tissues are well developed, resembling normal skin, epithelium,

TABLE 36-2

GERM CELL NEOPLASMS OF THE TESTIS

TYPE	(INCIDENCE %)	AGE (YEARS)	βHCG MARKER % ⊕	α-FP MARKER % ⊕	PROGNOSIS
Seminoma	(35)	30–50	10	0	Excellent
Non-seminoma					
• Embryonal	(20)	15–30	60	70	Good
• Teratoma	(5)	10–30	25	40	Fair
• Choriocarcinoma	(<1)	20–30	100 (high)	0	Poor
• Yolk sac (pure)	(<1)	1–3		100 (high)	Very good
• Mixed Cell	(40)	10–50	Depends on cell types	Depends on cell types	Variable

bone, and so on. In *immature* types, tissue resembles the more primitive germ layer tissues. Elevated levels of α-FP and βhCG are associated with these neoplasms. Metastases can occur via the lymphatic system or bloodstream.

Choriocarcinoma is a highly malignant, aggressive neoplasm that show trophoblastic (placental) differentiation, with cytotrophoblastic and syncytiotrophoblastic cells arranged much like those in a normal chorionic villus. The gross tumors are small, hemorrhagic, and often non-palpable. These cells secrete large amounts of βhCG, which aids in the diagnosis. Early, distant metastasis, due to hematologic spread, usually causes death within a year of diagnosis.

Yolk sac tumors show differentiation features of the yolk sac, forming lacy, delicate, and friable masses. Pure yolk sac tumors occur almost exclusively in very young boys. These tumors secrete large amounts of α-FP. Sometimes βhCG is also elevated.

Clinical Manifestations

The most frequent symptom of a testicular tumor is painless enlargement of the testis, sometimes accompanied by hydrocele. There may be complaints of scrotal heaviness, pulling, or a dull ache. About 10% of patients present with acute testicular pain. Another 10% present with symptoms of distant metastasis. On examination, the mass does not transilluminate, and swollen lymph nodes may be noted. Gynecomastia is an infrequent sign associated with tumors that produce βhCG and estrogen. Low back pain may be associated with retroperitoneal lymph node involvement. Other symptoms may be present that vary with the site of metastasis. The diagnosis and staging of testicular cancers are based on physical examination, protein biochemical markers in serum (α-FP and βhCG), CT scanning, and biopsy after orchiectomy, the removal of the entire testis. See Table 36-3 for staging of testicular cancer.

TABLE 36-3

STAGING OF TESTICULAR CANCER*

STAGE 0—CARCINOMA IN SITU	PREINVASIVE GERM CELL TUMOR
Stage I	No spread to lymph nodes or distant sites
Stage II	Spread to regional lymph nodes but not distant sites
Non-bulky	• No node is >5 cm
Bulky	• One or more node is >5 cm
Stage III	Spread to non-regional lymph nodes and/or distant sites
Non-bulky	• Metastasis limited to lymph nodes and lungs; no mass >2 cm
Bulky	• Large lymph node metastases and/or spread to other organs

* Adapted from American Cancer Society. The Testicular Cancer Resource Center, http://www.cancer.org/cancerinfo/main.

INFERTILITY

Abnormal spermatogenesis can result in male infertility. If the number of sperm drops below 20 million/mL, **infertility** (inability to conceive after 12 months of unprotected intercourse) or **sterility** (absolute inability to conceive) frequently results. Most common causes of male infertility result from problems associated with the testes. Less common causes of infertility result from diseases of the hypothalamus and pituitary and from obstructions in sperm outflow. Many problems of infertility are idiopathic, where no specific cause can be identified. In identifiable causes of male infertility the etiology can be classified according to (1) pretesticular, (2) testicular, or (3) post-testicular causes.[4] Sperm abnormalities vary with the conditions within these classifications, from azoospermia and oligospermia to abnormal morphology and abnormal motility, all of which may contribute to infertility.[3]

Pretesticular Infertility

Pretesticular infertility is associated with hypothalamic-pituitary disorders that result in testicular dysfunction due to decreased gonadotropin hormone production. Adrenal and thyroid disorders may also be associated with pretesticular infertility.

Testicular Infertility

Numerous conditions of the testes may be responsible for infertility, including injury, infections, varicocele, chromosomal abnormalities, cryptorchism, testicular atrophy, and drugs and toxins. Additionally, systemic disorders such as diabetes mellitus, cirrhosis, and uremia may decrease male fertility. The underlying mechanisms involved in infertility associated with systemic diseases are not clear.

Post-testicular Infertility

The most common cause of post-testicular infertility is an obstruction to the outflow of spermatozoa due to blockage of the excretory ducts. Other causes include genital tract infections, retrograde ejaculation, congenital and developmental abnormalities, and impotence.

Genital Ducts System

EPIDIDYMITIS

Epididymitis is an inflammation of the epididymis, usually due to infective organisms. The most common mechanism of infection is ascension from the bladder, urethra, prostate gland, or seminal vesicles. Epididymitis may result from sexually transmitted organisms such as *Neisseria gonorrhoeae* and *Chlamydia trachomatis*. Other common organisms are *Pseudomonas aeruginosa* or enteric bacteria. It may also occur as a complication of prostatectomy. Symptoms include pain, chills, fever, and malaise, with scrotal swelling so great that it interferes with ambulation and produces congestion of the testes. Necrosis and fibrosis may occlude the genital ducts and result in sterility.

Prostate Gland

The prostate gland maintains its normal size until about age 50. At this point, in some men, it begins to decrease in size. This atrophy is associated with a decrease in testosterone levels and usually produces no symptoms. Other alterations in prostate function normally occur in adult life and involve an enlargement of the prostate gland. These conditions include prostatitis, benign prostatic hyperplasia, and carcinoma.

PROSTATITIS

Prostatitis, inflammation of the prostate gland, is usually due to infection. Infection most often results due to ascension of organisms from the urethra. It may also result from descending infection from the bladder or kidneys; hematogenous spread from the teeth, skin, or gastrointestinal or respiratory system; or lymphogenous spread from rectal bacteria. The condition occurs in three forms: acute bacterial, chronic bacterial, and chronic abacterial.

Acute bacterial prostatitis is caused by the same organisms that produce urinary tract infections, the most frequent being *E. coli*, which ascends from the urethra. Manifestations of acute bacterial prostatitis include chills, fever, and urinary dysuria, frequency, urgency, and hematuria. It also may be associated with suprapubic, perineal, or scrotal pain and purulent urethral discharge. On rectal examination, the prostate is enlarged, tender, and warm. The seminal vesicles may also be palpable, because infection of these glands frequently accompanies prostatitis. Urinalysis may be positive for blood and pus. Urine cultures identify the specific organism. Although prostate massage can aid in identification of this condition, it should be used judiciously because it can precipitate bacteremia. Catheterization, if performed on a man with acute prostatitis, may be responsible for spreading the infection to the bladder. Appropriate antibiotics, analgesics, and sitz baths, if instituted early, usually resolve the condition. The infection may become chronic if it is not adequately treated.

Chronic bacterial prostatitis may represent a continuation of acute prostatitis that did not completely respond to antibiotics. Some men are asymptomatic, with diagnosis occurring with routine urinalysis. Clinical manifestations include low-grade fever, dull perineal pain, nocturia, and dysuria. Inflammatory cells and bacteria usually are found in prostatic secretions. The infection may be resistant to antibiotics because they do not adequately penetrate the prostate.

Abacterial prostatitis is the most common form of prostatitis.[16] Symptoms are mild and include low back pain, urinary frequency and urgency, and with rectal, urethral, or perineal discomfort. Physical examination usually reveals a nontender prostate with negative urine culture. Prostatic fluid reveals leukocytes. Symptoms may be exacerbated by excessive alcohol or caffeine intake.

BENIGN PROSTATIC HYPERPLASIA (BPH)

Benign prostatic hyperplasia (BPH) is an enlargement of the prostate gland that affects most men after age 50. Although there is no known cause for BPH, the incidence rises with age, with as many as 95% of men older than 70 affected. Unlike cancer of the prostate, which grows in the peripheral zones, BPH develops in the central and transitional zones of the prostate, which lie closest to the urethra. For this reason urinary symptoms appear early in BPH but not in prostate cancer. Figure 36-12 compares these two lesions.

Hyperplasia occurs in both glandular (epithelial) and smooth muscle (stromal) tissues. Glandular elements of the prostate are androgen dependent. Whereas testosterone levels remain stable or decline with age, symptoms of BPH develop in older males. It is now believed that this inconsistency is a result of increased sensitivity to androgens brought about by an age-related increase in estrogens that up-regulate, or increase, androgen receptors.[9] Hyperplasia due to stimulation of androgen-dependent glandular components increases prostate bulk and causes a *static* type of obstruction by physically blocking the prostatic portion of the urethra.[18]

Hyperplasia of smooth muscle also plays a role in the development of urinary obstruction. Here, obstruction comes about because hyperplastic smooth muscle causes a functional, or *dynamic*, form of obstruction, even in males with minimally enlarged prostates.[11,18]

CANCER OF THE PROSTATE

The American Cancer Society estimates an incidence of 184,500 new cases of prostate cancer in 1998, and 39,200 deaths due to it.[2] **Prostate cancer** is the most common invasive cancer, and the second leading cause of cancer deaths, in men. Age is the most significant risk factor, with more than 80% of all cases diagnosed in men older than 65. The incidence is 66%, and mortality 200%, greater in African-American males compared with white males. The incidence is increased within certain families. High dietary fat intake may also be a risk factor.

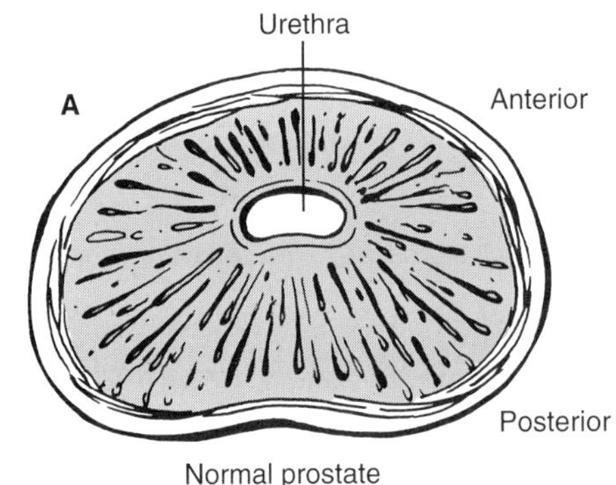

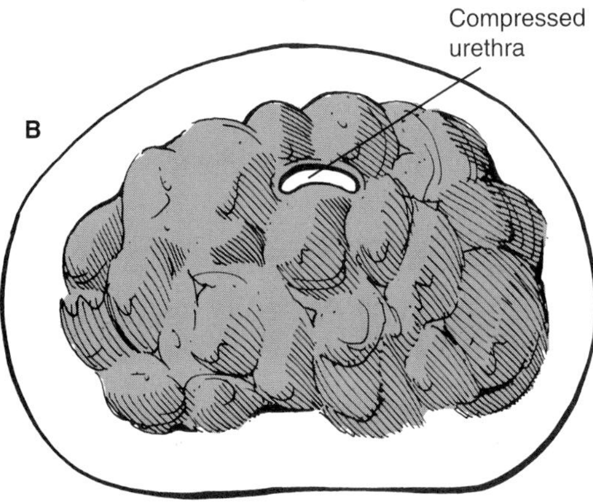

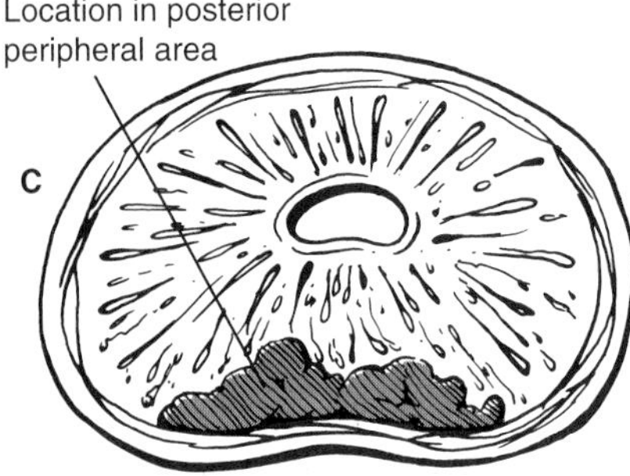

FIGURE 36-12. **Prostate gland. A. Normal B. Central zone enlargement is characteristic of BPH. C. Cancer of the prostate usually involves the peripheral zone.**

Etiology

The specific events that *initiate* changes in prostatic cells remain unknown. However, the fact that cell changes can be found in a large portion of very young men, and that prostate cancer is usually not diagnosed until the 60s, suggests a multiple-step promotion and progression process, with androgens stimulating growth of the altered cells.[13] Hereditary forms of prostate cancer, linked to the human prostate cancer gene on chromosome 1 (HPC1), account for only about 9% of all cases.[7]

Recent evidence suggests that many advanced tumors have cell clones with mutations in the gene that code for the testosterone receptor. Because these cells are androgen independent, they will thrive without androgens. The presence of such mutations has been implicated in progression of tumors after apparently successful ablation therapy.[15]

Clinical Manifestations

The most common (95%) type of prostate cancer is adenocarcinoma, which usually arises in the peripheral zones of the gland, facilitating its detection via digital rectal exam (DRE). When palpable, lesion are felt as hard, fixed nodules. As the tumor gains in aggressiveness, it spreads to other portions of the gland and then beyond its capsule to contiguous structures such as the seminal vesicles, bladder neck, and pelvic lymph nodes. In the early stages, it produces no symptoms. The first symptoms are those of urethral obstruction, but by the time they appear, metastasis is usually present. The most frequent sites of distant metastasis are the lymph nodes, bones, lungs, and liver.

Prostate-specific antigen (PSA) is a glycoprotein produced exclusively by epithelial cells of the prostate gland and may be elevated in prostatic carcinoma.[12] However, it is not specific for cancer as it can also increase with prostatitis, benign prostatic hyperplasia, and procedures that are traumatic to the gland. Therefore, annual screening is controversial among some clinicians.[1]

Grading of prostate cancer is important because a small aggressive tumor is thought to be a greater threat than large, indolent growths.[13] In order to stage the progress of the disease itself, a number of staging classifications are used. The AUA system for prostate cancer is shown in Table 36-4 and illustrated in Figure 36-13.

Exposure to Diethylstilbestrol

Diethylstilbestrol (DES) is a synthetic estrogenic hormone. The use of DES to treat threatened spontaneous abortion was widespread between 1947 and 1971, during which an estimated 2 to 3 million fetuses were exposed. The effects of in utero DES exposure on the female fetus had been known and publicized for years before evidence appeared that its use was associated with reproductive anomalies in male fetuses in the late 1970s. Reported reproductive system anomalies involve the urethra, penis, and testes and include urethral meatal stenosis, hypospadias, underdeveloped or undescended testes, and testicular cysts. Although exposure to DES has been associated with low sperm counts, abnormally-shaped sperm, and decreased volume of ejaculate,[6] more recently it has been shown that exposed males do not differ from unexposed males in rate of fertility.[19]

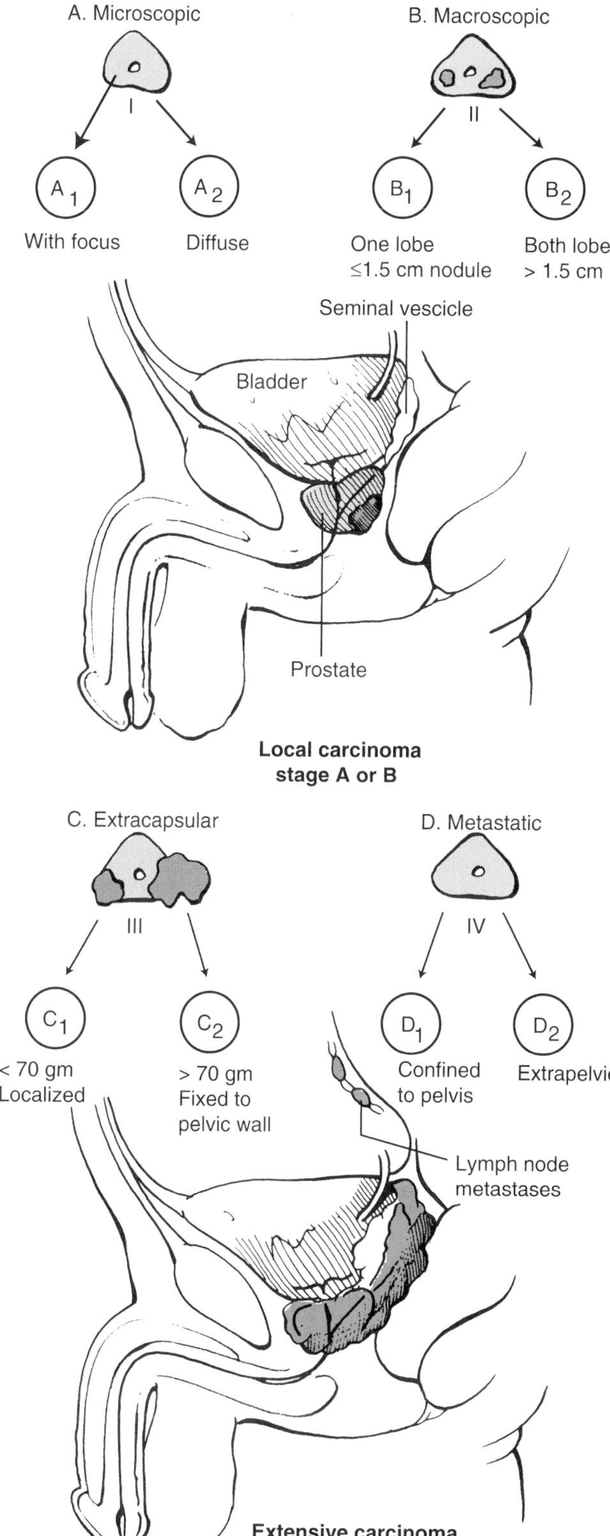

FIGURE 36-13. Prostate Cancer. **A.** Local carcinoma: stages A and B. **B.** Extensive carcinoma: stages C and D. (Adapted from Rubin, E. & Farber, J. [1999]. *Pathology* [3rd ed.]. Philadelphia: Lippincott-Raven; and Gittes, R. F. [1991]. Carcinoma of the prostate. *New England Journal of Medicine, 324*, 240.)

TABLE 36-4

STAGING OF PROSTATE CANCER*

STAGE	TUMOR
A	Clinically unsuspected but found on biopsy
A1	• Focal carcinoma, well differentiated
A2	• Diffuse carcinoma, poorly differentiated
B	Tumor confined to prostate gland
B1	• Small, discrete node in one lobe
B2	• Large or multiple nodules or areas of involvement
C	Tumor localized to periprostatic region
C1	• Outside prostatic capsule, estimated weight <70 g, seminal vesicles not involved
C2	• Outside prostatic capsule, estimated weight >70 g, seminal vesicles involved
D	Metastatic prostate cancer
D1	• Pelvic lymph node metastasis or ureteral obstruction with hydronephrosis, or both
D2	• Bone, soft tissue, organ, or distant lymph node involvement

* American Urologic Association (AUA).

REFERENCES

1. Albertsen, P. C. (1996). Screening for prostate cancer is neither appropriate nor cost-effective. *Urologic Clinics of North America, 23*(4), 521–530.
2. American Cancer Society (1998). *Cancer facts and figures–1998*. Atlanta: American Cancer Society.
3. Beckman, C., Ling, F., Barzansky, B., Bates, G., Herbert, W., Laube, D., & Smith, R. (1997). *Obstetrics and gynecology* (2nd ed.). Baltimore: Williams & Wilkins.
4. Chandrasoma, P. & Taylor, C. R. (1998). *Concise pathology* (3rd ed.). Norwalk, CT: Appleton & Lange.
5. Gill, B. & Kogan, S. (1997). Cryptorchidism—current concepts. *Pediatric Clinics of North America, 44*(5), 1211–1227.
6. Gill, W. B., Schumacher, G. F. B., Bibbo, M., Straus, F. H., & Schoenberg, H. W. (1979). Association of diethylstilbestrol exposure in utero with cryptorchidism, testicular hypoplasia and semen abnormalities. *Journal of Urology, 122*, 36–39.
7. Grönberg, H., Isaacs, S. D., Smith, J. R., Carpten, J. D., Bova, G. S., Freije, D., Xu, J., Meyers, D. A., Collins, F . S., Trent, J. M., Walsh, P. C. & Isaacs, W. B. (1997). Characteristics of prostate cancer in families linked to the hereditary prostate cancer 1 (HPC1) locus. *Journal of the American Medical Association, 278*(15), 1251–1255.
8. Kelley, W. (1997). *Textbook of internal medicine* (3rd ed.). Philadelphia: Lippincott-Raven.
9. Kumar, V., Cotran, R. S., & Robbins, S. L. (1997). *Basic pathology* (6th ed). Philadelphia: W.B. Saunders.
10. McAninch, J. W. (1995). Disorders of the testis, scrotum, and spermatic cord. In E. A. Tanagho & J. W. McAninch, *Smith's general urology* (14th ed.). Norwalk, CT: Appleton & Lange.
11. Oesterling, J. E. (1995). Benign prostatic hyperplasia. *New England Journal of Medicine, 332*(2), 99–108.
12. Partin, A. W. & Carter, H. B. (1996). The use of prostate-specific antigen and free/total prostate-specific antigen in the diagnosis of localized prostatic cancer. *Urologic Clinics of North America, 23*(4), 531–540.
13. Scher, H. I., Isaacs, J. T., Fuks, Z. & Walsh, P. C. (1995). Prostate. In M. D. Abeloff, J. O. Armitage, A.S. Lichter & J. E. Niederhuber (Eds.), *Clinical oncology*. New York: Churchill Livingstone.
14. Skakkebaek, N. E., Berthelsen, J. G. & Muller, J. (1982). Carcinoma in situ of the undescended testis. *Urologic Clinics of North America, 9*, 377.
15. Taplin, M. E., Bubley, G. J., Shuster, T. D., Frantz, M. E., Spooner, A. E., Ogata, G. K., Keer, H. N. & Balk, S. P. (1995). Mutation of the androgen-receptor gene in metastatic androgen-independent prostate cancer. *New England Journal of Medicine, 332*(21), 1393–1398.
16. Tierney, L. M., McPhee, S. J., & Papadakis, M. A. (1998). *Current medical diagnosis and treatment* (37th ed.). Stamford, CT: Appleton & Lange.
17. Tortora, G. J. & Grabowski, S. R. (1996). *Principles of anatomy and physiology* (8th ed.). New York: Harper Collins.
18. Walsh, P. C. (1996). Treatment of benign prostatic hyperplasia. *New England Journal of Medicine, 335*(8), 586–587.
19. Wilcox, J. A., Baird, D. D., Weinberg, C. R., Hornsby, P. P. & Herbst, A. L. (1995). Fertility in men exposed prenatally to diethylstilbestrol. *New England Journal of Medicine, 332*(21), 1411–1416.
20. Zaragosa, M. R. & Grossman, H. B. (1995). Penis and urethra. In M. D. Abeloff, J. O. Armitage, A. S. Lichter, & J. E. Niederhuber (Eds.), *Clinical oncology*. New York: Churchill Livingstone.

Chapter 37

Normal and Altered Female Reproductive Function

Susan P. Gauthier / Helen A. Carcio

KEY TERMS

adenomyosis
adrenopause
BRCA gene
carcinoma in situ
cervical eversion
cervical intraepithelial neoplasia (CIN)
chocolate cyst
climacteric
choriocarcinoma
ductal ectasia
dysfunctional uterine bleeding (DUB)
dysmenorrhea
ecoestrogen
endometrial hyperplasia
endometrioma
fibroadenoma
hydatidiform mole
hydrosalpinx
intraductal papilloma
mastitis
menopause
nabothian cyst
pelvic inflammatory disease (PID)
polyp
procidentia
squamous intraepithelial lesion (SIL)
uterine leiomyoma
uterine prolapse
xenoestrogen

The female reproductive system is designed for multiple activities, including the formation of gametes, the fertilization of an egg, the carrying of a fertilized egg to fetal maturity, and the nurturing of the newborn by means of milk production. Sexual functioning is important to the achievement of reproduction, nourishment of the newborn, and psychological well-being of the woman. Alterations may occur in the structure and function of the reproductive organs, at any age. This chapter provides an overview of the anatomy and physiology of the female reproductive structures, which is fundamental to understanding alterations in reproduction. Key concepts related to the etiology, pathophysiology, and clinical manifestations of the most common of these alterations are presented. Essential information related to the intricate interactions between endocrine organs and their many target tissues in relation to the menstrual cycle are explored.

Female reproductive structures include the internal and external organs and the breast. Additionally they include the exocrine glands, Bartholin's and Skene's, which are located in the genital tract, and the mammary glands, which are located in the breasts.

Diagnostic tests related to the female reproductive system are described in Appendix A of this unit.

NORMAL INTERNAL FEMALE STRUCTURES

The internal organs—the ovaries, uterus, and fallopian tubes—lie within the pelvis and include the vagina, which connects the internal organs to the external organs (Fig. 37-1). The internal organs are supported by the bony pelvis and ligaments.

Pelvic Support

The female reproductive organs are housed within a ring-shaped series of bones that form the bony pelvis. The pelvis consists of the innominate bones, the ilium, the ischium, the pubic bones, and the sacrum. These structures help support the pelvic organs in the upright position. The false, or greater, pelvis is the area situated above the iliopectineal line and bounded posteriorly by the lumbar vertebrae, laterally by the iliac fossa, and anteriorly by the anterior abdominal wall. The true, or lesser, pelvis is the pelvis below the iliopectineal line. The four different pelvic types include gynecoid, android, anthropoid, and platypelloid; they are compared in Figure 37-2.

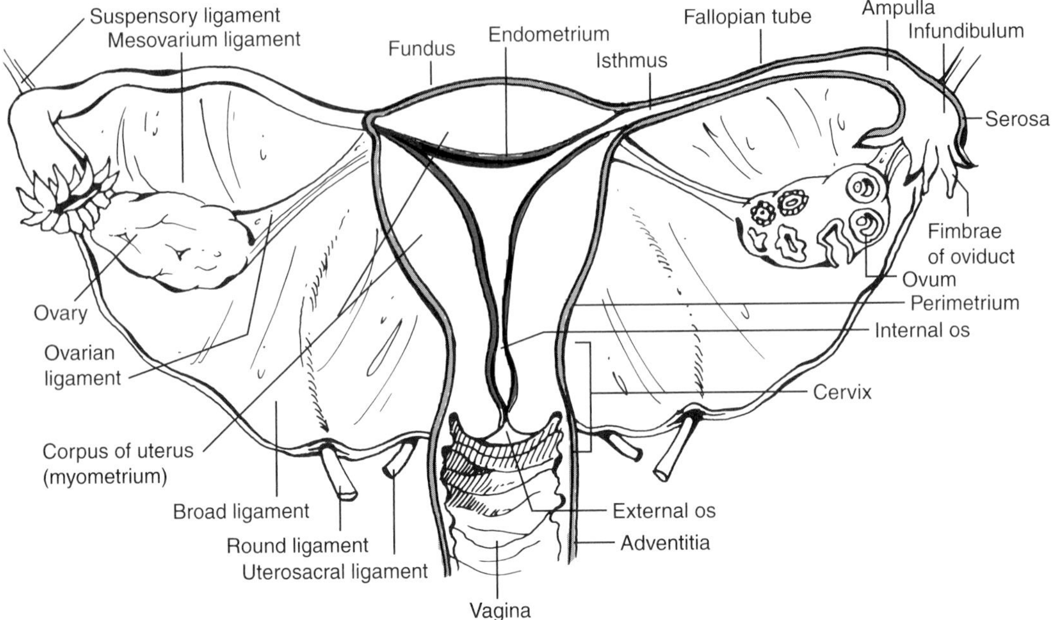

FIGURE 37-1. **Internal reproductive organs of the female: Anterior view of the female gonads, genital tract, and supporting structures. (Redrawn from Reeder, S. J., Martin, L. L., & Koniak, D. [1997].** ***Maternity nursing*** **[18th ed.]. Philadelphia: Lippincott-Raven.)**

All of the internal reproductive organs are supported in a slinglike fashion by ligaments and fascial structures. The ligaments and fascia are covered by folds of peritoneum and attached to the sidewalls of the pelvis. The pelvic diaphragm contains the levator ani and coccygeus muscle and forms a broad sling within the pelvis that swings forward at the pelvic outlet to surround the vagina and rectum as a form of sphincter. The pubovaginalis is the actual sphincter, which acts as a sling for the vagina and is the main muscular support for the pelvic organs. The urogenital diaphragm is the triangular area between the ischial tuberosities and the symphysis pubis. It contains urethral striated sphincter muscles, trigone fascia, and the inferior urogenital trigone fascia. The main function is to provide support for the lower urethra and the anterior wall of the vaginal canal.

The major uterine ligaments (see Fig. 37-1) are the broad ligaments and the round ligaments. The broad ligaments are two wormlike structures extending from the lateral margin of the uterus to the pelvic walls, dividing the uterine cavity into anterior and posterior compartments. These ligaments help the uterus remain supported in midpostion, acting as "guide wires." The cardinal ligaments are the lower portion, composed of dense connective tissue firmly joined to the supravaginal portion of the cervix. They support the vagina and prevent **uterine prolapse**.

Round ligaments are fibrous cords that attach to either side of the fundus, just below the fallopian tubes. They extend through the inguinal canal and terminate in the upper portion of the labia minora. They aid in holding the fundus tilted forward. The two uterosacral ligaments are cordlike structures that extend from the posterior cervical portion of the uterus to the sacrum and help support the cervix. The uterosacral ligaments include (1) the uterovesical ligament, which is a fold of peritoneum that passes over the fundus and extends to the bladder, and (2) the rectovaginal ligament, a fold of peritoneum that passes over the posterior surface of the uterus.

Ovaries

The ovaries, or female gonads, are paired glandular organs that lie in a depression in the lateral pelvic wall, on either side of the uterus. Each ovary is about the size of an almond. They vary considerably in size among women but usually measure between 3 to 5 cm long, 1.5 to 3 cm wide, and 1 to 1.5 cm thick—about the size of a thumbnail. They are pinkish-white to gray in appearance. They are not directly attached to the uterus and tubes but lie suspended in a strong, flexible structure, the round ligament, which anchors them to the uterus. (It is important to note that the uterine tubes, which consist of the oviducts and fallopian tubes, are not directly connected to the ovaries but open into the peritoneal cavity area near them.)

The inner ovary, or the medulla, is composed of blood and lymphatic tissues, connective tissue, and

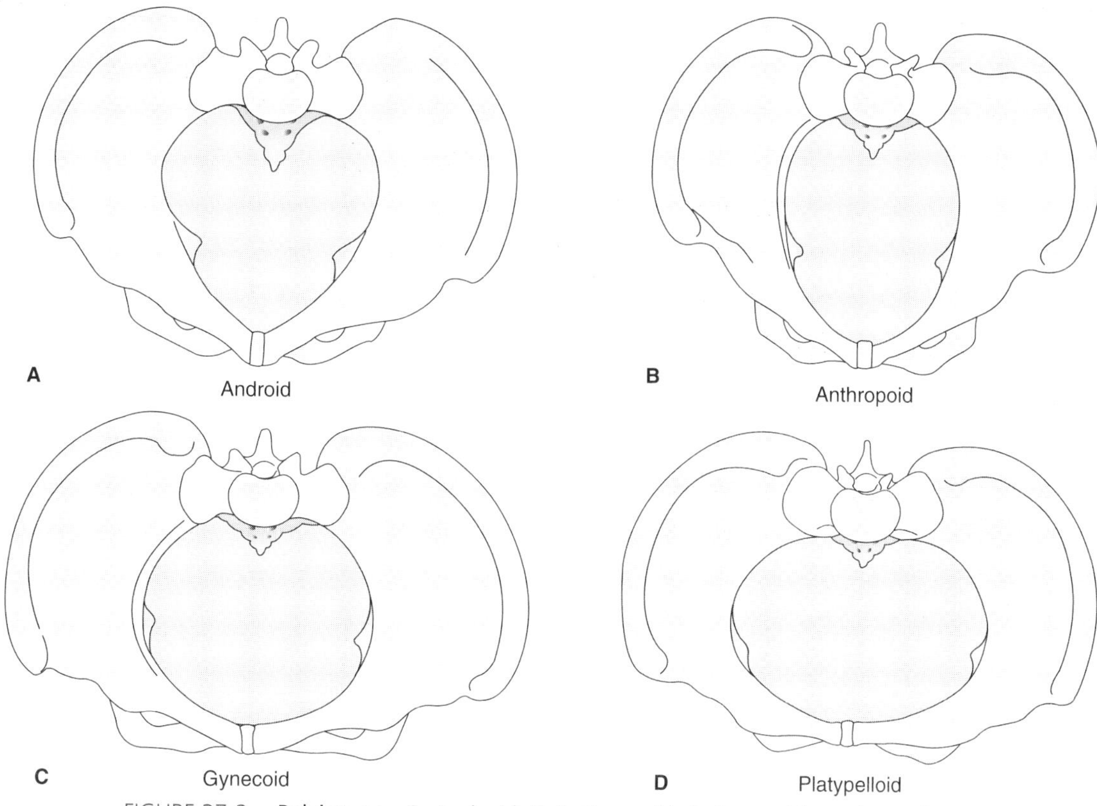

FIGURE 37-2. **Pelvic types. A. Android. B. Anthropoid. C. Gynecoid. D. Platypelloid.**

nerve fibers. The outer ovary, or cortex, contains the ovarian follicles and is under the influence of hormones.

The ovaries house the female sex gametes. They are the counterparts to the testes in the male in that they secret sex hormones. At birth each ovary contains about 400,000 primordial egg cells. These follicles are considered permanent cells because no more are produced after birth. At the time of puberty, between 30,000 and 50,000 of these primordial follicles remain. These follicles are oocytes that are in a sustained meiotic phase and surrounded by granulosa cells. They will either disintegrate or mature into eggs during the 30 reproductive years of active ovarian activity. During ovulation, the ovaries produce an ova (egg) in response to hormonal stimulation. They perform the vital functions of oogenesis, ovulation, and hormone secretion. The anterior pituitary glands regulate ovarian function and are discussed below (see menstrual cycle).

Uterus

The uterine corpus is a muscular, thick-walled, hollow organ, shaped like an inverted pear. It lies posterior to the bladder and anterior to the rectum. The size and shape vary but, in the nonpregnant state, is about 7.5 cm (3 in) long, 5 cm (2 in) wide, and 2.5 cm (1 in) in depth, a little smaller than a fist. It consists of two sections, the upper portion and the lower portion, roughly divided in the middle at the isthmus. The upper portion is the corpus, or the main body. The fundus is a dome-shaped portion located between the insertion points where the fallopian tubes enter the uterus. The doughnut-shaped cervix is the lower, narrower portion that opens into the vagina. The cervix is not a separate organ but is actually the lower half of the uterus. Figure 37-1 illustrates these aspects of the uterus. The functions of the uterus include menstruation, gestation, and parturition.

The uterus is not fixed. It is mobile and expands readily to accommodate a developing fetus. It is a freely movable organ suspended in the pelvic cavity, which varies as the woman changes her position. It is supported by the levator ani muscle and eight ligaments, as described above. The uterine artery is the main source of blood for the uterus.

The position of the uterus within the pelvis varies (Fig. 37-3). It can be anteverted (tilted toward the bladder), retroverted (tilted toward the rectum), or in midposition. The upper portion of the uterus is also described according to its relationship to the cervix. In an anteflexed uterus, the anterior surface is bent forward toward the cervix. Conversely, a retroflexed uterus is

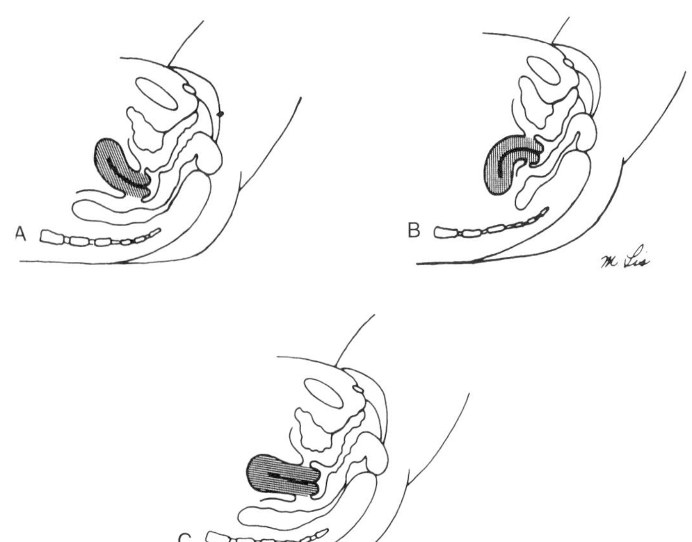

FIGURE 37-3. Positions of the uterine fundus and cervix. **A.** Anteversion. **B.** Midposition. **C.** Retroversion.

one in which the posterior surface bends backward toward the cervix. Consequently, a uterus can be anteverted (tilting toward the front) and anteflexed (the anterior portion bent).

UTERINE WALLS

The uterine walls are composed of three layers and include (1) the endometrium, (2) the myometrium, and (3) the perimetrium. The endometrium is the mucous membrane lining of the uterine cavity. Its ultimate purpose is to provide a suitable location for the implantation of a fertilized ovum and to establish, along with the developing embryo/fetus, a placenta during gestation. If pregnancy is not realized, menstruation occurs. The endometrium is divided into two layers: (1) the stratum functionalis, which is a superficial layer that is sloughed with each menstruation and after delivery, and (2) the stratum basalis, which is a deeper layer that is retained during menses and proliferates during the next menstrual cycle to regenerate the stratum functionalis.

The myometrium is the middle layer. It is thick and muscular; its function is to contract. Uterine contractions are necessary for normal vaginal delivery of the fetus during parturition and to aid in expelling menstrual secretions during menstruation. The myometrium is thickest in the fundus, which allows for more downward force during labor contractions, assisting in delivery. The perimetrium is a thin, serous, external peritoneal membrane that covers and protects the outside of the uterus.

UTERINE CERVIX

The uterine cervix is a knoblike structure. It is firmer upon palpation than the corpus because there is more connective tissue. It feels similar in consistency to the tip of the nose. The ectocervix is the external cervical portion that is visible and palpable in the upper vagina. It is covered by squamous epithelium, which is contiguous with the vaginal lining and is smooth, shiny, and pink. The squamous epithelium consists of four layers, similar to those of the skin (Fig. 37-4). The amount of cells in each layer varies in response to estrogen levels and to the presence of any inflammation or infection. The layers include (in order from the lower layer to the superficial layer):

- Basal: lies within the thin basement membrane; consists of one to two cell layers
- Parabasal: consists of three to four cell layers
- Intermediate: thicker than the previous two layers
- Superficial: mature cells that continuously shed; the thickest layer

The size of the cervical opening, or the external os, varies with the age, parity, and hormonal status of the woman. It is a tiny, round opening in women who have not borne children vaginally, and open, slitlike, and irregular in women who have delivered vaginally. It becomes tight and tiny in postmenopausal women due to cervical atrophy with decreasing estrogen levels. In ovulating women, in the presence of high estrogen levels it becomes open and even gaping at midcycle.

Columnar epithelium lines the endocervical canal and is darker red and granular appearing. It is mucus secreting. The squamocolumnar junction or transformation zone is the area where squamous epithelium and the columnar epithelium meet (Fig. 37-5). Squamous metaplasia occurs naturally in this area as columnar epithelium is changed to squamous epithelium in response to increasing estrogen levels as the woman matures. It becomes differentiated. This area of meta-

FOCUS ON CELLULAR PHYSIOLOGY

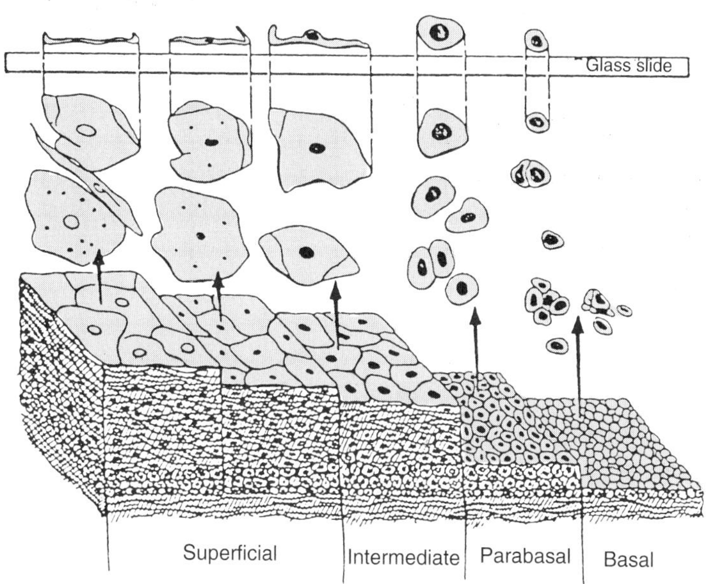

FIGURE 37-4. Layers of the vaginal epithelial cells.

FOCUS ON CELLULAR PHYSIOLOGY

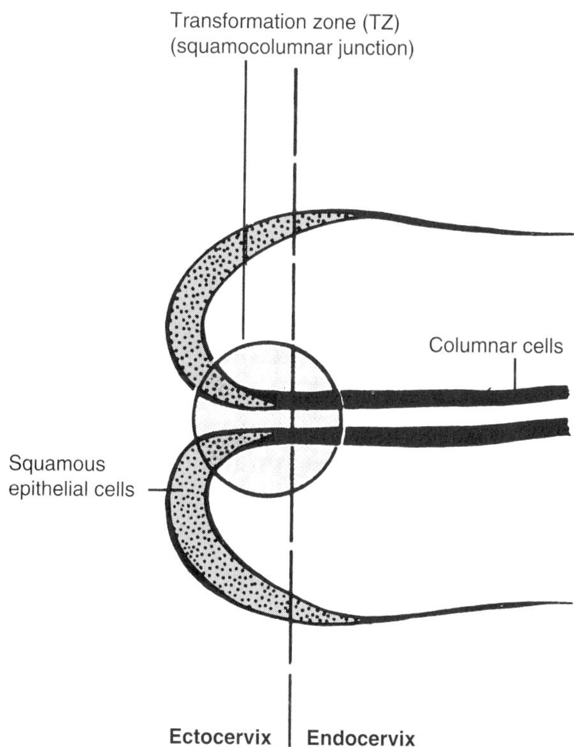

FIGURE 37-5. Transformation zone (TZ) is the area of metaplasia from which endocervical cells must be sampled. Location varies with estrogen level.

plasia is the area of "endocervical" cells, which is critical to sample during a routine Pap smear since it is particularly susceptible to neoplastic changes.

The actual location of this zone varies. In adolescents and women with high estrogen levels (for example, those on oral contraceptives), it is actually visible on the ectocervix. If present, it is termed a **cervical eversion**, ectropion, or ectomy. When this occurs, the ectocervix would contain both types of cells, an inner ring of columnar epithelium and an outer ring of squamous epithelium (Fig. 37-6). It extends up the canal with decreasing estrogen levels and may not be visible at all in a postmenopausal woman.

The surface of the extocervix normally has endocervical glands that secrete mucus. These ducts can become obstructed and appear cystic. They are called **Nabothian cysts**. Quite common, they are usually normal but may be increased in the presence of a vaginal infection. Their appearance varies from a few tiny cysts to large cysts covering the entire cervix.

Cervical Mucus

Cervical mucus is produced by the mucus-secreting cells of the endocervix. The cervical mucus also changes in response to hormonal variations. As ovulation approaches, ovarian secretion of estrogen rises, increasing the volume and water content of the mucus. Just prior to ovulation the cervical discharge changes from thick, scant mucus to become acellular, nonviscous, watery, and abundant, providing an environment that is conducive to sperm transport. At ovulation, nearly

FOCUS ON CELLULAR PHYSIOLOGY

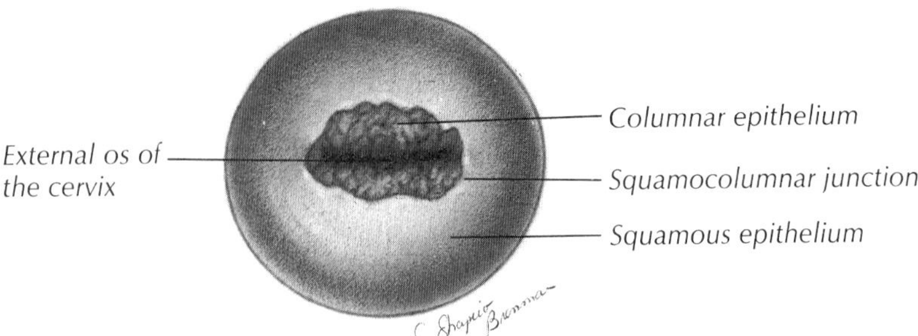

FIGURE 37-6. With cervical eversion, the ectocervix contains both columnar and squamous epithelium.

98% of the mucosal volume is water. If the mucus is thick it tends to "plug" the cervical os. Poor mucus is not an absolute barrier to fertility but may lower the possibility of conception.

The mucus usually remains clear for 2 to 3 days during ovulation. Table 37-1 compares ovulatory to non-ovulatory mucus. The ovulatory mucus should resemble the white of an uncooked egg. The mucus develops the ability to stretch as estrogen levels rise prior to ovulation; this is termed spinnbarkeit. It can be demonstrated when a sample of cervical mucus is grasped between the thumb and forefinger and stretched to 6 to 10 cm. Another interesting characteristic of ovulatory mucus is arborization or ferning, which can be seen microscopically when the cervical mucus is allowed to dry on a slide (Fig. 37-7). It is due to the crystallization of the mucus from electrolytes, mainly sodium chloride, interacting with glycoproteins in the mucus. Its presence indicates adequate estrogen production. Some writers suggest that the fernlike channels may actually provide a passageway for transport of sperm.

Fallopian tubes

Fallopian tubes extend outward from either side of the body of the uterus and act as a connecting tunnel between the ovary and the uterus. They attach at the upper uterus and run laterally for 10 to 12 cm to the ovaries. These narrow and muscular tubes act as oviducts and are lined with cilia (see Fig. 37-1). They are approximately 13 cm (5 in) long, rubbery in consistency, and less than half the diameter of a pencil (.05 to 1.0 cm). The tubes have two layers, inner and outer serous layers, surrounded by layers of involuntary muscle. The outer serosa is the smooth layer formed by part of the visceral peritoneum.

Tubes consist of four sections:

- Interstitial section: lies within the uterine wall
- Isthmus:
  - Narrowest section closest to the uterus
  - Opens into the cavity of the uterus
  - Has thick, muscular wall with narrow lumen
  - Is the usual site for a tubal ligation
- Ampulla:
  - Longest and widest section, about ⅔ of the total length
  - Widens progressively to the wide distal opening of the infundibulum
  - Thin-walled with a highly folded lining
  - Site of fertilization
- Infundibulum: fimbriated end, which lies in close proximity to the ovary

The main function of the fallopian tubes is the transportation of the sperm toward the ovary and, in the opposite direction, the egg towards the uterus. The inner wall of the tubes, the mucosa, is lined with cilia, which are hairlike projections. It is thought that the beating motion of these cilia has a role in transporting the fertilized egg along the tube to the uterus, where it

TABLE 37-1

COMPARISON OF FERTILE AND NONFERTILE CERVICAL MUCUS

OVULATORY "FERTILE" MUCUS	NONOVULATORY MUCUS
Clear, slightly cloudy	Opaque
Abundant	Scant
Stretchy, like raw egg white	Non-stretchy
Slippery	Rubbery
Dries without residue	Leaves white flakes when dry

FOCUS ON CELLULAR PHYSIOLOGY

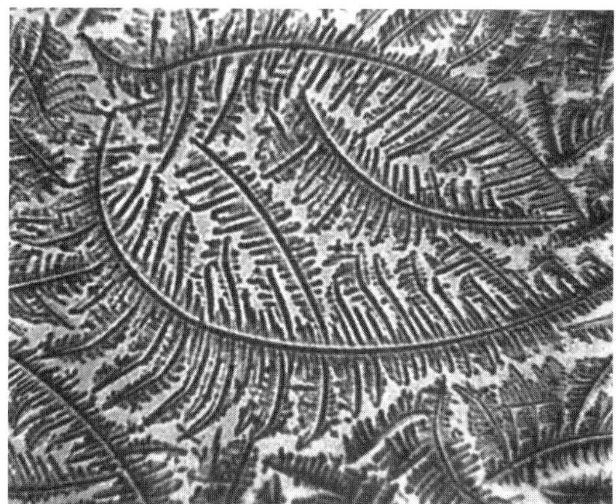

FIGURE 37-7. A ferning pattern of cervical mucus with high estrogen levels. (Magnification, X 40.)

is implanted. Muscle contractions in the muscularis layer assist in moving the egg along, much like intestinal peristalsis. Fallopian tubes have the unique ability to transport the ovum in one direction and the sperm in the opposite. Around the time of ovulation fingerlike projections, the fimbriae, bend down in closer proximity to the ovaries. The cilia, in the fimbriae, have adhesive sites. As the fimbriae sweep over the ovary, they create a current that scoops up the egg and propels it into the tube.

The Vagina

The vagina is a fibromuscular canal, located anterior to the rectum and posterior to the urethra, that connects the uterus to the outside of the body. It is normally pinkish red, about 9 cm long, and enters and protrudes into the upper vagina, causing the formation of a deeper ring posteriorly around the cervix, called the fornix. The fornix is comparatively thin walled, allowing for palpation of the ovaries and uterus during a bimanual pelvic examination. It may act to pool semen after ejaculation, allowing a "time release" effect as the sperm intermittently swim through the cervix.

The vagina is lined with squamous epithelium arranged in folds called rugae, extending from the cervix to the vestibule. The muscular coat of the vagina is much thinner than the uterus, allowing it to stretch and contract easily during intercourse or delivery. It is important to note that is does not contain any mucus-secreting glands; therefore, it needs to be moistened by cervical and glandular secretions. Additional fluids percolate into the vagina from other fluid compartments during sexual arousal. Vaginal branches of the uterine artery supply oxygenated blood to the vagina.

The opening at the inferior end of the vagina is called the vaginal orifice, which may be covered by a thin, vascularized membrane called the hymen. This membrane is usually incomplete, but if it entirely covers the orifice (imperforate hymen) it must be opened at puberty to allow the escape of menstrual fluids.

There are four major functions of the vagina. It acts as a passageway for menstrual flow to exit the uterus, for the fetus to be expelled from the uterus, and for sperm to travel towards the ovum. It also acts as a receptacle for the penis during sexual intercourse.

VAGINAL ECOLOGY

The vagina has minimal nerve endings; therefore, symptoms of vaginal disorders may only become evident when the vaginal discharge bathes and irritates the sensitive vulvar skin. The vaginal epithelium in a well-estrogenized woman contains large amounts of glycogen. Normal bacterial flora of the vagina consists of lactobacilli that metabolize the glycogen. Lactobacilli are pleomorphic, gram-positive, aerobic or facultative anaerobic, non–spore-forming organisms that usually dominate the flora of the normal vagina (96%). These elongated, rod-shaped bacilli appear as slightly motile straight rods that vary in length between 5 and 15 mm. Lactobacilli help maintain a low pH (3.8 to 4.2) of vaginal discharge by making lactic acid, which inhibits adherence of bacteria to epithelial cells. Normally the vagina cleanses itself by the discharge of acidotic secretions. Most organisms within the vagina live symbiotically in an acid environment.

Hormones play a major role in maintaining this environment. Estrogen causes glycogen to be deposited in the vagina, mainly in the epithelial cells. In the presence of estrogen, glycogen is produced and metabolized to become lactic acid. Glycogen present in the epithelial cells is utilized by the peroxide-producing lactobacilli to produce lactic acid, which maintains an acid environment. This level of acidotic secretions is antagonistic to harmful bacterial organisms. Progesterone causes shedding of these glycogen-rich cells into the vaginal pool. The number of glycogen-rich cells increases following menarche and markedly decrease following **menopause**, in response to declining estrogen levels.

Genital Tract Glands

Bartholin's (or greater vestibular) glands are two bean-shaped, mucus-secreting glands located on each side of the vaginal orifice (Fig. 37-8). Secretion is increased during sexual excitement and serves to moisten the inner surface of the labia in preparation for intercourse. Skene's glands are tiny, mucus-secreting glands located just posterior to the external urethral meatus

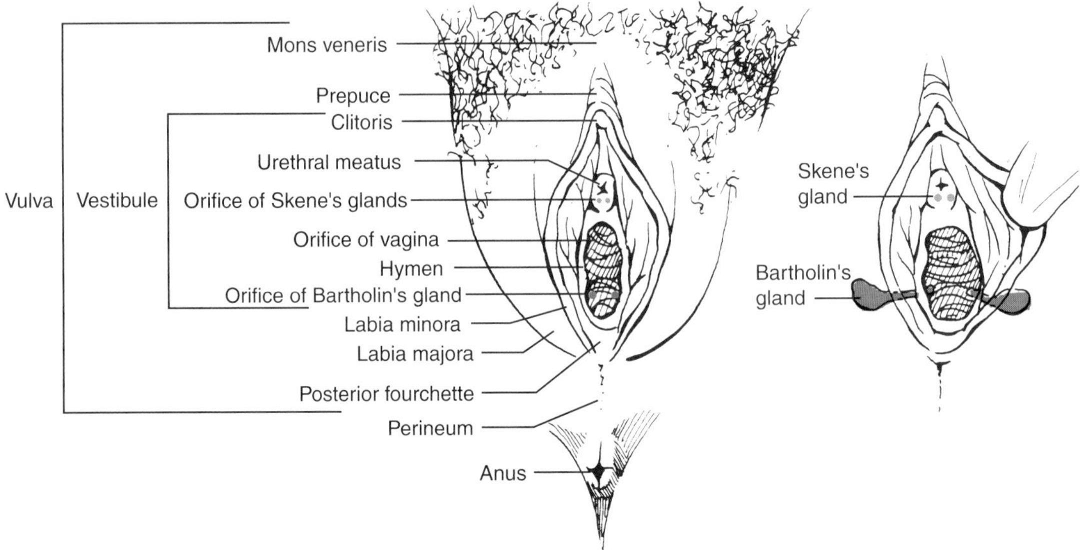

FIGURE 37-8. **External genitalia of the female. (Redrawn from Reeder, S. J., Martin, L. L. & Koniak, D. [1997]. *Maternity nursing* [18th ed.]. Philadelphia: Lippincott-Raven.)**

(see Fig. 37-8). The mucus from the Skene glands, together with that from glands in the urethra, keeps the urethral opening moist and lubricated.

NORMAL EXTERNAL GENITALIA

The external organs are those structures visible in the perineal area, which is the area that lies anterior to the symphysis pubis, posterior to the buttocks, and lateral to the thighs. The term *vulva* refers to these externally visible structures in the perineal region. The vulva is normally the same color as the skin covering the external parts of the rest of the body. This color is due to the fine network of superficial blood vessels located just below the thick epidermal layers of the skin and to the amount of melanin. The vulva area is always moist and actually sweats more than any area of the body except the axilla. The vulva contains the mons pubis; two sets of lips, the labia majora and labia minora; the clitoris; and the vestibule (which includes the urethral and vaginal orifices). The structures of the vulva are illustrated in Figure 37-8.

Mons Pubis

The mons pubis is a fatty tissue prominence overlying the bony symphysis. It contains hair follicles and is usually covered by coarse, curly pubic hair that appears as a flattened, inverted triangle over the symphysis. This is termed the escutcheon. The development of axillary and pubic hair coincides with the development of the secondary sexual characteristics. This development is influenced primarily by estrogen, although progesterone has an affect as well. The Tanner staging of sexual maturity, shown in Figure 37-9, details the development of pubic hair. The mons pubis protects the pubic bones from injury.

The Labia

The labia majora are two longitudinal folds of adipose tissues extending from the mons to enclose and protect the labia minora. The mons and labia majora are similar to skin in that they contain sweat glands, lymphatic and blood vessels, and nerves. The labia majora does not contain hair follicles. The labia minora lie inside and parallel to the labia majora. The labia minora are more like mucous membrane than skin. They fuse anteriorly to form the clitoral hood (the prepuce), split apart to surround the vestibule, and then join again posteriorly to form the slightly raised ridge of tissue called the fourchette.

The Vestibule

The vestibule is the area that lies within the labia minora, between the prepuce and the fourchette. It contains the clitoris, urethra meatus, vaginal introitus (opening or orifice), orifices to Skene's and Bartholin's glands (in which Bartholin's and Skene's glands are located), and hymen. The clitoris is a small, cylindrical, erectile organ approximately 1 to 2 cm long. It is located at the forward junction of the labia minora and covered by the prepuce. The center of sexual arousal and orgasm, the clitoris has many sensory nerve end-

Stage 1

Preadolescent—no pubic hair except for the fine body hair (vellus hair) similar to that on the abdomen

Stage 2

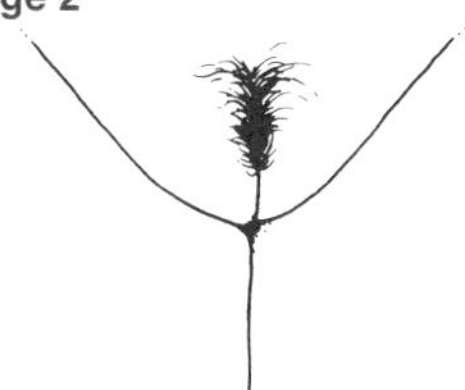

Sparse growth of long, slightly pigmented, downy hair, straight or only slightly curled, chiefly along the labia

Stage 3

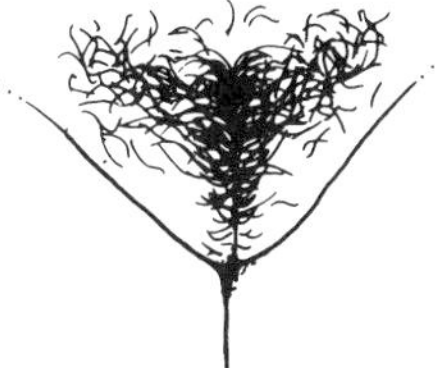

Darker, coarser, curlier hair, spreading sparsely over the pubic symphysis

Stage 4

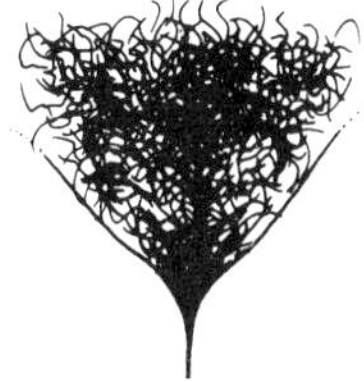

Coarse and curly hair as in adults; area covered greater than in stage 3 but not as great as in the adult and not yet including the thighs

Stage 5

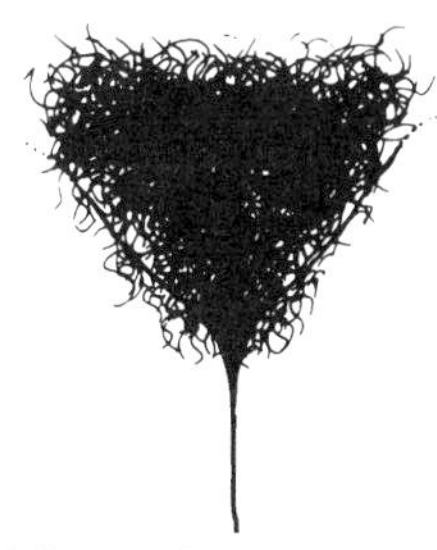

Hair adult in quantity and quality, spread on the medial surfaces of the thighs but not up over the abdomen

FIGURE 37-9. Tanner's sex maturity ratings in girls: pubic hair. (Illustration through the courtesy of W. A. Daniel, Jr., Division of Adolescent Medicine, University of Alabama, Birmingham.)

ings and a plentiful arterial blood supply. Thus, the clitoris is analogous to the penis in the male.

The perineal body lies between the fourchette and the anus. It is often the site of an episiotomy, which may be performed during childbirth to make the vaginal opening wider.

BLOOD SUPPLY AND NEURAL CONTROL

The blood supply of the pelvic structure is mainly derived from the internal iliac artery and its branches. The pelvic structures receive both sympathetic and parasympathetic nerve supplies. The sensory nerves fron the uterus travel with the sympathetic nerves to L2 and L4. The sensory nerves from the cervix generally transmit through the uterosacral ligaments and travel to S2, S3, and S4. Consequently, pain from the uterus is generally referred to the lower abdomen, and pain from the cervix to the lumbrosacral region.

BREASTS

The breasts are complex accessory organs of the female reproductive system, which respond to the hormonal changes of puberty, the menstrual cycle, pregnancy, and lactation. During puberty, breast development is controlled by multiple hormones, with estrogen playing a central role. Figure 37-10 shows the Tanner staging of breast development in the adolescent. Under the influence of prolactin, the mammary glands of the breast secrete milk necessary to nourish the newborn infant.

The two breasts are located over the pectoral muscles between the second and sixth ribs. The breasts extend from the second or third rib to the sixth or seventh rib, and from the sternal edge to the anterior axillary line. The breast tail, or tail of Spence, extends upward and laterally toward the axilla. The breasts are attached to the chest wall by a layer of connective tissue. As seen in Figure 37-11*A*, each breast consists of a nipple and surrounding areola, ducts, lobes, and fibrous and fatty tissue. The ridge of fat on the lower portion of the breast is called the inframammary ridge. The breast tissue here is often more dense. There is very little muscle in the breasts except a small amount in the areola and nipple, which causes it to contract, facilitating the emptying of the milk sinuses.

The nipple, a cylindrical projection near the center of the breast, is located approximately at the fourth intercostal space. It is surrounded by a pigmented, circular area, the areola, and is perforated by several duct openings. Sexual stimulation results in engorgement and muscle contraction, which causes the nipple to become erect.

Stage 1
Preadolescent. Elevation of nipple only

Stage 2

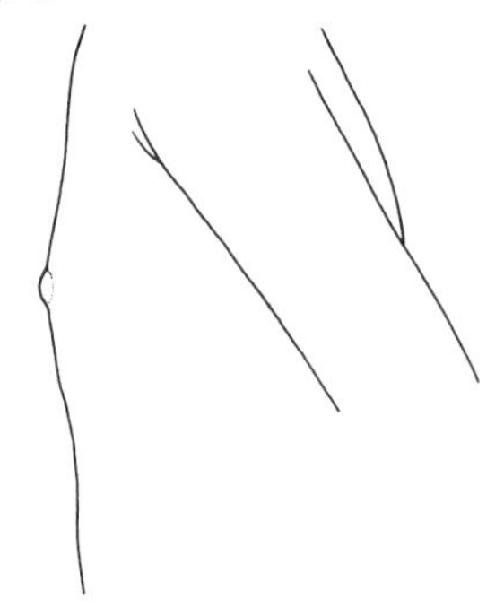

Breast bud stage. Elevation of breast and nipple as a small mound; enlargement of areolar diameter

Stage 3

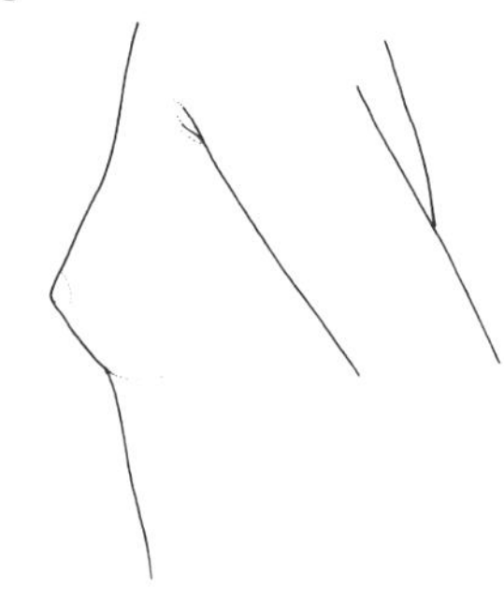

Further enlargement of elevation of breast and areola, with no separation of their contours

Stage 4

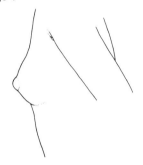

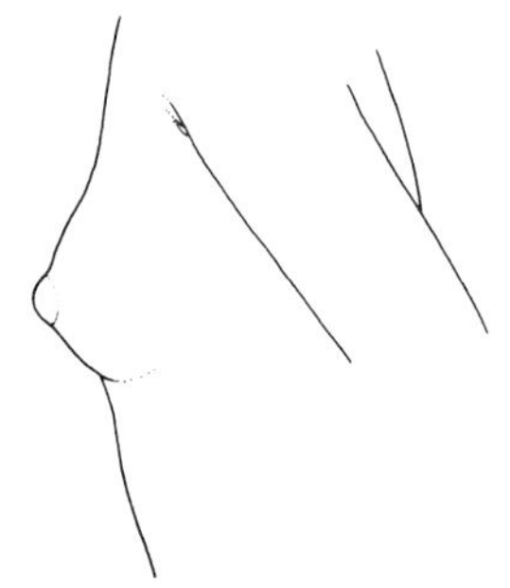

Projection of areola and nipple to form a secondary mound above the level of breast

Stage 5

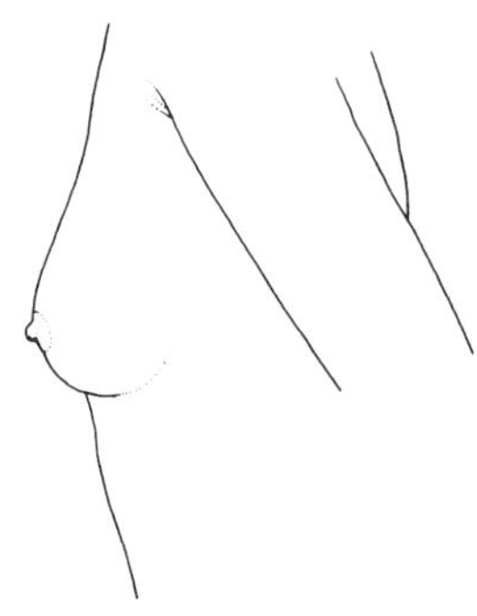

Mature stage; projection of nipple only. Areola has receded to general contour of the breast (although in some normal individuals the areola continues to form a secondary mound).

FIGURE 37-10. **Tanner's sex maturity ratings in girls: breasts. (Illustration through the courtesy of W. A. Daniel, Jr., Division of Adolescent Medicine, University of Alabama, Birmingham.)**

The mature female breast is made up of 15 to 20 lobes arranged around the nipple. These lobules (mammary glands) lie within the peripheral breast tissue and emerge at the nipple (the hub), like the spokes of a wheel. Each lobe is further composed of a number of lobules. Inside each lobule are the alveoli, which contain both acinar and myoepithelial cells. The acinar cells manufacture and secrete milk, and the myoepithelial cells contract to force milk into the ducts. Each lobule is drained by an intralobular duct that empties into a lactiferous duct. These ducts dilate, forming a reservoir called the lactiferous sinus (or ampulla) just before each opens in the nipple. Lobes and ducts are separated by fibrous tissue. Over half of the ducts are present in the upper outer breast quadrant (dividing the breast into four parts with the nipple at the center), in the tail of Spence. Breast tissue feels more firm in those areas. Breast cancers occurs more commonly in the ductal tissue within the upper outer quadrant.

Blood Supply and Neural Control

Blood reaches each breast by several arteries, the major one being a branch of the thoracic artery. Blood is drained by multiple veins, including the axillary and internal thoracic veins.

Lymph vessels are numerous in the breasts and provide drainage of the superficial, areolar, and glandular parts of the breast. They normally follow the lactiferous ducts, eventually draining into the axillary nodes. However, lymph flow is unpredictable, and many interconnecting channels make it possible for lymph to travel to subscapular or supraclavicular nodes or even to the contralateral breast or axillary

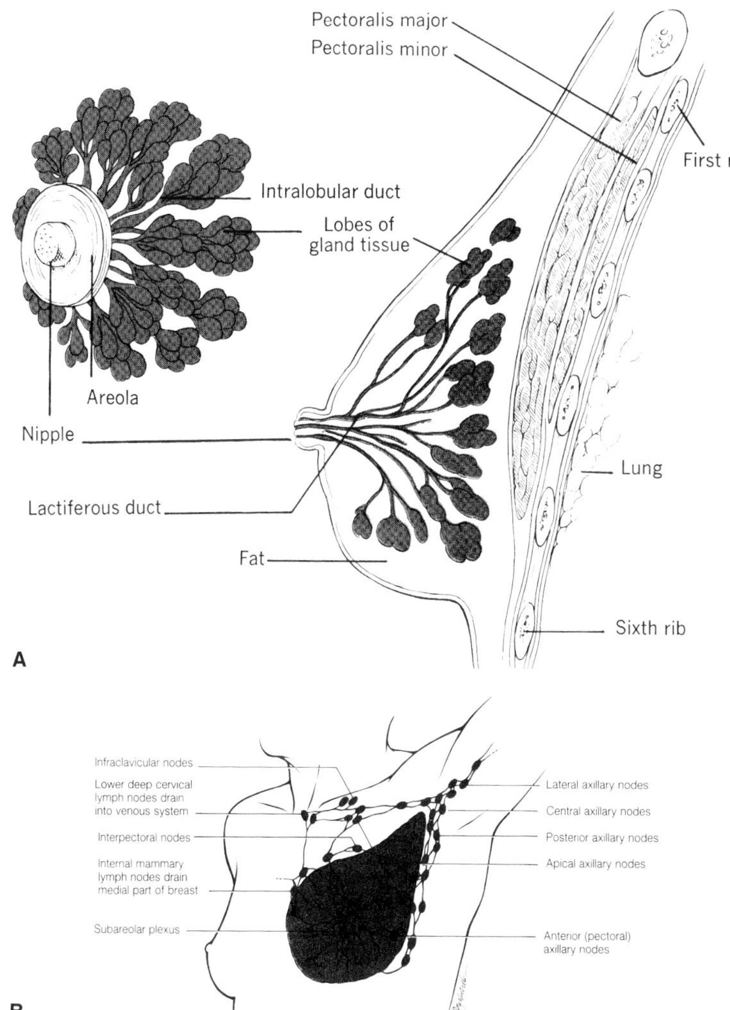

FIGURE 37-11. **Structure of the breast. A. Glandular tissues and ducts within the breast. (Redrawn from Reeder, C. J., Martin, L. I. & Koniak, D. [1997]. *Maternity nursing* [18th ed.]. Philadelphia: Lippincott-Raven.) B. Lymphatic pathways in the breast. (Redrawn from Smeltzer, S. C. & Bare, B. G. [1996]. *Brunner and Suddarth's textbook of medical-surgical nursing* [8th ed.]. Philadelphia: Lippincott.)**

nodes (see Fig. 37-11*B*). Lymph drainage of the breast is important, especially in considering the spread of breast cancer.

NORMAL FEMALE REPRODUCTIVE FUNCTION

Female reproductive function includes those processes that are related to creating gametes, preparing the uterus for pregnancy, carrying and delivering the fetus, and preparing the breasts for lactation. In the female, oogenesis and uterine preparation are periodic events that recur repeatedly, approximately once a month, in a complex sequence known as the menstrual cycle. If fertilization and implantation are successful, gestation, labor, delivery, and lactation normally follow. In order for normal reproductive functions to occur in the female, physiologic changes in multiple organs must be well coordinated. Such coordination relies heavily on hormones to direct the changes necessary during each menstrual cycle, throughout the period of gestation, and during lactation.

Hormonal Control

Estrogen and progesterone are the two gonadal (ovarian) sex hormones that control female reproductive system function. Both are necessary for the normal physical maturation of the female. Along with other hormones, estrogen and progesterone also provide for ovulation, implantation, pregnancy, parturition, and lactation. Secretion of the gonadal hormones is under the control of the hypothalamic gonadotropic releasing hormone (GnRH) and the pituitary gonadotropins (FSH and LH). Secretion of LH and FSH is inhibited by increasing progesterone levels after ovulation (negative feedback). Flowchart 37-1 diagrams the neuroen-

FLOWCHART 37-1 **Neuroendocrine Feedback Mechanisms**

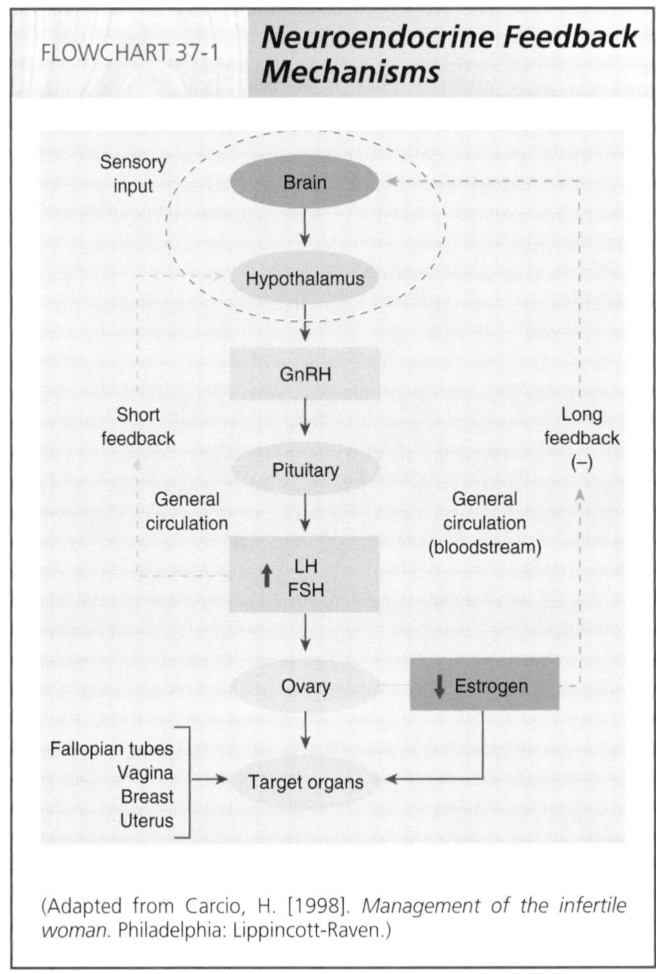

(Adapted from Carcio, H. [1998]. *Management of the infertile woman.* Philadelphia: Lippincott-Raven.)

docrine feedback mechanism. Other hormones such as androgens, prolactin, and the prostaglandins also play a role in female reproductive system function. The hormones involved in female reproduction are listed, along with their functions, in Table 37-2 and are discussed in subsequent sections.

The Menstrual Cycle

The menstrual cycle is a complicated monthly interaction between the hypothalamus, pituitary gland, ovaries, and endometrium that results in periodic fluctuations in hormone levels and changes in multiple body tissues, primarily the ovary and uterine endometrium. These modifications prepare the body for ovulation, conception, and gestation. Other tissues, such as the myometrium, vagina, and breasts, also respond to the monthly hormone surges. Changes in the ovaries during the menstrual cycle are referred to as the *ovarian cycle,* and changes in the endometrial tissue are called the *endometrial (or uterine) cycle.* Figure 37-12*A* shows the plasma hormone concentrations, ovarian events, and uterine changes during a menstrual cycle, which is repeated every 28 days (on average).

THE OVARIAN CYCLE

Many changes occur during the menstrual cycle. The ovarian cycle refers to those changes directly related to the hormonal response of the ovary. They include oogenesis, the follicular phase, ovulation, and the luteal phase.

Oogenesis

Oogenesis, or the creation of gametes (ova, eggs, oocytes) by the female, is very different from the process of spermatogenesis discussed in Chapter 36. A normally ovulating female usually generates one ovum per month, which is viable for only about 24 hours. The monthly development of an ovum begins when hormonal signals initiate a series of preparatory changes in the ovary during the first half of the menstrual cycle. The development of the follicle and ovum continues until

TABLE 37-2

HORMONES OF THE FEMALE REPRODUCTIVE SYSTEM

HORMONE	DESCRIPTION
Estrogens	A class of steroid hormones chiefly present in females that are secreted from ovarian follicular cells. Small amounts are also secreted by adrenal cortex. There are three major estrogens: 1. **Estradiol** (E_2) is the major estrogen in the non-pregnant female 2. **Estrone** (E_1) is also secreted in significant amounts but is much less potent 3. **Estriol** (E_3) is the major estrogen during pregnancy; secreted by placenta Estrogen is responsible for female secondary sex characteristics at puberty, and levels fluctuate during the menstrual cycle. Their primary effect is to promote proliferation of uterine endometrial cells, but they act on numerous other target tissues. Estrogens promote calcium and phosphate retention, strengthening bone. After menopause, when estrogen levels are reduced, bones weaken (osteoporosis) and may fracture.
Progesterone	A steroid hormone chiefly present in females. Progesterone works together with estrogen in coordinating events of the menstrual cycle and plays a major role in preparing the endometrium to receive and maintain an implanted embryo. Progesterone is produced almost exclusively by the corpus luteum in the non-pregnant female and during early pregnancy. Once the placenta forms, it secretes progesterone throughout the rest of pregnancy. During the menstrual cycle, progesterone promotes the differentiation of endometrial cells into glands that are capable of nourishing the early embryo.
GnRH (gonadotropic releasing hormone)	GnRH is a peptide hormone released from the hypothalamus. When GnRH is secreted, it is transported through the hypothalamic-hypophyseal portal system directly to the anterior pituitary gland, where it stimulates release of the pituitary gonadotropins (FSH/LH). GnRH secretion increases when gonadal hormone levels are low.
FSH (follicle stimulating hormone)	FSH is one of two gonadotropins (protein hormones secreted by the anterior pituitary gland that affect the ovaries). Secretion of FSH is increased by GnRH. FSH promotes proliferation and differentiation of ovarian follicular cells, increasing estrogen production by the follicle during the first half of the ovarian cycle. At the same time, it fosters development of the ovum within the follicle in preparation for ovulation.
LH (luteinizing hormone)	LH is the second gonadotropin. Secretion of LH is increased by GnRH. LH converts the empty follicle into a corpus luteum after ovulation. Cells of the corpus luteum then begin to secrete progesterone; a second peak of estrogen also occurs. If pregnancy occurs, the corpus luteum is maintained. If pregnancy does not occur, the corpus luteum degenerates.
PRL (prolactin)	PRL is a protein hormone secreted by the anterior pituitary gland. It is increased late in pregnancy and functions to stimulate production of milk by acinar cells in breast alveoli. Suckling during breastfeeding provides the stimulus for continued secretion. Pituitary gland tumors can cause hypersecretion of prolactin and cause milk production (galactorrhea), even in the absence of pregnancy.
OT (oxytocin)	OT is a protein hormone secreted by the posterior pituitary gland. Oxytocin increases uterine contractions during labor and moves milk from breast glands to nipples during suckling. It has also been found to rise during sexual intercourse and has been postulated to produce contraction of reproductive system smooth muscle during orgasm, in both males and females.[4]
Pgs (prostaglandins)	Pgs form a group of potent lipids that act as local hormones throughout the body. They are considered important in reproductive physiology. Specific prostaglandins have been separated into specific species designated by letters and subscripts (e.g., PgE_2, $PgF_{2\alpha}$). Each specific prostaglandin exerts distinct actions on different body tissues. Prostaglandins are degraded primarily in the lungs soon after they enter the circulation. For this reason, their actions are mainly local and short lived. Reproductive Pgs are primarily produced by endometrial cells, and their secretion varies during the menstrual cycle. Pgs rise after ovulation, with the highest levels produced during menses. Their major effects are vasoconstriction of endometrial blood vessels and contraction of the myometrium. Elevated levels of Pgs have been identified as a factor in primary dysmenorrhea. They are used clinically to induce labor contractions. Their effects are inhibited by anti-inflammatory agents.

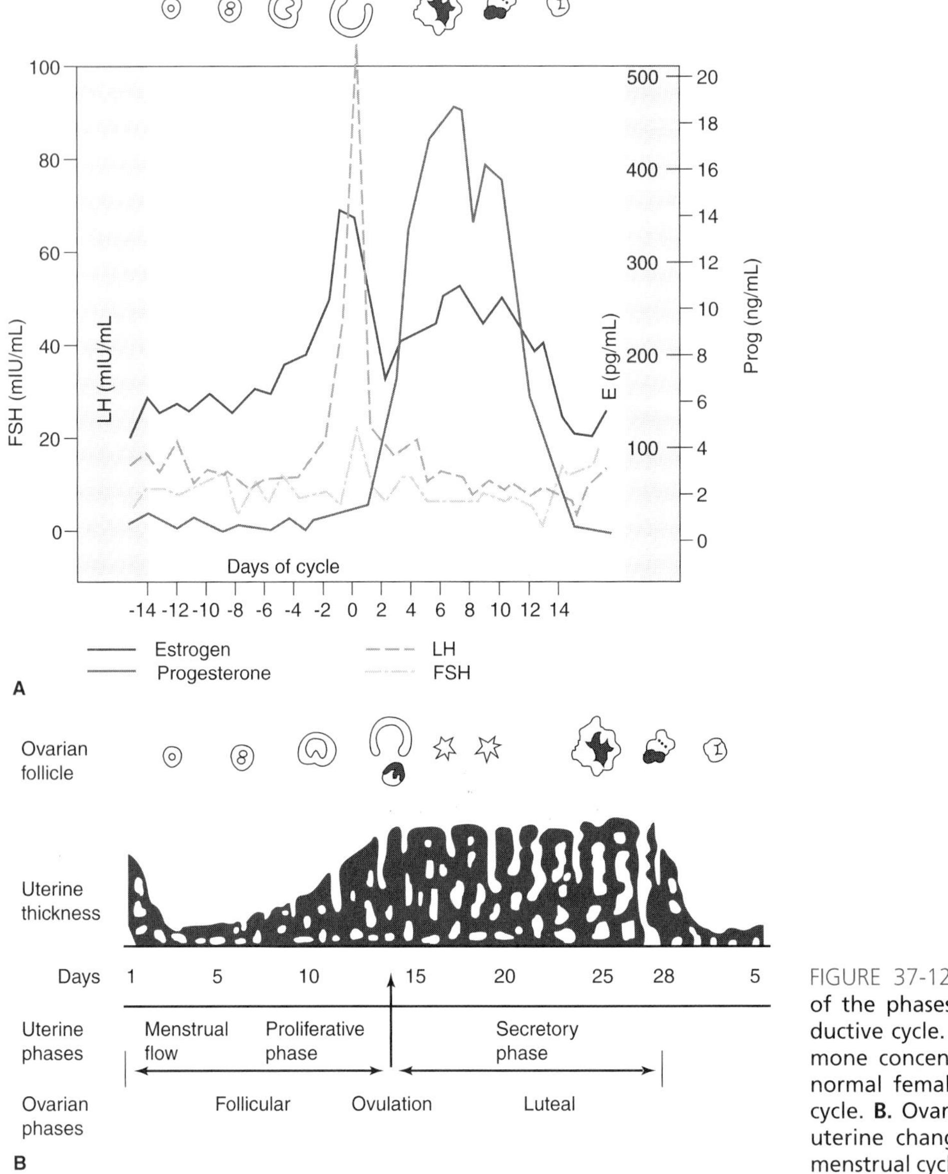

FIGURE 37-12. Comparison of the phases of the reproductive cycle. **A.** Plasma hormone concentrations in the normal female reproductive cycle. **B.** Ovarian events and uterine changes during the menstrual cycle.

ovulation, and a fully mature ovum is produced only if fertilization occurs. The maturation of one ovum during oogenesis is shown in Figure 37-13.

Just before ovulation, the primary oocyte completes its first meiotic division, resulting in a secondary oocyte, which contains 23 chromosomes and has received almost all of the cytoplasm. A second, smaller, cell is formed, which is called the first polar body. The first polar body receives 23 chromosomes but little cytoplasm. Meiosis is arrested at this phase if fertilization does not occur. If fertilized, the secondary oocyte executes a second meiotic division (see Fig. 37-13). Each of the newly formed cells again receives 23 chromosomes, but only one, called the mature ovum, receives the majority of cytoplasm. The other cell is the second polar body.

Follicular Phase

The ovaries enter their follicular phase, seen in Figure 37-12*B*, during which follicles develop and mature. By day 6 of the cycle, a dominant follicle has been selected, while the other recruited follicles undergo apoptosis. In the dominant follicle, the ovum enlarges and follicular cells proliferate and differentiate into estrogen-secreting cells. As the plasma estrogen level increases, it causes the cells of the endometrial stratum basalis to develop; hence, the term *proliferative phase* is applied to

FOCUS ON CELLULAR PHYSIOLOGY

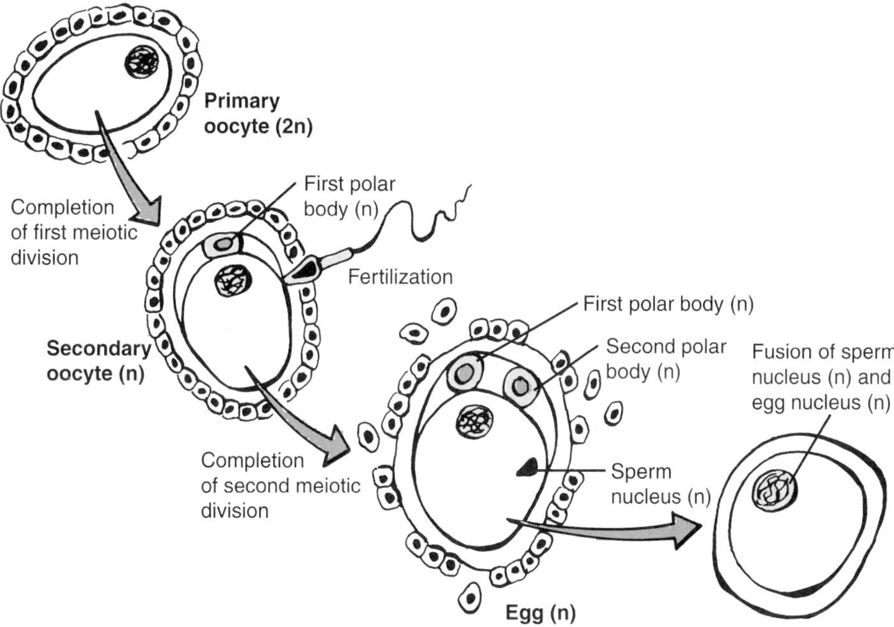

FIGURE 37-13. Oogenesis followed by fertilization results in second meiotic division, then a zygote.

this stage of uterine development (see Fig. 37-12*B*). As endometrial cells pile up, the endometrium thickens and arterioles grow longer and more coiled to supply the new tissue. At this time, blood levels of progesterone are low. Just before the end of the first half of the cycle FSH and LH rise sharply (gonadotropin surge), the estrogen level falls, and progesterone output by follicular cells begins to increase. The fully developed follicle, or graafian follicle, has gradually moved to the surface of the ovary, and the mid-cycle gonadotropin surge triggers ovulation about 18 hours after the gonadotropin peak.[9]

Ovulation

Ovulation divides the first and second halves of the menstrual cycle, but not necessarily evenly. The second half of the cycle is highly predictable in length, usually occurring 14 days before the onset of the next menses. The first half is much more variable, making ovulation timing difficult. During ovulation the graafian follicle thins and ruptures into the areas outside the ovary. The fimbriated edges of the fallopian tube draw the egg toward the tube. Ovulation may be accompanied by a low abdominal pain, termed mittelschmerz. The es-

TABLE 37-3

INDICATORS OF OVULATORY FUNCTION (MOLIMINIA)

OVULATION (MIDCYCLE)	FUNCTIONING CORPUS LUTEUM	MENSTRUATION
Pain (mittelschmerz) Biphasic basal body temperature Thin stretchy cervical mucus (spinnbarkeit)	Biphasic basal body temperature Premenstrual changes (correspond with adequate progesterone) Thick cervical mucus	Normal, regular pattern (absence of discernable dysfunction such as amenorrhea or oligomenorrhea

(Carcio, H. [1998]. *Management of the infertile woman.* Philadelphia: Lippincott-Raven.)

cape of fluid or blood from the follicle is believed to produce peritoneal irritation that causes the pain. The passage of blood vaginally during ovulation is termed Hartman's sign. Other predictive signs of ovulation are termed moliminia; Table 37-3 lists these symptoms. Ovulation is also accompanied by changes in cervical mucus, which increases in amount as it becomes clear and thin, to aid the journey of sperm.

Luteal Phase

Following ovulation, the ovary enters the luteal phase. The spot on the ovary where the egg ruptured transforms itself. The follicle walls collapse and some bleeding occurs into the cavity, forming a corpus hemorrhagica. Under the influence of LH, the cells hypertrophy, take on a yellow color, and become known as luteal cells, thus forming the corpus luteum (see Fig. 37-12). About 8 days after ovulation, the corpus luteum reaches full maturity and then begins to evolve into a white body called the corpus albican. If conception and pregnancy ensue, the copus luteum increases in size and governs hormonal requirements during gestation, particularly for the first 4 months. The primary function of the corpus luteum is to secrete progesterone and some estrogen. If conception does not occur, the progesterone secreted by the corpus luteum controls the postovulatory phase of the menstrual cycle for about 2 weeks.

THE ENDOMETRIAL CYCLE

The endometrial cycle refers to the cyclic changes in the cells lining the uterus (the endometrium). This is in contrast to the changes that occur in the ovary, which are termed the ovarian cycle. The endometrial cycle is divided into three phases: the proliferative and secretory phases and menses. These phases correspond directly to phases that are occurring in the ovary.

Proliferative Phase

At the end of menstruation the endometrium is thin and considered ischemic. By the second week of the cycle, hormonal production of estrogen increases and the endometrium becomes thicker. The cells undergo proliferatory growth and become taller as the glandular cells become deeper and wider. This thickness can increase up to eight times in height. The glands of the endometrium become more active, secreting, and nutritive.

During the same time, the follicles are producing more follicular fluid that contains estrogen. The proliferative phase is also called the follicular or estrogenic phase to signify that the dominant hormone is estrogen.

Secretory Phase

The second half of the uterine cycle is called the secretory phase. It usually comprises the last 2 weeks, or days 14 to 28 post-ovulation. During this period, the production of progesterone by the corpus luteum leads to changes in the endometrium that create a favorable environment for pregnancy. The endometrium becomes more vascular, with coiled spiral arteries located close to the surface. It becomes thicker as accumulation of nutrient fluids, rather than cellular proliferation, increases cell size. The lining is thrown into folds, forming glands. These changes produce a thick, succulent environment, rich in glycogen and ideal for implantation of the fertilized ovum. Progesterone also decreases myometrial contractions, which further aids the process of implantation. Increased levels of progesterone cause an increase in basal body temperature (BBT) during this phase of the menstrual cycle.

As noted in Figure 37-12*A*, high ovarian hormone secretion during the second half of the cycle initiates a negative feedback loop to the hypothalamus and pituitary gland, reducing their secretions, which prevents further follicle development and ovulation within the same cycle. In the absence of fertilization, luteal cells begin to degenerate, causing a decrease in estrogen and progesterone levels, which leads to an increase in GnRH and gonadotropins and hence a new cycle. The degenerating corpus luteum is eventually converted into the corpus albicans, which moves to the center of the ovary and finally disappears.

TABLE 37-4

COMPARISON OF NOMENCLATURE FOR THE VARIOUS PHASES OF THE REPRODUCTIVE CYCLE

	PREDOMINANT HORMONE	OVARIAN CYCLE	ENDOMETRIAL CYCLE	MENSTRUAL CYCLE
Day 1–14	Estrogenic phase	Follicular phase	Proliferative	Menstrual (1–7)
Day 14–28	Progestational	Luteal phase	Secretory	Premenstrual (21–28)

(Carcio, H. [1998]. *Management of the infertile woman.* Philadelphia: Lippincott-Raven.)

FOCUS ON CELLULAR PHYSIOLOGY

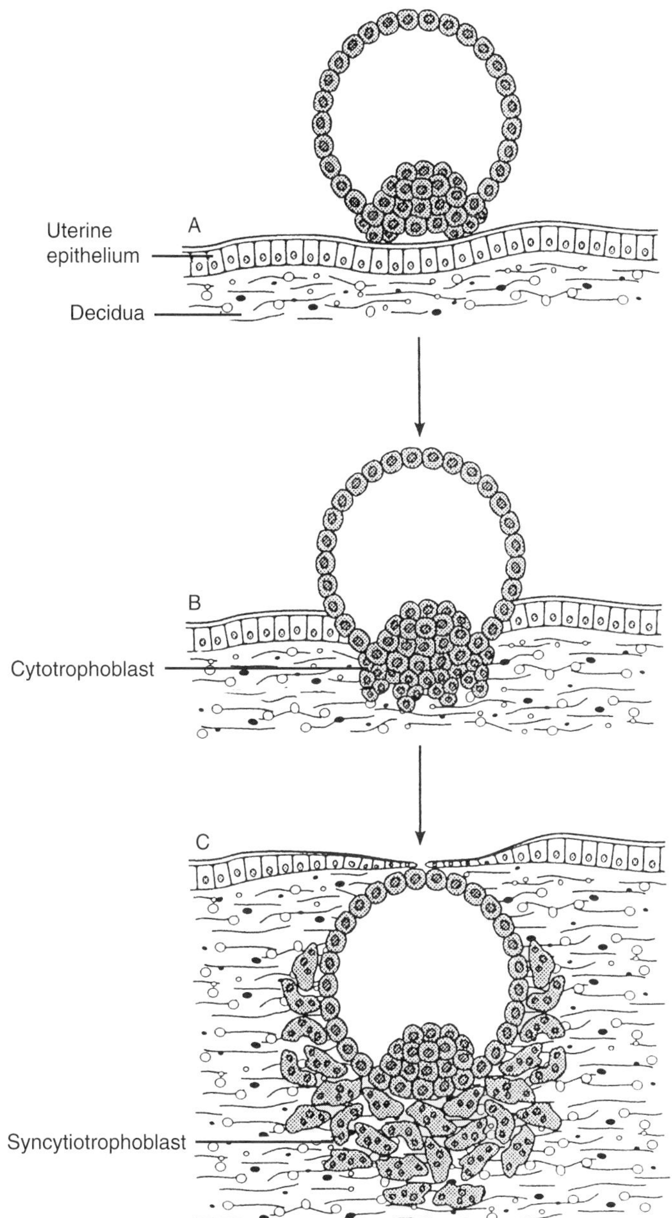

FIGURE 37-14. **Human implantation. The embryo attaches to the surface epithelium at the embryonic pole (A), penetrates the epithelium by intrusion led by cytotrophoblasts (B), and establishes a trophoblast bed in the decidua with fused syncytiotrophoblast (C).**

Other names for this phase are the luteal (referring to the ovary), progestational (referring to the dominant hormone), and premenstrual phase. Table 37-4 compares the nomenclature of the first half of the cycle with that of the second half.

Menses

If conception does not occur, the function of the corpus luteum wanes and levels of estrogen and progesterone drop, as does the basal body temperature. A new menstrual cycle begins when the lining of the endometrium becomes ischemic and cell degeneration occurs. Ultimately, as further cell degeneration occurs, the cells and subsequently small arterioles rupture. The deteriorating endometrium sloughs off the uterine wall and passes out the vagina in the form of menses (see Fig. 37-12*B*). Menstruation in effect allows the endometrial wall to be rebuilt with each month cycle, ensuring a fresh, new lining for each possible conception. Normal menstrual periods are, on average, repeated about every

28 days, last about 4 to 5 days, and have an average blood loss from 30 to 150 mL. Blood loss varies widely. However, normal periods can range from 21 to 35 days and last from 2 to 6 days. During menses, blood levels of both estrogen and progesterone are low, as noted in Figure 37-12*A*, and FSH is slightly elevated, which initiates recruitment of several primordial follicles.

Gestation

Gestation begins with fertilization and implantation of the ovum and continues as the conceptus develops into an embryo and then a fetus to complete its development. Conception can only occur when there is adequate maturing of an egg that becomes successfully implanted and then hormonally maintained by an adequately functioning corpus luteum. A full-term pregnancy, on average, lasts 40 weeks. The gestational period ends with parturition, or birth, which is normally preceded by a period of uterine contractions, or labor.

FERTILIZATION

As the egg matures and the fluid pressure increases, the egg and follicle are naturally moved toward the outside of the ovary. At some point the graafian follicle thins out to the outside edge of the ovary and ruptures into the area outside the ovary. The fimbriated edges of the fallopian tubes draw the egg toward the tube. Fertilization occurs in the distal upper third of the tube. After ovulation the ovum is captured in the distal portion of the fallopian tube, where fertilization takes place. About 4 days after ovulation, the developing zygote travels down the fallopian tube to enter the uterus. During embryonic cleavage the single-celled fertilized oocyte divides to produce two daughter cells (blastomeres). While the number of blastomeres is increasing, the embryo remains the size of the fertilized oocyte because no new cell growth is occurring during these first 4 days. Once it enters the uterus, the embryo differentiates into two distinct cell types: the inner cell mass, which becomes the embryo, and the outer cell mass, which becomes the placenta. The embryo enlarges as cell growth occurs after each cell division.

IMPLANTATION

Implantation is the process of embryonic attachment to the uterine wall. It occurs about 7 to 8 days after ovulation, allowing time for the embryo to pass along the fallopian tubes. The embryo does not simply attach itself to the wall but actually becomes embedded deep in the endometrium (Fig. 37-14). The embryo targets a site within the uterine cavity and attaches to the glandular crypts of the endometrium. As the embryo brushes the endometrium, the microvilli on the surface flatten and interdigitate with one another. Implantation usually occurs in the upper, posterior wall of the uterus. After implantation, additional blood vessels develop at the site. Implantation signals the pituitary to secrete additional luteinizing hormone (LH), which enlarges the granulosa cells of the corpus luteum. Human chorionic gonadotropin (HCG) is secreted by the placenta and stimulates the corpus luteum, after LH secretion is diminished, to produce progesterone. Progesterone production continues until about the 10th week of gestation.

EMBRYONIC AND FETAL PERIODS

From the third to the eighth week of gestation, the embryonic period ensues, during which all essential structures are developing and a definite form is being assumed. The fetal period lasts from the eighth week until the time of birth. During this period growth and maturation of the existing structure occurs.

Normally, around 40 weeks' gestation the fetus and placenta are expelled from the woman's body in a series of events termed *parturition* or *childbirth.* The mechanism by which parturition begins is still unknown. Once labor has begun, regular contractions increase in intensity and frequency under the influence of oxytocin. During the first stage of labor, these uterine contractions lead to the thinning and dilation of the cervix. Once the cervix is fully effaced (thinned) and dilated, the baby is delivered. This is referred to as the second stage of labor. The process of childbirth ends with the third stage of labor, which includes separation and expulsion of the placenta and the control of uterine bleeding (see also Chapter 4).

Lactation

Lactation is the period following parturition during which the breasts produce milk to nourish the newborn infant. Lactation involves hormonal and other stimuli, such as suckling, and can continue for extended periods of time. Lactation is initiated under the influence of the hormone prolactin (PRL) following the delivery of an infant. Myoepithelial cells within the breast contract in response to oxytocin in a reflex known as the milk ejection, or let-down, reflex. Oxytocin is a hormone manufactured in the hypothalamus and secreted from the posterior pituitary gland. Pregnancy and lactation produce hypertrophy of breast tissue.

Menopause

Menopause, or the last menstruation, is classically defined as occurring when the woman has experienced no menstrual cycles for a period of 1 year. It marks the end of female reproductive function. Other definitions surrounding menopause are shown in Box 37-1.

The age of menopause may be influenced by genetics, cigarette smoking, parity and nutritional status and varies according to geography. The average age of menopause for women in the United States is 51 years, although it can occur anywhere between the ages of 45 and 55. In some women menopause occurs abruptly, with complete cessation of menstruation after normal periods. In others, gradual cessation is characterized by increased or decreased amounts of bleeding with monthly cycles, periods of amenorrhea, and, finally, complete cessation of menses. Menopause is associated with atrophy of the breasts.

PHYSIOLOGY

The primary physiologic event associated with menopause is a reduced number of ovarian follicles (there are probably only a few hundred of the hundreds of thousands remaining) and a reduced sensitivity of the few remaining follicles to gonadotropins.[10] Without follicle development, the ovaries continue to produce androgen but production of all types of estrogen ceases. With menopause comes not only a decrease in the overall estrogen levels but also a change in the types of estrogen present in the body. The main estrogen secreted by the ovary before menopause is estradiol. The primary estrogen after menopause is estrone, which is converted from adrenally derived androstenedione in peripheral adipose (fat) tissues. Therefore, obese women have higher overall estrogen levels than thin women. During the **climacteric**, the gonadotropins, FSH and LH, rise due to loss of negative feedback by estrogen (see Flowchart 37-1).

BOX 37-1

DEFINITIONS RELATED TO MENOPAUSE

Premenopause: Reproductive years prior to menopause. Still having regular menstrual periods and not experiencing any symptoms.

Perimenopause: Transitional 5-year period surrounding menopause. Marks the beginning of the healthy aging process in women. Irregular menstrual periods (>25 days),beginning symptoms of menopause (hot flashes). Both ovulatory and anovulatory cycles.

Menopause: Absence of menses for the period of 1 year. End of reproductive capacity in women. Varying signs and symptoms of menopause. Average age is 51.8 years—has remained stable since medieval times.

Postmenopause: Begins 1 year after cessation of spontaneous menstrual cycles. Ovarian function has ceased.

Climacteric: Period of waning ovarian function.

Surgical menopause: Surgical removal of both ovaries or sterilization following radiation or chemotherapy.

ASSOCIATED MANIFESTATIONS

Menopause frequently is associated with physiologic changes and related symptomatology. These include menstrual disturbances, vasomotor symptoms such as hot flushes or flashes, atrophy of reproductive organs, and psychological symptoms such as nervousness and short-term memory loss. Hot flashes are the most common symptom. These begin as a feeling of warmth in the chest and progress upward over the neck and face. They may be accompanied by flushing of the skin in these areas and profuse diaphoresis. They often occur at night (night sweats) and can result in insomnia and fatigue. The exact cause has not been determined, but they are related to estrogen withdrawal and relieved by estrogen.

Changes in reproductive organs include atrophy of the labia and breasts; dryness and thinning of vaginal walls; decreased support of bladder, rectum, and uterus; and decreased size of the uterus and cervix. These changes are all associated with lower estrogen levels and account for such complaints as dyspareunia, stress incontinence, and vaginal itching or burning. Much evidence supports that the frequency of hypertension, stroke, and heart disease increases after menopause. Decreased estrogen levels are also linked to Alzheimer's dementia as well as osteoporosis, which causes bone fragility and fractures.

Psychological symptoms associated with menopause include sleep disturbance, nervousness, depression, headache, decreased sex drive, memory loss, vertigo, and feelings of worthlessness. Controversy remains concerning the relationship of these symptoms to decreasing estrogen levels. They may represent basic personality and/or cultural influences, or they may result from altered sleep patterns due to hot flashes.

Dehydroepiandrosterone

Dehydroepiandrosterone (DHEA) is an androgen. The four major androgens found in both men and women are testosterone, androstenedione, DHEAS (dehydroepiandrosterone sulfate), and DHEA. In the normal premenopausal women, androgens are produced by both the adrenal cortex and the ovary. DHEA is mainly produced by the adrenal gland. DHEA levels in both men and women peak around age 25 and then slowly decline by age 70. This decline has been termed **adrenopause**. In the postmenopausal woman the production of androgens, including DHEA, decreases and is approximately one half that found in premenopausal women. DHEA provides modest protection against heart disease and may additionally protect against breast cancer.

ALTERATIONS IN FEMALE REPRODUCTIVE FUNCTION

Menstrual Cycle Disorders

Alterations in menstrual cycles are a common female complaint and range from amenorrhea to heavy, frequent menses. Many factors are thought to influence this, including age, nutritional status, medications, endocrine status, and physiologic disturbances.

AMENORRHEA

Amenorrhea, or the absence of menses, is not a disease entity. It may be normal or a sign of a serious underlying problem. Primary amenorrhea refers to a failure to begin menstrual cycles or any sexual characteristics by age 14, the lack of menses by age 16½, or no menses in the 2 years after the breasts or pubic or axillary hair develop. Secondary amenorrhea, which occurs only in women who have previously menstruated, is the cessation of menstruation for at least 3 months in a woman with previous regular menses or for at least 6 to 12 months in a woman who normally experienced irregular cycles.

Etiology

Causes of amenorrhea may be (1) physiologic, (2) genetic, (3) anatomic, (4) endocrinologic, (5) constitutional, or (6) psychogenic. Physiologic amenorrhea is normal and occurs before puberty, during pregnancy and lactation, and after menopause. Genetic causes usually produce primary amenorrhea and include Turner syndrome and a multitude of other gonadal abnormalities, such as 17-hydroxylase deficiency and hermaphroditism. Anatomic factors that can cause amenorrhea include congenital anomalies, hysterectomy, and endometrial destruction. Endocrine dysfunction such as diabetes or disorders of the hypothalamus, pituitary, ovary, thyroid, or adrenal glands may also produce amenorrhea. Constitutional problems such as malnutrition, obesity, drug addiction, and anemia can interrupt menstrual periods. Psychogenic factors include psychosis and anorexia nervosa. Amenorrhea can also result from low body weight or excessive exercise; this can cause an alteration in the muscle/fat ratio that can affect the release of GnRH, returning the hypothalamus to a prepubertal state. Exercise can decrease gonadotropins and increase prolactin.

PREMENSTRUAL SYNDROME (PMS)

PMS represents a variety of temporary, cyclic emotional and physical changes that usually begin at midcycle, reach a crescendo premenstrually, and are, almost miraculously, relieved by the menstrual flow. The onset of PMS can occur at anytime during the reproductive years, but it seems most commonly (50%) to manifest itself in the early 30s. Women in the perimenopausal state often experience an exacerbation of PMS symptoms, which is very frightening to them.

Etiology

Speculative causes of PMS include an excess of estrogen, a progesterone deficiency, or an imbalance between the two. Recent research suggests that differences in sensitivity of cells to gonadal hormones may be the underlying mechanism.[28,33] Additionally, vitamin and mineral deficiencies, such as of vitamin B6, vitamin C, selenium, and magnesium, are suspected; these are all needed by the liver to metabolize estrogen. Excess prostaglandin, a hormone produced by the lining of the uterus, may be related to PMS, as it is with dysmenorrhea. Nutritional factors possibly causing PMS include excessive consumption of caffeine (soft drinks, caffeine, chocolate) or refined sugars (fruit juices) and alterations in carbohydrate metabolism causing hypoglycemia. Vegetarians tend to have a decreased incidence of PMS; this is thought to be related to a diet low in fat and high in fiber, which helps to excrete estrogen from the body.

Prolactin, a hormone that causes the milk let-down reflex, may also cause water retention in PMS. Emotional stress can cause cycles in which ovulation does not occur, leading to low levels of progesterone. Improper regulation of serotonin is known to be related to depression and anxiety. Since PMS shares many of the same symptoms, changing levels of serotonin may similarly cause the symptoms of PMS.

Clinical Manifestations

Symptoms and their severity vary among individuals but are usually quite consistent in the same woman. There are over 100 symptoms linked to PMS. The most common somatic symptoms include (1) edema, (2) weight gain, (3) bloating of the abdomen and breasts, (4) breast tenderness, (5) headache, and (6) food cravings. Emotional and behavioral symptoms include mood changes (depression, anxiety, anger), irritability, crying spells, changes in sex drive, decreased ability to concentrate, and insomnia. Numerous studies report the total incidence of PMS to be from 75% to 90% of all women. However, only 3% to 8% of these women have symptoms serious enough to disrupt their social or occupational functioning.[16] Symptoms do not all begin on the same day, nor are they always the same from month to month.

Women who have severe psychological symptoms may be diagnosed with premenstrual dysphoric disorder (PMDD) if they meet additional criteria that show that have no preexisting mental illness.[2] Women with preexisting mental disorders who show exacerbation of symptoms in the premenstrual period are said to have premenstrual magnification.

DYSMENORRHEA

Dysmenorrhea means painful menstruation, commonly referred to as "cramps." Dysmenorrhea may occur as a single entity or as part of premenstrual syndrome. There are two types of dysmenorrhea: (1) primary and (2) secondary. Primary dysmenorrhea refers to painful menses unrelated to a physical cause but is almost always associated with ovulatory cycles and the production of progesterone in the luteal phase.

Secondary dysmenorrhea is often associated with uterine or pelvic pathology and not directly related to menses. Painful menses may be produced by the following factors: endometriosis, adenomyosis, **pelvic inflammatory disease**, fibroid **polyps**, pelvic neoplasms, and IUD use. Pelvic diseases associated with secondary dysmenorrhea will be described later. The following discussion relates to primary dysmenorrhea.

Primary Dysmenorrhea

Primary dysmenorrhea does not usually begin at menarche, but only after regular ovulatory cycling has been established, usually 6 months to 2 years. It generally becomes more severe with time, peaking at ages 23 to 27. It is estimated that more than 50% of all post-adolescent, menstruating women are affected by dysmenorrhea, making it the most common gynecologic complaint.[6]

ETIOLOGY AND PATHOPHYSIOLOGY. It is now known that dysmenorrhea is produced by uterine vasoconstriction, ischemia, and smooth muscle spasms due to excessive amounts of prostaglandins.[6,7] Progesterone is produced during the second half of the menstrual cycle. Progesterone stimulates the production of prostaglandins in the endometrium. When the endometrium sloughs, excessive prostaglandins are produced in women with dysmenorrhea. Prostaglandins increase uterine activity, resulting in forceful uterine contractions. These forceful contractions lead to ischemia, and subsequently intensifying pain.

CLINICAL MANIFESTATIONS. Dysmenorrhea typically produces a sharp, cramping pain in the lower abdomen that may radiate to the lower back and/or inner thigh region. It may be accompanied by increased menstrual flow. Pain begins just prior to, or immediately following, the onset of menstrual flow and is usually most severe on the first 2 days of menses. It rarely lasts longer than 48 hours. Pain may be accompanied by nausea, vomiting, fatigue, diarrhea, or headache.

ABNORMAL VAGINAL BLEEDING

Abnormal bleeding is a symptom of some underlying pathophysiologic process. It may stem from systemic diseases, pregnancy complications, pelvic disorders, or reproductive endocrine dysfunction. The source of the bleeding may be uterine, cervical, or vaginal. Excessive menstrual bleeding is defined as a cycle length of less than 21 days, bleeding lasting more than 7 days, or a blood loss exceeding 150 mL. Menstrual periods that are greater than 35 days apart, last less than 2 days, or in which total blood loss is less than 20 mL are also considered abnormal. Terms useful to describe abnormal patterns of bleeding are listed in Box 37-2. The many types of abnormal bleeding can be grouped into four major pathologic categories as defined by their cause:

- Systemic disorders: diabetes mellitus, thyroid or adrenal gland disorders, blood dyscrasias, liver disease, or malnutrition
- Complications of pregnancy: abortion, ectopic pregnancy, placenta previa, abruptio placenta, or gestational trophoblastic disease
- Pelvic disorders: endometriosis, adenomyosis, infections, inflammation, polyps, or neoplasms, causing abnormal bleeding that can be uterine or stem from another location (e.g., cervicitis)
- Dysfunctional uterine bleeding: irregular uterine bleeding associated with anovulation

Dysfunctional Uterine Bleeding

Dysfunctional uterine bleeding (DUB) is a diagnosis of exclusion that is assigned when all possible pathologic causes of abnormal uterine bleeding have been ruled out. This irregular uterine bleeding is most often seen in women during puberty or the perimenopausal period. It is common with ectopic pregnancy and miscarriage. The exact cause remains unknown, but the irregular bleeding patterns seen with DUB probably represent some alteration in hypothalamic–pituitary–ovarian hormonal regulation.[29]

BOX 37-2 TERMS RELATED TO ABNORMAL UTERINE BLEEDING

Amenorrhea: Absence of menses
Hypermenorrhea: Excessive menstrual flow (>80 mL/period)
Hypomenorrhea: Deficient menstrual flow (<20 mL/period)
Menorrhagia: Excessive menstrual flow (>80 mL/period)
Metrorrhagia: Bleeding that occurs between menstrual periods (intermenstrual)
Oligomenorrhea: Abnormally infrequent menstrual periods (>35 days apart)
Polymenorrhea: Abnormally frequent menstrual periods (<21 days apart)
Perimenopausal: Irregular bleeding preceding menopause
Postmenopausal: Recurrence of bleeding after 1 full year of amenorrhea (menopause)

Dysfunctional uterine bleeding may be seen with a persistent corpus luteum cyst (see functional ovarian cysts, below) or a short luteal phase, but is usually associated with anovulation. In anovulatory cycles, no corpus luteum is formed, no progesterone is produced, and no secretory changes occur in the endometrium. The endometrium becomes hyperplastic due to estrogen. As estrogen levels decrease from degenerating follicles, withdrawal bleeding occurs that is prolonged and excessive. If ovulatory and anovulatory cycles are alternating, there is a pattern of menorrhagia alternating with oligomenorrhea. It is important to remember that not all abnormal bleeding originates in the uterus or even in the genital tract.

Dysfunctional uterine bleeding is commonly presented as bleeding that occurs outside of the normal menstrual cycles or menstrual bleeding that is either abnormally prolonged or increased in total amount. Symptoms vary depending on the hormonal state and age of the woman, whether she is prepubertal, perimenarchal, reproductive age, perimenopausal, or menopausal.

Postmenopausal Bleeding

Postmenopausal bleeding is uterine bleeding that resumes after 1 full year without a menstrual period. It can range from just a few drops or to what the woman describes as a menstrual period. This type of bleeding should be considered to be of pathologic origin until proved otherwise since endometrial cancer is found in 10% to 20% of women with postmenopausal bleeding. To evaluate postmenopausal bleeding it is critical to first determine that bleeding is originating from the uterus. Non-uterine causes of bleeding are vaginal atrophy (tearing of the delicate vaginal tissues), cervical polyps or infection, vulvovaginal disorders, and urethral lesions. If the woman is not on any hormone therapy that may induce bleeding, postmenopausal uterine bleeding may be due to endometrial atrophy, hyperplasia, or reproductive tract neoplasia. Women on unopposed estrogen replacement therapy are at the greatest risk since estrogen can stimulate the endometrium to develop hyperplasia without the regulating effects of progesterone. Obese women also are a risk since they still have estrogen production from the estrogen conversion in peripheral adipose tissue and no progesterone production.

POLYCYSTIC OVARIAN SYNDROME

Polycystic ovarian syndrome (PCOS) represents a heterogenous group of patients with a variety of underlying abnormalities. The lack of uniformity in criteria used for PCOS diagnosis further adds to the confusion surrounding this syndrome. Polycystic ovarian syndrome is a relatively common condition; up to 10% of reproductive-aged women have various components of the syndrome. There is strong evidence that it is hereditary. There may be many women with the syndrome within a generation for a series of generations.

The syndrome was first described in 1935 by Stein and Leventhal and until recently was named Stein-Leventhal syndrome. At that time it was associated with a specific medical history and characteristic findings upon physical examination (infertility, oligomenorrhea or amenorrhea, and masculinization). At present, findings are based on clinical symptoms and markers such as an elevated serum LH and high androgen levels. Other clinicians may use a combination of these two parameters. Chronic anovulation is a hallmark of the condition; it may have many causes, any one of which may result in PCOS.

Pathophysiology

PCOS is a condition in which there is increased production of estrogen and certain androgens, which causes a wide variety of symptoms. The main hormonal abnormality is increased LH levels, normal or low follicle stimulating hormone (FSH) levels, and increased levels of estrogen and androgens. These increased levels may lead to ovarian dysfunction. The exact cause is unknown, but it is related to hypothalamic–pituitary dysfunction. Many biochemical hormonal alterations are associated with PCOS; they are displayed in Table 37-5. The primary endocrine abnormalities are (1) altered gonadotropins, (2) ovarian hyperandrogenism, (3) adrenal hyperandrogenism, and (4) insulin resistance.[15] Whatever the cause, the net result is an elevated LH level and an inhibition of FSH. Eighty percent of the testosterone is normally bound to SHBP. However, with PCOS there is less SHBP available to bind with testosterone, freeing the testosterone. Hirsuitism is directly related to an increase in the amount of circulating free testosterone.

Clinical Manifestations

PCOS is characterized by three classic symptoms: irregular menstrual periods (80%), excessive hair growth, and acne (50% to 70%). Obesity may also occur. Additionally, since the woman does not ovulate, she is often infertile (75%). These symptoms usually first become apparent during adolescence. As the name implies, multiple follicular cysts develop on the ovaries, causing them to enlarge; however, enlarged or polycystic ovaries are not always present and are not necessary for the diagnosis, nor does their presence confirm the diagnosis of PCOS. Enlarged polycystic ovaries may also be associated with other conditions such as Cushing's syndrome, congenital adrenal hyperplasia, and adrenal and ovarian tumors. The polycystic ovary is actually a symptom of the disease rather than the cause of the symptoms. Thus, the name is confusing because it implies

TABLE 37-5

BIOCHEMICAL AND HORMONAL ALTERATIONS WITH POLYCYSTIC OVARIAN SYNDROME

ALTERATION	DESCRIPTION
Gonadotropins	LH levels are variable but often higher than normal, due to increased sensitivity of pituitary gonadotrophs to GnRH FSH levels are normal or low
Androgens	Androstenedione (A) and testosterone (T) levels are increased, due to gonadotropin-dependent secretion from ovary DHEA and DHEA-S levels are increased, due to excess secretion from adrenal cortex
Estrogens	Estrone (E_1) levels are elevated in early follicular phase in spite of normal estradiol (E_2) levels, due to enhanced peripheral conversion of A to E_1
Sex hormone binding protein (SHBP)	SHBP is decreased (which increases ratio of free androgen; causing virilism) due to hyperinsulinemia
Insulin resistance	Increased insulin levels with fasting or glucose tolerance test with normal blood glucose levels

that the ovary is the source of the syndrome, whereas the problem could be related to either the hypothalamic—pituitary, adrenal, or ovarian dysfunction. Polycystic ovaries develop as a result of stimulation of the ovarian follicles, which increase in size, maintaining this enlargement due to the continuous stimulation of low levels of FSH.

The increased growth of hair occurs gradually, usually 2 to 3 years after the onset of menses. Hair growth varies from fine to heavy, pigmented hair on the face (sideburns, upper lip, and chin) and may extend to the chest, lower abdomen, and inner thighs. Virilization to the degree of deepening of the voice, temporal hair loss, and clitoromegaly is uncommon and may suggest an androgen-producing tumor, which requires further diagnostic evaluation. PCOS is gradual.

The menstrual periods are irregular. Since most young women's cycles do not become regular until 1 to 2 years after menses begin, it may be difficult to differentiate this syndrome from the normal irregular periods that occur during adolescence. However, normally the menses become regular once the young woman matures and her cycles become ovulatory. With PCOS the cycles gradually become less regular. The periods may first be excessive or prolonged because of the increased hormonal stimulation of the uterus. Over a period of time they become infrequent, often skipping many months at a time, or absent altogether. Some young women with PCOS never begin to menstruate at puberty.

Early identification of women with PCOS is critical. Recent evidence suggests that hypertension, cholesterol abnormalities, and diabetes mellitus may result from the continuing effects of the excess androgens circulating in a woman's cardiovascular system. Additionally, the excessive amounts of estrogen increase the risk of developing endometrial cancer threefold.

ENDOMETRIOSIS

Endometriosis is a condition in which endometrial tissue is found in locations other than the inner surface of the uterus. As noted in Figure 37-15*A*, the most common ectopic sites are the ovaries; oviducts; peritoneal surfaces of the uterus, bladder, rectum, bowel, uterine ligaments, and cul-de-sac; and within the rectovaginal septum. Aberrant tissue may also be found within soft tissue in the vulva, vagina and umbilicus and in laparotomy scars. Rarely, it is located within other organs such as the lung or brain. Endometriosis is a common condition, affecting an estimated 10% of all women and up to 50% of infertile women during the reproductive years.[23] Adenomyosis (endometriosis internal) is thought to be a different entity and is discussed separately.

Etiology

The exact cause of endometriosis is unknown, but several theories have been advanced:

- Retrograde menstruation theory, first suggested by Sampson in 1927, proposes that during menstruation, endometrial tissue is regurgitated through the fallopian tubes into the pelvic cavity where it then develops into endometriosis.[27]
- Metastasis theory proposes that endometrial cells spread to other areas via the bloodstream or lymphatics.[12]
- Metaplasia theory suggests that the structures derived from embryonic coelomic epithelium, which includes the peritoneum, retain the ability to differentiate into endometrial tissue and do so under the influence of some unknown stimulus.

None of these theories is totally proved or disproved, nor are they mutually exclusive of one another. However, more recent studies are examining the role of genetic factors, inflammation, immune mechanisms, and cell biology in the development of endometriosis.

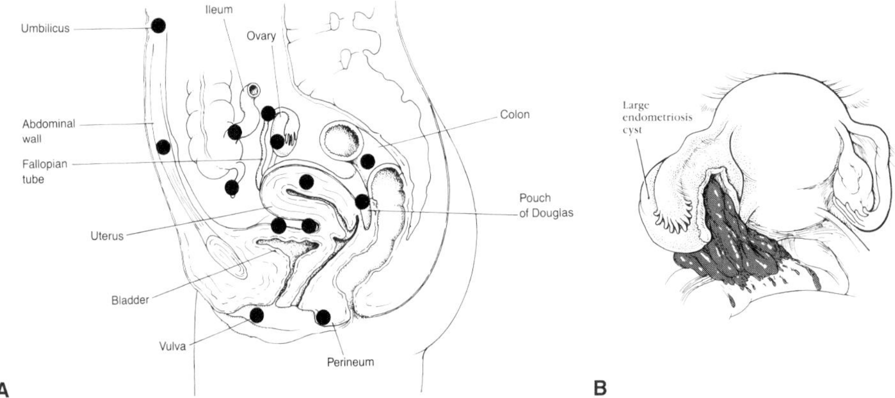

FIGURE 37-15. Endometriosis. **A.** Common sites of endometrial implants. (Rubin, E., & Farber, J. L. [1999]. *Pathology* [3rd ed.]. Philadelphia: Lippincott.) **B.** Endometrioma (chocolate cyst) of the ovary.

Pathophysiology

Although considered a benign disorder, ectopic endometrial cells behave much like cancer cells insofar as they must attach to new tissue, proliferate in a new location, and then foster a new blood supply.[25]

In endometriosis, implants respond to hormonal stimulation in the same way as normal uterine endometrium does. This tissue grows and thickens under cyclic hormonal influence and, as estrogen and progesterone are withdrawn, it reacts by bleeding. However, when bleeding occurs in visceral structures it cannot flow away from the tissue, and it then forms abnormal lesions. With progression, debris accumulates within, producing small dark (brown, black, blue) cystic lesions. These are usually located on the serosal layer of the involved organs. Bleeding within the ovary produces a cyst filled with a thick, chocolate-colored fluid called an **endometrioma** or **chocolate cyst** (see Fig. 37-15*B*). As serosal lesions become more numerous, increase in size, and coalesce, they eventually form adhesions, which lead to fixation of involved pelvic structures.

Clinical Manifestations

Clinical manifestations depend on the extent and location of lesions. It often consists of the "4 Ds": dysmenorrhea, dyschezia (painful defecation), dyspareunia (painful intercourse), and dysuria (painful urination). Pain characteristics vary widely from a dull, bearing-down type of pain to severely disabling. Pain severity is not correlated to the degree of endometriosis but is more closely related to location. The most common classic symptom is secondary dysmenorrhea, which in some women becomes progressively worse with time. Backache and cramps usually begin just before or with the onset of menses; the pain increases throughout menstruation and subsides afterward. Dyschezia is related to implants and adhension in the colorectal areas. Dyspareunia reflects involvement in the cul-de-sac, uterine ligaments, rectovaginal septum, or upper vagina. Dysuria reflects bladder involvement, and pain on defecation occurs with rectal involvement.

Infertility or sterility may result from mechanical obstruction due to extensive scarring of the ovaries and oviducts. In addition to the mechanical factors of scarring and adhesions, numerous other aspects of infertility related to endometriosis (such as immunologic factors) are being studied. Inflammatory mediators may be toxic to sperm, preventing fertilization, and alteration in cell adhesion molecules could prevent implantation of a fertilized ovum.[25] Alterations in hormones, prostaglandins, or immune function may negatively affect ovulation, ovum transport within the oviducts, or implantation.[7]

Pelvic examination may reveal small nodular masses on pelvic organs that are painful with palpation or a uterus that is retroverted and fixed due to adhesions. Laparoscopy positively identifies the lesions and adhesions themselves.

ADENOMYOSIS

In **adenomyosis**, endometrial tissue invades the myometrium (Fig. 37-16). It is sometimes referred to as internal endometriosis. The invasion may be diffuse or localized, with patches of endometrial cells surrounded by hypertrophied smooth muscle cells, which results in an enlarged uterus.[18] The incidence is estimated at approximately 10% of women. It is seen almost exclusively in multiparous women over 30 years of age, and it regresses after menopause. The cause is unknown, but causative factors may be similar to

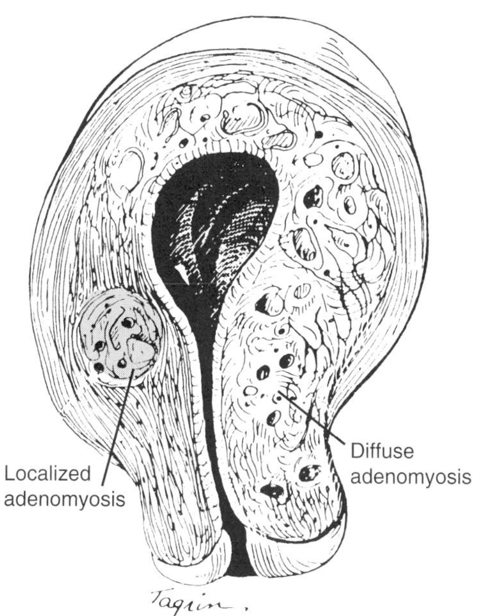

FIGURE 36-16. Appearance of adenomyosis of the uterus. It can be localized or diffuse.

those of endometriosis. The buried endometrium may respond to hormone changes of the menstrual cycle with bleeding, leaving insoluble iron deposits within myometrial tissues. Clinical manifestations include menorrhagia, progressively severe dysmenorrhea, dyspareunia, and generalized pelvic discomfort. The uterus becomes symmetrically enlarged—often the same size and consistency of an 8-week gestation. On bimanual exam, the uterus is soft and tender in the premenstrual and menstrual period, which is a positive Halban's sign.

Inflammation

Inflammatory conditions of the female reproductive system can affect the reproductive tract or the breast. Inflammation of the genital tract may be confined to one specific location or involve the entire reproductive tract, as in pelvic inflammatory disease (PID). It may also begin in the reproductive tract and then become systemic, as in toxic shock syndrome (TSS). The genital tract can be divided into the lower and upper segments, with the dividing line being the cervix. The upper genital tract is normally sterile, whereas the lower genital tract is normally colonized with floral organisms that protect it from infection. Infections of the upper genital tract are generally more serious than those of the lower. Figure 37-17 shows the female genital tract and defines the various site of inflammation.

VAGINITIS

All forms of vaginitis represent inflammation of the vaginal mucosa. Often the vulva is also inflamed (vulvovaginitis) due to the bathing of the vulvar tissue by vaginal secretions. Inflammation is most often the result of infection with fungal, protozoal, or bac-

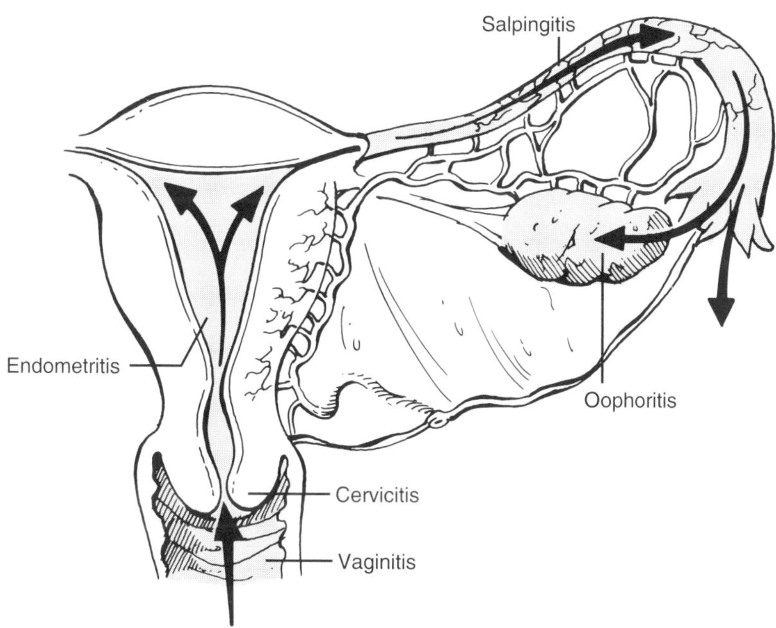

FIGURE 37-17. Sites and related terms of female genital tract inflammation.

terial organisms. However, it may be a manifestation of other processes, some of which are quite serious. Other causes of vaginitis include postmenopausal atrophy, chemical irritation, allergy, trauma, collagen vascular disease, or neoplasia. Clinical manifestations of specific types of vaginitis are distinguishable only from microscopic findings of the vaginal discharge. Table 37-6 compares various types of vaginitis.

Atrophic Vaginitis

Most menopausal women will experience atrophic changes in their vaginal epithelium to varying degrees. The vaginal rugae flatten as the epithelium thins. Lack of estrogen causes the vaginal epithelium to become thin, and remaining cells lack glycogen, which reduces the amount of lactic acid produced, resulting in an elevated pH. This, in turn, reduces the number of lactobacilli and increases the number of non-acidophilic bacteria. Lack of estrogen delays the maturation of the vaginal squamous epithelium. Maturation is manifested by an increase in the number of cellular layers, as shown in Figure 37-18. The thin vaginal wall loses some of its ability to support the bladder and rectum and may result in the formation of a cystocele or rectocele. Urinary incontinence can occur.

Most women do not have clinically significant symptoms.[30] With very severe atrophy, symptoms may include vaginal tenderness, dyspareunia, or postcoital burning or spotting. Minimal trauma with intercrouse may result in bleeding from the thin, friable tissues. There may be a watery vaginal discharge with pruritus, swelling, and secondary dyspareunia or dysuria. On examination the mucosa looks thin, lacks vaginal folds, and may show petechiae. Microscopic findings reveal a preponderance of parabasal cells.

CERVICITIS

Cervicitis refers to inflammation of the cervix, which may be acute or chronic. The causative factors and clinical manifestations of acute and chronic cervici-

TABLE 37-6

VAGINAL CONDITIONS

CONDITION	VULVOVAGINAL SYMPTOMS	VAGINAL DISCHARGE	LACTOBACILLI	PH
Candida albicans	Mild to severe itching Cyclic Marked vulvovaginal erythema	Increased amount White, curdy, cottage cheese like	Moderate	<5
glabrata	Mild to moderate burning/itching Chronic, cyclic Mild vulvovaginal erythema	Increased Unchanged to white	Moderate	<4.5
Bacterial vaginosis	Mild to moderate itching Absent to mild inflammation Mild vulvovaginal erythema	Adherent, homogenous discharge Appearance of milk poured into vagina Fish odor, particularly after intercourse	Rare	>4.5
Cytolytic vaginosis	Mild to moderate burning/itching Premenstrual, relieved with menses	Unchanged to increased, white	Excessive	3.5–4
Lactobacillosis	Vaginal itching/burning Chronic, cyclic	Thick White to creamy	Elongated Rare, short rods	4–5
Trichomonas	Severe vulvar itching Petechiae of cervix and vagina Vulvar erythema	Copious Yellow-green May be frothy Malodorous	Plus or minus	>5
Atrophic vaginitis	Pruritus, irritation Vaginal dryness and dyspareunia Smooth vaginal walls	Red, tender vestibule and vagina Scant discharge Lack of rugae	Rare	>5–6
Desquamative inflammatory vaginitis	Petechiae of vulva, vagina and cervix Dyspareunia Pruritus or irritation	Thick, profuse No odor	Rare	<4.5

(Carcio, H. [1999]. *Advanced health assessment of women.* Philadelphia: Lippincott Williams & Wilkins.)

FOCUS ON CELLULAR PHYSIOLOGY

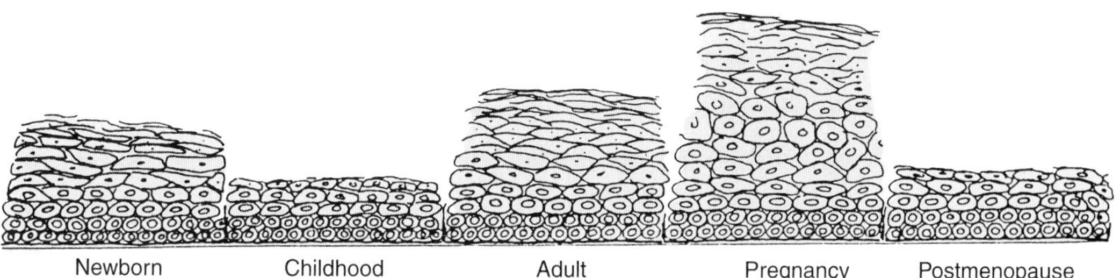

FIGURE 37-18. Schema showing the changes in the vaginal and cervical epithelium due to the hormonal milieu. *From left to right:* The newborn shows an estrogen effect from the mother. The prepubertal child has no estrogenic stimulation. The adult has normal estrogenic stimulation. The pregnant woman demonstrates an increased estrogen level. The postmenopausal woman shows an atrophic vaginal mucosa secondary to the loss of estrogenic stimulation. (Dunnihoo, D. R. [1992]. *Fundamentals of gynecology and obstetrics* [2nd ed.]. Philadelphia: J.B. Lippincott.)

tis may vary. Cervicitis is usually caused by cervical/vaginal infections, *Candida, Trichomonas,* and bacterial vaginosis, all common pathogens that involve the cervix.

Acute Cervicitis

Acute cervicitis usually occurs with sexually transmitted infections (discussed in Chapter 8). Nonsexually transmitted infections are much less common and may be due to *Escherichia coli, Staphylococcus* species, or *Streptococcus* species. These may follow childbirth, trauma, or surgery. Symptoms may include dyspareunia, backache, dull pain in the lower abdomen, and urinary frequency and urgency. The cervix appears congested, with a white purulent discharge with a foul odor. The cervix is reddened, eroded, and tender when moved. Vaginal microscopy will show many white blood cells.

Chronic Cervicitis

Many women exhibit some form of chronic cervicitis. It may occur after acute infection, childbirth trauma, or abortion. The endocervical os and cervical canal are primarily affected, but there are none of the findings seen with acute cervicitis. The only symptoms may be a vaginal discharge, which is less copious, varies in consistency, and is often irritating to the vulva. Metrorraghia may occur; this is also a sign of cervical cancer, which must be ruled out. Speculum examination may reveal redness and swelling with a granular appearance around the external margins of the cervical os. Cervical eversion of the mucus-secreting columnar cells, followed by inflammatory blockage of these glands, may produce nabothian cysts. Also, chronic inflammation may lead to cervical fibrosis and stenosis that can cause infertility. Chronic cervicitis, although not considered a primary cause of cervical cancer, may enhance the cancer-causing effect of the human papilloma viruses (HPV). Microscopic examination may reveal the presence of many white blood cells and the causative organism. The Pap smear will show inflammation.

PELVIC INFLAMMATORY DISEASE

Pelvic inflammatory disease (PID) is a general term used to refer to any infection of the upper reproductive tract. More precise terms such as endometritis, salpingitis, oophoritis, and pelvic peritonitis indicate specific areas of involvement (see Fig. 37-17). Infection of the upper genital tract is serious because organisms enter the peritoneal cavity, usually localizing to the pelvic area. The two most common causes of PID are the sexually transmitted infections chlamydia and gonorrhea (discussed in Chapter 8). Other causes include postpartum endometritis, the presence of an IUD, and abortion. It is less often caused by *Staphylococcus* or *Streptococcus* species. These infections most often occur after delivery or abortion or in women who use IUDs as a means of contraception. Figure 37-19 illustrates the etiology of PID.

Clinical Manifestations

Clinical manifestations of PID include the sudden onset of severe pelvic pain, chills and fever, nausea, vomiting, and a heavy, purulent vaginal discharge with foul odor. Vaginal itching and/or bleeding also may be present. On pelvic examination there is pelvic tenderness and cervical motion pain. An inflammatory mass (e.g., tubo-ovarian abscess) may be palpated or seen on ultrasonography. **Hydrosalpinx**, distention of the tube with fluid, may occur due to occlusion of the distal

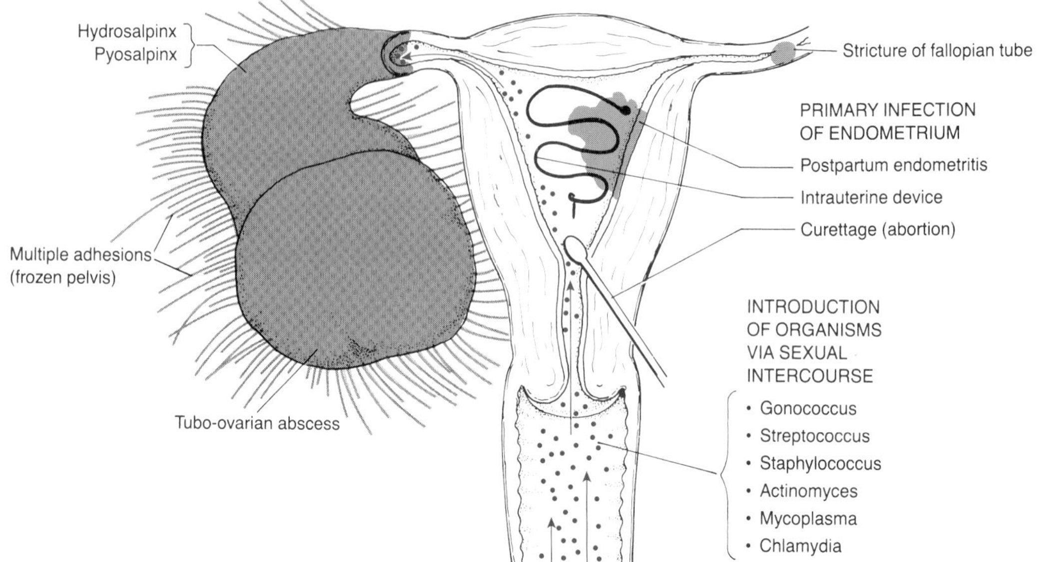

FIGURE 37-19. Etiology and manifestations of pelvic inflammatory disease. (Rubin, E., & Farber, J. L. [1999]. *Pathology* [3rd ed.]. Philadelphia: Lippincott Williams & Wilkins.)

portion (see Fig. 37-19). The white blood cell count may be elevated. Cultures of discharge are usually positive for the infectious agent. Complications in the acute phase include general abdominal peritonitis, paralytic ileus, pelvic abscess, and thrombophlebitis. Later, there may be intestinal obstruction due to adhesion formation. Untreated or inadequately treated PID may result in infertility due to scarring of the tubes, which may interfere with transport of the egg and/or sperm (see Fig. 37-19).

TOXIC SHOCK SYNDROME

Toxic shock syndrome (TSS) is a condition that affects many body systems and can be life threatening. The syndrome was first recognized and reported in 1978. The incidence of toxic shock is 6.2 to 14.2 per 100,000 menstruating women per year. It is caused by a toxin produced by the bacteria *Staphylococcus aureus*. Although it most frequently affects women under the age of 30 who use tampons, particularly those between the ages of 15 and 19, its incidence has increased in non-menstruating women, men, and children. In menstruating women, the risk is greatest among those using super-absorbent tampons. Cases of non-menstrual TSS have been linked to diaphragm contraceptives, soft tissue wounds, and osteomyelitis or following delivery or surgery. This is a serious infection, with a mortality rate of about 15%.

The absorbent nature of certain tampons and the chemicals used in them seem to provide a medium to foster the growth of *S. aureus*. Additionally, tampons may absorb the protective bacteria described above along with the menstrual flow. The warmth and moisture of the vaginal area may further encourge the growth of bacteria. Once the organism begins to grow, it produces dangerous toxins. The toxin may be absorbed into the body either through small tears in the vagina, which are thought to result from tampon use, or backward through the uterus, up the tubes, and out into the peritoneum. This reflux is possibly increased because of the blockage of the outward flow of blood by the tampon.

Clinical Manifestations

Clinical manifestations of TSS include (1) fever, (2) rash, (3) vomiting, (4) diarrhea, (5) hypotension, and (6) organ system (kidney, heart) symptoms. The elevated temperature is high (>102°F), of sudden onset, and accompanied by tachycardia. The macular rash is diffuse but especially prominent on the palms and soles, and progresses to peeling of palms and soles at about 10 days. Diarrhea is watery. The mucous membranes of the mouth and vagina also become reddened. Within 48 hours fluid protectively shifts away from the blood stream, causing the blood pressure to fall. Hypotension may lead to shock rapidly. Non-purulent conjunctivitis, sore throat, myalgia, and headache may also be present. Renal dysfunction may produce oliguria or anuria and rising creatinine. Additional complications include disseminated intravascular coagulation (DIC), adult respiratory distress syndrome (ARDS), congestive heart failure (CHF), and meningitis.

MASTITIS

Inflammation of the breast, or **mastitis**, occurs mainly in women in the postpartum period. The three types of mastitis include congestive, infective, and chronic.

Congestive Mastitis

In congestive mastitis, or breast engorgement, inflammation is not infectious but comes about due to accumulation fluid (milk, blood, lymph) as the breast shifts from producing colostrum to true milk at about the third to fourth postpartum day. At this time, both breasts abruptly become heavy, hard, warm, and tender. There may be a slight elevation in systemic temperature. This condition is entirely normal.

Infective Mastitis

Infective mastitis is an acute infection of the breast, usually due to *S. aureus*. Organisms enter the ducts to infect the mammary gland from the newborn's mouth via cracks in the nipple. It is a complication of breastfeeding, usually occurring more than 1 week postpartum. Infection is usually present in only one breast and may be confined to a breast quadrant or single lobule. Abscess formation is common. Symptoms are a breast that is red, hot, swollen, and tender, accompanied by fever and malaise. There may be a purulent nipple discharge, or pus may be aspirated from an abscess.

Chronic Mastitis

Chronic mastitis is a noninfectious breast inflammation that usually appears in perimenopausal women when lactiferous ducts become obstructed by secretions and cellular debris. Obstruction results in a dilation of the ducts, called **ductal ectasia**, as well as the development of a secondary inflammation in the ducts and periductal tissues. Small ducts may rupture into tissues, causing an inflammation. Induration and fibrosis can result in nipple retraction or a mass, and a greenish, gummy nipple secretion may be expressed. Clinical manifestations include breast pain, burning, and swelling. Each of these manifestations also may occur with breast cancer; thus, a thorough investigation is necessary to rule out carcinoma.

Non-neoplastic Growths

Many different types of benign growths can occur within the reproductive system. The ovaries can develop functional cysts in response to hormonal variations. Small growths in the form of polyps can occur on the cervix and endometrium. The breast can develop fibrocystic changes.

FUNCTIONAL OVARIAN CYSTS

Ovarian cysts may be functional or pathologic. Pathologic cysts may be (1) non-neoplastic or (2) neoplastic. Neoplastic cysts are discussed under neoplasms (below). Functional ovarian cysts are the result of normal ovarian function and account for more than 50% of all ovarian enlargements. The three types of functional ovarian cysts include follicular, lutein, and theca-luteal.

Follicular Cyst

A functional follicular cyst results when follicular fluid in regressing, non-ovulated follicles fails to be completely resorbed. They are seen only in menstruating women and may be associated with menstrual irregularities. Follicular cysts are generally less than 6 cm in size and usually resolve spontaneously within 60 days of formation. Symptoms can include pelvic pain, dyspareunia, and occasionally abnormal uterine bleeding patterns, but they are usually asymptomatic.

Lutein Cyst

A lutein cyst occurs when the corpus luteum fails to degenerate normally and instead develops into a persistent cyst. The lutein cyst continues to produce progesterone, prolonging the secretory stage of endometrial development. This may cause a prolonged period between menses or amenorrhea. Lutein cysts usually are small and regress spontaneously but occasionally they may rupture, causing ovarian torsion and hemorrhage.

Theca-luteal Cyst

Theca-luteal cysts develop from excessive hCG secretion, as with gestational trophoblastic growths (**hydatidiform mole**, choriocarcinoma) and polycystic ovarian syndrome, or they can result as a consequence of infertility treatment with gonadotropins or clomiphine. The cysts are usually small but bilateral. If the source of hCG is terminated, they regress within several months.

Clinical Manifestations and Complications

Functional ovarian cysts ordinarily produce no symptoms. They are usually unilateral, may be noted on periodic examination, and typically regress spontaneously within one to two menstrual cycles. If a functional cyst ruptures, it may tear an ovarian vessel. Intraperitoneal bleeding occurs, and the extent of symptoms is related to the amount of hemorrhage. With excessive bleeding, abdominal pain may be severe in onset, requiring hospitalization and surgery.

POLYPS

Polyps are spherical or cylindrical masses that jut out of the tissue from which they grow. As shown in Figure 37-20, they may be pedunculated (attached by a tiny stalk) or sessile (attached by a broad base). In the female reproductive tract, polyps can grow from the endometrium or on the cervix. They can also grow within the ducts of the breasts. The cause of polyps is unknown.

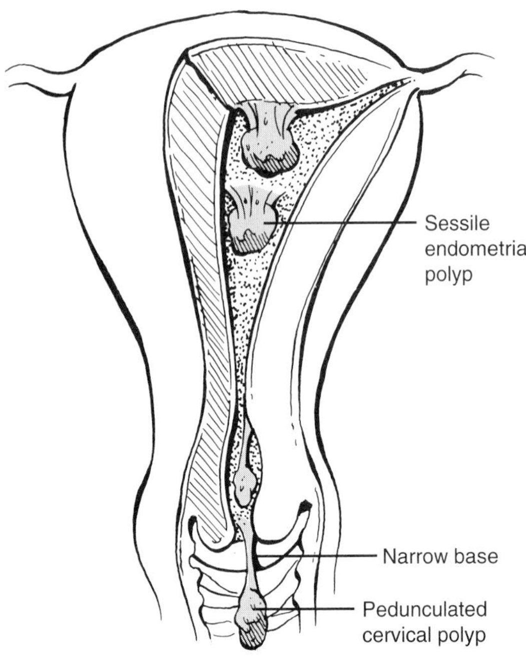

FIGURE 37-20. **Polyps of the female reproductive tract.**

Endometrial Polyps

Endometrial polyps are either pedunculated or sessile projections of the endometrium, ranging in size from 0.5 to 3 cm. They contain endometrial glands and may be singular or multiple. They may grow to become rather large, fleshy, smooth, reddish-brown tumors. The cause may be related to **endometrial hyperplasia.** Although they can form at any age, they mostly develop in the perimenopausal period. Endometrial polyps may be asymptomatic. They are often an incidental discovery during a sonohysterogram or hysterectomy. If symptomatic, they may cause recurrent menorrhagia and/or metrorrhagia. If a large polyp undergoes necrosis, there may be a sudden onset of significant bleeding along with intense, crampy pain. Endometrial polyps infrequently transform into cancer.

Cervical Polyps

Cervical polyps are pedunculated or sessile lesions that mostly arise in the endocervix. They are common, especially in multigravidas, and occasionally occur after menopause but very rarely before menarche. The cause is unknown, but they may develop from chronic cervicitis.[32] Cervical polyps appear as shiny, soft, red lesions that project from the cervical canal on pelvic examination. Clinical manifestations include metrorrhagia, postcoital bleeding, postmenopausal bleeding, leukorrhea, and hypermenorrhea. They have not been associated with a greater risk of developing cervical carcinoma, but the discovery of a polyp does not preclude investigation to rule out a concurrent malignancy. They can produce chronic bleeding and irritation, especially with intercourse.

FIBROCYSTIC CHANGES IN THE BREAST

The term *fibrocystic breast changes* is now used to describe a variety of non-neoplastic tissue changes within the breast, all of which produce lumps. In the past, these entities have been referred to as fibrocystic breast disease, mammary dysplasia, cystic mastitis, and cystic mastopathy; these names implied that these tissue variations are pathologic. Although some forms of fibrocystic changes are associated with an increased risk of breast cancer, most are of little clinical importance. They are present in about 50% of all women of childbearing age, but produce symptoms in only 10%. The exact cause is unknown, but it is thought that lesions arise from exaggerated response of breast tissue to cyclic hormonal stimulation. Fibrocystic changes span a wide spectrum of tissue alterations that are generally divided into two patterns, each of which is also heterogeneous.[18] These include nonproliferative and proliferative changes.

Nonproliferative fibrocystic changes show varying degrees of connective tissue fibrosis, cyst formation, and inflammation, with possibly some ductal metaplasia or mild hyperplasia of ductal or lobular cells (Fig. 37-21*A*). None of these changes are associated with an increased risk of breast cancer, although the nodularity produced may make it more difficult to identify an accompanying cancerous mass.

With proliferative fibrocystic changes (see Fig. 37-21*B*), there is a greater degree of hyperplastic cell growth, especially in the epithelial gland components comprising the acini, ducts, and lobules. Lesions may show degrees of cellularity, which range from a modest to severe increase in cell numbers, with cell changes ranging from mild to atypical hyperplasia. Atypical hyperplastic lesions resemble carcinoma in situ, and the greatest risk of malignancy is associated with the most atypical forms. Proliferative lesions may coexist with areas of nonproliferative changes in the same breast.

Fibrocystic changes may be asymptomatic, but on palpation there are lumps in both breasts. There may be complaints of tenderness or a dull, heavy pain and a sense of fullness, all of which tend to increase in the luteal phase, just before menstruation, as the cysts enlarge at this time. There may be a nipple discharge. Occasionally a large dominant cyst becomes noticeable. Such a nodule should be evaluated via mammography and/or needle aspiration with biopsy to rule out cancer.

FOCUS ON CELLULAR PATHOPHYSIOLOGY

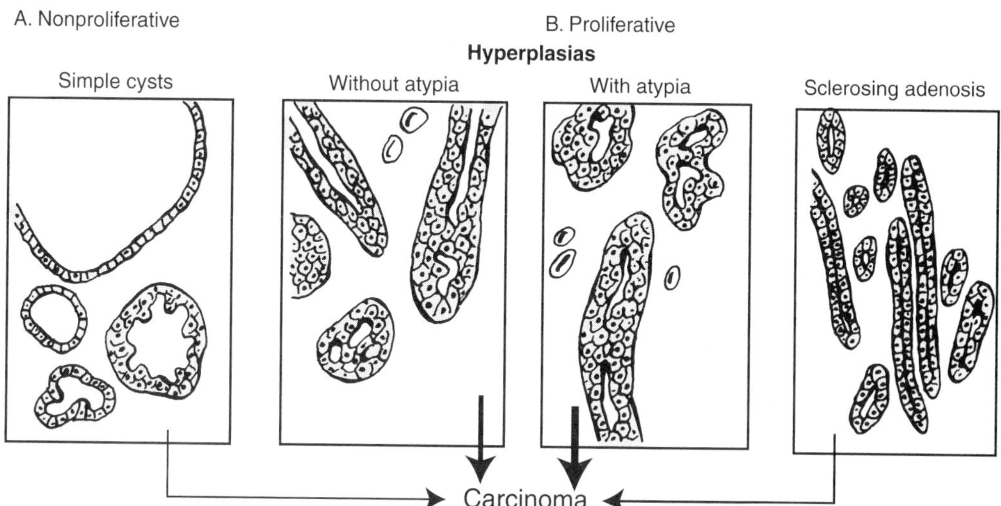

FIGURE 37-21. Fibrocystic breast changes (the size of the arrow indicates the risk of malignant transformation of the various patterns). **A.** Nonproliferative. **B.** Proliferative. (Redrawn from Kumar, V., Cotran, R. S., & Robbins, S. L. [1997]. *Basic pathology* [6th ed.]. Philadelphia: W.B. Saunders.)

Neoplasms

Female reproductive system neoplasms include benign and malignant tumors of the genital tract and breasts. Neoplasms of the genitalia can occur in any structure, but some, such as those of the vagina and oviduct, are quite rare. The usual locations for genital tract neoplasms are the ovary, uterine cervix, uterine endometrium, and vulva. Every year more than a quarter million women will learn they have a malignant neoplasm of the genital tract or breast. In the same year more than 70,000 will die.[1] Female reproductive system neoplasms are serious health problems resulting in untold fear, suffering, and death.

OVARIES

Neoplasms of the ovary are diverse, owing to the complexity of the cell types and growth potential of some of the cells located there. Benign neoplasms are much more common and much less harmful than malignancies, which tend to be advanced at diagnosis and carry a poor prognosis. All ovarian tumors may grow to be quite large because they grow in the abdominal cavity, which allows unrestricted growth. Both benign and malignant neoplasms can secrete hormones, which may manifest with symptoms of endocrine imbalance. Ovarian tumors may be secondary (metastatic), having developed at another site, seeded, and grown on the ovary, or they may be primary, having originated from ovarian cells.

Classification of Ovarian Neoplasms

It is difficult to classify ovarian tumors neatly into "benign" and "malignant" categories. Some are clearly benign; some are clearly malignant; yet others are defined as borderline types with "low malignant potential." It is preferable to categorize ovarian tumors by cell of origin and malignancy potential (grade) rather than as benign or malignant. There are three basic types of cell populations from which ovarian neoplasms arise: (1) surface (germinal) epithelial cells, (2) germ cells, and (3) gonadal stroma (sex cord) cells. From each of these cell types, multiple types of tumors can develop, as noted in Figure 37-22. Also, cells are graded by their degree of differentiation as Grade I (benign), Grade II (borderline), and Grade III (malignant). Figure 37-22 also shows the classification of ovarian neoplasms according to cell type and malignancy potential, along with their frequencies.

The clearly benign neoplasms are the most common of all ovarian tumors, accounting for 75% to 80%. Borderline tumors represent 10% to 15% of all ovarian tumors, and 5% to 15% are clearly malignant. Of all tissue types, surface epithelial tumors of the serous varieties are the most frequent.

Ovarian Cancer

In 1998 an estimated 25,400 new cases of ovarian cancer were diagnosed, and 14,500 deaths occurred. Although ovarian cancer accounts for only 32% of all

FOCUS ON CELLULAR PATHOPHYSIOLOGY

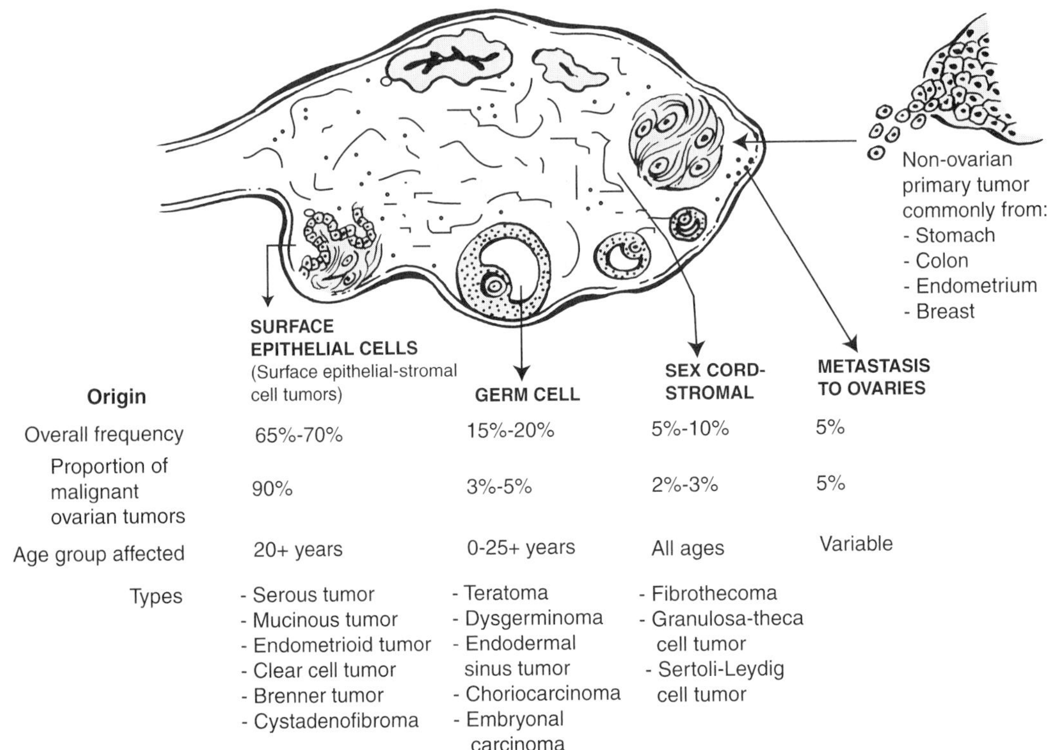

Origin	Surface epithelial cells (Surface epithelial-stromal cell tumors)	Germ cell	Sex cord-stromal	Metastasis to ovaries
Overall frequency	65%-70%	15%-20%	5%-10%	5%
Proportion of malignant ovarian tumors	90%	3%-5%	2%-3%	5%
Age group affected	20+ years	0-25+ years	All ages	Variable
Types	- Serous tumor - Mucinous tumor - Endometrioid tumor - Clear cell tumor - Brenner tumor - Cystadenofibroma	- Teratoma - Dysgerminoma - Endodermal sinus tumor - Choriocarcinoma - Embryonal carcinoma	- Fibrothecoma - Granulosa-theca cell tumor - Sertoli-Leydig cell tumor	

FIGURE 37-22. Histogenesis of ovarian neoplasms, showing derivation of various types and some data on their frequency and age distribution. (Redrawn from Kumar, V., Cotran, R. S., & Robbins, S. L. [1997]. *Basic pathology* [6th ed.]. Philadelphia: W. B. Saunders.)

gynecologic (genital tract) cancers among women, it causes 54% of the deaths, making it is the most lethal of all cancers affecting the female reproductive tract.[19] This lethality is attributed to the lack of both effective screening tools and early symptoms, which result in a delay in diagnosis and treatment. The American Cancer Society reports a 5-year survival rate of only 46% for all stages.[1] With early diagnosis and treatment, the survival rate may approach 93%. The survival rate associated with regional metastasis is 55% compared with only 25% with distant metastasis.

The exact cause of ovarian cancer remains largely unknown. Risk factors are displayed in Box 37-3. They can be categorized according to age, hormonal status, toxic agents, genetic factors, and miscellaneous influences.[3,14,22]

Clinical Manifestations. Most often ovarian cancer grows unimpeded and silently, producing no symptoms until there has been widespread dissemination. Before diagnosis, a woman may note vague complaints of bladder or bowel dysfunction, including stomachache, flatus, and/or distention. The presence of these complaints, especially in middle-aged women, without a definitive diagnosis may indicate the need for further study. The most common sign is abdominal enlargement, often associated with ascites. If the tumor is secreting excess amounts of estrogen, evidence of endocrine imbalance may be present, such as bleeding in postmenopausal women or precocious puberty in prepubescent females. If androgens are increased, menstrual irregularities and/or masculinization may result. Pain is a late symptom and usually only appears with an early lesion if rupture, torsion, or infection occurs. Enlarged ovaries may be palpated, but usually the disease is well advanced by that time.

Although not specific for ovarian carcinoma, CA 125 is elevated in 85% of women with some forms of advanced ovarian cancer. Measurement of CA 125 uses a monoclonal antibody to detect antigens in the blood. The markers, hCG and fetoprotein, will be present in germ cell tumors.

The BRCA Gene

Two genes have been identified that can signal whether a woman is at risk for developing the hereditary form of breast cancer or ovarian cancer. This discovery has been hailed as one of the most significant

BOX 37-3

OVARIAN CANCER RISK FACTORS

Increase Risk

Age: most develop after menopause; 50% after age 65

Reproductive history:
- Early menarche (before age 12)
- Late menopause (after age 50)
- Nulliparity
- Infertility
- Infertility treatment with clomiphene
- First pregnancy after age 30

Personal/family history:
- History of previous breast cancer
- History of ovarian cancer in members of mother's family
- History of ovarian cancer in female members of father's family

Genetics:
- BRCA1/BRCA2 mutation
- Lynch syndrome II

Environmental factors:
- High-fat/low-fiber diet
- Use of talcum powder

Reduce Risk

- Chronic anovulation
- Multiparity
- Lactation
- Oral contraceptive use

advances in medical science. The actual genes have been named BRCA1 and BRCA2. The "BRCA" stands for breast cancer, even though it has since been discovered that it also pertains to ovarian cancer. A positive BRCA1 or BRCA2 gene may be present, particularly in women with a strong familial history of breast or ovarian cancer.

Genes are blueprints for the makeup of the individual. Each person has two sets of genes, one inherited from the mother and one from the father. Genes determine hair and eye color, as well as other body composition. When cancer occurs, the genes are altered or mutated. It was recently discovered that two such altered genes are found in some families with a history of breast or ovarian cancer. Researchers have established that women who inherit **BRCA genes** appear to be more susceptible to environmental carcinogens, causings a significantly elevated risk of both breast and ovarian cancers compared with the general population.

When functioning properly, this gene is thought to help suppress the growth of cancerous cells. If one set (each individual gets two sets) of this tumor-suppressor gene becomes damaged, the other copy can act as a "brake" on uncontrolled cell growth. A woman born with one damaged version of the BRCA gene has only one working set of brakes. If her second BRCA gene (her second set of brakes) becomes damaged by exposure to environmental carcinogens, the woman can develop cancer. It must be pointed out that only 10% of breast and ovarian cancers are related to an alteration in these two genes.

Approximately 2 individuals per 1000 have inherited a clinically significant alteration in a BRCA gene. If either parent has the gene, each of their children has a 50% chance of inheriting the alteration. Interestingly, both men and women can have BRCA genes. This means that the alterations can be passed down either the mother's or the father's side of the family. It was previously thought that breast cancer could only be passed down the maternal side of the family.

If a woman is found to have inherited an altered gene, her risk of developing breast cancer may be increased by as much as sevenfold, from about 12% in the general population to as much as 40% to 85% by age 70. With ovarian cancer, her risk may be increased by as much as 28-fold, from about 1.8% to as much as 50% by age 70. An altered gene means that a woman is at risk for developing ovarian or breast cancer, but it does not necessarily mean that the woman will develop either form nor does it given any guidance as to when.

Opinions vary as to who, if anyone, should be tested. Most clinicians recommend testing only for woman at very high risk, and these women must be counseled regarding the impact of either a negative or positive result (Box 37-4).

CERVIX

Estimated new cases of invasive cervical cancer in 1998 were 13,700, or 17% of all gynecologic cancers, making it the ninth most common cancer in women. In the same year the number of deaths was about 4,900.[19] Both the incidence and mortality rates for cervical cancer have steadily declined since 1947.[7] These lowered rates reflect the effectiveness, and zealous use, of the Pap test (discussed in the Appendix of this unit) as a screening tool. The success of Pap screening is related to the accessibility of the cervix and the accuracy of the test to detect early cell changes that precede neoplastic cell changes. Invasive cervical cancer is usually diagnosed between the ages of 20 and 50 years. According to the American Cancer Society, the 5-year survival rate for cervical cancer in 1998 was 69% for all stages.[1] The survival rate associated with local disease was 91%; with regional spread, 49%; and with distant metastasis, only 9%.

Etiology

Most cases of cervical cancer are related to infection of cervical cells by the human papilloma virus

BOX 37-4 A WOMAN MIGHT CONSIDER BRCA EVALUATION IF SHE HAS ANY OF THE FOLLOWING:

- Personal history of breast cancer diagnosed before the age of 30
- Personal history of both breast and ovarian cancer
- Personal history of breast cancer or ovarian cancer and one or more close relative(s) with breast and/or ovarian cancer, especially breast cancer before the age of 50
- Women of Ashkenazi Jewish descent (eastern European) who have breast cancer before age 40 or ovarian cancer at any age (the mutation has been found in approximately 1% to 1.5% of Ashkenazi individuals)
- Multiple case of breast and/or ovarian cancer in blood relatives from the same family line across multiple generations. This would include two first- or second-degree relatives both diagnosed before age 50 if breast cancer, with at least one of the relatives a first-degree; or three first- or second-degree relatives with at least one relative diagnosed with breast cancer before age 50.
- Family history of ovarian cancer in at least two first- or second-degree relatives. (Ovarian cancer does not seem to be linked to age of onset of the condition, as does breast cancer.)
- Family history of both ovarian and breast cancer in at least one first- or second-degree relative
- Blood relative who has an altered BRAC gene

(HPV). Over 60 HPV viruses have been identified.[17] Many of the HPVs are sexually transmitted infections that cause condyloma acuminata on the cervix, as well as the vulva and anal regions. The HPV types 6 and 11 form wart (papilloma)-shaped lesions that are not very oncogenic. The HPV types 16, 18, 31, and 33 form flat lesions, and their DNA is frequently found inside cervical cancer cells.[5] The presence of oncogenic types of HPV imparts about a 15 times greater relative risk of developing carcinoma than in the general population. White women are more likely (54%) to be diagnosed at a localized stage than African-American women (40%).[19] This gap has been closing in recent years.

Most risk factors relate to spread of the virus and are listed in Box 37-5. Additionally, premalignant (dysplastic) cell changes are also more common in women

BOX 37-5 CERVICAL CANCER RISK FACTORS

Factors Related to HPV (Human Papillomavirus) Infection

- Intercourse beginning at an early age
- Multiple sexual partners
- Unprotected sex (at any age)

Other Factors

- HIV infection (especially with low CD4 count)
- Smoking
- Poor diet

who have a history of in utero exposure to DES or who are immunocompromised (transplant recipients, HIV infected).

Pathophysiology

Approximately 90% of all cervical cancers are epidermoid, developing from squamous cells of the exocervix and squamocolumnar junction. Because these cells are so easy to collect, assessing them via serial Pap smears has yielded much information regarding the development of cervical cancer. It is now known that the transformation of these cells to cancer takes from 7 to 10 years. During this long "latent" period cells display subtle, but progressive, cell changes, collectively referred to as **cervical intraepithelial neoplasia (CIN)**, or more recently as **squamous intraepithelial lesion (SIL)**. These progressive changes are displayed in Figure 37-23. Cells change both qualitatively and quantitatively.

Qualitative cell changes are manifested by alterations in the cytology, or appearance, of individual cells. As cells are transformed, nuclei become enlarged and stain darkly. Some cells may be multinucleated. Early, minimal changes are classified as mild dysplasia (CIN/SIL grade I); later, more severely altered cells are classified as severe dysplasia (CIN/SIL grade III).

As the cytologic changes progress, so too does the number of affected cells. Quantitative changes are best shown by serial biopsies. They demonstrate that, over years, accumulation of abnormal cells results in a disorderly cellular arrangement in a progressively greater proportion of the tissue until the entire epithelium contains only abnormal cells. At this point the disease becomes known as **carcinoma in situ**. Carcinoma in situ is distinguished from invasive cancer of the cervix only by the fact that abnormal cells have not yet pierced the basement membrane, a thin proteinaceous material that separates the epithelium from the connective

FOCUS ON CELLULAR PATHOPHYSIOLOGY

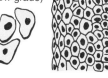

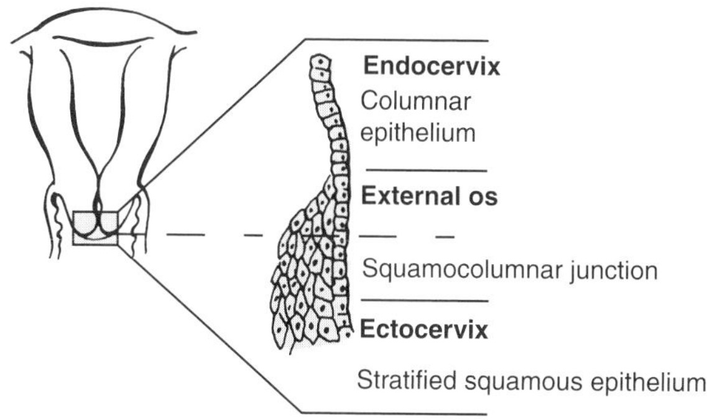

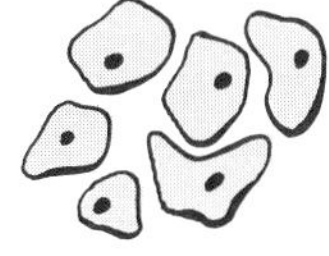

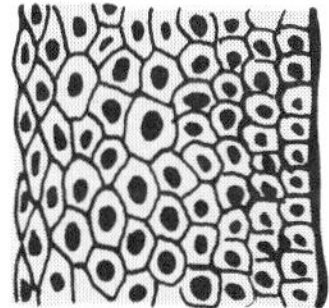
- Maturation disorderly
- Mild cytologic changes

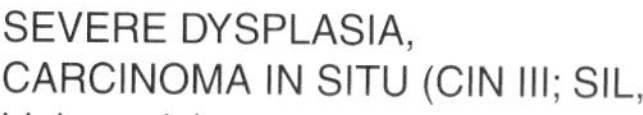
SEVERE DYSPLASIA, CARCINOMA IN SITU (CIN III; SIL, high grade)
- Basal type cells with very high nuclear: cytoplasmic ratio
- Marked hyperchromasia and chromatin abnormality

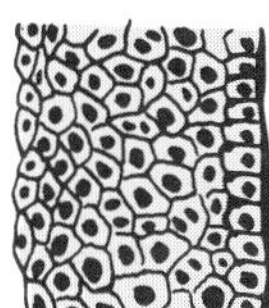
- Absent maturation
- Marked cytologic changes
- Mitosis near surface
INVASIVE CARCINOMA
- Marked pleomorphism
- Irregular nuclei with chromatin clumping and prominent nucleoli

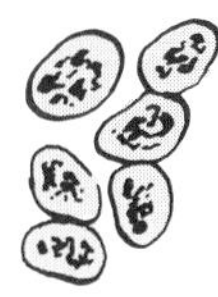

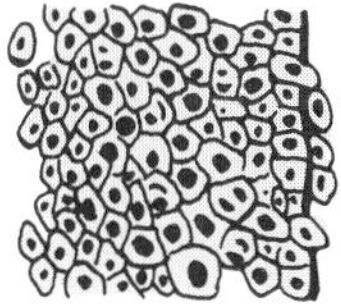
- Invasion through basement membrane

FIGURE 37-23. Cervical intraepithelial neoplasia. (Redrawn from Chandrasoma, P., & Taylor, C. R. [1998]. *Concise pathology* [3rd ed.]. Norwalk, CT: Appleton & Lange.)

tissue below. Once this barrier is breached, invasive cancer (carcinoma) is diagnosed.

Clinical Manifestations

Early cervical cancer is asymptomatic. Later, the most common symptoms are metrorrhagia and postcoital spotting, which result from cervical bleeding. There may be a foul serous or purulent discharge should inflammation occur. Bladder and/or rectal symptoms may result from larger tumors causing pressure to these areas. They are late symptoms, as is pain.

UTERUS

Uterine Leiomyoma

Uterine leiomyomas (myomas, fibromyomas, or fibroids) are benign smooth muscle tumors of the uterine body and/or cervix. They are the most common benign or malignant neoplasm of the female genital tract, being present in 20% to 25% of all women of reproductive age. They are three to nine times more common in African-American women than in white women,[7] suggesting a genetic influence.[18] Leiomyomas are second only to pregnancy as a cause of uterine enlargement, accounting for about 30% of all gynecologic hospital admissions, and they are one of the most common reasons for hysterectomy.[5]

Leiomyomas are thought to be dependent upon estrogen secretion and thus tend to regress in the postmenopausal period. Conversely, they tend to enlarge during pregnancy. The exact cause is unknown.

Although many estrogen receptors are present in the leiomyomas, a direct cause-and-effect relationship between estrogen and the development of leiomyomas has not been established. Their mass increases with pregnancy and decreases with menopause. They may occur singly but are more often multiple. Size varies widely, with most being less than 15 cm in diameter; however, there have been tumors as large as 100 lbs. They are firm, smooth, and spherical. Leiomyomas are classified by their position in the uterine wall, as shown in Figure 37-24. Certain manifestations and/or complications are associated with specific locations.

CLINICAL MANIFESTATIONS. Most leiomyomas are asymptomatic. Women with symptoms may experience excessive or prolonged bleeding during regular monthly cycles, metrorrhagia, dysmenorrhea, or pelvic tension. Enlargement of fibroids can put pressure on the bladder, urethra, rectum, or nerves, resulting in urinary frequency, constipation, abdominal fullness, or low abdominal pain. Extreme contortion of the uterus may result in infertility or habitual abortion. Complications of leiomyomas include acute abdominal pain, which is due to tumor torsion or degenerative changes; anemia, due to excessive bleeding; and urinary or bowel obstruction. Additionally, numerous complications of pregnancy, labor, and delivery may develop as a result of tumor growth during pregnancy.

On pelvic examination, the uterus may feel asymmetric and lumpy and may be distorted by one or more smooth, spherical masses. Ultrasonography, sonohysterography, MRI, radiography, hysterography, or hysteroscopy will determine the size and location of the leiomyoma.

Endometrial Cancer

Although other malignancies, such as leiomyosarcoma, are possible, they represent a small fraction of uterine cancers. The vast majority of uterine cancers are due to adenocarcinoma arising in the glandular endometrial tissue. Estimated new cases of endometrial cancer for 1998 were 36,100. This represents 49% of all gynecologic cancers and 6% of all cancers in women, making it the most common gynecologic cancer and the fourth most common of all cancers in women.[1] In the same year the number of deaths was about 6,300,[19] which represents 23% of all gynecologic cancer deaths and 2% of all cancer deaths in women, making it the ninth leading cause of cancer mortality. The incidence of endometrial cancer has remained stable since the mid-1980s.

Risk factors for endometrial cancer are listed in Box 37-6. Endometrial cancer is most often diagnosed in women 50 to 75 years of age.

The prognosis for endometrial cancer is much better than that for either ovarian or cervical cancer. According to the American Cancer Society, the 5-year survival rate for cervical cancer in 1998 was 84% for all stages. Survival rate associated with local disease was 96%; with regional spread, 66%; and with distant metastasis, 27%.[1]

ETIOLOGY. The exact mechanism by which endometrial cancer develops remains unknown. There now appear to be two distinct classifications of endometrial cancer, those associated with estrogen excess and those that are not. Each type has its own etiologic factors.[11] Types associated with excess estrogen stimulation are associated with the development of a low-grade lesion in perimenopausal white women. This type is frequently preceded by endometrial hyperplasia. Estrogen is known to produce proliferation of endometrial cells, and unopposed estrogen results in hyperplasia. The other classification has no known

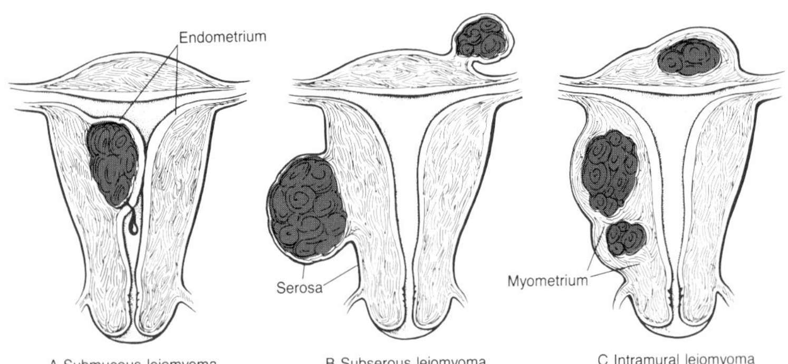

FIGURE 37-24. Appearance of uterine leiomyomas.

BOX 37-6

ENDOMETRIAL CANCER RISK FACTORS

Age: 95% in women over age of 40; average age = 60
Reproductive History:
- Early menarche (before age 12)
- Late menopause (after age 52)
- Nulliparity
- Infertility

Other risk factors:
- Obesity
- Diabetes
- Hypertension
- History of ERT (estrogen replacement therapy)
- High-fat diet
- High socioeconomic status
- History of breast or ovarian cancer
- History of previous pelvic irradiation
- History of tamoxifen use

predisposing factors but is seen more frequently in postmenopausal Asian or African-American women. It is a high-grade neoplasm and is more invasive. Additionally, genetic factors are increasingly being cited as a possible predisposing element, as oncogenes (HER2/neu) and tumor suppressor genes have been identified in endometrial cancer cells.[11]

COMMON MANIFESTATIONS. A common manifestation of endometrial cancer is abnormal uterine bleeding, which, due to the age of women affected, usually is postmenopausal. Bleeding may range from light, irregular bleeding with intermenstrual spotting to heavy or prolonged periods if it occurs before menopause. After menopause, any bleeding is suspicious. Abnormal bleeding is common enough to effect early treatment and an improved prognosis, but only if followed by proper evaluation. There may be other types of discharge, such as leukorrhea. Both bleeding and discharge are signs that reflect erosion and ulceration of the endometrium. Some women experience pelvic cramps when cell debris and blood become trapped behind a constricted cervix; infection may result. Later in the disease, symptoms include cramping, pelvic discomfort, lower abdominal or bladder pressure, bleeding after intercourse, and swollen lymph nodes. Pelvic examination may reveal an enlarged uterus, usually in an asymmetric pattern. Early tumors are usually soft, whereas more advanced tumors feel fixed.

VULVA

Cancer of the vulva can be located in one or more of these structures. In 1998, there were an estimated 3,200 new cases and 800 deaths. Vulvar cancer accounts for only about 4% of all gynecologic cancers and for less than 1% of all cancers in women.[19] Most types of vulvar cancer are diagnosed in women between 65 and 75 years of age. However, the incidence of vulvar cancer appears to be increasing, with the greatest increase appearing in a younger cohort of women. The increase in older women is believed to be the result of a rise in the percentage of older women in the population, whereas the increase in younger women is suspected as being due to a greater percentage who have HPV-associated lesions.[8] Additional risk factors are listed in Box 37-7. The American Cancer Society reported an overall 5-year survival rate of 90% for vulvar cancer cases in which lymph nodes were not involved and 50% to 60% if nodes were involved.[1]

Etiology and Pathophysiology

Malignant vulvar neoplasms may arise from varying cell origins. Since much of the vulva is composed of skin, any of the skin cancer types can develop there. The majority of vulvar cancers arise from squamous epithelial cells. The evolution of squamous cell carcinoma of the vulva may be like that of cervical cancer, and the premalignant cell changes of the vulva are classified in the same way except that they are referred to as *vulvar intraepithelial neoplasia* (VIN). Since CIN of the cervix, condyloma acuminata, and VIN of the vulvar have frequently been found to coexist in the same individuals, they are suspected of having as a common cause—infection by HPV.

Clinical Manifestations

Vulvar cancer presents in many ways. It may appear as white, red, blue, or brown pigmented lesions, oc-

BOX 37-7

RISK FACTORS FOR VULVAR CANCER

Age:
- 75% in women over age 50; average age is 65; but percentage in younger women is increasing

Factors related to HPV (human papillomavirus) infection:
- Intercourse beginning at an early age
- Multiple sexual partners
- Unprotected sex

Other factors:
- HIV infection
- Low socioeconomic status
- Smoking
- Chronic vulvar inflammation
- History of lichen sclerosis
- History of cervical cancer
- Atypical moles or melanoma anywhere on body

curring singly or as multiple macules, papules, nodules, or wartlike growths. They may be ulcerated. They usually occur on the labia majora, clitoris, and periurethral area. They may ulcerate as they enlarge. Most often, the patient is asymptomatic. If symptoms are present, they include pruritus, burning, bleeding, or pain. Large growths can interfere with urination or defecation or block blood or lymph drainage from the legs, resulting in thromboembolism or lymphedema.[7] Growth of most tumor types tends to be slow, with orderly spread to regional lymph nodes, but those involving the vagina, urethra, perineum, or anus may spread directly to deep pelvic nodes.

GESTATIONAL TROPHOBLASTIC NEOPLASMS

Gestational trophoblastic neoplasms (GTN) are tumors that develop abnormally from products of conception. There are three types: (1) hydatidiform mole, (2) invasive mole, and (3) choriocarcinoma. Hydatidiform mole is usually benign (but with malignant potential), whereas choriocarcinoma is a highly aggressive cancer. The invasive mole is intermediate between these two. All gestational trophoblastic neoplasms arise from trophoblasts, cells derived from the outer cell mass of a preimplantation embryo.[13] They all elaborate levels of hCG greater than would be expected in a normal pregnancy. Risk factors for the development of GTN include reproductive age, history of prior molar pregnancy, blood type B or AB, and possibly reduced carotene in the diet.[1]

Hydatidiform Mole

Hydatidiform mole, which represents a malformation of the placenta, is the most common of these neoplasms. The incidence of hydatidiform mole is approximately 1 in every 1,500 live births in the United States, but in developing countries the incidence can be as high as 1 in every 125 pregnancies. Two types are described, based on morphology, chromosomal pattern, and histopathology: (1) complete mole and (2) partial mole.

COMPLETE MOLE. A complete mole results from the fertilization of an anuclear (empty) ovum either by two different sperm or by an abnormal diploid sperm; therefore, all chromosomes are of paternal origin. In a complete mole there is total absence of embryo development and conversion of all chorionic villi into marked vesicles containing a clear, thick, sticky fluid (Fig. 37-25). The maternal serum hCG and level within molar cells is very high, and cells are atypical.[18] Complete moles are diploid, with either a 46,XX (more common) or 46,XY pattern.

Clinical manifestations of complete moles include intermittent first-trimester bleeding, with possible development of anemia; uterine size large for gestational date; and absence of fetal heart sounds by the 16th to 20th week. A dark-brown vaginal discharge may be accompanied by passage of watery fluid that contains characteristic vesicles. Hyperemesis gravidarum, bilateral ovarian cysts, and toxemia of pregnancy before the 24th week also have been observed with hydatidiform mole. There may be manifestations of hyperthyroidism (tachycardia, warm skin, tremor, nervousness). Ultrasonography reveals no fetal skeleton, and serum measurement of hCG shows markedly elevated hCG levels.

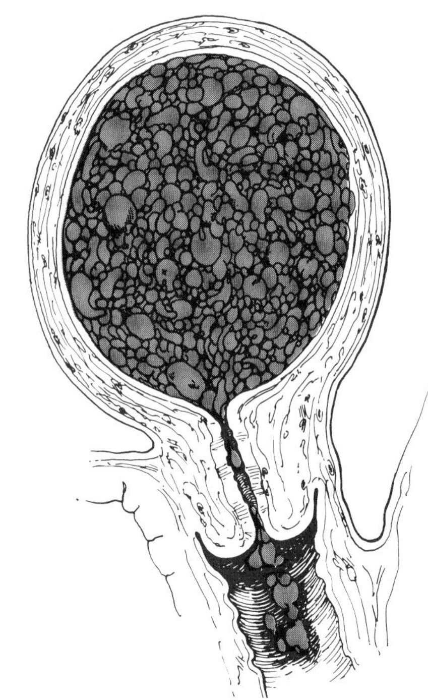

FIGURE 37-25. **Hydatidiform mole.**

PARTIAL MOLE. A partial mole forms when a normal ovum (23,X) is fertilized either by two spermatozoa or by an abnormal diploid (46,XY) sperm, so that the mother contributes a set of chromosomes. In a partial mole there is early embryo development, so fetal parts are present; only partial conversion of villi into vesicles; and lack of atypical cells. The blood levels and concentration of hCG are less elevated than with a complete mole. A partial mole is triploid, usually 69,XXY. Manifestations of partial moles are similar to, but less severe, than those of complete moles. Whereas about 3% of complete moles develop into choriocarcinoma, partial moles rarely do so.

Invasive Mole

Invasive mole is more aggressive than hydatidiform mole but much less aggressive than choriocarcinoma. Its etiology is unknown. With invasive mole, hCG levels remain elevated in the absence of pregnancy or development of metastatic disease, following a molar pregnancy. It is characterized by the presence of chorionic villi deep within the myometrium. Penetration of the uterine wall with rupture and hemorrhage is possible. Clinical manifestations include those of molar pregnancy, such as abnormal bleeding patterns and uterine size greater than gestational date. Other manifestations include a vaginal mass and signs and symptoms of infection or metastasis (cough, bloody sputum or stool, or headache or other central nervous system symptoms).

Choriocarcinoma

Choriocarcinoma is a rare, malignant tumor of the trophoblast that arises from gestational chorionic epithelium. Less often, non-gestational choriocarcinoma can arise from totipotential ovarian germ cells (see Ovarian Cancer). The etiology is unknown. The gestational form affects 1 in 20,000 to 40,000 pregnancies in the United States, about half of which follow a molar pregnancy. The other 50% arise from spontaneous or elective abortion, ectopic pregnancy, or after a normal pregnancy and delivery. Choriocarcinoma is much more common in Asia and Africa, where the incidence can reach as high as 1 per 2000 pregnancies. It primarily affects women younger than 20 or older than 40 years of age. Gestational choriocarcinoma is characterized by sheets of immature cells that invade the uterine wall, producing necrosis and hemorrhage. Chorionic villi are absent.

The only symptom noticed may be a bloody, brownish discharge associated with irregular bleeding or continual bleeding after a delivery or abortion. The first symptoms frequently are related to metastasis. Because the most common site of metastasis is the lung, hemoptysis may be the first complaint. Other metastatic sites include the vagina, brain, liver, oral cavity, and kidneys. Levels of hCG are markedly elevated. With appropriate chemotherapy the 5-year survival rate is now greater than 90%, even in those women with metastatic disease.[5]

BREAST

Fibroadenoma

Fibroadenoma is a benign breast neoplasm composed of connective tissue and glands. The most common of all breast neoplasms, fibroadenomas usually arise in young women between 15 and 40 years of age. They are slightly more common and tend to occur earlier in African-American compared with white women. The cause of this condition is unknown, but estrogen stimulation is suspected because (1) they primarily occur in menstruating women; (2) they tend to increase in size during the latter half of the menstrual cycle; (3) they regress with menopause; and (4) postmenopausal women receiving estrogen develop them.

Physical examination reveals a well-outlined, solid, firm lump that is freely moveable. Their usual size ranges from 1 to 5 cm. Multiple lesions are found in 10% of cases. They rarely transform into malignancy.

Intraductal Papilloma

Intraductal papilloma is a small benign neoplasm of the breast duct, most often located in the lactiferous ducts or sinuses. The etiology is unknown. They are usually solitary; however, they may be present in multiple ducts. Solitary lesions rarely undergo malignant transformation; multiple lesions may do so.

Possible manifestations of intraductal papilloma are a serous or bloody nipple discharge, a small nodule located under the areola, and possibly nipple retraction. All these signs can also be caused by cancer, so a thorough assessment is in order to rule out that disease.

Breast Cancer

Breast cancer is the most common site of cancer in women and is second only to lung cancer as a cause of cancer death in women.[19] Although breast cancer can occur in men, it is overwhelmingly a disease of women. The estimated number of new cases of breast cancer for 1998 was 180,300 (178,700 female, 1600 male); the number of deaths was about 43,900 (43,500 female, 400 male).[1] Breast cancer incidence had increased by 4% per year in the 1980s but has now reached a plateau. Currently, the overall lifetime risk of developing breast cancer is about 1 in 8. Box 37-8 lists risk factors for breast cancer.

According to the American Cancer Society, the 5-year survival rate for breast cancer in 1998 was 84% for all stages. Survival rate associated with local disease was 97%; with regional spread, 76%; and with distant metastasis, 21%. Although each passing year provides hope that a cure has been affected, some recurrences have appeared 15 years after the primary tumor was treated.

ETIOLOGY. Many factors that contribute to the risk of breast cancer are identified in Box 37-8. Some of these associations are well established, whereas others are more weakly linked. Sex is the strongest factor, with more than 99% of all breast cancer cases occurring in women. Genetic mutations in the BRCA1, BRCA2, and p53 (Li-Fraumeni syndrome) genes are strongly associated with the development of breast cancer (see previous section). Although responsible for only about 5% to 10% of all cases, the genetic forms tend to be bilateral and seen in younger women. Also, an extremely controversial factor proposed by some investigators is the presence of environmental pollutants (ecoestrogens; see below) that may act like estrogen to promote tumor growth.[21]

PATHOPHYSIOLOGY. Malignant neoplastic changes can occur in several different tissue types within the

BOX 37-8

RISK FACTORS FOR BREAST CANCER

Gender: female: male = 111 : 1
Age: risk increases with age
Race
- Incidence in white women slightly higher than in African American women
- Mortality in African American higher than in white women
- Asian and Hispanic women have lower risk

Personal history:
- Previous breast cancer
- Atypical hyperplastic fibrocystic breast changes
- Previous chest irradiation
- Estrogen replacement therapy

Reproductive history:
- Early menarche (before age 12)
- Late menopause (after age 50)
- Nulliparity
- Infertility
- First pregnancy after age 30

Genetic factors:
- Inherited mutations in BRCA1/BRCA2 genes
- Inherited mutations p53 gene

Family history:
- Breast cancer in members of mother's family
- Breast cancer in female members of father's family

Lifestyle factors:
- Alcohol use
- Smoking
- High-fat diet
- Obesity

Environmental pollutants:
- DDE
- PCBs

breast. These may be either in situ or invasive. The most common histologic types are ductal and lobular. Invasive types are much more common than in situ. Infiltrating (invasive) ductal carcinoma is the most common type, accounting for about 70% of all breast cancers. Approximately 10% are infiltrating lobular carcinomas. Prognosis is similar for both. Other histologic types include tubular, medullary, papillary, and mucinous carcinomas. Although these types are less common, each generally has a better prognosis than those of infiltrating ductal or lobular carcinomas.

The increased use of screening mammography has contributed to increased identification of in situ breast carcinomas. In these lesions, in situ intraductal or in situ intralobular carcinoma, all malignant cells grow atop the basement membrane and there is not yet invasion of breast tissue. They can be identified on mammogram because microcalcifications that form within them can be seen.

CLINICAL MANIFESTATIONS. Breast cancer presents clinically in a number of ways. It is most often discovered by the woman herself when she notes a breast lump. The "typical" breast cancer mass is found in the upper outer quadrant (Fig. 37-26) and is small, hard, and painless. However, different types of breast cancer produce different types of tumors; it is impossible to distinguish a benign versus malignant lesion by palpation alone. Most breast lumps are ultimately found to be benign, but this can only be determined through biopsy. A mass is not necessarily the first symptom noted. Nipple discharge may be watery, serous, or bloody. Breast distortion or a change in breast contour may be observed. With progression, many breast cancer tumors become fixed to the pectoral muscles or deep fascia to produce nipple retraction and/or skin dimpling. Peau d'orange skin, a peculiar skin change due to lymphedema around hair follicles that resembles the peel of an orange, may be noted. Vascular obstruction may lead to venous engorgement (Fig. 37-27). Manifestations of advanced breast cancer include breast edema, redness, ulceration, axillary or supraclavicular lymphadenopathy, ipsilateral arm edema, and signs of distant metastasis. Common sites of breast cancer metastasis are noted on Figure 37-28. Mammography may identify areas of density, or microcalcifications

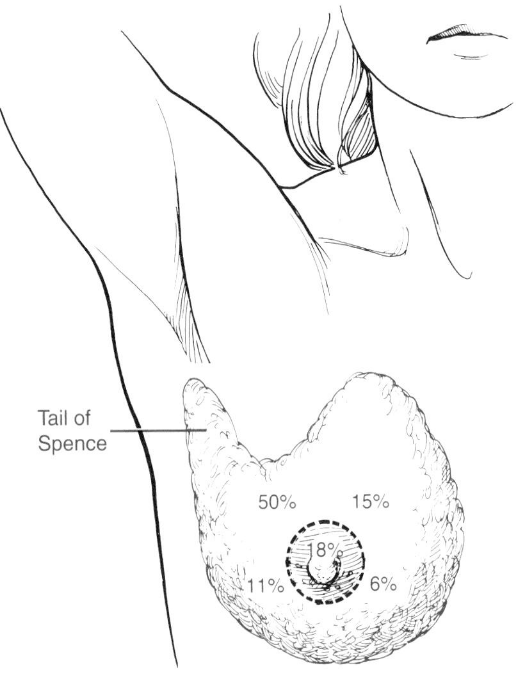

FIGURE 37-26. Breast cancer incidence per quadrant.

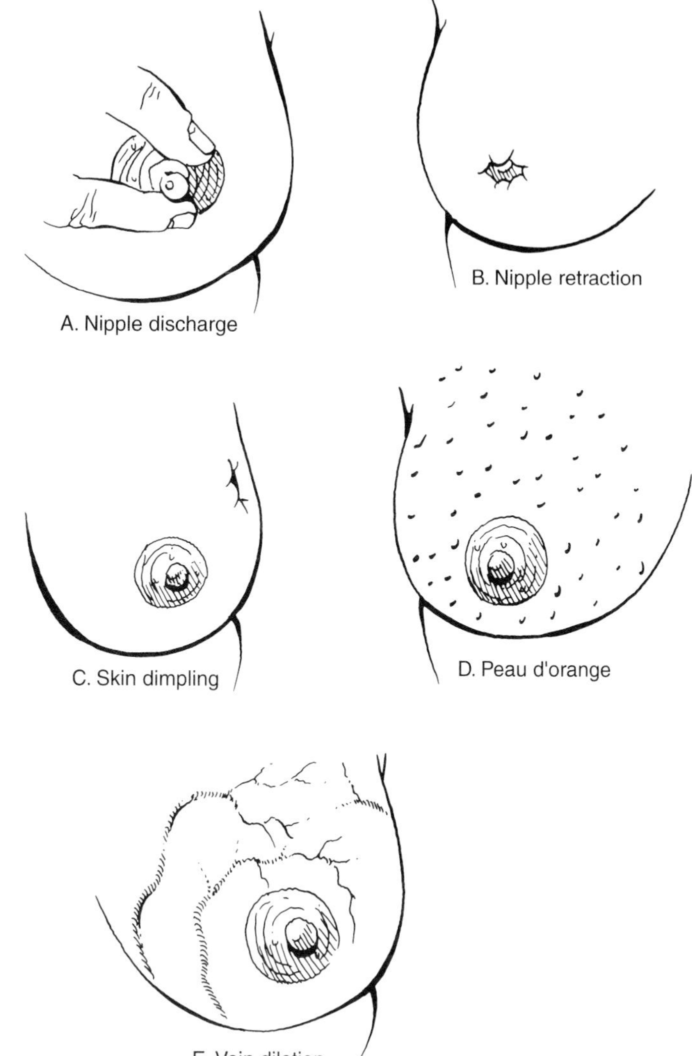

FIGURE 37-27. Clinical signs of breast cancer.

identified by mammography can be localized by use of fine wire placement for biopsy.

Exposure to Xenoestrogens

Xenoestrogens are synthetically produced chemicals that act at the estrogen receptor to produce estrogenic effects. Xenoestrogens may have the same effect as estrogen on reproductive tissue. They include drugs, such as the synthetic estrogen diethylstilbestrol (DES); phytoestrogens, which are found in certain foods; and ecoestrogens, environmental pollutants suspected to alter hormone-dependent body functions.

DIETHYLSTILBESTROL

DES, the first synthetic estrogen, was released in the 1940s. It was used to prevent miscarriage, to suppress lactation after delivery, and as hormonal therapy for dysfunctional uterine bleeding after menopause. In the late 1960s, it became linked with congenital abnormalities of both male and female offspring who were exposed to it in utero. Female anomalies included alterations in the structure of the uterus, cervix, and oviducts. Later, DES was related to certain reproductive cell changes, including cervical dysplasia, vaginal adenosis, squamous cell carcinoma of the cervix and vagina, and adenocarcinoma of the vagina.

Cancer of the vagina is a rare condition that occurs most commonly in women older than 50 years of age. It usually is the squamous cell type, but a rare adenocarcinoma was identified in a number of adolescent girls whose mothers received DES during pregnancy. Vaginal adenosis is a benign condition in which the transformation zone of the squamocolumnar junction

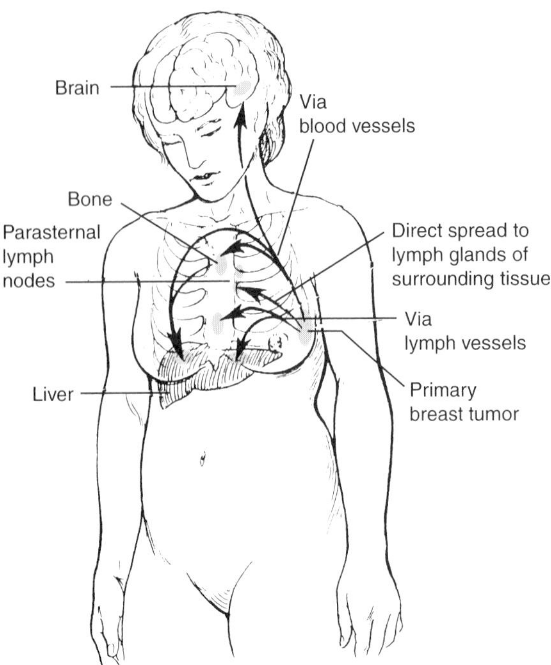

FIGURE 37-28. **Sites for metastasis of cancer of the breast.**

extends over the vaginal portion of the cervix and may involve the vaginal walls. This condition is extremely common in daughters of mothers who took DES and may predispose them to adenocarcinoma. A question also arises as to whether adenosis may progress to squamous cell cancer of the cervix or vagina. Additionally, DES has been associated with congenital anomalies in the male.

Lowered fertility rates have been linked in both male and female offspring of mothers who took DES. Irregular or infrequent menstrual periods as well as an increased incidence of incompetent cervix have been associated with in utero exposure of females to DES. There also is an increased rate of spontaneous abortion and premature delivery in women exposed to DES.

ECOESTROGENS

Recently, concern has arisen regarding the potential role of certain types of environmental pollutants on reproductive function in both animals and humans. Some researchers claim that these **ecoestrogens**, which include DDT, PCBs, kepone, and dioxin, exert estrogenic effects that alter fetal development and adult reproductive function.[21] These substances have been proposed as factors that may contribute to such conditions as alterations in lactation, reduced sperm counts, endometriosis, uterine leiomyoma, and breast or endometrial cancer. Other researchers refute such findings.[26] At present, the extent to which these compounds may contribute to reproductive pathology remains unknown.

Pelvic Organ Prolapse

The pelvic organs lie within the pelvis at the bottom of the abdominopelvic cavity. They are supported by a slinglike network of ligaments and fascial structures that normally prevent the pelvic organs from falling through the bony pelvis. As long as the pelvic floor musculature functions normally, the pelvic floor is closed and the supportive ligaments and fascia are under no tension. A problem exists when the pelvic floor muscles relax or are damaged. Conditions associated with pelvic organ prolapse include cystocele, urethrocele, rectocele, enterocele, and uterine prolapse.

CYSTOCELE

A cystocele occurs when there is (1) a defective support of the anterior vaginal wall or (2) herniation between the bladder and the vagina, with descent of a portion of the common wall between these structures (Fig. 37-29*A*). It occurs gradually with stretching, increased bladder capacity and development of atrophic vulvo-vaginitis. The major symptoms are stress urinary incontinence, which is caused by loss of urethral support of the lower vaginal wall. The woman experiences difficulty in emptying the bladder, caused by loss of support of the upper anterior vaginal wall and bladder. Urinary urgency and frequency are probably due to stretching of the bladder base associated with the prolapse, often less pronounced when supine. Development of recurrent cystitis or a stone from stagnant residual urine may occur.

RECTOCELE

A rectocele is the protrusion of the anterior rectal wall and posterior wall of the overlying vagina (see Fig. 37-29*B*). It may protrude below the hymenal ring to form a bulging mass originating from the posterior vaginal wall, causing the anterior rectal wall to balloon down through the vaginal ring. It is often caused by disruption of the rectovaginal fascia during childbirth or by chronic fecal constipation and straining. Symptoms associated with a rectocele include a feeling of rectal or pelvic pressure and difficulty emptying the rectum. A woman may state that she has to press between the vagina and rectum (to reduce the rectocele) or press in the vagina to help with defecation.

URETHROCELE

A urethrocele (see Fig. 37-29*C*) is caused by the descent of the lower anterior vaginal wall to the level of the hymenal ring. It is seen as a herniation between the urethra and vagina as the urethra prolapses into the anterior vaginal vault, out of the correct angle with the bladder. It is usually associated with stretch incontinence due to loss of urethral support. It often occurs with cystocele.

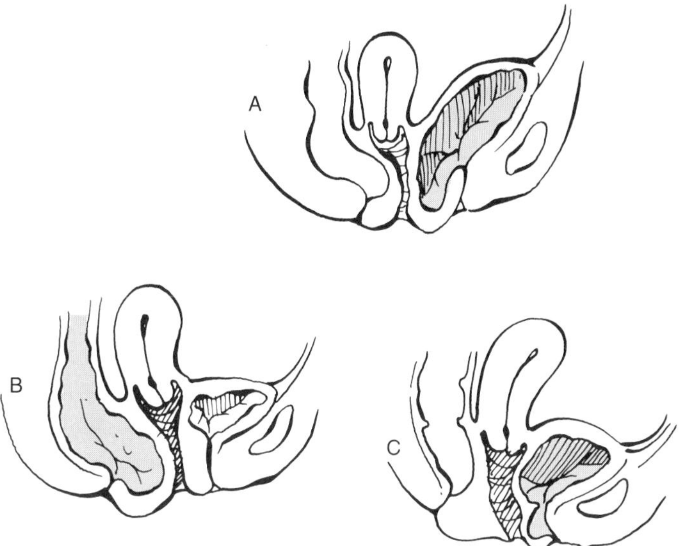

FIGURE 37-29. **A.** Cystocele. **B.** Rectocele. **C.** Urethrocele.

ENTEROCELE

An enterocele occurs when the cul-de-sac becomes distended with intestine and bulges the posterior vaginal wall outward. There is hernia of the fascia of the posterior vagina above the rectovaginal septum and below the cervix.

UTERINE PROLAPSE

Uterine prolapse is the descent of the uterus below its normal level high in the vagina. **Procidentia** is complete prolapse of the uterus to the extent that it falls outside of the vulva. The ligaments that normally support the uterus stretch, failing to hold the body of the uterus in position. An increase in intra-abdominal pressure will cause the uterus to descend down the vaginal canal (similar to the action of a piston in a cylinder) (Fig. 37-30). Symptoms include a dragging sensation, usually occurring in the groin and sacral and lumbar area. Discomfort improves when the woman lies flat, relieving the downward pressure. The sensation of peritoneal wetness is probably caused by protusion of moist vaginal walls rather than by leakage of urine. The woman may notice a mass protruding from her vagina, particularly after bearing down or with heavy lifting. Symptoms increase with advancing age and tissue atrophy during the postmenopausal years.

Grading systems are varied and very subjective. Types of uterine prolapse include:

1. First degree: without symptoms and mildly descended
2. Second degree: halfway into the vagina and usually asymptomatic
3. Third degree: at the level of the introitus and usually symptomatic
4. Fourth degree: out of the vagina even at rest and very symptomatic

Sexual Dysfunction

The sexual response is a complex process that may be affected by conditions of the reproductive tract, medications, responses of a woman's partner, or emotional aspects associated with her life. Most individuals experience some degree of sexual dysfunction at some point in their lives. Although it can occur at any time, occur once, and reoccur, it is most commonly seen in women in their late 20s or early 30s. Table 37-7 describes the five types of sexual dysfunction.

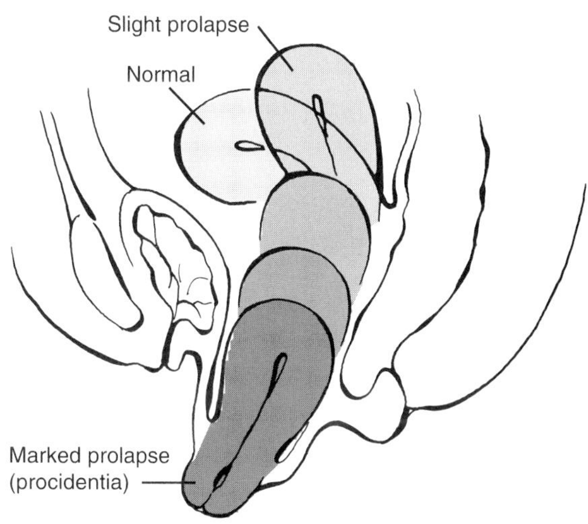

FIGURE 37-30. Stages of uterine prolapse (note piston-like progression).

TABLE 37-7

TYPES OF SEXUAL DYSFUNCTION

SEXUAL DYSFUNCTION	CAUSE	DESCRIPTION
Sexual desire disorders	Psychological factors	Absence of desire or aversion to sexual activity
Sexual excitement phase dysfunction	Psychological or physical factors	Impotence or frigidity
Orgasmic phase dysfunction	Psychological or medications (antihypertensives) or alcohol	Delayed or absent orgasm following a normal excitement phase
Interpretation of the sexual act	Psychological	Feelings of pleasure or displeasure following coitus Affects a woman's desire for the next sexual act (back to first phase)
Sexual pain disorder	Physical or psychological	Dyspareunia: pain with intercourse Vaginismus: spasm of the outer third of the vagina, preventing coitus

Infertility

Infertility is a major health care concern. Nearly 5.3 million American women are infertile. In fact, 25% of all women in the U.S. will have a concern related to fertility at some point during their reproductive years. The number of infertility clinics for assisted reproductive technique has increased 10-fold in the past 10 years. Contemporary therapy in the treatment of infertility is progressing faster than in any other field of medicine. More women than ever before are seeking diagnosis and treatment of fertility. There are many factors that cause this increase. Couples are putting off starting their families until later in their reproductive lives. Many women of today are over the age of 35, when reproductive potential begins to decline, before they even begin to attempt pregnancy. The number of women in the U.S. between 35 and 44 years of age is increasing and will continue to do so. More couples are aware of aspects surrounding infertility and the availability of techniques. Couples without male partners are taking advantage of various options available to them. The number of adoptable babies has decreased, probably because of improved contraceptive methods and treatments.

CAUSES OF INFERTILITY

Infertility affects 15% to 20% of all couples trying to conceive. The cause may be due to a female factor, a male factor, or both (Table 37-8). Female factors may involve any one of a variety of reproductive organs as described in the following:

Hypothalamus
Weight (either below 100 lbs or above 200 lbs)
Exercise, which decreases gonadotropins and increases prolactin
Polycystic ovarian syndrome, which increases luteinizing hormone

Pituitary Gland
Hyperprolactinemia, which causes anovulation
Hyperthyroidism, which may be associated with hyperprolactinemia and cause menstrual irregularities
Sheehan's syndrome, which can cause hypopituitarism

TABLE 37-8

CAUSES OF INFERTILITY

CAUSE	INCIDENCE
MALE FACTOR	35%–40%
FEMALE FACTOR	40%
Ovulatory	20%–40%
Tubal	20%–40%
Endometriosis	10%
Advanced age	18%–50%
Luteal phase defect	<10%
Uterine factors	10%
Fibroids	2%–3%
UNEXPLAINED	10%–15%
COMBINATION	10%–20%

(Carcio, H. [1998]. *Management of the infertile woman.* Philadelphia: Lippincott-Raven.)

Ovary
Premature ovarian failure, in which estrogen declines prior to menopause
Polycystic ovarian syndrome, which causes an increase in ovarian follicles
Luteal phase defect, which decreases progesterone levels

Cervix
Stenosis, which inhibits sperm motility through os
Poor cervical mucus during midcycle, creating a barrier to sperm

Fallopian tubes
Infection from *Chlamydia*, gonorrhea, or mycoplasma, especially if pelvic inflammatory disease occurred
Narrowing of the tubes in the presence of endometriosis

Uterus
Asherman's syndrome due to scarring of the uterine lining from a traumatic D & C may distort the shape and size of the uterus
Endometriosis, which causes adhesions in the tubes
Fibroids, which may distort the uterine contour

Other
Smoking, which causes a toxic effect on the follicles
Douching, which may upset the vaginal ecology

Assisted Reproductive Technology and Pregnancy Rates

Assisted reproductive technology (ART) is a group of different procedures designed to unite the sperm and egg in various ways, thus bypassing some of the natural obstacles to pregnancy that may be the cause of infertility. The most common procedures are in vitro fertilization (IVF), gamete intrafallopian transfer (GIFT), and zygote intrafallopian transfer (ZIFT). These procedures offer hope for those couples who are not able to conceive through natural methods or procedures such as intrauterine insemination. The pregnancy rates with ART vary, depending on the center, the procedure used, the cause of infertility, and the age of the woman. The chances of a pregnancy occurring naturally during each cycle is around 25%. This means that if 100 couples were attempting pregnancy in any one month, only 25 of them couples would conceive. The success of ART compares favorably with this, particularly if the woman is under age 40. However, this still means that only one in four or five couples will become pregnant with each ART attempt, which is certainly much more costly, financially and emotionally, than natural intercourse.

FOCUS ON THE WOMAN WITH PREMENOPAUSAL SYMPTOMS

Mrs. B. is a 52-year-old Caucasian woman. She is a grammar school teacher. Her three sons are all away at college. She is monogamous with her husband of 26 years, who has had a vasectomy. She presents to the clinic complaining of vaginal dryness and occasional hot flashes.

Her family history is negative for breast and ovarian cancer. Her parents are on antihypertensive medications. She denies any medication allergies. She has never smoked. She denies any chronic illness, and the only medication she is taking is a calcium supplement. Her last gynecological exam was 1 year ago and was normal. She has never had an abnormal Pap smear. She has gained a few pounds since her last visit but admits she should be exercising more.

Her menstrual periods are usually regular, occurring every 28 days, but have recently been progressively shorter and are now occurring every 25–26 days. The menstrual flow seems lighter. Her premenstrual moods have increased in intensity. During intercourse she notes a decrease in lubrication and often notes vaginal spotting immediately after intercourse. She denies any other vaginal spotting. She denies change in mentation or libido. Hot flashes occur almost daily, usually mid-morning. Face flushes for 1–2 minutes. Denies diaphoresis.

Questions

1. Define perimenopause. What is the average age of menopause?
2. Compare the phases of the ovarian cycle to those of the uterine endometrial cycle.
3. What mechanisms may cause the shortening of the interval between menstrual bleeding?
4. What factors affects the age of onset of menopause?
5. What effect do declining estrogen levels have on the vaginal epithelial cells?
6. What happens to the gonadotropin FSH after menopause?
7. List other symptoms that may indicate that Mrs. B. is perimenopausal.

REFERENCES

1. American Cancer Society. (1998). *Cancer facts and figures–1998*. Atlanta: American Cancer Society.
2. American Psychiatric Association. (1994). *Diagnostic and statistical manual of mental disorders* (4th ed.). Washington, DC: American Psychiatric Association.
3. Artini, P. G., Fasciani, A., Battaglia, C., deMicheroux, A. A. & D'Ambrogio, A. R. (1997). Fertility drugs and ovarian cancer. *Gynecologic Endocrinology, 11*(1), 59.
4. Carmichael, M. S., Humbert, R., Dixen, J., Palmisano, G., Greenleaf, W. & Davidson, J. M. (1987). Plasma oxytocin increases in the human sexual response. *Journal of Clinical Endocrinology and Metabolism, 64*, 27.
5. Chandrasoma, P. & Taylor, C. R. (1998). *Concise pathology* (3rd ed.). Norwalk, CT: Appleton & Lange.
6. Dawood, M. Y. (1998). Dysmenorrhea. In J. J. Sciarra, *Gynecology and obstetrics*, 5(6). Philadelphia: Lippincott-Raven.
7. DeCherney, A. H. & Pernoll, M. L. (1994). *Current obstetric and gynecologic diagnosis and treatment* (8th ed.). Norwalk, CT: Appleton & Lange.
8. DiSaia, P. J. & Creasman, W. T. (1997). *Clinical gynecologic oncology*. St. Louis: Mosby.
9. Ferin, M. (1998). The hypothalamic-hypophyseal-ovarian axis. In J. J. Sciarra, *Gynecology and obstetrics*, 5(6). Philadelphia: Lippincott-Raven.
10. Gass, M., Mezrow, G. & Rebar, R. W. (1998). Menopause. In J. J. Sciarra, *Gynecology and obstetrics*, 1(24). Philadelphia: Lippincott-Raven.
11. Gordan, M. D. & Ireland, K. (1998). Pathology of endometrial carcinoma. In J. J. Sciarra, *Gynecology and obstetrics*, 4(15). Philadelphia: Lippincott-Raven.
12. Halban, J. (1924). Metastatic hysteroadenosis. *Wiener Klinische Wochenschrift, 37*, 1205.
13. Hammond, C. B. & Spoer, J. T. (1998). Gestational trophoblastic diseases. In J. J. Sciarra, *Gynecology and obstetrics*, 5(48). Philadelphia: Lippincott-Raven.
14. Jacobs, A. (1996). Ovarian cancer. In *Clinical Symposia*, 48(2). New York: Ciba.
15. Kazer, R. R. (1998). Polycystic ovary syndrome. In J. J. Sciarra, *Gynecology and obstetrics*, 5(27). Philadelphia: Lippincott-Raven.
16. Korzweka, L. I. & Steiner, M. (1998). Premenstrual syndromes. In D. A. Baram, Psychosocial obstetrics and gynecology. *Clinical Obstetrics and Gynecology, 40*(3), 564.
17. Krebs, H. B. (1998). Human papillomavirus infections and genital tract cancers. In J. J. Sciarra, *Gynecology and obstetrics*, 4(2). Philadelphia: Lippincott-Raven.
18. Kumar, V., Cotran, R. S., & Robbins, S. L. (1997). *Basic pathology* (6th ed). Philadelphia: W. B. Saunders.
19. Landis, S. H., Murray, T., Bolden, S. & Wingo, P. A. (1998). Cancer statistics, 1998. *CA: A Cancer Journal for Clinicians, 48*(1), 6.
20. Marcoux, S., Maheux, R., Bérubé, S. & Canadian Collaborative Group on Endometriosis (1997). Laparoscopic surgery in infertile women with minimal or mild endometriosis. *New England Journal of Medicine, 337*(4), 217.
21. McLachlan, J. A. & Arnold, S. F. (1996). Environmental estrogens. *American Scientist, 84*, 452.
22. Nolte, S. (1996). Ovarian cancer. *Oncology nursing update, 3*(2), 1.
23. Nunley, W. C. & Kitchin, J. D. (1998). Endometriosis. In J. J. Sciarra, *Gynecology and obstetrics*, 1(20). Philadelphia: Lippincott-Raven.
24. Rossing, M. A., Daling, J. R., Weiss, N. S., Moore, D. E. & Self, S. G. (1997). Ovarian tumors in a cohort of infertile women. *New England Journal of Medicine, 331*(12), 771.
25. Ryan, I. P. & Taylor, R. N. (1997). Endometriosis and Infertility: New concepts. *Obstetrical and Gynecological Survey, 52*(6), 365.
26. Safe, S. H. (1997). Xenoestrogens and breast cancer. *New England Journal Of Medicine, 337*(18), 1303.
27. Sampson, J. A. (1927). Peritoneal endometriosis due to menstrual dissemination of endometrial tissue into the peritoneal cavity. *American Journal of Obstetrics and Gynecology, 14*, 422.
28. Schmidt, P. J., Nieman, L. K., Danaceau, R. N., Adams, L. F. & Rubinow, D. R. (1998). Differential effects of gonadal steroids in women with and those without premenstrual syndrome. *New England Journal of Medicine, 338*(4), 209.
29. Severino, M. F. (1998). Dysfunctional uterine bleeding. In J. J. Sciarra, *Gynecology and obstetrics*, 5(20). Philadelphia: Lippincott-Raven.
30. Sobel, J. D. (1997). Vaginitis. *New England Journal of Medicine, 337*(26), 1896.
31. Stein, I. F. & Leventhal, M. L. (1935). Amenorrhea associated with bilateral polycystic ovaries. *American Journal of Obstetrics and Gynecology, 29*, 181.
32. Tierney, L. M., McPhee, J., & Papadakis, M. A. (1998). *Current: Medical diagnosis and treatment* (37th ed.). Norwalk, CT: Appleton & Lange.
33. Yonkers, K. A., Halbreich, U., Freeman, E., Brown, C., Endicott, J., Frank, E., Parry, B., Pearlstein, T., Severino, S., Stout, A., Stone, A., & Harrison, W. (1997). Symptomatic improvement of premenstrual dysphoric disorder with sertraline treatment. *Journal of the American Medical Association, 278*(12), 983.

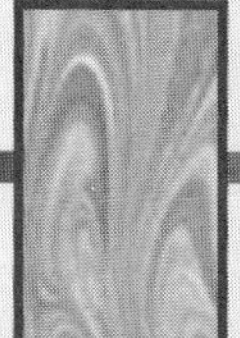

UNIT 12: CASE STUDY

The Woman With Abnormal Uterine Bleeding

Introduction to the Patient

C. K. is a 59-year-old Caucasian female who comes to the clinic complaining of uterine bleeding. She states, "I thought I was finished with my periods."

Present Illness

C. K. states that approximately 2 days ago, she noticed some vaginal spotting, which gradually increased over the next 2 days. Currently, C. K. reports that the bleeding is similar to a menstrual period. She also reports some slight, intermittent cramping. She denies any complaints of urinary frequency, constipation, or abdominal fullness or pain. She is 5 ft, 3 in tall and weighs 175 pounds.

Social History

C. K. is a single female (never married) who lives alone in a two-story home in the suburbs. She works full time as an assistant manager for a large drugstore chain. C. K. states that she is very active in her church and participates in a volunteer program at a local community center once a week.

Past Medical History

C. K. states that this is the third episode of bleeding in the last 7 months. The previous two episodes were just slight spotting, so "I really didn't think anything of it." She began menstruating at the age of 10, every 29 to 31 days with moderate flow lasting 3 to 4 days and minimal cramping. Menopause occurred at age 55, accompanied by severe "hot flashes" for which she was prescribed Premarin 1.25 mg daily for 25 days each month with relief. C. K. was also diagnosed with hypertension approximately 10 years ago, taking captopril 25 mg twice daily. She reports visiting her gynecologist yearly for a pelvic examination and Pap smear. "My last Pap smear was 10 months ago and it was normal." She denies any previous history of pregnancies, abortion, fibroids, or use of oral contraceptives.

Family History

C. K. is the oldest of two children. She has a sister, age 55, who is alive and relatively healthy. Both parents are deceased. Her father died at the age of 69 in a truck accident. Her mother died 3 years ago at the age of 79 from colon cancer.

Physical Examination

C. K. is alert and oriented to person, place, and time. Skin is pale, warm, and dry. Mucous membranes are pale. Her vital signs are as follows: temperature—98.4°F; pulse—92 and regular; respirations—20; blood pressure—140/86. Lungs are clear to auscultation. Heart sounds are normal. Abdomen is soft, non-tender, with positive bowel sounds in all four quadrants. Neurologic examination is unremarkable. Lymph nodes nonpalpable.

Perineal examination reveals moderate amount of dark red vaginal drainage without clots, saturating one perineal pad in the last 2 hours. Pelvic examination reveals slightly enlarged, asymmetrical uterus with a 2-cm soft, round mass palpated on lateral aspect of lower fundus.

Diagnostic Tests

Complete blood count: WBC—7000/µL; RBC—3.33 $\times 10^6$/µL; MCV—72µm^3; MCHC—31g/dL; hemoglobin—10.5 g/dL; hematocrit—33%
Pelvic ultrasound: small 2-cm mass identified in left lateral aspect of lower uterine wall
TSH—6 mU/L
APTT—33 seconds; PTT—64 seconds

CRITICAL THINKING QUESTIONS

1. Discuss the possible risk factors exhibited by C. K. that might lead you to suspect endometrial cancer.
2. Construct a chart to differentiate endometrial cancer from uterine leiomyomas. Include description, incidence, etiology, and clinical manifestations.
3. C.K. appears to be a little anemic. Identify the clinical and laboratory manifestations of her anemia. Discuss the type of anemia she has and your rationale for this. What is the likely intervention for her anemia?
4. Propose possible diagnostic tests that would be necessary to confirm and evaluate the diagnosis of endometrial cancer.
5. If the diagnosis of endometrial cancer is confirmed, describe how C. K. may be treated now and if a recurrence of the disease develops.

Besides your pathophysiology text, you'll need a good pharmacology text, a gynecology text, an oncology text, a diagnostic/laboratory test text, a medical-surgical nursing text, and current research to complete this case study. Suggested references follow:

DeVita, V. T. et al. (Eds.) (1997). *Cancer principles and practice of oncology,* (5th ed.). Philadelphia: Lippincott-Raven.

Fischbach, F. (1996). *Manual of laboratory and diagnostic tests,* (5th ed.). Philadelphia: Lippincott-Raven.

Karch, A. M. (1999). *Lippincott's nursing drug guide.* Philadelphia: Lippincott William & Wilkins.

Lambron, N. C., Morse, A. N., & Wallach, E. (1999). *The John Hopkins manual of gynecology and obstetrics.* Philadelphia: Lippincott-Raven.

Scott, J. et al. (Eds.) (1999). *Danforth's obstetrics and gynecology,* (8th ed.). Philadelphia: Lippincott Williams & Wilkins.

Smeltzer, S. & Bare, B. (2000). *Brunner and Suddarth's textbook of medical-surgical nursing,* (9th ed.). Philadelphia: Lippincott Williams & Wilkins.

Website resources

Abnormal Uterine Bleeding *http://www.obgyn.net/ah/patient/AUB.htm*

Diagnosing Abnormal Uterine Bleeding *http://www.gynalternatives.com/aubdiag.htm*

Dysfunctional Uterine Bleeding *http://www.emedicine.com/emerg/topic155.htm*

Women's Health Center *http://mayohealth.org/mayo/common/htm/womenpg.htm*

UNIT 12 APPENDIX A

DIAGNOSTIC TESTS

TEST	PURPOSE/ NORMAL FINDINGS	SIGNIFICANCE
Serum estrogen	Radioimmunoassay of the three estrogens (estradiol, estrone, and estriol) appearing in serum to evaluate female gonadal function Normal findings: Premenopausal females during days of menstrual cycle: • Days 1 to 10: 24–68 pg/mL • Days 11 to 20: 50–186 pg/mL • Days 21 to 30: 73–149 pg/mL Males: 12–34 pg/mL	Decreased levels may indicate primary hypogonadism, such as ovarian failure; secondary hypogonadism, such as hypopituitarism; or menopause. Increased levels may indicate estrogen-producing tumor, fibrocystic breast disease, or precocious puberty. Oral contraceptives may increase levels; clomiphene may decrease levels.
Serum progesterone	Radioimmunoassay of corpus luteum function Normal findings: Females (during phase of menstrual cycle): • Follicular phase: 0.1–1.5 ng/mL • Luteal phase: 2.5–28.1 ng/mL Females (during pregnancy): • First trimester: 9–47 ng/mL • Second trimester: 16.8–146 ng/mL • Third trimester: 55–255 ng/mL Females over age 60: 0–0.2 ng/mL Males: 0–0.4 ng/mL	Increased levels may suggest ovarian tumor or molar pregnancy. Decreased levels may be indicative of amenorrhea or threatened abortion. Higher levels usually are seen in twin, pregnancies when compared with single pregnancies
Serum human chorionic gonadotropin (hCG [beta subunit])	Qualitative evaluation of beta subunit of hCG to determine conception and changes in levels possibly secondary to a disorder Normal findings: Routine: negative Non-routine: • Nonpregnant females: less than 5.0 IU/L • Postmenopausal females: less than 9.0 IU/L • Pregnant females: increase in levels from 3 weeks after last menstrual period of 0–5 IU/L to 3640–117,000 IU/L at 25 to 40 weeks • Males: less than 2.5 IU/L	Increased levels are found in pregnancy, hydatiform mole, and ovarian and testicular teratomas. Decreased levels are usually seen with threatened abortion and ectopic pregnancy.
Serum prolactin	Evaluation of the level of pituitary hormone important for initiating and maintaining lactation Normal findings: Nonpregnant females: 0–17 ng/mL Pregnant females: 34–386 ng/mL Males: 0–15 ng/mL	Increased levels may indicate amenorrhea, prolactin-secreting tumors, primary hypothyroidism, or anorexia nervosa. Decreased levels may indicate Sheehan's syndrome. Drugs, such as estrogen, methyldopa, and tricyclic antidepressants, may increase levels.
Serum follicle stimulating hormone (FSH)	Evaluation of hormonal level to determine gonadal function Normal findings: Nonpregnant menstruating females (varies with phase of menstrual cycle) • Follicular phase: 5–20 mIU/mL • Luteal phase: 5–15 mIU/mL Postmenopausal females: 50–100 mIU/mL Males: 5–20 mIU/mL	Decreased levels may suggest aspermatogenesis, anovulation, or secondary hypogonadism. Increased levels in females may indicate ovarian failure or precocious puberty. Increased levels in males may indicate testicular destruction, testicular failure, seminoma, or male climacteric.

(continued)

UNIT 12 APPENDIX A

DIAGNOSTIC TESTS (Continued)

TEST	PURPOSE/ NORMAL FINDINGS	SIGNIFICANCE
Plasma luteinizing hormone (LH)	Quantitative evaluation of hormone involved with ovulation and transformation of ovarian follicle to corpus luteum Normal findings: Menstruating females (vary with the phase of menstrual cycle): • Follicular phase: 1–20 IU/L • Mid-cycle (ovulation): 25–100 IU/L • Luteal phase: 0.2–20 IU/L Postmenopausal females: 20–100 IU/L	Absence of midcycle peak may suggest anovulation. Decreased levels may suggest hypogonadism when accompanied by amenorrhea. Increased levels may suggest ovarian failure, menopause, or early-stage acromegaly.
Serum testosterone	Evaluation of total and unbound testosterone (active) responsible for male secondary sex characteristics Normal findings: Total: • Males: 300–1000 ng/mL • Nonpregnant females: 20–75 ng/mL • Pregnant females: 3 to 4 times higher • Postmenopausal females: 8–35 ng/mL Free (vary with age and sex; measured in pg/mL): • Age 20 to 29: 19–41 (males); 0.9–3.2 (females) • Age 30 to 39: 18–39 (males); 0.8–3.0 (females) • Age 40 to 49: 16–33 (males); 0.6–2.5 (females) • Age 50 to 59: 13–31 (males); 0.3–2.7 (females) • Age 60+: 9–26 (males); 0.2–2.2 (females)	Testosterone level is normal in cryptorchidism, azoospermia, and oligospermia. Decreased total levels may indicate pituitary failure, Klinefelter's syndrome, Down syndrome, or delayed puberty. Decreased free levels in males may suggest hypogonadism. Increased total levels in males may be seen with hyperthyroidism, adrenal tumors, or precocious puberty. Increased total levels in females may suggest adrenal tumors, benign or malignant ovarian tumors, gestational trophoblastic disease, or idiopathic hirsutism. Increased free levels may be seen with female hirsutism, polycystic ovarian disease, or virilization. Testosterone levels change during the day, with values highest in the morning and dropping in males by 30% to 50% (in females, by 20%) by mid-afternoon.
Serum glucoprotein CA 15-3	Marker used to diagnose and monitor treatment of breast cancer Normal findings: less than 22 U/mL	The test is more accurate in advanced breast cancer than early breast cancer. Abnormal results may also be seen in other benign and malignant conditions. Increased levels may indicate breast cancer.
Prostate-specific antigen (PSA)	Measurement of a marker for evaluating prostatic cancer and effectiveness of treatment Normal findings: 0 to 4.0 ng/mL	In most patients with prostatic cancer, PSA is increased. PSA is found in both normal epithelial and cancerous cells of the prostate. Level of 4–8 ng/mL suggest benign prostatic hypertrophy. Values greater than 8 ng/mL are highly suggestive of prostatic cancer.
Urine estrogen (total)	24-hour specimen collection to evaluate ovarian function Normal findings: Nonpregnant females (vary with phase of menstrual cycle): • Preovulatory phase: 5–25 μg • Ovulatory phase: 24–100 μg • Luteal phase: 12–80 μg Postmenopausal females: <10 μg Males: 4–25 μg	Decreased levels may suggest primary or secondary ovarian insufficiency or ovarian agenesis. Increased levels may suggest adrenocortical or ovarian tumor in females or testicular tumor in males. Rising levels are normal during pregnancy.
Urine FSH and LH	24-hour specimen collection to evaluate hormones produced by the anterior	Serial daily blood testing may also be obtained at the same time.

UNIT 12 APPENDIX A

DIAGNOSTIC TESTS (Continued)

TEST	PURPOSE/ NORMAL FINDINGS	SIGNIFICANCE
	pituitary gland to determine primary disorders or one due to insufficient pituitary hormone stimulation Normal findings (per 24 hours): FSH: • Nonpregnant females: 5–20 IU (mid cycle peak, 15–30 IU) • Postmenopausal females: 30–440 IU Male: 1–20 IU LH: • Nonpregnant females: 5–15 IU (mid cycle peak, 30–95 IU) • Postmenopousal females: 50 100 IU • Males: 5–20 IU	Decreased FSH levels may be associated with ovarian tumors, pituitary or hypothalamic failure, tumor of the testis or adrenal gland, polycystic ovarian disease, or pregnancy. Increased FSH levels may indicate Turner's syndrome, hypopituitarism, Sheehan's syndrome, Klinefelter's syndrome, or menopause. Increased FSH and LH levels may indicate hypogonadism, testicular feminization syndrome, congenital absence of testes, or menopause. Decreased FSH and LH levels may suggest pituitary or hypothalamic failure.
Urine pregnanediol	24-hour specimen collection to evaluate ovarian and placental function Normal findings (in 24 hours): Pregnant females (vary with trimester): • First trimester: 10–30 mg • Second trimester: 35–70 mg • Third trimester: 70–100 mg Postmenopausal females: 0.2–1 mg Males: 0–1 mg	Increased levels may indicate ovarian cysts, congenital adrenal hyperplasia, or malignant trophoblasts. Decreased levels may indicate amenorrhea, ovarian tumor, hydatiform mole, or eclampsia.
Urine hCG	Qualitative analysis of hormone to detect pregnancy Normal findings: Nonpregnant females: negative Pregnant females (vary with trimester): • First trimester: 500,000 IU • Second trimester: 10,000–25,000 IU • Third trimester: 5,000–15,000 IU Males: negative	Elevated levels during pregnancy may suggest multiple pregnancy. Positive levels in males or nonpregnant females may suggest choriocarcinoma, ovarian or testicular tumor, breast cancer, or other cancer, such as gastric, hepatic, or pancreatic.
Semen analysis	Examination of semen for number, appearance, and motility obtained usually via masturbation 2 to 4 days after sexual abstinence Normal findings: Amount: 2.5–5 mL Number: 20 million/mL (average of 50–200 million/mL pH: 7.3–7.9 Morphology: at least 40% normal Motility: 50% or more show progressive motility	Specimen must be analyzed within 1 hour of collection. Specimen must not be exposed to extremes of heat and cold. This is a common test for male infertility.
Antisperm antibody test	Evaluation for presence of sperm antibodies via semen, serum, or cervical mucus samples as a reason for infertility Normal findings: less than 20% sperm binding	Semen sampling is the preferred method of testing. The percentage of sperm binding is inversely proportional to sperm count. Greater than 20% binding may suggest infertility.
Basal body temperature (BBT)	Measurement of basal body temperature as an indication of ovulation Normal findings: BBT drops approximately 0.5 °; followed by a rise to a temperature no higher than normal body temperature and maintained for approximately 10 days	Increased BBT indicates the time of ovulation. BBT not maintained for 10 days suggests a luteal phase defect when progesterone production starts but is not sustained.

(continued)

UNIT 12 APPENDIX A

DIAGNOSTIC TESTS (Continued)

TEST	PURPOSE/ NORMAL FINDINGS	SIGNIFICANCE
Cervical mucus test	Evaluation of cervical mucus for changes indicative of high estrogen levels associated with ovulation Normal findings: fern pattern on drying; stretchable (+ spinnbarkeit)	Typically, cervical mucus is thin, watery, and copious with low viscosity under the influence of estrogen, possibly indicative that ovulation is about to occur. When progesterone is dominant, cervical mucus is thick and viscous.
Postcoital cervical mucus test	Combination of semen analysis and cervical mucus test to evaluate fertility with specimen obtained during female's fertile period and analyzed 2 to 8 hours after coitus Normal findings: Positive spinnbarkeit Ferning: 3+ or 4+ Viscosity: 1+ Sperm number high and motile	This test is not used as frequently as before because of scheduling difficulties.
Papanicolaou (Pap) smear	Aspiration of cervical secretions from cervical os for microscopic examination Normal findings: Class I; no abnormalities	Drugs such as tetracycline and digitalis may alter the results. Recent douching or using lubricating jelly in the vagina also may distort the findings. The ideal time for specimen collection is 2 weeks after the first day of the last menstrual period. Obtaining samples during menstruation should be avoided. Presence of abnormal cells does not confirm diagnosis of cancer but suggests need for further studies.
Colposcopy	Examination of the vagina and cervix with an optical instrument to visualize the cervix and obtain tissue samples if necessary Normal findings: absence of lesions in vagina, cervix; and genital areas	Abnormalities may include leukoplakia, varying degrees of dysplasia, abnormal blood vessels, or hyperkeratosis. An endocervical curettage may be done to evaluate if abnormalities have occurred in the cervical canal, subsequently requiring cryotherapy or cone biopsy.
Dilation and curettage (D&C)	Examination of cervical canal and endometrium via dilation and scraping with possible tissue sampling for cytology Normal findings: absence of abnormal tissue	This test may be used to control abnormal uterine bleeding and aids in further diagnosis of abnormal cells and dysmenorrhea.
Laparoscopy	Visualization of pelvic structures via a fiberoptic scope Normal findings: absence of abnormal tissue or secretions	Abnormal findings are seen with diseases of the uterus, fallopian tubes, and ovaries. This test may help identify tumors, cysts, endometriosis, causes of infertility, and infections; it is also used to stage gynecologic carcinomas. It is the most definitive test to diagnose PID.
Hysteroscopy (transcervical intrauterine endoscopy)	Direct visualization of entire uterine cavity Normal findings: absence of lesions, tumors, or occlusions	This test may be indicated for infection, unexplained bleeding, retained intrauterine device, or fibroid removal. Hysteroscopy is contraindicated in patients with cervical or endometrial cancer or acute pelvic inflammatory disease.
Hysterosalpingography	Radiographic evaluation of uterus and fallopian tubes using a contrast medium Normal findings:	This test may reveal bicornate uterus, tubal tortuosity, tubal obstruction, or evidence of tubal scarring or adhesions.

UNIT 12 APPENDIX A

DIAGNOSTIC TESTS (Continued)

TEST	PURPOSE/ NORMAL FINDINGS	SIGNIFICANCE
	Uterine cavity normal Patent fallopian tubes	
Mammography	Radiographic evaluation of soft tissue of the breast to screen for breast cancer Normal findings: Calcifications evenly distributed (if present) Ducts normal with gradual narrowing Absence of masses	This test can detect masses less than 1 cm in size. Benign tumors appear as round, smooth masses with definable edges. Malignant tumors appear irregular in shape, possibly extending to adjacent tissue and accompanied by an increase in the number of blood vessels. Diagnosis of breast cancer can only be confirmed by biopsy.
Pelvic ultrasound	Use of sound waves to evaluate the area from the umbilicus to the pubis for structure, size and location of possible masses Normal findings: normal image pattern of bladder, uterus, fallopian tubes and vagina	A transabdominal or transvaginal approach may be used. A transabdominal approach requires the patient to have a full bladder. This test determines uterine abnormalities such as fibroids, fluid collection, or structural variations. Masses are identified by size and consistency. Cysts typically appear as well-defined, smooth masses, showing an echo pattern similar to that of the bladder.
Breast ultrasound	Use of sound waves to evaluate the breast tissue for masses Normal findings: symmetric echo pattern bilaterally in all layers	Cysts; benign, solid, or malignant tumors; or metastasis to muscle or lymph nodes may be seen. This test is recommended for young women who have palpable masses.
Testicular scan	Radionuclide imaging of the scrotal structures Normal findings: Blood flow to scrotal structures intact Radioisotope evenly concentrated and distributed	This test is most commonly done as an emergency for acute testicular pain and swelling to evaluate for torsion secondary to epididymitis, injury, trauma, tumor, or mass. Abnormalities may indicate a tumor, hematoma, infection, or torsion.

UNIT BIBLIOGRAPHY

Abeloff, M. D., Armitage, J. O., Lichter, A. S. & Niederhuber, J. E. (Eds.) (1995). *Clinical oncology.* New York: Churchill Livingstone.

Allen, K. M. & Phillips, J. M. (1997). *Women's health across the lifespan. A comprehensive perspective.* Philadelphia: J. B. Lippincott.

American Cancer Society. (1999). *Cancer facts and figures.* Atlanta: American Cancer Society.

American College of Obstetricians and Gynecologists. (1996). *Guidelines for women's health care.* Washington, DC: ACOG.

Beckman, C., Ling, F., Barzansky, B., Bates, G., Herbert, W., Laube, D., & Smith, R. (1997). *Obstetrics and gynecology* (2nd ed.). Baltimore: Williams & Wilkins.

Borum, M. et al. (1998). Women's health issues. *Medical Clinics of North America, 82* (2), 189–401.

Carico, H. A. (1999). *Advanced health assessment of women.* Philadelphia: Lippincott Williams & Wilkins.

Cotran, R. S., Kumar, V., & Robbins, S. L. (1994). Robbins' pathologic basis of disease (5th ed.). Philadelphia: W. B. Saunders.

Cowan, B. D. & Seifer, D. B. (1997). *Clinical reproductive medicine.* Philadelphia: Lippincott-Raven.

DeVita, V. T., Hellman, S. & Rosenberg, S. A. (Eds.) (1997). *Cancer: Principles and practice of oncology,* (5th ed). Philadelphia: Lippincott-Raven.

Finan, S. (1997). Promoting healthy sexuality: Guidelines for early through older adulthood. *Nurse Practitioner 22*(12), 54–64.

Gill, B. & Kogan, S. (1997). Cryptorchidism—current concepts. *Pediatric Clinics of North America, 44*(5), 1211–1227.

Johnson, C. A. Johnson, B. E. Murrary, J. L. & Apgar, B. S. (1998). *Women's health care handbook.* Philadelphia: Hanley and Belfus.

Keller, M., Duerst, B., & Zimmerman, J. (1996). Adolescents' views of sexual decision making. *Image, 28*(2), 125–130.

Kelley, W. (1997). *Textbook of internal medicine* (3rd ed.). Philadelphia: Lippincott-Raven.

McPhee, S. I., Lingappa, V. R., Ganong, W. F. & Lange, J. D. (1997). *Pathophysiology of disease* (2nd ed.). Stamford, CT: Appleton & Lange.

Muscari, M. E. Adolescent health: The first gynecologic exam. *American Journal of Nursing, 99*(1), 66–67.

Rous, S. N. (1996). *Urology: A core textbook* (2nd ed.). Cambridge, MA: Blackwell Science.

Scott, J., Di Saia, P. J. et al. (1999). *Danforth's obstetrics and gynecology* (8th ed.). Philadelphia: Lippincott Williams & Wilkins.

Tanagho, E. A. & McAninch, J. W. (1995). *Smith's general urology* (14th ed.). Norwalk, CT: Appleton & Lange.

Walker, L., & Tinkle, M. (1996). Toward an integrative science of women's health. *JOGNN, 25*(5), 379–381.

Zaontz, M. R. & Packer, M. G. (1997). Abnormalities of the external genitalia. *Pediatric Clinics of North America, 44*(5), 1267–1297.

BENIGN PROSTATIC HYPERPLASIA

Agency for Health Care Policy and Research. (1994). *Benign prostatic hyperplasia: Diagnosis and treatment.* Clinical Practice Guidelines No. 8. Bethesda, MD; U.S. Department of Health and Human Services. AHCPR Publication No. 94-0582.

Barry, M. J. et al. (1997). The natural history of patients with benign prostatic hyperplasia as diagnosed by North American urologists. *Journal of Urology, 157*(1), 10–15.

Gerber, G. S. (1995). Lasers in the treatment of benign prostatic hyperplasia. *Urology, 45*(2), 193–195.

Gormley, G. J. et al. (1992). The effect of finesteride in men with benign prostatic hyperplasia. *New England Journal of Medicine, 327*(17), 1185–1191.

Keetch, D. W. et al. (1995). Cryosurgical ablation of the prostate. *AORN Journal 61*(5), 807–813.

Oesterling, J. E. (1995). Benign prostatic hyperplasia. *New England Journal of Medicine, 332*(2), 99–108.

Reilly, N. J. (1997). Benign prostatic hyperplasia in older men. *Lippincott's Primary Care Practice, 1*(4), 421–430.

Walsh, P. C. (1996). Treatment of benign prostatic hyperplasia. *New England Journal of Medicine, 335*(8), 586–587.

PROSTATITIS

Vetrosky, D. (1997). Prostatitis. *Lippincott's Primary Care Practice, 1*(4), 437–441.

PROSTATIC CANCER

Ahlering, T. et al. (1996). Practice guidelines for prostate cancer. *Cancer Journal Scientific American* 2(Suppl. to No. 3A), S77–S86.

Albertsen, P. C. (1996). Screening for prostate cancer is neither appropriate nor cost-effective. *Urologic Clinics of North America, 23*(4), 521–530.

Bolla, M. et al. (1997). Improved survival in patients with locally advanced prostate cancer treated with radiotherapy and goserelin. *New England Journal of Medicine, 337*(5), 295–300.

Cher, M. L. & Carroll, P. R. (1995). Screening for prostate cancer. *Western Journal of Medicine, 162*(3), 235–242.

Coley, C. M. et al. (1997). Early detection of prostate cancer. Part I: Prior probability and effectiveness of tests. American College of Physicians. *Annals of Internal Medicine, 126*(5), 394–406.

Coley, C. M. et al (1997). Early detection of prostate cancer. Part II: Estimating the risks, benefits, and costs. American College of Physicians. *Annals of Internal Medicines 126*(6), 468–479.

Collins, M. (1997). Increasing prostate cancer awareness in African American men. *Oncology Nursing Forum, 24*(1), 91–95.

Davison, B. J. et al. (1995) Information and decision-making preferences of men with prostate cancer. *Oncology Nursing Forum, 22*(9), 1401–1408.

Gelfand, D. E. et al. (1995). Digital rectal examinations and prostate cancer screening: Attitudes of African American men. *Oncology Nursing Forum, 22*(8), 1253–1263.

Grönberg, H., Isaacs, S. D., Smith, J. R., Carpten, J. D., Bova, G. S., Freije, D., Xu, J., Meyers, D. A., Collins, F. S., Trent, J. M., Walsh, P. C. & Isaacs, W. B. (1997). Characteristics of prostate cancer in families linked to the hereditary prostate cancer 1 *(HPC1)* locus. *JAMA, 278*(15), 1251–1255.

Haas, G. P. & Sakr, W. A. (1997). Epidemiology of prostate cancer. *CA: Cancer Journal for Clinicians, 47*(5), 273–287.

Held, J. L. et al. (1994). Cancer of the prostate: Treatment and nursing implications. *Oncology Nursing Forum, 21*(9), 1517–1529.

Herr, H. W. (1997). Quality of life in prostate cancer patients. *CA: Cancer Journal for Clinicians, 47*(4), 207–217.

Krongrad, A. et al. (1997). Survival after radical prostatectomy. *JAMA, 278*(1), 44–46.

McKee, J. M. (1994). Cues to action in prostate cancer screening. *Oncology Nursing Forum, 21*(7), 1171–1176.

Mettlin, C. (1997). The American Cancer Society National Prostate Cancer Detection Project and national patterns of prostate cancer detection and treatment. *CA: Cancer Journal for Clinicians, 47*(5), 365–372.

Middleton, R. G. (1996). The management of clinically localized prostate cancer: guidelines from the American Urological Association. *CA: Cancer Journal for Clinicians 46*(4), 249–253.

O'Rourke, M. E. & Germino, B. B. (1998). Prostate cancer treatment decisions: A focus group exploration, *Oncology Nursing Forum, 25*(1), 97–104.

Partin, A. W. & Carter, H. B. (1996). The use of prostate-specific antigen and free/total prostate-specific antigen in the diagnosis of localized prostatic cancer. *Urologic Clinics of North America,* 23(4), 531–540.

Partin, A. W. et al. (1997). Combination of prostate-specific antigen, clinical stage, and Gleason score to predict pathological stage of localized prostate cancer: a multi-institutional update. *JAMA, 277*(18), 1445–1451.

Society of Surgical Oncology. (1997). Prostate cancer surgical practice guidelines. *Oncology; 11*(6), 907–912.

Taplin, M. E., Bubley, G. J., Shuster, T. D., Frantz, M. E., Spooner, A. E., Ogata, G. K., Keer, H. N., & Balk, S. P. (1995). Mutation of the androgen-receptor gene in metastatic androgen-independent prostate cancer. *New England Journal of Medicine, 332*(21), 1393–1398.

von Eschenbach, A. et al. (1997). American Cancer Society guideline for the early detection of prostate cancer: Update 1997. *CA: Cancer Journal for Clinicians 47*(5), 261–264.

SCROTAL DISORDERS

Kass, E. J. & Lundak, B. (1997). The acute scrotum. *Pediatric Clinics of North America, 44*(5), 1251–1266.

Skoog, S. J. (1997). Benign and malignant pediatric scrotal masses. *Pediatric Clinics of North America, 44*(5), 1229–1249.

TESTICULAR CANCER

Brodsky, M. S. (1995). Testicular cancer survivors' impressions of the impact of the disease on their lives. *Qualitative Health Research, 5*(1), 78–96.

Hawkins, C. & Miaskowski, C. (1996). Testicular cancer: A review. *Oncology Nursing Forum, 23*(8), 1203–1211.

FERTILITY AND INFERTILITY (MALE AND FEMALE)

Alteneder, R. & Hartzell, D. (1997). Addressing couples' sexuality concerns during the childbearing years: Use of the PLISSIT Model. *JOGNN, 26*(6), 651–659.

Baker, H. W. (1994). Male infertility. *Endocrinology and Metabolism Clinics of North America, 23*(4), 783–793.

Carcio, H. A. (1998). *Management of the infertile woman.* Philadelphia: Lippincott-Raven.

Feldman, H. A. et al. (1994). Impotence and its medical and psychological correlates: Results of the Massachusetts male aging study. *Journal of Urology 151*(1), 54–61.

Goldstein, I. et al. (1998). Oral sildenafil in the treatment of erectile dysfunction. *New England and Journal of Medicine, 338*(20), 1397–1404.

Greenfeld, D. (1997). Infertility and assisted reproductive technology: The role of the perinatal social worker. *Social Work in Health Care, 24*(3–4), 39–46.

Hellstrom, W. J. G. (1997). *Male infertility and sexual dysfunction.* New York: Springer.

Lipshultz, L. I. & Howards, S. S. (Eds.) (1997). *Infertility in the male* (3rd ed.). St. Louis: Mosby.

Howards, S. S. (1995). Treatment of male infertility. *New England Journal of Medicine, 332*(5), 312–317.

Jansen, R. (1997). *Overcoming infertility: A compassionate resource for getting pregnant.* New York: W. H. Freeman.

Kennedy, H. P. (1998). Enabling conception and pregnancy. *Journal of Nursing Midwifery, 43*(3), 190–207.

LeMoncheck, L. (1996). Philosophy, gender politics and in vitro fertilization: A feminist ethics of reproductive health care. *Journal of Clinical Ethics, 7*(2), 160–176.

Lobo, R. A. et al. (1997). *Mishell's textbook of infertility, contraception, and reproductive endocrinology* (4th ed.). Malden, MA: Blackwell Science.

O'Keefe, M. & Hunt, D. K. (1995). Assessment and treatment of impotence. *Medical Clinics of North America; 79*(2), 415–434.

Padma-Nathan, H. et al. (1997). Treatment of men with erectile dysfunction with transurethral alprostadil. Medical Urethral System for Erection (MUSE) Study Group. *New England Journal of Medicine, 336*(1), 1–7.

Palermo, J., Cohen, J., & Rosenwaks, Z. (1997). Intracytoplasmic sperm injection: A powerful tool to overcome fertilization failure. *Fertility and Sterility, 67*(3), 583–584.

Seibel, M. M. (1997). *Infertility: A comprehensive text* (2nd ed.). Stamford, CT: Appleton & Lange.

Sundaram, C. P. et al. (1997). Long-term follow-up of patients receiving injection therapy for erectile dysfunction. *Urology 49*(6), 932–935.

MENOPAUSE

Aber, C. S., Arathuzik, D., & Righter, A. R. (1998). Women's perceptions and concerns about menopause. *Clinical Excellence for Nurse Practitioners, 2*(4), 232–238.

American Medical Association. (1998). *Essential guide to menopause.* New York: Pocket Books.

Barile, L. (1997). Theories of menopause: A brief, comparative synopsis. *Journal of Psychosocial Nursing and Mental Health Services, 35*(2), 36–41.

Bartman, B., & Moy, E. (1998). Racial differences in estrogen use among middle aged and older women. *Women's Health Issues, 8*(1), 32–44.

Colditz, G. A. et al. (1995). The use of estrogens and progestins and the risk of breast cancer in postmenopausal women. *New England Journal of Medicine, 332*(24), 1589–1593.

Kaplan, H., & Abisla, M. (1997). In transition: Empowering your menopausal patients. *Advance for Nurse Practitioners, 5*(6), 28–33.

Kwandala, S. (1998). Primary care of the perimenopausal woman. *Primary Care Update for OB/GYNs, 5*(1), 43–49.

MacPherson, K. (1997). Menopause on the Internet: Building knowledge and community on line. *Advances in Nursing Science, 20*(1), 66–78.

Moore, A., Furniss, K., & Garner, C. (1997). *Acute onset menopause: A self-study module.* (An educational module provided by AWHONN and NANPRH and published by MPE Communications.)

Norman, D. (1997). Variations on traditional HRT. *Advance for Nurse Practitioners, 5*(11), 34–37.

Norwitz, E. (1997). Managing the menopause without estrogen. *Female Patient, 22*(2), 62.

Perez, J. M. (1997). Development of the Menopause Symptom List: A factor analytic study of menopause associated symptoms. *Women & Health, 25*(1), 53–69.

Peters, S. (1998). Menopause: A new era. *Advance for Nurse Practitioners, 6*(7), 61–64.

Rabin, D. (1998). Understanding why women won't take HRT. *Contemporary Obstetrics and Gynecology, 43*(1), 133–141.

Scura, K., & Whipple, B. (1997). How to provide better care for the postmenopausal woman. *American Journal of Nursing, 97*(4), 36–43.

Smith, A. & Hughes, P. L. (1998). The estrogen dilemma. *American Journal of Nursing, 98*(4 Continuing Care extra ed.); 17–20.

Stewart, D. E. & Robinson G. E. (1997). *A clinician's guide to menopause.* Washington, DC: Health Press International.

Woods, N., Lentz, M., Mitchell, E. J., Heitkemper, M., & Shaver, J. (1997). PMS after 40: Persistence of a stress related symptom pattern. *Research in Nursing and Health, 20*(4), 329–340.

PREMENSTRUAL SYNDROME

Morse, G. (1997). Effect of positive reframing and social support on perception of permenstrual changes among women with premenstrual syndrome. *Health Care Women International, 18*(2), 175–193.

Peters, S. (1997). The puzzle of premenstrual syndrome. *Advance for Nurse Practitioners, 5*(10), 41–79.

Ugarizza, D. et al. (1998). Premenstrual syndrome. Diagnosis and intervention (consumer/patient teaching materials). *Nurse Practitioners, 23*(9), 40, 45, 49–50.

PAP SMEAR

Appleby, J. (1995). Management of the abnormal Papanicolaou smear. *Medical Clinics of North America, 72*(2), 345–360.

Foulks, M. (1998). The Papanicolou smear: Its impact on the promotion of women's health. *JOGNN, 27*(4), 367–373.

UTERINE AND MENSTRUAL CYCLE DISORDERS

Fogel, C. (1997). Endocrine causes of amenorrhea. *Lippincott's Primary Care Practice, 1*(5), 507–518.

Mehring, P. (1997). Dysfunctional uterine bleeding. *Advance for Nurse Practitioners, 5*(11), 27–32.

National Institutes of Health. (1996). Cervical cancer. *NIH Consensus Statement,* April 1–3, *14*(1), 1–38.

Smith-Bindman, R. et al. (1998). Endovaginal ultrasound to exclude endometrial cancer and other endometrial abnormalities. *JAMA, 280*(17), 1510–1517.

Stewart, E. & Nowak, R. (1998). New concepts in the treatment of uterine leoiomyomas. *Obstetrics and Gynecology, 92*(4), 624–627.

Wathen, P. I., Henderson, M. C., & Witz, C. A. (1995). Abnormal uterine bleeding. *Medical Clinics of North America, 79*(2), 329–333.

BREAST CANCER

Appling, S. (1996). One in nine: Risks and prevention strategies for breast cancer. *MEDSURG Nursing, 5*(1), 62–64.

Barron, C. R., Houfek, J. F. & Foxall, M. J. (1997). Coping style, health beliefs and breast self-examination. *Issues in Mental Health Nursing, 18*(4), 331–350.

Baron, R. H. & Borgen, P. I. (1997). Genetic susceptibility for breast cancer: Testing and primary prevention options. *Oncology Nursing Forum, 23*(4), 461–468.

Baron, R. H. & Walsh, A. (1995). Nine facts everyone should know about breast cancer. *American Journal of Nursing, 95*(7), 29–33.

Biesecker, B. B. (1997). Psychological issues in cancer genetics. *Seminars in Oncology Nursing, 13*(2), 129–134.

Bland, K. I. & Copeland, E. M. III (Ed.) (1998). *The breast: Comprehensive management of benign and malignant diseases.* Philadelphia: W.B. Saunders.

Bostwick, J. (1995). Breast reconstruction following mastectomy. *CA: Cancer Journal for Clinicians, 45,* 289–230.

Breast cancer screening for women ages 40–49 (1997). *NIH Consensus Statement* Jan. 21–23, *15*(1), 1–35.

Capriotti, T. (1998). Drug discoveries on the road to preventing breast cancer. *MEDSURG Nursing, 7*(5), 304–307.

Deane, K. A. & Degner, L. F. Determining the information needs of women after breast biopsy procedures. AORN J Apr; 65(4):767–776, 1997.

Deinger, M. J. & Llewellyn, J. (1995). Increasing compliance with breast self-examination. *MEDSURG Nursing, 4*(5), 359–366.

Dow, K. H. (1996). *Contemporary issues in breast cancer.* Boston; Jones and Bartlett.

Elston, C. W. & Ellis, I. O. (1998). *The breast.* New York: Churchill Livingstone.

Feig, S. A. (1997). Increased benefit from shorter screening mammography intervals for women ages 40–49 years. *Cancer, 80*(11), 2035–2039.

Fentiman, I. S. (1998). *Detection and treatment of breast cancer.* London: M. Dunitz.

Fisher, B. & Constantino, J. (1997). Highlights of the NSABP breast cancer prevention trial. *Cancer Control, 4*(1), 78–86.

Fleminging, I. D. & American Joint Committee on Cancer. (1997). *AJCC cancer staging manual.* Philadelphia: Lippincott-Raven.

Gross, R. E. & Major, M. (1997). Treatment options for breast cancer. *Gynecological Oncology Nursing, 7*(1), 13–22.

Gross, R. E. (1998). Current issues in the surgical treatment of early stage breast cancer. *Clinical Journal of Oncology Nursing, 2*(2), 55–63.

Gross, R. E. (1998). Women at high risk for breast cancer. *American Journal of Nursing, 98*(4), 55–58.

Harris, J. R., Lippman, M. E., Morrow, M. & Hellman, S. (1996). *Diseases of the breast.* Philadelphia; Lippincott-Raven.

Hartmann, L. C. et al. (1999). Efficacy of bilateral prophylactic mastectomy in women with a family history of breast cancer. *New England Journal of Medicine, 340*(2), 77–84.

Hortobagyi, G. N. (1998). Treatment of breast cancer *New England Journal of Medicine, 339*(14), 974–983.

Lessick, M. Wickham, R. & Rehwaldt, M. (1997). Breast and ovarian cancer: Genetic update and implications for nursing. *MEDSURG Nursing, 6*(6), 341–352.

Mansel, R. E. (Ed.) (1994). *Recent developments in the study of benign breast disease: The proceedings of the 5th International Symposium on benign breast disease.* New York; Parthenon.

Moore, G. (Ed.) (1997). *Women and cancer: A gynecologic oncology nursing perspective.* Boston; Jones & Bartlett.

Morrison, C. (1998). The significance of nipple discharge: Diagnosis and treatment regimes. *Primary Care Practice, 2*(2), 129–140.

National Institutes of Health. (1997). Consensus statement: Breast cancer screening for women ages. *Consensus Development Series, 15*(1), 40–49.

Northouse, L. L., Tocco, K. M. & West, P. (1997). Coping with a breast biopsy: How healthcare professionals can help women and their husbands. *Oncology Nursing Forum, 24*(3), 473–480.

Oktay, J. S. (1998). Psychosocial aspects of breast cancer. *Primary Care Practice, 2*(2), 149–159.

Osborne, C. K. (1998). Tamoxifen in the treatment of breast cancer. *New England Journal of Medicine, 339*(22), 1609–1618.

Rainsbury, P. A. & Viniker, D. A. (1997). *Practical guide to reproductive medicine.* New York: Parthenon.

Recht, A. et al. (1996). The sequencing of chemotherapy and radiation therapy after conservative surgery for early-stage breast cancer. *New England Journal of Medicine, 334*(21), 1356–1361.

Small, W. & Morrow, M. (1997). Local management of primary breast cancer. *Cancer Control, 4,* 201–210.

Tyler, T. (1998). The medical management of breast cancer. *Primary Care Practice, 2*(2), 176–183.

Van der Pompe, G., Antoni, M., Visser, A. & Garssen, B. (1996). Adjustment to breast cancer: The psychobiological effects of psychosocial interventions. *Patient Education and Counsel, 28*(2), 209–219.

Vogel, V. (1996). Assessing women's potential risk of developing breast cancer. *Oncology, 10*(10); 1451–1461.

Wagner, J. L. et al. (1995). Carcinoma of the male breast: Update 1994. *Medical Pediatric Oncology, 24*(2), 123–132.

Wasaff, B. (1997). Current status of hormonal treatments for metastatic breast cancer in postmenopausal women. *Oncology Nursing Forum, 24*(9), 1515–1520.

Weber, E. S. (1997). Questions and answers about breast cancer diagnosis. *American Journal of Nursing, 97*(10), 34–38.

Winchester, D. P. & Cox, J. D. (1998). Standards for diagnosis and management of invasive breast carcinoma. *CA: Cancer Journal for Clinicians, 48*(2), 83–107.

Winchester, D. P. & Strom, E. A. (1998). Standards for the diagnosis and management of ductal carcinoma in situ (DCIS) of the breast. *CA: Cancer Journal for Clinicians, 48*(2), 108–128.

Young-McCaughan, S. (1997). The impact of chemotherapy and endocrine therapy on sexual functioning in women with breast cancer. *Innovations Breast Cancer Care, 2*(3), 50–62.

Ziegfeld, C. R. (1998). Differential diagnosis of a breast mass. *Primary Care Practice, 2*(2), 121–128.

ON-LINE RESOURCES

American College of Obstetricians and Gynecologists *http://acog.org*
American Society for Colposcopy and Cervical Pathology *http://asccp.org*
American Board of Obstetrics and Gynecology (ACOG) *http://abog.org*
American Society for Reproductive Medicine (ASRM) *http://asrm.org*
Association of Reproductive Health Professionals *http://arhp.org*
Association of Women's Health Obstetric and Neonatal Nursing *http://awhonn.org*
Endometriosis Association *http://endometriosisassn.org*
International Pelvic Pain Society *http://pelvic pain.org*
National Association of Nurse Practitioners in Reproductive Health (NANPRH) *http://www.nurse.org/nanprh*
National Institute of Diabetes and Digestive and Kidney Diseases (NIDDK) *http:niddk.nih.gov*
Sexuality-Mayo Health Oasis *http://www.mayohealth.org/mayo-library/htm/sexual.htm*
Women's Health Center *http://mayohealth.org/mayo/common/htm/womenpg/htm*

FERTILITY AND INFERTILITY
Atlanta Reproductive Health Centre *http://ivf.com*
Impotence *http://www.niddk.nih.gov/Impotnce.html*
InterNational Council on Infertility Information Dissemination (INCIID) *http://inciid.org*
Planned Parenthood *http://plannedparenthood.org*
Serono Symposia (Clinical information on infertility) *http://www.springer-NY.com/serosym/serono.htm*

MENOPAUSE
Practical Guide to Hormone Replacement *http://ama-assn.org/insight/h_focus/wom_hlth/menopaus/hrt.htm*
Women's Health and Menopause *http://ama-assn.org/insight/h_focus/wom_hlth/menopaus/menopaus.htm*

BREAST CANCER
National Breast Cancer Coalition *http://www.natlbcc.org*
Clearing House for Information in breast cancer *http://nyser-net.org/bcic*

PROSTATITIS
Prostatitis *http://niddk.nih.gov/kusums/prstitis.htm*

PROSTATE CANCER
Prostate Cancer At-A-Glance-Centers for Disease Control: *http://www.cdc.gov/nccdphp/dcpc/prostate/pros95.htm*
The Prostate Cancer InfoLink: *http://www.cp.ed.com/prostate/*
US Too International, Inc. Prostate Cancer Survivor Support Group *http://www.ustoo.com*

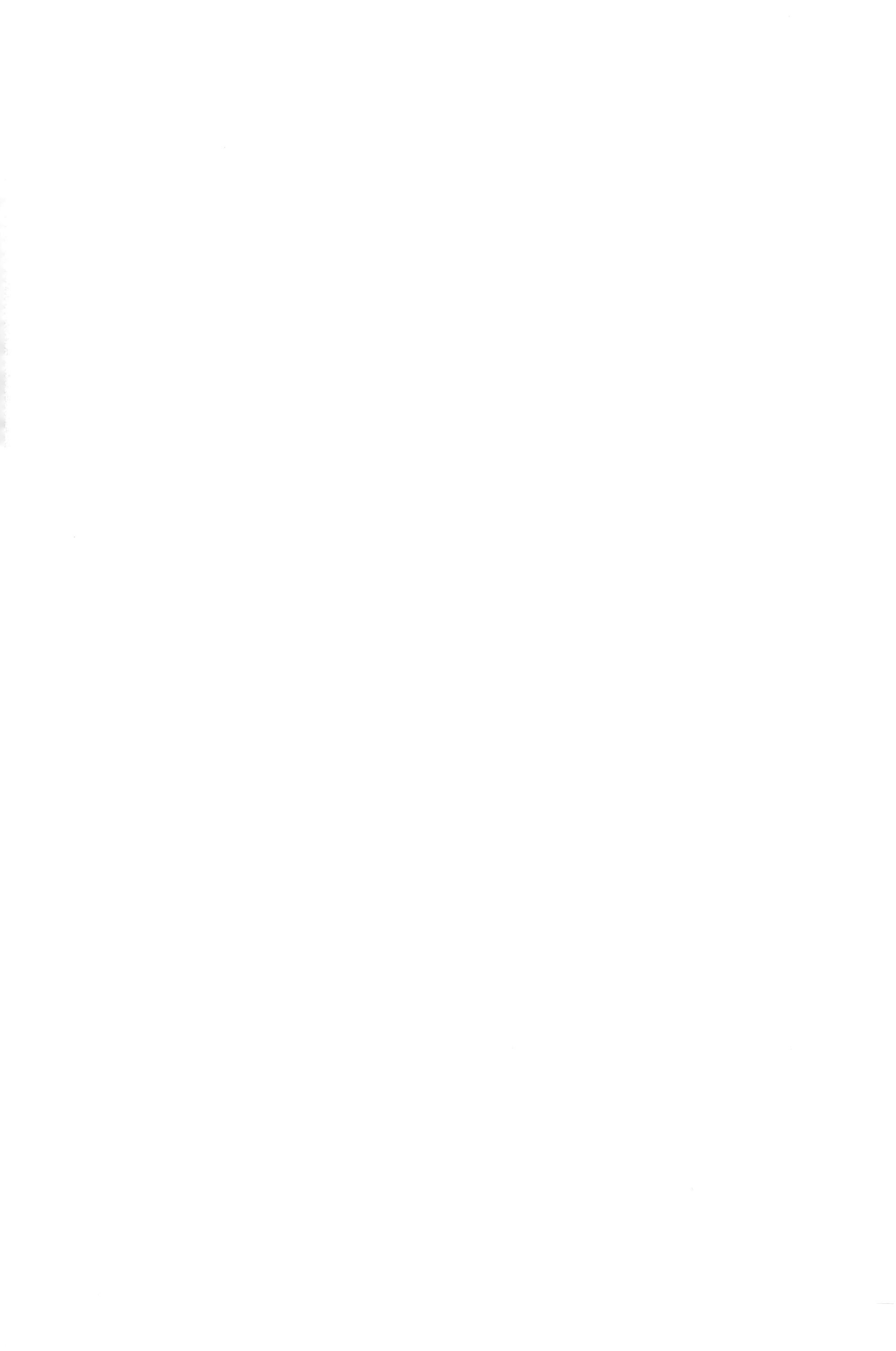

Appendix

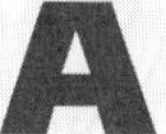

Answers to Case Studies

ANSWERS TO CASE STUDY 2-1

1. Hemophilia A is an X-linked recessive genetic disorder, with the recessive gene located on the X chromosome of the male. If Mrs. H. is not a carrier, then with each pregnancy, there is a 50% chance that female offspring would be carriers and a 50% change that a male child would not be affected. If the mother is a carrier, then there is a 25% chance that the female would be normal, a 25% that the female would be a carrier, a 25% chance that the male would be normal, and a 25% chance that the male would be affected with the disorder.
2. Karyotyping may be done before to pregnancy for both parents. Percutaneous umbilical blood sampling (removal of blood from the umbilical cord via amniocentesis) can be done to obtain a more rapid karyotype. Chorionic villi sampling (CVS) may be performed to karyotype cells. However, CVS detects only inherited disorders involving abnormal chromosomes or nondisjunction, or those disorders whose gene location on specific DNA is known.
3. His daughters should be told that there is a 50% chance that they are carriers for the disorder. However, if the mother is a carrier, then there is a 25% chance that each daughter is not a carrier and a 25% chance that each is a carrier. To be certain, genetic testing should be performed.
4. Mr. H. may experience an acute hemorrhage that could be life-threatening if it is not treated promptly. Also repeated use of factor VIII infusion may result in the development of antibodies, causing the factor to be ineffective, thus increasing his risk for life-threatening hemorrhage. Additionally, Mr. H. is at risk for long-term joint problems from hemarthrosis, leading to severe impairment in his ability to ambulate. The immobilization necessary during acute joint bleeding episodes may result in contractures, further limiting his mobility. Also, there is pain associated with acute bleeding episodes, further impairing his quality of life.

ANSWERS TO CASE STUDY 5-1

1. This is probably a disorder of excessive somnolence (DOES) that results from obstructive apnea. The obesity, constant sleepiness, snoring, nighttime restlessness, and nodding off during sedentary periods are characteristic of this form of sleep disorder.
2. A sleep log or sleep lab might be used to diagnose the problem.
3. The condition begins with progressive relaxation of the muscles of the chest, diaphragm, and throat, causing airway obstruction for as long as 30 seconds. The individual continues to attempt to breathe with chest and abdominal movements until the breath is strong enough to relieve the obstruction. Airway constriction causes the snoring. This condition would interrupt both REM and non-REM sleep.
4. DOES results from the effects of sleep pattern interruption. DIMS results from multiple factors that affect the ability to initiate and maintain sleep. Disorders of the sleep-wake cycle occur when the normal sleep cycle is interrupted, such as by working night shifts or traveling by air across multiple time zones. Dysfunctions associated with sleep or arousal include a diverse group of disturbances that may result from illnesses or may result in sleep walking or bedwetting.

ANSWERS TO CASE STUDY 5-2

1. Ms. J. can expect in the initial stages of her exercise program to suffer from muscle soreness and to be slowed by lactic acid accumulation in the muscles and shortness of breath. There is a gradual improvement of oxidative capacity and endurance.
2. The muscular factors for sprinting require a majority of white muscle fibers, which are the fast-twitch

type that tend to be mainly anaerobic. These muscles provide explosive power but fatigue easily. They have fewer mitochondria and fewer blood vessels than the slow-twitch type, which contain red muscle fibers. Obviously, there will be a combination of muscle fibers, and the predominance of one over the other is largely determined by genetics.

3. Aerobic training requires large amounts of ATP generated by oxidative phosphorylation. Anaerobic training requires ATP generated by glycolysis and creatine phosphate. Glycolysis provides a smaller number of ATP molecules than oxidative phosphorylation. Creatine phosphate provides ATP by donating a high-energy phosphate to ADP, and it functions for about 8 seconds of high-intensity exercise.
4. The adaptations that occur with regular exercise are gradual and include increased muscular strength, increased power, and increased endurance. Increased muscular strength involves muscular hypertrophy. Increased power is determined by strength, distance of contraction, and number of times the muscle contracts per minute. Increased endurance involves both strength and power but is dependent on proper nutritive support.

ANSWERS TO CASE STUDY 6-1

1. The fluid and electrolyte imbalance indicates dehydration and hypokalemia.
2. The contributing factors include vomiting and lack of oral intake. The history of alcoholism also contributes to the imbalance.
3. Hyponatremia is evident due to vomiting. Hypochloremia follows the sodium loss. The bicarbonate loss may indicate early metabolic acidosis. The hypokalemia has resulted from the lack of oral intake. Potassium levels are highly dependent on a continual dietary source to maintain normal levels. Potassium is poorly conserved by the body. The BUN is elevated due to the dehydration, and the kidneys are not able to clear the normal levels. The creatinine levels are only slightly elevated, which indicates that kidney function is not severely impaired.
4. Clinical manifestations of dehydration include a history of decreased fluid intake and vomiting. Dry mucous membranes are reflective of dehydration. A decreased blood pressure that is positional is characteristic of early loss of central blood volume and pressure.

ANSWERS TO CASE STUDY 6-2

1. Sodium levels are severely decreased. Potassium is elevated, probably the result of the decreased pH. The bicarbonate levels are decreased postoperatively. The pH is decreased also. Hypochloremia is evident preoperatively and severely depleted postoperatively.
2. The disorder presented is anion gap metabolic acidosis, probably lactic acidosis due to the seizure.
3. The seizure activity may have been caused by the depleted sodium levels.
4. The clinical manifestations that may be exhibited include those from hyponatremia, hyperkalemia, and metabolic acidosis. Hyponatremia may cause nausea and vomiting; muscular weakness; decreased thirst; peripheral, pulmonary, or cerebral edema; headache; stupor; and coma. Hyperkalemia may cause cardiac dysrhythmias, muscle weakness, intestinal colic, and diarrhea. Acidosis may lead to dysrhythmias, headache, CNS depression and coma, convulsions, increased serum potassium, and systemic vasodilation.
5. The anion gap (calculated by the formula sodium – [chloride + bicarbonate] is 112 – [74 + 16] = 22.

ANSWERS TO CASE STUDY 7-1

1. Hypoalbuminemic malnutrition or stressed starvation is indicated. Five percent of dextrose in water contains only 170 calories per liter. No intravenous protein has been given, and clear liquids administered orally do not provide adequate calories or protein to provide for basal needs, much less the needs for a reparative process.
2. In stressed starvation, the neuroendocrine control mechanisms are altered and increased levels of glucagon cause an increase in blood glucose. This hypermetabolism stimulates insulin release, but insulin resistance in the tissues allows hyperglycemia to persist. Gluconeogenesis from proteins occurs, and proteins are lost. Lipolysis occurs but ketones are not used for brain metabolism as they are in marasmus. The main calorie source is protein, and the administration of intravenous dextrose prevents ketoadaptation. Skeletal muscle is catabolized to provide energy sources. The liver, which normally produces albumin and other essential proteins, produces acute phase reactants such as interleukin. Alterations in the serum levels of the proteins can be used to assess the degree of nutritional depletion. Hypoalbuminemia alters wound healing and makes nutritional repletion difficult. Obese individuals often suffer greatly from this type of starvation, and the condition is not recognized because of their physical size.
3. Severe protein depletion is indicated with the albumin level of 2 g/dL or less.
4. Clinical manifestations include decreased wound strength, poor wound healing, altered coagulation, decreased immune response, and interstitial edema. Loss of muscle tone and increased incidence of infections are commonly seen. In marasmic individuals, there is a reduction in body weight but also a preservation of serum proteins and immune competence at the expense of the muscles and visceral

protein. Kwashiorkor is evidenced by a low ratio of protein to calories with dermatitis and hair changes. Body weight may not change, but protein is deficient.

5. Changes in the plasma levels of the branched-chain amino acids may be seen in repletion before albumin changes. Adequate protein must be given for repletion and to provide a source for anabolism.

ANSWERS TO CASE STUDY 9-1

1. The phases of wound healing depend on the initial clotting of the surgical wound, the process of inflammation to remove the clot, and, finally, the laying down of granulation tissue and formation of a scar.
2. In this case, there is superimposed infection, which delays healing and must be cleared before scarring can occur. This will require second intention healing, during which much more scar tissue must be made to seal the wound.
3. Factors to promote healing include clearing of infection by cleansing of the wound and probably the administration of antibiotics. After the wound is cleaned, the granulation of the wound may begin. Other factors that promote healing are an adequate blood supply and stabilization of the wound margins.
4. Delay in this case includes obesity, irregular wound margins, and presence of infection. Adipose tissue has less blood supply and does not heal as readily as lean tissue. A chainsaw injury will produce a wound with irregular margins that do not oppose well. Infection always delays healing since granulation tissue does not form well in the presence of infection and the wound may heal over the top, but if infection is present, the wound will reopen as occurred in the base of the wound.
5. Wound care teaching includes cleansing and dressing the wound and using an antiseptic solution and sterile dressings. The patient should be taught to assess the healing process. Diet and fluids should be encouraged to provide proteins to aid in healings.

ANSWERS TO CASE STUDY 9-2

1. The potential for wound complications should be considered in an obese, elderly, diabetic person. Each of these conditions has the potential for delaying wound healing. The wound should be assessed for healing prior to removal of staples. The diagnosis of a malignancy may alert you to nutritional depletion, which can interfere with healing.
2. Drainage on the binder was due to lack of wound healing and serous tissue fluid leakage. There is a great potential for complete dehiscence of the wound.
3. The thick, raised scar indicates excessive granulation that occurred in a previous scar. It can indicate difficulty in healing, or it may be a result of idiosyncratic healing.
4. Mrs. G. must be taught to assess healing of the wound. Redness, drainage and heat over the site are all warning signs that the wound may reopen and dehisce. She should be taught to cleanse the wound and dress the area as needed.

ANSWERS TO CASE STUDY 11-1

1. In 1993, the Centers for Disease Control and Prevention (CDC) included under Clinical Category B the presence of vulvovaginal candidiasis, which is persistent, frequent, or poorly responsive to treatment in women with laboratory evidence of human immunodeficiency virus (HIV) infection. It is important to rule out diabetes mellitus through the use of a fasting blood sugar test. A positive HIV-antibody test confirms the diagnosis of symptomatic HIV disease in women with persistent vulvovaginal candidiasis.
2. The incubation time is the time that has elapsed between infection with the HIV and the diagnosis of AIDS-related symptoms. The incubation time for HIV may be as long as 12 years. During this time, HIV replicates and increases in number in the infected person. Infected persons are able to transmit the virus regardless of whether or not they are symptomatic.
3. Seroconversion time is the time that the immune system requires to produce an antibody titer that is sufficiently high to be detected by antibody tests such as the enzyme-linked immunosorbent (ELISA) or the Western blot analysis. In the majority of cases, this time is 6 to 12 weeks. This concept should not be confused with that of incubation time. The ELISA is a screening test, and all persons who test positive must be confirmed by a diagnostic test such as Western blot analysis. The combination of two ELISAs and a Western blot analysis yield a high level of accuracy (99%) in detecting HIV-infected persons.
4. Acute retroviral syndrome (ARS) probably represents the first efforts of the immune system to combat an HIV infection. ARS is expressed by mononucleosis-like (or influenza-like) symptoms that occur between 2 and 4 weeks after exposure. Symptoms usually disappear in a few days. A diffuse rash may accompany this symptoms complex and may persist for 7 to 10 days. It is believed that a large percentage of infected persons experience these manifestations. However, because of its similarity to an influenza attack, many cases go unnoticed or unreported.
5. Three modes of transmission have been identified: unprotected sexual activity, blood-to-blood contact, and vertical (mother-to-child) transmission. The absence of transmission by casual contact has been well documented among family members of infected persons, health care providers, and others. If one believes the statement made by Ms. H. that her husband was the only sex partner she ever had, then her only risk factor was unprotected sexual ac-

tivity with her husband. Considering his extramarital sexual relationships, he was probably the source of her HIV infection. An incubation time of approximately 5 years falls within the norm as the range for HIV disease.

Assuming that Ms. H. acquired the virus from her husband before conceiving her daughter, the child would be at risk of being infected through vertical transmission. Every child born to an HIV-infected mother carries a 25% to 35% risk of being born infected, either through transplacental or intrapartum infection. The remaining 65% to 75% escape infection probably because of low maternal virus load. Because one does not know when Ms. H. became infected, her daughter either was born to an uninfected woman or escaped infection if her mother was already infected.

6. One of the consequences of HIV infection is a progressive loss of helper T cells, also referred to as T4 cells, which are very important cells in the regulation and modulation of immune function. Through the secretion of specialized lymphokines (such as interleukin 2), T4 cells are directly responsible for regulation of the cell-mediated immune response and indirectly for antibody secretion by B cells. Loss of T4 cells results in a compromised immune system and eventually renders most T4 cells unable to oppose a series of opportunistic infections and malignancies. One of the major causes of morbidity and mortality among HIV-infected individuals is *Pneumocystis carinii* pneumonia (PCP). Progressive loss of T4 cells greatly predisposes HIV-infected persons to develop PCP. This is especially true for individuals with a T4 cell count that is below 200 cells/mm^3, at which point prophylaxis against PCP should be instituted.
7. AZT is one of four approved antiretroviral agents in the United States. All agents act by blocking reverse transcription and arresting virus replication within infected cells. As such, AZT does not act directly on free viruses, which means that an infected person must remain in treatment for the duration of his or her life span. Any drug with such a requirement should have minimal (or tolerable) side effects. The major toxicity of AZT is to the bone marrow, resulting in anemia in many cases. In situations in which treatment with AZT becomes the only option, drugs that increase hematopoiesis may be used in conjunction with the antiretroviral agents. Another limitation of AZT is its limited efficacy. The earlier a person begins AZT treatments, the sooner it may have to be discontinued, because it loses its efficacy between 18 and 30 months of use. Until recently, this represented a serious life-threatening limitation. However, the development of other antiretroviral agents may allow for combination or sequential drug protocols, much like those used in cancer therapy.
8. Psychosocial interventions include safer sex practices such as the correct use of latex condoms. Maintaining an active lifestyle and decisions regarding disclosure of the patient's HIV status are essential. Identifying personal support systems and decisions relating to future care of the dependent child must be made. Health care costs are major and must be discussed before major expenses are incurred. Support groups and HIV clinics can aid the patient during the progression of the disease.

ANSWERS TO CASE STUDY 11-2

1. J. is experiencing Type I, immediate hypersensitivity with anaphylactic shock.
2. Antigen-specific allergic reactions are usually mediated primarily by IgE interactions with mast cells. The shock reaction occurs with a large systemic reaction in an individual who has been previously sensitized to the allergen. The mast cells release histamine and other mediators, causing increased vascular permeability and bronchoconstriction. The itching sensation is due to the hives that appear on the surface of the skin, usually first at the site of the bee sting. Angioneurotic edema follows, which results from the vasodilatation and swelling around the eyes. Acute anxiety, pruritus, dyspnea, wheezing, and hypotension are all physiologic manifestations the interaction.
3. Epinephrine is an effective bronchodilator for the bronchospasm. The hydrocortisone blocks the effects of the IgE interaction with the mast cells. Benadryl, an antihistamine drug, also is often given. The epinephrine response is immediate and, together with the hydrocortisone, may be life-saving.
4. Avoidance of areas where the patient could be stung may decrease the risk. Most highly allergic individuals are taught to carry a "bee sting" kit and to administer the drugs immediately after being stung.

ANSWERS TO CASE STUDY 12-1

1. Ms. P. is most likely experiencing iron deficiency anemia from increased blood loss secondary to heavy menstrual periods and a decreased intake from her dieting to lose 20 pounds. Serum iron and apoferritin levels are used to confirm the diagnosis of iron deficiency anemia. Red blood cell (RBC) count, hemoglobin, mean corpuscular volume (MCV), and mean corpuscular hemoglobin (MCH) also may be performed to provide additional support for the diagnosis.
2. Aplastic anemia results from reduced bone marrow function, with a decrease in the number of pluripotent stem cells, leading to nonformed or immature blood forming cells. Aplastic anemia results in normocytic, normochromic RBCs, and depleted leukocytes and platelets. Symptoms, which are variable and appear gradually, reflect progressive anemia and a decrease in oxygen transport. Weakness,

dyspnea, headache, and syncope are common. Recurrent infection and diminished immunologic defenses occur secondary to a decrease in white blood cells (WBCs). Bleeding tendencies from a decrease in platelets vary from small petechias to severe bleeding. Routine blood examination (smears) usually reveal normocytic, normochromic RBCs that are greatly reduced in number. Bone marrow aspiration typically shows hypocellular marrow. A bone marrow biopsy reveals large areas of fat with clusters of lymphocytic reticular cells and plasma cells. Marrow uptake of iron is decreased, and serum iron levels are elevated.

Hemolytic anemia results from intrinsic or extrinsic factors adversely affecting the cell, shortening its cycle and causing a normocytic, normochromic anemia characterized by an increase in the number of reticulocytes. Many different categories of hemolytic anemia occur, each with its own symptoms. Laboratory findings may include a positive direct and indirect Coombs' test, increased reticulocyte count, and changes in hemoglobin structure on microscopic examination.

Megaloblastic anemia is most commonly the result of a vitamin B_{12} or folic acid deficiency, causing a macrocytic anemia with a variation in the size and shape of RBCs. Pernicious anemia results from malabsorption of vitamin B_{12} due to a deficiency of the intrinsic factor, whereas folic acid anemia results form a lack of folic acid, commonly seen with alcoholism and chronic malnutrition. Signs and symptoms of pernicious anemia begin insidiously and may include anorexia, fatigue, shortness of breath, and irritability. Tongue soreness occurs early on and worsens with progression of the anemia. Folic acid anemia presents with similar findings. Laboratory findings of pernicious anemia include a macrocytic anemia with marked RBC size and shape variations and hyperbilirubinemia. Mild neutropenia and thrombocytopenia also may occur. With folic acid anemia, the RBCs are large and have fragile membranes.

Iron deficiency anemia is characterized by deficient hemoglobin synthesis secondary to a lack of iron, most commonly the result from increased loss such as with acute or chronic bleeding and decreased dietary intake. Signs and symptoms are nonspecific and insidious. They may include fatigue, tachycardia, irritability, and pallor with epithelial abnormalities. Spooning of the nails also may occur. Laboratory findings reflect decreased serum iron and apoferritin levels.

3. Most likely, oral iron therapy will be prescribed once the patient's gynecologic status is evaluated to determine the underlying cause (if any) of her heavy menstrual flow. If the patient's serum iron level is severely decreased, parenteral iron therapy may be necessary. Patient teaching should focus on the following: the medication therapy regimen, including use of citrus products to enhance absorption and produce changes in stool color and consistency, and dietary intake, including foods high in iron and the need for a well-balanced diet even with dieting. Ms. P. also should be urged to maintain follow-up, especially for laboratory testing to evaluate the effectiveness of therapy. She also needs instructions about her anemia and its causes, as well as information on important signs and symptoms, with emphasis on the need to call her physician with any problems.

ANSWERS TO CASE STUDY 13-1

1. Chronic myelogenous leukemia (CML), which is the same as chronic myelocytic leukemia, is characterized by granulocytic cells that cause a marked elevation in the leukocyte count. The chromosome marker Ph 1 (Philadelphia) is found in 90% of cases. CML is diagnosed by well-differentiated leukemic cells that are granulocytic. The spleen becomes very enlarged. The course of the disease is slowly progressive for about 3 years, and then it can enter an accelerated phase that terminates in acute leukemia. In comparison to acute myelocytic leukemia, the cells are more mature and proliferate more slowly. The WBC count is very high in patients with CML, from 50,000 to 500,000/L.
2. The clinical marker for CML is the Philadelphia chromosome.
3. Anemia, bleeding, and opportunistic infections develop late due to crowding out of the normal erythrocytes, platelets, and lymphocytes by the large number of myelocytes, which do not function well in themselves. The opportunistic organisms can be any that normally do not cause infection in the immune-competent individual.
4. The accelerated phase is heralded by rapid onset of anemia, hemorrhages, and often a disseminated intravascular coagulation (DIC)–type syndrome. The most common cause of death is infection resulting from marrow failure. Anorexia, weight loss, and weakness progress rapidly. Central nervous system (CNS) manifestations may result from leukemic infiltration of the meninges, CNS, and cranial nerves. These manifestations include headache and visual disturbances. Bone pain and hepatosplenomegaly are results of infiltration of the area with leukemic cells.
5. Chemotherapy, especially with oral alkylating agents, may decrease the WBC count and improve the condition for a period of time. Median survival is still only 3 to 4 years. Irradiation may be used for the splenomegaly or for bone marrow pain to decrease leukemic infiltration. Chemotherapy often causes neutropenia, stomatitis, and nausea and vomiting, which may increase the risk for infection and enhance the cachexia noted in the disease.

ANSWERS TO CASE STUDY 14-1

1. The coagulopathy described is DIC.
2. The portion of the retained placenta most likely resulted in a gram-negative infection, causing

endotoxemia and endothelial damage, possibly stimulating massive coagulation. Also, following the therapeutic abortion, Ms. P. was at risk for puerperal sepsis leading to vascular damage, which is a possible stimulus for massive coagulation as well.

3. DIC involves both bleeding and clotting. The clotting factors within the circulating blood are activated. These factors and platelets are consumed, resulting in severe hemorrhage accompanied by ischemic changes from microvascular thrombi.

   The clotting sequence is triggered by endothelial damage, activating the intrinsic coagulation cascade and release of thromboplastic substances. A large number of small peripheral vessels become occluded. The clotting sequence activates the fibrinolytic system, causing diffuse fibrinolysis. The conversion of plasminogen to plasmin inhibits proteolysis of fibrinogen by thrombi and possibly, platelet aggregation. Fibrin split products form, producing a complex with the fibrin monomer and preventing the laying down of fibrin thread and platelet aggregation.

   Bleeding occurs because the clotting factors are consumed. Cold, mottled fingers and toes result from tissue ischemia secondary to microvascular thrombosis. The patient's acute distress resulted from hypoxemia.

4. Surgery was performed to treat the underlying stimulus for the massive coagulation. Other treatment may include heparin to interrupt the clotting process, followed by replacement of clotting factors and platelets to prevent further bleeding.

ANSWERS TO CASE STUDY 16-1

1. Atherosclerotic lesions probably begin with the fatty streak composed of lipid droplets deposited on the intima of arteries. As the lesion expands, smooth muscle cells migrate into the intima. The atherosclerotic lesion is composed of fatty and fibrofatty material that protrudes into the artery and compromises blood flow. The altered intimal surface initiates the intrinsic coagulation system, and the final obstruction is usually due to a clot. Hemorrhage into the plaque itself may also occur.
2. Collateral circulation involves opening small arterial channels, which may help to sustain blood flow to the area for a time. In many cases, the blood flow is impaired but gangrene does not occur because of the collateral circulation.
3. The symptom of intermittent claudication occurs because of inadequate circulation to the limb, usually during exercise. Gradually, less and less exercise will produce the uncomfortable squeezing, aching pain. The pain is relieved by rest, when the circulation is restored to the limb. Loss of pulses usually indicates occlusion of the main vessels, as does the loss of color of the extremity.
4. Smoking has been closely associated with the acceleration of atherosclerotic changes. It enhances atheroma development and often causes spasm of the affected vessels. The carbon monoxide and nicotine in tobacco smoke are related to development of the disease.
5. Doppler studies use ultrasound waves to evaluate flow through both veins and arteries. The proximal and distal pressures of the suspected lesion are auscultated to determine the pressure gradient and are compared with the systemic blood pressure. The femoral arteriogram requires the use of contrast media injected into the artery. It shows the exact location of the lesion, the amount of obstruction, the presence of collateral circulation, and the vessels open below the lesion.
6. A femoral popliteal bypass operation usually involves the use of a piece of saphenous vein, which is inserted above the lesion and bypassed around the obstructed area, being inserted in the open vessel below the lesion.

ANSWERS TO CASE STUDY 17-1

1. Acute bacterial endocarditis (ABE) with mitral and aortic insufficiency is indicated.
2. Ms. J.'s clinical history of IV drug abuse and the sudden onset of the symptoms support the diagnosis of ABE. Blood cultures can be used to isolate the organism responsible. The loud systolic and diastolic murmurs would support mitral and aortic insufficiency, but an echocardiogram and a left-sided heart catheterization would be more definitive.
3. Acute bacterial endocarditis is most frequently caused by *Staphylococcus aureus,* an organism of high virulence that frequently resides on contaminated needles. The organisms cause sepsis and attach to the endocardial lining, forming large, septic vegetations that are friable and embolize through the arterial circuit. The vegetations settle on the cardiac valves and invade the leaflets, causing destruction and incomplete closure of the valves. Large insufficiency alters blood flow so that the symptoms of heart failure can rapidly result.
4. Without treatment, the prognosis for this condition is very poor. With treatment, the prognosis is good if lifestyle changes are made.
5. Treatment includes antibiotic therapy given intravenously. Emergency valve replacement is often performed to prevent death from congestive heart failure. Recurrence can be prevented by drug abuse therapy, prophylactic administration of antibiotics before any invasive procedure, improvement of the nutritional status, and anticoagulation therapy if artificial valves were placed. A significant amount of teaching and a high level of compliance are necessary for improvement of the prognosis.

ANSWERS TO CASE STUDY 18-1

1. D. M. is exhibiting signs and symptoms of hypovolemic shock.

2. D. M.'s shock is due to the following: large pelvic laceration from anus through the perineum to the left iliac crest; an open symphysis pubis fracture with a through-and-through 4-inch wooden stake protruding from the wound; multiple bony fractures apparent with exposed left iliac vessels; bowel visible through exposed peritoneum; large amounts of active bleeding; and multiple areas of soft tissue injury.
3. With hypovolemic shock, decreased circulating fluid volume decreases venous return, which reduces cardiac output and subsequently lowers blood pressure. Lowered blood pressure impedes tissue and organ perfusion as well as oxygen and nutrient blood delivery. This problem leads to ischemia and necrosis, with resulting organ malfunction and shock.
4. Signs and symptoms include pallor with obvious distress, vital signs such as blood pressure of 70/46, tachycardia (heart rate of 148) and respirations of 38; decreased hemoglobin (5.6) and hematocrit (17.1); confusion; active bleeding; and large amounts of soft tissue and long bone injury.
5. Expected treatment involves airway management and oxygenation, aggressive fluid resuscitation with intravenous fluids and blood replacement, and management of the patient's open and closed wounds.
6. D. M. is at risk for sepsis, possibly leading to a second shock episode.

ANSWERS TO CASE STUDY 20-1

1. D.'s history of hay fever, allergies, and eczema are all conditions commonly associated with asthma. Her family history of allergies is also a factor.
2. Exposure to her friend's cat raises the suspicion that D. may have developed a sensitivity to cats. Other environmental antigens could include grasses, pollens, and house dust mites.
3. The main pathophysiologic change associated with asthma is inflammation of the airways. Other features. including bronchospasm and excess mucus production, are thought to be due to the underlying inflammation.

ANSWERS TO CASE STUDY 20-2

1. Subtle changes such as memory changes, confusion, poor appetite and fatigue may have signaled a problem. Often, symptoms of pneumonia in the elderly are initially attributed to an exacerbation of the underlying disease, such as chronic heart or lung diseases. Absence of fever is common in the elderly.
2. Infiltration of the alveoli with inflammatory cells and fluid account for the auscultatory changes noted on examination. Changes in percussion notes may also be noted.

ANSWERS TO CASE STUDY 22-1

1. Damage to the kidney structures occurs gradually in many cases. Often, there is no reported history of disease at all, just the gradual onset of renal failure.
2. This case illustrates a probably immune-mediated glomerular disease. It could be a result of post-streptococcal glomerulonephritis, which would be unusual because the original disease occurred in childhood. This condition could be any of the chronic forms of glomerulonephritis or nephropathy. In any case, the result is chronic glomerulonephritis, which is a slowly progressive condition that may exhibit both nephrotic and nephritic characteristics.
3. The glomeruli become scarred and may be obliterated. The glomeruli and renal capsule are infiltrated with inflammatory cells. Vascular sclerosis contributes to the hypertension that is usually associated with the condition. Progressive renal dysfunction occurs, and nephrons are progressively lost. Retention of nitrogenous wastes, loss of protein in the urine, hypertension, and water balance problems gradually occur.
4. Delaying the chronic renal failure that results from this condition can be promoted by preventing infection, maintaining adequate nutritional balance, decreasing the protein intake, and maintaining fluid intake and output.
5. Treatment is not needed in early renal insufficiency. Dietary treatment and prevention of infection can be used during renal insufficiency and early chronic renal failure. In end-state renal failure, hemodialysis may be the only chronic form of treatment if surgical transplantation is not possible.

ANSWERS TO CASE STUDY 22-2

1. Acute renal failure due to ischemic tubular necrosis is the probable diagnosis. Nephrotoxic tubular necrosis also could be the result of the ingestion of drugs.
2. Low blood pressure leads to decreased renal perfusion. The drugs and alcohol consumed can cause nephrotoxic damage. Oliguria followed by anuria may result. Impaired renal function causes the retention of nitrogenous wastes and potassium, as well as other electrolytes. The tubular obstruction may result from swelling and necrosis of the tubular cells. The course varies with the duration of the renal insult. In the early stage, the initial insult is produced. The maintenance stage is characterized by oliguria and electrolyte imbalances. Recovery is characterized by a gradual increase of urine output with diuresis and early loss of electrolytes and water. Return of the ability to concentrate urine occurs gradually, and recovery does not always occur.

3. The level of the serum potassium could cause cardiac dysrhythmias and cardiac arrest. Some method to lower the serum potassium is essential. These methods could include potassium ion exchange resins, hemodialysis, and peritoneal dialysis.
4. The outcome depends on the success of the treatment for the electrolyte imbalances and the restoration of adequate blood pressure. Ms. J. is young and has a greater potential for recovery than an elderly person does. Renal function may be totally restored, or renal insufficiency or chronic renal failure may be the ultimate outcome.
5. Treatment options include potassium-decreasing drugs, hemodialysis, and peritoneal dialysis to help restore a more normal fluid and electrolyte balance. Fluid intake may be limited and dietary restriction of protein may be prescribed if the problem persists when Ms. J. is able to take a diet. If Ms. J. is anuric, she could suffer from fluid overload without fluid restriction. Restriction of protein decreases the amount of nitrogenous wastes that the kidneys must excrete.

ANSWERS TO CASE STUDY 24-1

1. D. W. has been on long-term steroid therapy, which can depress the neuroendocrine axis, promoting a relative adrenal insufficiency. The recent trauma and surgery have increased the need for glucocorticoids to greater than what is physiologically available.
2. The fracture of the femoral head results from osteoporosis due to long-term steroid therapy in combination with a sedentary lifestyle and age. Dehydration and elevated hematocrit and BUN occur because glucocorticoids have some mineralcorticoid activity. A reduction in this activity decreases sodium and water reabsorption. Hyperkalemia and hyponatremia are due to the reduction of mineralcorticoid activity. Hypoglycemia results from impaired gluconeogenesis due to decreased glucocorticoid activity. Hypotension is due to dehydration, and decreased vascular responsiveness results from the reduction in glucocorticoid activity. Weakness and lethargy are most likely the result of electrolyte imbalances.
3. Typically, primary adrenal insufficiency is a result of adrenocortical hypofunction, which causes a reduction in both mineralcorticoid and glucocorticoid activity. In secondary adrenal insufficiency, there is an alteration in the pituitary hypothalamic function, usually with just a reduction in glucocorticoid activity. Hyperpigmentation occurs in primary adrenal insufficiency as a result of an increased synthesis of adrenocorticotrophic hormone (ACTH), whereas in secondary adrenal insufficiency, there is no change in skin pigmentation. In both conditions, cortisol levels are decreased. Following ACTH stimulation, an increase in cortisol levels is seen only with secondary adrenal insufficiency. In primary adrenal insufficiency, ACTH levels are elevated, whereas in secondary adrenal insufficiency, they are decreased.

ANSWERS TO CASE STUDY 25-1

1. The colon cancer is in the left descending colon because it could undergo direct biopsy. The symptoms of melena, diarrhea, and constipation are common with left-sided lesions.
2. The carcinoembryonic antigen (CEA) is almost always positive with widespread metastasis. Normal levels are less than 2.5 ng/mL and may be elevated in nonmalignant inflammation of the gastrointestinal tract. Mr. F.'s CEA is markedly elevated, indicating probable metastasis.
3. Metastasis is due to invasion of the surrounding channels, especially the lymphatic, peritoneum, and venous channels. Distant areas of metastasis include the liver, lungs, bone, and brain.
4. Risk factors include increased dietary fat intake, heredity, previous colorectal cancer, smoking, alcohol abuse, inflammatory bowel disease, obesity, and polyposis of the colon. Fiber, intake of vegetables, aspirin or nonsteroidal antiinflammatory drugs (NSAIDS), physical activity, and calcium are probably factors that decrease the risk of colon cancer. Vitamins A, C, and E; selenium; and folate may decrease the risk of contracting colon cancer.

ANSWERS TO CASE STUDY 26-1

1. Alcohol abuse and biliary disease are the major risk factors for pancreatitis. In urban areas, alcoholism is the major cause. Mr. S. drinks alcoholic beverages, lives in an urban setting, and eats fried foods.
2. Clinical manifestations include pain, which results from edema that causes distention of the pancreatic capsule, pancreatic autodigestion from enzymes, and local peritonitis from the release of enzymes into the peritoneal area; nausea and vomiting, which are due to decreased intestinal motility and pain; vascular and cardiac dysfunction, which results from the release of vasoactive substances, causing capillary permeability, vasodilation, and hypotension; jaundice, which results from obstruction of the common bile duct secondary to edema; pleural effusion, which is caused by extension of the inflammatory process; and hyperglycemia, which results from damage to the islet cells.
3. The precise mechanism that triggers the sequence of enzymatic activity is unknown. A variety of factors, such as viral infections, trauma, and drugs have been implicated.
4. Exactly how the enzymes are activated remains unclear, but trypsin is believed to play a role.
5. A pseudocyst, an encapsulated collection of debris, tissue, fluid, blood, and high enzyme content, is usually within or adjacent to the pancreas. Pseudocysts may resolve or become infected. A pancreatic

abscess, a collection of necrotic tissue, is a suppurative process.

6. The elevation of the serum lipase and both the serum and urine amylase levels gives certainty to the diagnosis in conjunction with the other clinical findings. Damage to the acinar cells of the pancreas causes the release of amylase. Amylase is cleared by the kidneys and elevated levels are found in pancreatic disease. Lipase, like amylase, is secreted by the pancreas and appears in the serum following damage to the acinar cells.

ANSWERS TO CASE STUDY 26-2

1. The patient's current respiratory infections, failure to thrive, and steatorrhea suggest cystic fibrosis (CF). Laboratory findings of elevated sweat chlorides, absence of trypsin in duodenal aspirations, and low fat retention coefficient are characteristic of CF. The finding of atelectasis on x-ray, along with a positive history of CF, offer further supports the diagnosis.
2. The inheritance pattern is autosomal recessive. With each pregnancy, there is a 25% chance that the child will have CF, a 50% chance that the child will carry the trait, and a 25% chance that the child will neither carry the trait nor have the disease. Prenatal diagnosis is done by amniocentesis or CVS. Chromosomal studies are performed to identify the CF gene.
3. Dysfunction of the exocrine glands is the pathophysiologic mechanism in CF. Although CF is a multisystem disorder, the respiratory system and pancreas of the gastrointestinal tract are primarily affected. With pulmonary involvement, large amounts of thickened secretions are produced by the bronchial mucous gland along with decreased ciliary motility, which leads to chronic retention of secretions. Obstruction with thick mucus predisposes the lungs to infection. Chronic inflammation also leads to bronchiectasis, air trapping, and obstructive pulmonary disease.

   In the pancreas, obstruction of the pancreatic ducts with thick mucus blocks the flow of pancreatic enzymes, leading to degeneration and fibrosis of the pancreas. With deficiencies of pancreatic enzymes, there is an inadequate breakdown of proteins and fats. Malabsorption of nutrients occurs and results in nutritional abnormalities.
4. Progression of pulmonary disease follows chronic infection. Fibrosis with poor oxygen and carbon dioxide exchange results in changes in the pulmonary vasculature, pulmonary hypertension, and eventually cor pulmonale (right-sided heart failure).
5. Inadequate pancreatic enzymes lead to poor fat absorption, resulting in frothy, fatty, and foul-smelling stools.
6. With the CF gene, there is a defect in chloride conduction across epithelia. In a sweat electrolyte test, sweat is induced by electrical current (iontophoresis), collected, and analyzed for sodium and chloride content. This test is specific for CF.
7. Persons with CF have thick mucus that obstructs the pancreatic ducts. Thus, these enzymes are decreased or absent from the duodenum. Contents of the duodenum are aspirated, and the enzyme content is determined.
8. Obstruction of the pancreatic ducts by mucus plugs prevents enzymes that break down fats from entering the intestine. Without the enzymes, fat malabsorption occurs resulting in large, frothy, foul-smelling stools. A 72-hour collection would reflect fat absorption.
9. Advances in molecular genetic testing for CF offer a basis for risk counseling for family members with a history of CF.

ANSWERS TO CASE STUDY 27-1

1. Hyperuricemia is a major risk factor for gout. It may be primary or secondary. In some patients with primary gout, there is an abnormal urate metabolism, whereas in others, there is decreased renal clearance of uric acid. Some patients may have a combination of both. In certain rare cases, it is a genetically transmitted disease. Secondary gout results from excess breakdown of purines, which leads to increased uric acid synthesis. It is usually associated with other disease processes such as the leukemias. Other risk factors include excessive alcohol use, obesity, male gender, increasing age, a family history of gout, hypertension, renal insufficiency, and use of certain medications, such as diuretics and salicylates.
2. P. J. presents with the following known risk factors: male gender, increasing age, obesity, hypertension, and use of diuretic medication.
3. The four stages of gout are Stage I—asymptomatic; Stage II—acute gout arthritis; Stage III—intercritical gout; and Stage IV—chronic tophaceous gout. Stage I gout is an asymptomatic hyperuricemia. In Stage II, the patient presents with acute inflammation and usually monarticular involvement. The first joint in the big toe is most commonly involved in early presentation. Other common areas of involvement include ankles, heels, knees, wrists, and fingers. Stage III is a quiescent period without significant symptoms. Stage IV is associated with tophi and acute arthritis.

   P. J. is most likely in Stage II, as evidenced by his clinical manifestations of acute pain and inflammation.
4. The pathophysiology of gout evolves from the etiologic basis of hyperuricemia as described in answer #1. The deposition of urate crystals (monosodium urate) in the synovial membrane of joints causes an intense inflammation response. Kinins are activated, and neutrophils are attracted to the area. The monosodium urate crystals may be deposited in large amounts in tissues (particularly in the periph-

ery such as the helix of the ear, hands, and feet) and accumulate in masses called tophi.

5. Acute gout may present with monarticular joint inflammation with intense pain, swelling, and warmth. The individual usually is afebrile, but in rare situations, particularly with polyarticular involvement, may present with a fever. Uric acid levels are usually above 9 mg/dL, and leukocytosis may be present.

ANSWERS TO CASE STUDY 28-1

1. As with any trauma patient, assessment of airway, breathing, and circulation (ABCs) are the priorities in the immediate postburn phase. This patient most likely has some, if not severe, inhalation injury. His airway and breathing will become compromised very quickly owing to edema of the upper and lower airway. Intubation should be considered immediately to protect the airway. Owing to loss of fluids from the wounds and intravascular space due to capillary leakage, replacement with intravenous fluids (Lactated Ringer's solution) via large bore catheters can prevent burn shock, which can be life-saving.
2. The percentage of body surface area (BSA) burned would be left leg—18%; right leg—18%; face and neck—4.5%; right arm—9%; left arm—9%; and anterior chest (not abdomen)—9%, for a total of affected BSA burned of 67.5%.
3. The patient has a burn that is greater than 20% of total BSA, with inhalation injury and burns of the face and neck. Each of these factors is a criterion for transfer to a burn center.
4. In the first 24 hours after a burn, the amount of fluid replacement is calculated as 3 mL of lactated Ringer's solution $\times$ 67.5 $\times$ 80 kg, for a total of 16,200 mL. Half of this amount is given in the first 8 hours, then the other half is given over the following 16 hours.
5. The most frequent error in fluid resuscitation is inadequate fluid resuscitation.

ANSWERS TO CASE STUDY 30-1

1. S. is most likely exhibiting signs and symptoms of an anxiety disorder that interferes with his ability to function and interact with others.
2. The most probably diagnosis is obsessive compulsive disorder (OCD).
3. S. is exhibiting obsessions—checking to see if he hit anyone while driving—which are intrusive and anxiety producing, so much so that he is requesting projects to work on at home and leaving earlier each day to get to work. These obsessions lead to the performance of compulsions—stopping to check under the car wheels, asking bystanders if they see anyone near the car or hit by it, or asking police if anyone had been taken to the hospital. These compulsions are time consuming, as evidenced by his leaving earlier each day for work and arriving home hours after he is expected.
4. Major depression commonly occurs in almost one-half of patients with OCD. OCD is a chronic disorder. Treatment with medications and behavioral therapy are effective for controlling the symptoms, but they don't eliminate the disorder.

ANSWERS TO CASE STUDY 30-2

1. F. is most likely suffering from schizophrenia.
2. His appearance of being distracted may be reflective of disorganized thinking. Keeping scraps of paper in a shoebox and always carrying it with him possibly reflects grossly disorganized and inappropriate behavior. His difficulty interacting with customers may reflect affective flattening. Mumbling may indicate alogia. His reports of being told to document being followed by strangers reflect hallucinations, and his feelings of being followed are indicative of delusions. Delusions, hallucinations, disorganized thinking, and behavior are positive symptoms, whereas affective flattening and alogia are negative symptoms.
3. Schizophrenia is a chronic and deteriorating illness for many of those affected by it. The emotional and economic impact is great. After the disease onset, work, social relationships, and self may be compromised. Traditional antipsychotics used for treatment are associated with numerous side effects, leading to relapses when the patient decides to discontinue the medication. The newer atypical antipsychotics have fewer side effects and appear to decrease the number of relapses, leading to less disability overall.

ANSWERS TO CASE STUDY 30-3

1. M. is most likely experiencing post-traumatic stress disorder (PTSD).
2. M. experienced a trauma as a child, the death of her mother from a heart problem. She is re-experiencing the trauma through intrusive memories, exhibiting episodes of tension and irritability, and reflecting a heightened physiologic arousal in response to images or thoughts associated with the trauma. Autonomic hyperactivity is evidenced by pounding heart and tightness in her chest, very real complaints, requiring her to be transported to the emergency department. These symptoms reflect the physiologic reaction to cues that remind her of the trauma.
3. Her laboratory tests were normal because there is no indication of heart disease. Rather, her signs and symptoms are indicative of her responses to the memories of the trauma.

ANSWERS TO CASE STUDY 30-4

1. D. is most probably experiencing major depression, a mood disorder.
2. D. is exhibiting a change in mood that is persistent (greater than 2 weeks) and causing disruption in her personality and ability to function. Complaints of fatigue (no energy), increased sleeping, and feel-

ings of worthlessness (viewing the future as bleak) are characteristic of major depression. Also, she has withdrawn from her friends (being unable to experience pleasure from activities previously pleasurable [anhedonia]), feeling that she will not be able to control her emotions in front of them. All of these behaviors are characteristic of major depression.

ANSWERS TO CASE STUDY 31-1

1. C. seems to have suffered a sudden acceleration-deceleration injury, as evidenced by the circumstances of the accident (severe damage to the truck, broken glass in windshield). The picture here seems to reflect a coup-contrecoup injury in which there is injury not only at the site of impact (coup) but also at the opposite side of impact (contrecoup) as the buoyant brain shifts within the rigid skull.
2. Primary injuries are those that result from the physical insult to the brain and generally entail structural injury to the cranial contents. Secondary injuries result from the primary injury as the brain tissue responds to that insult. The primary injuries that threaten C.'s brain are contusions and lacerations as the brain shifts over the rough ridges within the cranial cavity. These injuries may be extensive and involve large areas of the cerebrum and brain stem. Brain stem injuries are associated with rotation of the cerebrum and usually result in loss of consciousness, which C. did not exhibit at this time. Therefore, C. has probably had only cerebral hemispheric involvement. The nature of C.'s injury also makes him a good candidate for a cervical cord injury. The secondary injuries that could be anticipated with C. include cerebral bleeds, cerebral edema, and increased intracranial pressure.
3. A concussion is a diffuse, transient, and reversible injury to the brain caused by a sudden blow to the head. It is a violent shaking of the brain that results in temporary changes in neuronal firing. Concussions range from very mild to severe interruptions in brain function. Some individuals experience very transitory changes in the level of consciousness, whereas others may be rendered unconscious for much longer. Usually, the individual who has suffered a concussion is amnesic to the event that caused the concussion. Other than the amnesia to the event, the individual does not present with significant neurologic deficits. Supporting data that might indicate that C. experienced a concussion was the fact that he was somewhat "dazed" at the scene of the accident, self-oriented, and unaware of what happened to him. No other neurologic deficits are noted early after injury. One could anticipate potential problems with C.'s attention span, memory, anxiety, and irritability on a longer term basis after this accident.
4. Contusion is a bruising of the brain as a result of a blow to the head. It usually is associated with structural damage to the parenchyma of the brain including small hemorrhages, edema, local acidosis, and changes in the electroencephalogram (EEG). In acceleration-deceleration injuries, the bruising may occur in the coup and contrecoup areas of the blow to the brain. Because there are bony irregularities within the cranium, it is not uncommon to see cerebral lacerations associated with cerebral contusions. Neurologic deficits vary with severity of injury and area of brain or brain stem involved. They frequently include changes in the level of consciousness and motor-sensory alterations.

   Diagnosis of brain contusions is based on the mechanism of injury, clinical presentation, and computed tomographic (CT) or magnetic resonance imaging (MRI) findings. EEG recordings over the contused area show abnormal waves. Though early after admission C. does not present specific neurological signs supporting a contusion, a brain contusion in C. at this point probably can be assumed based on the mechanism of injury and later deteriorating neurological findings. Additionally, the depressed area in the high forehead area may indicate a possible underlying brain contusion.
5. Major concerns post-injury would be extension of the primary injuries and development of secondary injuries. C. could very well have an associated neck injury given the circumstances of the accident. Therefore, neck immobilization is a critical intervention until this potential injury is ruled out. Additional potential problems for C. include cerebral bleed, cerebral edema, increased intracranial pressure, and seizures. An awareness for their potential development and astute neurological assessment are essential. All neurological complications of head injury cannot be prevented, but their detection and early intervention can prevent/minimize permanent neurological deficits.
6. The findings of bruising around the eyes (periorbital ecchymosis or raccoon eyes) and behind the ears, and on the mastoid bone area (Battle's sign) suggest basilar skull fracture. In C., there is a suggestion of involvement of both anterior and middle fossa skull. In addition to the periorbital ecchymosis and mastoid region bruising, anterior fossa involvement may reveal cranial nerve I, II, or III abnormalities, as well as cerebrospinal fluid (CSF) rhinorrhea. The presence of CSF otorrhea, hemotympanum, eighth cranial nerve deficits, and Battle's sign suggest a break in the integrity of the skull and put C. at risk for intracranial infection.
7. The change in the level of C.'s consciousness most likely resulted from an expanding cerebral lesion that has encroached on the reticular activating fibers. The reticular activating system is diffusely distributed in the cerebral hemispheres and brain stem. Its connection between higher and lower centers travel through the tentorial opening, a region that is frequently compressed as cranial contents shift medially with increasing intracranial pressure. Likewise, fibers controlling pupillary responses and

voluntary movement travel through the tentorial opening, and therefore, corresponding alteration in function would be noted. Changes in vital signs indicate compensatory responses in an attempt to maintain cerebral blood flow. The most important intervention at this time is to notify the physician immediately of the clinical changes because C. requires surgical intervention to ligate the bleeding vessel or vessels.

8. Depressed skull fractures are fractures that denote bony displacement into the brain parenchyma. They may result in secondary bleeds and increased intracranial pressure. The findings evident with depressed skull fractures relate to the region of the brain involved and the extent of brain tissue involvement. Hazards associated with depressed skull fractures may include increased intracranial pressure, brain tissue injury, alterations in venous return, secondary hemorrhages, and intracranial infections.

ANSWERS TO CASE STUDY 31-2

1. J. has spinal cord trauma that involves injury at the C5 level. This is one of the more commonly injured areas of the spinal cord. If sufficient injury has occurred to the spinal cord, the individual will be rendered quadriplegic. J. will retain neck, shoulder, and scapula movement because the innervation to the sternocleidomastoid muscle is intact. It would be anticipated that sensory perception is obliterated below the area innervated through the fifth cervical segment. Respiratory innervation is mediated through the diaphragmatic nerve, which evolves from C3 to C4, and through the intercostal nerves, which evolve from the region of T1 to T12. J.'s injury is above the thoracic spinal cord, and therefore, she has lost the intercostal innervation for respiration. However, J.'s diaphragmatic innervation is intact because her injury is slightly below the level of the origin of diaphragmatic innervation. Therefore, she has limited respiratory muscle function.
2. J. is at risk for developing spinal cord edema, which could extend the cord injury and result in respiratory arrest. J.'s cord injury is at level C5. Should the cord edema ascend to include C4 or higher, the only remaining respiratory muscle innervation may be obliterated. J. is at risk for other postinjury hazards, such as autonomic nervous system changes associated with spinal shock, gastrointestinal, bladder, and bowel atony, and emboli secondary to venous pooling associated with peripheral vasodilation.
3. Spinal shock results from a high spinal cord injury (above T6), where sympathetic nervous system innervation is obliterated and unopposed parasympathetic innervation from higher areas predominates. The modulation of sympathetic-parasympathetic innervation is inhibited by the cord lesion. In addition to flaccid paralysis and areflexia, the resulting findings associated with spinal shock relate to autonomic nervous system deficits. When its effects are unopposed, the parasympathetic nervous system results in hypotension, bradycardia, loss of sweating, piloerection, and poikilothermia (ambient temperature regulation). Additionally, bowel and bladder reflexes are lost during spinal shock. Clinical signs supporting spinal shock in J. include a blood pressure reading of 92/48, a temperature of 97.8, a pulse of 62, flaccid paralysis, and bowel atony.
4. A period of spinal shock or post-injury areflexia ensues for a period of time. Organized neural pathways are interrupted and reflex responses are inhibited below the level of the lesion. Bowel and bladder reflexes originate in the sacral regions and, therefore, are inhibited, and conscious control over their function is lost. Therefore, J. may need a Foley catheter inserted initially and assistance with bowel evacuation.
5. J. is prone to hazards of immobility due to major motor-sensory losses. The most significant of these hazards include skin breakdown, infections, muscle atrophy, bone demineralization, and thrombus formation.
6. J. most likely suffered an episode of autonomic dysreflexia or autonomic hyperreflexia. This is an exaggerated response of the sympathetic nervous system in individuals with high spinal cord injuries (above T6). A mass sympathetic discharge occurs in response to a specific noxious stimulus. This discharge occurs as a result of stimulation of sensory receptors, which, in turn, transmit to the spinal cord and continue ascending in the spinal cord via posterior columns and spinothalamic tracts, and reflexively stimulate the sympathetic nervous system neurons in the lateral areas of the cord. The parasympathetic modulation from higher centers is blocked by the injury, and the sympathetic nervous system effect continues unabated, resulting in arteriolar spasm and vasoconstriction below the level of the lesion. This situation results in severe hypertension, headache, and visceral changes. The high blood pressure is sensed by the higher centers, and the parasympathetic system is stimulated and results in bradycardia, and vasodilation above the level of the lesion. As a result, the individual presents with flushing and diaphoresis above the level of the lesion and pale skin with gooseflesh below the level of injury. The individual will be very anxious, restless, and may experience nausea.

   A cause of autonomic dysreflexia in J. could be a full bladder or bowel. A quick intervention that might be employed with J. is to raise the head of the bed quickly to obtain some postural hypotension. Then it is important to look for the underlying cause and eliminate it. Major hazards associated with this exaggerated sympathetic response are cerebral hemorrhage and myocardial infarction.

ANSWERS TO CASE STUDY 32-1

1. An astrocytoma is a tumor of neuroepithelial tissue (glioma). Glial cells are the supporting cells of the brain. These spider-shaped or star-shaped cells infiltrate brain tissue and are frequently associated with cysts of various sizes. Their invasive nature usually makes surgical removal difficult.

2. According to Laws (1993), cited in the reference list, the average age at diagnosis is 37 years. Prognostic factors in patients with astrocytomas of the brain are more favorable when the age of the patient is less than 40 years.
3. Because brain tumors eventually give rise to an increase in intracranial pressure, the three symptoms of brain tumors that often occur are headache, vomiting, and papilledema. Headache, a common symptom, is believed to result from local displacement and traction of pain-sensitive structures within the skull, such as cranial nerves, arteries, veins, and venous sinuses. As the tumor grows, the pain reflects generalized increased intracranial pressure. The headache may be dull and is usually temporary, often most severe on awakening and tending to improve throughout the day. It may be aggravated by stooping, coughing, or straining to have a bowel movement. Vomiting associated with tumors is not necessarily preceded by nausea and is not related to the ingestion of food. It often occurs before breakfast and is frequently projectile. Papilledema occurs as intracranial pressure increases. Blurring and an enlarged blind spot are associated with papilledema.

   Additionally, a person with a brain tumor may experience seizures, changes in mental function, and personality changes. The involvement of Mrs. M.'s dominant temporal lobe produced sensory aphasia, which begins with difficulty in naming objects. Also, the individual has difficulty comprehending the spoken word and speaks in jargon. Tinnitus occurs from irritation of the adjacent cortex or temporal auditory receptor.
4. The CT scan is the screening procedure of choice because it is noninvasive and not painful. The CT scan involves the use of a computer and produces a picture of the transverse sections of the brain through the various absorptive characteristics of brain tissue, blood, CSF, cyst fluid, and tumors. The MRI views the brain in successive layers within a powerful magnetic field, allowing for assessment of physiology, such as reactions to the tumor, including cerebral edema, as well as the nature and extent of blood flow.
5. Most likely, Mrs. M. will undergo a biopsy and radical excision if possible. Following the excision and biopsy report, radiotherapy and chemotherapy may be indicated. Often, these tumors are not radiosensitive. Prognosis is variable because astrocytomas have varying degrees of malignancy. Some are well differentiated and grow slowly for many years but may become more anaplastic over time. Other astrocytomas are very poorly differentiated and have a rapid rate of growth and poor prognosis. Mrs. M.'s prognosis is more favorable because she is younger than 40 years of age.

ANSWERS TO CASE STUDY 33-1

1. Amyotrophic lateral sclerosis (ALS) is a primary neurologic disease involving a loss of motor neurons of the cerebral cortex, brain, and spinal cord. It is a noninflammatory disease of the upper and lower motor neurons with demyelination secondary to axon degeneration. The disease leads to progressive muscle weakness and muscle wasting, and ultimately, to death, usually within 5 years from diagnosis. ALS typically occurs after age 50, being twice as prevalent in males than females. P. M. is a man who is older than 50 years of age, exhibiting muscle weakness in his face, palate, right hand, and left leg. He also has muscle wasting in these areas.
2. The exact cause of ALS is unknown. However, several possible causes have been postulated, including premature aging of the nerve cells from some environmental or genetic factor, nutritional deficiencies, heavy metal poisoning, an autoimmune response, metabolic defect, or a dormant virus. An autosomal dominant inheritance pattern is also seen in some cases.
3. When testing for fasiculations, a muscle is tapped or moved passively. In response, fasiculations, or small local muscle contractions, occur.
4. As P. M.'s condition progresses, weakness and atrophy also will continue to progress. Bulbar palsy, either spastic or flaccid, may occur from damage to the motor cranial nerves in the medulla. This palsy may lead to death. Brain stem involvement, evidenced by tongue fasiculations, may progress to slurred speech, difficulty swallowing (increasing the risk for aspiration), and unintelligible speech. As the disease continues, bladder and bowel sphincter control are affected. Eventually, paralysis of the trunk and respiratory muscles lead to death (if bulbar palsy has not already done so). Throughout the entire disease progression, intellectual function remains intact.

ANSWERS TO CASE STUDY 34-1

1. R. M.'s advancing age and loss of lens elasticity increase his risk for cataract formation. R. M.'s history of diabetes mellitus predisposes him to cataract formation secondary to elevated glucose levels in the aqueous humor. Patients with diabetes mellitus also are at increased risk for opacities of the lens. Also, R. M. is an avid golfer, exposing him to large amounts of ultraviolet radiation from the sun, which could possibly damage the lens and subsequently result in cataract formation.
2. With cataracts, the cells of the lens degenerate, leading to an increase in the cells' water content, causing a clouding of vision and interference with light transmission to the retina. Eventually, the entire lens is involved. The lens capsule degenerates and cellular debris escapes into the aqueous humor. Macrophages are called on to phagocytize the debris and remove it from the system.
3. Normally, intraocular pressure (IOP) is maintained by a balance between aqueous humor production and absorption. The ciliary epithelium produces aqueous humor, which flows from the posterior chamber through the pupil into the anterior chamber, out through the trabecular meshwork to the

canal of Schlemm and finally into the venous circulation of the eye for absorption.

4. R. M.'s development of acute glaucoma postoperatively is most likely related to an obstruction of the outflow of aqueous humor from edema secondary to surgery.

ANSWERS TO CASE STUDY 35-1

1. At the time of injury, the following alterations occurred. Cellular and tissue injury resulted from the release of K^+ and H^+ from cells, bradykinin from ruptured capillaries, and substance P release from unmyelinated nerve fibers, as well as synthesis of prostaglandins that sensitizes peripheral nerve endings. Injury leads to tissue changes due to inflammation. Organ and system functioning were altered in acute pain due to the transmission of the pain signal to the brain and the modulation of the pain signal. Stimulation of the autonomic nervous system is seen in acute pain. Diaphoresis and dizziness with a potential drop in pulse rate or blood pressure were reported. Muscle spasm related to the need to "guard" the area and edema related to increased vasodilatation and increased capillary permeability also occurred in the acute phase.
2. When the pain became chronic, pressure on the nerve roots leaving at the L4–L5 and L5–S1 levels caused neurogenic pain related to compression of the nerves. Chronic inflammation of the disks with the release of increased substance P is thought to contribute to the undergoing pain symptoms. Continuing muscle spasm leads to an increase in vasodilation, a tendency for tissue swelling and edema, and chronic muscle ischemia. The ischemia triggered muscle pain. At the systemic level, reduced physical activity led to poor conditioning, and changes in responsibilities at home and at work. Social relationships were at risk as the pain took control of her life. The patient experienced depression with feelings of helplessness and hopelessness related to multiple physical, psychological, and social losses.
3. Endogenous opioids (endorphins and enkephalins) are morphine-like substances that affect afferent nociceptive and descending responses. The opiate receptors are believed to provide presynaptic inhibition to nociceptors, and thus, diminish or eliminate secretion of substance P. In chronic pain, such as that experienced by J. J., there may be a deficient level of endogenous opiates. Additionally, unlike other sensory receptors, nociceptors adapt very little or not at all, leading to a lowering of the pain thresholds.
4. Transcutaneous electrical nerve stimulation (TENS) stimulates the large A afferent fibers in order to override the pain impulses traveling to the cord through small A-delta and small C fibers in someone with pain. An increase in the activity of large A fibers stimulates the substantia gelatinosa, thus "closing the gate" and decreasing the pain.

ANSWERS TO CASE STUDY 37-1

1. Perimenopause refers to the time surrounding the actual experience of menopause, that is, when menopausal changes are occurring. The age for menopause varies widely, ranging from 45 to 55 years. The average age for a woman in the United States is 51 years.
2. The ovarian cycle, those changes directly related to the hormonal response of the ovaries, consists of oogenesis, the follicular phase, ovulation, and the luteal phase. The endometrial cycle, the cyclic changes in uterine cell lining, consists of the proliferative and secretory phases and menses. The follicular phase of the ovarian cycle occurs, along with menses and the proliferative phase of the endometrial cycle. During this time, the ovarian follicle develops while the endometrium is being shed and then beginning its new growth. Ovulation occurs near the end of the proliferative phase. The luteal phase occurs after ovulation and occurs along with the secretory phase of the endometrial cycle. During this time, the corpus luteum reaches full maturity and the endometrial lining becomes highly vascular and thick. If conception does not occur, the corpus luteum regresses, with a decrease in progesterone and estrogen production. The decrease in progesterone causes the endometrium to degenerate, thus leading to menstruation.
3. The primary physiologic event associated with menopause is the reduced number of ovarian follicles and a reduced sensitivity of those few remaining to gonadotropins. With follicular development, the ovaries continue to produce androgens, but the productions of estrogen (all types) ceases. Therefore, a decrease in overall estrogen levels and a change in the type occur. With this decrease in estrogen, the endometrium does not proliferate to the extent that it did previously. Also, the neuroendocrine feedback mechanism is affected, thus altering the menstrual cycle.
4. Age of menopause may be influenced by genetics (familial patterns), cigarette smoking, parity, and nutritional status, and varies with geographic location.
5. Declining estrogen levels result in drying and thinning of the vaginal epithelium.
6. During menopause, gonadotropin follicle-stimulating hormone (FSH) rises owing to a loss of the negative feedback mechanism by estrogen.
7. Other symptoms suggesting perimenopause include progressively shorter menstrual periods with lighter flow; hot flashes and facial flushing; vaginal dryness; and decreased lubrication during intercourse. Additionally, vaginal spotting after intercourse may suggest trauma to the vaginal wall secondary to vaginal dryness and thinning of the vaginal wall.

Glossary

aberrant cellular growth: an alteration in normal cellular growth

abscess: a localized accumulation of pus in a cavity formed by tissue necrosis

acid: a substance that ionizes in water to release ions. Nonvolatile acids are those acids formed by the systemic cells that must be excreted by the kidney. Volatile acids are carbonic acids that can dissociate and be released through the lungs in the form of carbon dioxide

acidemia: an increase in acids in the blood

acidosis: an increase in acids in the body fluids

acinar cells: pancreatic cells that secrete pancreatic juice

acinus: respiratory bronchiole, alveolar duct, and alveoli

acrocentric chromosomes: a group of chromosomes in which the centromere is distally placed. Human chromosomes in groups D and G are acrocentric

actin: thin muscle filament that interacts with myosin to allow for muscle contraction

action potential: sequence of physiochemical events resulting in an alteration in the resting membrane potential

acute inflammation: the immediate and early response to an injurious agent. It involves the vascular and cellular changes that characterize the process

acute lung injury: a term often used interchangeably with adult respiratory distress syndrome that refers to diffuse alveolar capillary damage causing life-threatening respiratory insufficiency

acute pain: a complex constellation of unpleasant sensory, perceptual, and emotional experience associated with physiologic injury of less than 6 months' duration

acute tubular necrosis: a syndrome of destruction of renal tubules leading to acute impairment of renal function. It may be caused by ischemia or nephrotoxicity and is the most common cause of acute renal failure

adaptation: a change in function of an organ or tissue that allows it to function under new conditions

adenomyosis: invasion of endometrial tissue into the uterine myometrial layer

adherins: substances secreted by certain organisms, especially bacteria, that allow them to attach strongly to structures and penetrate to underlying tissues

adhesion: a carbohydrate-specific binding protein that projects from procaryotic cells; used for adherence. Also called ligand. It causes attachment of a microbe or phagocyte to another's plasma membrane

adhesion molecules: glycoproteins that assist in the process of adherence

adrenal insufficiency: a condition of decreased function of the gland resulting in decreased cortisol and aldosterone secretion

adrenopause: term used to denote the normal decline of dehydroepiandrosterone (DHEA) with aging

adult respiratory distress syndrome: a severe restrictive lung condition of widespread atelectasis that occurs secondary to another systemic conditions such as shock

aerobic capacity: the maximal amount of oxygen that can be consumed per minute

aerobic exercise: type of exercise that improves the efficiency of the aerobic energy–producing systems

afferent arteriole: arteriole delivering the blood supply to the glomerulus

afferent neuron: neurons that transmit sensory information from the periphery to the central nervous system

afterload: the load or resistance against which the ventricles must pump

ageusia: absence of taste; may occur as part of the aging process

agglutinins: antibody that participates in agglutination reaction

agglutinogens: antigens that participate in agglutination reactions. Agglutination reaction is one in which a particulate antigen or antibody reacts with soluble antibody or antigen to cause detectable clumping

agnosia: inability to recognize familiar objects or persons

agoraphobia: anxiety disorder characterized by the fear of being in an open, public, or crowded place where help might not be readily available if something alarming happens

agranulocytes: white blood cells that contain granules that do not pick up stain; includes monocytes and lymphocytes

air-trapping: condition in which small airways close prematurely during exhalation, thus preventing normal movement of air out of the lung

airway resistance: the opposition to air movement during ventilation caused by various factors, such as airway structures, inflammation, mucus, and patterns of airflow

algesic agent: biochemical substances such as potassium, hydrogen, and prostaglandins that cause pain

alimentary canal: term used to denote the gastrointestinal tract, which is a basic tubular structure that extends from the mouth to the anus; this is where food is ingested and processed, digested, and absorbed

alkalosis: an increase in the alkalinity of body fluids

allele: alternative expressions of a gene at a given locus. For example, the alleles H and h of the gene HexA would determine the synthesis (H), or nonsynthesis (h) of the enzyme hexosaminidase A, whose absence causes Tay-Sachs disease

allergen: an antigen that elicits a hypersensitivity or allergic reaction

allergy: usually refers to a Type I hypersensitivity reaction that involves IgE antibody and often manifests on second contact, usually with an environmental antigen

allodynia: pain produced by a stimulus (such as light touch) that normally does not cause pain

allosteric modulation: the binding of a ligand to a protein or changing the conformation of the protein

alogia: decreased ability to speak

alpha 1-antitrypsin: substance produced in liver that inhibits proteolytic enzymes in the lung

alpha 2-antiplasmin: an inhibitor of plasmin, thus preventing excessive fibrinolysis

alpha-delta fiber: a small-in-diameter, lightly myelinated nerve fiber associated with fast pain transmission

alveolar-capillary membrane: membrane between alveoli and pulmonary capillary where gas exchange takes place

alveolar dead space: alveoli that are not participating in gas exchange

alveolar ventilation: amount of gas that actually reaches the gas exchange area

alveolitis: inflammation of the walls of the alveoli

amniocentesis: prenatal diagnostic procedure that consists of transabdominally withdrawing a small sample of amniotic fluid for genetic analysis of embryonic cells

amphiarthrosis: joint with very limited movement such as the symphysis pubis

amphipathic phospholipid molecules: the most abundant of the lipids in the cell membrane

amylase: a pancreatic enzyme that hydrolyzes carbohydrates to disaccharides

anabolic: the phase of cellular repair and growth, especially of proteins; the constructive phase of metabolism

anaerobic glycolysis: the production of small quantities of energy-rich phosphate bonds in the absence of oxygen

anaerobic metabolism: metabolism of the body cells without oxygen. Used in shock situations to keep the cells alive

anaphase: the third stage of mitosis in which there is centromere division that allows the chromosomes to move to apposite poles of the spindle

anaphylactoid reaction: a reaction that has all of the features of the Type I reaction except that it is not IgE mediated

anaphylaxis: usually refers to a systemic reaction that causes circulatory collapse and respiratory distress due to the Type I hypersensitivity reaction

anaplasia: the loss of cellular differentiation

anatomic dead space: air in lung structures that do not come in contact with gas exchange surfaces

androgens: any of the steroid hormones that promote male sex characteristics

aneuploidy: an abnormal chromosome pattern in which the total number of chromosomes is not a multiple of the haploid number (n = 23). For instance, persons with 45 or 47 chromosomes, as in Turner or Down syndrome, respectively. Trisomies are examples of aneuploidy

angioedema: recurrent, large areas of subcutaneous edema of sudden onset, usually due to an allergic reaction. Also called angioneurotic edema

angiogenesis: also called neovascularization; involves the budding and sprouting of new vessels in a tissue to form a new blood supply

anion gap acidosis: a method for evaluating metabolic acidosis. Normal anion gap acidosis occurs when chloride ion increases to keep the ratio of anions in the normal range. High anion gap acidosis occurs when there is an accumulation of systemic acids that cause the normal gap to increase

anisocoria: unequal diameter size in two pupils

anorexia nervosa: clinical marasmus due to self-starvation

anosmia: loss of smell

anterior cord syndrome: incomplete cord lesion involving the anterior portion of the spinal cord and resulting in loss of motor function, touch, pain, and temperature sensation

antibody: protein produced as the result of introduction of an antigen; also called immunoglobulins; secreted by plasma cells (B lymphocytes)

anticipation: the occurrence of a hereditary disease at a younger age in successive generations

anticoagulants: natural or synthetic substances that inhibit the coagulation system

antigen: molecule that elicits an immune response in an immunocompetent host to whom it is foreign. Antigens can bind to T-cell receptors or to antibodies

antigen presenting cell (APC): cells that can process antigens by binding its epitope to an MHC II class protein. The processed antigen is then displayed on the APC's surface so it can be recognized by T-cell receptors

antigenic determinants: specific areas or combining sites on the surface of the membrane of an antigen; determine specificity of adaptive immune response

antistreptolysin O titer: serologic procedure used to detect reaction of body to infection caused by group A streptococci. Appears in serum 1 week to 1 month after infection

antithrombin III: a plasma protein that inactivates thrombin and inhibits clotting

aphasia: loss of neurologic capacity for language

apoferritin: a protein that combines with iron to form ferritin to regulate iron storage and transport

apoptosis (programmed cell death): physiologic process aimed at eliminating undesirable cells (as in progressive follicular cell atresia during female reproductive life) or a pathologic response due to certain external stimuli (as in HIV-induced T-cell destruction). Cell death results from activation of the internal lethal caspase enzyme cascade, which culminates in the destruction of the nuclear membrane, fragmentation of the genome, and formation of apoptotic bodies. Apoptosis activation is a genetically controlled form of cell suicide in both physiologic and pathologic processes

apraxia: inability to carry out a voluntary, purposeful motor skill such as brushing hair in spite of an intact conduction system, indicating cortical integrative impairment

arachidonic acid: fatty acid derived from membrane lipids; the products of its degradation are among the most important of the lipid mediators of inflammation and other biologic processes

arcus senilis: an opaque white ring seen at the periphery of the cornea in aged individuals

Arnold-Chiari malformation: a type of deformity associated with downward displacement of the cerebellum and brain stem through the foramen magnum. Associated anomalies establish this malformation into four classifications

arteriovenous malformation: developmental defect of connected cerebral veins and arteries without an intervening capillary bed, resulting in a thin, dilated, and weakened vascular area

arthritis: inflammation of a joint

ascites: accumulation of fluid in the peritoneal cavity

association neurons: neurons that relay messages between neurons in the central nervous system

asterixis: also known as "liver flap," a "flapping tremor" that occurs with dorsiflexion of the wrist

astigmatism: the refraction of parallel light rays spread over a diffuse area rather than being sharply focused on the retina

astrocytoma: a tumor derived from astrocytic glial cells; these cells infiltrate brain tissue and are frequently associated with cysts of various size

atelectasis: acute or chronic restrictive disorder of the lung that results from collapse of air spaces

atheroma: the raised area on the intimal surface of the artery that is composed of lipids, macrophages, and other substances that can lead to occlusion of the vessel; the causative lesion of atherosclerosis

athetosis: slow, writhing movements

athyreotic cretinism: congenital absence of the thyroid gland or suppression of its hormonal secretion

atopy: a genetic propensity to produce IgE (immune globulin), which is directed toward common environmental allergenic antigens such as pollens and the house dust mite

atrophy: decrease in muscle mass usually from disuse

autoantibodies: antibodies that react against "self" tissue and cause a destructive effect

autocoids: local short-range hormones that exert their effects locally and either decay spontaneously or are destroyed enzymatically
autoimmunity: immune reactions to self-antigens; represents a loss of self-tolerance
automaticity: the spontaneous property of generating an action potential; a feature of cardiac conduction tissue
autonomic dysreflexia: an exaggerated autonomic reflex response to stimuli in patients with spinal cord injuries above the level of T6, manifested by extremely elevated blood pressure, bradycardia, flushing, and diaphoresis above the level of the lesion and pale, cool skin below the lesion
autonomic nervous system: functional component of the nervous system that maintains the internal environment in a steady state. It is composed of the sympathetic and parasympathetic divisions
autoregulation: the intrinsic ability of the coronary and systemic vessels to regulate blood flow by constriction and dilation
autosome: the 22 pairs of chromosomes that do not greatly influence sex determination at conception. It does not include the sex chromosomes X and Y
avolition: inability to participate in goal-oriented activities
azotemia: the accumulation of nitrogenous waste products in the blood
balanitis: inflammation of the glans penis
balanoposthitis: inflammation of the glans penis and overlying prepuce
barotrauma: lung injury secondary to exertion of excess positive pressure
basal cell carcinoma: most common type of malignant lesion; it is slow growing
basal metabolic rate (BMR): the amount of energy used to maintain essential body function. It is expressed as a unit of calories per hour per square meter of body surface
base: a substance that ionized in water to release hydroxyl ions that combine with hydrogen ions
Bence Jones protein: abnormal proteins that appear in the urine or blood; derived from light chains of immunoglobulin molecules
benign: characterized by abnormal cell division but does not metastasize or invade surrounding tissue
benign prostatic hyperplasia (BPH): age-related hyperplasia of prostatic stromal and epithelial cells
benzodiazepines: class of sedative-hypnotic drugs that potentiate the inhibitory activity of gamma-aminobutyric acid (GABA); used for the treatment of anxiety
biliary colic: pain related to obstruction of the gallbladder by gallstones; it may be constant or excruciating spasmotic
bilirubin: a waste product primarily occurring from the breakdown of red blood cells that is excreted from the body in its conjugated form
bipolar disorder: a major psychological disorder characterized usually by alternating episodes of mania and depression
blood group: a genetically determined system of antigens located on the surface of a red blood cell; includes ABO and Rh systems
blood type: the specific blood group to which an individual belongs
Bouchard's nodes: bony enlargements or nodules of the joints of the hands that result from osteoarthritis or degenerative joint disease
Bowman's capsule: The part of the nephron that surrounds the glomerulus and receives glomerular filtrate
bradykinesia: slowed movement
bradykinin: a plasma kinin that mediates vasodilation, capillary permeability, smooth muscle contraction, and pain sensation
bradyphrenia: slowness in thinking without intellectual impairment
brain barriers: tight cellular junctions in the cerebral capillaries and choroid plexus that limit the passage of substances into the cerebrospinal fluid (CSF) and brain
brawny edema: a nonpitting swelling associated with thick, hardened skin and color changes that result from trapped and coagulated proteins in the tissue spaces
BRCA gene: BRCA1 and BRCA2 are tumor-suppressor genes that are probably involved in DNA repair. Mutations may cause an increased incidence of breast and other cancers
Broca's aphasia: impairment in expression of language resulting from lesions located in the posterior part of the inferior frontal gyrus. Also known as motor, expressive, or nonfluent aphasia
bronchoconstriction: narrowing of the bronchial airway lumen
bronchogenic: arising from the bronchi
Brown-Séquard syndrome: incomplete cord lesion in one half of the spinal cord, resulting in ipsilateral paralysis, loss of proprioception, touch, and vibratory sense, and contralateral loss of pain and temperature sensation
brownian movement: random movement of molecules due to thermal energy
buffer: any substance that prevents major changes in the pH of body fluids by reversibly binding hydrogen
bulbar palsy: progressive abnormalities of the muscles innervated by motor cranial nerves
bulimia nervosa: a disorder characterized by recurrent episodes of binge eating and self-induced purging behaviors

bursae: small, flat cavities filled with synovial fluid and used to prevent friction in the joint
C fiber: a smaller diameter, unmyelinated nerve fiber associated with slow, chronic pain transmission
C-reactive protein: a globulin that, in the presence of calcium ions, precipitates the C substance. It is an abnormal protein that is detectable in blood only during the active phase of certain acute illnesses
cancellous bone: spongy bone that has interlacing parts
cancer: malignant cellular growth with potential for invasion of surrounding tissues and metastasis to distant sites
capacitance vessels: blood vessels, especially veins, that have the capability to stretch and hold volumes of blood
capsid: a closed protein shell seen with viruses
capsomeres: protein subunits that make up the capsid
capsular hydrostatic pressure (CHP): the pressure exerted by the fluid in Bowman's capsule. This pressure opposes filtration
carbaminohemoglobin (CO_2Hgb): the result of a chemical combination of carbon dioxide and hemoglobin
carbon dioxide narcosis: an excessive accumulation of carbon dioxide in the arterial circuit that causes severe respiratory acidosis and symptoms of headache, blurred vision, and central nervous system effects, especially coma
carbuncles: large staphylococcal abscesses. May be composed of several furuncles
carcinogen: any substance or agent that is capable of producing cancer
carcinogenesis: the transformation of normal cells to malignant cells
carcinoma: malignant growth originating in epithelial tissue
carcinoma in situ: a malignant tumor that has not crossed the basement membrane; noninvasive
cardiogenic pulmonary edema: flooding of alveoli and lung tissue due to cardiac dysfunction
carotenoid pigment: pigment containing carotene that exhibits a bright yellow color
carpopedal spasm: spasm of both the wrist and foot, usually due to hypocalcemia
carrier state: a state exhibited by a person who harbors and can transmit a particular cicroorganism to others but exhibits no particular symptoms
catabolic: the breakdown of complex substances into simple ones; the destructive phase of metabolism
cataract: clouding of the lens with a loss of visual acuity
catecholamines: neurotransmitters of the sympathetic nervous system, including epinephrine, norepinephrine, and dopamine
cellulitis: a diffuse infection of the skin or subcutaneous tissue; usually refers to a process that extends along a tissue plane
central cord syndrome: incomplete cord lesion involving the central structures of the spinal cord, resulting in greater motor weakness in the upper extremities
central or neurogenic diabetes insipidus: inadequate amounts of antidiuretic hormone secretion, causing large amount of pale urine of low specific gravity
centromere: chromosomal region that separates the chromosome arms and unites the chromatids; attaches to spindle fibers during cell division
cerebral neuroblastoma: a tumor that is derived from precursor cells of neurons
cervical eversion: appearance of columnar cells, normally only within endocervix, on the exocervix; usually due to chronic inflammation (cervicitis)
cervical intraepithelial neoplasia (CIN): early tissue changes in the neoplastic transformation process (syn. squamous intraepithelial lesion)
cestodes: tapeworms of the helminth classification
chemoreceptive trigger zone: a group of neurons located on the dorsal surface of the floor of the fourth ventricle that sense stimuli that activate the vomiting center in the medulla
chemoreceptors: specialized tissue capable of monitoring pH, oxygen, and carbon dioxide levels in blood
chemotaxis: chemical stimulus, usually a cytokine, a bacterial toxin, or specific proteins of the complement system, that promotes cell movement toward the gradient produced
chief cells: cells in the stomach that secrete the proenzyme pepsinogen
chocolate cyst: an endometriomal cystic lesion that develops in endometriosis, usually covers ovary
cholecystokinin: a hormone secreted by the duodenal mucosa when fat moves through the duodenum
cholestasis: a biliary pigment that accumulates in the bile canaliculi and hepatocytes
chordae tendineae: the connective tissue strands that anchor the leaflets of the mitral and tricuspid valves to the papillary muscles, preventing prolapse of the valves into the atria during ventricular systole
chordoma: a congenital, malignant tumor derived from remnants of the primitive notochord

chorea: rapid, dancelike movement of the limbs, trunk, and face

choriocarcinoma: a malignant tumor of the products of conception or of the ovary

chromaffin cells: cells of the adrenal medulla and sympathetic paraganglion

chromatids: the two strands formed by duplication of a chromosome that become visible during prophase of mitosis or meiosis

chromatin: the deeply staining genetic material in the nucleus of a cell; mainly composed of uncoiled chromosomes

chromosome: filament-like nuclear structure, consisting of chromatin, that stores genetic information as base sequences in DNA, and whose number is constant in each species. Chromosomes are found in pairs in somatic cells (homologous chromosomes) and in single copies in germ cells. One member of a homologous pair is of paternal origin, and the other pair is of maternal origin. Homologous chromosomes have identical number and arrangement of genes

chromosome abnormalities: a group of genetic disorders that result from numeric or structural alterations of chromosomes

chronic analgesia nephritis: a syndrome of renal damage that occurs in persons who ingest large quantities of certain analgesic mixtures

chronic inflammation: a type of long-term inflammation that results in infiltration of the site with fibroblasts, increased amounts of collagen deposits, and varying amounts of scar tissue formation

chronic pain: pain that persists more or less continuously after 6 months or the normal time of healing, resulting in a pattern of physiologic, psychological, and social changes

chylomicron: the initial transport molecule for digested fat

chyme: semifluid mass of partly digested food; a thin, highly acidic liquid produced by the digestive action of the stomach

ciliata: the most complex of the protozoa; organisms have cilia distributed in rows or patches, and the shape of the organism varies

cicatrix: a scar left by a healed wound

cicatrization: the process of scar formation

circadian rhythm or pattern: biologic variations with a cycle of about 24 hours

cirrhosis: a condition in which the normal structure of the liver lobules is destroyed

climacteric: the perimenopausal period, during which female reproductive system activities are preparing for menopause

coagulopathy: a defect of the blood clotting system

cocaine: a drug that is abused for its nervous stimulant effect. Its abuse may lead to several complications such as cardiac dysrhythmias, convusions, and coma

codon: a genetic code composed of a sequence of three bases in a strand of DNA or mRNA

collateral circulation: an alternate arterial pathway that develops when there is an obstruction to blood flow through the vessel, commonly seen in coronary and systemic arteries when there is extensive atherosclerotic disease

collateral ventilation: movement of inspired gases between alveoli through the pores of Kohn

collecting duct: tubules that drain filtrate from the distal convoluted tubules of the nephrons

colony-forming units (CFUs): the first progenitor cell derived from the pluripotent hematopoietic stem cells that can give rise to granulocytes, erythrocytes, monocytes, and megakaryocytes

coma: disruption of conscious state, in which wakefulness and awareness are lacking

complement: series of enzymes and chemicals; normally inactive in the circulating blood, which when activated by an antigen or immune cell, assist in the inflammatory and specific immune responses

complement system: a group of serum proteins involved in phagocytosis, or lysis of bacteria, that produce widespread inflammatory effects

compliance: measurement of distensibility or the ease in which a tissue can be stretched

compulsions: persistent and irresistable impulse to perform an act that results in anxiety if not completed

concussion: diffuse, transient, and reversible injury to the brain from blows to the head

conducting airways: airways that do not participate in gas exchange (trachea, bronchi, bronchioles)

conductivity: the property of the heart muscle that allows the action potential in one cell to depolarize the adjacent cells

contractility: the force of contraction generated by the myocardial muscle; also referred to as the inotropic state

contusion: focal parenchymal injury (bruising and lacerations) of the brain resulting from blunt trauma

convergence: reception of neural input to a single neuron from many other neurons

cor pulmonale: right-sided heart failure secondary to high pulmonary pressures in moderate to severe lung or pulmonary vascular disease

cortical bone: bone with a hard surface that contains blood vessels and nerves

corticospinal tract: upper motor nerve fibers originating in the Betz cells of the motor cortex that transmit contralateral voluntary motor control through the basal ganglia and brainstem to the spinal cord. Most fibers cross at the level of the medulla and continue the descent into the spinal cord, where they synapse with lower motor neurons. Also known as the pyramidal tract

cortisol: a steroid hormone secreted by the adrenal cortex that functions in part as an insulin antagonist and elevates blood sugar

cotransport or symport: moving a transported soluted in the same direction as sodium through coupling of two different molecules

countercurrent exchanger: a system, dependent on the vasa recta, that protects the osmotic gradient of the renal medulla. The osmotic gradient is necessary for urine concentration

countercurrent mechanism: a system, composed of the countercurrent multiplier and the countercurrent exchanger, that promotes concentration of urine in the loop of Henle

countercurrent multiplier: a system for creating an osmotic gradient in the renal medulla around the loop of Henle

counter regulatory: action of hormones that produces opposite physiologic effects

counter-transport or antiport: the movement of two different molecules in opposite directions through a common carrier mechanism

covalent modification: formation of a chemical bond by electron sharing between atoms

craniopharyngioma (Rathke's pouch tumor): a tumor derived from Rathke's pouch, which is a pouch in the embryonic membrane that develops into the anterior lobe of the pituitary

creatine kinase (creatine phosphokinase): enzyme found predominantly in the heart muscle, skeletal muscle, and brain. Serum elevations occur with injury. Isoenzymes (CK—MB) are used to identify specifically if cardiac damage has occurred

cretinism: congenital hypothyroidism

critical oxygen tension: tissue oxygen level so low that it interferes with mitochondrial function

cross-bridge: connection of myosin to actin that pulls the fibers along and allows for muscle contraction

cryptorchidism: failure of one or both of the testes to descend into the scrotum

crypts of Lieberkühn: pitlike structures that lie in grooves between the villi of the intestinal wall; they are composed of absorptive cells and mucus-producing goblet cells

Cushing's disease: the pituitary form of Cushing syndrome; primary hypersecretion of adrenocorticotropic hormone (ACTH)

Cushing's syndrome: a condition that produces an elevation of glucocorticoid levels; hypercortisolism

cutaneous pain: pain that is localized to the skin and mucous membranes

cystitis: infection of the urinary bladder. It may be acute or chronic

cytogenetics: the study of chromosomes, with special focus on chromosome abnormalities

cytokine: a protein secreted by many cell types that regulates the intensity and duration of immune responses. A chemokine secreted by an activated lymphocyte is termed a lymphokine

cytolysis: the process of destruction of cell membranes that leads to cell death

cytosol: the fluid medium within the cytoplasm of the cell

cytotoxic edema: cerebral edema resulting from cellular injury or dysfunction associated with cerebral hypoxia

deamination: the removal of nitrogen or the amine group. The fate of the amine groups is primarily the conversion to ammonia and then to urea

decerebrate posturing: extension response of upper and lower extremities caused by brain stem lesions

decorticate posturing: flexion response of upper extremities caused by supratentorial brain lesions

decubitus ulcers: sores on the skin caused by prolonged pressure

deep somatic pain: pain originating from deep body structures resulting from mechanical trauma or a build up of algesic substances

degranulation: release of the contents of cellular granules into the extracellular fluid; a common activity of activated platelets

dehiscence: a bursting open; especially of a surgical abdominal wound

deletion: the loss of chromosomal material. An example of a terminal deletion is found in the cri-du-chat (cat's cry) syndrome, in which there is loss of a portion of the short arm of chromosome B(5)

delusions: false beliefs that persist despite obvious evidence or proof to the contrary

dementia: insidious, progressive neurologic degeneration, resulting in impairment of cognition

dendrites: projections from the neuron cell bodies that receive transmissions from other neurons

depression: a mood disorder characterized by sadness, despair and discouragement

dermatitis: inflammation of the skin

dermatome: area of skin receiving innervation from a single dorsal root. Dermatomes correspond with spinal cord segments, which give rise to the spinal nerve

dermis: the layer of skin directly under the epidermis that contains blood and lymphatic vessels, nerves, glands, and hair follicles

dermoid: a congenital cystic tumor that frequently arises in the ventricular system; filled with fluid or sebaceous matter

desmosomes: adhesive junctions found in tissues that are subjected to considerable mechanical stress

diabetic nephropathy: renal damage associated with diabetes mellitus

diaphysis: the shaft or long portion of the bone

diarthrosis: freely movable synovial joints such as the hip

diencephalon: component of the prosencephalon that includes the epithalamus, thalamus, hypothalamus, and subthalamus

diethylstilbestrol (DES): a synthetic estrogen

diffuse alveolar damage: a term used for extensive respiratory damage as a complication of other conditions; often used synonymously with adult respiratory distress syndrome

diffusion equilibrium: a condition in which there is no concentration gradient across a cell membrane

dihydrotestosterone (DHT): an androgen, or male sex hormone; steroid class

dilatation: enlargement of a cavity. In the heart, it refers to enlargement of a chamber of the heart

2,3-diphosphoglycerate (2,3-DPG): a low-energy side product of glycolysis that functions as a regulator for the affinity of hemoglobin for oxygen

diploid: a cell that contains two copies of each chromosome. The term is often extended to include an individual carrying such cells. The diploid number (2n) in humans is 46

disseminated intravascular coagulation: an acute coagulopathy that involves thrombosis and hemorrhage

distal convoluted tubule (DCT): a portion of the nephron active in secretion and reabsorption of substances from the filtrate

distensibility/compliance: a measure of the ease with which the chambers of the heart may be distended. Decreased compliance occurs when the chambers are stiff and restrict inflow

divergence: a single neuron making connections with many other neurons

diverticulum: a bulging or outpouching herniation through the muscular wall of any tubular organ, such as the esophagus or small intestine

DNA: abbreviation of deoxyribonucleic acid. Double-helix molecule consisting of an assembly of nucleotides (phosphate-sugar [deoxyribose]-nitrogenous base). DNA bases (cytosine, guanine, thymine, adenine) encode genetic information, which is *transcribed* into messenger RNA and further *translated* into proteins

dominant: an allele that is phenotypically expressed in a single copy (heterozygote) as well as in a double copy (homozygote). For example, polydactyly

ductal ectasia: dilation of ducts within the breast due to chronic inflammation (mastitis)

duodenum: the first part of the small intestine, which lies between the pyloric valve of the stomach to the jejunum; it is the shortest and widest piece of the small intestine

dysfunctional uterine bleeding (DUB): abnormal bleeding patterns of hormonal origin; usually due to anovulatory cycles

dyslipoproteinemias: a heterogenous group of hereditary defects in lipoprotein synthesis. Results in elevations of lipoprotein levels in the blood

dysmenorrhea: painful menstruation

dysmyelopoiesis: abnormal proliferation of blood cells, morphology or numbers may be changed

dysphagia: Difficulty in swallowing

dyssomnias: primary sleep disorders that cause difficulty in initiating and maintaining sleep or causing excessive daytime sleepiness

ecchymoses: large, irregular hemorrhagic areas, caused by blood extravasation into the skin or mucous membranes

eclampsia: a severe outcome of preeclampsia with hypertension, proteinuria, and edema. It is usually fatal if not treated

ecoestrogens: environmental pollutants that may act at estrogen receptors and promote reproductive pathologies

eczema: description of a symptom associated with inflammation of the skin (dermatitis)

efferent arteriole: arteriole emerging from the glomerulus that subdivides into a network of peritubular capillaries

efferent neuron: neurons that transmit motor information from the central nervous system

ejection fraction (EF): the relationship between the stroke volume and the end diastolic volume, expressed in terms of a precentage. Normally, ejection fraction is 67 +/− 9%

elastance: (1) measurement of forces that seek to return to the resting or relaxed position; (2) measurement of brain stiffness, indicating the brain's tolerance for increases in volume

electrothermal burns: damage to tissues due to the thermal injury produced by electrical current

ELISA (enzyme-linked immunosorbent assay): an assay method used to determine the presence of antibodies. Widely used as a screening test for HIV antibodies; the high sensitivity of the ELISA yields virtually no false-negative results, but produces a significant level of false-positive results, which precludes its use as a definitive test. Positive ELISA results must be confirmed by a confirmatory test, such as the Western blot

embolus: A traveling blood clot that lodges in a blood vessel

emigration: passage of white blood corpuscles through the walls of the capillaries and veins during inflammation

emmetropia: normal refraction of the eye
empty sella syndrome: an enlarged, empty sella turcica not filled with pituitary tissue
empyema: pus accumulation in a body cavity, usually the pleural space, resulting from a bacterial infection
encephalitis: a general term to denote infections of the brain parenchyma, most commonly caused by a virus but also possibly caused by bacteria, rickettsia, parasites, and fungi
endemic: refers to a disease that is routinely found among certain populations
endemic goiter: enlargement of thyroid gland due to lack of iodine in soil, water, and food supply; term used when goiters are present in more than 10% of the regional population
endogenous pyrogens: fever-producing substances arising from within the body
endometrial hyperplasia: overgrowth of endometrial tissue due to excess estrogen effect without progesterone effect
endometrioma: cystic lesions that develop in endometriosis
endorphins: endogenous opioids. Polypeptides that act as opiates and produce analgesia by binding to opiate receptor sites involved in pain perception
endosteum: thin lining of the marrow cavity of cancellous bone
endothelium: the inner lining of a vessel, also called the tunica intima. The layer is a very metabolically active area, with endothelium-derived factors that cause vasoconstriction and vasodilatation
endotoxins: toxins that are part of the cell wall of gram-negative bacteria; they are released during cell division or destruction
enkephalins: endogenous opioids. Polypeptides that act as opiates and produce analgesia by binding to opiate receptor sites involved in pain perception
enterobacteria: microorganisms (*Escherichia coli,* and Klebsiella and Proteus species) responsible for gram-negative bacteremia
eosinophilia: increased eosinophil count typically seen in helminth infections
ependymoma: a tumor derived from ependymal glial cells, which line the ventricalar walls and form the central canal of the spinal cord
epidemic: a significant increase in number of cases of a particular infection
epidemiology: the study of how disease is produced in a population
epidermis: the outermost major layer of the skin
epididymitis: inflammation of the epididymis
epidural hematoma: bleeding (generally arterial) into the extradural (epidural) space
epilepsy: general term for seizure disorders characterized by sudden, excessive discharges of neurons
epinephrine: A hormone secreted by the medulla of the adrenal gland that enhances myocardial contractility, increases heart rate, and increases venous return to the heart
epiphysis: knobby ends of long cancellous bone
epispadias: congenital anomaly in which the urethra opens on the dorsal surface of the penis
eponychium: the layer in direct contact with the nail root proximally or at the sides of the nail plate
erythroblastosis fetalis: a severe type of hemolytic disease of the fetus that results from maternal anti-Rh antibody that enters the fetal circulation and causes destruction of fetal red blood cells
erythropoietin: A hormone secreted by the kidney that stimulates erythropoieses
eschar: coagulated nonviable tissue
eumelanin: brown and black melanins in hair color
euploid: a cell (an by extension, an individual) whose chromosome number is a multiple of 23
exchange vessels: the vessels through whose walls nutrients and oxygen pass to systemic cells and waste products are removed
excitability: the property of cardiac muscle that allows it to respond to an action potential
exfoliation: detachment and shedding of superficial cells from a tissue surface
exotoxin: an antigenic, injurious substance released by certain bacteria
extraglandular disorders: those disorders in which the function of another organ influences the actions of an endocrine gland. For example, damage to the renal juxtaglomerular cells decreases renin release.
extramedullary intradural tumor: intraspinal tumor arising from the blood vessels, meninges, or nerve roots
extrapyramidal tract: highly complex component of the motor system that does not traverse the pyramid in the brain stem and facilitates fine tuning of voluntary movement
extravasation: the process of exuding or moving out of a vessel into the tissues; also refers to the process by which phagocytes move out of blood vessels; also called diapidesis
exudates: accumulation of a fluid in a cavity, or matter that penetrates through vessel walls, into adjoining tissue
facilitation: a neuron state that is above resting potential but below threshold value and very receptive to a stimulus
facultative intracellular parasites: organisms that are able to survive and grow within macrophages and emerge to infect the host
falx cerebi: extension of the dura mater between the cerebral hemispheres
fast pain: rapid transmission of nerve impulse along A-delta fibers. Felt as a sharp, stinging, pinprick sensation

fast-twitch fibers: type of anaerobic muscle fiber that has explosive power and fatigues easily
feedback—negative and positive: feedback is the process of self-regulation by which open systems determine and control the amount of input and output of the system. Negative feedback refers to returning to a state of equilibrium, whereas positive feedback indicates movement away from equilibrium
ferritin: form of storage iron in the body tissues
fibrin degradation products (FDPs): the result of the degradation of fibrin by plasmin. These products have an antithrombotic action and block fibrin-binding sites, thereby dissolving a clot
fibroadenoma: a benign breast neoplasm
flagellates: a classification of protozoa that have flagella or undulating membranes
flail chest: asynchronous chest wall movement due to fracture of several adjacent ribs
folliculitis: bacterial infection that originates in the hair follicle
furuncles: boils; frequently develop from a preceding staphylococcal folliculitis
gamete: a mature reproductive cell containing the haploid number of chromosomes ($n = 23$). In males, the spermatozoon; in females, the ovum
gametogenesis: a series of mitotic and meiotic divisions occurring in the gonads that lead to the production of gametes. In males, spermatogenesis; in females, oogenesis. Reduction in the number of chromosomes ($2n \rightarrow n$) during gametogenesis occurs in the first meiotic division (meiosis I)
ganglia: groups of neurons outside the central nervous system
ganglioglioma: a rare tumor composed of neuroglial tissue
gap or nexus junctions: specialized membrane junctions that are composed of proteins that form pores connecting adjacent cells and allow for rapid exchange of small molecules or ions between cells
gastrinomas: gastin-producing tumors of the stomach, duodenum, or pancreas
gastritis: an inflammation of the gastric mucosa
gastroesophageal reflux: movement of gastric contents into the esophagus
gene: a segment of nucleic acid that contains genetic information necessary to control a certain function, such as the synthesis of a polypeptide (structural gene). This segment is often referred to as a site, or locus, on a chromosome
generalized seizures: seizures involving both cerebral hemispheres, resulting in a variable period of unconsciousness
genetic counseling: the process by which genetic information is given to clients and their families. Such information about a genetic disease may include its natural history, risk figures, and management
genetic engineering: the processes involved in gene manipulation through recombinant DNA technology
genome: the individual's genetic material, often applied to the chromosome complement
genotype: the genetic constitution of an individual at any given locus
germinoma: a germ cell tumor found in the pineal and hypothalamic region
Ghon complex: a calcified lung tissue lesion that develops after infection with *Mycobacterium tuberculosis*
giant cells: large multinucleated cells often seen in granulomatous reactions; result from fusion of macrophages
gigantism: a condition of abnormal size or overgrowth of the entire body; often due to excessive growth hormone from pituitary before closure of epiphypes
gingivitis: inflamation of the borders surrounding the teeth
glaucoma: a group of eye diseases characterized by an increase in intraocular pressure, which results in atrophy of the optic nerve and may result in blindness. The two types of glaucoma are chronic simple and acute glaucoma
glioblastoma: extremely malignant, highly vascular tumors that frequently arise from undifferentiated astrocytomas
gliosis: an inflammatory or necrotic condition characterized by loss of neurons with a relative increase in glial cells
global aphasia: impairment of expressive and receptive speech, involving both Broca's and Wernicke's areas; caused by large lesions or disruption of blood through blood vessels serving these regions
glomerular blood hydrostatic pressure (GBHP): the pressure exerted by blood pressure in the glomerular capillary. This pressure promotes filtration
glomerular filtrate: a fluid, similar to plasma but nearly free of protein that passes from the glomerulus into Bowman's capsule of the nephron as the first step in urine formation
glomerular filtration rate: The rate of formation of glomerular filtrate, usually expressed in milliliters per minute
glomerulonephritis: a condition that primarily damages the glomeruli. It may be acute or chronic. There are many forms of acute glomerulonephritis, all of which can lead to chronic glomerulonephritis
glomerulus: a capillary tuft in the kidney that, along with Bowman's capsule, forms the renal corpuscle

glucagon: a pancreatic hormone that initiates the release of glucose by the liver

glucagonomas: a glucagon-secreting tumor

glucocorticoids: usually, a steroid hormone, especially cortisol

gluconeogenesis: a process by which the liver synthesizes glucose from noncarbohydrate substances, especially proteins

glycogen: the storage form of glucose in the liver

glycogenesis: promotion of the storage of glycogen when blood glucose levels are increased

glycogenolysis: breakdown of glycogen (stored carbohydrate) to glucose

glycolysis: the metabolism of glucose

goiter: enlargement of thyroid gland caused by hyperplasia of thyroid follicles

goitrogens: substances that can cause goiter formation

granulation tissue: precursor to scar tissue formed from injured tissue. Connective tissue that will become a scar

granulocytes: classification of white blood cells that have staining granules in their cytoplasm; a polymorphonuclear leukocyte (neutrophil, eosinophil, or basophil)

granuloma: an inflammatory lesion composed of granulation tissue

granulomatous disease: chronic inflammatory reactions characterized by persistent lesions containing mononuclear phagocytes

granulomatous hypersensitivity response: usually a reaction to persistent infectious agents that produces chronic inflammation, with a central area of macrophages fused into multinucleate giant cells, surrounded by T lymphocytes

granulomatous inflammation: a type of chronic inflammation characterized by the accumulation of modified macrophages and initiated by either infectious or noninfectious agents. The most predominant example is tuberculosis

hair shaft: the path a hair travels to emerge at the skin line

hallucinations: sensory perceptions occurring while awake that do not result from external stimuli

haploid: the number of chromosomes present in a gamete. Also, a cell that contains one copy of each chromosome. The haploid number (n) in humans is 23. The diploid number of chromosomes (46) is reconstituted in the zygote on fertilization of two haploid gametes

hapten: a molecule that cannot elicit an adaptive immune response until it is linked to a protein carrier. It then can become fully antigenic and elicit antibody and T-cell response

haptoglobin: a group of globulins in human serum that can combine with hemoglobin

Heberden's nodes: hard nodules or enlargement of the tubercles of the last joint of the fingers, seen in osteoarthritis

HELLP syndrome: severe preeclampsia characterized by hemolysis, elevated liver enzymes, and low platelet counts

helper T cell (T-h, T4, $CD4^+$ T cells): a population of T lymphocytes that display the CD4 antigen and secrete lymphokines necessary to cell-mediated (Th1) and humoral (Th2) immune responses. Thus, helper T cells are highly regulatory and their lymphokines coordinate various functions in the immune system

hemachromatosis: a disorder of iron metabolism characterized by excessive absorption of iron and deposition of hemosiderin in tissue

hemangioblastoma: a tumor made up of an aggregation of blood vessels that occurs most commonly in the cerebellum but also possibly in the cerebrum

hemangioma: benign tumor of newly formed blood vessels

hematogenous spread: spread of infection or malignancy via the bloodstream

hematopoiesis: the formation of the blood cells

hemianopia: blindness for half of the field of vision in one or both eyes

hemiparesis: muscular weakness in one half of the body

hemizygous: a condition in which an allele is present in a single copy. Males are hemizygous for all markers located on the X chromosome

hemoglobin: complex spheric molecule found in red blood cells that is made up of four heme groups; carries oxygen

hemorrhagic stroke: disruption of cerebral blood flow resulting from hemorrhage from rupture of parenchymal blood vessels, aneurysms, or arteriovenous malformations. Hypertension is the major cause of hemorrhagic strokes

heparin cofactor II: an enzyme inhibitor that resembles antithrombin III

hepatic encephalopathy: alteration in the neurologic status in persons with significant liver damage

hepatitis: a condition of inflammation and injury of the liver cells

hepatocytes: cells located in the parenchyma of the liver that process many substances in the organelles

herald patch: scaly lesion observed before the rash in pityriasis rosea

Hering-Breuer reflex: an intrinsic lung reflex that prevents overstretching

heterozygote: an individual who has two different alleles at a given locus on a pair of homologous chromosomes. For example, in the case of the *HexA* gene, above, +/– (or Hh)

hiatal hernia: a condition in which a part of the stomach protrudes through the opening of the diaphragm

histamine: a substance released by tissue cells that causes vasodilation, capillary permeability, and smooth muscle contraction

histocompatibility antigens: normal components of self that are genetically determined. It is important to test for these antigens in the transplantation of organs to prevent rejection of foreign material

HIV (human immune deficiency virus): non-oncogenic, cytopathic, retrovirus of the lentivirus subfamily with specificity for $CD4^+$ cells and whose long-term infection results in the progressive immune suppression characteristic of HIV disease and AIDS (acquired immune deficiency syndrome)

HIV nephropathy: a syndrome of renal impairment associated with infection by the human immunodeficiency virus (HIV)

homeostasis: the state of balance in the human body of chemical and fluids; the processes by which equilibrium is maintained

homocysteine: a sulfur-containing amino acid produced from the metabolism of methionine

homologous: refers to chromosomes with matching genes, or to those genes individually

hormone: substance that exerts a physiologic effect on other cells. Hormones are classified as peptides and proteins, amines and amino acids, and steroids

host: the larger organism that a pathogenic microorganism typically attaches to

hyaline: any alterations within cells or in the extracellular spaces that gives the appearance of a glassy, pink, homeogenous substance

hydatidiform mole: a benign, but potentially premalignant, growth that develops from abnormal fertilization

hydrocele: accumulation of fluid in the tunica vaginalis of the testis

hydrocephalus: increased quantity of CSF within the cerebral ventricular system resulting in enlarged or dilated ventricles and increased intracranial pressure

hydrogen hemoglobin: hemoglobin carrying an hydrogen ion

hydrophilic: a term for something that tends to associate with water

hydrophobic: a term for something that tends to repel water

hydrosalpinx: accumulation of serous fluid in the uterine tube

hypercalcemia: an elevated concentration of calcium ions in the blood

hypercalciuria: excretion of abnormally large amounts of calcium in the urine

hypercapnia: an increased pressure of carbon dioxide (greater than 45 mmHg) in arterial circulation

hypercystinuria: excretion of excessive amounts of cystine in urine

hyperkeratotic warts: an overgrowth of the horny layer of the epidermis, often seen in aged skin

hyperopia: parallel light rays focusing past the retina (farsightedness)

hyperoxaluria: presence of large amounts of oxalic acid (oxalates) in the urine

hyperparathyroidism: increased secretion of parathyroid hormone resulting in hypercalcemia

hyperplasia: an increased number of normal functioning cells

hypersensitivity reactions: states of heightened reactivity to antigens. They are genetically determined and cause symptomatic reactions on second exposure

hypertension: increase in blood pressure; usually refers to systemic arterial blood pressure

hypertonic fluid: fluid that contains a higher concentration of osmotically active particles than blood plasma and causes the red blood cells to shrink and shrivel

hypertrophy: an increase in the size of an individual cell; especially seen in mucle fibers. It may be physiologic as in muscle building or pathologic, as in cardiac hypertrophy

hyperuricemia: increased serum concentrations of uric acid

hyperuricosuria: increased concentration of uric acid in urine

hypervolemia: extracellular fluid volume excess

hypocapnia: a decreased pressure of carbon dioxide (less than 35 mmHg) in arterial circulation

hypocitraturia: decreased citrate excretion. Is associated with formation of calcium urinary stones

hypogeusia: a diminished sense of taste; may occur as part of the aging process

hypokinesis: in the heart, this refers to a decrease in the normal contractility of the myocardium. It may be due to ischemia, infarction, heart failure, or cardiomyopathies

hypomania: a less intense form of mania

hypospadias: congenital anomaly in which the urethra opens on the ventral surface of the penis

hypothalamic-pituitary-adrenal axis: a functional, neuroendocrine system that regulates the body's response to stress; composed of the hypothalamus, anterior pituitary, and adrenal glands

hypothalamus: located anterior to the brain stem; this structure controls appetite (hunger and satiety) and water balance, as well as regulates sexual function and temperature

hypothyroidism: decreased function of thyroid gland exhibited by decreased thyroid hormones
hypotonic fluid: fluid that contains a lower concentration of osmotically active particles that result in swelling and hemolysis of the red blood cells
hypovolemia: extracellular fluid volume deficit
hypoxemic: low oxygen level in blood ($PaO_2 < 50$ mmHg)
iatrogenic infection: an infection caused by medical personnel
ileum: the distal portion of the small intestine, which lies between the jejunum and the cecum
immunity: the process of protection of the body on a cellular level from agents that are foreign or potentially harmful to it; includes innate, nonspecific responses as well as the specific, adapative responses
immunocompetent cells: those cells that can recognize and react with antigen; usually referring to the cells of the specific immune responses (B and T lympohcytes)
immunocyte: cells that carry out specific immune functions; include T and B lymphocytes
immunogenicity: a molecule capable of stimulating an antigenic response. Often used to describe transplanted tissue
impetigo: bacterial infection that occurs superficially on skin
impotence: inability to achieve or maintain an erection
infarction: necrosis of an area due to lack of arterial or venous blood supply. In the heart, myocardial infarction refers to irreversible death of myocardium
infections: multiplication of parasitic organisms within the body
infertility: inability to conceive after 1 year of unprotected intercourse
inotropic state: refers to the contractility of the myocardium, with a positive inotropic state being one of increased contractility, whereas a negative inotropic state is one of decreased contractility
insufficiency (regurgitation): inability of the cardiac valves to close properly
insulin resistance: impaired biologic response by the tissues to endogenous or exogenous insulin. This impairment alters carbohydrate, protein, and fat metabolism
insulinitis: inflammation of cells of the islands of Langerhans that may result from viral infection
insulinomas: an islet cell adenoma that secrets insulin
intercalated disks: the tight junctions between cardiac cells that allow impulses to pass rapidly from one cell to the next
interferon: a family of antiviral proteins that inhibits viral spread from cell to cell
interleukins (IL): a group of cytokines produced by macrophages (eg, IL-1) and T cells (eg, IL-2, MAF, MIF) that modulate the activation, proliferation, and differentiation of various immune cells
intermittent claudication: characteristic pain of ischemic extremities; described as severe cramping on exercise and relieved by rest
interstitial edema: a type of edema in which fluid collects in intestitial tissue; may occur with cerebral tissues, lung, or systemic tissues. Cerebral edema can result from noncommunicating hydrocephalus
interstitial nephritis: disorders of the renal tubules and interstitium. It can be either acute or chronic
intracerebral hematoma: traumatic or spontaneous disruption of cerebral blood vessels within the parenchyma, potentially resulting in focal neurologic deficits
intraductal papilloma: a benign growth within the ducts of the breast; may cause nipple discharge
intramedullary intradural tumor: intraspinal tumor arising from the substance of the spinal cord
intrapleural pressure: pressure within pleural space
intrapulmonic pressure: pressure within the lung tissue
intrinsic factor: a glycoprotein secreted by the parietal cells of the gastric mucosa that binds to vitamin B_{12} to protect it from the digestive enzymes
ischemia: deprivation of tissue of blood and oxygen due to lack of blood supply to an area. It is a reversible condition that may progress to infarction if not relieved
ischemic damage: residual tissue damage from chronic ischemia
ischemic edema: cytotoxic and vasogenic cerebral edema associated with strokes
ischemic neuropathy: alterations in sensations of the extremities due to ischemia; there may be pain or paresthesias
ischemic stroke: cessation of cerebral blood flow to a region of the brain as a result of occlusion by thrombosis or emboli, leading to a cascade of detrimental biochemical, molecular, and cellular changes
isotonic fluid: fluids with the same osmotic pressure as serum, in which the cells will neither swell or shrink
jaundice: a yellowish staining of the skin, sclerae, and deeper tissues with bilirubin that is increased in the plasma
jejunum: the middle portion of the small intestine, which lies between the duodenum and the ileum
juxtaglomerular apparatus cells: a set of specialized cells in the nephron and adjacent capillaries that produce the hormone renin

karyotype: the chromosome constitution of an individual represented by a laboratory-made display in which chromosomes are arranged by size and centromere position

keloids: scar formation in the skin following trauma or surgical incision. Tissue response is out of proportion to the amount of scar tissue required for normal repair and healing. The result is a raised, firm, thickened red scar that may grow for a prolonged period of time. The increase in scar size is due to deposition of an abnormal amount of collagen into the tissues

keratocanthoma: benign nodule that resembles squamous cell carcinoma

keratinization: development of the keratin layer of skin

kernicterus: a condition that results from high levels of unconjugated bilirubin passing through the blood-brain barrier in infants. Causes degenerative lesions in basal ganglia and leads to mental retardation

ketosis: the accumulation of ketones caused by the rapid oxidation of fatty acids

kinin system: a general term for a group of polypeptides that have considerable biologic activity. They are capable of influencing smooth muscle contraction; inducing hypotension; increasing the blood flow and permeability of small blood capillaries; and inciting pain

koilonychia: deformation of the fingernails in which they appear thin and concave, often associated with iron deficiency anemia

Kupffer cells: part of the mononuclear phagocyte system; these cells remove bacteria from the portal venous blood

Kussmaul's breathing: rapid, gasping, deep respirations associated with diabetic (metabolic) acidosis

kyphoscoliosis: abnormal curvature of the spine and thoracic cage

kyphosis: a spinal deformity characterized by extensive flexion, as in humpback appearance

labile cells: cells that normally regenerate frequently

lactate: (1) a salt or ester of lactic acid; (2) to produce milk in the mammary gland

lactic acidosis: metabolic acidosis caused by accumulation of lactic acid, usually due to hypoxic condition

laminar flow: streamlined air flow through a tube

latent infection: episodes of disease that are interrupted by periods of no disease manifestation or infectivity

leukemoid reaction: a reaction characterized by leukocytosis like that occurring in leukemia but is not the result of leukemia

leukocidins: antiphagocytic substances secreted by certain bacteria that destroy phagocytes

leukocytosis: increased white blood cell count, often seen in infections

leukotrienes: a group of arachidonic acid metabolites that function as chemical mediators of inflammation. They are extremely powerful bronchial constrictors and vasodilators, and mediate the adverse vascular and bronchial effects of systemic anaphylaxis

Lewy bodies: spherical eosinophilic cytoplasmic inclusions in Parkinson's disease and other degenerative diseases

ligament: fibrous tissue that connects bones to bone or to cartilage

ligands: substances that bind selectively to cell-surface receptors for movement into the cell membrane channels or pores

limbic system: a more primitive portion of the brain that consists of the amygdala, the hippocampus, and the septal nuclei. It is associated with sexual behavior and the emotions of rage, fear, and motivation

linoleic acid: an essential fatty acid 18 carbons in length with two double bonds. The first double bond is located at the sixth carbon from the methyl end. This fatty acid is also considered an omega 6 fatty acid

lipase: a pancreatic enzyme that hydrolyzes fats, yielding glycerol and fatty acids

lipogenesis: the production of fats and lipids

lipolysis: the metabolism of fats and lipids

lipoproteins: a protein in which lipids form an integral part; mainly synthesized by the liver and the main way that lipids circulate in the plasma

locus: the chromosome location of a specific gene (site)

loop of Henle: a portion of the nephron active in the concentration of urine

lower motor neuron lesions: lesions of the cranial or spinal nerves and their nuclei that result in flaccid paralysis

lunula: the pale, arched area of base of nail plate

lymph: an alkaline fluid (usually transparent) that is found in the lymphatic vessels

lymphadenitis: inflammation of the lymph nodes

lymphadenopathy: enlarged lymph nodes. Nodes may be tender or nontender, movable, or fixed

lymphangitis: inflammation of lymph vessels

lymphocytes: the primary cells of the specific, adaptive, immune response; includes the classes of T lymphocytes and B lymphocytes

lymphocytosis: increased lymphocyte count that is often seen in chronic infections

major depression: synonymous with unipolar disorder

major histocompatability complex (the human leukocyte antigens): that portion of the genetic code within an individual that allows for immunocompetent cells to distinguish self-cells from non-self cells and thus to react only to foreign antigen

maladaptation: a disruptive disordering of the physiologic response

malformation: a primary morphologic defect occurring as a result of abnormal mo [illegible]

malignant: abnormal cell division wit [illegible] to invade, metastasize, and recur

malignant melanoma: malignant canc [illegible] from the melanin-producing cells

mania: a mood disorder characterized b [illegible] hyperexcitability, agitation, and overtal [illegible]

manic-depression: synonymous with bi [illegible] disorder

margination: the process by which phag [illegible] to the lining of blood vessels

mass effect: effect of a substance such as b [illegible] abscess, or edema that compresses surrou [illegible] tissue and causes possible neurologic defic [illegible]

mastitis: inflammation of breast tissue

maximal oxygen uptake (VO_2): functional [illegible] of a person's physical fitness; also called aer [illegible] capacity

mediastinum: space between lungs; houses, [illegible] airways, and lymphatics

medullary bone: central area of cancellous bone

medulloblastoma: a tumor derived primarily from the primitive cells in the cerebellum

megakaryocytes: large cells with single or multiple nuclei that give rise to platelets

meiosis: a reductional type of cell division, in which the chromosome number is halved. In humans, meiosis is one of the processes that lead to the formation of haploid gametes (n = 23)

melanin: a pigment found in the skin and hair

melanocytes: cells that originate in the basal layer of the epidermis and hair follicles, which synthesize pigment granules that give color to skin and hair

melatonin: a hormone secreted by the pineal gland that inhibits numerous endocrine functions and causes drowsiness

melena: the description of black tarry feces due to the action of intestinal secretions on free blood

mendelian inheritance: the mode of inheritance of single-gene traits. Term derived from Gregor Mendel, the pioneer of genetics

meninges: coverings of the brain composed of the dura mater, arachnoid mater, and pia mater

meningioma: a primary, extramedullary tumor that grows from the arachnoid membrane of the meninges

meningocele: a cystlike protrusion consisting of the meninges and CSF

menopause: the last menstrual period

mesencephalon: the midbrain region of the brain that connects the diencephalon with the pons and other lower structures

MET (metabolic equivalent): a measure used to determine the amount of energy expended during activity. 1 MET equals 50 Kcals per hour per square meter of body surface

metacentric chromosome: a group of chromosomes in which the centromere is placed approximately in the midpoint of the chromosome, resulting in arms of approximately equal length. Human chromosomes A(1), A(3), and E(16) exemplify this condition

[illegible]etaphase: the second stage of mitosis in which the pairs of chromatids align in a plane midway between the poles

[illegible]taphysis: location of the epiphyseal growth plate [illegible]n bone

[illegible]tastasis: ability to establish secondary tumor [illegible]owth at a new location away from the primary [illegible]mor

[illegible]hemoglobin: a form of hemoglobin generated [illegible] oxidation of the iron molecules to the ferric [illegible]te; has a very high oxygen affinity and does not [illegible]w oxygen to be delivered to the tissues

[illegible]onine: an essential amino acid, a sulfur-[illegible]ing compound

[illegible]locorticoids: a steroid hormone of adernal cortex that influences salt metabolism; aldosterone

mitosis: type of equational cell division in which the resulting daughter cells have the same number of chromosomes as the mother cell

modulation: modification of the pain transmission involving activation of descending nerve pathways that exert inhibitory effects on pain transmission

molecular mimicry: polypeptide sequence of a foreign antigen mimics (or is similar to) self-proteins.

monocyte-macrophage system (mononuclear phagocyte system; MPS): mononuclear phagocytic cells and tissues that participate in inflammation and immunity

monocytosis: increased monocyte count often seen in chronic infections

monorchidism: unilateral cryptorchidism

monosomy: the aneuploid condition of having a chromosome represented by a single copy in a somatic cell, ie, the absence of a chromosome from a given pair. Generally, monosomies are not compatible with life, except in the case of a missing X chromosome in Turner's syndrome (45, X0)

morbidity: a disease condition or state

morula: the mass of cells resulting from the early cleavage divisions of the zygote

mosaicism: the condition that results in an individual (mosaic) with two or more genetically different cell populations

mucociliary escalator system: defensive apparatus found in airways composed of mucous, cilia, and mucus secreting goblet cells found in the bronchi

multifactorial inheritance: the heritability of traits that result from interactions between genetic and environmental factors

multiple organ dysfunction syndrome: progressive loss of function in two or more organs; a sequela to a major body insult, such as shock

muscle fiber: muscle cell that contains myofibrils, the contractile units of muscles

mutation: an abrupt alteration in an individual that is transmitted to the offspring

mycosis (mycoses): fungal infections that may be systemic, subcutaneous, or superficial

myelin sheath: lipoprotein structure that insulates nerves

myelomeningocele: cystlike protrusion consisting of meninges, CSF, and a portion of the spinal cord

myeloproliferative disorders: conditions characterized by unusual proliferation of myelopoietic tissue

myocardial depressant factor: a general term for cytokine and secondary mediators that cause diminished myocardial contractility

myocardial oxygen consumption: the amount of oxygen consumed related to the amount of stress or tension developed in the ventricular wall

myocardial work: the amount of wall tension generated during systole to cause the ejection of blood

myoglobin: the oxygen-transporting and storage protein of muscle, similar to hemoglobin

myopathy: primary abnormality of muscles from inflammation and other causes

myopia: parallel light rays focus in front of the retina; nearsightedness

myosin: thick muscle myofilament that contains cross-bridges to connect with actin for muscle contraction

myositis: inflammation of muscle tissue

myotome: skeletal muscle innervation by a specific spinal root motor axon

myxedema: hypothyroidism characterized by decreased basal metabolism rate, edema, somnolence, slow mentation, and other symptoms

nabothian cyst: inclusion cyst formed when cervical glands are blocked; usually due to chronic inflammation (cervicitis)

natural killer (NK) cells: a subset of large granular lymphocytes, which are neither T nor B lymphocytes (null cells). NK cells respond to helper T-cell stimulation (via IL-2) and are capable of killing, by cell-to-cell cytotoxicity, malignant tumor cells, virus-infected cells, and cells infected with other endogenous parasites

near point: the closest point at which a person can clearly focus on an object

negative feedback: closed feedback loop whereby an elevated level in a specific hormone feeds back to its initiating signal to decrease further release. Most common mechanism is regulative hormone levels in the blood

negative nitrogen balance: a condition in which more nitrogen is lost than is consumed in food protein, which indicates that body tissue is breaking down faster than it is being replaced

nematodes: roundworms of the helminth classification

neocortex: specialized cortical region of the brain that is concerned with memory, learning, and the control of intellectual functions

neoplasia: abnormal cellular growth that is unresponsive to normal growth control mechanisms

neoplasm: a group or clump of neoplastic cells

nephritic disease: inflammation of the kidney, or parts of the kidney. Also called nephritis

nephritis: inflammation of the kidney, or parts of the kidney. Also called nephritic disease

nephrogenic diabetes insipidus: loss of renal responsiveness to antidiuretic hormone (ADH), resulting in the ability to concentrate urine and conserve water.

nephrolithiasis: calculi formation in the renal pelvis or calices

nephron: the functional unit of the kidney composed of the proximal convoluted tubule, the loop of Henle (in medullary nephrons), and the distal convoluted tubule

nephrosis: degeneration of kidney structures causing loss of protein in the urine and subsequent edema. Also called nephrotic syndrome

net bacterial clearance: rate of bacterial killing or removal exceeds the rate of bacterial growth

net filtration pressure (NFP): The effective pressure for formation of glomerular filtrate; the sum of all forces that promote filtration minus the forces that oppose filtration

neurilemmoma (schwannoma): a tumor derived from cells that ensheath cranial nerves, peripheral nerves, cauda equina, and nerve roots; cell types include Schwann cells, perineural cells, and fibroblasts

neuritic or senile plaque: core of amyloid beta-peptide surrounded by degenerated neurons, dendrites, and axons found in Alzheimer's disease, Down Syndrome, and to a much lesser extent, normal aging

neuroendocrine axis: the negative feedback relationship between the hypothalamus, the anterior pituitary gland, and the target organ

neurofibrillary tangles (NFTs): intracellular inclusions appearing as bundles and strands through the cytoplasm in the brains of persons with Alzheimer's and other degenerative diseases; consisting of paired helical filaments formed by hyperphosphorylation of tau protein

neurofibrils: delicate threads projecting into the axon from the cell body

neurofibroma: extramedullary tumor that grows in the nerve root and often forms an hourglass-like expansion that extends into the extradural space

neurogenic pain: severe, sharp pain due to altered nervous system function associated with neural injury along the course of a nerve within the peripheral or central nervous system

neuroglia: supporting structure to neurons of the central nervous system

neuroglycopenia: insufficient glucose for normal central nervous system function

neuroleptics: a class of antipsychotic drugs used to reduce agitation and psychotic symptoms of schizophrenia

neuron: functional and structural unit of the nervous system

neurotransmitter: substances released by the presynaptic neuron that has the potential to excite or inhibit the postsynaptic neuron

neutrophilia: an increased neutrophil count, seen in acute bacterial infections

nociception: activation of pain fibers and subsequent neural and reflex responses to noxious stimuli involving the four components of transduction, transmission, perception, and modulation

nociceptor: specialized group of sensory receptors (free nerve endings) responsible for transmitting painful stimuli

nocturia: excessive urination at night

noncardiogenic pulmonary edema: flooding of alveoli and lung tissue with fluid, resulting in impaired gas exchange secondary to toxic exposure, aspiration, infections, and other noncardiac conditions

nondisjunction: failure of homologous chromosomes or chromatids to separate properly during anaphase meiosis I and II, or mitosis, resulting in daughter cells with unequal chromosome numbers. Meiotic nondisjunction may result in gametes with abnormal chromosome number, which on fertilization, may produce aneuploidy. Mitotic nondisjunction occurring in a developing embryo may result in mosaicism

nonrapid eye movement sleep (NREM): a period of time of sleep characterized by slow regular respiration, absence of body movement, slow regular brain activity. It is one of four progressive stages of deep sleep

nontoxic goiter: diffuse enlargement of thyroid gland that involves the entire gland, with the follicles filled with colloid

nonvesicular hormone secretion: transport of hormone within the cell directly across the plasma membrane by a specific transporter or by diffusion

norepinephrine: a hormone released from the adrenal medulla that elevates blood pressure by constricting peripheral vessels, reduces gastric secretions, and dilates pupils

nosocomial infection: infection caused by exposure in the hospital or other medical setting

nuclei: (1) mass of protoplasm surrounded by a nuclear envelope containing chromosomes; (2) clusters of neurons within the central nervous system

nucleoplasm: the cytosol that resides within the nuclear envelope

obsessions: a recurrent, persistent thought or idea involuntarily arising and preoccupying a person

oculocephalic reflex: movement of the eyes in the opposite direction with head deviation, indicating intact brain stem structures in a coma patient

oculovestibular reflex: reflex response that results in nystagmus deviation of both eyes toward an irrigated ear, indicating intact brain stem structures

oligodendroglioma: a tumor derived from oligodendrocytic cells; vinelike processes present throughout the central nervous system

oncogene: a gene or group of genes, usually involved in cell division, whose malfunction (eg, a mutation) results in malignant transformation

oncogenic viruses: those viruses that have some relationship to the etiology of certain cancers

onycholysis: loosening of the nail usually beginning at the free border and incomplete

opioid system: an endogenous group of peptides that have analgesic properties, behavioral effects, and neurotransmitter and neuromodulator functions. Examples include are endorphins, enkephalins, and dynorphin

opportunistic infections: infections caused by organisms that are capable of causing disease only when the host resistance is lowered

opsonin: a substance that coats foreign antigens, making them more susceptible to macrophages and other leukocytes, thus increasing phagocytosis of the organism. Complement and antibodies are the two main opsonins in human blood

opsonization: the chemical targeting of antigen, usually by antibodies secreted from plasma cell, so it can be easily identified and engulfed by phagocytic cells

optic disk: physiologic blind spot

orchitis: inflammation of a testis

osmolality: the ionic concentration of plasma, expressed in osmoles of solute particles per kilogram of solvent
osmosis: the net diffusion of water through a selectively permeable membrane that separates two solutions with different solute concentrations. The water will diffuse toward the area of greater solute concentration
osmotic diuresis: excessive loss of water in urine due to osmotic gradient produced by a solute
osmotic pressure: the pressure created as water moves through the membrane toward the area of greater solute concentration. The magnitude depends on the number of particles in the solution toward which the water is moving
osteoarthritis: a type of arthritis characterized by progressive cartilage deterioration in the synovial joints and vertebrae
osteoblast: bone-forming cell
osteoclast: macrophage cells used in bone resorption
osteocytes: calcified cells involved in bone structure
osteomyelitis: an acute or chronic infection of the bone
osteopathy: any disease of bone
osteoporosis: loss of bone mass that interferes with the skeletal support of the body
oxidative phosphorylation: an aerobic reaction within the cellular mitochondria that provides the major supply of energy
oxyhemoglobin: form of hemoglobin when it is attached to oxygen
oxyhemoglobin dissociation curve: curve that plots the affinity of hemoglobin for oxygen
pain threshold: the point at which a stimulus is perceived as pain
pain tolerance: the highest amount of pain that one can tolerate
pancytopenia: a decrease in all of the bone marrow elements causing a decrease in all of the blood count numbers; usually due to severe suppression of the bone marrow
pandemic: a worldwide epidemic, such as acquired immune deficiency syndrome or certain flu outbreaks
pannus: a membrane of granulation tissue covering a normal surface. Seen in the articular cartilages in rheumatoid arthritis and in chronic granulomatous disease such as tuberculosis
papilledema: swelling of the optic disk; often seen with cerebral edema and increased intracranial pressure
paradoxical movement: abnormal movements of chest wall, opposite of those seen during normal ventilation
paraneoplastic syndrome: a systemic manifestation of malignant disease that is not directly related to invasion by the primary tumor or its metastases
paraphimosis: inability to return the foreskin to its normal position after it has been retracted
paraplegia: voluntary motor loss of lower extremities resulting from lesions of the thoracic and lumbar spinal cord
parapneumonic effusion: pleural effusion associated with pneumonia
paraproteinemias: the presence of abnormal immunoglobulins in the serum of persons with plasma cell dyscrasias
parasitism: the relationship between the host and a pathogenic microorganism
parasomnias: undersirable physical activities that occur during sleep or are exacerbated by sleep
paresthesias: a sensation of numbness, prickling or tingling of the body, especially the face hand and feet
parietal cells: cells in the stomach that secrete hydrochloric acid and possibly the intrinsic factor
partial seizures: seizures arising from a focal area in the brain
pathogen: an organism that can, under certain circumstances, produce a disease state in the host
pavementing: condition occuring during inflammation in which leukocytes adhere to the linings of capillaries
pectus carinatum (pigeon chest): abnormal bowing out deformity of the sternum and thoracic cage
pectus excavatum (funnel chest): depression deformity of lower sternum
pelvic inflammatory disease (PID): inflammation, usually due to infection, or upper genital tract structures (uterus, oviducts, ovaries, peritoneum)
penile carcinoma: malignant neoplasm of the penis; usually squamous cell carcinoma of glans or prepuce, or both
perception: processes involved in recognizing, defining, and responding to pain
perceptual dominance: pain that coexists in two areas, but the pain threshold for one location is higher than that of the other. When the more painful area is treated and pain is resolved, the second site becomes more painful
perfusion: blood flow through the tissues
perifolliculitis: inflammatory condition around the hair follicles
periosteum: hard outer covering of bone
peristalsis: waves of coordinated and rhythmic muscular contractions that force food to move through the alimentary canal

peritoneum: a serous membrane that lines the entire abdominal cavity. Consists of the parietal and visceral peritoneum

permanent cells: cells of the body that do not undergo mitosis

Peyronie's disease: idiopathic fibrosis of penile corpora cavernosa; produces painful erection

pH: the degree of acidity of alkalinity of a solution, in which below 7 is acid and above 7 is alkaline. In the arterial circulation, it is expressed as an alkaline number of a narrow range, 7.35 to 7.45

phagocytes: white blood cells whose purpose is to ingest and destroy foreign substances; includes neutrophils and macrophages

pharmacokinetic factors: the disposition of a drug in the body. Used to adjust dosage levels to maximum therapeutic results with minimal toxic effects

phenotype: any observable or measurable expression of gene function in an individual. For instance, eye color, and hemoglobin type are phenotypic expressions of specific genes

pheomelanin: amount and distribution of melanin that produces yellow color

phimosis: inability to retract the foreskin over the glans

phobia: an anxiety disorder characterized by irrational and intense fear of a physical situation (flying, heights), social activity (public speaking), or an object (blood, spiders, dogs)

Pick bodies: paired helical filaments formed by hyperphosphorylated tau protein (PHFtau)

pickwickian syndrome: syndrome of hypoventilation due to obesity

pilosebaceous ducts: involving hair follicles and sebaceous glands of the skin

pituitary adenoma: a special group of nervous system tumors that produces neurologic signs and symptoms from pressure on the hypothalamus, optic chiasm, third ventricle, and medial temporal lobe

pityriasis rosea: self-limiting acute disease of the skin, characterized by a herald patch, followed by pruritic smaller lesions

plasminogen activator inhibitor–1: an inhibitor of plasmin that prevents excess fibrinolysis

pleomorphic: refers to cells that can assume different shapes

pleural effusion: excess accumulation of fluid within the pleural space

pleuritis: inflammation of the pleura

pluripotential stem cells: cells in the bone marrow that can differentiate into various blood cell lines depending on the stimulation

pneumothorax: collapse of lung due to entry of air into the pleural space

polycythemia: an excessive number of red blood cells; often used interchangeably with erythrocytosis

polydipsia: excessive thirst

polygenic: referring to a trait whose phenotypic expression results from the cooperation of various genes

polyp: a growth on mucous membranes

polyphagia: excessive appetite and eating

polyploidy: chromosome abnormality in which the diploid chromosome number of a cell varies by increments of 23. For example, a triploid cell or individual would have 69 chromosomes (46 + 23); a tetraploid would have 92 (46 + 23 + 23)

polyuria: excessive excretion of urine

pores of Kohn: small openings between alveoli that allow collateral ventilation

porphyrin structure (heme): pigments that are important in biosynthesis of heme portion of hemoglobin

positive feedback: feedback loop in which a specific hormone stimulates increased secretion of the same or related hormone

preeclampsia: a progressive complication of pregnancy in which hypertension, proteinuria, and edema become progressively severe. It is a major cause of maternal morbidity and death

pregnancy induced hypertension (PIH): a complication of pregnancy characterized by systemic hypertension, proteinuria, and edema. It can progress to preeclampsia and the HELLP syndrome

preleukemic syndrome: like myelodysplastic syndrome, a proliferation of abnormal stem cells in the bone marrow that has the potential of developing into a specific type of leukemia

preload: the amount of myocardial stretch at the end of diastole which is related to the volume in the ventricles

presbyopia: a defect of vision related to aging that involves loss of accommodation or recession of the near point. Loss of elasticity of the crystalline lens also occurs

priapism: prolonged, usually painful erection; may lead to impotence

primary brain injury: injury occurring to the brain at the time of a traumatic event, includes diffuse axonal injury, concussion, contusion, and vascular injury

primary tuberculosis: infection with *Mycobacteria tuberculosis* causing an acute inflammatory reaction in lung tissue

prion disease: a group of encephalitis-inducing diseases characterized by a slow onset with a long latent period lasting from months to years before the manifestation of symptoms

procidentia: a prolapse of any organ or part
prolactinomas: a prolactin secreting adenoma
prophase: the first phase of cell division during which the chromatin condenses into distinct chromosomes that are visible as pairs of chromatids, joined at the centromere
prosencephalon: region of the brain encompassing the cerebral hemispheres, basal ganglia, and olfactory tracts
prostacyclin (PGI_2): a prostaglandin that is part of a large group of substances that are metabolites of arachidonic acid
prostaglandins: a large group of biologically active, carbon-20, unsaturated fatty acids that represent some of the metabolites of arachidonic acid. They are local short-range autocoids that are formed rapidly, exert their effects locally, and then decay or are destroyed enzymatically
prostate cancer: malignant neoplasm of the prostate gland; adenocarcinoma
prostate-specific antigen: glycoprotein produced by prostate gland in proportion to prostate mass; useful to diagnose prostate cancer, or other prostate disorders
prostatitis: inflammation of the prostate gland
protein C: a vitamin K–dependent plasma protein that degrades factor Va and VIIIa and functions as a natural anticoagulant
protein S: a vitamin K–dependent plasma protein that serves as a cofactor with protein C inhibiting the conversion reactions at the factor V and VIII levels in the clotting cascade
prothrominase: an enzyme responsible for the conversion of prothrombin to thrombin
protons: a positively charged particle forming the nucleus of hydrogen; present in the nuclei of all elements, with the atomic number indicating the number of protons present
proximal convoluted tubule (PCT): a portion of the nephron active in secretion and reabsorption of substances from the filtrate
pseudohermaphroditism: a state in which the individual has testes or ovaries but the external genitalia are ambiguous
pseudohypoaldosteronism: a syndrome most commonly associated with renal disease in which there is resistance to aldosterone hormonal activity. It is manifested by hyperkalemia and hyponatremia.
pseudotumor cerebri: benign intracranial hypertension of unknown origin associated with CSF increase
psoriasis: chronic, genetically determined epidermal disease that is characterized by sharply marginated erythematous plaques
psychogenic pain: pain whose origin has no physiologic cause
psychogenic polydipsia: increased drinking behavior stimulated by a psychological need
psychoneuroimmunology: a multidisciplinary field of study that proposes a model of ongoing bidirectional interactions between the central nervous, endocrine, and immune systems such that all are modulated by and influencing of the subjective experiences and psychological state of an individual. Thus, the patterns of biologic functioning and psychosocial functioning may be considered as reflections of shared processes
pulse pressure: the difference between the systolic and diastolic blood pressure
pulsus paradoxus: refers to an exaggeration of the normal respiratory fluctuation in systolic blood pressure so that a drop of greater than 10 mmHg is noted during inspiration. It may be seen in large pneumothorax or pericardial effusions, especially cardiac tamponade
pyelonephritis: inflammation of the renal pelvis, usually due to infection
pyothorax: pus in pleural cavity
pyramidal tract: nerve tract controlling voluntary motor activity. See *corticospinal tract*
pyrogenic: organisms that can produce fever and inflammation in the host
pyrogens: any substance that produces fever
quadriplegia: loss of voluntary motor function in upper and lower extremities resulting from cervical cord lesions
rapid eye movement sleep (REM): desynchronized or active sleep characterized by irregular respirations, rapid eye movement, and twitching of face and extremities
recessive: an allele whose phenotypic expression occurs in homozygous or hemizygous conditions. In heterozygosity, a recessive allele is masked by its dominant homologous counterpart. Example, cystic fibrosis
recognition: in immunology, the ability of an immunocompetent cell to determine that it can mount a response to a specific antigen
red blood cell aplasia: failure of regeneration of red blood cells; characterized by severe normocytic, normochromic anemia with no reticulocyte response
red fibers: slow-twitch muscle fibers with high myoglobin content used for sustained muscle activity
Reed-Sternberg cell: cell that specifically indicates the presence of Hodgkin's disease; the cell is thought to be a multinucleated, giant cell mutation of the T lymphocyte
referred pain: pain is felt a distance away from the noxious stimuli
reflex arc: chain of neuronal activity; impulse passes from receptor to effector, resulting in a quick response

refraction: bending of light rays
refractory period: the absolute refractory period is that time of depolarization and contraction of the heart during which it cannot respond to another stimulus. The relative refractory period is that time during repolarization when the heart will contract again when stimulated by a very strong impulse
regurgitation: backward flow of food, opposite its normal direction, after food is swallowed; the swallowed food moves upward into the mouth
relapse: the return of a disease after apparent recovery
remodeling: the process by which bone is formed and destroyed
renal artery: provides the blood supply to the kidney. It branches off the aorta and enters the kidney in the area of the hilum
renal corpuscle: the unit that forms glomerular filtrate, composed of a glomerulus surrounded by Bowman's capsule
renal failure: inability of the kidneys to remove the waste products of metabolism from the blood. It can be acute or chronic
renal osteodystrophy: faulty bone metabolism associated with chronic renal failure
renal tubular acidosis: a group of disorders characterized by normal glomerular filtration accompanied by impairment of renal acidification
renin: an enzyme that converts angiotensinogen to angiotensin I and initiates the renin-angiotensin-aldosterone cascade
renin-angiotensin-aldosterone system: A set of interacting hormone effects that play important roles in regulating blood pressure and sodium balance in the body
reperfusion: restoration of blood flow to a tissue that has been deprived of blood. Often seen in therapeutic intervention for myocardial infarction
respiratory acidosis: excessive carbon dioxide in blood that decreases the pH of arterial blood
respiratory alkalosis: abnormally reduced levels of carbon dioxide in blood that raises the pH of arterial blood
respiratory zone: Airways that participate in gas exchange (respiratory bronchiole, alveolar ducts, alveoli)
reticular activating system (RAS): a functional system in the brain essential for attention, concentration, and wakefulness. Includes fibers of the thalamus, hypothalamus, brain stem, and cerebral cortex
reticular formation: diffuse network of neurons evolving from the brain stem and projecting to the thalamus and cerebral cortex that is instrumental in activities associated with motor control, sleep and arousal, and certain autonomic functions
retinopathy: noninflammatory degenerative disease of the retina
rheumatoid factor: autoantibody found in many of the autoimmune diseases, especially rheumatoid arthritis and lupus erythematosus
rhombencephalon: region of the nervous system encasing the medulla oblongota, pons, cerebellum, and fourth ventricle
rhythmicity: the regular or rhythmic generation of an action potential by cardiac pacemakers
rubor: a characteristic redness of the skin. Occurs in ischemic vascular disease when there is long-term decrease in blood flow to the tissues
rugae: mucosal folds that line the interior of the stomach
saddle embolus: an embolus that lodges in a main vessel bifurcation, especially in pulmonary artery or terminal aorta
sarcodina: protozoa with typical ameboid characteristics
sarcoma: malignant growth originating in mesodermal tissues that form connective tissue, blood vessels, and lymphatic organs
sarcomere: The contractile unit of skeletal and cardiac muscle
sarcoplasmic reticulum: structure that transports calcium needed for muscle contraction into the cell
seborrheic keratosis: benign epithelial tumor; prolonged exposure to the sun is a strong predisposing factor
secondary brain injury: injury occurring to the brain as a sequela to primary injuries and includes cerebral edema, cerebral hypoxia, and increased intracranial pressure
selective serotonin reuptake inhibitors: class of antidepressant drugs that selectively inhibit the presynaptic reuptake of serotonin
sensory receptors: specialized nerve cells that respond to specific sensory information from the environment
serine proteases: a group of proteolytic enzymes
serotonin: (1) a chemical, 5-hydroxytryptamine, present in platelets, gastrointestinal mucosa, mast cells, and in carcinoid tumors. It is a potent vasoconstrictor; (2) acts as a neurotransmitter in the central nervous system
shock: a life-threatening condition that occurs from a combination of symptoms (loss of circulating volume, inadequate pump function, systemic infection, or generalized arteriolar or venous dilation) that result in circulatory failure and subsequent mismatch between oxygen supply and demand
shunting: in lung, blood in pulmonary capillary blood fails to become oxygenated as it passes by an airless alveoli

slow pain: dull, aching or burning sensation that takes about 1 second to get to the brain

slow wave sleep: the stages III and IV of NREM sleep that produce typical slow waves on the electroencephalogram (EEG)

somatostatinomas: a somatostatin-secreting tumor of the pancreas

somatic efferent system: transmission from the central nervous system to the striated skeletal muscles, tendons, and joints

somatogenic pain: pain whose origin has a known physiologic cause

sorbitol pathway: a sugar alcohol used as an alternative to sucrose for sweetening food products

specificity: the property in immunocompetent cells to react to only one type of antigen owing to the physical characteristics of that antigen

spermatogenesis: the process by which spermatogonia (sperm) are formed

sphincter ani: the external sphincter with which the rectum terminates; it opens to the outside of the body

spinal shock: depression of spinal cord reflex activity after higher acute cord injury

spirometry: pulmonary function testing limited to measures of volume and flow

splanchnic organ: abdominal or visceral organ

splenomegaly: enlargement of the spleen

splinting: intentional limitation of inspiratory effort for the purpose of avoiding pain

sporozoa: a protozoal classification of organisms that have a definite life cycle that usually involves two different hosts

squamous cell carcinoma: malignant lesion of epithelial tissue

squamous intraepithelial lesion (SIL): early tissue changes in the neoplastic transformation process (syn. cervical intraepithelial neoplasia)

stable cells: cells that undergo mitosis under specific stimulation

staphylococcal scalded skin syndrome (SSSS): skin sloughing syndrome caused by staphylococcal bacteria, usually less dramatic than toxic epidermal necrolysis syndrome (TENS)

Starling forces: net effect of physiologic forces that prevent undesired leakage of fluids between membranes

stasis dermatitis: pigmented appearance and edema of the legs due to chronic impairment of the circulation, especially the venous circulation

steady state: a state of balance; homeostasis

stem cell theory: the theory that all blood cells arise from pluripotential cells that can divide and differentiate into specific blood cells (eg, granulocytes, monocytes, erythrocytes, and megakaryocytes)

stenosis: a condition of being restricted. In the heart, it refers to a valve that is unable to open properly due to deformation or disease

sterility: absolute inability to conceive

stress: the nonspecific response of the body to any demand place on it

stressors: physiologic and psychological factors that may elicit the stress response

striae gravidarum: bands of thin wrinkled skin initially red but becoming purple and white owing to overextension of skin due to preganacy

subarachnoid hemorrhage: bleeding (generally from arterial sources) into the subarachnoid space resulting in meningeal irritation signs

subclavian steal: vigorous movement of the arm on the side of severe proximal subclavian arterial stenosis causes blood to be diverted from the cerebral circulation, and cerebral ischemia results

subcutaneous tissue: the tissue below the epidermis and the dermis

subdural hematoma: bleeding into the space between the dura mater and arachnoid mater, usually associated with torn cortical bridging veins

submetacentric chromosomes: a group of chromosomes in which the centromere is located closer to one telomere than to the other. Human B group chromosomes are submetacentric

substance P: polypeptide released from the nerve terminals that causes vasodilatation, increased blood flow, and edema

suffering: the emotional component of pain and anguish

suppressor T cells (T8, $CD8^+$ T cells): subset of T lymphocytes that express the CD8 marker and that act to inhibit the effector actions of other T cells

surface tension: tendency for a water drop to contract to a smaller size when in contact with air

surfactant: liquid phospholipid mixture secreted by alveolar type II epithelial cells for the purpose of creating a film across the alveolar to air-alveolar-air interface in an effort to lower surface tension and thus prevents collapse of the alveoli

synapse: area of contact between two neurons or a neuron and an effector organ

synarthrosis: joint with little movement, such as the skull

syncope: brief alteration in consciousness related to reduced cerebral perfusion

syncytia: in immune deficiency, designates fusion of cells, resulting in large masses of cytoplasm with multiple nuclei

syndrome: a collection of multiple primary malformations or defects all due to a single underlying cause. Examples include Down syndrome (chromosome abnormality) and Marfan's syndrome (single-gene disorder)

syringomyelia: presence of a syrinx in the spinal cord characterized by progressive motor deficits

syringomyelocele: outpouching of the spinal cord through a congenital defect in the spinal column containing cerebrospinal fluid but no spinal cord tissue

syrinx: an abnormal cavity in the spinal cord

systemic inflammatory response syndrome (SIRS): most severe manifestation of inflammation, usually triggered by systemic infection. The syndrome is manifested as hypermetabolism and shock, and often results in multiple organ failure

systemic vascular resistance: the resistance or impedance offered to blood flow by the systemic arterioles. It is a major determinant of diastolic blood pressure

systems theory: model frequently used for organizing and examining relationships among units

T tubule: channels used for ion exchange necessary for muscle contraction

telangiectasias: vascular lesions formed by dilatation of small blood vessels; may be seen as a birthmark or be caused by long-term sun exposure or aging

telencephalon: a subdivision of the brain that is encased in the prosencephalon. Cerebral hemispheres evolve from this region of the brain

telophase: the last phase of mitosis in which two daughter chromosomes are gathered at opposite poles and the nucleus and cytoplasm are divided equally into the newly formed daughter cells

tendons: extensions of muscles that attach muscle to bone

tentorium cerebelli: portion of the dura mater that divides the cerebrum from the cerebellum

teratoma: a rare germ-cell tumor arising from the pineal region

testicular cancer: malignant neoplasm of the testis; usually germ cell lines

testosterone: androgens, or male sex hormones, produced by the testes; steroid class

tetany: a neurologic syndrome characterized by muscle twiches, cramps, and carpopedal spasm usually relating to hypocalcemia

thermogenesis: physiologic metabolic production of body heat

threshold, renal: the plasma level at which a substance, such as glucose, is no longer fully absorbed by the kidney and begins to appear in the urine

thrombocythemia: an abnormal increase in the number of platelets

thrombocytopenia: an abnormal decrease in the number of platelets

thrombocytosis: an increase in the number of blood platelets

thrombophillia: an increased tendency to form blood clots

thromboxane A_2: a product of platelet and other cell synthesis, formed from a prostaglandin, that acts to aggregate platelets and also is a potent vasoconstrictor

thromboxane: an unstable compound synthesized in platelets and other cells from a prostaglandin. It acts to aggregate platelets

thrombus: a fibrinous blood clot that forms in a blood vessel and can obstruct blood flow

thymosins: a group of thymus proteins that assist in the differentiation and maturation of T cell precursors into immunocompetent T lymphocytes. Adequate concentrations of thymosins in humans begin to decline after age 40

thyroid dermopathy: scaly thickening and induration of the skin, especially over the shins; seen in Graves' disease

thyrotoxicosis: hyperthyroid state characterized by elevated basal metabolism from excessive thyroid hormones

tidal volume: volume of air inspired and expired with each breath at rest; approximately 500 mL in adults

tight junctions: regions of close association between adjacent membranes that limit movement of organic molecules through the spaces

tissue factor: a substance released from injured tissue that functions in the extrinsic coagulation pathway in a complex composed of factor VII, calcium, and phospholipids. This activates factor VII to tissue thromboplastin

tissue hypoxia: inadequate critical oxygen tension to meet the needs of the cell

tissue resistance: force exerted by the presence of lung and chest wall tissue

tissue thromboplastin: factor III of the blood coagulation system, which activates the final common coagulation pathway at factor X

tissue tropism: the affinity of an infectious organism to affect one organ system

TNM system: the most commonly used staging system for neoplastic diseases; reflects the extent of tumor (T), lymph node involvement (N), and presence of metastases (M)

torsion: rotation of the spermatic cord that reduces blood flow to the testis

total peripheral resistance: see systemic vascular resistance

toxic epidermal necrolysis syndrome (TENS): life-threatening syndrome characterized by skin and mucous membrane sloughing

trabeculae carnae: the bands of muscle projecting from the cardiac ventricular walls

transamination: the transfer of the amine group. The process is required in the synthesis of the nonessential amino acids

transduction: the changing of noxious stimuli in sensory nerve endings to electrical impulses
transferrin: a nonheme globulin of the plasma that can combine reversibly with iron and act as an iron-transporting protein
transient ischemic attack (TIA): temporary neurologic dysfunction resulting from diminished blood supply to an area of the brain
translocation: the misplacement of genetic material from one chromosome to another
transmission: the spread of impulses from the site of transduction through the sensory nervous system
transport maximum: the maximum amount of a substance, such as glucose, that an active transport system can move, usually determined by saturation of carrier sites
trematodes: flukes of the helminth classification
triglyceride: the major form of fat found in food and in adipose tissue. A triglyceride molecule consists of a glycerol backbone with three fatty acids attached
trinucleotide repeat amplifications: multiple copies of a specific trinucleotide in the DNA that increase with successive generations and cause anticipation
trisomy: an aneuploid condition caused by the presence of an extra chromosome that is added to a given chromosome pair and results in a total number of 47 chromosomes per cell. Down syndrome is the most common human autosomal trisomy
tropic hormone: hormones act selectively on a specific target gland to regulate and maintain normal function
troponin T and I: part of the sarcomere complex of myocardial muscle, released with myocardial injury. Becoming a reliable tool to gauge myocardial damage following infarction
tubercule: a fibrotic and calicified lung lesion that occurs in response to infection with *Mycobacterium tuberculosis*
tuberculous bacillemia: *Mycobacteria tuberculosis* in the blood
tubular reabsorption: movements of substances from the filtrate in the renal tubules back into the blood of the capillaries. It may involve active or passive transport
tubular secretion: movements of substances from the plasma of the capillaries into the filtrate in the renal tubules. It may involve active or passive transport
tumor: a neoplasm, may be benign or malignant
tumor necrosis factor: a protein produced by various cells in the body, often in response to tissue injury
tumor suppressor gene: a normal gene that has a negative effect on cellular growth; mutations that inactivate this gene can result in unregulated growth
turbulent flow: irregular and disrupted air flow in a tube
uncal herniation: displacement of the uncal gyrus of the temporal lobe resulting in compression of structures passing through the tentorial notch
unipolar disorder: a major psychological disorder characterized by episodes of depression
upper motor neuron lesions: lesions of the corticobulbar and corticospinal motor tracts resulting in spastic paralysis
uremia: symptomatic end-stage renal failure, with metabolic effects in all body systems. Also called uremic syndrome
uremic syndrome: symptomatic end-stage renal failure, with metabolic effects in all body systems. Also called uremia
urolithiasis: calculi anywhere in the urinary tract
urticaria: an eruption of pruritic wheals, usually due to an allergic reaction to some allergen. Also called hives. These wheals may cover parts or all of the body
uterine leiomyoma: a benign smooth muscle neoplasm of the uterus
uterine prolapse: descent of uterus from its normal position supported by ligaments due to relaxation of pelvic support, pulling with it the floor of the bladder
varicocele: dilated, tortuous veins within the venous plexus of the spermatic cord
vasa recta: a system of capillaries that surround the loop of Henle in the nephron
vascular redistribution: increase of blood flow to middle and upper lung lobes; often due to fluid overload and pulmonary edema
vasogenic edema: cerebral edema resulting from damage or dysfunction to cerebral blood vessels
ventilation-perfusion mismatching: reduced efficacy of gas exchange due to areas of compromised ventilation or perfusion, or both
ventricular remodeling: changes in the contour of the ventricles due to pressure or volume overload
verrucae: warts
vertigo: disturbance in equilibrium resulting in a sensation of whirling, rotation, weakness, lightheadedness, or faintness
vesicoureteral reflux: backflow of urine from the bladder toward the kidneys. It may be due to congenital defect or occur followng infection
vesicular hormone secretion: transport of hormone within the cell to the cell surface within a vesicle. Fusion of the vesicle with the cell surface causes release of the hormone (exocytosis)
Virchow's triad: risk factors for venous thrombus formation, including intimal injury of venous epithelium, venous stasis, and hypercoagulable state

virions: mature infective virus particles

virulence: the relative degree of pathogenicity exhibited by an organism

visceral efferent system: neural transmission to smooth muscles, cardiac muscle, and glands through the autonomic nervous system

visceral pain: pain that arises from internal organs

vitiligo: patchy areas of skin that lack pigmentation. Possibly due to decreased melanocyte-stimulating hormone activity

voltage-dependent calcium channels: the channels in the T tubules of the muscle that allow for the release of calcium into the myofibrils after an action potential

voltage-gated sodium channels: related to the leakiness of conduction system fibers, leading to the inward movement of sodium, which allows the action potential threshold to be reached

Von Willebrand's factor (vWF): a large plasma protein that binds receptors on the platelet membrane and that causes a bridge between activated platelets and the endothelial lining of the vessel

Wernicke's aphasia: impairment of language comprehension resulting from lesions in the superior temporal gyrus. Also known as receptive, sensory, or fluent aphasia

Western blot: an antibody test in which the test serum is matched to a preparation of antigens separated by electrophoresis and then blotted to a supportive medium where they bind and are subsequently identified. In the determination of HIV antibody, matching of one to three antigenic proteins is considered "inconclusive" (and should be repeated), matching of four or more is a "positive" test, whereas no matching is reported as a "negative" Western blot. Because of its high specificity, the Western blot is used as a confirmatory test for HIV antibody

white fiber: low myoglobin–containing muscle fibers used for activities requiring quick movements

Wilms' tumor: a malignant tumor of the kidney that occurs primarily in children

xenoestrogens: synthetic compound (drugs, foods, pollutants) with estrogenic effects

zone of coagulation: central area of burn injury composed of nonviable tissue.

zone of stasis: area surrounding the zone of coagulation that is vulnerable to becoming nonviable.

zone of hyperemia: outermost zone of burn injury that contains viable tissue.

zymogens: plasma proenzymes that must be activated to perform their function

Index

Note: Page numbers in italics indicate illustrations; t indicates a table, b indicates a box, and c indicates a flow chart.

B

E

F

G

J

K

M

N

Q

R

S

T